American DRUG INDEX

2006

50th Anniversary Edition

NORMAN F. BILLUPS, RPh, MS, PhD

Dean and Professor Emeritus
College of Pharmacy
The University of Toledo

Associate Editor

SHIRLEY M. BILLUPS, RN, LPC, MEd

Oncology Nurse
Licensed Professional Counselor

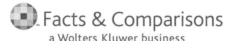 Facts & Comparisons
a Wolters Kluwer business

American Drug Index, Fiftieth Edition.

ISBN 1-57439-240-9

Library of Congress Catalog Card Number 55-6286

Printed in the United States of America

The information contained in *American Drug Index* is available for licensing as source data. For more information on data licensing, please call 1-800-223-0554.

Facts and Comparisons®
part of **Wolters Kluwer Health**
77 WestPort Plaza, Suite 450
St. Louis, Missouri 63146
(314) 216-2100 ● 800-223-0554
www.drugfacts.com

Facts and Comparisons® Staff

Cathy H. Reilly
vice president and
publisher

Angela J. Schwalm
managing editor

Carolee Ann Corrigan
assistant editor

Jennifer M. Reed
composition specialist

Heather L. Broad
purchasing specialist

Cathy A. Meives, PharmD
clinical manager

Linda M. Jones
senior sgml specialist

Renée M. Wickersham
senior managing editor,
content development

Jennifer A. Guimaraes
Joseph R. Horenkamp
associate editors

Julie A. Scott
senior managing editor,
quality control/print
production

Renée Rivard, PharmD
clinical director

Teri H. Burnham
director, referential product
management

Editorial Advisory Panel

Lawrence R. Borgsdorf, PharmD, FCSHP

Pharmacist Specialist-
Ambulatory Care
Kaiser Permanente

Dennis J. Cada, PharmD, FASHP, FASCP

Executive Director, *The Formulary*
Editor in Chief, *Hospital Pharmacy*

Michael Cirigliano, MD, FACP

Associate Professor of Medicine
University of Pennsylvania
School of Medicine

Timothy R. Covington, PharmD, MS

Bruno Professor of Pharmacy
Director, Managed Care Institute
McWhorter School of Pharmacy
Samford University

Joyce A. Generali, RPh, MS, FASHP

Director, Drug Information Center
Clinical Professor
University of Kansas
Medical Center

Contents

[•]   Denotes official name: Generic name or chemical name recognized by the
      USP, NF, or USAN.

Preface

The 50th Edition of the *American Drug Index (ADI)* has been prepared for the identification, explanation, and correlation of the many pharmaceuticals available to the medical, pharmaceutical, and allied health professions. The need for this index has become even more acute as the variety and number of drugs and drug products have continued to multiply. *ADI* should be useful to pharmacists, nurses, health care administrators, physicians, medical transcriptionists, dentists, sales personnel, students, and teachers in the fields incorporating pharmaceuticals.

Special note to medical transcriptionists: Generic names are in lowercase and all trade names are in upper/lowercase as appropriate to facilitate transcription. The names for officially designated products (eg, *United States Pharmacopeia* or *USP*) are preceded by a bullet (•) and should appear in lowercase in transcription.

The organization of *ADI* falls into 18 major sections:

Monographs of Drug Products
Standard Medical Abbreviations
Calculations
Common Systems of Weights and Measures
Approximate Practical Equivalents
International System of Units
Normal Laboratory Values
FDA Pregnancy Categories
Controlled Substances Summary
Medical Terminology Glossary
Oral Dosage Forms that Should Not Be Crushed or Chewed
Drug Names that Look Alike and Sound Alike
New Therapeutic Agents
Discontinued Drugs
Common Abbreviations of Chemotherapy Regimens
Radio-Contrast Media
Radio-Isotopes
Pharmaceutical Manufacturer and Drug Distributor Listing

MONOGRAPHS: The organization of the monograph section of *ADI* is alphabetical with extensive cross-indexing. Names listed are generic (also called nonproprietary, public name, or common name); brand (also called trademark, proprietary, or specialty); and chemical. Synonyms that are in general use also are included. All names used for a pharmaceutical appear in alphabetical order, with the pertinent data given under the brand name by which it is made available.

The monograph for a typical brand name product appears in upper/lowercase as appropriate, and consists of the manufacturer, generic name, composition and strength, available pharmaceutic dosage forms, package size, use, and appropriate legend designation (eg, *Rx, OTC, c-v*).

Generic names appear in lowercase in alphabetical order, followed by the pronunciation and the corresponding recognition of the drug to the *USP* (*United States Pharmacopeia*), *NF* (*National Formulary*), and USAN (*USP Dictionary of United States Adopted Names and International Drug Names*). Each of these official generic names is preceded by a bullet (•). The information is in accord with the *USP 28* and *NF 23*, which became official on January 1, 2005, and the 2005 *USP Dictionary of USAN and International Drug Names*.

To minimize medication errors, The Institute for Safe Medication Practices established Tall Man lettering for 16 look-alike generic pairs. Tall Man lettering was added to generic entries for the drugs involved in the name differentiation project.

Pronunciations have been included for many of the generic drugs. However, not every drug will have a corresponding pronunciation. Some of the most common pronunciations are not listed for every drug. The following list is included as a guide to very common names:

Acetate	ASS-eh-tate	Lactobionate	LACK-toe-BYE-oh-nate
Besylate	BESS-ih-late	Maleate	MAL-ee-ate
Borate	BOE-rate	Mesylate	MEH-sih-LATE
Bromide	BROE-mide	Monosodium	MAHN-oh-SO-dee-uhm
Butyrate	BYOO-tih-rate	Nitrate	NYE-trate
Calcium	KAL-see-uhm	Pendetide	PEN-deh-TIDE
Chloride	KLOR-ide	Pentetate	PEN-teh-tate
Citrate	SIH-trate	Phosphate	FOSS-fate
Dipotassium	die-poe-TASS-ee-uhm	Potassium	poe-TASS-ee-uhm
Disodium	die-SO-dee-uhm	Propionate	PRO-pee-oh-nate
Edetate	eh-deh-TATE	Sodium	SO-dee-uhm
Fosfatex	foss-FAH-tex	Succinate	SUCK-sih-nate
Fumarate	FEW-mah-rate	Sulfate	SULL-fate
Hydrobromide	HIGH-droe-BROE-mide	Tartrate	TAR-trate
Hydrochloride	HIGH-droe-KLOR-ide	Trisodium	try-SO-dee-uhm
Iodide	EYE-oh-dide		

Because of the multiplicity of brand names used for the same therapeutic agent or the same combination of therapeutic agents, it was apparent that some correlation could be done. As an example of this, please turn to aspirin. Here under the generic name are listed the various brand names. Following are combinations of aspirin organized in a manner to point out relationships among the many products. Reference then is made to the brand name or names having the indicated composition. Under the brand name are given manufacturer, composition, available forms, sizes, dosage, and use.

The multiplicity of generic names for the same therapeutic agent has complicated the nomenclature of these agents. Examples of multiple generic names for the same chemical substance are: (1) acetaminophen, N-acetyl-p-aminophenol; (2) guaifenesin, glyceryl guaiacolate, glyceryl guaiacolether, guaianesin, guayanesin; and (3) pyrilamine, pyranisamine, pyranilamine, pyraminyl, anisopyradamine.

The cross-indexing feature of *ADI* permits the finding of drugs or drug combinations when only one major ingredient is known. For example, a combination of aluminum hydroxide gel and magnesium trisilicate is available. This combination can be found by looking under the name of either of the two ingredients, and in each case the brand names are given. A second form of cross-indexing lists drugs under various therapeutic and pharmaceutical classes (ie, antacids, antihistamines, diuretics, laxatives).

ABBREVIATIONS: The listing of standard medical abbreviations is included as an aid in interpreting medical orders. The Latin or Greek word and abbreviation are given with the meaning.

CALCULATIONS: A listing of common formulas used to calculate weight, creatinine clearance, ideal body weight, and convert temperature between Celsius and Farenheit.

WEIGHTS AND MEASURES: Tables containing common systems of weights and measures are included to aid the practitioner in calculating dosages in the metric, apothecary, and avoirdupois systems.

CONVERSION FACTORS: A listing of approximate practical equivalents to aid in calculating and converting dosages among the metric, apothecary, and avoirdupois systems.

INTERNATIONAL SYSTEM OF UNITS: A modernized version of the metric system listed in tables for rapid reference.

NORMAL LABORATORY VALUES: Tables containing normal reference values for commonly requested laboratory tests are included as a guideline for the health care practitioner.

FDA PREGNANCY CATEGORIES: This table summarizes each of the pregnancy categories established by the FDA.

CONTROLLED SUBSTANCES SUMMARY: A brief summary explanation of the key points of the Controlled Substances Act of 1970.

MEDICAL TERMINOLOGY GLOSSARY: Commonly used terms are listed and defined as an aid in interpreting the use given for drug monographs included in *ADI.*

ORAL DOSAGE FORMS THAT SHOULD NOT BE CRUSHED OR CHEWED: This section has been added to alert the health care practitioner about oral dosage forms that should not be crushed, and to serve as an aid in consulting with patients. Examples of products falling into the non-crush category are extended-release, enteric-coated, encapsulated beads, wax matrix, sublingual dosage forms, and encapsulated liquid formulations.

DRUG NAMES THAT LOOK ALIKE AND SOUND ALIKE: A listing of common drugs that look alike and sound alike. Familiarity with this list may save the prescriber from making a dispensing error.

NEW THERAPEUTIC AGENTS: A table listing new therapeutic agents approved by the FDA.

DISCONTINUED DRUGS: A combined list of generic and brand products no longer available in the United States because they were withdrawn from the market or discontinued by the manufacturer.

COMMON ABBREVIATIONS OF CHEMOTHERAPY REGIMENS: This section describes the drugs, therapeutic uses, dosages, and dosing schedules of common acronyms used for combination chemotherapy regimens (eg, CHOP). Unlike many other quick references, the primary literature source for each regimen is cited. The combination regimens are listed in alphabetical order by acronym.

RADIO-CONTRAST MEDIA AND ISOTOPES: These tables provide the generic and trade names, doseform, packaging, and manufacturer information.

MANUFACTURER AND DRUG DISTRIBUTOR LISTING: The name, address, phone number, and Web site of virtually every American pharmaceutical manufacturer and drug distributor are listed in alphabetical order in this section.

Special appreciation and acknowledgment are given to my wife, Shirley, who served again this year as my associate editor. Special thanks are also extended to the manufacturers who supplied product information and to Dr. John F. Mitchell, Medication Safety Coordinator and Clinical Associate Professor at the University of Michigan, for the table on Oral Dosage Forms that Should Not Be Crushed or Chewed.

Correspondence or communication with reference to a drug or drug products listed in *ADI* should be directed to Editorial/Production, Attn: ADI, Wolters Kluwer Health, 77 Westport Plaza, Suite 450, St. Louis, Missouri 63146, or call 1-800-223-0554.

Norman F. Billups, RPh, MS, PhD

Monographs and
Reference Information

A

A and D Ointment. (Schering-Plough)
Fish liver oil, cholecalciferol. Oint. Tube
1.5 oz, 4 oz. Jar lb. *OTC.*
Use: Emollient.

A & D Tablets. (Barth's) Vitamins A
10,000 units, D 400 units. Tab. Bot.
100s, 500s. *OTC.*
Use: Vitamin supplement.

•**abacavir succinate.** (ab-ah-KAV-ear
SUCK-sih-nate) USAN.
Use: Antiviral.

abacavir sulfate.
Use: Antiviral; nucleoside reverse tran-
sciptase inhibitor.
See: Ziagen.
W/Lamivudine
See: Epzicom.
W/Lamivudine und Zidovudine
See: Trizivir.

•**abafilcon a.** (ab-ah-FILL-kahn) USAN.
Use: Contact lens material, hydrophilic.

•**abamectin.** (abe-ah-MEK-tin) USAN.
Use: Antiparasitic.

•**abarelix.** (ab-ah-RELL-ix) USAN.
Use: Gonadotropin-releasing hormone
antagonist; antineoplastic; infertility
therapy adjunct; antiendometriotic
agent.
See: Plenaxis.

•**abatacept.** (ab-a-TA-sept) USAN.
Use: Autoimmune diseases.

Abbokinase. (Abbott) Urokinase
250,000 units, mannitol 25 mg, albumin
(human) 250 mg, sodium chloride
50 mg/vial, preservative free. Pow. for
Inj., lyophilized. Vial. *Rx.*
Use: Thrombolytic.

Abbokinase Open-Cath. (Abbott) Urokinase for catheter clearance gelatin
5 mg, mannitol 15 mg, sodium chloride
1.7 mg, monobasic sodium phosphate
anhydrous/mL when reconstituted, preservative free. Single-dose *Univial*
1 mL, 1.8 mL. *Rx.*
Use: Thrombolytic.

Abbott AFP-EIA. (Abbott Diagnostics)
Enzyme immunoassay for the quanti-
tative measurement of alpha-fetoprotein
(AFP) in human serum and amniotic
fluid. Test kits 100s.
Use: Diagnostic aid.

Abbott AFP-EIA Monoclonal. (Abbott
Diagnostics) Enzyme immunoassay for
the quantitative measurement of alpha-
fetoprotein (AFP) in human serum and
amniotic fluid.
Use: Diagnostic aid.

Abbott Anti-Delta. (Abbott Diagnostics)
Radioimmunoassay for the detection
of antibody to hepatitis delta antigen
(HDAg) in human serum or plasma.
Use: For research only. Not for use in
diagnostic procedures.

Abbott Anti-Delta EIA. (Abbott Diagnostics) Enzyme immunoassay for the detection of antibody to hepatitis delta
antigen (HDAg) in human serum or
plasma.
Use: For research only. Not for use in
diagnostic procedures.

Abbott β-HCG 15/15. (Abbott Diagnostics) Enzyme immunoassay for the
quantitative determination of human
chorionic gonadotropin (hCG) in human
serum.
Use: Diagnostic aid.

Abbott CA125 EIA. (Abbott Diagnostics)
Enzyme immunoassay for the quantita-
tive measurement of cancer antigen
(CA) 125 in human serum.
Use: For research only. Not for use in
diagnostic procedures.

Abbott CEA-EIA Monoclonal. (Abbott
Diagnostics) Enzyme immunoassay for
the quantitative measurement of car-
cinoembryonic antigen (CEA) in human
serum or plasma to aid in the management of cancer patients and assessing
prognosis.
Use: Diagnostic aid.

Abbott CEA-RIA. (Abbott Diagnostics)
Solid phase radioimmunoassay for the
quantitative measurement of carcino-
embryonic antigen (CEA) in human serum or plasma to aid in the management of cancer patients and assessing
prognosis.
Use: Diagnostic aid.

Abbott CMV Total AB EIA. (Abbott Diagnostics) Enzyme immunoassay for the
detection of antibody to cytomegalovirus in human serum, plasma, and
whole blood. Test kits 100s.
Use: Diagnostic aid.

Abbott Diagnostic Reagents. (Abbott
Diagnostics) A series of diagnostic
tests for cancer, cardiovascular, hepatitis, infectious disease and immunology, metabolic and digestive disease,
OB/GYN, rubella, and thyroid.
Use: Diagnostic aid.

Abbott ER-EIA Monoclonal. (Abbott Diagnostics) Enzyme immunoassay for
the quantitative measurement of human
estrogen receptor in tissue cytosol.
Use: For research only. Not for use in
diagnostic procedures.

Abbott ER-ICA Monoclonal. (Abbott Diagnostics) Immunoassay for the detection of estrogen receptor.
Use: For research only. Not for use in diagnostic procedures.

Abbott HB-EIA. (Abbott Diagnostics) Enzyme immunoassay for the detection of hepatitis Be antigen or antibody to hepatitis Be antigen.
Use: Diagnostic aid.

Abbott HBe Test. (Abbott Diagnostics) Radioimmunoassay or enzyme immunoassay for detection of hepatitis Be antigen or antibody to hepatitis Be antigen. Test kits 100s.
Use: Diagnostic aid.

Abbott HIVAB HIV-1 EIA. (Abbott Diagnostics) Enzyme immunoassay for the antibody to human immunodeficiency virus type 1 (HIV-1) in serum or plasma. Test kits 100s, 1000s.
Use: Diagnostic aid.

Abbott HIVAG-1. (Abbott Diagnostics) Enzyme immunoassay for the human immunodeficiency virus type 1 (HIV-1) antigens in serum or plasma. Test kits 100s, 1000s.
Use: Diagnostic aid.

Abbott HTLV I EIA. (Abbott Diagnostics) To detect antibody to Human T-Lymphotropic Virus Type I in serum or plasma. Test kits 100s.
Use: Diagnostic aid.

Abbott HTLV III Antigen EIA. (Abbott Diagnostics) Enzyme immunoassay for the detection of Human T-Lymphotropic Virus Type III (HIV) antigens.
Use: For research only. Not for use in diagnostic procedures.

Abbott HTLV III Confirmatory EIA. (Abbott Diagnostics) Enzyme immunoassay for confirmation of specimens found to be positive to antibody to HTL VIII. Test kits 100s.
Use: Diagnostic aid.

Abbott HTLV III EIA. (Abbott Diagnostics) Enzyme immunoassay for the detection of antibody to Human T-Lymphotropic Virus Type III (HIV) in human serum or plasma. Test kits 1s.
Use: Diagnostic aid.

Abbott IGE EIA. (Abbott Diagnostics) Enzyme immunoassay for quantitative determination of IgE in human serum and plasma. Test kits 100s.
Use: Diagnostic aid.

Abbott PAP-EIA. (Abbott Diagnostics) Enzyme immunoassay for the measurement of prostatic acid phosphatase (PAP) in serum or plasma.
Use: Diagnostic aid.

Abbott RSV-EIA. (Abbott Diagnostics) Enzyme immunoassay for the detection of respiratory syncytial virus (RSV) in nasopharyngeal washes and aspirates.
Use: Diagnostic aid.

Abbott SCC-RIA. (Abbott Diagnostics) Radioimmunoassay for the quantitative measurement of squamous cell carcinoma-associated antigen in human serum.
Use: For research only. Not for use in diagnostic procedures.

Abbott TdT EIA. (Abbott Diagnostics) Enzyme immunoassay for the quantitative measurement of terminal deoxynucleotidyl transferase (TdT), in extracts of human whole blood or isolated mononuclear cells.
Use: Diagnostic aid.

Abbott Testpak hCG-Serum. (Abbott Diagnostics) Monoclonal antibody, enzyme immunoassay for the qualitative determination of human chorionic gonadotropin (hCG) in serum. No instrumentation required.
Use: Diagnostic aid.

Abbott Testpak hCG-Urine. (Abbott Diagnostics) Monoclonal antibody, enzyme immunoassay for the qualitative determination of human chorionic gonadotropin (hCG) in urine. No instrumentation required.
Use: Diagnostic aid.

Abbott Testpack-Strep A. (Abbott Diagnostics) A rapid screening and confirmatory test for the detection of group A beta-hemolytic streptococci from throat swabs. No instrumentation required.
Use: Diagnostic aid.

Abbott Toxo-G EIA. (Abbott Diagnostics) Enzyme immunoassay for the qualitative and quantitative determination of IgG antibody to toxoplasma gondii in human serum and plasma.
Use: Diagnostic aid.

Abbott Toxo-M EIA. (Abbott Diagnostics) Enzyme immunoassay for the qualitative determination of IgM antibody to toxoplasma gondii in human serum.
Use: Diagnostic aid.

•**abciximab.** (ab-SICK-sih-mab) USAN.
Use: Monoclonal antibody; antithrombotic; antiplatelet agent, glycoprotein IIb/IIIa inhibitor.
See: ReoPro.

ABC to Z. (NBTY) Iron 18 mg, Vitamins A 5000 units, D 400 units, E 30 units, B_1 1.5 mg, B_2 1.7 mg, B_3 20 mg, B_5 10 mg, B_6 2 mg, B_{12} 6 mcg, C 60 mg,

folic acid 0.4 mg, biotin 30 mcg, Ca, P, I, Mg, Cu, Mn, K, Cl, Cr, Mo, Se, Ni, Si, Sn, V, B, vitamin K, Zn 15 mg. Tab. Bot. 100s. *OTC.*
Use: Mineral, vitamin supplement.
Abelcet. (Enzon) Amphotericin B 100 mg/20 mL (as lipid complex). Susp. for Inj. Single-use Vial w/5-micron filter needles 10 mL, 20 mL. *Rx.*
Use: Antifungal.
•**abetimus sodium.** (a-BE-ti-mus) USAN.
Use: Investigational immunomodulator.
Abilify. (Bristol-Myers Squibb/Otsuka America) Aripiprazole. **Oral Soln.:** 1 mg/mL. Fructose, sucrose, parabens. Orange cream flavor. 50 mL, 150 mL, 480 mL. **Tab.:** 5 mg, 10 mg, 15 mg, 20 mg, 30 mg, lactose. Pkg. 30s, blister 100s. *Rx.*
Use: Antipsychotic.
Abitrexate. (International Pharm) Methotrexate sodium 25 mg/mL. Vial 2 mL, 4 mL, 8 mL. *Rx.*
Use: Antineoplastic.
•**ablukast.** (ab-LOO-kast) USAN.
Use: Antiasthmatic, leukotriene antagonist.
•**ablukast sodium.** (ab-LOO-kast) USAN.
Use: Antiasthmatic, leukotriene antagonist.
See: Ulpax.
abortifacients.
See: Mifepristone.
Prostaglandins
Abraxane. (Abraxis Oncology) Paclitaxel 100 mg. With human albumin 900 mg. Pow. for Inj., lyophilized (albumin-bound). Single-use vials. *Rx.*
Use: Antimitotic agent.
Abreva. (GlaxoSmithKline) Docosanol 10%, benzyl alcohol, light mineral oil. Cream. Tube 2 g. *OTC.*
Use: Cold sores; fever blisters.
•**abrineurin.** (aye-bri-NOOR-in) USAN.
Previously brineurin.
Use: Amyotrophic lateral sclerosis (ALS).
absorbable cellulose cotton or gauze.
See: Oxidized Cellulose.
absorbable dusting powder.
Use: Lubricant.
absorbable gelatin film.
Use: Hemostatic, topical.
See: Gelfilm.
Gelfilm Ophthalmic.
absorbable gelatin sponge.
Use: Hemostatic.
See: Gelfoam.
absorbable surgical suture.
Use: Surgical aid.

Absorbase. (Carolina Medical Products) Petrolatum, mineral oil, ceresin wax, wool wax, alcohol. Oint. Tube 114 g, 454 g. *OTC.*
Use: Pharmaceutical aid, emollient base.
absorbent gauze.
Use: Surgical aid.
Absorbent Rub Relief Formula. (DeWitt) Green soap 11.64%, camphor 1.63%, menthol 1.63%, pine tar soap 0.87%, wintergreen oil 0.71%, sassafras oil 0.54%, benzocaine 0.48%, capsicum 0.03%, wormwood oil 0.6%, isopropyl alcohol 75%. Bot. 2 oz. *OTC.*
Use: Analgesic, topical.
Absorbine Jr. (W. F. Young) Wormwood, thymol, chloroxylenol, menthol, acetone, zinc stearate, parachloroxylenol, aluminum chlorhydroxy, allantoate, benzethonium Cl, menthol. Liq. Bot. 1 oz, 2 oz, 4 oz, 12 oz w/applicator. *OTC.*
Use: Analgesic; antifungal, topical.
Absorbine Jr. Arthritis Strength. (W. F. Young) Natural menthol 4%, capsaicin 0.025%, acetone, calendula plant extracts, echinacea, wormwood. Liq. *OTC.*
Use: Liniment.
Absorbine Jr. Extra Strength. (W. F. Young) Natural menthol 4%; plant extracts of calendula, echinacea and wormwood; acetone; chloroxylenol iodine; potassium iodide; thymol; wormwood oil. Liq. Bot. 59 mL, 118 mL. *OTC.*
Use: Liniment.
Abuscreen. (Roche) An immunological and radiochemical assay for morphine and morphine glucuronide in nanogram levels. Utilizes I 125 labeled morphine requiring gamma scintillation equipment. Tests 100s.
Use: Diagnostic aid.
•**acacia syrup.** (ah-KAY-shah) *NF 23.*
Use: Pharmaceutic aid, suspending agent, viscosity agent.
•**acadesine.** (ack-AH-dess-een) USAN.
Use: Platelet aggregation inhibitor.
•**acamprosate calcium.** (a-kam-PROE-sate) USAN.
Use: Antialcoholic agent.
See: Campral.
•**acarbose.** (A-car-bose) USAN.
Use: Inhibitor, α-glucosidase.
See: Precose.
Accolate. (AstraZeneca) Zafirlukast 10 mg, 20 mg, lactose, povidone. Tab. Bot. 60s, UD 100s. *Rx.*
Use: Leukotriene receptor antagonist.

AccuHist. (PediaMed) Pseudoephedrine hydrochloride 12.5 mg, brompheniramine maleate 1 mg/mL. Saccharin, sorbitol. Cherry flavor. Drops. 30 mL with dropper. *Rx.*
Use: Decongestant, antihistamine.

AccuHist DM Pediatric. (PediaMed) **Drops:** Pseudoephedrine hydrochloride 15 mg, bromphinarmine maleate 1 mg, dextromethorphan HBr 4 mg/mL, saccharin, sorbitol, alcohol free, grape flavor. 30 mL. **Syrup:** Pseudoephedrine hydrochloride 30 mg, brompheniramine maleate 2 mg, dextromethorphan HBr 5 mg, guaifenesin 50 mg/5 mL, corn syrup, sucrose, alcohol free, grape flavor. 473 mL. *Rx.*
Use: Upper respiratory combination.

AccuHist LA. (PediaMed) Phenylephrine hydrochloride 20 mg, chlorpheniramine maleate 8 mg, hyoscyamine sulfate 0.19 mg, atropine sulfate 0.04 mg, scopolamine HBr 0.01 mg, lactose. SR Tab. 100s, 500s. *Rx.*
Use: Upper respiratory combination.

AccuHist PDX. (PediaMed) **Drops:** Pseudoephedrine hydrochloride 12.5 mg, brompheniramine maleate 1 mg, dextromethorphan HBr 3 mg/mL. Saccharin, sorbitol, grape flavor. 30 mL with dropper. **Syrup:** Phenylephrine hydrochloride 5 mg, dextromethorphan HBr 5 mg, guaifenesin 50 mg, brompheniramine maleate 2 mg/5 mL. Sucrose. Grape flavor. 473 mL. *Rx.*
Use: Pediatric antitussive combination; pediatric antitussive and expectorant combination.

AccuNeb. (Dey) Albuterol sulfate 0.63 mg/3 mL, 1.25 mg/3 mL, preservative free. Soln. for Inh. UD Vial 3 mL. *Rx.*
Use: Bronchodilator, sympathomimetic.

Accupep HPF. (Sherwood Davis & Geck) Hydrolyzed lactalbumin, maltodextrin, MCT oil, corn oil, mono- and diglycerides, vitamins A, B_1, B_2, B_3, B_5, B_6, B_{12}, C, D, E, K, Ca, Cl, Cu, Fe, I, Mg, Mn, P, Zn, biotin, and choline. Pks. 128 g. *OTC.*
Use: Nutritional supplement.

Accupril. (Pfizer) Quinapril hydrochloride 5 mg, 10 mg, 20 mg, 40 mg, lactose. Film-coated. Tab. Bot. 90s and UD 100s (except 40 mg). *Rx.*
Use: Antihypertensive.

Accurbron. (Hoechst) Theophylline, anhydrous 10 mg/mL. Bot. Pt. *Rx.*
Use: Bronchodilator.

Accuretic. (Parke-Davis) Quinapril hydrochloride 10 mg, hydrochlorothiazide 12.5 mg; quinapril hydrochloride 20 mg, hydrochlorothiazide 12.5 mg; quinapril hydrochloride 20 mg, hydrochlorothiazide 25 mg; lactose. Tab. Bot. 30s. *Rx.*
Use: Antihypertensive.

Accusens T Taste Function Kit. (Westport Pharmaceuticals, Inc.) Test for ability to distinguish among salty, sweet, sour, and bitter tastants. Kit contains 15 bottles (60 mL) tastants and 30 taste record forms.
Use: Diagnostic aid.

Accutane. (Roche) Isotretinoin 10 mg, 20 mg, 40 mg, soybean oil, parabens, EDTA. Cap. UD 100s. *Rx.*
Use: Retinoid.

Accuzyme. (Healthpoint) **Oint.:** Papain 8.3 × 10^5 units, urea 100 mg/g in a hydrophilic ointment base, parabens, glycerin. Tube 30 g. **Spray:** Papain 8.3 × 10^5 units, urea 10% per g. Anhydrous lactose, cetearyl alcohol, glycerin, mineral oil, parabens. 33 mL. *Rx.*
Use: Enzyme combination, topical.

A-C-D Solution. Sodium citrate, citric acid, and dextrose in sterile pyrogen-free solution. (Baxter Pharmaceutical Products, Inc.). Soln. 600 mL Bot. with 70 mL, 120 mL, 300 mL Soln.; 1000 mL Bot. with 500 mL Soln. (Bayer Biological). 500 mL Bot. with 75 mL, 120 mL Soln.; 650 mL Bot. with 80 mL, 130 mL Soln. (The Diamond Co.). 250 mL, 500 mL *Abbo-Vac. Rx.*
Use: Anticoagulant for preparation of plasma or whole blood.

A-C-D Solution Modified. (Bristol-Myers Squibb) Acid citrate dextrose anticoagulant solution modified. *Rx.*
Use: Anticoagulant, radiolabeled.

•**acebutolol hydrochloride.** (ass-cee-BYOO-toe-lahl) *USP 28.*
Use: Antiadrenergic/sympatholytic; beta-adrenergic blocking agent.
See: Sectral.

acebutolol hydrochloride. (Various Mfr.) Acebutolol hydrochloride 200 mg, 400 mg. Cap. Bot. 100s, 1000s. *Rx.*
Use: Antiadrenergic/sympatholytic, beta-adrenergic blocking agent.

•**acecainide hydrochloride.** (ASS-eh-CANE-ide) USAN.
Use: Cardiovascular agent.
See: NAPA.

•**aceclidine.** (ass-ECK-lih-DEEN) USAN.
Use: Cholinergic.

•**acedapsone.** (ASS-eh-DAP-sone) USAN.
Use: Antimalarial; antibacterial, leprostatic.

Acedoval. (Pal-Pak, Inc.) Dover's powder 15 mg, ipecac 1.5 mg, aspirin 162 mg, caffeine anhydrous 8.1 mg. Tab. Bot. 1000s, 5000s. *OTC.*
Use: Analgesic; antispasmodic; antiperistaltic.
●**aceglutamide aluminum.** (AH-see-GLUE-tah-mide ah-LOO-min-uhm) USAN.
Use: Antiulcerative.
acellular pertussis adsorbed, hepatitis B (recombinant) and inactivated poliovirus vaccine combined, diphtheria and tetanus toxoids.
Use: Active immunization, toxoid.
See: Diptheria and Tetanus Toxoids and Acellular Pertussis Adsorbed, Hepatitis B (Recombinant) and Inactivated Poliovirus Vaccine Combined.
acellular pertussis and Haemophilus influenzae type B conjugate vaccines (DTaP-HIB), diphtheria and tetanus toxoids.
Use: Active immunization, toxoid.
See: Diphtheria and Tetanus Toxoid, Acellular Pertussis and Haemophilus Influenzae Type B Conjugate Vaccines (DTaP-HIB).
acellular pertussis vaccine, adsorbed (DTaP), diphtheria and tetanus toxoids.
Use: Active immunization, toxoid.
See: Diphtheria and Tetanus Toxoids and Acellular Pertussis Vaccine, Adsorbed (DTaP).
●**acemannan.** (ah-see-MAN-an) USAN.
Use: Antiviral; immunomodulator.
See: Carrisyn.
acemannan hydrogel.
Use: Mouth and throat product.
See: Oral Wound Rinse.
Aceon. (Solvay Pharm) Perindopril erbumine 2 mg, 4 mg, 8 mg, lactose. Tab. Bot. 100s. *Rx.*
Use: Antihypertensive, angiotensin-converting enzyme inhibitor.
Acephen. (G & W) **Adult:** Acetaminophen 650 mg. Supp. Box 12s, 100s. **Pediatric:** Acetaminophen 120 mg. Supp. Box 12s, 100s. *OTC.*
Use: Analgesic.
●**acepromazine maleate.** (ASS-ee-PRO-mah-zeen) *USP 28.*
Use: Anxiolytic.
Acerola-C. (Barth's) Vitamin C 300 mg. Wafer. Bot. 30s, 90s, 180s, 360s. *OTC.*
Use: Vitamin supplement.
Acerola-Plex. (Barth's) Vitamin C 100 mg, bioflavonoids 50 mg. Tab. Bot. 100s, 500s. *OTC.*

Use: Vitamin supplement.
Aceta. (Century) Acetaminophen 325 mg or 500 mg. Tab. Bot. 100s, 1000s. *OTC.*
Use: Analgesic.
Acetadote. (Cumberland) Acetylcysteine 20% (200 mg/mL). EDTA 0.5 mg/mL. Preservative-free. Inj. Single-dose vials. 30 mL. *Rx.*
Use: Antidote.
Aceta Elixir. (Century) Acetaminophen 160 mg/5 mL, alcohol 7%. Elix. Bot. 120 mL, 1 gal. *OTC.*
Use: Analgesic.
Aceta-Gesic. (Rugby) Acetaminophen 325 mg, phenyltoloxamine citrate 30 mg. Tab. Bot. 24s, 1000s. *OTC.*
Use: Upper respiratory combination, analgesic, antihistamine.
●**acetaminophen.** (ass-cet-ah-MEE-noe-fen) *USP 20.* APAP
Use: Analgesic; antipyretic.
See: Acephen.
  Aceta.
  Anexsia 5/500.
  Anexsia 7.5/650.
  Anexsia 10/660.
  Children's Dynafed Jr.
  Dolono.
  Dynafed Jr., Children's.
  Extra Strength Dynafed E.X.
  FeverAll.
  Genapap.
  Genebs.
  Halenol.
  Infantaire.
  Liquiprin.
  Meda Cap.
  Meda Tab.
  Neopap.
  Panadol.
  Tempra.
  Tylenol.
  Tylenol Arthritis.
  Tylenol Extra-Strength.
  UN-Aspirin, Extra Strength.
W/Combinations:
  See: Aceta-Gesic.
  Aceta w/Codeine.
  Acid-X.
  Actifed Cold & Sinus Maximum Strength.
  Alka-Seltzer Plus Cold & Cough.
  Alka-Seltzer Plus Cold & Flu.
  Alka-Seltzer Plus Cold & Sinus.
  Alka-Seltzer Plus Cold Medicine.
  Alka-Seltzer Plus Liqui-Gels Flu Medicine.
  Alka-Seltzer Plus Night Time Cold.
  Alka-Seltzer Plus Nose & Throat.
  Allerest Allergy & Sinus Relief Maximum Strength.

All-Nite.
Americet.
Anacin Aspirin Free Extra Strength.
Anacin Aspirin Free Maximum
 Strength.
Anexsia.
Anexsia 5/500.
Anexsia 7.5/650.
Anexsia 10/660.
APAP-Plus.
Aspirin Free Anacin P.M.
Aspirin-Free Bayer Select Head &
 Chest Cold.
Benadryl Allergy & Cold.
Benadryl Allergy & Sinus Headache.
Benadryl Maximum Strength Severe
 Allergy & Sinus Headache.
Bromo Seltzer.
Bucet.
Bupap.
Butalbital, Acetaminophen, and Caf-
 feine.
Butex Forte.
Capital and Codeine.
Children's Dynafed Jr.
Codimal.
Cold Symptoms Relief Maximum
 Strength.
Comtrex Acute Head Cold & Sinus
 Pressure Relief, Multi-Symptom
 Maximum Strength.
Comtrex Allergy-Sinus Treatment,
 Maximum Strength.
Comtrex Cough and Cold Relief,
 Multi-Symptom Maximum Strength.
Comtrex Day & Night Cold & Cough
 Relief, Multi-Symptom Maximum
 Strength.
Comtrex Day/Night Flu Therapy Maxi-
 mum Strength Caplets.
Comtrex Maximum Strength Night-
 time Cold & Cough.
Comtrex Multi-Symptom Deep Chest
 Cold & Congestion Relief.
Comtrex Multi-Symptom Maximum
 Strength Non-Drowsy Cold &
 Cough Relief.
Contac Day & Night Allergy/Sinus Re-
 lief.
Contac Day & Night Cold & Flu.
Contac Severe Cold & Flu Maximum
 Strength.
Coricidin 'D' Cold, Flu & Sinus.
Coricidin HBP Cold & Flu.
Coricidin HBP Maximum Strength Flu.
Darvocet A500.
Darvocet-N 100.
Decodult.
DHC Plus.
Dimetapp Children's Nighttime Flu.
Dimetapp Children's Non-Drowsy Flu.

Dolgic.
Dristan Cold Multi-Symptom Formula.
Drixoral Allergy Sinus.
Dryphen, Multi-Symptom Formula.
Duradrin.
Duraflu.
Ed-Flex.
Endocet.
Esgic.
Esgic-Plus.
Excedrin Aspirin Free.
Excedrin Extra Strength.
Excedrin Migraine.
Extra Strength Dynafed E.X.
FemBack.
Fem-1.
Fioricet.
Fioricet with Codeine.
Flextra-DS.
Genacol Maximum Strength Cold &
 Flu Relief.
Good Sense Maximum Strength Dose
 Sinus.
Good Sense Maximum Strength Pain
 Relief Allergy Sinus.
Goody's Body Pain.
Goody's Extra Strength Headache.
Histenol-Forte.
Histex SR.
Hycet.
Hydrocet.
Hydrocodone Bitartrate and Aceta-
 minophen.
Hyflex 650.
Kolephrin/DM.
Levacet.
Liquiprin.
Lortab.
Lortab 10/500.
Major-gesic.
Mapap Cold Formula.
Margesic.
Marten-Tab.
Maxidone.
Medigesic.
Midol Maximum Strength Menstrual.
Midol Maximum Strength PMS.
Midol Teen Maximum Strength.
Midrin.
N-D Gesic.
Nite Time Cold Formula for Adults.
Norco.
Norco 5/325.
Nyquil.
Ornex No Drowsiness.
Ornex No Drowsiness Maximum
 Strength.
Painaid.
Painaid BRF Back Relief Formula.
Painaid ESF Extra-Strength Formula.
Painaid PMF Premenstrual Formula.

Pamprin Maximum Pain Relief.
Pamprin Multi-Symptom Maximum
Strength.
Panlor DC.
Panlor SS.
Pentazocine Hydrochloride and
Acetaminophen.
Percocet.
Percogesic.
Percogesic Extra Strength.
Phenylgesic.
Phrenilin.
Phrenilin Forte.
Prēmsyn PMS.
Propacet 100.
Relagesic.
Repan.
Repan CF.
Robitussin Cold, Multi-Symptom Cold
& Flu
Robitussin Cold Sinus & Congestion.
Robitussin Flu.
Robitussin Honey Flu Multi-Symp-
tom.
Robitussin Honey Flu NightTime.
Robitussin Honey Flu Non-Drowsy.
Robitussin Night Relief.
Saleto.
Sedapap.
Simplet.
Sine-Off Night Time Formula Sinus,
Cold & Flu Medicine.
Sine-Off Sinus Medicine.
Singlet for Adults.
Sinutab Sinus Allergy, Maximum
Strength.
666 Cold Preparation, Maximum
Strength.
Sudafed Maximum Strength Sinus
Nighttime Plus Pain Relief
Sudafed Multi-Symptom Cold &
Cough.
Sudafed Non-Drowsy Severe Cold
Formula Maximum Strength.
Summit Extra Strength.
Talacen.
Tavist Allergy/Sinus/Headache.
Tencon.
TheraFlu Cold & Cough Night Time.
TheraFlu Flu and Chest Congestion
Non-Drowsy Powder.
TheraFlu Flu & Cold Medicine for
Sore Throat, Maximum Strength.
TheraFlu Flu and Cold Medicine Origi-
nal Formula.
TheraFlu Flu & Cough Night Time,
Maximum Strength.
TheraFlu Flu & Sore Throat, Maxi-
mum Strength.
TheraFlu Flu & Sore Throat Night
Time, Maximum Strength.

TheraFlu Flu, Cold & Cough.
TheraFlu Flu, Cold & Cough and Sore
Throat, Maximum Strength.
TheraFlu Flu, Cold & Cough Night
Time, Maximum Strength.
TheraFlu Maximum Strength Flu &
Congestion Non-Drowsy.
TheraFlu Maximum Strength Night
Time Formula Flu, Cold & Cough
Medicine.
TheraFlu Non-Drowsy Flu, Cold &
Cough Maximum Strength.
TheraFlu Non-Drowsy Formula Maxi-
mum Strength.
TheraFlu Severe Cold & Congestion
Night Time, Maximum Strength.
TheraFlu Severe Cold & Congestion
Non-Drowsy, Maximum Strength.
Top Care LiquiCaps Night Time Multi-
Symptom Cold/Flu Relief.
Top Care Maximum Strength Flu, Cold
& Cough Medicine Night Time.
Top Care Multi-Symptom Pain Relief
Cold.
Triad.
Triaminicin Cold, Allergy, Sinus Medi-
cine.
Triaminic Cough & Sore Throat.
Triaminic Flu, Cough & Fever.
Triaminic Sore Throat Formula.
Triaminic Throat Pain and Cough Soft-
chews.
Trycet.
Tylenol.
Tylenol Allergy Sinus, Maximum
Strength.
Tylenol Children's Chewable Tablets.
Tylenol Children's Cold.
Tylenol Children's Cold Plus Cough.
Tylenol Children's Flu
Tylenol Children's Suspension.
Tylenol Cold Complete Formula
Tylenol Cold Non-Drowsy Formula.
Tylenol 8 Hour.
Tylenol Extended Relief.
Tylenol Flu, Maximum Strength.
Tylenol Flu Maximum Strength Non-
Drowsy.
Tylenol Flu Night Time, Maximum
Strength.
Tylenol Infants' Cold Decongestant &
Fever Reducer Plus Cough Con-
centrated.
Tylenol Multi-Symptom Cold Severe
Congestion.
Tylenol PM Extra Strength.
Tylenol Severe Allergy.
Tylenol Sinus NightTime, Maximum
Strength.
Tylenol Sinus Severe Congestion.
Tylenol w/Codeine.

Tylox.
Ultracet.
Vanquish.
Vicks DayQuil LiquiCaps Multi-Symptom Cold/Flu Relief.
Vicks DayQuil Multi-Symptom Cold/Flu Relief.
Vicks 44M Cough, Cold & Flu Relief.
Vicks NyQuil Multi-Symptom Cold & Flu Relief.
Vicodin.
Vicodin ES.
Vicodin HP.
Vitelle Lurline PMS.
Vopac.
Women's Tylenol Multi-Symptom Menstrual Relief.
Zydone.

- **acetaminophen and aspirin.** (ass-cet-ah-MEE-noe-fen and ASS-pihr-in) *USP 28.*
Use: Analgesic.
- **acetaminophen and caffeine.** (ass-cet-ah-MEE-noe-fen and KAF-een) *USP 28.*
Use: Analgesic.
See: Excedrin Extra Strength.
Excedrin QuickTabs.
Excedrin Tension Headache.
- **acetaminophen and codeine phosphate.** (ass-cet-ah-MEE-noe-fen and KOE-deen) *USP 28.*
Use: Analgesic.
- **acetaminophen and diphenhydramine citrate.** (ass-cet-ah-MEE-noe-fen and die-fen-HIGH-druh-meen) *USP 28.*
Use: Analgesic; antihistamine.
See: Excedrin PM.
Legatrin PM.
Midol PM.
- **acetaminophen and hydrocodone bitartrate.**
See: Hydrocodone bitartrate and acetaminophen.
- **acetaminophen and pseudoephedrine hydrochloride.** (ass-cet-ah-MEE-noe-fen and SUE-doe-eh-FED-rin HIGH-droe-KLOR-ide) *USP 28.*
Use: Analgesic; decongestant.
See: Alka-Seltzer Plus Cold & Sinus.
Cēpacol Sore Throat.
Coldrine.
Dilotab.
Dristan Cold Non-Drowsy Maximum Strength.
Mapap Sinus Maximum Strength.
Maximum Strength Dynafed Plus.
Nasal Decongestant Sinus Non-Drowsy.
Ornex No Drowsiness.

Ornex No Drowsiness Maximum Strength.
Phenapap.
Sine-Off No-Drowsiness Formula.
Sinus-Relief.
Sinus-Relief Maximum Strength.
Sinutab Sinus Without Drowsiness Maximum Strength.
Sinutab Sinus Without Drowsiness Regular Strength.
Sudafed Cold & Sinus Non-Drowsy.
Sudafed Sinus Headache Non-Drowsy.
SudoGest Sinus Maximum Strength.
Tavist Sinus Maximum Strength.
Tylenol Children's Sinus.
Tylenol Infant's Cold.
Tylenol Sinus Non-Drowsy Maximum Strength.

- **acetaminophen, aspirin, and caffeine.** (ass-cet-ah-MEE-noe-fen, ASS-pihr-in, and KAF-een) *USP 28.*
Use: Analgesic.
- **acetaminophen, diphenhydramine hydrochloride, and pseudoephedrine hydrochloride tablets.** *USP 28.*
Use: Analgesic, antihistamine, decongestant.
acetaminophen w/codeine. (Various Mfr.) **Tab.:** Codeine phosphate 15 mg, acetaminophen 300 mg. Bot. 100s, 500s, 1000s. Codeine phosphate 30 mg, acetaminophen 300 mg. Bot. 100s, 500s, 1000s, UD 100s, RN 100s. Codeine phosphate 60 mg, acetaminophen 300 mg. Bot. 100s, 500s, 1000s. *c-iii.* **Soln.:** Codeine phosphate 12 mg, acetaminophen 120 mg/5 mL. Bot. 120 mL, 500 mL, Pt, gal, UD 5 mL, 12.5 mL, 15 mL. *c-v.*
Use: Analgesic combination, narcotic.
acetaminophenol.
See: Acetaminophen.
acetanilid. (Various Mfr.) Acetylaminobenzene, acetylaniline, antifebrin.
Use: Analgesic (former use).
Acetasol HC Otic. (Ivax) Hydrocortisone 1%, acetic acid 2%. Bot. 10 mL. *Rx.*
Use: Anti-infective; corticosteroid, otic.
Acetasol Otic. (Ivax) Acetic acid (non-aqueous) 2%. Bot. 5 mL. *Rx.*
Use: Anti-infective, otic.
Aceta w/Codeine. (Century) Acetaminophen 300 mg, codeine phosphate 30 mg. Tab. Bot. 100s. *c-iii.*
Use: Analgesic combination, narcotic.
- **acetazolamide.** (uh-seet-uh-ZOLE-uh-mide) *USP 28.*
Tall Man: AcetaZOLAMIDE
Use: Carbonic anhydrase inhibitor; anticonvulsant.

acetazolamide. (Bedford Labs) Acetazolamide 500 mg. Pow. for Inj., lyophilized. Preservative-free. Vials. *Rx.*
Use: Anticonvulsant.
acetazolamide. (Various Mfr.) Acetazolamide 125 mg, 250 mg. May contain lactose. Tab. 50s, 100s, 250s, 500s, 1000s.
Use: Carbonic anhydrase inhibitor; anticonvulsant.
●acetazolamide sodium, sterile. (uhseet-uh-ZOLE-uh-mide SO-dee-uhm) *USP 28.*
Tall Man: AcetaZOLAMIDE
Use: Carbonic anhydrase inhibitor.
acet-dia-mer-sulfonamide. Sulfacetamide, sulfadiazine, and sulfamerazine. Susp. *Rx.*
Use: Antibacterial, sulfonamide.
Acetest Reagent. (Bayer Corp. (Consumer Div.)) Sodium nitroprusside, disodium phosphate, aminoacetic acid, lactose. Tab. Bot. 100s, 250s.
Use: Diagnostic aid.
●acetic acid. (ah-SEE-tick) *NF 23.*
Use: Pharmaceutic aid, acidifying agent.
See: Borofalr Otic.
Otic Domeboro.
●acetic acid, glacial. (ah-SEE-tick) *USP 28.*
Use: Pharmaceutic aid, acidifying agent.
W/Combinations
See: Fem ph.
acetic acid irrigation. (Abbott) Acetic acid 0.25% Soln. Glass Cont. 250 mL, 1000 mL.
Use: Irrigating solution.
acetic acid otic. (Various Mfr.) Acetic acid 2% with propylene glycol diacetate 3%, benzethonium chloride 0.02%, and sodium acetate 0.015%. Soln. Bot. 15 mL, 30 mL, 60 mL. *Rx.*
Use: Otic preparation.
acetic acid, potassium salt. (ah-SEEtick, poe-TASS-ee-uhm) Potassium Acetate.
●acetohexamide. (uh-seet-toe-HEX-uhmide) *USP 28.*
Tall Man: AcetoHEXAMIDE
Use: Antidiabetic.
See: Dymelor.
acetohexamide. (Various Mfr.) Acetohexamide 250 mg, 500 mg. Tab. Bot. 100s. *Rx.*
Use: Antidiabetic.
●acetohydroxamic acid. (ass-EE-toehigh-drox-AM-ik) *USP 28.*
Use: Enzyme inhibitor, urease.

See: Lithostat.
acetomeroctol.
Use: Antiseptic, topical.
●acetone. (ASS-eh-tone) *NF 23.*
Use: Pharmaceutic aid, solvent.
acetone or diacetic acid test. (ASS-ehtone)
See: Acetest.
acetophenetidin.
Use: Analgesic; antipyretic.
See: Phenacetin.
Ethoxyacetanilide.
acetorphan.
Use: Enkephalinase inhibitor.
●acetosulfone sodium. (ah-SET-ohSULL-fone SO-dee-uhm) USAN.
Use: Antibacterial, leprostatic.
acetoxyphenylmercury.
See: Phenylmercuric acetate.
acetylaniline.
See: Acetanilid.
acetyl-bromo-diethylacetyl-carbamide.
See: Acetylcarbromal.
acetylcarbromal. Acetyladalin, acetylbromodiethylacetylcarbamide. Pow. for manufacturing.
Use: Sedative.
See: Paxarel.
●acetylcholine chloride. (ah-SEH-tillKOE-leen KLOR-ide) *USP 28.*
Use: Cardiovascular agent; cholinergic; miotic; vasodilator, peripheral.
See: Miochol Ophthalmic.
Miochol E.
acetylcholine-like therapeutic agents.
See: Cholinergic agents.
●acetylcysteine. *USP 28.*
Use: Antidote; mucolytic.
See: Acetadote.
Mucomyst.
acetylcysteine. (Various Mfr.) Acetylcysteine 10%, 20%. EDTA. Oral Soln. Vial 4 mL, 10 mL, 30 mL. *Rx.*
Use: Antidote; mucolytic.
acetylcysteine.
Use: Treatment for severe acetaminophen overdose. [Orphan Drug]
See: Acetadote.
Mucomyst.
Mucomyst 10 IV.
●acetylcysteine and isoproterenol hydrochloride inhalation solution. (ASS-cee-till-SIS-teen and eye-so-proTER-uh-nahl) *USP 28.*
Use: Mucolytic.
acetylin.
See: Acetylsalicylic Acid.
n-acetyl-p-aminophenol. Acetaminophen.

acetylphenylisatin.
See: Oxyphenisatin Acetate.
acetylprocainamide-n.
Use: Cardiovascular agent.
See: Acecainide Hydrochloride.
NAPA.
acetylsalicylic acid.
Use: Analgesic; antipyretic; antirheu-
matic.
See: Aspirin.
n¹-acetylsulfanilamide.
Use: Sulfonamide therapy.
acetyl sulfisoxazole.
See: Sulfisoxazole Acetyl.
acetyltannic acid. Tannic acid acetate.
Use: Antiperistaltic.
AC Eye. (Walgreen) Tetrahydrozoline hy-
drochloride 0.05%, zinc sulfate
0.25%.Ophth. Drops. Bot. 0.75 oz.
OTC.
Use: Decongestant combination, oph-
thalmic.
achlorhydria therapy.
See: Glutamic Acid Hydrochloride.
Achol. (Enzyme Process) Vitamin A
4000 units, ketocholanic acids 62 mg.
Tab. Bot. 100s, 250s. OTC.
Use: Vitamin supplement.
acid acriflavine.
See: Acriflavine Hydrochloride.
**acid citrate dextrose anticoagulant
solution modified.**
See: A-C-D Solution Modified.
acid citrate dextrose solution.
See: A-C-D Solution.
acidifiers.
See: Ammonium Chloride.
K-Phos M.F.
Acid Jelly. (Hope Pharm) Oxyquinoline
sulfate 0.025%, ricinoleic acid 0.7%,
glacial acetic acid 0.921%, glycerin 5%,
propylparaben. Jelly. 85 g with applicator. OTC.
Use: Vaginal preparation.
Acid Mantle. (Doak Dermatologics) Water, cetearyl alcohol, sodium lauryl sulfate, sodium cetearyl sulfate, petrolatum, glycerin, synthetic beeswax, mineral oil, methylparaben, aluminum sulfate, calcium acetate, white potato
dextrin. Cream. Jar 4 oz. OTC.
Use: Ointment, lotion base.
acidophilus.
See: Bacid.
Lactinex.
More Dophilus.
acidophilus w/pectin. (Barth's) Lactobacillus acidophilus w/natural citrus
pectin 100 mg. Cap. Bot. 100s. OTC.
Use: Antidiarrheal.

acid trypaflavine.
See: Acriflavine Hydrochloride.
Acidulated Phosphate Fluoride. (Sch-
erer) Fluoride ion 0.31% in 0.1 molar
phosphate. Soln. Bot. 64 oz. (Office
Product).
Use: Dental caries agent.
Acid-X. (BDI) Acetaminophen 500 mg,
calcium carbonate 250 mg. Tab. Bot.
36s. OTC.
Use: Antacid.
•**acifran.** (ACE-ih-FRAN) USAN.
Use: Antihyperlipoproteinemic.
Aciphex. (Eisai) Rabeprazole sodium
20 mg, mannitol. DR Tab. Enteric
coated. Bot. 30s, 90s, UD 100s. Rx.
Use: Proton pump inhibitor.
Aclaro. (Harmony) Hydroquinone 4%. Al-
cohols, EDTA. Emulsion. Spray Bot.
50 mL. Rx.
Use: Pigment agent.
•**acitretin.** (ASS-ih-TREH-tin) USAN.
Use: Antipsoriatic; retinoid.
See: Soriatane.
•**acivicin.** (ace-ih-VIH-sin) USAN.
Use: Antineoplastic.
•**aclarubicin.** (ack-lah-ROO-bih-sin)
USAN. Formerly Aclacinomycin A.
Use: Antineoplastic.
Aclophen. (Nutripharm Laboratories,
Inc.) Phenylephrine hydrochloride
40 mg, chlorpheniramine maleate 8 mg,
acetaminophen 500 mg, dye free. SR
Tab. Bot. 100s. Rx.
Use: Analgesic; antihistamine; decon-
gestant.
Aclovate. (GlaxoSmithKline) Alclometa-
sone dipropionate 0.05%. Cream or
Oint. Tube 15 g, 45 g. Rx.
Use: Anti-inflammatory, topical.
A.C.N. (Person and Covey) Vitamin A
25,000 units, ascorbic acid 250 mg, nia-
cinamide 25 mg. Tab. Bot. 100s. OTC.
Use: Vitamin supplement.
Acnaveen.
See: Aveenobar Medicated.
Acna-Vite. (Cenci, H.R. Labs, Inc.) Vita-
mins A 10,000 units, C 250 mg, hes-
peridin 50 mg, niacinamide 25 mg. Cap.
Bot. 75s. OTC.
Use: Dermatologic, acne; vitamin
supplement.
Acno. (Baker Cummins Dermatologicals)
Micronized sulfur 3%. Lot. Bot. 120 mL.
OTC.
Use: Dermatologic, acne.
Acno Cleanser. (Baker Cummins Der-
matologicals) Isopropyl alcohol 60%,
laureth-23, tetrasodium EDTA. Bot.
240 mL. OTC.
Use: Dermatologic, acne.

Acnomel. (Numark) Sulfur 8%, resorcinol 2%, alcohol 11%. Cream. Tube 28 g. *OTC.*
Use: Keratolytic, acne product.
Acnotex. (C & M Pharmacal) Sulfur 8%, resorcinol 2%, isopropyl alcohol 20%, acetone. In lotion base. Bot. 60 mL. *OTC.*
Use: Dermatologic, acne.
• **acodazole hydrochloride.** (ah-KOE-dah-ZOLE) USAN.
Use: Antineoplastic.
• **acolbifene hydrochloride.** (aye-KOLE-bi-feen) USAN.
Use: Breast and uterine proliferation or cancer.
aconiazide. (Lincoln Diagnostics)
Use: Antituberculous. [Orphan Drug]
Acotus. (Whorton Pharmaceuticals, Inc.) Phenylephrine hydrochloride 5 mg, guaiacol glyceryl ether 100 mg, menthol 1 mg, alcohol by volume 10%/5 mL. Bot. 4 oz, 12 oz, gal. *OTC.*
Use: Antitussive; decongestant.
Acova. (GlaxoSmithKline) Argatroban 100 mg/mL. Inj. Single-use vial 2.5 mL. *Rx.*
Use: Anticoagulant.
ACR. (Western Research) Ammonium Cl 7.5 g. Tab. Handicount 28s (36 bags of 28 tab.). *Rx.*
Use: Diuretic.
acriflavine. (Eli Lilly) Acriflavine 1.5 g. Tab. Bot. 100s.
Use: Antiseptic.
acriflavine hydrochloride. (Various Mfr.) Hydrochloride form of acriflavine. Acid acriflavine, acid trypaflavine, flavine, trypaflavine. National Aniline-Pow., Bot. 1 g, 5 g, 10 g, 25 g, 50 g. Tab. 1.5 g. Bot. 50s, 100s. *Rx.*
Use: Anti-infective.
• **acrisorcin.** (ACK-rih-sahr-sin) USAN.
Use: Antifungal.
See: Akrinol.
• **acrivastine.** (ACK-rih-VASS-teen) USAN.
Use: Antihistamine.
acrivastine and pseudoephedrine hydrochloride.
Use: Upper respiratory combination, antihistamine, decongestant.
See: Semprex-D.
• **acronine.** (ACK-row-neen) USAN.
Use: Antineoplastic.
ACT. Dactinomycin.
Use: Antineoplastic.
See: Actinomycin D.
ACT. (J & J Merck Consumer Pharm.)
Rinse: 0.02% (from 0.05% sodium fluoride). **Mint:** Tartrazine, alcohol 8%.

Cinnamon: Alcohol 7%. Bot. 360 mL, 480 mL. *OTC.*
Use: Dentrifice.
Actacin. (Vangard Labs, Inc.) Triprolidine hydrochloride 2.5 mg, pseudoephedrine hydrochloride 60 mg. Tab. Bot. 100s, 1000s. *Rx-OTC.*
Use: Antihistamine; decongestant.
Actacin-C. (Vangard Labs, Inc.) Codeine phosphate 10 mg, triprolidine hydrochloride 2 mg, pseudoephedrine hydrochloride 20 mg, guaifenesin 100 mg/5 mL. Syr. Bot. Pt, gal. *c-v.*
Use: Antihistamine; antitussive; decongestant; expectorant.
Actal Plus. (Sanofi-Synthelabo) Aluminum hydroxide, magnesium hydroxide. Tab. *OTC.*
Use: Antacid.
Actal Suspension. (Sanofi-Synthelabo) Aluminum hydroxide. Susp. *OTC.*
Use: Antacid.
Actal Tablets. (Sanofi-Synthelabo) Aluminum hydroxide. Tab. *OTC.*
Use: Antacid.
Actamin. (Buffington) Acetaminophen 325 mg. Tab. *Dispens-A-Kit* 100s, 200s, 500s. *OTC.*
Use: Analgesic.
Actamine. (H.L. Moore Drug Exchange)
Tab.: Pseudoephedrine hydrochloride 60 mg, triprolidine hydrochloride 2.5 mg. Bot. 100s, 1000s. **Syr.:** Pseudoephedrine hydrochloride 30 mg, triprolidine hydrochloride 1.25 mg/5 mL. Bot. 120 mL, Pt, gal. *Rx-OTC.*
Use: Antihistamine; decongestant.
Actamin Extra. (Buffington) Acetaminophen 500 mg. Tab. Bot. 100s, 200s, 500s. *OTC.*
Use: Analgesic.
Actamin Super. (Buffington) Acetaminophen 500 mg, caffeine. Sugar, salt, and lactose free. Tab. *Dispens-A-Kit* 500s, *Medipak* 200s. *OTC.*
Use: Analgesic.
ACTH. Adrenocorticotrophic hormone. Adrenocorticotropin.
Use: Corticosteroid.
See: Corticotropin.
ACTH-Actest. (Forest) Repository corticotropin 40 units or 80 units/mL. Gel. Vial 5 mL. *Rx.*
Use: Corticosteroid.
ActHIB. (Aventis Pasteur) Purified capsular polysaccharide of *Haemophilus* b 10 mcg, tetanus toxoid 24 mcg/0.5 mL, sucrose 8.5%. Pow. for Inj., lyophilized. Single-dose Vial with 7.5 mL vials of diphtheria and tetanus toxoids and pertussis vaccine as diluents or 0.6 mL

vial containing 0.4% sodium chloride diluent. *Rx.*
Use: Vaccine.

ActHIB/DTP. (Aventis Pasteur) Diphtheria and tetanus toxoids and pertussis and *Haemophilus influenzae* type b vaccines. One package consists of one 7.5 mL vial of Connaught's DTwP and 10 single-dose vials of ActHIB vaccine. *Rx.*
Use: Immunization.

Acthrel. (Ferring) Corticorelin ovine triflutata 100 mcg. Cake, lyophilized. 5 mL single-dose vial w/diluent. *Rx.*
Use: Diagnostic aid.

ActiBath. (Andrew Jergens) Colloidal oatmeal 20%. Tab. Effervescent. Pkg. 4s. *OTC.*
Use: Emollient.

Acticin. (Bertek) Permethrin 5%. Coconut oil, lanolin alcohols, light mineral oil. Cream. Tube 60 g. *Rx.*
Use: Scabicide.

Acticort 100. (Baker Cummins Dermatologicals) Hydrocortisone 1%. Lot. Bot. 60 mL. *Rx.*
Use: Corticosteroid, topical.

Actidose. (Paddock) Activated charcoal. 25 g/120 mL or 50 g/240 mL. Soln. *OTC.*
Use: Antidote.

Actidose-Aqua. (Paddock) Activated charcoal. 25 g/120 mL or 50 g/240 mL. Aqueous susp. *OTC.*
Use: Antidote.

Actidose w/Sorbitol. (Paddock) Activated charcoal. 25 g in 120 mL susp. w/sorbitol, 50 g in 240 mL susp. w/sorbitol. Liq. *OTC.*
Use: Antidote.

Actifed Cold & Allergy. (Pfizer) Triprolidine hydrochloride 2.5 mg, pseudoephedrine hydrochloride 60 mg, sucrose, lactose. Tab. Pkg. 12s, 24s. *OTC.*
Use: Upper respiratory combination, antihistamine, decongestant.

Actifed Cold & Sinus Maximum Strength. (Pfizer) Pseudoephedrine hydrochloride 30 mg, chlorpheniramine maleate 2 mg, acetaminophen 500 mg. Tab. Pkg. 20s. *OTC.*
Use: Upper respiratory combination, analgesic, antihistamine, decongestant.

Actigall. (Watson) Ursodiol (Ursodeoxycholic acid) 300 mg. Cap. Bot. 100s. *Rx.*
Use: Gallstone solubilizing agent.

Actimmune. (Genentech) Interferon gamma-1b 100 mcg (3 million units)/vial. *Rx.*

Use: Anti-infective.

actinomycin c. Name previously used for Cactinomycin.

actinomycin d.
Use: Antineoplastic.
See: Dactinomycin.

•**actinoquinol sodium.** (ack-TIN-oh-kwih-nole SO-dee-uhm) USAN.
Use: Ultraviolet screen.

actinospectacin. Name previously used for Spectinomycin.

Actiq. (Cephalon) Fentanyl citrate (as base) transmucosal system 200 mcg, 400 mcg, 600 mcg, 800 mcg, 1,200 mcg, 1,600 mcg. Sugar (each unit contains ≈ 2 g), berry flavor. Loz. on a stick. 30s with carton blister packs. *c-II.*
Use: Opioid analgesic.

•**actisomide.** (ackt-EYE-so-MIDE) USAN.
Use: Cardiovascular agent.

Activase. (Genentech) Alteplase recombinant 50 mg (29 million U), 100 mg (58 million U). L-arginine, phosphoric acid, polysorbate 80. Pow. for Inj., lyophilized. Vials with diluent (50 mL sterile water for injection) and vacuum (50 mg only); vials with diluent (100 mL sterile water for injection) and 1 transfer device (100 mg only). *Rx.*
Use: Thrombolytic.

activated attapulgite. *OTC.*
Use: Dermatologic, acne.
W/Aluminum hydroxide, magnesium carbonate coprecipitate, compressed gel.
See: Hykasil.
W/Polysorbate 80, colloidal sulfur, salicylic acid, propylene glycol.
See: Sebasorb.

activated charcoal liquid. (Various Mfr.) Activated charcoal 12.5 g, 25 g with propylene glycol. Liq. Bot. 60 mL (12.5 g), 120 mL (25 g). *OTC.*
Use: Antidote.

activated charcoal powder. (Various Mfr.) Activated charcoal 15 g, 30 g, 40 g, 120 g, and 140 g. Pow. *OTC.*
Use: Antidote.

activated charcoal tablets. (Cowley) Activated charcoal 5 g. Tab. Bot. 1000s. *OTC.*
Use: Antidote.

activated ergosterol.
See: Calciferol.

activated 7-dehydrocholesterol.
See: Vitamin D-3.

active immunization agents.
See: BCG Vaccine.
Diphtheria and Tetanus Toxoids, Acellular Pertussis and Haemophilus In-

fluenzae Type B Conjugate Vaccines (DTaP-HIB).
Diphtheria and Tetanus Toxoids, Adsorbed (for Adult Use).
Diphtheria and Tetanus Toxoids, Adsorbed (for Pediatric Use).
Diphtheria and Tetanus Toxoids, Adult.
Diphtheria and Tetanus Toxoids and Acellular Pertussis Adsorbed, Hepatitis B (Recombinant) and Inactivated Poliovirus Vaccine Combined.
Diphtheria and Tetanus Toxoids and Acellular Pertussis Vaccine, Adsorbed (DTaP).
Haemophilus b Conjugate Vaccine
Haemophilus b Conjugate Vaccine with Hepatitis B Vaccine.
Hepatitis A, Inactivated and Hepatitis B, Recombinant Vaccine.
Hepatitis A Vaccine, Inactivated.
Hepatitis B Vaccine, Recombinant.
Influenza Virus Vaccine.
Measles Virus Vaccine, Live, Attenuated.
Meningococcal Vaccine.
Pneumococcal 7-Valent Conjugate Vaccine.
Pneumococcal Vaccine, Polyvalent.
Smallpox Vaccine.
Tetanus Toxoid, Fluid.
Toxoids.
Typhoid Vaccine.
Varicella Virus Vaccine.
viral vaccines.
• **actodigin.** (ACK-toe-dihj-in) USAN.
Use: Cardiovascular agent.
Actonel. (Procter & Gamble) Risedronate sodium 5 mg, 30 mg, 35 mg, lactose. Film coated Tab. Bot. 30s, 2000s (5 mg only); dose packs of 4s (35 mg only). *Rx.*
Use: Bisphosphonate.
actoquinol sodium.
Use: Ultraviolet screen.
Actos. (Takeda Pharm. America) Pioglitazone hydrochloride 15 mg, 30 mg, 45 mg, lactose. Tab. Bot. 30s, 90s, 500s. *Rx.*
Use: Antidiabetic.
Acucron. (Seatrace) Acetaminophen 300 mg, salicylamide 200 mg, phenyltoloxamine 20 mg. Tab. Bot. 100s, 1000s, 5000s. *OTC.*
Use: Analgesic; antihistamine.
Acu-Dyne. (Acme United Corp.)
Douche: Povidone-iodine. Pkt. 240 mL.
Oint.: Povidone-iodine. Jar. lb. Pkt. 1.2 g, 2.7 g (100s). **Perineal wash conc.:** Available iodine 1%. Bot. 40 mL.
Prep. Soln.: Povidone-iodine. Bot.

240 mL, Pt, qt, gal. Pkt. 30 mL, 60 mL.
Skin Cleanser: Povidone-iodine. Bot. 60 mL, 240 mL, Pt, qt, gal. **Soln., prep. swabs:** Available iodine 1%. Bot. 100s.
Soln., swabsticks: Povidone-iodine. Pkt. 1 or 3 in 25s. **Whirlpool conc.:** Available iodine 1%. Bot. gal. *OTC.*
Use: Antiseptic; antimicrobial.
Acular. (Allergan) Ketorolac tromethamine 0.5%. Benzalkonium Cl 0.01%, EDTA 0.1%, octoxynol 40, sodium chloride, hydrochloric acid, and/or sodium hydroxide. Ophth. Soln. Drop. Bot. 3 mL, 5 mL, 10 mL. *Rx.*
Use: Nonsteroidal anti-inflammatory drug, ophthalmic.
Acular LS. (Allergan) Ketorolac tromethamine 0.4%, benzalkonium chloride 0.006%, EDTA 0.015%, sodium chloride, hydrochloric acid, and/or sodium hydroxide. Soln. Drop. Bot. 5 mL. *Rx.*
Use: Nonsteroidal anti-inflammatory drug, ophthalmic.
Acular PF. (Allergan) Ketorolac tromethamine 0.5%. Sodium chloride, hydrochloric acid, and/or sodium hydroxide. Preservative free. Soln. Single-use vials. 0.4 mL. *Rx.*
Use: Nonsteroidal anti-inflammatory drug, ophthalmic.
• **acyclovir.** (A-SIKE-low-vir) *USP 28.*
Use: Antiviral.
See: Zovirax.
acyclovir. (Various Mfr.) Acyclovir. **Tab.:** 400 mg, 800 mg. Bot. 100s, 500s, 1000s (400 mg only). **Cap.:** 200 mg. Bot. 100s. **Susp.:** 200 mg/5 mL. 473 mL. *Rx.*
Use: Antiviral.
• **acyclovir sodium.** (A-SIKE-low-vir) USAN.
Use: Antiviral.
See: Zovirax.
acyclovir sodium. (Various Mfr.) Acyclovir sodium. **Inj.:** 50 mg/mL. Ctns. of 10.
Pow. for Inj.: 500 mg/vial, 1000 mg/vial. Vials. 10 mL (500 mg only), 20 mL (1000 mg only). *Rx.*
Use: Antiviral.
Adagen. (Enzon) Pegademase bovine 250 units/mL. Vial 1.5 mL. *Rx.*
Use: Enzyme (ADA) replacement therapy.
Adalat. (Bayer) Nifedipine 10 mg, 20 mg, saccharin (10 mg only). Cap. Bot. 100s, 300s, UD 100s. *Rx.*
Use: Calcium channel blocker.
Adalat CC. (Bayer) Nifedipine 30 mg, 60 mg, 90 mg, lactose. ER Tab. Bot. 100s, UD 100s. *Rx.*
Use: Calcium channel blocker.

●**adalimumab.** (ah-dah-LIM-you-mab) USAN.
Use: Immunomodulator.
See: Humira.

adamantanamine hydrochloride.
See: Amantadine Hydrochloride. Symmetrel.

●**adapalene.** (ADE-ah-PALE-een) USAN.
Use: Dermatologic, acne, retinoid.
See: Differin.

Adapettes. (Alcon) Povidone and other water-soluble polymers, sorbic acid, EDTA. Soln. Bot. 15 mL. *OTC.*
Use: Contact lens care.

Adapettes for Sensitive Eyes. (Alcon) Povidone and other water-soluble polymers, EDTA, sorbic acid. Pkg. 15 mL. *OTC.*
Use: Contact lens care.

Adapin. (Lotus Biochemical) Doxepin hydrochloride **10 mg, 75 mg, 100 mg:** Cap. Bot. 100s, 1000s, UD 100s. **25 mg, 50 mg:** Cap. Bot. 100s, 1000s, 5000s, UD 100s. **150 mg:** Cap. Bot. 50s, 100s. *Rx.*
Use: Antidepressant.

●**adaprolol maleate.** (ad-AH-prole-ole MAL-ee-ate) USAN.
Use: Antihypertensive, β-blocker, ophthalmic.

Adapt. (Alcon) Povidone, EDTA 0.1%, thimerosal 0.004%. Bot. 15 mL. *OTC.*
Use: Contact lens care.

Adapt Wetting Solution. (Alcon) Adsorbobase with thimerosal 0.004%, EDTA 0.1%. Soln. Bot. 15 mL. *OTC.*
Use: Contact lens care.

●**adatanserin hydrochloride.** (ahd-at-AN-ser-in HIGH-droe-KLOR-ide) USAN.
Use: Antidepressant; anxiolytic.

AdatoSil 5000. (Escalon Ophthalmics, Inc.) Polydimethylsiloxane oil. Inj. Vial 10 mL, 15 mL. *Rx.*
Use: Ophthalmic.

Adavite. (Hudson Corp.) Vitamins A 5000 units, D 400 units, E 30 mg, B_1 3 mg, B_2 3.4 mg, B_3 30 mg, B_5 10 mg, B_6 3 mg, B_{12} 90 mcg, C 90 mg, folic acid 0.4 mg, biotin 35 mcg, beta-carotene 1250 units. Tab. Bot. 130s. *OTC.*
Use: Mineral, vitamin supplement.

Adavite-M. (Hudson Corp.) Iron 27 mg, Vitamins A 5000 units, D 400 units, E 30 mg, B_1 3 mg, B_2 3.4 mg, B_3 20 mg, B_5 10 mg, B_6 3 mg, B_{12} 9 mcg, C 190 mg, folic acid 0.4 mg, Ca, Cl, Cr, Cu, I, K, Mg, Mn, Mo, P, Se, Zinc 15 mg, biotin 30 mcg. Tab. Bot. 130s. *OTC.*
Use: Mineral, vitamin supplement.

ADC with Fluoride. (Various Mfr.) Fluoride 0.5 mg, vitamins A 1500 units, D 400 units, C 35 mg, methylparaben/mL. Drops. Bot. 50 mL. *Rx.*
Use: Mineral, vitamin supplement.

Adderall. (Shire US) **5 mg:** Dextroamphetamine saccharate 1.25 mg, amphetamine aspartate monohydrate 1.25 mg, dextroamphetamine sulfate 1.25 mg, amphetamine sulfate 1.25 mg. **7.5 mg:** Dextroamphetamine saccharate 1.875 mg, amphetamine aspartate 1.875 mg, dextroamphetamine sulfate 1.875 mg, amphetamine sulfate 1.875 mg. **10 mg:** Dextroamphetamine sulfate 2.5 mg, dextroamphetamine saccharate 2.5 mg, amphetamine aspartate 2.5 mg, amphetamine sulfate 2.5 mg. **12.5 mg:** Dextroamphetamine saccharate 3.125 mg, amphetamine aspartate 3.125 mg, dextroamphetamine sulfate 3.125 mg, amphetamine sulfate 3.125 mg. **15 mg:** Dextroamphetamine saccharate 3.75 mg, amphetamine aspartate monohydrate 3.75 mg, dextroamphetamine sulfate 3.75 mg, amphetamine sulfate 3.75 mg. **20 mg:** Dextroamphetamine sulfate 5 mg, dextroamphetamine saccharide 5 mg, amphetamine aspartate 5 mg, amphetamine sulfate 5 mg. **25 mg:** Dextroamphetamine saccharate 6.25 mg, amphetamine aspartate monohydrate 6.25 mg, dextroamphetamine sulfate 6.25 mg, amphetamine sulfate 6.25 mg. **30 mg:** Dextroamphetamine saccharate 7.5 mg, amphetamine aspartate 7.5 mg, dextroamphetamine sulfate 7.5 mg, amphetamine sulfate 7.5 mg. Sucrose, lactose. Tab. Bot. 100s. *c-II.*
Use: CNS stimulant, amphetamine.

Adderall XR. (Shire) **5 mg:** Dextroamphetamine saccharate 1.25 mg, amphetamine aspartate monohydrate 1.25 mg, dextroamphetamine sulfate 1.25 mg, amphetamine sulfate 1.25 mg, talc. **10 mg:** Dextroamphetamine saccharate 2.5 mg, amphetamine aspartate monohydrate 2.5 mg, dextroamphetamine sulfate 2.5 mg, amphetamine sulfate 2.5 mg. **15 mg:** Dextroamphetamine saccharate 3.75 mg, amphetamine aspartate monohydrate 3.75 mg, dextroamphetamine sulfate 3.75 mg, amphetamine sulfate 3.75 mg, talc. **20 mg:** Dextroamphetamine saccharate 5 mg, amphetamine aspartate monohydrate 5 mg, dextroamphetamine sulfate 5 mg, amphetamine sulfate 5 mg. **25 mg:** Dextroamphetamine saccharate

6.25 mg, amphetamine aspartate monohydrate 6.25 mg, dextroamphetamine sulfate 6.25 mg, amphetamine sulfate 6.25 mg, talc. **30 mg:** Dextroamphetamine saccharate 7.5 mg, amphetamine aspartate monohydrate 7.5 mg, dextroamphetamine sulfate 7.5 mg, amphetamine sulfate 7.5 mg. Sugar spheres. Cap. Bot. 100s. *c-II.*
Use: CNS stimulant, amphetamine.

Adeecon. (CMC) Vitamins A 5000 units, D 1000 units. Cap. Bot. 1000s. *OTC.*
Use: Vitamin supplement.

●**adefovir dipivoxil.** (ah-DEF-fah-vihr die-pih-vox-ill) USAN.
Use: Antiviral, treatment of HIV and HBV infections.
See: Hepsera.

ADEKs. (Scandipharm, Inc.) Vitamins A 4000 units, D 400 units, E 150 units, vitamin K, C 60 mg, B_1 1.2 mg, B_2 1.3 mg, B_3 10 mg, B_6 1.5 mg, B_{12} 12 mcg, B_5 10 mg, folic acid 0.2 mg, biotin 50 mcg, beta-carotene 3 mg, Zn 1.1 mg, fructose. Tab. Bot. 60s. *OTC.*
Use: Mineral, vitamin supplement.

ADEKs Pediatric. (Scandipharm, Inc.) Vitamin A 1500 units, D 400 units, E 40 units, K_1 0.1 mg, C 45 mg, B_1 0.5 mg, B_2 0.6 mg, B_3 6 mg, B_5 3 mg, B_6 0.6 mg, B_{12} 4 mcg, biotin 15 mcg, Zn 5 mg, beta-carotene 1 mg per mL. Drops. Bot. 60 mL. *OTC.*
Use: Vitamin supplement.

●**adenine.** *USP 28.*
Use: Vitamin.

adeno-associated viral-based vector cystic fibrosis gene therapy. (Targeted Genetics)
Use: Cystic fibrosis. [Orphan Drug]

Adenocard. (Fujisawa Healthcare) Adenosine 3 mg/mL, NaCl 9 mg/mL. Preservative free. Inj. Vial. Syr. 2 mL, 5 mL. *Rx.*
Use: Antiarrhythmic.

Adenolin Forte. (Lincoln Diagnostics) Adenosine-5-monophosphate 25 mg, methionine 25 mg, niacin 10 mg/mL. Inj. Vial 15 mL. *Rx.*
Use: Anti-inflammatory.

Adenoscan. (Fujisawa Healthcare) Adenosine 3 mg/mL. Inj. Vial 30 mL. *Rx.*
Use: Diagnostic aid.

●**adenosine.** (ah-DEN-oh-seen) *USP 28.*
Use: Antiarrhythmic.
See: Adenocard.
  Adenoscan.

adenosine. (Medco Research)
Use: Antineoplastic. [Orphan Drug]

adenosine. (Various Mfr.) Adenosine 3 mg/mL. Sodium chloride 9 mg/mL. Preservative free. Inj. Vials. 2 mL, 4 mL. Disposable syringes. 2 mL. *Rx.*
Use: Antiarrhythmic agent.

adenosine in gelatin. (Forest) **Forte:** Adenosine-5-monophosphate 50 mg/mL. **Super:** Adenosine-5-monophosphate 100 mg/mL. *Rx.*
Use: Varicosity.

●**adenosine phosphate.** (ah-DEN-oh-seen) USAN. Adenosine monophosphate, AMP.
Use: Nutritional supplement.

adenosine phosphate. (Various Mfr.) Adenosine phosphate 25 mg/mL. May contain benzyl alcohol. Inj. vial. 10 mL, 30 mL. *Rx.*
Use: Treatment of statis dermatitis.

Adeno Twelve. (Forest) Adenosine-5-monophosphate 25 mg, methionine 25 mg, niacin 10 mg/mL. Gel. Inj. Vial 10 mL. *Rx.*
Use: Anti-inflammatory.

adenovirus vaccine type 4. (Wyeth) Adenovirus vaccine live type 4. At least 32,000 $TCID_{50}$. Tab. Bot. 100s. *Rx.*
Use: Immunization.

adenovirus vaccine type 7. (Wyeth) Adenovirus vaccine live type 7. At least 32,000 $TCID_{50}$. Tab. Bot. 100s. *Rx.*
Use: Immunization.

adepsine oil.
See: Petrolatum.

AdGVCFTR 10. (GenVec)
Use: Cystic fibrosis. [Orphan Drug]

●**adinazolam.** (AHD-in-AZE-oh-lam) USAN.
Use: Antidepressant, hypnotic, sedative.

●**adinazolam mesylate.** (AHD-in-AZE-oh-lam MEH-sih-LATE) USAN.
Use: Antidepressant.

Adipex-P. (Gate) **Cap.:** Phentermine hydrochloride 37.5 mg, lactose. Bot. 100s. **Tab.:** Phentermine hydrochloride 37.5 mg, lactose, sucrose. Bot. 30s, 100s, 1000s. *c-IV.*
Use: CNS stimulant, anorexiant.

●**adiphenine hydrochloride.** (ah-DIH-feh-neen HIGH-droe-KLOR-ide) USAN.
Use: Muscle relaxant.

Adisol. (Major) Disulfiram 250 mg, 500 mg. Tab. Bot. 50s (500 mg only), 100s (250 mg only). *Rx.*
Use: Antialcoholic.

Adlerika. (Last) Magnesium sulfate 4 g/15 mL. Bot. 12 oz. *OTC.*
Use: Laxative.

Adlone. (Forest) Methylprednisolone acetate 40 mg, 80 mg. Inj. Vial 5 mL. *Rx.*
Use: Corticosteroid, topical.

Adolph's Salt Substitute. (Adolphs) Potassium Cl 2480 mg/5 g, silicon dioxide, tartaric acid. Gran. Bot. 99.2 g. *OTC.*
Use: Salt substitute.

Adolph's Seasoned Salt Substitute. (Adolphs) Potassium Cl 1360 mg/5 g, silicon dioxide, tartaric acid. Gran. Bot. 92.1 g. *OTC.*
Use: Salt substitute.

Adonidine. (City Chemical Corp.) Bot. g. *Rx.*
Use: Cardiovascular agent.

Adoxa. (Bioglan) Doxycycline monohydrate 50 mg, 75 mg, 100 mg. Tab. Bot. 50s (100 mg only), 100s (except 100 mg), 250s (100 mg only), 500s (75 mg only). *Rx.*
Use: Anti-infective, tetracycline.

•**adozelesin.** (ADE-oh-ZELL-eh-sin) USAN.
Use: Antineoplastic.

Adprin-B. (Pfeiffer) Aspirin 325 mg, calcium carbonate, magnesium carbonate, magnesium oxide. Tab. Bot. 130s. *OTC.*
Use: Analgesic.

Adprin-B, Extra Strength. (Pfeiffer) Aspirin 500 mg w/calcium carbonate, magnesium carbonate, magnesium oxide. Tab. Bot. 130s. *OTC.*
Use: Analgesic.

ADR.
Use: Antineoplastic.
See: Doxorubicin Hydrochloride.

adrenal steroid inhibitors.
Use: Adrenocortical steroids.
See: Aminoglutethimide.

Adrenalin Chloride. (Monarch) **Soln. for Inh.:** Epinephrine hydrochloride 1:100 (10 mg/ml), benzethonium chloride, sodium bisulfite 0.2%. Bot. 7.5 mL. **Soln.:** Epinephrine hydrochloride 1:1000 (1 mg/mL). *Steri-Vials* 30 mL (chlorobutanol 0.5%, sodium bisulfite < 0.15%). Amp. 1 mL (sodium bisulfite < 0.1%). **Inj.:** Epinephrine hydrochloride 1:1000 (1 mg/mL). **Soln. Amp:** 1 mL, sodium bisulfite. *Steri-vial:* Chlorobutanol, sodium bisulfate. *Rx.*
Use: Bronchodilator, sympathomimetic; nasal decongestant, arylalkylamine.

adrenalin (e).
See: Epinephrine.

adrenaline hydrochloride.
See: Epinephrine Hydrochloride.

•**adrenalone.** (ah-DREN-ah-lone) USAN.
Use: Adrenergic, ophthalmic.

adrenamine.
See: Epinephrine.

adrenergic agents.
See: Sympathomimetic agents.

adrenergic-blocking agents.
See: Sympatholytic agents.

adrenine.
See: Epinephrine.

adrenocortical steroids.
See: Adrenal Steroid Inhibitors.
Betamethasone.
Betamethasone Sodium Phosphate.
Betamethasone Sodium Phosphate and Betamethasone Acetate.
Budesonide.
Corticotropin.
Corticotropin, repository injection.
Cosyntropin.
Fludrocortisone Acetate.
Glucocorticoids.
Mineralocorticoids.

adrenocorticotrophic hormone. ACTH acts by stimulating the endogenous production of cortisone. *Rx.*
See: ACTH.
Corticotropin.

Adrenomist Inhalant and Nebulizers. (Nephron) Epinephrine 1%. Bot. 0.5 oz, 1.25 oz. *Rx-OTC.*
Use: Bronchodilator.

Adrenucleo. (Enzyme Process) Vitamin C 250 mg, d-calcium pantothenate 12.5 mg, bioflavonoids 62.5 mg. Tab. Bot. 100s, 250s. *OTC.*
Use: Vitamin supplement.

Adriamycin PFS. (Pharmacia & Upjohn) Doxorubicin hydrochloride 2 mg/mL, preservative free. Inj. Single-dose vial. 5 mL, 10 mL, 25 mL, 37.5 mL; multi-dose vial 100 mL. *Rx.*
Use: Antibiotic.

Adriamycin RDF. (Pharmacia & Upjohn) Doxorubicin hydrochloride 10 mg, 20 mg, 50 mg, 150 mg; methylparaben, lactose 50 mg, 100 mg, 250 mg, 750 mg. Pow. for Inj., lyophilized. Single-dose vial, multiple-dose vial (150 mg only). Rapid dissolution formula. *Rx.*
Use: Antibiotic.

•**adrogolide hydrochloride.** USAN.
Use: Parkinson disease.

Adrucil. (Gensia Sicor) Fluorouracil 50 mg/mL. Inj. Vial 10 mL, 50 mL, 100 mL. *Rx.*
Use: Antineoplastic; antimetabolite.

Adsorbocarpine. (Alcon) Pilocarpine hydrochloride 1%, 2%, 4%. Bot. 15 mL. *Rx.*

Use: Miotic.

Adsorbonac. (Alcon) Sodium Cl 2%, 5%. Ophth. Soln. Vial 15 mL. *OTC.*
Use: Hyperosmolar preparation.

Adsorbotear. (Alcon) Hydroxyethylcellulose 0.4%, povidone 1.67%, watersoluble polymers, thimerosal 0.004%, EDTA 0.1%. Soln. Bot. dropper 15 mL. *OTC.*
Use: Artificial tears.

Adult Acnomel. (Numark) Sulfur 8%. resorcinol 2%, alcohol 15%, propylene glycol. Cream. Tube. 28 g. *OTC.*
Use: Keratolytic, acne product.

Advair Diskus. (GlaxoSmithKline) Fluticasone propionate 100 mcg, salmeterol 50 mcg; fluticasone propionate 250 mcg, salmeterol 50 mcg; fluticasone propionate 500 mcg, salmeterol 50 mcg. Lozenge. Pow. for Inh. Disp. device w/28 and 60 blisters. *Rx.*
Use: Respiratory inhalant combination.

Advance. (Ross) **Ready-to-Feed Infant Formula:** (16 cal/fl oz). Can 13 fl oz. **Conc. Liq:** 32 fl oz. *OTC.*
Use: Nutritional supplement.

Advanced Care Cholesterol Test. (Johnson & Johnson)
Use: At home cholesterol test.

Advanced Formula Centrum Liquid. (Wyeth) Vitamins A 2500 units, E 30 units, C 60 mg, B_1 1.5 mg, B_2 1.7 mg, B_3 20 mg, B_5 10 mg, B_6 2 mg, B_{12} 6 mcg, D 400 units, iron 9 mg, biotin 300 mcg, I, Zn 3 mg, Mn, Cr, Mo, alcohol 6.7%, sucrose. Bot. 236 mL. *OTC.*
Use: Mineral, vitamin supplement.

Advanced Formula Centrum Tablets. (Wyeth) Iron 18 mg, vitamins A 5000 units, D 400 units, E 30 units, B_1 1.5 mg, B_2 1.7 mg, B_3 20 mg, B_5 10 mg, B_6 2 mg, B_{12} 6 mcg, C 60 mg, folic acid 0.4 mg, biotin 30 mcg, B, Ca, Cl, Cr, Cu, I, K, Mg, Mn, Mo, Ni, P, Se, Si, Sn, V, Zn 15 mg, vitamin K. Bot. 60s, 130s, 200s. *OTC.*
Use: Mineral, vitamin supplement.

Advanced Formula Plax. (Pfizer) Tetrasodium pyrophosphate, alcohol, saccharin. Mouthwash. Bot. 120 mL, 240 mL, 473 mL, 720 mL, 1740 mL. *OTC.*
Use: Anti-infective.

Advanced Formula Zenate. (Solvay) Fe 65 mg, vitamins A 3000 units, D 400 units, E 10 units, C 70 mg, folic acid 1 mg, B_1 1.5 mg, B_2 1.6 mg, B_3 17 mg, B_6 2.2 mg, B_{12} 2.2 mcg, Ca 200 mg, I 175 mcg, Mg 100 mg, Zn 15 mg. Tab. UD 30s. *Rx.*

Use: Mineral, vitamin supplement.

Advanced-RF Natal Care. (Ethex) Ca 200 mg, Fe 90 mg, vitamin D_3 400 units, E 30 units, B_1 3 mg, B_2 3.4 mg, B_6 20 mg, B_{12} 12 mcg, folic acid 1 mg, C 120 mg, Cu 2 mg, docusate sodium 50 mg, niacinamide 20 mg, Mg 30 mg, zinc 25 mg. Dye-free. Tab. 90s. *Rx.*
Use: Multivitamin.

Advance Pregnancy Test. (Johnson & Johnson) Can be used as early as 3 days after a missed period. Gives results in 30 min. Test kit 1s.
Use: Diagnostic aid.

Advantage 24. (Women's Health Institute) Nonoxynol 93.5%. Gel. 1.5 g (3s, 6s). *OTC.*
Use: Contraceptive, spermicide.

Arivntn. (Bindor) Mannitol 38 mg, trehalose 10 mg, histidine 12 mM, tris 12 mM, calcium 1.9 mM, polysorbate 80 0.17 mg, glutathione 0.1 mg/mL, sodium 108 mEq/L, von Willebrand Factor ≤ 2 ng/unit recombinant antihemophilic factor (rAHF) when reconstituted. Preservative-free. Monoclonal purified and solvent-detergent treated. Pow. for Inj. 250, 500, 1000, 1500 IU per single-dose vials with 5 mL sterile water for inj., double-ended needle, filter needle, infusion set/blood collection set, and 10 mL sterile syringe. *Rx.*
Use: Antihemophilic agent.

Advera. (Ross) Protein 14.2 g, fat 5.4 g, carbohydrate 51.2 g, l-carnitine 30 mg, taurine 50 mg, vitamins A 2550 units, D 80 units, E 9 units, K 24 mcg, C 90 mg, folic acid 120 mcg, B, 0.75 mg, B_2 0.68 mg, B_6 9.5 mg, B_{12} 12 mcg, niacin 6 mg, choline 50 mg, biotin 50 mcg, B_5 3 mg, sodium 250 mg, potassium 670 mg, chloride 350 mg, Ca 260 mg, Ph 260 mg, Mg 50 mg, I 30 mcg, Mn 1.3 mg, Cu 0.5 mg, Zn 2 mg, Fe 4.5 mg, Se 14 mcg, chromium 17 mcg, Md 54 mcg/240 mL, 1.28 calories/mL, vanilla flavor. Liq. Bot. 273 mL. *OTC.*
Use: Nutritional supplement, enteral.

Advicor. (Kos) Lovastatin 20 mg; niacin (extended release) 500 mg or 1000 mg. Tab. Bot. 30s, 90s, 180s. *Rx.*
Use: Antihyperlipidemic.

Advil. (Wyeth) Ibuprofen 200 mg, sucrose. Tab. Bot. 8s, 24s, 50s, 72s, 100s, 165s, 250s. *OTC.*
Use: Analgesic; NSAID.

Advil Allergy Sinus. (Wyeth) Pseudoephedrine hydrochloride 30 mg, chlorpheniramine maleate 2 mg, ibuprofen

200 mg. Tab. 10s, 20s. *OTC.*
Use: Upper respiratory combination, decongestant, antihistamine, analgesic.

Advil, Children's. (Wyeth) **Susp.:** Ibuprofen 100 mg/5 mL, fruit flavor, sorbitol, sucrose, EDTA. Bot. 119 mL, 473 mL. **Chew. Tab.:** Ibuprofen 50 mg, aspartame, phenylalanine 2.1 mg, fruit and grape flavor. Bot. 24s, 50s. *Rx-OTC.*
Use: Analgesic; NSAID.

Advil Cold & Sinus. (Wyeth) Pseudoephedrine hydrochloride 30 mg, ibuprofen 200 mg, parabens, sucrose. Tab. Bot. 40s. *OTC.*
Use: Upper respiratory combination, analgesic, decongestant.

Advil Cold & Sinus Liqui-gels. (Wyeth) Pseudoephedrine hydrochloride 30 mg, ibuprofen 200 mg, sorbitol. Cap. 16s, 32s. *OTC.*
Use: Upper respiratory combination.

Advil Flu & Body Ache. (Wyeth) Pseudoephedrine hydrochloride 30 mg, ibuprofen 200 mg, parabens, sucrose. Tab. Pkg. 20s. *OTC.*
Use: Upper respiratory combination, analgesic, decongestant.

Advil, Junior Strength. (Wyeth) Ibuprofen 100 mg, aspartame, phenylalanine 4.2 mg, grape and fruit flavor. Chew. Tab. Bot. 24s. *OTC.*
Use: Analgesic; NSAID.

Advil Liqui-Gels. (Wyeth) Ibuprofen 200 mg, sorbitol. Cap. Bot. 4s, 20s, 40s, 80s. *OTC.*
Use: Analgesic; NSAID.

Advil Migraine. (Wyeth) Ibuprofen 200 mg, sorbitol. Cap. Bot. 20s. *OTC.*
Use: Analgesic; NSAID.

Advil Pediatric Drops. (Wyeth) Ibuprofen 100 mg/2.5 mL, sorbitol, sucrose, EDTA, glycerin, grape flavor. Susp. Bot. 7.5 mL. *OTC.*
Use: Analgesic; NSAID.

A.E.R. (Birchwood) Hamamelis water (witch hazel) 50%, glycerin 12.5%, methylparaben, benzalkonium chloride. Pads. Jar 40s. *OTC.*
Use: Dermatologic.

Aerdil. (Econo Med Pharmaceuticals) Triprolidine hydrochloride 1.25 mg, pseudoephedrine hydrochloride 30 mg/5 mL. Bot. Pt, gal. *OTC.*
Use: Antihistamine; decongestant.

Aeroaid. (Graham Field) Thimerosal 1:1000, alcohol 72%. Spray Bot. 90 mL.
Use: Antiseptic.

AeroBid. (Forest) Flunisolide approximately 250 mcg/actuation. Aerosol. Canister. 100 metered doses. *Rx.*

Use: Corticosteroid.

AeroBid-M. (Forest) Flunisolide approximately 250 mcg/actuation. Menthol flavor. Aerosol. Canister. 100 metered doses. *Rx.*
Use: Corticosteroid.

AeroCaine. (Health & Medical Techniques) Benzocaine 13.6%, benzethonium Cl 0.5%. Spray bot. 0.5 oz, 2.5 oz. *OTC.*
Use: Local anesthetic, topical.

Aerocell. (Health & Medical Techniques) Exfoliative cytology fixative spray. Bot. 3.5 oz.
Use: Exfoliative cytology fixative spray.

Aerofreeze. (Graham Field) Trichloromonofluoromethane and dichlorodifluoromethane 240 mL. Aerosol spray. Cont. 8 oz. (12s). *OTC.*
Use: Anesthetic, local.

AeroHist Plus. (Aero) Phenylephrine hydrochloride 20 mg, chlorpheniramine maleate 8 mg, methscopamine nitrate 2.5 mg. ER Tab. 100s. *Rx.*
Use: Upper respiratory combination.

AeroKid. (Aero) Phenylephrine hydrochloride 10 mg, chlorpheniramine maleate 4 mg, methscopamine nitrate 1.25 mg/5 mL. Glycerin, sorbitol, saccharin, raspberry flavor. Syrup. 20 mL, 120 mL, 480 mL. *Rx.*
Use: Upper respiratory combination.

Aerolate-III. (Fleming & Co.) Theophylline 65 mg/TD Cap. Bot. 100s, 1000s. *Rx.*
Use: Bronchodilator.

Aerolate Sr. & Jr. (Fleming & Co.) **Cap.:** Theophylline 4 g for Sr., 2 g for Jr. Cap. Bot. 100s, 1000s. **Syr.:** 160 mg/15 mL. Bot. Pt, gal. *Rx.*
Use: Bronchodilator.

Aeropin.
Use: Cystic fibrosis. [Orphan Drug]

Aeropure. (Health & Medical Techniques) Isopropanol 7.8%, triethylene glycol 3.9%, essential oils 3%, methyldodecyl benzyl trimethyl ammonium Cl 0.12%, methyldodecylxylene bis (trimethyl ammonium Cl) 0.03%, inert ingredients 85.15%. Bot. 0.8 oz, 4.5 oz.
Use: Antiseptic; deodorant.

Aeroseb-Dex. (Allergan) Dexamethasone 0.01%, alcohol 65.1%. Aerosol 58 g. *Rx.*
Use: Corticosteroid, topical.

Aerosil. (Health & Medical Techniques) Dimethylpolysiloxane. Bot. 4.5 oz.
Use: Lubricant; protectant.

aerosol ot.
See: Docusate Sodium.

aerosol talc, sterile. (Bryan)
Use: Malignant pleural effusion.
[Orphan Drug]
Aerosolv. (Health & Medical Techniques)
Isopropyl alcohol, methylene Cl, silicone. Aerosol 5.5 oz.
Use: Adhesive remover.
AeroZoin. (Health & Medical Techniques)
Benzoin compound tincture 30%, isopropyl alcohol 44.8%. Spray Bot. 3.5 oz.
OTC.
Use: Dermatologic, protectant.
Afaxin. (Sanofi-Synthelabo) Vitamin A Palmitate 10,000 units, 50,000 units.
Cap. Bot. *Rx-OTC.*
Use: Vitamin supplement.
Afeditab CR. (Watson) Nifedipine 30 mg, 60 mg. ER Tab. 100s. *Rx.*
Use: Calcium channel blocker.
A-Fil. (Medicis) Methyl anthranilate 5%, titanium dioxide 5% in vanishing cream base. Tube 45 g. Neutral or dark. *OTC.*
Use: Sunscreen.
Afko-Lube. (A.P.C.) Docusate sodium 100 mg. Cap. Bot. 100s. *OTC.*
Use: Laxative.
Afko-Lube Lax. (A.P.C.) Docusate sodium 100 mg, casanthranol 30 mg.
Cap. Bot. 100s. *OTC.*
Use: Laxative.
• **afovirsen sodium.** (aff-oh-VEER-sen SO-dee-uhm) USAN.
Use: Antiviral.
Afrin. (Schering-Plough) Oxymetazoline hydrochloride 0.05%. **Nose Drops:** Drop. Bot. 20 mL. **Nasal Spray:** Reg. Bot. 15 mL, 30 mL; Menthol. Bot. 15 mL. **Children's Nose Drops:** Oxymetazoline hydrochloride 0.025%.
Drop. Bot. 20 mL. *OTC.*
Use: Decongestant.
Afrin Children's. (Schering-Plough) Phenylephrine hydrochloride 0.25%, EDTA, benzalkonium chloride. Soln. Spray Bot. 15 mL. *OTC.*
Use: Nasal decongestant, arylalkylamine.
Afrin Moisturizing Saline Mist. (Schering-Plough) Sodium chloride 0.64%, benzalkonium chloride, EDTA. Soln. Bot. 30 mL. *OTC.*
Use: Decongestant.
Afrin No-Drip Sinus with Vapornase.
(Schering-Plough) Oxymetazoline hydrochloride 0.05%, carboxymethylcellulose sodium, microcrystalline cellulose, benzalkonium chloride, benzyl alcohol, camphor, EDTA, eucalyptol, menthol. Soln. Spray Bot. 15 mL. *OTC.*
Use: Nasal decongestant, imidazoline.

Afrin No-Drip 12-Hour. (Schering-Plough) Oxymetazoline hydrochloride 0.05%, carboxymethylcellulose sodium, microcrystalline cellulose, benzalkonium chloride, benzyl alcohol, EDTA. Soln. Spray Bot. 15 mL. *OTC.*
Use: Nasal decongestant, imidazoline.
Afrin No-Drip 12-Hour Extra Moisturizing. (Schering-Plough) Oxymetazoline hydrochloride 0.05%, carboxymethylcellulose sodium, microcrystalline cellulose, benzalkonium chloride, benzyl alcohol, EDTA, glycerin, Soln. Spray Bot. 15 mL. *OTC.*
Use: Nasal decongestant, imidazoline.
Afrin No-Drip 12-Hour Severe Congestion with Menthol. (Schering-Plough) Oxymetazoline hydrochloride 0.05%, carboxymethylcellulose sodium, microcrytalline cellulose, benzalkonium chloride, benzyl alcohol, camphor, EDTA, eucalyptol, menthol. Soln. Spray Bot. 15 mL. *OTC.*
Use: Nasal decongestant, imidazoline.
Afrinol Repetabs. (Schering-Plough) Pseudoephedrine sulfate 120 mg. Repeat Action Tab. Box 12s, bot. 100s, dispensary pack 48s. *OTC.*
Use: Decongestant.
Afrin Saline, Extra Moisturizing. (Schering-Plough) Sodium chloride, benzalkonium chloride, EDTA. Soln. Spray Bot. 45 mL. *OTC.*
Use: Nasal decongestant.
Afrin Severe Congestion with Menthol. (Schering Plough) Oxymetazoline hydrochloride 0.05%, benzalkonium chloride, benzyl alcohol, camphor, EDTA, eucalyptol, menthol. Soln. Spray Bot. 15 mL. *OTC.*
Use: Nasal decongestant, imidazoline.
Afrin Sinus. (Schering-Plough) Oxymetazoline hydrochloride 0.05%, benzyl alcohol. Spray. Bot. 15 mL. *OTC.*
Use: Decongestant.
Afrin Sinus with Vapornase. (Schering-Plough) Oxymetazoline hydrochloride 0.05%, benzalkonium chloride, benzyl alcohol, camphor, EDTA, eucalyptol, menthol. Soln. Spray Bot. 15 mL. *OTC.*
Use: Nasal decongestant, imidazoline.
Afrin 12-Hour Original. (Schering-Plough) Oxymetazoline hydrochloride 0.05%, benzalkonium chloride, EDTA. Soln. Spray Bot. 15 mL. *OTC.*
Use: Nasal decongestant, imidazoline.
After Bite. (Tender) Ammonium hydroxide 3.5% in aqueous solution. Pen-like dispenser. *OTC.*
Use: Analgesic; antipruritic, topical.
After Burn. (Tender) Lidocaine 0.5% in aloe vera 98% solution. *OTC.*

Use: Anesthetic, local.

● **agalsidase alfa.** (aye-GAL-si-days) USAN.
Use: Fabry disease.

● **agalsidase beta.** (aye-GAL-si-days) USAN.
Use: Fabry disease.
See: Fabrazyme.

● **agar.** (AH-gahr) *NF 23.*
Use: Pharmaceutical aid, suspending agent.
W/Mineral oil.
See: Agoral.

Agenerase. (GlaxoSmithKline) Amprenavir. **Cap.:** 50 mg (d-sorbitol, d-alpha tocopheryl polythylene glycol 1000 succinate, propylene glycol 19 mg). Bot. 480s. **Oral Soln.:** 15 mg/mL, acesulfame potassium, saccharin, propylene glycol 550 mg, vitamin E 46 units/mL, grape/bubblegum/peppermint flavor. Bot. 240 mL. *Rx.*
Use: Antiviral.

Aggrastat. (Merck) Tirofiban hydrochloride. **Inj.:** 50 mcg/mL, preservative-free. Single-dose *IntraVia* containers 250 mL (sodium chloride 2.25 g, sodium citrate dihydrate 135 mg), 500 mL (sodium chloride 4.5 g, sodium citrate dihydrate 270 mg). **Conc. Inj.:** 250 mcg/mL, preservative-free, sodium chloride 8 mg, sodium citrate dihydrate 2.7 mg. Vial 25 mL, 50 mL. *Rx.*
Use: Antiplatelet, glycoprotein IIb/IIIa inhibitor.

Aggrenox. (Boehringer Ingelheim) Dipyridamole 200 mg extended-release, aspirin 25 mg, lactose, sucrose. Cap. Bot. 60s. *Rx.*
Use: Antiplatelet.

aglucerase injection. (Genzyme Corp)
Use: Treatment of Type II and III Gaucher disease. [Orphan Drug]

Agoral. (Numark) Sennosides A and B 25 mg/15 mL, parabens. Liq. Bot. 473 mL. *OTC.*
Use: Laxative.

A/G-Pro. (Miller Pharmacal Group) Protein hydrolysate 542 mg, L-lysine 50 mg, L-methionine 12.5 mg, vitamin B_6 0.33 mg, C 16.7 mg, iron 1.66 mg, Cu, I, K, Mg, Mn, Zn. Tab. Bot. 180s. *OTC.*
Use: Nutritional supplement, amino acid.

Agrylin. (Roberts) Anagrelide hydrochloride 0.5 mg, 1 mg, lactose. Cap. Bot. 100s. *Rx.*
Use: Thrombocythemia; polycythemia vera; essential thrombocythemia; thrombocytosis in chronic myelogenous leukemia. [Orphan Drug]

agurin.
See: Theobromine Sodium Acetate.

AH-Chew. (WE Pharmaceuticals) **Chew. Tab.:** Chlorpheniramine maleate 2 mg, phenylephrine hydrochloride 10 mg, methscopolamine nitrate 1.25 mg, grape flavor. Bot. 100s. **Susp.:** Phenylephrine hydrochloride 10 mg, chlorpheniramine maleate 2 mg, methscopolamine nitrate 1.5 mg per 5 mL. Parabens. Grape flavor. 20 mL, 118 mL. *Rx.*
Use: Upper respiratory combination, anticholinergic, antihistamine, decongestant.

AH-Chew D. (WE Pharmaceuticals) Phenylephrine hydrochloride 10 mg, bubble gum flavor. Chew. Tab. Bot. 100s. *Rx.*
Use: Nasal decongestant, arylalkylamine.

AHF.
See: Antihemophilic factor.

A-Hydrocort. (Abbott Hospital Products) Hydrocortisone sodium succinate 100 mg/2 mL or 250 mg/2 mL, 500 mg/4 mL; 1000 mg/8 mL. *Rx.*
Use: Corticosteroid.

AIDS vaccine. (Various Mfr.) Phase I to III AIDS, HIV prophylaxis and treatment. *Rx.*
Use: Immunization.

air and surface disinfectant. (Health & Medical Techniques) Aerosol 16 oz.
Use: Antiseptic; deodorant.

Airet. (Medeva) Albuterol sulfate 0.083%. Soln. for Inhalation. Vial. *Rx.*
Use: Bronchodilator, sympathomimetic.

● **air, medical.** *USP 28.*
Use: Gas, medicinal.

Akarpine. (Akorn) Pilocarpine hydrochloride 1%, 2%, 4%. Soln. Bot. 15 mL. *Rx.*
Use: Miotic.

AK-Beta. (Akorn) Levobunolol hydrochloride 0.25%, 0.5%, polyvinyl alcohol 1.4%, benzalkonium chloride 0.004%, sodium metabisulfite, EDTA, dibasic sodium phosphate, monobasic potassium phosphate, NaCl, hydrochloric acid, sodium hydroxide. Ophth. Soln. Bot. 2 mL, 5 mL, 10 mL, 15 mL. *Rx.*
Use: Antiglaucoma.

AK-Chlor. (Akorn) **Oint.:** Chloramphenicol 10 mg/g. Tube 3.5 g. **Soln.:** Chloramphenicol 5 mg/mL. Bot. 7.5 mL, 15 mL. *Rx.*
Use: Anti-infective, ophthalmic.

AK-Con. (Akorn) Naphazoline hydrochloride 0.1%. Soln. Bot. 15 mL. *Rx.*

Use: Mydriatic, vasoconstrictor.
AK-Con-A. (Akorn) Naphazoline hydrochloride 0.025%, pheniramine maleate 0.3%, benzalkonium Cl 0.01%, EDTA. Soln. Bot. 15 mL. *Rx.*
Use: Antihistamine; decongestant, ophthalmic.
AK-Dilate. (Akorn) Phenylephrine hydrochloride 2.5%, 10%. Bot. 2 mL, 5 mL (10%), 15 mL (2.5%). *Rx.*
Use: Mydriatic, vasoconstrictor.
AK-Fluor. (Akorn) Fluorescein sodium. **10%:** Amp. 5 mL, Vial 5 mL. **25%:** Amp. 2 mL, Vial 2 mL.
Use: Diagnostic aid, ophthalmic.
Akineton. (Knoll) Biperiden hydrochloride 2 mg. Tab. Bot. 100s, 1000s. *Rx.*
Use: Antiparkinsonian.
Akineton Lactate. (Knoll) Biperiden lactate 5 mg in aqueous 1.4% sodium lactate soln/ml. Amp. 1 ml. Box 10s. *Rx.*
Use: Antiparkinsonian.
AK-NaCl. (Akorn) **Oint.:** Sodium Cl hypertonic 5%. Tube 3.5 g. **Soln.:** Sodium Cl hypertonic 5%. Bot. 15 mL. *OTC.*
Use: Ophthalmic.
Akne Drying Lotion. (Alto) Zinc oxide 12%, urea 10%, sulfur 6%, salicylic acid 2%, benzalkonium Cl 0.2%, isopropyl alcohol 70%, in a base containing menthol, silicon dioxide, iron oxide, perfume. Bot. ¾ oz, 2.25 oz. *OTC.*
Use: Dermatologic, acne.
Akne-Mycin. (Healthpoint) Erythromycin 2%. Cetostearyl alcohol, petrolatum, mineral oil. Oint. Tube 25 g. *Rx.*
Use: Dermatologic, acne.
AK-Neo-Dex. (Akorn) Dexamethasone sodium phosphate 0.1%, neomycin sulfate 0.35%. Ophth. Soln. Bot. 5 mL. *Rx.*
Use: Anti-infective; corticosteroid, ophthalmic.
Akne Scrub. (Alto) Povidone-iodine with polyethylene granules. Bot. ¾ oz. *OTC.*
Use: Dermatologic, acne.
AK-Pentolate. (Akorn) Cyclopentolate hydrochloride 1%, benzalkonium Cl 0.01%, EDTA. Soln. Bot. 2 mL, 15 mL. *Rx.*
Use: Cycloplegic, mydriatic.
AK-Poly-Bac. (Akorn) Polymyxin B sulfate 10,000 units, bacitracin zinc 500 units/g, white petrolatum, mineral oil. Oint. Tube 3.5 g. *Rx.*
Use: Anti-infective, ophthalmic.
AK-Pred. (Akorn) Prednisolone sodium phosphate 0.125% or 1%. Ophth. Soln. Bot. 5 mL, 10 mL, and 15 mL (1% only). *Rx.*

Use: Corticosteroid, ophthalmic.
AK-Pro. (Akorn) Dipivefrin hydrochloride 0.1%. Liq. Bot. 2 mL, 5 mL, 10 mL, 15 mL. *Rx.*
Use: Antiglaucoma agent.
AK-Ramycin. (Akorn) Doxycycline hyclate 100 mg. Cap. Bot. 50s, 100s, 200s, 250s, 500s, UD 100s. *Rx.*
Use: Anti-infective, tetracycline.
AK-Ratabs. (Akorn) Doxycycline hyclate 100 mg. Tab. Bot. 50s. *Rx.*
Use: Anti-infective, tetracycline.
Akrinol. (Schering-Plough) Acrisorcin.
Use: Antifungal.
AK-Rinse. (Akorn) Sodium carbonate, potassium Cl, boric acid, EDTA, benzalkonium Cl 0.01%. Soln. Bot. 30 mL, 118 mL. *OTC.*
Use: Irrigant, ophthalmic.
AK-Spore. (Akorn) Polymyxin B sulfate 10,000 units, neomycin (as sulfate) 3.5 mg, white petrolatum, mineral oil. Oint. Tube. 3.5 g. *Rx.*
Use: Anti-infective, ophthalmic.
AK-Sulf. (Akorn) **Soln.:** Sodium sulfacetamide 10%. Dropper Bot. 2 mL, 5 mL, 15 mL. **Oint.:** Sodium sulfacetamide 10%. Tube 3.5 g. *Rx.*
Use: Anti-infective, ophthalmic.
AK-Taine. (Akorn) Proparacaine hydrochloride 0.5%, glycerin, chlorobutanol, benzalkonium Cl. Dropper bot. 2 mL, 15 mL. *Rx.*
Use: Anesthetic, ophthalmic.
AK-Tate. (Akorn) Prednisolone acetate 1%, benzalkonium Cl, EDTA, polysorbate 80, polyvinyl alcohol, hydroxyethyl cellulose. Susp. Dropper bot. 5 mL, 10 mL, 15 mL. *Rx.*
Use: Corticosteroid, ophthalmic.
AK-Tob. (Akorn) Tobramycin 0.3%. Soln. Bot. 5 mL. *Rx.*
Use: Anti-infective, ophthalmic.
AK-Tracin. (Akorn) Bacitracin 500 units/g. Oint. Tube 3.5 g. *Rx.*
Use: Anti-infective, ophthalmic.
Akwa Tears. (Akorn) **Soln.:** Polyvinyl alcohol 1.4%, sodium Cl, sodium phosphate, benzalkonium Cl 0.01%, EDTA. Bot. 15 mL. **Oint.:** White petrolatum, mineral oil, lanolin. Tube 3.5 g. *OTC.*
Use: Artificial tears.
Ala-Bath. (Del-Ray) Bath oil. Bot. 8 oz. *OTC.*
Use: Emollient.
Alacol DM. (Ballay) Dextromethorphan HBr 10 mg, brompheniramine maleate 2 mg, phenylephrine hydrochloride 5 mg/5 mL, saccharin, sorbitol, black raspberry flavor, alcohol free. Syr. Bot. 473 mL. *Rx.*

Use: Upper respiratory combination, antitussive, antihistamine, decongestant.

Ala-Cort. (Del-Ray) Hydrocortisone 1%. **Cream:** Tube 1 oz, 3 oz. **Lot.:** Bot. 4 oz. *Rx.*
Use: Corticosteroid, topical.

Ala-Derm. (Del-Ray) Lot. Bot. 8 oz, 12 oz.
Use: Emollient.

Aladrine. (Scherer) Ephedrine sulfate 8.1 mg, secobarbital sodium 16.2 mg. Tab. Bot. 100s. *c-II.*
Use: Decongestant; hypnotic, sedative.

•**alagebrium chloride.** (al-A-je-BREE-um) USAN.
Use: Cardiovascular complications.

Alamag. (Ivax) Aluminum hydroxide 225 mg, magnesium hydroxide 200 mg, sorbitol, sucrose, parabens. Susp. Bot. 355 mL. *OTC.*
Use: Antacid.

Alamag Plus. (Ivax) Magnesium hydroxide 200 mg, aluminum hydroxide 225 mg, simethicone 25 mg/5 mL. Susp. Bot. 355 mL. *OTC.*
Use: Antacid.

•**alamecin.** (al-ah-MEE-sin) USAN.
Use: Anti-infective.

•**alanine.** (AL-ah-NEEN) *USP 28.*
Use: Amino acid.

•**alaproclate.** (AL-ah-PRO-klate) USAN.
Use: Antidepressant.

Ala-Quin 0.5%. (Del-Ray) Hydrocortisone, iodochlorhydroxyquinoline cream. Tube 1 oz. *Rx-OTC.*
Use: Corticosteroid, topical.

Ala-Scalp HP 2%. (Del-Ray) Hydrocortisone Lot. Bot. 1 oz. *Rx.*
Use: Corticosteroid, topical.

Ala-Seb. (Del-Ray) Shampoo. Bot. 4 oz, 12 oz. *OTC.*
Use: Antiseborrheic.

Ala-Seb T. (Del-Ray) Shampoo. Bot. 4 oz, 12 oz. *OTC.*
Use: Antiseborrheic.

Alasulf. (Major) Sulfanilamide 15%, aminacrine hydrochloride 0.2%, allantoin 2%. Vaginal Cream. Tube w/applicator 120 g. *Rx.*
Use: Anti-infective, vaginal.

Alatone. (Major) Spironolactone 25 mg. Tab. Bot. 100s, 250s, 500s, 1000s, UD 100s. *Rx.*
Use: Antihypertensive.

Alavert. (Wyeth) Loratadine 10 mg. Lactose. Orally Disintegrating Tab. 6s, 12s, 15s, 30s, 48s. *OTC.*
Use: Antihistamine, peripherally selective piperidine.

Alavert Allergy & Sinus D-12 Hour. (Wyeth) Pseudoephedrine 120 mg, loratadine 5 mg. Lactose. ER Tab. 12s. *OTC.*
Use: Decongestant, antihistamine.

Alavert Children's. (Wyeth) Loratadine 5 mg/5 mL. Sucrose. Syrup. 118 mL. *OTC.*
Use: Antihistamine.

Alaxin. (Delta Pharmaceutical Group) Oxyethlene oxypropylene polymer 240 mg. Cap. Bot. 100s. *OTC.*
Use: Laxative.

alazanine triclofenate.
Use: Anthelmintic.

Alazide. (Major) Spironolactone w/hydrochlorothiazide. Tab. Bot. 250s, 1000s. *Rx.*
Use: Antihypertensive, diuretic.

Alazine. (Major) Hydralazine 10 mg, 25 mg, 50 mg. Cap. Bot. 100s, 1000s. *Rx.*
Use: Antihypertensive.

Albalon. (Allergan) Naphazoline hydrochloride 0.1%. Bot. 15 mL. *Rx.*
Use: Vasoconstrictor, ophthalmic.

Albay. (Bayer Corp. (Consumer Div.)) Freeze-dried venom and venom protein. Vials of 550 mcg for each of honeybee, white-faced hornet, yellow hornet, yellow jacket, or wasp. Vials of 1650 mcg for mixed vespids (white-faced hornet, yellow hornet, yellow jacket). 10 mL. Inj. *Rx.*
Use: Antivenin.

•**albendazole.** (AL-BEND-ah-zole) *USP 28.*
Use: Anthelmintic.
See: Albenza.

Albenza. (GlaxoSmithKline) Albendazole 200 mg. Tab. Bot. 112s. *Rx.*
Use: Anthelmintic; hydatid disease. [Orphan Drug]

Albolene. (GlaxoSmithKline) Unscented or scented. Cream. Jar 6 oz, 12 oz.

Albuconn 25%. (Cryosan) Normal serum albumin (human) 12.5 g in 50 mL solution for IV administration. Vial 50 mL. *Rx.*
Use: Treatment of plasma or blood volume deficit, acute hypoproteinemia, oncotic deficit.

•**albumin, aggregated.** (al-BYOO-min AGG-reh-GAY-tuhd) USAN.
Use: Diagnostic aid, lung-imaging.
See: Technescan MAA.

•**albumin, aggregated iodinated I 131 injection.** (al-BYOO-min AGG-reh-GAY-tuhd) *USP 28.*
Use: Radiopharmaceutical.

●**albumin, aggregated iodinated I 131 serum.** (al-BYOO-min AGG-reh-GAY-tuhd) USAN. Blood serum aggregates of albumin labeled with iodine-131.
Use: Radiopharmaceutical.
See: Albumotope I-131.
Albuminar-5 and Albuminar-25. (Aventis Behring) Albumin (human).
5%: Solution with administration set. Bot. 50 mL, 1000 mL. **25%:** Solution. Vial 20 mL with administration set. *Rx.*
Use: Plasma protein fraction.
●**albumin, chromated Cr 51 serum.** (al-BYOO-min) USAN. Blood serum albumin labeled with chromium-51.
Use: Radiopharmaceutical.
●**albumin human.** (al-BYOO-MIN human) *USP 28.* Formerly Albumin, Normal Human Serum.
Use: Plasma protein fraction; blood volume supporter.
See: Albuminar-5 and Albuminar-25.
Albunex.
Albutein 5%.
Albutein 25%.
Buminate.
Plasbumin-5.
Plasbumin-25.
W/Combinations.
See: Monarc-M.
albumin human, 5%. (Baxter Healthcare) Normal serum albumin 5%. Inj. Vial 250 mL. *Rx.*
Use: Plasma protein fraction.
albumin human, 25%. (Baxter Healthcare) Normal serum albumin 25%. Inj. Vial 10 mL, 50 mL. *Rx.*
Use: Plasma protein fraction.
●**albumin, iodinated I 131 injection.** (al-BYOO-min) *USP 28.* Albumin labeled with iodine-131. Inj.
Use: Diagnostic aid, blood volume determination, intrathecal imaging; radiopharmaceutical.
●**albumin, iodinated I 131 serum.** (al-BYOO-min) *USP 28.*
Use: Diagnostic aid, blood volume determination, intrathecal imaging; radioactive agent.
●**albumin, iodinated I 125 injection.** (al-BYOO-min) *USP 28.* Albumin labeled with iodine-125.
Use: Diagnostic aid, blood volume determination; radiopharmaceutical.
●**albumin, iodinated I 125 serum.** (al-BYOO-min) *USP 28.*
Use: Diagnostic aid, blood volume determination; radiopharmaceutical.
albumin, normal serum 5%. (Baxter Healthcare) Albumin human 5%. Inj.

Vial 120 mL. *Rx.*
Use: Plasma protein fraction.
albumin, normal serum 25%. (Baxter Healthcare) Albumin human 25%. Inj. Vial 10 mL, 50 mL. *Rx.*
Use: Plasma protein fraction.
albumin-saline diluent. (Bayer Corp. (Consumer Div.)) Dilute allergenic extracts and venom products for patient testing and treating. Pre-measured vials 1.8 mL, 4 mL, 4.5 mL, 9 mL, 30 mL. Vial 2 mL, 5 mL, 10 mL, 30 mL.
Use: Pharmaceutical necessity, diluent.
Albumotope I-131. (Bristol-Myers Squibb) Albumin, iodinated I-131 serum (50 uCi).
Use: Diagnostic aid.
Albunex. (Mallinckrodt) Albumin (human) 5%, sonicated. Sodium acetyl tryptophanate 0.08 mmol, sodium caprylate 0.08 mmol/g albumin. Inj. Vial. 5 mL, 10 mL, 20 mL. Pkg. 6s. *Rx.*
Use: Plasma protein fraction.
Albustix Reagent Strips. (Bayer Corp. (Consumer Div.)) Firm paper reagent strips impregnated with tetrabromphenol blue, citrate buffer and a protein-adsorbing agent. Bot. 50s, 100s.
Use: Diagnostic aid.
Albutein 5%. (Alpha Therapeutic) Normal serum albumin 5%. Inj. Vial w/IV set 250 mL, 500 mL. *Rx.*
Use: Plasma protein fraction.
Albutein 25%. (Alpha Therapeutic) Normal serum albumin 25%. Inj. Vial w/IV set 50 mL. *Rx.*
Use: Plasma protein fraction.
●**albuterol.** (al-BYOO-ter-ahl) *USP 28.*
Use: Bronchodilator, sympathomimetic.
See: Proventil.
Ventolin.
albuterol. (Nephron) Albuterol sulfate 0.042% (1.25 mg/3 mL). Preservative free. Soln. for Inh. 3 mL UD vials. *Rx.*
Use: Bronchodilator.
albuterol. (Various Mfr.) Albuterol 90 mcg per actuation. Inh. Aer. Can. 6.8 g ($\geq$ 80 inhalations), 17 g ($\geq$ 200 inhalations). *Rx.*
Use: Bronchodilator, sympathomimetic.
Albuterol HFA. (Ivax) Albuterol 90 mcg per actuation. Contains no chlorofluorocarbons. Aerosol. 8.5 g (200 inhalations). *Rx.*
Use: Bronchodilator.
●**albuterol sulfate.** (al-BYOO-teh-rahl SULL-fate) *USP 28.*
Use: Bronchodilator, sympathomimetic.
See: AccuNeb.
Airet.
Proventil.

Proventil HFA.
Ventolin HFA.
VoSpire ER.
albuterol sulfate. (Various Mfr.) **Tab.:**
2 mg, 4 mg, may contain lactose. Bot.
100s, 500s, 600s. **Syr.:** 2 mg/5 mL, may
contain sorbitol. Bot. 473 mL. **Inh.
Soln.:** 0.083%, 0.5%. UD 0.5 mL (0.5%
only), 3 mL (0.083% only), Bot. 20 mL
(0.5% only). *Rx.*
Use: Bronchodilator, sympathomimetic.
**albuterol sulfate and ipratropium bro-
mide.** (al-BYOO-ter-ahl SULL-fate and
IH-pruh-TROE-pee-uhm BROE-mide)
Use: Chronic obstructive pulmonary
disease (COPD).
See: Combivent.
DuoNeb.
•**albutoin.** (al-BYOO-toe-in) USAN.
Use: Anticonvulsant.
Alcaine. (Alcon) Proparacaine hydrochlo-
ride 0.5%, glycerin, sodium Cl, benzal-
konium Cl. Bot. 15 mL. *Rx.*
Use: Anesthetic, ophthalmic.
Alcare. (GlaxoSmithKline) Ethyl alcohol
62%. Foam Bot. 210 mL, 300 mL,
600 mL. *OTC.*
Use: Antiseptic.
Alclear Eye. (Walgreen) Sterile isotonic
fluid. Lot. Bot. 8 oz. *OTC.*
Use: Anti-irritant, ophthalmic.
•**alclofenac.** (al-KLOE-feh-nak) USAN.
Use: Analgesic; anti-inflammatory.
See: Mervan.
•**alclometasone dipropionate.** (al-kloe-
MEH-tah-zone die-PRO-pee-oh-nate)
USP 28.
Use: Anti-inflammatory, topical.
See: Aclovate.
alclometasone dipropionate. (Taro)
Alclometasone dipropionate 0.05%.
Hexylene glycol, propylene glycol stea-
rate, petrolatum. Oint. 15 g, 45 g, 60 g.
Rx.
Use: Anti-inflammatory agent.
•**alcloxa.** (al-KLOX-ah) USAN.
Use: Astringent; keratolytic.
Alco-Gel. (Tweezerman) Ethyl alcohol
60%. Gel. Tube 60 g, 480 g. *OTC.*
Use: Dermatologic, cleanser.
•**alcohol.** (AL-koe-hol) *USP 28.* Ethanol,
ethyl alcohol.
Use: Anti-infective, topical; pharmaceu-
tic aid, solvent.
See: Anbesol.
Anbesol Maximum Strength.
Ru-Tuss.
Ru-Tuss Expectorant.
Ru-Tuss w/Hydrocodone.

alcohol, dehydrated.
Use: Solvent, vehicle.
•**alcohol, diluted.** (AL-koe-hol) *NF 23.*
Use: Pharmaceutic aid, solvent.
Alcohol 5% and Dextrose 5%. (Abbott
Hospital Products) Alcohol 5 mL, dex-
trose 5 g/100 mL. Bot. 1000 mL. *Rx.*
Use: Nutritional supplement, parenteral.
•**alcohol, rubbing.** (AL-koe-hol) *USP 28.*
Use: Rubefacient.
See: Lavacol.
Alcojet. (Alconox) Biodegradable ma-
chine washing detergent and wetting
agent. Ctn. 9 ×4 lb, 25 lb, 50 lb, 100 lb,
300 lb. *OTC.*
Use: Detergent, wetting agent.
Alcolec. (American Lecithin) Lecithin
w/choline base, cephalin, lipositol. Cap.
100s. Gran. 8 oz, lb. *OTC.*
Use: Nutritional supplement.
Alconefrin 12 and 50. (PolyMedica)
Phenylephrine hydrochloride 0.16%
w/benzalkonium Cl. Dropper bot.
30 mL. *OTC.*
Use: Decongestant.
Alconefrin 25. (PolyMedica) Phenyl-
ephrine hydrochloride 0.25% w/benzal-
konium Cl. Dropper bot. 30 mL. Spray
Pkg. 30 mL. *OTC.*
Use: Decongestant.
**Alcon Enzymatic Cleaning Tablets for
Extended Wear.** (Alcon) Pancreatin.
Tab. Pkg. 12s. *OTC.*
Use: Contact lens care.
**Alcon Opti-Pure Sterile Saline Solu-
tion.** (Alcon) Sterile unpreserved sa-
line solution. Aerosol 8 oz. *OTC.*
Use: Contact lens care.
Alconox. (Alconox) Biodegradable deter-
gent and wetting agent. Box 4 lb, Con-
tainer 25 lb, 50 lb, 100 lb, 300 lb. *OTC.*
Use: Contact lens care, detergent; wet-
ting agent.
**Alcon Saline Solution for Sensitive
Eyes.** (Alcon) Sodium Cl, edetate di-
sodium, borate buffer system, sorbic
acid. Bot. 360 mL. *OTC.*
Use: Contact lens care.
Alcortin. (Primus) Hydrocortisone 2%.
Alcohols, glycerin. Gel. Tubes. 2 g. *Rx.*
Use: Anti-inflammatory agent.
Alcotabs. (Alconox) Tab. Box 6s, 100s.
Use: Cleanser.
•**alcuronium chloride.** (al-cure-OH-nee-
uhm KLOR-ide) USAN. Diallyldinortox-
iferin dichloride.
Use: Muscle relaxant.
Aldactazide. (Pharmacia) Spirono-
lactone and hydrochlorothiazide.
25 mg/25 mg: Bot. 100s, 500s, 1000s,

2500s, UD 100s. **50 mg/50 mg:** Bot. 100s, UD 32s, UD 100s. Tab. *Rx.*
Use: Antihypertensive, diuretic.
Aldactone. (Pharmacia) Spironolactone. **25 mg. Tab.:** Bot. 100s, 500s, 1000s, UD 100s. **50 mg. Tab.:** Bot. 100s, UD 100s. **100 mg. Tab.:** Bot. 100s, UD 100s. *Rx.*
Use: Antihypertensive.
Aldara. (3M Pharm) Imiquimod 5%. Cetyl alcohol, stearyl alcohol, white petrolatum, benzyl alcohol, parabens. Cream. Boxes. 12s. Single-use packets. *Rx.*
Use: Topical immunomodulator.
●**aldesleukin.** (al-dess-LOO-kin) USAN. Recombinant form of interleukin-2.
Use: Biological response modifier; antineoplastic; immunostimulant.
See: Proleukin.
●**aldioxa.** (al-DIE-ox-ah) USAN. Aluminum dihydroxy allantoinate.
Use: Astringent; keratolytic.
Aldoclor 150. (Merck & Co.) Methyldopa 250 mg, chlorothiazide 150 mg. Tab. Bot. 100s. *Rx.*
Use: Antihypertensive.
Aldoclor 250. (Merck & Co.) Methyldopa 250 mg, chlorothiazide 250 mg. Tab. Bot. 100s. *Rx.*
Use: Antihypertensive.
Aldomet Ester Hydrochloride. (Merck & Co.) Methyldopate hydrochloride 250 mg/5 mL, citric acid anhydrous 25 mg, sodium bisulfite 16 mg, disodium edetate 2.5 mg, monothioglycerol 10 mg, sodium hydroxide to adjust pH, methylparaben 0.15%, propylparaben 0.02% w/water for inj. q.s. to 5 mL. Inj. Vial 5 mL. *Rx.*
Use: Antihypertensive.
Aldomet Oral Suspension. (Merck & Co.) Methyldopa 250 mg/5 mL, alcohol 1%, benzoic acid 0.1%, sodium bisulfite 0.2%. Oral Susp. Bot. 473 mL. *Rx.*
Use: Antihypertensive.
Aldomet Tablets. (Merck & Co.) Methyldopa. **125 mg Tab.:** Bot. 100s. **250 mg Tab.:** Bot. 100s, 1000s, UD 100s, unit-of-use 100s. **500 mg Tab.:** Bot. 100s, 500s, UD 100s, unit-of-use 60s, 100s. *Rx.*
Use: Antihypertensive.
W/Chlorothiazide.
See: Aldoclor.
W/Hydrochlorothiazide.
See: Aldoril.
Aldoril D30 & D50. (Merck & Co.) Methyldopa 500 mg, hydrochlorothiazide 30 mg or 50 mg. Tab. Bot. 100s.

Rx.
Use: Antihypertensive.
Aldoril-15. (Merck & Co.) Methyldopa 250 mg, hydrochlorothiazide 15 mg. Tab. Bot. 100s, 1000s. *Rx.*
Use: Antihypertensive.
Aldoril-25. (Merck & Co.) Methyldopa 250 mg, hydrochlorothiazide 25 mg. Tab. Bot. 100s, 1000s, UD 100s. *Rx.*
Use: Antihypertensive.
Aldosterone RIA Diagnostic Kit. (Abbott Diagnostics) Test kits 50s.
Use: Diagnostic aid.
Aldurazyme. (BioMarin) Laronidase 2.9 mg/5 mL, albumin (human) 0.1% after dilution, NaCl 43.9 mg, sodium phosphate monobasic monohydrate 63.5 mg, sodium phosphate dibasic heptahydrate 10.7 mg, preservative free. Inj. Single-use vials. 5 mL. *Rx.*
Use: Treatment of mucopolysaccharidosis.
ALEC. (Forum Products, Inc.) Dipalmitoyl phosphatidylcholine/phosphatidylglycerol.
Use: Neonatal respiratory distress syndrome. [Orphan Drug]
●**alefacept.** (ah-LEE-fah-sept) USAN.
Use: Immunologic agent, immunosuppressive.
See: Amevive.
●**alemcinal.** (al-EM-si-nal) USAN.
Use: Gastrointestinal prokinetic.
●**alemtuzumab.** (al-em-TUE-zue-mab) USAN.
Use: Antineoplastic; monoclonal antibody.
See: Campath.
●**alendronate sodium.** (al-LEN-droe-nate) USAN.
Use: Bone resorption inhibitor.
W/Cholecalciferol.
See: Fosamax Plus D.
Alenic Alka. (Rugby) **Liq.:** Aluminum hydroxide 31.7 mg, magnesium carbonate 137.3 mg, sodium alginate, EDTA, sodium 13 mg. Bot. 355 mL. **Chew. Tab.:** Aluminum hydroxide 80 mg, magnesium trisilicate 20 mg, sodium bicarbonate, calcium stearate, sugar. Bot. 100s. *OTC.*
Use: Antacid.
Alenic Alka, Extra Strength. (Rugby) Aluminum hydroxide 160 mg, magnesium carbonate 105 mg, sodium 29.9 mg. Chew. Tab. Bot. 100s. *OTC.*
Use: Antacid.
●**alentemol hydrobromide.** (al-EN-teh-mole HIGH-droe-BROE-mide) USAN.

Use: Antipsychotic; dopamine agonist.
Alersule. (Edwards) Chlorpheniramine maleate 8 mg, phenylephrine hydrochloride 20 mg. Cap. Bot. 100s. *Rx-OTC.*
Use: Antihistamine; decongestant.
Alert-Pep. (Health for Life Brands) Caffeine 200 mg. Cap. Bot. 16s. *OTC.*
Use: CNS stimulant.
Alesse. (Wyeth-Ayerst) Levonorgestrel 0.1 mg, ethinyl estradiol 20 mcg, lactose. Tab. Pkg. 28s. *Rx.*
Use: Sex hormone, contraceptive.
●**aletamine hydrochloride.** (al-ETT-ahmeen HIGH-droe-KLOR-ide) USAN.
Use: Antidepressant.
Aleve. (Bayer) Naproxen 200 mg (naproxen sodium 220 mg). Tab. Bot. 24s, 50s, 100s, 150s. Cap. Bot. 24s, 50s, 100s, 150s, 200s. Gelcap. Bot. 20s, 40s, 80s. *OTC.*
Use: NSAID.
Aleve Cold & Sinus. (Bayer) Pseudoephedrine hydrochloride 120 mg, naproxen sodium 220 mg (naproxen 200 mg), lactose. ER Tab. Pkg. 10s, 20s, 40s. *OTC.*
Use: Upper respiratory combination, analgesic, decongestant.
Aleve Sinus & Headache. (Bayer) Pseudoephedrine hydrochloride 120 mg, naproxen sodium 220 mg (naproxen 200 mg), lactose. ER Tab. Pkg. 10s. *OTC.*
Use: Upper respiratory combination, analgesic, decongestant.
●**alexidine.** (ah-LEX-ih-DEEN) USAN.
Use: Anti-infective.
alfa interferon-2a.
See: Roferon A.
alfa interferon-2b.
See: Intron A.
Alfenta. (Akorn) Alfentanil hydrochloride (as base) 500 mcg/mL. Preservative free. Inj. Amp. 2 mL, 5 mL, 10 mL, 20 mL. *c-II.*
Use: Opioid analgesic.
●**alfentanil hydrochloride.** (al-FEN-tuh-NILL HIGH-droe-KLOR-ide) USAN.
Use: Opioid analgesic.
See: Alfenta.
alfentanil hydrochloride. (Abbott) Alfentanil hydrochloride (as base) 500 mcg/mL. Preservative free. Inj. Amps. 2 mL, 5 mL, 10 mL. *c-II.*
Use: Opioid analgesic.
Alferon N. (Interferon Sciences) Interferon Alfa-N3 5 million units/mL, NaCl 8 mg, sodium phosphate dibasic 1.74 mg, potassium phosphate mono-

basic 0.2 mg, potassium chloride 0.2 mg. Inj. Vial 1 mL. *Rx.*
Use: Immunologic agent.
●**alfimeprase.** (AL-fi-me-prace) USAN.
Use: Thrombolytic.
●**alfuzosin hydrochloride.** (al-FEW-zoesin HIGH-droe-KLOR-ide) USAN.
Use: Antihypertensive, alpha-blocker.
See: Uroxatral.
Algel. (Faraday) Magnesium trisilicate 0.5 g, aluminum hydroxide 0.25 g. Tab. Bot. 100s. Susp. Bot. gal. *OTC.*
Use: Antacid.
●**algeldrate.** (AL-jell-drate) USAN.
Use: Antacid.
Algemin. (Thurston) Macrocystis pyrifera alga. Pow. Jar 8 oz. Tab. Bot. 300s. *OTC.*
Use: Dietary aid.
Algenic Alka. (Rugby) Aluminum hydroxide 31.7 mg/mL, magnesium carbonate 137 mg/mL, sodium alginate, sorbitol. Liq. Bot. 355 mL. *OTC.*
Use: Antacid.
Algenic Alka Improved. (Rugby) Aluminum hydroxide 240 mg, magnesium hydroxide 100 mg/Chew. Tab. Bot. 100s, 500s. *OTC.*
Use: Antacid.
●**algestone acetonide.** (al-JESS-tone ah-SEE-toe-nide) USAN.
Use: Anti-inflammatory.
●**algestone acetophenide.** (al-JESS-tone ah-SEE-toe-FEN-ide) USAN.
Use: Hormone, progestin.
Algex. (Health for Life Brands) Menthol, camphor, methylsalicylate, eucalyptus. Liniment. Bot. 4 oz. *OTC.*
Use: Analgesic, topical.
algin.
See: Sodium Alginate.
Algin-All. (Barth's) Sodium alginate from kelp. Tab. Bot. 100s, 500s.
●**alginic acid.** (al-JIN-ik) *NF 23.*
Use: Pharmaceutic aid, tablet binder, emulsifying agent.
W/Aluminum hydroxide dried gel, magnesium trisilicate, sodium bicarbonate.
See: Gaviscon Foamtabs.
W/Combinations.
See: Pretts Diet-Aid.
●**alglucerase.** (al-GLUE-ser-ACE) USAN.
Formerly Macrophage-targeted β-*glucocerebrosidase.*
Use: Enzyme replenisher, glucocerebrosidase. [Orphan Drug]
See: Ceredase.
●**alglucosidase alfa.** (al-gloo-KOSE-i-dase) USAN.
Use: Enzyme replacement therapy.

- **alicaforsen sodium.** (a-li-KA-for-sen)
  USAN.
  Use: Anti-inflammatory.
- **alidine dihydrochloride or phosphate.**
  See: Anileridine.
- **aliflurane.** (al-IH-flew-rane) USAN.
  Use: Anesthetic, inhalation.
- **Alikal.** (Sanofi-Synthelabo) Sodium bi-
  carbonate, tartaric acid powder. *OTC.*
  Use: Antacid.
- **Alimentum.** (Ross) Casein hydrolysate,
  sucrose, tapioca starch, MCT (fraction-
  ated coconut oil), safflower oil, soy oil.
  Qt. Ready-to-use. *OTC.*
  Use: Nutritional supplement-enteral.
- **Alimta.** (Eli Lilly) Pemetrexed 500 mg.
  Mannitol 500 mg. Pow. for Inj., lyophi-
  lized. Single-use vials. *Rx.*
  Use: Antimetabolite.
- **Alinia.** (Romark Laboratories)
  Nitazoxanide. **Pow. for Oral Susp.:**
  100 mg/5 mL (after reconstitution).
  Sugar, sucrose 1.48 mg/5 mL, straw-
  berry flavor. Bot. 60 mL. **Tab.:** 500 mg.
  Polyvinyl alcohol, sucrose, talc. Film
  coated. 60s, UD 6s. *Rx.*
  Use: Antiprotozoal.
- **alipamide.** (al-IH-pam-ide) USAN.
  Use: Antihypertensive; diuretic.
- **alisobumal.**
  See: Butalbital.
- **alitame.** (AL-ih-TAME) USAN.
  Use: Sweetener.
- **alitretinoin.** (a-li-TRET-i-noyn) USAN.
  Use: Antineoplastic, retinoid.
  See: Panretin.
- **alkalinizers, minerals and electrolytes.**
  See: Bicitra.
  Oracit
  Polycitra.
- **alkalinizers, urinary tract products.**
  See: Bicitra.
  Citrolith.
  Polycitra.
  Sodium Bicarbonate.
  Urocit-K.
- **Alkalol.** (Alkalol) Thymol, eucalyptol,
  menthol, camphor, benzoin, potassium
  alum, potassium chlorate, sodium bi-
  carbonate, sodium Cl, sweet birch oil,
  spearmint oil, pine and cassia oil, al-
  cohol 0.05%. Bot. Pt. Nasal douche cup
  pkg. 1s. *OTC.*
  Use: Eyes, nose, throat, and all in-
  flamed mucous membranes.
- **Alka-Med Liquid.** (Halsey Drug) Aluminum hydroxide 200 mg, magnesium
  hydroxide 200 mg/5 mL. Bot. 8 oz.
  OTC.
  Use: Antacid.

- **Alka-Med Tablets.** (Halsey Drug) Magne-
  sium hydroxide, aluminum hydroxide.
  Bot. 60s. *OTC.*
  Use: Antacid.
- **Alka-Mints.** (Bayer Corp. (Consumer
  Div.)) Calcium carbonate 850 mg/Chew.
  Tab. Carton 30s. *OTC.*
  Use: Antacid.
- **Alka-Seltzer.** (Bayer Corp. (Consumer
  Div.)) Heat treated sodium bicarbonate
  1,700 mg, citric acid 1,000 mg, aspirin
  325 mg. Eff. Tab. Bot. 36s. *OTC.*
  Use: Analgesic; antacid.
- **Alka-Seltzer, Advanced Formula.**
  (Bayer Corp. (Consumer Div.)) Heat
  treated sodium bicarbonate 465 mg, cit-
  ric acid 900 mg, acetaminophen
  325 mg, potassium bicarbonate
  300 mg, calcium carbonate 280 mg.
  Tab. Foil pack 36s. *OTC.*
  Use: Analgesic; antacid.
- **Alka-Seltzer, Extra Strength.** (Bayer
  Corp. (Consumer Div.)) Aspirin 500 mg,
  heat treated sodium bicarbonate
  1985 mg, citric acid 1000 mg, sodium
  588 mg. Tab. Bot. 12s, 24s. *OTC.*
  Use: Analgesic; antacid.
- **Alka-Seltzer Flavored Effervescent
  Antacid-Analgesic.** (Bayer Corp.
  (Consumer Div.)) Aspirin 325 mg, sodium bicarbonate 1700 mg, citric acid
  1000 mg, phenylalanine 9 mg, sodium
  506 mg, aspartame, lemon-lime flavor.
  Tab. Bot. 24s. *OTC.*
  Use: Analgesic; antacid.
- **Alka-Seltzer Gold.** (Bayer Corp. (Consumer Div.)) Heat treated sodium bi-
  carbonate 958 mg, citric acid 832 mg,
  potassium bicarbonate 312 mg, sodium
  311 mg. Tab. Bot. 20s, 36s. *OTC.*
  Use: Analgesic; antacid.
- **Alka-Seltzer Plus Cold & Sinus Effervescent.** (Bayer Corp. (Consumer
  Div.)) Phenylephrine hydrochloride
  5 mg, acetaminophen 250 mg, phenyl-
  alanine 4 mg, aspartame, acesulfame
  K, saccharin, sorbitol. Tab. Pkg. 20s.
  OTC.
  Use: Upper respiratory combination, analgesic, decongestant.
- **Alka-Seltzer Plus Cold & Sinus Liqui-
  Gels.** (Bayer Corp. (Consumer Div.))
  Pseudoephedrine hydrochloride 30 mg,
  acetaminophen 325 mg, sorbitol. Liqui-
  gel. Pkg. 12s, 20s. *OTC.*
  Use: Nasal decongestant, analgesic,
  decongestant.
- **Alka-Seltzer Plus Cough & Cold Effer-
  vescent.** (Bayer Corp. (Consumer
  Div.)) Dextromethorphan HBr 10 mg,
  chlorpheniramine maleate 2 mg,

phenylephrine hydrochloride 5 mg, aspartame, phenylalanine 11 mg, sorbitol. Effervescent Tab. Pkg. 20s. *OTC.*
Use: Upper respiratory combination, antitussive, antihistamine, decongestant.

Alka-Seltzer Plus Cough & Cold Liqui-Gels. (Bayer Corp. (Consumer Div.)) Dextromethorphan HBr 10 mg, pseudoephedrine hydrochloride 30 mg, chlorpheniramine maleate 2 mg, acetaminophen 325 mg, sorbitol. Liquigels Pkg. 12s, 20s. *OTC.*
Use: Upper respiratory combination, analgesic, antihistamine, antitussive, decongestant.

Alka-Seltzer Plus Flu Effervescent. (Bayer Corp. (Consumer Div.)) Dextromethorphan HBr 15 mg, chlorpheniramine maleate 2 mg, aspirin 500 mg, acesulfame K, aspartame, phenylalanine 6.7 mg, mannitol, saccharin, honey/orange flavor. Effervescent Tab. Pkg. 20s. *OTC.*
Use: Upper respiratory combination, antitussive, antihistamine, analgesic.

Alka-Seltzer Plus Flu Liqui-Gels. (Bayer Corp. (Consumer Div.)) Dextromethorphan HBr 10 mg, pseudoephedrine hydrochloride 30 mg, acetaminophen 325 mg, sorbitol. Liquigels. Pkg. 12s. *OTC.*
Use: Upper respiratory combination, antitussive, decongestant, analgesic.

Alka-Seltzer Plus Night-Time Effervescent. (Bayer Corp. (Consumer Div.)) Dextromethorphan HBr 10 mg, doxylamine succinate 6.25 mg, phenylephrine hydrochloride 5 mg, acelsulfame K, aspartame, phenylalanine 7.8 mg, sorbitol. Effervescent Tab. Pkg. 20s. *OTC.*
Use: Upper respiratory combination, antitussive, antihistamine, decongestant.

Alka-Seltzer Plus Night-Time Liqui-Gels. (Bayer Corp. (Consumer Div.)) Dextromethorphan HBr 10 mg, doxylamine succinate 6.25 mg, pseudoephedrine hydrochloride 30 mg, acetaminophen 325 mg, sorbitol, alcohol free. Liquigel. Pkg. 12s, 20s, 36s. *OTC.*
Use: Upper respiratory combination, antitussive, antihistamine, decongestant, analgesic.

Alkavite. (Vitality) Vitamins A 5000 units, C 250 mg, D 400 units, E 30 units, B_1 100 mg, B_6 3 mg, B_{12} 12 mcg, folic acid 1 mg, B_2 3 mg, niacin 20 mg, biotin 0.03 mg, Ca 68.5 mg, Fe 60 mg, Mg, Zn 4 mg, Se. ER Tab. UD 100s *OTC.*

Use: Vitamin supplement.

Alkeran. (Celgene) Melphalan. **Pow. for Inj., lyophilized:** 50 mg. Single-use vials (with povidone 20 mg) with 10 mL of sterile diluent (water for injection with sodium citrate 0.2 g, propylene glycol 6 mL, ethanol 0.52 mL). **Tab.:** 2 mg, lactose. Film-coated. Amber Glass Bot. 50s. *Rx.*
Use: Antineoplastic.

alkylamines, nonselective.
Use: Antihistamine
See: Brompheniramine Tannate.
Chlorpheniramine Maleate.
Dexchlorpheniramine Maleate.
Triprolidine Hydrochloride.

alkylating agents.
See: Alkyl Sulfonates.
Altretamine.
Busulfan.
Carmustine.
Chlorambucil.
Cyclophosphamide.
Dacarbazine.
Estramustine Phosphate Sodium.
Estrogen/Nitrogen Mustard.
Ethylenimines/Methylmelamines.
Ifosfamide.
Lomustine.
Mechlorethamine Hydrochloride.
Melphalan.
Nitrogen Mustards.
Nitrosureas.
Streptozocin.
Thiotepa.
Triazenes.

alkylbenzyldimethylammonium chloride. Benzalkonium Cl.

• **alkyl (C12-15) benzoate.** *NF 23.*
Use: Pharmaceutical aid, oleaginous vehicle emollient.

alkyl sulfonates.
Use: Alkylating agents.
See: Busulfan.

• **allantoin.** (al-AN-toe-in) USAN.
Use: Vulnerary, topical.
See: Cutemol.
W/Aminacrine, sulfanilamide.
See: Balmex Med.
Par.
W/p-Chloro-m-xylenol.
See: Cebum.
W/Coal tar extract, hexachlorophene, glycerin, lanolin.
See: Pso-Rite.
W/Coal tar in cream base.
See: Tegrin.
W/Coal tar solution, isopropyl myristate, psoralen.
See: Psorelief.
W/Dienestrol, sulfanilamide, aminacrine hydrochloride.

See: Tackle.
W/Salicylic acid, sulfur.
See: Neutrogena Disposables.
W/Sulfanilamide, 9-aminoacridine hydro-
chloride.
See: Nil Vaginal.
Sebical.
Vagisan.
Allay. (LuChem Pharmaceuticals, Inc.)
Acetaminophen 650 mg, hydrocodone
bitartrate 7.5 mg. Cap. Bot. 100s. *c-III.*
Use: Analgesic combination; narcotic.
Allbee C-800. (Wyeth) Vitamins E
45 units, C 800 mg, B_1 15 mg, B_2
17 mg, B_3 100 mg, B_5 25 mg, B_{12}
12 mcg. Tab. Bot. 60s. *OTC.*
Use: Vitamin supplement.
Allbee C-800 Plus Iron. (Wyeth) Vita-
mins E 45 units, C 800 mg, B_1 15 mg,
B_6 17 mg, niacin 100 mg, B_2 25 mg, B_{12}
12 mcg, pantothenic acid 25 mg, iron
27 mg, folic acid 0.4 mg. Tab. Bot. 60s.
OTC.
Use: Mineral, vitamin supplement.
Allbee-T. (Wyeth) Vitamins B_1 15.5 mg,
B_2 10 mg, B_6 8.2 mg, B_5 23 mg, B_3
100 mg, C 500 mg, B_{12} 5 mcg. Tab. Bot.
100s, 500s. *OTC.*
Use: Vitamin supplement.
Allbee w/C. (Wyeth) Vitamins B_1 15 mg,
B_6 5 mg, B_2 10.2 mg, B_3 50 mg, B_5
10 mg, C 300 mg. Cap. Bot. 30s. *OTC.*
Use: Vitamin supplement.
Allbex. (Health for Life Brands) Vitamins
B_1 5 mg, B_2 2 mg, B_6 0.25 mg, calcium
pantothenate 3 mg, niacinamide
20 mg, ferrous sulfate 194.4 mg, inositol 10 mg, choline 10 mg, B_{12} (concentrate) 3 mcg. Cap. Bot. 100s, 1000s.
OTC.
Use: Mineral, vitamin supplement.
All Clear. (Bausch & Lomb) Naphazoline
hydrochloride 0.012%, polyethylene gly
col 300 0.2%, benzalkonium chloride
0.01%, NaCl, EDTA, boric acid. Ophth.
Drops. Bot. 15 mL. *OTC.*
Use: Ophthalmic decongestant, vasoconstrictor.
All Clear AR. (Bausch & Lomb) Naphazoline hydrochloride 0.03%, hydroxypropyl methylcellulose 0.5%, benzalkonium chloride 0.01%, NaCl, boric
acid, EDTA. Ophth. Drops. Bot. 15 mL.
OTC.
Use: Ophthalmic decongestant, vasoconstrictor.
All-Day-C. (Barth's) Vitamin C 200 mg.
or 500 mg. Cap (200 mg). Tab
(500 mg). with rose hip extract. Bot.
30s, 90s, 180s, 360s. *OTC.*
Use: Vitamin supplement.

All-Day Iron Yeast. (Barth's) Iron 20 mg,
Vitamins B_1 2 mg, B_2 4 mg, niacin
0.57 mg. Cap. Bot. 30s, 90s, 180s.
OTC.
Use: Mineral, vitamin supplement.
All-Day-Vites. (Barth's) Vitamins A
10,000 units, D 400 units, B_1 3 mg, B_2
6 mg, niacin 1 mg, C 120 mg, B_{12}
10 mcg, E 30 units. Cap. Bot. 30s, 90s,
180s, 360s. *OTC.*
Use: Vitamin supplement.
Allegra. (Aventis) **Tab.:** Fexofenadine
30 mg, 60 mg, 180 mg. Film coated.
Bot. 100s, 500s, blister pack 100s
(60 mg only). **Cap.:** 60 mg, lactose. Bot.
60s, 100s, 500s, blisterpack 100s. *Rx.*
Use: Antihistamine, peripherally selective piperidine.
Allegra-D 12 Hour Tablets. (Aventis)
Fexofenadine 60 mg, pseudoephedrine
hydrochloride 120 mg. ER Tab. Bot.
60s, 100s, 500s, blister pack 100s. *Rx.*
Use: Upper respiratory combination,
antihistamine, decongestant.
Allegra-D 24 Hour. (Aventis) Pseudoephedrine hydrochloride 240 mg, fexofenadine hydrochloride 180 mg. Alcohols, talc. Film-coated. ER Tab. 30s,
100s, 500s. *Rx.*
Use: Decongestant and antihistamine.
allegron. Nortriptyline.
Use: Antidepressant.
Allent. (B.F. Ascher) Pseudoephedrine
hydrochloride 120 mg, brompheniramine maleate 12 mg. ER Cap. Bot.
100s. *Rx.*
Use: Antihistamine; decongestant.
Allerben. (Forest) Diphenhydramine
10 mg/mL. Inj. Vial 30 mL. *Rx.*
Use: Antihistamine.
Aller-Chlor. (Rugby) Chlorpheniramine
maleate. **Tab.:** 4 mg. Bot. 24s, 100s.
Syr.: 2 mg/5 mL, alcohol 5%, parabens,
sugar. Bot. 118 mL. *OTC.*
Use: Antihistamine, nonselective alkylamine.
Allercon. (Parmed Pharmaceuticals,
Inc.) Pseudoephedrine hydrochloride
60 mg, triprolidine hydrochloride
2.5 mg. Tab. Bot. 24s, 100s, 1000s.
OTC.
Use: Antihistamine; decongestant.
Allerest. (Novartis) **Eye Drops:** Naphazoline hydrochloride 0.012%. Bot.
0.5 oz. **Headache Strength Tab.:**
Acetaminophen 325 mg, pseudoephedrine hydrochloride 30 mg, chlorpheniramine maleate 2 mg. Tab. Pkg. 24s. **Nasal Spray:** Oxymetazoline hydrochloride 0.05%. Bot. 0.5 oz. *OTC.*
Use: Analgesic (Headache Strength

Tab. only); antihistamine; decongestant.

Allerest Allergy & Sinus Relief Maximum Strength. (Heritage) Pseudoephedrine hydrochloride 30 mg, acetaminophen 325 mg. Tab. 24s. *OTC.*
Use: Decongestant and analgesic.

Allerest Maximum Strength. (Heritage Consumer) Pseudoephedrine hydrochloride 30 mg, chlorpheniramine maleate 2 mg. Tab. Bot. 24s. *OTC.*
Use: Upper respiratory combination, antihistamine, decongestant.

Allerfrim. (Rugby) **Tab.**: Pseudoephedrine hydrochloride 60 mg, triprolidine hydrochloride 2.5 mg, lactose. Bot. 24s, 100s, 1000s. **Syr.**: Pseudoephedrine hydrochloride 30 mg, triprolidine hydrochloride 1.25 mg/5 mL, sucrose, methylparaben, sorbitol, corn syrup. Bot. 118 mL, 473 mL. *OTC.*
Use: Upper respiratory combination, antihistamine, decongestant.

Allerfrim OTC Syrup. (Rugby) Pseudoephedrine 30 mg, triprolidine 1.25 mg. Syr. Bot. Pt. *OTC.*
Use: Antihistamine; decongestant.

Allerfrim w/Codeine. (Rugby) Pseudoephedrine hydrochloride 30 mg, triprolidine hydrochloride 1.25 mg, codeine phosphate 10 mg, alcohol 4.3%. Syr. Bot. 120 mL, Pt, gal. *c-v.*
Use: Antihistamine; antitussive; decongestant.

Allergan Enzymatic. (Allergan) Papain, sodium Cl, sodium carbonate, sodium borate, edetate disodium. Kits 12s, 24s, 36s, 48s. *OTC.*
Use: Contact lens care.

Allergan Hydrocare Cleaning & Disinfecting Solution. (Allergan) tris (2-hydroxyethyl) tallow ammonium Cl 0.013%, thimerosal 0.002%, bis (2-hydroxyethyl) tallow ammonium Cl, sodium bicarbonate, dibasic, monobasic and anhydrous sodium phosphate, hydrochloric acid, propylene glycol, polysorbate 80, special soluble polyhema. Bot. 4 oz, 8 oz, 12 oz. *OTC.*
Use: Contact lens care.

Allergan Hydrocare Preserved Saline Solution. (Allergan) Sodium Cl, sodium hexametaphosphate, sodium hydroxide, boric acid, sodium borate, EDTA 0.01%, thimerosal 0.001%. Bot. 8 oz, 12 oz. *OTC.*
Use: Contact lens care.

Allergen Ear Drops. (Ivax) Benzocaine 1.4%, antipyrine 5.4%, glycerin, oxyquinoline sulfate. Bot. 0.5 oz. *Rx.*
Use: Otic.

allergenic extracts. (Various Mfr.) Allergenic extracts of pollens, foods, inhalants, epidermals, fungi, insects, miscellaneous antigens.
Use: Diagnostic aid, allergens.

allergenic extracts, alum-precipitated. *See:* Allpyral. Center-Al.

Allergen Patch Test Kit. (Healthpoint Medical) Box of tubes of semi-solid pastes or solutions. Allergens are either suspended in 4.5 g petrolatum, USP, or dissolved in 5.5 g water. Kit includes 20 reclosable syringes for topical use only (not for injection), each exuding sufficient allergen to test 150 patients, housed in a plastic case with two drawers. Allergens include benzocaine, mercaptobenzothiazole, colophony, p-phenylenediamine, imidazolidinyl urea (Germall115), cinnamon aldyhyde, lanolin alcohol (woolwax alcohols), carbarubber mix, neomycin sulfate, thiuram rubber mix, formaldehyde, ethylenediamine dihydrochloride, epoxyresin, quaternium 15, p-tert-butylphenol formalde hyderesin, mercapto rubber mix, black rubber p-phenylenediamine mix, potassium dichromate, balsam of Peru and nickel sulfate.

allergen test patches.
Use: Diagnostic aid; allergic dermatitis.
See: T.R.U.E. Test.

Allergex. (Bayer Corp. (Consumer Div.)) Silicones, polyethylene and triethylene glycol, antioxidants, mineral oil concentrate. Bot. Pt. Aerosol pt.
Use: Antiallergic.

Allergy. (Major) Chlorpheniramine maleate 4 mg, lactose. Tab. Bot. 24s, 100s. *OTC.*
Use: Antihistamine, non-selective alkylamine.

Allergy Drops. (Bausch & Lomb) Naphazoline hydrochloride 0.012%. Bot. 15 mL. *OTC.*
Use: Mydriatic; vasoconstrictor.

allergy preparations.
See: Antihistamine Preparations.

Allergy Relief. (Zee Medical) Chlorpheniramine maleate 4 mg. Tab. 12s. *OTC.*
Use: Antihistamine.

Allergy Tablets. (Major) Chlorpheniramine 4 mg. Tab. Bot. 24s and 100s. *OTC.*
Use: Antihistamine.

AllerMax. (Pfeiffer) Diphenhydramine hydrochloride 12.5 mg/5 mL, alcohol 0.5%, glucose, saccharin, sorbitol, sucrose, menthol, raspberry flavor. Liq.

Bot. 118 mL. *OTC.*
Use: Antihistamine, nonselective ethanolamine, nonnarcotic antitussive.
AllerMax Allergy & Cough Formula.
(Pfeiffer) Diphenhydramine hydrochloride 6.25 mg/5 mL, alcohol 0.5%, raspberry flavor, menthol, sucrose, glucose, saccharin, sorbitol. Bot. 118 mL. *OTC.*
Use: Antihistamine.
AllerMax Caplets, Maximum Strength.
(Pfeiffer) Diphenhydramine hydrochloride 50 mg, lactose. Tab. Bot. 24s. *OTC.*
Use: Antihistamine, nonselective ethanolamine.
Allersone. (Roberts) Hydrocortisone 0.5%, diperodon hydrochloride 0.5%, zinc oxide 5%, sodium lauryl sulfate, propylene glycol, cetyl alcohol, petrolatum, methyl- and propylparabens. Oint. Tube 15 g. *Rx-OTC.*
Use: Corticosteroid, topical.
Allersule Forte. (Edwards) Phenylephrine hydrochloride 20 mg, chlorpheniramine maleate 8 mg, methscopolamine nitrate 2.5 mg. Cap. Bot. 100s. *Rx-OTC.*
Use: Anticholinergic; antihistamine; decongestant.
AlleRx. (Adams) Phenylephrine tannate 5 mg, chlorpheniramine tannate 2 mg, pyrilamine tannate 12.5 mg/5 mL, methylparaben, saccharin, sucrose, raspberry flavor. Susp. 473 mL. *Rx.*
Use: Upper respiratory combination.
AlleRx-D. (Adams) Pseudoephedrine hydrochloride 120 mg, methscopolamine nitrate 2.5 mg. CR Tab. Bot. 60s. *Rx.*
Use: Upper respiratory combination, decongestant, anticholinergic.
AlleRx Dose Pack. (Adams) **AM:**
Pseudoephedrine hydrochloride 120 mg, methscopolamine nitrate 2.5 mg. **PM:** Chlorpheniramine maleate 8 mg, methscopolamine nitrate 2.5 mg. CR Tab. Pkg. 20s. *Rx.*
Use: Upper respiratory combination, anticholinergic, antihistamine, decongestant.
Allfen-DM. (MCR American) Dextromethorphan HBr 55 mg, guaifenesin 1000 mg, dye free. ER Tab. Bot. 100s. *Rx.*
Use: Upper respiratory combination, antitussive, expectorant.
Allfen Jr. (MCR American) Guaifenesin 400 mg, dye free. Tab. 100s. *Rx.*
Use: Expectorant.
All-Nite. (Major) Dextromethorphan HBr 5 mg, doxylamine succinate 2.1 mg, pseudoephedrine hydrochloride 10 mg,

acetaminophen 167mg/5 mL, alcohol 10%, saccharin, corn syrup, original and cherry flavors. Liq. Bot. 177 mL. *OTC.*
Use: Upper respiratory combination, antitussive, antihistamine, decongestant, analgesic.
All-Nite Cold Formula. (Major) Pseudoephedrine hydrochloride 10 mg, doxylamine succinate 1.25 mg, dextromethorphan HBr 5 mg, acetaminophen 167 mg/5 mL. Liq. Bot. 177 mL. *OTC.*
Use: Analgesic; antihistamine; antitussive; decongestant.
● **allobarbital.** (AL-low-BAR-bih-tal) USAN.
Formerly Diallylbarbituric acid.
Use: Hypnotic; sedative.
● **allopurinol.** (AL-oh-PURE-ee-nahl) *USP 28.*
Use: Antigout; xanthine oxidase inhibitor; antimetabolite.
See: Aloprim.
Zyloprim.
allopurinol. (Various Mfr.) Allopurinol 100 mg, 300 mg. Tab. Bot. 100s, 500s, 1000s, UD 100s. *Rx.*
Use: Antimetabolite.
allopurinol sodium. (Bedford Labs) Allopurinol sodium 500 mg. Preservative free. Pow. for Inj., lyophilized. Vials with rubber stopper. 30 mL. *Rx.*
Use: Antimetabolite.
Allpyral. (Bayer Corp. (Consumer Div.)) Allergenic extracts, alum-precipitated. For subcutaneous inj. pollens, molds, epithelia, house dust, other inhalants, stinging insects.
Use: Diagnostic aid, allergens.
allylamine antifungal.
Use: Antifungal agent.
See: Terbinafine hydrochloride.
allylbarbituric acid. (Various Mfr.) Allyl-isobutylbarbituric acid, butalbital. Tab.
Use: Sedative.
W/A.P.C.
See: Anti-Ten.
Fiorinal.
Tenstan.
W/Acetaminophen, homatropine methylbromide.
See: Panitol H.M.B.
allyl-isobutylbarbituric acid.
See: Allylbarbituric Acid.
allylisopropylmalonyl urea.
See: Aprobarbital.
● **allyl isothiocyanate.** *USP 28.*
Use: Counterirritant in neuralgia.
Almacone. (Rugby) **Chew Tab.:** Aluminum hydroxide 200 mg, magnesium hydroxide 200 mg, simethicone 20 mg. Bot. 100s, 1000s. **Liq.:** Aluminum

hydroxide 200 mg, magnesium hydroxide 200 mg, simethicone 20 mg, sodium 0.75 mg/5 mL. Bot. 360 mL, gal. *OTC.*
Use: Antacid.

Almacone II Double Strength Liquid. (Rugby) Aluminum hydroxide 400 mg, magnesium hydroxide 400 mg, simethicone 40 mg/5 mL. Bot. 360 mL, gal. *OTC.*
Use: Antacid.

• **almadrate sulfate.** (AL-ma-drate SULL-fate) USAN. Aluminum magnesium hydroxide-oxide-sulfate-hydrate.
Use: Antacid.

• **almagate.** (AL-mah-gate) USAN.
Use: Antacid.

almagucin. Gastric mucin, dried aluminum hydroxide gel, magnesium trisilicate. *OTC.*
Use: Antacid.

Almebex Plus B$_{12}$. (Dayton) Vitamins B$_1$ 1 mg, B$_2$ 2 mg, B$_3$ 5 mg, B$_6$ 0.4 mg, B$_{12}$ 5 mcg, choline 33 mg/5 mL. Bot. 473 mL (with B$_{12}$ in separate container). *OTC.*
Use: Vitamin supplement.

• **almond oil.** *NF 23.*
Use: Pharmaceutic aid, emollient, oleaginous vehicle, perfume.

• **almotriptan.** (al-moe-TRIP-tan) USAN.
Use: Antimigraine.

• **almotriptan maleate.** (al-moe-TRIP-tan MAL-ee-ate) USAN.
Use: Antimigraine, serotonin 5-HT$_1$ receptor agonist.
See: Axert.

• **alniditan dihydrochloride.** (al-nih-DIH-tan die-HIGH-droe-KLOR-ide) USAN.
Use: Antimigraine.

Alnyte. (Mayer Lab) Scopolamine aminoxide HBr 0.2 mg, salicylamide 250 mg. Tab. Pkg. 16s. *Rx.*
Use: Analgesic; anticholinergic.

Alocass Laxative. (Western Research) Aloin 0.25 g, cascara sagrada 0.5 g, rhubarb 0.5 g, ginger 1/32 g, powdered extract of belladonna g. Tab. Bot. 1000s. Pak 28s. *OTC.*
Use: Laxative.

Alocril. (Allergan) Nedocromil sodium 2% (20 mg/mL), benzalkonium Cl 0.01%, NaCl 0.5%, EDTA 0.05%. Ophth. Soln. Bot. 5 mL w/dropper tip. *Rx.*
Use: Ophthalmic agent, mast cell stabilizer.

• **aloe.** *USP 28.*
Use: See Compound Benzoin Tincture.

Aloe Grande Creme. (Gordon Laboratories) Aloe, vitamins E 1500 units, A 100,000 units/oz in cream base. Jar 2.5 oz. *OTC.*
Use: Emollient.

Aloe Vesta. (ConvaTec) Dimethicone 3%. Alcohols, aloe, glycerin, petrolatum. Lotion. 60 mL. *OTC.*
Use: Emollient.

Aloe Vesta Perineal. (GlaxoSmithKline) Solution of sodium C14-16 olefin sulfonate, propylene glycol, aloe vera gel, hydrolyzed collagen. Bot. 118 mL, 236 mL, gal. *OTC.*
Use: Perianal hygiene.

• **alofilcon a.** (AL-oh-FILL-kahn) USAN.
Use: Contact lens material, hydrophilic.

aloin. (J.T. Baker) A mixture of crystalline pentosides from various aloes. Bot. oz. *OTC.*
Use: Laxative.

Alomide. (Alcon) Lodoxamide tromethamine 0.1%. Soln. *Drop-tainers* 10 mL. *Rx.*
Use: Antiallergic, ophthalmic.

• **alonimid.** (ah-LAHN-ih-mid) USAN.
Use: Hypnotic; sedative.

Alophen. (Numark) Bisacodyl 5 mg, sugar. EC Tab. Bot. 100s. *OTC.*
Use: Laxative.

Aloprim. (Nabi) Allopurinol 500 mg. Preservative free. Pow. for Inj., lyophilized. Vial 30 mL with rubber stoppers. *Rx.*
Use: Antimetabolite.

Alora. (Watson) Estradiol 0.77 mg (0.025 mg/day), 1.5 mg (0.05 mg/day), 2.3 mg (0.075 mg/day), 3.1 mg (0.1 mg/day). Patch. Calendar packs 8 systems. *Rx.*
Use: Estrogen.

Alor 5/500. (Atley) Hydrocodone bitartrate 5 mg, aspirin 500 mg. Tab. Bot. 100s. *c-III.*
Use: Analgesic; narcotic.

• **alosetron hydrochloride.** (al-OH-seh-trahn HIGH-droe-KLOR-ide) USAN.
Use: Antiemetic.
See: Lotronex.

Alotone. (Major) Triamcinolone 4 mg. Tab. Bot. 100s. *Rx.*
Use: Corticosteroid.

• **alovudine.** (al-OHV-you-deen) USAN.
Use: Antiviral.

Aloxi. (MGI Pharma) Palonosetron hydrochloride 0.25 mg/5 mL. Mannitol 207.5 mg. Inj. Single-use vial. *Rx.*
Use: 5-HT$_3$ receptor antagonist.

• **alpertine.** (al-PURR-teen) USAN.
Use: Antipsychotic.

l-alpha-acetyl-methadol (LAAM). (Bio Development Corp.) *Rx.*
Use: Treatment of heroin addicts.

•**alpha amylase.** (AL-fah AM-ih-lace)
USAN. A concentrated form of alpha
amylase produced by a strain of non-
pathogenic bacteria.
Use: Digestive aid; anti-inflammatory.
See: Kutrase.
Ku-Zyme.
alpha-amylase w-100. W/Proteinase W-
300, cellase W-100, lipase, estrone,
testosterone, vitamins, minerals. *Rx.*
Use: Digestive aid.
alpha/beta-adrenergic blocking agent.
See: Carvedilol.
Labetolol Hydrochloride.
alpha-chymotrypsin.
See: Alpha Chymar (Centeon).
Alphaderm. (Teva) Hydrocortisone 1%.
Cream. Tube 30 g, 100 g. *Rx-OTC.*
Use: Corticosteroid, topical.
alpha-d-galactosidase.
Use: Antiflatulent.
Alpha-E. (Barth's) d-Alpha tocopherol.
50 units or 100 units: Cap. Bot. 100s,
500s, 1000s. **200 units:** Cap. Bot.
100s, 250s. **400 units:** Cap. Bot. 100s,
250s, 500s. *OTC.*
Use: Vitamin supplement.
alpha-estradiol. Known as beta-
estradiol.
See: Estradiol.
alpha-estradiol benzoate.
See: Estradiol benzoate.
Alpha Fast. (Eastwood) Bath oil. Bot.
16 oz. *OTC.*
Use: Emollient.
alpha-fetoprotein w/Tc-99m.
Use: Diagnostic aid.
•**alphafilcon a.** (al-fah-FILL-kahn) USAN.
Use: Contact lens material, hydrophillic.
alpha-galactosidase.
See: Aspergillus niger enzyme.
alpha-galactosidase a.
Use: Fabry disease. [Orphan Drug]
alpha-galactoside a.
Use: Treatment of Fabry disease.
Alphagan P. (Allergan) Brimonidine tar-
trate 0.15%, *Purite* 0.005%, boric acid,
potassium chloride, sodium borate, sodium chloride. Soln. Bot. 5 mL, 10 mL,
15 mL. *Rx.*
Use: Agent for glaucoma.
alpha-glucosidase inhibitor.
Use: Antidiabetic agent.
See: Acarbose.
Miglitol.
alpha-hypophamine.
See: Oxytocin.
alpha interferon-2a.
See: Roferon-A.

alpha interferon-2b.
See: Intron A.
•**alpha lipoic acid.** *NF 23.*
Use: Antioxidant.
Alpha-Keri. (Bristol-Myers Squibb)
Therapeutic Bath: Mineral oil, lanolin
oil, PEG-4-dilaurate, benzophenone-
3, D&C green #6, fragrance. Bot. 4 oz,
8 oz, 16 oz. **Cleansing Bar:** Bar containing sodium tallowate, sodium cocoate, water, mineral oil, fragrance,
PEG-75, glycerin, titanium dioxide,
lanolin oil, sodium Cl, BHT, EDTA, D&C
green #5, D&C yellow #10. 120 g. *OTC.*
Use: Emollient.
alpha-methyldopa. Name previously
used for Methyldopa.
Alphanate. (Grifols) Concentrate of human Factor VIII. When reconstituted,
contains FVIII:C/mg total protein
≥ 5 units, albumin (human) 0.3 to 0.9 g/
100 mL, calcium ≤ 5 mmol/L, glycine/
units ≤ 750 mcg, heparin ≤ 1 U/mL, histidine ≤ 10 to 40 mmol/L, imidazole
≤ 0.1 mg/mL, arginine ≤ 50 to
200 mmol/L, PEG and polysorbate
80 ≤ 1 mcg; solvent/detergent-and heat-
treated. Tri-n-butyl-phosphate
≤ 0.1 mcg/units FVIII:C. Inj., lyophilized.
Single-dose vials with diluent. Actual
number of AHF units are indicated on
the vials. *Rx.*
Use: Antihemophilic; treatment for von
Willebrand disease. [Orphan Drug]
AlphaNine. (Grifols) Purified heat-
treated/solvent preparation of coagulation Factor IX from human plasma.
With ≥ 50 units Factor IX per mg protein, < 5 units each Factor II (prothrombin) and Factor VII (proconvertin) per
100 IU Factor IX and < 20 units Factor
X (Stuart-Power Factor) per 100 IU
Factor IX. In single-dose vials with diluent, double-ended needle, and microaggregated filter. Pow. for Inj. *Rx.*
Use: Antihemophilic.
AlphaNine SD. (Grifols) Factor IX dried
plasma fraction (actual number of units
shown on each bottle), heparin, dextrose, solvent/detergent-treated, virus-
filtered. Pow. for Inj. Single-dose vials w/diluent, needle, and filter. *Rx.*
Use: Antihemophilic.
alpha-1-adrenergic blockers.
Use: Antihypertensives.
See: Cardura.
alpha-1-proteinase inhibitor.
Use: Treatment of alpha-1-antitrypsin
deficiency. [Orphan Drug]
See: Aralast.
Prolastin.
Zemaira

alphasone acetophenide. Name previously used for Algestone acetonide.

alpha-tocopherol.
See: Tocopherol, Alpha.

alpha-2 adrenergic agonist.
Use: Glaucoma agent.
See: Brimonidine tartrate.

Alpha Vee-12. (Schlicksup) Hydroxocobalamin 1000 mcg/mL. Vial 10 mL. *Rx.*
Use: Vitamin supplement.

Alphosyl. (Schwarz Pharma) Allantoin 1.7%, special crude coal tar extracts 5%. Lot.: Bot. 8 fl oz. **Cream:** 2 oz. *OTC.*
Use: Antipruritic.

•**alpidem.** (AL-PIH-dem) USAN.
Use: Antianxiety; anxiolytic.

•**alprazolam.** (al-PRAY-zoe-lam) *USP 28.*
Use: Hypnotic; sedative; antianxiety agent.
See: Niravam.
Xanax.
Xanax XR.

alprazolam. (al-PRAY-zoe-lam) (Various Mfr.) Alprazolam 0.25 mg, 0.5 mg, 1 mg, 2 mg. Tab. Bot. 100s, 500s, 1000s (except 2 mg), UD 100s (except 2 mg). *c-IV.*
Use: Management of anxiety disorders.

alprazolam intensol. (Roxane) Alprazolam 1 mg/mL. Oral Soln. 30 mL with calibrated dropper. *c-IV.*
Use: Antianxiety agent.

•**alprenolol hydrochloride.** (al-PREH-nolole HIGH-droe-KLOR-ide) USAN.
Use: Antiadrenergic; β-receptor.

•**alprenoxime hydrochloride.** (al-PREN-ox-eem) USAN.
Use: Antiglaucoma agent.

•**alprostadil.** (al-PRAHST-uh-dill) *USP 28.*
Formerly Prostaglandin E_1, PGE_1.
Use: Vasodilator; anti-impotence agent; arterial patency agent.
See: Caverject.
Edex.
Muse.
Prostin VR.
Prostin VR Pediatric.

•**alrestatin sodium.** (AHL-reh-STAT-in SO-dee-uhm) USAN.
Use: Enzyme inhibitor, aldose reductase.

Alrex. (Bausch & Lomb) Loteprednol etabonate 0.2%, benzalkonium chloride 0.01%, EDTA. Ophth. Susp. Bot. 5 mL, 10 mL. *Rx.*
Use: Corticosteroid, ophthalmic.

AL-721. (Matrix) Phase I/II AIDS, ARC, HIV positive.
Use: Antiviral.

Alsorb Gel. (Standex) Magnesium and aluminum hydroxide. Colloidal Susp. *OTC.*
Use: Antacid.

Alsorb Gel, C.T. (Standex) Calcium carbonate 2 g, glycine 3 g, magnesium trisilicate 3 g. Tab. *OTC.*
Use: Antacid.

Altace. (Monarch) Ramipril 1.25 mg, 2.5 mg, 5 mg, 10 mg. Cap. Bot. 100s, 500s (except 1.25 mg), 1000s (except 1.25 mg), UD 100s (except 10 mg), bulk pack 5000s (2.5 mg, 5 mg only). *Rx.*
Use: Antihypertensive; renin angiotensin system antagonist.

•**altanserin tartrate.** (AL-TAN-ser-in TAR-trate) USAN.
Use: Serotonin antagonist.

Altarussin. (Altaire) Guaifenesin 100 mg/5 mL. Alcohol-free. Corn syrup, menthol, saccharin. Syrup. 118 mL. *OTC.*
Use: Expectorant.

Altaryl Children's Allergy. (Altaire) Diphenhydramine (as hydrochloride) 12.5 mg per 5 mL. Alcohol free. Sodium 9 mg, glycerin, saccharin, sugar. Cherry flavor. Liq. 118 mL. *OTC.*
Use: Antihistamine.

•**alteplase, recombinant.** (AL-teh-PLACE) USAN.
Use: Plasminogen activator.
See: Activase.
Cathflo Activase.

AlternaGEL. (J & J Merck Consumer Pharm.) Aluminum hydroxide 600 mg/5 mL. Liq. Bot. 150 mL, 360 mL. *OTC.*
Use: Antacid.

•**althiazide.** (al-THIGH-azz-ide) USAN.
Use: Antihypertensive; diuretic.

•**altinicline maleate.** (AL-ti-ni-kleen) USAN.
Use: Antiparkinsonian agent.

Altocor. (Andryx) Lovastatin 10 mg, 20 mg, 40 mg, 60 mg, sugar, lactose. ER Tab. Bot. 30s. *Rx.*
Use: Antihyperlipidemic.

Altracin. (Alra) Bacitracin.
Use: Antibiotic. [Orphan Drug]

•**altretamine.** (ahl-TRETT-uh-meen) USAN.
Use: Antineoplastic.
See: Hexalen.

Alu-Cap. (3M) Aluminum hydroxide gel 400 mg. Cap. Bot. 100s. *OTC.*
Use: Antacid.

Al-U-Creme. (MacAllister) Aluminum hydroxide equivalent to 4% aluminum oxide. Susp. Bot. Pt, gal. *OTC.*
Use: Antacid.

Aludrox. (Wyeth) Aluminum hydroxide gel 307 mg, magnesium hydroxide 103 mg/5 mL. Susp. Bot. 355 mL. *OTC.*
Use: Antacid.

alukalin. Activated kaolin.
Use: Antidiarrheal.

Alulex. (Lexington) Magnesium trisilicate 3.25 g, aluminum hydroxide gel 3.5 g, phenobarbital ⅛ g, homatropine methylbromide g. Tab. Bot. 100s. *Rx.*
Use: Agent for peptic ulcer.

alum. Sulfuric acid, aluminum ammonium salt (2:1:1), dodecahydrate. Sulfuric acid, aluminum potassium salt (2:1:1), dodecahydrate.
Use: Astringent.

•**alum, ammonium.** (AL-um) *USP 28.*
Use: Astringent.

Alumate-HC. (Dermco) Hydrocortisone 0.125%, 0.25%, 0.5%, 1%. Cream. Pkg. 0.5 oz, 1 oz, 4 oz. *OTC.*
Use: Corticosteroid, topical.

Alumate Mixture. (Schlicksup) Aluminum hydroxide gel, milk of magnesia/ 5 mL. Bot. 12 oz, gal. *OTC.*
Use: Antacid.

alumina and magnesia.
Use: Antacid.

alumina and magnesium carbonate.
Use: Antacid.

alumina and magnesium trisilicate.
Use: Antacid.

alumina hydrated. W/Activated attapulgite, pectin. *OTC.*
Use: Antidiarrheal.

alumina, magnesia, and calcium carbonate.
Use: Antacid.

alumina, magnesia, and calcium chloride.
Use: Antacid.

alumina, magnesia, and simethicone. (Roxane) Aluminum hydroxide 213 mg, magnesium hydroxide 200 mg, simethicone 20 mg, parabens, sorbitol/5 mL. Susp. Bot. UD 15, 30 mL. *OTC.*
Use: Antacid.

alumina, magnesia, calcium carbonate, and simethicone.
Use: Antacid.

alumina, magnesium carbonate, and magnesium oxide.
Use: Antacid.

•**aluminum acetate topical solution.** (ah-LOO-min-uhm) *USP 28.*
Use: Astringent.
See: Bluboro.
  Buro-Sol.
  Domeboro.
  Domeboro Otic.

aluminum aminoacetate, dihydroxy.
See: Dihydroxy aluminum aminoacetate.

aluminum chlorhydroxide.
See: Aluminum chlorohydrate.

•**aluminum chloride.** (ah-LOO-min-uhm KLOR-ide) *USP 28.* Aluminum chloride hexahydrate.
Use: Astringent; drying agent.
See: Drysol.
  Xerac AC.

aluminum chloride (hexahydrate). (Glades) Aluminum chloride hexahydrate 20% in SD alcohol 40-2 88.5%. Soln. Bot. 37.5 mL, *Dab-O-Matic* applicator bottle 35 mL, 60 mL. *Rx.*
Use: Drying agent.

•**aluminum chlorohydrate.** (ah-LOO-min-uhm) *USP 28.* Formerly *Aluminum chlorhydroxide, aluminum hydroxychloride.*
Use: Anhidrotic.
See: Ostiderm.

•**aluminum chlorohydrex.** (ah-LOO-min-uhm) USAN. Formerly *Aluminum chlorhydroxide alcohol soluble complex, aluminum chlorohydrol propylene glycol complex.*
Use: Astringent.

•**aluminum chlorohydrex polyethylene glycol.** (ah-LOO-min-uhm) *USP 28.*
Use: Anhidrotic.

•**aluminum chlorohydrex propylene glycol.** (ah-LOO-min-uhm) *USP 28.*
Use: Anhidrotic.

•**aluminum dichlorohydrate.** (ah-LOO-min-uhm) *USP 28.*
Use: Anhidrotic.

•**aluminum dichlorohydrex polyethylene glycol.** (ah-LOO-min-uhm) *USP 28.*
Use: Anhidrotic.

•**aluminum dichlorohydrex propylene glycol.** (ah-LOO-min-uhm) *USP 28.*
Use: Anhidrotic.

aluminum dihydroxyaminoacetate. (ah-LOO-min-uhm)
See: Dihydroxy Aluminum Aminoacetate.

aluminum glycinate, basic.
See: Dihydroxy Aluminum Aminoacetate.
W/Aspirin, magnesium carbonate.
See: Bufferin.

aluminum hydroxide.
Use: Antacid.
W/Combinations.
See: Maalox Anti-Gas Extra Strength.
  Mylanta.

•**aluminum hydroxide gel.** (ah-LOO-min-uhm) *USP 28.*
Use: Antacid.
See: AlternaGEL.
   Alu-Cap.
   Al-U-Creme.
   Alu-Tab.
   Amphojel.
   Maalox HRF.
   Maalox Plus.
W/Aminoacetic acid, magnesium trisilicate.
See: Maracid-2.
W/Belladonna extract, magnesium hydroxide.
See: Trialka.
W/Calcium carbonate.
See: Alkalade.
W/Calcium carbonate, magnesium carbonate, magnesium trisilicate.
See: Marblen.
W/Clioquinol, methylcellulose, atropine sulfate, hyoscine HBr, hyoscyamine sulfate.
See: Enterex.
W/Dicyclomine hydrochloride, magnesium hydroxide, methylcellulose.
See: Triactin.
W/Gastric mucin, magnesium glycinate.
See: Mucogel.
W/Kaolin, pectin.
See: Metropectin.
W/Magnesium carbonate.
See: Algicon
   Estomul-M.
W/Magnesium carbonate, calcium carbonate, amino-acetic acid.
See: Glycogel.
W/Magnesium hydroxide.
See: Alsorb.
   Aludrox.
   Delcid.
   Gas Ban DS.
   Kolantyl.
   Maalox.
   Mylanta.
   Mylanta II.
   Neutralox.
   WinGel.
W/Magnesium hydroxide, aspirin.
See: Ascriptin.
   Ascriptin Extra Strength.
   Calciphen.
   Cama.
   Cama Inlay-Tab.
W/Magnesium hydroxide, calcium carbonate.
See: Camalox.
W/Magnesium hydroxide, simethicone.
See: Di-Gel.
   Gas-Ban DS.
   Maalox Plus.
   Mylanta.
   Mylanta-II.
   Silain-Gel.
   Simeco.
   Trial AG.
W/Magnesium trisilicilate.
See: Alsorb Gel, C.T.
   Arcodex Antacid.
   Gacid.
   Gaviscon.
   Maracid 2.
W/Phenindamine tartrate, phenylephrine hydrochloride, aspirin, caffeine, magnesium carbonate.
See: Dristan.
W/Phenol, zinc oxide, camphor, eucalyptol, ichthammol.
See: Almophen.
W/Prednisolone.
See: Fernisolone-B.
   Predoxine.
W/Sodium salicylate, acetaminophen, vitamin C.
See: Gaysal-S.
aluminum hydroxide gel. (Various Mfr.)
   Aluminum hydroxide 320 mg/5 mL.
   Susp. Bot. 360 mL, 480 mL, UD 15 and
   30 mL. *OTC.*
Use: Antacid.
aluminum hydroxide gel, concentrated. (Various Mfr.) Aluminum hydroxide 600 mg/5 mL. Liq. Bot. 30 mL, 180 mL, 480 mL. *OTC.*
Use: Antacid.
aluminum hydroxide gel, concentrated. (Roxane) Susp. **450 mg/5 mL:** Bot. 500 mL, UD 30 mL; **675 mg/5 mL:** Bot. 180 mL, 500 mL, UD 20 mL and 30 mL. *OTC.*
Use: Antacid.
W/Combinations.
See: AlternaGEL.
   Alu-Cap.
   Amphojel.
   Ascriptin.
   Di-Gel.
   Mylanta.
aluminum hydroxide gel, dried.
Use: Antacid.
W/Combinations.
See: Aludrox.
   Alurex.
   Banacid.
   Delcid.
   Eulcin.
   Gaviscon.
   Maalox.
   Maalox Plus
   Mylanta.
   Mylanta II.

Presalin.

aluminum hydroxide glycine.
See: Dihydroxyaluminum aminoacetate.

aluminum hydroxide magnesium carbonate.
Use: Antacid.
See: Aloxine.
Di-Gel.
Eugel.
W/Dicyclomine hydrochloride, magnesium trisilicate, methylcellulose.
See: Triactin.

●**aluminum monostearate.** (ah-LOO-min-uhm) *NF 23.*
Use: Pharmaceutic necessity for preparation of penicillin G procaine w/aluminum stearate suspension.
See: Penicillin G procaine w/aluminum stearate.

aluminum paste. (Paddock) Metallic aluminum 10%. Oint. Jar lb. *OTC.*
Use: Dermatologic, protectant.

●**aluminum phosphate gel.** (ah-LOO-min-uhm FOSS-fate) *USP 28.*
Use: Antacid.

●**aluminum sesquichlorohydrate.** (ah-LOO-min-uhm sess-kwih-KLOR-oh-HIGH-drate) *USP 28.*
Use: Anhidrotic.

●**aluminum sesquichlorohydrex polyethylene glycol.** (ah-LOO-min-uhm sess-kwih-KLOR-oh-HIGH-drex poli-eth-uh-leen gli-cawl) *USP 28.*
Use: Anhidrotic.

●**aluminum sesquichlorohydrex propylene glycol.** (ah-LOO-min-uhm sess-kwih-KLOR-oh-HIGH-drex) *USP 28.*
Use: Anhidrotic.

aluminum sodium carbonate hydroxide.
See: Dihydroxyaluminum sodium carbonate.

●**aluminum subacetate topical solution.** (ah-LOO-min-uhm) *USP 28.*
Use: Astringent.

●**aluminum sulfate.** (ah-LOO-min-uhm SULL-fate) *USP 28.*
Use: Pharmaceutic necessity for preparation of aluminum subacetate solution.
See: Aluminum subacetate.
Bluboro.
Ostiderm.

●**aluminum zirconium octachlorohydrate.** (ah-LOO-min-uhm zihr-KOE-nee-uhm) *USP 28.*
Use: Anhidrotic.

●**aluminum zirconium octachlorohydrex gly.** (ah-LOO-min-uhm zihr-KOE-nee-

uhm) *USP 28.*
Use: Anhidrotic.

●**aluminum zirconium pentachlorohydrate.** (ah-LOO-min-uhm zihr-KOE-nee-uhm) *USP 28.*
Use: Anhidrotic.

●**aluminum zirconium pentachlorohydrex gly.** (ah-LOO-min-uhm zihr-KOE-nee-uhm) *USP 28.*
Use: Anhidrotic.

●**aluminum zirconium tetrachlorohydrate.** (ah-LOO-min-uhm zihr-KOE-nee-uhm teh-trah-KLOR-oh-HIGH-drate) *USP 28.*
Use: Anhidrotic.

●**aluminum zirconium tetrachlorohydrex gly.** (ah-LOO-min-uhm zihr-KOE-nee-uhm teh-trah-KLOR-oh-HIGH-drex Gly) *USP 28.*
Use: Anhidrotic.

●**aluminum zirconium trichlorohydrate.** (ah-LOO-min-uhm zihr-KOE-nee-uhm try-KLOR-oh-HIGH-drate) *USP 28.*
Use: Anhidrotic.

●**aluminum zirconium trichlorohydrex gly.** (ah-LOO-min-uhm zihr-KOE-nee-uhm try-KLOR-oh-HIGH-drex Gly) *USP 28.*
Use: Anhidrotic.

●**alum, potassium.** (AL-um) *USP 28.*
Use: Astringent.

alum-precipitated allergenic extracts.
See: Allpyral.
Center-Al.

Alupent. (Boehringer Ingelheim) Metaproterenol sulfate. **Aer.:** 0.65 mg/actuation. Can 7 g (100 inhalations), 14 g (200 inhalations). Refills 14 g. **Inhalant Soln.:** 0.4%: 2.5 mL UD vial. **0.6%:** 2.5 mL UD vial. **5%:** Bot. 10 mL, 30 mL w/dropper. EDTA, benzalkonium chloride (5% only). 0.4% and 0.6% for use with an IPPB device. *Rx.*
Use: Bronchodilator, sympathomimetic.

Alurex. (Rexall Group) Magnesium-aluminum hydroxide. **Susp.:** 150 mg, 200 mg/5 mL. Bot. 12 oz. **Tab:** 300 mg, 400 mg. Box 50s. *OTC.*
Use: Antacid.

Alu-Tab. (3M) Aluminum hydroxide gel 500 mg. Tab. Bot. 250s. *OTC.*
Use: Antacid.

●**alvameline maleate.** (al-va-MEL-een) USAN.
Use: Partial M_1 agonist, M_2/M_3 antagonist.

Alvedil. (Luly-Thomas) Theophylline 4 g, pseudoephedrine hydrochloride 50 mg, butabarbital 15 mg. Cap. Bot. 100s.
Rx.

Use: Bronchodilator; decongestant; hypnotic; sedative.

●**alverine citrate.** (AL-ver-een SIH-trate) USAN.
Use: Anticholinergic.

●**alvimopan.** (al-VI-moe-pan) USAN.
Use: Peripherally restricted opioid receptor antagonist.

●**alvircept sudotox.** (AL-vihr-sept SOOD-ah-tox) USAN.
Use: Antiviral.

alvocidib. (al-voe-SID-ib) USAN.
Use: Antineoplastic.

Alzapam. (Major) Lorazepam 0.5 mg, 1 mg, 2 mg. Tab. Bot. 100s, 500s. *c-iv.*
Use: Antianxiety.

Ama. (Wampole) Antimitochondrial antibodies test by IFA. Test 48s.
Use: Diagnostic aid.

amacetam sulfate.
See: Pramiracetam sulfate.

●**amadinone acetate.** (aim-AD-ih-nohn ASS-eh-tate) USAN.
Use: Hormone, progestin.

●**amantadine hydrochloride.** (uh-MAN-tuh-deen) *USP 28.*
Use: Antiviral.
See: Symmetrel.

amantadine hydrochloride. (Various Mfr.) **Cap.:** 100 mg. Bot. 100s, 500s, UD 100s. **Syrup:** 50 mg/5 mL, may contain sorbitol and parabens. Bot. 480 mL. *Rx.*
Use: Antiviral; treatment of Parkinson disease.

amaranth.
Use: Color (Not for internal use).

Amaryl. (Hoechst) Glimepiride 1 mg, 2 mg, 4 mg, lactose. Tab. Bot. 100s, UD 100s (except 1 mg). *Rx.*
Use: Antidiabetic.

Amatine. (Roberts) Midodrine hydrochloride.
Use: Orthostatic hypotension. [Orphan Drug]

ambenonium chloride.
Use: Cholinergic for treatment of myasthenia gravis.
See: Mytelase.

Ambenyl Cough. (Forest) Codeine phosphate 10 mg, bromodiphenhydramine hydrochloride 12.5 mg/5 mL, alcohol 5%. Syr. Bot. 4 oz, Pt, gal. *c-v.*
Use: Antihistamine; antitussive.

Amberlite. (Rohm and Haas) I.R.P.-64. Polacrilin.

Ambien. (Sanofi) Zolpidem tartrate 5 mg, 10 mg. Tab. Bot. 100s, 500s, UD 100s. *c-iv.*
Use: Hypnotic; sedative.

AMBI 1000/55. (AMBI) Dextromethorphan HBr 55 mg, guaifenesin 1000 mg. Dye-free. ER Tab. 100s. *Rx.*
Use: Antitussive with expectorant.

AMBI 60/580. (AMBI) Pseudoephedrine hydrochloride 60 mg, guaifenesin 580 mg. Tab. 100s. *Rx.*
Use: Decongestant, antihistamine.

AMBI 60/580/30. (AMBI) Dextromethorphan HBr 30 mg, guaifenesin 580 mg, pseudoephedrine hydrochloride 60 mg. Dye-free. ER Tab. 100s. *Rx.*
Use: Antitussive, expectorant, decongestant.

AmBisome. (Fujisawa Healthcare) Amphotericin B 50 mg (as liposomal), sucrose. Pow. for Inj. Single-dose Vial w/5-micron filter. *Rx.*
Use: Antifungal.

Ambi 10 Cream. (Kiwi Brands) Benzoyl peroxide 10%, parabens. Cream. Tube 28.3 g. *OTC.*
Use: Antiacne.

Ambi 10 Soap. (Kiwi Brands) Triclosan, sodium tallouate, PEG-20, titanium dioxide. Soap. Bar 99 g. *OTC.*
Use: Antiacne.

●**ambomycin.** (AM-boe-MY-sin) USAN. Isolated from filtrates of *Streptomyces ambofaciens.*
Use: Antineoplastic.

●**ambruticin.** (am-brew-TIE-sin) USAN.
Use: Antifungal.

ambucaine. Ambutoxate hydrochloride.

●**ambuphylline.** (AM-byoo-fill-in) USAN. *Formerly Bufylline.*
Use: Diuretic; muscle relaxant.

●**ambuside.** (AM-buh-SIDE) USAN.
Use: Diuretic.

ambutonium bromide.
Use: Antispasmodic.

AMC. (Schlicksup) Ammonium Cl 7.5 g. Tab. Bot. 1000s. *Rx.*
Use: Diuretic; expectorant.

Amcill. (Parke-Davis) Ampicillin trihydrate. **Cap.:** 250 mg, 500 mg. Bot. 100s, 500s, UD 100s. **Oral Susp.:** 125 mg, 250 mg/5 mL. Bot. 100 mL, 200 mL.
Use: Anti-infective, penicillin.

●**amcinafal.** (am-SIN-ah-fal) USAN.
Use: Anti-inflammatory.

●**amcinafide.** (am-SIN-ah-fide) USAN.
Use: Anti-inflammatory.

●**amcinonide.** (am-SIN-oh-nide) *USP 28.*
Use: Corticosteroid, topical.
See: Cyclocort.

amcinonide. (Taro) **Cream:** Amcinonide 0.1%. 15 g, 30 g, 60 g. **Oint.:** 0.1%. Benzyl alcohol 2.2%, glycerin, white

petrolatum. 15 g, 30 g, 60 g. *Rx.*
Use: Corticosteroid, topical.
Amcort. (Keene Pharmaceuticals) Triamcinolone diacetate 40 mg/mL. Vial 5 mL. *Rx.*
Use: Corticosteroid.
•**amdinocillin.** (am-DEE-no-SILL-in) USAN.
Use: Anti-infective.
•**amdinocillin pivoxil.** (am-DEE-no-SILL-in pihv-OX-ill) USAN.
Use: Anti-infective.
•**amdoxovir.** (am-DOX-oh-veer) USAN.
Use: Antiviral; reverse transcriptase inhibitor.
ameban.
See: Carbarsone.
amebicides.
See: Acetarsone.
Carbarsone.
Chiniofon.
Chloroquine Hydrochloride.
Chloroquine Phosphate.
Emetine Hydrochloride.
Iodoquinol.
Metronidazole.
Paromomycin.
Amechol.
Use: Diagnostic aid.
See: Methacholine Cl.
•**amedalin hydrochloride.** (ah-MEH-dah-lin) USAN.
Use: Antidepressant.
•**ameltolide.** (AH I moll TOE lide) USAN.
Use: Anticonvulsant.
Amerge. (GlaxoSmithKline) Naratriptan hydrochloride 1 mg, 2.5 mg, lactose. Tab. Blister pack 9s. *Rx.*
Use: Antimigraine; serotonin 5-HT$_1$ receptor agonist.
Americaine. (Novartis) Benzocaine 20%. Spray Sol. 60 mL. *OTC.*
Use: Anesthetic, local.
Americaine Anesthetic Lubricant. (Fisons) Benzocaine 20%, benzethonium chloride 0.1%. Gel. Tube 30 g, UD 2.5 g. *Rx.*
Use: Anesthetic, local, topical.
Americaine First Aid Burn. (Novartis) Benzocaine 20%, benzethonium Cl 0.1% in a water-soluble polyethylene glycol base. Oint. Tube 0.75 oz. *OTC.*
Use: Anesthetic, local.
Americaine Hemorrhoidal. (Novartis) Benzocaine 20%. Oint. Tube 22.5 g w/rectal applicator. *OTC.*
Use: Anesthetic, local.
Americet. (MCR American) Acetaminophen 325 mg, caffeine 40 mg, butalbital 50 mg. Tab. 100s. *Rx.*

Use: Nonnarcotic analgesic combination with barbiturates.
Amerifed. (AMBI Pharm) Pseudoephedrine hydrochloride 15 mg/mL, brompheniramine maleate 1 mg/mL, parabens, aspartame, phenylalanine, alcohol free, raspberry flavor. Drops. 30 mL, 473 mL. *Rx.*
Use: Decongestant and antihistamine.
Amerigel. (Amerx Health Care Corp.)
Lot.: Glycerin, lemon oil, parabens, oak extract (Oakin). Bot. 228 g. **Oint.:** Meadowsweet extract, oakbark extract, polyethylene glycol 400, polyethylene glycol 3350, zinc acetate. Tube. 28.3 g. *OTC.*
Use: Diaper rash product.
Amerituss AD. (AMBI Pharm) Dextromethorphan HBr 15 mg, chlorpheniramine maleate 3 mg, phenylephrine hydrochloride 10 mg/5 mL, phenylalanine, aspartame, alcohol free. Liq. 473 mL. *Rx.*
Use: Upper respiratory combination.
Ames Dextro System Lancets. (Bayer Corp. (Consumer Div.)) Sterile disposable lancet. Box 100s.
Use: Diagnostic aid.
•**amesergide.** (am-eh-SIR-jide) USAN.
Use: Serotonin antagonist.
•**ametantrone acetate.** (am-ETT-an-TRONE) USAN.
Use: Antineoplastic.
A-Methapred Univial. (Abbott Hospital Products) Methylprednisolone sodium succinate 40 mg/mL, 500 mg/4 mL, 125 mg/2 mL, 1000 mg/8 mL. Pkg. 1s, 5s (except 40 mg/mL) 25s, 50s, 100s. *Rx.*
Use: Corticosteroid.
amethocaine hydrochloride.
Use: Anesthetic, local.
See: Tetracaine hydrochloride.
amethopterin.
Use: Antineoplastic.
See: Methotrexate.
Amevive. (Biogen) Alefacept 15 mg, sucrose 12.5 mg, preservative free. Pow. for Inj., lyophilized. Dose pack. 1s, 4s. *Rx.*
Use: Immunologic agent, immunosuppressive.
•**amfenac sodium.** (AM-fen-ack SO-dee-uhm) USAN.
Use: Anti-inflammatory.
•**amfilcon a.** (AM-FILL-kahn A) USAN.
Use: Contact lens material, hydrophilic.
•**amflutizole.** (am-FLEW-tih-zole) USAN.
Use: Treatment of gout.

amfodyne.
See: Imidecyl iodine.
•**amfonelic acid.** (am-fah-NEH-lick Acid) USAN.
Use: Central nervous system stimulant.
Amgenal Cough. (Ivax) Bromodiphenhydramine hydrochloride 12.5 mg, codeine phosphate 10 mg/5 mL, alcohol 5%. Syr. Bot. 120 mL, pt, gal. *c-v.*
Use: Antihistamine; antitussive.
amibiarson.
See: Carbarsone.
Amicar. (Xanodyne) **Tab.:** Aminocaproic acid 500 mg, 1,000 mg. Bot. 100s. **Syr.:** Aminocaproic acid 250 mg/mL, parabens, EDTA, sorbitol, saccharin, raspberry flavor. Bot. 473 mL. **Inj.:** Aminocaproic acid 250 mg/mL, benzyl alcohol 0.9%. Vial 20 mL. *Rx.*
Use: Hemostatic, systemic.
•**amicycline.** (AM-ee-SIGH-kleen) USAN.
Use: Anti-infective.
Amidate. (Abbott Hospital Products) Etomidate 2 mg/mL, propylene glycol 35%. Single-dose Amp 20 mg/10 mL, 40 mg/20 mL; Abboject syringe 40 mg/20 mL. *Rx.*
Use: Anesthetic, general.
amide local anesthetics.
See: Articaine Hydrochloride.
  Bupivacaine Hydrochloride.
  Bupivacaine Spinal.
  Bupivacaine Hydrochloride with Epinephrine 1:200,000.
  Carbocaine.
  Carbocaine with Neo-Cobefrin.
  Chirocaine.
  Citanest Forte.
  Citanest Plain.
  Levobupivacaine Hydrochloride.
  Lidocaine and Epinephrine.
  Lidocaine Hydrochloride.
  Lidocaine Hydrochloride and Epinephrine.
  Marcaine.
  Mepivacaine Hydrochloride.
  Mepivacaine Hydrochloride and Levonordefrin.
  Naropin.
  Octocaine.
  Polocaine.
  Polocaine MPF.
  Polocaine with Levonordefrin.
  Prilocaine Hydrochloride.
  Ropivacaine Hydrochloride.
  Sensorcaine.
  Sensorcaine MPF.
  Sensorcaine-MPF Spinal.
  Septocaine.
  Xylocaine.
  Xylocaine MPF.

•**amidephrine mesylate.** (AM-ee-DEH-frin MEH-sih-LATE) USAN.
Use: Adrenergic.
amidofebrin.
See: Aminopyrine.
amidone hydrochloride.
Use: Analgesic; narcotic.
See: Methadone hydrochloride.
amidopyrazoline.
See: Aminopyrine.
amidotrizoate, sodium.
See: Diatrizoate sodium.
•**amifloxacin.** (am-ih-FLOX-ah-SIN) USAN.
Use: Anti-infective.
•**amifloxacin mesylate.** (am-ih-FLOX-ah-SIN MEH-sih-LATE) USAN.
Use: Anti-infective.
•**amifostine.** (am-ih-FOSS-teen) USAN.
Formerly Ethiofos.
Use: Protectant, topical; radioprotector; cytoprotective agent.
See: Ethyol.
Amigen. (Baxter PPI) Protein hydrolysate. **5%, 10%:** Bot. 500 mL, 1000 mL; **5% w/dextrose 5%:** Bot. 500 mL, 1000 mL. **5% w/dextrose 5%, alcohol 5%:** Bot. 1000 mL. **5% w/fructose 10%:** Bot. 1000 mL. **5% w/fructose 12.5%, alcohol 2.4%:** Bot. 1000 mL. *Rx.*
Use: Nutritional supplement.
Amigesic. (Amide) Salsalate 500 mg. Cap or Tab. Salsalate 75 mg. Capl. Bot. 100s, 500s. *Rx.*
Use: Analgesic.
•**amikacin.** (am-ih-KAE-sin) *USP 28.*
Use: Anti-infective.
amikacin. (Bedford) Amikacin sulfate 250 mg, sodium metabisulfite 0.66%, sodium citrate dihydrate 2.5%/mL. Inj. Vial 2 mL, 4 mL. *Rx.*
Use: Anti-infective.
amikacin. (Various Mfr.) Amikacin 50 mg (as sulfate) per mL, sodium metabisulfite 0.13%, sodium citrate dihydrate 0.5%. Inj. Vial 2, 4 mL. 10s. *Rx.*
Use: Anti-infective.
•**amikacin sulfate.** (am-ih-KAE-sin) *USP 28.*
Use: Anti-infective.
amikacin sulfate. (Various Mfr.) Amikacin sulfate 50 mg/mL. Inj. Vial 2 mL, 4 mL (10s).
Use: Anti-infective.
See: Amikin.
Amikin. (Bristol-Myers Squibb) Amikacin sulfate. Inj. Vial 100 mg, 500 mg, 1 g, disposable syringes 500 mg. *Rx.*
Use: Anti-infective; aminoglycoside.

●**amiloride hydrochloride.** (uh-MILL-oh-ride) *USP 28.*
Use: Diuretic.
See: Midamor.
amiloride hydrochloride and hydrochlorothiazide.
Use: Antihypertensive; diuretic.
See: Moduretic.
●**amiloxate.** *USP 28. Formerly isoamyl methoxycinnamate.*
Use: Sunscreen.
●**aminacrine hydrochloride.** (ah-MEE-nah-kreen) USAN.
Use: Anti-infective, topical.
W/Dienestrol, sulfanilamide, allantoin.
See: AVC.
aminarsone.
See: Carbarsone.
Amina-21, (Miller Pharmacal Group)
Free-form amino acids 500 mg. Cap.
Bot. 100s, 300s. *OTC.*
Use: Dermatologic, wound therapy.
amine resin.
See: Polyamine Methylene Resin.
Aminess. (Clintec Nutrition) Essential amino acids. 10 Tab. = adult amino acid MDR. Jar 300s. *Rx.*
Use: Parenteral nutritional supplement
Aminess 5.2%. (Clintec Nutrition) Amino acids and electrolytes. *Rx.*
Use: Nutritional supplement, parenteral.
Aminicotin.
Use: Vitamin supplement.
See: Nicotinamide.
aminoacetic acid.
Use: Myasthenia gravis; irrigant.
See: Glycine.
W/Aluminum hydroxide, magnesium hydroxide, calcium carbonate.
See: Eugel.
W/Calcium carbonate.
See: Antacid pH
Eldamint.
W/Calcium carbonate, aluminum hydroxide, magnesium carbonate.
See: Glytabs.
W/Calcium carbonate, magnesium carbonate, bismuth subcarbonate, dried aluminum hydroxide gel.
See: Buffer-Tabs.
W/Magnesium trisilicate, aluminum hydroxide.
See: Maracid-2.
W/Phenylephrine hydrochloride, chlorpheniramine maleate, acetaminophen, caffeine.
See: Codimal.
amino acid and protein.
See: Aminoacetic Acid.
Glutamic Acid.
Histidine Hydrochloride.

Lysine.
Phenylalanine.
Thyroxine.
amino acid combinations.
See: A/G-Pro.
Amina-21.
Body Fortress Natural Amino.
Dequasine.
EMF.
Jets.
NeuRecover-DA.
NeuRecover-SA.
NeuroSlim.
PDP Liquid Protein.
PowerMate.
PowerSleep.
amino acid derivatives.
See: Carnitor.
L-Carnitine.
Levocarnitine.
amino acids.
Use: Amino acid supplement.
See: Aminosyn.
W/Estrone, testosterone, vitamins, minerals.
See: Stuart Amino Acids and B$_{12}$.
aminoacridine. (ah-MEE-no-ACK-rih-deen)
See: Aminacrine hydrochloride.
9-aminoacridine hydrochloride.
(Various Mfr.) Aminacrine hydrochloride.
Use: Anti-infective, vaginal.
See: Vagisec Plus.
W/Hydrocortisone acetate, tyrothricin, phenylmercuric acetate, polysorbate 80, urea, lactose.
See: Aquacort.
W/Phenylmercuric acetate, tyrothricin, urea, lactose.
See: Trinalis.
W/Polyoxyethylene nonyl phenol, sodium edetate, docusate sodium.
See: Vagisec Plus.
W/Pramoxine hydrochloride, acetic acid, parachlorometa-xylenol, methyl-dodecylbenzyltrimethyl ammonium Cl.
See: Drotic No. 2.
W/Sulfanilamide, allantoin.
See: AVC.
Nil Vaginal.
Par.
Vagisan.
p-aminobenzene-sulfonylacetylimide.
See: Sulfacetamide.
●**aminobenzoate potassium.** (ah-MEE-no-BEN-zoe-ate) *USP 28.*
Use: Analgesic, nutritional supplement.
See: Potaba.
W/Hydrocortisone, ammonium salicylate, ascorbic acid.

See: Neocylate Sodium Free.
W/Potassium salicylate.
See: Pabalate-SF.
aminobenzoate potassium. (Hope Pharm) Aminobenzoate potassium 500 mg. Cap. 250s. *Rx.*
Use: Nutritional supplement.
•**aminobenzoate sodium.** (ah-MEE-no-BEN-zoe-ate) *USP 28.*
Use: Analgesic.
See: PABA Sodium.
W/Phenobarbital, colchicine salicylate, Vitamin B₁, aspirin.
See: Doloral.
W/Salicylamide, sodium salicylate, ascorbic acid, butabarbital sodium.
See: Bisalate.
W/Sodium salicylate.
See: Pabalate.
•**aminobenzoic acid.** *USP 28. Formerly Para-aminobenzoic acid.*
Use: Ultraviolet screen.
See: Pabanol.
W/Mephenesin, salicylamide.
See: Sal-Phenesin.
•**aminocaproic acid.** (uh-mee-no-kuh-PRO-ik) *USP 28.*
Use: Hemostatic.
See: Amicar.
aminocaproic acid. (Orphan Medical)
Use: Topical treatment of traumatic hyphema of the eye.
aminocaproic acid. (Various Mfr.) Aminocaproic acid 250 mg/mL. Inj. Vial 20 mL. *Rx.*
Use: Antifibrinolytic; hemostatic, systemic.
aminocaproic acid. (VersaPharm) Aminocaproic acid. **Oral Soln.:** 250 mg/mL, saccharin, sorbitol, parabens, raspberry flavor. Bot. 237 mL, 473 mL. **Tab.:** 500 mg. 100s. *Rx.*
Use: Hemostatic.
aminocardol.
Use: Bronchodilator.
See: Aminophylline.
Amino-Cerv pH 5.5. (Milex) Urea 8.34%, sodium propionate 0.5%, methionine 0.83%, cystine 0.35%, inositol 0.83%, benzalkonium Cl, water miscible base. Tube with applicator 82.5 g. *Rx.*
Use: Vaginal agent.
2-aminoethanethiol.
Use: Urinary tract agent.
amino-ethyl-propanol.
See: Aminoisobutanol.
W/Bromotheophyllin.
See: Pamabrom.
Aminofen. (Dover Pharmaceuticals) Acetaminophen 325 mg. Sugar, lactose,

and salt free. Tab. UD Box 500s. *OTC.*
Use: Analgesic.
Aminofen Max. (Dover Pharmaceuticals) Acetaminophen 500 mg. Sugar, lactose, and salt free. Tab. UD Box 500s. *OTC.*
Use: Analgesic.
aminoform.
Use: Anti-infective, urinary.
See: Methenamine.
Aminogen. (Christina) Vitamin B complex, folic acid. Amp. 2 mL Box 12s, 24s, 100s. Vial 10 mL. *Rx.*
Use: Vitamin supplement.
•**aminoglutethimide.** (ah-MEE-no-glue-TETH-ih-mide) *USP 28.*
Use: Treatment of Cushing syndrome; adrenocortical suppressant; antineoplastic.
See: Cytadren.
aminohippurate sodium. (Merck & Co.) Aminohippurate sodium 0.2 g/10 mL. Amp 10 mL, 50 mL.
Use: IV diagnostic aid for renal plasma flow and function determination.
•**aminohippurate sodium injection.** (ah-MEE-no-HIP-your-ate) *USP 28.*
Use: Diagnostic aid, renal function determination.
•**aminohippuric acid.** (ah-MEE-no-hip-YOUR-ik) *USP 28.*
Use: Component of aminohippurate sodium (Inj.); diagnostic aid, renal function determination.
aminoisobutanol.
See: Butaphyllamine.
Pamabrom for combinations.
aminoisometradine.
See: Methionine.
•**aminolevulinic acid hydrochloride.** (ah-MEE-no-lev-you-LIN-ik ASS-id HIGH-droe-KLOR-ide) USAN.
Use: Antineoplastic.
See: Levulan Kerastick.
Amino-Min-D. (Tyson) Ca 250 mg, D 100 units, Fe 7.5 mg , Zn 5.6 mg, Mg, I, Mn, Cu, K, Cr, Se, betaine hydrochloride, glutamic acid hydrochloride. Cap. Bot. 100s. *OTC.*
Use: Mineral, vitamin supplement.
Aminonat. Protein hydrolysates (oral).
aminonitrozole.
Use: Antitrichomonal.
Amino-Opti-C. (Tyson) Vitamin C 1000 mg, lemon bioflavonoids 250 mg, rutin, hesperidin, rose hips powder, dicalcium phosphate, hydrogenated soybean oil. SR Tab. Bot. 100s. *OTC.*
Use: Vitamin supplement.

aminopenicillins.
Use: Anti-infective.
See: Amoxicillin.
Amoxicillin and Clavulanate Potassium.
Ampicillin.
Ampicillin Sodium and Sulbactam Sodium.
•**aminopentamide sulfate.** *USP 28.*
Use: Anticholinergic.
•**aminophylline.** (am-in-AHF-ih-lin)
USP 28. Formerly Theophylline ethylenediamine.
Use: Muscle relaxant.
W/Combinations.
See: Amesec.
Amphedrine Compound.
Asminorel.
Mudrane GG-2.
Orthoxine and Aminophylline.
Quinamm.
Quinite.
Ctroma.
aminophylline injection. (Abbott)
Aminophylline. Amp. 250 mg/10 mL,
500 mg/20 mL; Flip top vial 10 mg/
20 mL, 20 mg/50 mL.
Use: Bronchodilator.
aminophylline injection. (Various Mfr.)
Theophylline ethylenediamine 3 ¾ g,
7.5 g. Inj. Amp.
Use: Muscle relaxant.
aminophylline suppositories. (Various
Mfr.) Aminophylline 3⅜ g, 7.5 g. Supp.
Box.
Use: Muscle relaxant.
aminophylline tablets. (Various Mfr.)
Aminophylline 1.5 g, 3 g. Tab. Plain or
enteric coated. Bot.
Use: Muscle relaxant.
**aminophylline with phenobarbital
combinations.**
See: Amodrine.
Mudrane.
Mudrane GG.
Aminophyllin Injection. (Pharmacia)
Trademark for Aminophylline. Amp.
250 mg: 10 mL; 25s, 100s. **500 mg:**
20 mL; 25s, 100s. *Rx.*
Use: Bronchodilator.
Aminophyllin Tablets. (Pharmacia)
Trademark for Aminophylline. 100 mg,
200 mg. Tab. Bot. 100s, 1000s, UD
100s. *Rx.*
Use: Bronchodilator.
Aminoprel. (Taylor Pharmaceuticals) L-
lysine 60 mg, dl-methionine 15 mg, hydrolyzed protein 750 mg, iron 2 mg,
Cu, I, K, Mg, Mn, Zn. Cap. Bot. 180s.
Use: Nutritional supplement.
aminopromazine. (I.N.N.) Proquamezine.

4-aminopyridine.
Use: Relief of symptoms of multiple
sclerosis. [Orphan Drug]
aminopyrine.
Use: Antipyretic; analgesic.
See: Dipyrone.
4-aminoquinoline derivatives.
Use: Antimalarial.
See: Aralen hydrochloride.
Chloroquine Phosphate.
Plaquenil Sulfate.
8-aminoquinoline derivatives.
Use: Antimalarial.
See: Primaquine Phosphate.
Primaquine Phosphate.
•**aminorex.** (am-EE-no-rex) USAN.
Use: Anorexic.
aminosalicylate calcium. (Dumas-
Wilson) Aminosalicylate calcium 7.5 g.
Bot. 1000s.
Use: Tuberculosis therapy.
aminosalicylate potassium. Monopotassium 4-aminosalicylate.
Use: Antibacterial; tuberculostatic.
•**aminosalicylate sodium.** (uh-MEE-no-
suh-LIS-ih-LATE) *USP 28.*
Use: Anti-infective; tuberculostatic.
•**aminosalicylic acid.** (ah-MEE-no-sal-ih-
SILL-ik) *USP 28.*
Use: Anti-infective; tuberculostatic.
See: Paser.
4-aminosalicylic acid.
Use: Treatment of ulcerative colitis in
patients intolerant to sulfasalazine.
[Orphan Drug]
5-aminosalicylic acid.
See: Mesalamine.
p-aminosalicylic acid salts.
See: Aminosalicylate Calcium.
Aminosalicylate Potassium.
Aminosalicylate Sodium.
aminosidine.
Use: Mycobacterium avium complex;
tuberculosis; visceral leishmaniasism
(KALA-AZAR). [Orphan Drug]
See: Gabbromicina.
Paromomycin.
Aminosyn. (Abbott) Crystalline amino
acid solution. **3.5%:** 1000 mL; **5%:** Container 250 mL, 500 mL, 1000 mL; **7%:**
500 mL; 7% kit (cs/3); **8.5%:** Single-
dose container 500 mL, 1000 mL. **10%:**
500 mL, 1000 mL. W/Electrolytes. **7%:**
500 mL. **8.5%:** 500 mL. *Rx.*
Use: Nutritional supplement, parenteral.
Aminosyn-HBC 7%. (Abbott) Crystalline
amino acid infusion for high metabolic
stress. 500 mL, 1000 mL. *Rx.*
Use: Nutritional supplement, parenteral.

Aminosyn II. (Abbott) Crystalline amino acid infusion. **3.5%, 5%, 3.5% in 5% dextrose:** 1000 mL. **7%:** 500 mL. **8.5%, 10%:** 500 mL, 1000 mL. **W/Dextrose:** 3.5% in 25% dextrose, 5% in 25% dextrose: 1000 mL. **W/Dextrose and electrolytes:** 3.5% in 5% dextrose, 3.5% in 25% dextrose, 4.25% in 10% dextrose, 4.25% in 25% dextrose: 1000 mL. **W/Electrolytes:** 7%, 8.5%, 10%: 1000 mL. *Rx.*
Use: Nutritional supplement, parenteral.

Aminosyn II M. (Abbott) Crystalline amino acid infusion with maintenance electrolytes, 10% dextrose. Soln. 1000 mL. *Rx.*
Use: Nutritional supplement, parenteral.

Aminosyn M 3.5%. (Abbott) Crystalline amino acid infusion with electrolytes. 1000 mL. *Rx.*
Use: Nutritional supplement, parenteral.

Aminosyn-PF. (Abbott) Crystalline amino acid infusions for pediatric use. **7%:** 250 mL, 500 mL; **10%:** 1000 mL. *Rx.*
Use: Nutritional supplement, parenteral.

Aminosyn-RF. (Abbott) Crystalline amino acid infusion for renal failure patients. 5.2%. 300 mL. *Rx.*
Use: Nutritional supplement, parenteral.

Amino-Thiol. (Marcen) Sulfur 10 mg, casein 50 mg, sodium citrate 5 mg, phenol 5 mg, benzyl alcohol 5 mg/mL. Vial 10 mL, 30 mL. *Rx.*
Use: Treatment of arthritis; neuritis.

aminotrate phosphate. Trolnitratephosphate.
See: Triethanolamine.

Aminoxin. (Tyson & Assoc.) Pyridoxal-5′-phosphate 20 mg. EC Tab. Bot. 100s. *OTC.*
Use: Vitamin supplement.

aminoxytropine tropate hydrochloride. Atropine-N-oxide hydrochloride.

Amio-Aqueous. (Academic Pharmaceuticals) Amiodarone.
Use: Antiarrhythmic. [Orphan Drug]

• **amiodarone.** (A-MEE-oh-duh-rone) USAN.
Use: Cardiovascular agent; antiarrhythmic; ventricular.

amiodarone hydrochloride. (Various Mfr.) Amiodarone hydrochloride. **Inj.:** 50 mg/mL, may contain benzyl alcohol. 3 mL vials and amps. **Tab.:** 200 mg. Bot. 60s, 100s, 250s, 500s, UD 100s. *Rx.*
Use: Antiarrhythmic.
See: Amio-Aqueous.
  Cordarone.
  Pacerone.

Amipaque. (Sanofi-Synthelabo) Metrizamide 18.75%/20 mL Vial.
Use: Radiopaque agent.

• **amiprilose hydrochloride.** (ah-MIH-prih-LOHS) USAN.
Use: Anti-infective; antifungal; anti-inflammatory; antineoplastic; antiviral; immunomodulator.

• **amiquinsin hydrochloride.** (AM-ih-KWIN-sin) USAN. Under study.
Use: Antihypertensive.

Amitin. (Thurston) Vitamin C 200 mg, lemon bioflavonoid 100 mg, niacinamide 60 mg, methionine 100 mg. Tab. Bot. 100s, 500s. *Rx.*
Use: Vitamin supplement.

• **amitraz.** (AM-ih-trazz) *USP 28.*
Use: Scabicide.

• **amitriptyline hydrochloride.** (am-ee-TRIP-tih-leen) *USP 28.*
Use: Antidepressant.
See: Emitrip.
  Endep.
W/Chlordiazepoxide.
  See: Limbitrol.
W/Perphenazine.
  See: Etrafon.

amitriptyline hydrochloride. (Various Mfr.) Amitriptyline hydrochloride 10 mg, 25 mg, 50 mg, 75 mg, 100 mg, 150 mg. Tab. Bot. 100s, 500s (75 mg and 100 mg only), 1000s, UD 100s, blister pack 25s (25 mg and 50 mg), 100s, 600s (except 75 mg). *Rx.*
Use: Antidepressant.

AmLactin. (Upsher-Smith) Ammonium lactate 12%, parabens, light mineral oil. Cream, Lot. 140 g, 225 g, 400 g. *OTC.*
Use: Emollient.

AmLactin AP. (Upsher-Smith) Pramoxine hydrochloride 1%, lactic acid 12%, light mineral oil, cetyl alcohol, glycerin, parabens. Cream. 140 g. *OTC.*
Use: Local anesthetic, topical.

• **amlexanox.** (am-LEX-an-ox) USAN.
Use: Mouth and throat product.
See: Aphthasol.

• **amlintide.** (AM-lin-tide) USAN.
Use: Treatment of type I diabetes mellitus; antidiabetic.

amlodipine. (am-LOW-dih-PEEN)
Use: Calcium channel blocker.
See: Amvaz.
  Norvasc.

amlodipine and atorvastatin.
Use: Antihyperlipidemic.
See: Caduet.

amlodipine and benazepril hydrochloride. (am-LOW-dih-PEEN and BEN-AZE-eh-prill)
See: Lotrel.

•**amlodipine besylate.** (am-LOW-dih-PEEN) USAN.
Use: Antianginal; antihypertensive.
See: Norvasc.

amlodipine besylate/atorvastatin calcium.
Use: Antihyperlipidemic combination.
See: Caduet.

•**amlodipine maleate.** (am-LOW-dih-PEEN) USAN.
Use: Antianginal; antihypertensive.

Ammens Medicated. (Bristol-Myers Squibb) Boric acid 4.55%, zinc oxide 9.10%, talc, starch. Pow. Can 6.25 oz, 11 oz. *OTC.*
Use: Dermatologic; protectant.

ammoidin. Methoxsalen.
Use: Psoralen.

•**ammonia N 13 injection.** (uh MOE-nee-ah N13) USP 28.
Use: Diagnostic aid, cardiac imaging, liver imaging; radiopharmaceutical.

•**ammonia solution, strong.** (ah-MOE-nee-ah) NF 23.
Use: Pharmaceutic aid, solvent; source of ammonia.

•**ammonia spirit, aromatic.** (ah-MOE-nee-ah) USP 28.
Use: Respiratory.

•**ammonio methacrylate copolymer.** (ah-MOE-nee-oh meth-ah-KRILL-ate koe-PAHL-ih-mer) NF 23.
Use: Pharmaceutic aid, coating agent.

ammonium benzoate.
Use: Antiseptic, urinary.

ammonium biphosphate, sodium biphosphate, and sodium acid pyrophosphate.
Use: Genitourinary.

•**ammonium carbonate.** (ah-MOE-nee-uhm) NF 23
Use: Pharmaceutic aid, source of ammonia.

•**ammonium chloride.** (ah-MOE-nee-uhm) USP 28.
Use: Acidifier; diuretic.

ammonium chloride. (Various Mfr.) **Delayed Release Tab.:** Plain or E.C. 5 g, 7.5 g. (Bayer Corp. (Consumer Div.)). **Inj.:** 120 mEq/30 mL. Vial.
Use: Acidifier; diuretic; expectorant; alkalosis.

ammonium chloride. (Eli Lilly) Ammonium Cl. 7.5 g. Tab. Enseal Bot. 100s. *Rx.*
Use: Acidifier, urinary.

ammonium chloride. (Hospira) Ammonium chloride 26.75% (5 mEq/mL). To be diluted before infusion. Inj. Vials. 20 mL (100 mEq) with EDTA 2 mg. *Rx.*

Use: Intravenous nutritional therapy.

•**ammonium lactate.** (ah-MOE-nee-uhm LACK-tate) USAN.
Use: Antipruritic, topical.
See: AmLactin.
Lac-Hydrin.
LAC-Lotion.

ammonium lactate. (Glades) Ammonium lactate (equiv. to 12% lactic acid), cetyl alcohol, glycerin, glyceryl stearate, light mineral oil, parabens. Lot. 225 g, 400 g. *Rx.*
Use: Emollient.

ammonium mandelate. Ammonium salt of mandelic acid 8 g/fl oz. Syr. Bot. Pt, gal.
Use: Urinary antiseptic, oral.

•**ammonium molybdate.** (ah-MOE-nee-uhm) USP 28.

ammonium nitrate.
See: Reditemp-C.

•**ammonium phosphate.** (ah-MOE-nee-uhm) NF 23. Phosphoric acid diammonium salt. Diammonium phosphate.
Use: Pharmaceutic aid.

•**ammonium sulfate.** (ah-MOE-nee-uhm) USAN.
Use: Pharmaceutic aid.

ammonium tetrathiomolybdate.
Use: Treatment of Wilson disease. [Orphan Drug]

ammonium valerate.
Use: Sedative.

ammophyllin.
Use: Bronchodilator.
See: Aminophylline.

Amnesteem. (Bertek) Isotretinoin 10 mg, 20 mg, 40 mg. Cap. 30s, 100s. *Rx.*
Use: Retinoid.

•**amobarbital sodium.** (am-oh-BAR-bih-tahl) USP 28.
Use: Hypnotic; sedative.

amobarbital sodium. (Various Mfr.) **Cap. 1 g:** Bot. 100s, 500s; **3 g:** Bot. 100s, 500s, 1000s. (Various Mfr.) **Tab. 30 mg:** Bot. 100s; **50 mg:** Bot. 100s. **100 mg:** Bot. 100s. (Eli Lilly and Co.) Vial 250 mg, 500 mg. (Eli Lilly and Co.).
Use: Sedative; hypnotic.
W/Ephedrine hydrochloride, theophylline, chlorpheniramine maleate.
See: Amytal.
Theo-Span.
W/Secobarbital sodium.
See: Dusotal.
Tuinal.

Amoclan. (West-ward) Amoxicillin/clavulanic acid (as potassium salt) 200 mg/28.5 mg (potassium 0.143 mEq per 5 mL), 400 mg/57 mg (potassium

0.286 mEq per 5 mL) (after reconstitution) per 5 mL. Phenylalanine 7 mg, aspartame. Orange flavor. Pow. for Oral Susp. 50 mL, 75 mL, 100 mL. *Rx.*
Use: Penicillin.

•**amodiaquine.** (am-oh-DIE-ah-kwin) *USP 28.*
Use: Antiprotozoal.

•**amodiaquine hydrochloride.** (am-oh-DIE-ah-kwin) *USP 28.*
Use: Antimalarial.

Amodopa. (Major) Methyldopa 125 mg, 250 mg, 500 mg. Bot. 100s, 500s, (500 mg only), 1000s (250 mg only), UD 100s. *Rx.*
Use: Antihypertensive.

AMO Endosol. (Allergan) Sodium chloride 0.64%, potassium chloride 0.075%, calcium chloride dihydrate 0.048%, magnesium chloride hexahydrate 0.03%, sodium acetate trihydrate 0.39%, sodium citrate dihydrate 0.17%. Preservative free. Soln. Bot. 18 mL, 500 mL. *Rx.*
Use: Physiological irrigating solution.

AMO Endosol Extra. (Allergan) **Part I:** Water for injection with sodium chloride 7.14 mg, potassium chloride 0.38 mg, calcium chloride dihydrate 0.154 mg, magnesium chloride hexahydrate 0.2 mg, dextrose 0.92 mg, sodium hydroxide or hydrochloric acid/mL. Soln. Bot. 515 mL. **Part II:** Sodium bicarbonate 1081 mg, dibasic sodium phosphate anhydrous 216 mg, glutathione disulfide 95 mg. Soln. Bot. 60 mL. *Rx.*
Use: Ophthalmic irrigation solution.

Amol. (Mono-n-amyl-hydroquinone ether.)
See: B-F-I.

Amoline. (Major) Aminophylline 100 mg, 200 mg. Tab. Bot. 100s, 1000s, UD 100s. *Rx-OTC.*
Use: Bronchodilator.

amopyroquin hydrochloride.
See: Propoquin.

•**amorolfine.** (am-OH-role-feen) USAN.
Use: Antimycotic.

Amosan. (Oral-B) Sodium perborate, saccharin. Single-dose packet box. 1.76 g. 20s, 40s. *OTC.*
Use: Mouth and throat preparation.

•**amotosalen hydrochloride.** (a-moe-TOE-sa-len) USAN.
Use: Photochemical treatment for plasma.

Amotriphene. *Rx.*
Use: Coronary vasodilator.

AMO Vitrax. (Allergan) Sodium hyaluronate 30 mg/mL. Inj. Disp. syringe 0.65 mL. *Rx.*
Use: Viscoelastic, ophthalmic.

•**amoxapine.** (am-OX-uh-peen) *USP 28.*
Use: Antidepressant.
See: Asendin.

amoxapine. (Various Mfr.) Amoxapine 25 mg, 50 mg, 100 mg, 150 mg. Tab. Bot. 30s, 100s, 500s (50 mg only), 1000s, blister pack 100s (25 mg and 50 mg only). *Rx.*
Use: Antidepressant.

•**amoxicillin.** (a-MOX-ih-sil-in) *USP 28.*
Use: Anti-infective.
See: Amoxil.
  DisperMox.
  Trimox.

amoxicillin. (Ranbaxy) Amoxicillin. **Chew. Tab.:** 200 mg, 400 mg. Bot. 20s, 100s (400 mg only). **Pow. for Oral Susp.:** 200 mg/5 mL, 400 mg/5 mL, fruit flavor. 50 mL, 75 mL, 100 mL. *Rx.*
Use: Anti-infective.

amoxicillin and clavulanate potassium. (a-MOX-ih-sil-in and CLAV-you-lon-ate poe-TASS-ee-uhm)
Use: Anti-infective; penicillin.
See: Amoclan.
  Augmentin.

amoxicillin, clavulanate potassium. (Geneva) **Chew. Tab.:** Amoxicillin trihydrate 200 mg/clavulanic acid 28.5 mg, amoxicillin trihydrate 400 mg/clavulanic acid 57 mg. Bot. UD 20s. **Pow. for Oral Susp.:** Amoxicillin trihydrate 200 mg/clavulanic acid 28.5 mg, amoxicillin trihydrate 400 mg/clavulanic acid 57 mg. Vial. 100 mL. *Rx.*
Use: Anti-infective, penicillin.

amoxicillin, clavulanate potassium. (Various Mfr.) **Pow. for Oral Susp.:** Amoxicillin trihydrate 600 mg/clavulanic acid (as the potassium salt) 42.9 mg per 5 mL. Potassium 0.23 mEq per 5 mL. May contain aspartame or saccharin. 75 mL, 125 mL, 200 mL. **Tab.:** Amoxicillin trihydrate 500 mg/clavulanic acid 125 mg, amoxicillin trihydrate 875 mg/clavulanic acid 125 mg. Bot. 20s. *Rx.*
Use: Anti-infective, penicillin.

amoxicillin intramammary infusion.
Use: Anti-infective; penicillin.

•**amoxicillin sodium.** USAN.
Use: Antibiotic.

amoxicillin trihydrate. (Various Mfr.) Amoxicillin trihydrate. **Chew. Tab.:** 125 mg, 250 mg. Bot. 100s, 250s (250 mg only), 500s (250 mg only).

Tab.: 500 mg, 875 mg. Bot. 20s, 100s, 500s (875 mg only). **Cap.:** 250 mg, 500 mg. Bot. 50s (500 mg only), 100s, 500s, 1000s (250 mg only). **Pow. for Oral Susp.:** 125 mg/5 mL, 250 mg/mL when reconstituted. Bot. 80 mL, 100 mL, 150 mL. *Rx.*
Use: Anti-infective; penicillin.

Amoxil. (GlaxoSmithKline) Amoxicillin trihydrate. **Chew. Tab.:** 200 mg (phenylalanine 1.82 mg), 400 mg (phenylalanine 3.64 mg), aspartame, cherry-banana-peppermint flavor. Bot. 20s, 100s. **Cap.:** 500 mg. Bot. 500s. **Pow. for Oral Susp.:** 125 mg/5 mL, 200 mg/5 mL, 250 mg/5 mL, 400 mg/5 mL, sucrose, bubble gum flavor, strawberry flavor (125 mg). Bot. 50 mL (200 mg, 400 mg only), 75 ml (200 mg, 400 mg only), 80 mL (125 mg only), 100 mL (except 125 mg), 150 mL (125 mg, 250 mg only). **Tab.:** 500 mg, 875 mg. Bot. 20s, 100s, 500s. *Rx.*
Use: Anti-infective; penicillin.

Amoxil Pediatric Drops. (GlaxoSmith-Kline) Amoxicillin trihydrate 50 mg/mL when reconstituted, sucrose, bubble-gum flavor. Drops. Bot. 15 mL, 30 mL. *Rx.*
Use: Anti-infective; penicillin.

AMP. Adenosine Phosphate, USAN.
Use: Nutrient.

d-AMP. (Oxypure) Ampicillin trihydrate 500 mg. Cap. Bot. 100s. *Rx.*
Use: Anti-infective; penicillin.

amperil. (Armenpharm Ltd.) Ampicillin trihydrate 250 mg or 500 mg. Cap. Bot. 100s, 500s. *Rx.*
Use: Anti-infective; penicillin.

• **amphecloral.** (AM-feh-klahr-ahl) USAN.
Use: Sympathomimetic; anorexic.

amphenidone.
Use: CNS stimulant.

amphetamine aspartate combinations.
See: Adderall.
Adderall XR.
Amphetamine Salt Combo.

amphetamine hydrochloride. (am-FET-uh-meen) (Various Mfr.) Amphetamine hydrochloride 20 mg/mL, 1 mL. Amp. *Rx.*
Use: Vasoconstrictor; CNS stimulant.

amphetamine, levo.
Use: CNS stimulant.

amphetamine phosphate.
Use: CNS stimulant.

amphetamine phosphate, dextro.
(Various Mfr.) Dextroamphetamine phosphate. Tab.
Use: CNS stimulant.

amphetamine phosphate, dibasic.
(Various Mfr.) Racemic amphetamine phosphate 5 mg, 10 mg. Cap. or Tab. Bot. *Rx.*
Use: CNS stimulant.

amphetamines.
See: Desoxyephedrine.
Dextroamphetamine Sulfate.
Methamphetamine Hydrochloride.

amphetamine salt combo. (Barr) Amphetamine mixtures 5 mg, 10 mg, 20 mg, 30 mg (1.25 mg, 2.5 mg, 5 mg, 7.5 mg each of dextroamphetamine sulfate, dextroamphetamine saccharate, amphetamine aspartate, amphetamine sulfate). Tab. Bot. 50s, 100s, 500s. *c-II.*
Use: CNS stimulant, amphetamine.

• **amphetamine sulfate.** *USP 28.*
Use: CNS stimulant.

amphetamine sulfate. (Various Mfr.) Amphetamine sulfate 5 mg, 10 mg. Cap. Tab. Bot. Inj. 20 mg/mL. Vial.
Use: CNS stimulant.

amphetamine sulfate combinations.
See: Adderall.
Adderall XR.
Amphetamine Salt Combo.

amphetamine sulfate, dextro.
Use: CNS stimulant.
See: Dextroamphetamine Sulfate.

amphetamine with dextroamphetamine as resin complexes.
Use: Appetite depressant.

Amphidase. (Amphastar) Hyaluronidase (bovine source) 150 units/mL. Contains no more than 0.1 mg thimerosal. Soln. for Inj. Vials. 2 mL. *Rx.*
Use: Physical adjunct.

Amphocaps. (Halsey Drug) Ampicillin 250 mg, 500 mg. Cap. Bot. 100s. *Rx.*
Use: Anti-infective; penicillin.

Amphocin. (Gensia Sicor) Amphotericin B desoxylate 50 mg. Pow. for Inj. Vial. *Rx.*
Use: Antifungal.

Amphojel. (Wyeth) Aluminum hydroxide gel. 300 mg, 600 mg. Tab. Bot. 100s. *OTC.*
Use: Antacid.

• **amphomycin.** (AM-foe-MY-sin) USAN. An antibiotic produced by *Streptomyces canus.*
Use: Anti-infective.

Amphotec. (Sequus) Amphotericin B (as cholesteryl) 50 mg, 100 mg. Pow. for Inj. Single-use Vial 20 mL (50 mg), 50 mL (100 mg). *Rx.*
Use: Antifungal.

amphotericin. (am-foe-TER-ih-sin)
Use: Antifungal.

See: Fungizone.
- **amphotericin b.** (am-foe-TER-ih-sin B) *USP 28.*
Use: Antifungal.
See: Abelcet.
    Amphotec.
    Fungizone.
amphotericin b. (Pharma-Tek) Amphotericin B 50 mg as desoxycholate. Pow. for Inj. Vial. *Rx.*
Use: Antifungal.
amphotericin b desoxycholate.
Use: Antifungal.
See: Amphocin.
    Fungizone Intravenous.
amphotericin b, lipid-based.
Use: Antifungal.
See: Abelcet.
    AmBisome.
    Amphotec.
amphotericin b lipid complex.
Use: Invasive fungal infections. [Orphan Drug]
See: Abelcet.
- **ampicillin.** (am-pih-SILL-in) *USP 28.*
Use: Anti-infective.
See: Principen.
ampicillin and sulbactam. (ESI Lederle) Ampicillin sodium 1 g/sulbactam sodium 0.5 g, ampicillin sodium 2 g/sulbactam sodium 1 g. Pow. for Inj. Vials. *Rx.*
Use: Anti-infective, penicillin.
- **ampicillin sodium.** (am-pih-SILL-in) *USP 28.*
Use: Anti-infective.
See: Omnipen-N.
ampicillin sodium. (Various Mfr.) Ampicillin sodium 250 mg, 500 mg, 1 g, 2 g, sodium 2.9 mEq/g. Pow. for Inj. Vials. *Rx.*
Use: Anti-infective.
- **ampicillin sodium and sulbactam sodium.** (am-pih-SILL-in and sull-BAK-tam) *NF 23.*
Use: Anti-infective; penicillin.
See: Unasyn.
ampicillin trihydrate. (Various Mfr.) Ampicillin (as trihydrate) 250 mg, 500 mg. Cap. Bot. 100s, 500s. *Rx.*
Use: Anti-infective; penicillin.
Amplicor. (Roche) Kits 10s, 96s, 100s. *Rx.*
Use: Diagnostic aid, chlamydia.
Amplicor HIV-1 Monitor. (Roche) Reagent kit for plasma HIV-1 tests. Kit. 24 tests.
Use: Diagnostic aid.
Ampligen. (HEM Research) Poly I: Poly C12U. Phase II/III HIV.

Use: Immunomodulator.
amprenavir.
Use: Antiviral.
See: Agenerase.
- **ampyzine sulfate.** (AM-pih-zeen) USAN.
Use: Central nervous system stimulant.
- **amquinate.** (am-KWIN-ate) USAN.
Use: Antimalarial.
- **amrinone.** (AM-rih-nohn) *USP 28.*
Use: Cardiovascular agent.
See: Inocor.
- **amsacrine.** (AM-sah-KREEN) USAN.
Use: Investigational antineoplastic.
    [Orphan Drug]
Amvaz. (Reddy) Amlodipine 2.5 mg, 5 mg, 10 mg. Tab. 90s, 500s, UD 7s (except 2.5 mg). *Rx.*
Use: Calcium channel blocker.
Amvisc. (Bausch & Lomb) Sodium hyaluronate 12 mg/mL. Inj. Disp. syringe 0.5 mL, 0.8 mL. *Rx.*
Use: Viscoelastic.
Amvisc Plus. (Bausch & Lomb) Sodium hyaluronate 16 mg/mL. Inj. Disp. syringe 0.5 mL, 0.8 mL. *Rx.*
Use: Viscoelastic.
Am-Wax. (AmLab) Urea, benzocaine, propylene glycol, glycerin. Bot. 10 mL. *OTC.*
Use: Otic.
amyl. Phenyl phenol, phenyl mercuric nitrate.
See: Lubraseptic.
amylase.
W/Calcium carbonate, glycine, belladonna extract.
See: Trialka.
W/Lipase, protease.
See: Kutrase.
    Ku-Zyme.
    Lipram.
    Palcaps 10.
    Palcaps 20.
    Pancrelipase.
    Panocaps.
    Panocaps MT 16.
    Panocaps MT 20.
    PAN-2400.
    Ultrase.
    Ultrase MT 18.
    Viokase.
W/Pancreatin, protease, lipase.
See: Dizymes.
W/Pepsin, homatropine methyl bromide, lipase, protease, bile salts.
See: Gourmase.
- **amylene hydrate.** (AM-ih-leen HIGH-drate) *NF 23.*
Use: Pharmaceutic aid, solvent.

amylin analog.
Use: Antidiabetic agent.
See: Pramlintide Acetate.
•**amyl nitrite.** (A-mill NYE-trite) *USP 28.*
Use: Vasodilator.
W/Sodium nitrite, sodium thiosulfate.
See: Cyanide Antidote Pkg.
amyl nitrite. Isoamyl nitrite. Isopentylnitrite. (GlaxoSmithKline). Vaporole 0.18 mL or 0.3 mL. Box 12s. (Eli Lilly and Co.). Aspirols 0.3 mL. Box 12s.
Use: Inhalation, coronary vasodilator in angina pectoris.
amylolytic enzyme.
W/Butabarbital sodium, belladonna extract, cellulolytic enzyme, proteolytic enzyme, lipolytic enzyme, iron ox bile.
See: Butibel-Zyme.
W/Calcium carbonate, glycine, proteolytic and cellulolytic enzymes.
See: Converspaz.
W/Lipase, proteolytic, cellulolytic enzymes, phenobarbital, hyoscyamine sulfate, atropine sulfate.
See: Arco-Lipase Plus.
W/Proteolytic, cellulolytic, lipolytic enzymes.
See: Arco-Lase.
W/Proteolytic, cellulolytic, lipolytic enzymes, iron, ox bile.
See: Ku-Zyme.
Amytal Sodium. (Eli Lilly) Amobarbital sodium. 250 mg, 500 mg. Pow. for Inj. Vial. *c-II.*
Use: Hypnotic, sedative.
Ana. (Wampole) Antinuclear antibodies test by IFA. Test 54s.
Use: Diagnostic aid.
Ana-Guard. (Bayer Corp. (Consumer Div.)) Epinephrine 1:1000. Syr. 1 mL. *Rx.*
Use: Bronchodilator; sympathomimetic.
Ana Hep-2. (Wampole) Antinuclear antibodies test by IFA. Tests 60s.
Use: Diagnostic aid.
Ana-Kit. (Bayer Corp. (Consumer Div.)) Syringe, epinephrine 1:1000 in 1 mL; four (each 2 mg) chlorpheniramine maleate; two sterilized swabs, tourniquet, instructions/kit. *Rx.*
Use: Anaphylactic therapy.
anabolic agents. These agents stimulate constructive processes leading to retention of nitrogen and increasing the body protein.
See: Adroyd.
Anabolin-IM.
Anadrol.
Anavar.
Android.
Androlone.

Deca-Durabolin.
Di Genik.
Drolban.
Durabolin.
Halotestin.
Hybolin.
Maxibolin.
Nandrobolic.
Ora-Testryl.
anabolic steroids.
Use: Sex hormone.
See: Nandrolone Decanoate.
Oxandrolone.
Oxymetholone.
Anacaine. (Gordon Laboratories) Benzocaine 10%. Jar oz, lb. *OTC.*
Use: Anesthetic, local.
Anacin. (Whitehall-Robins) Aspirin 400 mg, caffeine 32 mg. Tab. Bot. 30s, 50s, 100s, 200s, 300s. Cap. Bot. 100s. *OTC.*
Use: Analgesic.
Anacin Aspirin Free Extra Strength. (Whitehall-Robins) Acetaminophen 500 mg. Tab. Bot. 60s. *OTC.*
Use: Analgesic.
Anacin Aspirin Free Maximum Strength. (Whitehall-Robins) Acetaminophen 500 mg. Gel Capl. Bot. 50s. Tab. Bot. 30s, 60s, 100s, 750s. *OTC.*
Use: Analgesic.
Anacin Maximum Strength. (Whitehall-Robins) Aspirin 500 mg, caffeine 32 mg. Tab. Bot. 20s, 40s, 75s. *OTC.*
Use: Analgesic.
Anadrol-50. (Unimed) Oxymetholone 50 mg. Lactose. Tab. Bot. 100s. *c-III.*
Use: Anabolic steroid.
anafebrina.
See: Aminopyrine.
Anafranil. (Novartis) Clomipramine hydrochloride 25 mg, 50 mg, 75 mg. Cap. Bot. 100s, UD 100s. *Rx.*
Use: Antidepressant.
•**anagestone acetate.** (AN-ah-JEST-ohn) USAN.
Use: Hormone, progestin.
anagrelide. (AN-AGG-reh-lide)
Use: Polycythemia vera; essential thrombocythemia; thrombocytosis in chronic myelogenous leukemia. [Orphan Drug]
See: Agrylin.
•**anagrelide hydrochloride.** (AN-AGG-reh-lide) USAN.
Use: Antithrombotic.
See: Agrylin.
anagrelide hydrochloride. (Mallinckrodt) Anagrelide hydrochloride 0.5 mg, 1 mg. Lactose. Cap. 100s. *Rx.*
Use: Antithrombotic.

• **anakinra.** (an-ah-KIN-rah) USAN.
Use: Anti-inflammatory, nonsteroidal; suppressant, inflammatory bowel disease; immunologic agent, immunomodulator.
See: Kineret.

Analbalm Improved Formula. (Schwarz Pharma) Methyl salicylate 10%, menthol 1.25%, camphor 3%. Liq. Bot. **Green:** 4 oz, gal. **Pink:** 4 oz, Pt, gal. *OTC.*
Use: Counterirritant.

analeptics. Usually a term applied to agents with stimulant action, particularly on the central nervous system.
See: Caffeine.
Doxapram Hydrochloride.
Modafinil.

Analgesia. (Rugby) Trolamine sulfate 10%. Cream. Tube 85 g. *OTC.*
Use: Liniment.

analgesic and antihistamine combinations.
Use: Upper respiratory combination.
See: Aceta-Gesic.
Coricidin HBP Cold & Flu.
Ed-Flex.
Major-gesic.
Percogesic
Percogesic Extra Strength.
Phenylgesic.
Tylenol PM Extra Strength.
Tylenol Severe Allergy.

analgesic and decongestant combinations.
Use: Upper respiratory combination.
See: Advil Cold & Sinus.
Advil Cold & Sinus Liqui-gels.
Advil Flu & Body Ache.
Aleve Cold & Sinus.
Aleve Sinus & Headache.
Alka-Seltzer Plus Cold & Sinus.
Allerest Allergy & Sinus Relief Maximum Strength.
Cēpacol Sore Throat.
Dristan Cold Non-Drowsy Maximum Strength.
Dristan Sinus.
Mapap Sinus Maximum Strength.
Motrin Children's Cold.
Motrin Sinus Headache.
Nasal Decongestant Sinus Non-Drowsy.
Ornex No Drowsiness.
Ornex No Drowsiness Maximum Strength.
Phenapap.
Sine-Off No-Drowsiness Formula.
Sinus-Relief Maximum Strength.
Sinutab Sinus Without Drowsiness Maximum Strength.

Sinutab Sinus Without Drowsiness Regular Strength.
Sudafed Cold & Sinus Non-Drowsy.
Sudafed Sinus Headache Non-Drowsy.
SudoGest Sinus Maximum Strength.
Tavist Sinus Maximum Strength.
Triaminic Softchews Allergy Sinus & Headache.
Tylenol Children's Sinus.
Tylenol Infant's Cold.
Tylenol Sinus Non-Drowsy Maximum Strength.

analgesic, antihistamine, and antitussive combinations.
Use: Upper respiratory combination.
See: Coricidin HBP Maximum Strength Flu.

analgesic, antihistamine, and decongestant combinations.
Use: Upper respiratory combination.
See: Actifed Cold & Sinus Maximum Strength.
Advil Allergy Sinus.
Alka-Seltzer Plus Cold Medicine.
Benadryl Allergy & Cold.
Benadryl Allergy & Sinus Headache.
Benadryl Maximum Strength Severe Allergy & Sinus Headache.
Comtrex Acute Head Cold & Sinus Pressure Relief, Multi-Symptom Maximum Strength.
Comtrex Allergy-Sinus Treatment, Maximum Strength.
Comtrex Flu Therapy & Fever Relief Day & Night, Multi-Symptom Maximum Strength.
Contac Day & Night Allergy/Sinus Relief.
Coricidin 'D' Cold, Flu, & Sinus.
Decodult.
Dristan Cold Multi-Symptom Formula.
Drixoral Allergy Sinus.
Dryphen, Multi-Symptom Formula.
Duadacin Extra Strength Cold and Flu.
Good Sense Maximum Strength Dose Sinus.
Good Sense Maximum Strength Pain Relief Allergy Sinus.
Kolephrin.
Scot-Tussin Original Clear 5-Action Cold and Allergy Formula.
Scot-Tussin Original 5-Action Cold and Allergy Formula.
Simplet.
Sine-Off Night Time Formula Sinus, Cold & Flu Medicine.
Sine-Off Sinus Medicine.
Singlet for Adults.
Sinutab Sinus Allergy, Maximum Strength.

Sudafed Maximum Strength Sinus Nighttime Plus Pain Relief.
Tavist Allergy/Sinus/Headache.
TheraFlu Flu & Cold Medicine for Sore Throat, Maximum Strength.
TheraFlu Flu & Cold Medicine Original Formula.
TheraFlu Flu & Sore Throat Night Time, Maximum Strength.
Triaminicin Cold, Allergy, Sinus Medicine.
Tylenol Allergy Sinus, Maximum Strength.
Tylenol Allergy Sinus Night Time, Maximum Strength.
Tylenol Children's Cold.
Tylenol Flu Night Time, Maximum Strength.
Tylenol Sinus Night Time, Maximum Strength.

analgesic, antihistamine, antitussive, and decongestant combinations.
Use: Upper respiratory combination.
See: Alka-Seltzer Plus Cold & Cough.
Alka-Seltzer Plus Flu Medicine.
Alka-Seltzer Plus Night Time Cold.
All-Nite.
Cold Symptoms Relief Maximum Strength.
Comtrex Cough & Cold Relief, Multi-Symptom Maximum Strength
Comtrex Day & Night Cold & Cough Relief, Multi-Symptom Maximum Strength.
Contac Day & Night Cold & Flu.
Contac Severe Cold & Flu Maximum Strength.
Dimetapp Children's Nighttime Flu.
Genacol Maximum Strength Cold & Flu Relief.
Kolephrin/DM.
Mapap Cold Formula.
Nite Time Cold Formula for Adults.
Robitussin Flu.
Robitussin Honey Flu Nighttime.
Robitussin Night Relief.
TheraFlu Cold & Cough NightTime.
TheraFlu Flu & Cough NightTime, Maximum Strength
TheraFlu Flu, Cold & Cough.
TheraFlu Flu, Cold & Cough and Sore Throat, Maximum Strength.
TheraFlu Flu, Cold & Cough Night-Time, Maximum Strength
TheraFlu Maximum Strength Night-Time Formula Flu, Cold, & Cough Medicine.
TheraFlu Severe Cold & Congestion Night Time, Maximum Strength
Top Care LiquiCaps Nite Time Multi-Symptom Cold/Flu Relief.

Top Care Maximum Strength Flu, Cold, & Cough Medicine Night Time.
Top Care Multi-Symptom Pain Relief Cold.
Triaminic Cold, Cough & Fever.
Tylenol Children's Cold Plus Cough.
Tylenol Children's Flu.
Tylenol Cold Complete Formula.
Tylenol Flu Night Time, Maximum Strength.
Vicks 44M Cough, Cold, & Flu Relief.
Vicks NyQuil Multi-Symptom Cold & Flu Relief.
Vicks NyQuil Multi-Symptom Cold/Flu Relief.

analgesic, antitussive, and decongestant combinations.
Use: Upper respiratory combination.
See: Alka-Seltzer Plus Cold & Flu.
Alka-Seltzer Plus Liqui-Gels Flu Medicine.
Comtrex Multi-Symptom Maximum Strength Non-Drowsy Cold & Cough Relief.
Dimetapp Children's Non-Drowsy Flu.
Duraflu.
Robitussin Honey Flu Multi-Symptom.
Robitussin Honey Flu Non-Drowsy.
666 Cold Preparation, Maximum Strength.
Sudafed Non-Drowsy Severe Cold Formula Maximum Strength.
TheraFlu Non-Drowsy Flu, Cold & Cough Maximum Strength.
TheraFlu Non-Drowsy Formula Maximum Strength.
TheraFlu Severe Cold & Congestion Non-Drowsy, Maximum Strength.
Top Care Multi-Symptom Pain Relief Cold.
Triaminic Cough & Sore Throat.
Triaminic Throat Pain & Cough.
Tylenol Cold Non-Drowsy Formula.
Tylenol Flu Maximum Strength Non-Drowsy.
Tylenol Infants' Cold Decongestant & Fever Reducer Plus Cough.
Vicks DayQuil LiquiCaps Multi-Symptom Cold/Flu Relief.
Vicks DayQuil Multi-Symptom Cold/Flu Relief.

analgesic, antitussive, decongestant, expectorant combinations.
Use: Upper respiratory combination.
See: Comtrex Multi-Symptom Deep Chest Cold & Congestion Relief.
Duraflu.
Robitussin Cold, Multi-Symptom Cold & Flu.
Sudafed Multi-Symptom Cold & Cough.

TheraFlu Maximum Strength Flu & Congestion Non-Drowsy.
TheraFlu Maximum Strength Flu, Cold & Cough.
Tylenol Multi-Symptom Cold Severe Congestion.

analgesic balm. (Various Mfr.) Menthol w/methylsalicylate in a suitable base. *OTC.*
Use: Counterirritant.
See: A.P.C.
Musterole.

Analgesic Liquid. (Weeks & Leo) Triethanolamine salicylate 20% in an alcohol base. Liq. Bot. 4 oz. *OTC.*
Use: Analgesic, topical.

Analgesic Lotion. (Weeks & Leo) Methyl nicotinate 1%, methyl salicylate 10%, camphor 0.1%, menthol 0.1%. Lot. Bot. 4 oz. *OTC.*
Use: Analgesic, topical.

analgesics, miscellaneous.
See: Ziconotide.

analgesics, opioid.
See: Opioid analgesics.

Analpram-HC. (Ferndale) Hydrocortisone acetate 1%, 2%, pramoxine hydrochloride 1%. Cream. Tube 30 g. *Rx.*
Use: Anesthetic; corticosteroid, local.

Analval. (Pal-Pak, Inc.) Aspirin 227 mg, acetaminophen 162 mg, caffeine 32 mg. Tab. Bot. 1000s. *OTC.*
Use: Analgesic combination.

AnaMantle HC. (Bradley) Hydrocortisone acetate 0.5%, lidocaine hydrochloride 3%, cetyl alcohol, light mineral oil, parabens, glycerin, stearyl alcohol, petrolatum. Cream. Kits. 7 g tubes w/single-use applicators (14s). *Rx.*
Use: Corticosteroid combination.

Anamine. (Merz) Pseudoephedrine hydrochloride 30 mg, chlorpheniramine maleate 2 mg/5 mL. Syr. Bot. 473 mL. *Rx.*
Use: Antihistamine; decongestant.

Anamine HD. (Merz) Phenylephrine hydrochloride 5 mg, chlorpheniramine maleate 2 mg, hydrocodone bitartrate 1.67 mg. Syr. Bot. *c-iii.*
Use: Antihistamine; antitussive; decongestant.

Anamine TD. (Merz) Chlorpheniramine maleate 8 mg, pseudoephedrine hydrochloride 120 mg. TD Cap. Bot. 100s. *Rx.*
Use: Antihistamine; decongestant.

Ananain, Comosain.
Use: Burn therapy. [Orphan Drug]
See: Vianain.

Anaplex DM. (ECR) Dextromethorphan HBr 30 mg, brompheniramine maleate 4 mg, pseudoephedrine hydrochloride 60 mg/5 mL, fruit flavor. Alcohol and dye free. Liq. Bot. 473 mL. *Rx.*
Use: Upper respiratory combination, antitussive, antihistamine, decongestant.

Anaplex HD. (ECR) Hydrocodone bitartrate 1.7 mg, pseudoephedrine hydrochloride 30 mg, brompheniramine maleate 2 mg/5 mL, alcohol and dye free, strawberry flavor. Liq. Bot. 118 mL, 473 mL. *c-iii.*
Use: Upper respiratory combination, antihistamine, antitussive, decongestant.

Anaprox. (Roche) Naproxen 250 mg (naproxen sodium 275 mg). Tab. Bot. 100s. *Rx.*
Use: NSAID.

Anaprox DS. (Roche) Naproxen 500 mg (naproxen sodium 550 mg). Tab. Bot. 100s, 500s. *Rx.*
Use: NSAID.

anarel. Guanadrel sulfate.

•**anaritide acetate.** (an-NAR-ih-TIDE) USAN.
Use: Antihypertensive; diuretic.

Anaspaz. (Ascher) L-hyoscyamine sulfate 0.125 mg. Tab. Bot. 100s, 500s. *Rx.*
Use: Anticholinergic; antispasmodic.

•**anastrozole.** (an-ASS-troe-zole) USAN.
Use: Antineoplastic; hormone.
See: Arimidex.

Anatrast. (Mallinckrodt) Barium sulfate 100%, simethicone, sorbitol, parabens. Paste. Tube 500 g, enema tip assemblies. *Rx.*
Use: Radiopaque agent, GI contrast agent.

Anatuss LA. (Merz) Guaifenesin 400 mg, pseudoephedrine hydrochloride 120 mg. Tab. Bot. 100s. *Rx.*
Use: Decongestant; expectorant.

Anavar. (Pharmacia) Oxandrolone 2.5 mg. Tab. Bot. 100s. *Rx.*
Use: Anabolic steroid.

anayodin.
See: Chiniofon.

•**anazolene sodium.** (an-AZZ-oh-leen) USAN. Sodium anoxynaphthonate.
Use: Diagnostic aid, blood volume, cardiac output determination.

Anbesol Baby Gel. (Whitehall-Robins) Benzocaine 7.5%. Gel. Tube 0.25 oz. *OTC.*
Use: Anesthetic, local.

Anbesol Gel. (Whitehall-Robins) Benzocaine 6.3%, phenol 0.5%, alcohol 70%. Gel. Tube 7.5 g. *OTC.*

Use: Anesthetic combination, topical.

Anbesol Liquid. (Whitehall-Robins) Benzocaine 6.3%, phenol 0.5%, povidone-iodine 0.04%, alcohol 70%. Liq. Bot. 9 mL, 22 mL. *OTC.*
Use: Anesthetic combination, topical.

Anbesol Maximum Strength. (Whitehall-Robins) **Gel:** Benzocaine 20%, alcohol 60%, carbomer 934P, polyethylene glycol, saccharin. Tube 7.2 g. **Liq.:** Benzocaine 20%, alcohol 60%, saccharin, polyethylene glycol. Bot. 9 mL. *OTC.*
Use: Anesthetic, local.

Ancef. (Hospira) Cefazolin sodium 500 mg, 1 g, 5 g, 10 g, 20 g. Sodium 2.1 mEq/g. Pow. for Inj. Vials and piggyback vials (500 mg, 1 g only). Bulk vials (5 g, 10 g). *Rx.*
Use: Anti-infective; cephalosporin.

Ancef. (SmithKline Beecham) Cefazolin sodium 500 mg, 1 g. Dextrose. Premixed, frozen. Inj. Plastic containers. 50 mL. *Rx.*
Use: Anti-infective; cephalosporin.

• **ancestim.** (an-SESS-tim) USAN.
Use: Investigational for treatment of anemia; hematopoietic adjuvant, stem cell factor.

Ancid. (Sheryl) Calcium aluminum carbonate, di-amino acetate complex. Tab. Bot. 100s. Susp. Bot. Pt. *OTC.*
Use: Antacid.

Ancobon. (ICN) Flucytosine 250 mg, 500 mg, lactose, parabens, talc. Cap. Bot. 100s. *Rx.*
Use: Anti-infective; antifungal.

• **ancrod.** (AN-krahd) USAN. An active principle obtained from the venom of the Malayan pit viper *Agkistrodonrhodostoma.*
Use: Anticoagulant.

ancrod. (Knoll)
Use: Antithrombotic in patients with heparin-induced thrombocytopenia orthrombosis who require immediate and continued anticoagulation.

Andehist DM NR. (Silarx) Pseudoephedrine hydrochloride 15 mg, carbinoxamine maleate 1 mg, dextromethorphan HBr 4 mg/mL, saccharin, sorbitol, grape flavor. Drops. 30 mL with dropper. *Rx.*
Use: Upper respiratory combination, decongestant, antihistamine, antitussive.

Andesterone. (Lincoln Diagnostics) Estrone 2 mg, testosterone 6 mg/mL. Susp. Vial 15 mL. **Forte:** Estrone 1 mg, testosterone 20 mg/mL. Inj. Vial 15 mL. *Rx.*

Use: Androgen, estrogen combination.

Andrest 90-4. (Seatrace) Testosterone enanthate 90 mg, estradiol valerate 4 mg/mL. Vial 10 mL. *Rx.*
Use: Androgen, estrogen combination.

Andro-Cyp 100. (Keene Pharmaceuticals) Testosterone cypionate 100 mg/mL. Vial 10 mL. *c-III.*
Use: Androgen.

Andro-Cyp 200. (Keene Pharmaceuticals) Testosterone cypionate 200 mg/mL. Vial 10 mL. *c-III.*
Use: Androgen.

Androderm. (Watson) Testosterone 2.5 mg, 5 mg. Patch. Pkg. 30s (5 mg only), 60s (2.5 mg only). *c-III.*
Use: Hormone, testosterone.

Andro-Estro 90-4. (Rugby) Estradiol valerate 4 mg, testosterone enanthate 90 mg/mL with chlorobutanol in sesame oil. Inj. Vial. 10 mL. *Rx.*
Use: Androgen, estrogen combination.

AndroGel-DHT. (Unimed Pharm) Dihydrotestosterone.
Use: AIDS. [Orphan Drug]

AndroGel 1%. (Unimed Pharm) Testosterone 1%, ethanol 68.9%. Gel. Pkt. UD 2.5 g, 5 g (30s). *c-III.*
Use: Sex hormone, androgen.

androgen-estrogen therapy.
See: Dienestrol with Methyltestosterone.
Estradiol Esters with Methyltestosterone.
Estradiol Esters with Testosterone.
Estrogenic Substance, Conjugated with Methyltestosterone.
Estrogenic Substance Mixed with Methyltestosterone.
Estrogenic Substance Mixed with Testosterone.
Estrone with Testosterone.

androgen hormone inhibitor.
See: Dutasteride.
Finasteride.

androgens. Substances that possess masculinizing activities.
Use: Sex hormone.
See: Fluoxymesterone.
Methyltestosterone.
Sex Hormones.
Teslac.
Testolactone.
Testosterone.
Testosterone, Buccal.
Testosterone Cyclopentylpropionate.
Testosterone Cypionate.
Testosterone Enanthate.
Testosterone Gel.
Testosterone Heptanoate.
Testosterone, Long-Acting.

Testosterone Pellets.
Testosterone Phenylacetate.
Testosterone Transdermal System.
W/Estrogen
See: Estratest.
Estratest H.S.
Syntest H.S.
Androlin. (Lincoln Diagnostics) Testosterone 100 mg/mL. Vial 10 mL. *c-III.*
Use: Androgen.
Andronaq-50. (Schwarz Pharma) Testosterone 50 mg/mL, sodium carboxymethylcellulose, methylcellulose, povidone, DSS, thimerosal. Inj. Vial. 10 mL. *c-III.*
Use: Androgen.
Andronaq LA. (Schwarz Pharma) Testosterone cypionate 100 mg, benzyl alcohol 0.9% in cottonseed oil. Vial 10 mL. Bot. 12s. *c-III.*
Use: Androgen.
Andronate 100. (Taylor Pharmaceuticals) Testosterone cypionate 100 mg/mL with benzyl alcohol in cottonseed oil. Vial 10 mL. *c-III.*
Use: Androgen.
Andronate 200. (Taylor Pharmaceuticals) Testosterone cypionate 200 mg/mL with benzyl alcohol, benzyl benzoate in cottonseed oil. Vial 10 mL. *c-III.*
Use: Androgen.
Andro 100. (Forest) Testosterone 100 mg/mL. Vial 10 mL. *c-III.*
Use: Androgen.
androstanazole.
See: Stanozolol.
androstanolone.
See: Stanolone.
androstenopyrazole. Anabolic steroid; pending release.
Androtest P.
See: Testosterone propionate.
Androvite. (Optimox) Iron 3 mg, vitamins A 4167 units, D 67 units, E 67 units, B_1 8.3 mg, B_2 8.3 mg, B_3 8.3 mg, B_5 16.7 mg, B_6 16.7 mg, B_{12} 20.8 mcg, C 167 mg, folic acid 0.06 mg, PABA, inositol, biotin, betaine, B, Cr, Cu, I, Mg, Mn, Se, Zn 8.3 mg, pancreatin, hesperidin, rutin. Tab. Bot. 180s. *OTC.*
Use: Mineral, vitamin supplement.
Andryl 200. (Keene Pharmaceuticals) Testosterone enanthate 200 mg/mL. Vial 10 mL. *c-III.*
Use: Androgen.
Andylate. (Vita Elixir) Sodium salicylate 10 g. Tab. *OTC.*
Use: Analgesic.
Andylate Forte. (Vita Elixir) Acetaminophen 3 g, salicylamide 3 g, caffeine 0.25 g. Tab. *OTC.*

Use: Analgesic combination.
Andylate Rub. (Vita Elixir) Methylnicotinate, methyl salicylate, camphor, dipropylene glycol salicylate, oil of cassia, oleo resin of capsicum, oleo resin of ginger. *OTC.*
Use: Analgesic, topical.
•**anecortave acetate.** (an-eh-CORE-tave ASS-eh-tate) USAN.
Use: Angiostatic steroid.
Anectine. (GlaxoSmithKline) Succinylcholine Cl. **Soln.:** 20 mg/mL. Multidose Vial 10 mL. **Sterile Pow.:** 500 mg, 1000 mg. Flo-Pak Box 12s. *Rx.*
Use: Muscle relaxant.
Anefrin Nasal Spray, Long Acting. (Walgreen) Oxymetazoline hydrochloride 0.05%. Bot. 0.5 oz. *OTC.*
Use: Decongestant.
Anemagen OB. (Ethex) Ca 200 mg, Fe (as ferrous fumarate) 28 mg, vitamin D_3 400 units, E (as d-alpha tocopherol) 30 units, B_1 1.6 mg, B_2 1.8 mg, B_6 20 mg, B_{12} 12 mcg, C 60 mcg, folic acid 1 mg, docusate calcium, parabens. Soft gelatin cap. Bot. 100s. *Rx.*
Use: Vitamin, mineral supplement.
Anergan 50. (Forest) Promethazine hydrochloride 50 mg/mL, EDTA, phenol. Vial 10 mL. *Rx.*
Use: Antihistamine.
anertan.
See: Testosterone propionate.
Anestacon. (PolyMedica) Lidocaine hydrochloride 20 mg/mL. Jelly. Tube. 15 mL, 240 mL. *Rx.*
Use: Anesthetic, local.
Anesthesin. (Ethyl-p-aminobenzoate.)
Use: Anesthetic, local.
See: Benzocaine.
anesthetics, combination local.
See: Duocaine.
anesthetics, general.
See: Diprivan.
Droperidol.
Inapsine.
Propofol.
Sevoflurane.
Ultane.
Volatile Liquids.
anesthetics, injectable local.
See: Amide Local Anesthetics.
Anesthetics, Combination Local.
Articaine Hydrochloride.
Bupivacaine Hydrochloride.
Chloroprocaine Hydrochloride.
Ester Local Anesthetics.
Levobupivacaine Hydrochloride.
Lidocaine Hydrochloride.
Mepivacaine Hydrochloride.
Prilocaine Hydrochloride.

Procaine Hydrochloride.
Ropivacaine Hydrochloride.
Tetracaine Hydrochloride.
anethaine.
See: Tetracaine Hydrochloride.
●**anethole.** (AN-eh-thole) *NF 23.*
Use: Pharmaceutic aid, flavor.
aneurine hydrochloride.
See: Thiamine hydrochloride.
Anexsia. (Andrx) Hydrocodone bitartrate
5 mg or 7.5 mg, acetaminophen
325 mg. Tab. Bot. 100s, 1000s. *c-III.*
Use: Analgesic combination, narcotic.
Anexsia 5/500. (Mallinckrodt) Hydro-
codone bitartrate 5 mg, acetaminophen
500 mg. Tab. Bot. 100s. *c-III.*
Use: Analgesic combination; narcotic.
Anexsia 7.5/650. (Mallinckrodt) Hydro-
codone bitartrate 7.5 mg, acetamino-
phen 650 mg. Tab. Bot. 1000s. *c-III.*
Use: Analgesic combination, narcotic.
Anexsia 10/660. (Mallinckrodt) Hydro-
codone bitartrate 10 mg, acetamino-
phen 660 mg. Tab. Bot. 100s, 1000s.
c-III.
Use: Analgesic combination, narcotic.
Angel Sweet. (Garrett) Vitamins A and
D_2. Cream. Tube 90 g. *OTC.*
Use: Dermatologic, protectant.
Angen. (Davis & Sly) Estrone 2 mg,
testosterone 25 mg/mL. Aqueous Susp.
Vial 10 mL. *Rx.*
Use: Androgen, estrogen combination.
Angerin. (Kingshay) Nitroglycerin 1 mg,
Cap. Bot. 60s. *Rx.*
Use: Coronary vasodilator.
Angex. (Janssen) Lidoflazine. *Rx.*
Use: Coronary vasodilator.
Angio-Conray. (Mallinckrodt) Iothala-
mate sodium 80% (48% iodine), EDTA.
Inj. Vial 50 mL.
Use: Radiopaque agent.
Angiomax. (Medicines Company) Bivali-
rudin 250 mg. Inj., lyophilized. Single-
use Vial. *Rx.*
Use: Anticoagulant.
●**angiotensin amide.** (an-JEE-oh-TEN-sin
AH-mid) USAN.
Use: Vasoconstrictor.
**angiotensin-converting enzyme inhibi-
tors.**
Use: Antihypertensive; congestive heart
failure.
See: Benazepril Hydrochloride.
Captopril.
Enalapril Maleate.
Fosinopril Sodium.
Lisinopril.
Moexipril Hydrochloride.
Perindopril Erbumine.
Quinapril Hydrochloride.

Ramipril.
Trandolapril.
angiotensin II receptor antagonists.
See: Candesartan Cilexetil.
Eprosartan Mesylate.
Irbesartan.
Losartan Potassium.
Telmisartan.
Valsartan.
Angiovist 370. (Berlex) Diatrizoate
meglumine 66%, diatrizoate sodium
10%, (iodine 37%). Vial 50 mL, 100 mL,
150 mL, or 200 mL. Box 10s.
Use: Radiopaque agent.
Angiovist 282. (Berlex) Diatrizoate
meglumine 60% (iodine 28%). Vial
50 mL, 100 mL, 150 mL. Box 10s.
Use: Radiopaque agent.
Angiovist 292. (Berlex) Diatrizoate
meglumine 52%, diatrizoate sodium 8%
(iodine 29.2%). Vial 30 mL, 50 mL,
100 mL. Box 10s.
Use: Radiopaque agent.
anhydrohydroxyprogesterone. Ethisterone.
●**anidoxime.** (AN-ih-DOX-eem) USAN.
Use: Analgesic.
●**anidulafungin.** USAN.
Use: Antifungal.
A-Nil. (Vangard Labs, Inc.) Codeine
phosphate 10 mg, bromodiphenhydramine hydrochloride 3.75 mg, diphenhydramine hydrochloride 8.75 mg,
ammonium Cl 80 mg, potassium
guaiacolsulfonate 80 mg, menthol
0.5 mg/5 mL, alcohol 5%. Bot. Pt. gal.
c-v.
Use: Antitussive; expectorant.
●**anileridine.** (an-ih-LURR-ih-deen)
USP 28.
Use: Analgesic, narcotic.
●**anileridine hydrochloride.** (an-ih-LURR-
ih-deen) *USP 28.*
Use: Analgesic, narcotic.
●**anilopam hydrochloride.** (AN-ih-low-
pam) USAN.
Use: Analgesic.
Animal Shapes. (Major) Vitamin A
2500 units, D 400 units, E 15 units, C
60 mg, B_1 1.05 mg, B_2 1.2 mg, B_3
13.5 mg, B_6 1.05 mg, B_{12} 4.5 mcg, folic
acid 0.3 mg. Chew. Tab. Bot. 100s,
250s. *OTC.*
Use: Vitamin supplement.
Animal Shapes + Iron. (Major) Vitamin
A 2500 units, D 400 units, E 15 units,
C 60 mg, B_1 1.05 mg, B_2 1.2 mg, B_3
13.5 mg, B_6 1.05 mg, B_{12} 4.5 mcg, folic
acid 0.3 mg, iron 15 mg. Chew. Tab.
Bot. 100s, 250s. *OTC.*

Use: Mineral, vitamin supplement.

Animi-3. (PBM Pharm) Omega-3 acids
500 mg (eicosapentaenoic acid [EPA]
35 mg and docosahexaenoic acid
[DHA] 350 mg), vitamin B_6 12.5 mg, B_{12}
500 mcg, folic acid 1 mg. Sunflower
oil. Cap. 60s. *Rx.*
Use: Dietary supplement.

anion exchange resins.
See: Polyamine-Methylene Resin.

•**aniracetam.** (AN-ih-RASS-eh-tam)
USAN.
Use: Mental performance enhancer.

•**anirolac.** (ah-NIH-role-ACK) USAN.
Use: Analgesic; anti-inflammatory.

•**anise oil.** (AN-is) *NF 23.*
Use: Flavoring.

anisopyradamine.
See: Pyrilamine Maleate.

•**anisotropine methylbromide.** (ah-NIH-
so-TROE-peen meth-ill-BROE-mide)
USAN.
Use: Anticholinergic.

•**anitrazafen.** (AN-ih-TRAY-zaff-en)
USAN.
Use: Anti-inflammatory, topical.

anodynon.
See: Ethyl Chloride.

Anodynos. (Buffington) Aspirin
420.6 mg, salicylamide 34.4 mg, caffeine 34.4 mg. Sugar, lactose, and salt
free. Tab. Dispens-A-Kit 500s, Bot.
100s, 500s, Medipak 200s. *OTC.*
Use: Analgesic combination.

Anodynos-DHC. (Buffington) Hydrocodone bitartrate 5 mg, acetaminophen
500 mg. Tab. Bot. 100s. *c-III.*
Use: Analgesic combination; narcotic.

Anorex. (Oxypure) Phendimetrazine
35 mg. Tab. Bot. 100s. *c-III.*
Use: Anorexiant.

anorexiants.
Use: Appetite suppressants.
See: Benzphetamine Hydrochloride.
Diethylpropion Hydrochloride.
Phendimetrazine Tartrate.
Phentermine Hydrochloride.
Sibutramine Hydrochloride.

anovlar. Norethindrone plus ethinyl estradiol. *Rx.*
Use: Contraceptive.

•**anoxomer.** (an-OX-ah-MER) USAN.
Use: Pharmaceutic aid, antioxidant;
food additive.

anoxynaphthonate sodium. Anazolene
sodium.

Ansaid. (Pharmacia) Flurbiprofen 50 mg,
100 mg, lactose. Tab. Bot. 100s, 500s,
2000s, UD 100s (100 mg only). *Rx.*
Use: Analgesic; NSAID.

Anspor. (GlaxoSmithKline) Cephradine
(a semisynthetic cephalosporin). **Cap.:**
250 mg, 500 mg. Bot. 20s (500 mg
only), 100s, UD 100s. **Oral Susp.:**
125 mg, 250 mg/5 mL. Bot. 100 mL.
Use: Anti-infective; cephalosporin.

Answer. (Carter-Wallace) Reagent in-
home pregnancy test kit for urine testing. Test kit box 1s.
Use: Diagnostic aid.

Answer One-Step Pregnancy Test.
(Carter-Wallace) Pregnancy test kit for
urine testing. Stick. Test kit box 1s.
OTC.
Use: Diagnostic aid.

Answer Plus. (Carter-Wallace) Reagent
in-home pregnancy test kit for urine
testing. Test kit box 1s.
Use: Diagnostic aid.

Answer Plus 2. (Carter-Wallace) Reagent in-home pregnancy test kit for
urine testing. Test kit box 2s.
Use: Diagnostic aid.

Answer Quick & Simple. (Carter-Wallace) Reagent in-home kit for urine
testing. Test kit box 1s.
Use: Diagnostic aid.

Answer 2. (Carter-Wallace) Reagent in-
home pregnancy test kit for urine testing. Test kit box 2s.
Use: Diagnostic aid.

Antabuse. (Odyssey) Disulfiram 250 mg.
Lactose. Tab. Bot. 50s *Rx.*
Use: Antialcoholic.

Antacid. (Walgreen) Calcium carbonate
500 mg. Tab. Bot. 75s. *OTC.*
Use: Antacid.

Antacid Extra Strength. (Various Mfr.)
Calcium carbonate 750 mg. Tab. Bot.
96s. *OTC.*
Use: Antacid.

Antacid M. (Walgreen) Aluminum oxide
225 mg, magnesium hydroxide
200 mg/5 mL. Liq. Bot. 12 oz, 26 oz.
OTC.
Use: Antacid.

Antacid No. 6. (Jones Pharma) Calcium
carbonate 0.42 g, glycine 0.18 g. Tab.
Bot. 100s. *OTC.*
Use: Antacid.

Antacid #2. (Global Source) Calcium
carbonate 5.5 g, magnesium carbonate
2.5 g. Tab. Bot. 100s. *OTC.*
Use: Antacid.

Antacid Relief. (Walgreen) Dihydroxy-
aluminum sodium carbonate 334 mg.
Tab. Bot. 75s. *OTC.*
Use: Antacid.

antacids. Drugs that neutralize excess
gastric acid.
See: Alka-Seltzer.

Alka-Seltzer Plus.
Alka-Seltzer Special Effervescent Antacid.
Aluminum Hydroxide Gel.
Aluminum Hydroxide Gel w/Combinations.
Aluminum Hydroxide Gel Dried.
Aluminum Hydroxide Gel Dried w/Combinations.
Aluminum Hydroxide Magnesium Carbonate.
Aluminum Phosphate Gel.
Aluminum Proteinate.
Amitone.
Calcium Carbonate.
Calcium Carbonate, Precipitated.
Ceo-Two.
Chooz.
Citrocarbonate.
Di Gel
Dicarbosil.
Dihydroxyaluminum Aminoacetate.
Dihydroxyaluminum Sodium Carbonate.
Magaldrate.
Magnesium Carbonate.
Magnesium Glycinate.
Magnesium Hydroxide.
Magnesium Oxide.
Magnesium Trisilicate.
Rolaids.
Romach.
Sodium Bicarbonate.
Tums.
Antacid Suspension. (Geneva) Aluminum hydroxide 225 mg, magnesium hydroxide 200 mg/5 mL. Bot. 360 mL. *OTC.*
Use: Antacid.
Antacid Tablets. (Ivax) Calcium carbonate 500 mg. Chew. Tab. Bot. 150s. *OTC.*
Use: Antacid.
Anta-Gel. (Halsey Drug) Aluminum hydroxide 200 mg, magnesium hydroxide 200 mg, simethicone 20 mg/5 mL. Bot. 12 oz. *OTC.*
Use: Antacid; antiflatulent.
antagonists of curariform drugs.
See: Neostigmine Methylsulfate.
Tensilon.
Antara. (Reliant) Fenofibrate (micronized) 43 mg, 87 mg, 130 mg. Sugar spheres. Cap. 30s, 100s. *Rx.*
Use: Antihyperlipidemic agent.
antazoline hydrochloride. Antastan.
● **antazoline phosphate.** *USP 28.*
Use: Antihistamine.
W/Naphazoline, boric acid, phenylmercuric acetate, sodium Cl, sodium carbonate anhydrous.

See: Vasocon-A Ophthalmic.
Antazoline-V. (Rugby) Naphazoline hydrochloride 0.05%, antazoline phosphate 0.5%, PEG 8000, polyvinyl alcohol, EDTA, benzalkonium chloride 0.01%. Soln. Drop. Bot. 5 mL, 15 mL. *Rx.*
Use: Ophthalmic decongestant combination.
anterior pituitary.
See: Pituitary, anterior.
anthelmintics.
Use: A remedy for worms.
See: Antiminth.
Betanaphthol Benzoate.
Biltricide.
Carbon Tetrachloride.
Gentian Violet.
Ivermectin.
Mintezol.
Piperazine.
Praziquantel.
Stromectol.
Terramycin.
Tetrachlorethylene.
Vermox.
● **anthelmycin.** (AN-thell-MY-sin) USAN.
Use: Anthelmintic.
Anthelvet. Tetramisole hydrochloride.
anthracenedione.
See: Mitoxantrone hydrochloride.
Novantrone.
anthracyclines.
See: Adriamycin PFS.
Adriamycin RDF.
Daunorubicin Citrate Liposomal.
Daunorubicin Hydrochloride.
Doxorubicin Hydrochloride.
Ellence.
Epirubicin Hydrochloride.
Idamycin.
Idamycin PFS.
Idarubicin Hydrochloride.
Valrubicin.
Valstar.
● **anthralin.** (AN-thrah-lin) *USP 28.*
Use: Antipsoriatic.
See: Dritho-Scalp.
Psoriatec Cream.
anthralin. (Rising Pharmaceuticals) Anthralin 1%. Cream. 50 g. *Rx.*
Use: Antipsoriatic agent.
● **anthramycin.** (an-THRAH-MY-sin) USAN.
Use: Antineoplastic.
anthraquinone of cascara.
See: Cascara Sagrada.
anthrax vaccine. (Michigan Biological Products Institute) Vial 5 mL. *Rx.*
Use: Immunization.

●**anthrax vaccine, adsorbed.** *USP 28.*
Use: Immunization.
anti-a blood grouping serum.
Use: Diagnostic aid, blood in vitro.
Antiacid. (Hillcrest North) Aluminum
hydroxide, magnesium trisilicate, cal-
cium carbonate. Tab. Bot. 100s. *OTC.*
Use: Antacid.
**antiadrenergic agents, peripherally
acting.**
Use: Antiadrenergic/sympatholytic.
See: Alfuzosin Hydrochloride.
Doxazosin Mesylate.
Guanadrel.
Guanethidine Monosulfate.
Prazosin Hydrochloride.
Reserpine.
Tamsulosin Hydrochloride.
Terazosin Hydrochloride.
antiadrenergics/sympatholytics.
See: Acebutolol Hydrochloride.
Alfuzosin Hydrochloride.
Alpha/Beta-Adrenergic Blocking
Agents.
Antiadrenergic Agents, Peripherally
Acting
Atenolol.
Beta-Adrenergic Blocking Agents.
Betaxolol Hydrochloride.
Bisoprolol Fumarate.
Carteolol Hydrochloride.
Carvedilol.
Doxazosin Mesylate.
Esmolol Hydrochloride.
Guanadrel.
Guanethidine Monosulfate.
Labetolol Hydrochloride.
Mecamylamine Hydrochloride.
Methyldopa.
Methyldopate Hydrochloride.
Metoprolol.
Metoprolol Tartrate.
Nadolol.
Penbutolol Sulfate.
Pindolol.
Prazosin Hydrochloride.
Propranolol Hydrochloride.
Reserpine.
Sotalol Hydrochloride.
Tamsulosin Hydrochloride.
Terazosin Hydrochloride.
Timolol Maleate.
Tolazoline Hydrochloride.
antialcoholic agents.
See: Acamprosate Calcium.
Disulfiram.
antiandrogen.
See: Bicalutamide.
Casodex.
Eulexin.
Flutamide.

Nilandron.
Nilutamide.
antianxiety agents.
See: Alprazolam.
Benzodiazepines.
Buspirone Hydrochloride.
Chlordiazepoxide Hydrochloride.
Clorazepate Dipotassium.
Diazepam.
Doxepin Hydrochloride.
Hydroxyzine.
Lorazepam.
Meprobamate.
Oxazepam.
antiarrhythmic agents.
See: Adenosine.
Amiodarone Hydrochloride.
Bretylium Tosylate.
Disopyramide.
Dofetilide.
Flecainide Acetate.
Ibutilide Fumarate.
Lidocaine Hydrochloride.
Mexilitine Hydrochloride.
Moricizine Hydrochloride.
Procainamide Hydrochloride.
Propafenone Hydrochloride.
Quinidine.
antiasthmatic combinations.
See: Cromolyn Sodium.
Decadron Respihaler.
Ephedrine Hydrochloride.
Ephedrine Sulfate.
Isoephedrine Hydrochloride.
Isoetharine.
Isoetharine Hydrochloride.
Isoetharine Mesylate.
Isoproterenol Hydrochloride.
Isoproterenol Sulfate.
Methoxyphenamine Hydrochloride.
Phenylephrine Hydrochloride.
Pseudoephedrine Hydrochloride.
Racephedrine Hydrochloride.
antiasthmatic inhalants.
See: AsthmaHaler.
AsthmaNefrin.
antibacterial antibodies.
See: Botulinum antitoxin.
Diphtheria antitoxin.
Immune globulin IM.
Immune globulin IV.
Tetanus immune globulin.
antibason.
See: Methylthiouracil.
anti-b blood grouping serum.
Use: Diagnostic aid, blood in vitro.
Antibiotic. (Parnell) **Otic Susp.:** Poly-
myxin B sulfate 10,000 units, neomycin
(as sulfate) 3.5 mg, hydrocortisone
10 mg/mL, thimerosal 0.01%. Bot.
10 mL w/dropper. **Otic Soln.:** Polymyxin

B sulfate 10,000 units, neomycin (as
sulfate) 3.5 mg, hydrocortisone 10 mg/
mL. Bot. 10 mL w/dropper. *Rx.*
Use: Anti-infective; anti-inflammatory.
antibiotic and steroid combinations.
See: AK-Trol.
Cortisporin.
Dexacidin.
Maxitrol.
NeoDecadron.
Neo-Dexameth.
Neomycin and Polymyxin B Sulfates
and Dexamethasone.
Poly-Pred Liquifilm.
Pred-G.
TobraDex.
antibiotics/anti-infectives.
See: Adriamycin PFS.
Adriamycin RDF.
Amobicidue, General.
Amikacin Sulfate.
Amoxicillin.
Amoxicillin and Clavulanate Potas-
sium.
Amoxicillin w/Comb.
Ampicillin.
Ampicillin w/Comb.
Anthelmintics.
Anthracyclines.
Antifungal agents.
Antimalarial agents.
Antiprotozoal agents.
Antituberculosis agents.
Antiviral agents.
Azithromycin.
Aztreonam.
Bacampicillin Hydrochloride.
Bacitracin.
Band-Aid Plus.
Betadine First Aid Antibiotics Plus
Moisturizer.
Betadine Plus First Aid Antibiotics and
Pain Reliever.
Bicillin C-R.
Blenoxane.
Bleomycin Sulfate.
Carbenicillin.
Capecitabine.
Cefaclor.
Cefadroxil.
Cefamandole Nafate.
Cefazolin Sodium.
Cefditoren Pivoxil.
Cefixime.
Cefmetazole Sodium.
Cefonicid Sodium.
Cefoperazone Sodium.
Cefotaxime Sodium.
Cefotetan Disodium.
Cefoxitin Sodium.
Cefpodoxime Proxetil.

Cefprozil.
Ceftazidime.
Ceftizoxime Sodium.
Ceftriaxone Sodium.
Cefuroxime.
Cephalexin.
Cephalexin Monohydrate.
Cephalothin Sodium.
Cephradine.
Chibroxin.
Chloramphenicol.
Ciclopirox.
Ciprofloxacin.
Clarithromycin.
Clindamycin.
Clioquinol.
Clofazimine.
Clotrimazole.
Cloxacillin Sodium.
Colistimethate Sodium.
Colistin Sulfate.
Cruex.
Dactinomycin.
Dapsone.
Daunorubicin Citrate Liposomal.
Daunorubicin Hydrochloride.
Demeclocycline.
Desenex.
Dicloxacillin.
Double Antibiotic.
Double Antibiotic Plus.
Doxil.
Doxorubicin Hydrochloride.
Doxycycline.
Econazole Nitrate.
Ellence.
Enoxacin.
Epirubicin Hydrochloride.
Erythromycin.
Erythromycin w/Comb.
Fungicides.
Fungoid.
Furazolidone.
Gentamicin Sulfate.
Gentian Violet.
Idamycin.
Idamycin PFS.
Idarubicin Hydrochloride.
Kanamycin Sulfate.
Keftab.
Lanabiotic.
Levofloxacin.
Lincomycin.
Lomefloxacin Hydrochloride.
Loprox.
Lorabid.
Lorcarbef.
Lotrimin.
Lotrimin AF.
Mandol.
Methacycline Hydrochloride.

Methenamine.
Methenamine w/Comb.
Methicillin Sodium.
Methylene Blue.
Metronidazole.
Mezlocillin Sodium.
Minocycline.
Mitomycin.
Nafcillin Sodium.
Nalidixic Acid.
Neomycin Sulfate.
Neosporin Original.
Neosporin Plus Pain Relief Maximum
  Strength.
Netilmicin Sulfate.
Nitrofurantoin.
Norfloxacin.
Novobiocin.
Ocuflox.
Ofloxacin.
Oxacillin Sodium.
Oxytetracycline.
Paromomycin.
Penicillin G Benzathine.
Penicillin G Benzathine w/Comb.
Penicillin G Potassium.
Penicillin G Potassium w/Comb.
Penicillin G Procaine.
Penicillin G Procaine w/Comb.
Penicillin G Sodium.
Penicillin V Potassium.
Penlac Nail Lacquer.
Pentamidine Isethionate.
Phenoxymethyl Penicillin.
Piperacillin Sodium.
Piperacillin Sodium w/Comb.
Polymyxin B Sulfate.
Polysporin.
Pyrimidine Analogs.
Quixin.
Rubex.
Spectazole.
Spectracef.
Spectinomycin.
Spectinmycin Sulfate.
Spectrocin Plus.
Sulfadiazine.
Sulfamethizole.
Sulfamethoxazole.
Sulfamethoxazole w/Comb.
Sulfasalazine.
Sulfasalazine w/Comb.
Sulfisoxazole.
Sulfonamides.
Tetracycline Hydrochloride.
Ticarcillin Disodium.
Ticarcillin w/Comb.
Tobramycin Sulfate.
Triacetyloleandomycin.
Tri-Biozene.
Triple Antibiotic.

Triple Antibiotic Plus.
Trimethoprim.
Trimethoprim w/Comb.
Trimetrexate Glucuronate.
Troleandomycin.
Valrubicin.
Valstar.
Vancomycin Hydrochloride.
Xeloda.
antibiotics, combinations.
  See: AK-Poly-Bac.
  AK-Spore.
  Bacitracin Zinc and Polymyxin B Sul-
    fate.
  Band-Aid Plus.
  Betadine Plus First Aid Antibiotics and
    Pain Reliever.
  Betadine First Aid Antibiotics Plus
    Moisturizer.
  Double Antibiotic.
  Double Antibiotic Plus.
  Lanabiotic.
  Neomycin and Polymyxin B Sulfates
    and Bacitracin Zinc.
  Neomycin and Polymyxin B Sulfates
    and Gramicidin.
  Neosporin.
  Neosporin Original.
  Neosporin Plus Pain Relief Maximum
    Strength.
  Polysporin.
  Polytrim.
  Spectrocin Plus.
  Terak with Polymyxin B Sulfate.
  Terramycin w/Polymyxin B Sulfate.
  Tri-Biozene.
  Triple Antibiotic.
  Triple Antibiotic Plus.
antibiotics, ophthalmic.
  See: Gatifloxacin.
  Moxifloxacin Hydrochloride.
antibodies, monoclonal.
  See: Alemtuzumab.
  Campath.
  Herceptin.
  Rituxan.
  Rituximab.
  Trastuzumab.
anticholinergic agents.
  Use: Antiemetic/antivertigo agents; anti-
    parkinson agents; bronchodilators.
  See: Antispasmodics.
  Belladonna Alkaloids.
  Benztropine Mesylate.
  Biperiden.
  Buclizine Hydrochloride.
  Cyclizine.
  Darifenacin Hydrobromide.
  Dimenhydrinate.
  Diphenhydramine.
  Flavoxate Hydrochloride.

Glycopyrrolate.
Ipratropium Bromide.
Ipratropium Bromide and Albuterol
  Sulfate.
Meclizine Hydrochloride.
Mepenzolate Bromide.
Methscopolamine Bromide.
Oxybutynin Chloride.
Procyclidine.
Propantheline Bromide.
Scopolamine.
Solifenacin Succinate.
Tiotropium Bromide.
Tolterodine Tartrate.
Trihexyphenidyl Hydrochloride.
Trimethobenzamide Hydrochloride.
Trospium Chloride.
**anticholinergic and antitussive combi-
nations.**
Use: Upper respiratory combination.
See: Hycodan.
  Hydromet.
  Hydromide.
  Hydropane.
  Tussigon.
**anticholinergic and decongestant
combinations.**
Use: Upper respiratory combination.
See: AlleRx-D.
  PSE 120/MSC 2.5.
**anticholinergic, antihistamine, and de-
congestant combinations.**
Use: Upper respiratory combination.
See: Accu list LA.
  AH-chew.
  AlleRx Dose Pack.
  CPM 8/PSE 90/MSC 2.5.
  D.A.
  D.A. II.
  Dallergy.
  Dallergy Extended Release.
  Dehistine.
  DriHist SR.
  Duradryl.
  Duradryl JR.
  Durahist.
  Dura-Vent/DA.
  Ex-Histine.
  Extendryl.
  Extendryl JR.
  Extendryl SR.
  Hista-Vent DA.
  Mescolor.
  OMNIhist L.A.
  Pannaz.
  Pannaz S.
  Pre-Hist-D.
  Rescon-MX.
  Respa A.R.
  Stahist.

●**anticoagulant citrate dextrose solution.** *USP 28.*
Use: Anticoagulant for storage of whole
blood.
See: A-C-D.
●**anticoagulant citrate phosphate dextrose adenine solution.** *USP 28.*
Use: Anticoagulant for storage of whole
blood.
●**anticoagulant citrate phosphate dex-
trose solution.** *USP 28.*
Use: Anticoagulant for storage of whole
blood.
●**anticoagulant heparin solution.**
USP 28.
Use: Anticoagulant for storage of whole
blood.
●**anticoagulant sodium citrate solution.**
USP 28.
Use: Anticoagulant for plasma and
blood fractionation.
anticoagulants.
See: Anisindione.
  Antithrombin Agents.
  Ardeparin sodium.
  Argatroban.
  Bivalirudin.
  Dalteparin Sodium.
  Danaparoid Sodium.
  Desirudin.
  Diphenadione.
  Enoxaparin Sodium.
  Ethyl Biscoumacetate.
  Fondaparinux Sodium.
  Heparin.
  Lepirudin.
  Low Molecular Weight Heparins.
  Selective Factor Xa Inhibitor.
  Thrombin Inhibitor.
  Tinzaparin Sodium.
  Warfarin.
●**anticoagulant sodium citrate solution.**
USP 28.
Use: Anticoagulant for plasma and
blood fractionation.
anticonvulsants.
See: Acetazolamide.
  Benzodiazepines.
  Carbamazepine.
  Clonazepam.
  Clorazepate Dipotassium.
  Diazepam.
  Felbamate.
  Gabapentin.
  Lamotrigine.
  Levetiracetam.
  Lorazepam.
  Magnesium Sulfate.
  Mephobarbital.
  Methsuximide.

Oxcarbazepine.
Phenobarbital.
Phenytoin.
Phenytoin Sodium.
Primidone.
Tiagabine Hydrochloride.
Topiramate.
Valproic Acid.
Zonisamide.
anticytomegalovirus monoclonal antibodies.
Use: Treatment of cytomegalovirus.
antidepressants.
See: Amitriptyline Hydrochloride.
Amoxapine.
Bupropion Hydrochloride.
Citalopram Hydrobromide.
Clomipramine Hydrochloride.
Desipramine Hydrochloride.
Doxepin Hydrochloride.
Duloxetine Hydrochloride.
Escitalopram Oxalate.
Fluoxetine Hydrochloride.
Fluvoxamine Maleate.
Imipramine Hydrochloride.
Imipramine Pamoate.
Isocarboxazid.
Maprotiline Hydrochloride.
Mirtazapine.
Monoamine Oxidase Inhibitors.
Nefazodone Hydrochloride.
Nortriptyline Hydrochloride.
Paroxetine.
Phenelzine Sulfate.
Protriptyline Hydrochloride.
Selective Serotonin Reuptake Inhibitors.
Sertraline Hydrochloride.
Tetracyclic Compounds.
Tranylcypromine Sulfate.
Trazodone Hydrochloride.
Tricyclic Compounds.
Trimipramine Maleate.
Venlafaxine Hydrochloride.
antidiabetic combinations.
See: Glipizide and Metformin Hydrochloride.
Glyburide and Metformin Hydrochloride.
Rosiglitazone Maleate and Metformin Hydrochloride.
antidiabetics.
See: Acarbose.
Acetohexamide.
Alpha-Glucosidase Inhibitors.
Amylin Analog.
Biguanides.
Chlorpropamide.
Exenatide.
Glimepiride.
Glipizide.

Glyburide.
Glipizide/Metformin Hydrochloride.
Glyburide/Metformin Hydrochloride.
Incretin Mimetic Agents.
Insulin.
Insulin Analog.
Insulin Glargine.
Insulin Glulisine.
Insulin Zinc, Extended (Ultralente).
Insulin Zinc (Lente).
Isophane Insulin.
Meglitinides.
Metformin Hydrochloride.
Miglitol.
Nateglinide.
Pioglitazone Hydrochloride.
Pramlintide Acetate.
Repaglinide.
Rosiglitazone Maleate.
Rosiglitazone Maleate/Metformin Hydrochloride.
Sulfonylureas.
Thiazolidinediones.
Tolazamide.
Tolbutamide.
antidiarrheals.
See: Attapulgite, Activated.
Cantil.
Coly-Mycin S.
Diasorb.
Diphenoxylate Hydrochloride w/Atropine Sulfate.
Furoxone.
Imodium.
Imodium A-D.
K-Pek.
Kaodene Non-Narcotic.
Kaolin.
Kaolin Colloidal.
Kaopectate.
Kao-Spen.
Kapectolin.
K-C.
Lactinex.
Lactobacillus acidophilus and *bulgaricus* mixed culture.
Lactobacillus acidophilus, viable culture.
Logen.
Lomanate.
Lomotil.
Lonox.
Loperamide.
Milk of Bismuth.
Motofen.
Mycifradin Sulfate.
Pepto-Bismol.
Pepto Diarrhea Control.
Pink Bismuth.
Rheaban Maximum Strength.

antidiuretics.
See: Pitressin.
Pitressin Tannate In Oil.
Pituitary Post. Inj.
antidotes.
See: Acetylcysteine.
Charcoal, Activated.
Digoxin Immune Fab (Ovine).
Flumazenil.
Fomepizole.
Ipecac Syrup.
Methylene Blue.
Nalmefene Hydrochloride.
Naltrexone Hydrochloride.
Narctotic Antagonists.
Physostigmine Salicylate.
Pralidoxime Chloride.
antiemetic/antivertigo agents.
See: Alosetron Hydrochloride.
Anticholinergics.
Aprepitant.
Dimenhydrinate.
Dolasetron Mesylate.
Dronabinol.
Dymenate.
Granisetron Hydrochloride.
Meclizine Hydrochloride.
Metoclopramide.
Ondansetron Hydrochloride.
Phosphorated Carbohydrate Solution.
Prochlorperazine.
Scopolamine.
Trimethobenzamide Hydrochloride.
antiepilepsirine.
Use: Treatment for drug-resistant generalized tonic-clonic epilepsy.
[Orphan Drug]
antiepileptic agents.
See: Anticonvulsants.
antiestrogen.
Use: Hormone for cancer therapy.
See: Fulvestrant.
Tamoxifen Citrate.
Toremifene Citrate.
antifebrin.
See: Acetanilid.
antiflatulents.
See: Di-Gel.
Simethicone.
Antifoam A Compound. (Hoechst)
Use: Antiflatulent.
See: Simethicone.
antifolic acid.
See: Methotrexate.
Antiformin. Sodium hypochlorite in sodium hydroxide 7.5%, available chlorine 5.2%; may be colored with meta cresol purple.
Use: Antiseptic; antimicrobial.
antifungal agents.
See: Allylamine Antifungals.

Amphotericin B Desoxycholate.
Amphotericin B, Lipid-based.
Butenafine Hydrochloride.
Caspofungin Acetate.
Ciclopirox.
Clioquinol.
Clotrimazole.
Echinocandins.
Econazole Nitrate.
Fluconazole.
Flucytosine.
Fungicides.
Gentian Violet.
Griseofulvin.
Imidazole Antifungals.
Itraconazole.
Ketoconazole.
Micafungin Sodium.
Nystatin.
Polyene Antifungals.
Sertaconazole Nitrate.
Terbinafine Hydrochloride.
Triazole Antifungals.
Voriconazole.
antiglaucoma agents.
See: AKBeta.
Betagan Liquifilm.
Betaxolol Hydrochloride.
Betaxon Hydrochloride.
Betimol.
Betoptic.
Betoptic S.
Bimatoprost.
Carteolol Hydrochloride.
Levobetaxolol Hydrochloride.
Levobunolol.
Levobunolol Hydrochloride.
Lumigan.
Metipranolol Hydrochloride.
Ocupress.
OptiPranolol.
Rescula.
Timolol.
Timolol Maleate.
Timoptic.
Timoptic-XE.
Travatan.
Travoprost.
Unoprostone Isopropyl.
antihemophilic agents.
See: Antihemophilic Factor (Factor VIII; AHF).
Anti-Inhibitor Coagulant Complex.
Coagulation Factor VIIa (Recombinant).
Factor IX Concentrates.
Kogenate.
•**antihemophilic factor (factor VIII; AHF).**
USP 28.
Use: Antihemophilic.
See: Advate.
Alphanate.

Bioclate.
Helixate FS.
Hemofil M.
Hyate:C (Porcine).
Koate-DVI.
Koate HP.
Kogenate FS.
Monoclate-P.
Monarc-M.
Recombinate.
ReFacto.
W/von Willebrand Factor Complex.
See: Humate-P.
antihemophilic factor, human.
Use: Treatment of von Willebrand disease. [Orphan Drug]
See: Alphanate.
Humate P.
antihemophilic factor (recombinant).
Use: Prophylaxis/treatment of bleeding in hemophilia A. [Orphan Drug]
See: Kogenate FS.
antiheparin.
See: Protamine Sulfate.
antiherpes virus agents.
Use: Antiviral.
See: Acyclovir.
Famciclovir.
Valacyclovir Hydrochloride.
antihistamine, analgesic, and decongestant combinations.
Use: Upper respiratory combination.
See: Analgesic, Antihistamine, and Decongestant Combinations.
antihistamine and analgesic combinations.
Use: Upper respiratory combination.
See: Analgesic and antihistamine combinations.
antihistamine and antitussive combinations.
Use: Upper respiratory combination.
See: Coricidin HBP Cough & Cold.
Prometh w/Codeine Cough.
Scot-Tussin DM.
S-T Forte 2.
Tannic-12.
Tricodene Cough & Cold.
Tricodene Sugar Free.
Trionate.
Tussionex Pennkinetic.
Tussi-12.
Tussi-12 S.
antihistamine and decongestant combinations.
Use: Upper respiratory combination.
See: AccuHist Pediatric.
Actifed Cold & Allergy.
Allegra-D.
Allerest Maximum Strength.
Allerfrim.

AlleRx.
Amerifed.
Andehist.
Aprodine.
Benadryl Allergy & Sinus.
Benadryl Children's Allergy & Cold.
Benadryl Children's Allergy & Sinus.
Biohist-LA.
Brofed.
Bromanate.
Bromfed.
Bromfed-PD.
Bromfenex.
Bromfenex PD.
Brompheniramine Maleate and Pseudoephedrine Hydrochloride.
Carbinoxamine.
Cardec-S.
Cenafed Plus.
Chlorpheniramine Maleate/Pseudoephedrine Hydrochloride ER.
Chlorpheniramine Tannate/Pseudoephedrine Tannate.
Chlor-Trimeton Allergy•D 4 Hour.
Chlor-Trimeton Allergy•D 12 Hour.
Claritin-D 12 Hour.
Claritin-D 24 Hour.
Coldec D.
Colfed-A.
C-PHED Tannate.
CP-TANNIC.
Cydec.
Dallergy-JR.
Deconomed SR.
Deconamine.
Deconamine SR.
Dimaphen.
Dimetapp Cold & Allergy.
Drixomed.
Drixoral Cold & Allergy.
Duonate-12.
Dytan-D.
Ed A-Hist.
Genac.
Histab Plus.
Histade.
Histex.
Histex SR.
Kronofed-A.
Kronofed-A Jr.
Lodrane.
Lodrane LD.
N D Clear.
Palgic-D.
Palgic DS.
PediaCare Children's Cold & Allergy.
Pediatex-D.
Phenylephrine Tannate/Chlorpheniramine Tannate/Pyrilamine Tannate Pediatric.

Promethazine Hydrochloride and Phenylephrine Hydrochloride.
Prometh VC Plain.
Quadra-Hist D.
Quadra-Hist D PED.
Rescon Jr.
Rescon 12 Hour.
Respahist.
Rhinatate Pediatric.
Rinade B.I.D.
Rondec.
Rondec-TR.
R-Tanna 12.
R-Tannic-S A/D.
Ryna.
Rynatan.
Rynatan Pediatric.
Ryna-12.
Ryna-12 S.
Ucot Tussin Huylubrol.
Semprex-D.
Silafed.
Sudafed Cold & Allergy Maximum Strength.
Sudafed Sinus Nighttime Maximum Strength.
Tanafed.
Thera Hist Cold & Allergy.
Time-Hist.
Touro Allergy.
Triacting Cold & Allergy.
Tri-Acting Cold & Allergy.
Triaminic.
Triaminic Cold & Allergy.
Trinalin Repetabs.
Triotann Pediatric.
Triotann-S Pediatric.
Triprolidine Hydrochloride w/Pseudoephedrine Hydrochloride.
ULTRAbrom.
ULTRAbrom PD.
Zyrtec-D 12 Hour.

antihistamine, anticholinergic, and decongestant combinations.
Use: Upper respiratory combination.
See: Anticholinergic, Antihistamine, and Decongestant Combinations.

antihistamine, antitussive, analgesic, and decongestant combinations.
Use: Upper respiratory combination.
See: Analgesic, Antihistamine, Antitussive, and Decongestant Combinations.

antihistamine, antitussive, and analgesic combinations.
Use: Upper respiratory combination.
See: Analgesic, Antihistamine, and Antitussive Combinations.

antihistamine, antitussive, and decongestant combinations.
Use: Upper respiratory combination.

See: AccuHist DM Pediatric.
All-Nite Children's Cold/Cough Relief.
Anaplex-DM.
Anaplex HD.
Andehist-DM.
Atuss HD.
Atuss MS.
Balamine DM.
Bellahist-D LA.
Bromanate DM Cold & Cough.
Bromatane DX.
Bromfed DM Cough.
Carbinoxamine Compound.
Carbofed DM.
Cardec DM.
Children's Elixir DM Cough & Cold.
Codal-DH.
Codimal DH.
Codimal PH.
Coldec DM.
Comtussin HC.
C.P.-DM.
Cydec-DM.
Cytuss HC.
Decohistine DH.
Dicomal-DH.
Dihistine DH.
Dimaphen DM Cold & Cough.
Dimetapp DM Children's Cold & Cough.
ED-TLC.
ED Tuss HC.
Endagen-HD.
Histinex HC.
Histinex PV.
Histussin HC.
Hydrocodone CP.
Hydrocodone HD.
Hydro-PC.
Hydro-Tussin HC.
Hyphed
Kid Kare Children's Cough/Cold.
Maxi-Tuss HC.
Nite Time Children's.
Pancof-HC.
Pedia Care Cough-Cold.
Pedia Care Multi-Symptom Cold.
Pedia Care NightRest Cough & Cold.
Pediatex-DM.
Promethazine VC w/Codeine Cough.
Prometh VC w/Codeine Cough.
P-V Tussin.
Quad Tann.
Robitussin Allergy & Cough.
Robitussin Pediatric Night Relief Cough & Cold.
Rondec-DM.
Rynatuss.
Rynatuss Pediatric.
Sildec-DM.
Statuss Green.
Tannic-12.

Thera-Hist Cold & Cough.
Triacin-C Cough.
Tri-Acting Cold & Cough.
Triaminic Cold & Cough.
Triaminic Cold & Night Time Cough.
Triaminic Cough.
Tussafed.
Tussend.
Vanex HD.
Vicks Children's NyQuil Cold/Cough
Relief.
Vicks Pediatric 44M Cough & Cold
Relief.
Z-Cof HC.

antihistamine, antitussive, decongestant, expectorant combinations.
Use: Upper respiratory combination.
See: Donatussin.
Tussirex.
Tussirex Sugar Free.
ZTuss Expectorant.

Antihistamine Cream. (Towne) Methapyrilene hydrochloride 10 mg, pyrilamine maleate 5 mg, allantoin 2 mg, diperodon hydrochloride 2.5 mg, benzocaine 10 mg, menthol 2 mg/g. Cream. Jar 2 oz. *OTC.*
Use: Antihistamine, topical.

antihistamine, decongestant, and expectorant combinations.
Use: Upper respiratory combination.
See: Decolate.
Donatussin.
Polaramine Expectorant.

antihistamines.
See: Alkylamines, Nonselective.
Azatadine Maleate.
Azelastine Hydrochloride.
Brompheniramine Tannate.
Carbinoxamine Maleate.
Cetirizine Hydrochloride.
Chlorpheniramine Maleate.
Clemastine Fumarate.
Cyproheptadine Hydrochloride.
Desloratadine.
Dexchlorpheniramine Maleate.
Diphenhydramine Hydrochloride.
Doxylamine Succinate.
Efidac 24 Chlorpheniramine.
Ethanolamines, Nonselective.
Fexofenadine Hydrochloride.
Hydroxyzine.
Hydroxyzine Hydrochloride.
Hydroxyzine Pamoate.
Loratadine.
Phenindamine Tartrate.
Phenothiazines, Nonselective.
Phthalazinones, Peripherally-selective.
Piperazine, Peripherally-selective.
Piperazines, Nonselective.
Piperidines, Nonselective.
Piperidines, Peripherally-selective.
Promethazine Hydrochloride.
Prophenpyridamine Maleate.
Pyrilamine Maleate.
Tripelennamine Hydrochloride.
Triprolidine Hydrochloride.

Antihist-1. (Various Mfr.) Clemastine fumarate 1.34 mg. Tab. Pkg. 16s. *OTC.*
Use: Antihistamine.

antihyperlipidemics.
See: Atorvastatin Calcium.
Cholestyramine.
Clofibrate.
Colesevelam Hydrochloride.
Colestipol Hydrochloride.
Ezetimibe.
Ezetimibe/Simvastatin.
Fenofibrate.
Fluvastatin Sodium.
Gemfibrozil.
HMG-CoA Reductase Inhibitors.
Lovastatin.
Niacin.
Niacin (Extended Release)/Lovastatin.
Pravastatin Sodium.
Simvastatin.

antihyperlipidemic combinations.
See: Amlodipine Besylate/Atorvastatin Calcium.
Aspirin/Pravastatin.
Ezetimibe/Simvastatin.
Niacin (Extended Release)/Lovastatin.

antihypertensives.
See: Accupril.
Acebutolol Hydrochloride.
Aceon.
Adaprolol Maleate.
Alazide.
Alazine.
Aldactazide.
Aldactone.
Aldoclor 250.
Aldomet.
Aldoril.
Alfuzosin Hydrochloride.
Alpha$_1$-Adrenergic Blockers.
Altace.
Althiazide.
Amiquinsin Hydrochloride.
Amlodipine Besylate.
Amlodipine Maleate.
Amodopa.
Anaritide Acetate.
ACE Inhibitors.
Apresazide.
Apresodex.
Apresoline.
Aprozide.

Arcum R-S.
Arlix.
Artarau.
Atenolol/Chlorthalidone.
Atiprosin Maleate.
Belfosdil.
Bendacalol Mesylate.
Bendroflumethiazide.
Betaxolol Hydrochloride.
Bethanidine Sulfate.
Bevantolol Hydrochloride.
Biclodil Hydrochloride.
Bisoprolol Humarate.
Bucindolol Hydrochloride.
Cam-Ap-Es.
Candoxatril.
Candoxatrilat.
Capoten.
Capozide.
Cuplupril.
Captopril and Hydrochlorothiazide.
Cardura.
Carvedilol.
Catapres.
Ceronapril.
Chlorothiazide Sodium.
Chlorthalidone.
Cicletanine
Cilazapril.
Cithal.
Citrin.
Clentiazem Maleate.
Clonidine.
Clonidine Hydrochloride.
Clonidine Hydrochloride and Chlor-
thalidone.
Clopamide.
Combipres.
Coreg.
Corzide.
Cyclothiazide.
De Serpa.
Debrisoquin Sulfate.
Delapril Hydrochloride.
Demser.
Diaserp.
Diazoxide.
Diazoxide Parenteral.
Dibenzyline.
Dilevalol Hydrochloride.
Diovan.
Ditekiren.
Diucardin.
Diulo.
Diurigen w/Reserpine.
Diuril.
Diuril Sodium.
Diutensen-R.
Doxazosin Mesylate.
Elserpine.
Enalaprilat.

Enalapril Maleate.
Enalkiren.
Endralazine Mesylate.
Enduronyl.
Enduronyl Forte.
Eprosartan.
Eprosartan Mesylate.
Eserdine.
Eserdine Forte.
Esidrix.
Esimil.
Exna.
Fenoldopam Mesylate.
Flavodilol Maleate.
Flolan.
Flordipine.
Flosequinan.
Forasartan.
Fosinopril.
Fosinoprilat
Fosinopril Sodium.
Guanabenz.
Guanabenz Acetate.
Guanacline Sulfate.
Guanadrel Sulfate.
Guancydine.
Guanethidine Monosulfate.
Guanethidine Sulfate.
Guanfacine Hydrochloride.
Guanisoquin.
Guanisoquin Sulfate.
Guanocitine Hydrochloride.
Guanoclor Sulfate.
Guanoxabenz.
Guanoxan Sulfate.
Guanoxyfen Sulfate.
Harbolin.
H.H.R.
Hiwolfia.
Hydralazine.
Hydralazine Hydrochloride.
Hydralazine Polistirex.
Hydrap-ES.
Hydraserp.
Hydra-Zide.
Hydrazide.
Hydrochloroserpine.
Hydrochlorothiazide/Hydralazine.
Hydroflumethiazide.
Hydromox-R.
Hydropine.
Hydropine H.P.
Hydropres-50.
Hydroserp.
Hydroserp-50.
Hydroserpine #1, #2.
Hydrosine 25, 50.
Hydrotensin-50.
Hydroxyisoindolin.
Hylorel.
Hyperstat.

Hytrin.
Hyzaar.
Indacrinone.
Indapamide.
Inderide.
Indolapril Hydrochloride.
Indoramin.
Indoramin Hydrochloride.
Indorenate Hydrochloride.
Ingadine.
Inhibace.
Inversine.
Irbesartan.
Ismelin.
Labetalol Hydrochloride.
Leniquinsin.
Levcromakalim.
Lexxel.
Lofexidine Hydrochloride.
Loniten.
Lopressor HCT.
Losartan Potassium.
Losulazine Hydrochloride.
Lotensin.
Lotrel.
Lozol.
Marpres.
Mavik.
Maxzide.
Mebutamate.
Mecamylamine Hydrochloride.
Medroxalol.
Medroxalol Hydrochloride.
Metatensin.
Methalthiazide.
Methyclodine.
Methylclothiazide.
Methyldopa.
Methyldopa and Chlorothiazide.
Methyldopa and Hydrochlorothiazide.
Methyldopate Hydrochloride.
Metipranolol.
Metipranolol Hydrochloride.
Metolazone.
Metoprolol Fumarate.
Metoprolol Succinate.
Metoprolol Tartrate and Hydrochloro-
    thiazide.
Metyrosine.
Midamor.
Minipress.
Minizide.
Minoxidil.
Moduretic.
Moexipril Hydrochloride.
Monopril.
Muzolimine.
Nadolol.
Nadolol and Bendroflumethiazide.
Natrico.
Nebivolol.

Nitrendipine.
Nitropress.
Nitroprusside Sodium.
Normodyne.
Normotensin.
Pargyline Hydrochloride.
Pelanserin Hydrochloride.
Pentina.
Pentolinium Tartrate.
Perindoprll Erbumine.
Pheniprazine Hydrochloride.
Phenoxybenzamine Hydrochloride.
Phentolamine Hydrochloride.
Pinacidil.
Pivopril.
Prazosin Hydrochloride.
Prinivil.
Prinzide.
Priscoline.
Prizidilol Hydrochloride.
Propanolol Hydrochloride and Hydro-
    chlorothiazide.
Quinaprilat.
Quinapril Hydrochloride.
Quinazosin Hydrochloride.
Quinelorane Hydrochloride.
Quinuclium Bromide.
Ramipril.
Rauneed.
Raunescine.
Raurine.
Rautina.
Rauval.
Rauwolfia/Bendroflumethiazide.
Rauwolfia Serpentina.
Rauwolscine.
Rauzide.
Rawfola.
Regroton.
Regroton Demi.
Renese.
Renese-R.
Reserpaneed.
Reserpine.
Reserpine and Chlorothiazide.
Reserpine and Hydrochlorothiazide.
Reserpine, Hydralazine Hydrochlo-
    ride, and Hydrochlorothiazide.
R-HCTZ-H.
Salazide.
Salazide-Demi.
Salutensin.
Salutensin-Demi.
Saprisartan Potassium.
Saralasin Acetate.
Sectral.
Ser-A-Gen.
Ser-Ap-Es.
Serpasil-Apresoline.
Serpasil-Esidrix.
Serpazide.

Sertabs.
Sertina.
Sodium Nitroprusside.
Sulfinalol Hydrochloride.
Tarka.
Teludipine Hydrochloride.
Temocapril Hydrochloride.
Tenex.
Tenoretic.
Tenormin.
Terazosin Hydrochloride.
Tiamenidine Hydrochloride.
Ticrynafen.
Timolide 10-25.
Timolol Maleate.
Timolol Maleate and Hydrochloride.
Tinabinol.
Tipentosin Hydrochloride.
Tolazoline Hydrochloride.
Toprol XL.
Trandate.
Trandate Hydrochlorothiazide.
Tri-Hydroserpine.
Trimazosin Hydrochloride.
Trimethamide.
Trimoxamine Hydrochloride.
T-Sert.
Univasc.
Valsartan.
Vaseretic.
Vasotec.
Visken.
Xipamide.
Zankiren Hydrochloride.
Zepine.
Zestoretic.
Zestril.
Ziac.
Zofenoprilat Arginine.
anti-infectives.
See: Antibiotics/Anti-infectives.
anti-infectives, miscellaneous.
See: Clindamycin Phosphate.
Metronidazole.
anti-infectives, topical.
See: Amphotericin B.
Antifungal Agents.
Band-Aid Plus.
Betadine Plus First Aid Antibiotics and
Pain Reliever.
Betadine First Aid Antibiotics Plus
Moisturizer.
Butenafine Hydrochloride.
Double Antibiotic.
Double Antibiotic Plus.
Econazole Nitrate.
Fungizone.
Gentian Violet.
Lanabiotic.
Mentax.
Neosporin Original.

Neosporin Plus Pain Relief Maximum
Strength.
Polysporin.
Sertaconazole Nitrate.
Spectrocin Plus.
Tri-Biozene.
Triple Antibiotic.
Triple Antibiotic Plus.
anti-inhibitor coagulant complex.
Use: Antihemophilic agent.
See: Autoplex T.
Feiba VH Immuno.
Anti-Itch. (Taro) Diphenhydramine 2%,
zinc acetate 0.1%. Cetyl alcohol, para-
bens. Cream. 28.4 g. OTC.
Use: Topical antihistamine.
Anti-Itch Gel. (Band-Aid) Camphor
0.45%, SD alcohol 23 A 37%. Gel. 60 g.
OTC.
Use: Poison ivy treatment.
Antilerge. (Merz) Chlorpheniramine
maleate 8 mg, phenylephrine hydro-
chloride 12 mg. Tab. Bot. 30s. OTC.
Use: Antihistamine; decongestant.
antileukemia.
See: Antineoplastic agents.
Antilirium. (Forest) Physostigmine sa-
licylate 1 mg/mL, benzyl alcohol 2%,
sodium bisulfite 0.1%. 2 mL. Rx.
Use: Antidote. [Orphan Drug]
antimalarial agents.
See: Atovaquone and Proguanil Hydro-
chloride.
Folic Acid Antagonists.
Halofantrine Hydrochloride.
Hydroxychloroquine Sulfate.
Mefloquine Hydrochloride.
Pyrimethamine.
Quinine Sulfate.
Sulfadoxine and Pyrimethamine.
antimetabolites.
See: Allopurinol.
Capecitabine.
Cladribine.
Clofarabine.
Cytarabine.
Floxuridine.
Fludarabine Phosphate.
Fluorouracil.
Folic Acid Antagonists.
Gemcitabine.
Mercaptopurine.
Methotrexate.
Pemetrexed.
Pentostatin.
Purine Analogs and Related Agents.
Pyrimidine Analogs.
Rasburicase.
Thioguanine.
antimigraine agents.
See: Almotriptan Maleate.

Amerge.
Axert.
Frova.
Frovatriptan Succinate.
Imitrex.
Maxalt.
Maxalt-MLT.
Midrin.
Naratriptan Hydrochloride.
Rizatriptan Benzoate.
Serotonin 5-HT$_1$Receptor Agonists.
Sumatriptan Succinate.
Zolmitriptan.
Zomig.
Zomig ZMT.
antimitotic agents.
 See: Docetaxel.
 Paclitaxel.
 Taxoids.
 Vinblastine Sulfate (VLB).
 Vinca Alkaloids.
 Vincristine Sulfate.
 Vinorelbine Tartrate.
•**antimony potassium tartrate.** *USP 28.*
 Use: Antischistosomal; leishmaniasis;
 expectorant; emetic.
 W/Cocillana, euphorbia pilulifera, squill,
 senega.
 See: Cylana.
 W/Guaifenesin, codeine phosphate.
 See: Cheracol.
 W/Guaifenesin, dextromethorphan HBr.
 See: Cheracol D.
antimony preparations.
 See: Antimony Potassium Tartrate.
 Antimony Sodium Thioglycollate.
 Tartar Emetic.
•**antimony sodium tartrate.** *USP 28.*
 Use: Antischistosomal.
antimony sodium thioglycollate.
 (Various Mfr.). *Rx.*
 Use: Schistosomiasis; leishmaniasis;
 filariasis.
•**antimony trisulfide colloid.** USAN.
 Use: Pharmaceutic aid.
anti-my9-blocked ricin.
 Use: Leukemia treatment.
antinauseants.
 See: Antiemetic/antivertigo agents
antineoplastic agents.
 See: Adriamycin.
 Allopurinol Sodium.
 Aloprim.
 Amifostine.
 Amsacrine.
 Arsenic Trioxide.
 Azacitidine.
 Blenoxane.
 Cosmegen.
 Elspar.

Emcyt.
Estinyl.
Ethyol.
FUDR.
Gefitinib.
Herceptin.
Hexalen.
Hydrea.
Idamycin.
Leukeran.
Lysodren.
Matulane.
Medroxyprogesterone Acetate.
Megace.
Mercaptopurine
Methotrexate.
Methotrexate Sodium.
Mithracin.
Mitotane.
Mustargen.
Myleran.
Nolvadex.
Oncovin.
Purinethol.
Tamoxifen.
Temodar.
Temozolomide.
Thioguanine.
Thio Tepa.
Trastuzumab.
Trisenox.
antineoplastics, miscellaneous.
 See: Mitotane.
 Porfimer Sodium.
 Talc Powder, Sterile.
antiobesity agents.
 See: Acutrim.
 Adderall.
 Adipex-P.
 Amphetamine.
 Anorex.
 Bontril.
 Control.
 Dexatrim Pre-Meal.
 Dextroamphetamine.
 Didrex.
 Diethylpropion Hydrochloride.
 Dieutrim T.D.
 Fastin.
 Ionamin.
 Levo-Amphetamine.
 Maximum Strength Dexatrim.
 Mazanor.
 Methamphetamine.
 Obe-Nix 30.
 Phendimetrazine Tartrate.
 Phentermine Hydrochloride.
 Phentermine Resin.
 Prelu-2.
 Sanorex.
 Tenuate.

Tenuate Dospan.
Tepanil.
Trimstat.
Wehless Timecelles.
Xenical.
Antiox. (Merz) Vitamin C 120 mg, vitamin E 100 units, beta-carotene 25 mg. Cap. Bot. 60s. *OTC.*
Use: Vitamin supplement.
Anti-Pak Compound. (Lowitt) Phenylephrine hydrochloride 5 mg, salicylamide 0.23 g, acetophenetidin 0.15 g, caffeine 0.03 g, ascorbic acid 50 mg, hesperidin complex 50 mg, chlorprophenpyridamine maleate 2 mg. Tab. Bot. 30s, 100s. *OTC.*
Use: Analgesic; antihistamine; decongestant combination.
antiparasympathomimetics.
See: Parasympatholytic agents.
antiparkinson agents.
See: Anticholinergics.
Amantadine Hydrochloride.
Apomorphine Hydrochloride.
Belladonna Alkaloids.
Benztropine Mesylate.
Biperiden.
Bromocriptine Mesylate.
Carbidopa.
Carbidopa, Levodopa, and Entacapone.
Diphenhydramine.
Dopaminergics.
Entacapone.
Levodopa.
Levodopa and Carbidopa.
Pergolide Mesylate.
Pramipexole.
Procyclidine.
Ropinirole Hydrochloride.
Selegiline Hydrochloride.
Tolcapone.
Trihyexyphenidyl Hydrochloride.
antipellagra vitamin.
See: Nicotinic acid.
antipernicious anemia principle.
See: Vitamin B$_{12}$.
Antiphlogistine. (Denver Chemical [Puerto Rico] Inc.) Medicated poultice. Jar 5 oz, lb. Tube 8 oz. Can 5 lb.
antiplatelet agents.
See: Abciximab.
Anagrelide Hydrochloride.
Clopidogrel.
Dipyridamole.
Eptifibatide.
Glycoprotein IIb/IIIa Inhibitors.
Tirofiban Hydrochloride.
Treprostinil Sodium.
W/Combinations.

See: Dipyridamole and Aspirin.
antiprotozoal agents.
See: Antimony.
Arsenic.
Bismuth.
Diiodohydroxyquinoline.
Emetine Hydrochloride.
Furazolidone.
Levofuraltadone.
Nitazoxanide.
Quinoxyl.
Suramin Sodium.
Tinidazole.
anti-psoriatic agents.
See: Methotrexate.
Selenium Sulfide.
antipsychotics.
See: Aripiprazole.
Benzisoxazole Derivatives.
Chlorpromazine Hydrochloride
Clozapine.
Dibenzapine Derivatives.
Dihydroindolone Derivatives.
Fluphenazine.
Haloperidol.
Lithium.
Loxapine.
Molindone Hydrochloride.
Nucleoside Reverse Transcriptase Inhibitors.
Nucleotide Analog Reverse Transcriptase Inhibitors.
Olanzapine.
Perphenazine.
Phenothiazine Derivatives.
Phenylbutylpiperadine Derivatives.
Pimozide.
Prochlorperazine.
Quetiapine Fumarate.
Quinolinone Derivatives.
Risperidone.
Tenofovir Disoproxil Fumarate.
Thioridazine Hydrochloride.
Thiothixene.
Thioxanthene Derivatives.
Trifluoperazine Hydrochloride..
Ziprasidone.
•**antipyrine.** *USP 28.*
Use: Analgesic; antipyretic.
W/Benzocaine, chlorobutanol.
See: G.B.A.
W/Carbamide, benzocaine, cetyldimethylbenzylammonium hydrochloride.
See: Auralgesic.
W/Phenylephrine hydrochloride, benzocaine.
See: Tympagesic.
antipyrine and benzocaine.
Use: Anesthetic, local.
See: Auro Ear Drops.

antipyrine, benzocaine, and phenylephrine hydrochloride.
Use: Anesthetic, local; decongestant eardrop.
antiretroviral agents.
See: Abacavir/Lamivudine.
Abacavir Sulfate.
Abacavir Sulfate/Lamivudine/Zidovudine.
Amprenavir.
Atazanavir Sulfate.
Delavirdine Mesylate.
Didanosine.
Efavirenz.
Emtricitabine.
Emtricitabine/Tenofovir Disoproxil Fumarate.
Enfuvirtide.
Fosamprenavir Calcium.
Indinavir Sulfate.
Lamivudine (3TC).
Lamivudine/Zidovudine.
Lopinavir/Ritonavir.
Nevirapine.
Non-Nucleoside Reverse Transcriptase Inhibitors.
Nucleoside Analog Reverse Transcriptase Inhibitor Combination.
Nucleoside Reverse Transcriptase Inhibitors.
Nucleotide Analog Reverse Transcriptase Inhibitor.
Protease Inhibitors.
Ritonavir.
Saquinavir.
Stavudine
Tenofovir Disoproxil Fumarate.
Zalcitabine.
Zidovudine.
antirheumatic agents.
See: Arava.
Azulfidine.
Azulfidine EN-tabs.
Hydroxychloroquine Sulfate.
Leflunomide.
Plaquenil.
Sulfasalazine.
antirickettsial agents.
See: p-Aminobenzoic Acid.
Aureomycin.
Chloromycetin.
Terramycin.
antiscorbutic vitamin.
See: Ascorbic Acid.
antiseptic, chlorine, active.
See: Antiseptic, N-Chloro Compounds, Hypochlorite.
antiseptic, dyes.
See: Acriflavine.
Aminoacridine Hydrochloride.
Bismuth Violet.

Crystal Violet.
Fuchsin.
Gentian Violet.
Methylrosaniline Cl.
Methyl Violet.
Pyridium.
antiseptic, mercurials.
See: Merthiolate.
Phenylmercuric Acetate.
Phenylmercuric Borate.
Phenylmercuric Nitrate.
Phenylmercuric Picrate.
Thimerosal.
antiseptic, n-chloro compounds.
See: Chloramine-T.
Chlorazene.
Dichloramine T.
Halazone.
antiseptic, phenols.
See: Anthralin.
Bithionol.
Coal Tar Products.
Creosote.
Guaiacol.
Hexachlorophene.
Hexylresorcinol.
Methylparaben.
Oxyquinoline Salts.
Parachlorometaxylenol.
Phenol.
o-Phenylphenol.
Picric Acid.
Propylparaben.
Pyrogallol.
Resorcinol.
Resorcinol Monoacetate.
Thymol.
Trinitrophenol.
antiseptics.
See: Furacin.
Iodine Products.
Phenols.
antiseptic, surface-active agents.
See: Bactine.
Bactine Pain Relieving Cleansing.
Benzalkonium Cl.
Benzethonium Cl.
Ceepryn.
Cēpacol.
Cetylpyridinium Cl.
Diaparene Cl.
Methylbenzethonium Cl.
Zephiran Cl.
antisickling agents.
See: Droxia.
Hydroxyurea.
Antispas. (Keene Pharmaceuticals) Dicyclomine hydrochloride 10 mg/mL. Vial 10 mL. *Rx.*
Use: Antispasmodic.
antispasmodics. Parasympatholytic agents.

See: Anticholinergic Agents.
Belladonna Alkaloids.
Dicyclomine Hydrochloride.
Spasmolytic Agents.
Antispasmodic Capsules. (Teva)
Phenobarbital 16.2 mg, hyoscyamine
sulfate 0.1037 mg, atropine sulfate
0.0194 mg, scopolamine HBr
0.0065 mg. Cap. Bot. 1000s. *Rx.*
Use: Anticholinergic; antispasmodic;
hypnotic; sedative.
Antispasmodic Elixir. (Various Mfr.)
Atropine sulfate 0.0194 mg, scopol-
amine HBr 0.0065 mg, hyoscyamine
HBr or SO₄ 0.1037 mg, phenobarbital
16.2 mg/mL w/alcohol 23%. Elix. Bot.
120 mL, Pt, gal, and UD 5 mL. *Rx.*
Use: Anticholinergic; antispasmodic;
hypnotic; sedative.
antisterility vitamin.
See: Vitamin E.
antistreptolysin-O.
Use: Titration procedure.
Anti-Tac, Humanized. (Roche)
Use: Prevention of acute renal allograft
rejection. [Orphan Drug]
Anti-Ten. (Century) Allylisobutylbarbituric
acid ¾ g, aspirin 3 g, phenacetin 2 g,
caffeine g. Tab. Bot. 100s, 1000s. *Rx.*
Use: Analgesic; sedative; stimulant.
antithrombin agents.
Use: Anticoagulant.
See: Antithrombin III (Human).
antithrombin III concentrate IV.
Use: Prophylaxis/treatment of thrombo-
embolic episodes in AT-III deficiency.
[Orphan Drug]
•**antithrombin III human.** *USP 28.*
Use: Thromboembolic.
See: Thrombate III.
•**antithymocyte globulin (equine).**
Use: Immune globulin.
See: Atgam.
antithymocyte globulin (rabbit).
Use: Immunosuppressant.
See: Thymoglobulin.
antithyroid agents.
See: Iothiouracil Sodium.
Methimazole.
Methylthiouracil.
Propylthiouracil.
Tapazole.
antitoxins.
See: Botulism Antitoxin.
Diphtheria Antitoxin.
Tetanus Immune Globulin.
antitrypsin, alpha 1.
See: Alpha-1-antitrypsin.
antituberculosis agents.
See: Aminosalicylic Acid.
Capreomycin.

Cycloserine.
Ethambutol Hydrochloride.
Ethionamide.
Isoniazid.
Pyrazinamide.
Rifabutin.
Rifampin.
Rifapentine.
Streptomycin Sulfate.
Anti-Tuss DM. (Century) Guaifenesin
100 mg, dextromethorphan HBr 15 mg/
5 mL. Syr. Bot. 120 mL, 3.8 L. *OTC.*
Use: Antitussive; expectorant.
**antitussive, analgesic, antihistamine,
and decongestant combinations.**
Use: Upper respiratory combination.
See: Analgesic, Antihistamine, Antitus-
sive, and Decongestant Combina-
tions.
**antitussive, analgesic, decongestant,
expectorant combinations.**
Use: Upper respiratory combination.
See: Analgesic, Antitussive, Deconges-
tant, Expectorant Combinations.
**antitussive and anticholinergic combi-
nations.**
Use: Upper respiratory combination.
See: Anticholinergic and Antitussive
Combinations.
**antitussive and antihistamine combi-
nations.**
Use: Upper respiratory combination.
See: Antihistamine and Antitussive
Combinations.
**antitussive and decongestant combi-
nations.**
Use: Upper respiratory combination.
See: Detussin.
Dimetapp Decongestant Plus Cough
Infants.
Histussin D.
Pedia Care Infants' Decongestant &
Cough.
Pedia Relief Decongestant Plus
Cough Infants
P-V-Tussin.
St. Joseph Cough Syrup for Children.
Sudafed Children's Non-Drowsy Cold
& Cough.
Tussend.
**antitussive and expectorant combina-
tions.**
Use: Upper respiratory combination.
See: AccuHist DM Pediatric.
Allfen-DM.
Aquatab DM.
Atuss Ex.
Benylin Expectorant.
Cheracol Cough.
Cheracol D Cough Formula.
Cheracol Plus.

Codeine Phosphate and Guaifenesin.
Codiclear DH.
Coricidin HBP Chest Congestion &
Cough.
Dex GG TR.
Diabetic Tussin DM.
Diabetic Tussin Maximum Strength
DM.
Dilaudid Cough.
Duratuss DM.
Extra Action Cough.
Fenesin DM.
Gani-Tuss-DM NR.
Gani-Tuss NR.
Genatuss DM.
GFN 1200/DM 60.
Guaifenesin DM.
Guaifenesin-DM NR.
Guaifenesin 1000 mg and Dextro-
methorphan HBr 60 mg LA.
Guaifenex DM
Guiadrine DM.
Guiatuss AC.
Guiatuss DM.
Halotussin AC.
Humidid DM.
Hycosin Expectorant.
Hycotuss Expectorant.
Hydrocodone Bitartrate and Guaifen-
esin.
Hydrocodone GF.
Hydron KGS.
Hydro-Tussin DM.
Iobid DM.
Kolephrin GG/DM.
Kwelcof.
Marcof Expectorant.
Maxi-tuss DM.
Muco-Fen-DM.
Mytussin AC Cough.
Mytussin DM.
Naldecon Senior DX.
Phanatuss DM Cough.
Pneumotussin.
Pneumotussin 2.5 Cough.
Prolex DH.
Protuss.
Protuss DH.
Respa-DM.
Robitussin Cough & Congestion For-
mula.
Robitussin DM.
Robitussin DM Infant.
Robitussin Sugar Free Cough.
Romilar AC.
Safe Tussin.
Scot-Tussin Senior Clear.
Siltussin DM Cough.
Sudal-DM.
SU-TUSS DM.
Tolu-Sed DM.

Touro DM.
Tuss-DM.
TUSSI-bid.
Tussi-Organidin-DM NR.
Tussi-Organidin NR.
Tussi-Organidin-S NR.
Vicks 44E Cough & Chest Conges-
tion Relief.
Vicks Pediatric 44e Cough & Chest
Congestion Relief.
Vicodin Tuss.
Vitussin.
Z-Cof LA.

**antitussive, antihistamine, and decon-
gestant combinations.**
Use: Upper respiratory combination.
See: Antihistamine, Antitussive, and
Decongestant Combinations.
**antitussive, antihistamine, deconges-
tant, expectorant combinations.**
Use: Upper respiratory combination.
See: Antihistamine, Antitussive, Decongestant, Expectorant Combinations.
Antitussive Cough Syrup. (Weeks &
Leo) Chlorpheniramine 2 mg, phenylephrine hydrochloride 5 mg, dextromethorphan 15 mg, ammonium Cl
50 mg/5 mL. Syr. Bot. *OTC.*
Use: Antitussive; antihistamine; decon-
gestant; expectorant.
**Antitussive Cough Syrup with Co-
deine.** (Weeks & Leo) Chlorphenir-
amine maleate 2 mg, phenylephrine
hydrochloride 5 mg, codeine phosphate
10 mg, ammonium Cl 50 mg/5 mL. Syr.
Bot. 4 oz. *c-v.*
Use: Antihistamine; antitussive; decon-
gestant; expectorant.
**antitussive, decongestant, expecto-
rant combinations.**
Use: Upper respiratory combination.
See: Aquatab C.
Atuss-G.
Cold & Cough Tussin.
Dihistine Expectorant.
Donatussin DC.
Duratuss HD.
Endal Expectorant.
Entex HC.
GFN 1200/DM 60/PSE 120.
Guaifenex-Rx DM.
Guiatuss CF.
Guiatuss DAC.
Halotussin DAC.
Hydro-Tussin HD.
Levall.
Levall 5.0.
Maxifed DM.
Medent-DM.
MED-Rx DM.
Mytussin DAC.

Novagest Expectorant with Codeine.
Nucofed Expectorant.
Nucofed Pediatric Expectorant.
Nucotuss Expectorant.
Nucotuss Pediatric Expectorant.
Pancof-XP.
Panmist-DM.
Profen Forte DM.
Profen II DM.
Protuss-D.
Protuss DM.
Robafen CF.
Robitussin CF.
Robitussin Cold, Cold & Congestion.
Robitussin Cold, Cold & Cough.
Robitussin Cough & Cold Infant.
Touro CC.
Tussafed HC.
Tussafed LA.
Tussafed Ex.
Tussex Cough.
Su-Tuss HD.
Z-Cof DM.
antitussives, narcotic.
 See: Narcotic antitussives.
antivenin Centruroides sculpturatus.
 (Arizona State University) Available in
 Arizona only. 5 mL vials. *Rx.*
 Use: Antivenin.
•**antivenin (Crotalidae) polyvalent.**
 USP 28.
 Use: Immunization.
antivenin (Crotalidae) polyvalent. (Wy-
 eth) Antivenin (Crotalidae) polyvalent
 (equine origin), phenol 0.25%, thi-
 merosal 0.005%, phenylmercuric nitrate
 0.001%. Pow. for Inj., lyophilized.
 Single-use Vial with 1 vial diluent (Bacteriostatic Water for Injection, USP
 10 mL). *Rx.*
 Use: Bites of crotalid snakes of North,
 Central, and South America.
•**antivenin (Latrodectus mactans).**
 *USP 28. Formerly Widow spider spe-
 cies antivenin (Latrodectus mactans).*
 Use: Immunization.
antivenin (Latrodectus mactans).
 (Merck) Black widow spider antivenin
 (equine origin) at least 6000 antivenin
 units/vial, thimerosal 1:10,000. Pow.
 for Inj. Single-use Vial with 1 vial diluent (Sterile Water for Injection 2.5 mL)
 and normal horse serum 1 mL (1:10
 dilution) for sensitivity testing. *Rx.*
 Use: Treatment of black widow spider
 bites.
•**antivenin (Micrurus fulvius).** *USP 28.*
 Use: Immunization.
antivenin (Micrurus fulvius). North
 American coral snake antivenin (equine

origin), phenol 0.25%, thimerosal
0.005%, phenylmercuric nitrate
1:100,000. Pow. for Inj., lyophilized.
Single-use Vial with 1 vial diluent (Wa-
ter for Injection 10 mL). *Rx.*
Use: Bites of North American coral
 snake and Texas coral snake.
**antivenin, polyvalent crotalid (ovine)
fab.**
 Use: Bites of North American crotalid
 snakes. [Orphan Drug]
 See: CroFab.
antivenins.
 See: Antivenin (Crotalidae) Polyvalent.
 Antivenin (Latrodectus mactans).
 Antivenin (Micrurus fulvius).
 Crotalidae Polyvalent Immune Fab
 (Ovine origin).
**antivenom (Crotalidae) purified
(avian).** (Ophidian Pharmaceuticals,
 Inc.)
 Use: Bites of snakes of the Crotalidae
 family. [Orphan Drug]
Antivert. (Pfizer US) Meclizine hydro-
 chloride 12.5 mg. Tab. Bot. 100s,
 1000s, UD 100s. *Rx.*
 Use: Antiemetic/antivertigo agent.
Antivert/50. (Pfizer US) Meclizine hydro-
 chloride 50 mg, Tab. Bot. 100s. *Rx.*
 Use: Antiemetic/antivertigo agent.
Antivert/25. (Pfizer US) Meclizine hydro-
 chloride 25 mg. Tab. Bot. 100s, 1000s,
 UD 100s. *Rx.*
 Use: Antiemetic/antivertigo agent.
antiviral agents.
 See: Abacavir Sulfate.
 Acyclovir.
 Adefovir Dipivoxil.
 Amantadine Hydrochloride.
 Antiherpes Virus Agents.
 Cidofovir.
 Entecavir.
 Famciclovir.
 Foscarnet Sodium.
 Ganciclovir (DHPG).
 Oseltamivir Phosphate.
 Ribavirin.
 Rimantadine Hydrochloride.
 Valacyclovir Hydrochloride.
 Valganciclovir Hydrochloride.
 Zanamivir.
antiviral antibodies.
 See: Cytomegalovirus Immune Glob-
 ulin.
 Hepatitis B Immune Globulin.
 Immune Globulin IM.
 Immune Globulin IV.
 Rabies Immune Globulin.
 Vaccinia Immune Globulin.
 Varicella-Zoster Immune Globulin.

antixerophthalmic vitamin.
See: Vitamin A.
Antizol. (Orphan Medical) Fomepizole 1 g/mL. Preservative free. Inj. Conc. Vial 1.5 mL. Rx.
Use: Antidote.
Antril. (Amgen) Interleukin-1 receptor antagonist (human recombinant).
Use: Arthritis; organ rejection. [Orphan Drug]
Antrizine. (Major) Meclizine hydrochloride 12.5 mg. Tab. Bot. 100s, 500s, 1000s. Rx.
Use: Antiemetic/antivertigo agent.
Antrocol. (ECR) Atropine sulfate 0.195 mg, phenobarbital 16 mg, alcohol 20%/5 mL. Sugar free. Elix. Bot. Pt. Rx.
Use: Anticholinergic; antispasmodic; hypnotic; sedative.
Antrypol. Suramin. Rx.
Use: CDC anti-infective agent.
Anturane. (Novartis) Sulfinpyrazone, U.S.P. 100 mg. Tab. Bot 100s. 200 mg. Cap. Bot. 100s. Rx.
Use: Antigout agent.
Anucaine. (Calvin) Procaine 50 mg, butyl-p-aminobenzoate 200 mg, benzyl alcohol 265 mg in sweet almond oil/ 5 mL. Amp. 5 mL. Box 6s, 24s, 100s. OTC.
Use: Anorectal preparation.
Anucort-HC. (G & W) Hydrocortisone acetate 25 mg in a hydrogenated vegetable oil base. Supp. Box 12s, 24s, 100s. Rx.
Use: Anorectal preparation.
Anuject. (Roberts) Procaine. Soln. Vial 5 mL, 10 mL. Rx.
Use: Anorectal preparation.
Anumed. (Major) Bismuth subgallate 2.25%, bismuth resorcin compound 1.75%, benzyl benzoate 1.2%, zinc oxide 11%, balsam Peru 1.8% in a hydrogenated vegetable oil base. Supp. Box 12s. OTC.
Use: Anorectal preparation.
Anumed HC. (Major) Hydrocortisone acetate 10 mg. Supp. Box 12s. Rx.
Use: Anorectal preparation.
Anuprep HC. (Great Southern) Hydrocortisone acetate 25 mg. Supp. Box 12s.
Use: Anorectal preparation.
Anuprep Hemorrhoidal. (Great Southern) Bismuth subgallate 2.25%, bismuth resorcin compound 1.75%, benzyl benzoate 1.2%, peruvian balsam 1.8%, and zinc oxide 11% in a hydrogenated vegetable oil base. Supp. Box 12s, 24s. Rx.

Use: Anorectal preparation.
Anusol-HC. (Salix) Hydrocortisone 2.5%. Cream. Tube 30 g. Rx.
Use: Corticosteroid, topical.
Anusol-HC-1. (Warner) Hydrocortisone 1%, diazolidinyl urea, parabens, mineral oil, sorbitan sesquioleate, white petrolatum. Oint. Tube 21 g. OTC.
Use: Corticosteroid, topical.
Anusol Ointment. (Warner) Pramoxine hydrochloride 1%, zinc oxide 12.5%/g, benzyl benzoate 1.2%, pramoxine hydrochloride 1% in mineral oil and cocoa butter. Oint. Tube 30 g. OTC.
Use: Anorectal preparation.
Anusol Suppository. (Salix) Topical starch 51%, benzyl alcohol, soybean oil, tocopheryl acetate. Supp. Pkg. 12s. OTC.
Use: Anorectal preparation.
Anzemet. (Aventis) Dolasetron mesylate. **Tab.:** 50 mg, 100 mg, lactose. Pkg. 5s, blister pack 5s, UD 10s. **Inj.:** 20 mg/ mL, mannitol 38.2 mg/mL. Single-use amp. 0.625 mL, 0.625 mL fill in 2 mL Carpu-ject, single-use vial 5 mL. Rx.
Use: Antiemetic; antivertigo.
A1cNow. (Metrika) Reagent kit for blood tests. Box 1s, 2s with lancet(s), monitor, dilution kit. Rx.
Use: In vitro diagnostic aid.
AOSEPT. (Ciba Vision) Hydrogen peroxide 3%, sodium Cl 0.85%, phosphonic acid, phosphate buffer. Soln. Bot. 120 mL, 240 mL, 360 mL. OTC.
Use: Contact lens care.
Apacet. (Parmed Pharmaceuticals, Inc.) Acetaminophen 80 mg. Chew. Tab. Bot. 100s. OTC.
Use: Analgesic.
•**apafant.** (APP-ah-fant) USAN.
Use: Platelet activating factor antagonist; antiasthmatic.
•**apalcillin sodium.** (APE-al-SIH-lin) USAN.
Use: Anti-infective.
APAP.
See: Acetaminophen.
APAP-Plus. (Textilease Medique) Acetaminophen 500 mg, caffeine 65 mg. Bot. 100s, 200s, 500s. OTC.
Use: Analgesic.
•**apaxifylline.** (A-pock-SIH-fih-leen) USAN.
Use: Selective adenosine A_1 antagonist.
•**apaziquone.** (a-PA-zi-kwone) USAN.
Use: Antineoplastic.
•**apazone.** (APP-ah-zone) USAN.
Use: Anti-inflammatory.

A.P.C. (Various Mfr.) Aspirin, phenacetin, caffeine. Cap., Tab.
Use: Analgesic combination.
See: A.S.A. Compound (Eli Lilly).
Pan-APC (Panray).
Phensal (Hoechst).
W/Codeine phosphate. (Various Mfr.).
See: Anexsia D (GlaxoSmithKline).
Anexsia w/Codeine (SmithKline Beecham Pharmaceuticals).

Apcogesic. (Apco) Sodium salicylate 5 g, colchicine 1/320 g, calcium carbonate 65 mg, dried aluminum hydroxide gel 130 mg, phenobarbital ⅛ g. Tab. Bot. 100s. *Rx.*
Use: Antigout; hypnotic; sedative.

Apcoretic. (A.P.C) Caffeine anhydrous 100 mg, ammonium Cl 325 mg. Tab. Bot. 90s. *Rx.*
Use: Diuretic.

Ap Creme. (T.E. Williams Pharmaceuticals) Hydrocortisone 0.5%, iodochlorhydroxyquin 3%. Tube. *Rx-OTC.*
Use: Antifungal; corticosteroid, topical.

A.P.C. w/gelsemium combinations.
See: Valacet (Pal-Pak, Inc.).

Apetil. (Kenwood) B₁ 1.7 mg, B₂ 0.3 mg, B₃ 6.7 mg, B₆ 2.5 mg, B₁₂ 5 mcg, Zn 14.6 mg, Mg, Mn, I-lysine. Liq. Bot. 237 mL. *OTC.*
Use: Mineral, vitamin supplement.

ApexiCon. (PharmaDerm) Diflorasone diacetate 0.05%. Oint. 30 g, 60 g. *Rx.*
Use: Anti-inflammatory.

ApexiCon E. (PharmaDerm) Diflorasone diacetate 0.05%. Stearyl alcohol, cetyl alcohol. Cream. 30 g, 60g. *Rx.*
Use: Anti-inflammatory.

APF. (Whitehall-Robins)
Use: Analgesic.
See: Arthritis Pain Formula (Whitehall-Robins).

Aphco Hemorrhoidal Combination.
(A.P.C) Combination package of Aphco Hemorrhoidal ointment 1.5 oz tube, Aphco Hemorrhoidal supp. Box 12s, 1000s. *OTC.*
Use: Anorectal preparation.

Aphen. (Major) Trihexyphenidyl 2 mg, 5 mg. Tab. Bot. 250s, 1000s. *Rx.*
Use: Antiparkinsonian.

Aphrodyne. (Star) Yohimbine hydrochloride 5.4 mg. Tab. Bot. 100s, 1000s. *Rx.*
Use: Anti-impotence agent, alpha-adrenergic blocker.

Aphthasol. (Access) Amlexanox 5%, benzyl alcohol, mineral oil, petrolatum. Paste. Tube. 5 g. *Rx.*
Use: Mouth and throat product.

Apicillin.
See: Ampicillin.

Apidra. (Aventis) Insulin glulisine (rDNA) 100 units/mL. Inj. Vials. 10 mL. *Rx.*
Use: Antidiabetic agent.

APL 400-020. (Apollon)
Use: Treatment of cutaneous T-cell lymphoma. [Orphan Drug]

•**aplindore fumarate.** (AP-lin-dor) USAN.
Use: Antischizophrenic.

Aplisol. (Monarch) Tuberculin purified protein derivative 5 units/0.1 mL, polysorbate 80, potassium and sodium phosphates, phenol 0.35%. Vial 1 mL (10 tests), 5 mL (50 tests). *Rx.*
Use: Diagnostic aid.

Aplitest. (Parke-Davis) Purified tuberculin protein derivative buffered with potassium and sodium phosphates, phenol 0.5%/single-use, multipuncture unit. 25s. *Rx.*
Use: Diagnostic aid.

Apokyn. (Mylan Bertek) Apomorphine hydrochloride 10 mg/mL. Sodium metabisulfite. Inj. Glass Amps. 2 mL. Cartridges. 3 mL. *Rx.*
Use: Antiparkinson agent.

•**apolizumab.** (ap-ol-IZ-yoo-mab) USAN.
Use: Anti-cancer agent.

•**apomorphine hydrochloride.** (ah-poh-MORE-feen) *USP 28.*
Use: Treatment of Parkinson disease.
See: Apokyn.

aporphine-10, 11-diol hydrochloride.
See: Apomorphine hydrochloride.

appetite-depressants.
See: Anorexiant agents.

APPG.
See: Penicillin G, Procaine, Aqueous.

Apra. (Altaire) Acetaminophen 160 mg/ 5 mL. Alcohol-free. Sorbitol, sucrose. Grape flavor. Elix. 118 mL. *OTC.*
Use: Analgesic.

•**apraclonidine hydrochloride.** (app-rah-KLOE-nih-deen) *USP 28.*
Use: Adrenergic, α₂-agonist.
See: Iopidine.

•**apramycin.** (APP-rah-MY-sin) USAN.
Use: Anti-infective.

Aprazone. (Major) Sulfinpyrazone 100 mg. Tab. Bot. 100s. *Rx.*
Use: Antigout agent.

•**aprepitant.** (ap-REH-pih-tant) USAN.
Use: Antiemetic.
See: Emend.

Apresazide. (Novartis) **25/25:** Hydralazine hydrochloride 25 mg, hydrochlorothiazide 25 mg. **50/50:** Hydralazine hydrochloride 50 mg, hydrochlorothiazide 50 mg. **100/50:** Hydralazine 100 mg, hydrochlorothiazide 50 mg. Cap. Bot. 100s. *Rx.*

Use: Antihypertensive.

Apresodex. (Rugby) Hydrochlorothiazide 15 mg, hydralazine hydrochloride 25 mg. Tab. Bot. 100s, 1000s. *Rx.*
Use: Antihypertensive.

Apresoline. (Novartis) Hydralazine hydrochloride. **Amp.:** 20 mg w/propylene glycol, methyl and propyl parabens/mL. Pkg. 5s. **Tab.:** 10 mg Bot. 100s, 1200s; 25 mg or 50 mg Bot. 100s, 1000s; 100 mg Bot. 100s. Consumer pack 100s. *Rx.*
Use: Antihypertensive.
W/Serpasil.
See: Serpasil (Novartis).

Apresoline-Esidrix. (Novartis) Hydralazine hydrochloride 25 mg, hydrochlorothiazide 15 mg. Tab. Bot. 100s. *Rx.*
Use: Antihypertensive.

Apri. (Barr) Desogestrel 0.15 mg, ethinyl estradiol 30 mcg, lactose. Tab. Blister cards 28s. *Rx.*
Use: Sex hormone, contraceptive.

•**aprindine.** (APE-rin-deen) USAN.
Use: Cardiovascular agent.

•**aprindine hydrochloride.** (APE-rindeen) USAN.
Use: Cardiovascular agent.

•**aprinocarsen sodium.** (ap-ri-NOE-karsen) USAN.
Use: Protein kinase inhibitor.

Aprobee w/C. (Health for Life Brands) Vitamins B₁ 15 mg, B₂ 10 mg, B₆ 5 mg, niacinamide 50 mg, calcium pantothenate 10 mg, C 250 mg. Cap. Bot. 100s, 1000s. Tab. Bot. 50s, 100s, 1000s. *OTC.*
Use: Mineral, vitamin supplement.

Aprodine. (Major) **Tab.:** Pseudoephedrine hydrochloride 60 mg, triprolidine hydrochloride 2.5 mg, lactose. Bot. 24s. **Syr.:** Pseudoephedrine hydrochloride 30 mg, triprolidine hydrochloride 1.25 mg/5 mL. Bot. 118 mL. *OTC.*
Use: Upper respiratory combination, antihistamine, decongestant.

Aprodine w/Codeine. (Major) Pseudoephedrine hydrochloride 30 mg, triprolidine hydrochloride 1.25 mg, codeine phosphate 10 mg. Syr. Bot. Pt, gal. *c-v.*
Use: Antihistamine; decongestant.

•**aprotinin.** (app-row-TIE-nin) USAN.
Use: Enzyme inhibitor, proteinase.
See: Trasylol.

Aprozide 50/50. (Major) Hydrochlorothiazide 50 mg, hydralazine 50 mg. Cap. Bot. 100s, 250s. *Rx.*
Use: Antihypertensive.

Aprozide 25/25. (Major) Hydralazine 25 mg, hydrochlorothiazide 25 mg. Cap.

Bot. 100s, 250s. *Rx.*
Use: Antihypertensive.

A.P.S. Aspirin, phenacetin, and salicylamide.

APSAC. Thrombolytic enzyme.
See: Eminase (SmithKline Beecham Pharmaceuticals).

•**aptazapine maleate.** (app-TAZZ-ah-PEEN MAL-ee-ate) USAN.
Use: Antidepressant.

•**aptiganel hydrochloride.** (app-tih-GAN-ehl) USAN.
Use: Stroke and traumatic brain injury treatment (NMDA ion channel blocker).

Aptivus. (Boehringer Ingelheim) Tipranavir 250 mg. Cap. Unit-of-use Bot. 120s. *Rx.*
Use: Antiretroviral treatment for HIV.

apyron.
See: Magnesium acetylsalicylate.

AQ-4B. (Western Research) Trichlormethiazide 4 mg. Tab. Bot. 1000s. *Rx.*
Use: Diuretic.

AquaBalm. (Quintessa) Petrolatum, methyl glucate dioleate, propylene glycol, DMDM hydantoin, iodopropynyl butylcarbamate, fragrance free. Cream. Tube. 114 g. *OTC.*
Use: Emollient.

Aqua-Ban. (Thompson Medical) Caffeine 100 mg, ammonium Cl 325 mg. Tab. Bot. 60s. *OTC.*
Use: Diuretic.

Aqua-Ban, Maximum Strength.
See: Maximum Strength Aqua-Ban.

Aqua-Ban Plus. (Thompson Medical) Ammonium Cl 650 mg, caffeine 200 mg, iron 6 mg. Tab. Bot. 30s. *OTC.*
Use: Diuretic; mineral supplement.

Aquabase. (Pal-Pak, Inc.) Cetyl alcohol, propylene glycol, sodium lauryl sulfate, white wax, purified water. Jar lb. *OTC.*
Use: Pharmaceutic aid; ointment base.

Aquacare Cream. (Allergan) Urea 2%, benzyl alcohol, carbomer 934, cetyl esters wax, fragrance, glycerin, oleth-3 phosphate, petrolatum, phenyldimethicone, water, sodium hydroxide. Cream. Tube 2.5 oz. *OTC.*
Use: Emollient.

Aquacare/HP. (Allergan) Urea 10%, benzyl alcohol. **Cream:** Tube 2.5 oz. **Lot.:** Bot. 8 oz, 16 oz. *OTC.*
Use: Emollient.

Aquacare Lotion. (Allergan) Benzyl alcohol, oleth-3 phosphate, phenyldimethicone, fragrance. Lot. Bot. 8 oz. *OTC.*
Use: Emollient.

Bot. 100s, 250s. *Rx.*
Use: Antihypertensive.

Aquachloral Supprettes. (PolyMedica) Chloral hydrate 324 mg (tartrazine), 648 mg. Supp. 12s. *c-iv.*
Use: Sedative/hypnotic, nonbarbiturate.
Aquacillin G. (Armenpharm Ltd.) Penicillin G. *Rx.*
Use: Anti-infective, penicillin.
Aquacycline. (Armenpharm Ltd.) Tetracycline hydrochloride. *Rx.*
Use: Anti-infective, tetracycline.
Aquaderm. (C & M Pharmacal) Purified water, glycerin 25%, salicylic acid 0.1%, octoxynol-9 0.03%, FD&C Red #40 0.0001%. Bot. 2 oz. *OTC.*
Use: Emollient.
Aquaderm. (Baker Norton) Octyl methoxycinnamate 7.5%, oxybenzone 6%. SPF 15. Cream. Tube. 105 g. *OTC.*
Use: Sunscreen.
Aquaflox Ultrasound Gel Pad. (Parker) Clear, solid, flexible, moist, standoff gel pad for use where transducer movement is impeded by bony or irregular body surfaces. 2 cm × 9 cm.
Use: Ultrasound aid.
Aquafuren. (Armenpharm Ltd.) Nitrofurantoin. *Rx.*
Use: Anti-infective, urinary.
Aquagen. (ALK) Allergenic extracts. Vials.
aquakay.
See: Menadione.
Aqua Lacten. (Allergan) Demineralized water, urea, petrolatum, propylene glycol monostearate, sorbitan monostearate, lactic acid. Lot. Bot. 8 oz. *OTC.*
Use: Emollient.
AquaMEPHYTON. (Merck & Co.) Phytonadione 10 mg/mL, polyoxyethylated fatty acid derivative, dextrose, benzyl alcohol. Inj. Amp. 1 mL. *Rx.*
Use: Coagulant.
Aqua Mist. (Faraday) Nasal spray. Squeeze Bot. 20 mL.
Aquamycin. (Armenpharm Ltd.) Erythromycin. *Rx.*
Use: Anti-infective, erythromycin.
Aquanil. (Sigma-Tau) Mersalyl 100 mg, theophylline (hydrate) 50 mg, methylparaben 0.18%, propylparaben 0.02%. Vial 10 mL. *OTC.*
Use: Bronchodilator; diuretic.
Aquanil Cleanser. (Person and Covey) Glycerin, cetyl, stearyl, and benzyl alcohol, sodium laureth sulfate, xanthan gum. Lipid free. Lot. Bot. 240 mL, 480 mL. *OTC.*
Use: Dermatologic, cleanser.
Aquanine. (Armenpharm Ltd.) Quinine hydrochloride. *Rx.*
Use: Antimalarial.

Aquaoxy. (Armenpharm Ltd.) Oxytetracycline hydrochloride. *Rx.*
Use: Anti-infective, tetracycline.
Aquaphenicol. (Armenpharm Ltd.) Chloramphenicol. *Rx.*
Use: Anti-infective.
Aquaphilic Ointment. (Medco Lab) Hydrated hydrophilic oint. Jar 16 oz. *OTC.*
Use: Emollient; ointment base.
Aquaphilic Ointment with Carbamide 10% and 20%. (Medco Lab) Stearyl alcohol, white petrolatum, sorbitol, propylene glycol, sodium lauryl sulfate, lactic acid, methylparaben, propylparaben.
Use: Prescription compounding; emollient.
Aquaphor. (Beiersdorf) Cholesterolized anhydrous petrolatum ointment base. Tube 1.75 oz, 3.25 oz, 16 oz, Jar 5 lb, Bar 3 oz. *OTC.*
Use: Pharmaceutic aid; ointment base.
See: Eucerin (Duke).
Aquaphor Antibiotic. (Beiersdorf) Polymyxin B sulfate 10,000 units, bacitracin zinc 500 units/g in a cholesterolized ointment base. Oint. Tube 15 g. *OTC.*
Use: Anti-infective, topical.
Aquaphor Healing Ointment. (Beiersdorf) Petrolatum, mineral oil, lanolin, alcohol, panthenol, glycerin. Oint. Tubes. 10 g, 50 g. Jars. 99 g, 396 g. *OTC.*
Use: Emollient.
Aquapool Concentrate. (Parker) Color additive for hydrotherapy to control foaming. Bot. Pt, gal.
Aquasol A. (AstraZeneca) Vitamin A palmitate 50,000 units/mL, chlorobutanol 0.5%, polysorbate 80, butylated hydroxyanisole, butylated hydroxytoluene. Inj. Vial 2 mL. *Rx.*
Use: Vitamin supplement.
Aquasonic 100. (Parker) Water-soluble, viscous, contact medium gel for ultrasonic transmission. Bot. 250 mL, 1 L, 5 L.
Use: Ultrasound aid.
Aquasonic 100 Sterile. (Parker) Water-soluble, sterile gel for ultrasonic transmission. Overwrapped Foil Pouches 15 g, 50 g.
Use: Ultrasound aid.
Aquasulf. (Armenpharm Ltd.) Triple sulfa tablet. *Rx.*
Use: Anti-infective.
Aquatab C. (Adams) Guaifenesin 1200 mg, pseudoephedrine hydrochloride 60 mg, dextromethorphan HBr 60 mg. ER Tab. Bot. 100s. *Rx.*
Use: Upper respiratory combination, expectorant, decongestant, antitussive.

Aquatab D. (Adams) Guaifenesin 1200 mg, pseudoephedrine hydrochloride 75 mg. ER Tab. Bot. 100s. *Rx.*
Use: Upper respiratory combination, expectorant, decongestant.

Aquatab D Dose Pack. (Adams) Pseudoephedrine hydrochloride 60 mg, guaifenesin 600 mg. SR Tab. Bot. 56s. *Rx.*
Use: Upper respiratory combination, decongestant, expectorant.

Aquatab DM. (Adams) **ER Tab.:** Guaifenesin 1200 mg, dextromethorphan HBr 75mg. Bot. 100s. **Syr.:** Guaifenesin 200 mg, dextromethorphan HBr 10 mg/5 mL, acesulfame K, aspartame, menthol, methylparaben, phenylalanine. 473 mL. *Rx.*
Use: Upper respiratory combination, expectorant, antitussive.

Aquavite. (Armenpharm Ltd.) Soluble multivitamin.
Use: Vitamin supplement.

Aquavit-E. (Cypress) Dl-alpha tocopheryl acetate 15 units/0.3 mL. Drops. Bot. 30 mL. *OTC.*
Use: Vitamin supplement.

Aquazide. (Western Research) Trichlormethiazide 4 mg. Tab. Bot. 100s. *Rx.*
Use: Antihypertensive; diuretic.

Aquazide H. (Western Research) Hydrochlorothiazide 50 mg. Tab. Bot. 1000s. *Rx.*
Use: Diuretic.

Aquazol. (Armenpharm Ltd.) Sulfisoxazole.
Use: Anti-infective.

Aqueous Allergens. (Bayer Corp. (Consumer Div.))
Use: Antiallergic.

aquinone.
See: Menadione.

Aquol Bath Oil. (Lamond) Vegetable oil, olive oil. Bot. 4 oz, 6 oz, 16 oz, qt, gal. *OTC.*
Use: Antipruritic; emollient.

ARA-C.
See: Cytarabine.

Aralast. (Baxter) Alpha₁-proteinase inhibitor (human) 400 mg, 800 mg (≥ 16 mg alpha₁-PI per mL when reconstituted). Preservative free, polyethylene glycol, sodium, albumin. Pow. for Inj., lyophilized. Single-dose vial with 25 mL diluent (400 mg only), single-dose vial with 50 mL diluent (800 mg only). *Rx.*
Use: Respiratory enzyme.

Aralen Hydrochloride. (Sanofi-Synthelabo) Chloroquine hydrochloride 50 mg/mL. Inj. Amp. 5 mL. *Rx.*

Use: Amebicide; antimalarial.

Aralen Phosphate. (Sanofi-Synthelabo) Chloroquine phosphate 500 mg. Tab. Bot. 25s. *Rx.*
Use: Amebicide; antimalarial.

Aralis. (Sanofi-Synthelabo) Glycobiarsol, chloroquine phosphate. Tab. *Rx.*
Use: Amebicide.

Aramine. (Merck & Co.) Metaraminol bitartrate 10 mg/mL, methylparaben 0.15%, propylparaben 0.02%, sodium bisulfite 0.2%. Inj. Vial 10 mL. *Rx.*
Use: Antihypotensive.

Aranelle. (Barr) **Phase 1:** Norethindrone 0.5 mg, ethinyl estradiol 35 mcg. **Phase 2:** Norethindrone 1 mg, ethinyl estradiol 35 mcg. **Phase 3:** Norethindrone 0.5 mg, ethinyl estradiol 35 mcg. Lactose. Tab. 28s. *Rx.*
Use: Contraceptive hormone.

Aranesp. (Amgen) **Inj.:** 25 mcg/0.42 mL, 40 mcg/0.4 mL, 60 mcg/0.3 mL, 100 mcg/0.5 mL, 150 mcg/0.3 mL, 200 mcg/0.4 mL, 300 mcg/0.6 mL, 500 mcg/1 mL. Single-dose prefilled syringe. **Soln. for Inj.:** Darbepoetin alfa 25 mcg/mL, 40 mcg/mL, 60 mcg/mL, 100 mcg/mL, 150 mcg/mL, 200 mcg/mL, 300 mcg/mL, 500 mcg/mL, preservative-free. In polysorbate or albumin solutions (150 mcg/mL, 300 mcg/mL, 500 mcg/mL in albumin only solution). The polysorbate solution contains polysorbate 80 0.05 mg, sodium phosphate monobasic monohydrate 2.12 mg, sodium phosphate dibasic anhydrous 0.66 mg, sodium chloride 8.18 mg. The albumin solution contains human albumin 2.5 mg, sodium phosphate monobasic monohydrate 2.23 mg, sodium phosphate dibasic anhydrous 0.53 mg, sodium chloride 8.18 mg. Single-dose vial 1 mL. *Rx.*
Use: Hematopoietic agent, recombinant human erythropoietin.

●**aranotin.** (AR-ah-NO-tin) USAN.
Use: Antiviral.

Arava. (Hoechst) Leflunomide 10 mg, 20 mg, 100 mg, lactose. Tab. Bot. 30s, 100s. Blister pack 3 count (100 mg only). *Rx.*
Use: Antirheumatic.

●**arbaprostil.** (ahr-bah-PRAHST-ill) USAN.
Use: Antisecretory, gastric.

Arbolic. (Burgin-Arden) Methandriol dipropionate 50 mg/mL. Vial 10 mL. *Rx.*
Use: Anabolic steroid.

Arbutal. (Arcum) Butalbital 0.75 g, phenacetin 2 g, aspirin 3 g, caffeine g. Tab. Bot. 100s, 1000s. *Rx.*
Use: Analgesic; hypnotic; sedative.

• **arbutamine hydrochloride.** (ahr-BYOO-tah-meen) USAN.
Use: Cardiovascular agent.
See: GenESA.

Arcet. (Econo Med Pharmaceuticals) Butalbital 50 mg, acetaminophen 325 mg, caffeine 40 mg. Tab. Bot. 100s. *Rx.*
Use: Analgesic; hypnotic; sedative.

• **arcitumomab.** (ahr-sigh-TOO-moe-mab) USAN.
Use: Monoclonal antibody.
See: CEA-Scan.

• **arclofenin.** (AHR-kloe-FEN-in) USAN.
Use: Diagnostic aid for hepatic function determination.

Arcoban. (Arcum) Meprobamate 400 mg. Tab. Bot. 50s, 1000s. *Rx.*
Use: Anxiolytic.

Arcobee w/C. (NBTY) Vitamins B_1 15 mg, B_2 10.2 mg, B_3 60 mg, B_5 10 mg, B_6 5 mg, C 300 mg, tartrazine. Cap. Box 100s. *OTC.*
Use: Vitamin supplement.

Arcodex Antacid. (Arcum) Magnesium trisilicate 500 mg, aluminum hydroxide 250 mg. Tab. Bot. 100s, 1000s. *OTC.*
Use: Antacid.

Arco-Lase. (Arco) Trizyme 38 mg (amylase 30 mg, protease 6 mg, cellulase 2 mg), lipase 25 mg. Tab. Bot. 50s. *Rx.*
Use: Digestive aid.

Arcosterone. (Arcum) Methyltestosterone. **Oral:** 10 mg, 25 mg. Tab. Bot. 100s, 1000s. **Sublingual Tab.:** 10 mg. Bot. 100s, 1000s. *Rx.*
Use: Androgen.

Arco-Thyroid. (Arco) Thyroid 1.5 g. Tab. Bot. 1000s. *Rx.*
Use: Hormone, thyroid.

Arcotrate. (Arcum) Pentaerythritol tetranitrate 10 mg. Tab. **No. 2:** Pentaerythritol tetranitrate 20 mg. **No. 3.** Pentaerythritol tetranitrate 20 mg, phenobarbital ⅛ g. Bot. 100s, 1000s. *Rx.*
Use: Antianginal.

Arcoval Improved. (Arcum) Vitamin A palmitate 10,000 units, D 400 units, thiamine mononitrate 15 mg, B_2 10 mg, nicotinamide 150 mg, B_6 5 mg, calcium pantothenate 10 mg, B_{12} 5 mcg, C 150 mg, E 5 units. Cap. Bot. 100s, 1000s. *OTC.*
Use: Mineral, vitamin supplement.

Arcum R-S. (Arcum) Reserpine 0.25 mg. Tab. Bot. 100s, 1000s. *Rx.*
Use: Antihypertensive.

Arcum V-M. (Arcum) Vitamin A palmitate 5000 units, D 400 units, B_1 2.5 mg, B_2 2.5 mg, B_6 0.5 mg, B_{12} 2 mcg, C 50 mg, niacinamide 20 mg, calcium

pantothenate 5 mg, iron 18 mg. Cap. Bot. 100s, 1000s. *OTC.*
Use: Mineral, vitamin supplement.

A-R-D. (Birchwood) Anatomically shaped dressing. Dispenser 24s.
Use: Antipruritic; counterirritant, rectal.

Ardeben. (Burgin-Arden) Diphenhydramine hydrochloride 10 mg, chlorobutanol 0.5%. Inj. Vial 30 mL. *Rx.*
Use: Antihistamine.

Ardecaine 1%. (Burgin-Arden) Lidocaine hydrochloride 1%. Inj. Vial 30 mL. *Rx.*
Use: Anesthetic, local.

Ardecaine 1% w/Epinephrine. (Burgin-Arden) Lidocaine hydrochloride 1%, epinephrine. Inj. Vial 30 mL. *Rx.*
Use: Anesthetic, local.

Ardecaine 2%. (Burgin-Arden) Lidocaine hydrochloride 2%. Inj. Vial 30 mL. *Rx.*
Use: Anesthetic, local.

Ardecaine 2% w/Epinephrine. (Burgin-Arden) Lidocaine hydrochloride 2%, epinephrine. Inj. Vial 30 mL. *Rx.*
Use: Anesthetic, topical.

Ardefem 40. (Burgin-Arden) Estradiol valerate 40 mg/mL. Vial 10 mL. *Rx.*
Use: Estrogen.

Ardefem 10. (Burgin-Arden) Estradiol valerate 10 mg/mL. Vial 10 mL. *Rx.*
Use: Estrogen.

Ardefem 20. (Burgin-Arden) Estradiol valerate 20 mg/mL. Vial 10 mL. *Rx.*
Use: Estrogen.

• **ardenermin.** (ar-den-ER-min) USAN.
Use: Tumor necrosis factor

• **ardeparin sodium.** (ahr-dee-PA-rin) USAN.
Use: Anticoagulant.

Ardepred Soluble. (Burgin-Arden) Prednisolone 20 mg, niacinamide 25 mg, disodium edetate 0.5 mg, sodium bisulfite 1 mg, phenol 5 mg/mL. Vial 10 mL. *Rx.*
Use: Corticosteroid combination.

Arderone 100. (Burgin-Arden) Testosterone enanthate 100 mg/mL. Vial 10 mL. *c-III.*
Use: Androgen.

Arderone 200. (Burgin-Arden) Testosterone enanthate 200 mg/mL. Vial 10 mL. *c-III.*
Use: Androgen.

Ardevila. (Sanofi-Synthelabo) Inositol hexanicotinate. Tab. *Rx.*
Use: Vasodilator.

Ardiol 90/4. (Burgin-Arden) Testosterone enanthate 90 mg, estradiol valerate 4 mg/mL. Vial 10 mL. *Rx.*
Use: Androgen, estrogen combination.

Aredia. (Novartis) Pamidronate disodium 30 mg (470 mg mannitol), 90 mg

(375 mg mannitol). Pow. for Inj., lyophilized. Vial. *Rx.*
Use: Bisphosphonate, antihypercalcemic.

Arestin. (Cord Logistics) Minocycline hydrochloride 1 mg. SR Microspheres. UD 12s. *Rx.*
Use: Mouth and throat product.

●**arformoterol tartrate.** (ar-for-MOE-terole) USAN.
Use: Bronchodilator.

●**argatroban.** (ahr-GAT-troe-ban) USAN.
Use: Anticoagulant.
See: Acova.

Argatroban. (GlaxoSmithKline) Argatroban 100 mg/mL. D-sorbitol 750 mg, dehydrated alcohol 1000 mg. Inj. Singleuse vial 2.5 mL. *Rx.*
Use: Anticoagulant.

Argesic-SA. (Econo Med Pharmaceuticals) Disalicylic acid 500 mg. Tab. Bot. 100s. *Rx.*
Use: Analgesic, topical.

Arginaid Extra. (Novartis Nutrition) Protein (whey protein isolate, L-arginine, L-cysteine) 25.3 g, carbohydrate (sugar, hydrolyzed corn starch) 219.4 g/L, vitamins A, B_1, B_2, B_3, B_5, B_6, B_{12}, C, D, E, K, biotin, folic acid, Cu, Fe, I, Mn, P, Zn, Na < 295 mg, K < 93 mg/L, 1.05 cal/mL, orange and wild berry flavors. Liq. *Tetra Brik Paks. OTC.*
Use: Enteral nutritional therapy.

●**arginine.** (AHR-jih-neen) *USP 28.*
Use: Ammonia detoxicant; diagnostic aid, pituitary function determination.

arginine butyrate. (AHR-jih-neen)
Use: Sickle cell disease; beta-thalassemia. [Orphan Drug]

●**arginine glutamate.** (AHR-jih-neen GLUE-tah-mate) USAN.
Use: Ammonia detoxicant.

●**arginine hydrochloride.** (AHR-jih-neen) *USP 28.*
Use: Ammonia detoxicant.

arginine hydrochloride. (AHR-jih-neen)
Use: Diagnostic aid.
See: R-Gene 10.

8-arginine-vasopressin.
See: Vasopressin.

●**argipressin tannate.** (AHR-JIH-press-in TAN-ate) USAN.
Use: Antidiuretic.

argyn.
See: Mild Silver Protein.

Aricept. (Eisai/Pfizer) Donepezil hydrochloride 5 mg, 10 mg. Tab. 30s, 90s, UD blister pack 100s. *Rx.*
Use: Treatment of mild to moderate dementia associated with Alzheimer disease.

Aricept ODT. (Eisai/Pfizer) Donepezil hydrochloride 5 mg, 10 mg. Orally Disintegrating Tab. UD blister pack 30s. *Rx.*
Use: Treatment of mild to moderate dementia associated with Alzheimer disease.

Aridol. (MPL) Pamabrom 52 mg, pyrilamine maleate 30 mg, homatropine methylbromide 1.2 mg, hyoscyamine sulfate 0.10 mg, scopolamine HBr 0.02 mg, methamphetamine hydrochloride 1.5 mg. Tab. Bot. 100s. *Rx.*
Use: Anticholinergic; antispasmodic; diuretic; stimulant.

●**arildone.** (AR-ill-dohn) USAN.
Use: Antiviral.

Arimidex. (AstraZeneca) Anastrozole 1 mg, lactose. Tab. Bot. 30s. *Rx.*
Use: Hormone; aromatase inhibitor.

●**aripiprazole.** (a-rih-PIP-ray-zole) USAN.
Use: Antipsychotic; antischizophrenic.
See: Abilify.

Aris Phenobarbital Reagent Strips. (Bayer Corp. (Consumer Div.)) Box 25s.
Use: Diagnostic aid.

Aris Phenytoin Reagent Strips. (Bayer Corp. (Consumer Div.)) Box 25s.
Use: Diagnostic aid.

Aristo-Pak. (Wyeth) Triamcinolone 4 mg. Tab. 16s. *Rx.*
Use: Corticosteroid.

Aristocort. (Fujisawa Healthcare) Triamcinolone. **Tab.:** 1 mg Bot. 50s; 2 mg Bot. 100s; 4 mg Bot. 30s, 100s; 8 mg Bot. 50s. **Syr.:** Diacetate (w/methylparaben 0.08%, propylparaben 0.02%) 2 mg/5 mL. Bot. 4 oz. *Rx.*
Use: Corticosteroid.

Aristocort Acetonide, Sodium Phosphate Salt. (Fujisawa Healthcare)
Use: Corticosteroid, topical.
See: Aristocort.
Sodium Phosphate Triamcinolone Acetonide.

Aristocort A Cream. (Fujisawa Healthcare) Triamcinolone acetonide w/emulsifying wax, isopropyl palmitate, glycerin, sorbitol, lactic acid, benzyl alcohol. **0.025% w/Aquatain:** Tube 15 g, 60 g. **0.1%:** Tube 15 g, 60 g, Jar 240 g. **0.5%:** Tube 15 g. *Rx.*
Use: Corticosteroid, topical.

Aristocort A Ointment. (Fujisawa Healthcare) Triamcinolone acetonide 0.1%. Tube 15 g, 60 g. *Rx.*
Use: Corticosteroid, topical.

Aristocort Cream. (Fujisawa Healthcare) Triamcinolone acetonide w/emulsifying wax, polysorbate 60, mono and diglycerides, squalane, sorbitol soln., sorbic acid, potassium sorbate. **LP: 0.025%:**

Tube 15 g, 60 g; Jar 240 g, 480 g. **R:**
0.1%: Tube 15 g, 60 g; Jar 240 g,
480 g. **HP: 0.5%:** Tube 15 g, Jar 240 g.
Rx.
Use: Corticosteroid, topical.
Aristocort Intralesional. (Fujisawa
Healthcare) Triamcinolone diacetate
25 mg/mL. Vial 5 mL. *Rx.*
Use: Corticosteroid.
Aristocort Ointment. (Fujisawa Healthcare) Triamcinolone acetonide. **R:**
0.1%: Tube 15 g, 60 g; Jar 240 g. **HP:**
0.5%: Tube 15 g; Jar 240 g. *Rx.*
Use: Corticosteroid, topical.
Aristospan Intra-articular. (Wyeth) Triamcinolone hexacetonide 20 mg/mL
micronized susp., polysorbate 80 0.4%
w/v, sorbitol soln. 64% w/v, water q.s.,
benzyl alcohol 0.9% w/v. Vial 1 mL,
5 mL. *Rx.*
Use: Corticosteroid.
Aristospan Intralesional. (Wyeth) Triamcinolone hexacetonide 5 mg/mL,
polysorbate 80 0.2% w/v, sorbitol soln.
64% w/v, water q.s., benzyl alcohol
0.9% w/v. Vial 5 mL. *Rx.*
Use: Corticosteroid.
Arixtra. (GlaxoSmithKline) Fondaparinux
sodium 2.5 mg per 0.5 mL, 5 mg per
0.4 mL, 7.5 mg per 0.6 mL, 10 mg per
0.8 mL. Preservative free. Inj. Single-
dose prefilled syringes with 27-gauge
needle. 10s. *Rx.*
Use: Anticoaqulant, selective factor Xa
inhibitor.
Arlacel C. (AstraZeneca) Sorbitan sesquioleate. Mixture of oleate esters of
sorbitol and its anhydrides.
Use: Surface active agent.
Arlacel 83. (AstraZeneca) Sorbitan sesquioleate.
Use: Surface active agent.
Arlacel 165. (AstraZeneca) Glyceryl
monostearate, PEG-100 stearate nonionic self-emulsifying.
Use: Surface active agent.
Arlamol E. (AstraZeneca) Polyoxypropyl-
ene (15), stearyl ether, BHT 0.1%.
Use: Emollient.
Arlatone 507. (AstraZeneca) Padimate
O. *OTC.*
Use: Sunscreen.
Arm-a-Med Metaproterenol Sulfate.
(Centeon) Metaproterenol sulfate 0.4%,
0.6%, sodium Cl, EDTA. Soln. for
nebulization. Vial UD 2.5 mL for use
with IPPB device. *Rx.*
Use: Bronchodilator.
Arm-a-Vial. (Centeon) Sterile water, so-
dium Cl 0.45%, 0.9%. Box 100s. Plas-
tic vial 3 mL, 5 mL.

Use: Electrolyte supplement.
• **armodafinil.** (ar-moe-DAF-in-il) USAN.
Use: Analeptic.
Armour Thyroid. (Forest) Thyroid desiccated 15 mg (¼ gr), 30 mg (½ gr),
60 mg (1 gr), 90 mg (1 ½ gr), 120 mg
(2 gr), 180 mg (3 gr), 240 mg (4 gr),
300 mg (5 gr), dextrose. Tab. Bot. 100s,
1000s (except 15 mg, 90 mg, 240 mg,
300 mg), 5000s (30 mg, 60 mg only),
50,000s (60 mg, 120 mg only), UD 100s
(30 mg, 60 mg, 120 mg only). *Rx.*
Use: Thyroid hormone.
Arnica Tincture. (Eli Lilly) Arnica 20% in
alcohol 66%. Bot. 120 mL, 480 mL.
OTC.
Use: Analgesic, topical.
• **arofylline.** (ah-ROE-fih-lin) USAN.
Use: Bronchodilator; asthma prophyl-
actic.
Aromasin. (Pharmacia) Exemestane
25 mg, mannitol, methylparaben, poly-
vinyl alcohol. Tab. Bot. 30s. *Rx.*
Use: Hormone, breast cancer.
aromatase inhibitors.
See: Anastrozole.
Arimidex.
Aromasin.
Exemestane.
Femara.
Letrozole.
Aromatic Ammonia Vaporole. (Glaxo-
SmithKline) Inhalant. Vial 5 min. Box
10s, 12s, 100s. *Rx.*
Use: Respiratory.
Aromatic Cascara Fluidextract.
(Various Mfr.) Cascara sagrada, alco-
hol 19%. Liq. Bot. 473 mL. *OTC.*
Use: Laxative.
• **aromatic elixir.** *NF 23.*
Use: Pharmaceutic aid, vehicle, fla-
vored, sweetened.
aromatic elixir. (Eli Lilly) Alcohol 22%.
Bot. 16 fl. oz.
Use: Pharmaceutic aid, flavoring.
AR-121. (Argus) Phase I/II HIV. *Rx.*
Use: Antiviral.
• **arprinocid.** (ahr-PRIN-oh-sid) USAN.
Use: Coccidiostat.
arseclor.
See: Dichlorophenarsine hydrochloride.
arsenic compounds.
Use: Rarely employed in modern medi-
cine; there are no longer any official
compounds.
See: Acetarsone.
Arsphenamine.
Carbarsone.
Dichlorophenarsine Hydrochloride.
Ferric Cacodylate.

Glycobiarsol.
Neoarsphenamine.
Oxophenarsine Hydrochloride.
Sodium Cacodylate.
Tryparsamide.
• **arsenic trioxide.** (AR-se-nik) USAN.
Use: Antineoplastic.
See: Trisenox.
arsenobenzene.
See: Arsphenamine.
arsenphenolamine.
See: Arsphenamine.
Arsobal. Melarsoprol (Mel B).
Use: CDC anti-infective agent.
arsphenamine. Arsenobenzene, arseno-
benzol, arsenophenolamine, Ehrlich
606, salvarsan.
Use: Formerly used as antisyphilitic.
arsthinol. Cyclic.
Use: Antiprotozoal.
Artarau. (Archer-Taylor) Rauwolfia ser-
pentina 50 mg, 100 mg. Tab. Bot.
100s, 1000s. *Rx.*
Use: Antihypertensive.
Arta-Vi-C. (Archer-Taylor) Multivitamins
with Vitamin C 100 mg. Tab. Bot. 100s.
OTC.
Use: Vitamin supplement.
Artazyme. (Archer-Taylor) Bot. 13 mL.
Use: Autolyzed proteolytic enzyme.
• **arteflene.** (AHR-teh-fleen) USAN.
Use: Antimalarial.
• **artegraft.** (AHR-teh-graft) USAN. Arterial
graft composed of a section of bovine
carotid artery that has been subjected to
enzymatic digestion with ficin and
tanned with dialdehyde starch.
Use: Prosthetic aid, arterial.
arterenol.
See: Norepinephrine bitartrate.
• **artesunate.** (ar-TES-oo-nate) USAN.
Use: Investigational antimalarial agent.
Artha-G. (T.E. Williams Pharmaceuticals)
Salsalate 750 mg. Tab. Bot. 120s. *Rx.*
Use: Analgesic.
Arthralgen. (Wyeth) Salicylamide
250 mg, acetaminophen 250 mg. Tab.
Bot. 30s, 100s, 500s. *OTC.*
Use: Analgesic combination.
ArthriCare Daytime Formula. (Del)
Menthol 1.25%, methyl nicotinate
0.25%, capsaicin 0.025%, with aloe
vera gel, carbomer 940, DMDM hydan-
toin, glyceryl stearate SE, myristyl pro-
pionate, propylparaben, triethanol-
amine. Cream. Jar 90 g. *OTC.*
Use: Analgesic, topical.
ArthriCare Double Ice. (Del) Menthol
4%, camphor 3.1%, with aloe vera gel,
carbomer 940, dioctyl sodium sulfo-

succinate, propylene glycol, triethanolamine. Gel. Jar 90 g. *OTC.*
Use: Analgesic, topical.
ArthriCare Odor Free Rub. (Del) Menthol 1.25%, methyl nicotinate 0.25%,
capsaicin 0.025%, aloe vera gel, carbomer 940, DMDM hydantoin, emulsifying wax, glyceryl stearate SE, isopropyl alcohol, myristyl propionate, propylparaben, triethanolamine. Oint. Jar
90 g. *OTC.*
Use: Liniment.
ArthriCare Triple Medicated. (Del)
Methyl salicylate 30%, menthol 1.25%,
methyl nicotinate 0.7%, dioctyl sodium
sulfosuccinate, hydroxypropyl methylcellulose, isopropyl alcohol, propylene
glycol. Gel. Tube 3 oz. *OTC.*
Use: Analgesic, topical.
Arthritic Pain. (Walgreen) Triethanolamine salicylate 10%. Lot. Bot. 6 oz.
OTC.
Use: Analgesic, topical.
Arthritis Bayer Timed Release Aspirin.
(Bayer Corp. (Consumer Div.)) Aspirin
650 mg. TR Tab. Bot. 30s, 72s, 125s.
OTC.
Use: Analgesic.
Arthritis Hot Creme. (Thompson Medi-
cal) Methyl salicylate 15%, menthol
10%, glyceryl stearate, carbomer 934,
lanolin, PEG-100 stearate, propylene
glycol, trolamine, parabens. Cream. Jar
90 g. *OTC.*
Use: Liniment.
Arthritis Pain Formula. (Whitehall-Rob-
ins) Aspirin 486 mg, aluminum hydrox-
ide gel 20 mg, magnesium hydroxide
60 mg. Tab. Bot. 40s, 100s, 175s. *OTC.*
Use: Analgesic combination.
Arthritis Pain Formula, Aspirin Free.
(Whitehall-Robins) Acetaminophen
500 mg. Tab. Bot. 30s, 75s. *OTC.*
Use: Analgesic.
Arthropan. (Purdue) Choline salicylate
870 mg/5 mL. Liq. Bot. 8 oz, 16 oz. *Rx.*
Use: Analgesic.
Arthrotec. (Pharmacia) Diclofenac so-
dium 50 mg/misoprostol 200 mcg,
diclofenac sodium 75 mg/misoprostol
200 mcg, lactose. Tab. Bot. 60s, 90s
(50 mg only). *Rx.*
Use: Analgesic.
Arthrotrin. (Whiteworth Towne) Enteric-
coated aspirin 325 mg. Tab. Bot. 100s.
Use: Analgesic.
• **articaine.** (AR-ti-kane) USAN.
Use: Anesthetic, injectable local amide.
See: Septocaine.
Articulose L.A. (Seatrace) Triamcinolone diacetate 40 mg/mL. Vial 5 mL.

Rx.
Use: Corticosteroid.
artificial tanning agent.
See: Sudden Tan.
artificial tear insert.
See: Lacrisert.
artificial tears. (Various Mfr.) Benzalkonium Cl 0.01%. May also contain EDTA, NaCl, polyvinyl alcohol, hydroxypropyl methylcellulose Soln. Bot. 15 mL, 30 mL. *OTC.*
Use: Lubricant, ophthalmic.
artificial tears. (Rugby) White petrolatum, anhydrous liquid lanolin, mineral oil. Ophth. Oint. Tube 3.5 g. *OTC.*
Use: Lubricant, ophthalmic.
artificial tear solutions.
Use: Lubricant, ophthalmic.
See: Akwa Tears.
Aquasite
Artificial Tears.
Artificial Tears Plus.
Celluvisc.
Comfort Tears.
Dry Eyes.
Preservative Free Moisture Eyes.
Puralube Tears.
Refresh Plus.
Teargen.
Tears Naturale Forte.
TheraTears.
Visine Pure Tears.
Visine Tears.
Visine Tears Preservative Free.
Artificial Tears Plus. (Various Mfr.) Polyvinyl alcohol 1.4%, povidone 0.6%, chlorobutanol 0.5%, NaCl. Soln. Bot. 15 mL. *OTC.*
Use: Lubricant, ophthalmic.
• **artilide fumarate.** (AHR-tih-lide) USAN.
Use: Cardiovascular agent.
Artra Beauty Bar. (Schering-Plough) Triclocarban 1% in soap base. Cake 3.6 oz. *OTC.*
Use: Dermatologic; cleanser.
Artra Skin Tone Cream. (Schering-Plough) Hydroquinone 2%. Oint. Tube 1 oz (normal only), 2 oz, 4 oz.
Use: Dermatologic.
arylalkylamines.
Use: Nasal decongestant.
See: Adrenalin Chloride.
Afrin Children's Pump Mist.
AH-chew D.
Cenafed.
Decofed.
Dimetapp Decongestant Pediatric.
Dimetapp, Maximum Strength, Non-Drowsy.
Dimetapp, Maximum Strength 12-Hour, Non-Drowsy.

Drixoral 12 Hour Non-Drowsy Formula.
Efidac 24 Hour Relief.
Ephedrine Sulfate.
Epinephrine Hydrochloride.
4-Way Fast Acting.
Genaphed.
Kid Kare.
Little Colds for Infants and Children.
Little Noses Gentle Formula, Infants & Children.
Medi-First Sinus Decongestant.
Nasal Decongestant, Children's Non-Drowsy.
Nasal Decongestant Oral.
Neo-Synephrine 4-Hour Extra Strength.
Neo-Synephrine 4-Hour Mild Formula.
Neo-Synephrine 4-Hour Regular Strength.
PediaCare Decongestant, Infants'.
Phenylephrine Hydrochloride.
Pretz-D.
Pseudoephedrine Hydrochloride.
Pseudoephedrine Sulfate.
Rhinall.
Silfedrine, Children's.
Simply Stuffy.
Sinustop.
Sudafed, Children's Non-Drowsy.
Sudafed Non-Drowsy, Maximum Strength.
Sudafed Non-Drowsy 12 Hour Long-Acting.
Sudafed Non-Drowsy 24 Hour Long-Acting.
Sudodrin.
Triaminic Allergy Congestion.
Vicks Sinex Ultra Fine Mist.
Arzol Silver Nitrate Applicators. (Arzol) Silver nitrate 75% and potassium nitrate 25%. Applicator. 100s. *Rx.*
Use: Topical anti-infective.
• **arzoxifene hydrochloride.** (ar-ZOX-ifeen) USAN.
Use: Uterine fibroids; endometriosis; dysfunctional uterine bleeding; breast cancer.
5-asa. Mesalamine.
See: Asacol.
Rowasa.
ASA. (Wampole) Anti-skin antibodies test by IFA. Test 48s.
Use: Diagnostic aid.
A.S.A. (Eli Lilly) Aspirin. Acetylsalicylic acid. **Enseal:** 5 g, 10 g. Bot. 100s, 1000s. **Supp.:** 5 g, 10 g. Pkg. 6s, 144s. *OTC.*
Use: Analgesic.
Asacol. (Procter & Gamble) Mesalamine 400 mg. Tab. DR Bot. 100s. *Rx.*

Use: Anti-inflammatory.

asafetida, emulsion of. Milk of Asafetida.

Asaped. (Sanofi-Synthelabo) Acetylsalicylic acid. Tab. *OTC.*
Use: Analgesic.

Asawin. (Sanofi-Synthelabo) Acetylsalicylic acid. Tab. *OTC.*
Use: Analgesic.

A.S.B. (Femco) Calcium carbonate, magnesium carbonate, bismuth subcarbonate, sodium bicarbonate, kaolin. Pow. Can 3 oz. Tab. Bot. 50s. *OTC.*
Use: Antacid.

Asclerol. (Spanner) Liver injection crude (2 mcg/mL) 50%, Vitamins B_1 20 mg, B_2 3 mg, B_6 1 mg, B_{12} 30 mcg, niacinamide 100 mg, panthenol 2.8 mg, choline Cl 20 mg, inositol 10 mg/mL. Multiple dose vial 10 mL. *Rx.*
Use: Vitamin supplement.

ASC Lotionized. (Geritrex) Triclosan 0.3%. Aloe vera gel, sweet almond oil, parabens, tartrazine. Liq. 8 oz. *OTC.*
Use: Topical anti-infective.

Asco-Caps. (Key Company) Ascorbic acid 500 mg. Cap. 100s, 500s. *OTC.*
Use: Vitamin.

Ascomp with Codeine. (Breckenridge) Codeine phosphate 30 mg, aspirin 325 mg, caffeine 40 mg, butalbital 50 mg. Cap. Bot. 100s, 500s. *c-iii.*
Use: Narcotic analgesic combination.

ascorbate sodium. Antiscorbutic vitamin.

•**ascorbic acid.** (ASS-kor-bik) *USP 28.*
Use: Vitamin, antiscorbutic; acidifier, urinary.
See: Asco-Caps.
　Ascor L 500.
　Ascorbineed.
　Cecon.
　Cenolate.
　Cevalin.
　Cevi-Bid.
　Ce-Vi-Sol.
　Dull-C
　Neo-Vadrin.
　N'ice Vitamin C Drops.
　Sunkist Vitamin C.
　Vita-C
W/Combinations.
See: Chewable Vitamin C.
　C-Max.
　Fruit C 500.
　Fruit C 100.
　Fruit C 200.
　Sunkist Vitamin C.
　Vicks Vitamin C Drops.

ascorbic acid. (Various Mfr.) Vitamin C.
　Tab.: 250 mg, 500 mg, 1000 mg, 1500 mg. Bot. 100s, 250s (500 mg, 1000 mg only), 1000s (500 mg only), UD 100s (250 mg, 500 mg only). **TR Tab.:** 500 mg, 1000 mg. Bot. 100s, 250s, 500s. **Cap.:** 500 mg. Bot. 100s. **Pow.:** 60 mg/¼ tsp. Bot. 454 g. **Liq.:** 500 mg/5 mL. Bot. 120 mL, 480 mL. *OTC.*
Use: Vitamin supplement.

ascorbic acid injection.
Use: Vitamin supplement.
See: Cevalin.

ascorbic acid salts.
See: Bismuth Ascorbate.
　Calcium Ascorbate.
　Sodium Ascorbate.

Ascorbineed. (Hanlon) Vitamin C 500 mg. T-Cap. Bot. 100s. *OTC.*
Use: Vitamin supplement.

Ascorbin/11. (Taylor Pharmaceuticals) Lemon bioflavonoids 110 mg, Vitamin C 1 g, rosehips powder 50 mg, rutin 25 mg. SR Tab. Bot. 100s. *OTC.*
Use: Vitamin supplement.

Ascorbocin. (Paddock) Vitamin C 500 mg, niacin 500 mg, B_1 50 mg, B_6 50 mg, d-α-tocopheryl, polyethylene glycol 1000 succinate 50 units, lactose/ 3 g. Pow. Bot. lb. *OTC.*
Use: Vitamin supplement.

•**ascorbyl palmitate.** (ah-SCORE-bill PAL-mih-tate) *NF 23.*
Use: Preservative; pharmaceutic aid, antioxidant.

Ascor L 500. (McGuff) Ascorbic acid 500 mg/mL, EDTA 0.025%, preservative free. Inj. 50 mL. *Rx.*
Use: Vitamin.

Ascorvite S.R. (Eon Labs) Vitamin C 500 mg. SR Cap. *OTC.*
Use: Vitamin supplement.

Ascriptin. (Aventis) Aspirin 325 mg, magnesium hydroxide 50 mg, aluminum hydroxide 50 mg. Tab. Bot. 50s, 100s, 225s, 500s. *OTC.*
Use: Analgesic; antacid.

Ascriptin A/D. (Aventis) Acetylsalicylic acid 325 mg with magnesium hydroxide 75 mg, aluminum hydroxide and calcium carbonate 75 mg. Tab. Bot. 225s. *OTC.*
Use: Analgesic; antacid.

Ascriptin Extra Strength. (Aventis) Aspirin 500 mg with magnesium hydroxide 80 mg, aluminum hydroxide and calcium carbonate 80 mg. Tab. Bot. 50s. *OTC.*
Use: Analgesic; antacid.

•**asenapine maleate.** (ay-SEN-a-peen) USAN.
Use: Serotonin antagonist.

Asendin. (Wyeth) Amoxapine 25 mg, 50 mg, 100 mg, 150 mg. Tab. Bot. 30s (150 mg only), 100s (except 150 mg), 500s (50 mg only), UD 100s (50 mg and 100 mg only). *Rx.*
Use: Antidepressant.
aseptichrome.
See: Merbromin.
Aslum. (Drug Products) Carbolic acid 1%, aluminum acetate, ichthammol, zinc oxide, aromatic oils in a petrolatum-stearin base. Tube. Jar.
Use: Astringent.
Asma. (Wampole) Anti-smooth muscle antibody test by IFA. Test 48.
Use: Diagnostic aid.
Asmalix. (Century) Theophylline 80 mg, alcohol 20%/15 mL. Bot. qt, gal. *Rx.*
Use: Bronchodilator.
Asmanex Twisthaler. (Schering) Mometasone furoate 220 mg/actuation. Lactose. Pow. for Inh. Inhalation device. 14 units, 30 units, 60 units, 120 units. *Rx.*
Use: Corticosteroid.
Asma-Tuss. (Halsey Drug) Phenobarbital 4 mg, theophylline 15 mg, ephedrine sulfate 12 mg, guaifenesin 50 mg/5 mL. Bot. 4 oz. *Rx.*
Use: Bronchodilator.
Asolectin. (Associated Concentrates) Chemical lecithin 25%, chemical cephalin 22%, inositol phosphatides 16%, soybean oil 2.5%, other miscellaneous sterols and lipids 34.5%. *OTC.*
Use: Diet supplement.
• **asoprisnil.** (as-oh-PRIS-nil) USAN.
Use: Endometriosis.
• **asparaginase.** (ass-PAR-uh-jin-aze) USAN.
Use: Antineoplastic.
See: Elspar.
• **aspartame.** (ass-PAR-tame) *NF 23.*
Use: Sweetener.
• **aspartic acid.** (ass-PAR-tick) *USP 28.* Aspartic acid; aminosuccinic acid.
Use: Management of fatigue; amino acid.
• **aspartocin.** (ass-PAR-toe-sin) USAN.
Use: Anti-infective.
A-Spas S/L. (Hyrex) Hyoscyamine sulfate 0.125 mg. Tab., sublingual. Bot. 100s. *Rx.*
Use: Antispasmodic/anticholinergic.
Aspercreme. (Thompson Medical) Triethanolamine salicylate 10% in cream base. *OTC.*
Use: Analgesic, topical.
aspergillus niger enzyme. Alpha-galactosidase. *OTC.*

See: Beano.
aspergillus oryzae enzyme. Diastase.
Aspergum. (Schering-Plough) Aspirin 227.5 mg/1 Gum. Tab. Orange or cherry flavor. Box 16s, 40s. *OTC.*
Use: Analgesic.
asperkinase. Proteolytic enzyme mixture derived from aspergillus oryzae.
• **asperlin.** (ASS-per-lin) USAN.
Use: Anti-infective; antineoplastic.
Aspermin. (Buffington) Aspirin 325 mg. Sugar, caffeine, lactose, and salt free. Tab. *Dispens-A-Kit* 500s. *OTC.*
Use: Analgesic.
Aspermin Extra. (Buffington) Aspirin 500 mg. Sugar, caffeine, lactose, and salt free. Tab. *Dispens-A-Kit* 500s. *OTC.*
Use: Analgesic.
• **aspirin.** (ASS-pihr-in) *USP 28.*
Use: Analgesic; antipyretic; antirheumatic. Prophylactic to reduce risk of death or non-fatal MI in patients with a previous infarction or unstable angina pectoris.
See: A.S.A.
  Aspergum.
  Asprimox.
  Bayer Buffered Aspirin.
  Bayer Children's Aspirin.
  Bayer, 8-Hour Timed-Release.
  Bayer Extra Strength Back & Body Pain.
  Bayer Low Adult Strength.
  Bayer Women's Aspirin Plus Calcium.
  Darvon Compound 32.
  Easprin.
  Ecotrin.
  Ecotrin Adult Low Strength.
  Ecotrin Maximum Strength.
  Genprin.
  Genuine Bayer Aspirin.
  Halfprin 81.
  Heartline.
  Maximum Bayer Aspirin.
  Norwich Aspirin.
  St. Joseph.
  ZORprin.
W/Combinations.
  See: Adprin-B.
  Alka Seltzer.
  Alka Seltzer Plus.
  Anacin.
  Anacin Maximum Strength.
  A.P.C.
  Arthritis Foundation Pain Reliever.
  Arthritis Strength BC Powder.
  Ascriptin.
  Ascriptin A/D.
  Ascriptin, Extra Strength.
  Asprimox Extra Protection for Arthritis Pain.

Bayer Aspirin.
Bayer Buffered Aspirin.
Bayer Extra Strength Back & Body
   Pain.
Bayer Low Adult Strength.
Bayer Plus Extra Strength.
Bayer PM Extra Strength Aspirin Plus
   Sleep Aid.
Bayer Women's Aspirin Plus Calcium.
BC.
BC Powder Arthritis Strength.
BC Powder Original Formula.
Buffaprin.
Cama.
Cama Arthritis Pain Reliever.
Cope.
Darvon Compound 32.
Ecotrin Adult Low Strength.
Equagesic.
Excedrin.
Extra Strength Adprin-B.
Extra Strength Bayer Plus.
4-Way.
Goody's Headache.
Halfprin 81.
Heartline.
Levacet.
Micrainin.
Midol.
Mobigesic.
Momentum.
Night-Time Effervescent.
Orphengesic.
Orphengesic Forte.
P-A-C Analgesic.
Painaid.
Painaid ESF Extra-Strength Formula.
Presalin.
Saleto.
Salocol.
Sine-Off.
St. Joseph Adult Chewable Aspirin.
St. Joseph Cold Tablets For Children.
Vanquish.
Zee-Seltzer.
aspirin, alumina, and magnesia.
   Use: Analgesic; antacid.
**aspirin, alumina, and magnesium
   oxide.**
   Use: Analgesic; antacid.
aspirin and barbiturate combinations.
   Use: Analgesic; sedative; hypnotic.
   See: BAC.
   Butalbital.
   Fiorinal.
   Lanorinal.
aspirin and codeine phosphate.
   Use: Analgesic.
aspirin and codeine phosphate. (Vin-
   tage Pharmaceuticals) Codeine phos-
   phate 15 mg/aspirin 325 mg. Tab. 100s,

500s, 1,000s. *c-III.*
   Use: Analgesic, narcotic.
aspirin and dipyridamole.
   Use: Antiplatelet.
   See: Aggrenox.
aspirin and narcotic combinations.
   See: Alor 5/500.
   Ascomp with Codeine.
   Butalbital, Aspirin, and Caffeine.
   Butalbital Compound.
   Florinal with Codeine.
aspirin and oxycodone. (Various Mfr.)
   Oxycodone hydrochloride 4.5 mg, oxy-
   codone terephthalate 0.38 mg, aspirin
   325 mg. Tab. Bot. 100s, 500s, 1000s,
   UD 25s. *c-II.*
   Use: Analagesic combination, narcotic.
aspirin and pravastatin.
   Use: Antihyperlipidemic combination.
   See: Pravigard PAC.
aspirin, butalbital, and caffeine.
   See: Butalbital, Aspirin, and Caffeine.
**aspirin, caffeine, and dihydrocodeine
   bitartrate.**
   Use: Analgesic.
aspirin, caffeine, and orphenadrine.
   Use: Analgesic.
   See: Orphengesic.
   Orphengesic Forte.
**aspirin, codeine, phosphate alumina,
   and magnesia.**
   Use: Analgesic.
**Aspirin Free Anacin Maximum
   Strength.** (Whitehall-Robins) Aceta-
   minophen 500 mg. Capl., Gel Capl. Bot.
   100s. Tab. Bot. 60s. *OTC.*
   Use: Analgesic.
Aspirin Free Anacin P.M. (Whitehall-
   Robins) Diphenhydramine hydrochlo-
   ride 25 mg, acetaminophen 500 mg.
   Tab. Bot. 20s. *OTC.*
   Use: Sleep aid.
**Aspirin-Free Bayer Select Allergy Si-
   nus.** (Bayer Corp. (Consumer Div.))
   Pseudoephedrine hydrochloride 30 mg,
   chlorpheniramine maleate 2 mg, aceta-
   minophen 500 mg. Cap. Pkg. 16s. *OTC.*
   Use: Analgesic; antihistamine; decon-
   gestant.
Aspirin-Free Bayer Select Headache.
   (Bayer Corp. (Consumer Div.)) Aceta-
   minophen 500 mg, caffeine 65 mg. Cap.
   Bot. 50s. *OTC.*
   Use: Analgesic combination.
**Aspirin-Free Bayer Select Head &
   Chest Cold.** (Bayer Corp. (Consumer
   Div.)) Pseudoephedrine hydrochloride
   30 mg, dextromethorphan HBr 10 mg,
   guaifenesin 100 mg, acetaminophen
   325 mg. Capl. Bot. 16s. *OTC.*
   Use: Analgesic; decongestant; expecto-
   rant.

Aspirin Free Excedrin. (Bristol-Myers Squibb) Acetaminophen 500 mg, caffeine 65 mg. Tab., Capl. Bot. 20s, 40s, 80s. *OTC.*
Use: Analgesic combination.
Aspirin Free Pain Relief. (Hudson Corp.) Acetaminophen 325 mg. Tab. Bot. 100s. *OTC.*
Use: Analgesic.
Aspirin Plus. (Walgreen) Aspirin 400 mg, caffeine 32 mg. Tab. Bot. 100s. *OTC.*
Use: Analgesic combination.
aspirin salts.
See: Calcium Acetylsalicylate.
Aspirin Uniserts. (Upsher-Smith) Aspirin 125 mg, 300 mg, 650 mg. Supp. Ctn. 12s, 50s. *OTC.*
Use: Analgesic.
aspirin w/codeine no. 4. (Various Mfr.) Codeine phosphate 60 mg, aspirin 325 mg Tab. Bot. 100s, 500s, 1000s. *c-III.*
Use: Analgesic combination, narcotic.
aspirin w/codeine no. 3. (Various Mfr.) Codeine phosphate 30 mg, aspirin 325 mg. Tab. Bot. 100s, 1000s. *c-III.*
Use: Analgesic combination, narcotic.
Aspirtab. (Dover Pharmaceuticals) Aspirin 325 mg. Sugar, lactose, and salt free. Tab. UD Box 500s. *OTC.*
Use: Analgesic.
Aspirtab Max. (Dover Pharmaceuticals) Aspirin 500 mg. Sugar, lactose, and salt free. Tab. UD Box 500s. *OTC.*
Use: Analgesic.
Asprimox. (Invamed) Aspirin 325 mg (buffered). Capl. Bot. 100s, 500s. *OTC.*
Use: Analgesic.
Asprimox Extra Protection for Arthritis Pain. (Invamed) Aspirin 325 mg, aluminum hydroxide gel (dried) 75 mg, magnesium hydroxide 75 mg, calcium carbonate. Capl. Bot. 100s, 500s. *OTC.*
Use: Analgesic.
Astaril. (Sanofi-Synthelabo) Theophylline anhydrous, ephedrine sulphate. Tab. *Rx.*
Use: Bronchodilator.
Astelin. (Medpointe) Azelastine 137 mcg/spray, benzalkonium chloride, EDTA. Nasal Spray. Bot. 17 mg (100 metered sprays) per bottle. 2s. *Rx.*
Use: Antihistamine, peripherally selective phthalazinone.
•**astemizole.** (ASS-TEM-ih-zole) USAN.
Use: Antihistamine; antiallergic.
asterol.
Use: Antifungal.
Asthmalixir. (Reese) Theophylline 45 mg, ephedrine sulfate 36 mg, guaifenesin 150 mg, phenobarbital 12 mg/

15 mL, alcohol 19%. Bot. *Rx.*
Use: Bronchodilator; expectorant; hypnotic; sedative.
AsthmaNefrin. (Numark) Racepinephrine hydrochloride 2.25%. Soln. for Inh. Bot. 15 mL. *OTC.*
Use: Sympathomimetic.
AsthmaNefrin Solution & Nebulizer. (Numark) Racepin (racemic epinephrine) as hydrochloride equivalent to epinephrine base 2.25%, chlorobutanol 0.5%. Bot. 0.5 fl oz. With sodium bisulfite. Bot. 1 fl oz. *OTC.*
Use: Bronchodilator.
•**astifilcon a.** (ASS-tih-FILL-kahn) USAN.
Use: Contact lens material, hydrophilic.
Astramorph PF. (AstraZeneca) Morphine sulfate 0.5 mg/mL, 1 mg/mL, preservative free. Inj. Amp. 2 mL, 10 mL. Single-use vial 10 mL, c-II.
Use: Analgesic, narcotic agonist.
Astroglide. (Biofilm) Purified water, glycerin, propylene glycol, parabens. Vaginal gel. Bot 66.5 mL. Travel pks. 5 mL. *OTC.*
Use: Lubricant.
•**astromicin sulfate.** (ASS-troe-MY-sin) USAN.
Use: Anti-infective.
Astro-Vites. (Faraday) Vitamins A 3500 units, D 400 units, C 60 mg, B_1 0.8 mg, B_2 1.3 mg, niacinamide 14 mg, B_6 1 mg, B_{12} 2.5 mcg, folic acid 0.05 mg, pantothenic acid 5 mg, iron 12 mg. Tab. Bot. 100s, 250s. *OTC.*
Use: Mineral, vitamin supplement.
AST/SGOT Reagent Strips. (Bayer Corp. (Consumer Div.)) Seralyzer reagent strip. A quantitative strip test for aspartate transaminase/serum glutamic oxaloacetic transaminase in serum or plasma. Bot. Strip 25s.
Use: Diagnostic aid.
Asupirin. (Suppositoria Laboratories, Inc.) Aspirin 60 mg, 120 mg, 200 mg, 300 mg, 600 mg, 1.2 g. Supp. Box 12s, 100s, 1000s. *OTC.*
Use: Analgesic.
Atabee TD. (Defco) Vitamins C 500 mg, B_1 15 mg, B_2 10 mg, B_6 2 mg, nicotinamide 50 mg, calcium pantothenate 10 mg. Cap. Bot. 30s, 1000s. *OTC.*
Use: Vitamin supplement.
Atacand. (AstraZeneca) Candesartan cilexetil 4 mg, 8 mg, 16 mg, 32 mg, lactose. Tab. Bot. Unit-of-use 30s, 90s; UD 100s (only 16 mg, 32 mg). *Rx.*
Use: Antihypertensive.
Atacand HCT. (AstraZeneca) Candesartan cilexetil 16 mg, 32 mg, hydrochlorothiazide 12.5 mg, lactose. Tab. Bot.

1000s, UD 100s, unit-of-use 30s, 90s. *Rx.*
Use: Antihypertensive.

• **atazanavir sulfate.** (AT-ah-zah-NAH-veer) USAN.
Use: Antiretroviral, protease inhibitor.
See: Reyataz.

• **atenolol.** (ah-TEN-oh-lahl) *USP 28.*
Use: Beta-adrenergic blocker.
See: Tenormin.

atenolol. (Various Mfr.) Atenolol. **Tab.:** 25 mg, 50 mg, 100 mg. Bot. 100s, 500s (25 mg only), 1000s. **Robot Ready:** 25s, UD 100s (25 mg only). *Rx.*
Use: Antiadrenergic/sympatholytic; beta-adrenergic blocking agent.

atenolol/chlorthalidone. (Various Mfr.) Atenolol 50 mg, 100 mg, chlorthalidone 25 mg. Tab. Bot. 50s, 100s, 250s, 500s, 1000s. *Rx.*
Use: Antihypertensive.

• **atevirdine mesylate.** (at-TEH-vihr-DEEN) USAN.
Use: Antiviral.

Atgam. (Pharmacia) Lymphocyte immune globulin, antithymocyte globulin horse gamma globulin 50 mg/mL, glycine 0.3 M. Inj. Amp. 5 mL. *Rx.*
Use: Immunosuppressant.

Athlete's Foot. (Walgreen) Zinc undecylenate 20%, undecylenic acid 5%. Oint. Tube 1.5 oz. *OTC.*
Use: Antifungal, topical.

• **atilmotin.** (A-til-MOE-tin) USAN.
Use: Gastrointestinal agent.

• **atipamezole.** (AT-ih-pam-EH-zole) USAN.
Use: Antagonist, α_2-receptor.

• **atiprimod dihydrochloride.** (at-TIH-prih-mahd) USAN.
Use: Antiarthritic, immunomodulator, suppressor cell inducing agent; antiinflammatory; antirheumatic, disease-modifying.

• **atiprimod dimaleate.** (at-TIH-prih-mahd) USAN.
Use: Antiarthritic; anti-inflammatory; immunomodulator; antirheumatic, disease-modifying.

• **atiprosin maleate.** (ah-TIH-pro-SIN) USAN.
Use: Antihypertensive.

Ativan. (Baxter) Lorazepam 2 mg/mL, 4 mg/mL. Inj. Multidose vials. Single and 10 mL (PEG400, propylene glycol, benzyl alcohol 2%), boxes of 10 *Tubex. c-iv.*
Use: Anxiolytic.

• **atlafilcon a.** (at-LAH-FILL-kahn A) USAN.

Use: Contact lens material, hydrophilic.

ATnativ. (Bayer Corp. (Biological and Pharmaceutical Div.)) Antithrombin III (human), lyophilized powder/500 units. Inj. Bot. 50 mL w/10 L sterile water. *Rx.*
Use: Thromboembolic. [Orphan Drug]

• **atolide.** (ATE-oh-lide) USAN. Under study.
Use: Anticonvulsant.

Atolone. (Major) Triamcinolone 4 mg. Tab. Bot. 100s, *Uni-Pak* 16s. *Rx.*
Use: Corticosteroid.

• **atomoxetine hydrochloride.** (AT-oh-mox-ah-teen) USAN.
Use: Psychotherapeutic agent.
See: Strattera.

atorvastatin and amlodipine.
Use: Antihyperlipidemic.
See: Caduet.

• **atorvastatin calcium.** (a-TORE-va-statin) USAN.
Use: HMG-CoA reductase inhibitor; antihyperlipidemic.
See: Lipitor.

• **atosiban.** (at-OH-sih-ban) USAN.
Use: Antagonist; oxytocin.

• **atovaquone.** (uh-TOE-vuh-KWONE) *USP 28.*
Use: Antipneumocystic.
See: Mepron.

atovaquone and proguanil hydrochloride.
Use: Antimalarial.
See: Malarone.
   Malarone Pediatric.

Atozine. (Major) Hydroxyzine hydrochloride. 10 mg, 25 mg, 50 mg. Tab. Bot. 100s, 250s, 500s (50 mg only), 1000s (except 50 mg), UD 100s. *Rx.*
Use: Anxiolytic.

Atpeg. (AstraZeneca) Polyethylene glycol available as 300, 400, 600, or 4000.
Use: Humectant; surfactant.

• **atracurium besylate.** (AT-rah-CUE-ree-uhm BESS-ih-late) *USP 28.*
Use: Neuromuscular blocker; muscle relaxant.
See: Tracrium.

atracurium besylate. (Bedford Labs) Atracurium besylate 10 mg/mL. Inj. Single-dose vials. 5 mL. Multidose vials (benzyl alcohol 0.9%). 10 mL. *Rx.*
Use: Muscle relaxant.

Atragen. (Hannan Ophthalmic) Tretinoin.
Use: Antineoplastic. [Orphan Drug]

• **atrasentan.**
Use: Investigational selective endothelin-A receptor antagonist.

●**atreleuton.** (at-reh-LOO-tuhn) USAN.
Use: Antiasthmatic.

Atridine. (Henry Schein) Triprolidine
2.5 mg, pseudoephedrine hydrochloride
60 mg. Tab. Bot. 100s, 1000s. *OTC.*
Use: Antihistamine; decongestant.

Atridox. (CollaGenex) Doxycycline
42.5 mg (as hyclate, 10%). Inj. 2-
syringe mixing system and blunt cannula. *Rx.*
Use: Mouth and throat product.

Atrocap. (Freeport) Atropine sulfate
0.06 mg, hyoscyamine sulfate 0.3 mg,
hyoscine hydrobromide 0.02 mg,
phenobarbital 50 mg. TR Cap. Bot.
1000s. *Rx.*
Use: Anticholinergic; antispasmodic;
hypnotic; sedative.

Atrocholin. (GlaxoSmithKline) Dehydro-
cholic acid 130 mg. Tab. Bot. 100s.
OTC.
Use: Laxative.

Atrofed. (Genetco, Inc.) Pseudoephedrine hydrochloride 60 mg, triprolidine
hydrochloride 2.5 mg. Tab. Bot. 24s,
100s, 1000s. *OTC.*
Use: Antihistamine; decongestant.

Atrohist LA. (Medeva) Pseudoephedrine
hydrochloride 120 mg, brompheni-
amine maleate 4 mg, phenyltoloxamine
citrate 50 mg. SR Tab with atropine
sulfate 0.0242 mg available for immediate release. Bot. 100s. *Rx.*
Use: Antihistamine; decongestant.

Atrohist Pediatric Capsules. (Medeva)
Chlorpheniramine maleate 4 mg,
pseudoephedrine hydrochloride 60 mg.
SR Cap. Bot. 100s. *Rx.*
Use: Antihistamine; decongestant.

Atrohist Pediatric Suspension.
(Medeva) Phenylephrine tannate 5 mg,
chlorpheniramine tannate 2 mg, pyrilamine tannate 12.5 mg. Susp. Bot.
473 mL. Unit-of-use 118 mL. *Rx.*
Use: Antihistamine; decongestant.

Atrohist Sprinkle. (Medeva) Pseudoephedrine hydrochloride 120 mg, brompheniramine maleate 2 mg, phenyto-
loxamine citrate 25 mg. SR Cap. Bot.
100s. *Rx.*
Use: Antihistamine; decongestant.

AtroPen. (Meridian Medical Technologies) Atropine sulfate 0.5 mg, 1 mg,
2 mg. Glycerin, phenol. Inj. Auto-injectors prefilled. *Rx.*
Use: Gastrointestinal anticholinergic/
antispasmodic.

●**atropine.** (AT-troe-peen) *USP 28.*
Use: Anticholinergic.

**atropine-hyoscine-hyoscyamine com-
binations.** (Also see Belladonna Products).

See: Barbella.
Barbeloid.
Belbutal No. 2 Kaptabs.
Brobella-P.B.
Donnatal #2.
Nilspasm.
Sedamine.
Sedapar.
Spabelin.
Spasmolin.
Urogesic.

atropine-n-oxide hydrochloride.
See: Atropine Oxide Hydrochloride.

Atropine-1. (Optopics) Atropine sulfate
1%. Soln. Bot. 2 mL, 5 mL, 15 mL. *Rx.*
Use: Cycloplegic; mydriatic.

●**atropine oxide hydrochloride.** (AT-row-
peen OX-ide) USAN.
Use: Anticholinergic
See: X-Tro.

●**atropine sulfate.** (AT-row-peen) *USP 28.*
Use: Anticholinergic/antispasmodic,
ophthalmic.
See: AtroPen.
Atropine-1.
Atropine Sulfate S.O.P.
Bellahist-D LA.
Isopto-Atropine.
Lyopine.
Parasympatholytic and antispas-
modic.
Sal-Tropine.
W/Combinations.
See: Donnatal.
Donnatal Extentabs.

atropine sulfate. (Abbott) Atropine sulfate 0.05 mg/mL, 0.1 mg/mL. *Abboject*
syringes. 5 mL, 10 mL (0.1 mg/mL
only). *Rx.*
Use: Anticholinergic/antispasmodic.

atropine sulfate. (Various Mfr.). **Pediatric Inj.:** 0.05 mg/mL 5 mL *Abboject.*
Tab, Hypodermic: 0.3 mg, 0.4 mg,
0.6 mg. Tab. Bot. 100s. **Inj.:** 0.3 mg/mL.
Vial 1 mL, 30 mL; 0.4 mg/mL. Amp.
1 mL, vial 20 mL, 30 mL; 0.5 mg/mL.
Vials. 1 mL, 30 mL. Syringes. 5 mL;
0.8 mg/mL. Amp. 0.5 mL, 1 mL. Syringes. 0.5 mL; 1 mg/mL. Amp., vial
1 mL, syringe 10 mL; 1.2 mg/mL. Vial
1 mL syringe. **Lyophilized:** Lyopine
(Hyrex Pharmaceuticals). **Ophth. Oint:**
1%. Tube 3.5 g, UD 1 g. **Ophth. Soln:**
1%. Bot. UD 1 mL, 2 mL, 5 mL, 15 mL;
2%. Bot. 2 mL.
Use: Anticholinergic, ophthalmic.

**atropine sulfate and edrophonium
chloride.** Anticholinesterase muscle
stimulant.
See: Enlon-Plus.

atropine sulfate combinations.
See: Bellatal.
Stahist.

atropine sulfate S.O.P. (Allergan) Atropine sulfate 0.5%, 1%. Oint. Tube 3.5 g. *Rx.*
Use: Cycloplegic; mydriatic.

atropine sulfate w/phenobarbital.
See: Antrocol.
Arco-Lase Plus.
Barbeloid.
Brobella-P.B.
Donnatal.
Donnatal #2.
Palbar No. 2.
Spabelin.

Atrosed. (Freeport) Atropine sulfate 0.0195 mg, hyoscine HBr 0.0065 mg, hyoscyamine sulfate 0.104 mg, phenobarbital 0.25 g. Tab. Bot. 1000s, 5000s. *Rx.*
Use: Anticholinergic; antispasmodic; hypnotic; sedative.

Atrosept. (Geneva) Methenamine 40.8 mg, phenylsalicylate 18.1 mg, atropine sulfate 0.03 mg, hyoscyamine 0.03 mg, benzoic acid 4.5 mg, methylene blue 5.4 mg. Tab. Bot. 100s, 1000s. *Rx.*
Use: Anti-infective, urinary.

Atrovent. (Boehringer Ingelheim) Ipratropium bromide. **Aerosol:** 18 mcg/dose. Metered dose inhaler 14 g (200 inhalations). **Nasal Spray:** 0.03% (21 mcg/spray). Bot. 30 mL (345 sprays); 0.06% (42 mcg/spray). Bot. 15 mL (165 sprays). *Rx.*
Use: Bronchodilator.

Atrovent HFA. (Boehringer Ingelheim) Ipratropium bromide 17 mcg per actuation. Aerosol. 12.9 g metered-dose inhaler with mouthpiece (200 inhalations). *Rx.*
Use: Bronchodilator.

A/T/S Gel. (Medicis) Erythromycin 2%. Gel. Tube 30 g. *Rx.*
Use: Dermatologic; acne.

AT-Solution. (Sanofi-Synthelabo) Dihydrotachysterol solution.
Use: Antihypocalcemic.

A/T/S Topical Solution. (Medicis) Erythromycin 2%. Top. Soln. Bot. 60 mL. *Rx.*
Use: Dermatologic; acne.

Attain. (Sherwood Davis & Geck) Sodium caseinate, calcium caseinate, maltodextrin, corn oil, soy lecithin. Liq. Can 250 mL and 1000 mL closed system. *OTC.*
Use: Nutritional supplement.

• **attapulgite, activated.** (at-ah-PULL-gyte) *USP 28.*
Use: Antidiarrheal; pharmaceutic aid, suspending agent.
W/Pectin, hydrated alumina.
See: Sebasorb.

A.T. 10.
See: Dihydrotachysterol.

Attenuvax. (Merck & Co.) Measles virus vaccine, live, attenuated $\geq$ 1000 TCID$_{50}$ (tissue culture infectious doses) per 0.5 mL dose, neomycin 25 mcg, sorbitol 14.5 mg, sucrose 1.9 mg, hydrolyzed gelatin 14.5 mg, human albumin 0.3 mg, fetal bovine serum < 1 ppm per dose, preservative free. Single-dose vial w/diluent, 50-dose vial w/30 mL diluent. *Rx.*
Use: Immunization.
W/Meruvax.
See: M-R-Vax-II (Merck & Co.).
W/Mumpsvax, Meruvax.
See: M-M-R II (Merck & Co.).

Atuss DM. (Atley) Dextromethorphan 15 mg, phenylephrine hydrochloride 10 mg, chlorpheniramine maleate 2 mg/5 mL, sucrose, saccharin, menthol, methylparaben, strawberry flavor, alcohol free. Syr. Bot. 473 mL. *Rx.*
Use: Upper respiratory combination, antihistamine, antitussive, decongestant.

Atuss G. (Atley) Hydrocodone bitartrate 2 mg, phenylephrine hydrochloride 10 mg, guaifenesin 100 mg/5 mL, sucrose, saccharin, menthol, grape flavor. Syr. Bot. 473 mL. *c-III.*
Use: Upper respiratory combination, antitussive, decongestant, expectorant, narcotic.

Atuss HC. (Atley) Hydrocodone bitartrate 2.5 mg, chlorpheniramine maleate 2 mg, phenylephrine hydrochloride 10 mg/5 mL. Menthol, sucrose. Cherry flavor. Liq. 473 mL. *c-III.*
Use: Antitussive combination.

Atuss HD. (Atley) Hydrocodone bitartrate 2.5 mg, phenylephrine hydrochloride 10 mg, chlorpheniramine maleate 4 mg/5 mL, menthol, sucrose, cherry flavor. Liq. Bot. 473 mL. *c-III.*
Use: Upper respiratory combination, antihistamine, antitussive, decongestant.

Atuss MS. (Atley) Hydrocodone bitartrate 5 mg, chlorpheniramine maleate 2 mg, phenylephrine hydrochloride 10 mg/5mL, menthol, sucrose, pineapple/orange flavor. Liq. Bot. 473 mL. *c-III.*

Use: Upper respiratory combination, antitussive, antihistamine, decongestant.

Atuss-12 DM. (Atley) Pseudoephedrine hydrochloride (as polistirex) 30 mg, chlorpheniramine maleate (as polistirex) 6 mg, dextromethorphan HBr (as polistirex) 30 mg/5 mL. Corn syrup, parabens. ER Susp. 20 mL, 473 mL. *Rx.*
Use: Pediatric antitussive combination.

Atuss-12 DX. (Atley) Dextromethorphan polistirex (equiv. to dextromethorphan HBr 30 mg), guaifenesin 200 mg/5 mL. Parabens, honey. Honey-lemon flavor. ER Susp. 20 mL, 473 mL. *Rx.*
Use: Antitussive, expectorant.

A-200. (Hogil) Pyrethrins 0.33%, piperonyl butoxide 4%. Shampoo. 59 mL, 118 mL with comb; 118 mL kits containing comb and lice control spray. *OTC.*
Use: Pediculicide.

augmented betamethasone dipropionate.
Use: Corticosteroid, topical.
See: Diprolene.

Augmentin. (GlaxoSmithKline) **Tab.:** Amoxicillin trihydrate 250 mg, 500 mg, 875 mg; clavulanic acid (as the potassium salt) 125 mg, potassium 0.63 mEq. Film coated (except 875 mg). Bot. 20s (except 250 mg), 30s (250 mg only), UD 100s. **Chew. Tab.:** Amoxicillin trihydrate 125 mg, clavulanic acid 31.25 mg (potassium 0.16 mEq, mannitol, saccharin, lemon-lime flavor), amoxicillin trihydrate 200 mg, clavulanic acid 28.5 mg (potassium 0.14 mEq, mannitol, phenylalanine 2.1 mg, saccharin, aspartame, cherry-banana flavor), amoxicillin trihydrate 250 mg, clavulanic acid 62.5 mg (potassium 0.32 mEq, mannitol, saccharin, lemon-lime flavor), amoxicillin 400 mg, clavulanic acid 57 mg (potassium 0.29 mEq, mannitol, phenylalanine 4.2 mg, saccharin, aspartame, cherry-banana flavor). Bot. 20s (200 mg, 400 mg only), 30s (125 mg, 250 mg only). **Pow. for Oral Susp.:** Amoxicillin 125 mg, clavulanic acid 31.25 mg/5 mL (potassium 0.16 mEq, mannitol, saccharin, banana flavor), amoxicillin 200 mg, clavulanic acid 28.5 mg/5 mL (potassium 0.14 mEq, mannitol, phenylalanine 7 mg/5 mL, saccharin, aspartame, orange-raspberry flavor), amoxicillin 250 mg, clavulanic acid 62.5 mg/5 mL (potassium 0.32 mEq, mannitol, saccharin, orange flavor), amoxicillin 400 mg, clavulanic acid 57 mg/5 mL (potassium 0.29 mEq,

mannitol, phenylalanine 7 mg/5 mL, saccharin, aspartame, orange-raspberry flavor). Bot. 50 mL (200 mg, 400 mg only), 75 mL, 100 mL, 150 mL (125 mg, 250 mg only). *Rx.*
Use: Anti-infective, penicillin.

Augmentin ES-600. (GlaxoSmithKline) Amoxicillin trihydrate 600 mg/clavulanic acid 42.9 mg/5 mL, potassium 0.23 mEq/ 5 mL, aspartame, phenylalanine 7 mg/5 mL, orange-raspberry flavor. Pow. for Oral Susp. Bot. 75 mL. *Rx.*
Use: Anti-infective, penicillin.

Augmentin XR. (GlaxoSmithKline) Amoxicillin 1000 mg, clavulanic acid 62.5 mg, potassium 0.32 mEq, sodium 1.27 mEq. Film coated. ER Tab. Pkg. 28s (7-day XR pack), 40s (10-day XR pack). *Rx.*
Use: Anti-infective, penicillin.

Auralgan Otic Solution. (Wyeth) Antipyrine 54 mg, benzocaine 14 mg/mL w/oxyquinoline sulfate in dehydrated glycerin (contains not more than 0.6% moisture). Bot. Dropper 15 mL. *Rx.*
Use: Otic.

Auralgesic. (Wesley) Carbamide 10%, antipyrine 5%, benzocaine 2.5%, cetyldimethylbenzylammonium hydrochloride 0.2%. Bot. 0.5 oz. *Rx.*
Use: Otic.

•**auranofin.** (or-RAIN-oh-fin) USAN.
Use: Antirheumatic.
See: Ridaura.

Aureoquin Diamate. Name previously used for Quinetolate.

Aurinol Ear Drops. (Various Mfr.) Chloroxylenol and acetic acid, w/benzalkonium chloride and glycerin. Soln. Bot. 15 mL. *Rx.*
Use: Otic.

Aurocein. (Christina) Gold naphthyl sulfhydryl derivative 5%, 12.5%. Inj. Amp. 10 mL. *Rx.*
Use: Antirheumatic.

Auro-Dri. (Del) Boric acid 2.75% in isopropyl alcohol. Bot. oz. *OTC.*
Use: Otic.

Auro Ear Drops. (Del) Carbamide peroxide 6.5% in a specially prepared base. Bot. Drops. 15 mL. *OTC.*
Use: Otic.

Auroguard Otic. (SDA) Benzocaine 1.4%, antipyrine 5.4%/mL, glycerin, oxyquinolone sulfate. Otic Soln. 15 mL. *Rx.*
Use: Otic preparation.

Aurolate. (Taylor Pharmaceuticals) Gold sodium thiomalate 50 mg, benzyl alcohol 0.5%/mL. Inj. Vial 2 mL, 10 mL. *Rx.*
Use: Antirheumatic.

aurolin.
See: Gold sodium thiosulfate.
auropin.
See: Gold sodium thiosulfate.
aurosan.
See: Gold sodium thiosulfate.
•**aurothioglucose.** (or-oh-THIGH-oh-GLUE-kose) USP 28.
Use: Antirheumatic.
aurothioglucose injection.
See: Sterile aurothioglucose.
aurothiomalate, sodium.
See: Gold Sodium Thiomalate.
Ausab. (Abbott Diagnostics) Radioimmunoassay or enzyme immunoassay for detection of antibody to hepatitis B surface antigen. Test kit 100s.
Use: Diagnostic aid.
Ausab EIA. (Abbott Diagnostics) Enzyme immunoassay for the detection of antibody to hepatitis B surface antigen.
Use: Diagnostic aid.
Auscell. (Abbott Diagnostics) Reverse passive hemagglutination test for hepatitis B surface antigen. Test kit 110s, 450s, 1800s.
Use: Diagnostic aid.
Ausria II-125. (Abbott Diagnostics) Radioimmunoassay for detection of hepatitis B surface antigen. Test kit 100s, 500s, 600s, 700s, 800s, 900s, 1000s.
Use: Diagnostic aid.
Auszyme II. (Abbott Diagnostics) Enzyme immunoassay for detection of hepatitis B surface antigen (HBsAg) in human serum or plasma. Test kit 100s, 500s.
Use: Diagnostic aid.
Auszyme Monoclonal. (Abbott Diagnostics) Qualitative third generation enzyme immunoassay for the detection of hepatitis B surface antigen (HBsAg) in human serum or plasma.
Use: Diagnostic aid.
Autoantibody Screen. (Wampole) Autoantibody screening system. To screen serum for the presence of a variety of autoantibodies. Test 48s.
Use: Diagnostic aid.
Autolet Kit. (Bayer Corp. (Consumer Div.)) Automatic bloodletting spring-loaded device to obtain capillary blood samples from fingertips, ear lobes, or heels.
Use: Diagnostic aid.
autolymphocyte therapy; ALT. (Cellcor, Inc.)
Use: Treatment of renal cancer.
[Orphan Drug]
Autoplex T. (NABI) Dried anti-inhibitor coagulant complex. With a maximum of heparin 2 units and polyethylene glycol 2 mg per mL reconstituted material, sodium ≈ 177 mEq/L. Heat-treated. Inj. Vial with diluent and needles. Each bottle is labeled with the units of Factor VIII correctional activity it contains. Rx.
Use: Antihemophilic agent.
Autrinic. Intrinsic factor concentrate. Rx.
Use: To increase absorption of vitamin B_{12}.
Auxotab Enteric 1 & 2. (Colab) Rapid identification of enteric bacteria and Pseudomonas. Test contains capillary units with selective biochemical reagents.
Use: Diagnostic aid.
Avage. (Allergan) Tazarotene 0.1%, benzyl alcohol 1%, EDTA, medium chain triglycerides, mineral oil. Cream. 15 g, 30 g. Rx.
Use: Retinoid.
Avail. (Menley & James Labs, Inc.) Iron 18 mg, vitamin A 5000 units, D 400 units, E 30 mg, B_1 2.25 mg, B_2 2.55 mg, B_3 20 mg, B_6 3 mg, B_{12} 9 mcg, C 90 mg, folic acid 0.4 mg, Ca, Cr, I, Mg, Se, Zn 22.5 mg. Tab. Bot. 60s. OTC.
Use: Mineral, vitamin supplement.
Avalgesic. (Various Mfr.) Methyl salicylate, menthol, camphor, methylnicotinate, dipropylene glycol salicylate, oil of cassia, oleoresins capsicum, ginger. Bot. 120 mL, Pt, gal. OTC.
Use: Analgesic, topical.
Avalide. (Bristol-Myers Squibb) Irbesartan/hydrochlorothiazide 150 mg/ 12.5 mg, 300 mg/12.5 mg, 300 mg/ 25 mg. Lactose. Tab. Bot. 30s, 90s; 500s, blister pack 100s (except 300 mg/ 25 mg). Rx.
Use: Antihypertensive.
A-Van. (Stewart-Jackson Pharmacal) Dimenhydrinate 50 mg. Cap. Bot. 100s.
Use: Antivertigo.
•**avanafil.** (av-AN-a-fil) USAN.
Use: Erectile dysfunction.
Avandamet. (GlaxoSmithKline) Rosiglitazone maleate/metformin hydrochloride. 1 mg/500 mg, 2 mg/500 mg, 4 mg/ 500 mg, 2 mg/1000 mg, 4 mg/1000 mg. Lactose. Tab. Bot. 60s, 100s, SUP 100s (except 2 mg/1000 mg and 4 mg/ 1000 mg). Rx.
Use: Antidiabetic.
Avandia. (GlaxoSmithKline) Rosiglitazone maleate 2 mg, 4 mg, 8 mg, lactose. Tab. Bot. 30s, 60s (except 8 mg), 100s, 500s (except 75 mg), SUP 100s (150 mg only). Rx.

Use: Antidiabetic.

Avapro. (Bristol-Myers Squibb Sanofi-Synthelabo Partnership) Irbesartan 75 mg, 150 mg, 300 mg, lactose. Tab. Bot. 30s, 90s, 500s (except 75 mg), UD 100s (150 mg only). *Rx.*
Use: Antihypertensive.

Avar. (Sirius) **Cleanser:** Sulfur 5%, sodium sulfacetamide 10%, cetyl alcohol, stearyl alcohol. 226.8 g. **Gel:** Sulfur 5%, sodium sulfacetamide 10%, EDTA, benzyl alcohol. 45 g. *Rx.*
Use: Keratolytic agent.

Avar Green. (Sirius) Sulfur 5%, sodium sulfacetamide 10%, EDTA, benzyl alcohol. Gel. 45 g. *Rx.*
Use: Keratolytic agent.

•**avasimibe.** (av-ASS-ih-mibe) USAN.
Use: Antiatherosclerotic; hypolipidemic (acylCoA: Cholesterol acyltransferase [ACAT] inhibitor).

Avastin. (Genentech) Bevacizumab 25 mg/mL. Preservative-free. Inj. Single-use vials. 4 mL, 16 mL. *Rx.*
Use: Monoclonal antibody.

Aveenobar Medicated. (Rydelle) Aveeno colloidal oatmeal 50%, sulfur 2%, salicylic acid 2%, in soap-free cleansing bar. *Formerly Acnaveen.* Bar 3.5 oz. *OTC.*
Use: Antipruritic.

Aveenobar Oilated. (Rydelle) Vegetable oils, lanolin derivative, glycerine 29%, aveeno colloidal oatmeal 30% in soap-tree base. *Formerly Emulave.* Bar. 3 oz. *OTC.*
Use: Emollient.

Aveenobar Regular. (Rydelle) Colloidal oatmeal 50%, an ionic sulfonate, hypoallergenic lanolin. *Formerly Aveeno Bar.* Bar 3.2 oz., 4.4 oz. *OTC.*
Use: Dermatologic; cleanser.

Aveeno Bath. (Rydelle) Colloidal oatmeal. Box 1 lb, 4 lb. *OTC.*
Use: Emollient.

Aveeno Cleansing for Acne Prone Skin. (Rydelle) Sulfur 2%, salicylic acid 2%, colloidal oatmeal 50%, glycerin, titanium dioxide. Soap Bar 90 g. *OTC.*
Use: Antiacne.

Aveeno Cleansing Bar. (Rydelle) **Combination Skin:** Soap free. Colloidal oatmeal 51%, sodium cocoyl isethionate, glycerin, lactic acid, sodium lactate, petrolatum, magnesium aluminum silicate, potassium sorbate, titanium dioxide, PEG 14M. Bar 90 g. **Dry Skin:** Soap free. Colloidal oatmeal 51%, sodium cocoyl isethionate, vegetable oil and shortening, glycerin, PEG-75, lauramide DEA, lactic acid, sodium lactate, sorbic acid, titanium dioxide. Bar 90 g. *OTC.*
Use: Dermatologic; cleanser.

Aveeno Colloidal Oatmeal. (Rydelle) Colloidal oatmeal. Box 1 lb, 4 lb. *OTC.*
Use: Emollient.

Aveeno Dry. (Rydelle) Dry skin formula, soap free, emollient colloidal oatmeal, vegetable oils, lanolin derivative, and glycerin 29% in mild surfactant base. Cleansing bar 90 g. *OTC.*
Use: Dermatologic; cleanser.

Aveeno Lotion. (Rydelle) Colloidal oatmeal 1%, glycerin, petrolatum, dimethicone, phenylcarbinol. Lot. Bot. 354 mL. *OTC.*
Use: Emollient.

Aveeno Moisturizing Cream. (Rydelle) Colloidal oatmeal, glycerin, petrolatum, dimethicone, phenylcarbinol. Cream. Tube 120 g. *OTC.*
Use: Emollient.

Aveeno Normal. (Rydelle) Normal to oily skin formula, soap free. Colloidal oatmeal 50%, lanolin derivative and mild surfactant. Cleansing bar 96 g, 132 g. *OTC.*
Use: Dermatologic; cleanser.

Aveeno Oilated. (Rydelle) Aveeno colloidal oatmeal impregnated with 35% liquid petrolatum, refined olive oil. Box 8 oz, 2 lb. *OTC.*
Use: Emollient.

Aveeno Shave. (Rydelle) Oatmeal flour Gel. Can 210 g. *OTC.*
Use: Emollient.

Aveeno Shower & Bath. (Rydelle) Colloidal oatmeal, 5% mineral oil, laureth-4, silica benzaldehyde. Oil. Bot. 240 mL. *OTC.*
Use: Emollient.

Avelox. (Bayer) Moxifloxacin hydrochloride 400 mg, lactose. Tab. Bot. 30s, UD 50s, *ABC* Packs of 5. *Rx.*
Use: Anti-infective; fluoroquinolone.

Avelox I.V. (Bayer) Moxifloxacin hydrochloride 400 mg, sodium chloride 0.8%, preservative free. Premix Inj. Flexible bag (latex free) 250 mL. *Rx.*
Use: Anti-infective, fluoroquinolone.

Aventyl Hydrochloride Pulvules. (Eli Lilly) Nortriptyline hydrochloride 10 mg, 25 mg. Cap. Bot. 100s, 500s. *Rx.*
Use: Antidepressant.

Aviane. (Barr) Ethinyl estradiol 20 mcg, levonorgestrel 0.1 mg, lactose. Tab. Pkg. 28s. *Rx.*
Use: Sex hormone, contraceptive.

•**avilamycin.** (ah-VILL-ah-MY-sin) USAN.
Use: Anti-infective.

Avinar. Uredepa.
Use: Antineoplastic.

Avinza. (Ligand) Morphine sulfate 30 mg, 60 mg, 90 mg, 120 mg, sugar starch spheres, fumaric acid. ER Pellets Cap. 100s. *c-II.*
Use: Opioid analgesic.

Avita. (Bertek) Tretinoin. **Cream:** 0.025%, stearyl alcohol. Tube 20 g, 45 g. **Gel:** 0.025%, ethanol 83%. Tube. 20 g, 45 g. *Rx.*
Use: Dermatologic, retinoid.

Avitene Hemostat. (Davol) Hydrochloric acid salt of purified bovine corium collagen. **Fibrous Form:** Jar 1 g, 5 g. **Web Form:** Blister Pak. Sheets of 70 mm × 70 mm, 70 mm × 35 mm, 35 mm × 35 mm. *Rx.*
Use: Hemostatic, topical.

•**avitriptan fumarate.** (av-ih-TRIP-tan FEW-mah-rate) USAN.
Use: Antimigraine.

•**avobenzone.** (AV-ah-BENZ-ohn) USAN.
Use: Sunscreen.
W/Combinations.
See: PreSun Ultra.

Avodart. (GlaxoSmithKline) Dutasteride 0.5 mg. Cap. Bot. 100s, UD 100s. *Rx.*
Use: Sex hormone, androgen hormone inhibitor.

Avonex. (Biogen Idec) **Pow. for Inj., lyophilized:** Interferon beta-1A 33 mcg (6.6 million units), albumin human 16.5 mg, sodium chloride 6.4 mg, dibasic sodium phosphate 6.3 mg, monobasic sodium phosphate 1.3 mg. Preservative free. In Administration Dose Packs (single-use vial w/diluent [Sterile Water for Injection], alcohol wipes, gauze pad, syringe, *MicroPin* vial access pin, needle, and bandage). **Prefilled Syringe:** 30 mcg/0.5 mL. Albumin-free. Sodium acetate trihydrate 0.79 mg, glacial acetic acid 0.25 mg, arginine hydrochloride 15.8 mg, polysorbate 20 0.025 mg in water for injection. Administration dose packs (single-use syringe, needle, reclosable accessory pouch, alcohol wipes, gauze pads, and bandages). *Rx.*
Use: Immunologic agent, immunomodulator.

Avonique. (Armenpharm Ltd.) Vitamins A 4000 units, D 400 units, B_1 1 mg, B_2 1.2 mg, B_6 2 mg, B_{12} 2 mcg, calcium pantothenate 5 mg, B_3 10 mg, C 30 mg, calcium 100 mg, phosphorus 76 mg, iron 10 mg, manganese 1 mg, magnesium 1 mg, zinc 1 mg. *OTC.*
Use: Mineral, vitamin supplement.

•**avoparcin.** (AVE-oh-PAR-sin) USAN.
Use: Anti-infective.

•**avridine.** (AV-rih-deen) USAN.
Use: Antiviral.

Awake. (Walgreen) Caffeine 100 mg. Tab. Bot. 36s. *OTC.*
Use: CNS stimulant.

axerophthol.
See: Vitamin A.

Axert. (Ortho-McNeil) Almotriptan malate 6.25 mg, 12.5 mg. Tab. UD 6s. *Rx.*
Use: Antimigraine, serotonin 5-HT_1 receptor agonist.

Axid. (Reliant) Nizatidine 15 mg/mL. Parabens, saccharin, sucrose. Bubble gum flavor. Oral Soln. 480 mL. *Rx.*
Use: Histamine H_2 antagonist.

Axid AR. (Wyeth Consumer) Nizatidine 75 mg. Tab. Bot. 12s, 30s. *OTC.*
Use: Histamine H_2 antagonist.

Axid Pulvules. (Reliant) Nizatidine 150 mg, 300 mg. Cap. Bot. 30s, (300 mg only); 60s, 500s, *Indenti-Dose* 100s, 620s (150 mg only). *Rx.*
Use: Histamine H_2 antagonist.

•**axitirome.** (ax-i-TYE-rome) USAN.
Use: Hypolipidemic.

Axsain.
See: Zostrix (Medicis Pharmaceutical Corp.).

Aygestin. (Barr) Norethindrone acetate 5 mg, lactose. Tab. Bot. 50s. *Rx.*
Use: Hormone, progestin.

Ayr Saline. (B.F. Ascher) Sodium Cl 0.65%, benzalkonium chloride, EDTA. Soln. **Drops:** Bot. 5 mL. **Gel:** Aloe vera gel, glycerin, parabens. Tube. 14 g. **Mist:** Bot. 50 mL. *OTC.*
Use: Dermatologic; moisturizer.

•**azabon.** (AZE-ah-bahn) USAN.
Use: CNS stimulant.

•**azacitidine.** (AZE-ah-SIGH-tih-deen) USAN. *Formerly Ladakamycin.*
Use: Antineoplastic.
See: Vidaza.

•**azaclorzine hydrochloride.** (AZE-ah-KLOR-zeen) USAN. *Formerly Nonachlazine.*
Use: Coronary vasodilator.

•**azaconazole.** (AZE-ah-CONE-ah-zole) USAN. *Formerly Azoconazole.*
Use: Antifungal.

AZA-CR. NCI Investigational agent.
See: Azacitidine.

Azactam. (Bristol-Myers Squibb) Aztreonam 500 mg, 1 g, 2 g ($\approx$ 780 mg L-arginine/g of aztreonam). Pow. for Inj. (lyophilized cake). Single-dose vial 15 mL (500 mg, 1 g), 30 mL (2 g only); Single-dose infusion bot. 100 mL (1 g

and 2 g). *Rx.*
Use: Anti-infective.

●**azalanstat dihydrochloride.** (aze-ah-LAN-stat) USAN.
Use: Hypolipidemic.

Azaline. (Major) Sulfasalazine 500 mg. Tab. Bot. 100s, 500s, 1000s.
Use: Anti-inflammatory.

●**azaloxan fumarate.** (aze-ah-LOX-ahn) USAN.
Use: Antidepressant.

●**azanator maleate.** (AZE-an-nay-tore) USAN.
Use: Bronchodilator.

●**azanidazole.** (AZE-ah-NIH-dah-zole) USAN.
Use: Antiprotozoal.

●**azaperone.** (AZE-app-eh-RONE) *USP 28.*
Use: Antipsychotic.

●**azaribine.** (aze-ah-RYE-bean) USAN.
Use: Dermatologic.

●**azarole.** (AZE-ah-role) USAN.
Use: Immunoregulator.

Azasan. (Various Mfr.) Azathioprine 25 mg, 50 mg, 75 mg, 100 mg. Lactose. Tab. 100s. *Rx.*
Use: Immunosuppressant.

●**azaserine.** (AZE-ah-SER-een) USAN.
Use: Antifungal.

●**azatadine maleate.** (aze-AT-ad-EEN) *USP 28.*
Use: Antihistamine.
See: Optimine.
W/Combinations.
See: Rynatan.

●**azathioprine.** (AZE-uh-THIGH-oh-preen) *USP 28.*
Use: Immunosuppressant.
See: Azasan.
Imuran.

azathioprine. (aaiPharma) Azathioprine 50 mg. Tab. 100s. *Rx.*
Use: Immunosuppressant.

azathioprine sodium. (Various Mfr.) Azathioprine sodium 100 mg. Pow. for Inj. Vial. 20 mL. *Rx.*
Use: Antileukemic.

●**azathioprine sodium for injection.** (AZE-uh-THIGH-oh-preen) *USP 28.*
Use: Immunosuppressant.

5-aza-2′-deoxycytidine.
Use: Treatment of acute leukemia. [Orphan Drug]

5-azc.
See: Azacitidine.

Azdone. (Schwarz Pharma) Hydrocodone bitartrate 5 mg, aspirin 500 mg. Tab. Bot. 100s, 1000s. *c-III.*

Use: Analgesic combination, narcotic.

●**azelaic acid.** (aze-eh-LAY-ik) USAN.
Use: Dermatologic; acne.
See: Azelex.
Finacea.
Finevin.

●**azelastine.** (ah-ZELL-ass-teen) USAN.
Use: Antiallergic, antiasthmatic, antihistamine, peripherally selective phthalazinone.
See: Astelin.
Optivar.

Azelex. (Allergan) Azelaic acid 20%, glycerin, cetearyl alcohol, benzoic acid. Cream. Tube 30 g, 50 g. *Rx.*
Use: Dermatologic, acne.

●**azepindole.** (AZE-eh-PIN-dole) USAN.
Use: Antidepressant.

●**azetepa.** (AZE-eh-teh-pah) USAN.
Use: Antineoplastic.

●**3-azido-2, 3 dideoxyuridine.** USAN.
Use: Antiviral, HIV.

azidothymidine.
See: Zidovudine.

Azidouridine. (Berlex) Phase I HIV-positive symptomatic, ARC, AIDS. *Rx.*
Use: Antiviral.

●**azimilide dihydrochloride.** (azz-IM-ih-lide die-HIGH-droe-KLOR-ide) USAN.
Use: Cardiovascular agent.

●**azipramine hydrochloride.** (aze-IPP-RAH-meen) USAN.
Use: Antidepressant.

●**azithromycin.** (UHZ-lth-row-MY-sin) *USP 28.*
Use: Anti-infective, macrolide.
See: Zithromax.

●**azlocillin.** (AZZ-low-SILL-in) USAN.
Use: Anti-infective.

Azma-Aid. (Purepac) Theophylline 118 mg, ephedrine 24 mg, phenobarbital 8 mg. Tab. Bot. 100s, 250s, 1000s. *Rx.*
Use: Bronchodilator.

Azmacort. (Aventis Pharm) Triamcinolone acetonide 100 mcg/actuation. Inhaler 20 g (triamcinolone acetonide 60 mg) w/actuator (≥ 240 metered doses). *Rx.*
Use: Respiratory inhalant, corticosteroid.

azoconazole.
See: Azaconazole.

Azodyne Hydrochloride.
See: Pyridium.

●**azolimine.** (aze-OLE-ih-meen) USAN.
Use: Diuretic.

AZO Negacide. (Sanofi-Synthelabo) Nalidixic acid, phenazopyridine hydrochloride. Tab. *Rx.*

Use: Anti-infective, urinary.
AZO-100. (Scruggs) Phenylazodiamino-pyridine hydrochloride 100 mg. Tab. Bot. 100s, 1000s. *OTC.*
Use: Analgesic, urinary.
Azopt. (Alcon) Brinzolamide 1%. Benzalkonium chloride 0.01%, mannitol, carbomer 974P tyloxapol, sodium chloride, hydrochloric acid and/or sodium hydroxide, and EDTA. Ophth. Susp. *Drop-Tainers* 2.5 mL, 5 mL, 10 mL, 15 mL. *Rx.*
Use: Glaucoma treatment.
AZO-Standard. (PolyMedica) Phenazopyridine hydrochloride 100 mg. Tab. Bot. 360s. *OTC.*
Use: Analgesic, urinary.
Azostix Reagent Strips. (Bayer Corp. (Consumer Div.)) Bromthymol blue, urease, buffers. Colorimetric test for blood urea nitrogen level. Bot 25 strips.
Use: Diagnostic aid.
azo-sulfisoxazole. (Various Mfr.) Sulfisoxazole 500 mg, phenazopyridine hydrochloride 50 mg. Tab. Bot. 100s, 1000s. *Rx.*
Use: Anti-infective, urinary.
•**azotomycin.** (aze-OH-toe-MY-sin) USAN. Antibiotic isolated from broth filtrates of *Streptomyces ambofaciens.*
Use: Antineoplastic.

Azovan Blue.
See: Evans Blue Dye (City Chemical; Harvey).
AZO Wintomylon. (Sanofi-Synthelabo) Nalidixic acid, phenazopyridine hydrochloride. *Rx.*
Use: Anti-infective, urinary.
•**azosemide.** (AZE-oh-SEH-mide) USAN.
Use: Diuretic.
AZT.
See: Zidovudine.
AZT-P-ddi. (Baker Norton) Phase I AIDS.
Use: Antiviral.
•**aztreonam.** (AZZ-TREE-oh-nam) *USP 28.*
Use: Antimicrobial.
See: Azactam.
Azulfidine. (Pharmacia) Sulfasalazine 500 mg. Tab. Bot. 100s, 300s, UD 100s. *Rx.*
Use: Anti-inflammatory.
Azulfidine EN-tabs. (Pharmacia) Sulfasalazine 500 mg. DR Tab. Bot. 100s, 300s. *Rx.*
Use: Anti-inflammatory.
•**azumolene sodium.** (AH-ZUH-moe-leen) USAN.
Use: Muscle relaxant.

B

B_1. Thiamine hydrochloride.
B_2. Riboflavin.
B_3. Niacin, nicotinamide.
B_5. Calcium pantothenate.
B_6. Pyridoxine hydrochloride.
B_6 50. (Western Research) Vitamin B_6 50 mg. Tab. Bot. 1000s. *OTC.*
Use: Vitamin supplement.
B_{12}. Cyanocobalamin. *OTC.*
Babee Teething. (Pfeiffer) Benzocaine 2.5%, cetalkonium Cl 0.02%, alcohol, eucalyptol, menthol, camphor. Soln. Bot. 15 mL. *OTC.*
Use: Anesthetic, local.
Baby Anbesol. (Whitehall-Robins) Benzocaine 7.5%, saccharin. Gel. Tube 7.2 g. *OTC.*
Use: Mouth and throat preparation
BabyBIG. (California Dept. of Health Sciences) Botulism immune globulin IV (human) 100 ± 20 mg (50 mg/mL when reconstituted). Sucrose 5%, albumin (human) 1%. Solvent/detergent-treated. Preservative-free. Pow. for Inj., lyophilized. Single-dose vial with 2 mL vial of diluent. *Rx.*
Use: Infant botulism, immune globulin.
Baby Cough. (Towne) Ammonium Cl 300 mg, sodium citrate 600 mg/oz w/citric acid. Syr. Bot. 4 oz.
Use: Antitussive.
Baby Orajel. (Del) Benzocaine 7.5%, saccharin, sorbitol, alcohol free. Gel. Tube 9.45 g. *OTC.*
Use: Mouth and throat preparation.
Baby Orajel Nighttime Formula. (Del) Benzocaine 10%, saccharin, sorbitol, alcohol free. Gel. Tube 6 g. *OTC.*
Use: Mouth and throat preparation.
Baby Orajel Teeth & Gum Cleanser. (Del) Poloxamer 407 2%, simethicone 0.12%, parabens, saccharin, sorbitol. Gel. Tube 14.2 g. *OTC.*
Use: Mouth and throat preparation.
Baby Vitamin. (Ivax) Vitamins A 1500 units, D 400 units, E 5 units, B_1 0.5 mg, B_2 0.6 mg, B_3 8 mg, B_6 0.4 mg, B_{12} 2 mcg, C 35 mg/mL. Drop. Bot. 50 mL. *OTC.*
Use: Vitamin supplement.
Baby Vitamin Drops with Iron. (Ivax) Iron 10 mg, vitamins A 1500 units, D 400 units, E 5 units, B_1 0.5 mg, B_2 0.6 mg, B_3 8 mg, B_6 0.4 mg, C 35 mg/mL. Bot. 50 mL. *OTC.*
Use: Mineral, vitamin supplement.
BAC. Benzalkonium Cl.
•**bacampicillin hydrochloride.** (BACK-am-PIH-sill-in) *USP 28.*

Use: Anti-infective.
See: Spectrobid.
Bacco-Resist. (Vita Elixir) Lobeline sulfate $1/64$ g.
Use: Smoking deterrent.
Bacid. (Novartis) A specially cultured strain of human *Lactobacillus acidophilus*, sodium carboxymethylcellulose 100 mg, sodium 0.5 mEq. Cap. Bot. 50s, 100s. *OTC.*
Use: Antidiarrheal; nutritional supplement.
Bacillus Calmette-Guérin.
See: BCG vaccine.
•**bacitracin.** (bass-ih-TRAY-sin) *USP 28.*
Use: Anti-infective.
See: AK-Tracin.
   Altracin.
   W/Neomycin, polymyxin B sulfate.
See: BPN.
   Mycitracin.
   Neosporin.
   Neo-Thrycex.
   Tigo.
   Tri-Biotic.
   Triple Antibiotic.
   W/Neomycin sulfate.
See: Bacimycin.
   Bacitracin-neomycin.
   W/Neomycin sulfate, polymyxin B sulfate, diperodon hydrochloride.
See: Polysporin.
   W/Polymyxin B sulfate and neomycin sulfate.
See: Trimixin.
   W/Polymyxin B sulfate, neomycin sulfate, and hydrocortisone-free alcohol.
See: Biotic-Ophth.
   HC.
   W/Polymyxin B sulfate, neomycin sulfate, lidocaine.
See: Triliotic Plus.
bacitracin. (Various Mfr.) An antibiotic produced by a strain of *Bacillus subtilis.* Diagnostic Tabs., Oint., Ophth. Oint. 500 units/g. Tube 3.5 g, 3.75 g. Soluble Tab., Systemic Use, Vial, Topical Use, Vial, Troche. Vaginal Tab.
Use: Anti-infective. [Orphan Drug]
bacitracin. (Various Mfr.) Bacitracin 500 units/g. May contain mineral oil or white petrolatum. Oint. 14 g, 28 g, 120 g, 454 g, UD 144s. *OTC.*
Use: Anti-infective, topical.
bacitracin-neomycin ointment. (Various Mfr.) Neomycin sulfate equivalent to 3.5 mg base, bacitracin 500 units/g. Topical Oint. Tube 0.5 oz, 1 oz, Ophth. Oint. $1/8$ oz. *OTC.*
Use: Anti-infective, topical.

bacitracin/neomycin/polymyxin B ointment. (Various Mfr.) Polymyxin B sulfate 10,000 units/g, neomycin sulfate 3.5 mg/g, bacitracin zinc 400 units/g. Tube 3.5 g. *Rx.*
Use: Anti-infective, ophthalmic.

• **bacitracin zinc.** (bass-ih-TRAY-sin) *USP 28.*
Use: Anti-infective.
W/Neomycin sulfate, polymyxin B, benzalkonium Cl.
See: Coracin.
W/Neomycin sulfate, polymyxin B sulfate.
See: AK-Poly-Bac.
Bacitracin zinc and polymyxin B sulfate.
Neomycin and polymyxin B sulfates and bacitracin zinc.
Neosporin Original.
Neotal.
Ocutricin.
Triple Antibiotic.
W/Polymyxin B sulfate.
See: Betadine First Aid Antibiotics Plus Moisturizer.
Double Antibiotic.
Polysporin.
W/Polymyxin B sulfate, neomycin, pramoxine hydrochloride.
See: Band-Aid Plus.
Lanabiotic.
Neosporin Plus Pain Relief Maximum Strength.
Tri-Biozene.
Triple Antibiotic Plus.

bacitracin zinc. (Pharmacia) Bacitracin zinc 10,000 units, 50,000 units. Sterile pow. Vial.
Use: Anti-infective.

bacitracin zinc and polymyxin B sulfate. (Roerig) Polymyxin B sulfate 10,000 units, bacitracin zinc 500 units/g, white petrolatum, mineral oil. Ophth. Oint. Tube 3.5 g. *Rx.*
Use: Antibiotic.

bacitracin zinc/neomycin sulfate/polymyxin B sulfate/hydrocortisone. (Various Mfr.) Hydrocortisone 1%, neomycin sulfate 0.35%, bacitracin zinc 400 units, polymyxin B sulfate 10,000 units. Tube 3.5 g. *Rx.*
Use: Anti-infective; corticosteroid ophthalmic.

bacitracin zinc ointment. (Alpharma) Bacitracin zinc is an anhydrous ointment base. Polymyxin B sulfate 10,000 units, bacitracin zinc 500 units. Oint. Tube 3.5 g.
Use: Anti-infective, topical.

Bacit White. (Whiteworth Towne) Bacitracin. Oint. Tube 0.5 oz, 1 oz. *OTC.*
Use: Anti-infective, topical.

Backache Maximum Strength Relief. (Bristol-Myers Squibb) Magnesium salicylate anhydrous (as tetrahydrate) 467 mg. Cap. Bot. 24s, 50s. *OTC.*
Use: Analgesic.

• **baclofen.** (BACK-low-fen) *USP 28.*
Use: Muscle relaxant.
See: Kemstro.
Lioresal.

baclofen. (Various Mfr.) Baclofen 10 mg, 20 mg. Tab. Bot. 30s, 100s, 250s, 500s, 1000s, UD 100s.
Use: Muscle relaxant.

baclofen, l-baclofen. *Rx.*
Use: Treatment of muscle spasticity. [Orphan Drug]

Bacmin. (Marnel) Iron 27 mg, Vitamin A 5000 units, E 30 units, C 500 mg, B_1 20 mg, B_2 20 mg, B_3 100 mg, B_5 25 mg, B_6 25 mg, B_{12} 50 mcg, biotin 0.15 mg, folic acid 0.8 mg, Cr, Cu, Mg, Mn, Zn 22.5 mg. Tab. Bot. 100s. *Rx.*
Use: Mineral, vitamin supplement.

Bac-Neo-Poly. (Burgin-Arden) Bacitracin 400 units, neomycin sulfate 5 mg, polymyxin B sulfate 5000 units/g. Oint. Tube 5 oz. *OTC.*
Use: Anti-infective, topical.

Bactal Soap. (Whittaker General) Triclosan 0.5%, anhydrous soap 10%. Liq. Bot. 240 mL, ½ gal. *OTC.*
Use: Antiseptic; cleaner.

bacteriostatic sodium chloride. (Various Mfr.) Sodium Cl 0.9%. Benzyl alcohol, parabens. Inj. Bot. 10 mL, 20 mL, 30 mL. *Rx.*
Use: Parenteral diluent.

• **bacteriostatic water for injection.** *USP 28.*
Use: Pharmaceutic aid, diluting and dissolving drugs for injection.

bacteriostatic water for injection. (Abbott) 30 mL. Multiple-dose fliptop vial (plastic).
Use: Pharmaceutic aid, diluting and dissolving drugs for injection.

bacteriuria tests. In vitro diagnostic aids.
See: Isocult for bacteriuria.
Microstix-3.
Uricult.

Bacti-Cleanse. (Pedinol Pharmacal) Benzalkonium Cl, mineral oil, isopropyl palmitate, cetyl alcohol, glycerine, glyceryl stearate, PEG-100 stearate, dimethicone, diazolidinyl urea, parabens, DMDM hydantoin, EDTA. Liq. Bot. 453.6 g. *OTC.*
Use: Dermatologic cleanser.

Bacticort. (Rugby) Hydrocortisone 1%, neomycin sulfate equivalent to 0.35% neomycin base, polymyxin B sulfate 10,000 units/mL, benzalkonium Cl, cetyl alcohol, glyceryl monostearate, mineral oil, polyoxyl 40 stearate, propylene glycol. Ophth. Soln. Bot. 7.5 mL. *Rx. Use:* Anti-infective; corticosteroid, ophthalmic.

Bactigen Group A Streptococcus. (Wampole) Latex agglutination slide test for the qualitative detection of group A streptococcal antigen directly from throat swabs. Test kit 60s.
Use: Diagnostic aid.

Bactigen Group A Streptococcus with Gast Trak Slides. (Wampole) Latex agglutination slide test for qualitative detection of group A streptococcal antigen directly from throat swabs. Test 24s. Kit 48s.
Use: Diagnostic aid.

Bactigen H. Influenzae. (Wampole) Rapid latex agglutination slide test for the qualitative detection of *Haemophilus influenzae* type b antigen in cerebrospinal fluid, serum, and urine. Test kit 15s, 30s.
Use: Diagnostic aid.

Bactigen Meningitis Panel. (Wampole) Rapid latex agglutination slide test for the qualitative detection of *Haemophilus influenzae* type b, *Neisseria meningitidis* A/B/C/Y/W135, and *Streptococcus pneumoniae* antigens in cerebrospinal fluid, serum, and urine. Test kit 18s.
Use: Diagnostic aid.

Bactigen Salmonella-Shigella. (Wampole) Latex agglutination slide test for the qualitative detection of *Salmonella* or *Shigella* from cultures. Test kit 96s.
Use: Diagnostic aid.

Bactine Antiseptic/Anesthetic First Aid Spray. (Bayer Corp. (Consumer Div.)) Benzalkonium Cl 0.13%, lidocaine 2.5%. Spray. **Squeeze Bot.:** 2 oz, 4 oz. **Liq.:** 16 oz. **Aerosol:** 3 oz. *OTC. Use:* Anesthetic; antiseptic, topical.

Bactine First Aid Antibiotic. (Bayer Corp. (Consumer Div.)) Polymyxin B sulfate 5000 units, bacitracin 500 units, neomycin sulfate 5 mg/g in mineral oil, white petrolatum. Oint. Tube 15 g. *OTC. Use:* Anti-infective, topical.

Bactine Hydrocortisone Skin Cream. (Bayer Corp. (Consumer Div.)) Hydrocortisone 0.5%. Tube 0.5 oz. *OTC. Use:* Corticosteroid, topical.

Bactine Maximum Strength. (Bayer Corp. (Consumer Div.)) Hydrocortisone 1%, glycerin, mineral oil, methylpara-

ben, white petrolatum. Cream. Tube 30 g. *OTC. Use:* Corticosteroid, topical.

Bactine Pain Relieving Cleansing. (Bayer Corp. (Consumer Div.)) **Spray:** 2.5% lidocaine, 0.13% benzalkonium chloride, EDTA. 150 mL. **Wipes:** 1% pramoxine hydrochloride, 0.13% benzalkonium chloride, EDTA.16s. *OTC. Use:* Anesthetic; antiseptic, topical.

Bactocill. (GlaxoSmithKline) Oxacillin sodium 500 mg, 1 g, 2 g, 4 g, 10 g. Pow. for Inj. Vial (except 10 g); piggyback and *ADD-Vantage* vial (only 1 g and 2 g); Bulk vial (10 g only). *Rx. Use:* Anti-infective; penicillin.

Bacto Shield Foam. (Steris) Chlorhexidine gluconate 4%, isopropyl alcohol 4%. Foam. Aerosol. 180 mL. *OTC. Use:* Dermatologic, cleanser.

Bacto Shield Solution. (Steris) Chlorhexidine gluconate 4%, isopropyl alcohol 4%. Soln. Bot. 960 mL. *OTC. Use:* Dermatologic, cleanser.

Bacto Shield 2. (Steris) Chlorhexidine gluconate 2%, isopropyl alcohol 4%. Soln. Bot. 960 mL. *OTC. Use:* Preoperative skin preparation, cleanser.

Bactrim. (Roche) Sulfamethoxazole 400 mg, trimethoprim 80 mg. Tab. Bot. 100s. *Rx. Use:* Anti-infective.

Bactrim DS. (Roche) Trimethoprim 160 mg, sulfamethoxazole 800 mg. Tab. Bot. 100s, 200s, 500s. *Rx. Use:* Anti-infective.

Bactrim IV Infusion. (Roche) Sulfamethoxazole 400 mg, trimethoprim 80 mg/5 mL. Inj. Multidose vials. 10 mL, 30 mL. *Rx. Use:* Anti-infective.

Bactrim Pediatric. (Roche) Trimethoprim 40 mg, sulfamethoxazole 200 mg/5 mL. Susp. Bot. 480 mL. *Rx. Use:* Anti-infective.

Bactrim Suspension. (Roche) Sulfamethoxazole 200 mg, trimethoprim 40 mg/5 mL. Susp. Bot. 16 oz. *Rx. Use:* Anti-infective.

Bactroban. (GlaxoSmithKline) Mupirocin. **Oint.:** 2% in a polyethylene glycol base. Tube 22 g. **Cream:** Mupirocin calcium 2.15%. Oil/water base, benzyl alcohol, cetyl alcohol, stearyl alcohol. Tube 15 g, 30 g. *Rx. Use:* Anti-infective, topical.

Bactroban Nasal. (GlaxoSmithKline) Mupirocin calcium 2.15%, glycerin esters. Oint. 1 g. *Rx. Use:* Anti-infective used in adult patients and health care workers during institutional outbreaks.

Bacturcult. (Wampole) A urinary bacteria culture medium diagnostic urine culture system for urine collection, bacteriuria screening, and presumptive bacterial identification. Test kit 10s, 100s.
Use: Diagnostic aid.

B.A. Gradual. (Federal) Theophylline 260 mg, pseudoephedrine hydrochloride 50 mg, butabarbital 15 mg. Gradual. Bot. 50s, 1000s. *Rx.*
Use: Bronchodilator; decongestant; hypnotic; sedative.

Bain de Soleil All Day For Kids SPF 30. (Procter & Gamble) Ethylhexyl p-methoxycinnamate, 2-ethylhexyl 2-cyano-3, 3-diphenyl acrylate, oxybenzone, titanium dioxide, stearyl alcohol, tocopheryl acetate, EDTA. PABA free. Waterproof. Lot. Bot. 120 mL. *OTC.*
Use: Sunscreen.

Bain de Soleil All Day Waterproof Sunblock. (Procter & Gamble) SPF 15, 30. Ethylhexyl p-methoxycinnamate, 2-ethylhexyl 2-cyano-3, 3-diphenyl acrylate, oxybenzone, titanium dioxide, stearyl alcohol, vitamin E, EDTA. Lot. Bot. 120 mL. *OTC.*
Use: Sunscreen.

Bain de Soleil All Day Waterproof Sunfilter. (Procter & Gamble) SPF 4, 8. 2-ethylhexyl 2-cyano-3, 3-diphenyl acrylate, ethylhexyl p-methoxycinnamate, titanium dioxide, stearyl alcohol, vitamin E, EDTA. Lot. Bot. 120 mL. *OTC.*
Use: Sunscreen.

Bain de Soleil Body Silkening Creme. (Procter & Gamble) Padimate O, ethylhexyl p-methoxycinnamate, oxybenzone, benzyl alcohol. Waterproof. Cream. Bot. 94 g. *OTC.*
Use: Sunscreen.

Bain de Soleil Body Silkening Spray. (Procter & Gamble) Padimate O, oxybenzone, ethylhexyl p-methoxycinnamate. Waterproof. Lot. Bot. 240 mL. *OTC.*
Use: Sunscreen.

Bain de Soleil Body Silkening Stick. (Procter & Gamble) Padimate O, ethylhexyl p-methoxycinnamate, oxybenzone, dioxybenzone. Stick 53 g. *OTC.*
Use: Sunscreen.

Bain de Soleil Face Creme. (Procter & Gamble) Padimate O, ethylhexyl p-methoxycinnamate, oxybenzone. Waterproof. Cream. Bot. 60 g. *OTC.*
Use: Sunscreen.

Bain de Soleil Kids Sport. (Procter & Gamble) SPF 25. Ethylhexyl p-methoxycinnamate, 2-ethylhexyl 2-cyano-3, 3-diphenyl acrylate, titanium dioxide, PVP/eicosene copolymer, dimethicone, cyclomethicone, triethanolamine, glyceryl tribehenate, tocopheryl acetate, carbomer, EDTA, DMDM hydantoin. PABA free. Waterproof, all day protection. Lot. Bot. 120 mL. *OTC.*
Use: Sunscreen.

Bain de Soleil Lip Protecteur. (Procter & Gamble) Ethylhexyl p-methoxycinnamate, oxybenzone, 2-ethylhexyl salicylate, oleyl alcohol, petrolatum. PABA free. Lip balm 3 g. *OTC.*
Use: Sunscreen.

Bain de Soleil Megatan. (Procter & Gamble) Ethylhexyl p-methoxycinnamate, 2-ethylhexyl salicylate, lanolin, cocoa butter, palm oil, aloe, DMDM hydantoin, xanthan gum, shea butter, EDTA. Lot. Bot. 120 mL. *OTC.*
Use: Sunscreen.

Bain de Soleil Orange Gelee SPF 4. (Procter & Gamble) Ethylhexyl p-methoxycinnamate, 2-ethylhexyl salicylate. PABA free. Gel. Tube 93.75 g. *OTC.*
Use: Sunscreen.

Bain de Soleil SPF 8+ Color. (Procter & Gamble) Octyl methoxycinnamate, octocrylene, mineral oil, cetyl alcohol, EDTA. Lot. Bot. 118 mL. *OTC.*
Use: Sunscreen.

Bain de Soleil SPF 15+ Color. (Procter & Gamble) Octyl methoxycinnamate, octocrylene, oxybenzone, mineral oil, cetyl alcohol, EDTA. Lot. Bot. 118 mL. *OTC.*
Use: Sunscreen.

Bain de Soleil SPF 30+ Color. (Procter & Gamble) Octocrylene, octyl methoxycinnamate, oxybenzone, mineral oil, cetyl alcohol, EDTA. Lot. Bot. 118 mL. *OTC.*
Use: Sunscreen.

Bain de Soleil Sport. (Procter & Gamble) SPF 15. 2-ethylhexyl 2-cyano-3, 3-diphenyl acrylate, ethylhexyl p-methoxycinnamate, titanium dioxide, dimethicone, cyclomethicone, panthenol, tocopheryl acetate, carbomer, EDTA, DMDM hydantoin. PABA free. Waterproof, sweatproof, all day protection. Lot. Bot. 180 mL. *OTC.*
Use: Sunscreen.

Bain de Soleil Tropical Deluxe SPF 4. (Procter & Gamble) Ethylhexyl p-methoxycinnamate, 2-ethylhexyl salicylate, cetyl alcohol, EDTA. PABA free. Waterproof. Lot. Bot. 240 mL. *OTC.*
Use: Sunscreen.

Bain de Soleil Under Eye. (Procter & Gamble) Ethylhexyl p-methoxycinnamate, oxybenzone, 2-ethylhexyl salicylate. Stick 1.5 g. *OTC.*
Use: Sunscreen.

Bakers Best. (Scherer) Water, alcohol 38%, propylene glycol, extract of capsicum, glycerin, boric acid, Tween 80, diethylphthalate, rose oil, pyrilamine maleate, glacial acetic acid, Uvinul MS 40, hexetidine, benzalkonium Cl 50%, sodium hydroxide 76%. Bot. 8 oz. *OTC.*
Use: Antipruritic; antiseborrheic, topical.

●**balafilcon A.** (ba-lah-FILL-kahn A) USAN.
Use: Contact lens material, hydrophilic.

Balamine DM Oral Drops. (Ballay) Pseudoephedrine hydrochloride 25 mg, carbinoxamine maleate 2 mg, dextromethorphan HBr 3.5 mg/mL, menthol, grape flavor. Oral Drops. Bot. 30 mL w/dropper. *Rx.*
Use: Upper respiratory combination, decongestant, antihistamine, antitussive.

Balamine DM Syrup. (Ballay) Dextromethorphan HBr 12.5 mg, carbinoxamine maleate 4 mg, pseudoephedrine hydrochloride 60 mg/5 mL, menthol, grape flavor. Syr. Bot. 473 mL. *Rx.*
Use: Upper respiratory combination, antitussive, antihistamine, decongestant.

Balanced B₁₀₀. (Fibertone) Vitamins B₁ 100 mg, B₂ 100 mg, B₃ 100 mg, B₅ 100 mg, B₆ 100 mg, B₁₂ 100 mcg, folic acid 0.1 mg, PABA 100 mg, inositol 100 mg, d-biotin 100 mcg. SR Tab. Bot. 50s.
Use: Mineral, vitamin supplement.

Balanced Salt Solution. (Various Mfr.) Sodium Cl 0.64%, potassium Cl 0.075%, calcium Cl 0.048%, magnesium Cl 0.03%, sodium acetate 0.39%, sodium citrate 0.17%, sodium hydroxide or hydrochloric acid. Soln. *Drop-Tainer* 18 mL, 500 mL.
Use: Irrigant, ophthalmic.

Baldex Ophthalmic. (Bausch & Lomb) Dexamethasone phosphate. **Oint.:** 0.05%. Tube 3.75 g. **Soln.:** 0.01%. Dropper Bot. 5 mL. *Rx.*
Use: Corticosteroid, ophthalmic.

BAL in Oil. (Becton Dickinson & Co.) 2, 3-dimercaptopropanol 100 mg, benzylbenzoate 210 mg, peanut oil 680 mg/mL. Amp. 3 mL. Box 10s. *Rx.*
Use: Antidote.

Balmex. (Block Drug) Zinc oxide 11.3%, aloe vera gel, parabens, mineral oil.

Tube 30 g, 60 g, 120 g, 454 g. *OTC.*
Use: Emollient.

Balmex Baby Powder. (Block Drug) Specially purified balsam Peru, zinc oxide, starch, calcium carbonate. Shaker top can. 4 oz. *OTC.*
Use: Adsorbent, emollient.

Balneol Perianal Cleansing. (Solvay) Mineral oil, lanolin oil, methylparaben. Bot. 120 mL. *OTC.*
Use: Anorectal preparation.

Balnetar. (Westwood Squibb) Coal tar 2.5% in mineral oil, lanolin oil. Liq. 221 mL. *OTC.*
Use: Dermatologic.

●**balsalazide disodium.** (bahl-SAL-ah-zide) USAN.
Use: Anti-inflammatory, gastrointestinal.
See: Colazal.

Balsan. Specially purified balsam Peru.
See: Balmex.

●**bambermycins.** (BAM-ber-MY-sinz) USAN.
Use: Anti-infective.

●**bamethan sulfate.** (BAM-eth-an) USAN.
Use: Vasodilator.

●**bamifylline hydrochloride.** (BAM-ih-FILL-in) USAN.
Use: Bronchodilator.

●**bamnidazole.** (bam-NIH-DAH-zole) USAN.
Use: Antiprotozoal, trichomonas.

Banacid. (Buffington) Magnesium trisilicate 220 mg. Tab. Bot. 100s, 200s, 500s. *OTC.*
Use: Antacid.

Banadyne-3. (Norstar Consumer) Lidocaine 4%, menthol 1%, alcohol 45%. Soln. Bot. 7.5 mL. *OTC.*
Use: Mouth and throat preparation.

Banalg. (Forest) Methyl salicylate 4.9%, camphor 2%, menthol 1%. Lot. Bot. 60 mL, 480 mL. *OTC.*
Use: Analgesic, topical.

Banalg Hospital Strength Liniment. (Forest) Methyl salicylate 14%, menthol 3%. Bot. 60 mL. *OTC.*
Use: Analgesic, topical.

Bancap HC. (Forest) Acetaminophen 500 mg, hydrocodone bitartrate 5 mg. Cap. Bot. 100s, 500s. *c-iii.*
Use: Analgesic combination, narcotic.

B & A. (Eastern Research) Sodium bicarbonate, potassium, aluminum, borax. Hygienic pow. Jar 8 oz, 5 lb. *Rx.*
Use: Vaginal agent.

●**bandage, adhesive.** *USP 28.*
Use: Surgical aid.

●**bandage, gauze.** *USP 28.*
Use: Surgical aid.

B and O Supprettes No. 15A & No. 16A. (PolyMedica) Opium 30 mg, 60 mg, belladonna extract 16.2 mg. Supp. Jar 12s. *c-II.*
Use: Analgesic; antispasmodic; narcotic.

Banflex. (Forest) Orphenadrine citrate 30 mg/mL. Inj. Vial 10 mL. *Rx.*
Use: Muscle relaxant.

Bangesic. (H.L. Moore Drug Exchange) Menthol, camphor, methyl salicylate, eucalyptus oil in nongreasy base. Bot. 2 oz, gal. *OTC.*
Use: Analgesic, topical.

Banocide.
See: Diethylcarbamazine citrate.

Banophen. (Major) Diphenhydramine hydrochloride. **Tab.:** 25 mg. Bot. 24s, 100s. **Cap.:** 25 mg. Bot. 24s, 100s. *OTC.*
Use: Antihistamine, nonselective ethanolamine.

Banophen Allergy. (Major) Diphenhydramine hydrochloride 12.5 mg/5 mL, sugar. Elixir. Bot. 118 mL. *OTC.*
Use: Antihistamine, nonselective ethanolamine.

Banophen Decongestant. (Major) Diphenhydramine 25 mg, pseudoephedrine 60 mg. Cap. Bot. 24s. *OTC.*
Use: Antihistamine; decongestant.

Bansmoke. (Thompson Medical) Benzocaine 6 mg, corn syrup, dextrose, lecithin, sucrose. Gum. Pack 24s. *OTC.*
Use: Smoking deterrent.

Baraclude. (Bristol-Myers Squibb Company) Entecavir. **Oral Soln.:** 0.05 mg/mL. Parabens. Orange flavor. 210 mL. **Tab.:** 0.5 mg, 1 mg. Lactose. Film coated. 30s, 90s (0.5 mg only). *Rx.*
Use: Antiviral agent.

Barbased. (Major) **Tab.:** Butabarbital 0.25 g, 0.5 g. Tab. Bot. 1000s. **Elix.:** Butabarbital 30 mg/5 mL, alcohol 7%. Bot. 480 mL. *Rx.*
Use: Hypnotic; sedative.

Barbatose No. 2. (Pal-Pak, Inc.) Barbital 64.8 mg, hyoscyamus sulfate, passiflora, valerian. Tab. Bot. 1000s. *Rx.*
Use: Sedative.

Barbella Elixir. (Forest) Phenobarbital 0.25 g, hyoscyamine sulfate 0.1037 mg, atropine sulfate 0.0194 mg, scopolamine HBr 0.0065 mg, alcohol 24%/5 mL. Elix. Bot. 4 oz, gal. *Rx.*
Use: Anticholinergic; antispasmodic; hypnotic; sedative.

Barbella Tablets. (Forest) Phenobarbital 16.2 mg, atropine sulfate 0.0194 mg, hyoscyamine sulfate 0.1037 mg, hyoscine HBr 0.0065 mg. Tab. Bot. 100s,

1000s, 5000s. *Rx.*
Use: Anticholinergic; antispasmodic; hypnotic; sedative.

Barbeloid. (Pal-Pak, Inc.) Phenobarbital 16.2 mg, hyoscyamine sulfate 0.1037 mg, atropine sulfate 0.0194 mg, scopolamine HBr 0.0065 mg. Tab. Bot. 100s, 1000s. *Rx.*
Use: Anticholinergic; antispasmodic; hypnotic; sedative.

Barbenyl.
See: Phenobarbital.

Barbiphenyl.
See: Phenobarbital.

barbital. Barbitone, Deba, Dormonal, Hypnogene, Malonal, Sedeval, Uronal, Veronal, Vesperal, diethylbarbituric acid, diethylmalonylurea.
Use: Hypnotic; sedative.

barbital sodium. Barbitone sodium, diethylbarbiturate monosodium, diethylmalonylurea sodium, Embinal, Medinal, Veronal sodium.
Use: Hypnotic; sedative.

barbitone.
See: Barbital.

barbitone sodium.
See: Barbital sodium.

barbiturate-aspirin combinations.
See: Aspirin-barbiturate combinations.

barbiturates, intermediate duration.
See: Butabarbital.
   Butethal.

barbiturates, long duration.
See: Barbital.
   Mebaral.
   Mephobarbital.
   Phenobarbital.
   Phenobarbital sodium.

barbiturates, short duration.
See: Amobarbital.
   Amobarbital sodium.
   Butalbital.
   Butallylonal.
   Cyclobarbital.
   Pentobarbital salts.
   Sandoptal.
   Secobarbital.

barbiturates, ultrashort duration.
See: Hexobarbital.
   Neraval.
   Pentothal sodium.
   Thiopental sodium.

Baricon. (Mallinckrodt) Barium sulfate 98%, simethicone, sorbitol, sucrose, lemon-vanilla flavor. Pow. for Susp. UD 340 g. *Rx.*
Use: Radiopaque agent, GI contrast agent.

Baridium. (Pfeiffer) Phenazopyridine hydrochloride 100 mg. Tab. Bot. 32s.

OTC.
Use: Analgesic, urinary.
Bari-Stress M. (Alpharma) Vitamins B₁ 10 mg, B₂ 10 mg, niacinamide 100 mg, C 300 mg, B₆ 2 mg, B₁₂ 4 mcg, folic acid 1.5 mg, calcium pantothenate 20 mg. Cap. Bot. 30s, 100s, 1000s. Tab. Bot. 100s, 1000s. *Rx.*
Use: Mineral, vitamin supplement.
●**barium hydroxide lime.** (BA-ree-uhm) *USP 28.*
Use: Carbon dioxide absorbent.
●**barium sulfate.** *USP 28.* Paste; For suspension; Suspension; Tablets.
Use: Diagnostic aid, radiopaque medium.
See: Anatrast.
  Baricon.
  Burobag.
  Baro-cat.
  Barosperse.
  Bear-E-Yum CT.
  Bear-E-Yum GI.
  Cheetah.
  Enecat CT.
  Enhancer.
  Entrobar.
  EntroEase.
  EntroEase Dry.
  Epi-C.
  Flo-Coat.
  HD 85.
  HD 200 Plus.
  Imager ac.
  Intropaste.
  Liqui-Coat HD.
  Liquid Barosperse.
  Medebar Plus.
  Medescan.
  Prepcat.
  Tomocat.
  Tonopaque.
barium sulfate. (Various Mfr.) Barium sulfate. Pow. for Susp. Pkg. 1 lb. *Rx.*
Use: Radiopaque agent, GI contrast agent.
barium sulfate preparation.
See: Fleet.
Barlevite. (Barth's) Vitamins B₆ 0.6 mg, B₁₂ 3 mcg, pantothenic acid 0.6 mg, D 3 units, l-lysine 20 mg/0.6 mL. 100-day supply. *OTC.*
Use: Vitamin, mineral supplement.
●**barmastine.** (BAR-mast-een) USAN.
Use: Antihistamine.
BarnesHind Cleaning and Soaking Solution. (PBH Wesley Jessen) Cleaning and buffering agents, benzalkonium Cl 0.01%, disodium edetate 0.2%. Soln. Bot. 1.2 oz, 4 oz. *OTC.*

Use: Contact lens care.
BarnesHind Saline for Sensitive Eyes. (PBH Wesley Jessen) Potassium sorbate 0.13%, EDTA 0.025%. Soln. Bot. 360 mL (2s). *OTC.*
Use: Contact lens care.
BarnesHind Wetting & Soaking Solution. (PBH Wesley Jessen) Polyvinyl alcohol, povidone, hydroxyethyl cellulose, octylphenoxy (oxyethylene) ethanol, benzalkonium Cl, edetate disodium. Soln. Bot. 4 oz. *OTC.*
Use: Contact lens care.
BarnesHind Wetting Solution. (PBH Wesley Jessen) Polyvinyl alcohol, edetate disodium 0.02%, benzalkonium Cl 0.004%. Soln. Bot. 35 mL, 60 mL. *OTC.*
Use: Contact lens care.
Barobag. (Mallinckrodt) Barium sulfate W/%, simethicone. Pow. for Susp. Kit 340 g, 454 g. *Rx.*
Use: Radiopaque agent, GI contrast agent.
Baro-cat. (Mallinckrodt) Barium sulfate 1.5%, simethicone, sorbitol, pineapple-banana flavor. Susp. Bot. 300 mL, 900 mL, 1900 mL. *Rx.*
Use: Radiopaque agent, gastrointestinal.
Baroset. (Lafayette) Air contrast stomach. Unit-of-use kit. Case 12s.
Use: Radiopaque agent.
barosmin.
See: Diosmin.
Barosperse. (Mallinckrodt) Barium sulfate 95%, simethicone, vanilla flavor. Pow. for Susp. UD Bot. 225 g, 900 g. Enema kit 340 g, 454 g. Bulk 25 lb. *Rx.*
Use: Radiopaque agent, GI contrast agent.
Basa. (Freeport) Acetylsalicylic acid 324 mg. Tab. Bot. 1000s. *OTC.*
Use: Analgesic.
basic aluminum carbonate.
See: Basaljel.
basic aluminum glycinate.
See: Dihydroxyaluminum aminoacetate.
basic bismuth carbonate.
See: Bismuth subcarbonate.
basic bismuth gallate.
See: Bismuth subgallate.
basic bismuth nitrate.
See: Bismuth subnitrate.
basic bismuth salicylate.
See: Bismuth subsalicylate.
basic fuchsin.
See: Carbol-Fuchsin.
●**basifungin.** (bass-ih-FUN-jin) USAN.
Use: Antifungal.

• **basiliximab.** (bass-ih-LICK-sih-mab) USAN.
Use: Immunosuppressant.
See: Simulect.

Basis, Glycerin Soap. (Beiersdorf) Tallow, coconut oil, glycerin. Sensitive and normal to dry. Bar 90 g, 150 g. *OTC.*
Use: Dermatologic, cleanser.

Basis, Superfatted Soap. (Beiersdorf) Sodium tallowate, sodium cocoate, petrolatum, glycerin, zinc oxide, sodium Cl, titanium dioxide, lanolin, alcohol, beeswax, BHT, EDTA. Bar 99 g, 225 g. *OTC.*
Use: Dermatologic, cleanser.

• **batabulin sodium.** (bat-a-BUE-lin) USAN.
Use: Antineoplastic agent.

• **batanopride hydrochloride.** (bah-TAN-oh-pride) USAN.
Use: Antiemetic.

• **batelapine maleate.** (bat-EH-lap-EEN) USAN.
Use: Antipsychotic.

• **batimastat.** (bat-IM-ah-stat) USAN.
Use: Antineoplastic.

Bayer Aspirin, Genuine. (Bayer Corp. (Consumer Div.)) Aspirin 325 mg. Tab. Bot. 50s, 100s, 200s, 300s. Pkg. 12s, 24s. *OTC.*
Use: Analgesic.

Bayer Aspirin, Maximum. (Bayer Corp. (Consumer Div.)) Aspirin 500 mg. Tab. Bot. 30s, 60s, 100s. *OTC.*
Use: Analgesic.

Bayer Buffered Aspirin. (Bayer Corp. (Consumer Div.)) Buffered aspirin 325 mg. Tab. Bot. 100s. *OTC.*
Use: Analgesic.

Bayer Children's Chewable Aspirin. (Bayer Corp. (Consumer Div.)) Aspirin 1.25 g (81 mg). Chew. Tab. Bot. 30s. *OTC.*
Use: Analgesic.

Bayer 8-Hour Timed-Release Aspirin. (Bayer Corp. (Consumer Div.)) Aspirin 10 g (650 mg). TR Tab. Bot. 30s, 72s, 125s. *OTC.*
Use: Analgesic.

Bayer Enteric Coated Caplets, Regular Strength. (Bayer Corp. (Consumer Div.)) Aspirin 325 mg. EC Tab. Bot. 50s, 100s. *OTC.*
Use: Analgesic.

Bayer Enteric 500 Aspirin, Extra Strength. (Bayer Corp. (Consumer Div.)) Aspirin 500 mg. EC Tab. Bot. 60s. *OTC.*
Use: Analgesic.

Bayer Extra Strength Back & Body Pain. (Bayer Corp. (Consumer Div.)) Aspirin 500 mg, caffeine 32.5 mg. Tab. 50s, 100s. *OTC.*
Use: Analgesic; CNS stimulant.

Bayer Low Adult Strength. (Bayer Corp. (Consumer Div.)) Aspirin 81 mg, lactose. DR Tab. Bot. 120s. *OTC.*
Use: Analgesic.

Bayer Muscle & Joint Cream. (Bayer Corp. (Consumer Div.)) Menthol 10%, camphor 4%, methyl salicylate 30%. EDTA, glyceryl, lanolin, stearyl alcohol. Cream 56 g, 114 g. *OTC.*
Use: Rub and liniment.

Bayer Plus Extra Strength. (Bayer Corp. (Consumer Div.)) Aspirin 500 mg, calcium carbonate 250 mg. Cap. Bot. 50s. *OTC.*
Use: Analgesic.

Bayer PM Extra Strength Aspirin Plus Sleep Aid. (Bayer Corp. (Consumer Div.)) Aspirin 500 mg, diphenhydramine hydrochloride 25 mg. Cap. Bot. 24s. *OTC.*
Use: Analgesic.

Bayer Select Chest Cold. (Bayer Corp. (Consumer Div.)) Dextromethorphan HBr 15 mg, acetaminophen 500 mg. Cap. Pkg. 16s. *OTC.*
Use: Analgesic; antitussive.

Bayer Select Maximum Strength Backache. (Bayer Corp. (Consumer Div.)) Magnesium salicylate tetrahydrate 580 mg. Cap. Bot. 24s, 50s. *OTC.*
Use: Analgesic.

Bayer Select Maximum Strength Night Time Pain Relief. (Bayer Corp. (Consumer Div.)) Acetaminophen 500 mg, diphenhydramine hydrochloride. Tab. Bot. 24s, 50s. *OTC.*
Use: Antihistamine.

Bayer Select Maximum Strength Sinus Pain Relief. (Bayer Corp. (Consumer Div.)) Acetaminophen 500 mg, pseudoephedrine hydrochloride 30 mg. Tab. Bot. 50s. *OTC.*
Use: Analgesic; decongestant.

Bayer Women's Aspirin Plus Calcium. (Bayer Corp. (Consumer Div.)) Aspirin 81 mg, calcium 300 mg, lactose, mineral oil, polydextrose. Tab. 60s, 90s. *OTC.*
Use: Analgesic; mineral supplement.

BayGam. (Bayer) Immune globulin (human) 15% to 18% protein, glycine 0.21 to 0.32 M, solvent/detergent treated, preservative free. Soln. for Inj. Single-dose vial 2 mL, 10 mL. *Rx.*
Use: Immune globulin.

BayHep B. (Bayer) Hepatitis B immune globulin (human) 15% to 18% protein,

0.21 to 0.32 M glycine, solvent/detergent treated, preservative free. Soln. for Inj. Single-dose vial 1 mL, 5 mL; Neonatal single-dose syringe 0.5 mL. *Rx.*
Use: Immunization.
Baylocaine 4%. (Bay Labs) Lidocaine 4% w/methylparaben. Soln. Bot. 50 mL, 100 mL.
Use: Anesthetic, local.
Baylocaine 2% Viscous. (Bay Labs) Lidocaine 2% w/sodium carboxymethylcellulose. Soln. Bot. 100 mL. *OTC.*
Use: Local anesthetic, topical.
BayRab. (Bayer Pharmaceutical) Rabies immune globulin (human) 150 IU/mL. Preservative free. Glycine 0.21 to 0.32 M. Solvent/detergent treated. Inj. Single-dose vial 2 mL, 10 mL. *Rx.*
Use: Immunization.
BayRho D. (Bayer) Rh₀(D) immune globulin (human). Prefilled single-dose syringe. Single-dose syringe. Single-dose vial. *Rx.*
Use: Immunization.
BayRho-D Full Dose. (Bayer) Rh₀(D) immune globulin 15% to 18% protein, glycine 0.21 to 0.32 M, solvent/detergent treated, preservative free. Soln. for Inj. Individual and multiple-pack single-dose syringes w/attached needles and vials. *Rx.*
Use: Immune globulin.
BayRho D Mini Dose. (Bayer) Rh₀(D) immune globulin micro-dose 15% to 18% protein, glycine 0.21 to 0.32 M, solvent/detergent treated, preservative free. Single-dose Syr. 10s. *Rx.*
Use: Immune globulin.
BayTet. (Bayer) Tetanus immune globulin (human) 15% to 18% protein, glycine 0.21 to 0.32 M, solvent/detergent treated, preservative free. Vial 250 units. Syringe 250 units. *Rx.*
Use: Immunization.
● **bazedoxifene acetate.** (bay-ze-DOX-i-feen) USAN.
Use: Osteoporosis; estrogen receptor modulator.
BCAD 2. (Mead Johnson Nutritionals) Protein 24 g (L-glutamine, potassium aspartate, L-lysine hydrochloride, L-tyrosine, L-proline, L-alanine, L-arginine, L-phenylalanine, L-threonine, L-serine, glycine, L-histidine, L-methionine, L-tryptophan, L-cystine, L-carnitine, taurine), carbohydrate 57 g (corn syrup solids, sugar, modified corn starch), fat 8.5 g (soy oil)/100 g, vitamins A, B₁, B₂, B₃, B₅, B₆, B₁₂, C, D, E, K, biotin, choline, folic acid, inositol, Ca, chloride,

Cr, Cu, Fe, I, Mg, Mn, Mo, P, Se, Zn, Na 610 mg, K 1220 mg/g, 410 cal/100 g. Pow. Can 1 lb. *OTC.*
Use: Enteral nutritional therapy.
BC Arthritis Strength. (Block Drug) Aspirin 742 mg, salicylamide 222 mg, caffeine 36 mg. Pow. Bot. 6s, 24s, 50s. *OTC.*
Use: Analgesic combination.
BCG, intravesical.
Use: Biological response modifier.
See: TheraCys.
Tice BCG.
● **BCG vaccine.** *USP 28.*
Use: Immunization.
See: BCG vaccine.
Tice BCG.
BCG vaccine. (Organon) Prepared from Tice strain of BCG bacillus (1 to 8 × 10⁸ CFU equiv. to ≈ 50 mg) Preservative-free. Pow. for Inj., lyophilized. Vials. *Rx.*
Use: Immunization against tuberculosis, active.
BCNU.
Use: Antineoplastic.
See: BiCNU.
BCO. (Western Research) Vitamins B₁ 10 mg, B₂ 2 mg, B₆ 1.5 mg, B₁₂ 25 mcg, niacinamide 50 mg. Tab. Bot. 1000s. *OTC.*
Use: Vitamin supplement.
B-Com. (Century) Vitamins B₁ 3 mg, B₂ 3 mg, B₆ 0.5 mg, niacinamide 20 mg, calcium pantothenate 5 mg, B₁₂ 1 mcg, desiccated liver (undefatted) 60 mg, debittered brewer's dried yeast 60 mg. Cap. Bot. 100s, 1000s. *OTC.*
Use: Mineral, vitamin supplement.
● **B Complex and B₁₂.** (NBTY) Vitamins B₁ 7 mg, B₂ 14 mg, B₃ 4.5 mg, B₁₂ 25 mcg, protease 10 mg. Tab. Bot. 90s. *OTC.*
Use: Vitamin supplement.
B-Complex Capsules. (Arcum) Vitamins B₁ 1.5 mg, B₂ 2 mg, niacinamide 10 mg, B₆ 0.1 mg, calcium pantothenate 1 mg, desiccated liver 70 mg, dried yeast 100 mg. Cap. Bot. 100s, 1000s. *OTC.*
Use: Mineral, vitamin supplement.
B-Complex Capsules J.F. (Bryant) Vitamins B₁ 1 mg, B₂ 0.3 mg, nicotinic acid 0.3 mg, B₆ 0.25 mg, desiccated liver 0.15 g, yeast powder, dried 0.15 g. Cap. Bot. 100s, 1000s. *OTC.*
Use: Mineral, vitamin supplement.
B-Complex Elixir. (Nion Corp.) B₁ 2.3 mg, B₂ 1 mg, B₃ 6.7 mg, B₆ 0.3 mg, alcohol 10%. Elix. Bot. 240 mL, 480 mL. *OTC.*
Use: Mineral, vitamin supplement.

B-Complex-50. (Nion Corp.) Vitamins B$_1$ 50 mg, B$_2$ 50 mg, B$_3$ 50 mg, B$_5$ 50 mg, B$_6$ 50 mg, B$_{12}$ 50 mcg, FA 0.4 mg, biotin 50 mcg, PABA 50 mg, choline bitartrate 50 mg, inositol 50 mg. SR Tab. Bot. 100s. *OTC.*
Use: Mineral, vitamin supplement.

B-Complex "50". (Vitaline) Vitamins B$_1$ 50 mg, B$_2$ 50 mg, B$_3$ 50 mg, B$_4$ 50 mg, B$_5$ 50 mg, B$_6$ 50 mg, B$_{12}$ 50 mcg, FA 0.1 mg, PABA 30 mg, inositol 50 mg, biotin 50 mcg, choline bitartrate 50 mg. Reg. or TR Tab. Bot. 90s, 1000s. *OTC.*
Use: Vitamin supplement.

B-Complex Injection with Vitamin C.
Use: Vitamin supplement.
See: Cplex.

B-Complex 100. (Rabin-Winters) Vitamins B$_1$ 100 mg, B$_2$ 2 mg, B$_6$ 2 mg, niacinamide 125 mg, panthenol 10 mg/mL. Inj. Vial 30 mL. *Rx.*
Use: Vitamin supplement.

B-Complex-150. (Nion Corp.) Vitamins B$_1$ 150 mg, B$_2$ 150 mg, B$_3$ 150 mg, B$_5$ 150 mg, B$_6$ 150 mg, B$_{12}$ 1 mcg, FA 0.4 mg, biotin 150 mcg, PABA 100 mg, choline bitartrate 150 mg, inositol 150 mg. SR Tab. Bot. 30s. *OTC.*
Use: Mineral, vitamin supplement.

B-Complex 100/100. (Sandia) Vitamins B$_1$ 100 mg, B$_2$ 2 mg, B$_6$ 2 mg, niacinamide 100 mg/mL. Inj. Vial 30 mL. *Rx.*
Use: Vitamin supplement.

B Complex + C. (Various Mfr.) Vitamins B$_1$ 15 mg, B$_2$ 10 mg, B$_3$ 100 mg, B$_5$ 20 mg, B$_6$ 5 mg, B$_{12}$ 10 mcg, C 500 mg. Tab. Bot. 100s. *OTC.*
Use: Vitamin supplement.

B-Complex + C. (NBTY) Vitamins C 200 mg, B$_1$ 10 mg, B$_2$ 10 mg, B$_3$ 50 mg, B$_5$ 10 mg, B$_6$ 5 mg. Tab. Bot. 100s. *OTC.*
Use: Vitamin supplement.

B-Complex 25-25. (Forest) Niacinamide 100 mg, vitamins B$_1$ 25 mg, B$_2$ 1 mg, B$_6$ 2 mg, pantothenic acid 2 mg/mL. Inj. Vial 30 mL. *Rx.*
Use: Vitamin supplement.

B-Complex/Vitamin C Caplets. (Geneva) Vitamins B$_1$ 15 mg, B$_2$ 10.2 mg, B$_3$ 50 mg, B$_5$ 10 mg, B$_6$ 5 mg, C 300 mg. Cap. Bot. 100s. *OTC.*
Use: Vitamin supplement.

B-Complex with B-12. (Ivax) B$_1$ 1.5 mg, B$_2$ 1.7 mg, B$_3$ 20 mg, B$_5$ 10 mg, B$_6$ 2 mg, B$_{12}$ 6 mcg, FA 0.4 mg. Tab. Bot. 100s. *OTC.*
Use: Mineral, vitamin supplement.

B Complex with B$_{12}$ Capsules. (Bryant) Vitamins B$_1$ 2 mg, B$_2$ 2 mg, B$_6$ 0.5 mg, niacinamide 10 mg, B$_{12}$ 2 mcg, biotin 10 mcg, calcium pantothenate 1.5 mg, choline dihydrogen citrate 40 mg, inositol 30 mg, desiccated liver 1 g, brewer's yeast 3 g. Cap. Bot. 100s, 1000s. *OTC.*
Use: Mineral, vitamin supplement.

B Complex with C and B-12. (Ivax) Vitamins B$_1$ 50 mg, B$_2$ 5 mg, B$_3$ 125 mg, B$_5$ 6 mg, B$_6$ 5 mg, B$_{12}$ 1000 mcg, C 50 mg. Inj. Vial 10 mL. *Rx.*
Use: Vitamin supplement.

B-Complex with Vitamin C and B$_{12}$-10,000. (Fujisawa Healthcare) Vitamins B$_1$ 20 mg, B$_2$ 3 mg, B$_3$ 75 mg, B$_5$ 5 mg, B$_6$ 5 mg, B$_{12}$ 1000 mcg, C 100 mg. Covial. 10 mL multiple dose. *Rx.*
Use: Vitamin supplement.

BC-1000. (Solvay) Vitamins B$_1$ 50 mg, B$_2$ 5 mg, B$_{12}$ 1000 mcg, B$_6$ 5 mg, d-panthenol 6 mg, niacinamide 125 mg, ascorbic acid 50 mg, benzyl alcohol 1%/mL. Vial 10 mL. *OTC.*
Use: Vitamin supplement.

BC Powder, Arthritis Strength. (Block Drug) Aspirin 742 mg, salicylamide 222 mg, caffeine 38 mg, lactose. Pow. Pkg. 50s. *OTC.*
Use: Analgesic combination.

BC Powder Original Formula. (Block Drug) Aspirin 650 mg, salicylamide 195 mg, caffeine 33.3 mg, lactose. Pow. Pkg. 50s. *OTC.*
Use: Analgesic combination.

BC Tablets. (Block Drug) Aspirin 325 mg, salicylamide 95 mg, caffeine 16 mg. Tab. Pkg 4s. Bot. 50s, 100s. *OTC.*
Use: Analgesic combination.

B-C w/Folic Acid. (Geneva) Vitamins B$_1$ 15 mg, B$_2$ 15 mg, B$_3$ 100 mg, B$_5$ 18 mg, B$_6$ 4 mg, B$_{12}$ 5 mcg, C 500 mg, folic acid 0.5 mg. Tab. Bot. 100s. *Rx.*
Use: Mineral, vitamin supplement.

B-C w/Folic Acid Plus. (Geneva) Fe 27 mg, vitamins A 5000 units, E 30 units, B$_1$ 20 mg, B$_2$ 20 mg, B$_3$ 100 mg, B$_5$ 25 mg, B$_6$ 25 mg, B$_{12}$ 50 mcg, C 500 mg, FA 0.8 mg, biotin 0.15 mg, Cr, Cu, Mg, Mn, Zn 22.5 mg. Tab. Bot. 100s. *Rx.*
Use: Mineral, vitamin supplement.

B-Day. (Barth's) Vitamins B$_1$ 7 mg, B$_2$ 14 mg, niacin 4.67 mg, B$_{12}$ 5 mcg. Tab. Bot. 100s, 500s. *OTC.*
Use: Vitamin supplement.

B-D Glucose. (Becton Dickinson & Co.) Glucose 5 g. Chew. Tab. Bot. 36s. *OTC.*
Use: Hyperglycemic.

B Dozen. (Standex) Vitamin B$_{12}$ 25 mcg Tab. Bot. 1000s. *OTC.*
Use: Vitamin supplement.

B-Dram w/C Computabs. (Dram) Vitamins B_1 5 mg, B_2 10 mg, B_6 5 mg, nicotinamide 50 mg, calcium pantothenate 20 mg. Tab. Bot. 100s. OTC.
Use: Mineral, vitamin supplement.

Beano. (AKPharma) Alpha-D-galactosidase derived from *Aspergillus niger*, a fungal source in carrier of water and glycerol. Liq. Bot. 75 serving size at 5 drops per dose. Tab. Pkg. 12s. Bot. 30s, 100s. OTC.
Use: Antiflatulent.

Bear-E-Yum CT. (Mallinckrodt) Barium sulfate 1.5%, simethicone, sorbitol. Susp. Bot. 200 mL, 1900 mL. Rx.
Use: Radiopaque agent, GI contrast agent.

Bear-E-Yum GI. (Mallinckrodt) Barium sulfate 60%, simethicone. Susp. Bot. 200 mL. Rx.
Use: Radiopaque agent, GI contrast agent.

Bebatab No. 2. (Freeport) Belladonna ⅙ g, phenobarbital 0.25 g. Tab. Bot. 1000s. Rx.
Use: Anticholinergic; antispasmodic; hypnotic; sedative.

Bebulin VH. (Baxter Healthcare) Purified freeze-dried concentrate of coagulation Factor IX, II, and X. Heat-treated. Actual number of units shown on each bottle. Pow. for Inj. Single-dose vials with Sterile Water for Injection, double-ended needle, and filter needle. Rx.
Use: Antihemophilic agent.

• **becanthone hydrochloride.** (BEE-kanthone) USAN.
Use: Antischistosomal.

• **becaplermin.** (beh-kah-PLER-min) USAN.
Use: Chronic dermal ulcers treatment.
See: Regranex.

• **becatecarin.** (BE-Ka-TEK-ar-in) USAN.
Use: Antineoplastic.

Beceevite. (Halsey Drug) Vitamins C 300 mg, B_1 15 mg, B_2 10 mg, niacin 50 mg, B_6 5 mg, pantothenic acid 10 mg. Cap. Bot. 100s. OTC.
Use: Vitamin supplement.

• **beclomethasone dipropionate.** (BEK-low-METH-uh-zone die-PRO-peo-uh-NATE) USP 28.
Use: Corticosteroid; intranasal steroid.
See: Beclovent.
  Beconase AQ.
  QVAR.
  Vanceril.
  Vanceril Double Strength.

beclomycin dipropionate.
Use: Corticosteroid.

Beclovent. (GlaxoSmithKline) Beclomethasone dipropionate 42 mcg/actuation. Canister 6.7 g (80 metered doses), 16.8 g (200 metered doses), adapter. Refill canister 16.8 g. Rx.
Use: Respiratory inhalant, corticosteroid.

Becomp-C. (Cenci, H.R. Labs, Inc.) Vitamins C 250 mg, B_1 25 mg, B_2 10 mg, nicotinamide 50 mg, B_6 2 mg, calcium pantothenate 10 mg, hesperidin complex 50 mg. Cap. Bot. 100s, 500s. OTC.
Use: Mineral, vitamin supplement.

Beconase AQ. (GlaxoSmithKline) Beclomethasone dipropionate 0.042% (42 mcg/actuation), dextrose, polysorbate 80, benzalkonium chloride, 0.25% w/w phenylethyl alcohol. Spray. Bot. 25 g (180 metered doses per bottle) with metering pump and nasal adaptor. Rx.
Use: Corticosteroid; intranasal steroid.

Becotin-T. (Eli Lilly) Vitamins B_1 15 mg, B_2 10 mg, B_6 5 mg, niacinamide 100 mg, pantothenic acid 20 mg, B_{12} 4 mcg, C 300 mg. Tab. Bot. 100s, 1000s, Blister pkg. 10 × 10s. OTC.
Use: Vitamin supplement.

• **bectumomab.** (beck-TYOO-moe-mab) USAN.
Use: Monoclonal antibody, diagnosis of non-Hodgkin lymphoma and detection of AIDS-related lymphoma.

Bedoce. (Lincoln Diagnostics) Crystalline anhydrous vitamin B_{12} 1000 mcg/mL. Vial 10 mL. Rx.
Use: Vitamin supplement.

Bedoce-Gel. (Lincoln Diagnostics) Vitamin B_{12} 1000 mcg/mL in 17% gelatin gel. Vial 10 ml. Rx.
Use: Vitamin supplement.

Bedside Care. (Sween) Bot. 8 oz, gal.
Use: Dermatologic.

beechwood creosote.
See: Creosote.

Bee-Forte w/C. (Rugby) Vitamins B_1 25 mg, B_2 12.5 mg, B_3 50 mg, B_5 10 mg, B_6 3 mg, B_{12} 2.5 mcg, C 250 mg. Cap. Bot. 100s. OTC.
Use: Vitamin supplement.

beef peptones. (Sandia) Water-soluble peptones derived from beef 20 mg/2 mL. Inj. Vial 30 mL. Rx.
Use: Nutritional supplement, parenteral.

Beelith. (Beach) Pyridoxine hydrochloride 20 mg, magnesium oxide 600 mg. Tab. Bot. 100s. OTC.
Use: Mineral, vitamin supplement.

Beepen-VK. (GlaxoSmithKline) Penicillin V. **Tab.:** 250 mg, Bot. 1000s; 500 mg, Bot. 500s. **Pow. for Oral Soln.:**

125 mg/5 mL; 250 mg/5 mL. Bot.
100 mL, 200 mL. *Rx.*
Use: Anti-infective; penicillin.
Bee-Thi. (Burgin-Arden) Cyanoco-
balamin 1000 mcg, thiamine hydrochlo-
ride 100 mg in isotonic soln. of sodium
Cl/mL. Vial 10 mL, 20 mL. *Rx.*
Use: Vitamin supplement.
Bee-Twelve 1000. (Burgin-Arden)
Cyanocobalamin 1000 mcg/mL. Vial
10 mL, 30 mL. *Rx.*
Use: Vitamin supplement.
Bee-Zee. (Rugby) Vitamins E 45 mg,
B_1 15 mg, B_2 10.2 mg, B_3 100 mg, B_5
25 mg, B_6 10 mg, B_{12} 6 mcg, C 600 mg,
zinc 5.2 mg. Tab. Bot. 60s. *OTC.*
Use: Mineral, vitamin supplement.
Behepan.
See: Vitamin B_{12}.
Belatol Elixir. (Cenci, H.R. Labs, Inc.)
Phenobarbital 20 mg, belladonna
6.75 mg/5 mL w/alcohol 45%. Bot. Pt,
gal. *Rx.*
Use: Anticholinergic; antispasmodic;
hypnotic; sedative.
Belatol No. 1; No. 2. (Cenci, H.R. Labs,
Inc.) **No. 1:** Belladonna leaf extract
⅛ g, phenobarbital 0.25 g. Tab. Bot.
100s, 1000s. **No. 2:** Belladonna leaf ex-
tract, phenobarbital 0.5 g. Tab. Bot.
100s, 1000s. *Rx.*
Use: Anticholinergic; antispasmodic;
hypnotic; sedative.
Belbutal No. 2 Kaptabs. (Churchill)
Phenobarbital 32.4 mg, hyoscyamine
sulfate 0.1092 mg, atropine sulfate
0.0215 mg, hyoscine HBr 0.0065 mg.
Tab. Bot. 100s. *Rx.*
Use: Anticholinergic; antispasmodic;
hypnotic; sedative.
Beldin. (Halsey Drug) Diphenhydramine
hydrochloride 12.5 mg/5 mL w/alcohol
5%. Bot. Gal. *OTC.*
Use: Antihistamine.
Belexal. (Pal-Pak, Inc.) Vitamins B_1
1.5 mg, B_2 2 mg, B_6 0.167 mg, calcium
pantothenate 1 mg, niacinamide
10 mg, brewer's yeast. Tab. Bot. 1000s,
5000s. *OTC.*
Use: Mineral, vitamin supplement.
Belexon Fortified Improved. (A.P.C.)
Liver fraction No. 2, 3 g, yeast extract
3 g, vitamins B_1 5 mg, B_2 6 mg, niacinamide 10 mg, calcium pantothenate
2 mg, cyanocobalamin 1 mcg, iron
10 mg. Cap. Bot. 100s. *OTC.*
Use: Mineral, vitamin supplement.
Belfer. (Forest) Vitamins B_1 2 mg, B_2
2 mg, B_{12} 10 mcg, B_6 2 mg, C 50 mg,
iron 17 mg. Tab. Bot. 100s. *OTC.*
Use: Mineral, vitamin supplement.

●**belfosdil.** (bell-FOSE-dill) USAN.
Use: Antihypertensive; calcium channel
blocker.
Belganyl. CDC anti-infective agent. *Rx.*
See: Suramin.
●**belimumab.** (bel-LIM-oo-mab) USAN.
Use: Monoclonal antibody.
●**belladonna.** (bell-a-DON-a) *USP 28.*
Use: Gastrointestinal anticholinergic/an-
tispasmodic.
See: Belladonna Tincture.
belladonna alkaloids.
Use: Anticholinergic; antispasmodic.
W/Combinations.
See: Atropine Sulfate.
Belladonna.
L-Hyoscyamine Sulfate.
belladonna alkaloids w/phenobarbital.
(Various Mfr.) Atropine sulfate
0.0194 mg, scopolamine HBr
0.0065 mg, hyoscyamine HBr or SO_4
0.1037 mg, phenobarbital 16.2 mg. Tab.
Bot. 20s, 1000s, UD 100s. *Rx.*
Use: Anticholinergic; antispasmodic;
hypnotic; sedative.
**belladonna and phenobarbital combi-
nations.**
Use: Anticholinergic; antispasmodic;
hypnotic; sedative.
See: Atrocap.
Atrosed.
Bebatab.
Belatol.
Bellamine.
Bellergal.
Chardonna.
Donnatal.
Donnatal #2.
Donnazyme.
Phenobarbital and Belladonna.
Sedapar.
Spabelin.
Spabelin No. 2.
●**belladonna extract.** (bell-a-DON-a)
USP 28.
Use: Antispasmodic.
belladonna extract. (Eli Lilly) Belladonna
extract 15 mg (0.187 mg belladonna).
Tab.
Use: Antispasmodic.
belladonna extract combinations.
Use: Anticholinergic; antispasmodic.
See: B & O Supprettes.
Butibel.
●**belladonna leaf.** *USP 28.*
Use: Antispasmodic.
**belladonna leaf, phenobarbital, and
benzocaine.**
Use: Anticholinergic.

• **belladonna tincture.** *USP 28.*
Use: Antispasmodic.

belladonna tincture. (Various Mfr.) Belladonna alkaloids 27 to 33 mg/100 mL. Alcohol 65% to 70%. Liq. 120 mL, pint, gallon. *Rx.*
Use: Gastrointestinal anticholinergic/ antispasmodic.

Bellahist-D LA. (Cypress) Phenylephrine hydrochloride 20 mg, chlorpheniramine maleate 8 mg, hyoscyamine sulfate 0.19 mg, atropine sulfate 0.04 mg, scopolamine HBr 0.01 mg. Alcohol, sugar, and dye free. ER Tab. 100s. *Rx.*
Use: Upper respiratory combination, decongestant, antihistamine, anticholinergic.

Bellamine. (Major) Levorotatory alkaloids of belladonna 0.2 mg, phenobarbital 40 mg, ergotamine tartrate 0.6 mg. Tab. 100s. *Rx.*
Use: Anticholinergic; sedative.

Bellaneed. (Hanlon) Belladonna, phenobarbital 16 mg. Cap. Bot. 100s. *Rx.*
Use: Anticholinergic; antispasmodic; hypnotic; sedative.

Bell/ans. (C.S. Dent & Co.) Sodium bicarbonate 520 mg (sodium content 144 mg). Tab. Bot. 30s, 60s. *OTC.*
Use: Antacid.

Bellastal. (Wharton) Atropine sulfate 0.0194 mg, scopolamine HBr 0.0065 mg, hyoscyamine HBr or SO₄ 0.1037 mg, phenobarbital 16.2 mg. Cap. Bot. 1000s. *Rx.*
Use: Anticholinergic; antispasmodic.

Bellatal. (Richwood Pharmaceuticals) Phenobarbital 16.2 mg, hyoscyamine sulfate 0.1037 mg, atropine sulfate 0.0194 mg, scopolamine HBr 0.0065 mg, lactose. Tab. Bot. 100s, 500s. *Rx.*
Use: Hypnotic; sedative.

• **beloxamide.** (bell-OX-ah-mid) USAN.
Use: Antihyperlipoproteinemic.

• **beloxepin.** (beh-LOX-eh-pin) USAN.
Use: Antidepressant.

Bel-Phen-Ergot SR. (Ivax) Phenobarbital 40 mg, ergotamine tartrate 0.6 mg, l-alkaloids of belladonna 0.2 mg. Tab. Bot. 100s. *Rx.*
Use: Anticholinergic.

• **bemarinone hydrochloride.** (BEH-mah-rih-NOHN) USAN.
Use: Cardiovascular agent, positive inotropic, vasodilator.

• **bemesetron.** (beh-meh-SET-rone) USAN.
Use: Antiemetic.

Beminal 500. (Whitehall-Robins) Vitamins B₁ 25 mg, B₂ 12.5 mg, B₃ 100 mg, B₆ 10 mg, B₅ 20 mg, C 500 mg, B₁₂ 5 mcg. Tab. Bot. 100s. *OTC.*
Use: Vitamin supplement.

• **bemitradine.** (beh-MIH-trah-DEEN) USAN.
Use: Antihypertensive; diuretic.

• **bemoradan.** (beh-MOE-rah-DAN) USAN.
Use: Cardiovascular agent.

• **bemotrizinol.** (be-MOE-trye-zi-nol) USAN.
Use: Sunscreen.

Benacen. (Cenci, H.R. Labs, Inc.) Probenecid 0.5 g. Tab. Bot. 100s, 1000s. *Rx.*
Use: Antigout.

Benacol. (Cenci, H.R. Labs, Inc.) Dicyclomine hydrochloride 20 mg. Tab. Bot. 100s, 1000s. *Rx.*
Use: Anticholinergic; antispasmodic.

benactyzine hydrochloride. 2-Diethylaminoethyl benzilate hydrochloride.
Use: Anxiolytic.

benactyzine/meprobamate. Psychotherapeutic combination.

Benadryl. (Parke-Davis) Diphenhydramine hydrochloride. **Cream:** 1%. Tube 1 oz. **Elix. (w/alcohol 14%):** 12.5 mg/ 5 mL. Bot. 4 oz, pt, gal, UD 5 mL (100s). **Spray:** 1%. Bot. 2 oz. **Tab.:** 25 mg. Bot. 100s. *OTC.*
Use: Antihistamine.

Benadryl. (Parke-Davis) Diphenhydramine hydrochloride 50 mg/mL. Amps 1 mL; *Steri-vials* (with benzethonium chloride) 1 mL, 10 mL; *Steri-dose* syringe 1 mL. *Rx.*
Use: Antihistamine.

Benadryl Allergy. (Pfizer) Diphenhydramine hydrochloride. **Chew. Tab.:** 12.5 mg, aspartame, phenylalanine 4.2 mg, grape flavor. Pkg. 24s. **Tab.:** 25 mg. Pkg. 24s. Bot. 100s. **Liq.:** 12.5 mg/5 mL. Bot. 118 mL. *OTC.*
Use: Antihistamine, nonselective ethanolamine.

Benadryl Allergy & Cold. (Warner Lambert) Pseudoephedrine hydrochloride 30 mg, diphenhydramine hydrochloride 12.5 mg, acetaminophen 500 mg. Tab. Pkg. 24s. *OTC.*
Use: Upper respiratory combination, decongestant, antihistamine, analgesic.

Benadryl Allergy & Sinus Fastmelt Dissolving Tablets. (Warner Lambert) Pseudoephedrine hydrochloride 30 mg, diphenhydramine citrate 19 mg (diphenhydramine hydrochloride

12.5 mg), phenylalanine 4.6 mg, aspartame, mannitol. Dissolving Tab. Pkg. 20s. *OTC.*
Use: Upper respiratory combination, decongestant, antihistamine.

Benadryl Allergy & Sinus Headache Tablets and Gelcaps. (Warner Lambert) Pseudoephedrine hydrochloride 30 mg, diphenhydramine hydrochloride 12.5 mg, acetaminophen 500 mg. Tab., Gelcap. Bot. 24s, 48s. *OTC.*
Use: Upper respiratory combination, analgesic, antihistamine, decongestant.

Benadryl Allergy & Sinus Liquid. (Warner Lambert) Pseudoephedrine hydrochloride 30 mg, diphenhydramine hydrochloride 12.5 mg/5 mL, saccharin, sorbitol, grape flavor. Liq. Bot. 118 mL. *OTC.*
Use: Upper respiratory combination, decongestant, antihistamine.

Benadryl Allergy & Sinus Tablets. (Warner Lambert) Pseudoephedrine hydrochloride 60 mg, diphenhydramine hydrochloride 25 mg. Tab. Pkg. 24s. *OTC.*
Use: Upper respiratory combination, decongestant, antihistamine.

Benadryl Allergy Kapseals. (Pfizer) Diphenhydramine hydrochloride 25 mg, lactose. Cap. Pkg. 24s, 48s. *OTC.*
Use: Antihistamine, nonselective ethanolamine.

Benadryl Allergy Ultratabs. (Pfizer) Diphenhydramine hydrochloride 25 mg. Tab. Bot. 24s, 48s, 100s. *OTC.*
Use: Antihistamine, nonselective ethanolamine.

Benadryl Children's Allergy. (Pfizer) Diphenhydramine hydrochloride 12.5 mg/5 mL, sugar, cherry flavor. Liq. Bot. 118 mL, 236 mL. *OTC.*
Use: Antihistamine, nonselective ethanolamine.

Benadryl Children's Allergy & Cold Fastmelt Tablets. (Warner Lambert) Pseudoephedrine hydrochloride 30 mg, diphenhydramine citrate 19 mg (diphenhydramine hydrochloride 12.5 mg), phenylalanine 4.6 mg, aspartame, mannitol. *Fastmelt* Tab. Pkg. 20s. *OTC.*
Use: Upper respiratory combination, decongestant, antihistamine.

Benadryl Children's Allergy Fastmelt. (Pfizer) Diphenhydramine citrate 19 mg, phenylalanine 4.5 mg. Aspartame. Orally Disintegrating Tab. 20s. *OTC.*
Use: Antihistamine.

Benadryl Children's Allergy & Sinus Liquid. (Warner Lambert) Pseudoephedrine hydrochloride 30 mg, diphenhydramine hydrochloride 12.5 mg/5 mL, saccharin, sorbitol, grape flavor, alcohol free. Liq. Bot. 118 mL. *OTC.*
Use: Upper respiratory combination, decongestant, antihistamine.

Benadryl Children's Dye-Free Allergy. (Pfizer) Diphenhydramine 12.5 mg/5 mL, saccharin, sorbitol, alcohol free, bubble-gum flavor. Liq. Bot. 118 mL. *OTC.*
Use: Antihistamine, nonselective ethanolamine.

Benadryl Dye-Free Allergy Liqui Gels. (Pfizer) Diphenhydramine hydrochloride 25 mg, sorbitol. Cap. Bot. 24s. *OTC.*
Use: Antihistamine, nonselective ethanolamine.

Benadryl Elixir. (Parke-Davis) Diphenhydramine hydrochloride 12.5 mg/5 mL w/alcohol 14%. Bot. 4 oz, pt, gal, UD (5 mL) 100s. *OTC.*
Use: Antihistamine.

Benadryl Injection. (Parke-Davis) Diphenhydramine hydrochloride 50 mg/mL. Amp. 1 mL, *Steri-Vials* 10 mL, *Steri-dose* syringe 1 mL. *Rx.*
Use: Antihistamine.

Benadryl Itch Relief. (GlaxoSmithKline) Diphenhydramine hydrochloride 1%, zinc acetate 0.1%, alcohol 73.6%, aloe vera. Spray. Bot. 59 mL. *OTC.*
Use: Antihistamine.

Benadryl Itch Relief Children's. (GlaxoSmithKline) **Cream:** Diphenhydramine hydrochloride 1%, zinc acetate 0.1%, aloe vera, cetyl alcohol, parabens. Jar 14.2 g. **Spray:** Diphenhydramine hydrochloride 1%, zinc acetate 0.1%, alcohol 73.6%, aloe vera, povidone. Can. 59 mL. *OTC.*
Use: Antihistamine.

Benadryl Itch Relief, Maximum Strength. (GlaxoSmithKline) **Cream:** Diphenhydramine hydrochloride 2%, zinc acetate 0.1%, parabens, aloe vera. Tube 14.2 g. **Stick:** Diphenhydramine hydrochloride 2%, zinc acetate 0.1%, alcohol 73.5%, aloe vera. Tube 14 mL.

Benadryl Itch Stopping Gel Children's Formula. (GlaxoSmithKline) Diphenhydramine hydrochloride 1%, zinc acetate 1%, camphor, parabens. Gel. Tube 118 mL. *OTC.*
Use: Antihistamine.

Benadryl Itch Stopping Gel Maximum Strength. (GlaxoSmithKline) Diphenhydramine hydrochloride 2%, zinc ace-

tate 1%, camphor, parabens. Tube 118 g. *OTC.*
Use: Antihistamine.

Benadryl Itch Stopping Spray, Extra Strength. (Warner Lambert) Diphenhydramine hydrochloride 2%, zinc acetate 0.1%, alcohol 73.5%, glycerin, tromethamine. Spray. Bot. 59 mL. *OTC.*
Use: Antihistamine.

Benadryl Itch Stopping Spray, Original Strength. (Warner Lambert) Diphenhydramine hydrochloride 1%, zinc acetate 0.1%, alcohol 73.6%, glycerin, tromethamine. Spray. Bot. 59 mL. *OTC.*
Use: Antihistamine.

Benadryl Maximum Strength. (Parke-Davis) **Cream:** Diphenhydramine hydrochloride 2% and parabens in a greaseless base in 15 g. Nonaerosol **spray:** Diphenhydramine hydrochloride 2%, alcohol 85% in 60 mL. *OTC.*
Use: Dermatologic.

Benadryl Maximum Strength Severe Allergy & Sinus Headache. (Warner Lambert) Pseudoephedrine hydrochloride 30 mg, diphenhydramine hydrochloride 25 mg, acetaminophen 500 mg. Tab. Pkg. 20s. *OTC.*
Use: Upper respiratory combination, decongestant, antihistamine, analgesic.

Benahist 50. (Keene Pharmaceuticals) Diphenhydramine 50 mg/mL. Vial 10 mL. *Rx.*
Use: Antihistamine.

Benahist 10. (Keene Pharmaceuticals) Diphenhydramine 10 mg/mL. Vial 30 mL. *Rx.*
Use: Antihistamine.

benanserin hydrochloride.
Use: Serotonin antagonist.

Benaphen Caps. (Major) Diphenhydramine 25 mg, 50 mg. Cap. Bot. 100s, 1000s. *OTC.*
Use: Antihistamine.

•**benapryzine hydrochloride.** (BEN-ah-PRY-zeen) USAN.
Use: Anticholinergic.

Benase. (Ferndale) Proteolytic enzymes extracted from Carica papaya 20,000 units enzyme activity. Tab. Bot. 1000s. *Rx.*
Use: Reduction of edema, relief of episiotomy.

benazepril and amlodipine.
Use: Antihypertensive.
See: Lotrel.

•**benazeprilat.** (BEN-AZE-eh-prill-at) USAN.
Use: Angiotensin-converting enzyme inhibitor.

•**benazepril hydrochloride.** (BEN-AZE-eh-prill) USAN.
Use: Angiotensin-converting enzyme inhibitor.
See: Lotensin.

benazepril hydrochloride. (Various Mfr.) Benazepril hydrochloride 5 mg, 10 mg, 20 mg, 40 mg. May contain lactose, maltodextrin. Tab. 100s, 500s, 1,000s, 2,500s (except 5 mg), 5,000s (except 5 mg), UD 100s (except 5 mg). *Rx.*
Use: Angiotensin-converting enzyme inhibitor.

benazepril hydrochloride and hydrochlorothiazide. (Sandoz) Hydrochlorothiazide/benazepril hydrochloride 6.25 mg/5 mg, 12.5 mg/10 mg, 12.5 mg/20 mg, 25 mg/20 mg. Castor oil (except 6.25 mg/5 mg), lactose. Tab. 100s. *Rx.*
Use: Antihypertensive.

•**bendacalol mesylate.** (ben-DACK-ah-LOLE) USAN.
Use: Antihypertensive.

•**bendazac.** (BEN-dah-ZAK) USAN.
Use: Anti-inflammatory.

•**bendroflumethiazide.** (ben-droe-floo-meth-EYE-a-zide) *USP 28.*
Use: Antihypertensive; diuretic.
See: Naturetin.
W/Potassium Cl.
See: Naturetin W-K.
W/Rauwolfia serpentina.
See: Rauzide.

Benefiber. (Novartis Nutritional) Partially hydrolyzed guar gum (3 g dietary fiber/pkt or tbsp). Flavor free. Pkt. (14s). 102 g, 180 g. *OTC.*
Use: Laxative.

BeneFix. (Genetics Institute) Nonpyrogenic lyophilized powder preparation. Purified protein produced by recombinant DNA for use in Factor IX deficiency. Actual number of units shown on each bottle. Single-dose vial with diluent needle, filter, infusion set, and alcohol swabs. 250 units, 500 units, 1000 units. *Rx.*
Use: Antihemophilic agent.

Benemid. (Merck & Co.) Probenecid 0.5 g. Tab. Bot. 100s, 1000s, UD 100s. *Rx.*
Use: Antigout.

Benephen Antiseptic Medicated Powder. (Halsted) Methylbenzethonium Cl 1:1800, magnesium carbonate in corn starch base. Pow. Shaker can 3.56 oz. *OTC.*
Use: Antiseptic; deodorant.

Benephen Antiseptic Ointment w/Cod Liver Oil. (Halsted) Methylbenzethonium Cl 1:1000, water-repellent base of zinc oxide, corn starch. Oint. Tube 1.5 oz. Jar lb. *OTC.*
Use: Antiseptic.

Benephen Antiseptic Vitamin A & D Cream. (Halsted) Methylbenzethonium Cl 1:1000, cod liver oil w/vitamins A and D in petrolatum and glycerin base. Cream. Tube 2 oz. Jar lb. *OTC.*
Use: Antiseptic.

Benepro Tabs. (Major) Probenecid 500 mg. Tab. Bot. 100s, 1000s. *Rx.*
Use: Antigout.

bengal gelatin.
See: Agar.

Bengay Children's Vaporizing Rub. (Pfizer) Camphor, menthol, w/oils of turpentine, eucalyptus, cedar leaf, nutmeg, thyme in stainless white base. Jar 1.125 oz. *OTC.*
Use: Analgesic, topical.

Bengay Extra Strength. (Pfizer) Methyl salicylate 30%, menthol 8%. Balm. Jar 3.75 oz. *OTC.*
Use: Analgesic, topical.

Bengay Extra Strength Sports. (Pfizer) Methyl salicylate 28%, menthol 10%. Balm. Tube 1.25 oz, 3 oz. *OTC.*
Use: Analgesic, topical.

Bengay Gel. (Pfizer) Methyl salicylate 15%, menthol 7%, alcohol 40%. Gel. Tube 1.25 oz, 3 oz. *OTC.*
Use: Analgesic, topical.

Bengay Greaseless. (Pfizer) Methyl salicylate 18.3%, menthol 16%. Oint. Tube 1.25 oz, 3 oz, 5 oz. *OTC.*
Use: Analgesic, topical.

Bengay Lotion. (Pfizer) Methyl salicylate 15%, menthol 7% in lotion base. Lot. Bot. 2 oz, 4 oz. *OTC.*
Use: Analgesic, topical.

Bengay Ointment. (Pfizer) Methyl salicylate 15%, menthol 10% in ointment base. Oint. Tube 1.25 oz, 3 oz, 5 oz. *OTC.*
Use: Analgesic, topical.

Bengay Original. (Pfizer) Methyl salicylate 18.3%, menthol 16%. Oint. Tube. 37.5 g, 90 g, 150 g. *OTC.*
Use: Analgesic, topical.

Bengay Patch. (Pfizer) Menthol 1.4%. Glycerin. Patch, regular and large size. 1s. *OTC.*
Use: Liniment.

Bengay Sportsgel. (Pfizer) Methyl salicylate, menthol, alcohol 40%. Gel. Tube 1.25 oz, 3 oz. *OTC.*
Use: Analgesic, topical.

Benicar. (Sankyo Pharm) Olmesartan medoxomil 5 mg, 20 mg, 40 mg, lactose. Tab. Bot. 30s, 90s (except 5 mg), blister card 100s (except 5 mg). *Rx.*
Use: Antihypertensive.

Benicar HCT. (Sankyo Pharma) Hydrochlorothiazide/olmesartan medoxomil. 12.5 mg/20 mg, 12.5 mg/40 mg, 25 mg/40 mg. Lactose. Tab. 30s, 90s, 100s, blister card 10s. *Rx.*
Use: Antihypertensive.

Benoquin. (ICN) Monobenzone 20% in a water washable base. Cetyl alcohol, propylene glycol. Cream. 35.4 g. *Rx.*
Use: Pigment agent.

•**benorterone.** (bee-NAHR-ter-ohn) USAN.
Use: Antiandrogen.

•**benoxaprofen.** (ben-OX-ah-PRO-fen) USAN.
Use: Anti-inflammatory; analgesic.

•**benoxinate hydrochloride.** (ben-OX-ih-nate) *USP 28.*
Use: Anesthetic, topical.
See: Flurate.
    Fluress.

•**benperidol.** (BEN-peh-rih-dahl) USAN.
Use: Antipsychotic.

•**bensalan.** (BEN-sal-an) USAN. Under study.
Use: Disinfectant.

Bensal HP. (7 Oaks) Benzoic acid 6%, salicyclic acid 3%, extract of oak bark. Oint. Tube 15 g, 30 g. Jar 30 g, 60 g. *Rx.*
Use: Anti-infective, topical.

•**benserazide.** (ben-SER-ah-zide) USAN.
Use: Inhibitor, decarboxylase; antiparkinson.

Bensulfoid. (ECR) Sulfur 8%, resorcinol 2%, alcohol 12%. Cream. Tube 15 g. *OTC.*
Use: Antiacne.

Ben-Tann. (Midlothian) Diphenhydramine tannate 25 mg per 5 mL. Sucrose, saccharin. Strawberry flavor. Susp. 118 mL. *Rx.*
Use: Antihistamine.

•**bentazepam.** (BEN-tay-zeh-pam) USAN.
Use: Hypnotic; sedative.

Bentical. (Lamond) Bentonite, zinc oxide, zinc carbonate, titanium dioxide. Bot. 4 oz, 6 oz, 8 oz, 16 oz, 32 oz, 0.5 gal, gal.
Use: Emollient.

•**bentiromide.** (ben-TIRE-oh-mide) USAN.
Use: Diagnostic aid, pancreas function determination.
See: Chymex.

• **bentonite.** (BEN-tun-ite) *NF 23.*
Use: Pharmaceutic aid, suspending agent.

bentonite magma.
Use: Pharmaceutic aid, suspending agent.

bentonite, purified.
Use: Pharmaceutic aid.

• **bentoquatam.** (BEN-toe-KWAH-tam) USAN.
Use: Barrier for prevention of allergic contact dermatitis.
See: Ivy Block.

Bentyl. (Axcan Scandipharm) Dicyclomine hydrochloride. **Cap.:** 10 mg. Bot. 100s, 500s, UD 100s. **Tab.:** 20 mg. Bot. 100s, 500s, 1000s, UD 100s. **Syr.:** 10 mg/5 mL. Bot. Pt. **Inj.:** 10 mg/mL. Amp. 2 mL, syringe 2 mL. Vial 10 mL (also contains chlorobutanol) Rx
Use: Anticholinergic; antispasmodic.

• **benurestat.** (BEN-YOU-reh-stat) USAN.
Use: Enzyme inhibitor, urease.

Benylin Adult. (Pfizer) Dextromethorphan HBr 15 mg/5 mL, saccharin, sorbitol, alcohol free. Liq. Bot. 118 mL. *OTC.*
Use: Antitussive.

Benylin Expectorant. (Pfizer) Dextromethorphan HBr 5 mg, guaifenesin 100 mg, saccharin, sorbitol, raspberry flavor, alcohol free. Bot. Liq. 118 mL. *OTC.*
Use: Upper respiratory combination, antitussive, expectorant.

Benylin Pediatric. (Pfizer) Dextromethorphan HBr 7.5 mg/5 mL, saccharin, sorbitol, alcohol free, grape flavor. Liq. Bot. 118 mL. *OTC.*
Use: Antitussive.

Benza. (Century) Benzalkonium Cl 1:5000, 1:750. Bot. 2 oz, 4 oz.
Use: Antimicrobial; antiseptic.

Benzac AC 2.5, 5, & 10. (Galderma) Benzoyl peroxide 2.5%, 5%, 10%, glycerine and EDTA in water base. Gel. Tube 60 g, 90 g. *Rx.*
Use: Antiacne.

Benzac AC Wash 2.5, 5, & 10. (Galderma) Benzoyl peroxide 2.5%, 5%, 10%, glycerin. Liq. Bot. 240 mL. *Rx.*
Use: Antiacne.

Benzac 5 & 10. (Galderma) Benzoyl peroxide 5%, 10%, alcohol 12%. Tube 60 g, 90 g. *Rx.*
Use: Antiacne.

BenzaClin. (Dermik) Clindamycin 1%, benzoyl peroxide 5%. Gel. Tube 25 g. *Rx.*
Use: Anti-infective, antibiotic, topical.

Benzac W/2.5, 5 & 10. (Galderma) Benzoyl peroxide 2.5%, 5%, 10%. EDTA.

Tube 60 g, 90 g. *Rx.*
Use: Antiacne.

Benzac W Wash 5 & 10. (Galderma) Benzoyl peroxide 5%, 10%, Bot. 120 mL (5% only), 240 mL. *Rx.*
Use: Antiacne.

Benzagel Wash. (Dermik) Benzoyl peroxide 10%, alcohol 14%. Gel. 60 g. *Rx.*
Use: Dermatologic, acne.

• **benzalkonium chloride.** (benz-al-KOE-nee-uhm) USAN.
Use: Surface antiseptic; pharmaceutical aid, preservative.
See: Bacti-Cleanse.
Benz-All.
Econopred.
Eye-Stream.
Germicin.
Hyramino 3500.
Mycocide NS.
Otrivin.
Ultra Tears.
Zephiran Chloride.
W/Combinations.
See: Aerocaine.
Alochor Styptic.
Barseb Thera-Spray.
Bactine Pain Relieving Cleansing.
Bite Rx.
Boro.
Computer Eye.
Cydonol Massage.
Dacriose.
E-Pilo.
Epinal.
Garamycin.
Goniosol.
Ionax.
Isopto Plain & Tears.
Medicone.
Mediotic-HC.
Mycomist.
Ocusol.
Oxyzal Wet Dressing.
Prefrin-A.
Rescula.
Salinex.
Swim-Eye.
Tearisol.
Unguentine.

Benzamycin. (Dermik) Benzoyl peroxide 5%, erythromycin 3%, alcohol 20%. Gel. 8 g, 23 g, 46 g. *Rx.*
Use: Anti-infective, topical.

Benzamycin Pak. (Dermik) Benzoyl peroxide 5%, erythromycin 3%, SD alcohol 40B. Gel. 0.8 g pouches. 60s. *Rx.*
Use: Anti-infectives, topical.

• **benzbromarone.** (BENZ-brome-ah-rone) USAN.

Use: Uricosuric.

Benzedrex. (B.F. Ascher) Propylhexedrine 250 mg, menthol, lavender oil. Inhaler. *OTC.*
Use: Nasal decongestant.

•**benzethonium chloride.** (benz-eth-OH-nee-uhm) *USP 28.* Topical solution; Tincture.
Use: Anti-infective, topical; pharmaceutic aid, preservative.

•**benzetimide hydrochloride.** (benz-ETT-ih-mide) USAN.
Use: Anticholinergic.

•**benzilonium bromide.** (BEN-zill-oh-nih-uhm) USAN.
Use: Anticholinergic.

•**benzindopyrine hydrochloride.** (BENZ-in-doe-pie-reen) USAN.
Use: Antipsychotic.

benzisoxazole derivatives.
Use: Antipsychotic.
See: Risperidone.
  Ziprasidone.

benzoate and phenylacetate.
Use: Treatment of hyperammonemia. [Orphan Drug]

Benzo-C. (Freeport) Benzocaine 5 mg, cetalkonium Cl 5 mg, ascorbic acid 50 mg. Troche. Bot. 1000s, cello-packed boxes 1000s. *OTC.*
Use: Anesthetic, local.

•**benzocaine.** (BEN-zoe-kane) *USP 28.* Ethyl-p-aminobenzoate. Anesthesin, orthesin, parathesin.
Use: Anesthetic, topical.
See: Bansmoke.
  Cēpacol Maximum Strength.
  Orajel P.M. Nighttime Formula Toothache Pain Relief.
  SensoGARD.
  Trocaine.
W/Combinations.
See: Aerocaine.
  Americaine.
  Anacaine.
  Auralgan.
  Auralgesic.
  Benzo-C.
  Benzodent.
  Bicozene.
  Boil-Ease Anesthetic.
  Bowman Drawing Paste.
  Cēpacol.
  Cetacaine.
  Chiggerex.
  Chigger-Tox.
  Chloraseptic Children's.
  Dent's.
  Dent's Dental Poultice.
  Dent's Toothache.
  Derma Medicone.
  Derma Medicone-HC.
  Dermoplast.
  Detane.
  Foille.
  Foille Medicated First Aid.
  Foille Plus.
  Formula 44 Cough Control.
  GBA.
  Hurricaine.
  Jiffy.
  Lanacane.
  Listerine Cough Control.
  Maximum Strength Anbesol.
  Medicone.
  Off-Ezy Corn Remover.
  Orabase.
  Orajel Mouth-Aid.
  Pazo.
  Pyrogallic Acid.
  Rectal Medicone.
  Rectal Medicone-HC.
  Rectal Medicone Unguent.
  Solarcaine.
  Spec-T Sore Throat-Decongestant.
  Sucrets Cold Control.
  Sucrets Cold Decongestant.
  Tanac.
  Toothache.
  Tympagesic.
  Unguentine.
  Unguentine Maximum Strength.
  Vicks Cough Silencers.
  Vicks Formula 44 Cough Control.
  Vicks Medi-Trating Throat.
  Vicks Oracin.
  Zilactin-B Medicated.

benzochlorophene sodium. Sodium salt of ortho-benzyl-para-chlorophenol.

•**benzoctamine hydrochloride.** (benz-OCK-tah-meen) USAN.
Use: Hypnotic; muscle relaxant; sedative.

Benzodent. (Procter & Gamble) Benzocaine 20%. Tube 30 g. *OTC.*
Use: Anesthetic, local.

•**benzodepa.** (BEN-zoe-DEH-pah) USAN.
Use: Antineoplastic.

benzodiazepines.
Use: Antianxiety agents; anticonvulsants; sedative/hypnotics, nonbarbiturates.
See: Alprazolam.
  Clonazepam.
  Clorazepate dipotassium.
  Chlordiazepoxide Hydrochloride.
  Diazepam.
  Estazolam.
  Flurazepam Hydrochloride.
  Lorazepam.

Oxazepam.
Quazepam.
Temazepam.
Triazolam.
• **benzoic acid.** (ben-ZOE-ik) *USP 28.*
Use: Pharmaceutic aid, antifungal.
W/Boric acid, zinc oxide, zinc stearate.
See: Whitfield's.
benzoic acid. (Various Mfr.) Benzoic
acid. Pkg. 0.25 lb, 1 lb. *OTC.*
Use: Antifungal; fungistatic.
benzoic acid, 2-hydroxy. Salicylic acid.
benzoic and salicylic acids.
Use: Antifungal, topical.
See: Whitfield's.
• **benzoin.** (BEN-zoyn) *USP 28.*
Use: Protectant, topical; expectorant.
See: Methagual.
W/Podophyllum rosin
See: Podoben.
W/Polyoxyethylene dodecanol, aro-
matics.
See: Vicks Vaposteam.
benzoin. (Morton International) Benzoin,
tolu balsam, styrax, alcohol w/propel-
lant. Aerosol. Can 7 oz. *OTC.*
Use: Skin protectant.
benzol. Usually refers to benzene.
Benzo-Menth. (Pal-Pak, Inc.) Benzo-
caine 2.2 mg. Tab. Bot. 1000s. *OTC.*
Use: Anesthetic, topical.
• **benzonatate.** (ben-ZOE-nah-tate)
USP 28.
Use: Antitussive.
See: Tessalon.
Tessalon Perles.
benzonatate softgels. (Various Mfr.)
Benzonatate 100 mg, 200 mg. Cap.
Bot. 100s, 500s. *Rx.*
Use: Antitussive.
benzophenone.
See: Pan Ultra.
W/Oxybenzone, dioxybenzone.
See: Solbar.
benzoquinonium chloride. (Various
Mfr.) *Rx.*
Use: Muscle relaxant.
benzosulfimide.
See: Saccharin.
benzosulphinide sodium. Name previ-
ously used for saccharin sodium.
• **benzoxiquine.** (benz-OX-ee-kwine)
USAN.
Use: Disinfectant.
• **benzoylpas calcium.** (benz-oe-ILL-pass)
USAN.
Use: Anti-infective, tuberculostatic.
• **benzoyl peroxide.** (BEN-zoyl per-OX-
ide) *USP 28.*
Use: Keratolytic.

See: Benoxyl.
Benzac AC Wash.
Benzac W Wash.
Brevoxyl Creamy Wash.
Brevoxyl Cleansing.
Clearasil Maximum Strength Acne
Treatment.
Clinac BPO.
Dermoxyl.
Desquam-E.
Desquam-X.
Neutrogena Clear Pore.
Oxy Oil-Free Maximum Strength Acne
Wash.
PanOxyl.
PanOxyl AQ.
Persadox.
Persadox HP.
Theroxide.
Triaz.
Zoderm.
W/Chlorhydroxyquinoline, hydrocorti-
sone.
See: Vanoxide-HC.
W/Clindamycin.
See: Duac.
W/Polyoxyethylene lauryl ether.
See: Benzac 5 & 10.
Desquam-X.
W/Sulfur.
See: Sulfoxyl.
benzoyl peroxide. (Various Mfr.) Ben-
zoyl peroxide. **Mask:** 5%. In 30 mL.
Lot: 5%, 10%. Bot. 30 mL. **Gel:** 2.5%,
5%, 10%. Tube 60 g, 90 g (except
2.5%). *Rx.*
Use: Keratolytic.
**benzoyl peroxide wash, 2.5%, 5%, &
10%.** (Various Mfr.) Benzoyl peroxide
2.5%, 5%, 10%. Liq. Bot. 118 mL
(5% only) 148 mL (except 2.5%),
237 mL. *Rx.*
Use: Keratolytic.
n'-benzoylsulfanilamide.
See: Sulfabenzamide.
W/Sulfacetamide, sulfathiazole, urea.
See: Sultrin.
benzphetamine hydrochloride. (benz-
FET-uh-meen)
Use: CNS stimulant, anorexiant.
See: Didrex.
• **benzquinamide.** (benz-KWIN-ah-mid)
USAN.
Use: Antiemetic.
benztropine mesylate. (BENZ-troe-
peen) *USP 28.*
Use: Parasympatholytic, antiparkinso-
nian.
W/Sodium Cl.
See: Cogentin.

benztropine mesylate. (Various Mfr.)
Benztropine mesylate 0.5 mg, 1 mg,
2 mg. Tab. 100s, 1000s (except
0.5 mg), UD 100s. *Rx.*
Use: Antiparkinson agent, anticholinergic.

benztropine methanesulfonate.
See: Benztropine mesylate.

•**benzydamine hydrochloride.** (ben-ZIH-
dah-meen) USAN.
Use: Analgesic; anti-inflammatory; antipyretic.

benzydroflumethiazide.
See: Bendroflumethiazide.

•**benzyl alcohol.** (BEN-zil) *NF 23.* Phenyl-
carbinol.
Use: Anesthetic; antiseptic, topical;
pharmaceutic aid, antimicrobial.
See: Topic.
Vicks Blue Mint, Regular, & Wild
Cherry Medicated Cough.

•**benzyl benzoate.** *USP 28.*
Use: Pharmaceutical necessity for
Dimercaprol Inj.

benzyl benzoate saponated. Triethanolamine 20 g, oleic acid 80 g, benzyl benzoate q.s. 1000 mL.

benzyl carbinol.
See: Phenylethyl alcohol.

**benzylpenicillin, benzylpenicilloic,
benzylpenilloic acid.** (Kremers Urban)
Use: Assessment of penicillin sensitivity. [Orphan Drug]
See: Pre-Pen/MDM.

benzyl penicillin-C-14. (Nuclear-Chi-
cago) Carbon-14 labelled penicillin.
Vacuum-sealed glass vial 50 microcu-
ries, 0.5 millicuries.
Use: Radiopharmaceutical.

benzyl penicillin G, potassium.
See: Penicillin G potassium.

benzyl penicillin G, sodium.
See: Penicillin G sodium.

•**benzylpenicilloyl polylysine concentrate.** *USP 28.*
Use: Diagnostic aid, penicillin sensitivity.
See: Pre-Pen.

bepanthen.
See: Panthenol.

bephedin. Benzyl ephedrine.

bephenium hydroxynaphthoate.
Use: Anthelmintic, hookworms.

•**beractant.** (ber-ACT-ant) USAN.
Use: Lung surfactant. [Orphan Drug]
See: Survanta.

beractant intrathecal suspension.
Use: Lung surfactant. [Orphan Drug]
See: Survanta.

•**beraprost.** (BEH-reh-prahst) USAN.
Use: Platelet aggregation inhibitor, improves ischemic syndromes.

•**beraprost sodium.** (BEH-reh-prahst)
USAN.
Use: Platelet aggregation inhibitor, im-
proves ischemic action.

berberine.
W/Hydrastine, glycerin.
See: Murine.

berberine hydrochloride.
W/Borax, sodium Cl, boric acid, camphor
water, cherry laurel water, rose water,
thimerosal.
See: Lauro.

•**berefrine.** (BEH-reh-FREEN) USAN. *Formerly* Burefrine.
Use: Mydriatic.

Ber-Ex. (Dolcin) Calcium succinate 2.8 g,
acetyl salicylic acid 3.7 g. Tab. Bot.
100s, 500s. *OTC.*
Use: Antiarthritic; antirheumatic.

Berinert P. (Aventis Behring) C1-Ester-
ase-inhibitor, human, pasteurized.
Use: Hereditary angioedema. [Orphan
Drug]

Berocca Plus. (Roche) Vitamins A
5000 units, E 30 units, C 500 mg, B₁
20 mg, B₂ 20 mg, B₃. Tab. Bot. 100s.
Rx.
Use: Iron, vitamin supplement.

•**berythromycin.** (beh-RITH-row-MY-sin)
USAN.
Use: Antiamebic; anti-infective.

Beserol. (Sanofi-Synthelabo) Acetaminophen, chlormezanone. Tab. *Rx.*
Use: Analgesic; tranquilizer; muscle relaxant.

•**besipirdine hydrochloride.** (beh-SIH-
pihr-deen) USAN.
Use: Cognition enhancer; Alzheimer
disease.

•**besonprodil.** (be-son-PROE-dil) USAN.
Use: Parkinson disease.

Besta. (Roberts) Vitamins B₁ 20 mg, B₂
15 mg, niacinamide 100 mg, calcium
pantothenate 20 mg, E 50 units, magnesium sulfate 70 mg, zinc 18.4 mg, B₁₂
4 mcg, B₆ 25 mg, C 300 mg. Cap. Bot.
100s. *OTC.*
Use: Vitamin, mineral supplement.

Best C. (Roberts) Ascorbic acid 500 mg.
TR Cap. Bot. 100s. *OTC.*
Use: Vitamin supplement.

Bestrone. (Bluco) Estrone in aqueous
susp. 2 mg/mL, 5 mg/mL. Inj. Vial
10 mL. *Rx.*
Use: Hormone, estrogen.

beta-adrenergic blockers, ophthalmic.
See: AKBeta.
Betagan Liquifilm.

Betaxolol hydrochloride.
Betimol.
Betoptic.
Betoptic S.
Carteolol hydrochloride.
Levobunolol.
Levobunolol hydrochloride.
Metipranolol hydrochloride.
Ocupress.
OptiPranolol.
Timolol.
Timolol Maleate.
Timoptic.
Timoptic in Ocudose.
Timoptic-XE.
beta-adrenergic blocking agents.
See: Acebutolol Hydrochloride.
Atenolol.
Betaxolol Hydrochloride.
Bisoprolol Fumarate.
Carteolol Hydrochloride.
Esmolol Hydrochloride.
Metoprolol.
Nadolol.
Penbutolol Sulfate.
Pindolol.
Propranolol Hydrochloride.
Sotalol Hydrochloride.
Timolol Maleate.
beta alethine.
Use: Antineoplastic. [Orphan Drug]
See: Betathine.
●**beta carotene.** (BAY-tah CARE-oh-teen)
USP 28.
Use: Ultraviolet screen.
beta carotene. (Various Mfr.) Beta caro-
tene 15 mg (vitamin A 25,000 units).
Softgel cap. Bot. 60s, 100s. *OTC.*
Use: Vitamin supplement.
●**beta cyclodextrin.** (BAY-tah sigh-kloe-
DEX-trin) *NF 23.*
See: Betadex.
●**betadex.** (BAY-tah-dex) *USAN. Formerly
beta cyclodextrin.*
Use: Pharmaceutical aid.
Betadine. (Purdue) Povidone-iodine.
Available as: Aerosol Spray, Bot. 3 oz.
Antiseptic Gz. Pads 3" × 9". Box 12s.
Antiseptic Lubricating Gel, Tube 5 g.
Disposable Medicated Douche, concen-
trated packette w/cannula and 6 oz wa-
ter. Douche, Bot. 1 oz, 4 oz, 8 oz.
Douche Packette, 0.5 oz (6 per carton).
Helafoam Solution Canister 250 g.
Mouthwash/Gargle, Bot. 6 oz. Oint.
Tube 1 oz. Jar 1 lb, 5 lb. Oint., Pack-
ette. Perineal Wash Conc. Kit, Bot. 8 oz
w/dispenser. Skin Cleanser, Bot. 1 oz,
4 oz. Skin Cleanser Foam, Canister
6 oz. Solution, 0.5 oz, 8 oz, 16 oz,

32 oz, gal. Solution Packette, oz. Solution Swab Aid, 100s. Solution Swabsticks, 1s Box 200s; 3s Box 50s. Surgical Scrub, Bot. Pt w/dispenser, qt, gal,
packette 0.5 oz. Surgi-prep Sponge-
Brush 36s. Vaginal Suppositories, Box
7s w/vaginal applicator. Viscous Formula Antiseptic Gauze Pads: 3" × 9",
5" × 9". Box 12s. Whirlpool Concentrate, Bot. Gal. *OTC.*
Use: Antiseptic.
Betadine Antiseptic. (Purdue) Povidone-
iodine 10%. Vaginal gel. 18 g with applicator. *OTC.*
Use: Vaginal agent.
Betadine Cream. (Purdue) Povidone-
iodine 5% mineral oil, polyoxyethylene
stearate, polysorbate, sorbitan mono-
stearate, white petrolatum. Cream.
Tube 14 g. *OTC.*
Use: Antimicrobial; antiseptic.
**Betadine First Aid Antibiotics Plus
Moisturizer.** (Purdue) Polymyxin B sul-
fate 10,000 units/g, bacitracin zinc
500 units/g. Cholesterolized ointment
base. Tube 14 g. *OTC.*
Use: Anti-infective, topical.
**Betadine 5% Sterile Ophthalmic Prep
Solution.** (Alcon) Povidone-iodine 5%.
Soln. Bot. 50 mL. *Rx.*
Use: Antiseptic, ophthalmic.
**Betadine Medicated Disposable
Douche.** (Purdue) Povidone-iodine
10%. Soln (0.3% when diluted). Vial
5.4 mL with 180 mL bot. Sanitized wa-
ter. 1 and 2 packs. *OTC.*
Use: Vaginal agent.
Betadine Medicated Douche. (Purdue)
Povidone-iodine 10% (0.3% when di-
luted). Soln. in 15 mL (6s) packettes
and 240 mL. *OTC.*
Use: Vaginal agent.
**Betadine Medicated Premixed Dispos-
able Douche.** (Purdue) Povidone-
iodine 10%. Soln. (0.3% when diluted).
Bot. 180 mL. 1s, 2s. *OTC.*
Use: Vaginal agent.
**Betadine Medicated Vaginal Gel and
Suppositories.** (Purdue) **Gel:** Povi-
done-iodine 10%. Tube 18 g, 85 g
w/applicator. **Supp:** Povidone-iodine
10%. In 7s w/applicator. *OTC.*
Use: Vaginal agent.
**Betadine Plus First Antibiotics and
Pain Reliever.** (Purdue) Polymyxin B
sulfate 10,000 units/g, bacitracin zinc
500 units/g, pramoxine 10 mg/g. Cho-
lesterolized ointment base. Tube 14 g.
OTC.
Use: Anti-infective, topical.

Betadine PrepStick. (Purdue) Povidone-iodine 10%. Soln. Prep Swab. Box 150s, 600s. *OTC.*
Use: Anti-infective, topical.

Betadine PrepStick Plus. (Purdue) Povidone-iodine 10%, alcohol. Soln. Prep Swab. Box 150s, 600s. *OTC.*
Use: Anti-infective, topical.

Betadine Shampoo. (Purdue) Povidone-iodine 7.5%. Shampoo. Bot. 118 mL. *OTC.*
Use: Antiseborrheic.

beta-estradiol.
See: Estradiol.

beta eucaine hydrochloride. Name previously used for Eucaine hydrochloride.

Betagan Liquifilm. (Allergan) Levobunolol hydrochloride 0.25%, 0.5%. Liquifilm. Bot. 2 mL (0.5%), 5 mL, 10 mL, 15 mL (0.5%) w/B.I.D. C Cap and Q.D. C Cap (0.5%). *Rx.*
Use: Antiglaucoma, beta-adrenergic blocker.

Betagen. (Enzyme Process) Vitamins B_1 1 mg, B_2 1.2 mg, niacin 15 mg, B_6 18 mg, pantothenic acid 18 mg, choline 1.8 g, betaine 96 mg. 6 Tab. Bot. 100s, 250s. *OTC.*
Use: Mineral, vitamin supplement.

Betagen Ointment. (Ivax) Povidone-iodine. Oint. Tube oz. Jar lb. *OTC.*
Use: Antiseptic.

Betagen Solution. (Ivax) Povidone-iodine. Soln. Bot. Pt, gal. *OTC.*
Use: Antiseptic.

Betagen Surgical Scrub. (Ivax) Povidone-iodine. Bot. Pt, gal. *OTC.*
Use: Antiseptic.

•**betahistine hydrochloride.** (BEE-tah-HISS-teen) USAN.
Use: Vasodilator, Meniere disease; diamine oxidase inhibitor, increase microcirculation.

beta-hypophamine.
See: Vasopressin.

betaine anhydrous. (Orphan Medical)
Use: Treatment of homocystinuria.
[Orphan Drug]
See: Cystadane.

•**betaine hydrochloride.** (BEE-tane)
USP 28. Acidol hydrochloride, lycine hydrochloride.
Use: Replenisher adjunct, electrolytes.
W/Ferrous fumarate, docusate sodium, desiccated liver, vitamins, minerals.
See: Hemaferrin.

Betalin S. (Eli Lilly) Thiamine hydrochloride 50 mg, 100 mg. Tab. Bot. 100s. *OTC.*
Use: Vitamin supplement.

•**betamethasone.** (BAY-tuh-METH-uh-zone) *USP 28.*
Use: Adrenocortical steroid, glucocorticoid.
See: Celestone.

•**betamethasone acetate.** *USP 28.*
Use: Corticosteroid, topical.

•**betamethasone dipropionate.** *USP 28.*
Use: Corticosteroid, topical.
See: Diprolene.
Diprosone.
Psorion.

betamethasone dipropionate and clotrimazole.
See: Clotrimazole and betamethasone diproprionate.

betamethasone dipropionate, augmented. (Various Mfr.) Betamethasone (augmented). **Cream:** 0.05%, propylene glycol, sorbitol solution, white petrolatum. 15 g, 50 g. **Gel:** 0.05%, propylene glycol. 15 g, 50 g. *Rx.*
Use: Anti-inflammatory.

•**betamethasone sodium phosphate.**
USP 28.
Use: Adrenocortical steroid, glucocorticoid.
See: Celestone Phosphate.

betamethasone sodium phosphate and betamethasone acetate.
Use: Adrenocortical steroid, glucocorticoid.
See: Celestone Soluspan.

•**betamethasone valerate.** *USP 28.*
Use: Corticosteroid, topical.
See: Beta-Val.
Luxiq.
Valisone.
Valnac.

•**betamicin sulfate.** (bay-tah-MY-sin) USAN.
Use: Anti-infective.

betanaphthol. 2-Naphthol.
Use: Parasiticide.

Betapace. (Berlex) Sotalol hydrochloride 80 mg, 120 mg, 160 mg, 240 mg, lactose. Tab. Bot. 100s, UD 100s. *Rx.*
Use: Antiadrenergic/sympatholytic, beta-adrenergic blocker.

Betapace AF. (Berlex) Sotalol hydrochloride 80 mg, 120 mg, 160 mg, lactose. Tab. UD 60s, 100s. *Rx.*
Use: Antiadrenergic/sympatholytic, beta-adrenergic blocker.

Betapen-VK. (Bristol-Myers Squibb) Penicillin V potassium. **Oral Soln.:** 125 mg/mL, 250 mg/5 mL Bot. 100 mL, 200 mL (250 mg/5mL only). **Tab.:** 250 mg, 500 mg. Tab. Bot. 100s, 1000s (250 mg only). *Rx.*

Use: Anti-infective, penicillin.

beta-phenyl-ethyl-hydrazine. Phenelzine dihydrogen sulfate.
See: Nardil.

beta-pyridyl-carbinol. Nicotinyl alcohol. Alcohol corresponding to nicotinic acid.

BetaRx. (VivoRx, Inc.) Encapsulated porcine islet preparation.
Use: Type I diabetic patients already on immunosuppression. [Orphan Drug]

Betasept. (Purdue) Chlorhexidine gluconate 4%, isopropyl 4%, alcohol. Liq. Bot. 946 mL. *OTC.*
Use: Dermatologic.

Betaseron. (Berlex) Interferon beta-1b 0.3 mg, albumin human 15 mg, mannitol 15 mg, preservative free. Pow. for Inj. lyophilized, single-use vial (capacity 3 mL) w/1.2 mL prefilled syringe of diluent (sodium chloride 0.54%), alcohol prep pads, and vial adaptor with attached needle for each drug vial. Blister units. 15s. *Rx.*
Use: Immunologic agent, immunomodulator.

Betathine. (Dovetail Technologies, Inc.) Beta alethine.
Use: Antineoplastic. [Orphan Drug]

Beta-2. (Nephron) Isoetharine hydrochloride 1% with glycerin, sodium bisulfite, parabens. Liq. Bot. 10 mL, 30 mL. *Rx.*
Use: Respiratory product.

Beta-Val. (Teva) Betamethasone valerate equivalent to 0.1% betamethasone base in cream base. Cream. Tube 15 g, 45 g. *Rx.*
Use: Corticosteroid, topical.

• **betaxolol hydrochloride.** (BAY-TAX-oh-lahl) *USP 28.*
Use: Antiadrenergic/sympatholytic, beta-adrenergic blocking agent.
See: Betoptic.
Betoptic S.
Kerlone.

betaxolol hydrochloride. (Various Mfr.) Betaxolol hydrochloride 5.6 mg (equiv. to 5 mg base)/mL (0.5%). Ophth. Soln. Bot. 2.5 mL, 5 mL, 10 mL, 15 mL. *Rx.*
Use: Antiglaucoma, beta-adrenergic blocker.

betaxolol ophthalmic solution.
Use: Beta-adrenergic blocker.

Betaxon. (Alcon) Levobetaxolol hydrochloride 5.6 mg/mL, benzalkonium chloride 0.01%, EDTA, hydrochloric acid, boric acid. Ophth. Susp. *Drop-Tainers* 5 mL, 10 mL, 15 mL. *Rx.*
Use: Antiglaucoma, beta-adrenergic blocker.

• **bethanechol chloride.** (beth-AN-ih-kole) *USP 28.*
Use: Cholinergic.
See: Myotonachol.
Urabeth.
Urecholine.

bethanechol chloride. (Various Mfr.) Bethanechol chloride 5 mg, 10 mg, 25 mg, 50 mg. Tab. Bot. 100s, 250s (10 mg, 25 mg only), 500s (50 mg only), 1000s, UD 100s. *Rx.*
Use: Urinary cholinergic.

bethanidine.
Use: Hypotensive.

• **bethanidine sulfate.** (beth-AN-ih-deen) *USAN.*
Use: Antihypertensive.

Bethaprim. (Major) Trimethoprim 40 mg, sulfamethoxazole 200 mg/5 mL, alcohol 0.26%, saccharin, sorbitol. Susp. *Rx.*
Use: Anti-infective.

Bethaprim DS Tabs. (Major) Trimethoprim 160 mg, sulfamethoxazole 800 mg. Tab. Bot. 100s, 500s, UD 100s. *Rx.*
Use: Anti-infective.

Bethaprim SS Tabs. (Major) Trimethoprim 80 mg, sulfamethoxazole 400 mg. Tab. Bot. 100s, 500s. *Rx.*
Use: Anti-infective.

• **betiatide.** (BEH-tie-ah-tide) *USAN.*
Use: Pharmaceutic aid.

Betimol. (Novartis Ophthalmics) Timolol maleate (as hemihydrate) 0.25%, 0.5%, benzalkonium Cl 0.01%, monosodium and disodium phosphate dihydrate. Soln. Bot. 2.5 mL, 5 mL, 10 mL, 15 mL. *Rx.*
Use: Antiglaucoma, beta-adrenergic blocker.

Betoptic. (Alcon) Betaxolol hydrochloride 5.6 mg (equiv. to 5 mg base) per mL (0.5%), benzalkonium chloride 0.01%, sodium chloride, hydrochloric acid and/or sodium hydroxide, EDTA. Soln. *Drop-Tainer* dispenser 2.5 mL, 5 mL, 10 mL, 15 mL. *Rx.*
Use: Antiglaucoma, beta-adrenergic blocker.

Betoptic S. (Alcon) Betaxolol hydrochloride 2.8 mg (equiv. to 2.5 mg base) per mL (0.25%), benzalkonium chloride 0.01%, mannitol, polysulfonic acid, hydrochloric acid or sodium hydroxide, EDTA. Susp. *Drop-Tainer* dispenser 2.5 mL, 5 mL, 10 mL, 15 mL. *Rx.*
Use: Antiglaucoma, beta-adrenergic blocker.

●**bevacizumab.** (beh-vuh-SIZ-uh-mab) USAN.
Use: Antiangiogenic; monoclonal antibody.
See: Avastin.

●**bevantolol hydrochloride.** (beh-VAN-toe-LOLE) USAN.
Use: Antianginal; antihypertensive; cardiac depressant, antiarrhythmic.

●**bexarotene.** (bex-AIR-oh-teen) USAN.
Use: Antineoplastic; antidiabetic; rexinoid.
See: Targretin.

●**bexlosteride.** (bex-LOW-ster-ide) USAN.
Use: Prostate cancer.

Bexomal-C. (Roberts) Vitamins B_1 6 mg, B_2 7 mg, B_3 80 mg, B_5 10 mg, B_6 5 mg, B_{12} 6 mcg, C 250 mg. Tab. Bot. 50s. *OTC.*
Use: Vitamin supplement.

Bexxar Dosimetric Packaging. (Corixa/GlaxoSmithKline) **Nonradioactive Component:** Tositumomab 14 mg/mL. Maltose (w/v) 10%. Preservative-free. Inj. Single-use vials 35 mg, 225 mg. **Radioactive Component:** Iodine ^{131}I-tositumomab 0.1 mg/mL (0.61 mCi/mL at calibration). Preservative-free. Inj. Single-use vials (contains povidone 5% to 6%, maltose 1 to 2 mg/mL, sodium chloride 0.85 to 0.95 mg/mL, ascorbic acid 0.9 to 1.3 mg/mL). *Rx.*
Use: Monoclonal antibody.

Bexxar Therapeutic Packaging. (Corixa/GlaxoSmithKline) **Nonradioactive Component:** Tositumomab 14 mg/mL. Maltose (w/v) 10%. Preservative-free. Inj. Single-use vials 35 mg, 225 mg. **Radioactive Component:** Iodine ^{131}I-tositumomab 1.1 mg/mL (5.6 mCi/mL at calibration). Preservative-free. Inj. Single-use vials (contains povidone 5% to 6%, maltose 9 to 15 mg/mL, sodium chloride 0.85 to 0.95 mg/mL, ascorbic acid 0.9 to 1.3 mg/mL). *Rx.*
Use: Monoclonal antibody.

●**bezafibrate.** (BEH-zah-FIE-brate) USAN.
Use: Antihyperlipoproteinemic.

Bezon. (Whittier) Vitamins B_1 5 mg, B_2 3 mg, niacinamide 20 mg, pantothenic acid 3 mg, B_6 0.5 mg, C 50 mg, B_{12} 1 mcg. Cap. Bot. 30s, 100s. *OTC.*
Use: Vitamin supplement.

Bezon Forte. (Whittier) Vitamins B_1 25 mg, B_2 12.5 mg, niacinamide 50 mg, pantothenic acid 10 mg, B_6 5 mg, C 250 mg. Cap. Bot. 30s, 100s. *OTC.*
Use: Vitamin supplement.

B-F-I. (GlaxoSmithKline) Bismuth-formic-iodide, zinc phenolsulfonate, bismuth subgallate, amol, potassium alum, boric acid, menthol, eucalyptol, thymol, and inert diluents. Pow. Can. 0.25 oz, 1.25 oz, 8 oz. *OTC.*
Use: Antiseptic, topical.

B-50. (NBTY) Vitamins B_1 50 mg, B_2 50 mg, B_3 50 mg, B_5 50 mg, B_6 50 mg, B_{12} 50 mcg, folic acid 0.1 mg, d-biotin 50 mcg, PABA, choline bitartrate, inositol. Tab. Bot. 50s, 100s. *OTC.*
Use: Mineral, vitamin supplement.

B-50 Time Release. (NBTY) Vitamins B_1 50 mg, B_2 50 mg, B_3 50 mg, B_5 50 mg, B_6 50 mg, B_{12} 50 mcg, folic acid 0.1 mg, d-biotin 50 mcg, PABA 50 mg, choline bitartrate 50 mg, inositol 50 mg, lecithin. Tab. Bot. 100s. *OTC.*
Use: Mineral, vitamin supplement.

B.G.O. (Calotabs) Iodoform, salicylic acid, sulfur, zinc oxide, phenol (liquefied) 1%, calamine, menthol, petrolatum, lanolin, mineral oil, undecylenic acid 1%. Jar 7/8 oz, Tube 1 oz. *OTC.*
Use: Antifungal, topical; antiseptic.

●**bialamicol hydrochloride.** (bye-AH-lam-IH-KAHL) USAN.
Use: Antiamebic.

●**biapenem.** (bye-ah-PEN-en) USAN.
Use: Anti-infective.

biaphasic insulin. A suspension of insulin crystals in a solution of insulin buffered at pH 7. Insulin Novo Rapitard. Inj.

Biavax II. (Merck & Co.) Rubella and mumps virus vaccine, live. See details under *Meruvax-II* and *Mumpsvax.* Single-dose vial w/diluent. Pkg. 1s, 10s. *Rx.*
Use: Immunization.

Biaxin. (Abbott) Clarithromycin 250 mg, 500 mg. Tab. Bot. 60s, *ABBO-PAC* UD 100s. Clarithromycin 125 mg/5 mL, 250 mg/5 mL. Sucrose, fruit punch flavor. Gran. for Oral Susp. Bot. 50 mL, 100 mL. *Rx.*
Use: Anti-infective, erythromycin, macrolide.

Biaxin XL. (Abbott) Clarithromycin 500 mg, lactose. ER Tab. Bot. 60s, *BIAXIN XL PAC* blister pack 4 × 14s. *Rx.*
Use: Anti-infective, macrolide.

●**bibapcitide.** (bib-APP-sih-tide) USAN.
Use: Radionuclide carrier; detection and localization of deep vein thrombosis.

●**bicalutamide.** (bye-kah-LOO-tah-mide) USAN.
Use: Antineoplastic; antiandrogen.
See: Casodex.

- **bicifadine hydrochloride.** (bye-SIGH-fah-deen) USAN.
  Use: Analgesic.
- **Bicillin C-R.** (Monarch) **600,000 units/dose:** Penicillin G benzathine 300,000 units, penicillin G procaine 300,000 units. *Tubex* 1 mL.
  1,200,000 units/dose: Penicillin G benzathine 600,000, penicillin G procaine 600,000. *Tubex* 2 mL.
  2,400,000 units/dose: Penicillin G benzathine 1,200,000 penicillin G procaine 1,200,000. Syr. 4 mL. Parabens, lechithin, povidone. Inj. *Rx.*
  Use: Anti-infective.
- **Bicillin C-R 900/300.** (Monarch) 1,200,000 units/dose (penicillin G benzathine 900,000, penicillin G procaine 300,000). parabens, lecithin, povidone. *Tubex* 2 mL. *Rx.*
  Use: Anti-infective.
- **Bicillin L-A.** (Monarch) Penicillin G benzathine 600,000 units/dose, 1,200,000 units/dose, 2,400,000 units/dose, povidone, parabens. Inj. *Tubex* 1 mL (600,000 only), 2 mL (1,200,000 only); Prefilled syringes 4 mL (2,400,000 only). *Rx.*
  Use: Anti-infective.
- **biciromab.** (bye-SIH-rah-mab) USAN.
  Use: Monoclonal antibody, antifibrin.
- **Bicitra.** (Alza) Sodium citrate dihydrate 500 mg, citric acid monohydrate 334 mg, 5 mEq sodium ion/5 mL. Shohl's Solution. Bot. 4 oz, pt, gal. UD 15 mL, 30 mL. *Rx.*
  Use: Systemic alkalinizer.
- **biclodil hydrochloride.** (BYE-kloe-DILL) USAN.
  Use: Antihypertensive, vasodilator.
- **BiCNU.** (Bristol Labs Oncology) Carmustine (BCNU) 100 mg, sterile diluent 3 mL. Pow. for Inj., lyophilized. Preservative free. Single-dose vial. *Rx.*
  Use: Antineoplastic, alkylating agent.
- **Bicozene.** (Novartis) Benzocaine 6%, resorcinol 1.66% in cream base. Cream. Tube 30 g. *OTC.*
  Use: Anesthetic, topical.
- **Bicycline.** (Knight) Tetracycline hydrochloride 250 mg. Cap. Bot. 100s.
  Use: Anti-infective.
- **Bidhist.** (PharmaFab) Brompheniramine maleate 6 mg. ER Tab. 100s. *Rx.*
  Use: Antihistamine.
- **bidisomide.** (bye-DIH-so-mide) USAN.
  Use: Cardiovascular agent, antiarrhythmic.
- **bifonazole.** (BYE-FONE-ah-zole) USAN.
  Use: Antifungal.

Big Shot B-12. (Naturally) Cyanocobalamin (vitamin B_{12}) 5000 mcg. Tab. Bot. 30s, 60s. *OTC.*
  Use: Vitamin supplement.
biguanides.
  Use: Antidiabetic agent.
  See: Metformin Hydrochloride.
bile acids, oxidized. Note also dehydrocholic acid.
  W/Atropine methyl nitrate, ox and hog bile extract, phenobarbital.
  See: G.B.S.
  W/Bile whole (desiccated), desiccated whole pancreas, homatropine methylbromide.
  See: Pancobile.
bile acid sequestrants.
  See: Cholestyramine.
  Cholestyramine Light.
  Colesevelam Hydrochloride.
  Colestid.
  Colestipol hydrochloride.
  LoCHOLEST.
  LoCHOLEST Light.
  Prevalite.
  Questran.
  Questran Light.
  Welchol.
bile extract. (Various Mfr.) Bile extract. Pow. 0.25 lb, 1 lb.
  W/Cascara sagrada, dandelion root, podophyllin, nux vomica.
  See: Neocholan.
bile extract, ox. Purified ox gall. (Eli Lilly) Enseal 5 g, Bot. 100s, 500s, 1000s. (C.D. Smith) Tab. 5 g, Bot. 1000s. (Stoddard) Tab. 3 g, Bot. 100s, 500s, 1000s.
  W/Cellulase, pepsin, glutamic acid hydrochloride, pancreatin.
  See: Kanumodic.
  W/Dehydrocholic acid, homatropine methylbromide, phenobarbital.
  See: Bilamide.
  W/Dehydrocholic acid, pepsin, homatropine methylbromide.
  See: Biloric.
  W/Desoxycholic acid, oxidized bile acids, pancreatin.
  See: Bilogen.
  W/Enzyme concentrate, pepsin, dehydrocholic acid, belladonna extract.
  See: Konzyme.
bilein. Bile salts obtained from ox bile.
bile-like products. Bile products.
  See: Bile salts.
  Dehydrocholic acid.
bile salts. Sodium glycocholate and taurocholate. Note also Bile extract, ox, and oxidized bile acids. (Eli Lilly) Enseal 5 g. Bot. 100s.

See: Bilein.
Bisol.
Bile extract, ox.
Bile acids, oxidized.
W/Cascara sagrada, phenolphthalein, capsicum oleoresin, peppermint oil.
See: Torocol.
W/Cellulase, calcium carbonate, pancrelipase.
See: Progestive.
W/Pancrelipase, cellulase.
See: Torocol Compound.
W/Pepsin, homatropine, methylbromide, amylase, lipase, protease.
See: Bile Anthus Compound.
bile salts and belladonna. Belladonna, nux vomica compound bile salts 60 mg, belladonna leaf extract 5 mg, nux vomica extract 2 mg, phenolphthalein 30 mg, sodium salicylate 15 mg, aloin 15 mg. Tab. Bot. 1000s.
Use: Laxative; antispasmodic.
bile, whole desiccated.
W/Pancreatin, mycozyme diastase, pepsin, nux vomica extract.
See: Enzobile.
Bili-Labstix Reagent Strips. (Bayer Corp. (Consumer Div.)) Reagent strips. Test for pH, protein, glucose, ketones, bilirubin, and blood in urine. Bot. 100s.
Use: Diagnostic aid.
Bili-Labstix SG Reagent Strips. (Bayer Corp. (Consumer Div.)) Urinalysis reagent strip test for specific gravity, pH, protein, glucose, ketone, bilirubin, and blood. Bot. 100s.
Use: Diagnostic aid.
Bilirubin Reagent Strips. (Bayer Corp. (Consumer Div.)) Seralyzer reagent strip. Quantitative strip test for total bilirubin serum or plasma. Bot. 25s.
Use: Diagnostic aid.
Bilirubin Test.
See: Ictotest.
Bilivist. (Berlex) Ipodate sodium 500 mg. Cap. Bot. 120s. *Rx.*
Use: Radiopaque agent.
Biloric. (Arcum) Pepsin 9 mg, ox bile 160 mg. Cap. Bot. 100s, 1000s. *OTC.*
Use: Antispasmodic.
Bilstan. (Standex) Bile salts 0.5 g, cascara sagrada powder extract 0.5 g, phenolphthalein 0.5 g, aloin ⅛ g, podophyllin g. Tab. Bot. 100s. *OTC.*
Use: Laxative.
Biltricide. (Bayer Corp. (Consumer Div.)) Praziquantel 600 mg. Tab. Bot. 6s. *Rx.*
Use: Anthelmintic.
● **bimatoprost.** (bi-MA-toe-prost) USAN.
Use: Antiglaucoma; prostaglandin agonist.

See: Lumigan.
● **bimosiamose disodium.** (bye-moh-SYE-a-mose) USAN.
Use: Anti-inflammatory agent.
● **bindarit.** (BIN-dah-rit) USAN.
Use: Antirheumatic.
● **binetrakin.** (bih-NEH-trah-kin) USAN.
Use: Gastrointestinal carcinoma; rheumatoid arthritis; dendritic cell activation; immunomodulatory.
● **biniramycin.** (bih-NEER-ah-MY-sin) USAN.
Use: Anti-infective.
● **binodenoson.** (bi-NOE-den-oh-son) USAN.
Use: Vasodilator.
● **binospirone mesylate.** (bih-NO-spy-rone) USAN.
Use: Anxiolytic.
Bintron. (Madland) Liver fraction 4.6 g, ferrous sulfate 5 g, vitamins B_1 3 mg, B_2 0.5 mg, B_6 0.15 mg, C 20 mg, calcium pantothenate 0.3 mg, niacinamide 10 mg. Tab. Bot. 100s, 1000s. *OTC.*
Use: Mineral, vitamin supplement.
Biobrane. (Sanofi-Synthelabo) Temporary skin substitute available in various sizes. *OTC.*
Use: Dermatologic.
Biocal 500. (Bayer Corp. (Consumer Div.)) Calcium 500 mg. Tab. Bot. 75s. *OTC.*
Use: Mineral supplement.
Biocal 250. (Bayer Corp. (Consumer Div.)) Calcium 250 mg. Chew. Tab. Bot. 75s. *OTC.*
Use: Calcium supplement.
Biocef. (International Ethical Labs) Cephalexin monohydrate 500 mg. Cap. Bot. 100s. Cephalexin monohydrate 125 mg/mL, 250 mg/mL. Pow. for susp. Bot. 100 mL. *Rx.*
Use: Anti-infective, cephalosporin.
Bioclate. (Aventis) Concentrated recombinant antihemophilic factor. After reconstitution, also contains albumin (human) 12.5 mg/mL, PEG 3350 1.5 mg/mL, sodium 180 mEq/L, histidine 55 mM, calcium 0.2 mg/mL, preservative free. Monoclonal purified. Pow. for Inj., lyophilized. Bot. 250, 500, 1,000 IU per single-dose bottle with diluent, double-ended needle, and filter needle. *Rx.*
Use: Antihemophilic agent.
Biocult-GC. (Orion) Swab test for gonorrhea. For endocervical, urethral, rectal, and pharyngeal cultures. Box 1 test per kit.
Use: Diagnostic aid.

biodegradable polymer implant containing carmustine.
Use: Antineoplastic. [Orphan Drug]
See: Biodel Implant/BCNU.
Biodel Implant/BCNU. (Scios Nova) Biodegradable polymer implant containing carmustine. *Rx.*
Use: Antineoplastic.
Biodine. (Major) Iodine 1%. Soln. Bot. Pt, gal. *OTC.*
Use: Antimicrobial; antiseptic.
bio-flavonoid compounds.
See: Amino-Opti-C.
  C Factors "1000" Plus.
  Ester-C Plus 500 mg Vitamin C.
  Ester-C Plus Multi-Mineral.
  Ester-C Plus 1000 mg Vitamin C.
  Flavons.
  Flavons-500
  Pan-C Ascorbate.
  Pan C-500.
  Peridin-C.
  Quercetin.
  Span C.
  Super Flavons.
  Super Flavons 300.
  Tri-Super Flavons 1000.
Biogastrone.
See: Carbenoxolone.
Biohist-LA. (IVAX) Chlorpheniramine maleate 12 mg, pseudoephedrine hydrochloride 120 mg. SR Tab. Bot. 100s. *Rx.*
Use: Upper respiratory combination, antihistamine, decongestant.
• **biological indicator for dry-heat sterilization, paper strip.** *USP 28.*
Use: Biological indicator, sterilization.
• **biological indicator for ethylene oxide sterilization, paper strip.** *USP 28.*
Use: Biological indicator, sterilization.
• **biological indicator for steam sterilization, paper strip.** *USP 28.*
Use: Biological indicator, sterilization.
• **biological indicator for steam sterilization, self-contained.** *USP 28.*
Use: Biological indicator, sterilization.
biological response modifiers.
See: Aldesleukin.
  BCG, Intravesical.
  Denileukin Diftitox.
  Levamisole Hydrochloride.
  Ontak.
  Pacis.
  TheraCys.
  TICE BCG.
Bionate 50-2. (Seatrace) Testosterone cypionate 50 mg, estradiol cypionate 2 mg/mL. Vial 10 mL. *Rx.*
Use: Androgen; estrogen combination.

Bion Tears. (Alcon) Dextran 70 0.1%, hydroxypropyl methylcellulose 2910 0.3%, NaCl, KCl, sodium bicarbonate. Preservative free. Soln. In single-use 0.45 mL containers (28s). *OTC.*
Use: Artificial tears.
Bioral.
See: Carbenoxolone.
Bio-Rescue. (Biomedical Frontiers) Dextran and deferoxamine.
Use: Acute iron poisoning. [Orphan Drug]
Bios I.
See: Inositol.
Biosynject. (Chembiomed, Inc.) Trisaccharides A and B.
Use: Hemolytic disease of the newborn. [Orphan Drug]
Bio-Tab. (International Ethical Labs) Doxycycline hyclate 100 mg. Tab. Bot. 50s, 100s, 500s. *Rx.*
Use: Anti-infective, tetracycline.
Biotel Diabetes. (Biotel Corp.) In vitro diagnostic test for diabetes and other metabolic disorders by screening for glucose in the urine. Test kit 12s.
Use: Diagnostic aid.
Biotel Kidney. (Biotel Corp.) In vitro diagnostic test for early detection of diseases of the kidneys, bladder, and urinary tract by screening for hemoglobin, red blood cells, and albumin in the urine. Test kit 12s.
Use: Diagnostic aid.
Biotel U.T.I. (Biotel Corp.) In vitro diagnostic home test to detect urinary tract infections by screening fornitrate in urine. Test kit 12s.
Use: Diagnostic aid.
Biotexin.
See: Novobiocin.
Biothesin. (Pal-Pak, Inc.) Phosphorated carbohydrate solution ceriumoxalate 120 mg, bismuth subnitrate 120 mg, benzocaine 15 mg, aromatics. Tab. 1000s. *OTC.*
Use: Antiemetic; antivertigo.
Bio-Throid. (Bio-Tech) Thyroid desiccated 7.5 mg (⅛ g), 15 mg (¼ g), 30 mg (½ g), 60 mg (1 g), 90 mg (1½ g), 120 mg (2 g), 150 mg (2½ g), 180 mg (3 g), 240 mg (4 g). Cap. Bot. 100s, 1,000s. *Rx.*
Use: Hormone, thyroid.
Bio-Tytra. (Health for Life Brands) Neomycin sulfate 2.5 mg, gramicidin 0.25 mg, benzocaine 10 mg. Troche. Box 10s. *Rx.*
Use: Anti-infective.
• **bipenamol hydrochloride.** (bye-PEN-ah-MAHL) USAN.

Use: Antidepressant.

●**biperiden.** (by-PURR-ih-den) *USP 28.*
Use: Anticholinergic; antiparkinson.

●**biperiden hydrochloride.** (by-PURR-ih-den) *USP 28.*
Use: Anticholinergic; antiparkinson.

biperiden hydrochloride and lactate.
Use: Anticholinergic; antiparkinson.
See: Akineton.

●**biperiden lactate, injection.** (by-PURR-ih-den) *USP 28.*
Use: Anticholinergic; antiparkinsonian.

biphasic oral contraceptives.
See: Jenest-28.
Mircette.
Necon 10/11.
Nelova 10/11.
Ortho-Novum 10/11.

●**biphenamine hydrochloride.** (bye-FEN-ah-meen) USAN.
Use: Anesthetic, local; anti-infective; antimicrobial.

Bipole-S. (Spanner) Testosterone 25 mg, estrone 2 mg/mL. Inj. Vial. 10 mL. *Rx.*
Use: Androgen, estrogen combination.

●**biricodar dicitrate.** (BYE-rih-koe-dahr die-SIH-trate) USAN.
Use: Chemotherapy agent, multidrug resistance inhibitor.

Bisac-Evac. (G & W) Bisacodyl. **EC Tab.:** 5 mg. Bot. 25s. **Supp.:** 10 mg. Pkg. 8s, 12s, 50s, 100s, 500s, 1000s. *OTC.*
Use: Laxative.

bisacetoxphenyl oxindol.
See: Oxyphenisatin.

●**bisacodyl.** (BISS-uh-koe-dill) *USP 28.*
Use: Laxative.
See: Alophen.
Bisac-Evac.
Bisacodyl Uniserts.
Bisa-Lax.
Caroid.
Correctol.
Dacodyl.
Deficol.
Delco-Lax.
Dulcagen.
Dulcolax.
Feen-a-mint.
Fleet Laxative.
Modane.
Reliable Gentle Laxative.
Women's Gentle Laxative.

bisacodyl. (Various Mfr.) Bisacodyl.
EC Tab.: 5 mg. Bot. 25s, 50s, 100s, 1000s, UD 100s. **Supp.:** 10 mg. Pkg. 12s, 16s, 100s. *OTC.*
Use: Laxative.

●**bisacodyl tannex.** (BISS-uh-koe-dill) USAN.

Use: Laxative.

Bisacodyl Uniserts. (Upsher-Smith) Bisacodyl 10 mg. Supp. Pack. 12s. *OTC.*
Use: Laxative.

Bisalate. (Allison) Sodium salicylate 5 g, salicylamide 2.5 g, sodium paramino-benzoate 5 g, ascorbic acid 50 mg, butabarbital sodium ⅛ g. Tab. Bot. 100s, 1000s. *Rx.*
Use: Antirheumatic.

Bisa-Lax. (Bergen Brunswig) **Supp.:** Bisacodyl 10 mg. Hydrogenated vegetable oil. 50s. **EC Tab.:** Bisacodyl 5 mg. 25s, 50s. *OTC.*
Use: Laxative.

●**bisantrene hydrochloride.** (BISS-an-TREEN) USAN.
Use: Antineoplastic.

bisatin.
See: Oxyphenisatin.

bishydroxycoumarin.
See: Dicumarol.

Bismapec. (Pal-Pak, Inc.) Bismuth hydroxide 137.7 mg, colloidal kaolin 648 mg, citrus pectin 129.6 mg. Tab. Bot. 1000s. *OTC.*
Use: Antidiarrheal.

Bismu-Kino. (Denver Chemical (Puerto Rico) Inc.) Bismuth oxycarbonate 10 g, eucalyptus gum 6 g, phenyl salicylate, camphor, menthol, carminative oils of nutmeg, and clove in soothing, demulcent base w/alcohol 2%/fl oz. Bot. 4 oz, pt. *OTC.*
Use: Gastrointestinal.

●**bismuth aluminate.** (BISS-muth) USAN.
Aluminum bismuth oxide.

●**bismuth carbonate.** USAN.
Use: Protectant, topical.

●**bismuth citrate.** *USP 28.*

bismuth glycolylarsanilate.
Use: Antiamebic.
See: Glycobiarsol.

bismuth hydroxide.
See: Bismuth, milk of.

bismuth, insoluble products.
See: Bismuth subgallate.
Bismuth subsalicylate.
Bismuth tribromophenate.

bismuth, magma. Name previously used for Milk of Bismuth.

●**bismuth, milk of.** *USP 28. Formerly Bismuth Magma.*
Use: Astringent; antacid.

bismuth oxycarbonate.
See: Bismuth subcarbonate.

bismuth potassium tartrate. Basic bismuth potassium bismuthotartrate. (Brewer) 25 mg/mL. Amp. 2 mL.

(Miller Pharmacal Group) 0.016 g/mL.
Amp. 2 mL. Box 12s, 100s; Bot. 30 mL,
60 mL. (Raymer) 2.5%. Amp. 2 mL.
Box 12s, 100s. *Rx.*
Use: Agent for syphilis.
bismuth resorcin compound.
W/Bismuth subgallate, balsam Peru,
benzocaine, zinc oxide, boric acid.
See: Bonate.
W/Bismuth subgallate, balsam Peru, zinc
oxide, boric acid.
See: Versal.
bismuth sodium tartrate.
Use: I.M., syphilis.
bismuth subbenzoate.
Use: Dusting powder for wounds.
•**bismuth subcarbonate.** *USP 28.*
Use: Protectant, topical.
bismuth subcarbonate.
Use: Gastroenteritis, diarrhea.
W/Benzocaine, zinc oxide, boric acid.
See: Aracain.
W/Calcium carbonate, magnesium carbo-
nate, aminoacetic acid, dried aluminum
hydroxide gel.
See: Bufferlabs.
W/Charcoal and ginger.
See: Harv-a-carbe.
W/Ephedrine sulfate, belladonna extract,
zinc oxide, boric acid, bismuth oxyio-
dide, balsam Peru.
See: Wyanoids.
W/Hydrocortisone acetate, belladonna
extract, ophedrine sulfate, zinc oxide,
boric acid, balsam Peru, cocoa butter.
See: K-C.
W/Pectin, kaolin, opium powder.
See: Bismuth, salol, zinc compound.
W/Phenyl salicylate, chloroform, eucalyp-
tus gum, camphor.
See: Bismu-Kino.
•**bismuth subgallate.** *USP 28.* (Various
Mfr.) Dermatol.
Use: Topically for skin conditions; orally
as an antidiarrheal.
See: Devrom.
W/Benzocaine, resorcin, cod liver oil,
lanolin, zinc oxide.
See: Biscolan.
W/Benzocaine, zinc oxide, boric acid, bal-
sam Peru.
See: Bonate.
W/Bismuth resorcin compound, balsam
Peru, benzocaine, zinc oxide, boric
acid.
See: Bonate.
W/Bismuth resorcin compound, zinc ox-
ide, boric acid, balsam Peru.
See: Versal.
W/Cod liver oil, benzocaine, lanolin, zinc
oxide, resorcin, balsam Peru, hydro-
cortisone.

See: Anusol-HC.
W/Diethylaminoacet-2,6-xylidide, zinc ox-
ide, aluminum subacetate, balsam
Peru.
See: Xylocaine.
W/Kaolin, colloidal.
See: Diastop.
W/Kaolin colloidal, calcium carbonate,
magnesium trisilicate, papain, atropine
sulfate.
See: Kaocasil.
W/Kaolin, opium, zinc phenolsulfonate,
pectin.
See: Cholactabs.
W/Kaolin, pectin, zinc phenolsulfonate,
opium powder.
See: Diastay.
W/Opium powder, pectin, kaolin, zinc
phenolsulfonate.
See: Diamuth, Pectin, Paregoric.
W/Zinc oxide, bismuth resorcin com-
pound, balsam Peru, benzyl benzoate.
See: Anusol.
bismuth subiodide.
See: Bismuth oxyiodide.
•**bismuth subnitrate.** *USP 28.*
Use: Pharmaceutic necessity; gastroen-
teritis; amebic dysentery; locally for
wounds.
W/Calcium carbonate, magnesium carbo-
nate.
See: Antacid No. 2.
•**bismuth subsalicylate.** *USP 28.* Basic
bismuth salicylate. Agent for syphilis.
Used in combination with metronidazole
and tetracycline hydrochloride to treat
active duodenal ulcer associated with
H. pylori infection.
Use: Antidiarrheal; antacid; antiulcer-
ative.
See: Kaopectate.
Kaopectate Children's.
Kaopectate Extra Strength.
Kapectolin.
K-Pek.
Peptic Relief.
W/Calcium carbonate, glycocoll.
See: Pepto-Bismol.
W/Pectin, salol, kaolin, zinc sulfocarbo-
late, aluminum hydroxide.
See: Pepto-Bismol.
bismuth tannate. (Various Mfr.) Tan bis-
muth. *OTC.*
Use: Astringent and protective in GI dis-
orders.
bismuth tribromophenate.
Use: Intestinal antiseptic.
bismuth violet. (Table Rock) Bismuth
Violet. **Oint.:** 1%. Jar oz, lb. **Soln.:**
0.5%. Bot. 0.5 oz, 6 oz, pt, gal. **Tr.:**
0.5%. Bot. 6 oz, pt, also 1% w/benzoic

and salicylic acid. Bot. 0.5 oz, 6 oz, pt. *OTC.*
Use: Anti-infective, topical.
bismuth, water-soluble products.
See: Bismuth potassium tartrate.
•**bisnafide dimesylate.** (BISS-nah-fide die-MEH-sih-late) USAN.
Use: Antineoplastic.
•**bisobrin lactate.** (BISS-oh-brin LACK-tate) USAN.
Use: Fibrinolytic.
•**bisoctrizole.** (bis-OK-trye-zole) USAN.
Use: Sunscreen.
•**bisoprolol.** (bih-SO-pro-lahl) *USP 28.*
Use: Antiadrenergic/sympatholytic, beta-adrenergic blocking agent.
•**bisoprolol fumarate.** *USP 28.*
Use: Antiadrenergic/sympatholytic, beta-adrenergic blocking agent.
See: Zebeta.
Ziac.
bisoprolol fumarate. (Eon) Bisoprolol fumarate 5 mg, 10 mg. Tab. Bot. 30s, 100s. *Rx.*
Use: Antihypertensive, beta-blocker.
bisoprolol fumarate and hydrochlorothiazide. (Various Mfr.) Bisoprolol fumarate 2.5 mg, 5 mg, 10 mg; hydrochlorothiazide 6.25 mg. Tab. Bot. 30s (10 mg only), 100s, 500s, 1000s. *Rx.*
Use: Antihypertensive, diuretic.
•**bisoxatin acetate.** (biss-OX-at-in) USAN.
Use: Laxative.
bispecific antibody 520C9x22. (Medarex)
Use: Antineoplastic; serotherapy.
[Orphan Drug]
bisphosphonates.
Use: Antihypercalcemic; bone resorption inhibitor.
See: Alendronate Sodium.
Alendronate Sodium/Cholecalciferol.
Etidronate Disodium.
Ibandronate Sodium.
Pamidronate Disodium.
Risedronate Sodium.
Tiludronate Disodium.
Zoledronic Acid.
•**bispyrithione magsulfex.** (BISS-PIHR-ih-thigh-ohn mag-sull-fex) USAN.
Use: Antidandruff; anti-infective; antimicrobial.
bis-tropamide. Tropicamide.
See: Mydriacyl.
Bite & Itch Lotion. (Weeks & Leo) Pramoxine hydrochloride 1%, pyrilamine maleate 2%, pheniramine maleate 0.2%, chlorpheniramine maleate 0.2%. Bot. 4 oz. *OTC.*
Use: Dermatologic, topical.

Bite Rx. (International Lab. Tech.) Aluminum acetate 0.5%, benzalkonium chloride. Soln. Bot. 120 mL. *OTC.*
Use: Astringent.
•**bithionolate, sodium.** (bye-THIGH-oh-noe-late) USAN.
Use: Topical anti-infective.
Bitin. CDC anti-infective agent.
See: Bithionol.
•**bitolterol mesylate.** (by-TOLE-tor-ole) USAN.
Use: Bronchodilator, sympathomimetic.
See: Tornalate.
Bitrate. (Arco) Phenobarbital 15 mg, pentaerythritol tetranitrate 20 mg. Tab. Bot. 100s. *Rx.*
Use: Antianginal; hypnotic; sedative.
•**bivalirudin.** (bye-VAL-ih-ruh-din) USAN.
Use: Anticoagulant; antithrombotic.
See: Angiomax.
•**bizelesin.** (bye-ZELL-eh-sin) USAN.
Use: Antineoplastic.
B-Ject 100. (Hyrex) Vitamins B_1 100 mg, B_2 2 mg, B_3 100 mg, B_5 2 mg, B_6 2 mg/mL. Inj. Vial 10 mL, 30 mL. *Rx.*
Use: Vitamin supplement.
Black and White Bleaching Cream. (Schering-Plough) Hydroquinone 2%. Cream. Tube 0.75 oz, 1.5 oz. *Rx.*
Use: Dermatologic.
Black and White Ointment. (Schering-Plough) Resorcinol 3%. Oint. Tube 0.62 oz, 2.25 oz.
Use: Antiseptic; dermatologic, topical.
Black Draught. (Lee Pharmaceuticals) Sennosides. **Chew. Tab.:** 10 mg. Sugar. 30s. **Tab.:** 6 mg, sucrose. Bot. 30s. **Gran.:** 20 mg/5 mL, tartrazine, sucrose. Bot. 22.5 g. *OTC.*
Use: Laxative.
black widow spider, antivenin.
See: Antivenin (*Lactrodectus mactens*).
Blairex Hard Contact Lens Cleaner. (Blairex) Anionic detergent. Liq. Bot. 60 mL. *OTC.*
Use: Contact lens care.
Blairex Lens Lubricant. (Blairex) Isotonic. Sorbic acid 0.25%, EDTA 0.1%, borate buffer, NaCl, hydroxypropyl methylcellulose, glycerin. Soln. Bot. 15 mL. *OTC.*
Use: Contact lens care.
Blairex Sterile Saline Solution. (Blairex) Sodium Cl, boric acid, sodium borate. Soln. Bot. Aerosol. 90 mL, 240 mL, 360 mL. *OTC.*
Use: Contact lens care.
Blairex System. (Blairex) Sodium Cl 135 mg. Tab. 200s, 365s w/15 mL bot. *OTC.*

Use: Contact lens care.
Blairex System II. (Blairex) Sodium Cl
250 mg. Tab. 90s, 180s w/27.7 mL bot.
OTC.
Use: Contact lens care.
Blaud Strubel. (Strubel) Ferrous sulfate
5 g. Cap. Bot. 100s. *OTC.*
Use: Mineral supplement.
Blefcon. (Madland) Sodium sulfacet-
amide 30%. Oint. Tube ⅛ oz. *Rx.*
Use: Anti-infective, ophthalmic.
Blenoxane. (Bristol-Myers Oncology)
Bleomycin sulfate 15 units, 30 units.
Pow. for Inj. Vial. *Rx.*
Use: Antineoplastic; antibiotic.
bleomycin. (Various Mfr.) Bleomycin
15 units, 30 units. Pow. for Inj. Vial. *Rx.*
Use: Antineoplastic; antibiotic.
bleomycin sulfate. Various Mfr. Bleo-
mycin sulfate 15 units, 30 units. Pow.
for Inj. Vial. *Rx.*
Use: Antineoplastic.
●**bleomycin sulfate, sterile.** (BLEE-oh-
MY-sin) *USP 28.* Antibiotic obtained
from cultures of *Streptomyces verti-*
cillus.
Use: Antineoplastic; antibiotic.
See: Blenoxane.
Blephamide. (Allergan) Sulfacetamide
sodium 10%, prednisolone acetate
0.2%. Susp. Bot. 2.5 mL, 5 mL, 10 mL.
Rx.
Use: Anti-inflammatory; anti-infective,
ophthalmic.
Blephamide Ophthalmic Ointment.
(Allergan) Prednisolone acetate 0.2%,
sulfacetamide sodium 10%. Ophth.
Oint. Tube 3.5 g. *Rx.*
Use: Anti-inflammatory; anti-infective,
ophthalmic.
Bleph-10. (Allergan) Sulfacetamide so-
dium 10%. Dropper Bot. 2.5 mL, 5 mL,
15 mL. *Rx.*
Use: Anti-infective, ophthalmic.
Bleph-10 Sterile Ophthalmic Ointment.
(Allergan) Sulfacetamide sodium 10%.
Tube 3.5 g. *Rx.*
Use: Anti-infective, ophthalmic.
Blinx. (Akorn) Sodium Cl, potassium Cl,
sodium phosphate, benzalkonium Cl
0.005%, EDTA 0.02%. Soln. Bot.
120 mL. *OTC.*
Use: Irrigant, ophthalmic.
Blis. (Del) Boric acid 47.5%, salicylic acid
17%. Bot. 7 oz. *OTC.*
Use: Antifungal, topical.
BlisterGard. (Medtech) Alcohol 6.7%, py-
roxylin solution, oil of cloves, B-hydroxy-
quinolone. Liq. Bot. 30 mL. *OTC.*
Use: Dermatologic, protectant.

Blistex. (Blairex) Camphor 0.5%, phenol
0.5%, allantoin 1%, lanolin, mineral oil.
Tube 4.2 g, 10.5 g. *OTC.*
Use: Lip protectant.
Blistex Lip Balm. (Blairex) SPF 10.
Camphor 0.5%, phenol 0.5%, allantoin
1%, dimethicone 2%, pamidate 0.25%,
oxybenzone, parabens, petrolatum.
Tube 4.5 g. *OTC.*
Use: Lip protectant.
Blistex Ultra Protection. (Blairex) Octyl
methoxycinnamate, oxybenzone, octyl-
salicylate, menthylanthranilate, homo-
salate, dimethicone. Tube 4.2 g. *OTC.*
Use: Lip protectant.
Blistik. (Blairex) Padimate O 6.6%, oxy-
benzone 2.5%, dimethicone 2%. Lip-
balm stick 4.5 g. *OTC.*
Use: Lip protectant.
Blis-To-Sol. (Chattem) **Liq.:** Tolnaftate
1%. Bot. 30 mL. **Pow.:** Zinc undecy-
lenate 12%. Bot. 60 g. **Soln.:** Tolnaftate
1% Bot. 30 mL, 55.5 mL. *OTC.*
Use: Antifungal, topical.
BLM.
See: Bleomycin sulfate.
Blocadren. (Merck & Co.) Timolol
maleate 5 mg, 10 mg, 20 mg. Tab. Bot.
100s. *Rx.*
Use: Antiadrenergic/sympatholytic,
beta-adrenergic blocker.
Block Out by Sea & Ski. (Carter-
Wallace) Padimate O, octyl methoxycin-
namate, oxybenzone. Cream. Tube
120 g. *OTC.*
Use: Sunscreen.
Block Out Clear by Sea & Ski. (Carter-
Wallace) Padimate O, octyl methoxy-
cinnamate, octyl salicylate, SD alcohol
40. Lot. Bot. 120 mL. *OTC.*
Use: Sunscreen.
blood, anticoagulants.
See: Anticoagulants.
●**blood cells, red.** *USP 28. Formerly*
Blood cells, human red.
Use: Blood replenisher.
blood coagulation.
See: Hemostatics.
blood fractions.
See: Albumin (human) Salt-Poor.
blood glucose concentrator.
See: Glucagon.
blood glucose test.
See: Chemstrip bG.
Dextrostix Reagent Strips.
First Choice.
Glucostix.
●**blood grouping serum, anti-A.** *USP 28.*
Use: Diagnostic aid, blood, in vitro.
●**blood grouping serum, anti-B.** *USP 28.*
Use: Diagnostic aid, blood, in vitro.

•**blood grouping serums anti-D, anti-C, anti-E, anti-c, anti-e.** *USP 28.* Formerly *Anti-Rh typing serums.*
Use: Diagnostic aid, blood, in vitro.

blood group specific substances A, B and AB. Formerly *Blood Grouping specific substances A and B.*
Use: Blood neutralizer.

•**blood, whole.** *USP 28.* Formerly *Blood, whole human.*
Use: Blood replenisher.

Bluboro. (Allergan) Aluminum sulfate 53.9%, calcium acetate 43% w/boric acid, FD&C Blue 1. Pow. Packet 1.9 g. Box 12s. *OTC.*
Use: Astringent.

Bludex. (Burlington) Methenamine 40.8 mg, methylene blue 5.4 mg, phenylsalicylate 18.1 mg, atropine sulfate 0.03 mg, hyoscyamine 0.03 mg, benzoic acid 4.5 mg. Tab. Bot. 100s, 1000s. *Rx.*
Use: Antiseptic; antispasmodic, urinary.

Blue. (Various Mfr.) Pyrethrins 0.3%, piperonyl butoxide 3%, petroleum distillate 1.2%. Gel. Bot. 30 g, 480 g. *OTC.*
Use: Pediculicide.

Blue Gel Muscular Pain Reliever. (Rugby) Menthol in a specially formulated base. Gel. Tube 240 g. *OTC.*
Use: Liniments.

Blue Star. (McCue Labs.) Salicylic acid, benzoic acid, methyl salicylate, camphor, lanolin, petrolatum. Oint. Jar 2 oz. *OTC.*
Use: Dermatologic, counterirritant.

Blu-12 100. (Bluco) Cyanocobalamin 100 mcg/mL. Vial 30 mL. *Rx.*
Use: Vitamin supplement.

Blu-12 1000. (Bluco) Cyanocobalamin 1000 mcg/mL. Vial 30 mL. *Rx.*
Use: Vitamin supplement.

B-Major. (Barth's) Vitamins B_1 7 mg, B_2 14 mg, niacin 2.35 mg, B_{12} 7.5 mcg, B_6 0.15 mg, pantothenic acid 0.37 mg, choline 85 mg, inositol 6 mg, biotin, folic acid, aminobenzoic acid. Cap. Bot. 1s, 3s, 6s, 12s. *Rx-OTC.*
Use: Mineral, vitamin supplement.

B-N. (Eric, Kirk & Gary) Bacitracin 500 units, neomycin sulfate 5 mg. Oint. Tube 0.5 oz. *OTC.*
Use: Anti-infective, topical.

b-naphthyl salicylate. Betol, naphthosalol, salinaphthol.
Use: gastrointestinal and genitourinary, antiseptic.

Bo-Cal. (Fibertone) Calcium 250 mg, magnesium 125 mg, vitamin D_3 100 units, boron 0.75 mg. Tab. Bot. 120s. *OTC.*

Use: Mineral, vitamin supplement.

Bodi Kleen. (Geritrex) Triethanolamine lauryl sulfate, 2-phenoxy-ethanol, hexylene glycol, aloe vera gel. Spray. 8 oz. *OTC.*
Use: Anorectal preparation.

Body Fortress Natural Amino. (Nature's Bounty) Protein 1.67 g, lactalbumin hydrolysate 1500 mg, yeast and preservative free. Tab. Bot. 150s. *OTC.*
Use: Amino acid.

Boil-Ease Salve. (Del) Benzocaine 20%, camphor, eucalyptus oil, menthol, petrolatum, phenol. Oint. 30 g. *OTC.*
Use: Anesthetic drawing salve.

BoilnSoak. (Alcon) Sodium Cl 0.7%, boric acid, sodium borate, thimerosal 0.001%, disodium edetate 0.1%. Bot. 8 oz, 12 oz. *OTC.*
Use: Contact lens care.

•**bolandiol dipropionate.** (bole-AN-die-ole die-PRO-pee-oh-nate) *USAN.*
Use: Anabolic.

•**bolasterone.** (BOLE-ah-STEE-rone) *USAN.*
Use: Anabolic.

Bolax. (Boyd) Docusate sodium 240 mg, phenolphthalein 30 mg, dihydrocholic acid ¾ g. Cap. Bot. 100s. *OTC.*
Use: Laxative.

•**boldenone undecylenate.** (BOLE-deen-ohn uhn-deh-sih-LEN-ate) *USAN.* Parenabol. Under study.
Use: Anabolic.

•**bolenol.** (BOLE-ee-nahl) *USAN.*
Use: Anabolic.

•**bolmantalate.** (BOLE-MAN-tah-late) *USAN.*
Use: Anabolic.

Bonacal Plus. (Kenwood) Vitamins A 5000 units, D 400 units, C 100 mg, B_1 3 mg, B_2 3 mg, B_6 10 mg, B_{12} 4 mcg, niacinamide 20 mg, d-calcium pantothenate 3.3 mg, iron 42 mg, calcium 350 mg, manganese 0.33 mg, zinc 0.1 mg, magnesium 1.67 mg, potassium 1.67 mg. Tab. Bot. 100s. *OTC.*
Use: Mineral, vitamin supplement.

Bonamil Infant Formula with Iron. (Wyeth) Protein 2.3 g (from nonfat milk, taurine), fat 5.4 g (from soybean and coconut oils, soy lecithin), carbohydrate 10.7 g (from lactose), linoleic acid 1300 mg, vitamin A 300 units, D 60 units, E 2.85 units, K 8 mcg, B_1 100 mcg, B_2 150 mcg, B_6 63 mcg, B_{12} 0.2 mcg, B_3 750 mcg, folic acid 7.5 mcg, B_5 315 mcg, biotin 2.2 mcg, vitamin C 8.3 mg, choline 15 mg, Ca 69 mg, P 54 mg, Mg 6 mg, Fe 1.8 mg,

Zn 0.75 mg, Mn 15 mcg, Cu 70 mcg, I 5 mcg, Na 27 mg, K 93 mg, Cl 63 mg/100 cal (5.3 cal/g). Conc., Liq. Bot. 453 g. Conc. 384 mL. Ready-to-feed liq. 946 mL. *OTC.*
Use: Nutritional supplement, enteral.

Bonate. (Suppositoria Laboratories, Inc.) Bismuth subgallate, balsam Peru, benzocaine, zinc oxide. Supp. Box 12s, 100s, 1000s. *OTC.*
Use: Anorectal preparation.

Bonefos. (Leiras) Disodium clodronate tetrahydrate.
Use: Bone resorption inhibitor. [Orphan Drug]

B 100. (Fibertone) Vitamins B_1 100 mg, B_2 100 mg, B_3 100 mg, B_5 100 mg, B_6 100 mg, B_{12} 100 mcg, FA 0.4 mg, biotin 50 mcg, PABA 100 mg, choline bitartrate 100 mg, inositol 100 mg, FR Tab. Bot. 100s. *OTC.*
Use: Vitamin supplement.

B-100. (NBTY) Vitamins B_1 100 mg, B_2 100 mg, B_3 100 mg, B_5 100 mg, B_6 100 mg, B_{12} 100 mcg, folic acid 0.1 mg, d-biotin 100 mcg, PABA 100 mg, choline bitartrate, inositol, lecithin. Tab. Bot. 50s, 100s. *OTC.*
Use: Mineral, vitamin supplement.

B150. (NBTY) Vitamins B_1 150 mg, B_2 150 mg, B_3 150 mg, B_5 150 mg, B_6 150 mg, B_{12} 150 mcg, folic acid 0.1 mg, d-biotin 150 mcg, PABA 150 mg, choline bitartrate 150 mg, inositol 150 mg, lecithin. Tab. Bot. 100s. *OTC.*
Use: Mineral, vitamin supplement.

B125. (NBTY) Vitamins B_1 125 mg, B_2 125 mg, B_3 125 mg, B_5 125 mg, B_6 125 mg, B_{12} 125 mcg, folic acid 0.1 mg, d-biotin 105 mcg, PABA 125 mg, choline bitartrate 125 mg, inositol 125 mg, lecithin. Tab. Bot. 100s. *OTC.*
Use: Mineral, vitamin supplement.

Bone Meal w/Vitamin D. (Natures Bounty) Calcium 220 mg, vitamin D 100 units, phosphorus 100 mg, iron 0.45 mg, copper 3.25 mg, zinc 20 mcg, manganese 2.75 mcg, magnesium 0.925 mg. Tab. Bot. 100s, 250s. *OTC.*
Use: Mineral, vitamin supplement.

Boniva. (Roche) Ibandronate sodium (as base) 2.5 mg, 150 mg. Lactose. Film coated. Tab. 30s (2.5 mg only), unit-dose 1s (150 mg only). *Rx.*
Use: Bisphosphonate.

Bontril PDM. (Valeant) Phendimetrazine tartrate 35 mg, sugar, isopropyl alcohol, lactose. Tab. Bot. 100s, 1000s. *c-III.*
Use: CNS stimulant, anorexiant.

Bontril Slow Release. (Valeant) Phendimetrazine tartrate 105 mg. SR Cap.

Bot. 100s. *c-III.*
Use: CNS stimulant, anorexiant.

Boost. (Mead Johnson Nutritionals) Protein 10 mg, fat 7 g, carbohydrate 35 g, sodium 130 mg, potassium 400 mg, vitamins A, C, D, E, B_1, B_2, B_3, B_5, B_6, B_9, B_{12}, biotin, Ca, P, I, Mg, Zn, Cu, sugar, corn syrup. Liq. Bot. 247 mL. *OTC.*
Use: Nutritional supplement, enteral.

Boost Nutritional Pudding. (Mead Johnson Nutritionals) Protein 7 g, fat 9 g, carbohydrate 32 g, sodium 120 mg, potassium 320 mg, calories 240/serving, vitamins A, C, D, E, K, B_6, B_{12}, B_1, B_2, B_3, B_5, Ca, Fe, folic acid, biotin, P, I, Mg, Zn, Se, Cu, Mn, Cr, Mo, sugar. Pudding Cont. 142 g. *OTC.*
Use: Nutritional supplement.

Bopen-VK. (Boyd) Potassium phenoxymethyl penicillin 400,000 units. Tab. Bot. 100s.
Use: Anti-infective, penicillin.

borax. Sodium borate.

● **boric acid.** (BOR-ik) *NF 23.*
Use: Antiseptic, pharmaceutic necessity.
See: Borofax.
W/Combinations.
See: Saratoga.

boric acid. (Various Mfr.) Boric acid. **Top. Oint.:** 5%, 10%. Tube, Jar 30 g, 52.5 g, 60 g; 120 g, 454 g. **Ophth. Oint.:** 0.5%, 10%. Tube, Jar 3.5 g, 3.75 g, 30 g, 60 g, 480 g. *Rx-OTC.*
Use: Dermatologic, counterirritant.

2-bornanone. Camphor.

● **bornelone.** (BORE-neh-LONE) *USAN.*
Use: Ultraviolet screen.

● **bornyl acetate.** *USAN.*

● **borocaptate sodium 10.** (bore-oh-CAP-tate) *USAN.*
Use: Antineoplastic; radiopharmaceutical.

Borocell. (Neutron Technology) Sodium monomercaptoundecahdrocloso-dodecaborate.
Use: Boron neutron capture therapy (BNCT) in glioblastoma multiforme.

Borofair Otic. (Major) Acetic acid 2% in aluminum acetate. Soln. Bot. 60 mL. *Rx.*
Use: Otic preparation.

Borofax Skin Protectant. (Warner Lambert) Zinc oxide 15%, petrolatum 68.6%, lanolin, mineral oil. Oint. Tube 50 g. *OTC.*
Use: Dermatologic, counterirritant.

boroglycerin. (Emerson) Glycerol borate. Bot. Pt.

Use: Agent for dermatitis.

boroglycerin glycerite. Boric acid 31 parts, glycerin 96 parts.
Use: Agent for dermatitis.

Boropak. (Glenwood) Aluminum sulfate and calcium acetate. One packet dissolved in a pint of water yields a 1:40 dilution. Pow. Packs 2.4 g. 100s. *OTC.*
Use: Anti-inflammatory, topical.

borotannic complex. Boric acid 31 mg, tannic acid 50 mg.

●**bortezomib.** (bore-TEZZ-oh-mib) USAN.
Use: Antineoplastic.
See: Velcade.

●**bosentan.** (boe-SEN-tan) USAN.
Use: Vasodilator, endothelin receptor antagonist.
See: Tracleer.

Boston Advance Cleaner. (Polymer Technology) Concentrated homogenous surfactant with friction-enhancing agents. Soln. Bot. 30 mL. *OTC.*
Use: Contact lens care.

Boston Advance Comfort Formula. (Polymer Technology) Buffered, slightly hypertonic. Polyaminopropyl biguanide 0.00015%, EDTA 0.05%, cationic cellulose derivative polymer. Soln. Bot. 120 mL. *OTC.*
Use: Contact lens care.

Boston Advance Conditioning Solution. (Polymer Technology) Sterile, buffered, slightly hypertonic. Polyaminopropyl biguanide 0.0015%, EDTA 0.05%. Soln. Bot. 120 mL or with cleaner in a convenience pack. *OTC.*
Use: Contact lens care.

Boston Advance Rewetting Drops. (Polymer Technology) Buffered, slightly hypertonic. Polyaminopropyl biguanide 0.0015%, EDTA 0.05%. Drops. Bot. 10 mL. *OTC.*
Use: Contact lens care.

Boston Cleaner. (Polymer Technology) Concentrated homogeneous surfactant with friction-enhancing agents, sodium Cl. Soln. Bot. 30 mL. *OTC.*
Use: Contact lens care.

Boston Conditioning Solution. (Polymer Technology) Sterile, buffered, slightly hypertonic, low viscosity. EDTA 0.05%, chlorhexidine gluconate 0.006%. Soln. Bot. 120 mL. *OTC.*
Use: Contact lens care.

Boston Reconditioning Drops. (Polymer Technology) Hydrophilic polyelectrolyte, polyvinyl alcohol, hydroxyethylcellulose, chlorhexidine gluconate, EDTA. Soln. Bot. 120 mL. *OTC.*
Use: Contact lens care.

Boston Rewetting Drops. (Polymer Technology) Buffered, slightly hypertonic. Chlorhexidine gluconate 0.006%, EDTA 0.05%, cationic cellulose derivative polymer. Soln. Bot. 10 mL. *OTC.*
Use: Contact lens care.

Boston Simplicity Multi-Action. (Polymer Technology) PEO sorbitan monolaurate, silicone glycol copolymer, cellulosic viscoslfler, derivatized PEG, chlorhexidine gluconate, polyaminopropyl biguanide, EDTA. 0.05%. Soln. Bot. 60 mL, 90 mL, 120 mL. *OTC.*
Use: Contact lens product.

Botox. (Allergan) Vacuum-dried *Clostridium botulinum* toxin type A neurotoxin complex 100 units (one unit corresponds to the calculated median lethal intraperitoneal dose [LD_{50}] in mice), human albumin 0.5 mg, sodium chloride 0.9 mg, preservative free. Inj. (vacuum dried). Single-use vial. *Rx.*
Use: Ophthalmic; treatment of cervical dystonia; axillary hyperhidrosis, strabismus and blepharospasm.

Botox Cosmetic. (Allergan) Vacuum-dried *Clostridium botulinum* toxin type A neurotoxin complex 100 units (one unit corresponds to the calculated median lethal intraperitoneal dose (LD_{50}) in mice), human albumin 0.5 mg, sodium chloride 0.9 mg, preservative free. Pow. for Inj. (vacuum dried). Single-use vial. *Rx.*
Use: Treatment of glabellar lines.

Bottom Better. (InnoVisions) Petrolatum 49%, lanolin 15.5%, beeswax, sodium borate, lanolin alcohols, methyl salicylate, sorbitan sesquioleate, parabens, oxyquinolone, EDTA. Oint. Pkg. 18s. *OTC.*
Use: Diaper rash preparation.

botulinum toxins.
See: Botox.
Botox Cosmetic.
Botulinum toxin type A.
Botulinum toxin type B.
Botulinum toxin type F.
Myobloc.

botulinum toxin type A.
Use: Ophthalmic; treatment of cervical dystonia, glabellar lines; axillary hyperhidrosis, strabismus and blepharospasm.
See: Botox.
Botox Cosmetic.

botulinum toxin type B. (Athena Neurosciences)
Use: Cervical dystonia.
See: Myobloc.

botulinum toxin type F. (Porton Product Limited)

Use: Cervical dystonia; essential blepharospasm. [Orphan Drug]

• **botulism antitoxin.** (BOT-yoo-lism) *USP 28.*
Use: Prophylaxis and treatment of the toxins of C botulinum, types A or B; passive immunizing agent.

botulism immune globulin.
Use: Infant botulism.
See: BabyBIG.

Bounty Bears. (NBTY) Vitamins A 2500 units, D 400 units, E 15 units, C 60 mg, B₁ 1.05 mg, B₂ 1.2 mg, B₃ 13.5 mg, B₆ 1.05 mg, B₁₂ 4.5 mcg, folic acid 0.3 mg. Tab. Bot. 100s. *OTC.*
Use: Mineral, vitamin supplement.

Bounty Bears Plus Iron. (NBTY) Vitamins A 2500 units, D 400 units, E 15 units, C 60 mg, B₁ 1.05 mg, B₂ 1.2 mg, B₃ 13.5 mg, B₆ 1.05 mg, B₁₂ 4.5 mcg, folic acid 0.3 mg, iron 15 mg. Tab. Bot. 100s. *OTC.*
Use: Mineral, vitamin supplement.

bourbonal.
See: Ethyl Vanillin.

bovine colostrum.
Use: AIDS-related diarrhea. [Orphan Drug]

bovine immunoglobulin concentrate, Cryptosporidium parvum.
Use: Anti-infective. [Orphan Drug]

bovine whey protein concentrate.
Use: Treatment of cryptosporidiosis. [Orphan Drug]
See: Immuno-C.

bowel evacuants.
Use: Laxative.
See: CoLyte.
Fleet Prep Kit 1.
Fleet Prep Kit 3.
Fleet Prep Kit 2.
GoLYTELY.
HalfLytely
MiraLax.
NuLytely.
OCL.
Polyethylene Glycol-Electrolyte Solution (PEG-ES).
Tridate Bowel Cleansing System.
X-Prep Bowel Evacuant Kit-1.
X-Prep Bowel Kit-2.
X-Prep Liquid.

Bowman's Poison Antidote Kit. (Jones Pharma) Syrup of ipecac 1 oz, 1 bottle; activated charcoal liquid 2 oz, 3 bottles. *OTC.*
Use: Antidote.

Bowsteral. (Jones Pharma) Isopropanol 60%. Bot. Pt, gal.
Use: Disinfectant.

• **boxidine.** (BOX-ih-deen) USAN.
Use: Adrenal steroid blocker; antihyperlipoproteinemic.

Boylex. (Health for Life Brands) Diperodon, hexachlorophene, rosin cerate, ichthammol, carbolic acid, thymol, camphor, juniper tar. Tube oz. *OTC.*
Use: Drawing salve.

B-Pap. (Wren) Acetaminophen 120 mg, sodium butabarbital 15 mg/5 mL. Bot. Pt, gal. *Rx.*
Use: Analgesic; sedative.

b-pas.
See: Calcium Benzoyl PAS.

B-Plex. (Ivax) Vitamins B₁ 15 mg, B₂ 15 mg, B₃ 100 mg, B₅ 18 mg, B₆ 4 mg, B₁₂ 5 mcg, C 500 mg, folic acid 0.5 mg. Tab. Bot. 100s. *Rx.*
Use: Mineral, vitamin supplement.

BP-Papaverine (Burlington) Papaverine hydrochloride 150 mg. SR Cap. Bot. 50s. *Rx.*
Use: Vasodilator.

Brace. (GlaxoSmithKline) Denture adhesive. Tube 1.4 oz, 2.4 oz.

Bradosol Bromide. (Novartis) Domiphen bromide.

BranchAmin 4%. (Baxter PPI) Isoleucine 1.38 g, leucine 1.38 g, valine 1.25 g, phosphate 31.6 mOsm/100 mL. Bot. 500 mL. *Rx.*
Use: Adjunct to regular TPN therapy for highly stressed or traumatized patients.

branched chain amino acids.
Use: Nutritional supplement; amyotrophic lateral sclerosis agent. [Orphan Drug]

Brasivol Fine, Medium, and Rough. (Stiefel) Aluminum oxide scrub particles in a surfactant cleansing base. **Fine:** Jar 153 g. **Medium:** Jar 180 g. **Rough:** Jar 195 g. *OTC.*
Use: Scrub cleanser.

• **brasofensine maleate.** (brah-so-FEN-seen MAL-ee-ate) USAN.
Use: Antiparkinsonian.

Bravelle. (Ferring) Urofollitropin 75 units FSH activity. Contains up to 2% luteinizing hormone activity. Pow. for Inj., lyophilized. Vials with NaCl 2 mL as diluent and lactose monohydrate 23 mg. *Rx.*
Use: Ovulation stimulant.

Breatheasy. (Pascal Co. Inc.) Racemic epinephrine hydrochloride 2.2%. Soln. inhaled by use of nebulizer. Bot. 0.25 oz, 0.5 oz, 1 oz. *OTC.*
Use: Bronchodilator.

Breathe Free. (Thompson Medical) Sodium chloride 0.65%, benzalkonium

chloride. Soln. Spray Bot. 45 mL. *OTC.*
Use: Nasal decongestant.

Breathe Right Children's Cold Nasal Strips. (CNS Inc.) Menthol. Strip. Pkg. 10s. *OTC.*
Use: Upper respiratory combination, topical.

Breathe Right Colds Nasal Strips. (CNS Inc.) Menthol. Strip. Pkg. 10s. *OTC.*
Use: Upper respiratory combination, topical.

Breezee Mist. (Pedinol Pharmacal) Aluminum chlorhydrate, undecylenic acid, menthol. Aerosol. Bot. 4 oz. *OTC.*
Use: Antifungal; deodorant; antiperspirant; foot powder.

Breezee Mist Antifungal. (Pedinol Pharmacal) Miconazole nitrate 2%, isobutane, talc, aluminum chlorhydrate, cyclomethicone, isopropyl myristate, propylene carbonate, menthol. Pow. Tube 113 g. *OTC.*
Use: Anti-infective, topical.

Breezee Mist Foot Powder. (Pedinol) Isobutane, talc, aluminum chlorhydrate, cyclomethicone, isopropyl myristate, propylene carbonate, stearalkonium hectorite, undecylenic acid, menthol. Pow. Aerosol can. 113 g. *OTC.*
Use: Antifungal, topical.

•**brequinar sodium.** (BREh-kwih-NAHR) USAN.
Use: Antineoplastic.

•**bretazenil.** (bret-AZZ-eh-nill) USAN.
Use: Anxiolytic.

Brethancer. (Novartis)
Use: Inhaler, complete unit to be used with *Brethaire.*

Brethine. (aaiPharma) Terbutaline sulfate. **Tab.:** 2.5 mg, 5 mg, lactose. Bot. 100s, 1000s, UD 100s. **Inj.:** 1 mg/mL. Amp. 2 mL w/1 mL fill. *Rx.*
Use: Bronchodilator, sympathomimetic.

•**bretylium tosylate.** (bre-TILL-ee-uhm TAH-sill-ate) *USP 28.*
Use: Hypotensive; antiadrenergic; cardiovascular agent, antiarrhythmic.

bretylium tosylate. (Various Mfr.) Bretylium tosylate 50 mg/mL. Inj. Amps 10 mL, vials, syringes. *Rx.*
Use: Antiarrhythmic agent.

bretylium tosylate in 5% dextrose. (Various Mfr.) Bretylium tosylate 2 mg/mL (500 mg/vial), 4 mg/mL (1,000 mg/vial). Inj. Vial 250 mL. *Rx.*
Use: Antiarrhythmic agent.

Brevibloc. (Baxter) Esmolol hydrochloride 10 mg/mL, 250 mg/mL. Inj. **10 mg/mL:** Vial 10 mL. **250 mg/mL:** Amp 10 mL, propylene glycol 25%, alcohol 25%. *Rx.*
Use: Antiadrenergic/sympatholytic, beta-adrenergic blocker.

Brevibloc Double Strength. (Baxter) Esmolol hydrochloride 20 mg/mL. Preservative-free. Inj. Ready-to-use 5 mL vials. 100 mL bags. *Rx.*
Use: Beta-adrenergic blocking agent.

Brevicon. (Watson) Norethindrone 0.5 mg, ethinyl estradiol 35 mcg, lactose. Tab. Wallette 28s. *Rx.*
Use: Sex hormone, contraceptive.

Brevital Sodium. (Monarch) Methohexital sodium. **Vial:** 2.5 g/250 mL. **Amp.:** 2.5 g. *Rx.*
Use: Anesthetic, general.

Brevoxyl Creamy Wash. (Stiefel) Benzoyl peroxide 4%, 8%. Glycerin, castor oil, parabens, mineral oil. Liq. Tube 170 g. *Rx.*
Use: Anti-infective, antibiotic, topical.

Brevoxyl-8. (Stiefel) Benzoyl peroxide 8%. Cetyl alcohol, stearyl alcohol. Gel. Tube 42.5 g, 90 g. *Rx.*
Use: Anti-infective, antibiotic, topical.

Brevoxyl 8 Cleansing. (Stiefel) Benzoyl peroxide 8%. Cetyl alcohol. Lot. Bot. 297 g. *Rx.*
Use: Anti-infective, antibiotic, topical.

Brevoxyl-4. (Stiefel) Benzoyl peroxide 4%. Cetyl alcohol, stearyl alcohol. Gel. Tube 42.5 g, 90 g. *Rx.*
Use: Antiacne.

Brevoxyl 4 Cleansing. (Stiefel) Benzoyl peroxide 4%. Cetyl alcohol. Lot. Bot. 297 g. *Rx.*
Use: Anti-infective, antibiotic, topical.

brewer's yeast. (NBTY) Vitamins B_1 0.06 mg, B_2 0.02 mg, B_3 0.2 mg. Tab. Bot. 250s. *OTC.*
Use: Vitamin supplement.

Brexin EX. (Savage) **Liq.:** Pseudoephedrine hydrochloride 30 mg, guaifenesin 200 mg/5 mL. **Tab.:** Pseudoephedrine hydrochloride 60 mg, guaifenesin 400 mg. Bot. 100s. *OTC.*
Use: Decongestant, expectorant.

Bricanyl. (Hoechst) Terbutaline sulfate. **Tab.:** 2.5 mg, 5 mg. Bot. 100s. **Inj.:** 1 mg/mL. Amp. 2 mL w/1 mL fill. *Rx.*
Use: Bronchodilator.

•**brifentanil hydrochloride.** (brih-FEN-tah-NILL) USAN.
Use: Analgesic; narcotic.

Brigen-G. (Grafton) Chlordiazepoxide 5 mg, 10 mg, 25 mg. Tab. Bot. 500s. *c-iv.*
Use: Anxiolytic.

Brij 96 and 97. (ICI) Polyoxyl 10 oleyl ether available as 96 and 97.

Use: Surface active agent.
Brij-721. (ICI) Polyoxyethylene 21 stearyl ether (100% active).
Use: Surface active agent.
●**brimonidine tartrate.** (brih-MOE-nih-DEEN) USAN.
Use: Agent for glaucoma.
See: Alphagan P.
brimonidine tartrate. (Various Mfr.) Brimonidine tartrate 0.2%. Soln. 5 mL, 10 mL, 15 mL. *Rx.*
Use: Agent for glaucoma.
brineurin.
See: Abrineurin.
●**brinolase.** (BRIN-oh-laze) USAN. Fibrinolytic enzyme produced by *Aspergillus oryzae.*
Use: Fibrinolytic.
●**brinzolamide.** (brln ZOE luh mlduu) *USP 28.*
Use: Antiglaucoma agent.
See: Azopt.
Bristoject. (Bristol-Myers Squibb) Prefilled disposable syringes w/needle.
Available with: Aminophylline: 250 mg/10 mL. Atropine sulfate: 5 mg/5 mL or 1 mg/mL. 10s. Calcium Cl: 10%. 10 ml 10s. Dexamethasone: 20 mg/5 mL. Dextrose: 50%. 50 mL. 10s. Diphenhydramine: 50 mg/5 mL. Dopamine hydrochloride: 200 mg/5 mL, 400 mg/10 mL. Ephedrine: 50 mg/10 mL. Epinephrine: 1:10,000. 10 mL. 10s. Lidocaine hydrochloride: 1%: 5 mL, 10 mL; 2%: 5 mL; 4%: 25 mL, 50 mL; 20%: 5 mL, 10 mL. Magnesium sulfate: 5 g/10 mL, 10s. Metaraminol: 1%. 10 mL. Sodium bicarbonate: 75%: 50 mL; 84%: 50 mL. 10s.
Use: Medical device.
british anti-lewisite. Dimercaprol.
See: BAL.
Brobella-P.B. (Brothers) Atropine sulfate 0.0195 mg, hyoscine HBr 0.0065 mg, hyoscyamine sulfate 0.1040 mg, phenobarbital 0.25 g. Tab. Bot. 100s, 1000s. *Rx.*
Use: Anticholinergic; antispasmodic; hypnotic; sedative.
●**brocresine.** (broe-KREE-seen) USAN.
Use: Histidine decarboxylase inhibitor.
●**brocrinat.** (BROE-krih-NAT) USAN.
Use: Diuretic.
Brocycline. (Brothers) Tetracycline hydrochloride 250 mg. Cap. Bot. 100s, 1000s. *Rx.*
Use: Anti-infective, tetracycline.
Brofed. (Marnel) Pseudoephedrine hydrochloride 30 mg, brompheniramine maleate 4 mg/5 mL, parabens, saccha-rin, sorbitol, sucrose, corn syrup, menthol, mint flavor. Liq. Bot. 473 mL. *Rx.*
Use: Upper respiratory combination, antihistamine, decongestant.
●**brofoxine.** (BROE-fox-een) USAN.
Use: Antipsychotic.
●**bromadoline maleate.** (BROE-mah-DOE-leen) USAN.
Use: Analgesic.
bromaleate.
See: Pamabrom.
Bromanate. (Alpharma) Brompheniramine maleate 1 mg/5 mL, pseudoephedrine hydrochloride 15 mg, alcohol free, grape flavor. Elix. Bot. 118 mL, 237 mL, 473 mL, gal. *OTC.*
Use: Upper respiratory combination, antihistamine, decongestant.
Bromanate DM Cold & Cough. (Alpharma) Pseudoephedrine hydrochloride 15 mg, brompheniramine maleate 1 mg, dextromethorphan HBr 5 mg/5 mL, alcohol free, grape flavor. Elixir. Bot. 118 mL. *OTC.*
Use: Upper respiratory combination, decongestant, antihistamine, antitussive.
Bromanyl. (Various Mfr.) Bromodiphenhydramine hydrochloride 12.5 mg, codeine phosphate 10 mg, alcohol 5%. Syr. Bot. Pt, gal. *c-v.*
Use: Antihistamine; antitussive.
Bromarest DX. (Warner Chilcott) Pseudoephedrine hydrochloride 30 mg, brompheniramine maleate 2 mg, dextromethorphan HBr 10 mg, alcohol 0.95%. Butterscotch flavor. Syr. Bot. 480 mL. *Rx.*
Use: Antihistamine; antitussive; decongestant.
Bromatane DX. (Ivax) Pseudoephedrine hydrochloride 30 mg, brompheniramine maleate 2 mg, dextromethorphan HBr 10 mg, alcohol 0.95%. Bot. 473 mL. *Rx.*
Use: Upper respiratory combination, antihistamine, antitussive, decongestant.
Bromatap. (Ivax) Brompheniramine maleate 2 mg, phenylephrine hydrochloride 12.5 mg, alcohol 2.3%/5 mL. Liq. Bot. 4 oz, 8 oz, pt, gal. *OTC.*
Use: Antihistamine; decongestant.
bromauric acid. Hydrogen tetrabromoaurate.
●**bromazepam.** (broe-MAY-zeh-pam) USAN.
Use: Anxiolytic.
Brombay. (Rosemont) Brompheniramine maleate 2 mg/5 mL, alcohol 3%. Elix. Bot. 4 oz, pt, gal. *OTC.*

Use: Antihistamine.

●**bromchlorenone.** (brome-KLOR-ee-nohn) USAN.
Use: Anti-infective, topical.

●**bromelains.** (BROE-meh-lanes) USAN.
Use: Anti-inflammatory.
See: Dayto-Anase.

bromethol.
See: Avertin.

Bromfed. (Verum Pharm.) Brompheniramine maleate. **Cap.:** 12 mg, phenylephrine hydrochloride 15 mg, parabens, sucrose. ER Cap. Bot. 100s. **Tab.:** 4 mg, pseudoephedrine hydrochloride 60 mg, lactose. Bot. 100s. *Rx.*
Use: Upper respiratory combination, antihistamine, decongestant.

Bromfed DM Cough. (Verum Pharm.) Brompheniramine maleate 2 mg, pseudoephedrine hydrochloride 30 mg, dextromethorphan HBr 10 mg/5 mL, saccharin, sorbitol, sucrose, methylparaben, cherry flavor. Syr. Bot. 473 mL. *Rx.*
Use: Upper respiratory combination, antihistamine, antitussive, decongestant.

Bromfed-PD. (Verum Pharm.) Brompheniramine maleate 6 mg, phenylephrine hydrochloride 7.5 mg, parabens, sucrose. ER Cap. Bot. 100s. *Rx.*
Use: Upper respiratory combination, antihistamine, decongestant.

bromfenac.
Use: Nonsteroidal anti-inflammatory agent, ophthalmic.
See: Xibrom.

Bromfenex. (Ethex) Brompheniramine maleate 12 mg, pseudoephedrine hydrochloride 120 mg, sucrose. ER Cap. Bot. 100s. *Rx.*
Use: Upper respiratory combination, antihistamine, decongestant.

Bromfenex PD. (Ethex) Brompheniramine maleate 6 mg, pseudoephedrine hydrochloride 60 mg, sucrose. ER Cap. Bot. 100s. *Rx.*
Use: Upper respiratory combination, antihistamine, decongestant.

bromhexine. (Boehringer Ingelheim)
Use: Mild/moderate keratoconjunctivitis sicca. [Orphan Drug]

●**bromhexine hydrochloride.** (brome-HEX-een) USAN.
Use: Expectorant; mucolytic.

Bromhist-DM. (Cypress) Pseudoephedrine hydrochloride 30 mg, brompheniramine maleate 2 mg, dextromethorphan hydrobromide 5 mg, guaifenesin 50 mg/5 mL. Alcohol free, dye free.

Saccharin, sorbitol. Grape flavor. Syrup. 473 mL. *Rx.*
Use: Pediatric antitussive and expectorant.

Bromhist-NR. (Cypress) Pseudoephedrine hydrochloride 12.5 mg, brompheniramine maleate 1 mg per mL. Alcohol free. Saccharin, sorbitol. Cherry flavor. Drops. 30 mL with dropper. *Rx.*
Use: Pediatric decongestant and antihistamine.

Bromhist PDX Drops. (Cypress) Pseudoephedrine hydrochloride 12.5 mg, brompheniramine maleate 1 mg, dextromethoprhan hydrobromide 3 mg per mL. Alcohol free. Saccharin, sorbitol. Grape flavor. Drops. 30 mL with dropper. *Rx.*
Use: Pediatric antitussive combination.

Bromhist-PDX Syrup. (Cypress) Phenylephrine hydrochloride 5 mg, dextromethorphan hydrobromide 5 mg, guaifenesin 50 mg, brompheniramine maleate 2 mg/5 mL. Alcohol free. Parabens, sugar. Grape flavor. Syrup. 473 mL. *Rx.*
Use: Pediatric antitussive and expectorant.

bromides.
See: Peacock's Bromides.

bromide salts.
See: Calcium bromide.
Ferrous bromide.
Potassium bromide.
Sodium bromide.
Strontium bromide.

Bromi-Lotion. (Gordon Laboratories) Aluminum hydroxychloride 20%, emollient base. Lot. Bot. 1.5 oz, 4 oz. *OTC.*
Use: Antiperspirant.

●**bromindione.** (BROME-in-die-ohn) USAN.
Use: Anticoagulant.

Bromi-Talc. (Gordon Laboratories) Potassium alum, bentonite, talc. Shaker can 3.5 oz, 1 lb, 5 lb. *OTC.*
Use: Bromidrosis; hyperhidrosis.

●**bromocriptine.** (BROE-moe-KRIP-teen) USAN.
Use: Enzyme inhibitor, prolactin.

●**bromocriptine mesylate.** (BROE-moe-KRIP-teen) *USP 28.*
Use: Enzyme inhibitor, prolactin.
See: Parlodel.

●**bromocriptine mesylate.** (Mylan) Bromocriptine mesylate 2.5 mg. Lactose, EDTA. Tab. 30s, 100s. *Rx.*
Use: Enzyme inhibitor, prolactin; antiparkinson agent.

bromodeoxyuridine. (NeoPharm, Inc.) *Use:* Radiation sensitizer in treatment of primary brain tumors. [Orphan Drug]
bromodiethylacetylurea. *See:* Carbromal.
• **bromodiphenhydramine hydrochloride.** (BROE-moe-die-feu-HIGH-drahmeen) *USP 28.* *Use:* Antihistamine.
• **bromodiphenhydramine hydrochloride/codeine phosphate.** *USP 28.* Antitussive combination.
bromodiphenhydramine hydrochloride/codeine phosphate. (Rosemont) Bromodiphenhydramine hydrochloride 12.5 mg, codeine phosphate 10 mg. Syr. Bot. 480 mL. *c-v.* *Use:* Antitussive combination.
bromoform. Tribromomethane.
bromoisovaleryl urea. Alpha, bromoisovaleryl urea.
Bromophin. *See:* Apomorphine hydrochloride.
Bromo Seltzer. (Warner Lambert) Acetaminophen 325 mg, sodium bicarbonate 2.78 g, citric acid 2.22 g (when dissolved, forms sodium citrate 2.85 g)/ dose. Large (2 ⅝ oz), King (4.25 oz), Giant (9 oz), Foil pack, single-dose 48s. *OTC.* *Use:* Antacid; analgesic.
bromotheophyllinate aminoisobutanol. *See:* Pamabrom.
bromotheophyllinate pyranisamine. *See:* Pyrabrom.
bromotheophyllinate pyrilamine. *See:* Pyrabrom.
8-bromotheophylline. *See:* Pamabrom.
Bromotuss w/Codeine. (Rugby) Bromodiphenhydramine hydrochloride 12.5 mg, codeine phosphate 10 mg, alcohol 5%. Syr. Bot. 120 mL, pt, gal. *c-v.* *Use:* Antihistamine; antitussive.
• **bromoxanide.** (broe-MOX-ah-nide) USAN. *Use:* Anthelmintic.
• **bromperidol.** (brome-PURR-ih-dahl) USAN. *Use:* Antipsychotic.
• **bromperidol decanoate.** (brome-PURRih-dole deh-KAN-oh-ate) USAN. *Use:* Antipsychotic.
Bromphen DX. (Rugby) Pseudoephedrine hydrochloride 30 mg, brompheniramine maleate 2 mg, dextromethorphan HBr 10 mg, alcohol 0.95%. Syr. Bot.

480 mL. *Rx.* *Use:* Antihistamine; antitussive; decongestant.
brompheniramine. *Use:* Antihistamine, nonselective aklylamine. *See:* Bidhist. BröveX. BröveX CT. Lodrane D. Lodrane 24. Lodrane XR. LoHist 12 Hour. VaZol.
Brompheniramine Cough. (Geneva) Pseudoephedrine hydrochloride 30 mg, brompheniramine maleate 2 mg, dextromethorphan HBr 10 mg, alcohol 0.95%. Syr. Bot. 480 mL. *Rx.* *Use:* Antihistamine; antitussive; decongestant.
• **brompheniramine maleate.** (brome-fenAIR-uh-meen) *USP 28.* *Use:* Antihistamine.
brompheniramine maleate/pseudoephedrine hydrochloride. (Cypress) Pseudoephedrine hydrochloride 60 mg, brompheniramine maleate 4 mg/5 mL, saccharin, sorbitol, raspberry flavor. Syr. Bot. 473 mL. *Rx.* *Use:* Upper respiratory combination, decongestant, antihistamine.
brompheniramine maleate w/combinations. *See:* AccuHist. AccuHist DM Pediatric. AccuHist PDX. Alacol DM. Anaplex-DM. Anaplex HD. Brofed. Bromanate. Bromanate DM Cold & Cough. Bromatane DX. Bromfed. Bromfed DM Cough. Bromfed-PD. Bromfenex. Bromfenex PD. Bromhist-DM. Bromhist-NR. Bromhist PDX. Carbodex DM. Carbofed DM. Children's Elixir DM Cough & Cold. Coldec DM. Comtrex Acute Head Cold & Sinus Pressure Relief, Multi-Symptom Maximum Strength. Cortane. DALLERGY-JR.

Dimaphen.
Dimaphen DM Cold & Cough.
Dimetapp Children's Nighttime Flu.
Dimetapp Cold & Allergy.
Dimetapp DM Children's Cold & Cough.
Histacol DM.
Histex SR.
Lodrane.
Lodrane LD.
Lodrane 12 D.
Lortuss DM.
Pediahist DM.
Robitussin Allergy & Cough.
Rondamine DM.
Rondec.
Rondec DM.
Sildec-DM.
Touro Allergy.

Brompton's Cocktail. Heroin or morphine 10 mg, cocaine 10 mg, alcohol, chloroform water, syrup. *c-II.*
Use: Analgesic, narcotic.

Bronchial. (Various Mfr.) Theophylline 150 mg, guaifenesin 90 mg. Cap. Bot. 100s, 1000s. *Rx.*
Use: Antiasthmatic; expectorant.

bronchodilators.
See: Albuterol.
Anticholinergics.
Bitolterol mesylate.
Diluents.
Ephedrine sulfate.
Epinephrine.
Formoterol fumarate.
Ipratropium bromide and albuterol sulfate.
Isoetharine hydrochloride.
Isoproterenol hydrochloride.
Levabuterol hydrochloride.
Metaproterenol sulfate.
Pirbuterol acetate.
Salmeterol.
Sodium chloride.
Sympathomimetics.
Terbutaline sulfate.
Tiotropium bromide.
Xanthine derivatives.

Broncholate. (Sanofi-Synthelabo) Ephedrine hydrochloride 12.5 mg, guaifenesin 200 mg. **Cap.:** Bot. 100s, 1000s. **Softgels:** Bot. 100s. *Rx.*
Use: Bronchodilator; expectorant.

Broncholate Syrup. (Sanofi-Synthelabo) Ephedrine hydrochloride 6.25 mg, guaifenesin 100 mg/5 mL, orange flavor. Syr. Bot. 473 mL. *Rx.*
Use: Bronchodilator; upper respiratory combination, decongestant, expectorant.

Brondecon. (Parke-Davis) **Tab.:** Oxtriphylline 200 mg, guaifenesin 100 mg. Bot. 100s. **Elix.:** Oxtriphylline 100 mg, guaifenesin 50 mg/5 mL w/alcohol 20%. Bot. 8 oz, 16 oz. *Rx.*
Use: Bronchodilator; expectorant.

Brondelate. (Various Mfr.) Oxtriphylline 300 mg, guaifenesin 150 mg/5 mL. Elix. Bot. 480 mL, gal. *Rx.*
Use: Bronchodilator; expectorant.

Bronitin. (Whitehall-Robins) Theophylline hydrous 120 mg, guaifenesin 100 mg, ephedrine hydrochloride 24.3 mg, pyrilamine maleate 16.6 mg. Tab. Bot. 24s, 60s. *OTC.*
Use: Bronchodilator.

Bronitin Mist. (Whitehall-Robins) Epinephrine bitartrate in inhalation aerosol. Each spray releases 0.3 mg epinephrine bitartrate equivalent to 0.16 mg epinephrine base. Bot. 15 mL or 15 mL refills. *OTC.*
Use: Bronchodilator.

Bronkaid Dual Action. (Bayer Corp. (Consumer Div.)) Ephedrine sulfate 25 mg, guaifenesin 400 mg. Tab. Bot. 24s. *OTC.*
Use: Bronchodilator; upper respiratory combination, decongestant, expectorant.

Bronkodyl. (Sanofi-Synthelabo) Theophylline 100 mg, 200 mg. Cap. Bot. 100s. Theophylline 300 mg. SR Cap. Bot. 100s. *Rx.*
Use: Bronchodilator.

Bronkometer. (Sanofi-Synthelabo) Isoetharine mesylate 0.61%, saccharin, menthol, alcohol 30%. Metered dose of 340 mcg isoetharine in fluorohydrocarbon propellant. Bot. w/nebulizer 10 mL, 15 mL. Refill 10 mL, 15 mL. *Rx.*
Use: Bronchodilator.

Bronkosol. (Sanofi-Synthelabo) Isoetharine hydrochloride 1% w/glycerin, sodium bisulfite, parabens for oral inhalation. Bot. 10 mL, 30 mL. *Rx.*
Use: Bronchodilator.

Bronkotuss. (Hyrex) Chlorpheniramine maleate 4 mg, guaifenesin 100 mg, ephedrine sulfate 8.216 mg, hydriodic acid syrup 1.67 mg/5 mL w/alcohol 5%. Bot. Pt, gal. *Rx.*
Use: Antihistamine; decongestant; expectorant.

Brontex Liquid. (Procter & Gamble) Codeine phosphate 2.5 mg, guaifenesin 75 mg/5 mL, methylparaben, saccharin, sucrose. Liq. Bot. 473 mL. *c-v.*
Use: Antitussive expectorant; narcotic.

Brontex Tablets. (Procter & Gamble) Codeine phosphate 10 mg, guaifenesin 300 mg. Tab. Bot. 100s. *c-III.*

Use: Antitussive expectorant; narcotic.
•**broperamole.** (BROE-PURR-ah-mole)
USAN.
Use: Anti-inflammatory.
•**bropirimine.** (broe-PIE-rih-MEEN)
USAN.
Use: Antineoplastic; antiviral.
Broserpine. (Brothers) Reserpine
0.25 mg. Tab. Bot. 250s, 100s.
Use: Antihypertensive.
•**brotizolam.** (broe-TIE-zoe-LAM) USAN.
Use: Hypnotic; sedative.
Bro-T's. (Brothers) Bromisovalum 0.12 g,
carbromal 0.2 g. Tab. Bot. 100s, 1000s.
Rx.
Use: Sedative; anxiolytic.
Bro-Tuss. (Brothers) Dextromethorphan
HBr 15 mg, chlorpheniramine maleate
2 mg, phenylephrine hydrochloride
5 mg, ammonium Cl 100 mg, sodium
citrate 150 mg, vitamin C 30 mg/10 mL.
Bot. 4 oz, pt, gal. OTC.
Use: Antihistamine; antitussive; decongestant; expectorant.
Bro-Tuss A.C. (Brothers) Acetaminophen
120 mg, codeine phosphate 10 mg,
phonylephrine hydrochloride 5 mg,
chlorpheniramine maleate 2 mg, menthol 1 mg, alcohol 10%/5 mL. Bot. Pt,
gal. c-v.
Use: Analgesic; antihistamine; antitussive; decongestant.
BröveX (Athlon) Brompheniramine tannate 12 mg/5 mL, methylparaben, saccharin, sucrose, tartrazine, banana flavor. Oral Susp. Bot. 20 mL, 118 mL.
Rx.
Use: Antihistamine, nonselective alkylamine.
BröveX CT. (Athlon) Brompheniramine
tannate 12 mg, sucrose, banana flavor. Chew. Tab. Bot. 60s. Rx.
Use: Antihistamine, nonselective alkylamine.
Bryrel. (Sanofi-Synthelabo) Piperazine
citrate anhydrous 110 mg/mL. Syr. Bot.
oz. Rx.
Use: Anthelmintic.
B-Scorbic. (Pharmics) Vitamins C
300 mg, B₁ 25 mg, B₂ 10 mg, calcium
pantothenate 10 mg, niacinamide
50 mg, lemon flavored complex 200 mg.
Tab. Bot. 100s, 1000s. OTC.
Use: Mineral, vitamin supplement.
BSS. (Alcon) Sodium Cl 0.64%, potassium Cl 0.075%, magnesium Cl 0.03%,
calcium Cl 0.048%, sodium acetate
0.39%, sodium citrate 0.17%, sodium
hydroxide or hydrochloric acid. Bot.
15 mL, 30 mL, 250 mL, 500 mL. Rx.

Use: Irrigant, ophthalmic.
BSS Plus. (Alcon) **Part I:** Sodium Cl
7.44 mg, potassium Cl 0.395 mg, dibasic sodium phosphate 0.433 mg, sodium bicarbonate 2.19 mg, hydrochloric acid, or sodium hydroxide/mL. Soln.
Bot. 240 mL. **Part II:** Calcium chloride dihydrate 3.85 mg, magnesium
chloride hexahydrate 5 mg, dextrose
24 mg, glutathione disulfide 4.5 mg/mL.
Soln. Bot. 10 mL. Rx.
Use: Irrigant, ophthalmic.
BTA Rapid Urine Test. (Bard) Reagent
kit for detection of bladder tumor associated analytes in urine to aid in management of bladder cancer. Kits of
15 and 30 tests. Rx.
Use: Diagnostic aid.
•**bucainide maleate.** (hyoo-CANE-ido)
USAN.
Use: Cardiovascular agent, antiarrhythmic.
Bucet. (Forest) Butalbital 50 mg, acetaminophen 650 mg, benzyl alcohol,
EDTA, parabens. Cap. Bot. 20s, 100s,
500s. Rx.
Use: Analgesic.
buchu.
See: Barosmin.
•**bucindolol hydrochloride.** (BYOO-SIN-
doe-lole) USAN.
Use: Investigative; antihypertensive.
Bucladin-S. (AstraZeneca) Buclizine hy-
drochloride 50 mg. Softab Tab. Bot.
100s. Rx.
Use: Antiemetic; antivertigo.
•**buclizine hydrochloride.** (BYOO-klih-
zeen) USAN.
Use: Antiemetic; antinauseant.
See: Bucladin-S.
•**bucromarone.** (byoo-KROE-mah-rone)
USAN.
Use: Cardiovascular agent, antiar-
rhythmic.
•**bucrylate.** (BYOO-krih-late) USAN.
Use: Surgical aid, tissue adhesive.
Budeprion SR. (Impax) Bupropion hy-
drochloride 100 mg. SR Tab. 100s. Rx.
Use: Antidepressant.
•**budesonide.** (BYOO-DESS-oh-nide)
USAN.
Use: Anti-inflammatory; adrenocortical
steroid, glucocorticoid; corticosteroid,
intranasal steroid.
See: Entocort EC.
Pulmicort Respules.
Pulmicort Turbuhaler.
Rhinocort Aqua.
Buf Acne Cleansing Bar. (3M) Salicylic
acid 1%, sulfur 1% in detergent cleans-

ing bar. 3.5 oz. *OTC.*
Use: Antiacne.
Buf-Bar. (3M) Sulphur 3% and titanium dioxide. Bar 105 g. *OTC.*
Use: Antiacne.
Buf Body Scrub. (3M) Round cleansing sponge on plastic handles. *OTC.*
Use: Cleansing sponge.
Buff-A. (Merz) Aspirin acid 5 g buffered w/magnesium hydroxide, aluminum hydroxide dried gel. Tab. Bot. 100s, 1000s. *OTC.*
Use: Analgesic; antacid.
Buffaprin. (Buffington) Aspirin 325 mg buffered with magnesium oxide. Sugar, caffeine, lactose, salt free. Tab. *Dispens-A-Kit* 500s. *OTC.*
Use: Analgesic.
Buffasal. (Dover Pharmaceuticals) Aspirin 325 mg, magnesium oxide. Sugar, lactose, salt free. Tab. UD Box 500s. *OTC.*
Use: Analgesic.
Buffasal Max. (Dover Pharmaceuticals) Aspirin 500 mg, magnesium oxide. Sugar, lactose, salt free. Tab. *OTC.*
Use: Analgesic.
Bufferin AF Nite Time. (Bristol-Myers Squibb) Acetaminophen 500 mg, diphenhydramine citrate 38 mg, simethicone. Tab. Bot. 24s, 50s. *OTC.*
Use: Analgesic; sedative.
Buffered Aspirin. (Various Mfr.) Aspirin 325 mg with buffers. Tab. Bot. 100s, 500s, 1000s, UD 100s and 200s. *OTC.*
Use: Analgesic.
buffered intrathecal electrolyte/dextrose injection.
Use: Diluent. [Orphan Drug]
See: Elliot's B.
Buffex. (Roberts) Aspirin 325 mg w/dihydroxyaluminum aminoacetate. Tab. Bot. 1000s, *Sanipack* 1000s. *OTC.*
Use: Analgesic.
Buf Foot Care Kit. (3M) Cleansing system for the feet. *OTC.*
Use: Foot preparation.
Buf Foot Care Lotion. (3M) Moisturizing lotion for feet. *OTC.*
Use: Foot preparation.
Buf Foot Care Soap. (3M) Bar 3.5 oz. *OTC.*
Use: Foot preparation.
•**bufilcon A.** (BYOO-fill-kahn A) USAN.
Use: Contact lens material, hydrophilic.
Buf Kit for Acne. (3M) Cleansing sponge, cleansing bar 3.5 oz w/booklet, holding tray. *OTC.*
Use: Antiacne.
Buf Lotion. (3M) Moisturizing lotion. *OTC.*

Use: Emollient.
•**buformin.** (BYOO-FORE-min) USAN.
Use: Antidiabetic.
Bufosal. (Table Rock) Sodium salicylate 15 g/dram w/calcium carbonate, sodium bicarbonate as granulated effervescent powder. Bot. 4 oz. *OTC.*
Use: Analgesic; antacid.
Buf-Ped Non-Medicated Cleansing Sponge. (3M) Abrasive cleansing sponge. *OTC.*
Use: Cleansing skin or feet.
Buf-Puf Bodymate. (3M) Oval two-sided cleansing sponge. Abrasive/gentle. *OTC.*
Use: Cleansing all areas of the body.
Buf-Puf Medicated. (3M) Water-activated. Salicylic acid 0.5% (reg. strength), alcohols, benzoate, EDTA, triethanolamine, and vitamin E acetate. Salicylic acid 2% (max. strength). Pads. Jar 30s. *OTC.*
Use: Antiacne.
Buf-Puf Non-Medicated Cleansing Sponge. (3M) Abrasive cleansing sponge. *OTC.*
Use: Skin cleansing.
Buf-Sul Tablets and Suspension. (Sheryl) Sulfacetamide 167 mg, sulfadiazine 167 mg, sulfamerazine 167 mg. Tab. Bot. 100s. Susp. Bot. Pt. *Rx.*
Use: Anti-infective, sulfonamide.
Buf-Tabs. (Halsey Drug) Aspirin 5 g. Tab. w/aluminum hydroxide, glycine magnesium carbonate. Bot. 100s. *OTC.*
Use: Analgesic; antacid.
Bugs Bunny Chewable Vitamins and Minerals. (Bayer Corp. (Consumer Div.)) Vitamins A 5000 units, D 400 units, E 30 units, C 60 mg, folic acid 0.4 mg, B_1 1.5 mg, B_2 1.7 mg, niacin 20 mg, B_6 2 mg, B_{12} 6 mcg, biotin 40 mcg, pantothenic acid 10 mg, iron 18 mg, calcium 100 mg, phosphorus 100 mg, iodine 150 mcg, magnesium 20 mg, copper 2 mg, zinc 15 mg. Chew. Tab. Bot 60s. *OTC.*
Use: Mineral, vitamin supplement.
Bugs Bunny Complete. (Bayer Corp. (Consumer Div.)) Ca 100 mg, iron 18 mg, vitamins A 5000 units, D 400 units, E 30 mg, B_1 1.5 mg, B_2 1.7 mg, B_3 20 mg, B_5 10 mg, B_6 2 mg, C 60 mg, folic acid 0.4 mg, biotin 40 mcg, Cu, I, Mg, P, aspartame, phenylalanine, Zn 15 mg. Tab. Bot 60s. *OTC.*
Use: Mineral, vitamin supplement.
Bugs Bunny Plus Iron. (Bayer Corp. (Consumer Div.)) Vitamins A 2500 units, E 15 units, C 60 mg, folic acid 0.3 mg,

B_1 1.05 mg, B_2 1.2 mg, niacin 13.5 mg, B_6 1.05 mg, B_{12} 4.5 mcg, D 400 units, iron 15 mg. Chew. Tab. Bot. 60s. *OTC.*
Use: Mineral, vitamin supplement.

Bugs Bunny With Extra C. (Bayer Corp. (Consumer Div.)) Vitamins A 2500 units, D 400 units, E 15 units, C 250 mg, folic acid 0.3 mg, B_1 1.05 mg, B_2 1.2 mg, niacin 13.5 mg, B_6 1.05 mg, B_{12} 4.5 mcg. Tab. Bot. 60s. *OTC.*
Use: Mineral, vitamin supplement.

Bulk Forming Fiber Laxative. (Goldline Consumer) Calcium polycarbophil 625 mg (equiv. to polycarbophil 500 mg). Tab. Bot. 60s. *OTC.*
Use: Laxative.

bulkogen. A mucin extracted from the seeds of *Cyanopsis tetragonaloba.*

bulk-producing laxatives
See: Bulk Forming Fiber Laxative.
Citrucel.
Citrucel Sugar Free.
Equalactin.
Fiber-Lax.
Fiberall Orange Flavor.
Fiberall Tropical Fruit Flavor.
FiberCon.
FiberNorm.
Genfiber.
Genfiber, Orange Flavor.
Hydrocil Instant.
Konsyl.
Konsyl-D.
Konsyl Easy Mix Formula.
Konsyl Fiber.
Konsyl-Orange.
Maltsupex.
Metamucil.
Metamucil Orange Flavor, Original Texture.
Metamucil Orange Flavor, Smooth Texture.
Metamucil Original Texture.
Metamucil, Sugar Free, Orange Flavor, Smooth Texture.
Metamucil, Sugar Free, Smooth Texture.
Mitrolan.
Modane Bulk.
Natural Fiber Laxative.
Perdiem Fiber Therapy.
Polycarbophil.
Psyllium.
Reguloid.
Reguloid, Orange.
Reguloid, Sugar Free Orange.
Reguloid, Sugar Free Regular.
Serutan.
Syllact.
Unifiber.

Bullfrog. (Chattem) Benzophenone-3, octyl methoxycinnamate, isostearyl alcohol, aloe, hydrogenated vegetable oil, vitamin E. Waterproof. Stick 16.5 g. *OTC.*
Use: Sunscreen.

Bullfrog Extra Moisturizing. (Chattem) Benzophenone-3, octocrylene, octyl methoxycinnamate, vitamin E, aloe. SPF 18. Gel. Tube 90 g. *OTC.*
Use: Sunscreen.

Bullfrog for Kids. (Chattem) SPF 18. Octocrylene, octyl methoxycinnamate, octyl salicylate, vitamin E, aloe, alcohols, benzoate. Gel. Tube 60 g. *OTC.*
Use: Sunscreen.

Bullfrog Sport. (Chattem) SPF 18. Benzophenone-3, octocrylene, octyl methoxycinnamate, octyl salicylate, titanium dioxide, diazolidinyl urea, EDTA, parabens, vitamin A, aloe. Lot. Bot. 120 mL. *OTC.*
Use: Sunscreen.

Bullfrog Sunblock. (Chattem) SPF 18, 36. Benzophenone-3, octocrylene, octyl methoxycinnamate, aloe, vitamin E, isostearyl alcohol. PABA free. Waterproof. Gel. Tube 120 g. *OTC.*
Use: Sunscreen.

• **bumetanide.** (BYOO-MET-uh-hide) *USP 28.* Injection; Tablets.
Use: Diuretic.
See: Bumex.

bumetanide. (Various Mfr.) Bumetanide. **Tab:** 0.5 mg, 1 mg, 2 mg. Bot. 100s. **Inj.:** 0.25 mg/mL. Amp. 2 mL. Vial 2 mL, 4 mL, 10 mL; 4 mL fill in 5 mL. *Rx.*
Use: Diuretic.

• **bumetrizole.** (BYOO-meh-TRY-zole) USAN.
Use: Ultraviolet screen.

Bumex. (Roche) Bumetanide 0.5 mg, 1 mg, 2 mg. Tab. Bot. 100s, 500s (except 2 mg), UD 100s. *Rx.*
Use: Diuretic.

Buminate. (Baxter PPI) Normal serum albumin (human). **25%:** Soln. in 20 mL w/o administration set; 50 mL and 100 mL w/administration set. **5%:** Soln. in 250 mL, 500 mL w/administration set. *Rx.*
Use: Albumin replacement.

• **bunamidine hydrochloride.** (BYOO-NAM-ih-deen) USAN.
Use: Anthelmintic.

bunamiodyl sodium.
Use: Diagnostic aid, radiopaque medium.

• **bunaprolast.** (BYOO-nah-PROLE-ast) USAN.
Use: Antiasthmatic.

●**bunolol hydrochloride.** (BYOO-no-lole) USAN.
Use: Antiadrenergic, β-receptor.

Bun Reagent Strips. (Bayer Corp. (Consumer Div.)) Seralyzer reagent strips. A quantitative strip test for BUN in serum or plasma. Bot. 25s.
Use: Diagnostic aid.

Bupap. (ECR) Butalbital 50 mg, acetaminophen 650 mg. Tab. Bot. 100s. *Rx.*
Use: Analgesic.

Buphenyl. (Ucyclyd Pharma) Sodium phenylbutyrate. **Tab.:** 500 mg. Bot. 250s, 500s. **Pow.:** 3.2 g (3 g sodium phenylbutyrate)/tsp and 9.1 g (8.6 g sodium phenylbutyrate)/tsp. Bot. 500 mL, 950 mL. *Rx.*
Use: Antihyperammonemic.

●**bupicomide.** (byoo-PIH-koe-mide) USAN.
Use: Antihypertensive.

bupivacaine and epinephrine.
Use: Anesthetic, local.
See: Marcaine w/epinephrine.

bupivacaine hydrochloride. (Abbott) Bupivacaine hydrochloride 0.25%, 0.5%, 0.75%. Inj. Amp. 20 mL, 30 mL, 50 mL (0.25% only). Vial 10 mL, 30 mL. Multidose vial 50 mL (except 0.75%) with methylparaben 1 mg/mL. *Abboject* 30 mL (0.5% only), 50 mL (0.25% only). *Rx.*
Use: Anesthetic, local.

bupivacaine hydrochloride with epinephrine 1:200,000. (Hospira) Bupivicaine hydrochloride 0.25%, 0.5%, 0.75% with epinephrine 1:200,000. Inj. Amp. 30 mL (except 0.25%), 50 mL (0.25% only). Vial 10 mL, 30 mL (except 0.75%). Fliptop multidose vial 50 mL (except 0.75%). *Rx.*
Use: Anesthetic, local.

●**bupivacaine hydrochloride.** (byoo-PIH-vah-cane) *USP 28.*
Use: Anesthetic, local.
See: Bupivacaine hydrochloride.
  Bupivacaine hydrochloride with epinephrine 1:200,000.
  Bupivacaine Spinal.
  Marcaine.
  Marcaine w/epinephrine.
  Sensorcaine.
  Sensorcaine MPF.
  Sensorcaine MPF Spinal.

bupivacaine in dextrose.
Use: Anesthetic, local.

Bupivacaine Spinal. (Abbott) Bupivacaine hydrochloride 0.75% in dextrose 8.25%, preservative-free. Inj. Amp. 2 mL. *Rx.*
Use: Anesthetic, local.

Buprenex. (Reckitt & Benckiser) Buprenorphine hydrochloride 0.3 mg/mL w/50 mg anhydrous dextrose. Inj. Amp. 1 mL. *c-III.*
Use: Analgesic; narcotic.

●**buprenorphine hydrochloride.** (BYOO-preh-NAHR-feen) *USP 28.*
Use: Analgesic.
See: Buprenex.
  Subutex.
W/Naloxone.
See: Suboxone.

buprenorphine hydrochloride. (Abbott) Buprenorphine hydrochloride 0.3 mg/mL with anhydrous dextrose 50 mg. Inj. *Carpu-ject* 1 mL. *c-III.*
Use: Analgesic.

●**bupropion hydrochloride.** (byoo-PRO-pee-ahn) USAN.
Tall Man: BuPROPion.
Use: Antidepressant; smoking deterrent.
See: Budeprion SR.
  Wellbutrin.
  Wellbutrin SR.
  Wellbutrin XL.
  Zyban.

bupropion hydrochloride. (Global) Bupropion hydrochloride 200 mg. SR (12-hour) Tab. 60s, 180s. *Rx.*
Use: Antidepressant.

bupropion hydrochloride. (Reckitt & Colman)
Use: Treatment of opiate addiction. [Orphan Drug]

bupropion hydrochloride. (Various Mfr.) Bupropion hydrochloride 75 mg, 100 mg. Tab. Bot. 100s. *Rx.*
Use: Antidepressant.

bupropion hydrochloride. (Eon Labs) Bupropion hydrochloride 100 mg. ER Tab. 60s, 100s, 500s, Film-coated. *Rx.*
Use: Antidepressant.

bupropion hydrochloride sustained-release. (Watson) Bupropion hydrochloride 100 mg, 150 mg. Film-coated. ER Tab. 60s, 250s (150 mg only). *Rx.*
Use: Antidepressant.

●**buramate.** (BYOO-rah-mate) USAN.
Use: Anticonvulsant; antipsychotic; anxiolytic.

Burdeo. (Hill Dermaceuticals) Aluminum subacetate 100 mg, boric acid 300 mg/oz. Bot. 3 oz. Roll-on 8 oz. *OTC.*
Use: Deodorant.

Burn-a-Lay. (Ken-Gate) Chlorobutanol 0.75%, oxyquinoline benzoate 0.025%, zinc oxide 2%, thymol 0.5%. Cream. Tube oz. *OTC.*
Use: Burn therapy.

Burnate. (Burlington) Vitamins A 4000 units, D₂ 400 units, thiamine hydrochloride 3 mg, riboflavin 2 mg, niacinamide 10 mg, pyridine hydrochloride 2 mg, cyanocobalamin 5 mcg, calcium pantothenate 0.5 mg, folic acid 0.4 mg, ascorbic acid 50 mg, ferrous fumarate 300 mg, calcium 200 mg, iodine 0.15 mg, copper 1 mg, magnesium 5 mg, zinc 1.5 mg. Tab. Bot. 100s. *OTC.*
Use: Mineral, vitamin supplement.
Burn-Quel. Halperin aerosol dispenser 1 oz, 2 oz.
Use: Burn therapy.
burn therapy.
See: Americaine.
  Burn-A-Lay.
  Burn-Quel.
  Butesin Picrate.
  Foille.
  Nupercainal.
  Silvadene.
  Solarcaine.
  Sulfamylon.
  Unguentine.
Buro-Sol Antiseptic. (Doak Dermatologics) Contents make a diluted Burow's Solution. Aluminum acetate topical soln. plus benzethonium Cl. Pow. Pkg. (2.36 g) 12s, 100s. Bot. Pow. 4 oz, 1 lb, 5 lb. *OTC.*
Use: Astringent.
Bursul. (Burlington) Sulfamethizole 500 mg. Tab. Bot. 100s. *Rx.*
Use: Anti-infective; sulfonamide.
Bur-Zin. (Lamond) Aluminum acetate solution 2%, zinc oxide 10%. Bot. 4 oz, 8 oz, pt, qt, gal. Also w/o lanolin. *OTC.*
Use: Antipruritic, counterirritant.
●**buserelin acetate.** (BYOO-seh-REH-lin ASS-eh-tate) USAN.
Use: Gonad-stimulating principle.
BuSpar. (Bristol-Myers Squibb) Buspirone hydrochloride 5 mg, 10 mg, 15 mg, 30 mg, lactose. Tab. Bot. 100s, 500s (5 mg, 10 mg); *DIVIDOSE* 60s (15 mg, 30 mg); *DIVIDOSE* 180s (15 mg). *Rx.*
Use: Anxiolytic.
●**buspirone hydrochloride.** (byoo-SPY-rone) *USP 28.*
Tall Man: BusPIRone.
Use: Anxiolytic.
See: BuSpar.
buspirone hydrochloride. (Par) Buspirone hydrochloride 7.5 mg. May contain lactose. Tab. 100s, 500s. *Rx.*
Use: Anxiolytic.
buspirone hydrochloride. (Mylan) Buspirone hydrochloride 30 mg. Tab. Bot. 60s, 100s, 180s. *Rx.*
Use: Anxiolytic.

buspirone hydrochloride. (Various Mfr.) Buspirone hydrochloride 5 mg, 10 mg, 15 mg. May contain lactose. Tab. Bot. 100s, 500s. *Rx.*
Use: Anxiolytic.
●**busulfan.** (byoo-SULL-fate) *USP 28.*
Use: Alkylating agent.
See: Busulfex.
  Myleran.
Busulfex. (ESP Pharma) Busulfan 6 mg/mL. Inj. Single-use amp 10 mL w/syr. filters. *Rx.*
Use: Alkylating agent.
●**butabarbital.** (byoo-tah-BAR-bih-tahl) *USP 28.*
Use: Hypnotic; sedative.
See: BBS.
  Butisol.
  Da Sed.
  Expansatol.
  Medarsed.
W/Combinations
See: Airet R.
  Airet Y.
  Aludrox.
  Banatil.
  Bontril Timed No. 2.
  Broncholate.
  Butabell HMB.
  Cystospaz-SR.
  Dapco.
  Monosyl.
  Pedo-Sol.
  Petn Plus.
  Phenazopyridine Plus.
  Pyridium Plus.
  Quad-Set.
  Quibron Plus.
  Quiess.
  Sedapap.
  Sedapap-10.
  T-Caps.
●**butabarbital sodium.** (byoo-tah-BAR-bih-tahl) *USP 28.*
Use: Hypnotic; sedative.
See: BBS.
  Butalan.
  Butisol Sodium.
  Expansatol.
  Quiebar.
  Renbu.
W/Combinations.
See: Amino-Bar.
  Bancaps-C.
  Banesin Forte.
  Bisalate.
  Bontril.
  Butibel.
  Decholin-BB.
  Dolor Plus.

Dularin-TH.
Eulcin.
Hexett.
Hyonatol.
Hyonatol B.
Indogesic.
Metrogesic.
Minotal.
Monosyl.
Nidar.
Phrenilin.
Quiebel.
Sidonna.
Trio-Bar.
butabarbital sodium. Butabarbital sodium. **Tab.:** 15 mg, 30 mg. Bot. 100s (30 mg only), 1000s. **Elixir:** 30 mg/5 mL Bot. Pt.
Use: Sedative; hypnotic.
butacaine.
Use: Anesthetic, local.
•**butacetin.** (byoot-ASS-ih-tin) USAN.
Use: Analgesic; antidepressant.
•**butaclamol hydrochloride.** (byoo-tah-KLAM-ole) USAN.
Use: Antipsychotic.
Butagen Caps. (Ivax) Phenylbutazone 100 mg. Cap. Bot. 100s, 500s. *Rx.*
Use: Antirheumatic; hypnotic; sedative.
Butalan. (Lannett) Sodium butabarbital 0.2 g/30 mL. Elix. Bot. Pt, gal.
Use: Hypnotic; sedative.
•**butalbital.** (BYOO-TAL-bih-tuhl) *USP 28.* *Formerly Allybarbituric acid.*
Use: Hypnotic; sedative. .
See: Buff-A-Comp #3.
  Sandoptal.
W/Acetaminophen.
See: Bucet.
  Bupap.
  Butex Forte.
  Dolgic.
  Marten-Tab.
  Phrenilin.
  Phrenilin Forte.
  Promacet.
  Repan CF.
  Sedapap.
  Tencon.
W/Acetaminophen, caffeine.
See: Arbutal.
  Buff-A-Comp.
  Cefinal.
  Dolgic LQ.
  Esgic.
  Esgic-Plus.
  Fioricet.
  Fiorinal.
  Florpap.

Margesic.
Medigesic.
Protension.
Repan.
Triad.
W/Acetaminophen, codeine.
See: Phrenilin w/Codeine.
W/Aspirin, caffeine.
See: Amaphen.
  Americet.
  Arcet.
  Axotal.
  BAC.
  Bancap.
  Bucet.
  Butalbital Compound.
  Duogesic.
  Endolor.
  Esgic.
  Esgic-Plus.
  Fioricet.
  Fiorinal.
  G-1.
  Lanorinal.
  Lorprin.
  Margesic.
  Medigesic Plus.
  Phrenilin Forte.
  Repan.
  Sedapap-10.
  Tencon.
  Triad.
W/Aspirin, caffeine, codeine phosphate.
See: Ascomp with Codeine.
  Buff-A-Comp.
  Fiorinal with Codeine.
  Floricet with Codeine.
butalbital, acetaminophen, and caffeine. (Various Mfr.) Acetaminophen 325 mg, 500 mg, caffeine 40 mg, butalbital 50 mg, Tab. Bot. 30s, 50s, 100s, 500s, 1000s, UD 100s. *Rx.*
Use: Analgesic.
butalbital, acetaminophen, caffeine, and codeine phosphate. (Breckenridge) Codeine phosphate 30 mg, acetaminophen 325 mg, caffeine 40 mg, butalbital 50 mg. Cap. 100s, 500s. *c-III.*
Use: Narcotic analgesic.
butalbital and aspirin.
Use: Analgesic; sedative.
butalbital, aspirin, & caffeine. (Various Mfr.) **Tab.:** Aspirin 325 mg, caffeine 40 mg, butalbital 50 mg. Bot. 30s, 50s, 100s, 500s, 1000s, UD 100s. **Cap.:** Aspirin 325 mg, caffeine 40 mg, butalbital 50 mg. Bot. 100s, 1000s. *c-III.*
Use: Analgesic combination.

butalbital compound. (Various Mfr.) Aspirin 325 mg, caffeine 40 mg, butalbital 50 mg. Tab., Cap. Bot. 100s, 1000s (Tab. only). *c-iii.*
Use: Analgesic.

butalgin.
See: Methadone hydrochloride.

butallylonal. (Pernocton)
Use: Hypnotic.

•**butamben.** (BYOO-tam-ben) *USP 28.*
Formerly Butyl aminobenzoate.
Use: Anesthetic, local.

•**butamirate citrate.** (byoo-tah-MY-rate SIH-trate) USAN.
Use: Antitussive.

•**butane.** *NF 23.*
Use: Aerosol propellant.

•**butaperazine.** (BYOO-tah-PURR-ah-zuun) USAN.
Use: Antipsychotic.

•**butaperazine maleate.** USAN.
Use: Antipsychotic.

butaphyllamine. Ambuphylline. Theophylline aminoisobutanol. Theophylline with 2-amino-2-methyl-1-propanol.

Butapro. (Health for Life Brands) Butabarbital sodium 0.2 g/30 mL. Elix. Bot. pt, gal. *c-v.*
Use: Hypnotic; sedative.

•**butaprost.** (BYOO-tah-PRAHST) USAN.
Use: Bronchodilator.

Butazone. (Major) Phenylbutazone 100 mg. Cap. Tab. Bot. 100s (Cap. only), 500s. *Rx.*
Use: Antirheumatic.

•**butedronate tetrasodium.** (BYOO-teh-DROE-nate TET-rah-SO-dee-uhm) USAN.
Use: Diagnostic aid, bone imaging.

butelline.
See: Butacaine Sulfate.

•**butenafine hydrochloride.** (byoo-TEN-ah-feen) USAN.
Use: Topical anti-infective, antifungal.
See: Lotrimin Ultra.
Mentax.

butenafine hydrochloride. (Penederm)
Use: Treatment of interdigital tinea pedis, athlete's foot.

•**buterizine.** (byoo-TER-ih-ZEEN) USAN.
Use: Vasodilator, peripheral.

butethal. (Various Mfr.) *Rx.*
Use: Hypnotic; sedative.

butethanol.
See: Tetracaine.

Butex Forte. (Athlon) Acetaminophen 650 mg, butalbital 50 mg, benzyl alcohol, EDTA, parabens. Cap. Bot. 100s. *Rx.*
Use: Analgesic.

•**buthiazide.** (byoo-THIGH-azz-IDE) USAN.
Use: Antihypertensive; diuretic.

Butibel. (Wallace) Butabarbital sodium 15 mg, belladonna extract 15 mg. Tab.: Bot. 100s. Elix.: (w/alcohol 7%) 5 mL. Bot. Pt. *Rx.*
Use: Anticholinergic; antispasmodic; hypnotic; sedative.

•**butikacin.** (BYOO-tih-KAY-sin) USAN.
Use: Anti-infective.

•**butilfenin.** (BYOO-till-FEN-in) USAN.
Use: Diagnostic aid, hepatic function determination.

•**butirosin sulfate.** (byoo-TIHR-oh-sin) USAN. A mixture of the sulfates of the A and B forms of an antibiotic produced by Bacillus circularis.
Use: Anti-infective.

Butisol Sodium. (Wallace) Butabarbital sodium. Elix.: 30 mg/5 mL. Bot. Pt, gal. Tab.: 15 mg, 30 mg, 50 mg, 100 mg. Bot. 100s, 1000s (15 mg, 30 mg only). *c-iii.*
Use: Hypnotic; sedative.

•**butixirate.** (BYOO-TIX-ih-rate) USAN.
Use: Analgesic; antirheumatic.

•**butoconazole nitrate.** (BYOO-toe-KOE-nuh-zole) *USP 28.*
Use: Antifungal.
See: Gynazole-1.
Mycelex-3.

butolan. Benzylphenyl carbamate.

•**butonate.** (BYOO-tahn-ate) USAN.
Use: Anthelmintic.

•**butopamine.** (BYOO-TOE-pah-meen) USAN.
Use: Cardiovascular agent.

•**butoprozine hydrochloride.** (byoo-TOE-pro-ZEEN) USAN.
Use: Cardiovascular agent, antiarrhythmic; antianginal.

butopyronoxyl. (Indalone) Butylmesityl oxide.
Use: Insect repellant.

•**butorphanol.** (BYOO-TAR-fan-ahl) USAN.
Use: Analgesic; antitussive.

•**butorphanol tartrate.** (BYOO-TAR-fan-ahl) *USP 28.*
Use: Analgesic; antitussive.
See: Stadol.

butorphanol tartrate. (Various Mfr.) Butorphanol tartrate. Inj.: 1 mg/mL, 2 mg/mL. Vials 1 mL (1 mg/mL only), 2 mL. Nasal Spray: 10 mg/mL. Vials 2.5 mL. *c-iv.*
Use: Analgesic; antitussive.

•**butoxamine hydrochloride.** (byoo-TOX-ah-meen) USAN.
Use: Antidiabetic; antihyperlipoproteinemic.

•**butriptyline hydrochloride.** (BYOO-TRIP-till-een) USAN.
Use: Antidepressant.

•**butyl alcohol.** *NF 23.* Butyl alcohol is n-butyl alcohol.
Use: Pharmaceutic aid, solvent.

butyl aminobenzoate. n-butyl p-aminobenzoate. Scuroforme.
Use: Anesthetic, local.
W/Benzocaine, tetracaine hydrochloride.
See: Cetacaine.
W/Benzyl alcohol, phenylmercuric borate, benzocaine.
See: Dermathyn.
W/Procaine, benzyl alcohol, in sweet almond oil.
See: Anucaine.
W/Tetracaine.
See: Pontocaine.

•**butylated hydroxyanisole.** (hye-drox-ee-AN-i-sole) *NF 23.*
Use: Pharmaceutic aid, antioxidant.

•**butylated hydroxytoluene.** (hye-drox-ee-TOL-yoo-een) *NF 23.*
Use: Pharmaceutic aid, antioxidant.

•**butylparaben.** (byo-till-PAR-ah-ben) *NF 23.*
Use: Pharmaceutic aid, antifungal.

butylphenylsalicylamide.
See: Butylphenamide.

butyrophenone. Class of antipsychotic agents. *Rx.*
See: Haloperidol.

butyrylcholinesterase. (Pharmavene)
Use: Treat cocaine overdose; postsurgical apnea. [Orphan Drug]

B vitamins, parenteral.
See: B-Ject-100.

B vitamins with vitamin C, parenteral.
See: Key-Plex.
Neurodep.
Vicam.

B-Vite Injection. (Bluco) Vitamins B_1 50 mg, B_2 5 mg, B_6 5 mg, niacinamide 125 mg, B_{12} 1000 mcg, dexpanthenol 6 mg, C 50 mg/10 mL. Mono vial w/benzyl alcohol 1% in water for injection. *Rx.*
Use: Vitamin supplement.

Byclomine w/Phenobarbital. (Major)
Cap.: Dicyclomine hydrochloride 10 mg, phenobarbital 15 mg. Bot. 250s, 1000s. **Tab.:** Dicyclomine hydrochloride 20 mg, phenobarbital 15 mg. Bot. 100s, 250s, 1000s. *Rx.*
Use: Antispasmodic; sedative; hypnotic.

Byetta. (Amylin Pharmaceuticals, Inc.) Exenatide 5 mcg/dose, 10 mcg/dose. Subcutaneous Inj. Prefilled pens. 1.2 mL (60 doses) (5 mcg/dose only), 2.4 mL (60 doses) (10 mcg/dose only). *Rx.*
Use: Antidiabetic agent.

C

●**cabergoline.** (cab-ERR-go-leen) USAN.
Use: Antidyskinetic; antihyperprolactinemic; antiparkinsonian; dopamine agonist; hyperprolactinemic disorders treatment.
See: Dostinex.

●**cabufocon a.** (cab-YOU-FOE-kahn A) USAN.
Use: Contact lens material, hydrophobic.

●**cabufocon b.** (cab-YOU-FOE-kahn B) USAN.
Use: Contact lens material.

Cachexon. (Telluride) L-Glutathione.
Use: AIDS-associated cachexia.
[Orphan Drug]

cacodylic acid salts.
See: Ferric Salt.
Iron Salt.
Sodium Salt.

●**cactinomycin.** (KACK-tih-no-MY-sin) USAN. Antibiotic produced by *Streptomyces chrysomallus.* Formerly Actinomycin c.
Use: Antineoplastic.

cade oil.
See: Juniper Tar.

●**cadexomer iodine.** (kad-EX-oh-mer) USAN.
Use: Antiseptic; antiulcerative.

Caduet. (Pfizer) Amlodipine besylate/ atorvastatin calcium. 2.5 mg/10 mg, 2.5 mg/20 mg, 2.5 mg/40 mg, 5 mg/ 10 mg, 5 mg/20 mg, 5 mg/40 mg, 5 mg/80 mg, 10 mg/10 mg, 10 mg/ 20 mg, 10 mg/40 mg, 10 mg/80 mg. calcium carbonate. Film-coated. Tab. 30s. *Rx.*
Use: Antihyperlipidemic.

Cafatine. (Major) Ergotamine tartrate 2 mg, caffeine 100 mg. Supp. Box 12s. *Rx.*
Use: Antimigraine.

Cafatine-PB. (Major) Ergotamine tartrate 2 mg, caffeine 100 mg, belladonna alkaloids 0.25 mg, pentobarbital 60 mg. Supp. Box foil 10s. *Rx.*
Use: Antimigraine.

Cafcit. (Mead Johnson Nutritionals.) Caffeine citrate. **Oral Soln.:** 20 mg/mL.
Inj.: 20 mg/mL (caffeine citrate 2 mg equivalent to caffeine base 1 mg). Preservative free. Vial 3 mL. *Rx.*
Use: CNS stimulant.

Cafenol. (Sanofi-Synthelabo) Aspirin, caffeine. *OTC.*
Use: Analgesic combination.

Cafergot P-B Suppositories. (Novartis) Ergotamine tartrate 2 mg, caffeine 100 mg, bellafoline 0.25 mg, pentobarbital 60 mg. Supp. Box 12s. *Rx.*
Use: Antimigraine.

Cafergot P-B Tablets. (Novartis) Ergotamine tartrate 1 mg, caffeine 100 mg, bellafoline 0.125 mg, pentobarbital sodium 30 mg. Tab. *SigPak* dispensing pkg. of 90s, 250s. *c-iv.*
Use: Antimigraine.

Cafergot Suppositories. (Novartis) Ergotamine tartrate 2 mg, caffeine 100 mg in cocoa butter base. Supp. Box 12s. *Rx.*
Use: Antimigraine.

Cafergot Tablets. (Novartis) Ergotamine tartrate 1 mg, caffeine 100 mg. SC Tab. Bot. 250s. *SigPak* dispensing pkg. of 00s. *Rx.*
Use: Antimigraine.

Caffedrine. (Various Mfr.) Caffeine 200 mg. Tab. Pkg. 16s. *OTC.*
Use: CNS stimulant.

●**caffeine.** (ka-FEEN) *USP 28.*
Use: CNS stimulant; apnea of prematurity.
See: Cafcit.
Caffedrine.
Enerjets.
Fastlene.
.44 Magnum.
Keep Alert.
Keep Going.
Lucidex.
Maximum Strength NoDoz.
Overtime.
Stay Alert.
Stay Awake.
Stim 250.
357 HR Magnum.
20-20.
Valentine.
Vivarin.
W/Combinations.
See: Americet.
Anacin.
Anacin Maximum Strength.
APAP-Plus.
Ascomp with Codeine.
BC Powder Arthritis Strength.
BC Powder Original Formula.
Butalbital, Aspirin, and Caffeine.
Butalbital Compound.
Caffeine and Sodium Benzoate.
Esgic.
Esgic-Plus.
Excedrin Aspirin Free.
Excedrin Extra Strength.
Excedrin Migraine.
Excedrin QuickTabs.

Excedrin Tension Headache.
Fiorinal with Codeine.
Floricet with Codeine.
Goody's Extra Strength Headache.
Levacet.
Margesic.
Medigesic.
Midol Maximum Strength Menstrual.
Orphengesic.
Orphengisic Forte.
Painaid.
Painaid ESF Extra-Strength Formula.
Panlor DC.
Panlor SS.
Saleto.
Summit Extra Strength.
Triad.
Vanquish.
caffeine and sodium benzoate. (Bedford, American Regent) Caffeine and sodium benzoate 250 mg/mL (121 mg caffeine, 129 mg sodium benxoate). Inj. Single-use vial. 2 mL. *Rx.*
Use: CNS stimulant.
•**caffeine citrate.** *USP 28.*
Use: CNS stimulant.
W/Combinations.
See: Scot-Tussin Original Clear 5-Action Cold and Allergy Formula.
Scot-Tussin Original 5-Action Cold and Allergy Formula.
caffeine citrated.
Use: CNS stimulant.
caffeine sodio-benzoate.
See: Caffeine Sodium Benzoate.
caffeine sodium salicylate. (Various Mfr.) Caffeine sodium salicylate Bot. 1 oz; Pkg. 0.25 lb, 1 lb. *OTC.*
Use: CNS stimulant.
Cagol. (Harvey) Guaiacol 0.1 g, eucalyptol 0.08 g, iodoform 0.2 g, camphor 0.05 g/2 mL in olive oil. Vial 30 mL. *Rx.*
Use: Expectorant.
Caladryl. (Pfizer) Calamine 8%, pramoxine hydrochloride 1%, alcohol, camphor, diazolidinyl urea, parabens. Lot. Bot. 177 mL. *OTC.*
Use: Antipruritic, topical; poison ivy treatment.
Caladryl Clear. (Pfizer) Pramoxine hydrochloride 1%, zinc acetate 0.1%, alcohol, camphor, diazolidinyl urea, parabens. Lot. Bot. 177 mL. *OTC.*
Use: Antipruritic, topical; poison ivy treatment.
Calafol. (Alaven) Vitamin B$_6$ 25 mg, vitamin B$_{12}$ 425 mg, FA 1.6 mg, Ca 400 mg, D$_3$ 400 units. Tab. 90s. *Rx.*
Use: Nutritional product.
Calaformula. (Eric, Kirk & Gary) Ferrous gluconate 130 mg, calcium lactate

130 mg, vitamins A 1000 units, D 400 units, B$_1$ 2 mg, B$_2$ 2 mg, niacinamide 5 mg, ascorbic acid 20 mg, folic acid 0.13 mg, Mg 0.25 mg, Cu 0.25 mg, Zn 0.25 mg, Mn 0.25 mg, K 0.075 mg. Cap. Bot. 50s, 100s, 500s, 1000s, 5000s. *OTC.*
Use: Mineral, vitamin supplement.
Calaformula F. (Eric, Kirk & Gary) Calaformula plus fluorine 0.333 mg. Tab. Bot. 100s. *Rx.*
Use: Mineral, vitamin supplement; dental caries agent.   ,
Calahist. (Walgreen) Diphenhydramine hydrochloride 1%, calamine 8.1%, camphor 0.1%. Lot. Bot. 6 oz. *OTC.*
Use: Antipruritic, topical.
•**calamine.** (kal-a-MINE) *USP 28.*
Use: Protectant, topical.
W/Combinations.
See: Caladryl.
Ivarest Maximum Strength.
calamine. (Various Mfr.) Calamine 6.97%, zinc oxide 6.97%, glycerin. Lot. Bot. 118 mL, 240 mL, 480 mL. *OTC.*
Use: Antiseptic; astringent; poison ivy treatment.
calamine, phenolated. (Humco) Calamine, zinc oxide, glycerin, liquefied phenol 1%. Lot. Bot. 177 mL. *OTC.*
Use: Antiseptic; astringent; poison ivy treatment.
Calamycin. (Pfeiffer) Pyrilamine maleate, zinc oxide 10%, calamine 10%, benzocaine, chloroxylenol, zirconium oxide, isopropyl alcohol 10%. Lot. Bot. 120 mL. *OTC.*
Use: Antipruritic, topical.
Calan. (Searle) Verapamil hydrochloride 40 mg, 80 mg, 120 mg. Film-coated. Tab. Bot. 100s, 500s (80 mg only), 1000s (80 mg, 120 mg only). *Rx.*
Use: Calcium channel blocker.
Calan SR. (Searle) Verapamil hydrochloride 120 mg, 180 mg, 240 mg. Film-coated. SR Tab. Bot. 100s, 500s (240 mg only), UD 100s. *Rx.*
Use: Calcium channel blocker.
Cal-Bid. (Roberts) Elemental calcium 250 mg, ascorbic acid 100 mg, vitamin D 125 units. Tab. Bot. 100s. *OTC.*
Use: Mineral, vitamin supplement.
Cal-Carb Forte. (Vitaline) Calcium carbonate. **Tab.:** 1250 mg (elemental calcium 500 mg). Bot. 100s. **Chew Tab.:** 1250 mg (elemental calcium 500 mg), mint flavor. Bot. 100s. *OTC.*
Use: Mineral.
Calcarb 600 with Vitamin D. (Ivax) Calcium carbonate 1.5 g (elemental calcium 600 mg), vitamin D 125 units. Tab.

Bot. 60s. *OTC.*
Use: Vitamin, mineral supplement.
Calcet. (Mission Pharmacal) Elemental calcium 153 mg, vitamin D 100 units. Tab. Bot. 100s. *OTC.*
Use: Mineral, vitamin supplement.
Calcet Plus. (Mission Pharmacal) Elemental calcium 152.8 mg, elemental iron 18 mg, vitamins A 5000 units, D 400 units, E 30 mg, B$_1$ 2.25 mg, B$_2$ 2.55 mg, B$_3$ 30 mg, B$_5$ 15 mg, B$_6$ 3 mg, B$_{12}$ 9 mcg, C 500 mg, folic acid 0.8 mg, zinc 15 mg, sugar. Tab. Bot 60s. *OTC.*
Use: Mineral, vitamin supplement.
Calcibind. (Mission Pharmacal) Inorganic phosphate content 34%, sodium content 11%. Packets: Cellulose sodium phosphate 25 g. Single-dose 90 packets, 000 g bulk pack. *Rx.*
Use: Genitourinary.
CalciCaps. (Nion Corp.) Calcium (dibasic calcium phosphate, calcium gluconate, calcium carbonate) 125 mg, vitamin D 67 units, phosphorus 60 mg. Tab. Bot. 100s, 500s. *OTC.*
Use: Mineral, vitamin supplement.
CalciCaps M-Z. (Nion Corp.) Ca 400 mg, Mg 133 mg, Zn 5 mg, vitamin A 1667 mg, D 133 units, Se. Tab. Bot. 90s. *OTC.*
Use: Mineral, vitamin supplement.
CalciCaps, Super. (Nion Corp.) Calcium 400 mg, phosphorus 41.7 mg, vitamin D 100 units. Tab. Bot. 90s. *OTC.*
Use: Mineral, vitamin supplement.
CalciCaps with Iron. (Nion Corp.) Calcium 125 mg, phosphorus 60 mg, vitamin D 67 units, ferrous gluconate 7 mg, iodine. Tab. Bot. 100s. *OTC.*
Use: Mineral, vitamin supplement.
Calci-Chew. (Watson) Calcium carbonate 1250 mg (elemental calcium 500 mg), sugar, cherry and assorted flavors. Chew. Tab. Bot. 100s. *OTC.*
Use: Mineral supplement.
Calcidrine. (Abbott) Codeine 8.4 mg, calcium iodide anhydrous 152 mg, alcohol 6%/5 mL. Syr. Bot. 120 mL, 480 mL. *c-v.*
Use: Antitussive; expectorant.
•**calcifediol.** (KAL-sih-feh-DIE-ahl) *USP 28.*
Use: Calcium regulator.
See: Calderol.
calciferol. (Schwarz Pharma) Ergocalciferol (Vitamin D$_2$). **Liq.:** 8000 units/mL. Bot. 60 mL. **Inj.:** 500,000 units/mL. Amp. 1 mL. *Rx-OTC.*
Use: Refractory rickets; familial hypophosphatemia; hypoparathyroidism.

Calcijex. (Abbott) Calcitriol 1 mcg, 2 mcg/mL, polysorbate 20 4 mg, sodium chloride 1.5 mg, sodium ascorbate 10 mg, dibasic sodium phosphate 7.6 mg, anhydrous, EDTA. Inj. Amp. 1 mL. *Rx.*
Use: Antihypocalcemic; antihypoparathyroid.
Calcimar. (Aventis) Calcitonin solution (salmon origin), phenol/200 units/mL. Inj. Vial 2 mL. *Rx.*
Use: Treatment of Paget disease.
Calci-Mix. (Watson) Calcium carbonate 1250 mg (elemental calcium 500 mg). Cap. Bot. 100s. *OTC.*
Use: Mineral supplement.
Calcionate. (Various Mfr.) Calcium glubionate 1.8 g/5 mL. Syr. Bot. 473 mL. *OTC.*
Use: Mineral supplement.
•**calcipotriene.** (kal-sih-POE-try-een) USAN.
Use: Antipsoriatic.
See: Dovonex.
Calciquid. (Breckenridge) Calcium glubionate 1.8 g/5 mL. Syr. Bot. 473 mL. *OTC.*
Use: Mineral supplement.
•**calcitonin.** (kal-sih-TOE-nin) USAN.
Use: Treatment of Paget disease, calcium regulator.
See: Calcimar.
Cibacalcin.
Miacalcin.
calcitonin-human for injection. Hormone from thyroid gland.
Use: Plasma hypocalcemic hormone; symptomatic Paget disease of bone. [Orphan Drug]
See: Cibacalcin.
calcitonin-salmon.
Use: Antihypercalcemic.
See: Calcimar.
Miacalcin.
Osteocalcin.
Cal-Citrate-250. (Bio-Tech) Elemental calcium 250 mg. Tab. Bot. 250s. *OTC.*
Use: Mineral supplement.
Cal-Citrate-225. (Bio-Tech) Elemental calcium 225 mg. Cap. Bot. 100s, 250s. *OTC.*
Use: Mineral.
•**calcitriol.** (KAL-sih-TRY-ole) USAN.
Use: Antihypocalcemic, calcium regulator.
See: Calcijex.
Rocaltrol.
calcitriol. (Roxane) Calcitriol 1 mcg/mL. Oral Soln. 15 mL with 20 single-use graduated oral dispensers. *Rx.*

Use: Antihypocalcemic, calcium regulator.

calcitriol. (Teva) Calcitriol 0.25 mcg, 0.5 mcg. Mannitol, sorbitol. Cap. 100s. *Rx.*
Use: Vitamin.

Calcitriol Injection. (aaiPharma) Calcitriol 1 mcg/mL, 2 mcg/mL, sodium chloride, EDTA. Inj. 1 mL vial. *Rx.*
Use: Antihypocalcemic, calcium regulator.

calcium.
Use: Mineral.
See: Calcium Acetate.
Calcium Citrate.
Calcium Carbonate.
Calcium Gluconate.
Calcium Lactate.
Tricalcium Phosphate.

•**calcium acetate.** *USP 28.*
Use: Pharmaceutic aid, buffering agent; hyperphosphatemia; mineral.
See: PhosLo.

calcium acetate mineral/electrolytes.
See: Phos-Ex 62.5 Mini-Tabs.
PhosLo.

calcium acetylsalicylate. Kalmopyrin, kalsetal, soluble aspirin, tylcalsin.
Use: Analgesic.

calcium aluminum carbonate. W/DI-Amino Acetate Complex.
See: Ancid.

calcium aminosalicylate. *NF 23.* Aminosalicylate calcium.

calcium amphomycin.
See: Amphomycin.

calcium and magnesium carbonates.
Use: Mineral; antacid.

•**calcium and vitamin D with minerals.** *USP 28.*
Use: Mineral, vitamin supplement.

Calcium Antacid Extra Strength. (Various Mfr.) Calcium carbonate 750 mg (elemental calcium 300 mg). Chew. Tab. Bot. 96s. *OTC.*
Use: Mineral; antacid.

•**calcium ascorbate.** (KAL-see-uhm a-skor-bate) *USP 28.*
Use: Nutritional supplement.

calcium ascorbate. (Freeda) **Tab.:** Calcium ascorbate 500 mg, calcium 75 mg. Buffered. Bot. 100s, 250s, 500s. **Pow.:** Calcium ascorbate 814 mg, calcium 100 mg per ¼ tsp. Buffered. Bot. 120 g, 1 lb. *OTC.*
Use: Mineral supplement.

calcium 4-benzamidosalicylate. Calcium aminacyl B-PAS. Benzoylpas calcium.
See: Benzopas.

calcium benzoyl-p-aminosalicylate.
See: Benzoylpas Calcium.

calcium benzoylpas.
See: Benzoylpas Calcium.

calcium bis-dioctyl sulfosuccinate.
See: Dioctyl Calcium.

calcium carbimide. Calcium cyanamide. Sulfosuccinate.
See: Alka-Mints.
Amitone.
Antacid.
Chooz.
Dicarbosil.
Extra Strength Antacid.
Mallamint.
Mylanta.
Tums.

•**calcium carbonate.** *USP 28. Formerly calcium carbonate, precipitated.*
Use: Antacid; mineral; hyperphosphatemia.
See: Cal-Carb Forte.
Calcarb 600 with Vitamin D.
Calci-Chew.
Calci-Mix.
Calcium Antacid Extra Strength.
Calcium 600.
Caltrate 600.
Extra Strength Alkets Antacid.
Florical.
Maalox Antacid/Calcium Supplement.
Maalox Maximum Strength Quick Dissolve.
Maalox Quick Dissolve.
Nephro-Calci.
Os-Cal 500.
Oysco 500.
Oyst-Cal 500.
Oyster Shell Calcium.
R&D Calcium Carbonate/600.
Rolaids Extra Strength Softchews
Surpass.
Surpass Extra Strength.
Trial Antacid.
Tums.
Tums Calcium for Life Bone Health.
Tums Calcium for Life PMS.
Tums E-X.
Tums Smooth Dissolve.
Tums Ultra.
W/Combinations.
See: Acid-X.
Ca-Plus.
Gas Ban.
Gas-X with Maalox.
Lactocal.
MagneBind 400 Rx.
MagneBind 300.
MagneBind 200.
Mylanta Supreme.
Natabec.

Pepcid Complete.
Rolaids.
Rolaids Extra Strength.
Rolaids Multi-Symptom.
Titralac.
calcium carbonate. (Roxane) **Tab.:**
1250 mg. Bot. 100s, UD 100s. **Susp.:**
1250 mg/5 mL. Bot. 500 mL, UD 5 mL.
OTC.
Use: Antacid; calcium supplement.
calcium carbonate. (Various Mfr.) Precipitated chalk; carbonic acid, calcium salt (1:1).
Use: Antacid.
calcium carbonate. (Various Mfr.) Calcium carbonate. **Tab.:** 648 to 650 mg (elemental calcium 260 mg), 1250 mg (elemental calcium 500 mg), 1500 mg (elemental calcium 600 mg). Bot. 60s (1500 mg only), 100s (unsupl 1500 mg), 150s (1500 mg only), 1000s (648 to 650 mg only). **Chew Tab.:** 1250 mg (elemental calcium 500 mg). Bot. 60s. **Oral Susp.:** 1250 mg/5 mL (elemental calcium 500 mg). Bot. 500 mL, UD 5 mL. **Pow.:** Bot. 454 g. *OTC.*
Use: Mineral.
calcium carbonate. (Various Mfr.) Calcium carbonate 648 to 650 mg (elemental calcium 260 mg), original and mint flavors. Tab. Bot. 100s, 250s, 500s. *OTC.*
Use: Mineral.
calcium carbonate, aromatic. (Fli l illy) Calcium carbonate 10 g. Tab. Bot. 100s, 1000s. *OTC.*
Use: Antacid.
Calcium Carbonate 600 mg + Vitamin D. (Major) Ca 600 mg, D 125 units. Tab. Bot. 60s. *OTC.*
Use: Mineral, vitamin supplement.
calcium carbonate, sodium chloride, and potassium chloride.
Use: Salt replacement.
See: Sustain.
calcium caseinate.
See: Casec.
calcium channel blockers.
Use: Angina pectoris; vasospastic and unstable angina.
See: Amlodipine.
 Diltiazem hydrochloride.
 Felodipine.
 Isradipine.
 Nicardipine Hydrochloride.
 Nifedipine.
 Nimodipine.
 Nisoldipine.
 Verapamil hydrochloride.
Calcium Chel 330. (Novartis)
Use: Antidote, heavy metals.

See: Calcium Trisodium Pentetate.
●**calcium chloride.** *USP 28.*
Use: Electrolyte, calcium replenisher.
calcium chloride. (Pharmacia) Calcium chloride. 1 g. Inj. Amp. 10 mL, 25s. (Torigian) 1 g. Inj. Amp. 10 mL 12s, 25s, 100s. (Trent) 10%. Inj. Amp. 10 mL. (Bayer Corp. (Consumer Div.)) 13.6 mEq/10 mL Inj. Vial.
Use: Antihypocalcemic.
●**calcium chloride Ca 45.** USAN.
Use: Radiopharmaceutical.
●**calcium chloride Ca 47.** USAN.
Use: Radiopharmaceutical.
●**calcium citrate.** *USP 28.*
Use: Mineral supplement.
See: Cal-Citrate-250.
 Cal-Citrate-225.
 Citrunul.
 Citracal Liquitab.
calcium citrate. (Various Mfr.) **Tab.:** Elemental calcium 250 mg. Bot. 100s, 120s, 250s, 500s, 1000s. Calcium citrate 950 mg. Bot. 100s. **Pow.:** Elemental calcium 760 mg/5 mL. Pow. Bot. 454 g. *OTC.*
Use: Mineral.
calcium cyclamate. Calcium cyclohexanesulfamate.
calcium cyclobarbital.
Use: Central depressant.
calcium cyclohexanesulfamate.
See: Calcium Cyclamate.
●**calcium dioctyl sulfosuccinate.** (KAL-see-uhm die-OC-tuhl sul-foe-SUCK-sih-nate) *USP 28.* Docusate calcium.
See: Surfak.
●**calcium disodium edathamil.** (KAL-see-uhm die-SO-dee-uhm eh-DATH-ah-mil) *USP 28.*
See: Edetate calcium disodium.
●**calcium disodium edetate.** (KAL-see-uhm die-SO-dee-uhm ed-deh-TATE) *USP 28.* Edetate calcium disodium.
Use: Antidote for acute and chronic lead poisoning, lead encephalopathy.
See: Calcium Disodium Versenate.
calcium disodium versenate. (3M) Calcium disodium edetate 200 mg/mL. Inj. Amp 5 mL. *Rx.*
Use: IV or IM for lead poisoning and lead encephalopathy.
●**calcium dl-pantothenate.** (KAL-see-uhm dl pan-toe-THEH-nate) *USP 28.* Calcium Pantothenate, Racemic.
calcium edetate sodium.
See: Calcium Disodium Edetate.
calcium EDTA.
See: Calcium Disodium Versenate.

●**calcium glubionate.** (KAL-see-uhm
glue-BYE-oh-nate) *USP 28.*
Use: Calcium replenisher.
calcium glucoheptonate. (Various Mfr.)
Cal. D-glucoheptonate O. *OTC.*
Use: Nutritional supplement.
●**calcium gluconate.** (KAL-see-uhm glue-
KAHN-nate) *USP 28.*
Use: Mineral supplement.
calcium gluconate. (Freeda) Elemental
calcium 346.7 mg/15 mL. Pow. Bot.
454 g. *OTC.*
Use: Mineral supplement.
calcium gluconate. (Various Mfr.) Elemental calcium 50 mg. Tab. Bot. 100s,
500s. calcium gluconate 500 mg (elemental calcium 45 mg), 648 to 650 mg
(elemental calcium 58.5 to 60 mg),
972 to 975 mg (elemental calcium
87.75 to 90 mg). Tab. Bot. 1000s. *OTC.*
Use: Mineral supplement.
calcium gluconate gel 2.5%. (LTR Pharmaceuticals, Inc.)
Use: Topical treatment of hydrogen fluoride burns. [Orphan Drug]
See: H-F.
calcium glycerophosphate. Neurosin.
(Various Mfr.)
●**calcium hydroxide.** (KAL-see-uhm high-
DROX-ide) *USP 28.*
Use: Astringent; pharmaceutic necessity for calamine lotion.
calcium hydroxide. (Eli Lilly) Calcium
hydroxide. Powder Bot. 4 oz.
Use: Lime water.
calcium hypophosphite. (N.Y. Quinine
& Chem. Works)
calcium iodide.
W/Codeine Phosphate.
See: Calcidrine.
W/Chloral Hydrate, Ephedrine hydrochlo-
ride.
See: Iophen.
calcium iodized.
See: Cal-Lime-1.
W/Calcium Creosote.
See: Niocrese.
calcium iodobehenate. Calioben.
(Various Mfr.).
●**calcium ipodate.** (KAL-see-uhm ip-OH-
date) *USP 28.* Ipodate calcium.
See: Oragrafin calcium.
calcium kinate gluconate. Kinate is
hexahydrotetrahydroxybenzoate. Cal-
cium quinate.
●**calcium lactate.** *USP 28.*
Use: Mineral supplement.
See: Cal-Lac.
W/Calcium glycerophosphate.
See: Calphosan.

W/Calcium glycerophosphate, phenol, sodium Cl.
See: Calpholac.
Calphosan.
W/Niacinamide, folic acid, ferrous gluconate, vitamins.
See: Pergrava No. 2.
W/Theobromine sodium salicylate,
phenobarbital.
See: Zinc-220.
calcium lactate. (Various Mfr.) Calcium
lactate 648 to 650 mg (elemental calcium 84.5 mg). Tab. Bot. 100s, 1000s.
Elemental calcium 100 mg. Tab. Bot.
100s, 250s. *OTC.*
Use: Mineral supplement.
●**calcium lactobionate.** *USP 28.*
Use: Mineral supplement.
calcium lactophosphate. Lactic acid hy-
drogen phosphate calcium salt.
calcium leucovorin.
Use: For overdosage of folic acid an-
tagonists; megaloblastic anemias.
See: Leucovorin calcium.
Wellcovorin.
●**calcium levulinate.** (KAL-see-uhm LEV-
you-lih-nate) *USP 28.*
Use: Calcium replenisher.
Calcium Magnesium Chelated. (NBTY)
Ca 500 mg, Mg 250 mg. Tab. Bot. 50s,
100s. *OTC.*
Use: Mineral supplement.
Calcium Magnesium Zinc. (NBTY) Ca
333 mg, Mg 133 mg, Zn 8.3 mg. Tab.
Bot. 100. *OTC.*
Use: Mineral supplement.
calcium novobiocin. Calcium salt of an
antibacterial substance produced by
Streptomyces niveus.
Use: Anti-infective.
●**calcium oxytetracycline.** (KAL-see-uhm
ox-EE-tet-rah-SYE-kleen) *NF 23.* Oxy-
tetracycline calcium.
●**calcium pantothenate.** (KAL-see-uhm
pan-toe-THEH-nate) *USP 28.*
Use: Pantothenic acid (B$_5$) deficiency;
coenzyme A precursor; vitamin, en-
zyme cofactor.
W/Ascorbic Acid, viacinamide, vitamins
B$_1$, B$_2$, B$_6$, B$_{12}$, A, D, E.
See: Tota-Vi-Caps.
W/Calcium carbonate.
See: Ilomel.
W/Calcium carbonate, ferrous fumarate,
niacinamide.
See: Prenatag.
W/Danthron.
See: Modane.
Parlax.

W/Docusate sodium.
See: Pantyl.
W/Methoscopolamine nitrate, mephobarbital.
See: Ilocalm.
W/Niacinamide and vitamins.
See: Allbee C-800.
Allbee T.
Allbee with C.
Ferrovite.
Fumatinic.
Maintenance Vitamin Formula.
Mulvidren.
OB-Tabs.
Probec.
Probec-T.
Stuart Hematinic.
Stuart Therapeutic Multivitamin.
W/Niacinamide, vitamins B_1, B_2, B_6
See: Noviplex.
W/Vitamin C, niacinamide, zinc sulfate, magnesium sulfate, vitamins B_1, B_2, B_6.
See: Vicon-C.
W/Vitamin C, niacin, zinc sulfate, vitamins E, B_1, B_2, B_6, B_{12}.
See: Z-Bec.
W/Vitamin complex, iron.
See: Vita-iron.
W/Vitamins A, E, C, zinc sulfate, magnesium sulfate, niacinamide, B_1, B_2, manganese Cl, B_6, folic acid, B_{12}.
See: Vicon Forte.
W/Vitamins D_1, D_2, D_6, D_{12}, niacinamide, choline Cl, inositol, dl-methionine, testosterone, estrone, procaine.
See: Geriatric Vitamin Formula.
W/Vitamins, minerals, methyltestosterone, ethinyl estradiol, niacinamide.
See: Geritag.
W/Vitamins, minerals, niacinamide.
See: Arcum-VM.
Capre.
Orovimin.
Os-Cal Forte.
Os-Vim.
Stuartinic.
Theramin.
Uplex.
W/Zinc sulfate, niacinamide, magnesium sulfate, manganese sulfate, vitamin complex.
See: Vicon Plus.
calcium pantothenate. (Various Mfr.) Calcium pantothenate 100 mg (equiv. to 92 mg pantothenic acid), 218 mg (equiv. to 200 mg pantothenic acid), 545 mg (equiv. to 500 mg pantothenic acid). Tab. Bot. 100s, 250s. *OTC.*
Use: Pantothenic acid deficiency.

●**calcium pantothenate, racemic.** (KAL-see-uhm pan-toe-THEH-nate, ray-SEE-mik) *USP 28.*
Use: Vitamin B, enzyme cofactor.
●**calcium phosphate, dibasic.** *USP 28.*
Use: Calcium replenisher; pharmaceutic aid, tablet base.
W/Dicalcium Phosphate.
See: Diostate D.
calcium phosphate, monocalcium.
See: Dicalcium Phosphate.
●**calcium phosphate, tribasic.** *NF 23.*
Use: Mineral supplement.
See: Posture.
calcium-phosphorus-free.
See: Fosfree.
●**calcium polycarbophil.** (KAL-see-uhm PAHL-ee-CAR-boe-fill) *USP 28.*
Use: Laxative.
See: Equalactin.
Fibercon.
FiberNorm.
Konsyl Fiber.
calcium polysulfide.
Use: Wet dressing, soak.
See: Vlemasque.
calcium quinate.
See: Calcium Kinate Gluconate.
calcium receptor agonists.
See: Cinacalcet hydrochloride
●**calcium saccharate.** (KAL-see-uhm SACK-uh-rate) *USP 28.*
Use: Pharmaceutic aid, sweetener, stabilizer.
calcium saccharin. Saccharin calcium.
Use: Pharmaceutic aid, sweetener.
●**calcium silicate.** (KAL-see-uhm SILL-eh-cate) *NF 23.*
Use: Pharmaceutic aid, tablet excipient.
Calcium 600. (Rugby) Calcium carbonate 1500 mg (elemental calcium 600 mg). Tab. Bot. 60s. *OTC.*
Use: Mineral supplement.
Calcium 600 + D. (NBTY) Calcium 600 mg, vitamin D 125 units. Film coated. Tab. Bot. 60s. *OTC.*
Use: Mineral, vitamin supplement.
Calcium 600/Vitamin D. (Schein) Ca 600 mg, D 125 units. Tab. Bot. 60s. *OTC.*
Use: Mineral, vitamin supplement.
●**calcium stearate.** (KAL-see-uhm STEE-uh-rate) *NF 23.*
Use: Pharmaceutic aid, tablet and capsule lubricant.
calcium succinate.
W/Aspirin.
See: Ber-Ex.
Dolcin.

•**calcium sulfate.** *NF 23.*
Use: Pharmaceutic aid, tablet and capsule diluent.

calcium thiosulfate.
Use: Wet dressing, soak.
See: Vlemasque.

calcium trisodium pentetate.
Use: Antidote, heavy metals.
See: Calcium Chel 330.

•**calcium undecylenate.** (KAL-see-uhm un-DES-eye-lie-nate) *USP 28.*
Use: Antifungal.

calcium undecylenate. Calcium undecylenate 10% Powder.
Use: Antifungal, topical.
See: Cruex Squeeze.

Caldecort. (Novartis) Hydrocortisone 0.5%. Spray. Aerosol Can 1.5 oz. *OTC.*
Use: Corticosteroid, topical.

Calderol. (Organon Teknika) Calcifediol 20 mcg, 50 mcg, propylparabens. Cap. Bot. 60s. *Rx.*
Use: Antihypocalcemia.

•**caldiamide sodium.** (KAL-DIE-ah-MIDE) USAN.
Use: Pharmaceutic aid.

Cal-D-Mint. (Enzyme Process) Ca 800 mg, Mg 150 mg, Fe 18 mg, iodine 0.1 mg, Cu 2 mg, vitamin D 200 units. Tab. Bot. 100s, 250s. *OTC.*
Use: Mineral, vitamin supplement.

Cal-D-Phos. (Archer-Taylor) Dicalcium phosphate 4.5 g, calcium gluconate 3 g, vitamin D. Tab. Bot. 1000s. *OTC.*
Use: Mineral, vitamin supplement.

calfactant.
Use: Lung surfactant.
See: Infasurf.

Cal-Gest. (Rugby) Calcium carbonate 500 mg (elemental calcium 200 mg), dextrose, assorted flavors. Chew. Tab. Bot. 150s. *OTC.*
Use: Mineral supplement.

Calicylic. (Gordon Laboratories) Salicylic acid 10%, mineral oil, cetyl alcohol, propylene glycol, white wax, sodium lauryl sulfate, oleic acid, methyl- and propylparabens, triethanolamine. Cream. Tube. 60 g. *OTC.*
Use: Keratolytic.

Cal-Im. (Standex) Calcium glycerophosphate 1%, calcium levulinate 1.5%. Vial 30 mL. *Rx.*
Use: Mineral supplement.

Calinate-FA. (Solvay) Ca 250 mg, vitamins A 4000 units, D 400 units, B_1 3 mg, B_2 3 mg, B_6 5 mg, B_{12} 1 mcg, folic acid 1 mg, C 50 mg, B_3 (niacinamide) 20 mg, B_5 (d-panthenol) 1 mg, Fe 60 mg, I 0.02 mg, Mn 0.2 mg, Mg 0.2 mg, Zn 0.1 mg, Cu 0.15 mg. Tab.

Bot. 100s. *Rx.*
Use: Mineral, vitamin supplement.

calioben.
See: Calcium Iodobehenate.

Calivite. (Apco) Calcium carbonate 885 mg, ferrous sulfate 199 mg, vitamins A 3600 units, D 400 units, C 75 mg, B_1 1.5 mg, B_2 1.95 mg, B_6 0.75 mg, nicotinic acid 15 mg, B_{12} activity 0.025 mcg, choline 1500 mcg, inositol 2500 mcg, pantothenic acid 75 mcg, folic acid 25 mcg, p-aminobenzoic acid 12 mcg, K 10 mg, Mg 1 mg, Zn 0.075 mg, Mn 0.02 mg, Cu 0.01 mg, cobalt 0.02 mcg. Tab. Bot. 100s. *OTC.*
Use: Mineral, vitamin supplement.

Cal-Lac. (Bio-Tech) Calcium lactate 500 mg (elemental calcium 96 mg). Cap. Bot. 100s. *OTC.*
Use: Mineral supplement.

Cal-Lime-1. (Scrip) Calcium iodized 1 g. Tab. Bot. 1000s.

Calmol 4. (Mentholatum Co.) Cocoa butter 80%, zinc oxide 10%, parabens. Supp. Box 12s, 24s. *OTC.*
Use: Anorectal preparation.

Calmosin. (Spanner) Calcium gluconate, strontium bromide. Amp. 10 mL. 100s.

Cal-Nate. (Ethex) Ca 125 mg, Fe 27 mg, vitamin A 2700 units, D_3 400 units, E 30 units, B_1 3 mg, B_2 3.4 mg, B_3 20 mg, B_6 20 mg, C 120 mg, folic acid 1 mg, Zn 25 mg, iodine 150 mcg, Cu 2 mg, docusate sodium 50 mg. Tab. 100s. *Rx.*
Use: Multivitamin.

Cal-Nor. (Vortech Pharmaceuticals) Calcium glycerophosphate 100 mg, calcium levulinate 150 mg/10 mL. Inj. Vial 100 mL. *Rx.*
Use: Mineral supplement.

Calocarb. (Pal-Pak, Inc.) Calcium carbonate 648 mg, cinnamon flavor. Tab. Bot. 1000s. *OTC.*
Use: Antacid.

calomel. Mercurous Cl.
Use: Cathartic.

Calotabs. (Calotabs) Docusate sodium 100 mg, casanthranol 30 mg. Tab. Box 10s. *OTC.*
Use: Laxative.

caloxidine (iodized calcium).
See: Calcium Iodized.

Calphosan. (Glenwood) Calcium glycerophosphate 50 mg, calcium lactate 50 mg/10 mL sodium Cl solution. Contains calcium 0.08 mEq/mL. Inj. Amp. 10 mL, Vial 60 mL. *Rx.*
Use: Mineral supplement.

Calsan. (Burgin-Arden) Calcium glycerophosphate 10 mg, calcium levulinate 15 mg, chlorobutanol 0.5% mL. Inj. Vial

100 mL. *Rx.*
Use: Calcium supplement.
Cal Sup Instant 1000. (3M) Elemental calcium 1000 mg, vitamins D 400 units, C 60 mg. Pow. Packet 12s. *OTC.*
Use: Mineral, vitamin supplement.
Cal Sup 600 Plus. (3M) Elemental calcium 600 mg, vitamins D 200 units, C 30 mg. Tab. Bot. 60s. *OTC.*
Use: Mineral, vitamin supplement.
●**calteridol calcium.** (KAL-TER-ih-dahl KAL-see-uhm) USAN.
Use: Pharmaceutic aid.
Caltrate Plus. (Wyeth) Vitamin D 200 units, Ca 600 mg, Zn 7.5 mg, Mg, Cu, Mn, B. Sugar free. Tab. Bot. 60s. *OTC.*
Use: Mineral, vitamin supplement.
Caltrate 600. (Wyoth) Caloium oarbo nate 1500 mg (elemental calcium 600 mg), preservative free. Tab. Bot. 60s. *OTC.*
Use: Mineral supplement.
Caltrate 600 + D. (Wyeth) Vitamin D 200 units, Ca 600 mg. Sugar free. Tab. Bot. 60s. *OTC.*
Use: Mineral, vitamin supplement.
Caltrate 600 + Iron. (Wyeth) Calcium carbonate 600 mg, iron 18 mg, vitamin D 125 units. Tab. Bot. 60s. *OTC.*
Use: Mineral, vitamin supplement.
Caltro. (Geneva) Elemental calcium 250 mg, vitamin D 125 units. Tab. Bot. 100s, 1000s. *OTC.*
Use: Mineral, vitamin supplement.
●**calusterone.** (kal-YOO-ster-ohn) USAN.
Use: Antineoplastic.
Cam-Ap-Es. (Camall) Hydrochlorothiazide 15 mg, reserpine 0.1 mg, hydralazine hydrochloride 25 mg. Tab. Bot. 100s. *Rx.*
Use: Antihypertensive.
Cama Arthritis Pain Reliever. (Novartis) Aspirin 500 mg, magnesium oxide 150 mg, aluminum hydroxide 125 mg, methylparaben. Tab. Bot. 100s. *OTC.*
Use: Analgesic; antacid.
●**cambendazole.** (kam-BEND-ah-zole) USAN.
Use: Anthelmintic.
Camellia. (O'Leary) Moisturizer for face, hands and body. For normal to oily skin. Lot. Bot. 4 oz. *OTC.*
Use: Emollient.
Cameo. (Medco Lab) Mineral oil, isopropyl myristate, lanolin oil, PEG-8-Dioleate. Oil. Plastic Bot. 8 oz, 16 oz, 32 oz. *OTC.*
Use: Emollient.

●**camiglibose.** (kah-mih-GLIE-bose) USAN.
Use: Antidiabetic, glucohydrolase inhibitor.
Camila. (Barr) Norethindrone 0.35 mg, lactose. Tab. 28s. *Rx.*
Use: Sex hormone, contraceptive hormone.
Camouflage Crayon. (O'Leary) Coverup for minor skin discolorations, under eye concealer, lipstick fixer. Available in 6 shades. Crayon 0.05 oz. *OTC.*
Use: Skin coverup.
Campath. (Berlex) Alemtuzumab 30 mg/ mL. Sodium chloride 8 mg, dibasic sodium phosphate 1.44 mg, potassium chloride 0.2 mg, monobasic potassium phosphate 0.2 mg, polysorbate 80 0.1 mg, EDTA 0.0187 mg. Preservative free. Soln. for Inj. Single use vials. *Rx.*
Use: Monoclonal antibody.
Campho-Phenique. (Bayer) Camphor 10.8%, phenol 4.7%. **Liq.:** Bot. 22.5 mL, 45 mL, 120 mL. **Gel:** Tube. 6.9 g, 15 g. *OTC.*
Use: Analgesic; antiseptic, local.
Campho-Phenique Cold Sore Treatment and Scab Relief. (Bayer) Pramoxine hydrochloride 1%. Petrolatum 30%, alcohol, EDTA, glycerin, parabens, ureas. Mint flavor. Cream. 6.5 g. *OTC.*
Use: Local anesthetics, topical.
●**camphor.** (KAM-fore) *USP 28.*
Use: Topical antipruritic; anti-infective; pharmaceutic necessity for camphorated phenol; paregoric and flexible collodion; antitussive; expectorant, local counterirritant; nasal decongestant.
See: Anti-Itch Gel.
　Itch Relief Gel Spritz
　TheraFlu Vapor Stick.
　TheraFlu Vapor Stick Cough & Muscle Aches.
　Vicks Cough.
　Vicks Sinex.
　Vicks Vapor Inhaler.
　Vicks VapoRub.
　Vicks VapoSteam.
W/Combinations.
See: Bayer Muscle & Joint Cream.
　Ivy Super Dry.
camphorated, parachlorophenol.
Use: Anti-infective, dental.
camphoric acid ester. Ester of p-Tolylmethylcarbinol as Diethanolamine Salt.
Campral. (Forest) Acamprosate calcium 333 mg. DR Tab. 180s, 1,080s, Dose pak 180s. *Rx.*
Use: Antialcoholic agent.

Camptosar. (Pharmacia) Irinotecan hydrochloride 20 mg/mL, sorbitol 45 mg. Inj. Vial. 2 mL, 5 mL. *Rx.*
Use: Antineoplastic, DNA topoisomerase inhibitor.

Canasa. (Axcan Scandipharm) Mesalamine 500 mg, 1,000 mg (in base of hard fat). Supp. 30s. *Rx.*
Use: Anti-inflammatory.

Cancidas. (Merck) Caspofungin acetate 50 mg, 70 mg. Pow. for Inj., lyophilized. Single-use Vial. *Rx.*
Use: Antifungal, echinocandins.

C & E Capsules. (NBTY) Vitamins C 500 mg, E 400 mg. Cap. Bot. 50s, 100s. *OTC.*
Use: Vitamin supplement.

•**candesartan.** (kan-deh-SAHR-tan) USAN.
Use: Antagonist, angiotensin II receptor; antihypertensive.

•**candesartan cilexetil.** (kan-deh-SAHR-tan sigh-LEX-eh-till) USAN.
Use: Antagonist, angiotensin II receptor; antihypertensive.
See: Atacand.
W/Hydrochlorothiazide.
See: Atacand HCT.

C & E Softgels. (NBTY) Vitamins E 400 mg, C 500 mg. Cap. Bot. 50s.
Use: Vitamin supplement.

•**candicidin.** (KAN-dih-SIDE-in) *USP 28.*
An antifungal antibiotic derived from *Strepomyces griseus.*
Use: Antifungal.

candida albicans skin test antigen.
Use: Diagnostic aid.
See: Candin.

candida test. (SmithKline Diagnostics) Culture test for *Candida.* Box 4s.
Use: Diagnostic aid.

Candin. (ALK) *Candida albicans* skin test antigen prepared from the culture filtrate and cells of 2 strains of *Candida albicans.* Vial 1 mL. *Rx.*
Use: Evaluation of cell-mediated immunity; diagnostic aid.

•**candoxatril.** (kan-DOXE-at-trill) USAN.
Use: Antihypertensive.

•**candoxatrilat.** (kan-DOXE-at-trill-at) USAN.
Use: Antihypertensive.

Candycon. (Allison) Chlorprophenpyridamine maleate 2 mg, phenylephrine hydrochloride 5 mg. Tab. Bot. 50s. *OTC.*
Use: Antihistamine; decongestant.

•**canertinib dihydrochloride.** (can-ER-tin-ib) USAN.
Use: Epithelial tumors.

•**canfosfamide hydrochloride.** (kan-FOS-fa-mide) USAN.
Use: Antineoplastic.

Cankaid Liquid. (Dickinson) Carbamide peroxide 10% in anhydrous glycerol, EDTA. Soln. 22.5 mL. *OTC.*
Use: Mouth and throat product.

cannabinoids.
Use: Antiemetic; antivertigo agent.
See: Dronabinol.

cannabis.
Use: Antiemetic; antivertigo.
See: Dronabinol.

•**canrenoate potassium.** (kan-REN-oh-ate) USAN.
Use: Aldosterone antagonist.

•**canrenone.** (kan-REN-ohn) USAN.
Use: Aldosterone antagonist.

cantharidin.
Use: Keratolytic.

Cantil. (Hoechst Marion Roussel) Mepenzolate bromide 25 mg. Tab. Bot. 100s. *Rx.*
Use: Anticholinergic; antispasmodic.

•**cantuzumab mertansine.** (can-TUE-zue-mab mer-TAN-seen) USAN.
Use: Colorectal and pancreatic cancer.

Ca-Orotate. (Miller Pharmacal Group) Calcium (as calcium orotate) 50 mg. Tab. Bot. 100s. *OTC.*
Use: Mineral supplement.

C-A-P. (Eastman Kodak) Cellulose acetate phthalate.

Capastat Sulfate. (Dura) Capreomycin 1 g/10 mL. Vial 10 mL. *Rx.*
Use: Antituberculosis agent.

•**capecitabine.** (cap-eh-SITE-ah-bean) USAN.
Use: Antineoplastic, antimetabolite.
See: Xeloda.

Capex. (Galderma) Fluocinolone acetonide 0.01%, dibasic calcium phosphate dihydrate 5.48 mg. Shampoo. In 12 mg capsule with shampoo base to be mixed by pharmacist before dispensing. *Formerly Fs Shampoo (Hill) Rx.*
Use: Anti-inflammatory; corticosteroid, topical.

•**capimorelin tartrate.** (CAP-eh-mohr-lyn) USAN.
Use: Prevention of frailty; congestive heart failure; catabolic illness.

Capital with Codeine. (Carnrick) Acetaminophen 120 mg, codeine phosphate 12 mg/5 mL. Susp. Bot. 473 mL. *c-v.*
Use: Analgesic combination, narcotic.

Capital with Codeine. (Carnrick) Codeine phosphate 30 mg, acetaminophen 325 mg, Tab. Bot. 100s. *c-III.*
Use: Analgesic combination, narcotic.

Capitrol Cream Shampoo. (Bristol-Myers Squibb) Chloroxine 2%. Shampoo. Bot. 120 mL. *Rx.*
Use: Antiseborrheic.
Ca-Plus-Protein. (Miller Pharmacal Group) Calcium (as contained in a calcium-protein complex made with specially isolated soy protein) 280 mg. Tab. Bot. 100s. *OTC.*
Use: Mineral supplement.
Capnitro. (Freeport) Nitroglycerin 6.5 mg. TR Cap. Bot. 100s. *Rx.*
Use: Antianginal agent.
●**capobenate sodium.** (CAP-oh-BEN-ate) USAN.
Use: Cardiovascular agent, antiarrhythmic.
●**capobenic acid.** (CAP-oh-BEN-ik) USAN
Use: Cardiovascular agent, antiarrhythmic.
Capoten. (PAR) Captopril 12.5 mg, 25 mg, 50 mg, 100 mg, lactose. Tab. Bot 100s, 1,000s (except 12.5 mg and 100 mg), UD 100s (except 100 mg). *Rx.*
Use: Antihypertensive; angiotensin-converting enzyme inhibitor.
Capozide. (Bristol-Myers Squibb) Captopril/hydrochlorothiazide 25/15 mg, 25/25 mg, 50/15 mg, 50/25 mg. Tab. Bot. 100s. *Rx.*
Use: Antihypertensive; angiotensin-converting enzyme inhibitor.
●**capravirine.** (cap-ruh-VYE-reen) USAN.
Use: Antiviral.
●**capreomycin.** (CAP-ree-oh-MY-sin) *USP 28.* An antibiotic derived from *Streptomyces capreolus. Capreomycin*
Use: Antituberculosis agent.
See: Capastat Sulfate.
●**capromab pendetide.** (KAP-row-mab PEN-deh-TIDE) USAN.
Use: Monoclonal antibody.
See: ProstaScint.
●**capromorelin tartrate.** (kap-roe-moor-lyn) USAN.
Use: Prevention of frailty; congestive heart failure; carabolic illness.
caprylate, salts.
See: Sodium Caprylate.
Zinc Caprylate.
caprylate sodium. (Ingram) Caprylate sodium 33%. Inj. Amp. 1 mL. Pkg. 12s, 25s, 100s.
Use: Antifungal.
See: Sodium Caprylate.
●**capsaicin.** (kap-SAY-uh-sin) *USP 28.*
Use: Analgesic, topical; antineuralgic; specific pain syndromes, topical.

See: Capsin.
Capzasin-P.
Dolorac.
No Pain-HP.
Pain Doctor.
Pain-X.
R-Gel.
Rid-a-Pain-HP.
Zostrix.
capsaicin. (Various Mfr.) Capsaicin 0.025%, 0.075%. Cream. Tube. 45 g (0.025% only), 60 g. *OTC.*
Use: Analgesic, topical; antineuralgic; specific pain syndromes, topical.
●**capsicum.** (KAP-see-kum) *USP 28.*
Use: Carminative; counterirritant, external; stomachic.
●**capsicum oleoresin.** (KAP-see-kum OH-leo oh RES in) *USP 28.*
Use: Carminative; counterirritant, external; stomachic.
Capsin. (Fleming & Co.) Capsaicin 0.025%, 0.075%, benzyl alcohol, propylene glycol, denatured alcohol. Lot. Bot. 59 mL. *OTC.*
Use: Analgesic, topical.
capsules, empty gelatin. (Eli Lilly) Lilly markets clear empty gelatin capsules in sizes 000, 00, 0, 1, 2, 3, 4, 5.
●**captamine hydrochloride.** (KAP-tam-een) USAN.
Use: Depigmentor.
●**captopril.** (KAP-toe-prill) *USP 28.*
Use: Antihypertensive; angiotensin-converting enzyme inhibitor.
See: Capoten.
captopril. (Various Mfr.) Captopril 12.5 mg, 25 mg, 50 mg, 100 mg. Tab. Bot. 100s, 500s, 1000s, 5000s (except 100 mg), UD 100s, blister 600s. *Rx.*
Use: Antihypertensive; angiotensin-converting enzyme inhibitor.
captopril and hydrochlorothiazide. (Various Mfr.) Captopril 25 mg, 50 mg, hydrochlorothiazide 15 mg; captopril 25 mg, 50 mg, hydrochlorothiazide 25 mg. Tab. Bot. 100s. *Rx.*
Use: Antihypertensive; diuretic.
●**capuride.** (CAP-you-ride) USAN.
Use: Hypnotic; sedative.
Capzasin-P. (Thompson Medical) Capsaicin 0.025%, benzyl and cetyl alcohols. Cream. Tube 42.5 g. *OTC.*
Use: Analgesic, topical.
Carac. (Dermik) Fluorouracil 0.5%, glycerin, parabens. Cream. Tube 30 g. *Rx.*
Use: Pyrimidine antagonist, topical.
●**caracemide.** (car-ASS-eh-MIDE) USAN.
Use: Antineoplastic.

Carafate. (Axcan Scandipharm) **Tab.:**
Sucralfate 1 g. Bot. 100s, 120s, 500s.
Susp.: Sucralfate 1 g/10 mL, sorbitol,
methylparaben. Bot. 415 mL. *Rx.*
Use: Antiulcerative.
•**caramel.** (KAR-uh-mel) *NF 23.*
Use: Pharmaceutic aid, color.
caramiphen ethanedisulfonate.
W/Phenylephrine hydrochloride, Phen-
indamine Tartrate.
See: Dondril.
caramiphen hydrochloride.
Use: Proposed antiparkinson.
•**caraway.** (KAR-uh-way) *NF 23.*
Use: Flavoring.
•**caraway oil.** (KAR-uh-way oil) *NF 23.*
Use: Flavoring.
•**carbachol.** (KAR-bah-kole) *USP 28.*
Use: Parasympathomimetic; choliner-
gic, ophthalmic.
See: Carbastat.
Miostat Intraocular.
Murocarb.
W/Methylcellulose.
See: Isopto Carbachol.
carbacrylamine resins.
Use: Cation-exchange resin.
•**carbadox.** (KAR-bah-dox) USAN.
Use: Anti-infective.
•**carbamazepine.** (KAR-bam-AZE-uh-
peen) *USP 28.*
Use: Analgesic; anticonvulsant.
See: Carbatrol.
Epitol.
Equetro.
Tegretol.
carbamazepine. (Alpharma) Carba-
mazepine 200 mg/10 mL. Sorbitol, sucrose, citrus/vanilla flavor. Susp. Dose
cups. 10 mL. *Rx.*
Use: Anticonvulsant.
carbamazepine. (Various Mfr.) Carba-
mazepine. **Chew. Tab.:** 100 mg. May
contain corn starch, sorbitol, sucrose.
Bot. 100s, 500s, UD 50s, UD 100s.
Tab.: 200 mg. May contain corn starch,
lactose. Bot. 100s, 500s, 1000s, UD
100s, 300s. **Susp.:** 100 mg/5 mL. May
contain saccharin, sorbitol, sucrose,
parabens. Bot. 450 mL, UD 10 mL. *Rx.*
Use: Treatment of epilepsy and tri-
geminal neuralgia.
carbamide.
Use: Emollient.
See: Aquacare.
Carmol 20.
Nutraplus.
Rea-Lo.
Ultra Mide Moisturizer.
Ureacin-20.

carbamide compounds.
See: Acetylcarbromal.
Carbromal.
•**carbamide peroxide.** (CAR-bah-mide
purr-ox-ide) *USP 28.* Urea compound
w/hydrogen peroxide (1:1).
Use: Anti-inflammatory; mouth and
throat product.
See: Cankaid Liquid.
Gly-Oxide.
Orajel Perioseptic.
carbamide peroxide 6.5% in glycerin.
Use: Otic.
See: Murine Ear.
Murine Ear Wax Removal System.
carbamylcholine chloride.
See: Carbachol.
carbamylmethylcholine chloride.
See: Urecholine.
•**carbantel lauryl sulfate.** (CAR-ban-tell
LAH-ruhl) USAN.
Use: Anthelmintic.
carbapenem.
Use: Anti-infective.
See: Ertapenem.
Invanz.
carbarsone. (Various Mfr.) N-carbam-
oylarsanilic acid. Amabevan, ameban,
amibiarson, arsambide, fenarsone, leu-
carsone, aminarsone, amebarsone. p-
Ureidobenzenearsonic acid. Caps.
Use: Acute and chronic amebiasis and
trichomoniasis.
•**carbaspirin calcium.** (kar-ba-SPEER-in)
USAN.
Use: Analgesic.
Carbastat. (Novartis Ophthalmics)
Carbachol 0.1%, sodium Cl 0.64%, potassium Cl 0.075%, calcium Cl dihydrate 0.048%, magnesium Cl hexahydrate 0.03%, sodium acetate trihydrate 0.39%, sodium citrate dihydrate
0.17%. Soln. Vial 1.5 mL. *Rx.*
Use: Antiglaucoma.
Carbatrol. (Shire) Carbamazepine
100 mg, 200 mg, 300 mg, lactose. ER
Cap. Bot. 14s (100 mg only), 30s (except 100 mg), 120s. *Rx.*
Use: Anticonvulsant.
•**carbazeran.** (KAR-BAY-zeh-ran) USAN.
Use: Cardiovascular agent.
•**carbenicillin disodium, sterile.** (KAR-
ben-ih-SILL-in die-SO-dee-uhm,
STEER-ill) *USP 28.*
Use: Anti-infective.
See: Geopen.
•**carbenicillin indanyl sodium.** (car-BEN-
ih-SILL-in IN-duh-nil) *USP 28.*
Use: Anti-infective.
See: Geocillin.

- **carbenicillin phenyl sodium.** (CAR-ben-ih-SILL-in FEN-ill) USAN.
  Use: Anti-infective.
- **carbenicillin potassium.** (CAR-ben-ih-SILL-in) USAN.
  Use: Anti-infective.
- **carbenoxolone sodium.** (CAR-ben-ox-ah-lone) USAN.
  Use: Corticosteroid, topical.
  carbetapentane citrate.
  Use: Antitussive.
  W/Combinations.
  See: Levall.
  Tussar SF.
  Tussar-2.
  carbetapentane tannate.
  Use: Antitussive.
  W/Combinations.
  See' C-Tanna 12D
  Dytan-CS.
  Exratuss.
  Quad Tann.
  Rynatuss.
  Rynatuss Pediatric.
  Tannic-12
  Trionate.
  Tussi-12.
  Tussi-12D.
  Tussi-12D S.
  Tussi-12 S.
  Tussizone-12 RF.
  Tuss-Tan.
  Tuss-Tan Pediatric.
- **carbetimer.** (kar-BEH-tih-MER) USAN.
  Use: Antineoplastic.
  Carbex. (DuPont) Selegiline hydrochloride 5 mg, lactose. Tab. Bot. 60s. *Rx.*
  Use: Used in combination with levo-dopa/carbidopa for treatment of Parkinson disease.
- **carbidopa.** (KAR-bih-doe-puh) *USP 28.*
  Use: Decarboxylase inhibitor.
  See: Lodosyn.
  W/Levodopa.
  See: Parcopa.
  Sinemet CR.
  Sinemet-10/100.
  Sinemet-25/100.
  Sinemet-25/250.
  W/Levodopa and Entacapone.
  See: Stalevo.
  carbidopa and levodopa. (Various Mfr.)
  ER Tab.: Carbidopa 25 mg, levodopa 100 mg. 100s, 500s. **Tab.:** Carbidopa 10 mg, levodopa 100 mg; carbidopa 25 mg, levodopa 100 mg; carbidopa 25 mg, levodopa 250 mg; carbidopa 50 mg, levodopa 200 mg. Bot. 100s, 500s, 1000s. *Rx.*
  Use: Antiparkinsonian.

carbinoxamine.
  Use: Antihistamine.
  See: Histex CT.
  Histex I/E.
  Histex Pd.
  Pediatex.
  Palgic.
  W/Combinations.
  See: Andehist DM.
  Andehist DM NR.
  Balamine DM.
  Carbofed DM.
  DMax.
  DMax Pediatric.
  Histex HC.
  Hydrocodone Bitartrate 5 mg/Pseudo-ephedrine hydrochloride 30 mg/Carbinoxamine Maleate 2 mg.
  Norel LA.
  Pannaz S
  Pediatex-DM.
  Rondec-DM.
  Sildec-DM.
  Tussafed.
  W/Pseudoephedrine hydrochloride.
  See: Biohist-LA.
  Carbodex DM.
  Cardec DM.
  Cardec-S.
  Coldec D.
  C.P.-DM.
  Cydec.
  Cydec-DM.
  Palgic-D.
  Palgic DS.
  Pannaz.
  Pediatex-D.
  Rondec.
  Rondec-TR.
  carbinoxamine maleate
  Use: Antihistamine, nonselective ethanolamine.
  See: Histex CT.
  Histex PD.
  Pediatex.
  carbinoxamine maleate, pseudoephedrine hydrochloride, dextromethorphan HBr. (Cypress) **Syr.:** Carbinoxamine maleate 4 mg, pseudoephedrine hydrochloride 60 mg, dextromethorphan HBr 15 mg/5 mL. Bot. 120 mL, pt, gal. **Drops:** Carbinoxamine maleate 2 mg, pseudoephedrine hydrochloride 25 mg, dextromethorphan HBr 4 mg/mL. Bot. 30 mL w/dropper. *Rx.*
  Use: Antihistamine; decongestant; antitussive.
  carbinoxamine oral drops. (Morton Grove) Carbinoxamine maleate 2 mg, pseudoephedrine hydrochloride 25 mg/mL, sorbitol, parabens, alcohol free,

raspberry, fruit flavors. Bot. 30 mL w/calibrated dropper. *Rx.*
Use: Upper respiratory combination, antihistamine, decongestant.

carbinoxamine syrup. (Morton Grove) Carbinoxamine maleate 4 mg, pseudoephedrine hydrochloride 60 mg/5 mL, sorbitol, parabens, alcohol free, raspberry, fruit flavors. Bot. 118 mL, 237 mL, 473 mL. *Rx.*
Use: Upper respiratory combination, antihistamine, decongestant.

● **carbiphene hydrochloride.** (KAR-bih-FEEN) USAN.
Use: Analgesic.

Carbiset. (Nutripharm Laboratories, Inc.) Pseudoephedrine 60 mg, carbinoxamine maleate 4 mg. Tab. Bot. 100s, 500s. *Rx.*
Use: Antihistamine; decongestant.

Carbiset-TR. (Nutripharm Laboratories, Inc.) Pseudoephedrine hydrochloride 120 mg, carbinoxamine maleate 8 mg. Tab. Bot. 100s. *Rx.*
Use: Antihistamine; decongestant.

Carbocaine. (Eastman-Kodak) Mepivacaine hydrochloride. **1%:** Methylparaben. Inj. Single-dose vial 30 mL. Multidose vial 50 mL. **1.5%:** Inj. Single-dose vial 30 mL. **2%:** Inj. Single-dose vial 20 mL. Multidose vial 50 mL, methylparaben. **3%:** Acetone sodium bisulfite. Inj. Dental Cartridge 1.8 mL. *Rx.*
Use: Anesthetic, local amide, injectable.

Carbocaine with Neo-Cobefrin. (Eastman-Kodak) Mepivacaine hydrochloride 2% with levonordefrin 1:20,000, acetone sodium bisulfite. Inj. Dental cartridge 1.8 mL. *Rx.*
Use: Anesthetic, local amide, injectable.

● **carbocloral.** (KAR-boe-KLOR-uhl) USAN.
Use: Hypnotic; sedative.
See: Chloralurethane.

● **carbocysteine.** (kar-boe-SIS-teen) USAN.
Use: Mucolytic.

Carbodec DM. (Rugby) **Syr.:** Pseudoephedrine hydrochloride 60 mg, carbinoxamine maleate 4 mg, dextromethorphan HBr 15 mg, alcohol < 0.6%/5 mL. Bot. 30 mL, 120 mL, pt, gal.
Drops: (Pediatric Pharmaceuticals) Pseudoephedrine hydrochloride 25 mg, carbinoxamine maleate 2 mg, dextromethorphan HBr 4 mg, alcohol 0.6%/mL. Bot. 30 mL. *Rx.*
Use: Antihistamine, antitussive, decongestant.

Carbodec Syrup. (Rugby) Pseudoephedrine hydrochloride 60 mg, carbinoxamine maleate 4 mg/5 mL. Syr. Bot. 473 mL. *Rx.*
Use: Antihistamine, decongestant.

Carbodec Tablets. (Rugby) Pseudoephedrine hydrochloride 60 mg, carbinoxamine maleate 4 mg. Tab. Bot. 100s. *Rx.*
Use: Antihistamine, decongestant.

Carbodec TR. (Rugby) Pseudoephedrine hydrochloride 120 mg, carbinoxamine maleate 8 mg. Tab. Bot. 100s. *Rx.*
Use: Antihistamine, decongestant.

Carbodex DM Drops. (Tri-Med) Carbinoxamine maleate 2 mg, pseudoephedrine hydrochloride 15 mg, dextromethorphan HBr 4 mg/mL. Drops. Bot. 30 mL. *Rx.*
Use: Upper respiratory combination, antihistamine, antitussive, decongestant.

Carbodex DM Syrup. (Tri-Med) Dextromethorphan HBr 15 mg, brompheniramine maleate 4 mg, pseudoephedrine hydrochloride 45 mg/5 mL, menthol, sorbitol. Syr. Bot. 473 mL. *Rx.*
Use: Upper respiratory combination, antihistamine, antitussive. decongestant.

Carbofed DM Oral Drops. (Hi-Tech) Pseudoephedrine hydrochloride 15 mg, carbinoxamine maleate 1 mg, dextromethorphan HBr 4 mg/mL, alcohol free. Drops. Bot. 30 mL w/dropper. *Rx.*
Use: Upper respiratory combination, antihistamine, antitussive, decongestant.

Carbofed DM Syrup. (Hi-Tech Pharmacal) Dextromethorphan HBr 15 mg, brompheniramine maleate 4 mg, pseudoephedrine hydrochloride 45 mg/5 mL, sorbitol, grape flavor. Syr. Bot. 473 mL. *Rx.*
Use: Upper respiratory combination, antihistamine, antitussive, decongestant.

carbol-fuchsin paint. Original fuchsin formula known as Castellani's Paint. Basic Fuchsin 0.3%, phenol 4.5%, resorcinol 10%, acetone 5%, alcohol 10%. Paint. Bot. 30 mL, 120 mL, 480 mL.
Use: Antifungal, topical.
See: Castellani's Paint.

● **carbol-fuchsin, topical solution.** (KAR-buhl-FOOK-sin) *USP 28.*
Use: Antifungal.

● **carbomer.** (KAR-boe-mer) *NF 23.* A polymer of acrylic acid, crosslinked with a polyfunctional agent.

Use: Pharmaceutic aid, emulsifying, suspending agent.
●**carbomer copolymer.** (KAR-boe-mer) *NF 23.*
Use: Pharmaceutic aid.
●**carbomer interpolymer.** (KAR-boe-mer) *NF 23.*
Use: Pharmaceutic aid; emulsifying, suspending agent.
●**carbomer 940.** (KAR-boe-mer 940) *NF 23.*
Use: Pharmaceutic aid, emulsifying, suspending agent.
●**carbomer 941.** (KAR-boe-mer 941) *NF 23.*
Use: Pharmaceutic aid, emulsifying, suspending agent.
●**carbomer 910.** (CAR-boe-mer 910) *NF 23.*
Use: Pharmaceutic aid, emulsifying, suspending agent.
●**carbomer 934.** (KAR-boe-mer 934) *NF 23.*
Use: Pharmaceutic aid, emulsifying, suspending agent.
●**carbomer 934p.** (KAR-boe-mer 934) *NF 23. Formerly carpolene.*
Use: Pharmaceutic aid, emulsifying, suspending, viscosity, thickening agent.
●**carbomer 1342.** (CAR-boe-mer 1342) *NF 23.*
Use: Pharmaceutic aid, emulsifying, suspending agent.
carbomycin. An antibiotic from *Streptomyces halstedii.*
Use: Anti-infective.
●**carbon dioxide.** (KAR-bahn dye-OX-ide) *USP 28.*
Use: Inhalation, respiratory.
See: Ceo-Two (Beutlich).
●**carbonic acid, dilithium salt.** (KAR-bahn-ik acid, dye-LITH-ee-uhm) *USP 28.* Lithium Carbonate.
●**carbonic acid, disodium salt.** (KAR-bahn-ik) *USP 28.* Sodium Carbonate.
●**carbonic acid, monosodium salt.** (KAR-bahn-ik) *USP 28.* Sodium Bicarbonate.
carbonic anhydrase inhibitors.
See: Acetazolamide.
Brinzolamide.
Daranide.
Dazamide.
Diamox.
Dorzolamide Hydrochloride.
●**carbon monoxide c 11.** (KAR-bahn moe-NOX-ide C11) *USP 28.*
Use: Diagnostic aid, blood volume de-

termination; radiopharmaceutical.
Carbonis Detergens, Liquor.
See: Coal Tar Solution.
●**carbon tetrachloride.** (KAR-bahn teh-truh-KLOR-ide) *NF 23.* Benzinoform.
Use: Pharmaceutic aid, solvent.
carbonyl diamide.
See: Chap Cream.
carbonyl iron.
Use: Mineral supplement.
See: Feosol.
Icar.
Ircon.
●**carboplatin.** (kar-boe-PLATT-in) *USP 28.*
Use: Antineoplastic.
See: Paraplatin.
carboplatin. (Mayne) Carboplatin 10 mg/mL. Inj. Single-use vials. 5 mL, 15 mL, 45 mL. *Rx.*
Use: Antineoplastic.
carboplatin. (Various Mfr.) Carboplatin 50 mg, 150 mg, 450 mg. Mannitol. Pow. for Inj., lyophilized. Single-dose vials. *Rx.*
Use: Antineoplastic.
●**carboprost.** (KAR-boe-prahst) USAN.
Use: Oxytocic.
●**carboprost methyl.** (KAR-boe-prahst METH-ill) USAN.
Use: Oxytocic.
●**carboprost tromethamine.** (KAR-boe-prahst troe-METH-ah-meen) *USP 28.*
Use: Oxytocic.
See: Prostin.
Carboptic. (Optopics) Carbachol 3%. Soln. Bot. 15 mL. *Rx.*
Use: Ophthalmic.
carbose d.
See: Carboxymethylcellulose sodium.
carbowax. Polyethylene glycol 300, 400, 1540, 4000.
carboxymethylcellulose.
Use: Ocular lubricant.
See: Refresh Tears.
●**carboxymethylcellulose calcium.** *NF 23.*
Use: Pharmaceutic aid, tablet disintegrant.
carboxymethylcellulose salt of dextroamphetamine. Carboxyphen.
See: Bontril.
●**carboxymethylcellulose sodium.** (kar-BOX-ee-meth-ill-SELL-you-lohs) *USP 28.*
Use: Pharmaceutic aid, suspending agent, tablet excipient, viscosity-increasing agent; cathartic.
W/Belladonna extract, kaolin, pectin, zinc phenosulfonate.
See: Foxalin.

W/Docusate sodium.
See: Dialose.
W/Methylcellulose.
See: Ex-Caloric.
•**carboxymethylcellulose sodium 12.**
(car-BOX-ee-meth-ill-SELL-you-lohs)
NF 23.
Use: Pharmaceutic aid, suspending,
viscosity-increasing agent; mucolytic
agent.
carboxyphen.
W/Butabarbital.
See: Bontril.
Carbromal. (Various Mfr.) Bromodiethylacetylurea, bromadel, nyctal, planada-
lin, uradal. *Rx.*
Use: Sedative; hypnotic.
W/Bromisovalum (Bromural).
See: Bro-T's.
carbutamide.
Use: Hypoglycemic.
•**carbuterol hydrochloride.** (kar-BYOO-
ter-ole) USAN.
Use: Bronchodilator.
•**cardamon.** (KAR-duh-mohn) *NF 23.* Oil,
seed, Cpd. Tincture.
Use: Flavoring.
Cardec DM Drops. (Various Mfr.) Carbinoxamine maleate 2 mg, pseudoephedrine hydrochloride 25 mg, dextromethorphan HBr 4 mg, alcohol < 0.6%/
mL. Drop. Bot. 30 mL. *Rx.*
Use: Antihistamine; antitussive; decongestant.
Cardec DM Pediatric Syrup. (Schein)
Pseudoephedrine hydrochloride 60 mg,
dextromethorphan HBr 15 mg, carbinoxamine maleate 4 mg, < 0.6% alcohol. Bot. Pt. *Rx.*
Use: Antihistamine; antitussive; decongestant.
Cardene. (Roche) Nicardipine 20 mg,
30 mg. Cap. Bot. 100s, 500s. *Rx.*
Use: Calcium channel blocker.
Cardene I.V. (Roche) Nicardipine hydrochloride 2.5 mg/mL, sorbitol 48 mg. Inj.
10 mL amp. *Rx.*
Use: Calcium channel blocker.
Cardene SR. (Roche) Nicardipine hydrochloride 30 mg, 45 mg, 60 mg, lactose.
SR Cap. Bot. 60s, 200s (except
60 mg). *Rx.*
Use: Calcium channel blocker.
Cardenz. (Miller Pharmacal Group) Vitamins C 25 mg, E 5 mg, inositol 30 mg,
p-aminobenzoic acid 9 mg, A
2000 units, B_6 1.5 mg, B_{12} 1 mcg, D
100 units, niacinamide 20 mg, Mg
23 mg, I 0.05 mg, K 8 mg. Tab. Bot.
100s. *OTC.*

Use: Mineral, vitamin supplement.
cardiac glycosides.
Use: Inotropic agent.
See: Digitek.
Digoxin.
Lanoxicaps.
Lanoxin.
Cardilate. (GlaxoSmithKline) Erythrityl
tetranitrate 10 mg. Tab. Bot. 100s.
Use: Antianginal.
Cardio-Green Disposable Unit. (Becton
Dickinson & Co.) Cardio-Green 10 mg.
Vial. Amp. Aqueous solvent and cali-
brated syringe.
Use: Diagnostic aid.
Cardi-Omega 3. (Thompson Medical)
EPA 180 mg, DHA 120 mg, cholesterol
5 mg, < 2% RDA of vitamins A, B_1, B_2,
B_3, C, D, Fe, Ca. Cap. Bot. 60s. *OTC.*
Use: Mineral, vitamin supplement.
cardioplegic solution.
Use: During open heart surgery.
See: Plegisol.
Cardiotek Rx. (Stewart-Jackson) Vita-
min B_6 50 mg, B_{12} 500 mcg, FA 2 mg.
With L-arginine hydrochloride. Coated.
Tab. 30s. *Rx.*
Use: Nutritional product.
Cardiotrol-CK. (Roche) Lyophilized hu-
man serum containing 3 CK isoen-
zymes from human tissue source.
10 × 2 mL.
Use: Diagnostic aid, quality control.
Cardiotrol-LD. (Roche) Lyophilized human serum containing all LD isoen-
zymes from human tissue source.
10 × 1 mL.
Use: Diagnostic aid, quality control.
Cardizem. (Biovail) **Tab.:** Diltiazem hydrochloride 30 mg, 60 mg, 90 mg,
120 mg. Bot. 90s (60 mg, 90 mg only),
100s, 500s (30 mg, 60 mg only), UD
100s. **Inj.:** 5 mg/mL. Single-use vial.
5 mL, 10 mL. **Pow. for Inj.:** 25 mg.
Cartons. 6 *Lyo-Ject* syringes with diluent (25 mg only). *Rx.*
Use: Calcium channel blocker.
Cardizem CD. (Biovail) Diltiazem hydrochloride 120 mg, 180 mg, 240 mg,
300 mg, 360 mg, sucrose. ER Cap. Bot.
30s (except 360 mg), 90s, UD 100s
(except 360 mg). *Rx.*
Use: Calcium channel blocker.
Cardizem LA. (Biovail) Diltiazem hydrochloride 120 mg, 180 mg, 240 mg,
300 mg, 360 mg, 420 mg. Sucrose. ER
Tab. Bot. 7s, 30s, 90s, 1000s. *Rx.*
Use: Calcium channel blocker.
Cardophyllin.
See: Aminophylline.

Cardoxin. (Vita Elixir) Digoxin 0.25 mg. Tab. *Rx.*
Use: Cardiovascular agent.
Cardura. (Roerig) Doxazosin mesylate 1 mg, 2 mg, 4 mg, 8 mg. Tab. Bot. 100s, UD 100s. *Rx.*
Use: Antihypertensive.
carena.
See: Aminophylline.
•**carfentanil citrate.** (kar-FEN-tah-NILL SIH-trate) USAN.
Use: Analgesic; narcotic.
Cargentos.
See: Silver protein, mild.
Carimune NF. (ZLB Bioplasma) Immune globulin IV 1 g, 3 g, 6 g, 12 g. Preservative-free. With 1.67 g sucrose/g protein. Pow. for Inj., lyophilized. Vials. 1 g, 3 g, 6 g, 12 g. *Rx.*
Use: Immune globulin.
•**cariporide mesylate.** (kar-ee-POR-ide) USAN.
Use: Cardiovascular agent.
•**carisoprodol.** (car-eye-so-PRO-dole) *USP 28.*
Use: Muscle relaxant.
See: Soma.
carisoprodol. (Various Mfr.) Carisoprodol 350 mg. Tab. Bot. 30s, 60s, 100, 500s, 1000s, UD 100s.
Use: Muscle relaxant.
carisoprodol and aspirin.
Use: Analgesic; muscle relaxant.
See: Soma Compound.
carisoprodol, aspirin, and codeine phosphate.
Use: Analgesic; muscle relaxant.
See: Soma Compound w/Codeine.
carisoprodol, aspirin, and codeine phosphate. (Amide) Carisoprodol 200 mg, aspirin 325 mg, codeine phosphate 16 mg. Tab. 100s, 500s. *c-III.*
Use: Skeletal muscle relaxant.
carisoprodol compound. (Various Mfr.) Carisoprodol 200 mg, aspirin 325 mg. Tab. Bot. 15s, 30s, 40s, 100s, 500s, 1000s. *Rx.*
Use: Analgesic; muscle relaxant.
Cari-Tab. (Jones Pharma) Fluoride 0.5 mg, vitamins A 2000 units, D 200 units, C 75 mg. Softab. Bot. 100s. *Rx.*
Use: Vitamin supplement; dental caries agent.
•**carmantadine.** (kar-MAN-tah-deen) USAN.
Use: Antiparkinsonian.
Carmol 40. (Doak Dermatologics) Urea 40%. **Cream:** Mineral oil, petrolatum,

cetyl alcohol. Tube. 28.35 g, 85 g. **Gel:** Glycerin, EDTA. Tube. 15 mL *Rx.*
Use: Emollient.
Carmol HC Cream 1%. (Doak Dermatologics) Micronized hydrocortisone acetate 1%, urea 10% in water-washable base. Tube 1 oz, Jar 4 oz. *Rx.*
Use: Corticosteroid, topical.
Carmol 10. (Doak Dermatologics) Urea (carbamide) 10% in hypoallergenic water-washable lotion base. Bot. 6 fl oz. *OTC.*
Use: Emollient.
Carmol 20. (Doak Dermatologics) Urea (carbamide) 20% in hypoallergenic vanishing cream base. Tube 3 oz, Jar lb. *OTC.*
Use: Emollient.
•**carmustine.** (KAR-muss-teen) USAN. BCNU.
Use: Antineoplastic, alkylating agent.
See: BiCNU.
 Gliadel.
Carnation Follow-Up. (Carnation) Protein (from nonfat milk) 18 g, carbohydrate (from lactose and corn syrup) 89.2 g, fat 27.7 g, vitamins A, D, E, K, C, B_1, B_2, B_3, B_6, B_{12}, B_5, biotin, choline, Ca, P, Cl, Mg, I, Mn, Cu, Zn, Fe 13 mg, inositol, cholesterol 11.4 mg, taurine, Na 264 mg, K 913 mg. Pow. 360 g. Conc. 390 mL. *OTC.*
Use: Nutritional supplement.
Carnation Good-Start. (Carnation) Protein 16 g, carbohydrate 74.4 g, fat 34.5 g, vitamins A, D, E, K, B_1, B_2, B_3, B_5, B_6, B_{12}, C, biotin, choline, inositol, cholesterol 68 mg, taurine, Ca, P, Mg, Fe 10 mg, Zn, Mn, Cu, I, Cl, Na, 162 mg, K 663 mg. Pow 360 g. Conc. 390 mL. *OTC.*
Use: Nutritional supplement.
Carnation Instant Breakfast. (Carnation) Nonfat instant breakfast containing 280 K calories w/15 g protein and 8 oz whole milk. Pkt. 35 g, Ctn. 6s. Six flavors. *OTC.*
Use: Nutritional supplement.
•**carnidazole.** (kar-NIH-dah-zole) USAN. Methylnitroimidazole.
Use: Antiparasitic; antiprotozoal.
Carnitor. (Sigma-Tau) Levocarnitine. **Soln.:** 100 mg/mL, sucrose, parabens, cherry flavor. Bot. 118 mL. **Tab.:** 330 mg. Bot. 90s. **Inj.:** 200 mg/mL, preservative-free. Single-dose vial, amp. *Rx.*
Use: Amino acid derivative.
•**caroxazone.** (kar-OX-ah-zone) USAN.
Use: Antidepressant.

•**carphenazine maleate.** (kar-FEN-azz-een) USAN.
Use: Antipsychotic.

•**carprofen.** (car-PRO-fen) USAN.
Use: Investigational analgesic, NSAID.

•**carrageenan.** (ka-rah-GEE-nan) *NF 23.*
Use: Pharmaceutic aid, suspending, viscosity-increasing agent.

Carrasyn. (Carrington) Phase I AIDS, ARC. *Rx.*
Use: Antiviral, immunomodulator.

•**carsatrin succinate.** (car-SAT-rin) USAN.
Use: Cardiovascular agent.

•**cartazolate.** (kar-TAZZ-oh-late) USAN.
Use: Antidepressant.

•**carteolol hydrochloride.** (KAR-tee-oh-lahl) *USP 28.*
Use: Antiadrenergic, beta-receptor; antiglaucoma.
See: Cartrol.

carteolol hydrochloride. (Various Mfr.) Carteolol hydrochloride 1%. Soln. Bot. 5 mL, 10 mL, 15 mL. *Rx.*
Use: Antiglaucoma; beta-adrenergic blocker.

Carter's Little Pills. (Carter-Wallace) Bisacodyl 5 mg. Bot. 30s, 85s. *OTC.*
Use: Laxative.

Cartia XT. (Andrx) Diltiazem hydrochloride 120 mg, 180 mg, 240 mg, 300 mg, sucrose. ER Cap. Box 30s, 90s, 500s, 1000s. *Rx.*
Use: Calcium channel blocker.

Cartrol. (Abbott) Carteolol hydrochloride 2.5 mg, 5 mg, lactose. Tab. Bot. 100s. *Rx.*
Use: Antiadrenergic, sympatholytic; beta-adrenergic blocker.

Cartucho Cook with Ravocaine. (Sanofi-Synthelabo) Ravocaine, novacaine, levophed, or neo-cobefrin. *Rx.*
Use: Anesthetic.

•**carubicin hydrochloride.** (kah-ROO-bih-sin) USAN. *Formerly carminomycin hydrochloride.*
Use: Antineoplastic.

•**carumonam sodium.** (kah-roo-MOE-nam) USAN.
Use: Anti-infective.

•**carvedilol.** (CAR-veh-DILL-ole) USAN.
Use: Antianginal; antihypertensive.
See: Coreg.

Car-Vit. (Mericon Industries) Ascorbic acid 60 mg, vitamins A acetate 4000 units, D-2 400 units, ferrous fumarate 90 mg (elemental iron 30 mg), oyster shell 600 mg (calcium 230 mg). Cap. Bot. 90s, 1000s. *OTC.*
Use: Mineral, vitamin supplement.

•**carvotroline hydrochloride.** (car-VAH-trah-leen) USAN.
Use: Antipsychotic.

•**carzelesin.** (car-ZELL-eh-sin) USAN.
Use: Antineoplastic, site-selective DNA binding.

carzenide.
Use: Carbonic anhydrase inhibitor.

casa-dicole. (Halsey Drug) Docusate sodium 100 mg, casanthrol 30 mg. Cap. Bot. 100s. *OTC.*
Use: Laxative.

•**casanthranol.** (kass-AN-thrah-nole) *USP 28.* A purified mixture of the anthranol glycosides derived from cascara sagrada.
Use: Laxative.
See: Black Draught.
W/Docusate sodium.
See: Bu-Lax-Plus.
　Calotabs.
　Diolax.
　Dio-Soft.
　Disulans.
　Docusate w/Casanthranol.
　Doxidan.
　Easy-Lax Plus.
　Genericace.
　Laxative & Stool Softener.
　Neo-Vardin D-S-S-C.
　Nuvac.
　Peri-Dos.
W/Docusate sodium, sodium carboxymethylcellulose.
See: Dialose Plus.
　Tri-Vac.

Cascara. (Eli Lilly) Cascara 150 mg. Tab. Bot. 100s. *OTC.*
Use: Laxative.

Cascara Aromatic. (Humco Holding Group) Cascara sagrada, alcohol 18%. Liq. Bot. 120 mL, 473 mL. *OTC.*
Use: Laxative.

cascara fluid extract, aromatic.
Use: Laxative.

cascara glycosides.
Use: Laxative.

•**cascara sagrada.** (kass-KA-rah sah-GRAH-dah) *USP 28.*
Use: Cathartic.
See: Aromatic Cascara Fluid Extract.
　Cascara Aromatic.
　Nature's Remedy.
W/Bile Salts, Papain, Phenolphthalein, Capsicum Oleoresin.
See: Torocol Compound.
W/Bile Salts, Phenolphthalein, Capsicum Oleoresin, Peppermint Oil.
See: Torocol.

W/Ox Bile (Desiccated), Phenolphthalein, Aloin, Podophyllin.
See: Bocresin.
cascara sagrada. (Various Mfr.) Cascara sagrada 325 mg. Tab. Bot. 100s, 1000s. OTC.
Use: Cathartic.
cascara sagrada fluid extract. (Parke-Davis) Alcohol 18%/5 mL. Bot. Pt, gal, UD 5 mL.
Use: Laxative. [Orphan Drug]
See: Bilstan.
cascarin.
See: Casanthranol.
Casec. (Bristol-Myers Squibb) Calcium caseinate (derived from skim milk curd and calcium carbonate). Pow. Can 2.5 oz. OTC.
Use: Mineral supplement.
Uasodex. (AstraZeneca) Bicalutamide 50 mg, lactose. Tab. Bot. 30s, 100s, UD 30s. Rx.
Use: Antineoplastic; hormone, antimutagenic.
●**caspofungin acetate.** (KASS-poe-FUN-jin) USAN.
Use: Antifungal.
See: Cancidas.
CAST. (Biomerica) Reagent test for immunoglobulin E in serum. Tube Kit 25s.
Use: Diagnostic aid.
Castellani Paint Modified. (Pedinol Pharmacal) Basic fuchsin, phenol resorcinol, acetone, alcohol. Bot. 30 mL, 120 mL, 480 mL. Also available as colorless solution without basic fuchsin. Bot. 30 mL, 120 mL, 480 mL. Rx.
Use: Antifungal, topical.
Castellani's Paint. (Penta) Carbol-fuchsin solution. Fuchsin 0.3%, phenol 4.5%, resorcinol 10%, acetone 1.5%, alcohol 13%. Bot. 1 oz, 4 oz, pt. Rx.
Use: Antifungal, topical.
●**castor oil.** (KASS-ter oil) USP 28.
Use: Laxative; pharmaceutic aid, plasticizer.
See: Emusoil.
Neoloid.
castor oil. (Various Mfr.) Castor oil. Liq. Bot. 60 mL, 120 mL, 480 mL. OTC.
Use: Laxative; pharmaceutic aid, plasticizer.
castor oil, hydrogenated.
Use: Laxative.
Cataflam. (Novartis) Diclofenac 50 mg (as potassium), sucrose. Tab. Bot. 100s, UD 100s. Rx.
Use: Analgesic, NSAID.
Catapres. (Boehringer Ingelheim) Clonidine hydrochloride 0.1 mg, 0.2 mg,

0.3 mg. Tab. Bot. 100s, 1000s, UD 100s (except 0.3 mg). Rx.
Use: Antihypertensive.
Catapres-TTS. (Boehringer Ingelheim) Clonidine 2.5 mg, 5 mg, 7.5 mg. Transdermal patch. Pkg. 4s, 12s. Rx.
Use: Antihypertensive.
Catatrol. (AstraZeneca) Viloxazine.
Use: Antidepressant.
Cathflo Activase. (Genentech) Alteplase 2 mg, L-arginine, phosphoric acid, polysorbate 80. Pow. for Inj., lyophilized. Vials. Rx.
Use: Thrombolytic.
cathomycin calcium. Calcium novobiocin.
Use: Anti-infective.
cathomycin sodium. Novobiocin sodium.
Use: Anti-infective.
cationic resins.
See: Resins, sodium-Removing.
Caverject. (Pharmacia & Upjohn) Alprostadil. **Inj., aqueous:** 10 mcg/mL, 20 mcg/mL, 40 mcg/2 mL Amps. 1 mL and kit with 2 mL Luer-lock syringe, 2½-inch needles (one 27-gauge and one 30-gauge) alcohol swab. **Pow. for Inj., lyophilized:** 5 mcg/mL, 10 mcg/mL, 20 mcg/mL, 40 mcg/mL, benzyl alcohol 8.4 mg, lactose. Vials, vials with diluent syringes (except 40 mcg/mL). Rx.
Use: Anti-impotence agent.
Caverject Impulse. (Pharmacia & Upjohn) Alprostadil 10 mcg/0.5 mL, 20 mcg/0.5 mL, benzyl alcohol 4.45 mg, lactose. Blister tray containing 1 dual chamber syringe system, 1 needle, 2 alcohol swabs. Rx.
Use: Anti-impotence agent.
Cav-X Fluoride Treatment. (Palisades Pharmaceuticals) Stannous fluoride 0.4%. Gel. Bot. 121.9 g. Rx.
Use: Dental caries agent.
C-Bio. (Barth's) Vitamin C 150 mg, citrus bioflavonoid complex 100 mg, rutin 50 mg. Tab. Bot. 100s, 500s, 1000s. OTC.
Use: Vitamin supplement.
C-B Time. (Arco) Vitamins C 300 mg, B_1 15 mg, B_2 10 mg, B_3 100 mg, B_5 20 mg, B_6 5 mg, B_{12} 5 mcg. Liq. Bot. 120 mL. OTC.
Use: Vitamin supplement.
CCD 1042. (Cocensys, Inc.)
Use: Treatment of infantile spasms. [Orphan Drug]
CC-Galactosidase. Alpha-galactosidase A.
Use: Fabry disease. [Orphan Drug]

CCNU. Lomustine.
Use: Antineoplastic.
See: CeeNU.

C-Crystals. (NBTY) Vitamin C 5000 mg/
tsp. Crystals. Bot. 180 g. *OTC.*
Use: Vitamin supplement.

CDDP.
Use: Antineoplastic.
See: Cisplatin.

CD-45 monoclonal antibodies.
Use: Prevent graft rejection in organ
transplants. [Orphan Drug]

**CD4, recombinant soluble human
(rCD4).**
Use: Antiviral, HIV. [Orphan Drug]

C.D.P. (Ivax) Chlordiazepoxide hydrochloride 5 mg, 10 mg, 25 mg. Cap. Bot.
100s, 500s, 1000s. *c-iv.*
Use: Anxiolytic.

Cea. (Abbott Diagnostics) Radioimmunoassay or enzyme immunoassay for
quantitative measurement of carcino-
embryonic antigen in human serum or
plasma. Test Kit 100s.
Use: Diagnostic aid.

Cea-Roche. (Roche) Radioimmunoassay
capable of detecting and measuring
plasma levels of CEA in the nanogram
range. Sensitivity-0.5 ng/mL of CEA.
Use: Diagnostic aid.

Cea-Roche Test Kit. (Roche) Carcino-
embryonic antigen, a glycoprotein
which is a constituent of the glycocalyx
of embryonic entodermal epithelium.
Test Kit.
Use: Diagnostic aid.

CEA-Scan. (Immunomedics; Mallinckrodt-Baker) Arcitumomab 1.25 mg. Re-
constitute with Tc 99m sodium pertechnetate in NaCl for Inj. Inj. Single-dose
Vial. *Rx.*
Use: For detection of recurrent or metastatic colorectal carcinoma of the liver,
extrahepatic abdomen and pelvis; radioimmunoscintigraphy.

Ceb Nuggets. (Scot-Tussin) Vitamins B_1
15 mg, B_2 15 mg, B_6 5 mg, B_{12} 5 mcg,
C 600 mg, niacinamide 100 mg, E
40 units, calcium pantothenate 20 mg,
folic acid 0.1 mg. Nugget. Bot. 60s.
OTC.
Use: Mineral, vitamin supplement.

Cebo-Caps. (Forest) Placebo capsules.
OTC.

Ceclor. (Eli Lilly) **Pulv.:** Cefaclor 250 mg,
500 mg. Bot. 15s, 30s, 100s, UD 100s.
Oral Susp.: Cefaclor 125 mg, 187 mg,
250 mg, 375 mg/5 mL. Bot. 50 mL,
75 mL, 100 mL, 150 mL. 375 mg/5 mL.
Use: Anti-infective, cephalosporin.

Cecon. (Abbott) Ascorbic acid 100 mg/
mL. Soln. Bot. w/dropper 50 mL. *OTC.*
Use: Vitamin supplement.

Cedax. (Schering-Plough) **Cap.:** Ceftibuten 400 mg, parabens. Bot 20s, UD
40s. **Pow. for Oral Susp.:** Ceftibuten
90 mg/5 mL, sucrose. Cherry flavor.
Bot 30 mL, 60 mL, 90 mL, 120 mL. *Rx.*
Use: Anti-infective, cephalosporin.

•**cedeflngol.** (seh-deh-FIN-gole) USAN.
Use: Antineoplastic, adjunct; antipsoriatic.

•**cedelizumab.** (sed-eh-LIE-zoo-mab)
USAN.
Use: Monoclonal antibody; immuno-
suppressant.

Ceebevim. (NBTY) Vitamins B_1 15 mg,
B_2 10.2 mg, B_3 50 mg, B_5 10 mg, B_6
5 mg, C 300 mg. Cap. Bot. 100s, 300s.
OTC.
Use: Vitamin supplement.

CeeNU. (Bristol Labs Oncology) Lomustine (CCNU) 10 mg, 40 mg, 100 mg,
mannitol. Cap. 20s, dose pk. of 2 cap.
each of all 3 strengths. *Rx.*
Use: Antineoplastic, alkylating agent.

Ceepa. (Geneva) Theophylline 130 mg,
ephedrine hydrochloride 24 mg, phenobarbital 8 mg. Tab. Bot. 100s, 1000s.
Rx.
Use: Bronchodilator; decongestant;
hypnotic; sedative.

Ceepryn. Cetylpyridinium Cl. *OTC.*
Use: Antiseptic.
See: Cēpacol.

Cee with Bee. (Wesley) Vitamins B_1
15 mg, B_2 10.2 mg, B_3 50 mg, B_5
10 mg, B_6 5 mg, C 300 mg, tartrazine.
Bot. 100s, 1000s. *OTC.*
Use: Vitamin supplement.

•**cefaclor.** (SEFF-uh-klor) *USP 28.*
Use: Anti-infective, cephalosporin.
See: Ceclor.
Raniclor.

cefaclor. (Ivax) Cefaclor 500 mg. ER Tab.
Bot. 100s. *Rx.*
Use: Anti-infective.

cefaclor. (Various Mfr.) Cefaclor. **Cap.:**
250 mg, 500 mg. Bot. 15s (500 mg),
30s (250 mg), 100s, 500s (250 mg),
1000s (250 mg), UD 100s (500 mg).
Pow. for Oral Susp.: 125 mg/5 mL,
187 mg/5 mL, 250 mg/5 mL, 375 mg/
5 mL, Bot. 50 mL, 75 mL, 100 mL,
150 mL. *Rx.*
Use: Anti-infective.

•**cefadroxil.** (SEFF-uh-DROX-ill) *USP 28.*
Use: Anti-infective, cephalosporin.
See: Duricef.

cefadroxil. (Various Mfr.) Cefadroxil.
Cap.: 500 mg. Bot 100s. **Tab.:** 1 g. Bot

24s, 50s, 100s, 500s. *Rx.*
Use: Anti-infective, cephalosporin.
• **cefamandole.** (SEFF-ah-MAN-dole)
USAN.
Use: Anti-infective.
• **cefamandole sodium for injection.**
(SEFF-ah-MAN-dole) *USP 28.*
Use: Anti-infective, cephalosporin.
Cefanex. (Apothecon) Cephalexin mono-
hydrate 250 mg, 500 mg. Cap. Bot.
100s. *Rx.*
Use: Anti-infective, cephalosporin.
• **cefaparole.** (SEFF-ah-pah-ROLE)
USAN.
Use: Anti-infective.
• **cefatrizine.** (SEFF-ah-TRY-zeen) USAN.
Use: Anti-infective, cephalosporin.
• **cefazaflur sodium.** (seff-AZE-ah-flure)
USAN.
Use: Anti-infective, cephalosporin.
• **cefazolin sodium.** (seff-AH-zoe-lin)
USP 28.
Use: Anti-infective, cephalosporin.
See: Ancef
Zolicef
cefazolin sodium. (Apothecon) Cefazolin sodium 500 mg, 1 g, 5 g, 10 g,
20 g. Sodium 2.1 mEq/g. Pow. for Inj.
Vials and piggyback vials (500 mg, 1 g,
5 g only); pharmacy bulk packages
(10 g, 20 g only).
Use: Anti-infective, cephalosporin.
• **cefbuperazone.** (SEFF-byoo-PURR-ah
zone) USAN.
Use: Anti-infective, cephalosporin.
• **cefdinir.** (SEFF-dih-ner) USAN.
Use: Anti-infective, cephalosporin.
See: Omnicef.
• **cefditoren pivoxil.** (SEFF-dih-TOR-en
pih-VOX-ill) USAN.
Use: Anti-infective.
See: Spectracef.
• **cefepime.** (SEFF-eh-pim) USAN.
Use: Anti-infective.
• **cefepime hydrochloride.** (SEFF-eh-pim)
USAN.
Use: Anti-infective.
See: Maxipime.
• **cefetecol.** (seff-EH-teh-kahl) USAN.
Use: Antibacterial, cephalosporin.
Cefinal II. (Alto) Salicymide 150 mg,
acetaminophen 250 mg, doxylamine
succinate 25 mg. Tab. Bot. 100s. *OTC.*
Use: Analgesic combination.
• **cefixime.**
Use: Cephalosporin.
See: Suprax.
Cefizox. (GlaxoSmithKline) Ceftizoxime
sodium. **Pow. for Inj.:** 500 mg (single-

dose fliptop vials 10 mL); 1 g, 2 g (vial
20 mL, piggyback vial 100 mL); 10 g
(bulk pkg). **Inj.:** 1 g, 2 g. Frozen, pre-
mixed, single-dose plastic containers
50 mL. *Rx.*
Use: Anti-infective, cephalosporin.
• **cefmenoxime hydrochloride, sterile.**
(SEFF-men-ox-eem) *USP 28.*
Use: Anti-infective, cephalosporin.
• **cefmetazole.** (seff-MET-ah-zole)
USP 28.
Use: Anti-infective, cephalosporin.
• **cefmetazole for injection.** (seff-MET-ah-
zole) *USP 28.*
Use: Anti-infective, cephalosporin.
• **cefmetazole sodium.** (seff-MET-ah-zole)
USP 28.
Use: Anti-infective, cephalosporin.
See: Zefazone
Cefobid. (Roerig) Cefoperazone sodium.
Pow. for Inj.: 1 g, 2 g. Piggyback unit.
Inj.: 1 g, 2 g. Premixed, frozen, 50 mL
plastic container 10 g Pharmacy bulk
package. *Rx.*
Use: Anti-infective, cephalosporin.
Cefol Filmtab. (Abbott) Vitamins B$_1$
15 mg, B$_2$ 10 mg, B$_6$ 5 mg, B$_{12}$ 6 mcg,
C 750 mg, E 30 mg, B$_5$ 20 mg,
B$_3$100 mg, folic acid 0.5 mg. Tab. Bot.
100s. *OTC.*
Use: Mineral, vitamin supplement.
• **cefonicid monosodium.** (seh-FAHN-ih-
SID MAHN-oh-SO-dee-uhm) USAN.
Use: Anti-infective, cephalosporin.
• **cefoperazone sodium.** (SEFF-oh-PUR-
uh-zone) *USP 28.*
Use: Anti-infective, cephalosporin.
See: Cefobid.
• **cefexranide for injection.** (seh-FAR-ah-
NIDE) *USP 28.*
Use: Anti-infective, cephalosporin.
Cefotan. (AstraZeneca) Cefotetan di-
sodium. **Pow. for Inj.:** 1 g, 2 g (*ADD-
Vantage* and piggyback vials); 10 g (vial
100 mL). **Inj.:** 1 g/50 mL, 2 g/50 mL,
dextrose. Frozen, iso-osmotic, pre-
mixed single-dose *Galaxy* containers
50 mL. *Rx.*
Use: Anti-infective, cephalosporin.
• **cefotaxime sodium.** (seff-oh-TAX-eem)
USP 28.
Use: Anti-infective, cephalosporin.
See: Claforan.
• **cefotetan.** (SEFF-oh-tee-tan) *USP 28.*
Use: Anti-infective.
• **cefotetan disodium.** (SEFF-oh-tee-tan
die-SO-dee-uhm) *USP 28.*
Use: Anti-infective.
See: Cefotan.

●**cefotiam hydrochloride sterile.** (SEFF-oh-TIE-am) *USP 28.*
Use: Anti-infective, cephalosporin.
●**cefovecin sodium.** (sef-OH-vee-sin) USAN.
Use: Antibacterial (veterinary).
●**cefoxitin.** (seff-OX-ih-tin) USAN.
Use: Anti-infective, cephalosporin.
See: Mefoxin.
cefoxitin. (American Pharmaceutical Partners) Cefoxitin (as sodium) 1 g, 2 g, 10 g. Pow. for Inj. Vials and infusion bottles (1 g, 2 g); pharmacy bulk packages (10 g). *Rx.*
Use: Anti-infective, cephalosporin.
●**cefoxitin sodium.** (seff-OX-ih-tin) *USP 28.*
Use: Anti-infective, cephalosporin.
●**cefpimizole.** (seff-PIH-mih-zole) USAN.
Use: Anti-infective, cephalosporin.
●**cefpimizole sodium.** (seff-PIH-mih-zole) USAN.
Use: Anti-infective, cephalosporin.
See: Mefoxin.
●**cefpiramide.** (SEFF-PIHR-am-ide) USAN.
Use: Anti-infective, cephalosporin.
●**cefpiramide sodium.** (SEFF-PIHR-am-ide) USAN.
Use: Anti-infective, cephalosporin.
●**cefpirome sulfate.** (SEFF-pihr-ome) USAN.
Use: Anti-infective, cephalosporin.
●**cefpodoxime proxetil.** (SEFF-pode-OX-eem PROX-uh-til) *USP 28.*
Use: Anti-infective, cephalosporin.
See: Vantin.
●**cefprozil.** (SEFF-pro-zill) *USP 28.*
Use: Anti-infective, cephalosporin.
See: Cefzil.
●**cefroxadine.** (SEFF-ROX-ah-deen) USAN.
Use: Anti-infective, cephalosporin.
●**cefsulodin sodium.** (SEFF-SULL-oh-din) USAN.
Use: Anti-infective, cephalosporin.
●**ceftazidime.** (seff-TAZE-ih-deem) *USP 28.*
Use: Anti-infective, cephalosporin.
See: Ceptaz.
Fortaz.
Tazicef.
Tazidime.
●**ceftibuten.** (seff-TIE-byoo-ten) USAN.
Use: Anti-infective.
See: Cedax.
Ceftin. (GlaxoSmithKline) Cefuroxime axetil. **Tab.:** 125 mg, 250 mg, 500 mg. Tab. Bot. 20s, 60s, UD 50s, 100s.

Susp.: 125 mg/5 mL, 250 mg/5 mL, sucrose. Bot. 50 mL, 100 mL. *Rx.*
Use: Anti-infective, cephalosporin.
●**ceftizoxime sodium.** (SEFF-tih-ZOX-eem) *USP 28.*
Use: Anti-infective, cephalosporin.
See: Cefizox.
●**ceftriaxone sodium.** (SEFF-TRY-AXE-own) *USP 28.*
Use: Anti-infective, cephalosporin.
See: Rocephin.
●**cefuroxime.** (SEFF-yur-OX-eem) USAN.
Use: Anti-infective, cephalosporin.
See: Ceftin.
●**cefuroxime axetil.** (SEFF-your-OX-eem ACK-seh-TILL) *USP 28.*
Use: Anti-infective, cephalosporin.
See: Ceftin.
cefuroxime axetil. (Ranbaxy) Cefuroxime (as axetil) 125 mg, 250 mg, 500 mg. Tab. 20s (250 mg, 500 mg), 60s, 100s. *Rx.*
Use: Anti-infective, cephalosporin.
●**cefuroxime pivoxetil.** (SEFF-your-OX-eem pih-VOX-eh-till) USAN.
Use: Anti-infective, cephalosporin.
●**cefuroxime sodium.** (SEFF-your-OX-eem) *USP 28.*
Use: Anti-infective, cephalosporin.
See: Zinacef.
cefuroxime sodium. (Various Mfr.) Cefuroxime sodium 750 mg, 1.5 g in 10 mL (750 mg only), 20 mL (1.5 g only), 100 mL piggyback vials; 7.5 g/vial pharmacy bulk package. *Rx.*
Use: Anti-infective, cephalosporin.
cefuroxime sodium, sterile.
Use: Anti-infective, cephalosporin.
See: Kefurox.
Zinacef.
Cefzil. (Bristol-Myers Squibb) Cefprozil. **Tab.:** 250 mg, 500 mg. Bot. 50s, 100s, and UD 100s. **Pow. for Oral Susp.:** 125 mg/5 mL, 250 mg/5 mL, sucrose, aspartame, phenylalanine 28 mg/5 mL. Bot. 50 mL, 75 mL, 100 mL. *Rx.*
Use: Anti-infective, cephalosporin.
Celebrex. (Searle) Celecoxib 100 mg, 200 mg, 400 mg, lactose. Cap. Bot. 60s, 100s, 500s, UD 100s. *Rx.*
Use: Nonsteroidal anti-inflammatory agent.
●**celecoxib.** (cell-ih-COX-ib) USAN.
Use: Anti-inflammatory; analgesic, NSAID.
See: Celebrex.
Celestone. (Schering) Betamethasone 0.6 mg/5 mL, alcohol < 1%, sorbitol, sugar. Syrup. Bot. 118 mL. *Rx.*
Use: Adrenocortical steroid, glucocorticoid.

Celestone Phosphate. (Schering) Betamethasone sodium phosphate 4 mg/mL (equivalent to betamethasone alcohol 3 mg). EDTA, phenol, sodium bisulfite. Inj. Multidose vials. 5 mL. *Rx.*
Use: Adrenocortical steroid, glucocorticoid.

Celestone Soluspan. (Schering) Betamethasone sodium phosphate 3 mg, betamethasone acetate 3 mg/mL, EDTA, benzalkonium Cl. Multidose vials. 5 mL. *Rx.*
Use: Adrenocortical steroid, glucocorticoid.

Celexa. (Forest) Citalopram hydrobromide. **Tab.:** 10 mg, 20 mg, 40 mg, lactose. Bot. 100s, UD 100s (except 10 mg). **Oral Soln.:** 10 mg/5 mL, sorbitol, parabono, puppurmint flavor. 240 mL. *Rx.*
Use: Antidepressant, SSRI.

●**celgosivir hydrochloride.** (sell-GO-sih-vihr) USAN.
Use: Antiviral; inhibitor, alpha-glucoside.

●**celiprolol hydrochloride.** (SEE-lih-PRO-lahl) USAN.
Use: Investigational beta-adrenergic blocking agent.

Cellaburate. (Eastman Kodak) Cellulose acetate butyrate.
Use: Pharmaceutic aid, plastic-filming agent.

cellacefate.
Use: Pharmaceutic aid, tablet coating agent.
See: Cellulose Acetate Phthalate.

CellCept. (Roche) Mycophenolate mofetil. **Cap.:** 250 mg. Bot. 100s, 500s. Pkg. containing 12 bottles of 120s. **Tab.:** 500 mg, alcohols. Film coated. Bot. 100s, 500s. **Pow. for Oral Susp.:** 200 mg/mL (reconstituted), aspartame, methylparaben, sorbitol, phenylalanine 0.56 mg/mL, mixed fruit flavor. Bot. 225 mL. **Pow. for Inj., lyophilized:** 500 mg, preservative free. Vial 20 mL. *Rx.*
Use: Immunosuppressant.

Cellepacbin. (Arthrins) Vitamins A 1200 units, B_1 1.5 mg, B_2 1.5 mg, B_6 0.75 mg, niacinamide 7.5 mg, panthenol 3 mg, C 20 mg, B_{12} 2 mcg, E 1 units. Cap. Bot. 180s. *OTC.*
Use: Vitamin supplement.

Cellothyl. (Numark) Methylcellulose 0.5 g. Tab. Bot. 100s, 1000s. *OTC.*
Use: Laxative.

●**cellulase.** (SELL-you-lace) USAN. A concentrate of cellulose-splitting enzymes

derived from *Aspergillus niger* and other sources.
Use: Enzyme, digestive adjunct.
W/Bile Salts, Mixed Conjugated, Pancrelipase.
See: Zylase.
W/Mylase, Prolase, Lipase.
See: Ku-Zyme.

cellulose.
W/Hexachlorophene.
See: Zeasorb.

●**cellulose acetate.** (SELL-you-lohs) *NF 23.*
Use: Pharmaceutic aid, coating agent; polymer membrane, insoluble.

●**cellulose acetate phthalate.** (SELL-you-lohs ASS-eh-tate THAL-ate) *NF 23.*
Use: Pharmaceutic aid, tablet coating agent
See: Cellacefate.

●**cellulose, carboxymethyl, sodium salt.** (SELL-you-lohs kar-BOX-ee-meth-ill) *USP 28.* Carboxymethylcellulose sodium.

●**cellulose, hydroxypropyl methyl ether.** (SELL-you-lohs, hi-DROX-ee-pro-pill meth-ill E-thur) *USP 28.* Hydroxypropyl methylcellulose.

cellulose methyl ether.
See: Methylcellulose.

●**cellulose microcrystalline.** (SELL-you-lohs my-KROE-cris-tahl-een) *NF 23.*
Use: Pharmaceutic aid, tablet and capsule diluent.

cellulose, nitrate. Pyroxylin.

●**cellulose, oxidized.** (SELL-you-lohs, OX-ih-dized) *USP 28.*
Use: Hemostatic.

●**cellulose, oxidized, regenerated.** (SELL-you-lohs, OX-ih-dized) *USP 28.*
Use: Hemostatic.

cellulose, powdered.
Use: Tablet and capsule diluent.

●**cellulose sodium phosphate.** (SELL-you-lohs) *USP 28.*
Use: Antiurolithic.
See: Calcibind.

cellulosic acid.
See: Oxidized cellulose.

cellulolytic enzyme.
See: Cellulase.
W/Amylolytic, proteolytic enzymes, lipase, phenobarbital, hyoscyamine sulfate, atropine sulfate.
See: Arco-Lipase Plus.
W/Amylolytic enzyme, proteolytic enzyme, lipolytic enzyme, butisol sodium, belladonna.
See: Butibel-zyme.
W/Calcium carbonate, glycine, amylolytic

and proteolytic enzymes.
See: Ku-Zyme.

Celluvisc. (Allergan) Carboxymethylcellulose 1%, NaCl, KCl, sodium lactate. Ophth. Soln. Single-use containers 0.3 mL (UD 30s). *OTC.*
Use: Artificial tears.

Celontin. (Parke-Davis) Methsuximide 150 mg, 300 mg. Cap. Bot. 100s. *Rx.*
Use: Anticonvulsant.

Cenafed Plus. (Century) Pseudoephedrine hydrochloride 60 mg, triprolidine hydrochloride 2.5 mg. Tab. Bot. 30s, 100s. *OTC.*
Use: Upper respiratory combination; antihistamine; decongestant.

Cenafed Syrup. (Century) Pseudoephedrine hydrochloride 30 mg/5 mL, methylparaben. Liq. Bot. 120 mL, 480 mL, 3.8 L. *OTC.*
Use: Nasal decongestant, arylalkylamine.

Cenafed Tablets. (Century) Pseudoephedrine hydrochloride 60 mg. Tab. Bot. 100s. *OTC.*
Use: Nasal decongestant, arylalkylamine.

Cena-K. (Century) Potassium and Cl 20 mEq/15 mL (10% KCl), saccharin. Bot. Pt, gal. *Rx.*
Use: Electrolyte supplement.

Cenalax. (Century) Bisacodyl. **Tab.:** 5 mg. Bot. 100s, 1000s. **Supp.:** 10 mg. Pkg. 12s, 1000s. *OTC.*
Use: Laxative.

Cenestin. (Barr/Duramed) Synthetic conjugated estrogens A 0.3 mg, 0.45 mg, 0.625 mg, 0.9 mg, 1.25 mg, lactose. Tab. Bot. 30s, 100s, 1000s. *Rx.*
Use: Estrogen.

CenogenUltra. (US Pharm.) Fe (as ferrous sulfate) 106 mg, B_1 10 mg, B_2 6 mg, B_3 30 mg, B_5 10 mg, B_6 5 mg, B_{12} 15 mcg, C 200 mg, folic acid 1 mg, Cu, Mn. Cap. UD 100s. *Rx.*
Use: Vitamin, mineral supplement.

Cenolate. (Abbott Hospital Products) Sodium ascorbate 562.5 mg/mL (equivalent to 500 mg/mL ascorbic acid), sodium hydrosulfate 0.5%. Inj. Amp. 1 mL, 2 mL. *Rx.*
Use: Vitamin supplement.

Centany. (OrthoNeutrogena) Mupirocin 2% in a base containing castor oil and hard fat. Oint. 15 g, 30 g. *Rx.*
Use: Anti-infective.

Centeon Thyroid. (Aventis) Desiccated animal thyroid glands (active thyroid hormones) T-4 thyroxine, T-3 thyronine 0.25 g, 0.5 g, 1 g, 1.5 g, 2 g, 3 g, 4 g, 5 g. Tab. Bot. 100s, 1000s. Handy Hundreds, Carton Strip 100s. *Rx.*
Use: Hormone, thyroid.

Center-Al. (Center) Allergenic extracts, alum precipitated 10,000 PNU/mL, 20,000 PNU/mL. Vial 10 mL, 30 mL. *Rx.*
Use: Antiallergic.

Centoxin. (Centocor) Nebacumab.
Use: Antibacterial. [Orphan Drug]

Centrafree. (NBTY) Iron 27 mg, vitamins A 5000 units, D 400 units, E 30 units, B_1 2.25 mg, B_2 2.6 mg, B_3 20 mg, B_5 10 mg, B_6 3 mg, B_{12} 9 mcg, C 90 mg, folic acid 0.4 mg, biotin 45 mcg, Ca, Cl, Cr, Cu, I, K, Mg, Mn, Mo, P, Se, Zn. Tab. Bot. 100s. *OTC.*
Use: Mineral, vitamin supplement.

central nervous system depressants.
See: Sedative/Hypnotic Agents.

central nervous system stimulants.
See: Amphetamine Mixtures.
Amphetamines.
Analeptics.
Anorexiants.
Benzphetamine Hydrochloride.
Caffeine.
Dexmethylphenidate Hydrochloride.
Dextroamphetamine Sulfate.
Diethylpropion Hydrochloride.
Doxapram Hydrochloride.
Methamphetamine Hydrochloride.
Methylphenidate Hydrochloride.
Modafinil.
Pemoline.
Phendimetrazine Tartrate.
Phentermine Hydrochloride.
Sibutramine Hydrochloride.

Centrovite Advanced Formula. (Rugby) Fe 18 mg, A 5000 units, D 400 units, E 30 units, B_1 1.5 mg, B_2 1.7 mg, B_3 20 mg, B_5 10 mg, B_6 2 mg, B_{12} 6 mcg, C 60 mg, Fa 0.4 mg, biotin 30 mcg, Ca, Cl, Cr, Cu, I, vitamin K, Mg, Mn, Mo, Ni, P, Se, Si, Sn, V, Zn, K. Tab. Bot. 100s. *OTC.*
Use: Mineral, vitamin supplement.

Centrovite Jr. (Rugby) Iron 18 mg, vitamins A 5000 units, D 400 units, E 15 units, B_1 1.5 mg, B_2 1.7 mg, B_3 20 mg, B_5 10 mg, B_6 2 mg, B_{12} 6 mcg, C 60 mg, folic acid 0.4 mg, biotin 45 mcg, Cr, Cu, I, Mg, Mn, Mo, Zn. Chew. Tab. Bot. 60s. *OTC.*
Use: Mineral, vitamin supplement.

Centrum. (Wyeth) Vitamins A 5000 units, E 30 units, C 90 mg, folic acid 400 mcg, B_1 2.25 mg, B_2 2.6 mg, B_6 3 mg, niacinamide 20 mg, B_{12} 9 mcg, D 400 units, biotin 45 mcg, pantothenic acid 10 mg, Ca 162 mg, P 125 mg, I 150 mcg, Fe 27 mg, Mg 100 mg, K

30 mg, Mn 5 mg, chromium 25 mcg, Se 25 mcg, Mo 25 mcg, Zn 15 mg, Cu 2 mg, vitamin K 25 mcg, Cl 27.2 mg. Tab. *OTC.*
Use: Mineral, vitamin supplement.
Centrum, Advanced Formula. (Wyeth) Vitamins A 2500 units, E 30 units, C 60 mg, B_1 1.5 mg, B_2 1.7 mg, B_3 20 mg, B_5 10 mg, B_6 2 mg, B_{12} 6 mcg, D_2 400 units, Fe 9 mg, biotin 300 mcg per 15 mL. With I, Zn, Mn, Cr, Mo, alcohol. 6.6%. Liq. Bot. 236 mL. *OTC.*
Use: Mineral, vitamin supplement.
Centrum Jr. (Wyeth) Vitamins A 5000 units, D 400 units, E 30 units, C 60 mg, folic acid 400 mcg, B_1 1.5 mg, B_6 2 mg, B_{12} 6 mcg, riboflavin 1.7 mg, niacinamide 20 mg, Fe 18 mg, Mg 25 mg, Cu 2 mg, Zn 10 mg, biotin 45 mcg, pantothenic acid 10 mg, Mo 20 mcg, chromium 20 mcg, I 150 mcg, Mn 1 mg. Chew. Tab. Bot. 60s. *OTC.*
Use: Mineral, vitamin supplement.
Centrum Jr. + Extra C. (Wyeth) Vitamins A 5000 units D 400 units, E 30 units, C 300 mg, folic acid 400 mcg, biotin 45 mcg, B_1 1.5 mg, B_5 10 mg, B_2 1.7 mg, B_3 20 mg, B_6 2 mg, B_{12} 6 mcg, K, Fe 18 mg, Mg, I, Cu, P, Ca 108 mg, Zn 15 mg, Mn, Mo, Cr, biotin 45 mcg, sugar, lactose. Chew. Tab. Bot. 60s. *OTC.*
Use: Mineral, vitamin supplement.
Centrum Jr. + Extra Calcium. (Wyeth) Calcium 160 mg, iron 18 mg, vitamins A 5000 units, D 400 units, E 30 mg, B_1 1.5 mg, B_2 1.7 mg, B_3 20 mg, B_5 10 mg, B_6 2 mg, B_{12} 6 mcg, C 60 mg, folic acid 400 mcg, Cr, Cu, I, Mn, Mg, Mo, P, Zn 15 mg, vitamin K, biotin 45 mcg, sugar. Chew. Tab. Bot. 60s. *OTC.*
Use: Mineral, vitamin supplement.
Centrum Jr. + Iron. (Wyeth) Iron 18 mg, vitamins A 5000 units, D 400 units, E 30 units, B_1 1.5 mg, B_2 1.7 mg, B_3 20 mg, B_5 10 mg, B_6 2 mg, B_{12} 6 mcg, C 60 mg, folic acid 0.4 mg, Ca, Cr, Cu, I, Mg, Mn, Mo, P, Zn 15 mg, biotin 45 mcg, vitamin K. Chew. Tab. Bot. 60s. *OTC.*
Use: Mineral, vitamin supplement.
Centrum Performance. (Wyeth) Ca 100 mg, Fe 18 mg, A 5000 units, D 400 units, E 60 units, B_1 4.5 mg, B_2 5.1 mg, B_3 40 mg, B_5 10 mg, B_6 6 mg, B_{12} 18 mcg, C 120 mg, folic acid 400 mcg, K 25 mcg, biotin 40 mcg, chloride 72 mcg, Ginkgo biloba leaf 60 mg, ginseng root 50 mg, B, Cr, Cu, I, K, Mg, Mn, Mo, Ni, P, Se, Si, Sn, V,

Zn 15 mg, glucose, lactose, maltodextrin, sucrose. Tab. Bot. 120s. *OTC.*
Use: Mineral, vitamin supplement.
Centrum Silver. (Wyeth) Vitamin A 3500 units, D 400 units, E 45 units, B_1 1.5 mg, B_2 1.7 mg, B_3 20 mg, B_5 10 mg, B_6 3 mg, B_{12} 25 mcg, C 60 mg, folic acid 400 mcg, Zn 15 mg, vitamin K 10 mcg, biotin 30 mcg, chloride, lutein 250 mcg, B, Ca, Cr, Cu, I, K, Mg, Mn, Mo, Ni, P, Se, Si, V, sucrose, glucose. Tab. Bot. 220s. *OTC.*
Use: Mineral, vitamin supplement.
Centrum Silver Gel-Tabs. (Wyeth) Vitamins A 6000 units, D 400 units, E 45 units, B_1 1.5 mg, B_2 1.7 mg, B_3 20 mg, B_5 10 mg, B_6 3 mg, B_{12} 25 mcg, C 60 mg, K 10 mcg, biotin 30 mcg, folic acid 200 mcg, Fe 9 mg. With Ca 200 mg, Cu, I, Mg, P, Zn, Cl, Cr, Mn, Mo, Ni, K, Se, Si, V. Tab. Bot. 60s. *OTC.*
Use: Mineral, vitamin supplement.
Centurion A-Z. (Mission Pharmacal) Vitamins A 5000 units, D 400 units, E 27 mg, A 5000 units, D 400 units, E 30 units, B_1 2.25 mg, B_2 2.6 mg, B_3 20 mg, B_5 10 mg, B_6 3 mg, B_{12} 9 mcg, C 90 mg, FA 0.4 mg, biotin 0.45 mg, Ca, Cl, Cr, Cu, I, K, Mg, Mn, Mo, P, Se, Zn, vitamin K. Tab. Bot. 130s. *OTC.*
Use: Mineral, vitamin supplement.
Ceo-Two. (Beutlich) Potassium bitartrate, sodium bicarbonate in polyethylene glycol base. Supp. Box 10s. *OTC.*
Use: Laxative.
Cepacol. (J.B. Williams Company) cetyl pyridinium Cl 0.05%, alcohol 14%, tartrazine, saccharin. Liq. Bot. 360 mL, 540 mL, 720 mL, 960 mL. *OTC.*
Use: Antiseptic.
Cepacol Anesthetic Lozenges. (J.B. Williams Company) Benzocaine 10 mg, cetylpyridinium Cl 0.07%, tartrazine. Pkg. 18s, 24s. *OTC.*
Use: Anesthetic, local.
Cepacol Maximum Strength. (J.B. Williams Company) Benzocaine 10 mg, menthol, cool mint, cherry flavors. Loz. Pkg. 16s. *OTC.*
Use: Mouth and throat product.
Cepacol Sore Throat. (J.B. Williams Company) Pseudoephedrine hydrochloride 10 mg, acetaminophen 106.7 mg/5 mL, tartrazine, honey, saccharin, sorbitol, honey flavor, alcohol free. Liq. Bot. 237 mL. *OTC.*
Use: Upper respiratory combination, decongestant, analgesic.
Cepacol Throat Lozenges. (J.B. Williams Company) cetylpyridinium Cl 0.07%, benzyl alcohol 0.3%, tartrazine. Loz. Pkg. 27s, 40s. *OTC.*

Use: Antiseptic.

Cēpacol Viractin. (J.B. Williams Company) **Cream:** Tetracaine 2%, hydrochloric acid, methylparaben. Tube 7.1 g. **Gel:** Tetracaine 2%, parabens. Tube 7.1 g. *OTC.*
Use: Anesthetic, local.

Cēpastat Cherry Lozenges. (GlaxoSmithKline) Phenol 14.5 mg, menthol, sorbitol, saccharin. Sugar free. Loz. Box 18s. *OTC.*
Use: Anesthetic.

Cēpastat Extra Strength. (GlaxoSmithKline) Phenol 29 mg, menthol, sorbitol, eucalyptus oil. Sugar free. Loz. Pkg. 18s. *OTC.*
Use: Anesthetic.

●**cephacetrile sodium.** (SEFF-ah-seh-TRILE) USAN.
Use: Anti-infective, cephalosporin.

●**cephalexin.** (SEFF-ah-LEX-in) *USP 28.*
Use: Anti-infective, cephalosporin.
See: Biocef.
Keflex.

cephalexin. (Various Mfr.) Cephalexin. **Cap.:** 250 mg, 500 mg. Bot. 100s, 250s (500 mg), 500s, 1000s, UD 20s, 100s. **Tab.:** 250 mg, 500 mg, 1 g. Bot. 20s, 100s, 500s. Pkg. 24s (1 g only). **Pow. for Oral Susp.:** 125 mg/5 mL, 250 mg/5 mL. Bot. 100 mL, 200 mL. *Rx.*
Use: Anti-infective, cephalosporin.

cephalin.
W/Lecithin with Choline Base, Lipositol.
See: Alcolec.

●**cephaloglycin.** (SEFF-ah-low-GLIE-sin) USAN.
Use: Anti-infective.

●**cephaloridine.** (SEFF-ah-lor-ih-deen) USAN.
Use: Anti-infective, cephalosporin.

cephalosporins and related antibiotics.
Use: Antibiotics.
See: Cefaclor.
Cefadroxil.
Cefazolin Sodium.
Cefdinir.
Cefditoren Pivoxil.
Cefepime Hydrochloride.
Cefixime.
Cefmetazole Sodium.
Cefoperazone Sodium.
Cefotaxime Sodium.
Cefotetan Disodium.
Cefoxitin Sodium.
Cefpodoxime Proxetil.
Cefprozil.
Ceftazidine.
Ceftibutin.
Ceftizoxime Sodium.
Ceftriaxone Sodium.
Cefuroxime.
Cephalexin.
Cephradine.
Loracarbef.

●**cephalothin sodium.** (seff-AY-low-thin) *USP 28.*
Use: Anti-infective, cephalosporin.

●**cephapirin benzathine.** (SEFF-uh-PIE-rin BEN-zuh-theen) *USP 28.*
Use: Anti-infective.

●**cephapirin sodium.** (SEFF-uh-PIE-rin) *USP 28.*
Use: Anti-infective.

cephazolin sodium.
See: Cefazolin.

●**cephradine.** (SEFF-ruh-deen) *USP 28.*
Use: Anti-infective, cephalosporin.
See: Velosef.

cephradine. (Various Mfr.) Cephradine. **Cap.:** 250 mg, 500 mg. Bot. 24s, 40s, 100s, 500s, UD 100s. **Pow. for Oral Susp.:** 125 mg/5 mL, 250 mg/5 mL when reconstituted. Bot. 100 mL, 200 mL. *Rx.*
Use: Anti-infective, cephalosporin.

Cephulac. (Hoechst) Lactulose 10 g/15 mL (< galactose 1.6 g, lactose 1.2 g, other sugars 1.2 g). Soln. Bot. 473 mL, 1.9 L, UD 30 mL. *Rx.*
Use: Laxative.

Ceptaz. (GlaxoSmithKline) Ceftazidime pentahydrate with L-arginine 1 g, 2 g. Vial. Infusion packs (1 g, 2 g). Pharmacy bulk packages (10 g). *Rx.*
Use: Anti-infective, cephalosporin.

ceramide trihexosidase/alpha-galactosidase a. (Genzyme)
Use: Fabry disease. [Orphan Drug]

Cerapon. (Purdue) Triethanolamine polypeptide oleate condensate.
See: Cerumenex.

Cerebyx. (Parke-Davis) Fosphenytoin 150 mg (100 mg phenytoin sodium) in 2 mL vials and 750 mg (500 mg phenytoin sodium) in 10 mL vials. *Rx.*
Use: Treatment of certain types of seizures.

Ceredase. (Genzyme) Alglucerase 10 units/mL, 80 units/mL. Inj. Bot. 50 units with 5 mL fill volume (10 units), 400 units with 5 mL fill volume (80 units). *Rx.*
Use: Enzyme replacement for Gaucher disease.

Cerefolin. (Pan American Labs) Vitamin B_2 5 mg, vitamin B_6 50 mg, vitamin B_{12} 1 mg. L-methylfolate 5.635 mg. Tab. 90s. *Rx.*

Use: Nutritional product.

cerelose.
See: Glucose.

Ceretex. (Enzyme Process) Iron 15 mg, vitamins B_{12} 10 mcg, B_1 2 mg, B_6 1 mg, niacinamide 1 mg, pantothenic acid 0.15 mg, B_2 2 mg, iodine 15 mg/ 2 mL. Bot. 60 mL, 240 mL. *OTC.*
Use: Mineral, vitamin supplement.

Cerezyme. (Genzyme) Imiglucerase 212 units (equiv. to a withdrawal dose of 200 units). Pow. for Inj. Vials. *Rx.*
Use: Treatment for Gaucher disease.

Cernevit-12. (Baxter Healthcare) Vitamin A 3500 units, D_3 200 units, E (as dl-alpha tocopheryl) 11.2 units, C 125 mg, B_3 46 mg, B_5 17.25 mg, B_6 4.53 mg, B_2 4.14 mg, B_1 3.51 mg, folic acid 414 mcg, d-biotin 60 mcg, B_{12} 5.5 mcg. Pow. for Inj., lyophilized. Single-dose vial 5 mL. *Rx.*
Use: Vitamin supplement.

• **ceronapril.** (seh-ROE-nap-rill) USAN.
Use: Antihypertensive.

Cerovite. (Rugby) Iron 18 mg, vitamins A 5000 units, D 400 units, E 30 units, B_1 1.5 mg, B_2 1.7 mg, B_3 20 mg, B_5 10 mg, B_6 2 mg, B_{12} 6 mcg, C 60 mg, folic acid 0.4 mg, Ca, Cl, Cr, Cu, I, Mg, Mn, Mo, Ni, P, Se, Si, SN, V, biotin 30 mcg, vitamin K, Zn 15 mg. Tab. Bot. 130s. *OTC.*
Use: Mineral, vitamin supplement.

Cerovite Advanced Formula. (Rugby) Iron 18 mg, A 5000 units, D 400 units, E 30 units, B_1 1.5 mg, B_2 1.7 mg, B_3 20 mg, B_5 10 mg, B_6 2 mg, B_{12} 6 mcg, C 60 mg, folic acid 0.4 mg, biotin 30 mcg, Ca, P, I, Mg, Cu, Mn, K, Cl, Cr, Mo, Se, Ni, Si, Sn, V, vitamin K, Zn 15 mg. Tab. Bot. 130s, 200s. *OTC.*
Use: Iron with vitamin supplement.

Cerovite Jr. (Rugby) Iron 18 mg, vitamins A 5000 units, D 400 units, E 15 units, B_1 1.5 mg, B_2 1.7 mg, B_3 20 mg, B_5 10 mg, B_6 2 mg, B_{12} 6 mcg, C 60 mg, folic acid 0.4 mg, Cu, I, Mg, Zn, Mn, Mo, biotin 45 mcg, Cr, sugar. Tab. Bot. 60s. *OTC.*
Use: Mineral, vitamin supplement.

Cerovite Senior. (Rugby) Vitamins A 6000 units, D 400 units, E 45 units, B_1 1.5 mg, B_2 1.7 mg, B_3 20 mg, B_5 10 mg, B_6 3 mg, B_{12} 25 mcg, C 60 mg, iron 9 mg, folic acid 0.2 mg, Cu, I, Mg, P, Cl, Cr, Mn, Mo, Ni, Se, Si, V, vitamin K. Tab. Bot. 60s. *OTC.*
Use: Mineral, vitamin supplement.

Certagen Liquid. (Ivax) Vitamins A 2500 units, B_1 1.5 mg, B_2 1.7 mg, B_3

20 mg, B_5 10 mg, B_6 2 mg, B_{12} 6 mcg, C 60 mg, D_3 400 units, E 30 units, biotin 300 mcg, iron 9 mg, Zn 3 mg, Cr, I, Mn, Mo/15 mL. Alcohol 6.6%. Liq. Bot. 237 mL. *OTC.*
Use: Mineral, vitamin supplement.

Certagen Senior. (Ivax) Vitamin A 6000 units, B_1 1.5 mg, B_2 1.7 mg, B_6 3 mg, B_{12} 25 mcg, C 60 mg, D 400 units, E 45 units, vitamin K, biotin 30 mcg, folic acid 200 mcg, B_3 20 mg, B_5 10 mg, Ca 80 mg, Cl, Cr, Cu, I, Fe 3 mg, Mg, Mn, Mo, Ni, P, K, Se, Si, V, Zn 15 mg. Tab. Bot. 60s. *OTC.*
Use: Mineral, vitamin supplement.

Certagen Tablets. (Ivax) Iron 18 mg, A 5000 units, D 400 units, E 30 units, B_1 1.5 mg, B_2 1.7 mg, B_3 20 mg, B_5 10 mg, B_6 2 mg, B_{12} 6 mcg, C 60 mg, folic acid 0.4 mg, biotin 30 mcg, Ca, P, I, Mg, Cu, Mn, K, Cl, Cr, Mo, Se, Ni, Si, Sn, V, vitamin K, Zn 15 mg. Tab. Bot. 130s, 1000s. *OTC.*
Use: Mineral, vitamin supplement.

Certa-Vite. (Major) Vitamin A 5000 units, D 400 units, E 30 units, K_1, C 60 mg, B_1 1.5 mg, B_2 1.7 mg, B_3 20 mg, B_6 2 mg, B_{12} 6 mcg, B_5 10 mg, folic acid 0.4 mg, biotin 30 mcg, Fe 18 mg, Ca, P, I, Mg, Cu, Zn, Mn, K, Cl, Cr, Mo, Se, Ni, Si, V, B. Tab. Bot. 130s, 300s. *OTC.*
Use: Mineral, vitamin supplement.

Certa-Vite Golden. (Major) Vitamin A 6000 units, D 400 units, E 45 units, B_1 1.5 mg, B_2 1.7 mg, B_3 20 mg, B_5 10 mg, B_6 3 mg, B_{12} 25 mcg, C 60 mg, vitamin K, Ca 200 mg, Zn 15 mg, biotin 30 mcg, Cl, Cr, Cu, I, K, Mg, Mn, Mo, Ni, P, Se, Si, V. Tab. Bot. 60s. *OTC.*
Use: Mineral, vitamin supplement.

Cerubidine. (Bedford) Daunorubicin hydrochloride 21.4 mg (equivalent to daunorubicin 20 mg), mannitol 100 mg. Pow. for Inj., lyophilized. Single-dose vial. *Rx.*
Use: Antibiotic, anthracycline.

• **ceruletide.** (seh-ROO-leh-tide) USAN.
Use: Stimulant, gastric secretory.

• **ceruletide diethylamine.** (seh-ROO-leh-tide die-ETH-ill-ah-meen) USAN.
Use: Stimulant, gastric secretory.

Cerumenex. (Purdue) Triethanolamine polypeptide oleate-condensate 10%, chlorobutanol in propylene glycol 0.5%. Liq. Dropper bot. 6 mL, 12 mL. *Rx.*
Use: Otic.

cervical ripening agents.
See: Dinoprostone.
Prepidil.

Cervidil. (Forest) Dinoprostone 10 mg. Insert. 1s. *Rx.*

Use: Cervical ripening.
Ces. (ICN) Conjugated estrogens 0.625 mg, 1.25 mg, 2.5 mg. Tab. *Rx.*
Use: Estrogen.
Cesia. (Prasco) **Phase 1:** Desogestrel 0.1 mg, ethinyl estradiol 25 mcg. **Phase 2:** Desogestrel 0.125 mg, ethinyl estradiol 25 mcg. **Phase 3:** Desogestrel 0.15 mg, ethinyl estradiol 25 mcg. Lactose. Tab. 28s. *Rx.*
Use: Contraceptive.
•**cesium chloride Cs 131.** (SEE-zee-uhm KLOR-ide) USAN.
Use: Radiopharmaceutical agent.
Ceta. (C & M Pharmacal) Soap-free. Propylene glycol, hydroxyethylcellulose, cetyl and cetearyl alcohols, sodium lauryl sulfate, parabens. Liq. Bot. 240 mL. *OTC.*
Use: Dermatologic cleanser.
•**cetaben sodium.** (SEE-tah-ben) USAN.
Use: Antihyperlipoproteinemic.
Cetacaine. (Cetylite Industries) Benzocaine 14%, butyl aminobenzoate 2%, tetracaine hydrochloride 2%, benzalkonium Cl 0.5%, cetyl dimethyl ethyl ammonium bromide 0.005%. **Aerosol Spray:** 56 g. **Liq.:** 56 g. **Oint.:** Jar 37 g, flavored. **Hosp. Gel:** 29 g. *Rx.*
Use: Anesthetic, local.
Cetacort. (Galderma) Hydrocortisone 0.25%, 0.5%, 1% w/cetyl alcohol, propylene glycol, stearyl alcohol, sodium lauryl sulfate, butylparaben, methylparaben, propylparaben, purified water. Bot. 120 mL (0.25% only), 60 mL (0.5%, 1% only). *Rx.*
Use: Corticosteroid, topical.
•**cetalkonium chloride.** (SEET-al-KOE-nee-uhm) USAN.
Use: Anti-infective, topical.
W/Phenylephrine, pyrilamine maleate, thimerosal.
See: Anti-B Mist.
Cetamide. (Alcon) Sulfacetamide sodium 10%. Sterile ophth. oint. Tube 3.5 g. *Rx.*
Use: Anti-infective, ophthalmic.
•**cetamolol hydrochloride.** (SEET-AM-oh-lahl) USAN.
Use: Anti-adrenergic, beta-receptor.
Cetaphil. (Galderma) **Cream, Lot.:** Cetyl alcohol, stearyl alcohol, propylene glycol (cream only), sodium lauryl sulfate, methylparaben, propylparaben, butylparaben. Bot. 480 g (cream), 120 mL, 240 mL, 480 mL (lotion). **Antibacterial Bar:** Triclosan, petrolatum. Soap-free. 127 g. **Bar:** Petrolatum. Soap-free. 127 g. **Cleanser:** Cetyl alcohol, stearyl alcohol, parabens. Bot. 236 mL. *OTC.*

Use: Dermatologic cleanser.
Ceta-Plus. (Seatrace) Hydrocodone bitartrate 5 mg, acetaminophen 500 mg. Cap. Bot. 100s. *c-III.*
Use: Analgesic combination, narcotic.
Cetazol. (Professional Pharmacal) Acetazolamide 250 mg. Tab. Bot. 100s. *Rx.*
Use: Anticonvulsant; diuretic.
•**cethromycin.** (ceth-roe-MYE-sin) USAN.
Use: Antibacterial.
•**cetiedil citrate.** (see-TIE-eh-DILL SIH-trate) USAN.
Use: Vasodilator, peripheral.
•**cetirizine.** (seh-TIH-rih-zeen) USAN.
Use: Antihistamine, peripherally selective piperazine.
See: Zyrtec.
W/Pseudoephedrine hydrochloride.
See: Zyrtec-D 12 Hour.
•**cetocycline hydrochloride.** (SEE-toe-SIGH-kleen) USAN. *Formerly cetotetrine hydrochloride.*
Use: Anti-infective.
•**cetophenicol.** (see-toe-FEN-ih-kole) USAN.
Use: Antibacterial.
•**cetostearyl alcohol.** *NF 23.*
Use: Pharmaceutic aid, emulsifying agent.
•**cetraxate hydrochloride.** (seh-TRAX-ate) USAN.
Use: Antiulcerative; gastrointestinal.
cetrorelix acetate.
Use: Sex hormone; gonadotropin-releasing hormone antagonist.
See: Cetrotide.
Cetrotide. (ASTA Medica) Cetrorelix acetate 0.25 mg, 3 mg. Inj. Trays containing 1 vial of 0.26 to 0.27 mg or 3.12 to 3.24 mg cetrorelix acetate, 1 mL or 3 mL syr. of Sterile Water for Inj., 20-gauge needle, 27-gauge needle, alcohol swabs. 1s, 7s (0.25 mg only). *Rx.*
Use: Sex hormone; gonadotropin-releasing hormone antagonist.
•**cetuximab.** (seh-TUCKS-ih-mab) USAN.
Use: Monoclonal antibody.
See: Erbitux.
•**cetyl alcohol.** (SEE-till) *NF 23.*
Use: Pharmaceutic aid, emulsifying and stiffening agent.
Cetylcide Solution. (Cetylite Industries) Cetyldimethylethyl ammonium bromide 6.5%, benzalkonium Cl 6.5%, isopropyl alcohol 13%. Inert ingredients 74%, including sodium nitrite. Bot. 16 oz, 32 oz.
Use: Disinfectant.

cetyldimethyl benzyl ammonium chloride.
W/Benzocaine, ascorbic acid.
See: Locane.
●**cetyl esters wax.** (SEE-till ess-ters) *NF 23. Formerly synthetic spermacet.*
Use: Pharmaceutic aid, stiffening agent.
●**cetylpyridinium chloride.** (SEE-till-pihr-ih-DIH-nee-uhm) *USP 28.*
Use: Anti-infective, topical; pharmaceutic aid, preservative.
See: Bactalin.
W/Benzocaine.
See: Axon.
Cēpacol.
Cēpacol Antiseptic.
Coirex.
Semets.
Spec-T Sore Throat
W/d-Methorphan HBr, phenyltoloxamine dihydrogen citrate, sodium citrate.
See: Exo-Kol.
W/Phenylephrine hydrochloride, methapyrilene hydrochloride, menthol, eucalyptol, camphor, methyl salicylate.
See: Vicks Sinex.
cetyltrimethyl ammonium bromide.
(Bioline Labs) Cetrimide B.P., Cetavlon, CTAB.
Use: Antiseptic.
Cevi-Bid. (Lee) Ascorbic acid 500 mg. Tab. Bot. 100s, 500s, UD 12s, 96s. *OTC.*
Use: Vitamin supplement.
●**cevimeline hydrochloride.** (seh-vih-MEH-leen) USAN.
Use: Treatment of Alzheimer disease, adjunct; dry mouth.
See: Evoxac.
cevitamic acid.
See: Ascorbic acid.
cevitan.
See: Ascorbic acid.
Cewin. (Sanofi-Synthelabo) Ascorbic acid. *OTC.*
Use: Vitamin supplement.
Ceylon gelatin.
See: Agar.
Cezin. (Forest) Vitamins B_1 20 mg, B_2 10 mg, B_3 100 mg, B_5 20 mg, B_6 5 mg, C 300 mg, magnesium sulfate 70 mg, zinc sulfate 80 mg. Cap. Bot. 100s. *OTC.*
Use: Vitamin supplement.
Cezin-S. (Forest) Vitamins A 10,000 units, D 50 units, E 50 units, B_1 10 mg, B_2 5 mg, B_3 50 mg, B_5 10 mg, B_6 2 mg, C 200 mg, folic acid 0.5 mg, Zn 18 mg, Mg, Mn. Cap. Bot. 100s. *Rx.*
Use: Vitamin supplement.

C Factors "1000" Plus. (Solgar) Vitamin C 1000 mg, rose hips 25 mg, citrus bioflavonoids complex 250 mg, rutin 50 mg, hesperidin 25 mg. Tab. Bot. 50s. *OTC.*
Use: Vitamin supplement.
C.G. (Sigma-Tau) Chorionic gonadotropin (lyophilized) 10,000 units, mannitol 100 mg, supplied with diluent. Univial 10 mL. *Rx.*
Use: Hormone, chorionic gonadotropin.
CG Disposable Unit.
See: Cardio Green.
CG Ria. (Abbott Diagnostics) Radioimmunoassay for the quantitative measurement of total circulating serum cholylglycine.
Use: Diagnostic aid.
Chap Cream. (Ar-Ex) Carbonyl diamide. Cream. Tube 1.5 oz, 3.25 oz. Jar 4 oz, 9 oz, 18 oz. *OTC.*
Use: Emollient.
Chapoline Cream Lotion. (Wade) Glycerin, boric acid, chlorobutanol 0.5%, alcohol 10%. Lot. Bot. 4 oz, pt, gal. *OTC.*
Use: Emollient.
Chapstick Medicated Lip Balm. (Wyeth) **Jar:** Petrolatum 60%, camphor 1%, menthol 0.6%, phenol 0.5%, microcrystalline wax, mineral oil, cocoa butter, lanolin, paraffin wax, parabens 7 g. **Squeezable tube:** Petrolatum 67%, camphor 1%, menthol 0.6%, phenol 0.5%, microcrystalline wax, mineral oil, cocoa butter, lanolin, parabens 10 g. **Stick:** Petrolatum 41%, camphor 1%, menthol 0.6%, phenol 0.5%, paraffin wax, mineral oil, cocoa butter, 2-octyl dodecanol, arachidyl propionate, polyphenyl methylsiloxane 556, white wax, oleyl alcohol, isopropyl lanolate, carnuba wax, isopropyl myristate, lanolin, cetyl alcohol, parabens. 4.2 g. *OTC.*
Use: Mouth and throat preparation.
Chapstick Sunblock 15. (Wyeth) Padimate O 0.7%, oxybenzone 3%. Stick 4.25 g. *OTC.*
Use: Lip protectant.
Chapstick Sunblock 15 Petroleum Jelly Plus. (Wyeth) White petrolatum 89%, padimate O 7%, oxybenzone 3%, aloe, lanolin. Stick 10 g. *OTC.*
Use: Lip protectant.
CharcoAid. (Requa, Inc.) Activated charcoal 15 g/120 mL, 30 g/150 mL, sorbitol. Susp. Bot. *OTC.*
Use: Antidote.
CharcoAid 2000. (Requa, Inc.) Activated charcoal 15 g/120 mL, 50 g/240 mL with and without sorbitol. Liq. 15 g/240 mL.

Granules. Bot. *OTC.*
Use: Antidote.
charcoal. (Various Mfr.) Cap., Tab. *OTC.*
Use: Antiflatulent.
•**charcoal, activated.** (CHAR-kole)
USP 28.
Use: Antidote, general purpose; pharmaceutic aid, adsorbent.
See: Actidose-Aqua.
CharcoAid.
Charcoal Plus.
Liqui-Char.
W/Nux vomica, bismuth subgallate, pepsin, berberis, diastase, pancreatin, hydrastis, papain.
See: Charcocaps.
charcoal and simethicone. Antiflatulent.
See: Charcoal Plus.
Flatulex.
Charcoal Plus. (Kramer) Activated charcoal 250 mg, sugar. EC Tab. Bot. 120s.
OTC.
Use: Antiflatulent.
CharcoCaps. (Requa, Inc.) Activated charcoal 260 mg. Cap. Bot. 36s. *OTC.*
Use: Antiflatulent.
Chardonna-2. (Kremers Urban) Belladonna extract 15 mg, phenobarbital 15 mg. Tab. Bot. 100s. *Rx.*
Use: Anticholinergic; antispasmodic; hypnotic; sedative.
Charo Scatter-Paks. (Requa, Inc.) Activated charcoal 5 g. Packet.
Use: Odor absorbent.
Chaz Scalp Treatment Dandruff Shampoo. (Revlon) Zinc pyrithione 1% in liquid shampoo. *OTC.*
Use: Antiseborrheic.
Chealamide. (Vortech Pharmaceuticals) Disodium edetate 150 mg/mL. Inj. Vial. 20 mL. *Rx.*
Use: Chelating agent.
Checkmate. (Oral-B) Acidulated phosphate fluoride 1.23%. Bot. 2 oz, 16 oz. *Rx.*
Use: Dental caries agent.
Cheetah. (Mallinckrodt) Barium sulfate 2.2%, simethicone, sorbitol, saccharin, sodium benzoate. Susp. Bot. 250 mL, 450 mL, 900 mL, 1900 mL. *Rx.*
Use: Radiopaque agent, GI contrast agent.
Chek-Stix Urinalysis Control Strips. (Bayer Corp. (Consumer Div.)) Bot. 25s.
Use: Diagnostic aid.
chelafrin.
See: Epinephrine.
Chelated Calcium Magnesium. (NBTY) Ca++ 500 mg, Mg 250 mg. Tab. Protein coated. Bot. 50s. *OTC.*

Use: Mineral supplement.
Chelated Calcium Magnesium Zinc. (NBTY) Ca++ 333 mg, Mg 133 mg, Zn 8.3 mg. Tab. Bot. 100s. *OTC.*
Use: Mineral supplement.
Chelated Manganese. (Freeda) Manganese 20 mg, 50 mg. Tab. Bot. 100s, 250s, 500s. *OTC.*
Use: Mineral supplement.
chelating agents.
See: BAL.
Deferoxamine Mesylate.
Dimercaprol.
Edetate Calcium Disodium.
Pentetate Calcium Trisodium.
Pentetate Zinc Trisodium.
Succimer (DMSA).
Trientine Hydrochloride.
chelen.
See: Ethyl Chloride.
Chemet. (Ovation) Succimer 100 mg. Cap. Bot. 100s. *Rx.*
Use: Chelating agent.
Chemipen. Potassium phenethicillin.
Use: Anti-infective, penicillin.
Chemovag. (Forest) Sulfisoxazole 0.5 g. Supp. Bot. 12s w/applicators. *Rx.*
Use: Anti-infective, sulfonamide.
Chemozine. (Tennessee Pharmaceutic) Sulfadiazine, 0.167 g, sulfamerazine 0.167 g, sulfamethazine 0.167 g. Tab. Bot. 100s, 1000s. Susp. Bot. Pt, gal. *Rx.*
Use: Anti-infective, sulfonamide.
Chemstrip bG. (Boehringer Mannheim) Reagent strips for testing blood sugar. Strip Bot. 50s.
Use: Diagnostic aid.
Chemstrip 8. (Boehringer Mannheim) Broad range urine test for glucose, protein, pH, blood, ketones, bilirubin, urobilinogen, leukocytes. Strip Bot. 100s.
Use: Diagnostic aid.
Chemstrip 4 the OB. (Boehringer Mannheim) Broad range test for glucose, protein, blood, leukocytes in urine. Strip Bot. 100s.
Use: Diagnostic aid.
Chemstrip-K. (Boehringer Mannheim) Reagent papers for ketones in urine. Paper Bot. 25s, 100s.
Use: Diagnostic aid.
Chemstrip Micral. (Boehringer Mannheim) In vitro reagent strips to detect albumin in urine. Strip Pkg. 5s, 30s.
Use: Diagnostic aid.
Chemstrip Mineral. (Boehringer Mannheim) In vitro reagent strips used to detect albumin in urine. Strip Pkg. 5s, 30s.
Use: In vitro diagnostic aid.

Chemstrip 9. (Boehringer Mannheim) Broad range test for glucose, protein, pH, blood, ketones, bilirubin, urobilinogen, nitrite, leukocytes in urine. Strip Bot. 100s.
Use: Diagnostic aid.

Chemstrip 7. (Boehringer Mannheim) Broad range test for glucose, protein, pH, blood, ketones, bilirubin, leukocytes. Strip Bot. 100s.
Use: Diagnostic aid.

Chemstrip 6. (Boehringer Mannheim) Broad range test for glucose, protein, pH, blood, ketones, leukocytes. Strip Bot. 100s.
Use: Diagnostic aid.

Chemstrip 10 SG. (Boehringer Mannheim) Broad range test for glucose, protein, pH, blood, ketones, bilirubin, urobilinogen, nitrite, leukocytes in urine. Strip Bot. 100s.
Use: Diagnostic aid.

Chemstrip 2 GP. (Boehringer Mannheim) Broad range test for glucose and protein. Strip Bot. 100s.
Use: Diagnostic aid.

Chemstrip 2 LN. (Boehringer Mannheim) Broad range test for nitrite and leukocytes. Strip Bot. 100s.
Use: Diagnostic aid.

Chemstrip uG. (Boehringer Mannheim) Reagent strips for glucose in urine. Strip Bot. 100s.
Use: Diagnostic aid.

Chemstrip uGK. (Boehringer Mannheim) Broad range test for glucose and ketones. Strip Bot. 50s, 100s.
Use: Diagnostic aid.

Chenatal. (Miller Pharmacal Group) Calcium 580 mg, Mg 200 mg, vitamins C 100 mg, folic acid 0.4 mg, A 5000 units, D 400 units, B_1 3 mg, B_2 3 mg, B_6 5 mg, B_{12} 9 mcg, niacinamide 30 mg, pantothenic acid 5 mg, tocopherols (mixed) 10 mg, Fe 20 mg, Cu 1 mg, Mn 2 mg, K 10 mg, Zn 25 mg, I 0.1 mg. 2 Tabs. Bot. 100s. *OTC.*
Use: Mineral, vitamin supplement.

Chenix. (Solvay) Chenodil.
Use: Anticholelithogenic. [Orphan Drug]

chenodeoxycholic acid.
Use: Urolithic.
See: Chenodiol.

•**chenodiol.** (KEEN-oh-DIE-ahl) USAN.
Formerly chenic acid.
Use: Anticholelithogenic. [Orphan Drug]

Cheracol. (Lee) Codeine phosphate 10 mg, guaifenesin 100 mg/5 mL, alcohol 4.75%. Bot. 2 oz, 4 oz, pt. *c-v.*
Use: Antitussive; expectorant.

Cheracol Cough. (Lee) Codeine phosphate 10 mg, guaifenesin 100 mg/5 mL, alcohol 4.75%, fructose, sucrose. Syr. Bot. 60 mL, 120 mL, 480 mL. *c-v.*
Use: Upper respiratory combination, antitussive, expectorant.

Cheracol D. (Lee) Dextromethorphan HBr 10 mg, guaifenesin 100 mg/5 mL, alcohol 4.75%. Bot. 2 oz, 4 oz, 6 oz. *OTC.*
Use: Antitussive, expectorant.

Cheracol D Cough Formula. (Lee) Dextromethorphan HBr 10 mg, guaifenesin 100 mg/5 mL, alcohol 4.75%, fructose, sucrose. Syr. Bot. 118 mL, 177 mL. *OTC.*
Use: Upper respiratory combination, antitussive, expectorant.

Cheracol Plus. (Lee) Dextromethorphan HBr 10 mg, guaifenesin 100 mg/5 mL, alcohol 4.75%, fructose, sucrose. Liq. Bot. 118 mL. *OTC.*
Use: Upper respiratory combination, antitussive, expectorant.

Cheracol Sore Throat. (Lee) Phenol 1.4%, saccharin, sorbitol, alcohol 12.5%. Spray Bot. 180 mL. *OTC.*
Use: Mouth and throat product.

Chero-Trisulfa-V. (Vita Elixir) Sulfadiazine 0.166 g, sulfacetamide 0.166 g, sulfamerazine 0.166 g, sodium citrate 0.5 g/5 mL. Susp. Bot. Pt.
Use: Anti-infective, sulfonamide.

•**cherry juice.** *NF 23.*
Use: Flavoring.

•**cherry syrup.** *NF 23.*
Use: Pharmaceutic aid, vehicle.

Chest Throat. (Lane) Eucalyptol, anise, horehound, tolu balsam, benzoin tincture, sugar, corn syrup. Loz. Pkg. 30s. *OTC.*
Use: Antiseptic.

Chewable Multivitamins w/Fluoride. (H.L. Moore Drug Exchange) Fluoride 1 mg, vitamins A 2500 units, D 400 units, E 15 units, B_1 1.05 mg, B_2 1.2 mg, B_3 13.5 mg, B_6 1.05 mg, B_{12} 4.5 mcg, C 60 mg, folic acid 0.3 mg, sucrose. Tab. Bot. 100s. *Rx.*
Use: Mineral, vitamin supplement; dental caries agent.

Chewable Vitamin C. (Various Mfr.) Vitamin C (as sodium ascorbate and ascorbic acid) 250 mg, 500 mg. Chew. Tab. Bot. 100s. *OTC.*
Use: Vitamin supplement.

Chew-C. (Key Company) Vitamin C (as ascorbic acid and sodium ascorbate) 500 mg. Sugar. Orange flavor. Chew. Tab. 100s. *OTC.*
Use: Vitamin.

Chew-Vims. (Barth's) Vitamins A 5000 units, D 400 units, B_1 3 mg, B_2 6 mg, niacin 1.71 mg, C 100 mg, B_{12} 5 mcg, E 5 units. Tab. Bot. 30s, 90s, 180s, 360s. *OTC.*
Use: Vitamin supplement.

Chew-Vi-Tab. (Halsey Drug) Vitamins A 2500 units, D 400 units, E 15 units, C 60 mg, folic acid 0.3 mg, B_1 1.05 mg, B_2 1.2 mg, niacin 13.5 mg, B_6 1.05 mg, B_{12} 4.5 mcg. Tab. Bot. 100s. *OTC.*
Use: Vitamin supplement.

Chew-Vi-Tab with Iron. (Halsey Drug) Vitamins A 5000 units, C 60 mg, E 15 units, folic acid 0.4 mg, $B_1$1.5 mg, B_2 1.7 mg, niacin 20 mg, B_6 2 mg, B_{12} 6 mcg, D 400 units, iron 18 mg. Tab. Bot. 100s. *OTC.*
Use: Mineral, vitamin supplement.

chicken pox vaccine.
See: Varivax.

Chiggerex. (Scherer) Benzocaine 0.02%, camphor, menthol, peppermint oil, olive oil, clove oil, pegosperse, methylparaben. Oint. Jar 50 g. *OTC.*
Use: Anesthetic, counterirritant.

Chigger-Tox. (Scherer) Benzocaine 2.1%, benzyl benzoate 21.4%, soft soap, isopropyl alcohol. Liq. Bot. 30 mL. *OTC.*
Use: Anesthetic, topical.

Children's Advil Suspension. (Wyeth) Ibuprofen 100 mg/5 mL, sorbitol, sucrose, EDTA, fruit flavor. Susp. Bot. 119 mL, 473 mL. *Rx.*
Use: Analgesic, NSAID.

Children's Advil Tablets. (Whitehall-Robins) Ibuprofen 50 mg, aspartame, phenylalanine 2.1 mg, fruit and grape flavor. Chew. Tab. Bot. 24s, 50s. *OTC.*
Use: Analgesic, NSAID.

Children's Benadryl Allergy Fastmelt. (Pfizer) Diphenhydramine 12.5 mg (equiv. to 19 mg citrate). Aspartame, mannitol, phenylalanine 4.5 mg. Orally Disintegrating Tab. 20s. *OTC.*
Use: Antihistamine.

Children's Dramamine. (Pharmacia) Dimenhydrinate 12.5 mg/5 mL, alcohol 5%, sucrose. Liq. Bot. 120 mL. *OTC.*
Use: Antiemetic; antivertigo.

Children's Dynafed Jr. (BDI) Acetaminophen 80 mg, fruit flavor. Chew. Tab. Bot. 36s. *OTC.*
Use: Analgesic.

Children's Elixir DM Cough & Cold. (AmerisourceBergen) Pseudoephedrine hydrochloride 15 mg, brompheniramine maleate 1 mg, dextromethorphan HBr 5 mg/5 mL, saccharin, sorbitol, grape flavor, alcohol free. Elixir. Bot. 118 mL.

OTC.
Use: Upper respiratory combination, decongestant, antihistamine, antitussive.

Children's Feverall. (Upsher-Smith) Acetaminophen 120 mg, 325 mg. Supp. Pkg. 6s. *OTC.*
Use: Analgesic.

Children's Formula Cough. (Pharmakon) Guaifenesin 50 mg, dextromethorphan HBr 5 mg/5 mL, sucrose, corn syrup. Alcohol free. Grape flavor. Syr. Bot. 118 mL, 236 mL. *OTC.*
Use: Expectorant; antitussive.

Children's Ibuprofen Cold. (Major) Pseudoephedrine hydrochloride 15 mg, ibuprofen 100 mg/5 mL. Alcohol-free. Corn syrup. Berry flavor. Susp. 120 mL. *OTC.*
Use: Decongestant, analgesic.

Children's Kaopectate. (Pharmacia) Attapulgite 600 mg/5 mL. Liq. Bot. 180 mL. *OTC.*
Use: Antidiarrheal.

Children's Loratadine. (Taro) Loratadine 5 mg per 5 mL. Fruit flavor. Syrup. 120 mL. *OTC.*
Use: Antihistamine.

Children's Mapap. (Major) Acetaminophen 160 mg/5 mL, alcohol free. Elix. Bot. 120 mL. *OTC.*
Use: Analgesic.

Children's Motrin. (Ortho-McNeil) Ibuprofen. **Chew. Tab.:** 50 mg, aspartame, phenylalanine 3 mg, orange flavor. Bot. 24s. **Susp.:** 100 mg/5 mL; sucrose; berry, grape, and bubble gum flavors. Bot. 60 mL, 120 mL. *OTC.*
Use: Analgesic, NSAID.

Children's Motrin Cold. (McNeil Consumer) Ibuprofen 100 mg, pseudoephedrine hydrochloride 15 mg/5 mL, sucrose, alcohol free, berry and grape flavors. Ped. Susp. Bot. 4 oz. *OTC.*
Use: Analgesic, decongestant.

Children's NasalCrom. (Pharmacia) Cromolyn sodium 40 mg/mL (cromolyn sodium 5.2 mg/spray), benzalkonium chloride 0.01%, EDTA 0.01%. Spray. Bot. 13 mL, 26 mL. *OTC.*
Use: Analgesic; prophylactic.

Children's No Aspirin Elixir. (Walgreen) Acetaminophen 80 mg/2.5 mL. Nonalcoholic. Elix. Bot. 4 oz. *OTC.*
Use: Analgesic.

Children's No-Aspirin Tablets. (Walgreen) Acetaminophen 80 mg. Tab. Bot. 30s. *OTC.*
Use: Analgesic.

Children's Nyquil. (Procter & Gamble) Pseudoephedrine hydrochloride 10 mg,

chlorpheniramine maleate 0.6 mg, dextromethorphan HBr 5 mg/5 mL. Bot. 120 mL, 240 mL. *OTC.*
Use: Decongestant, antihistamine, antitussive.
Children's Nyquil Nighttime Head Cold, Allergy Formula. (Procter & Gamble) Pseudoephedrine hydrochloride 10 mg, chlorpheniramine maleate 0.67 mg/5 mL. Alcohol free. Sorbitol, sucrose. Grape flavor. Liq. Bot. 120 mL. *OTC.*
Use: Decongestant, antihistamine.
Children's Silapap. (Silarx) Acetaminophen 80 mg/2.5 mL, sugar free, alcohol free. Liq. Bot. 237 mL. *OTC.*
Use: Analgesic.
Children's Silfedrine. (Silarx) Pseudoephedrine hydrochloride 30 mg/5 mL. Liq. Bot. 111 ml. *OTC.*
Use: Decongestant, nasal.
Children's Sunkist Multivitamins Complete. (Novartis) Iron 18 mg, vitamin A 5000 units, D_3 400 units, E 30 units, B_1 1.5 mg, B_2 1.7 mg, B_3 20 mg, B_5 10 mg, B_6 2 mg, B_{12} 6 mcg, C 60 mg, folic acid 0.4 mg, Ca, Cu, I, K, Mg, Mn, P, Zn 10 mg, biotin 40 mcg, vitamin K, sorbitol, aspartame, phenylalanine, tartrazine. Chew. Tab. Bot. 60s. *OTC.*
Use: Mineral, vitamin supplement.
Children's Sunkist Multivitamins + Extra C. (Novartis) Vitamin A 2500 units, E 15 units, D_3 400 units, B_1 1.05 mg, B_2 1.2 mg, B_3 13.5 mg, B_6 1.05 mg, B_{12} 4.5 mcg, C 250 mg, folic acid 0.3 mg, vitamin K_1 5 mcg, sorbitol, aspartame, phenylalanine, tartrazine. Chew. Tab. Bot. 60s. *OTC.*
Use: Mineral, vitamin supplement.
Children's Tylenol Cold Liquid. (McNeil Consumer) Pseudoephedrine hydrochloride 15 mg, chlorpheniramine maleate 1 mg, acetaminophen 160 mg/ 5 mL, sorbitol, sucrose. Alcohol free. Grape flavor. Liq. Bot. 120 mL. *OTC.*
Use: Decongestant, antihistamine, analgesic.
Children's Tylenol Cold Multi Symptom Plus Cough. (McNeil Consumer) Acetaminophen 160 mg, dextromethorphan HBr 5 mg, chlorpheniramine maleate 1 mg, pseudoephedrine hydrochloride 15 mg/5 mL. Liq. Bot. 120 mL. *OTC.*
Use: Analgesic, antitussive, antihistamine, decongestant.
Children's Tylenol Cold Tablets. (McNeil Consumer) Pseudoephedrine hydrochloride 7.5 mg, chlorpheniramine maleate 0.5 mg, acetaminophen 80 mg,

aspartame, sucrose, phenylalanine 4 mg. Grape flavor. Chew. Tab. Bot. 24s. *OTC.*
Use: Decongestant, antihistamine, analgesic.
Children's Tylenol Elixir. (McNeil Consumer) Acetaminophen 160 mg/5 mL. Elix. Bot. 60 mL, 120 mL. *OTC.*
Use: Analgesic.
Children's Ty-Tabs. (Major) Acetaminophen 80 mg. Tab. Bot. 100s, 1000s. *OTC.*
Use: Analgesic.
chimeric A2 (human-murine) IgG monoclonal anti-TNF antibody (CA2). (Centocor)
Use: Crohn disease. [Orphan Drug]
chimeric (murine variable, human constant) Mab (C2B8) to CD20. (IDEC)
Use: Treatment of non-Hodgkin B-cell lymphoma. [Orphan Drug]
chinese gelatin.
See: Agar.
chinese isinglass.
Use: Amebicide.
chiniofon.
Use: Amebicide.
Chinosol. (Vernon) 8-Hydroxyquinoline sulfate 7.5 g. Tab. Vial 6s. Trit. Tab. (600 mg) Bot. 50s. Vial 110s. Pow. 1 oz.
Use: Antiseptic.
Chirocaine. (Purdue) Levobupivacaine hydrochloride 2.5 mg, 5 mg, 7.5 mg/ mL, sodium chloride. Preservative free. Inj. Single-dose vial 10 mL, 00 mL. *Rx.*
Use: Anesthetic, local amide, injectable.
chlamydia trachomatis test.
Use: Diagnostic aid.
See: MicroTrak.
Chlamydiazyme. (Abbott Diagnostics) Enzyme immunoassay for detection of *Chlamydia trachomatis* from urethral or urogenital swabs. Test Kit 100s.
Use: Diagnostic aid.
Chlo-Amine. (Hollister-Stier) Chlorpheniramine maleate 2 mg, sugar, orange flavor. Chew. Tab. Bot. 96s. *OTC.*
Use: Antihistamine, nonselective alkylamine.
•**chlophedianol hydrochloride.** (KLOE-fee-DIE-ah-nole) USAN.
Use: Antitussive.
Chloracol 0.5%. (Horizon) Chloramphenicol 5 mg/mL with chlorobutanol, hydroxypropyl methylcellulose. Dropper bot. 7.5 mL. *Rx.*
Use: Anti-infective, ophthalmic.
Chlorafed. (Roberts) Chlorpheniramine maleate 2 mg, pseudoephedrine hydrochloride 30 mg/5 mL, alcohol, dye,

sugar, and corn free. Liq. Bot. 120 mL, 480 mL. *OTC.*
Use: Antihistamine; decongestant.
Chlorafed H.S. Timecelles. (Roberts) Chlorpheniramine maleate 4 mg, pseudoephedrine hydrochloride 60 mg. SR Cap. Bot. 100s. *Rx.*
Use: Antihistamine; decongestant.
Chlorafed Timecelles. (Roberts) Chlorpheniramine maleate 8 mg, pseudoephedrine hydrochloride 120 mg. SA Timecelles. Bot. 100s. *Rx.*
Use: Antihistamine; decongestant.
Chlorahist. (Evron) Chlorpheniramine maleate. **Tab:** 4 mg. Bot. 100s, 1000s. **Cap:** 8 mg, 12 mg. Bot. 250s, 1000s. **Syr:** 2 mg/4 mL. Bot. qt. *Rx-OTC.*
Use: Antihistamine.
●**chloral betaine.** (KLOR-uhl BEE-tah-een) USAN.
Use: Hypnotic; sedative.
●**chloral hydrate.** (KLOR-uhl HIGH-drate) *USP 28.*
Use: Hypnotic/sedative, nonbarbiturate.
See: Aquachloral Supprettes.
Somnote.
chloral hydrate. (Various Mfr.) Chloral hydrate. **Cap.:** 500 mg. 100s, 500s, 1,000s, UD 100s. **Syrup:** 250 mg/5 mL, 500 mg/5 mL. Pt., gal., UD 5 mL (100s) (500 mg/5 mL only); UD 10 mL (40s and 100s). *c-IV.*
Use: Hypnotic/sedative, nonbarbiturate.
chloral hydrate betaine (1:1) compound. Chloral Betaine.
chloralpyrine dichloralpyrine.
See: Dichloralantipyrine.
chloralurethane. Name used for Carbochloral.
●**chlorambucil.** (klor-AM-byoo-sill) *USP 28.*
Use: Antineoplastic; alkylating agent; nitrogen mustard.
See: Leukeran.
Chloramine-T. Sodium paratoluenesulfan chloramide, chloramine, chlorozone. **Eli Lilly:** Tab. (0.3 g), Bot. 100s, 1000s. **Robinson:** Pow., 1 oz.
Use: Antiseptic; deodorant.
See: Chlorazene.
●**chloramphenicol.** (KLOR-am-FEN-ih-kole) *USP 28.*
Use: Anti-infective; antirickettsial; treatment of superficial ocular infections involving the conjunctiva or cornea caused by susceptible organisms.
See: AK-Chlor.
Chloromycetin.
Chloromyxin.
Econochlor.

Mychel.
Ophthochlor.
W/Hydrocortisone Acetate.
See: Chloromycetin.
W/Hydrocortisone Acetate, Polymyxin B Sulfate.
See: Chloromycetin.
W/Prednisolone.
See: Chloromycetin.
chloramphenicol. (Various Mfr.) **Soln.:** 5 mg/mL. Bot. 7.5 mL, 15 mL. **Oint.:** 10 mg/g. Tube 3.5 g.
Use: Anti-infective; antirickettsial.
●**chloramphenicol palmitate.** (KLOR-am-FEN-ih-kahl pal-mih-tate) *USP 28.*
Use: Anti-infective; antirickettsial.
See: Chloromycetin Palmitate.
●**chloramphenicol pantothenate complex.** (KLOR-am-FEN-ih-kahl PAN-toe-THEH-nate) USAN.
Use: Anti-infective; antirickettsial.
●**chloramphenicol sodium succinate.** (KLOR-am-FEN-ih-kahl) *USP 28.*
Use: Anti-infective; antirickettsial.
See: Chloromycetin Succinate.
Mychel-S.
chloramphenicol sodium succinate. (Various Mfr.) Chloramphenicol sodium succinate 100 mg/mL. Inj. Vial. 1 g in 15 mL.
Use: Anti-infective; antirickettsial.
Chloraseptic Children's. (Procter & Gamble) Benzocaine 5 mg. Loz. Pkg. 18s. *OTC.*
Use: Anesthetic, local.
Chloraseptic Liquid. (Procter & Gamble) Total phenol 1.4% as phenol and sodium phenolate, saccharin. Menthol and cherry flavors. Liq. Bot. 180 mL, 360 mL (mouthwash/gargle); 45 mL, 240 mL, 360 mL (throat spray). *OTC.*
Use: Anesthetic; antiseptic, local.
Chloraseptic Lozenge. (Procter & Gamble) Total phenol 32.5 mg as phenol and sodium phenolate. Menthol and cherry flavors. Pkg. 18s, 36s. *OTC.*
Use: Anesthetic; antiseptic.
Chlorazene. (Badger) Chloramine-T, sodium p-toluene-sulfonchloramide. **Pow.:** UD Pkg. 20 g, 38 g, 50 g, 88 g, 200 g, 240 g, 320 g, Bot. 1 lb, 5 lb. **Aromatic Pow. (5%):** Bot. 1 lb, 5 lb. **Tab. (0.3 g):** Bot. 20s, 100s, 1000s, 5000s. *OTC.*
Use: Antiseptic; deodorant.
chlorazepate dipotassium.
See: Clorazepate dipotassium.
chlorazepate monopotassium.
See: Clorazepate monopotassium.
Chlorazine. (Major) Prochlorperazine 5 mg, 10 mg. Tab. Bot. 100s.

Use: Antiemetic; antipsychotic; antivertigo.
Chlor Mal w/Sal + APAP S.C. (Global Source) Chlorpheniramine maleate 2 mg, acetaminophen 150 mg, salicylamide 175 mg. Tab. Bot. 1000s. *OTC.*
Use: Analgesic; antihistamine.
Chlor-Niramine Allergy Tabs. (Whiteworth Towne) Chlorpheniramine maleate 4 mg. Tab. Bot. 24s, 100s. *OTC.*
Use: Antihistamine.
chlorbutanol.
See: Chlorobutanol.
chlorbutol.
See: Chlorobutanol.
•**chlorcyclizine hydrochloride.** (klor-SIK-lih-zeen) *NF 23.*
Use: Antihistamine.
•**chlordantoin.** (KLOR-dan-toe-in) USAN.
Use: Antifungal.
•**chlordiazepoxide.** (klor-DIE-aze-ee-POX-side) *USP 28.*
Use: Anxiolytic.
See: Brigen-G.
Libritabs.
W/Amitriptyline.
See: Limbitrol.
chlordiazepoxide and amitriptyline hydrochloride.
Use: Anxiolytic.
See: Limbitrol.
chlordiazepoxide and clindinium bromide. (Various Mfr.) Clindinium 2.5 mg, chlordiazepoxide hydrochloride 5 mg. Cap. Bot. 30s, 100s, 500s, 1000s, UD 100s. *c-iv.*
Use: Gastrointestinal; anticholinergic.
chlordiazepoxide and clindinium bromide. (Chelsea) Clindinium bromide 2.5 mg, chlordiazepoxide hydrochloride 5 mg. Cap. Bot. 100s, 500s, 1000s.
Formerly Clindex (Rugby Labs, Inc.). *Rx.*
Use: Anticholinergic; antispasmodic.
•**chlordiazepoxide hydrochloride.** (klor-DIE-aze-ee-POX-ide) *USP 28.*
Use: Hypnotic; sedative; anxiolytic.
See: Librium.
Screen.
Zetran.
W/Methscopolamine Nitrate.
See: Librax.
chlordiazepoxide hydrochloride. (Various Mfr.) Chlordiazepoxide hydrochloride 5 mg, 10 mg, 25 mg. Cap. 20s, 100s, 500s, 1000s, UD 100s. *c-iv.*
Use: Anxiolytic.
Chlordrine S.R. (Rugby) Pseudoephedrine hydrochloride 120 mg, chlorphenir-

amine maleate 8 mg. SR Cap. Bot. 100s. *Rx.*
Use: Antihistamine; decongestant.
Chloren 8 T.D. (Wren) Chlorpheniramine maleate 8 mg. Tab. Bot. 100s, 1000s. *OTC.*
Use: Antihistamine.
Chloren 12 T.D. (Wren) Chlorpheniramine maleate 12 mg. Tab. Bot. 100s, 1000s. *Rx-OTC.*
Use: Antihistamine.
Chloresium. (Rystan) Oint.: Chlorophyllin copper complex 0.5% in hydrophilic base. Tube 1 oz, 4 oz, Jar lb.
Soln.: Chlorophyllin copper complex 0.2% in isotonic saline soln. Bot. 60 mL, 240 mL, qt. *OTC.*
Use: Deodorant; healing agent.
Chloresium Tablets. (Rystan) Chlorophyllin copper complex 14 mg. Tab. 100s, 1000s. *OTC.*
Use: Deodorant, oral.
Chloresium Tooth Paste. (Rystan) Chlorophyllin copper complex. Tube 3.25 oz. *OTC.*
Use: Deodorant, oral.
chlorethyl.
See: Ethyl Chloride.
chlorguanide hydrochloride.
See: Chloroguanide hydrochloride.
chlorhexidine. *OTC.*
Use: Antiseptic.
See: Bacto Shield.
Bacto Shield 2.
Hibiclens.
•**chlorhexidine gluconate.** (klor-HEX-ih-deen GLUE-koe-nate) USAN.
Use: Antimicrobial.
See: Bacto Shield.
Bacto Shield 2.
Hibiclens.
Hibistat.
Peridex.
PerioChip.
PerioGard.
chlorhexidine gluconate mouthrinse.
Use: Amelioration of oral mucositis associated with cytoreductive therapy for conditioning patients for bone marrow transplantation. [Orphan Drug]
See: Peridex.
PerioGard.
•**chlorhexidine hydrochloride.** (klor-HEX-ih-deen) USAN.
Use: Anti-infective, topical.
•**chlorhexidine phosphanilate.** (klor-HEX-ih-deen FOSS-fah-nih-LATE) USAN.
Use: Anti-infective.
chlorinated and iodized peanut oil.
Chloriodized oil.

•**chlorindanol.** (klor-IN-dah-nahl) USAN.
Use: Antiseptic, spermaticide.
chlorine compound, antiseptic. Antiseptic, chlorine.
chloriodized oil. Chlorinated and iodized peanut oil.
•**chlormadinone acetate.** (klor-MAD-ih-nohn) USAN.
Use: Hormone, progestin.
chlormerodrin. Mercloran. *Rx.*
Use: Diuretic.
•**chlormerodrin Hg 197.** USAN.
Use: Diagnostic aid, renal function determination; radiopharmaceutical.
•**chlormerodrin Hg 203.** USAN.
Use: Diagnostic aid, renal function determination; radiopharmaceutical.
chlormezanone. Chlormethazanone.
Use: Anxiolytic.
See: Trancopal.
•**chlorobutanol.** (Klor-oh-BYOO-tah-nole) *NF 23.*
Use: Anesthetic; antiseptic; hypnotic; pharmaceutic aid, antimicrobial.
See: Cerumenex.
Pre-Sert.
W/Calcium glycerophosphate, calcium levulinate.
See: Cal San.
W/Cetyltrimethylammonium Br, methapyrilene hydrochloride, phenylephrine hydrochloride, hydrocortisone.
See: T-Spray.
W/Desmopressin Acetate.
See: Minirin.
W/Diphenhydramine hydrochloride.
See: Ardeben.
W/Ephedrine hydrochloride, sodium Cl.
See: Efedron hydrochloride.
W/Estradiol cypionate, testosterone cypionate.
See: Depo-Testadiol.
Depotestogen.
W/Glycerin, anhydrous.
See: Ophthalgan.
W/Liquifilm.
See: Liquifilm Tears.
W/Methylcellulose.
See: Lacril.
W/Myristyl-gamma-picolinium Cl.
See: Wet Tone.
W/Nonionic lanolin derivative.
See: Lacri-Lube.
W/Polyethylene glycol, polyoxyl 40 stearate.
See: Ocean.
•**chlorocresol.** (KLOR-oh-KREE-sole) *NF 23.*
Use: Antiseptic; disinfectant.

chloroethane.
Use: Anticholinergic; antispasmodic.
See: Ethyl Chloride.
Chlorofair. (Bausch & Lomb) **Soln.:** Chloramphenicol 5 mg/mL. Bot. 7.5 mL. **Oint.:** Chloramphenicol 10 mg/g in white petrolatum base with mineral oil, polysorbate 60. Tube 3.5 g. *Rx.*
Use: Anti-infective, ophthalmic.
chloroguanide hydrochloride. (Various Mfr.) Proguanil hydrochloride. *Rx.*
Use: Antimalarial.
Chlorohist-LA. (Roberts) Xylometazoline hydrochloride 0.1%. Soln. Spray 15 mL. *OTC.*
Use: Decongestant.
chloro-iodohydroxyquinoline.
See: Clioquinot.
chloromethapyrilene citrate.
See: Chlorothen Citrate.
Chloromycetin. (Parke-Davis) Chloramphenicol. **Oint.:** 10 mg/g. With liquid petrolatum and polyethylene base. Preservative-free. Tube 3.5 g. **Pow. for Soln.:** 25 mg/vial. Preservative-free. In 15 mL with diluent. *Rx.*
Use: Anti-infective.
Chloromycetin/Hydrocortisone. (Parke-Davis) Hydrocortisone acetate 0.5% (2.5% as powder), chloramphenicol 0.25% (1.25% as powder). Pow. Bot. with dropper 5 mL. *Rx.*
Use: Anti-infective, ophthalmic.
Chloromycetin Sodium Succinate I.V. (Monarch) Chloramphenicol sodium succinate dried powder which when reconstituted contains chloromycetin 100 mg/mL. *Steri-vial* 1 g, 10s. *Rx.*
Use: Anti-infective.
chlorophenothane.
Use: Pediculicide.
chlorophyll. (Freeda) Chlorophyll 20 mg, sugar free. Tab. Bot. 100s, 250s, 500s. *OTC.*
Use: Deodorant, oral.
Chlorophyll "A".
See: Chloresium.
chlorophyll derivatives, systemic.
See: Chlorophyll.
Derifil.
Chloresium.
chlorophyll derivatives, topical.
See: Chloresium.
chlorophyllin.
Use: Deodorant; healing agent.
•**chlorophyllin copper complex.** (KLOR-oh-FILL-in KAHP-uhr) USAN.
Use: Deodorant.
See: PALS.
•**chlorophyllin copper complex sodium.** (KLOR-oh-FILL-in KAHP-uhr) *USP 28.*
Use: Deodorant.

W/Combinations.
See: Panafil.
chlorophyll tablets.
See: Derifil.
chlorophyll, water-soluble. Chloro-
phyllin.
See: Chloresium.
Derifil.
●**chloroprocaine hydrochloride.** (klor-oh-
PRO-cane) *USP 28.*
Use: Anesthetic, local ester, injectable.
See: Nesacaine.
Nesacaine-MPF.
chloroprocaine hydrochloride. (Bedford) Chloroprocaine hydrochloride 2%,
3%, preservative-free. Inj. Single-dose
vials. 20 mL. *Rx.*
Use: Anesthetic, local ester, injectable.
●**chloroquine.** (KLOR-oh-kwin) *USP 28.*
Use: Antiamebic; antimalarial.
See: Aralen hydrochloride.
●**chloroquine phosphate.** (KLOR-oh-
kwin) *USP 28.*
Use: Antiamebic; antimalarial; lupus
erythematosus agent.
See: Aralen Phosphate.
chloroquine phosphate. (Various Mfr.)
Cloroquine phosphate 250 mg (equiv.
to 150 mg base). Tab. Bot. 20s, 22s,
30s, 100s, 1000s, UD 100s. *Rx.*
Use: Amebicide.
chlorothen.
Use: Antihistamine.
chlorothen citrate. (Whittier) Chlorothen
citrate. Tab. Bot. 100s.
Use: Antihistamine.
W/Pyrilamine, thenylpyramine.
See: Derma-Pax.
chlorothenylpyramine. Chlorothen.
chlorotheophyllinate w/Benadryl.
See: Dramamine.
●**chlorothiazide.** (KLOR-oh-THIGH-uh-
zide) *USP 28.*
Use: Diuretic.
See: Diuril.
W/Methyldopa.
See: Aldoclor.
●**chlorothiazide sodium for injection.**
(KLOR-oh-THIGH-uh-zide) *USP 28.*
Use: Antihypertensive; diuretic.
See: Sodium Diuril.
chlorothymol.
Use: Anti-infective.
●**chlorotrianisene.** (klor-oh-try-AN-ih-
seen) *USP 28.*
Use: Estrogen.
See: Placidyl.
●**chloroxine.** (KLOR-ox-een) USAN.
Use: Antiseborrheic.

●**chloroxylenol.** (KLOR-oh-ZIE-len-ole)
USP 28.
Use: Antibacterial.
W/Benzocaine, menthol, lanolin.
See: Unburn.
W/Hexachlorophene.
See: Desitin.
W/Hydrocortisone, pramoxine.
See: Cortic.
Mediotic-HC.
Otomar-HC.
W/Methyl salicylate, menthol, camphor,
thymol, eucalyptus oil, isopropyl
alcohol.
See: Gordobalm.
W/Pramoxine hydrochloride, hydrocorti-
sone.
See: Oti-Med.
Tri-Otic.
Zoto-I IC.
chlorozone.
See: Chloramine-T.
Chlorpazine. (Major) Prochlorperazine
maleate 5 mg, 10 mg, 25 mg. Tab. Bot.
100s, UD 100s (5 mg, 10 mg only). *Rx.*
Use: Antipsychotic.
Chlorphed. (Roberts) Brompheniramine
maleate 10 mg/mL. Inj. Vial 10 mL. *Rx.*
Use: Antihistamine.
Chlorphed-LA. (Roberts) Oxymetazoline
0.05%. Soln. Spray 15 mL. *OTC.*
Use: Decongestant.
Chlorphedrine SR. (Ivax) Chlorphenir-
amine maleate 8 mg, pseudoephed-
rine hydrochloride 120 mg. Cap. Bot.
100s. *Rx.*
Use: Antihistamine; decongestant.
●**chlorphenesin carbamate.** (KLOR-fen-
ee-sin CAR-bah-mate) USAN.
Use: Muscle relaxant.
See: Maolate.
●**chlorpheniramine maleate.** (klor-fen-
IHR-ah-meen) *USP 28.*
Use: Antihistamine, nonselective alkyl-
amine.
See: Aller-Chlor.
Allergy.
Allergy Relief.
Chlo-Amine.
Chlor-Trimeton Allergy 8 Hour.
Chlor-Trimeton Allergy 12 Hour.
Efidac 24.
Polaramine.
W/Combinations.
See: AccuHist LA.
Actifed Cold & Sinus Maximum
Strength.
Advil Allergy Sinus.
AeroHist Plus.
AeroKid.
AH-chew.

Alka-Seltzer Plus Cold & Cough Medicine.
Alka-Seltzer Plus Cold Medicine.
Alka-Seltzer Plus Flu Medicine.
Alka-Seltzer Plus Nose & Throat.
Allerest.
Allerest Maximum Strength.
AlleRx.
All-Nite Children's Cold/Cough Relief.
Amerituss AD.
Atuss DM.
Atuss HC.
Atuss HD.
Atuss MS.
Bellahist-D LA.
Biohist-LA.
Chlorpheniramine Maleate/Pseudoephedrine hydrochloride.
Chlor-Trimeton Allergy•D 4 Hour.
Chlor-Trimeton Allergy•D 12 Hour.
Clorfed.
Codimal.
Cold Symptoms Relief Maximum Strength.
Colfed-A.
Comtrex Allergy-Sinus Treatment, Maximum Strength.
Comtrex Cough and Cold Relief, Multi-Symptom Maximum Strength.
Comtrex Day & Night Cold & Cough Relief, Multi-Symptom Maximum Strength.
Comtrex Day/Night Flu Therapy Maximum Strength Caplets.
Comtrex Maximum Strength Nighttime Cold & Cough.
Comtussin HC.
Contac Severe Cold & Flu Maximum Strength.
Coricidin 'D' Cold, Flu, & Sinus.
Coricidin HBP Cold & Flu.
Coricidin HBP Cough & Cold.
Coricidin HBP Maximum Strength Flu.
CPM 8/PSE 90/MSC 2.5.
Cytuss HC.
D.A.
D.A. II.
Dallergy.
Dallergy-JR.
Decodult.
Decohistine DH.
Decolate.
Deconamine.
Deconamine SR.
Deconomed SR.
Dehistine.
Derma-Pax.
Dihistine DH.
Donatussin.
DriHist SR.
Dristan.

Dristan Cold Multi-Symptom Formula.
Dryphen, Multi-Symptom Formula.
Duradryl.
Durahist.
Ed A-Hist.
ED-TLC.
ED Tuss HC.
Efidac 24.
Endagen-HD.
Ex-Histine.
Extendryl.
Extendryl JR.
Extendryl SR.
Father John's Medicine Plus.
Genacol Maximum Strength Cold & Flu Relief.
Good Sense Maximum Strength Dose Sinus.
Good Sense Maximum Strength Pain Relief Allergy Sinus.
Histade.
Histatab Plus.
Hista-Vent DA.
Histinex HC.
Histinex PV.
Histussin HC.
Hydrocodone CP.
Hydrocodone HD.
Hydron CP.
Hydron PSC.
Hydro-PC.
Hydro-PC II.
Hydro-Tussin HC.
Hyphed.
Kid Kare Children's Cough/Cold.
Kolephrin/DM.
Kronofed-A.
Kronofed-A Jr.
Lemotussin-DM.
Mapap Cold Formula.
Maxi-Tuss HC.
Maxi-Tuss HCX.
Nalex-A.
Nite Time Children's.
Norel DM.
OMNIhist L.A.
Pancof.
Pancof-HC.
Pancof PD.
PediaCare Children's Cold & Allergy.
PediaCare Children's Multi-Symptom Cold.
PediaCare Cough-Cold.
PediaCare Multi-Symptom Cold.
PediaCare NightRest Cough & Cold.
Pediox.
Poly-Tussin.
Pre-Hist-D.
PSE CPM.
P-V-Tussin.
QDALL.

Quelidrine.
Rescon-DM.
Rescon-Jr.
Rescon-MX.
Robitussin Flu.
Robitussin Honey Flu Nighttime.
Robitussin Pediatric Night Relief
  Cough & Cold.
Robitussin PM Cough & Cold.
Scot-Tussin DM.
Scot-Tussin Hayfebrol.
Simplet.
Sine-Off Sinus Medicine.
Singlet for Adults.
Sinutab Sinus Allergy, Maximum
  Strength.
Stahist.
Statuss Green.
S-T Forte 2.
Sudafed Cold & Allergy Maximum
  Strength.
TheraFlu Cold & Cough Night Time.
TheraFlu Flu & Cold Medicine for
  Sore Throat, Maximum Strength.
TheraFlu Flu and Cold Medicine Origi-
  nal Formula.
TheraFlu Flu & Cough Night Time,
  Maximum Strength.
TheraFlu Flu & Sore Throat, Maxi-
  mum Strength.
TheraFlu Flu & Sore Throat Night
  Time, Maximum Strength.
TheraFlu Flu, Cold, & Cough and
  Sore Throat, Maximum Strength.
TheraFlu Flu, Cold & Cough Night-
  Time, Maximum Strength.
TheraFlu Maximum Strength Night-
  Time Formula Flu, Cold, & Cough
  Medicine.
TheraFlu Severe Cold & Congestion
  Night Time, Maximum Strength.
Thera-Hist Cold & Allergy.
Thera-Hist Cold & Cough.
Time-Hist.
Top Care Maximum Strength Flu, Cold
  & Cough Medicine Night Time.
Top Care Multi-Symptom Pain Relief
  Cold.
Triacting Cold & Allergy.
Tri-Acting Cold & Allergy.
Tri-Acting Cold & Cough.
Triaminic Cold, Allergy, Sinus Medi-
  cine.
Triaminic Cold & Allergy.
Triaminic Cold & Cough.
Triaminic Cough.
Triaminic Flu, Cough & Fever.
Triaminic Night Time Cough & Cold.
Triaminic Softchews.
Tricodene Sugar Free.
Tussend.

Tylenol Allergy Sinus, Maximum
  Strength.
Tylenol Children's Cold.
Tylenol Children's Cold Plus Cough.
Tylenol Children's Flu.
Tylenol Cold Complete Formula.
Vanex HD.
Vicks Children's NyQuil Cold/Cough
  Relief.
Vicks 44M Cough, Cold, & Flu Relief.
Vicks Pediatric 44M Cough & Cold
  Relief.
Z-Cof HC.
ZTuss Expectorant.
d-chlorpheniramine maleate.
  See: Polaramine Expectorant.
chlorpheniramine maleate. (Various
  Mfr.) Chlorpheniramine maleate. 4 mg.
  Tab. Bot. 24s, 100s, 1000s. *OTC.*
  Use: Antihistamine, nonselective alkyl-
  amine.
chlorpheniramine maleate. (Various
  Mfr.) Chlorpheniramine maleate 8 mg,
  10 mg. SR Cap. Bot. 100s, 1000s. *Rx.*
  Use: Antihistamine, nonselective alkylamine.
chlorpheniramine maleate. (Various
  Mfr.) Chlorpheniramine maleate 10 mg/
  mL, benzyl alcohol 1.5%. Inj. Multidose
  vial. *Rx.*
  Use: Antihistamine, nonselective alkylamine.
• **chlorpheniramine maleate w/pseudo-
  ephedrine hydrochloride.** (klor-fen-
  IHR-ah-meen MAL-ee-ate with OOO
  do-ee-fed-rin) *USP 28.*
  Use: Antihistamine, decongestant.
**chlorpheniramine maleate w/pseudo-
  ephedrine hydrochloride.** (Eon Labs)
  Pseudoephedrine hydrochloride
  120 mg, chlorpheniramine maleate
  8 mg. Cap. Bot. 100s, 250s, 1000s.
  OTC.
  Use: Antihistamine; decongestant.
• **chlorpheniramine polistirex.** (klor-fen-
  IHR-ah-meen pahl-ee-STIE-rex) *USAN.*
  Use: Antihistamine.
  W/Combinations.
  See: Atuss-12 DM.
**chlorpheniramine polistirex and
  hydrocodone polistirex combina-
  tions.**
  Use: Upper respiratory combination, an-
  tihistamine, antitussive.
  See: Tussionex PennKinetic.
chlorpheniramine tannate.
  See: Ed-Chlor-Tan.
  W/Combinations.
  See: AlleRx.
  Chlorpheniramine Tannate/Pseudo-
  ephedrine Tannate.

C-PHED Tannate.
CP-TANNIC.
Dallergy-Jr.
Exratuss.
Gelhist Pediatric.
Nalex-A 12.
Nuhist.
Phenylephrine Tannate/Chlorpheniramine Tannate/Pyrilamine Tannate Pediatric.
Quad Tann.
Rhinatate-NF Pediatric.
Rhinatate Pediatric.
R-Tanna.
R-Tanna S Pediatric.
Rynatan.
Rynatan Pediatric.
Rynatuss.
Rynatuss Pediatric.
Tannic-12.
Triaminic Severe Cold & Fever.
Trionate.
Triotann Pediatric.
Triotann-S Pediatric.
Tussi-12.
Tussi-12 S.
Tussizone-12 RF.
Tuss-Tan.
Tuss-Tan Pediatric.
chlorpheniramine tannate/pseudoephedrine tannate. (Various Mfr.) Pseudoephedrine tannate 75 mg, chlorpheniramine tannate 4.5 mg/5 mL, strawberry/banana flavor, alcohol free. Susp. Bot. 118 mL, 473 mL. *Rx.*
Use: Upper respiratory combination, decongestant, antihistamine.

• **chlorphentermine hydrochloride.** (klor-FEN-ter-meen) USAN.
Use: Anorexic.

chlorphthalidone.
See: Chlorthalidone.

• **chlorpromazine.** (klor-PRO-muh-zeen) *USP 28.*
Tall Man: ChlorproMAZINE
Use: Antiemetic; antipsychotic.

• **chlorpromazine hydrochloride.** (klor-PRO-muh-zeen) *USP 28.*
Tall Man: ChlorproMAZINE
Use: Antiemetic; antipsychotic.
See: Promachlor.
Promaz.
Thorazine.

chlorpromazine hydrochloride injection. (Various Mfr.) Chlorpromazine hydrochloride 25 mg/mL. sodium metabisulfite, sodium sulfite. Amp. 1 mL, 2 mL. *Rx.*
Use: Antipsychotic.

chlorpromazine hydrochloride intensol oral solution. (Roxane) Chlorpromazine hydrochloride 100 mg/mL. Parabens, sulfites, sorbitol, saccharin. Oral concentrate. 237 mL with calibrated dropper graduated in 25 mg increments. *Rx.*
Use: Antiemetic; antipsychotic.

chlorpromazine hydrochloride tablets. (Various Mfr.) Chlorpromazine hydrochloride 10 mg, 25 mg, 50 mg, 100 mg, 200 mg. Tab. Bot. 100s, 1000s, UD 100s. *Rx.*
Use: Antipsychotic.

• **chlorpropamide.** (klor-PRO-puh-mide) *USP 28.*
Tall Man: ChlorproPAMIDE
Use: Antidiabetic.
See: Diabinese.

chlorpropamide. (Various Mfr.) Chlorpropamide 100 mg, 250 mg. Tab. Bot. 100s, 250s (250 mg only), 500s, 1000s, UD 100s, 600s. *Rx.*
Use: Antidiabetic.

chlorprophenpyridamine maleate.
See: Chlorpheniramine maleate.

Chlor-Pro 10. (Schein) Chlorpheniramine maleate 10 mg/mL, benzyl alcohol. Inj. Vial 30 mL. *Rx.*
Use: Antihistamine.

chlorquinol. Mixture of the chlorinated products of 8-hydroxyquinoline containing about 65% of 5,7-dichloro-8-hydroxyquinoline.

chlortetracycline and sulfamethazine bisulfates.
Use: Anti-infective.

• **chlortetracycline bisulfate.** (klor-the-trah-SIGH-kleen) *USP 28.*
Use: Anti-infective; antiprotozoal.

• **chlorthalidone.** (klor-THAL-ih-dohn) *USP 28.*
Use: Antihypertensive; diuretic.
See: Hygroton.
Thalitone.
W/Reserpine.
See: Demi-Regroton.
Regroton.

chlorthalidone. (Various Mfr.) Chlorthalidone 25 mg, 50 mg, 100 mg. Tab. Bot. 100s (25 mg); 100s, 250s, 1000s (50 mg); 100s, 500s, 1000s (100 mg). *Rx.*
Use: Diuretic; antihypertensive.

Chlor-Trimeton Allergy. (Schering-Plough) Chlorpheniramine maleate 4 mg, lactose. Tab. Box. 24s. *OTC.*
Use: Antihistamine.

Chlor-Trimeton Allergy•D 4 Hour. (Schering-Plough) Pseudoephedrine sulfate

60 mg, chlorpheniramine maleate 4 mg, lactose. Tab. Box. 24s. *OTC.*
Use: Upper respiratory combination, decongestant, antihistamine.

Chlor-Trimeton Allergy•D 12 Hour. (Schering-Plough) Pseudoephedrine sulfate 120 mg, chlorpheniramine maleate 8 mg, butylparaben, sugar, lactose. Tab. Bot. 24s. *OTC.*
Use: Upper respiratory combination, decongestant, antihistamine.

Chlor-Trimeton Allergy 8 Hour. (Schering-Plough Healthcare) Chlorpheniramine maleate 8 mg. ER Tab. Box. 15s. *OTC.*
Use: Antihistamine, nonselective alkylamine.

Chlor-Trimeton Allergy 12 Hour. (Schering-Plough Healthcare) Chlorpheniramine maleate 12 mg. ER Tab. Box. 10s. *OTC.*
Use: Antihistamine, nonselective alkylamine.

Chlor-Trimeton 4 Hour Relief. (Schering-Plough) Chlorpheniramine maleate 4 mg, pseudoephedrine sulfate 60 mg. Tab. Box 24s, 48s. *OTC.*
Use: Antihistamine; decongestant.

Chlor-Trimeton 12 Hour Allergy. (Schering-Plough) Chlorpheniramine maleate 8 mg, pseudoephedrine sulfate 120 mg. SR Tab. Box 24s, 48s. UD 96s. *OTC.*
Use: Antihistamine; decongestant.

Chlor-Trimeton 12 Hour Relief. (Schering-Plough) Chlorpheniramine 8 mg, pseudoephedrine sulfate 120 mg. Tab. Box 12s. Bot. 36s. *OTC.*
Use: Antihistamine; decongestant.

Chlor-Trimeton w/Combinations. (Schering-Plough) Chlorpheniramine maleate.
W/Acetaminophen.
See: Coricidin.
W/Phenylephrine hydrochloride.
See: Demazin.
W/Pseudoephedrine sulfate.
See: Chlor-Trimeton Decongestant.
  Chlor-Trimeton 12 Hour Allergy.
W/Salicylamide, phenacetin, caffeine, vitamin C.
See: Coriforte.
W/Sodium salicylate, amino acetic acid.
See: Corilin.

Chlorzide. (Foy Laboratories) Hydrochlorothiazide 50 mg. Tab. Bot. 1000s. *Rx.*
Use: Diuretic.

•**chlorzoxazone.** (klor-ZOX-uh-zone) *USP 28.*
Use: Muscle relaxant.

See: Paraflex.
  Parafon Forte DSC.
  Remular-S.

chlorzoxazone. (Various Mfr.) Chlorzoxane 250 mg, 500 mg. Tab. Bot. 100s, 500s (500 mg only), 1000s.
Use: Muscle relaxant.

chlorzoxazone and acetaminophen.
Use: Analgesic; muscle relaxant.

•**chocolate.** *NF 23.*
Use: Flavoring.

Choice DM. (Bristol-Myers Squibb) Kit for blood samples. 1 single-use test kit. *OTC.*
Use: In vitro diagnostic aid.

Choice 10. (Whiteworth Towne) Potassium Cl 10%. Soln., unflavored. Bot. Gal. *Rx.*
Use: Electrolyte supplement.

Choice 20. (Whitoworth Towne) Potassium Cl 20%. Soln., unflavored. Bot. Gal. *Rx.*
Use: Electrolyte supplement.

Cholac. (Alra) Lactulose 10 g/15 mL (< galactose 1.6 g, lactose 1.2 g, other sugars 1.2 g). Soln. Bot. 30 mL, 240 mL, 480 mL, 960 mL, 1920 mL, 3785 mL. *Rx.*
Use: Laxative.

cholacrylamine resin. Anion exchange resin consisting of a water-soluble polymer having a molecular weight equivalent between 350 and 360 in which aliphatic quaternary amine groups are attached to an acrylic backbone by ester linkages.

cholalic acid.
See: Cholic Acid.

Cholan-DH. (Medeva) Dehydrocholic acid 250 mg. Tab. Bot. 100s.
Use: Laxative.

cholanic acid. Dehydrodesoxycholic acid.

Cholebrine. (Mallinckrodt) Iocetamic acid (62% iodine) 750 mg. Tab. Bot. 100s, 150s.
Use: Radiopaque agent.

•**cholecalciferol.** (kole-eh-kal-SIH-fer-ole) *USP 28.* Formerly 7-Dehydrocholesterol, activated.
Use: Vitamin D₃ (antirachitic).
See: A and D Ointment.
  Decavitamin.
  Delta-D.
  Vitamin D₃.
W/Alendronate Sodium.
See: Fosamax Plus D.

cholecystography agents.
See: Bilopaque.
  Iodized Oil.
  Iopanoic Acid.

Iophendylate.
Pantopaque.
Telepaque.
choleretic. Bile salts.
See: Bile Preps and Forms.
Dehydrocholic Acid.
Tocamphyl.
cholesterin.
See: Cholesterol.
●**cholesterol.** (koe-LESS-ter-all) *NF 23.*
Use: Pharmaceutic aid, emulsifying agent.
cholesterol reagent strips. (Bayer Corp. (Consumer Div.)) A quantitative strip test for cholesterol in serum. Seralyzer reagent strips. Bot. 25s.
Use: Diagnostic aid.
cholestyramine. (Various Mfr.) Anhydrous cholestyramine resin 4 g/9 g powder. Pow. for Susp. 9 g Packet 42s, 60s; Can 378 g. *Rx.*
Use: Antihyperlipidemic; bile acid sequestrant.
cholestyramine light. (Various Mfr.) Anhydrous cholestyramine resin 4 g/dose. Pow. for Susp. 5 g and 5.7 g Packets, 60s; Can 210 g, 231 g, 239 g. *Rx.*
Use: Antihyperlipidemic; bile acid sequestrant.
cholestyramine powder. (Ivax) 4 g (as anhydrous resin), phenylalanine 14.1 mg/5.5 g powder, aspartame. Pow. Single-dose 5.5 g Pkt. 42s, 60s. *Rx.*
Use: Bile acid sequestrant.
●**cholestyramine resin.** (koe-less-TEER-uh-meen) *USP 28.*
Use: Antihyperlipidemic; ion-exchange resin, bile salts.
See: Cholestyramine Light.
LoCHOLEST.
LoCHOLEST Light.
Prevalite.
Questran.
Questran Light.
Cholidase. (Freeda) Choline 450 mg, inositol 150 mg, vitamins B_6 2.5 mg, B_{12} 5 mcg, E 7.5 mg. Tab. Bot. 100s, 250s, 500s. *OTC.*
Use: Lipid, vitamin supplement.
choline. (Various Mfr.) Choline. 250 mg, 500 mg, 650 mg. Tab. Bot. 90s (650 mg only); 100s, 250s, 500s (except 500 mg); 1000s (250 mg only). *OTC.*
Use: Lipotropic.
●**choline bitartrate.** (koe-leen bye-TAR-trait) *USP 28.*
W/Bile extract, pancreatic substance, dl-methionine.
See: Ilopan-Choline.

●**choline chloride.** (koe-leen) *USP 28.* (Various Mfr.).
Use: Liver supplement. [Orphan Drug]
choline chloride, carbamate. Carbachol.
choline chloride succinate.
See: Succinylcholine chloride.
choline dihydrogen citrate. 2-Hydroxyethyl trimethylammonium citrate US vitamin 0.5 g. Bot. 100s, 500s.
Use: Lipotropic.
choline magnesium trisalicylate. (Sidmak) Choline magnesium trisalicylate 500 mg, 750 mg, 1000 mg. Tab. Bot. 100s, 500s. *Rx.*
Use: Analgesic.
cholinergic agents.
Use: Parasympathomimetic agents.
See: Mecholyl Cl.
Mestinon.
Mytelase.
Pilocarpine Nitrate.
Tensilon.
Urecholine.
Urinary Cholinergics.
cholinergic blocking agents.
See: Parasympatholytic agents.
●**choline salicylate.** (koe-leen suh-lih-sih-late) USAN.
Use: Analgesic.
cholinesterase inhibitors. Agents that inhibit the enzyme cholinesterase and enhance the effects of endogenous acetylcholine.
Use: Glaucoma therapy; Alzheimer disease; muscle stimulant.
See: Donepezil Hydrochloride.
Eserine Salicylate.
Eserine Sulfate.
Exelon.
Galantamine HBr.
Isopto Eserine.
Neostigmine Methylsulfate.
Rivastigmine Tartrate.
Tacrine Hydrochloride.
choline theophyllinate.
See: Oxtriphylline.
Cholinoid. (Ivax) Choline 111 mg, inositol 111 mg, vitamins B_1 0.33 mg, B_2 0.33 mg, B_3 3.33 mg, B_5 1.7 mg, B_6 0.33 mg, B_{12} 1.7 mcg, C 100 mg, lemon bioflavonoid complex 100 mg. Cap. Bot. 100s. *OTC.*
Use: Lipid, vitamin supplement.
Chol Meth in B. (Esco) Choline bitartrate 235 mg, inositol 112 mg, methionine 70 mg, betaine anhydrous 50 mg, vitamins B_{12} 6 mcg, B_1 6 mg, B_6 3 mg, niacin 10 mg. Cap. Bot. 500s, 1000s. *OTC.*
Use: Vitamin supplement.

Cholografin Meglumine. (Bracco Diagnostics) Iodipamide meglumine 520 mg, iodine 257 mg/mL, EDTA. Inj. Vial 20 mL. *Rx.*
Use: Radiopaque agent; parenteral agent.

cholylglycine.
See: CG RIA.

chondodendron tomentosum.
See: Curare.

•**chondroitin sulfate and sodium hyaluronate.** (kon-DRO-ih-tin SULL-fate and SO-dee-uhm HIGH-ah-loo-rohn-ate) *USP 28.* Surgical aid in anterior segment procedures including cataract extraction and intraocular lens implantation. *Rx.*
See: Viscoat.

•**chondroitin sulfate sodium.** (kon-DRO-ih-tin SULL-fate SO-dee-uhm) *NF 23.*
Use: Dietary supplement.

chondrus. Irish Moss. W/Petrolatum.
See: Kondremul.

Chooz. (Schering-Plough) Calcium carbonate 500 mg. Gum Tab. Pkg. 16s. *OTC.*
Use: Antacid.

. **Chorex 5.** (Hyrex) Chorionic gonadotropin 5,000 units per vial with 10 mL diluent (500 units per mL), mannitol, benzyl alcohol 0.9%. Pow. for Inj. Vials. 10 mL. *Rx.*
Use: Ovulation stimulant.

•**choriogonadotropin alfa.** (kore-ee-oh-goe-NAD-oh-troe-pin) USAN.
Use: Sex hormone, ovulation stimulant.
See: Ovidrel.

chorionic gonadotropin.
Use: Ovulation stimulant.
See: A.P.L.
  Chorex-5.
  Choron-10.
  Gonic.
  Pregnyl.
  Profasi.

chorionic gonadotropin. (Various Mfr.) Chorionic gonadotropin 5,000 units per vial with 10 mL diluent (500 units per mL), 10,000 units per vial with 10 mL diluent (1,000 units per mL), 20,000 units per vial with 10 mL diluent (2,000 units per mL). Pow. for Inj. Vials. 10 mL. *Rx.*
Use: Ovulation stimulant.

Choron 10. (Forest) Chorionic gonadotropin 10,000 units/vial with diluent 10 mL (1,000 units per mL), mannitol, benzyl alcohol 0.9%. Pow. for Inj. Vials. 10 mL. *Rx.*
Use: Ovulation stimulant.

Chromagen. (Ther-Rx) Fe (as elemental iron) 70 mg, vitamins C 150 mg, B_{12} 10 mcg, desiccated stomach substance 100 mg. Cap. UD 100s. *Rx.*
Use: Mineral, vitamin supplement.

Chromagen FA. (Ther-Rx) Fe (as elemental iron) 70 mg, vitamin C 150 mg, folic acid 1 mg, B_{12} 10 mcg. Parabens. Cap. UD 100s. *Rx.*
Use: Mineral, vitamin supplement.

Chromagen Forte. (Ther-Rx) Fe (as elemental iron) 151 mg, vitamin C 60 mg, folic acid 1 mg, B_{12} 10 mcg. Parabens. Cap. UD 100s. *Rx.*
Use: Mineral, vitamin supplement.

Chromagen OB. (Savage) Ca 200 mg, Cu, folic acid 1 mg, Fe 28 mg, Mn, B_2 1.8 mg, B_1 1.6 mg, B_6 20 mg, C 60 mg, D 400 units, Zn 25 mg, E 30 units, niacinamide 5 mg, B_{12} 12 mcg, docusate calcium 25 mg. Cap. Bot. 100s. *Rx.*
Use: Vitamin supplement.

Chroma-Pak. (SoloPak Pharmaceuticals, Inc.) Chromium **4 mcg/mL:** Vial 10 mL, 30 mL. **20 mcg/mL:** Vial 5 mL. *Rx.*
Use: Nutritional supplement, parenteral.

chromargyre.
See: Merbromin.

chromated. Solution (Cr^{51}).
See: Chromitope sodium.

Chromelin Complexion Blender. (Summers) Dihydroxyacetone 5%, isopropyl alcohol, propylene glycol. Susp. 30 mL. *OTC.*
Use: Hyperpigmenting.

chromic acid, disodium salt. Sodium Chromate Cr^{51}.

•**chromic chloride.** (kroe-MIK) *USP 28.*
Use: Supplement, trace mineral.

•**chromic chloride Cr^{51}.** (kroe-MIK) USAN.
Use: Radiopharmaceutical.
See: Chromitope Cl.

•**chromic phosphate Cr^{51}.** (kroe-MIK) USAN.
Use: Radiopharmaceutical.

•**chromic phosphate P^{32} suspension.** (kroe-MIK) *USP 28.*
Use: Radiopharmaceutical.

Chromitope sodium. (Bristol-Myers Squibb) Chromate Cr^{51}, sodium for Inj. 0.25 mCi.
Use: Radiopharmaceutical.

chromium. A trace metal used in IV nutritional therapy that helps maintain normal glucose metabolism and peripheral nerve function.
See: Chroma-Pak.
  Chromic Chloride.
  Chromium.

Chromium Chloride.
Chromium Trace Metal Additive.
Concentrated Chromic Chloride.
•**chromium Cr 51 edetate.** (KRO-me-um) *USP 28.*
Use: Radiopharmaceutical.
•**chromonar hydrochloride.** (kroe-moe-NAHR) USAN.
Use: Coronary vasodilator.
Chronulac. (Hoechst) Lactulose 10 g/15 mL (< galactose 1.6 g, lactose 1.2 g, other sugars 1.2 g). Soln. Bot. 240 mL, 960 mL. *Rx.*
Use: Laxative.
Chur-Hist. (Churchill) Chlorpheniramine 4 mg. Kaptab. Bot. 100s.
Use: Antihistamine.
Cialis. (Lilly) Tadalafil 5 mg, 10 mg, 20 mg. Lactose. Film-coated. 30s. *Rx.*
Use: Erectile dysfunction.
Cibacalcin. (Novartis) Calcitonin-human for injection.
Use: Paget disease. [Orphan Drug]
CI basic violet 3. Gentian Violet.
Ciba Vision Cleaner. (Ciba Vision) Cocoamphocarboxyglycinate, sodium lauryl sulfate, sorbic acid 0.1%, hexylene glycol, EDTA 0.2%. Soln. 5 mL, 15 mL. *OTC.*
Use: Contact lens care.
Ciba Vision Saline. (Ciba Vision) Buffered, isotonic with NaCl, boric acid. Soln. Bot. 90 mL, 240 mL, 360 mL. *OTC.*
Use: Contact lens care, rinsing, storage.
cibenzoline.
See: Cifenline succinate.
•**ciclafrine hydrochloride.** (SIK-lah-freen) USAN.
Use: Antihypotensive.
•**ciclazindol.** (sigh-CLAY-zin-dole) USAN.
Use: Antidepressant.
•**ciclesonide.** (sik-lih-SON-ide) USAN.
Use: Asthma
•**cicletanine.** (sik-LET-ah-neen) USAN.
Use: Antihypertensive.
•**ciclopirox.** (sigh-kloe-PEER-ox) USAN.
Use: Antifungal.
See: Loprox.
Penlac Nail Lacquer.
ciclopirox. (Fougera) Ciclopirox. **Cream:** 0.77%. Water miscible base. Benzyl alcohol 1%, cetyl alcohol, mineral oil, stearyl alcohol, myristyl alcohol. 15 g, 30 g, 90 g. **Susp., topical:** 0.77%. Alcohols, mineral oil. 30 mL, 60 mL. *Rx.*
Use: Antifungal agent.
•**ciclopirox olamine.** (sigh-kloe-PEER-ox OLE-ah-meen) *USP 28.*

Use: Antifungal.
See: Loprox.
•**cicloprofen.** (SIK-low-pro-fen) USAN.
Use: Anti-inflammatory.
•**cicloprolol hydrochloride.** (SIGH-kloe-PRO-lahl) USAN.
Use: Antiadrenergic, beta-receptor.
Cidex. (Johnson & Johnson) Activated dialdehyde. Soln. Bot. Qt, gal, 2.5 gal.
Use: Disinfectant, sterilizing.
Cidex Plus. (Johnson & Johnson) Glutaraldehyde 3.2%. Soln. Gal.
Use: Disinfectant, sterilizing.
Cidex-7. (Johnson & Johnson) Glutaraldehyde 2% and vial of activator with aqueous potassium salt as buffer and sodium nitrite as a corrosive inhibitor. Soln. Bot. Qt, gal, 5 gal.
Use: Disinfectant, sterilizing.
C.I. direct blue 53 tetrasodium salt. Evans Blue. *Rx.*
•**cidofovir.** (sigh-DAH-fah-vihr) USAN.
Use: Antiviral.
See: Vistide.
•**cidoxepin hydrochloride.** (sih-DOX-eh-PIN) USAN.
Use: Antidepressant.
•**cifenline.** (sigh-FEN-leen) USAN. *Formerly cibenzoline.*
Use: Cardiovascular, antiarrhythmic.
•**cifenline succinate.** (sigh-FEN-leen) USAN.
Use: Cardiovascular agent, antiarrhythmic.
•**ciglitazone.** (sigh-GLIE-tah-ZONE) USAN.
Use: Antidiabetic.
cignolin.
See: Anthralin.
•**ciladopa hydrochloride.** (SIGH-lah-doe-pah) USAN.
Use: Antiparkinsonian, dopaminergic.
cilastatin-imipenem. A formulation of imipenem, a thienamycin antibiotic, and cilastatin sodium, the inhibitor of the renal dipeptidase, dehydropeptidase-1.
Use: Anti-infective.
See: Primaxin I.M.
Primaxin I.V.
•**cilastatin sodium.** (SIGH-lah-STAT-in) *USP 28.*
Use: Enzyme inhibitor.
W/Imipenem.
See: Primaxin.
•**cilazapril.** (sile-AZE-ah-PRILL) USAN.
Use: Investigational antihypertensive.
•**cilengitide.** (sye-LEN-gi-tide) USAN.
Use: Angiogenesis inhibitor.

●**cilexetil.** (sigh-LEX-eh-till) USAN.
Use: Anti-infective.

Cilfomide. (Sanofi-Synthelabo) Inositol
hexanicotinate. Tab. *Rx.*
Use: Hypolipidimic, peripheral vasodilator.

Cillium. (Whiteworth Towne) Psyllium
seed husk 4.94 g, 14 calories/rounded
tsp. Pow. Bot. 420 g, 630 g. *OTC.*
Use: Laxative.

●**cilmostim.** (SILL-moe-stim) USAN. *Formerly rhM-CSF, M-CSF, CSF-1.*
Use: Hematopoietic, macrophage
colony-stimulating factor.

●**cilobamine mesylate.** (SIGH-low-BAM-
een) USAN. *Formerly clobamine mesylate.*
Use: Antidepressant.

●**cilofungin.** (SIGH-low-FUN-jin) USAN.
Use: Antifungal.

●**cilomilast.** (sill-OH-mih-last) USAN.
Use: Investigational drug for asthma;
COPD; arthritis; atopic dermatitis;
multiple sclerosis.

●**cilostazol.** (sill-OH-stah-zole) USAN.
Use: Antithrombotic; platelet inhibitor;
vasodilator.
See: Pletal.

cilostazol. (Various Mfr.) Cilostazol
50 mg, 100 mg. Tab. 60s. *Rx.*
Use: Antiplatelet agent.

Ciloxan. (Alcon) Ciprofloxacin hydrochloride 3.33 mg (equivalent to 3 mg base)/
g, mineral oil, white petrolatum. Oint.
Tube. 3.5 g. *Rx.*
Use: Anti-infective.

●**ciluprevir.** (sigh-loo-PRAH-veer) USAN.
Use: Hepatitis C.

●**climaterol.** (sigh-MAT-toh-role) USAN.
Use: Repartitioning agent.

●**cimetidine.** (sigh-MET-ih-deen) *USP 28.*
Use: Histamine H₂ antagonist.
See: Tagamet.
Tagamet HB 200.

cimetidine. (Endo) Cimetidine (as hydrochloride) 150 mg per mL, phenol 5 mg/
mL. Inj. Vials. 2 mL. Multidose vials.
8 mL. *Rx.*
Use: Histamine H₂ receptor antagonist.

cimetidine. (Various Mfr.) Cimetidine
200 mg, 300 mg, 400 mg, 800 mg. Tab.
Bot. 100s, 500s, 1,000s. *Rx.*
Use: Histamine H₂ receptor antagonist.

cimetidine. (Zenith Goldline) Cimetidine
200 mg. Tab. Bot. 30s, 50s. *OTC.*
Use: Histamine H₂ receptor antagonist.

●**cimetidine hydrochloride.** (sigh-MET-ih-
deen) USAN.
Use: Histamine H₂ receptor antagonist.

cimetidine hydrochloride. (Endo)
Cimetidine hydrochloride 150 mg, phenol 5 mg/mL. Inj. Vial 2 mL, Multidose
vial 8 mL. *Rx.*
Use: Histamine H₂ antagonist.

cimetidine oral solution. (Barre-
National) Cimetidine 300 mg (as hydrochloride)/5 mL. Alcohol 2.8%, parabens, saccharin, sorbitol. Mint-peach
flavor. Bot. 240 mL, 470 mL. *Rx.*
Use: Histamine H₂ antagonist.

●**cinacalcet hydrochloride.** (sin-a-KAL-
set) USAN.
Use: Hyperparathyroidism agent.
See: Sensipar.

Cinacort Span. (Foy Laboratories) Triamcinolone acetonide 40 mg/mL. Vial
5 mL. *Rx.*
Use: Corticosteroid.

●**cinalukast.** (sin-ah-LOO-kast) USAN.
Use: Antiasthmatic; leukotriene antagonist.

●**cinanserin hydrochloride.** (sin-AN-ser-
in) USAN.
Use: Serotonin inhibitor.

cinchona alkaloid.
Use: Antimalarial.
See: Quinine Sulfate.

cinchona bark. (Various Mfr.).
Use: Antimalarial, tonic.
W/Anhydrous quinine, cinchonidine, cin-
chonine, quinidine, quinine.
See: Totaquine.

cinchonine salts. (Various Mfr.).
Use: Quinine dihydrochloride.

cinchophen.
Use: Analgesic.

●**cinepazet maleate.** (SIN-eh-PAZZ-ett)
USAN.
Use: Antianginal.

●**cinflumide.** (SIN-flew-mide) USAN.
Use: Muscle relaxant.

●**cingestol.** (sin-JESS-tole) USAN.
Use: Hormone, progestin.

●**cinnamedrine.** (sin-am-ED-reen) USAN.
Use: Muscle relaxant.
See: Midol.

cinnamic aldehyde. Name previously
used for Cinnamaldehyde.

cinnamon.
Use: Flavoring.

cinnamon oil. (Various Mfr.).
Use: Pharmaceutic aid.

●**cinnarizine.** (sin-NAHR-ih-zeen) USAN.
Use: Antihistamine.

cinnopentazone. INN for Cintazone.

Cinobac. (Oclassen) Cinoxacin 250 mg.
Cap. Bot. 40s. *Rx.*
Use: Anti-infective, urinary.

●**cinoxate.** (sin-OX-ate) USAN.
Use: Ultraviolet screen.

•**cinperene.** (SIN-peh-reen) USAN.
Use: Antipsychotic.
Cin-Quin. (Solvay) Quinidine sulfate.
(Contains 83% anhydrous quinidine al-
kaloid.) **Tab.:** 100 mg, 200 mg,
300 mg. Bot. 100s, 1000s, UD 100s.
Cap.: 200 mg. Bot. 100s. 300 mg. Bot.
100s, 1000s, UD 100s. *Rx.*
Use: Antiarrhythmic.
•**cinromide.** (SIN-row-mide) USAN.
Use: Anticonvulsant.
•**cintazone.** (SIN-tah-zone) USAN.
Use: Anti-inflammatory.
•**cintriamide.** (sin-TRY-ah-mid) USAN.
Use: Antipsychotic.
•**cioteronel.** (SIGH-oh-TEH-row-nell)
USAN.
Use: Dermatologic, acne; androgenic
alopecia and keloid, antimutagenic.
•**cipamfylline.** (sigh-PAM-fih-lin) USAN.
Use: Antiviral.
Cipralan. (Roche) Cifenline succinate.
Formerly cibenzoline. Rx.
Use: Antiarrhythmic.
•**cipralisant maleate.** (ci-PRAL-is-ant)
USAN.
Use: Histamine H$_3$ antagonist; ADHD.
•**ciprefadol succinate.** (sih-PREH-fah-
dahl) USAN.
Use: Analgesic.
Cipro. (Bayer) Ciprofloxacin. **Tab.:**
100 mg, 250 mg, 500 mg, 750 mg. Bot.
50s, 100s, UD 100s; 100 mg in *Cipro
Cystitis Packs* 6s only. **Pow. for Oral
Susp.:** 250 mg/5 mL (5%), 500 mg/
5 mL (10%) when reconstituted, sucrose, strawberry flavor. Bot. of micro-
capsules, bot. of diluent, and a teaspoon. *Rx.*
Use: Anti-infective, fluoroquinolone.
•**ciprocinonide.** (sih-PRO-SIN-oh-nide)
USAN.
Use: Adrenocortical steroid.
Ciprodex. (Alcon) Ciprofloxacin 0.3%,
dexamethasone 0.1%. Benzalkonium
chloride, boric acid, sodium chloride,
hydroxyethyl cellulose, tyloxapol, acetic
acid, sodium acetate, EDTA. Otic
Susp. 5 mL, 7.5 mL. *Drop-Tainer. Rx.*
Use: Steroid and antibiotic combination.
•**ciprofibrate.** (sip-ROW-FIE-brate)
USAN.
Use: Antihyperlipoproteinemic.
•**ciprofloxacin.** (sip-ROW-FLOX-ah-sin)
USP 28.
Use: Anti-infective, fluoroquinolone.
See: Cipro.
   Cipro I.V.
   Cipro XR.
W/Dexamethasone.
See: Ciprodex.

ciprofloxacin. (Barr) Ciprofloxacin hydrochloride. **Tab.:** 250 mg, 500 mg,
750 mg. 50s (750 mg), 100s (250 mg,
500 mg). **Pow. for Oral Susp:** 250 mg/
5 mL (5%), 500 mg/5mL (10%) (when
reconstituted), sucrose, strawberry flavor. Bot. of microcapsules, diluent, and
a teaspoon. *Rx.*
Use: Anti-infective, fluoroquinolone.
ciprofloxacin. (Dr. Reddy's) Ciprofloxacin 100 mg. Film-coated. Tab. 6s. *Rx.*
Use: Fluoroquinolone.
ciprofloxacin. (Various Mfr.) Ciprofloxacin 3.5 mg/mL (equiv. to 3 mg base),
benzalkonium chloride 0.006%, mannitol, and EDTA. Dropper Bot. 2.5 mL,
5 mL, 10 mL. *Rx.*
Use: Antibiotic.
•**ciprofloxacin hydrochloride.** (sip-ROW-
FLOX-ah-sin) *USP 28.*
Use: Anti-infective.
See: Ciloxan.
Cipro HC Otic. (Bayer) Ciprofloxacin
2 mg, hydrocortisone 10 mg/mL, benzyl
alcohol. Susp. Bot. 10 mL. *Rx.*
Use: Otic preparation.
Cipro I.V. (Bayer) Ciprofloxacin 200 mg,
400 mg, with lactic acid. Inj. **200 mg:**
Vial 20 mL (1%); Flexible cont. 100 mL
in 5% dextrose (0.2%), 120 mL. Bulk
packages. **400 mg:** Vial 40 mL (1%);
Flexible cont. 200 mL in 5% dextrose
(0.2%), 120 mL. Bulk packages. *Rx.*
Use: Anti-infective, fluoroquinolone.
•**ciprostene calcium.** (sigh-PRAHS-teen)
USAN.
Use: Platelet aggregation inhibitor.
Cipro XR. (Bayer) Ciprofloxacin 500 mg,
1000 mg. ER Tab. Bot. 50s, 100s, UD
30s (1000 mg only). *Rx.*
Use: Fluoroquinolone.
•**ciramadol.** (sihr-AM-ah-dole) USAN.
Use: Analgesic.
•**ciramadol hydrochloride.** (sihr-AM-ah-
dole) USAN.
Use: Analgesic.
Cirbed. (Boyd) Papaverine hydrochloride
150 mg. Cap. Bot. 100s. *Rx.*
Use: Antispasmodic.
Circavite-T. (Circle) Iron 12 mg, vitamins
A 10,000 units, D 400 units, E 15 mg,
B$_1$ 10.3 mg, B$_2$ 10 mg, B$_3$ 100 mg, B$_5$
18.4 mg, B$_6$ 4.1 mg, B$_{12}$ 5 mcg, C
200 mg, Cu, I, Mg, Mn, Zn 1.5 mg. Bot.
100s. *OTC.*
Use: Mineral, vitamin supplement.
•**cirolemycin.** (sih-ROW-leh-MY-sin)
USAN.
Use: Anti-infective; antineoplastic.

●**cisapride.** (SIS-uh-PRIDE) USAN.
Note: Withdrawn from US market.
Available from the manufacturer on a
limited-access protocol.
Use: Gastrointestinal; stimulant, peristaltic.
See: Propulsid.
●**cisatracurium besylate.** (sis-ah-trah-
CURE-ee-uhm BESS-ih-late) USAN.
Use: Nondepolarizing neuromuscular
blocking agent; muscle relaxant.
See: Nimbex.
●**cisconazole.** (SIS-KOE-nah-zahl) USAN.
Use: Antifungal.
●**cisplatin.** (SIS-plat-in) *USP 28.* Formerly
cis-Platinum II.
Use: Antineoplastic.
See: Platinol-AQ.
cisplatin (Various Mfr.) Cisplatin 1 mg/
mL. Inj. Multidose vial 50 mL, 100 mL,
200 mL. *Rx.*
Use: Antineoplastic.
cis-retinoic acid. (13-cis-Retinoic Acid).
Rx.
Use: Antiacne.
See: Accutane.
Isotretinoin.
9-cis retinoic acid. (Allergan)
Use: Promyelocytic leukemia treatment;
prevention of retinal detachment
caused by proliferative vitreoretinopa-
thy. [Orphan Drug]
●**citalopram hydrobromide.** (sih-TAHL-
oh-pram) USAN.
Use: Antidepressant.
See: Celexa.
citalopram hydrobromide. (Roxane)
Citalopram (as hydrobromide) 10 mg
per 5 mL. Sorbitol, parabens. Peppermint flavor. Oral Soln. 240 mL. *Rx.*
Use: Antidepressant.
citalopram hydrobromide. (Various Mfr.)
Citalopram hydrobromide 10 mg,
20 mg, 40 mg. May contain lactose.
Tab. 30s, 100s, 500s, 1,000s, UD 100s
(except 10 mg). *Rx.*
Use: Antidepressant.
Citanest Plain. (AstraZeneca) Prilocaine
hydrochloride 4%. Inj. Dental Cartridge.
1.8 mL. *Rx.*
Use: Anesthetic, local amide, injectable.
Citanest Forte. (AstraZeneca) Prilocaine
hydrochloride 4% with epinephrine
1:200,000, sodium metabisulfite. Inj.
Dental cartridge 1.8 mL. *Rx.*
Use: Anesthetic, local amide, injectable.
●**citenamide.** (sigh-TEN-ah-MIDE) USAN.
Use: Anticonvulsant.

Cithal. (Table Rock) Watermelon seed
extract 2 g, theobromine 4 g, phenobarbital 0.25 g. Cap. Bot. 100s, 500s.
Rx.
Use: Antihypertensive.
●**citicoline sodium.** (SIGH-tih-koe-leen)
USAN.
Use: Poststroke and posthead trauma
treatment.
Citracal. (Mission) Elemental calcium
200 mg. Tab. Bot. 100s. *OTC.*
Use: Calcium supplement.
Citracal Liquitab. (Mission) Elemental
calcium 500 mg, aspartame, phenyl-
alanine 12 mg, saccharin, orange fla-
vor. Effervescent Tab. Pkg. 30s. *OTC.*
Use: Mineral.
Citracal 1500 + D. (Mission) Calcium cit-
rate 1500 mg, vitamin D 200 units. Tab.
Bot. 60s. *OTC.*
Use: Mineral, vitamin supplement.
Citracal Plus with Magnesium. (Mis-
sion) Ca 250 mg, vitamin D 125 units,
B₆ 5 mg, B, Cu, Mg, Mn, Zn. Tab. Bot.
150s. *OTC.*
Use: Mineral, vitamin supplement.
Citra Forte. (Boyle and Co. Pharm.)
Hydrocodone bitartrate 5 mg, ascorbic
acid 30 mg, pheniramine maleate
2.5 mg, pyrilamine maleate 3.33 mg,
potassium citrate 150 mg/5 mL. Bot. Pt,
gal. *c-III.*
Use: Antihistamine; antitussive; vitamin
supplement.
Citranox. (Alconox)
Use: Liquid acid detergent for manual
and ultrasonic washers.
Citra pH. (ValMed, Inc.) Sodium citrate
dihydrate 450 mg/30 mL. Soln. 30 mL.
OTC.
Use: Antacid.
Citrasan B. (Sandia) Lemon bioflavonoid
complex 300 mg, vitamins C 300 mg,
B₁ 30 mg, B₂ 10 mg, B₆ 5 mg, B₁₂
4 mcg, calcium pantothenate 10 mg,
niacinamide 50 mg. Tab. Bot. 100s,
1000s. *OTC.*
Use: Mineral, vitamin supplement.
Citrasan K. (Sandia) Vitamins C 125 mg,
K 0.66 mg, lemon bioflavonoid complex
125 mg/5 mL. Liq. Bot. Pt, gal. *OTC.*
Use: Vitamin supplement.
Citrasan K-250. (Sandia) Vitamins C
250 mg, K 1 mg, lemon bioflavonoid
250 mg. Tab. Bot. 100s, 1000s. *OTC.*
Use: Vitamin supplement.
citrate acid.
See: Bicitra.
citrate and citric acid.
Use: Alkalinizer.
See: Bicitra.

Oracit.
Polycitra.
Polycitra K.
Polycitra LC.
W/Combinations.
See: Zee-Seltzer.
citrated normal human plasma.
See: Plasma, Normal Human.
Citresco-K. (Esco) Vitamins C 100 mg, K 0.7 mg, citrus bioflavonoid complex 100 mg. Cap. Bot. 100s, 500s, 1000s. *OTC.*
Use: Vitamin supplement.
•**citric acid.** (SI-trik) *USP 28.*
Use: Component of anticoagulant solutions and drug products.
citric acid and d-gluconic acid irrigant.
Use: Irrigant, genitourinary. [Orphan Drug]
See: Renacidin.
citric acid, glucono-delta-lactone and magnesium carbonate.
Use: Renal and bladder calculi of the apatite or struvite variety. [Orphan Drug]
citric acid, magnesium oxide, and sodium carbonate irrigation.
Use: Irrigant, ophthalmic.
citrin.
See: Vitamin P.
Citrin Capsules. (Table Rock) Watermelon seed extract 4 g. Bot. 100s, 500s. *Rx.*
Use: Antihypertensive.
Citrocarbonate. (Pharmacia) Sodium bicarbonate 0.78 g, sodium citrate anhydrous 1.82 g/3.9 g. Bot. 4 oz, 8 oz. *OTC.*
Use: Antacid.
Citrocarbonate Effervescent Granules. (Roberts) Sodium bicarbonate 780 mg, sodium citrate anhydrous 1820 mg, sodium 700.6 mg/5 mg. Bot. 150 g. *OTC.*
Use: Analgesic; antacid.
Citro Cee, Super. (Marlyn Nutraceuticals) Bioflavonoids 500 mg, rutin 50 mg, vitamin C 500 mg, rose hips powder 500 mg. Tab. Bot. 50s, 100s. *OTC.*
Use: Vitamin supplement.
Citrolith. (Beach) Potassium citrate 50 mg, sodium citrate 950 mg. Tab. Bot. 100s, 500s. *Rx.*
Use: Alkalinizer, urinary.
Citroma. (Century) Magnesium citrate. Oral Soln. Bot. 10 oz. *OTC.*
Use: Laxative.
Citroma Low Sodium. (National Magnesia) Magnesium citrate, lemon or cherry flavor in sugar-free vehicle. Oral soln. Bot. 10 oz. *OTC.*
Use: Laxative.

Citrotein. (Novartis) Sucrose, pasteurized egg white solids, amino acids, maltodextrin, citric acid, natural and artificial flavors, mono- and diglycerides, partially hydrogenated soybean oil, 0.66 cal/mL, protein 40.7 g, carbohydrate 120.7 g, fat 1.55 g, Na 698 mg, K 698 mg/L. Tartrazine (orange flavor only). Orange, grape, and punch flavors. Pow. 1.57 oz. Pkt., Can 14.16 oz. *OTC.*
Use: Nutritional supplement, enteral.
•**citrovorum factor.** (sih-troe-VOHR-uhm) *USP 28.*
See: Leucovorin calcium.
Citrucel. (GlaxoSmithKline) Methylcellulose. **Pow.:** 2 g/heaping tbsp., sucrose, orange flavor. Can. 480 g, 846 g. **Tab.:** 500 g. Maltodextrin. 164s. *OTC.*
Use: Laxative
Citrucel Sugar Free. (GlaxoSmithKline) Methylcellulose 2 g, aspartame, phenylalanine 52 mg/levelled scoop. Pow. Can. 245 g, 480 g. *OTC.*
Use: Laxative.
citrus bioflavonoid compound.
See: Bioflavonoid Compounds.
C.V.P.
Vitamin P.
CKA Canker Aid. (Pannett Prod.) Benzocaine, aluminum hydrate, magnesium trisilicate, sodium acid carbonate. Pow. *OTC.*
Use: Cancer; cold sores.
CK (CPK) Reagent Strips. (Bayer Corp. (Consumer Div.)) Seralyzer reagent strips for creatinine phosphokinase in serum or plasma. Bot. 25s.
Use: Diagnostic aid.
•**cladribine.** (KLAD-rih-BEAN) USAN.
Use: Antineoplastic.
See: Leustatin.
cladribine. (Bedford) Cladribine 1 mg/mL, sodium chloride 9 mg/mL. Soln. for Inj. Single-use Vial 20 mL w/10 mL fill. *Rx.*
Use: Antineoplastic.
Claforan. (Hoechst) Cefotaxime sodium. **Pow. for Inj.:** 500 mg. Vial Pkg. 10s. 1 g, 2 g Vial. Pkg. 10s, 25s, 50s. Infusion bot. 10s, *ADD-Vantage* system Vial 25s. 10 g. Bot. **Inj.:** 1 g, 2 g. Premixed, frozen. 50 mL Pkg. 12s. *Rx.*
Use: Anti-infective, cephalosporin.
•**clamoxyquin hydrochloride.** (KLAM-OX-ee-kwin) USAN.
Use: Amebicide.
Claravis. (Barr Laboratories) Isotretinoin 10 mg, 20 mg, 40 mg. Cap. 30s, 100s. *Rx.*

Use: Retinoid.

Clarinex. (Schering) Desloratadine.
Syrup: 2.5 mg/5 mL. Sugar, EDTA.
Bubble gum flavor. 480 mL. **Tab.:** 5 mg,
lactose. Film coated. Bot. 100s, 500s,
unit-of-use 30s, UD hospital pack 100s.
Rx.
Use: Antihistamine, peripherally selective piperidine.

Clarinex-D 24 Hour. (Schering) Pseudoephedrine sulfate 240 mg, desloratadine 5 mg. EDTA. ER Tab. 100s. **Rx.**
Use: Decongestant and antihistamine.

Clarinex RediTabs. (Schering) Desloratadine 5 mg, mannitol, aspartame, phenylalanine 1.75 mg per tab., tutti frutti flavor. Rapidly disintegrating Tab. Bot. 30s. **Rx.**
Use: Antihistamine, peripherally selective piperidine.

Claripel. (Steifel) Hydroquinone 4%, cetostearyl alcohol, EDTA, parabens, octyl methoxycinnamate, avobenzone, oxybenzone, sodium metabisulfite, stearyl alcohol, glycerin. Cream. Tube. 45 g. **Rx.**
Use: Pigment agent.

• **clarithromyoin.** (kluh-RITH-row-MY-sin) **USP 28.**
Use: Anti-infective.
See: Biaxin.
Biaxin XL.

Claritin. (Schering) Loratadine 5 mg/ 5 ml , sugar, sucrose, EDTA. Fruit flavor. Syrup. Bot. 120 mL. **OTC.**
Use: Antihistamine, peripherally selective piperidine.

Claritin-D. (Schering-Plough) Loratadine 5 mg, pseudoephedrine sulfate 120 mg, Tab , CR Tab. Bot. 30s (except Tab.), 100s, unit-of-use 10s, 30s (except SR Tab.), UD 100s. **OTC.**
Use: Antihistamine, decongestant.

Claritin-D 12 Hour. (Schering-Plough) Pseudoephedrine sulfate 120 mg, loratadine 5 mg, lactose, sugar, butylparaben. ER Tab. Bot. 100s, unit of use 30s, UD 100s. **OTC.**
Use: Upper respiratory combination, decongestant, antihistamine.

Claritin-D 24-Hour. (Schering-Plough) Loratadine 10 mg, pseudoephedrine sulfate 240 mg, sugar. ER Tab. Bot. 100s, UD 100s. **OTC.**
Use: Upper respiratory combination, antihistamine, decongestant.

Claritin Hives Relief. (Schering) Loratadine 10 mg. Lactose. Tab. 10s. **OTC.**
Use: Antihistamine.

Claritin Reditabs. (Schering) Loratadine 10 mg, mannitol, mint flavor. Rapidly disintegrating Tab. 4, 10s, 20s, 30s. **OTC.**
Use: Antihistamine, peripherally selective piperidine.

Claritin 24-Hour Allergy. (Schering-Plough) Loratadine 10 mg. Lactose. Tab. 1s, 2s, 5s, 10s, 20s, 30s, 40s. **OTC.**
Use: Antihistamine.

• **clavulanate potassium.** (CLAV-you-lah-nate) **USP 28.**
Use: Inhibitor, β-lactamase.

clavulanate potassium and ticarcillin.
Use: Anti-infective, penicillin.
See: Timentin.

clavulanic acid/amoxicillin.
Use: Anti-infective, penicillin.
See: Augmentin.

clavulanic acid/ticarcillin.
Use: Anti-infective, penicillin.
See: Timentin.

• **clazolam.** (CLAY-zoe-lam) USAN.
Use: Anxiolytic.

• **clazolimine.** (clay-ZOLE-ih-meen) USAN.
Use: Diuretic.

Clean-N-Soak. (Allergan) Cleaning agent with phenylmercuric nitrate 0.004%. Bot. 120 mL. **OTC.**
Use: Contact lens care.

Clearasil Adult Care Cream. (Procter & Gamble) Sulfur, resorcinol, alcohol 10%, parabens. Cream. Tube. 17 g. **OTC.**
Use: Dermatologic, acne.

Clearasil Adult Care Medicated Blemish Stick. (Procter & Gamble) Sulfur 8%, resorcinol 1%, bentonite 4%, laureth-4, titanium dioxide. Stick ⅛ oz **OTC.**
Use: Dermatologic, acne.

Clearasil Antibacterial Soap. (Procter & Gamble) Triclosan 0.75%. Bar 92 g. **OTC.**
Use: Dermatologic, acne.

Clearasil Clearstick for Sensitive Skin, Maximum Strength. (Procter & Gamble) Salicylic acid 2%, alcohol 39%, aloe vera gel, menthol, EDTA. Liq. 35 mL. **OTC.**
Use: Dermatologic, acne.

Clearasil Clearstick, Maximum Strength. (Procter & Gamble) Salicylic acid 2%, alcohol 39%, menthol, EDTA. Liq. 35 mL. **OTC.**
Use: Dermatologic, acne.

Clearasil Clearstick, Regular Strength. (Procter & Gamble) Salicylic acid 1.25%, alcohol 39%, aloe vera gel, menthol, EDTA. Liq. 35 mL. **OTC.**

Use: Dermatologic, acne.

Clearasil Daily Face Wash. (Procter & Gamble) Triclosan 0.3%, glycerin, aloe vera gel, EDTA. Liq. Bot. 135 mL. *OTC.*
Use: Dermatologic, acne.

Clearasil Double Clear. (Procter & Gamble) **Pads, maximum strength:** Salicylic acid 2%, alcohol 40%, witch hazel distillate, menthol. Jar 32s. **Pads, regular strength:** Salicylic acid 1.25%, alcohol 40%, witch hazel distillate, menthol. Jar 32s. *OTC.*
Use: Dermatologic, acne.

Clearasil Double Textured Pads. (Procter & Gamble) **Pads, regular strength:** Salicylic acid 2%, alcohol 40%, glycerin, aloe vera gel, EDTA. Pkg. 32s, 40s. **Pads, maximum strength:** Salicylic acid 2%, alcohol 40%, menthol, aloe vera gel, EDTA. Pkg. 32s, 40s. *OTC.*
Use: Dermatologic, acne.

Clearasil Maximum Strength Acne Treatment. (Boots Healthcare) Benzoyl peroxide 10%, parabens in vanishing base. Cream. Tube 18 g. *OTC.*
Use: Dermatologic, acne.

Clearasil Medicated Deep Cleanser. (Procter & Gamble) Salicylic acid 0.5%, alcohol 42%, menthol, EDTA, aloe vera gel, hydrogenated castor oil. Liq. Bot. 229 mL. *OTC.*
Use: Dermatologic, acne.

Clearasil 10%. (Procter & Gamble) Benzoyl peroxide 10%. Bot. oz. *OTC.*
Use: Dermatologic, acne.

Clear-Atadine. (Major) Loratadine 10 mg. Lactose. Tab. 10s. *OTC.*
Use: Antihistamine.

Clear Away. (Schering-Plough) Salicylic acid 40%. Disc Pck. 18s. *OTC.*
Use: Dermatologic, acne.

Clear Away Plantar. (Schering-Plough) Salicylic acid 40%. Disc (for feet) Pck. 24s. *OTC.*
Use: Dermatologic, acne.

Clearblue Easy. (Unipath Diagnostics) Dipstick for in-home pregnancy test. Kit 1s, 2s.
Use: Diagnostic aid.

Clearblue Easy Ovulation Test. (Unipath Diagnostics) For urine test. Kit. Contains 7 test sticks. *OTC.*
Use: Ovulation test.

Clearblue Pregnancy Test. (VLI) Dip stick for pregnancy test. Kit 2s.
Use: Diagnostic aid.

Clearex Acne. (Health for Life Brands) Allantoin, sulfur, resorcinol, d-panthenol, isopropanol. Cream. Tube 1.5 oz. *OTC.*

Use: Dermatologic, acne.

Clear Eyes ACR Eye Drops. (Ross) Naphazoline hydrochloride 0.012%. Bot. 15 mL, 30 mL. *OTC.*
Use: Mydriatic, vasoconstrictor.

Clear Eyes Eye Drops. (Ross) Naphazoline hydrochloride 0.012%. Bot. 15 mL, 30 mL. *OTC.*
Use: Mydriatic, vasoconstrictor.

Clearly Cala-Gel. (Tec) Diphenhydramine hydrochloride, zinc acetate, menthol, EDTA. Gel. Tube. 180 g. *OTC.*
Use: Antipruritic, topical.

Clearplan. (VLI) Ovulation prediction test. Box 10s.
Use: Diagnostic aid.

●**clebopride.** (KLEH-boe-PRIDE) USAN.
Use: Antiemetic.

●**clemastine.** (KLEM-ass-teen) USAN.
Use: Antihistamine.
See: Tavist.

●**clemastine fumarate.** (KLEM-ass-teen) *USP 28.*
Use: Antihistamine, nonselective ethanolamine.
See: Dayhist-1.
Tavist.
Tavist Allergy.
W/Combinations.
See: Antihist-D.
Tavist Allergy/Sinus/Headache.

clemastine fumarate. (Various Mfr.) Clemastine fumarate. 0.67 mg/5 mL, may contain alcohol. Syr. Bot. 118 mL, 120 mL. *Rx.*
Use: Antihistamine, nonselective ethanolamine.

clemastine fumarate. (Various Mfr.) Clemastine fumarate 1.34 mg, 2.68 mg. Tab. Bot. 100s. *OTC.*
Use: Antihistamine, nonselective ethanolamine.

Clenia. (Upsher-Smith) Sodium sulfacetamide 10%, sulfur 5%, parabens, EDTA. **Cream:** Tube. 28 g. **Foam:** Bot. 170 mg, 340 mg. *Rx.*
Use: Keratolytic.

Clens. (Alcon) Cleansing agent with benzalkonium Cl 0.02%, EDTA 0.1%. Soln. Bot. 60 mL. *OTC.*
Use: Contact lens care.

●**clentiazem maleate.** (klen-TIE-ah-zem) USAN.
Use: Antianginal; antihypertensive; antagonist, calcium channel.

Cleocin. (Pfizer) Clindamycin phosphate. **Cream:** 2%. Benzyl alcohol, cetostearyl alcohol, mineral oil. Tube. 40 g with 7 disposable applicators. **Supp.:** 100 mg (as base). Cartons of 3 with

applicator. *Rx.*
Use: Vaginal preparation; anti-infective.
Cleocin. (Pfizer) Clindamycin hydrochloride. **Cap.:** 75 mg, 150 mg, 300 mg, tartrazine, lactose. Bot. 100s (75 mg); 16s, 100s, UD 100s (150 mg, 300 mg). **Vag. Supp.:** 100 mg/2.5 g. Box 3s w/applicator. *Rx.*
Use: Anti-infective.
Cleocin Pediatric. (Pfizer) Clindamycin palmitate 75 mg/5 mL. Gran. for Oral Soln. Bot. 100 mL. *Rx.*
Use: Anti-infective.
Cleocin Phosphate. (Pfizer) Clindamycin phosphate 150 mg/mL. Vial 2 mL, 4 mL, 6 mL; *ADD-Vantage* Vial 4 mL, 6 mL; *Galaxy* Plastic Cont. 50 mL; Bulk pkg. 60 mL. *Rx.*
Use: Anti-infective.
Cleocin T. (Pfizer) Clindamycin phosphate. **Gel:** 1%. Methylparaben. 30 g, 60 g. **Lotion:** 1%. Cetostearyl alcohol 2.5%, glycerin, isostearyl alcohol 2.5%, methylparaben 0.3%. 60 mL. **Top.**
Susp.: 1%. Isopropyl alcohol 50%. 30 mL, 60 mL, single-use pledget applicators. *Rx.*
Use: Anti-infective.
Cleocin Vaginal. (Pfizer) Clindamycin phosphate 2%, mineral oil, benzyl alcohol, propylene glycol, polysorbate 60, sorbitan, monostearate. Cream. Tube with 7 disposable applicators 40 g. *Rx.*
Use: Anti-infective, vaginal.
Clerz Drops for Hard Lenses. (Alcon) Hypertonic solution with hydroxyethylcellulose, sorbic acid, poloxamer 407, EDTA 0.1%, thimerosal 0.001%. Soln. Bot. 25 mL. *OTC.*
Use: Contact lens care.
Clerz Drops for Soft Lenses. (Alcon) Hypertonic solution with hydroxyethylcellulose, sodium borate, poloxamer 407, sorbic acid, thimerosal 0.001%, EDTA 0.1%. Soln. Bot. 25 mL. *OTC.*
Use: Contact lens care.
Clerz Plus. (Alcon) Buffered, isotonic, citrate buffer, NaCl, EDTA 0.05%, polyquaternium-1 0.001%, PEG-11. Drops. Bot. 5 mL, 8 mL, 10 mL. *OTC.*
Use: Contact lens product.
Clerz 2 for Hard Lenses. (Alcon) Isotonic solution with hydroxyethylcellulose, poloxamer 407, sodium Cl, potassium Cl, sodium borate, boric acid, sorbic acid, EDTA. Soln. Bot. 5 mL, 15 mL, 30 mL. *OTC.*
Use: Contact lens care.
Clerz 2 for Soft Lenses. (Alcon) Isotonic solution with sodium Cl, potassium Cl, hydroxyethylcellulose, poloxamer

407, sodium borate, boric acid, sorbic acid, EDTA. Soln. Bot. 5 mL (2s), 15 mL, 30. *OTC.*
Use: Contact lens care.
●**clevudine.** (cleh-VOO-deen) USAN.
Use: Antiviral.
Climara. (Berlex) Estradiol 2 mg (0.025 mg/day), 2.85 mg (0.0375 mg/day), 3.8 mg (0.05 mg/day), 4.55 mg (0.06 mg/day), 5.7 mg (0.075 mg/day), 7.6 mg (0.1 mg/day). Transdermal Patch. Box 4s. *Rx.*
Use: Estrogen.
ClimaraPro. (Berlex) Estradiol 0.045 mg/levonorgestrel 0.015 mg/day. Transdermal Patch. 4s. *Rx.*
Use: Sex hormone.
Clinac BPO. (Ferndale) Benzoyl peroxide 7%, EDTA. Gel. Tube. 45 g, 90 g. *Rx.*
Use: Anti-infective, topical.
●**clinafloxacin hydrochloride.** (klin-ah-FLOX-ah-sin) USAN.
Use: Anti-infective.
Clindagel. (Galderma) Clindamycin phosphate 1%, methylparaben. Gel. Tube. 7.5 g, 42 g, 77 g. *Rx.*
Use: Anti-infective, topical.
ClindaMax. (PharmaDerm) Clindamycin phosphate. **Cream:** 2%. Benzyl alcohol, cetostearyl alcohol, mineral oil. 40 g tube with 7 disposable applicators. **Gel:** 1%, methylparaben. 30 g, 60 g. **Lot.:** 1%, cetostearyl alcohol 2.5%, glycerin, isostearyl alcohol 2.5%, methylparaben 0.3%. Top. Susp. 60 mL. *Rx.*
Use: Anti-infective, topical.
●**clindamycin.** (KLIN-dah-MY-sin) USAN.
Use: Anti-infective; dermatologic, acne. Oral as antibiotic. Vaginal as anti-infective. AIDS-associated pneumonia. [Orphan Drug]
See: BenzaClin.
Cleocin.
Cleocin T.
Cleocin Vaginal.
Clindagel.
ClindaMax.
Clindets.
Evoclin.
●**clindamycin hydrochloride.** (KLIN-dah-MY-sin) *USP 28.*
Use: Anti-infective.
See: Cleocin hydrochloride A.D.T.
clindamycin hydrochloride. (Various Mfr.) Clindamycin hydrochloride 75 mg, 150 mg, 300 mg. Cap. Bot. 16s (300 mg only), 100s. *Rx.*
Use: Lincosamide.

•**clindamycin palmitate hydrochloride.**
(KLIN-dah-MY-sin PAL-mih-tate)
USP 28.
Use: Anti-infective.
See: Cleocin Pediatric.
Cleocin T.
•**clindamycin phosphate.** (KLIN-dah-MY-sin) *USP 28.*
Use: Anti-infective.
See: Cleocin.
Clindesse.
W/Benzoyl peroxide.
See: Duac.
clindamycin phosphate. (Various Mfr.)
Clindamycin phosphate. **Inj.:** 150 mg/mL. Vial 2 mL, 4 mL, 6 mL, 60 mL, 100 mL. **Top. Susp.:** 1%. Bot. 30 mL, 60 mL. **Gel:** 1%. Tube 30 g, 60 g. **Lot.:** 1%. Bot. 60 mL. *Rx.*
Use: Lincosamide; dermatologic, acne.
Clindesse. (KV Pharma) Clindamycin phosphate 2%. EDTA, mineral oil, parabens. Cream. Carton of 1 single-dose, prefilled, disposable applicator. *Rx.*
Use: Vaginal preparation.
Clindets. (Stiefel Labs) Clindamycin 1%. Isopropyl alcohol 52%. Pledgets. 1 mL. *Rx.*
Use: Anti-infective.
Clindex. (Rugby)
See: Chlordiazepoxide and clindinium bromide.
Clinistix Reagent Strips. (Bayer Corp. (Consumer Div.)) Glucose oxidase, peroxidase and orthotolidine. Diagnostic test for glucose in urine. Bot. 50s.
Use: Diagnostic aid.
Clinitest. (Bayer Corp. (Consumer Div.)) 2-drop and 5-drop combination packages w/color charts for both 2-drop and 5-drop use. Reagent tablets containing copper sulfate, sodium hydroxide, heat-producing agents. Patient's plastic set; Tab. refills. **Box:** 100s, 500s, sealed in foil. **Child-resistant bot.:** 36s, 100s.
Use: Diagnostic aid.
clinocaine hydrochloride.
See: Procaine hydrochloride.
Clinoril. (Merck) Sulindac 150 mg, 200 mg. Tab. Bot. 100s. *Rx.*
Use: Analgesic; NSAID.
Clinoxide. (Geneva) Clidinium bromide 2.5 mg, chlordiazepoxide hydrochloride, 5 mg. Cap. Bot. 100s, 500s. *c-IV.*
Use: Gastrointestinal; anticholinergic.
•**clioquinol.** (Klye-oh-KWIN-ole) *USP 28.*
Formerly Iodochlorhydroxyquin.
Use: Antiamebic; anti-infective, topical.
W/Aluminum acetate solution, hydrocortisone.

See: Hysone.
W/Hydrocortisone.
See: Hysone.
•**clioxanide.** (klie-OX-ah-nide) USAN.
Use: Anthelmintic.
Clipoxide. (Schein) Clidinium bromide 2.5 mg, chlordiazepoxide hydrochloride 5 mg. Cap. Bot. 100s, 500s. *c-v.*
Use: Anticholinergic; antispasmodic.
•**cliprofen.** (klih-PRO-fen) USAN.
Use: Anti-inflammatory.
clobamine mesylate. Name previously used. See cilobamine mesylate.
Use: Antidepressant.
•**clobazam.** (KLOE-bazz-am) USAN.
Use: Investigational anxiolytic.
•**clobetasol propionate.** (kloe-BEE-tah-sahl PRO-ee-oh-nate) *USP 28.*
Use: Anti-inflammatory.
See: Clobex.
Cormax.
Embeline.
Embeline E.
Olux.
Temovate.
clobetasol propionate. (Various Mfr.)
Clobetasone propionate 0.05%. **Gel:** Tube. 15 g, 30 g, 60 g. **Cream:** Tube. 15 g, 30 g, 45 g. **Ointment:** White petrolatum. Tube. 15 g, 30 g, 45 g. *Rx.*
Use: Anti-inflammatory; corticosteroid, topical.
•**clobetasone butyrate.** (kloe-BEE-tih-sone BYOO-tah-rate) USAN.
Use: Corticosteroid; anti-inflammatory.
•**clocortolone acetate.** (kloe-CORE-toe-lone) USAN.
Use: Corticosteroid, topical.
Clobex. (Galderma) Clobetasol propionate 0.05%. **Lot.:** Mineral oil. 15 mL, 30 mL, 59 mL, 118 mL. **Shampoo:** Alcohol. 118 mL. *Rx.*
Use: Anti-inflammatory; corticosteroid, topical.
•**clocortolone pivalate.** (kloe-CORE-toe-lone PIH-vah-late) *USP 28.*
Use: Corticosteroid, topical.
Clocream. (Pharmacia) Vitamins A and D in vanishing base. Tube oz. *OTC.*
Use: Emollient.
•**clodanolene.** (Kloe-DAN-oh-leen) USAN.
Use: Muscle relaxant.
•**clodazon hydrochloride.** (KLOE-dah-zone) USAN.
Use: Antidepressant.
Cloderm. (Healthpoint Medical) Clocortolone pivalate 0.1%. Cream. Tube 15 g, 45 g. *Rx.*
Use: Corticosteroid, topical.

●**clodronate disodium.** (kloe-DRAHN-ate) USAN.
Use: Bone calcium regulator.

●**clodronic acid.** (kloe-DRAHN-ik) USAN.
Use: Calcium regulator.

●**clofarabine.** (kloe-FAR-a-bine) USAN.
Use: Antimetabolite.
See: Clolar.

●**clofazimine.** (kloe-FAZZ-ih-meen) *USP 28.*
Use: Investigational tuberculostatic, leprostatic. [Orphan Drug]
See: Lamprene.

●**clofilium phosphate.** (KLOE-FILL-ee-uhm) USAN.
Use: Cardiovascular agent, antiarrhythmic.

●**cloflucarban.** (KLOE-flew-CAR-ban) USAN.
Use: Antiseptic; disinfectant.

●**clogestone acetate.** (kloe-JESS-tone) USAN. Under study.
Use: Hormone, progestin.

Clolar. (Genzyme Corporation) Clofarabine 1 mg/mL. Preservative free. Soln. for Inj. Vials. 20 mL. *Rx.*
Use: Antimetabolite.

●**clomacran phosphate.** (KLOE-mah-KRAN) USAN. Under study.
Use: Antipsychotic.

●**clomegestone acetate.** (KLOE-meh-JESS-tone) USAN. Under study.
Use: Hormone, progestin.

●**clometherone.** (kloe-METH-ehr-OHN) USAN.
Use: Antiestrogen.

Clomid. (Aventis Pasteur) Clomiphene citrate 50 mg. Tab. Bot. 30s. *Rx.*
Use: Sex hormone, ovulation stimulant.

●**clominorex.** (kloe-MEE-no-rex) USAN.
Use: Anorexic.

●**clomiphene citrate.** (KLOE-mih-feen SIH-trate) *USP 28.*
Tall Man: ClomiPHENE
Use: Antiestrogen; sex hormone, ovulation stimulant.
See: Clomid.
Milophene.
Serophene.

clomiphene citrate. (Various Mfr.) Clomiphene citrate 50 mg. Tab. Bot. 10s, 30s. *Rx.*
Use: Sex hormone, ovulation stimulant.

●**clomipramine hydrochloride.** (kloe-MIH-pruh-meen) USAN.
Tall Man: ClomiPRAMINE
Use: Antidepressant.
See: Anafranil.

clomipramine hydrochloride. (Various Mfr.) Clomipramine hydrochloride 25 mg, 50 mg, 75 mg. Cap. Bot. 100s, 1000s. *Rx.*
Use: Antidepressant.

●**clonazepam.** (kloe-NAY-ze-pam) *USP 28.*
Use: Anticonvulsant; antianxiety agent.
See: Klonopin.

clonazepam. (Various Mfr.) Clonazepam 0.5 mg, 1 mg, 2 mg. May contain lactose. Tab. Bot. 100s, 500s, 1000s (except 2 mg), UD 100s. *c-iv.*
Use: Anticonvulsant; antianxiety agent.

●**clonidine.** (KLOE-nih-DEEN) USAN.
Use: Antihypertensive.
See: Catapres.

●**clonidine hydrochloride.** (KLOE-nih-DEEN) *USP 28.*
Use: Antihypertensive. Epidural use for pain in cancer patients.
See: Catapres.
Duraclon.
W/Chlorthalidone
See: Clorpress.
Combipres.

clonidine hydrochloride and chlorthalidone. (Various Mfr.) Clonidine hydrochloride 0.1 mg, 0.2 mg, 0.3 mg, chlorthalidone 15 mg. Tab. Bot. 100s, 500s, 1000s.
Use: Antihypertensive; diuretic.

●**clonitrate.** (KLOE-nye-trate) USAN.
Use: Coronary vasodilator.

●**clonixeril.** (kloe-NIX-ehr-ill) USAN.
Use: Analgesic.

●**clonixin.** (kloe-NIX-in) USAN.
Use: Analgesic.

●**clopamide.** (kloe-PAM-id) USAN.
Use: Antihypertensive; diuretic.

●**clopenthixol.** (KLOE-pen-THIX-ole) USAN.
Use: Antipsychotic.

●**cloperidone hydrochloride.** (KLOE-per-ih-dohn) USAN.
Use: Hypnotic; sedative.

clophenoxate hydrochloride.
Use: Cerebral stimulant.

●**clopidogrel bisulfate.** (kloe-PIH-doe-grell bye-SULL-fate) *USP 28.*
Use: Platelet inhibitor.
See: Plavix.

●**clopimozide.** (KLOE-PIM-oh-zide) USAN.
Use: Antipsychotic.

●**clopipazan mesylate.** (KLOE-pip-ah-ZAN) USAN.
Use: Antipsychotic.

●**clopirac.** (KLOE-pih-rack) USAN.
Use: Anti-inflammatory.

•**cloprednol.** (kloe-PRED-nahl) USAN.
Use: Corticosteroid, topical.
•**cloprostenol sodium.** (kloe-PROSTE-
een-ole) USAN.
Use: Prostaglandin.
•**clorazepate dipotassium.** (klor-AZE-eh-
PATE DIE-poe-TASS-ee-uhm) *USP 28.*
Use: Anxiolytic; anticonvulsant.
See: Tranxene.
clorazepate dipotassium. (Various Mfr.)
Clorazepate dipotassium 3.75 mg,
7.5 mg, 15 mg. Tab. Bot. 100s, 500s,
1000s, UD 100s. *c-iv.*
Use: Anxiolytic; anticonvulsant.
•**clorazepate monopotassium.** (clor-
AZE-eh-PATE MAHN-oh-poe-TASS-ee-
uhm) USAN.
Use: Anxiolytic.
•**clorethate.** (klahr-ETH-ate) USAN.
Use: Hypnotic; sedative.
•**clorexolone.** (KLOR-ex-oh-LONE)
USAN.
Use: Diuretic.
Clorfed. (Stewart-Jackson Pharmacal)
Pseudoephedrine hydrochloride 60 mg,
chlorpheniramine maleate 4 mg. ER
Tab. 100s. *Rx.*
Use: Decongestant, antihistamine.
Clorfed Capsules. (Stewart-Jackson
Pharmacal) Chlorpheniramine 8 mg,
pseudoephedrine 120 mg. Bot. 100s.
Rx-OTC.
Use: Antihistamine; decongestant.
Clorfed Expectorant. (Stewart-Jackson
Pharmacal) Pseudoephedrine 30 mg,
guaifenesin 100 mg, codeine 10 mg/
5 mL. Bot. Pt. *c-v.*
Use: Antitussive; decongestant; expec-
torant.
Clorfed II. (Stewart-Jackson Pharmacal)
Chlorpheniramine 4 mg, pseudoephed-
rine 60 mg. Tab. Bot. 100s. *OTC.*
Use: Antihistamine; decongestant.
•**cloroperone hydrochloride.** (KLOR-oh-
PURR-ohn) USAN.
Use: Antipsychotic.
•**clorophene.** (KLOR-oh-feen) USAN.
Use: Disinfectant.
Clorpactin WCS-90. (Guardian Labora-
tories) Sodium oxychlorosene 2 g. Bot.
5s.
Use: Antiseptic.
•**clorprenaline hydrochloride.** (klor-
PREN-ah-leen) USAN.
Use: Bronchodilator.
Clorpress. (Bertek) Clonidine hydrochlo-
ride/chlorthalidone. 0.1 mg/15 mg,
0.2 mg/15 mg, 0.3 mg/15 mg. Tab.
100s. *Rx.*
Use: Antihypertensive.

•**clorsulon.** (KLOR-sull-ahn) *USP 28.*
Use: Antiparasitic; fasciolicide.
•**clortermine hydrochloride.** (klor-TER-
meen) USAN.
Use: Anorexic.
•**closantel.** (KLOSE-an-tell) USAN.
Use: Anthelmintic.
•**closiramine aceturate.** (kloe-SIH-rah-
meen ah-SEE-tur-ate) USAN.
Use: Antihistamine.
clostridial collagenase.
Use: Dupuytren disease. [Orphan Drug]
•**clothiapine.** (KLOE-THIGH-ah-peen)
USAN.
Use: Antipsychotic.
•**clothixamide maleate.** (kloe-THIX-ah-
mid) USAN.
Use: Antipsychotic.
•**cloticasone propionate.** (kloe-TIK-ah-
SONE PRO-pee-oh-nate) USAN.
Use: Anti-inflammatory.
•**clotrimazole.** (kloe-TRIM-uh-zole)
USP 28.
Use: Antifungal.
See: Cruex.
Desenex.
Gyne-Lotrimin.
Gyne-Lotrimin 7.
Gyne-Lotrimin 3.
Gyne-Lotrimin 3 Combination Pack.
Lotrimin.
Lotrimin AF.
Mycelex.
Mycelex-7.
Mycelex-7 Combination Pack.
clotrimazole. (Alra) Clotrimazole 1%,
benzyl alcohol. Vaginal cream. In 45 g
with 7 disposable applicators. *OTC.*
Use: Antifungal, vaginal.
clotrimazole. (Roxane) Clotrimazole
10 mg. Troches. 70s, 140s, 500s, UD
70s. *Rx.*
Use: Mouth and throat product.
clotrimazole. (Various Mfr.) Clotrima-
zole. **Cream:** 1% in a vanishing base,
benzyl alcohol 1%, cetostearyl alcohol.
Tube 15 g, 30 g, 45 g, 2 × 45 g. **Top.
Soln.:** 1%, PEG 400. Bot. 30 mL.
Rx-OTC.
Use: Antifungal, topical.
clotrimazole. (Various Mfr.) Clotrimazole. **Vaginal Insert.:** 200 mg. Box 3s
with applicator. **Vaginal Cream:** 2%.
Tube 21 g with 3 disp. applicators. 1%.
Tube 15 g, 30 g. 45 g with applicators.
Rx-OTC.
Use: Antifungal, *Candida* infections.
**clotrimazole and betamathasone di-
propionate.** (Fougera) Clotrimazole
1%, betamethasone dipropionate

0.05%, mineral oil, white petrolatum, cetearyl alcohol, benzyl alcohol. Cream. 15 g. 45 g. *Rx.*
Use: Antifungal; anti-inflammatory.
clotrimazole combination pack. (Various Mfr.) Clotrimazole. **Vag. Supp.:** 200 mg. 3s w/applicator. **Top. Cream:** 1%. Tube. Pack. *OTC.*
Use: Antifungal.
clotrimidazole. (Fujisawa Healthcare) *Use:* Sickle cell disease. [Orphan Drug]
●**clove oil.** *NF 23.*
Use: Pharmaceutic aid, flavor.
Cloverine. (Medtech) White salve. Tin Oz. *OTC.*
Use: Dermatologic, counterirritant.
●**clover, red.** *NF 23.*
Use: Dietary supplement.
Clovocain. (Vita Elixir) Benzocaine, oil of cloves. *OTC.*
Use: Anesthetic, local.
●**cloxacillin benzathine.** (KLOX-ah-SILL-in BENZ-ah-theen) *USP 28.*
Use: Anti-infective.
●**cloxacillin sodium.** (KLOX-ah-SILL-in) *USP 28.*
Use: Anti-infective, penicillin.
See: Cloxapen.
cloxacillin sodium. (Various Mfr.) Cloxacillin sodium. **Cap.:** 250 mg, 500 mg. Bot. 100s, UD 100s (250 mg only). **Pow. for Oral Soln.:** 125 mg/5 mL when reconstituted. Bot. 100 mL, 200 mL. *Rx.*
Use: Anti-infective, penicillin.
Cloxapen. (GlaxoSmithKline) Cloxacillin sodium 250 mg, 500 mg. Cap. Bot. 30s (500 mg only), 100s, UD 100s (500 mg only). *Rx.*
Use: Anti-infective, penicillin.
●**cloxyquin.** (KLOX-ee-kwin) *USAN.*
Use: Anti-infective.
●**clozapine.** (KLOE-zuh-PEEN) *USP 28.*
Use: Antipsychotic.
See: Clozaril.
Fazalco.
clozapine. (Various Mfr.) Clozapine 12.5 mg, 25 mg, 100 mg. Tab. Bot. 30s (12.5 mg only), 100s, 500s (except 12.5 mg). *Rx.*
Use: Antipsychotic.
Clozaril. (Novartis) Clozapine 25 mg, 100 mg, lactose, talc. Tab. 100s, 500s, UD 100s. *Rx.*
Use: Antipsychotic.
C-Max. (Bio-Technology General) Vitamin C 1000 mg, Mg 40 mg, Zn 5 mg, K 10 mg, Mn 1 mg, pectin 10 mg. Gradual release Tab. Bot. 100s. *OTC.*
Use: Mineral, vitamin supplement.

C.M.C. Cellulose Gum.
See: Carboxymethylcellulose sodium.
CMV. (Wampole) Cytomegalovirus antibody test system for the qualitative and semi-quantitative detection of CMV antibody in human serum. Test 100s.
Use: Diagnostic aid.
CMV-IGIV.
Use: Immunization.
See: Cytogam.
Cytomegalovirus Immune Globulin Intravenous.
CNS stimulants.
Use: Central Nervous System Stimulants.
Coadvil. (Whitehall-Robins) Ibuprofen 200 mg, pseudoephedrine hydrochloride 30 mg. Tab. Bot. 100s. *OTC.*
Use: Analgesic; decongestant.
coagulants.
See: Hemostatics.
Protamine Sulfate.
coagulation factor IX.
Use: Antihemophilic. [Orphan Drug]
See: Factor IX Complex, Vapor Heated Bebulin VH Immuno.
Mononine.
coagulation factor IX (human).
Use: Antihemophilic. [Orphan Drug]
See: AlphaNine.
coagulation factor IX (recombinant).
Use: Antihemophilic. [Orphan Drug]
See: BeneFix.
coagulation factor VIIa (recombinant).
Use: Antihemophilic.
See: NovoSeven.
●**coal tar.** *USP 28.*
Use: Topical antieczematic; antipsoriatic.
See: Balnetar.
Creamy Tar.
L.C.D. Compound
PC-Tar.
Polytar Bath.
Protar Protein.
Tarbonis.
Tera-Gel.
Zetar.
W/Allantoin, hydrocortisone.
See: Alphosyl-HC.
W/Hydrocortisone.
See: Doak Oil Forte.
Ze Tar-Quin.
W/Iodoquinol, hydrocortisone.
See: Tarcotin.
W/Zinc oxide.
See: Tarpaste.
coal tar, distillate.
Use: Dermatologic, topical.
See: Lavatar.
Syntar.

W/Sulfur, salicylic acid.
See: Pragatar.
coal tar extract.
Use: Dermatologic, topical.
W/Allantoin, hexachlorophene.
See: Sebical.
W/Allantoin, hexachlorophene, glycerin, lanolin.
See: Pso-Ritc.
W/Allantoin, salicylic acid, perhydrosqualene.
See: Skaylos.
W/Salicylic acid.
See: Neutrogena T/Sal.
coal tar paste.
Use: Dermatologic, topical.
W/Zinc paste.
See: Tarpaste.
coal tar topical solution. Liquor Carbonis Detergens. L.C.D.
Use: Antieczematic, topical.
See: Balnetar.
Creamy Tar.
Estar.
L.C.D. Compound.
MG217 Medicated Tar.
Psorigel.
PsoriNail.
Wright's.
Zetar.
W/Allantoin, psorilan, myristate.
See: Iocon.
Psorelief.
W/Hydrocortisone alcohol, clioquinololine, diperodon hydrochloride, vitamins A, D.
See: Pentarcort.
W/Hydrocortisone, iodoquinol.
See: Cor-Tar-Quin.
W/Robane (perhydrosqualene).
See: Skaylos.
W/Salicylic acid.
See: Ionil T.
W/Salicylic acid, sulfur, protein.
See: Vanseb-T Tar.
Co-Apap. (Various Mfr.) Pseudoephedrine hydrochloride 30 mg, chlorpheniramine maleate 2 mg, dextromethorphan HBr 15 mg, acetaminophen 325 mg. Tab. Bot. 24s, 50s, 1000s. *OTC.*
Use: Analgesic; antihistamine; antitussive; decongestant.
•**cobalamine concentrate.** (koe-BALL-uh-meen kahn-SEN-trate) *USP 28.*
Use: Hematopoietic vitamin.
See: Vitamin B_{12}.
cobalt chloride.
W/Ferrous gluconate, vitamin B_{12}, duodenum whole desiccated.
See: Bitrinsic-E.

cobalt gluconate.
W/Ferrous gluconate, vitamin B_{12} activity, desiccated stomach substance, folic acid.
See: Chromagen.
cobalt-labeled vitamin B_{12}.
See: Rubratope-57.
•**cobaltous chloride Co 57.** (koe-BALL-tuss) USAN.
Use: Radiopharmaceutical.
See: Cobatope-57
•**cobaltous chloride Co 60.** (koe-BALL-tuss) USAN.
Use: Radiopharmaceutical.
cobalt standards for vitamin B_{12}.
See: Cobatope-57 and Cobatope-60.
Cobatope-57. (Bristol-Myers Squibb) Cobaltous Cl Co 57.
cobex 1000. (Standex) Vitamin B_{12} 1000 mcg/10 mL. Vial 30 mL. *Rx.*
Use: Vitamin supplement.
Co-Bile. (Western Research) Hog bile 64.8 mg, pancreas substance 64.8 mg, papain-pepsin complex 97.2 mg, diatase malt 16.2 mg, papain 48.6 mg, pepsin 48.6 mg. Tab. Bot. 1000s. *Пx-OTC.*
Use: Digestive enzyme.
•**cocaine.** (koe-CANE) *USP 28.*
Use: Anesthetic, local.
•**cocaine hydrochloride.** (koe-KANE) *USP 28.*
Use: Anesthetic, local.
cocaine hydrochloride. top. soln.: (Various Mfr.). Cocaine hydrochloride 4%, 10%. Bot. 10 mL, UD 4 mL. **Pow.:** (Mallinckrodt). Cocaine hydrochloride 5 g, 25 g. *c-ii.*
Use: Mucosal anesthetic.
cocaine viscous. (Various Mfr.) Cocaine viscous 4%, 10%. Soln. Top. Bot. 10 mL, UD 4 mL. *c-ii.*
Use: Anesthetic, local.
•**coccidioidin.** (cox-id-ee-OY-din) *USP 28.*
Use: Diagnostic aid, dermal reactive indicator.
See: Spherulin.
cocculin.
See: Picrotoxin.
Cocilan. (Health for Life Brands) Euphorbia, wild lettuce, cocillana, squill, senega, cascarin (bitterless). Syr. Bot. Gal. Available w/codeine. Bot. Gal.
cocoa.
Use: Pharmaceutic aid, flavored vehicle.
•**cocoa butter.** (koe-koe) *NF 23.*
Use: Pharmaceutic aid, suppository base.

Codal-DH. (Cypress) Hydrocodone bitartrate 1.66 mg, pyrilamine maleate 8.33 mg, phenylephrine hydrochloride 5 mg/5 mL. Syr. Bot. 473 mL. *c-III.*
Use: Upper respiratory combination, antitussive, antihistamine, decongestant.

Codal-DM. (Cypress) Dextromethorphan HBr 10 mg, pyrilamine maleate 8.33 mg, phenylephrine hydrochloride 5 mg/5 mL, alcohol and dye free. Syr. Bot. 473 mL. *OTC.*
Use: Upper respiratory combination, antitussive, antihistamine, decongestant.

Codanol. (A.P.C.) Vitamins A, D, hexachlorophene, zinc oxide. Oint. Tube 1.5 oz, 4 oz. Jar lb. *OTC.*
Use: Dermatologic, counterirritant.

Codap (Solvay) Codeine phosphate 32 mg, acetaminophen 325 mg. Tab. Bot. 250s. *c-III.*
Use: Analgesic combination.

Codehist DH. (Geneva) Pseudoephedrine 30 mg, chlorpheniramine maleate 2 mg, codeine phosphate 10 mg/5 mL, alcohol 5.7%. Elix. Bot. 120 mL, 480 mL. *c-V.*
Use: Antihistamine; antitussive; decongestant.

●**codeine.** (KOE-deen) *USP 28.*
Use: Opioid analgesic.
See: Codeine Phosphate.
Codeine Sulfate.

codeine combinations.
See: Actifed.
Anexsia w/Codeine.
APAP w/Codeine.
A.P.C. w/Codeine.
Aspriptin w/Codeine No. 3
Ascriptin w/Codeine No. 2.
Brontex.
Calcidrine.
Capital w/Codeine.
Cheracol.
Chlor-Trimeton Expectorant.
Cycofed Pediatric.
Deconsal Pediatric.
Drucon w/Codeine.
Empirin No. 1, No. 2, No. 3, No. 4.
Fiorinal w/Codeine.
Golacol.
Guaifenesin DAC.
Nucofed.
Partuss AC.
Pediacof.
Phenergan Expectorant w/Codeine.
Proval No. 3.
Robitussin A-C, DAC.
Tolu-Sed.
Tussar-2.

Tussar SF.
Tussi-Organidin.
Tylenol w/Codeine No. 2, No. 3, No. 4.
Tylenol w/Codeine.
Vasotus.
codeine methylbromide. Eucodin.
Use: Antitussive.
●**codeine phosphate.** (KOE-deen) *USP 28.*
Use: Analgesic; antitussive, narcotic. W/Combinations.
See: Ascomp with Codeine.
Cheracol Cough.
Codeine Phosphate and Guaifenesin.
Codimal PH.
Cycofed.
Decohistine DH.
Dihistine DH.
Dihistine Expectorant.
Endal Expectorant.
Fiorinal with Codeine.
Floricet with Codeine.
Gani-Tuss NR.
Guiatuss AC.
Guiatuss DAC.
Mytussin AC Cough.
Mytussin DAC.
Novagest Expectorant with Codeine.
Nucofed.
Nucofed Expectorant.
Nucofed Pediatric Expectorant.
Nucotuss Expectorant.
Nucotuss Pediatric Expectorant.
Promethazine hydrochloride w/Codeine.
Promethazine VC w/Codeine Cough.
Prometh VC w/Codeine Cough.
Prometh w/Codeine Cough.
Romilar AC.
Triacin-C Cough.
Tricodene Cough & Cold.
Tussi-Organidin NR.
Tussirex.
Tussirex Sugar Free.
Vopac.
codeine phosphate. (Roxane) Codeine phosphate 15 mg/5 mL. Parabens. Oral. Soln. Bot. 500 mL, UD 5 mL. *c-II.*
Use: Opioid analgesic.
codeine phosphate. (Various Mfr.) Codeine phosphate 15 mg/mL, 30 mg/mL. May contain sulfites. Inj. *Carpuject* syringe system. 2 mL. *c-II.*
Use: Opioid analgesic.
codeine phosphate and aspirin.
See: Aspirin and Codeine Phosphate.
codeine phosphate and guaifenesin. (Ethex) Codeine phosphate 10 mg, guaifenesin 300 mg, sugar. Tab. Bot. 100s. *c-III.*

Use: Upper respiratory combination, expectorant, narcotic, antitussive.

● **codeine polistirex.** (KOE-deen pahl-ee-STIE-rex) USAN.
Use: Antitussive.

codeine resin complex combinations.
See: Omni-Tuss.

● **codeine sulfate.** (KOE-deen) *USP 28.*
Use: Analgesic; antitussive, narcotic.

codeine sulfate. (Various Mfr.) Codeine sulfate 15 mg, 30 mg, 60 mg. Tab. Bot. 100s (except 15 mg), UD 100s (except 60 mg). *c-II.*
Use: Opioid analgesic.

codelcortone.
See: Prednisolone.

Codiclear DH. (Schwarz Pharma) Hydrocodone bitartrate 5 mg, guaifenesin 100 mg/5 mL, saccharin, sorbitol, alcohol and dye free. Syr. Bot. 118 mL, 473 mL. *c-III.*
Use: Upper respiratory combination, antitussive, expectorant.

Codimal. (Schwarz Pharma) Chlorpheniramine maleate 2 mg, pseudoephedrine hydrochloride 30 mg, acetaminophen 325 mg. Cap.Tab. Bot. 24s, 100s, 1000s. *OTC.*
Use: Antihistamine, decongestant, analgesic.

Codimal DH. (Schwarz Pharma) Hydrocodone bitartrate 1.66 mg, phenylephrine hydrochloride 5 mg, pyrilamine maleate 8.33 mg/5 mL, alcohol free, menthol, sucrose. Syr. Bot. 118 mL, 473 mL. *c-III.*
Use: Upper respiratory combination, antitussive, decongestant, antihistamine.

Codimal DM. (Schwarz Pharma) Dextromethorphan HBr 10 mg, phenylephrine hydrochloride 5 mg, pyrilamine maleate 8.33 mg/5 mL, saccharin, sorbitol, menthol, alcohol and dye free. Syr. Bot. 120 mL, 473 mL, 3.8 mL. *OTC.*
Use: Upper respiratory combination, antitussive, decongestant, antihistamine.

Codimal-L.A. (Schwarz Pharma) Chlorpheniramine maleate 8 mg, pseudoephedrine hydrochloride 120 mg. SR Cap. Bot. 100s, 1000s. *Rx.*
Use: Antihistamine, decongestant.

Codimal-L.A. Half Capsules. (Schwarz Pharma) Pseudoephedrine hydrochloride 60 mg, chlorpheniramine maleate 4 mg, sucrose. Cap. Bot. 100s. *Rx.*
Use: Antihistamine; decongestant.

Codimal PH. (Schwarz Pharma) Codeine phosphate 10 mg, phenylephrine hydrochloride 5 mg, pyrilamine maleate 8.33 mg/5 mL, sucrose, alcohol free. Bot. 118 mL, 473 mL. *c-v.*

Use: Upper respiratory combination, antihistamine, antitussive, decongestant.

● **cod liver oil.** *USP 28.* Emulsion.
Use: Vitamin A and D therapy.
See: Cod Liver Oil Concentrate.
W/Anesthesin, zinc oxide, hydroxyquinoline.
See: Medicone Dressing.
W/Benzocaine.
See: Morusan.
W/Malt extract.
See: Vitamins A, D.
W/Methylbenzethonium Cl.
See: Benephen.
W/Viosterol.
See: Vitamins A, D.
W/Zinc oxide.
See: Desitin.

cod liver oil concentrate. (Schering-Plough) Concentrate of cod liver oil with vitamins A and D added. **Cap.:** Bot. 40s, 100s. **Tab.:** Bot. 100s, 240s. Also w/vitamin C. Bot. 100s. *OTC.*
Use: Vitamin supplement.

codorphone hydrochloride. (KOE-dahr-fone) Name previously used for Conorphone hydrochloride.
Use: Analgesic.
See: Conorphone hydrochloride.

● **codoxime.** (CODE-ox-eem) USAN.
Use: Antitussive.

codoxy. (Halsey Drug) Oxycodone hydrochloride 4.5 mg, oxycodone terephthalate 0.38 mg, aspirin 325 mg. Tab. Bot. 100s.
Use: Analgesic combination.

Coease. (Advance Medical) Sodium hyaluronate 12 mg/mL, NaCl 9 mg/mL. Inj. Disp. syringe. 0.5 mL, 0.8 mL. *Rx.*
Use: Ophthalmic surgical adjunct.

Cogentin. (Merck & Co.) Benztropine mesylate. **Tab.:** 0.5 mg Bot. 100s; 1 mg Bot. 100s, UD 100s; 2 mg Bot. 100s, 1000s, UD 100s. **Inj.:** Benztropine mesylate 1 mg/mL w/sodium Cl 9 mg and water for injection q.s. to 1 mL Amp. 2 mL, Box 6s. *Rx.*
Use: Antiparkinsonian.

Co-Gesic. (Schwarz Pharma) Hydrocodone bitartrate 5 mg, acetaminophen 500 mg. Tab. Bot. 100s, 500s. *c-III.*
Use: Analgesic combination.

Cognex. (Parke-Davis) Tacrine hydrochloride 10 mg, 20 mg, 30 mg, 40 mg. Lactose. Cap. Bot. 120s, UD 100s. *Rx.*
Use: Psychotherapeutic.

Co-Hep-Tral. (Davis & Sly) Folic acid 10 mg, vitamin B$_{12}$ 100 mcg, liver injection q.s./mL. Vial 10 mL. *Rx.*
Use: Mineral, vitamin supplement.

Co-Hist. (Roberts) Pseudoephedrine hydrochloride 30 mg, chlorpheniramine 2 mg, acetaminophen 325 mg. Tab. Bot. 500s, 1000s. *OTC.*
Use: Analgesic; antihistamine; decongestant.

Colabid. (Major) Probenecid 500 mg, colchicine 0.5 mg. Tab. Bot. 100s, 1000s. *Rx.*
Use: Antigout.

Colace. (Purdue) Docusate sodium. **Cap.:** 50 mg, 100 mg. Bot. 30s, 60s, 250s (100 mg only), 1000s (100 mg only), UD 100s. **Syr.:** 60 mg/15 mL with alcohol less than 1%, menthol, parabens, sucrose. Bot. 237 mL, 473 mL. **Liq.:** 150 mg/15 mL, parabens. Bot. 30 mL, 480 mL. *OTC.*
Use: Laxative.

Colace. (Purdue) Glycerin. Supp. Bot. 12s, 24s, 48s, 100s. *OTC.*
Use: Laxative.

Colace Infant/Child Suppositories. (Purdue) Glycerin. Supp. 12s, 24s. *OTC.*
Use: Laxative.

Colagyn. (Smith & Nephew) Zinc sulfocarbolate, potassium, oxyquinoline sulfate, lactic acid, boric acid. Jelly. Tube w/applicator and refill 6 oz. Douche Pow. 3 oz, 7 oz, 14 oz. *OTC.*

Colana. (Hance) Euphorbia pilulifera tincture 8 mL, wild lettuce syrup 8 mL, coaillana tincture 2.5 ml, squill compound syrup 1.5 mL, cascara 0.25 g, menthol 4.8 mg/fl oz. Bot. 4 fl oz, gal. Also w/Dionin 15 mg/fl oz. Syr. Bot. gal.

Colazal. (Salix) Balsalazide disodium 750 mg, sodium ≈ 86 mg. Cap. Bot. 280s. *Rx.*
Use: Ulcerative colitis.

• **colchicine.** (KOHL-chih-seen) *USP 28.*
Use: Gout suppressant. Treat multiple sclerosis [Orphan Drug]
W/Benemid.
See: Benn-C.
Col-Probenecid.
W/Sodium salicylate, calcium carbonate, dried aluminum hydroxide gel, phenobarbital.
See: Apcogesic.

colchicine. (Abbott) Colchicine 0.6 mg (1/100 g), lactose. Tab. Bot. 100s. *Rx.*
Use: Gout suppressant.

colchicine. (Bedford) Colchicine 0.5 mg/mL. Inj. Vials. 2 mL. *Rx.*
Use: Gout suppressant.

colchicine. (Various Mfr.) Colchicine 0.6 mg (1/100 g). Tab. Bot. 30s, 60s, 100s, 100s. *Rx.*

Use: Gout suppressant. Treat multiple sclerosis [Orphan Drug]

colchicine salicylate.
W/Phenobarbital, sodium p-aminobenzoate, vitamin B_1, aspirin.
See: Doloral.

Cold & Cough Tussin. (Amerisource Bergen) Dextromethorphan HBr 10 mg, guaifenesin 200 mg, pseudoephedrine hydrochloride 30 mg, sorbitol. Softgels. Pkg. 12s. *OTC.*
Use: Upper respiratory combination, antitussive, expectorant, decongestant.

• **cold cream.** *USP 28.*
Use: Emollient; water in oil emulsion ointment base.

Coldec D. (Breckenridge) Pseudoephedrine hydrochloride 80 mg, carbinoxamine maleate 8 mg. ER Tab. Bot. 100s. *Rx.*
Use: Upper respiratory combination, decongestant, antihistamine.

Coldec DM. (Silarx) Dextromethorphan HBr 15 mg, brompheniramine maleate 4 mg, pseudoephedrine hydrochloride 60 mg/5 mL, saccharin, sorbitol, grape flavor, alcohol free. Syr. Bot. 480 mL. *Rx.*
Use: Upper respiratory combination, antitussive, antihistamine, decongestant.

Cold-Gest Cold. (Major) Chlorpheniramine maleate 8 mg, pseudoephedrine hydrochloride 75 mg. Cap. Pkg. 10s, 20s. *OTC.*
Use: Antihistamine, decongestant.

Coldmist JR. (Breckenridge) Pseudoephedrine hydrochloride 48 mg, guaifenesin 595 mg. ER Tab. Bot. 100s. *Rx.*
Use: Upper respiratory combination, decongestant, expectorant.

Coldmist LA. (Breckenridge) Pseudoephedrine hydrochloride 85 mg, guaifenesin 795 mg. ER Tab. Bot. 100s. *Rx.*
Use: Upper respiratory combination, decongestant, expectorant.

Coldonyl. (Dover Pharmaceuticals) Acetaminophen, phenylephrine hydrochloride. Tab. Sugar, lactose, salt free. UD 500s. *OTC.*
Use: Analgesic, decongestant.

Coldran. (Halsey Drug) Phenylephrine hydrochloride 5 mg, chlorpheniramine maleate 2 mg, salicylamide 1.5 g, acetaminophen 0.5 g, caffeine. Tab. Bot. 30s. *OTC.*
Use: Decongestant, analgesic, antihistamine.

Coldrine. (Roberts) Acetaminophen 325 mg, pseudoephedrine hydrochloride 30 mg, sodium metabisulfite. Tab.

Bot. 1000s, 500s (packets), 4-dose boxes. *OTC.*
Use: Analgesic, decongestant.
Cold Sore. (Purepac) Camphor, benzoin, aluminum Cl. Lot. Bot. 0.5 oz.
Use: Cold sores, fever blisters.
Cold Symptoms Relief. (Major) Pseudoephedrine hydrochloride 30 mg, chlorpheniramine maleate 2 mg, dextromethorphan HBr 10 mg, acetaminophen 325 mg. Tab. Bot. 50s. *OTC.*
Use: Decongestant, antihistamine, antitussive, analgesic.
Cold Symptoms Relief Maximum Strength. (Major) Dextromethorphan HBr 15 mg, chlorpheniramine maleate 2 mg, pseudoephedrine hydrochloride 30 mg, acetaminophen 500 mg. Tab. Pkg. 24s. *OTC.*
Use: Upper respiratory combination, antitussive, antihistamine, decongestant, analgesic.
Cold Tablets. (Walgreen) Phenylephrine hydrochloride 5 mg, chlorpheniramine maleate 2 mg, acetaminophen 325 mg. Tab. Bot. 50s. *OTC.*
Use: Decongestant, analgesic, antihistamine.
Cold Tablets Multiple Symptom. (Walgreen) Acetaminophen 500 mg, pseudoephedrine hydrochloride 30 mg, chlorpheniramine maleate 2 mg, dextromethorphan HBr 10 mg. Tab. Bot. 50s. *OTC.*
Use: Analgesic, decongestant, antihistamine, antitussive.
• **colesevelam hydrochloride.** (koe-leh-SEH-veh-lam) USAN.
Use: Antihyperlipidemic; bile acid sequestrant.
See: Welchol.
Colestid. (Pharmacia) Colestipol hydrochloride. **Unflavored Gran.:** 5 g/dose. Bot. 300 g, 500 g. Pkt. 5 g (30s, 90s). **Flavored Gran.:** 5 g/7.5 g pow, aspartame, mannitol, orange flavor. Bot. 450 g (60 doses). Pkt. 7.5 g (60s). **Tab.:** 1 g. Bot. 120s, 500s. *Rx.*
Use: Antihyperlipidemic; bile acid sequestrant.
• **colestipol hydrochloride.** (koe-LESS-tih-pole) *USP 28.*
Use: Antihyperlipidemic.
See: Colestid.
• **colestolone.** (koe-LESS-toe-LONE) USAN.
Use: Hypolipidemic.
Col-Evac. (Forest) Potassium bitartrate, bicarbonate of soda and a blended base of polyethylene glycols. Supp. Box. 2s, 12s.

Use: Laxative.
Colfed-A. (Breckenridge) Pseudoephedrine hydrochloride 120 mg, chlorpheniramine maleate 8 mg. ER Cap. Bot 100s. *Rx.*
Use: Upper respiratory combination, decongestant, antihistamine.
• **colforsin.** (kole-FAR-sin) USAN.
Use: Antiglaucoma agent.
colfosceril palmitate, cetyl alcohol, tyloxapol.
Use: Hyaline membrane disease; adult respiratory distress syndrome. [Orphan Drug]
See: Exosurf Neonatal for Intrathecal Suspension.
colimycin sodium methanesulfonate. (Parke-Davis)
See: Colistimethate sodium.
colimycin sulfate.
See: Coly-Mycin.
• **colistimethate sodium.** (koe-LISS-tih-METH-ate) *USP 28.*
Use: Anti-infective.
See: Coly-Mycin M Parenteral.
colistin and neomycin sulfates and hydrocortisone acetate.
Use: Anti-infective; anti-inflammatory.
colistin base.
W/Neomycin base, hydrocortisone acetate, thonzonium bromide, polysorbate 80, acetic acid, sodium acetate.
See: Coly-Mycin Otic W/Neomycin and Hydrocortisone. Cortisporin-TC.
colistin methanesulfonate.
See: Colistimethate sodium.
Co-Liver. (Standex) Folic acid 1 mg, vitamin B$_{12}$ 100 mcg, liver 10 mcg/mL. Inj. Vial 10 mL. *Rx.*
Use: Mineral, vitamin supplement.
Colladerm. (C & M Pharmacal) Glycerin, soluble collagen, hydrolysed elastin, allantoin, ethylhydroxycellulose, sorbic, octoxynol-9. Bot. 2.3 oz. *OTC.*
Use: Emollient.
collagenase.
Use: Enzyme preparation.
See: Collagenase Santyl.
collagenase ABC. (Advance Biofactures) Collagenase 250 units/g in white petrolatum. Oint. Tube. 25 g, 50 g. *OTC.*
Use: Enzyme, topical.
collagenase (lyophilized) for injection.
Use: Peyronie disease. [Orphan Drug]
Collagenase Santyl. (Ross) Collagenase enzyme 250 units/g, white petrolatum. Oint. Tube. 15 g, 30 g. *Rx.*
Use: Enzyme preparation.
collagen implant. (Lacrimedics) Collagen 0.2 mm, 0.3 mm, 0.4 mm, 0.5 mm,

0.6 mm. Box 12s. *Rx.*
Use: Collagen implant, ophthalmic.
See: Zyderm I.
Zyderm II.
• **collodion.** (kah-LOW-dee-uhm) *USP 28.*
Use: Topical protectant.
colloidal aluminum hydroxide.
See: Aluminum Hydroxide Gel.
colloidal oatmeal.
Use: Emollient.
See: Actibath.
Aveeno.
colloidal sulfur.
Use: Antiseborrheic.
W/Combinations.
See: MG217 Medicated Tar-Free
Colloral. (AutoImmune) Purified type II collagen.
Use: Juvenile rheumatoid arthritis.
[Orphan Drug]
Collyrium for Fresh Eyes. (Wyeth) Boric acid, sodium borate, benzalkonium Cl. Bot. 120 mL. *OTC.*
Use: Irrigant, ophthalmic.
Collyrium Fresh Eye Drops. (Wyeth) Tetrahydrozoline hydrochloride 0.05%. Drop. Bot. 15 mL. *OTC.*
Use: Mydriatic, vasoconstrictor.
ColoCARE. (Helena Laboratories) In-home fecal test. Kit. 3s.
Use: Diagnostic aid.
Coloctyl. (Eon Labs) Docusate sodium 100 mg. Cap. Bot. 100s, 1000s, UD 1000s. *OTC.*
Use: Laxative.
Cologel. (Eli Lilly) Methylcellulose 450 mg/5 mL, alcohol 5%, saccharin. Bot. 16 fl oz. *OTC.*
Use: Laxative.
colony stimulating factor.
Use: Hematopoietic agent.
See: Filgrastim.
Pegfilgrastim.
Sargramostim.
color allergy screening test.
See: CAST.
ColoScreen. (Helena Laboratories) Occult blood screening test. Kit 12s, 25s, 50s. 3 tests per kit.
Use: Diagnostic aid.
ColoScreen/VPI. (Helena Laboratories) Occult blood screening test. Box 100s, 1000s.
Use: Diagnostic aid.
Coltab Children's. (Roberts) Phenylephrine hydrochloride 2.5 mg, chlorpheniramine maleate 1 mg. Chew. Tab. Bot. 30s. *OTC.*
Use: Antihistamine; decongestant.
• **colterol mesylate.** (KOLE-ter-ole) USAN.

Use: Bronchodilator.
Columbia Antiseptic Powder. (F.C. Sturtevant) Zinc oxide, talc, carbolic acid, borid acid. Pow. 30 g, 420 g. *OTC.*
Use: Topical combination.
Coly-Mycin M Parenteral. (Monarch) Colistimethate sodium equivalent to 150 mg colistin base. Inj. Vial. *Rx.*
Use: Anti-infective.
Coly-Mycin S Otic Drops w/Neomycin and Hydrocortisone. (Parke-Davis) Colistin base as the sulfate 3 mg, neomycin base as the sulfate 3.3 mg, hydrocortisone acetate 10 mg, thonzonium bromide 0.5 mg/mL, polysorbate 80, acetic acid, sodium acetate, thimerosal. Dropper bot. 5 mL, 10 mL. *Rx.*
Use: Anti-infective.
Colyte. (Schwarz Pharma) Polyethylene glycol-electrolyte 3350 **Gal:** PEG 3350 227.1 g, sodium sulfate 21.5 g, sodium bicarbonate 6.36 g, sodium Cl 5.53 g, potassium Cl 2.82 g. **4 L:** PEG 3350 240 g, sodium sulfate 22.72 g, sodium bicarbonate 6.72 g, sodium chloride 5.84 g, potassium chloride 2.98 g. Soln. Bot. 1 gal, 4 L. *Rx.*
Use: Bowel evacuant.
ComBgen. (Ethex) Vitamin B$_6$ 25 mg, vitamin B$_{12}$ 500 mcg, FA 2.2 mg. Tab. 100s. *Rx.*
Use: Nutritional product.
Combichole. (Trout) Dehydrocholic acid 2 g, desoxycholic acid 1 g. Tab. Bot. 100s, 1000s. *Hx.*
Use: Hydrocholeretic.
CombiPatch. (Aventis) **Transdermal Patch 9 cm²:** Estradiol 0.05 mg, norethindrone acetate 0.14 mg. **Transdermal Patch 16 cm²:** Estradiol 0.05 mg, norethindrone acetate 0.25 mg. Box. 8s. *Rx.*
Use: Sex hormone, estrogen and progestin combination.
Combipres. (Boehringer Ingelheim) 0.1 mg, 0.2 mg, 0.3 mg, chlorthalidone 15 mg. Tab. Bot. 100s, 1000s (except 0.3 mg). *Rx.*
Use: Antihypertensive.
Combistix. (Bayer Corp. (Consumer Div.)) Urine test for glucose, protein and pH. In 100s.
Use: Diagnostic aid.
Combistix Reagent Strips. (Bayer Corp. (Consumer Div.)) Protein test area: tetrabromphenol blue, citrate buffer, protein-absorbing agent; glucose test area: glucose oxidase, orthotolidin and a catalyst; pH test area methyl red and bromthymol blue. Strip Box 100s.
Use: Diagnostic aid.

Combivent. (Boehringer Ingelheim) Ipratropium bromide 18 mcg, albuterol sulfate 103 mcg/actuation (equivalent to albuterol base 90 mcg). Aer. Metered dose inhaler 14.7 g (200 inhalations) w/mouthpiece. *Rx.*
Use: Bronchodilator, anticholinergic.
Combivir. (GlaxoSmithKline) Lamivudine 150 mg, zidovudine 300 mg. Tab. Bot. 60s, UD 120s. *Rx.*
Use: Antiviral, nucleoside analog reverse transcriptase inhibitor combination.
Combunox. (Forest) Oxycodone hydrochloride 5 mg, ibuprofen 400 mg. Film coated. Tab. 100s. *c-II.*
Use: Narcotic analgesic.
ComfortCare GP Wetting & Soaking. (PBH Wesley Jessen) Buffered, isotonic. Chlorhexidine gluconate 0.005%, EDTA 0.02%, octylphenoxy (oxyethylene) ethanol, povidone, polyvinyl alcohol, propylene glycol, hydroxyethylcellulose, NaCl. Soln. Bot. 120 mL, 240 mL. *OTC.*
Use: Contact lens care.
Comfort Drops. (PBH Wesley Jessen) Isotonic solution containing naphazoline 0.03%, benzalkonium Cl 0.005%, edetate disodium 0.02%. Bot. 15 mL. *OTC.*
Use: Contact lens care.
Comfort Eye Drops. (PBH Wesley Jessen) Naphazoline hydrochloride 0.03%. Bot. 15 mL. *OTC.*
Use: Decongestant, ophthalmic.
Comfort Gel Liquid. (Walgreen) Aluminum hydroxide compressed gel 200 mg, magnesium hydroxide 200 mg, simethicone 20 mg/5 mL. Gel. Bot. 12 oz. *OTC.*
Use: Antacid; antiflatulent.
Comfort Gel Tablets. (Walgreen) Magnesium hydroxide 85 mg, simethicone 25 mg, aluminum hydroxide-magnesium carbonate co-dried gel 282 mg. Tab. Bot. 100s. *OTC.*
Use: Antacid; antiflatulent.
Comfort Tears. (Allergan) Hydroxyethylcellulose, benzalkonium Cl 0.005%, edetate disodium 0.02%. Soln. Bot. 15 mL. *OTC.*
Use: Artificial tear solution.
Comhist. (Roberts) Phenylephrine hydrochloride 10 mg, chlorpheniramine maleate 2 mg, phenyltoloxamine citrate 25 mg. Tab. Bot. 100s. *Rx.*
Use: Antihistamine; decongestant.
Comhist L.A. (Roberts) Phenylephrine hydrochloride 20 mg, chlorpheniramine maleate 4 mg, phenyltoloxamine citrate

50 mg. Cap. Bot. 100s. *Rx.*
Use: Antihistamine; decongestant.
Commit. (GlaxoSmithKline) Nicotine polacrilex 2 mg, 4 mg, aspartame, phenylalanine 3.4 mg, mannitol. Lozenge. 72s. *OTC.*
Use: Smoking deterrent.
Compal. (Solvay) Dihydrocodeine 16 mg, acetaminophen 356.4 mg, caffeine 30 mg. Cap. Bot. 100s. *c-III.*
Use: Analgesic combination.
Compat Nutrition Enteral Delivery System. (Novartis) Top fill feeding containers 600 mL, 1400 mL. Gravity delivery set. Pump delivery set. Compat enteral feeding pump.
Use: Nutritional supplement.
Compazine. (GlaxoSmithKline) Prochlorperazine. **Tab.:** As maleate 5 mg, 10 mg, lactose. Bot. 100s, UD 100s. **Inj.:** As edisylate 5 mg/mL, sodium saccharin, benzyl alcohol, sodium biphosphate, sodium tartrate. Vial. 2 mL, 10 mL. **SR Spansule:** As maleate 10 mg, 15 mg. Bot. 50s. **Supp.:** 2.5 mg, 5 mg, 25 mg, glycerin. Coconut oil. Box 12s. **Syr.:** As edisylate salt 5 mg/5 mL, sucrose, fruit flavor. Bot. 120 mL. *Rx.*
Use: Antiemetic; antipsychotic.
Compete. (Mission Pharmacal) Iron 27 mg, vitamins A 5000 units, D 400 units, E 45 units, B$_1$ 2 mg, B$_2$ 2.6 mg, B$_3$ 30 mg, B$_6$ 20.6 mg, B$_{12}$ 9 mcg, C 90 mg, folic acid 0.4 mg, Zn 22.5 mg. Tab. Bot. 100s. *OTC.*
Use: Mineral, vitamin supplement.
Compleat B Meat Base Formula. (Novartis) Beef, nonfat milk, hydrolyzed cereal solids, maltodextrin, pureed fruits and vegetables, corn oil, mono- and diglycerides. Bot. 250 mL, Can 250 mL.
Use: Nutritional supplement, eternal.
Compleat Modified Formula Meat Base. (Novartis) Hydrolyzed cereal solids, calcium caseinate, pureed fruits and vegetables, corn oil, beef puree, mono- and diglycerides. Can 250 mL. *OTC.*
Use: Enteral nutritional supplement.
Compleat Regular Formula. (Novartis) Deionized water, beef puree, hydrolyzed cereal solids, green bean puree, pea puree, nonfat milk, corn oil, maltodextrin, peach puree, orange juice, mono- and diglycerides, carrageenan, vitamins, minerals. Bot. 250 mL, Can 250 mL. *OTC.*
Use: Nutritional supplement, eternal.
Complete All-In-One. (Allergan) Buffered, isotonic. sodium Cl, polyhexa-

methylene biguanide, EDTA. Soln. Bot. 60, 120, 360 mL. *OTC.*
Use: Contact lens care.

Complete Solution. (Allergan) Buffered, isotonic. sodium Cl, polyhexamethylene biguanide 0.0001%, tromethamine, tyloxapol, EDTA. Soln. Bot. 15 mL. *OTC.*
Use: Contact lens care.

Complete Vitamins. (Mission Pharmacal) Vitamins A 5000 units, D 400 units, E 45 units, C 90 mg, B_1 2.25 mg, folic acid 0.4 mg, B_2 2.6 mg, B_3 30 mg, B_6 25 mg, B_{12} 9 mcg, ferrous gluconate 233 mg, zinc 22.5 mg. Tab. Bot. 100s, 1000s. *OTC.*
Use: Mineral, vitamin supplement.

Complete Weekly Enzymatic Cleaner. (Allergan) Effervescing, buffering and tableting agents, Sublitisin A. Tab. Pkg 8s. *OTC.*
Use: Contact lens care.

Completone Elixir Fort. (Sanofi-Synthelabo) Ferrous gluconate.
Use: Mineral supplement.

Complex 15 Cream. (Baker Cummins Dermatologicals) Jar 4 oz. *OTC.*
Use: Emollient.

Complex 15 Lotion. (Baker Cummins Dermatologicals) Bot. 8 oz. *OTC.*
Use: Emollient.

Complex Zinc Carbonates.
See: Zinc (Pharmaceutical Labs).

Comply Liquid. (Sherwood Davis & Geck) sodium caseinate, calcium caseinate, hydrolyzed cornstarch, sucrose, corn oil, soy lecithin, vitamins A, B_1, B_2, B_3, B_5, B_6, B_{12}, C, D, E, K, folic acid, biotin, choline, Ca, Cl, Cu, Fe, I, Mg, Mn, P, Zn. Can 250 mL, Bot. 200 mL. *OTC.*
Use: Nutritional supplement, enteral.

compound cb3025.
See: Alkeran.

compound e.
See: Cortisone acetate.

compound f.
See: Hydrocortisone.

compound 42.
See: Warfarin.

compound q.
Use: Antiviral.

compound s.
Use: Antiviral.
See: Retrovir.
Zidovudine.

Compound 347. (Minrad) Enflurane. Liq. for Inh. 250 mL. *Rx.*
Use: General anesthetic.

Compound W. (Medtech) Salicylic acid 17% w/w in flexible collodion vehicle

w/ether 63.5%. Bot. 0.31 oz. *OTC.*
Use: Keratolytic.

Compound W for Kids. (Medtech) Salicylic acid 40% in a plaster vehicle, lanolin, rubber. Pad. Box. 12s. *OTC.*
Use: Keratolytic.

Compound W One Step Wart Remover for Kids. (Medtech) Salicylic acid 40% in a plaster vehicle, lanolin, rubber. Pad. Box 12s. *OTC.*
Use: Keratolytic.

Compoz. (Medtech) **Tab.:** Diphenhydramine hydrochloride 50 mg. Pkg. 12s, 24s. **Cap.:** Diphenhydramine hydrochloride 25 mg. Pkg. 16s. *OTC.*
Use: Sleep aid.

comprecin.
See: Penetrex.

Compro. (Paddock) Prochlorperazine 25 mg, glycorin, coconut oil. Supp. Box 12s. *Rx.*
Use: Antiemetic; antivertigo agent; antidopaminergic; antipsychotic.

Computer Eye. (Bausch & Lomb) Glycerin 1%, benzalkonium chloride 0.01%, NaCl, boric acid, EDTA. Drops. Bot. 15 mL. *OTC.*
Use: Artificial tears.

Comtan. (Novartis) Entacapone 200 mg, mannitol, sucrose. Tab. Bot. 10s, 100s, 500s. *Rx.*
Use: Antiparkinsonian.

Comtrex Acute Head Cold & Sinus Pressure Relief, Multi-Symptom Maximum Strength. (Bristol-Myers Squibb) Pseudoephedrine hydrochloride 30 mg, brompheniramine maleate 2 mg, acetaminophen 500 mg, parabens. Tab. Pkg. 24s. *OTC.*
Use: Upper respiratory combination, decongestant, antihistamine; analgesic.

Comtrex Allergy-Sinus Treatment, Maximum Strength. (Bristol-Myers Squibb) Pseudoephedrine hydrochloride 30 mg, chlorpheniramine maleate 2 mg, acetaminophen 500 mg, parabens. Tab. Bot. 24s, 50s. *OTC.*
Use: Upper respiratory combination, decongestant, antihistamine, analgesic.

Comtrex Cough and Cold Relief, Multi-Symptom Maximum Strength. (Bristol-Myers Squibb) Dextromethorphan HBr 15 mg, chlorpheniramine maleate 2 mg, pseudoephedrine hydrochloride 30 mg, acetaminophen 500 mg, parabens. Tab. Pkg. 24s. *OTC.*
Use: Upper respiratory combination, antitussive, antihistamine, decongestant, analgesic.

Comtrex Cough Formula. (Bristol-Myers Squibb) Pseudoephedrine hydro-

chloride 15 mg, dextromethorphan 7.5 mg, guaifenesin 50 mg, acetaminophen 125 mg/5 mL, alcohol 20%. Bot. 120 mL, 240 mL. *OTC.*
Use: Decongestant; antitussive; expectorant; analgesic.

Comtrex Day & Night Cold & Cough Relief, Multi-Symptom Maximum Strength. (Bristol-Myers Squibb) Dextromethorphan HBr 15 mg, chlorpheniramine maleate 2 mg, pseudoephedrine hydrochloride 30 mg, acetaminophen 500 mg. Tab. Pkg. 24s (18 day, 6 night). *OTC.*
Use: Upper respiratory combination, antitussive, antihistamine, decongestant, analgesic.

Comtrex Day-Night. (Bristol-Myers Squibb) **Night:** Pseudoephedrine hydrochloride 30 mg, chlorpheniramine maleate 2 mg, dextromethorphan HBr 10 mg, acetaminophen 325 mg. Tab. Pkg. 6s. **Day:** Pseudoephedrine hydrochloride 30 mg, dextromethrophan HBr 10 mg, acetaminophen 500 mg. Tab. Pkg. 18s. *OTC.*
Use: Decongestant, antihistamine, antitussive, analgesic.

Comtrex Day/Night Flu Therapy Maximum Strength Caplets. (Bristol-Myers Squibb) **Day:** Pseudoephedrine hydrochloride 30 mg, acetaminophen 500 mg. **Night:** Pseudoephedrine hydrochloride 30 mg, chlorpheniramine maleate 2 mg, acetaminophen 500 mg, parabens. Tab. Pkg. 24s (18 day, 6 night). *OTC.*
Use: Upper respiratory combination, decongestant, antihistamine, analgesic.

Comtrex Maximum Strength Nighttime Cold & Cough. (Bristol-Myers Squibb) Dextromethorphan 5 mg, chlorpheniramine maleate 0.67 mg, pseudoephedrine hydrochloride 10 mg, acetaminophen 166.7 mg per 5 mL. Alcohol 10%, glycerin, saccharin, sucrose. Orange flavor. Liq. 240 mL. *OTC.*
Use: Antitussive combination.

Comtrex Maximum Strength Non-Drowsy. (Bristol-Myers Squibb) Pseudoephedrine hydrochloride 30 mg, dextromethorphan HBr 15 mg, acetaminophen 500 mg. Capl. Pkg. 24s. *OTC.*
Use: Analgesic; antitussive; decongestant.

Comtrex Multi-Symptom Deep Chest Cold & Congestion Relief. (Bristol-Myers Squibb) Dextromethorphan HBr 10 mg, guaifenesin 100 mg, pseudoephedrine hydrochloride 30 mg, aceta-

minophen 250 mg, sorbitol. Softgels. Pkg. 24s. *OTC.*
Use: Upper respiratory combination, antitussive, expectorant, decongestant, analgesic.

Comtrex Multi-Symptom Maximum Strength Non-Drowsy Cold & Cough Relief. (Bristol-Myers Squibb) Dextromethorphan HBr 15 mg, pseudoephedrine hydrochloride 30 mg, acetaminophen 500 mg, parabens. Tab. Pkg. 24s. *OTC.*
Use: Upper respiratory combination, antitussive, decongestant, analgesic.

Comtussin HC. (Econolab) Hydrocodone bitartrate 2.5 mg, chlorpheniramine maleate 2 mg, phenylephrine hydrochloride 5 mg/5 mL, sorbitol, saccharin. Syr. Bot. 473 mL. *c-III.*
Use: Upper respiratory combination, antitussive, antihistamine, decongestant.

Comvax. (Merck) *Haemophilus* b PRP capsular polysaccharide 7.5 mcg, *Neisseria meningitidis* OMPC 125 mcg, hepatitis B surface antigen 5 mcg, aluminum hydroxide ≈ 225 mcg, sodium borate decahydrate 35 mcg/0.5 mL, sodium chloride 0.9%. Inj. Single-dose vial. 0.5 mL *Rx.*
Use: Vaccine.

Concentraid. (Ferring) Desmopressin acetate 0.1 mg/mL (0.1 mg equals 400 units arginine vasopressin). Soln. Disposable intranasal pipettes containing 20 mcg/2 mL. *Rx.*
Use: Hormone.

Concentrated Cleaner. (Bausch & Lomb) Anionic sulfate surfactant with friction-enhancing agents and sodium chlorine. Soln. Bot. 30 mL. *OTC.*
Use: Contact lens care.

Concentrated Milk of Magnesia-Cascara. (Roxane) Milk of magnesia-cascara 15 mL equivalent to milk of magnesia 30 mL and aromatic cascara fluid extract 5 mL, alcohol 7%. *OTC.*
Use: Laxative.

Concentrated Multiple Trace Element. (American Regent) Zinc (as sulfate) 5 mg, copper (as sulfate) 1 mg, manganese (as sulfate) 0.5 mg, chromium (as chloride) 10 mcg. Vial. 10 mL. *Rx.*
Use: Trace element supplement.

concentrated oleovitamin a & d.
See: Oleovitamin A & D, Concentrated.

Concentrated Phillips' Milk of Magnesia. (Roxane) Magnesium hydroxide 800 mg/5 mL, sorbitol, and sugar. Strawberry and orange vanilla creme flavors. Liq. 8 fl. oz. *OTC.*

Use: Antacid; laxative.

Concentrin. (Parke-Davis) Dextromethorphan HBr 15 mg, pseudoephedrine hydrochloride 30 mg, guaifenesin 100 mg. Cap. Bot. 12s. *OTC.*
Use: Antitussive; decongestant; expectorant.

Conceptrol Disposable Contraceptive. (Johnson & Johnson) Nonoxynol-9 4%. Vaginal gel. Tube. 2.7 mL (6s, 10s). *OTC.*
Use: Contraceptive, spermicide.

Concerta. (McNeil) Methylphenidate hydrochloride 18 mg, 27 mg, 36 mg, 54 mg, lactose. ER Tab. Bot. 100s. *c-II.*
Use: CNS stimulant.

Condol Suspension. (Sanofi-Synthelabo) Dipyrone, chlormezanone. *Rx.*
Use: Analgesic; muscle relaxant.

Oondol Tablets. (Sanofi Synthelabo) Dipyrone, chlormezanone. *Rx.*
Use: Analgesic; muscle relaxant.

condylox. (Oclassen) Podofilox 0.5%, alcohol 95%. Soln. Bot. 3.5 mL. *Rx.*
Use: Keratolytic.

c1-esterase-inhibitor, human, pasteurized. (Alpha Therapeutic)
Use: Prevention, treatment of angio edema. [Orphan Drug]

c1-esterase-inhibitor, human, pasteurized.
Use: Prevention, treatment of angioedema.
See: Berinert P.

c1-inhibitor. (Osterreichisches Baxter Healthcare)
Use: Treatment of angioedema. [Orphan Drug]

c1-inhibitor (human) vapor heated. (Immuno Therapoutics)
Use: Treatment of angioedema. [Orphan Drug]

Conest. (Grafton) Conjugated estrogens 0.625 mg, 1.25 mg, 2.5 mg. Tab. Bot. 100s, 1000s. *Rx.*
Use: Estrogen.

Confide. (Direct Access Diagnostics) Reagent kit for HIV blood tests. Kit contains materials to draw a blood sample, a test card, and a protective mailer for 1 test. *OTC.*
Use: Diagnostic aid.

Confident. (Block Drug) Carboxymethylcellulose gum, ethylene oxide polymer, petrolatum/mineral oil base. Tube 0.7 oz, 1.4 oz, 2.4 oz. *OTC.*
Use: Denture adhesive.

Congess. (Fleming & Co.) **Sr.:** Guaifenesin 250 mg, pseudoephedrine hydrochloride 120 mg. SR Cap. **Jr.:** Guaifenesin 125 mg, pseudoephedrine hy-

drochloride 60 mg. TR Cap. Bot. 100s, 1000s. *Rx-OTC.*
Use: Decongestant; expectorant.

Congestac. (B.F. Ascher) Pseudoephedrine hydrochloride 60 mg, guaifenesin 400 mg. Tab. Bot. 12s, 24s. *OTC.*
Use: Upper respiratory combination, decongestant, expectorant.

Congestaid. (Zee Medical) Pseudoephedrine hydrochloride 30 mg. Tab. 24s. *OTC.*
Use: Decongestant.

congo red. Injection.
Use: Hemostatic in hemorrhagic disorders.

• **conivaptan.** (kahn-ih-VAP-tahn) USAN.
Use: Investigational hyponatremia; congestive heart failure.

conjugated estrogens.
Use: Estrogen.
See: Estrogens, Conjugated.

Conjunctamide. (Horizon) Prednisolone acetate 0.5%, sodium sulfacetamide 10%, hydroxypropyl methylcellulose, polysorbate 80, sodium thiosulfate, benzalkonium Cl 0.01%. Susp. Dropper bot. 5 mL, 15 mL. *Rx.*
Use: Anti infective; corticosteroid, ophthalmic.

• **conorphone hydrochloride.** (KOE-nahr-fone) USAN. *Formerly Codorphone.*
Use: Analgesic.

Consin Compound Salve. (Wisconsin Pharmacal Co.) Carbolic acid ointment. Jar 2 oz, lb. *OTC.*
Use: Minor skin irritations.

Constilac. (Alra) Lactulose 10 g/15 mL (< galactose 1.6 g, lactose 1.2 g, other sugars 1.2 g). Soln. Bot. 30 mL, 946 mL, 1000 mL, 3785 mL. *Rx.*
Use: Laxative.

Constonate 60. Docusate sodium 100 mg, 250 mg. Cap. Bot. 100s, 1000s. *OTC.*
Use: Laxative.

Constulose. (Alra) Lactulose 10 g/15 mL (< galactose 1.6 g, lactose 1.2 g, other sugars). Soln. Bot. 237 mL, 946 mL. *Rx.*
Use: Analgesic; laxative.

Contac Cough & Chest Cold. (GlaxoSmithKline) Pseudoephedrine hydrochloride 15 mg, dextromethorphan HBr 5 mg, guaifenesin 50 mg, acetaminophen 125 mg/5 mL, alcohol 10%, saccharin, sorbitol. Liq. Bot. 4 fl. oz. *OTC.*
Use: Analgesic; antitussive; decongestant; expectorant.

Contac Cough and Sore Throat Formula. (GlaxoSmithKline) Dextromethor-

phan HBr 5 mg, acetaminophen 125 mg/5 mL, alcohol 10%. Bot. 120 mL. *OTC.*
Use: Analgesic; antitussive.
Contac Day & Night Allergy/Sinus Relief. (GlaxoSmithKline) **Day:** Pseudoephedrine hydrochloride 60 mg, acetaminophen 650 mg. Capl. **Night:** Pseudoephedrine hydrochloride 60 mg, diphenhydramine hydrochloride 50 mg, acetaminophen 650 mg. Tab. Pkg. 20 (15 day; 5 night). *OTC.*
Use: Upper respiratory combination, decongestant, antihistamine, analgesic.
Contac Day & Night Cold & Flu. (GlaxoSmithKline) **Day:** Pseudoephedrine hydrochloride 60 mg, dextromethorphan HBr 30 mg, acetaminophen 650 mg. **Night:** Pseudoephedrine hydrochloride 60 mg, diphenhydramine hydrochloride 50 mg, acetaminophen 650 mg. Tab. Pkg. 20s (15 day, 5 night). *OTC.*
Use: Upper respiratory combination, decongestant, antihistamine, antitussive, analgesic.
Contac Nighttime Cold. (GlaxoSmithKline) Acetaminophen 167 mg, dextromethorphan HBr 5 mg, pseudoephedrine hydrochloride 10 mg, doxylamine succinate 1.25 mg/5 mL, alcohol 25%. Bot. 177 mL. *OTC.*
Use: Analgesic, decongestant, antitussive, antihistamine.
Contac Non-Drowsy Formula Sinus. (GlaxoSmithKline) Pseudoephedrine hydrochloride 30 mg, acetaminophen 500 mg. Capl. Tab. Pkg. 24s. *OTC.*
Use: Decongestant, analgesic.
Contac Severe Cold & Flu Maximum Strength. (GlaxoSmithKline) Dextromethorphan HBr 15 mg, chlorpheniramine maleate 2 mg, pseudoephedrine hydrochloride 30 mg, acetaminophen 500 mg. Tab. Bot. 30s. *OTC.*
Use: Upper respiratory combination, antitussive, antihistamine, decongestant, analgesic.
Contac Severe Cold & Flu Nighttime. (GlaxoSmithKline) Pseudoephedrine hydrochloride 10 mg, chlorpheniramine maleate 0.67 mg, dextromethorphan HBr 5 mg, acetaminophen 167 mg, alcohol 18.5%, saccharin, sorbitol, glucose. Liq. Bot. 180 mL. *OTC.*
Use: Antihistamine; antitussive; decongestant.
contact lens products, disinfectant. *OTC.*
See: Allergan Hydrocare Cleaning and Disinfecting.
Aosept.

Disinfecting Solution.
Flex-Care.
Lens Plus Oxysept System.
Lensept.
MiraSept System.
Opti-Free.
contact lens products, enzymatic cleaners. *OTC.*
See: Allergan Enzymatic.
Extenzyme Protein Cleaner.
Opti-zyme Enzymatic Cleaner.
ReNu Effervescent Enzymatic Cleaner.
ReNu Thermal Enzymatic Cleaner.
Ultrazyme Enzymatic Cleaner.
contact lens products, rewetting solutions. *OTC.*
See: Adapettes for Sensitive Eyes.
Clerz.
Clerz 2.
Comfort Tears.
Lens.
Lens Fresh.
Lens Lubricant.
Lens Plus Rewetting.
Lens-Wet.
Murine Sterile Lubricating and Rewetting.
Opti-Tears.
Sensitive Eye Drops.
Soft Mate Comfort.
Soft Mate Lens.
Sterile Lens Lubricant.
contact lens products, soft. *OTC.*
Use: Contact lens care, rinsing, storage.
See: Allergan Hydrocare Preserved Saline.
Allergan Sorbi-Care Saline.
BoilnSoak.
Blairex Sterile Saline.
Ciba Vision Saline.
Hypo-Clear.
Lens Plus Preservative Free.
Lensrins.
Murine Preserved All-Purpose Saline Solution.
Opti-Soft.
ReNu Saline.
Saline Solution, Sterile Preserved.
Sensitive Eyes Plus.
Sensitive Eyes Saline.
Soft Mate Saline for Sensitive Eyes.
Soft Mate Saline Preservative-Free.
Sterile Saline.
Unisol.
Unisol 4.
contact lens products, soft, salt tablets for normal saline. *OTC.*
Use: Salt tablets for normal saline.
See: Amcon 250.

Easy Eyes.
Marlin Salt System II.
Soft Rinse 135.
Soft Rinse 250.
**contact lens products, surfactant
cleaning solutions.** *OTC.*
See: Ciba Vision Cleaner.
Daily Cleaner.
DURAcare II.
LC-65.
Lens Clear.
Lens Plus Daily Cleaner.
Mira Flow Extra Strength.
Murine Contact Lens Cleaner.
Opti-Clean II.
Pliagel.
Preflex for Sensitive Eyes.
Sensitive Eyes Saline/Cleaning Solu-
tion
Sof/Pro-Clean.
Soft Mate Daily Cleaning for Sensi-
tive Eyes.
Soft Mate Hands Off Daily Cleaner.
Soft Mate Protein Remover.
contraceptive hormones.
Use: Sex hormone.
See: Biphasic Oral Contraceptives.
Contraceptives, Emergency.
Etonogestrel/Ethinyl Estradiol Vaginal
Ring.
Intrauterine Progesterone Contracep-
tive System.
Levonorgestrel Implants.
Levonorgestrel-Releasing Intrauterine
System.
Medroxyprogesterone Acetate/Estra-
diol Cypionate.
Medroxyprogesterone Contraceptive
Injection.
Monophasic Oral Contraceptives.
Norelgestromin/Ethinyl Estradiol
Transdermal System.
Progestin-Only Products.
Triphasic Oral Contraceptives.
contraceptives, emergency.
See: Plan B.
Preven.
contraceptives, intrauterine system.
See: Mirena.
Progestasert.
contraceptives, miscellaneous.
See: Depo-Provera.
Lunelle.
Norplant.
Oral Contraceptives.
VCF.
contraceptives, vaginal foams.
See: Delfen.
Emko.

**contraceptives, vaginal jellies and
creams.**
See: Colagyn.
Conceptrol.
Gynol II.
Immolin.
Koromex.
Koromex-A.
Ortho-Gynol.
contraceptives, vaginal suppositories.
See: Intercept.
Lorophyn.
Contrin. (Geneva) Iron (from ferrous
fumarate) 110 mg, B_{12} 15 mcg, IFC (in-
trinsic factor as concentrate or from
stomach preparations) 240 mg, C
75 mg, folic acid 0.5 mg. Cap. Bot.
100s. *Rx.*
Use: Mineral, vitamin supplement.
ControlRx (Omnii Oral) Neutral sodium
fluoride 1.1%, *Microdent* (emulsion of
dimethicone and poloxamer 407) 2%.
Sorbitol, saccharin. Berry and vanilla
mint flavors. Paste. 56 g. *Rx.*
Use: Prevention of dental caries.
Converspaz. (B.F. Ascher) Cellulase
5 mg, protease 10 mg, amylase 30 mg,
lipase 13 mg, l-hyoscamine sulfate
0.0625 mg. Cap. Bot. 100s. *Rx.*
Use: Decongestant; expectorant.
Cool-Mint Listerine. (Warner Lambert)
Thymol, eucalyptol, methyl salicylate,
menthol, alcohol 21.6%. Liq. Bot.
90 mL, 180 mL, 360 mL, 540 mL,
720 mL, 960 mL. *OTC.*
Use: Mouthwash.
CooperVision Balanced Salt. (Ciba Vision) Sterile intraocular irrigation soln.
Bot. 15 mL, 500 mL.
Use: Irrigant, ophthalmic.
Copavin Pulvules. (Eli Lilly) Codeine sulfate 15 mg, papaverine hydrochloride
15 mg. Cap. Bot. 100s. *c-v.*
Use: Antitussive.
Copaxone. (Teva) Glatiramer acetate
20 mg/mL, mannitol 40 mg. Preserva-
tive free. Inj. Single-use premixed pre-
filled syringes. *Rx.*
Use: Multiple sclerosis agent; immuno-
suppressant.
COPE. (Mentholatum Co.) Aspirin
421 mg, magnesium hydroxide 50 mg,
aluminum hydroxide 25 mg, caffeine
32 mg. Tab. Bot. 36s, 60s. *OTC.*
Use: Analgesic; antacid.
Copegus. (Roche) Ribavirin 200 mg.
Tab. Bot. 168s. *Rx.*
Use: Antiviral agent.
copolymer 1, (cop 1).
Use: Treat multiple sclerosis. [Orphan
Drug]

copper. (Abbott) Copper 0.4 mg/mL (as 0.85 mg cupric Cl.) Inj. Vial 10 mL, 30 mL. *Rx.*
Use: Nutritional supplement, parenteral.

•**copper gluconate.** (KAHP-er GLUE-kohn-ate) *USP 28.*
Use: Supplement, trace mineral.

copperhead bite therapy.
See: Antivenin, (Crotalidae) Polyvalent.

Copperin. (Vernon) Iron ammonium citrate, copper (6 g). "A" adult dose, "B" children dose. Bot. 30s, 100s, 500s.
Use: Mineral supplement.

Coppertone. (Schering-Plough) A series of sun-care products marketed under the Coppertone name including Waterproof Lotions SPF 4, 6, 8, 15, and 25. Bot. 4 fl oz, 8 fl oz. Oil SPF 2: Bot. 4 fl oz, 8 fl oz; Lite Formula Oil SPF 2: Bot. 4 fl oz; Lite Lotion SPF 4: Bot. 4 fl oz; Dark Tanning Body Mousse SPF 4: Tube 4 oz; Suntanning Gel SPF 4: Tube 3 oz; Noskote SPF 8: Tube 0.44 oz, Jar 1 oz; Noskote SPF-15, Jar 1 oz. Contain one or more of the following ingredients: Padimate O, oxybenzone, homosalate, ethylhexyl p-methocinnamate. *OTC.*
Use: Sunscreen.

Coppertone Bug and Sun Adult Formula. (Schering-Plough) Ethylhexyl p-methoxycinnamate, oxybenzone, 2-ethylhexyl salicylate, homosalate. SPF 15. Waterproof. PABA-free. Aloe vera. Lot. Bot. 237 mL. *OTC.*
Use: Sunscreen; insect repellant.

Coppertone Bug and Sun Kid's Formula. (Schering-Plough) Octocrylene, ethylhexyl p-methoxycinnamate, oxybenzone. SPF 30. Waterproof. PABA-free. Hypoallergenic. Aloe vera. Lot. Bot. 237 mL. *OTC.*
Use: Sunscreen; insect repellant.

Coppertone Dark Tanning. (Schering-Plough) Padimate O in spray base (SPF 2). Spray. Bot. 8 fl oz. *OTC.*
Use: Sunscreen.

Coppertone Face. (Schering-Plough) A series of sunscreen lotions with SPF 2, 4, 6 and 15 in a nongreasy base with padimate O, oxybenzone (SPF 15 only). *OTC.*
Use: Sunscreen.

Coppertone Kids Sunblock. (Schering-Plough) **SPF 15:** Ethylhexyl p-methoxycinnamate, oxybenzone, 2-ethylhexyl salicylate, homosalate. Lot. Bot. 120 mL, 240 mL. **SPF 30:** Octocrylene, ethylhexyl p-methoxycinnamate, oxybenzone, 2-ethylhexyl salicylate. Lot. Bot. 120 mL, 240 mL. *OTC.*
Use: Sunscreen.

Coppertone Lipkote. (Schering-Plough) Ethylhexyl p-methoxycinnamate, oxybenzone. SPF 15. Stick 4.5 g. *OTC.*
Use: Sunscreen.

Coppertone Moisturizing Sunblock. (Schering-Plough) **SPF 45:** Ethylhexyl p-methoxycinnamate, 2-ethylhexyl salicylate, octocrylene, oxybenzone. Lot. Bot. 120 mL, 300 mL. **SPF 25, 30:** Ethylhexyl p-methoxycinnamate, oxybenzone, 2-ethylhexyl salicylate, homosalate. Lot. Bot. SPF 30: 120 mL, 240 mL; SPF 25: 120 mL. **SPF 15:** Ethylhexyl p-methoxycinnamate, oxybenzone. Lot. Bot. 120 mL, 240 mL, 300 mL. *OTC.*
Use: Sunscreen.

Coppertone Moisturizing Sunscreen. (Schering-Plough) Ethylhexyl p-methoxycinnamate, oxybenzone, benzyl alcohol, vitamin E, aloe. PABA free. SPF 6, 8. Waterproof. Lot. Bot. 120 mL, 240 mL. *OTC.*
Use: Sunscreen.

Coppertone Moisturizing Suntan. (Schering-Plough) **SPF 2:** homosalate, vitamin E, aloe. PABA free. Waterproof. Oil. Bot. 120 mL. **SPF 4:** Ethylhexyl p-methoxycinnamate, oxybenzone, benzyl alcohol, vitamin E, aloe. PABA free. Waterproof. Lot. Bot. 120 mL, 240 mL. *OTC.*
Use: Sunscreen.

Coppertone Noskote. (Schering-Plough) Homosalate 8%, oxybenzone 3%. (SPF 8) Oint. Jar 13.2 g, 30 g. *OTC.*
Use: Sunscreen.

Coppertone SPF-25 Sunblock Lotion. (Schering-Plough) Ethylhexyl p-methoxycinnamate, oxybenzone, padimate O in lotion base (SPF 25). Bot. 120 mL. *OTC.*
Use: Sunscreen.

Coppertone Sport. (Schering-Plough) Ethylhexyl p-methoxycinnamate, oxybenzone. SPF 4, 8, 15, 30. Lot. Bot. 120 mL. *OTC.*
Use: Sunscreen.

Coppertone Tan Magnifier Suntan. (Schering-Plough) **SPF 2:** Triethanolamine salicylate. Oil Bot. 120 mL. **SPF 4 Lotion:** Ethylhexyl p-methoxycinnamate. Bot. 120 mL. **Gel:** 2-phenylbenzimidazole-5-sulfonic acid. Tube 120 g. *OTC.*
Use: Sunscreen.

Coppertone Water Babies. (Schering-Plough) SPF 30, SPF 45. Ethylhexyl p-methoxycinnamate, 2-ethylhexyl salicylate, oxybenzone, homosalate, alco-

hol, aloe, parabens. PABA free. Waterproof. Lot. Bot. 118 mL. *OTC.*
Use: Sunscreen.
copper trace metal additive. (I.M.S., Ltd.) Copper 1 mg. Inj. Vial 10 mL. *Rx.*
Use: Copper supplement.
•**copper undecylenate.** (KAHP-er undeh-sil-EN-ate) USAN.
Use: Copper supplement.
Co-Pyronil 2. (Eli Lilly) Chlorpheniramine maleate 4 mg, pseudoephedrine hydrochloride 60 mg. Pulvule. Bot. 100s. *OTC.*
Use: Antihistamine, decongestant.
Corab. (Abbott Diagnostics) Radioimmunoassay for detection of antibody to hepatitis B core antigen. Test kit 100s.
Use: Diagnostic aid.
Corab-M. (Abbott Diagnostics) Radioimmunoassay for the qualitative determination of specific Ig antibody to hepatitis B virus core antigen (Anti-HBc Ig) in human serum or plasma and may be used as an aid in the diagnosis of acute or recent hepatitis B infection.
Use: Diagnostic aid.
Corace. (Forest) Cortisone acetate 50 mg/mL. Inj. Vial 10 mL. *Rx.*
Use: Corticosteroid, topical.
Coracin. (Roberts) Hydrocortisone acetate 1%, neomycin sulfate 0.5%, bacitracin zinc 400 units, polymyxin B sulfate 10,000 units/g in white petrolatum and mineral oil base. Oint. Tube 3.5 g. *Rx.*
Use: Anti-infective; corticosteroid, ophthalmic.
Coral. (Young Dental) Fluoride ion 1.23%, 0.1 molar phosphate. Jar 250 g, Coral II: 180 disposable cup units/carton. *Rx.*
Use: Fluoride, dental.
Coral/Plus. (Young Dental) Free fluoride ion 2.2%, recrystallized kaolinite. Tube 250 g. *Rx.*
coral snake antivenin. (NABI)
See: Antivenin (*Micrurus fulvius*).
Cordarone. (Wyeth) **Tab.:** Amiodarone hydrochloride 200 mg, lactose. Bot. 60s, UD 100s. **Inj.:** Amiodarone 50 mg/mL, benzyl alcohol 20.2 mg/mL. Amp. 3 mL. *Rx.*
Use: Antiarrhythmic.
Cordran. (Eli Lilly) Flurandrenolide 0.05% in emulsified petrolatum base/g. Tube 15 g (0.05% only), 30 g, 60 g, Jar 225 g. *Rx.*
Use: Corticosteroid, topical.
Cordran Lotion. (Eli Lilly) Flurandrenolide 0.05%, cetyl alcohol, benzyl alcohol, stearic acid, glyceryl monostearate,

polyoxyl 40 stearate, glycerin, mineral oil, menthol, purified water. Squeeze bot. 15 mL, 60 mL. *Rx.*
Use: Corticosteroid, topical.
Cordran SP. (Eli Lilly) Flurandrenolide 0.05% in emulsified base w/cetyl alcohol, stearic acid, polyoxyl 40 stearate, mineral oil, propylene glycol, sodium citrate, citric acid, purified water. Tube 15 g (0.05% only), 30 g, 60 g, Jar 225 g. *Rx.*
Use: Corticosteroid, topical.
Cordran Tape. (Eli Lilly) Flurandrenolide 4 mcg/sq. cm. Roll 7.5 cm × 60 cm, 7.5 cm × 200 cm. *Rx.*
Use: Corticosteroid, topical.
Cordrol. (Vita Elixir) Prednisolone 5 mg, 10 mg, 20 mg. Tab. Bot. 100s. *Rx.*
Use: Corticosteroid.
CO₂-releasing suppositories.
See: Ceo-Two.
Coreg. (GlaxoSmithKline) Carvedilol 3.125 mg, 6.25 mg, 12.5 mg, 25 mg, lactose, sucrose. Tab. Bot. 100s. *Rx.*
Use: Antihypertensive.
Corgard. (Monarch) Nadolol 20 mg, 40 mg, 80 mg, 120 mg, 160 mg. Tab. Bot. 100s, 1000s (except 20 mg), 160 mg), *Unimatic* 100s (except 120 mg, 160 mg). *Rx.*
Use: Antiadrenergic/sympatholytic, beta-adrenergic blocker.
•**coriander oil.** (kor-ee-ANN-der oil)
NF 23.
Use: Pharmaceutic aid, flavor.
Coricidin 'D' Cold, Flu, & Sinus. (Schering-Plough) Pseudoephedrine sulfate 30 mg, chlorpheniramine maleate 2 mg, acetaminophen 325 mg, lactose. Tab. Pkg. 24s. *OTC.*
Use: Upper respiratory combination, decongestant, antihistamine, analgesic.
Coricidin HBP Chest Congestion & Cough. (Schering-Plough) Dextromethorphan HBr 10 mg, guaifenesin 200 mg, sorbitol. Softgel Cap. 20s. *OTC.*
Use: Upper respiratory combination, antitussive, expectorant.
Coricidin HBP Cold & Flu. (Schering-Plough) Chlorpheniramine maleate 2 mg, acetaminophen 325 mg, sugar, lactose, butylparaben. Tab. Bot. 24s. *OTC.*
Use: Upper respiratory combination, antihistamine, analgesic.
Coricidin HBP Cough & Cold. (Schering-Plough) Dextromethorphan HBr 30 mg, chlorpheniramine maleate 4 mg, sugar. Tab. Pkg. 16s. *OTC.*

Use: Upper respiratory combination, antitussive, antihistamine.

Coricidin HBP Maximum Strength Flu. (Schering-Plough) Dextromethorphan HBr 15 mg, chlorpheniramine maleate 2 mg, acetaminophen 500 mg, lactose. Tab. Pkg. 20s. *OTC.*
Use: Upper respiratory combination, antitussive, antihistamine, analgesic.

Corilin Infant. (Schering-Plough) Chlorpheniramine maleate 0.75 mg, sodium salicylate 80 mg/mL, alcohol <1%. Liq. Bot. 30 mL. *OTC.*
Use: Analgesic; antihistamine.

Corlopam. (Hospira) Fenoldopam mesylate 10 mg/mL, sodium metabisulfite. Inj. Single-dose Amp. 5 mL. *Rx.*
Use: Antihypertensive.

Cormax. (Oclassen) Clobetasol propionate 0.05%, white petrolatum, sorbitan sesquioleate. Oint. Tube. 15 g, 45 g. *Rx.*
Use: Corticosteroid, topical.

•**cormethasone acetate.** (core-METH-ahsone) USAN.
Use: Anti-inflammatory, topical.

Corn Huskers. (Warner Lambert) Glycerin 6.7%, SD alcohol, algin, TEA-oleoyl sarcosinate, guar gum, methylparaben, calcium sulfate, calcium Cl, TEA-fumarate, TEA-borate. Bot. 4 oz, 7 oz. *OTC.*
Use: Emollient.

•**corn oil.** *NF 23.*
Use: Pharmaceutic aid, solvent, oleaginous vehicle.
See: G. B. Prep Emulsion.

Corotrope. (Sanofi-Synthelabo) Milrinone for IV use. *Rx.*
Use: Cardiovascular agent.

corpus luteum, extract (water soluble).
See: Progesterone.

Corque. (Geneva) Hydrocortisone 1%, iodochlorhydroxyquin 3%. Cream. Tube 20 g. *Rx.*
Use: Corticosteroid, topical.

Correctol. (Schering-Plough) Bisacodyl 5 mg, talc, lactose, sugar. EC Tab. Bot. 30s, 60s, 90s. *OTC.*
Use: Laxative.

Cortaid, Maximum Strength. (Pharmacia) Hydrocortisone in parabens 1%, cetyl and stearyl alcohols, glycerin, white petrolatum. Cream. Tube 15 g, 30 g. *OTC.*
Use: Corticosteroids, topical.

Cortaid Maximum Strength Spray. (Pharmacia) Hydrocortisone 1%, alcohol 55%, glycerin, methylparaben. Liq: Pump spray 45 mL. *OTC.*
Use: Corticosteroid, topical.

Cortan. (Halsey Drug) Prednisone 5 mg. Tab. Bot. 1000s. *Rx.*
Use: Corticosteroid.

Cortane-B. (Blansett) Hydrocortisone 1%, pramoxine hydrochloride 1%, chlorxylenol 0.1%, benzalkonium chloride. Lot. 60 mL. *Rx.*
Use: Corticosteroid, topical.

Cortane-B Aqueous. (Blansett) Hydrocortisone 1%, pramoxine hydrochloride 1%, chloroxylenol 0.1%. Drops. Vial. 10 mL. *Rx.*
Use: Otic preparation.

Cortane-B Otic. (Blansett) Hydrocortisone 1%, pramoxine hydrochloride 1%, chloroxylenol 0.1%. Drops. Vial. 10 mL. *Rx.*
Use: Otic preparation.

Cortatrigen Ear. (Ivax) Hydrocortisone 1%, neomycin sulfate 5 mg, polymyxin B sulfate 10,000 units/mL. Susp. Bot. 10 mL. *Rx.*
Use: Anti-infective; corticosteroid, otic.

Cortatrigen Modified Ear Drops. (Ivax) Hydrocortisone 1%, neomycin sulfate 5 mg/mL, polymyxin B 10,000 units/mL, propylene glycol, glycerin, potassium metabisulfite. Drops. Bot. 10 mL. *Rx.*
Use: Anti-infective; corticosteroid, otic.

Cort-Dome. (Bayer Corp. (Consumer Div.)) Hydrocortisone alcohol. **Cream:** 0.25%: 1 oz, 4 oz; 0.5%, 1%: 1 oz. **Lot.:** 0.25%, 0.5%: 4 oz; 1%: 1 oz. *Rx.*
Use: Corticosteroid, topical.

Cort-Dome High Potency. (Bayer Corp. (Consumer Div.)) Hydrocortisone acetate 25 mg in a monoglyceride base. *Rx.*
Use: Corticosteroid, topical.

Cortef. (Pfizer) Hydrocortisone. Tab. **5 mg:** Bot. 50s. **10 mg, 20 mg:** Bot. 100s. *Rx.*
Use: Corticosteroid.

cortenil.
See: Desoxycorticosterone Acetate.

cortical hormone products.
See: Adrenal Cortex Extract.
Aristocort.
Betamethasone.
Betamethasone Sodium Phosphate.
Betamethasone Sodium Phosphate and Betamethasone Acetate.
Budesonide.
Celestone.
Celestone Phosphate.
Celestone Soluspan.
Corticotropin.
Cortisone Acetate.
Decadron.
Decadron LA.
Desoxycorticosterone Acetate.

Dexamethasone.
Entocort EC.
Fludrocortisone.
Hydeltrasol.
Hydrocortisone.
Hydrocortone Acetate.
Hydrocortone Phosphate.
Medrol.
Methylprednisolone.
Prednisolone.
Prednisone.
Triamcinolone.
Cortic Ear. (Everett) Hydrocortisone 10 mg, pramoxine hydrochloride 10 mg, chloroxylenol 1 mg/mL. Drops. Vial 10 mL. *Rx.*
Use: Otic preparation.
Cortic-ND. (Everett) Hydrocortisone 1%, pramoxine hydrochloride 0.1%, chloroxylenol 0.1%, benzalkonium chloride. Drops. Vial. 15 mL. *Rx.*
Use: Otic preparation.
•**corticorelin acetate.** (core-tih-kah-REH-lin) USAN.
Use: Hormone
•**corticorelin ovine triflutate.** (core-tih-kah-REH-lin OH-vine TRY-flew-TATE) USAN.
Use: Hormone, corticotropin-releasing; diagnostic aid, adrenocortical insufficiency; Cushing syndrome. [Orphan Drug]
See: Acthrel.
corticosteroid/mydriatic combo, ophthalmics. Prednisolone acetate 0.25%, atropine sulfate 1%. *Rx.*
Use: Treatment of anterior uveitis.
corticosteroids.
Use: Respiratory inhalant.
See: Beclomethasone Dipropionate.
Budesonide.
Flunisolide.
Fluocinolone Acetonide.
Fluticasone Propionate.
Mometasone Furoate Inhalation.
Triamcinolone Acetonide.
•**corticotropin.** (core-tih-koe-TROE-pin) *USP 28.*
Use: Adrenocortical steroids.
See: Corticotropin Injection, Repository. Cosyntropin.
•**corticotropin, repository, injection.** (core-tih-koe-TROE-pin) *USP 28.*
Use: Hormone, adrenocorticotrophic; corticosteroid, topical; diagnostic aid, adrenocortical insufficiency.
See: H.P. Acthar Gel.
Cortifoam. (Schwarz Pharma) Hydrocortisone acetate 10% in an aerosol foam w/propylene glycol, emulsifying wax, steareth 10, cetyl alcohol, methyl-

paraben, propylparaben, trolamine, inert propellants. Container 20 g w/rectal applicator for 14 applicatorsful. *Rx.*
Use: Corticosteroid, topical.
cortisol.
Note: Cortisol was the official published name for hydrocortisone in *USP 24.* The name was changed back to Hydrocortisone, *USP.* in Supplement 1 to the *USP 24.*
See: Hydrocortisone.
cortisol cyclopentylpropionate.
See: Cortef Fluid.
cortisone.
Use: Adrenocortical steroid, glucocorticoid.
See: Cortisone Acetate.
•**cortisone acetate.** (CORE-tih-sone) *USP 28.*
Use: Corticosteroid, topical.
See: Cortistan.
Cortone Acetate.
cortisone acetate. (Various Mfr.) Cortisone acetate 25 mg. Tab. 8s, 100s, 500s, 1,000s, UD 100s. *Rx.*
Use: Adrenocortical steroid, anti-inflammatory.
Cortisporin Cream. (GlaxoSmithKline) Polymyxin B sulfate 10,000 units, neomycin sulfate 5 mg, hydrocortisone acetate 5 mg/g, methylparaben 0.25%. Cream. Tube 7.5 g. *Rx.*
Use: Anti-infective; corticosteroid, topical.
Cortisporin Ointment. (GlaxoSmithKline) Polymyxin B sulfate 5000 units, bacitracin zinc 400 units, neomycin sulfate 5 mg, hydrocortisone (1%) 10 mg/g in petrolatum base. Oint. Tube 30 g. *Rx.*
Use: Anti-infective; corticosteroid, topical.
Cortisporin Ophthalmic Ointment. (GlaxoSmithKline) Polymyxin B sulfate 10,000 units, bacitracin 400 units, neomycin sulfate 0.35%, hydrocortisone 0.1%. Ophth. Oint. Tube 3.5 g. *Rx.*
Use: Anti-infective; corticosteroid, ophthalmic.
Cortisporin Ophthalmic Suspension. (Monarch) Polymyxin B sulfate 10,000 units, neomycin sulfate 0.35%, hydrocortisone 1%/mL, thimerosal 0.001%, cetyl alcohol, glyceryl monostearate, mineral oil, propylene glycol. Ophth. Susp. *Drop Dose* 7.5 mL. *Rx.*
Use: Anti-infective; corticosteroid, ophthalmic.
Cortisporin Otic Solution Sterile. (GlaxoSmithKline) Polymyxin B sulfate 10,000 units, neomycin sulfate 5 mg,

hydrocortisone 10 mg/mL, glycerin, propylene glycol, vitamin K metabisulfite 0.1%. Otic. Soln. Dropper bot. 10 mL Sterile. *Rx.*
Use: Anti-infective; corticosteroid, otic.
Cortisporin Otic Suspension. (GlaxoSmithKline) Polymyxin B sulfate 10,000 units, neomycin sulfate 5 mg, hydrocortisone free alcohol 10 mg/mL, cetyl alcohol, propylene glycol, polysorbate 80, thimerosal. Otic. Susp. Dropper bot. 10 mL Sterile. *Rx.*
Use: Anti-infective; corticosteroid, otic.
Cortisporin-TC. (Monarch) Colistin sulfate 3 mg, neomycin sulfate 3.3 mg, hydrocortisone acetate 10 mg, thonzonium bromide 0.5 mg, polysorbate 80, acetic acid, sodium acetate. Otic Susp. Bot. 10 mL w/dropper. *Rx.*
Use: Otic preparation.
Cortistan. (Standex) Cortisone 25 mg/10 mL. *Rx.*
Use: Corticosteroid.
•**cortivazol.** (core-TIH-vah-zole) USAN.
Use: Corticosteroid, topical.
Cortizone•5. (Pfizer Consumer) Hydrocortisone 0.5%, glycerin, mineral oil, white petrolatum. Tube 30 g. *OTC.*
Use: Corticosteroid, topical.
Cortizone Kids. (Pfizer) Hydrocortisone 0.5%, parabens, cetearyl alcohol, glycerin, white petrolatum. Cream. Tube 14 g. *OTC.*
Use: Corticosteroid, topical.
Cortizone-S, Maximum Strength. (Pfizer) Hydrocortisone 0.5%. Tube. *OTC.*
Use: Corticosteroid, topical.
Cortizone•10 Plus. (Pfizer) Hydrocortisone 1%. Alcohol, aloe, glycerin, mineral oil, parabens, petrolatum. Cream. 28 g, 57 g. *OTC.*
Use: Anti-inflammatory agent.
Cortizone•10 Quick Shot. (Pfizer) Hydrocortisone 1%. Alcohols. Spray. 44 mL. *OTC.*
Use: Anti-inflammatory agent.
•**cortodoxone.** (CORE-toe-dox-OHN) USAN.
Use: Anti-inflammatory.
Cortone Acetate. (Merck & Co.) Cortisone acetate 50 mg/mL, sodium chloride, sodium carboxymethylcellulose, benzyl alcohol. Susp. Inj. Vial 10 mL. *Rx.*
Use: Corticosteroid.
Cortril Topical Ointment 1%. (Pfizer) Hydrocortisone 1%, cetyl and stearyl alcohol, propylene glycol, sodium lauryl sulfate, petrolatum, cholesterol, mineral oil, methyl- and propylparabens in

ointment base. Oint. Tube 0.5 oz.
Use: Corticosteroid, topical.
Cortrosyn. (Amphastar) Cosyntropin 0.25 mg, mannitol 10 mg, Pow. for Inj., lyophilized. Vials with diluent. *Rx.*
Use: Corticosteroid.
Corubeen. (Spanner) Vitamin B_{12} crystalline 1000 mcg/mL. Vial 10 mL. *Rx.*
Use: Vitamin supplement.
Corvert. (Pharmacia) Ibutilide fumarate 0.1 mg/mL. Soln. Vial. 10 mL. *Rx.*
Use: Antiarrhythmic.
Coryza Brengle. (Roberts) Pseudoephedrine hydrochloride 30 mg, acetaminophen 200 mg. Cap. Bot. 1000s. *OTC.*
Use: Analgesic; decongestant.
Corzide. (Monarch) Nadolol 40 mg, bendroflumethiazide 5 mg. Tab. Nadolol 80 mg, bendroflumethiazide 5 mg. Tab. Bot. 100s. *Rx.*
Use: Antihypertensive.
Corzyme. (Abbott Diagnostics) Enzyme immunoassay for detection of antibody to hepatitis B core antigen in serum or plasma. Test kit 100s.
Use: Diagnostic aid.
Corzyme-M. (Abbott Diagnostics) Enzyme immunoassay for the detection of Ig antibody to hepatitis B core antigen (Anti-HBc Ig). In human serum or plasma. Test kit 100s.
Use: Diagnostic aid.
Cosmegen. (Merck) Actinomycin D (dactinomycin) 500 mcg. Mannitol 20 mg. Pow. for Inj., lyophilized. Vials. *Rx.*
Use: Antineoplastic; antibiotic.
Cosmoline.
See: Petrolatum.
Cosopt. (Merck & Co.) Dorzolamide 2%, timolol maleate 0.5%, benzalkonium chloride 0.0075%, mannitol. Ophth. Soln. Ocumeters 5 mL, 10 mL. *Rx.*
Use: Antiglaucoma agent.
Cosulid. (Novartis) Sulfachloropyridazine.
•**cosyntropin.** (koe-sin-TROE-pin) USAN.
Use: Hormone, adrenocorticotrophic.
See: Cortrosyn.
Cotaphylline. (Major) Oxtriphylline 100 mg, 200 mg. Tab. Bot. 100s, 500s. *Rx.*
Use: Bronchodilator.
cotarnine chloride. Cotarnine hydrochloride.
Use: Astringent.
cotarnine hydrochloride.
See: Cotarnine Chloride.
•**cotinine fumarate.** (koe-TIH-neen) USAN.

Use: Antidepressant; psychomotor stimulant.

Cotolate. (Major) Benztropine 1 mg, 2 mg. Tab. Bot. 100s, 1000s. *Rx.*
Use: Antiparkinsonian.

Cotrim. (Teva) Sulfamethoxazole 400 mg, trimethoprim 80 mg. Tab. Bot. 100s, 500s. *Rx.*
Use: Anti-infective.

Cotrim DS. (Teva) Sulfamethoxazole 800 mg, trimethoprim 160 mg. Tab. Bot. 100s, 500s. *Rx.*
Use: Anti-infective.

Cotrim Pediatric. (Teva) Sulfamethoxazole 200 mg, trimethoprim 40 mg/ 5 mL. Oral Susp. Bot. 473 mL. *Rx.*
Use: Anti-infective.

●**cotton, purified.** (KAHT-uhn) *USP 28.*
Use: Surgical aid

●**cottonseed oil.** (KAHT-uhn-seed oil) *NF 23.*
Use: Pharmaceutic aid; solvent, oleaginous vehicle.

Co-Tuss V. (Rugby) Hydrocodone bitartrate 5 mg, guaifenesin 100 mg. Liq. Bot. 480 mL. *c-III.*
Use: Antitussive; expectorant.

Cotylenol Children's Chewable Cold Tablet. (McNeil Consumer) Acetaminophen 80 mg, chlorpheniramine maleate 0.5 mg, pseudoephedrine hydrochloride 7.5 mg. Chew. Tab. Bot. 24s. *OTC.*
Use: Analgesic; antihistamine; decongestant.

Cotylenol Children's Liquid Cold Formula. (McNeil Consumer) Acetaminophen 160 mg, chlorpheniramine maleate 1 mg, pseudoephedrine hydrochloride 15 mg, sorbitol/5 mL. Bot. 4 oz. *OTC.*
Use: Analgesic; antihistamine; decongestant.

Cotylenol Cold Formula. (McNeil Consumer) Chlorpheniramine maleate 2 mg, dextromethorphan HBr 15 mg, pseudoephedrine hydrochloride 30 mg, acetaminophen 325 mg. **Tab.:** Box 24s, Bot. 50s, 100s. **Capl.:** Bot. 24s, 50s. *OTC.*
Use: Analgesic; antihistamine; antitussive; decongestant.

Cotylenol Liquid Cold Formula. (McNeil Consumer) Acetaminophen 650 mg, chlorpheniramine maleate 4 mg, pseudoephedrine hydrochloride 60 mg, dextromethorphan hydrochloride 30 mg/30 mL, alcohol 7.5%, sorbitol. Bot. 5 oz. *OTC.*
Use: Analgesic; antihistamine; antitussive; decongestant.

Cough Formula Comtrex. (Bristol-Myers Squibb) Pseudoephedrine hydrochloride 15 mg, dextromethorphan HBr 7.5 mg/5 mL, guaifenesin, saccharin, sucrose. Liq. Bot. 120 mL, 240 mL. *OTC.*
Use: Antitussive; expectorant.

Cough Syrup. (Ivax) Phenylephrine hydrochloride 5 mg, dextromethorphan HBr 10 mg, guaifenesin 100 mg, alcohol free. Bot. 120 mL. *OTC.*
Use: Antitussive; decongestant; expectorant.

Cough-X. (B.F. Ascher) Dextromethorphan 5 mg, benzocaine 2 mg, dye free, menthol-eucalyptus flavor. Loz. Pkg. 9s. *OTC.*
Use: Anesthetic; antitussive.

Coumadin. (Bristol-Myers Squibb) Warfarin sodium. **Tab.:** 1 mg, 2 mg, 2.5 mg, 3 mg, 4 mg, 5 mg, 6 mg, 7.5 mg, 10 mg, dye-free (10 mg only), lactose. Bot. 100s, 1000s (except 7.5 mg, 10 mg), UD 100s. **Pow. for Inj., lyophilized:** Warfarin sodium 5.4 mg (2 mg/mL when reconstituted), mannitol, preservative-free. Vial. 5 mg. *Rx.*
Use: Anticoagulant.

coumarin.
Use: Anticoagulant; treat renal cell carcinoma. [Orphan Drug]

coumarin and indandione derivatives.
Use: Anticoagulant.
See: Coumadin.
Miradon.
Warfarin sodium.

●**coumermycin.** (KOO-mer-MY-sin) USAN.
Use: Anti-infective.

●**coumermycin sodium.** (KOO-mer-MY-sin) USAN.
Use: Anti-infective.

Counterpain Rub. (Bristol-Myers Squibb) Methylsalicylate, eugenol, menthol. Oint. Tube 1 oz. *OTC.*
Use: Analgesic, topical.

Covera-HS. (Searle) Verapamil hydrochloride 180 mg, 240 mg. Film-coated. ER Tab. Bot. 100s, UD 100s. *Rx.*
Use: Calcium channel blocker.

Covermark. (O'Leary) Neutral cream, hypoallergenic, opaque, greaseless. Jar 1 oz, 3 oz, available in 11 shades. *OTC.*
Use: Conceals birthmarks and skin discolorations.

Covermark Stick. (O'Leary) For normal to oily skin, available in 7 shades. *OTC.*
Use: Conceals birthmarks and skin discolorations.

Co-Xan. (Schwarz Pharma) Theophylline anhydrous 150 mg, ephedrine hydro-

chloride 25 mg, guaifenesin 100 mg, codeine phosphate 15 mg, alcohol 10%/ 15 mL. Syr. Bot. Pt. *Rx.*
Use: Antitussive; bronchodilator; decongestant; expectorant.

Cozaar. (Merck) Losartan potassium 25 mg (potassium 2.12 mg), 50 mg (potassium 4.24 mg), 100 mg (potassium 8.48 mg), lactose. Tab. Bot. 1000s (50 mg only); unit-of-use 30s (except 25 mg), 90s (except 100 mg), 100s; UD 100s. *Rx.*
Use: Antihypertensive.

C.P.-DM. (Hi-Tech) Pseudoephedrine hydrochloride 15 mg, carbinoxamine maleate 1 mg, dextromethorphan HBr 4 mg/mL, saccharin, sorbitol, grape flavor. Drops. Bot. 30 mL w/dropper. *Rx.*
Use: Upper respiratory combination, decongestant, antihistamine, antitussive.

C-Phed Tannate. (Morton Grove) Pseudoephedrine tannate 75 mg, chlorpheniramine tannate 4.5 mg/5 mL, strawberry/banana flavor. Susp. Bot. 118 mL. *Rx.*
Use: Upper respiratory combination, decongestant, antihistamine.

Cplex. (Arcum) Vitamins B$_1$ 10 mg, B$_2$ 10 mg, B$_6$ 5 mg, B$_{12}$ 10 mcg, niacinamide 100 mg, calcium pantothenate 25 mg, C 150 mg, liver 50 mg, dried yeast 50 mg. Cap. Bot. 100s, 1000s. *OTC.*
Use: Mineral, vitamin supplement.

C.P.M. (Ivax) Chlorpheniramine 4 mg. Tab. Bot. 1000s. *OTC.*
Use: Antihistamine.

CPM 8/PSE 90/MSC 2.5. (Cypress) Pseudoephedrine hydrochloride 90 mg, chlorpheniramine maleate 8 mg, methscopolamine nitrate 2.5 mg. SR Tab. Bot. 100s. *Rx.*
Use: Upper respiratory combination, decongestant, antihistamine, anticholinergic.

CP-TANNIC. (Cypress) Pseudoephedrine tannate 75 mg, chlorpheniramine tannate 4.5 mg/5 mL, strawberry/banana flavor. Susp. Bot. 473 mL. *Rx.*
Use: Upper respiratory combination, decongestant, antihistamine.

Crantex ER. (Breckenridge) Phenylephrine hydrochloride 10 mg, guaifenesin 300 mg. Sugar. ER Cap. 100s. *Rx.*
Use: Decongestant and expectorant.

c-reactive protein test.
See: LA Test-CRP.

Cream Camellia. (O'Leary) Jar 2 oz. *OTC.*
Use: Emollient.

Creamy Tar. (Genesis) Coal tar solution 6.65%, crude coal tar 0.67%. Shampoo. Bot. 240 mL. *OTC.*
Use: Antiseborrheic.

•**creatinine.** (kree-OT-ih-nihn) *NF 23.*
Use: Bulking agent for freeze drying.

creatinine reagent strips. (Bayer Corp. (Consumer Div.)) Seralyzer reagent strips. A quantitative strip test for creatinine in serum or plasma. Bot. 25s.
Use: Diagnostic aid.

Cremagol. (Cremagol) Emulsion of liquid petrolatum, agar agar, acacia, glycerin. Bot. 14 oz. W/cascara 11 g/oz, Bot. 14 oz. W/phenolphthalein 2 g/oz, Bot. 14 oz. *OTC.*
Use: Laxative.

Creomulsion Cough Medicine. (Summit) Beechwood creosote, cascara, ipecac, menthol, white pine, wild cherry w/alcohol. For adults. Liq. Bot. 4 fl oz, 8 fl oz. *OTC.*
Use: Cough preparation.

Creomulsion for Children. (Summit) Beechwood creosote, cascara, ipecac, menthol, white pine, wild cherry w/alcohol. For children. Liq. Bot. 4 fl oz, 8 fl oz. *OTC.*
Use: Cough preparation.

Creon. (Solvay) Lipase 8000 units, amylase 30,000 units, protease 13,000 units, pancreatin 300 mg. Cap. Bot. 100s, 250s. *Rx.*
Use: Digestive enzyme.

Creon 5. (Solvay) Lipase 5000 units, protease 18,750 units, amylase 16,600 units. DR Cap. Bot. 100s, 250s. *Rx.*
Use: Digestive enzyme.

Creon 10. (Solvay) Lipase 10,000 units, amylase 33,200 units, protease 37,500 units. DR Cap. Bot. 100s, 250s. *Rx.*
Use: Digestive enzyme.

Creon 20. (Solvay) Lipase 20,000 units, amylase 66,400 units, protease 75,000 units. DR Cap. Bot. 100s, 250s. *Rx.*
Use: Digestive enzyme.

creosote. Wood creosote, creosote, beechwood creosote.

Creo-Terpin. (Lee) Dextromethorphan HBr 10 mg/15 mL, tartrazine, alcohol 25%, saccharin, corn syrup. Liq. Bot. 120 mL. *OTC.*
Use: Antitussive.

Crescormon. (Pharmacia) Somatotropin 4 units. Vial. IM administration. *Rx.*
Note: Crescormon will be available only for patients who qualify for treatment. Apply to Kabi Group Inc. for approval.

Use: Hormone, growth.

•**cresol.** (KREE-sole) *NF 23.*
Use: Antiseptic; disinfectant.

cresol preparations.
Use: Antiseptic; disinfectant.
See: Saponated Cresol.

Crestor. (AstraZeneca) Rosavastatin calcium 5 mg, 10 mg, 20 mg, 40 mg. Lactose. 30s (40 mg only), 90s (except 40 mg), UD 100s (except 5 mg). *Rx.*
Use: HMG-CoA reductase inhibitors.

m-cresyl-acetate.
See: Cresylate.

Cresylate. (Recsei) M-cresyl-acetate 25%, isopropanol 25%, chlorobutanol 1%, benzyl alcohol 1%, castor oil 5%, propylene glycol/15 mL. Bot. 15 mL, pt. *Rx.*
I /9e' Ollti

cresylic acid. Same as Cresol.

•**crilvastatin.** (krill-vah-STAT-in) USAN.
Use: Antihyperlipidemic.

Crinone. (Serono) Progesterone 4% (45 mg), glycerin, mineral oil, hydrogenated palm oil. Vag. gel. Single-dose disposable applicator. *Rx.*
Use: Assisted reproductive technology treatment.

Crinone 8%. (Serono) Progesterone 8% (90 mg). Mineral oil, glycerin. Gel. Single-use, one piece 1.125 g applicators. *Rx.*
Use: Assisted reproductive technology treatment.

•**crisnatol mesylate.** (KRISS-nah-tole) USAN.
Use: Antineoplastic.

Criticare HN. (Bristol-Myers Squibb) High nitrogen elemental diet. Protein 14%, fat 4.3%, carbohydrate 81.5%. Bot. 8 oz. *OTC.*
Use: Nutritional supplement, enteral.

Crixivan. (Merck & Co.) Indinavir sulfate 100 mg, 200 mg, 333 mg, 400 mg (corresponding to 125 mg, 250 mg, 416.3 mg, 500 mg indinavir sulfate, respectively), lactose. Cap. Unit-of-use 18s, 90s, 120s (400 mg only); 135s (333 mg only); 180s (100 mg, 400 mg only); 360s 200 mg only). *Rx.*
Use: Antiretroviral agent, protease inhibitor.

CroFab. (Protherics) Crotalidae polyvalent immune fab (ovine origin). Total protein 1 g, thimerosal (mercury 0.11 mg)/Vial. Single-use Vial. Diluent not included. *Rx.*
Use: Antivenin.

Croferrin. (Forest) Iron peptonate 50 mg, liver injection 2.5 mcg, vitamin

B_{12}12.5 mcg, lidocaine hydrochloride 1%, phenol 0.5%, sodium citrate 0.125%, sodium bisulfite 0.009%/mL. Vial 10 mL, 30 mL. *Rx.*
Use: Mineral, vitamin supplement.

•**crofilcon A.** (kroe-FILL-kahn A) USAN.
Use: Contact lens material, hydrophilic.

Crolom. (Dura) Cromolyn sodium 4%. Soln. Bot. 2.5 mL, 10 mL w/controlled drop tip. *Rx.*
Use: Antiallergic, ophthalmic.

Cro-Man-Zin. (Freeda) Cr 200 mcg, Mn 5 mg, Zn 25 mg, kosher, sugar free. Tab. Bot. 100s, 250s. *OTC.*
Use: Electrolyte, mineral supplement.

•**cromitrile sodium.** (KROE-mih-TRILE) USAN.
Use: Antiasthmatic.

•**cromolyn sodium.** (KI IUL moe lin) *USP 28.*
Use: Antiasthmatic; prophylactic; mastocytosis. [Orphan Drug]
See: Children's NasalCrom.
Gastrocrom.
Intal.
NasalCrom.

cromolyn sodium. (Various Mfr.) Cromolyn sodium **Inhalation:** 20 mg/2 mL. Vial or Amps. 60 mL, 120 mL. **Soln. for Nebulization:** 20 mg. Vial. 2 mL. *Rx.*
Use: Antiasthmatic; prophylactic.

cromolyn sodium 4% ophthalmic solution.
Use: Antiallergic, ophthalmic.
See: Crolom.

Cronetal.
See: Disulfiram.

•**croscarmellose sodium.** (KRAHS-CAR-mell-ose) *NF 23.* Formerly *Cross-linked Carboxymethylcellulose Sodium and Modified Cellulose Gum.*
Use: Pharmaceutic aid, tablet disintegrant.

•**crospovidone.** (krahs-PAV-ih-dohn) *NF 23.*
Use: Pharmaceutic aid, tablet excipient.

Cross Aspirin. (Cross) Aspirin 325 mg. Sugar, salt and lactose free. Tab. Bot. 100s, 1000s. *OTC.*
Use: Analgesic.

CroTAb. (CroFab)

Crotalidae antivenin polyvalent. (Wyeth) 1 vial of lyophilized serum, 1 vial of bacteriostatic water 10 mL, USP, 1 vial normal horse serum. Inj. Vial Combination Pkg. *Rx.*
Use: Antivenin.

Crotalidae polyvalent immune fab (ovine origin).
Use: Antivenin.
See: CroFab.

•**crotaline antivenin, polyvalent.** (kroe-TAHL-een an-tee-VEH-nen pahl-ee-VAY-lent) *USP 28.* Antivenin Crotalidae Polyvalent, North and South American antisnakebite serum. *Rx.*
Use: Immunizing agent.

•**crotamiton.** (kroe-TAM-ih-tuhn) *USP 28.*
Use: Scabicide.
See: Eurax.

CRPA Latex Test. (Laboratory Diagnostics) Rapid latex agglutination test for the qualitative determination of C-reactive protein. CRPA, 1 mL CRP Positest Control, 0.5 mL CRPA Latex Test Kit.
Use: Diagnostic aid.

Cruex Cream. (Novartis) Clotrimazole 1%, benzyl alcohol 1%, cetostearyl alcohol. Cream. Tube. 15 g. *OTC.*
Use: Antifungal, topical.

Cruex Spray Powder. (Novartis) Undecylenic acid 2% and zinc undecylenate 20%. Pow. Aerosol can 1.8 oz, 3.5 oz, 5.5 oz. *OTC.*
Use: Antifungal, topical.

Cruex Squeeze Powder. (Novartis) Calcium undecylenate 10%. Pow. Plastic squeeze bot. 1.5 oz. *OTC.*
Use: Antifungal, topical.

cryptosporidium hyperimmune bovine colostrum IgG concentrate. (Immucell)
Use: Treat diarrhea in AIDS patients. [Orphan Drug]

cryptosporidium parvum bovine immunoglobulin concentrate.
Use: Treat infection of GI tract in immunocompromised patients. [Orphan Drug]

Cryselle. (Barr) Norgestrel 0.3 mg, ethinyl estradiol 30 mcg. Packs. 21s. 28s. *Rx.*
Use: Sex hormone, contraceptive hormone.

crystalline trypsin. Highly purified preparation of enzyme as derived from mammalian pancreas glands.

crystal violet.
See: Methylrosaniline chloride.

Crystamine. (Oxypure) Cyanocobalamin 100 mcg, 1000 mcg/mL, benzyl alcohol. Vial 10 mL, 30 mL. *Rx.*
Use: Vitamin supplement.

Crysti-Liver. (Roberts) Liver injection (equivalent to B_{12} 10 mcg), crystalline B_{12} 100 mcg, folic acid 0.4 mg. Inj. Vial 10 mL. *Rx.*

Use: Mineral, vitamin supplement.

Crysti 1000. (Roberts) Cyanocobalamin crystalline 1000 mcg/mL. Inj. Vial 10 mL, 30 mL. *Rx.*
Use: Vitamin B_{12}.

Crystodigin. (Eli Lilly) Digitoxin 0.05 mg, 0.1 mg. Tab. Bot. 100s. *Rx.*
Use: Cardiovascular agent.

CTab.
See: Cetyl Trimethyl Ammonium Bromide.

C-Tanna 12D. (Prasco) **Susp.:** Carbetapentane tannate 30 mg, pyrilamine tannate 5 mg per 5 mL. Glycerin, methylparaben, sucrose. Purple, strawberry flavor. 118 mL. **Tab.:** Carbetapentane tannate 60 mg, pyrilamine tannate 40 mg, phenylephrine tannate 10 mg. Corn starch. Tab. 100s. *Rx.*
Use: Antitussive combination.

C-Tussin. (Century) Codeine phosphate 10 mg, pseudoephedrine hydrochloride 30 mg, guaifenesin 100 mg/5 mL, alcohol 7.5%. Bot. 120 mL, gal. *c-iv.*
Use: Antitussive; decongestant; expectorant.

Cubicin. (Cubist) Daptomycin 250 mg, 500 mg. Preservative free. Pow. for Inj., lyophilized. Vials, single-use. *Rx.*
Use: Anti-infective.

Culminal. (Culminal) Benzocaine 3% in water-miscible cream base. Tube 1 oz. *OTC.*
Use: Anesthetic, local.

Culturette 10 Minute Group A Step ID. (Hoechst) Latex slide agglutination test for group A streptococcal antigen on throat swabs. Kit 55 determinations.
Use: Diagnostic aid.

•**cupric acetate Cu 64.** (koo-PRIK) USAN.
Use: Radioactive agent.

•**cupric chloride.** (koo-PRIK) *USP 28.*
Use: Supplement, trace mineral.

•**cupric sulfate.** (koo-PRIK) *USP 28.*
Use: Antidote to phosphorus.

Cuprid. (Merck & Co.) Trientine hydrochloride 250 mg. Cap. Bot. 100s. *Rx.*
Use: Chelating agent.

Cuprimine. (Merck & Co.) Penicillamine 125 mg, 250 mg. Cap. Bot. 100s. *Rx.*
Use: Chelating agent.

•**cuprimyxin.** (KUH-prih-mix-in) USAN.
Use: Antifungal.

Cupri-Pak. (SoloPak Pharmaceuticals, Inc.) Copper. **0.4 mg/mL:** Vial 10 mL, 30 mL. **2 mg/mL:** Vial 5 mL. *Rx.*
Use: Nutritional supplement, parenteral.

curare.
Use: Muscle relaxant.

curare antagonist.
See: Neostigine Methylsulfate.
Tensilon.
Curel. (Bausch & Lomb) Glycerin, petrolatum, dimethicone, parabens. Lot. 180, 300, 390 mL. Cream. Tube. 90 g.
Rx-OTC.
Use: Emollient.
Curosurf. (Dey) Poractant alfa (porcine origin). Phospholipids 80 mg/mL (including phosphatidylcholine 54 mg, of which 30.5 mg is dipalmitoyl phosphatidylcholine and 1 mg of protein, including 0.3 mg of SP-B), preservative free. Intratracheal Susp. Single-use vials. 1.5 mL, 3 mL. *Rx.*
Use: Lung surfactant; respiratory distress syndrome.
curral.
See: Diallyl Barbituric Acid.
Cutar Emulsion. (Summers) LCD 7.5% (coal tar 1.5%) in mineral oil, lanolin alcohols extract, parabens. Liq. 177 mL, 1 gal. *OTC.*
Use: Dermatologic.
Cutemol Emollient. (Summers) Allantoin 0.2%, liquid petrolatum, acetylated lanolin, lanolin alcohols extract, isopropyl myristate, water. Cream. Jar 2 oz. *OTC.*
Use: Emollient.
Cuticura Medicated Shampoo. (DEP Corp.) Sodium lauryl sulfate, sodium stearate, salicylic acid, protein, sulfur. Shampoo. Tube 3 oz. *OTC.*
Use: Antidandruff.
Cuticura Medicated Soap. (DEP Corp.) Triclocarban 1%, petrolatum, sodium tallowate, sodium cocoate, glycerin, mineral oil, sodium Cl, tetrasodium EDTA, sodium bicarbonate, magnesium silicate, iron oxides. Soap. Bar 3.5 oz, 5.5 oz. *OTC.*
Use: Anti-infective, topical.
Cutivate. (GlaxoSmithKline) Fluticasone propionate. **Cream:** 0.05%. Jar 15 g, 30 g, 60 g. **Oint.:** 0.005%. Jar 15 g, 30 g, 60 g. *Rx.*
Use: Corticosteroid, topical.
Cutter Insect Repellent. (Bayer Corp. (Consumer Div.)) N,N-Diethyl-meta-toluamide 28.5%, other isomers 1.5%. Vial 1 oz; Foam, Can 2 oz; Spray 7 oz, Aerosol can 14 oz; Assortment Pack; First Aid Kits, Trial Pack, 6s; Marine Pack 3s; Camp Pack 4s; Pocket Pack, Travel Pack.
Use: Insect repellent.
c vitamin.
See: Ascorbic Acid.
CY 1503. (Cytel Corp.)
Use: Antithromboembolic. [Orphan Drug]

CY 1899. (Cytel Corp.)
Use: Antiviral, hepatitis B. [Orphan Drug]
Cyanide Antidote Package. (Various Mfr.) 2 amp. (300 mg/10 mL) sodium nitrite; 2 vials (12.5 g/50 mL), sodium thiosulfate; 12 amps amyl nitrite inhalant 5 minim/0.3 mL, disposable syringes, stomach tube, tourniquet, and instructions. *Rx.*
Use: Antidote, cyanide poisoning.
Cyanocob. (Paddock) Vitamin B$_{12}$ 1000 mcg/mL. Bot. 1000 mL, Vial 10 mL. *Rx.*
Use: Vitamin supplement.
●**cyanocobalamin.** (sigh-an-oh-koe-BAL-uh-min) *USP 28.* Formerly Vitamin B$_{12}$.
Use: Vitamin, hematopoietic.
See: Big Shot B-12.
Nascobal.
Twelve Resin-K.
Vitamin B$_{12}$.
W/Combinations.
See: Folgard.
FOLTX.
●**cyanocobalamin Co 57.** (sigh-an-oh-koe-BAL-uh-min) *USP 28.*
Use: Diagnostic aid, pernicious anemia; radioactive agent.
●**cyanocobalamin Co 58.** (sigh-an-oh-koe-BAL-uh-min) *USP 28.*
Use: Diagnostic aid, pernicious anemia; radioactive agent.
●**cyanocobalamin Co 60.** (sigh-an-oh-koe-BAL-uh-min) *USP 28.*
Use: Diagnostic aid, pernicious anemia; radioactive agent.
cyanocobalamin crystalline. *Rx-OTC.*
Use: Vitamin B$_{12}$ supplement.
See: Betalin 12.
Cobex.
Crystamine.
Crysti 1000.
Cyanoject.
Cyomin.
Vitamin B$_{12}$.
Cyanoject. (Merz) Vitamin B$_{12}$ 1000 mcg/mL, benzyl alcohol. Vial 10 mL, 30 mL. *Rx.*
Use: Vitamin supplement.
Cyanover. (Research Supplies) Cyanocobalamin 100 mcg, liver injection 10 mcg, folic acid 10 mg/mL. *Lyo-layer* vial 10 mL with vial of diluent 10 mL. *Rx.*
Use: Mineral, vitamin supplement.
●**cyclacillin.** (SIGH-klah-SILL-in) *USP 28.*
Use: Anti-infective.
cyclamate sodium. Cyclohexanesulfamate dihydrate salt.

•**cyclamic acid.** (sigh-KLAM-ik) USAN.
Use: Sweetener, nonnutritive.

•**cyclazocine.** (SIGH-CLAY-zoe-seen) USAN. Under study.
Use: Analgesic.

Cyclessa. (Organon) **Phase 1:** Desogestrel 0.1 mg, ethinyl estradiol 25 mcg. **Phase 2:** Desogestrel 0.125 mg, ethinyl estradiol 25 mcg. **Phase 3:** Desogestrel 0.15 mg, ethinyl estradiol 25 mcg. Tab. 28s. *Rx.*
Use: Sex hormone, contraceptive hormone.

•**cyclindole.** (sigh-KLIN-dole) USAN.
Use: Antidepressant.

Cyclinex-1. (Ross) Protein 7.5 g (from carnitine, cystine, histidine, isoleucine, leucine, lysine, methionine, phenylalanine, taurine, threonine, tryptophan, tyrosine, valine), fat 27 g (from palm oil, hydrogenated coconut oil, soy oil), carbohydrate 52 g (from hydrolyzed corn starch), linoleic acid 2000 mg, Fe 10 mg, Na 215 mg, K 760 mg, Ca, vitamins A, B_1, B_2, B_3, B_5, B_6, B_{12}, C, D, E, K, biotin, choline, folic acid, inositol, Cl, Cu, I, Mg, Mn, P, Se, Zn and 515 Cal per 100 g. Nonessential amino acid free. Pow. Can 350 g. *OTC.*
Use: Nutritional supplement.

Cyclinex-2. (Ross) Protein 15 g (from carnitine, cystine, histidine, isoleucine, leucine, lysine, methionine, phenylalanine, taurine, threonine, tryptophan, tyrosine, valine), fat 20.7 g (from palm oil, hydrogenated coconut oil, soy oil), carbohydrate 40 g (from hydrolyzed cornstarch), Fe 17 mg, Na 1175 mg, K 1830 mg, Ca, vitamins A, B_1, B_2, B_3, B_5, B_6, B_{12}, C, D, E, K, biotin, choline, folic acid, inositol, Cl, Cu, I, Mg, Mn, P, Se, Zn and 480 Cal per 100 g. Nonessential amino acid free. Pow. Can 325 g. *OTC.*
Use: Nutritional supplement.

•**cycliramine maleate.** (SIGH-klih-rah-meen) USAN.
Use: Antihistamine.

•**cyclizine.** (SIGH-klih-zeen) *USP 28.*
Use: Antihistamine.

•**cyclizine hydrochloride.** (SIGH-klih-zeen) *USP 28.*
Use: Antiemetic.
See: Marezine hydrochloride and Lactate.

•**cyclizine lactate injection.** (SIGH-klih-zeen LACK-tate) *USP 28.*
Use: Antihistamine; antinauseant.

cyclobarbital.
Use: Central depressant.

cyclobarbital calcium.
Use: Hypnotic; sedative.

•**cyclobendazole.** (SIGH-kloe-BEN-dah-zole) USAN.
Use: Anthelmintic.

•**cyclobenzaprine hydrochloride.** (SIGH-kloe-BEN-zuh-preen) *USP 28.*
Use: Muscle relaxant.
See: Flexeril.

cyclobenzaprine hydrochloride. (Various Mfr.) Cyclobenzaprine hydrochloride 10 mg. Tab. Bot. 30s, 100s, 1000s.
Use: Muscle relaxant.

Cyclocort Cream. (Wyeth) Amcinonide 0.1% in Aquatain hydrophilic base. Cream. Tube. 15 g, 30 g, 60 g. *Rx.*
Use: Corticosteroid, topical.

Cyclocort Ointment. (Wyeth) Amcinonide 0.1% in ointment base. Oint. Tube 15 g, 30 g, 60 g. *Rx.*
Use: Corticosteroid, topical.

cyclocumarol.
Use: Anticoagulant.

•**cyclofilcon a.** (SIGH-kloe-FILL-kahn A) USAN.
Use: Contact lens material, hydrophilic.

Cyclogen. (Schwarz Pharma) Dicyclomine hydrochloride 10 mg, sodium Cl 0.9%, chlorobutanol hydrate 0.5%. Vial 10 mL, Box 12s. *Rx.*
Use: Antispasmodic.

•**cycloguanil pamoate.** (SIGH-kloe-GWAHN-ill PAM-oh-ate) USAN.
Use: Antimalarial.

Cyclogyl. (Alcon) Cyclopentolate hydrochloride 0.5%, 1%, 2%. Soln. Droptainer 2 mL, 5 mL, 15 mL. *Rx.*
Use: Cycloplegic; mydriatic.

•**cycloheximide.** (sigh-KLOE-HEX-ih-mid) USAN.
Use: Antipsoriatic.

•**cyclomethicone.** (sigh-kloe-METH-ih-cone) *NF 23.*
Use: Pharmaceutic aid, wetting agent.

cyclomethycaine and methapyrilene.
Use: Anesthetic, local.

cyclomethycaine sulfate.
Use: Anesthetic, local.

Cyclomydril. (Alcon) Phenylephrine hydrochloride 1%, cyclopentolate hydrochloride 0.2%. Droptainer 2 mL, 5 mL. *Rx.*
Use: Mydriatic.

Cyclonil. (Seatrace) Dicyclomine hydrochloride 10 mg/mL. Vial 10 mL. *Rx.*
Use: Anticholinergic; antispasmodic.

Cyclopar. (Parke-Davis) Tetracycline hydrochloride. Cap. **250 mg:** Bot. 100s, 1000s. **500 mg:** Bot. 100s, UD 100s.

Rx.
Use: Anti-infective, tetracycline.
● **cyclopentamine hydrochloride.** (SIGH-kloe-PEN-teh-meen) *USP 28.*
Use: Adrenergic, vasoconstrictor.
See: Clopane Hydrochloride.
W/Aludrine.
See: Aerolone Compound.
● **cyclopenthiazide.** (SIGH-kloe-pen-THIGH-ah-zide) USAN.
Use: Antihypertensive; diuretic.
● **cyclopentolate hydrochloride.** (sigh-kloe-PEN-toe-tate) *USP 28.*
Use: Anticholinergic, ophthalmic.
See: AK-Pentolate.
Cyclogyl.
W/Phenylephrine hydrochloride.
See: Cyclomydril.
cyclopentolate hydrochloride. (Various Mfr.) Cyclopentolate hydrochloride 1% Soln. Bot. 2 mL, 15 mL.
Use: Anticholinergic, ophthalmic.
8 cyclopentyl 1,3-dipropylxanthine. (SciClone)
Use: Cystic fibrosis. [Orphan Drug]
cyclopentylpropionate.
See: Depo-Testosterone.
● **cyclophenazine hydrochloride.** (SIGH-kloe-FEH-nazz-een) USAN.
Use: Antipsychotic.
● **cyclophosphamide.** (sigh-kloe-FOSS-fuh-mide) *USP 28.*
Use: Antineoplastic, immunosuppressant, alkylating agent; nitrogen mustard.
See: Cytoxan.
Neosar.
cyclophosphamide. (Gensia Sicor) Cyclophosphamide 25 mg, 50 mg. Lactose. Tab. 100s, UD 100s. *Rx.*
Use: Antineoplastic, immunosuppressant; alkylating agent; nitrogen mustard.
● **cyclopropane.** (sigh-kloe-PRO-pane) *USP 28.*
Use: Anesthetic, general.
● **cycloserine.** (sigh-kloe-SER-een) *USP 28.*
Tall Man: CycloSERINE
Use: Antituberculosis agent.
See: Seromycin Pulvules.
l-cycloserine.
Use: Treat Gaucher disease. [Orphan Drug]
cyclosporin a.
Use: Immunosuppressant.
See: Cyclosporine.
● **cyclosporine.** (SIGH-kloe-spore-EEN) *USP 28. Formerly Cyclosporin A.*
Tall Man: CycloSPORINE

Use: Immunosuppressant.
See: Gengraf.
Neoral.
Sandimmune.
cyclosporine. (Pliva) Cyclosporine 100 mg/mL. Oral Soln. Bot. 50 mL. *Rx.*
Use: Immunosuppressant.
cyclosporine. (Various Mfr.) Cyclosporine 25 mg, 100 mg, castor oil, sorbitol, alcohol. Soft gelatin Cap. UD 30s. *Rx.*
Use: Immunosuppressant.
cyclosporine injection. (Bedford Labs) Cyclosporine 50 mg/mL. Inj. Single-use vials. 5 mL. *Rx.*
Use: Immunosuppressant.
cyclosporine ophthalmic.
Use: Severe keratoconjunctivitis sicca; graft rejection following keratoplasty. [Orphan Drug]
cyclosporine ophthalmic emulsion.
Use: Immunologic agent.
See: Restasis.
cyclosporine 2% ophthalmic ointment. (Allergan)
Use: Treatment of graft rejection after keratoplasty and corneal melting syndromes. [Orphan Drug]
● **cyclothiazide.** (SIGH-kloe-thigh-AZZ-ide) USAN.
Use: Antihypertensive; diuretic.
Cycofed. (Cypress) Codeine phosphate 20 mg, pseudoephedrine hydrochloride 60 mg/5 mL, spearmint flavor. Syr. Bot. 473 mL. *c-III.*
Use: Upper respiratory combination, antitussive, decongestant.
Cycofed Pediatric. (Cypress) Codeine phosphate 10 mg, pseudoephedrine hydrochloride 30 mg, guaifenesin 100 mg/5 mL, alcohol 6%. Syr. Bot. 480 mL. *c-v.*
Use: Antitussive, decongestant, expectorant.
Cydec-DM Drops. (Cypress) Pseudoephedrine hydrochloride 25 mg, carbinoxamine maleate 2 mg, dextromethorphan HBr 4 mg/mL, grape flavor. Drops. Bot. 30 mL w/dropper. *Rx.*
Use: Upper respiratory combination, decongestant, antihistamine, antitussive.
Cydec-DM Syrup. (Cypress) Dextromethorphan HBr 15 mg, carbinoxamine maleate 4 mg, pseudoephedrine hydrochloride 60 mg/5 mL, grape flavor. Syr. Bot. 118 mL, 473 mL, 3.8 L. *Rx.*
Use: Upper respiratory combination, antitussive, antihistamine, decongestant.

Cydec Oral. (Cypress) Pseudoephedrine hydrochloride 25 mg, carbinoxamine maleate 2 mg/mL, raspberry flavor. Drops. Bot. 30 mL. *Rx.*
Use: Upper respiratory combination, decongestant, antihistamine.

Cydonol Massage Lotion. (Gordon Laboratories) Isopropyl alcohol 14%, methyl salicylate, benzalkonium Cl. Lot. Bot. 4 oz, gal. *OTC.*
Use: Counterirritant.

•**cyheptamide.** (sigh-HEP-tah-mid) USAN.
Use: Anticonvulsant.

Cyklokapron. (Pharmacia) Tranexamic acid. **Tab.:** 500 mg. Bot. 100s. **Inj.:** 100 mg/mL. Amp. 10 mL. *Rx.*
Use: Hemostatic.

Cylert. (Abbott) Pemoline. **Chew. Tab.:** 27.5 mg, mannitol. Bot. 100s. **Tab.:** 18.75 mg, 37.5 mg, 75 mg, lactose. Tab. Bot. 100s. *c-iv.*
Use: CNS stimulant.

Cylex Sugar Free. (Pharmakon) Benzocaine 15 mg, cetylpyridinium Cl 5 mg, sorbitol. Loz. Pkg. 12s. *OTC.*
Use: Antiseptic; analgesic, topical.

Cylex Throat. (Pharmakon) Benzocaine 15 mg, cetylpyridinium Cl 5 mg, sorbitol. Loz. Pkg. 12s. *OTC.*
Use: Antiseptic; analgesic, topical.

Cymbalta. (Eli Lilly) Duloxetine hydrochloride (as base) 20 mg, 30 mg, 60 mg. Sucrose, sugar spheres. Enteric-coated pellets. Cap. 30s (except 20 mg), 60s (20 mg only), 90s (except 20 mg), 1,000s (except 20 mg), unit-dose 100s. *Rx.*
Use: Antidepressant.

Cynobal. (Arcum) Cyanocobalamin 10 mcg, 1000 mcg/mL. Inj. Vial 10 mL (1000 mcg only), 30 mL. *Rx.*
Use: Vitamin supplement.

Cyomin. (Forest) Cyanocobalamin 1000 mcg/mL. Inj. Vial 10 mL, 30 mL. *Rx.*
Use: Vitamin B_{12} supplement.

•**cypenamine hydrochloride.** (sigh-PEN-ah-meen) USAN.
Use: Antidepressant.

•**cyprazepam.** (sigh-PRAY-zeh-pam) USAN.
Use: Hypnotic; sedative.

•**cyproheptadine.** (sip-row-HEP-tuh-deen) *USP 28.*
Use: Antihistamine, nonselective piperidine; antipruritic.
See: Periactin.

cyproheptadine. (Various Mfr.) Cyproheptadine hydrochloride. **Tab.:** 4 mg.

Bot. 100s, 1,000s, UD 100s. **Syr.:** 2 mg/ 5 mL. May contain alcohol. Bot. 473 mL. *Rx.*
Use: Antihistamine, nonselective piperidine; antipruritic.

•**cyprolidol hydrochloride.** (sigh-PRO-lih-dahl) USAN.
Use: Antidepressant.

•**cyproterone acetate.** (sigh-PRO-ter-ohn) USAN.
Use: Antiandrogen.

•**cyproximide.** (sigh-PROX-ih-MIDE) USAN.
Use: Antidepressant; antipsychotic.

cyren a.
See: Diethylstilbestrol.

Cyronine. (Major) Liothyronine sodium 25 mcg. Tab. Bot. 100s. *Rx.*
Use: Hormone, thyroid.

Cystadane. (Orphan Medical) Betaine anhydrous 1 g/1.7 mL. Pow. for Inj. Bot. 180 g. *Rx.*
Use: Treatment of homocystinuria.

Cystagon. (Mylan) Cysteamine bitartrate 50 mg, 150 mg. Cap. Bot. 100s, 500s. *Rx.*
Use: Urinary tract agent.

Cystamin.
See: Methenamine.

Cystamine. (Tennessee Pharmaceutic) Methenamine 2 g, phenyl salicylate 0.5 g, phenazopyridine hydrochloride 10 mg, benzoic acid ⅛ g, hyoscyamine sulfate g, atropine sulfate g. SC Tab. Bot. 100s, 1000s. *Rx.*
Use: Anti-infective, urinary.

•**cysteamine.** (sis-TEE-ah-MEEN) USAN.
Use: Antiurolithic, cystine calculi; nephropathic cystinosis. [Orphan Drug]

•**cysteamine hydrochloride.** (sis-TEE-ah-MEEN) USAN.
Use: Antiurolithic, cystine calculi; nephropathic cystinosis.
See: Cystagon.

•**cysteine hydrochloride.** (SIS-teh-een) *USP 28.*
Use: Amino acid for replacement therapy, treatment of photosensitivity in erythropoietic protoporphyria. [Orphan Drug]
See: Cysteine hydrochloride.

Cystex. (Numark) Methenamine 162 mg, sodium salicylate 162.5 mg, benzoic acid 32 mg. Tab. Bot. 40s, 100s. *OTC.*
Use: Anti-infective, urinary.

cystic fibrosis gene therapy. (Genzyme)
Use: Cystic fibrosis. [Orphan Drug]

cystic fibrosis TR gene therapy (recombinant adenovirus). (Gerac)
Use: Cystic fibrosis. [Orphan Drug]
See: AdGVCFTR 10.

•**cystine.** (SIS-TEEN) USAN.
Use: Amino acid replacement therapy, an additive for infants on TPN.

Cysto. (Freeport) Methenamine 40.8 mg, methylene blue 5.4 mg, phenyl salicylate 18.1 mg, atropine sulfate 0.03 mg, hyoscyamine 0.03 mg, benzoic acid 4.5 mg. Tab. Bot. 1000s. *Rx.*
Use: Anti-infective, urinary.

Cystografin. (Bracco Diagnostics) Diatrizoate meglumine 300 mg, iodine 141 mg/mL, EDTA. Inj. Bot. 100 mL in 200 mL, 300 mL fill in 400 mL. *Rx.*
Use: Radiopaque agent.

Cystografin Dilute. (Bracco Diagnostics) Diatrizoate meglumine 100 mg, iodine 85 mg/mL, EDTA. Inj. Bot. 300 mL w/or without administration sets. *Rx.*
Use: Radiopaque agent.

Cystospaz. (PolyMedica) l-hyoscyamine 0.15 mg. Tab. Bot. 100s. *Rx.*
Use: Anticholinergic; antispasmodic.

Cystospaz-M. (PolyMedica) Hyoscyamine sulfate 375 mcg. Cap. Bot. 100s. *Rx.*
Use: Anticholinergic; antispasmodic.

Cytadren. (Novartis) Aminoglutethimide 250 mg. Tab. Bot. 100s. *Rx.*
Use: Adrenal steroid inhibitor; treatment of Cushing syndrome.

•**cytarabine.** (SIGH-tar-ah-bean) *USP 28.*
Use: Antineoplastic; antiviral.
See: DepoCyt.
Tarabine PFS.

cytarabine. (Mayne Pharma) Cytarabine 20 mg/mL, preservative free. Inj. Single and multidose vials 5 mL, bulk pkg. vial 50 mL. *Rx.*
Use: Antineoplastic; antiviral.

cytarabine. (Various Mfr.) Cytarabine 100 mg, 500 mg, 1 g, 2 g. Pow. for Inj. Vials. *Rx.*
Use: Antineoplastic; antiviral.

cytarabine, depofoam encapsulated.
Use: Neoplastic meningitis. [Orphan Drug]

•**cytarabine hydrochloride.** (SITE-ah-rah-been) USAN. *Formerly Cytosine Arabinoside Hydrochloride.*
Use: Antiviral management of acute leukemias.
See: Cytosar-U.

CytoGam. (MedImmune) Cytomegalovirus immune globulin IV (human) 50 ± 10 mg/mL, sucrose 5%, human albumin 1%, preservative free, solvent/deter-

gent treated. Soln. for Inj. Vial 20 mL, 50 mL. *Rx.*
Use: Antiviral, cytomegalovirus; immune globulin.

cytomegalovirus immune globulin (human).
Use: Antiviral, cytomegalovirus. [Orphan Drug]
See: CytoGam.

cytomegalovirus immune globulin (human) intravenous.
Use: CMV pneumonia in bone marrow transplants.
See: CytoGam.

cytomegalovirus immune globulin intravenous (human). (Bayer Corp. (Biological and Pharmaceutical Div.))
Use: With ganciclovir sodium for the treatment of CMV pneumonia in bone marrow transplant patients. [Orphan Drug]

Cytomel. (Monarch) Liothyronine sodium 5 mcg, 25 mcg, 50 mcg, sucrose. Tab. Bot. 100s. *Rx.*
Use: Hormone, thyroid.

cytoprotective agents.
See: Allopurinol sodium.
Amifostine.
Dexrazoxane.
Mesna.

cytosine arabinoside hydrochloride.
Cytarabine hydrochloride.
See: Cytosar-U.

Cytosol. (Cytosol) Calcium chloride 48 mg, magnesium chloride 30 mg, potassium chloride 75 mg, sodium acetate 390 mg, sodium chloride 640 mg, sodium citrate 170 mg/100 mL. Soln. Bot. 200 mL, 500 mL. *Rx.*
Use: Irrigant.

Cytospaz. (PolyMedica) L-hyoscyamine sulfate 0.15 mg. Tab. 100s. *Rx.*
Use: Anticholinergic/antispasmodic.

Cytotec. (Pfizer) Misoprostol 100 mcg, 200 mcg. Tab. Bot. UD 100s, unit-of-use 60s, 100s (200 mcg only), 120s (100 mcg only). *Rx.*
Use: Prostaglandins, antiulcerative.

Cytovene. (Roche) Ganciclovir. **Cap.:** 250 mg, 500 mg. Bot. 180s. **Inj. (as sodium):** 500 mg, sodium 46 mg. Pow, lyophilized. Vial. 10 mL. *Rx.*
Use: Antiviral.

Cytox. (MPL) Cyanocobalamin 500 mcg, vitamins B_6 20 mg, B_1 100 mg, benzyl alcohol 2% in isotonic solution of sodium Cl/mL. Inj. Vial 10 mL. *Rx.*
Use: Vitamin supplement.

Cytoxan. (Mead Johnson Oncology) Cyclophosphamide 25 mg, 50 mg. Lactose. Tab. Bot. 100s, 1,000s (50 mg

only). *Rx.*
Use: Antineoplastic; alkylating agent.
Cytoxan Lyophilized. (Mead Johnson Oncology) Cyclophosphamide 100 mg, mannitol 75 mg. Pow. for Inj. Vial 100 mg, 200 mg, 500 mg, 1 g, 2 g. *Rx.*
Use: Antineoplastic; alkylating agent.
Cytoxan Powder. (Bristol-Myers Squibb Oncology/Virology) Cyclophosphamide 100 mg, 200 mg, 500 mg, 1 g, 2 g. Pow. Vial. *Rx.*
Use: Antineoplastic.
Cytra-K. (Cypress) Potassium citrate monohydrate 1100 mg, citric acid monohydrate 334 mg/5 mL. Soln. Bot. 473 mL. *Rx.*
Use: Alkalinizer, systemic.
Cytra-LC. (Cypress) Potassium citrate monohydrate 550 mg, sodium citrate dihydrate 500 mg, citric acid mono-

hydrate 334 mg/5 mL. Soln. Bot. 473 mL. *Rx.*
Use: Alkalinizer, systemic.
Cytra-3. (Cypress) Potassium citrate monohydrate 550 mg, sodium citrate dihydrate 500 mg, citric acid monohydrate 334 mg/5 mL. Syr. Bot. 480 mL. *Rx.*
Use: Alkalinizer, systemic.
Cytra-2. (Cypress) Sodium citrate dihydrate 500 mg, citric acid monohydrate 334 mg/5 mL. Soln. Bot. 16 oz. *Rx.*
Use: Alkalinizer, systemic.
Cytuss HC. (Cypress) Hydrocodone bitartrate 2.5 mg, chlorpheniramine maleate 2 mg, phenylephrine hydrochloride 5 mg/5 mL. Liq. Bot. 473 mL. *c-III.*
Use: Upper respiratory combination.

D

daa.
See: Dihydroxy Aluminum Aminoacetate.

DAB₃₈₉ IL-2. (Seragen)
Use: Cutaneous T-cell lymphoma.
[Orphan Drug]

•**dabuzalgron hydrochloride.** (da-bue-ZAL-gron) USAN.
Use: Urinary agent

•**dacarbazine.** (da-CAR-buh-zeen) USP 28.
Use: Antineoplastic.
See: DTIC-Dome.

dacarbazine. (Various Mfr.) Dacarbazine 100 mg, 200 mg. May contain mannitol. Pow. for Inj. Vials. Rx.
Use: Alkylating agent, antineoplastic.

D.A. Chewable Tabs. (Biovail) Phenylephrine hydrochloride 10 mg, chlorpheniramine 2 mg, methscopolamine nitrate 1.25 mg, orange flavor. Chew. Tab. Bot. 100s. Rx.
Use: Upper respiratory combination, anticholinergic, antihistamine, decongestant.

•**daclizumab.** (dac-KLYE-zue-mab) USAN.
Use: Immunosuppressant.
See: Zenapax.

Dacodyl. (Major) **Tab.:** Bisacodyl 5 mg. Bot. 100s, 250s, 1000s. UD 100s. **Supp.:** Bisacodyl 10 mg. Box 12s, 100s. OTC.
Use: Laxative.

Dacriose. (Novartis Ophthalmics) Sodium chloride, potassium chloride, sodium hydroxide, sodium phosphate, benzalkonium chloride 0.01%, EDTA. Bot. 15 mL, 120 mL. OTC.
Use: Irrigant, ophthalmic.

•**dactinomycin.** (DAK-tih-no-MY-sin) USP 28.
Use: Antineoplastic; antibiotic.
See: Cosmegen.

Daily Cleaner. (Bausch & Lomb) Isotonic solution with sodium Cl, sodium phosphate, tyloxapol, hydroxyethylcellulose, polyvinyl alcohol with thimerosal 0.004%, EDTA 0.2%. Soln. Bot. 45 mL. OTC.
Use: Contact lens care.

Daily Conditioning Treatment. (Blairex) Padimate O 7.5%, oxybenzone 3.5%, petrolatum. Stick 11.4 g. SPF 15. OTC.
Use: Lip protectant.

Daily Vitamins. (Rugby) Vitamins A 2500 units, D 400 units, E 15 units, C 60 mg, B₁ 1.2 mg, B₂ 1.2 mg, B₆ 1.05 mg, B₁₂ 4.5 mcg, niacinamide 13.5 mg/5 mL. Bot. 273 mL, 473 mL. OTC.
Use: Vitamin supplement.

Daily Vitamins Tablets. (Kirkman) Vitamins A 5000 units, D 400 units, C 50 mg, B₁ 3 mg, B₂ 2.5 mg, B₆ 1 mg, B₁₂ 1 mcg, niacinamide 20 mg, d-calcium pantothenate 1 mg. Tab. Bot. 100s. OTC.
Use: Vitamin supplement.

Daily Vitamins w/Iron. (Kirkman) Vitamins A 5000 units, D 400 units, B₁ 2 mg, B₂ 2.5 mg, B₆ 1 mg, B₁₂ 1 mcg, niacinamide 20 mg, d-calcium pantothenate 1 mg, iron 18 mg. Tab. Bot. 100s. OTC.
Use: Vitamin supplement.

Daily-Vite w/Iron & Minerals. (Rugby) Iron 18 mg, vitamins A 5000 units, D 400 units, E 30 mg, B₁ 1.5 mg, B₂ 1.7 mg, B₃ 20 mg, B₅ 10 mg, B₆ 2 mg, B₁₂ 6 mcg, C 60 mg, folic acid 0.4 mg, Ca, Cl, Cr, Cu, I, K, Mg, Mn, Mo, P, Se, zinc 15 mg, biotin, vitamin K. Tab. Bot. 100s. OTC.
Use: Mineral, vitamin supplement.

Dairy Ease. (Blistex) Lactase 3300 FCC units, mannitol, sucrose. Tab. Bot. 60s, 100s. OTC.
Use: Digestive enzyme.

Dakin's Solution.
See: Sodium Hypochlorite Solution Diluted.

Dakin's Solution Full Strength. (Century) Sodium hypochlorite 0.5%. Soln. Bot. Pt, gal. OTC.
Use: Anti-infective, topical.

Dakin's Solution Half Strength. (Century) Sodium hypochlorite 0.25%. Soln. Bot. Pt. OTC.
Use: Anti-Infective, topical.

Dalalone. (Forest) Dexamethasone sodium phosphate 4 mg/mL, parabens, sodium bisulfite. Vial 5 mL. Rx.
Use: Corticosteroid.

Dalalone DP. (Forest) Dexamethasone acetate 16 mg/mL, polysorbate 80, carboxymethylcellulose, sodium bisulfite, EDTA, benzyl alcohol. Vial 1 mL, 5 mL. Rx.
Use: Corticosteroid.

d-ala-peptide t.
Use: Antiviral.

•**dalbavancin.** (dal-ba-VAN-sin) USAN.
Use: Antibiotic.

•**daledalin tosylate.** (dah-LEH-dah-lin TAH-sill-ate) USAN.
Use: Antidepressant.

•**dalfopristin.** (dal-FOE-priss-tin) USAN.
Use: Anti-infective.
W/Quinupristin.
See: Synercid.

Dallergy. (Laser) **Syr.**: Chlorpheniramine maleate 2 mg, phenylephrine hydrochloride 10 mg, methscopolamine nitrate 0.625 mg/5 mL. Bot. 473 mL. **Tab.**: Chlorpheniramine maleate 4 mg, phenylephrine hydrochloride 10 mg, methscopolamine nitrate 1.25 mg. Bot. 100s. **ER Tab.**: Chlorpheniramine maleate 12 mg, phenylephrine hydrochloride 20 mg, methscopolamine nitrate 2.5 mg. ER Tab. Bot. 100s. *Rx.*
Use: Upper respiratory combination, anticholinergic, antihistamine, decongestant.

Dallergy-D Syrup. (Laser) Chlorpheniramine maleate 2 mg, phenylephrine hydrochloride 5 mg/5 mL. Bot. 118 mL. *OTC.*
Use: Antihistamine, decongestant.

Dallergy-Jr. (Laser) **ER Cap.**: Phenylephrine hydrochloride 20 mg, chlorpheniramine maleate 4 mg, sucrose. Bot. 100s. **Susp.**: Phenylephrine tannate 20 mg, chlorpheniramine tannate 4 mg per 5 mL. 473 mL. *Rx.*
Use: Upper respiratory combination, antihistamine, decongestant.

Dalmane. (Valeant) Flurazepam hydrochloride 15 mg, 30 mg. Cap. Bot. 100s, 500s. *c-IV.*
Use: Sedative/hypnotic, nonbarbiturate.

•**dalteparin sodium.** (dal-TEH-puh-rin) USAN.
Use: Anticoagulant; antithrombotic; low molecular weight heparin.
See: Fragmin.

•**daltroban.** (DAL-troe-ban) USAN.
Use: Platelet aggregation inhibitor; immunosuppressant.

•**dalvastatin.** (DAL-vah-STAT-in) USAN.
Use: Antihyperlipidemic.

Damacet-P. (Mason) Hydrocodone bitartrate 5 mg, acetaminophen 500 mg. Tab. Bot. 100s, 500s. *c-III.*
Use: Analgesic combination; narcotic.

Damason-P. (Mason) Hydrocodone bitartrate 5 mg, aspirin 500 mg. Tab. Bot. 100s, 500s, 1000s. *c-III.*
Use: Analgesic combination; narcotic.

Dambose.
See: Inositol.

Danatrol. (Sanofi-Synthelabo) Danazol. Cap. *Rx.*
Use: Gonadotropin inhibitor.

•**danazol.** (DAN-uh-ZOLE) *USP 28.*
Use: Anterior pituitary suppressant, sex hormone.

danazol. (Various Mfr.) Danazol 50 mg, 100 mg, 200 mg. Cap. Bot. 60s (200 mg only), 100s, 500s (200 mg only). *Rx.*
Use: Anterior pituitary suppressant, sex hormone.

Dandruff Shampoo. (Walgreen) Zinc pyrithione 2 g/100 mL. Bot. 11 oz. Tube 7 oz. *OTC.*
Use: Antiseborrheic.

•**daniplestim.** (dan-ih-PLEH-stim) USAN.
Use: Antineutropenic; hematopoietic stimulant; treatment of chemotherapy-induced bone marrow suppression.

Danogar Tablets. (Sanofi-Synthelabo) Danazol. *Rx.*
Use: Gonadotropin inhibitor.

Danol Capsules. (Sanofi-Synthelabo) Danazol. *Rx.*
Use: Gonadotropin inhibitor.

Dantrium. (Procter & Gamble) Dantrolene sodium. Cap. **25 mg:** Bot. 100s, 500s, UD 100s; **50 mg:** Bot. 100s; **100 mg:** Bot. 100s, UD 100s. *Rx.*
Use: Muscle relaxant.

Dantrium IV. (Procter & Gamble) Dantrolene sodium 20 mg. Vial. 70 mL. *Rx.*
Use: Muscle relaxant.

•**dantrolene.** (dan-troe-LEEN) USAN.
Use: Muscle relaxant.

•**dantrolene sodium.** (dan-troe-LEEN) USAN.
Use: Muscle relaxant.
See: Dantrium.

Dapa Extra Strength Tablets. (Ferndale) Acetaminophen 500 mg. Bot. 50s, 100s, 1000s, UD 100s. *OTC.*
Use: Analgesic.

Dapco. (Schlicksup) Salicylamide 300 mg, butabarbital 15 mg. Tab. Bot. 100s, 1000s. *c-III.*
Use: Analgesic; hypnotic; sedative.

•**dapiprazole hydrochloride.** (DAP-ih-PRAY-zole) USAN.
Use: Alpha-adrenergic blocker; antiglaucoma agent; neuroleptic; psychotherapeutic agent.
See: Rēv-Eyes.

•**dapoxetine hydrochloride.** (dap-OX-eh-teen) USAN.
Use: Antidepressant.

•**dapsone.** (DAP-sone) *USP 28. Formerly Diaminodiphenylsulfone.*
Use: Leprostatic.

dapsone. (Jacobus) Dapsone 25 mg, 100 mg. Tab. Bot. 100s. *Rx.*
Use: Leprostatic.

Daptacel. (Aventis Pasteur) Diphtheria toxoid 15 Lf, tetanus toxoid 5 Lf, per-

tussis toxoid 10 mcg, hemagglutinin 5 mcg, pertactin 3 mcg, fimbriae types 2 and 3 5 mcg/0.5 mL. Inj. Single-dose vials. 2-phenoxyethanol 3.3 mg, aluminum 0.33 mg. *Rx.*
Use: Immunization.

●**daptomycin.** (DAP-toe-MY-sin) USAN.
Use: Anti-infective.
See: Cubicin.

Daragen. (Galderma) Collagen polypeptide, benzalkonium Cl in a mild amphoteric base. Shampoo. Bot. 8 oz. *OTC.*
Use: Dermatologic.

Daraprim. (GlaxoSmithKline) Pyrimethamine 25 mg. Lactose. Tab. Bot. 100s. *Rx.*
Use: Antimalarial.

Dara Soapless Shampoo. (Galderma) Purified water, potassium coco hydrolyzed protein, sulfated castor oil, pentasodium triphosphate, sodium benzoate, sodium lauryl sulfate, fragrance. Shampoo. Bot. 8 oz, 16 oz. *OTC.*
Use: Dermatologic, scalp.

darbepoetin alfa.
Use: Hematopoietic agent, recombinant human erythropoietin.
See: Aranesp.

●**darbufelone mesylate.** (DAR-byoo-fehlone MEH-sih-late) USAN.
Use: Anti-inflammatory; antiarthritic.

Darco G-60. (AstraZeneca) Activated carbon from lignite.
Use: Purifier.

●**darglitazone sodium.** (dahr-GLIH-tahzone) USAN.
Use: Oral hypoglycemic.

●**darifenacin hydrobromide.** (dar-ih-FEN-ah-sin)
Use: Treatment of overactive bladder.
See: Enablex.

●**darodipine.** (DA-row-dih-PEEN) USAN.
Use: Antihypertensive; bronchodilator; vasodilator.

Darvocet A500. (aaiPharma) Propoxyphene napsylate 100 mg, acetaminophen 500 mg. Tab. 100s. *c-iv.*
Use: Narcotic analgesic.

Darvocet-N 50. (aaiPharma) Propoxyphene napsylate 50 mg, acetaminophen 325 mg. Tab. *RxPak* 100s, 500s, UD 100s. *c-iv.*
Use: Narcotic analgesic.

Darvocet-N 100. (aaiPharma) Propoxyphene napsylate 100 mg, acetaminophen 650 mg. Tab. Bot. 100s (Rx Pak) 500s, UD 100s, 500s, RN 500s. *c-iv.*
Use: Analgesic combination; narcotic.

Darvon. (Eli Lilly) Propoxyphene hydrochloride 65 mg. Pulv. Bot. 100s. Rx

Pak 500s; Blister pkg. 10 × 10s; UD 20 rolls 25s. *c-iv.*
Use: Analgesic combination; narcotic.

Darvon Compound 65 Pulvules. (Eli Lilly) Propoxyphene hydrochloride 65 mg, aspirin 389 mg, caffeine 32.4 mg. Pulv. Bot. 100s, Rx Pak 500s. *c-iv.*
Use: Analgesic combination; narcotic.

Darvon Compound 32 Pulvules. (aaiPharma) Propoxyphene hydrochloride 32 mg, aspirin 389 mg, caffeine 32.4 mg. Cap. 100s. *c-iv.*
Use: Analgesic combination; narcotic.

Darvon-N. (aaiPharma) Propoxyphene napsylate 100 mg, lactose. Film coated. Tab. Bot. 100s, 500s, UD 100s. *c-iv.*
Use: Opioid analgesic.

Darvon Pulvules. (aaiPharma) Propoxyphene hydrochloride 65 mg. Cap. Bot. 100s, 500s. *c-iv.*
Use: Opioid analgesic.

●**dasantafil.** (da-SAN-ta-fil) USAN.
Use: Erectile dysfunction.

Da-Sed. (Sheryl) Butabarbital 0.5 g. Tab. Bot. 100s. *c-iii.*
Use: Hypnotic; sedative.

Dasin. (GlaxoSmithKline) Ipecac 3 mg, acetylsalicylic acid 130 mg, camphor 15 mg, caffeine 8 mg, atropine sulfate 0.13 mg. Cap. Bot. 100s, 500s. *Rx.*
Use: Analgesic; anticholinergic; antispasmodic.

daturine hydrobromide.
See: Hyoscyamine Salts.

D.A. II. (Biovail) Chlorpheniramine maleate 4 mg, phenylephrine hydrochloride 10 mg, methscopolamine nitrate 1.25 mg. SR Tab. Bot. 100s. *Rx.*
Use: Upper respiratory combination, anticholinergic, antihistamine, decongestant.

daunorubicin citrate liposomal.
Use: Antibiotic.
See: DaunoXome.

daunorubicin citrate liposome.
Use: Treatment of advanced HIV-associated Kaposi sarcoma. [Orphan Drug]
See: DaunoXome.

●**daunorubicin hydrochloride.** (DAW-no-RUE-bih-sin) *USP 28.*
Tall Man: DAUNOrubicin
Use: Antineoplastic.
See: Cerubidine.

daunorubicin hydrochloride. (Various Mfr.) Daunorubicin hydrochloride 20 mg, 50 mg, mannitol 100 mg, 250 mg. Pow. for Inj., lyophilized. Single-dose vial 10 mL (20 mg only),

20 mL (50 mg only). *Rx.*
Use: Antineoplastic.

daunorubicin hydrochloride for injection. (Various Mfr.) Daunorubicin hydrochloride for Injection 5 mg/mL (equivalent to 5.34 mg daunorubicin hydrochloride), preservative free. Single-use vial. 4 mL, 10 mL. *Rx.*
Use: Antibiotic.

DaunoXome. (Gilead Sciences) Daunorubicin citrate liposomal 2 mg/mL (equivalent to daunorubicin base 50 mg). Inj. Single-use vials and single-unit packs. *Rx.*
Use: Antibiotic; treatment of advanced HIV-associated Kaposi sarcoma.

Davitamon K.
See: Menadione.

Davosil. (Colgate Oral) Silicon carbide in glycerin base. Jar 8 oz, 10 oz. *OTC.*
Use: Agent for oral hygiene.

Dayalets + Iron. (Abbott) Vitamins B_1 1.5 mg, B_2 1.7 mg, B_6 2 mg, B_{12} 6 mcg, C 60 mg, A 5000 units, D 400 units, E 30 units, iron 18 mg, folic acid 0.4 mg, niacinamide 20 mg. Filmtab. Bot. 100s. *OTC.*
Use: Mineral, vitamin supplement.

Daycare. (Procter & Gamble) Pseudoephedrine hydrochloride 10 mg, dextromethorphan HBr 3.3 mg, guaifenesin 33.3 mg, acetaminophen 108 mg, alcohol 10%, saccharin. Expectorant Liq. Bot. 180 mL, 300 mL. *OTC.*
Use: Analgesic, antitussive, decongestant, expectorant.

Dayhist-1. (Major) Clemastine fumarate 1.34 mg (equivalent to clemastine 1 mg), lactose. Tab. Pkg. 8s. *OTC.*
Use: Antihistimine, non-selective ethanolamine.

Day-Night Comtrex. (Bristol-Myers Squibb) Pseudoephedrine hydrochloride 30 mg, chlorpheniramine maleate 2 mg, dextromethorphan HBr 10 mg, acetaminophen 325 mg. Tab. Pkg. 6s. *OTC.*
Use: Analgesic, antihistamine, antitussive, decongestant.

Daypro. (Pharmacia) Oxaprozin 600 mg. Capl. Bot. 100s, 500s, UD 100s. *Rx.*
Use: Analgesic; NSAID.

Daypro ALTA. (Pharmacia) Oxaprozin potassium 678 mg (equivalent to 600 mg oxaprozin). FC Tab. Bot. 100s, 500s, UD 100s. *Rx.*
Use: Analgesic; NSAID.

Day Tab. (Towne) Vitamins A 5000 units, D 400 units, B_1 15 mg, B_2 10 mg, B_6 5 mg, B_{12} 5 mcg, folic acid 400 mcg, pantothenic acid 10 mg, zinc 15 mg,

copper 2 mg, C 600 mg, niacinamide 20 mg. Tab. Bot. 100s, 200s. *OTC.*
Use: Mineral, vitamin supplement.

Day Tab Essential. (Towne) Vitamins A 5000 units, D 400 units, E 15 units, C 60 mg, folic acid 0.4 mg, B_1 1.5 mg, B_2 1.7 mg, B_6 2 mg, B_{12} 6 mcg, niacin 20 mg. Tab. Bot. 200s. *OTC.*
Use: Vitamin supplement.

Day Tab Plus Iron. (Towne) Iron 18 mg, vitamins A 5000 units, D 400 units, B_1 1.5 mg, B_2 1.7 mg, B_6 2 mg, B_{12} 6 mcg, pantothenic acid 10 mg, folic acid 0.1 mg, niacinamide 20 mg, C 60 mg. Tab. Bot. 100s. *OTC.*
Use: Mineral, vitamin supplement.

Day Tabs, New. (Towne) Vitamins A 5000 units, E 15 units, D 400 units, C 60 mg, folic acid 0.4 mg, B_1 1.5 mg, B_2 1.7 mg, B_6 20 mg, B_{12} 6 mcg, niacin 20 mg. Tab. Bot. 100s, 250s. *OTC.*
Use: Vitamin supplement.

Day Tabs Plus Iron, New. (Towne) Vitamins A 5000 units, E 15 units, D 400 units, C 60 mg, folic acid 0.4 mg, B_1 1.5 mg, B_2 1.7 mg, B_6 20 mg, B_{12} 6 mcg, niacin 20 mg, iron 18 mcg. Tab. Bot. 250s. *OTC.*
Use: Mineral, vitamin supplement.

Day Tab Stress Complex. (Towne) Vitamins A 5000 units, C 600 mg, B_1 15 mg, B_2 10 mg, B_6 5 mg, B_{12} 6 mcg, niacin 100 mg, D 400 units, E 30 units, folic acid 400 mcg, pantothenic acid 20 mg, iron 18 mg, zinc 15 mg, copper 2 mg. Tab. Bot. 60s. *OTC.*
Use: Mineral, vitamin supplement.

Day Tab with Iron. (Towne) Vitamins A 5000 units, D 400 units, E 15 units, C 60 mg, folic acid 1.5 mg, B_1 15 mg, B_2 1.7 mg, B_6 2 mg, B_{12} 6 mcg, niacin 20 mg, iron 18 mg. Tab. Bot. 200s. *Rx.*
Use: Mineral, vitamin supplement.

Dayto-Anase. (Dayton) Bromelains 50,000 units (protease activity). Tab. Bot. 60s. *OTC.*
Use: Enzyme.

Dayto Himbin. (Dayton) Yohimbine 5.4 mg. Tab. Bot. 60s. *Rx.*
Use: Alpha-adrenergic blocker.

•**dazadrol maleate.** (DAY-zah-drole) USAN.
Use: Antidepressant.

•**dazepinil hydrochloride.** (dahz-EH-pih-NILL) USAN.
Use: Antidepressant.

•**dazmegrel.** (DAZE-meh-grell) USAN.
Use: Inhibitor (thromboxane synthetase).

•dazopride fumarate. (DAY-zoe-PRIDE) USAN.
Use: Peristaltic stimulant.
•dazoxiben hydrochloride. (DAZE-OX-ih-ben) USAN.
Use: Antithrombotic.
Dbed. Dibenzylethylenediamine dipenicillin G.
Use: Anti-infective; penicillin.
DB Electrode Paste. (Day-Baldwin) Tube 5%.
DCA.
See: Desoxycorticosterone Acetate.
DCF.
Use: Anti-infective.
See: Nipent.
DCP. (Towne) Calcium 180 mg, phosphorus 105 mg, vitamins D 66.7 units. Tab. Bot. 100s. *OTC*
Use: Mineral, vitamin supplement.
DC Softgels. (Ivax) Docusate calcium 240 mg. Softgel Cap. Bot. 100s, 500s. *OTC.*
Use: Laxative.
DC 240. (Ivax) Docusate calcium 240 mg. Cap. Bot. 100s, 500s. *OTC.*
Use: Laxative.
DDAVP. (Aventis) Desmopressin acetate.
Tab.: 0.1 mg, 0.2 mg, lactose. Bot. 100s. **Nasal Soln.:** 0.1 mg/mL (0.1 mg equals ≈ 400 units arginine vasopressin). Nasal Spray Pump. Citric acid monohydrate 1.7 mg, disodium phosphate dihydrate 3 mg, benzalkonium chloride solution (50%) 0.2 mg/mL, sodium chloride 7.5mg/mL. Bot. 5 mL w/spray pump (50 doses of 10 mcg). Rhinal tube delivery system. Chlorobutanol 5 mg/mL, sodium chloride 9 mg, chlorobutanol 5 mg/mL. Vial 2.5 mL w/2 applicator tubes. **Inj.:** 4 mcg/mL, sodium chloride 9 mg/mL. Amp. 1 mL, multidose vial 10 mL. *Rx.*
Use: Posterior pituitary hormone.
DDAVP Spray. (Aventis) Desmopressin acetate 0.1 mg, chlorobutanol 5 mg/mL. Bot. 5 mL. Vial 2.5 mL w/applicator tubes for nasal administration. *Rx.*
Use: Antidiuretic.
ddC. Dideoxycytidine.
Use: Antiviral.
See: HIVID.
ddl. Didanosine.
Use: Antiviral.
DDS.
See: Dapsone.
DDT.
See: Chlorophenothane.
deacetyllanatoside C.
See: Deslanoside.

deadly nightshade leaf.
See: Belladonna Leaf.
1-deamino-8-d-arginine vasopressin. Desmopressin acetate.
Use: Hormone.
See: Concentraid. DDAVP.
deba.
See: Barbital.
Debacterol. (Epien Medical) Sulfuric acid 30%, sulfonated phenolics 50%. Liq. 1.5 mL *Rx.*
Use: Mouth and throat product.
Debrisan. (Johnson & Johnson) Dextranomer. **Beads:** Spherical hydrophilic 0.1 to 0.3 mm diameter. Bot. 25 g, 60 g, 120 g. Pk. 7 × 4 g, 14 × 14 g. **Paste:** 10 g. Foil packets 6s. *OTC.*
Use: Dermatologic, wound therapy.
•debrisoquin sulfate. (deh-RICE-oh-kwin) USAN.
Use: Antihypertensive.
Debrox. (Hoechst) Carbamide peroxide 6.5% in anhydrous glycerol. Plastic squeeze bot. 0.5 oz, 1 oz. *OTC.*
Use: Otic preparation.
Deca-Bon. (Barrows) Vitamins A 3000 units, D 400 units, C 60 mg, B_1 1 mg, B_2 1.2 mg, B_6 1 mg, B_{12} 1 mcg, niacinamide 8 mg, panthenol 3 mg, biotin 30 mcg/0.6 mL. Drops. Bot. 50 mL. *OTC.*
Use: Vitamin supplement.
Decaderm. (Merck & Co.) Dexamethasone 0.1% w/isopropyl myristate gel, wood alcohols, refined lanolin alcohol, microcrystalline wax, anhydrous citric acid, anhydrous sodium phosphate dibasic. Tube 30 g. *Rx.*
Use: Corticosteroid.
Decadron. (Merck) Dexamethasone 0.5 mg, 0.75 mg. Lactose. Tab. 12s (0.75 mg only), 100s. *Rx.*
Use: Adrenocortical steroid, glucocorticoid.
Decadron Phosphate. (Merck & Co.) Dexamethasone sodium phosphate 0.1%. Ophth. Soln. Ocumeter dispenser 5 mL. *Rx.*
Use: Corticosteroid, ophthalmic.
Decadron Phosphate Injection. (Merck & Co.) Dexamethasone sodium phosphate 4 mg/mL, 24 mg/mL, creatinine 8 mg, sodium citrate 10 mg, EDTA 0.5 mg (24 mg/mL only), sodium hydroxide to adjust pH, sodium bisulfite 1 mg, methylparaben 1.5 mg, propylparaben 0.2 mg/mL. **4 mg/mL:** Vial 1 mL, 5 mL, 25 mL. **24 mg/mL (for IV use only):** Vial 5 mL, 10 mL. *Rx.*
Use: Corticosteroid.

Decagen. (Ivax) Iron 18 mg, vitamins A 5000 units, D 400 units, E 30 units, B_1 1.7 mg, B_2 2 mg, B_3 20 mg, B_5 10 mg, B_6 3 mg, B_{12} 6 mcg, C 60 mg, folic acid 0.4 mg, Ca, Cl, Cr, Cu, B, I, K, Mg, Mn, Mo, Ni, P, Se, Si, Sn, V, Zn 15 mg, vitamin K, biotin 30 mcg. Tab. Bot. 130s. *OTC.*
Use: Mineral, vitamin supplement.
Decaject. (Merz) Dexamethasone sodium phosphate 4 mg/mL. Vial 5 mL, 10 mL. *Rx.*
Use: Corticosteroid.
Decaject-L.A. (Merz) Dexamethasone acetate 8 mg/mL suspension, polysorbate 80, carboxymethylcellulose, sodium bisulfite, EDTA, benzyl alcohol. Inj. Vial 5 mL. *Rx.*
Use: Corticosteroid.
Decalix. (Pharmed) Dexamethasone 0.5 mg/5 mL. Bot. 100 mL. *Rx.*
Use: Corticosteroid.
Decameth. (Foy Laboratories) Dexamethasone sodium phosphate injection 4 mg/5 mL Inj. Vial. *Rx.*
Use: Corticosteroid.
Decameth L.A. (Foy Laboratories) Dexamethasone sodium phosphate injection 8 mg/mL. Inj. Vial 5 mL. *Rx.*
Use: Corticosteroid.
Decameth Tablets. (Foy Laboratories) Dexamethasone 0.75 mg. Bot. 1000s. *Rx.*
Use: Corticosteroid.
Decapryn. (Hoechst) Doxylamine succinate 12.5 mg. Tab. Bot. 100s. *OTC.*
Use: Antihistamine.
Decasone Injection. (Forest) Dexamethasone sodium phosphate equivalent to dexamethasone phosphate 4 mg/mL. Vial 5 mL. *Rx.*
Use: Corticosteroid.
Decavac. (Aventis Pasteur) Diphtheria 2 Lf units and tetanus 5 Lf units per 0.5 mL dose. Preservative free. Inj. 0.5 mL *Luer-Lok* syringe (with not more than 0.28 mg of aluminum and trace thimerosal [up to 0.3 mcg mercury/dose]). *Rx.*
Use: Agent for active immunization.
•**decavitamin.** (dek-a-VYE-ta-min) *USP 28.* Vitamins A 4000 units, D 400 units, C 70 mg, calcium pantothenate 10 mg, B_1 2 mg, B_2 2 mg, B_6 2 mg, B_{12} 5 mcg, folic acid 100 mcg, nicotinamide 20 mg. Cap. or Tab. *OTC.*
Use: Vitamin supplement.
Decholin. (Bayer Corp. (Consumer Div.)) Dehydrocholic acid 250 mg. Tab. Bot. 100s, 500s. *OTC.*
Use: Hydrocholeretic.

Decicain. Tetracaine hydrochloride.
•**decitabine.** (deh-SIGH-tah-BEAN) USAN.
Use: Antineoplastic.
declaben. (DEH-klah-BEN) *Formerly lodelaben.*
Use: Antiarthritic; emphysema therapy adjunct.
Declomycin. (ESP Pharma) Demeclocycline hydrochloride 150 mg, 300 mg. Tab. Bot. 100s (150 mg only), 48s (300 mg only). *Rx.*
Use: Anti-infective; tetracycline.
Decodult. (Wesley Pharmacal) Phenylephrine hydrochloride 5 mg, chlorpheniramine maleate 2 mg, acetaminophen 300 mg. Tab. Bot. 1000s. *OTC.*
Use: Upper respiratory combination, decongestant, antihistamine, analgesic.
Decofed. (Various Mfr.) Pseudoephedrine hydrochloride 30 mg/5 mL. Syr. Bot. 118 mL, 473 mL. *OTC.*
Use: Nasal decongestant, aryalkylamine.
Decohistine DH. (Morton Grove) Pseudoephedrine hydrochloride 30 mg, chlorpheniramine maleate 2 mg, codeine phosphate 10 mg, alcohol 5.8%, sugar, menthol, parabens, sorbitol, grape/honey flavor. Liq. Bot. 118 mL, 473 mL, 3.8 L. *c-v.*
Use: Upper respiratory combination, antihistamine, antitussive, decongestant.
Decolate. (Wesley) Phenylephrine hydrochloride 5 mg, chlorpheniramine maleate 4 mg, guaifenesin 100 mg. Tab. Bot. 1000s. *Rx.*
Use: Upper respiratory combination, decongestant, antihistamine, expectorant.
Deconamine. (Kenwood) **Syr.:** Chlorpheniramine maleate 2 mg, pseudoephedrine hydrochloride 30 mg/5 mL, sorbitol, sucrose, grape flavor, alcohol and dye free. Bot. 473 mL. **Tab.:** Chlorpheniramine maleate 4 mg, pseudoephedrine hydrochloride 60 mg, lactose. Bot. 100s. *Rx.*
Use: Upper respiratory combination, antihistamine, decongestant.
Deconamine SR Capsules. (Kenwood) Chlorpheniramine maleate 8 mg, pseudoephedrine hydrochloride 120 mg, sugar. SR Cap. Bot. 100s, 500s, 1000s. *Rx.*
Use: Upper respiratory combination, antihistamine, decongestant.
decongestant, analgesic, antihistamine, antitussive combinations.
Use: Upper respiratory combination.

See: Analgesic, Antihistamine, Antitussive, Decongestant Combinations.

decongestant, analgesic, antihistamine combinations.
Use: Upper respiratory combination.
See: Analgesic, Antihistamine, and Decongestant combinations.

decongestant, analgesic, antitussive, expectorant combinations.
Use: Upper respiratory combination.
See: Analgesic, Antitussive, Decongestant, Expectorant Combinations.

decongestant and analgesic combinations.
Use: Upper respiratory combination.
See: Analgesic and Decongestant Combinations.

decongestant and antihistamine combinations.
Use: Upper respiratory combination.
See: Antihistamine and Decongestant combinations.

decongestant and expectorant combinations.
Use: Upper respiratory combination.
See: AquatabD.
Broncholate.
Bronkaid Dual Action.
Coldmist JR.
Coldmist LA.
Congestac.
Deconsal II.
Defen-LA.
Durasal II.
Duratuss.
Duratuss GP.
Dynafed Asthma Relief.
Dynex.
Endal.
Entex.
Entex LA.
Entex PSE.
GFN/PSE.
GFN 600/Phenylephrine 20.
GP-500.
G/P 1200/60.
Guaifed.
Guaifed-PD.
Guaifenesin/Pseudoephedrine hydrochloride.
Guaifenex GP.
Guaifenex PSE 120.
Guaifenex PSE 60.
Guaifenex-Rx
GuaiMAX-D.
Guaipax PSE.
Guai-Vent/PSE.
Guiatuss PE.
H 9600 SR.
Iosal II.
KIE.

Liquibid-D.
Maxifed.
Maxifed-G.
Miraphen PSE.
Mini Two-Way Action.
Nasatab LA.
PanMist JR.
PanMist LA.
PanMist-S.
Primatene.
Profen Forte.
Profen II.
Pseudovent.
Pseudovent-PED.
Refenesen Plus Severe Strength Cough & Cold Medicine.
Rescon-GG.
Respa-1st.
Respaire-120 SR.
Roopairo 60 SR.
Robafen PE.
Robitussin Cold Sinus & Congestion.
Robitussin PE.
Robitussin Severe Congestion.
Severe Congestion Tussin.
Sinutab Non-Drying.
Stamoist E.
Cudafed Non Drowsy Non-Drying Sinus.
Sudal 60/500.
Thera-Hist Expectorant Chest Congestion.
Touro LA.
Triacting
Triaminic Chest Congestion.
V-Dec-M.
Versacaps.

decongestant, anticholinergic, antihistamine, antitussive combinations.
Use: Upper respiratory combination.
See: Anticholinergic, Antihistamine, Antitussive, Decongestant Combinations.

decongestant, anticholinergic, antihistamine combinations.
Use: Upper respiratory combination.
See: Anticholinergic, Antihistamine, Decongestant Combinations.

decongestant, antihistamine, and analgesic combinations.
Use: Upper respiratory combination.
See: Analgesic, Antihistamine, and Decongestant Combinations.

decongestant, antihistamine, and antitussive combinations.
Use: Upper respiratory combination.
See: Antihistamine, Antitussive, Decongestant Combinations.

decongestant, antihistamine, and expectorant combinations.
Use: Upper respiratory combination.

See: Antihistamine, Decongestant, and Expectorant Combinations.

decongestant, antihistamine, antitussive, expectorant combinations.
Use: Upper respiratory combination.
See: Antihistamine, Antitussive, Decongestant, Expectorant Combinations.

decongestant, antitussive, and expectorant combinations.
Use: Upper respiratory combination.
See: Antitussive, Decongestant and Expectorant Combinations.

Decongestant Formula Mediquell.
(Parke-Davis) Dextromethorphan HBr 30 mg, pseudoephedrine hydrochloride 60 mg. Square.
Use: Antitussive, decongestant.

decongestant, nasal.
See: Nasal decongestants.

Deconomed. (Iomed) Chlorpheniramine maleate 8 mg, pseudoephedrine hydrochloride 120 mg, sucrose, parabens. SR Cap. Bot. 100s, 500s. *Rx.*
Use: Upper respiratory combination, antihistamine, decongestant.

Deconsal II. (Cornerstone Biopharma) Phenylephrine hydrochloride 20 mg, guaifenesin 375 mg. Sucrose. ER Tab. Bot. 30s, 100s. *Rx.*
Use: Upper respiratory combination, decongestant, expectorant.

●**dectaflur.** (DECK-tah-flure) USAN.
Use: Dental caries agent.

Decubitex. (I.C.P. Pharmaceuticals)
Oint.: Biebrich scarlet red sulfonated 0.1%, balsam Peru, castor oil, zinc oxide, starch, sodium propionate, parabens. Jar 15 g, 60 g, 120 g, lb. **Pow.:** Biebrich scarlet red sulfonated 0.1%, starch, zinc oxide, sodium propionate, parabens. Bot. 30 g, UD 1 g. *OTC.*
Use: Antipruritic; dermatologic, wound therapy; emollient.

Decylenes. (Rugby) Undecylenic acid, zinc undecylenate. Oint. Tube 30 g, lb. *OTC.*
Use: Antifungal, topical.

Deep-Down Pain Relief Rub. (GlaxoSmithKline) Methyl salicylate 15%, menthol 5%, camphor 0.5%. Tube 1.25 oz, 3 oz. *OTC.*
Use: Analgesic, topical.

Deep Strength Musterole. (Schering-Plough) Methyl salicylate 30%, menthol 3%, methyl nicotinate 0.5%. Tube 1.25 oz, 3 oz. *OTC.*
Use: Analgesic, topical.

●**deferasirox.** (de-FER-a-sir-ox) USAN.
Use: Iron chelator.

●**deferoxamine.** (DEE-fer-OX-ah-meen) USAN.
Use: Chelating agent (iron).

●**deferoxamine hydrochloride.** (DEE-fer-OX-ah-meen) USAN.
Use: Chelating agent for iron.

●**deferoxamine mesylate.** (DEE-fer-OX-ah-meen) *USP 28.*
Use: Iron depleter; antidote to iron poisoning; chelating agent.
See: Desferal Mesylate.

deferoxamine mesylate. (Hospira) Deferoxamine mesylate 500 mg, 2 g. Pow. for Inj., lyophilized. Vials. *Rx.*
Use: Detoxification agent, chelating agent.

defibrotide. (Crinos International)
Use: Thrombotic thrombocytopenic purpura. [Orphan Drug]

Deficol. (Vangard Labs, Inc.) Bisacodyl 5 mg. Tab. Bot. 100s, 1000s. *OTC.*
Use: Laxative.

Definity. (Bristol-Myers Squibb) Octafluoropropane 6.52 mg/mL in lipid-coated microspheres, preservative free. Inj. Single-use vial 2 mL. Requires activation with a *Vialmix* (not included). *Rx.*
Use: Radiopaque agent, parenteral agent.

●**deflazacort.** (deh-FLAZE-ah-cart) USAN.
Use: Anti-inflammatory.

Degas. (Invamed) Simethicone 80 mg, sucrose, mannitol. Chew. Tab. Bot. 100s. *OTC.*
Use: Antiflatulent.

Degest 2. (Akorn) Naphazoline hydrochloride 0.012%. Bot. 15 mL. *OTC.*
Use: Decongestant, ophthalmic.

Dehistine. (Cypress) Phenylephrine hydrochloride 10 mg, chlorpheniramine maleate 2 mg, methscopolamine nitrate 1.25 mg/5 mL, root beer flavor, alcohol free. Syr. Bot. 473 mL. *Rx.*
Use: Upper respiratory combination, decongestant, antihistamine, anticholinergic.

dehydrex. (Holles)
Use: Recurrent corneal erosion. [Orphan Drug]

dehydrocholate sodium inj. *USP 28.*
Use: Relief of liver congestion; diagnosis of cardiac failure.
See: Decholin Sodium.

7-dehydrocholesterol, activated. (Various Mfr.) Vitamin D-3.
Use: Vitamin supplement.

●**dehydrocholic acid.** (dee-HIGH-droe-KOLE-ik) *USP 28.*
Use: Orally, hydrocholeretic and choleretic.

See: Atrocholin.
Cholan-DH.
Decholin.
Dilabil.
Ketocholanic Acid.
Neocholan.
Procholon.
W/Amylolytic and proteolytic enzymes, desoxycholic acid.
See: Bilezyme.
W/Bile, homatropine methylbromide, pepsin.
See: Biloric.
W/Bile, homatropine methylbromide, phenobarbital.
See: Bilamide.
W/Bile extract, pepsin, pancreatin.
See: Progestive.
W/Desoxycholic acid.
See: Combichole.
Ketosox.
W/Docusate sodium.
See: Dubbalax-B.
Dubbalax-N.
Neolax.
W/Docusate sodium, phenolphthalein.
See: Bolax.
Tripalax.
W/Homatropine methylbromide.
See: Cholan V.
Homachol.
W/Methscopolamine, ox bile, amobarbital.
See: Hydrochol Plus.
W/Ox bile, homatropine methylbromide, phenobarbital.
See: Bilamide.
W/Pancreatin, pepsin, ox bile, belladonna extract.
See: Canz.
W/Pepsin, pancreatin enzyme concentrate, cellulase.
See: Cholan-HMB.
W/Phenobarbital, homatropine methylbromide, gerilase, geriprotase, desoxycholic acid.
See: Bilezyme Plus.
dehydrocholin.
Use: Hydrocholeretic.
See: Dehydrocholic acid.
dehydrodesoxycholic acid.
See: Cholanic acid.
dehydroepiandrosterone. (Genelabs Technologics, Inc.)
Use: Treatment of systemic lupus erythematosus (SLE). [Orphan Drug]
dehydroepiandrosterone sulfate sodium. (Pharmadigm)
Use: Treat serious burns; accelerate re-epithelialization of donor sites in autologous skin grafting. [Orphan Drug]

DEKA. (Dayton) Dextromethorphan hydrobromide 15 mg, guaifenesin 100 mg, pseudoephedrine hydrochloride 15 mg, dexbrompheniramine maleate 0.5 mg per 5 mL. Alcohol free. EDTA, saccharin, sucrose, parabens. Grape flavor. Liq. 120 mL. Rx.
Use: Antitussive and expectorant.
DEKA Pediatric. (Dayton) Pseudoephedrine hydrochloride 12.5 mg, dextromethorphan hydrobromide 4 mg, guaifenesin 40 mg, dexbrompheniramine maleate 0.5 mg per mL. Alcohol free. EDTA, parabens, saccharin, sucrose. Grape flavor. Drops. 30 mL with dropper. Rx.
Use: Pediatric antitussive and expectorant.
Dekasol. (Seatrace) Dexamethasone phosphate 4 mg/ml Vial 5 mL, 10 mL. Rx.
Use: Corticosteroid.
Dekasol L.A. (Seatrace) Dexamethasone acetate 8 mg/mL. Vial 5 mL. Rx.
Use: Corticosteroid.
De-Koff. (Whiteworth Towne) Terpin hydrate w/dextromethorphan. Elix. Bot. 4 oz. OTC.
Use: Antitussive, expectorant.
Delacort Lotion. (Mericon Industries) Hydrocortisone 0.5%. Bot. 4 oz. OTC.
Use: Corticosteroid, topical.
•**delapril hydrochloride.** (DELL-ah-prill) USAN.
Use: Antihypertensive; angiotensin-converting enzyme inhibitor.
Del Aqua-10. (Del-Ray) Benzoyl peroxide 10%. 42.5 g. Rx.
Use: Dermatologic, acne.
Delaquin. (Schlicksup) Hydrocortisone 0.5%, iodoquin 3%. Lot. Bot. 3 oz. Rx.
Use: Antifungal; corticosteroid.
Delatest. (Dunhall Pharmaceuticals, Inc.) Testosterone enanthate 100 mg/mL, chlorobutanol in sesame oil. Amp. 10 mL. c-III.
Use: Androgen.
Delatestadiol. (Dunhall Pharmaceuticals, Inc.) Testosterone enanthate 90 mg, estradiol valerate 4 mg/mL, chlorobutanol in sesame oil. Amp. 10 mL. Rx.
Use: Androgen, estrogen combination.
Delatestryl. (Savient) Testosterone enanthate 200 mg/mL in sesame oil, chlorobutanol 5 mg. Inj. Multidose vial 5 mL, single dose syr. w/needle 1 mL. c-III.
Use: Sex hormone, androgen.
•**delavirdine mesylate.** (de-la-VIR-deen) USAN.
Use: Antiretroviral, non-nucleoside reverse transcriptase inhibitor.

See: Rescriptor.

Delcid. (GlaxoSmithKline) Aluminum hydroxide 600 mg, magnesium hydroxide 665 mg/5 mL, alcohol 0.3%, saccharin. Bot. 8 oz. *OTC.*
Use: Antacid.

Del-Clens. (Del-Ray) Soapless cleanser. Bot. 8 oz. *OTC.*
Use: Dermatologic, cleanser.

Delco-Lax. (Delco) Bisacodyl 5 mg. Tab. Bot. 1000s. *OTC.*
Use: Laxative.

Delcort. (Lee) Hydrocortisone 0.5%, 1%. Cream. Pack. 1 g, 20 g, 1 lb. (1% only). *OTC.*
Use: Corticosteroid, topical.

Delcozine. (Delco) Phendimetrazine tartrate 70 mg. Tab. Bot. 1000s, 5000s. *c-III.*
Use: Anorexiant.

• **delequamine hydrochloride.** (deh-LEH-kwah-meen) USAN.
Use: Anti-impotence agent.

Delestrec. Estradiol 17-undecanoate. *Rx.*
Use: Estrogen.

Delestrogen. (Monarch) Estradiol valerate. **10 mg/mL:** In sesame oil, chlorobutanol. Multidose Vial 5 mL. **20 mg/mL, 40 mg/mL:** In castor oil, benzyl benzoate, benzyl alcohol. Multidose Vial 5 mL. *Rx.*
Use: Estrogen.

Delfen Contraceptive Foam. (Johnson & Johnson) Nonoxynol-9 12.5% in an oil-in-water emulsion at pH 4.5 to 5. Starter can with applicator 20 g. Refill 20 g, 42 g. *OTC.*
Use: Contraceptive, spermicide.

• **deligoparin sodium.** (de-li-GOE-pa-rin) USAN.
Use: Inflammatory bowel disease.

delinal. Propenzolate hydrochloride.

• **delmadinone acetate.** (del-MAD-ih-nohn ASS-eh-tate) USAN.
Use: Antiandrogen; antiestrogen; hormone, progestin.

Del-Mycin. (Del-Ray) Erythromycin 2%, ethyl alcohol 66%. Topical soln. Bot. 60 mL. *Rx.*
Use: Dermatologic, acne.

Del-Stat. (Del-Ray) Abradant cleaner. Jar 2 oz. *OTC.*
Use: Dermatologic, acne.

Delsym. (Celltech) Dextromethorphan HBr 30 mg/5 mL, alcohol 0.26%, sodium 5 mg/5 mL, corn syrup, sucrose, parabens, orange flavor. ER Oral Susp. Bot. 89 mL. *OTC.*
Use: Antitussive.

Delta-Cortef. (Pharmacia) Prednisolone 5 mg. Tab. Bot. 100s, 500s. *Rx.*
Use: Corticosteroid.

Deltacortone. Prednisone.
Use: Corticosteroid.

Delta-Cortril. Prednisolone.
Use: Corticosteroid.

Delta-D. (Freeda) Cholecalciferol (Vitamin D₃) 400 units. Tab. Bot. 250s, 500s. *OTC.*
Use: Vitamin supplement.

• **deltafilcon a.** (DELL-tah-FILL-kahn A) USAN.
Use: Contact lens material, hydrophilic.

• **deltafilcon b.** (DELL-tah-FILL-kahn B) USAN.
Use: Contact lens material, hydrophilic.

delta-1-cortisone.
Use: Corticosteroid.
See: Deltasone.

delta-1-hydrocortisone.
Use: Corticosteroid.
See: Prednisolone.

Deltasone. (Pharmacia) Prednisone. **2.5 mg:** Tab. Bot. 100s. **5 mg:** Tab. Bot. 100s, 500s, UD 100s, Dosepak 21s. **10 mg, 20 mg:** Tab. Bot. 100s, 500s, UD 100s. *Rx.*
Use: Corticosteroid.

Deltastab.
Use: Corticosteroid.
See: Prednisolone.

• **deltibant.** (DELL-tih-bant) USAN.
Use: Antagonist (bradykinin).

Del-Trac. (Del-Ray) Acne lotion. Bot. 2 oz. *OTC.*
Use: Dermatologic, acne.

• **delucemine hydrochloride.** (de-LOO-se-meen) USAN.
Use: Neuroprotector.

Delysid. Lysergic acid diethylamide.
Use: Potent psychotogenic.

Demadex. (Roche) Torsemide **Tab.:** 5 mg, 10 mg, 20 mg, 100 mg. Bot. UD 100s. **Inj.:** 10 mg/mL. Amp. 2 mL, 5 mL. *Rx.*
Use: Diuretic.

• **demeclocycline.** (DEH-meh-kloe-SIGH-kleen) *USP 28.* Formerly Demethylchlortetracycline.
Use: Anti-infective.
See: Declomycin.

• **demeclocycline hydrochloride.** (DEH-meh-kloe-SIGH-kleen) *USP 28.*
Use: Anti-infective, tetracycline.
See: Declomycin hydrochloride.

demeclocycline hydrochloride. (Impax) Demeclocycline hydrochloride 150 mg, 300 mg. Lactose. Tab. 48s (300 mg only), 100s, 500s. *Rx.*

Use: Anti-infective.

demeclocycline hydrochloride and nystatin tablets.
Use: Anti-infective.

●**demecycline.** (DEH-meh-SIGH-kleen) USAN.
Use: Anti-infective.

Demerol. (Abbott) Meperidine hydrochloride 25 mg/mL, 50 mg/mL, 75 mg/mL, 100 mg/mL. Inj. Amp. 0.5 mL (50 mg only) (preservative free), 1 mL (50 mg and 100 mg only); 1.5 mL and 2 mL (50 mg only). Multidose vial (contains metocresol as preservative) 20 mL (100 mg only), 30 mL (50 mg only). *Carpuject* syringe. 1 mL (preservative free). *c-ii.*
Use: Analgesic, narcotic agonist.

Demerol (Sanofi Synthelabo) Meperidine hydrochloride. **Syrup:** 50 mg/ 5 mL, saccharin, glucose, alcohol free, banana flavor. Bot. 473 mL. **Tab.:** 50 mg, 100 mg. Bot. 100s; 500s, UD 25s (50 mg only). *c-ii.*
Use: Opioid analgesic.

demethylchlortetracycline hydrochloride.
Use: Anti-infective; tetracycline.
See: Demeclocycline hydrochloride.

●**demoxepam.** (dem-OX-eh-pam) USAN.
Use: Anxiolytic.

Demser. (Merck & Co.) Metyrosine 250 mg. Cap. Bot. 100s. *Rx.*
Use: Antihypertensive.

Demulen 1/50. (Searle) Ethynodiol diacetate 1 mg, ethinyl estradiol 50 mcg, lactose. *Compack* tablet dispensers 21s, 28s. *Rx.*
Use: Sex hormone, contraceptive hormone.

Demulen 1/35. (Searle) Ethynodiol diacetate 1 mg, ethinyl estradiol 35 mcg, lactose. *Compack* tablet dispensers 21s, 28s. *Rx.*
Use: Sex hormone, contraceptive hormone.

Denalan Denture Cleanser. (Whitehall-Robins) Sodium percarbonate 30%. Bot. 7 oz., 13 oz. *OTC.*
Use: Agent for oral hygiene.

●**denatonium benzoate.** (DEE-nah-TOE-nee-uhm BEN-zoh-ate) *NF 23.*
Use: Pharmaceutic aid (flavor, alcohol denaturant).

Denavir. (GlaxoSmithKline) Penciclovir 10 mg/g. Cream. Tube 2 g. *Rx.*
Use: Cold sores.

Dencorub. (Last) Methyl salicylate 20%, menthol 0.75%, camphor 1%, eucalyptus oil 0.5%. Tube 1.25 oz, 2.75 oz.

OTC.
Use: Analgesic, topical.

Dencorub Analgesic Liquid. (Last) Oleoresin capsicum suspension in aqueous vehicle. Bot. 6 oz. *OTC.*
Use: Analgesic, topical.

●**denileukin diftitox.** (deh-nih-LOO-kin DIFF-tih-tox) USAN.
Use: Treatment of proliferative malignant diseases and autoimmune diseases expressing interleukin 2 receptors. Biological response modifier; antineoplastic.
See: Ontak.

●**denofungin.** (DEE-no-FUN-jin) USAN.
Use: Antifungal; antibacterial.

Denorex Everyday Dandruff. (Medtech) Pyrithione zinc 2%, propylene glycol, menthol. Shampoo. 110 mL, 240 ml *OTC.*
Use: Antiseborrheic.

Denorex Mountain Fresh. (Whitehall-Robins) Coal tar solution 9%, menthol 1.5%. Bot. 4 oz, 8 oz. *OTC.*
Use: Antiseborrheic.

Denorex with Conditioners. (Whitehall-Robins) Coal tar solution 9%, menthol 1.5%. Bot 4 oz, 8 oz. *OTC.*
Use: Antiseborrheic.

Denquel. (Procter & Gamble) Potassium nitrate 5%, calcium carbonate, glycerin, flavors. Tube 1.6 oz, 3 oz, 4.5 oz. *OTC.*
Use: Dentifrice.

Denta 5000 Plus. (Rising Pharmaceuticals) Sodium fluoride 1.1%, spearmint flavor. Cream. 51 g (2s). *Rx.*
Use: Dental caries agent.

DentaGel. (Rising Pharmaceuticals) Sodium fluoride 1.1%, saccharin, parabens, sorbitol, fresh mint flavor. Gel. 56 g. *Rx.*
Use: Dental caries agent.

Dental Caries Preventive. (Colgate Oral) Fluoride ion 1.2%, alumina abrasive. 2 g Box 200s, Jar 9 oz. *Rx.*
Use: Dental caries agent.

DentiPatch. (Noven) Lidocaine 23 mg, 46.1 mg[2] patch, aspartame. Patch. Box 50s, 100s. *Rx.*
Use: Anesthetic, local.

Dentrol. (Block Drug) Carboxymethylcellulose, polyethylene oxide homopolymer, peppermint and spearmint in mineral oil base. Bot. 0.9 oz, 1.8 oz. *OTC.*
Use: Denture adhesive.

Dent's Dental Poultice. (C.S. Dent & Co.) Glycerin, mineral oil, polyoxyethylene sorbitan monooleate. Bot. 0.125 oz, 0.25 oz. *OTC.*
Use: Dental poultice.

Dent's Ear Wax Drops. (C.S. Dent & Co.) Glycerin, mineral oil, polyoxyethylene sorbitan monooleate. Bot. 0.125 oz, 0.25 oz. *OTC.*
Use: Otic.

Dent's Extra Strength Toothache Gum. (C.S. Dent & Co.) Benzocaine. Box. 1 g. *OTC.*
Use: Anesthetic, local.

Dent's Lotion-Jel. (C.S. Dent & Co.) Benzocaine in special base. Tube 2 oz. *OTC.*
Use: Anesthetic, local.

Dent's Maximum Strength Toothache Drops. (C.S. Dent & Co.) Benzocaine, alcohol 74%, chlorobutanol anhydrous 0.09%. Liq. Bot. 3.7 mL. *OTC.*
Use: Anesthetic, local.

Dent's Toothache Drops Treatment. (C.S. Dent & Co.) Alcohol 60%, chlorobutanol anhydrous (chloroform derivative) 0.09%, propylene glycol, eugenol. Bot. 3.75 mL. *OTC.*
Use: Anesthetic, local.

Dent's Toothache Gum. (C.S. Dent & Co.) Benzocaine, eugenol, petrolatum in base of cotton and wax. Box 1.05 g. *OTC.*
Use: Anesthetic, local.

Denture Orajel. (Del) Benzocaine 10%, saccharin. Gel. Tube. 9.45 g. *OTC.*
Use: Anesthetic, local.

Dent-Zel-Ite. (Last) Oral Mucosal Analgesic: Benzocaine 5%, alcohol, glycerin. Bot. 1.875 g. **Temporary Dental Filling:** Sandarac gum, alcohol. Bot. 1 oz. **Toothache Drops:** Eugenol 85% in alcohol. Bot. 1 oz. *OTC.*
Use: Anesthetic, local.

•**denufosol tetrasodium.** (den-ue-FOE-sol) USAN.
Use: Cystic fibrosis.

denyl sodium.
Use: Anticonvulsant.
See: Diphenylhydantoin Sodium.

deodorizers, systemic. Chlorophyll derivatives (chlorophyllin). *OTC.*
Use: Oral: Control of fecal and urinary odors in colostomy, ileostomy, or incontinence. Topical: Reduce pain and inflammation (wounds, burns, surface ulcers, skin irritation).
See: Chloresium.
  Chlorophyll.
  Derifil.

deoxyadenosine, 2-chloro-2¹. (St. Jude Medical)
Use: Antineoplastic. [Orphan Drug]

2′deoxycoformycin. Pentostatin.
Use: Antibiotic; antineoplastic.
See: Nipent.

deoxycytidine (5-AZA-2′). (Pharmachemie USA, Inc.)
Use: Antineoplastic. [Orphan Drug]

deoxynojirimycin. (Pharmacia) Butyl-DNJ. *Rx.*
Use: Antiviral.

Depacon. (Abbott) Valproate sodium 100 mg/mL, EDTA, preservative-free. Inj. Single-dose Vial 5 mL. *Rx.*
Use: Anticonvulsant.

Depakene. (Abbott) **Cap.:** Valproic acid 250 mg, parabens, corn oil. Bot. 100s. **Syr.:** Sodium valproate 250 mg/5 mL, sorbitol, parabens, sucrose. Bot. 473 mL. *Rx.*
Use: Anticonvulsant.

Depakote. (Abbott) Divalproex sodium. **DR Tab.:** 125 mg, 250 mg, 500 mg. Talc. Bot. 100s, 500s (except 125 mg), *Abbo-Pac* UD 100s. **Sprinkle Cap.:** 125 mg. Bot. 100s, *Abbo-Pac* UD 100s. *Rx.*
Use: Anticonvulsant.

Depakote ER. (Abbott) Divalproex sodium 250 mg, 500 mg, lactose, polydextrose (500 mg only). ER Tab. Bot. 60s, 100s, 500s, *Abbo-Pac* UD 100s. *Rx.*
Use: Anticonvulsant.

Depa-Syrup. (Alra) Valproic acid syrup 250 mg/5 mL. Bot. 4 oz, 16 oz. *Rx.*
Use: Anticonvulsant.

•**depelestat.** (dep-EL-e-stat) USAN.
Use: Cystic fibrosis.

Depen. (Wallace) Penicillamine 250 mg. Tab. Bot. 100s. *Rx.*
Use: Chelating agent.

depepsen. Amylosulfate sodium.
Use: Digestive aid.

depGynogen. (Forest) Estradiol cypionate in cottonseed oil 5 mg/mL, cottonseed oil, chlorobutanol. Inj. Vial 10 mL. *Rx.*
Use: Estrogen.

depMedalone 80. (Forest) Methylprednisolone acetate 80 mg/mL, polyethylene glycol, myristyl-gamma-picolinium Cl. Vial 5 mL. *Rx.*
Use: Corticosteroid.

depMedalone 40. (Forest) Methylprednisolone acetate in aqueous suspension 40 mg/mL, polyethylene glycol, myristyl-gamma-picolinium Cl. Vial 5 mL. *Rx.*
Use: Corticosteroid.

DepoCyt. (Enzon) Cytarabine, liposomal 10 mg/mL, preservative free, sodium chloride 0.9%. Inj. Vial. 5 mL. *Rx.*
Use: Antimetabolite.

DepoDur. (Endo) Morphine sulfate 10 mg/mL. ER Liposomal Inj. Single-

use vials in cartons of 5. 1 mL, 1.5 mL, 2 mL. c-II.
Use: Opioid analgesic.
Depoestra. (Tennessee Pharmaceutic) Estradiol cypionate 5 mg/mL. Vial 10 mL. Rx.
Use: Estrogen.
Depo-Estradiol. (Pharmacia) Estradiol cypionate 5 mg/mL, chlorobutanol 5.4 mg, cottonseed oil. Inj. Vial 5 mL. Rx.
Use: Estrogen.
Depofoam encapsulated cytarabine. (DepoTech)
Use: Neoplastic meningitis. [Orphan Drug]
DepoGen. (Hyrex) Estradiol cypionate 5 mg/mL, cottonseed oil, chlorobutanol. Inj. Vial 10 mL. Rx.
Use: Estrogen.
Depo-Medrol. (Pharmacia) Methylprednisolone acetate 20 mg, 40 mg. Inj. Vial. 5 mL, 10 mL. 80 mg. Vial. 1 mL, 5 mL. Rx.
Use: Corticosteroid.
Depopred-80. (Hyrex) Methylprednisolone acetate 80 mg. Inj. Vial. 5 mL. Rx.
Use: Corticosteroid.
Depopred-40. (Hyrex) Methylprednisolone acetate suspension 40 mg/mL, polyethylene glycol, myristyl-gamma-picolinium Cl. Vial 5 mL, 10 mL. Rx.
Use: Corticosteroid.
Depo-Provera. (Pharmacia) Medroxyprogesterone acetate 400 mg/mL, polyethylene glycol 3350, sodium sulfate anhydrous, myristyl-gamma-picolinium Cl. Vial 2.5 mL, 10 mL, 1 mL U-Ject. Rx.
Use: Hormone, progestin.
Depo-Provera Contraceptive Injection. (Pharmacia) Medroxyprogesterone acetate 150 mg/mL, with PEG-3350 28.9 mg, polysorbate 80 2.41 mg, sodium Cl 8.68 mg, methylparaben 1.37 mg, propylparaben 0.15 mg. Vial. 1 mL. Rx.
Use: Contraceptive.
Depo-Sub Q Provera 104. (Pfizer) Medroxyprogesterone acetate 104 mg (160 mg/mL). Sodium chloride 5.2 mg, parabens, polythylene glycol. Inj. Pre-filled single-use syringes. 0.65 mL. Rx.
Use: Contraceptive hormone.
Depo-Testadiol. (Pharmacia) Testosterone cypionate 50 mg, estradiol cypionate 2 mg/mL, chlorobutanol in cottonseed oil. Inj. (in oil). Vial 10 mL. Rx.
Use: Androgen, estrogen combination.
Depo-Testosterone. (Pharmacia) Testosterone cypionate. Inj. **100 mg/mL:** In

benzyl alcohol 9.45 mg, cottonseed oil 736 mg/mL, benzyl benzoate 0.1 mL. Vial 10 mL. **200 mg/mL:** In benzyl benzoate 0.2 mL, benzyl alcohol 9.45 mg, cottonseed oil 560 mg/mL. Vial 1 mL, 10 mL. c-III.
Use: Sex hormone, androgen.
deprenyl. Selegiline hydrochloride.
See: Eldepryl.
• **depreotide.** (deh-PREE-oh-tide) USAN.
Use: Diagnostic aid.
Deproist Expectorant/Codeine. (Geneva) Pseudoephedrine hydrochloride 30 mg, codeine phosphate 10 mg, guaifenesin 100 mg/5 mL. Bot. 120 mL, 480 mL. c-v.
Use: Antitussive, decongestant, expectorant.
• **deprostil.** (deh-PRAHS I-ill) USAN.
Use: Antisecretory, gastric.
Dep-Test. (Sigma-Tau) Testosterone cypionate 100 mg/mL. Vial 10 mL. c-III.
Use: Androgen.
Dequasine. (Miller Pharmacal Group) L-lysine 20 mg, l-cysteine 50 mg, DL-methionine 150 mg, N-acetyl cysteine 50 mg, vitamin C 200 mg, Ca 40 mg, Cu 1 mg, Fe 5 mg, I 0.015 mg, K 20 mg, Mg 40 mg, Mn 5 mg, Mo 150 mcg, Zn 5 mg. Tab. Bot. 100s. OTC.
Use: Amino acid; vitamin, mineral supplement.
• **deracoxib.** (der-ah-KOX-ib) USAN.
Use: Anti-inflammatory; analgesic.
Derifil. (Rystan) Chlorophyllin copper complex 100 mg. Tab. Bot. 30s, 100s, 1000s. OTC.
Use: Deodorant, oral.
Dermabase. (Paddock) Mineral oil, petrolatum, cetostearyl alcohol, propylene glycol, sodium lauryl sulfate, isopropyl palmitate, imidazolidinyl urea, methyl- and propylparabens. Cream. Jar 1 lb. OTC.
Use: Emollient.
Dermacoat Aerosol Spray. (Century) Benzocaine 4.5%. Bot. 7 oz. OTC.
Use: Anesthetic, local.
Dermacort. (Solvay) Hydrocortisone. **Cream:** 0.5%, 1% in a water soluble cream of stearyl alcohol, cetyl alcohol, isopropyl palmitate, citric acid, polyoxyethylene 40 stearate, sodium phosphate, propylene glycol, water, benzyl alcohol, buffered to pH 5. 0.5% in 30 g tube, 1% in 1 lb jar. **Lot.:** 1% in lotion base, buffered to pH 5. Paraben free. Bot. 120 mL. Rx.
Use: Corticosteroid, topical.

Derma-Cover. (Scrip) Sulfur, salicylic acid, hyamine 10x, isopropyl alcohol 22%, in powder film forming base. Bot. 2 oz. *OTC.*
Use: Keratolytic.

Dermadrox. (Geritrex) Aluminum hydroxide gel, zinc chloride, lanolin, calcium carbonate, vitamin A in a hydrophilic ointment base. Oint. 113 g. *OTC.*
Use: Topical combination.

DermaFlex. (Zila) Lidocaine 2.5%, alcohol 79%. Gel. Tube 15 g. *OTC.*
Use: Anesthetic, local.

Derma-Guard. (Greer) Protective adhesive pow. Can w/sifter top, 4 oz. Spray Top Bot. 4 oz, pkg. 1 lb. Rings. Pkg. 5s, 10s. *OTC.*
Use: Dermatologic, protectant.

Dermal-Rub Balm. (Roberts) Menthol racemic 7%, camphor 1%, methyl salicylate 1%, cajuput oil 1%. Cream. Jar 1 oz, 1 lb. *OTC.*
Use: Analgesic, topical.

Dermamycin. (Pfeiffer) **Cream:** Diphenhydramine hydrochloride 2% in a base of parabens, polyethylene glycol monostearate and propylene glycol. Tube 28.35 g. **Spray:** Diphenhydramine hydrochloride 2%, menthol 1%, alcohol, methylparaben. Bot. 60 mL. *OTC.*
Use: Antihistamine, topical.

Dermaneed. (Hanlon) Zirconium oxide 4.5%, calamine 6%, zinc oxide 4%, actamer 0.1% in bland lotionized base. Bot. 4 oz. *OTC.*
Use: Antipruritic, topical.

Derma-Pax. (Recsei) Methapyrilene hydrochloride 0.22%, chlorothenylpyramine maleate 0.06%, pyrilamine maleate 0.22%, benzyl alcohol 1%, chlorobutanol 1%, isopropyl alcohol 40%. Liq. 4 oz, pt. *OTC.*
Use: Antihistamine, topical; antipruritic, topical.

Derma-Pax HC. (Recsei) Hydrocortisone 0.5%, pyrilamine maleate 0.2%, pheniramine maleate 0.2%, chlorpheniramine 0.06%, benzyl alcohol 1%. Liq. Bot. 60 mL, 120 mL, 480 mL.
Use: Antihistamine, topical; corticosteroid, topical.

Dermarest. (Del) Diphenhydramine hydrochloride 2%, resorcinol 2%, aloe vera gel, benzalkonium chloride, EDTA, menthol, methylparaben, propylene glycol. Gel. Tube 29.25 g, 56.25 g. *OTC.*
Use: Antihistamine, topical.

Dermarest Dricort. (Del) Hydrocortisone 1%, white petrolatum. Cream. Bot. 14 g. *OTC.*

Use: Corticosteroid, topical.

Dermarest Plus. (Del) **Gel:** Diphenhydramine hydrochloride 2%, menthol 1%, aloe vera gel, benzalkonium chloride, isopropyl alcohol, methylparaben, propylene glycol. Tube 15 g, 30 g. **Spray:** Diphenhydramine hydrochloride 2%, menthol 1%, aloe vera gel, benzalkonium chloride, methylparaben propylene glycol, SDA 40 alcohol, EDTA. Bot. 60 mL. *OTC.*
Use: Antihistamine, topical.

Dermasept Antifungal. (Pharmakon) Tannic acid 6.098%, zinc Cl 5.081%, benzocaine 2.032%, methylbenzethonium hydrochloride, tolnaftate 1.017%, undecylenic acid 5.081%, ethanol 38B 58.539%, phenol, benzyl alcohol, benzoic acid, coal tar, camphor, menthol. Liq. Bot. 30 mL. *OTC.*
Use: Antifungal, topical.

Dermasil. (Chesebrough-Ponds USA) Glycerin and dimethicone in a base containing cyclomethicone, sunflower oil, petrolatum, borage oil, lecithin, vitamin E acetate, vitamin A palmitate, vitamin D_3, corn oil, EDTA, methylparaben. Lot. Bot. 120 mL, 240 mL. *OTC.*
Use: Emollient.

Derma-Smoothe/FS Oil. (Hill Dermaceuticals) Fluocinolone acetonide 0.01%. Oil. Bot. 4 oz. *Rx.*
Use: Antipsoriatic; antiseborrheic, topical.

Derma-Smoothe Oil. (Hill Dermaceuticals) Refined peanut oil, mineral oil in lipophilic base. *OTC.*
Use: Antipruritic; dermatologic, protectant.

Derma Soap. (Ferndale) Dowicil 0.1%. 4 oz w/dispenser. *OTC.*
Use: Antiseptic.

Derma-Soft. (Vogarell) Salicylic acid, castor oil, triethanolamine. Medicated cream. Tube ¾ oz. *OTC.*
Use: Keratolytic.

Derma-Sone 1%. (Hill Dermaceuticals) Hydrocortisone 1%, pramoxine hydrochloride 1%, cetyl alcohol, glyceryl monostearate, isopropyl myristate, potassium sorbate, furcelleran. *Rx-OTC.*
Use: Anesthetic; corticosteroid, local.

Dermasorcin. (Lamond) Resorcin 2%, sulfur 5%. Bot. 1 oz, 2 oz, 4 oz, 8 oz, pt, 32 oz, 0.5 gal. *OTC.*
Use: Dermatologic, acne; antiseborrheic, topical.

Dermastringe. (Lamond) Bot. 4 oz, 6 oz, 8 oz, pt, 32 oz, gal. *OTC.*
Use: Dermatologic, cleanser.

Dermasul. (Lamond) Sulfur 5%. Bot. 1 oz, 2 oz, 4 oz, 8 oz, pt, 32 oz, 0.5 gal, gal. *OTC.*
Use: Dermatologic, acne; antiseborrheic, topical.

Dermathyn. (Davis & Sly) Benzyl alcohol 3%, benzocaine 3.5%, butyl-p-aminobenzoate 1%, phenylmercuric borate. Tube 1 oz. *OTC.*
Use: Anesthetic, local.

Dermatic Base. (Whorton Pharmaceuticals, Inc.) Compounding cream base. Bot. 16 oz.
Use: Pharmaceutical aid, emollient base.

Dermatol.
See: Bismuth subgallate (Various Mfr.).

Dermatop E. (Dermik) Prednicarbate 0.1%. **Cream:** White petrolatum, lanolin alcohols, mineral oil, cetostearyl alcohol, EDTA, lactic acid. Tube. 15 g, 60 g. **Oint.:** Glycerin. Tube. 15 g, 60 g. *Rx.*
Use: Corticosteroid, topical.

DermaVite. (Stiefel) Vitamin A 3500 units (29% as beta carotene), E 60 units, B_2 8.5 mg, B_6 10 mg, C 120 mg, folate 400 mcg, Zn 45 mg, biotin 600 mcg, lycopene 5 mg, Ca, Cr, Cu, Mn, Se, Si, sucrose. Tab. Bot. 60s. *OTC.*
Use: Vitamin, mineral supplement.

Dermazine. (Dermalogix) Pyrithione zinc 0.25%, parabens. Shampoo. 240 mL. *OTC.*
Use: Antiseborrheic.

Dermed. (Holloway) Vitamins A and D with hydrogenated vegetable oil. Cream. Tube 60 g, 120 g. *OTC.*
Use: Emollient.

Dermeze. (Premo) Thenylpyramine hydrochloride 2%, benzocaine 2%, tyrothricin 0.25 mg/g. Massage Lot. Bot. 5¾ oz. *OTC.*
Use: Anesthetic; antihistamine; antiinfective.

Dermolate Anti-Itch. (Schering-Plough) Hydrocortisone 0.5% petrolatum, mineral oil, chlorocresol. Cream. Tube 15 g, 30 g. *OTC.*
Use: Corticosteroid, topical.

Dermol HC. (Dermol Pharmaceuticals, Inc.) **Cream:** Hydrocortisone 1%, 2.5%. Tube 30 g. **Oint.:** Hydrocortisone 1%. Tube 30 g. *Rx.*
Use: Anorectal preparation.

Dermolin. (Roberts) Menthol racemic, methyl salicylate, camphor, mustard oil, isopropyl alcohol 8%. Bot. 3 oz, pt, gal. *OTC.*
Use: Liniment.

Dermoplast. (Whitehall-Robins) **Spray:** Benzocaine 20%, menthol, methylparaben, aloe, lanolin. Bot. 82.5 mL. **Lot.:** Benzocaine 8%, menthol, aloe, glycerin, parabens, lanolin. Bot. 90 mL. *OTC.*
Use: Anesthetic, local.

Dermovan. (Galderma) Glyceryl stearate, spermaceti, mineral oil, glycerin, cetyl alcohol, butylparaben, methylparaben, propylparaben, purified water. Vanishing-type base, Jar 1 lb. *OTC.*
Use: Dermatologic, protectant.

Dermtex HC. (Pfeiffer) Hydrocortisone 0.5% in a glycerin base. Tube 15 g. *OTC.*
Use: Corticosteroid, topical.

Dermuspray. (Warner Chilcott) Trypsin 0.1 mg, balsam Peru 72.5 mg, castor oil 650 mg/0.82 mL. Aer. Bot. 120 g. *Rx.*
Use: Enzyme, topical.

DES.
See: Diethylstilbestrol.

desacchromin. A nonprotein bacterial colloidal dispersion of polysaccharide.

•**desciclovir.** (DESS-sigh-kloe-veer) USAN.
Use: Antiviral.

•**descinolone acetonide.** (DESS-SIN-oleohn ah-SEE-toe-nide) USAN.
Use: Corticosteroid, topical.

Desenex. (Novartis) Total undecylenate (as undecylenic acid and zinc undecylenate). **Aer. Spray Pow.:** 25%, menthol, talc. Can 81 g. **Cream:** Clotrimazole 1%, benzyl alcohol 1%, cetostearyl alcohol. Tube 15 g, 30 g. **Oint.:** 25%, parabens, white petrolatum, lanolin. Tube 14 g. **Pow.:** 25%, talc. Bot. 45 g. **Foam:** Total undecylenate (as undecylenic acid) 10% isopropyl alcohol 29.2%. Can 45 g. *OTC.*
Use: Antifungal, topical.

Desenex Antifungal, Maximum. (Novartis) Miconazole nitrate 2%. Pow. Tube 14 g. *OTC.*
Use: Antifungal, topical.

Desenex Foot & Sneaker Spray. (Novartis) Aluminum chlorhydrex w/alcohol 89.3%. Aerosol Can 2.7 oz. *OTC.*
Use: Foot deodorant; antiperspirant.

Desenex Max. (Novartis) Terbinafine hydrochloride 1%, benzyl alcohol, stearyl alcohol, cetyl alcohol. Cream. 24 g. *OTC.*
Use: Antifungal, topical.

De Serpa. (de Leon) Reserpine 0.25 mg, 0.5 mg. Tab. Bot. 100s, 500s, 1000s (0.25 mg only). *Rx.*
Use: Antihypertensive.

•**deserpidine.**
Use: Antihypertensive.

W/Methyclothiazide.
See: Enduronyl.
Desert Pure Calcium. (CalWhite Mineral Co.) Calcium (from mineral calcite) 500 mg, vitamin D 125 units. Tab. Bot. 200s. *OTC.*
Use: Mineral, vitamin supplement.
Desferal. (Novartis) Deferoxamine mesylate 500 mg/5 mL. Amp. 4s. *Rx.*
Use: Antidote.
•**desflurane.** (dess-FLEW-rane) *USP 28.*
Use: Anesthetic.
See: Suprane.
•**desipramine hydrochloride.** (dess-IPP-ruh-meen high-droe-KLOR-ide) *USP 28.*
Use: Antidepressant.
See: Norpramin.
desipramine hydrochloride. (Various Mfr.) Desipramine hydrochloride 10 mg, 25 mg, 50 mg, 75 mg, 100 mg, 150 mg. Tab. Bot. 50s (150 mg), 100s, 500s (except 10 mg, 150 mg), 1000s, UD 100s (25 mg, 50 mg, 75 mg only); blister pack 100s, 600s (25 mg, 50 mg, 75 mg). *Rx.*
Use: Antidepressant.
•**desirudin.** (deh-SIHR-uh-din) USAN.
Use: Anticoagulant.
See: Iprivask.
Desitin. (Pfizer) **Pow.:** Talc. Can 3 oz, 7 oz, 10 oz. **Oint.:** Cod liver oil, zinc oxide 40%, talc, petrolatum, lanolin. Tube 1 oz, 2 oz, 4 oz, 8 oz, Jar 1 lb. *OTC.*
Use: Astringent; skin protectant.
Desitin Creamy. (Pfizer) Zinc oxide 10%, mineral oil, white petrolatum, parabens. Oint. Tube 57 g. *OTC.*
Use: Antifungal, topical.
Desitin with Zinc Oxide. (Pfizer) Cornstarch 88.2%, zinc oxide 10%. Pow. Bot. 28 g, 397 g. *OTC.*
Use: Diaper rash preparation.
•**deslanoside.** (dess-LAN-oh-side) *USP 28.*
Use: Cardiovascular agent.
•**desloratadine.** (dess-lore-AT-ah-deen) USAN.
Use: Antihistamine, peripherally-selective piperidine.
See: Clarinex.
Clarinex RediTabs.
W/Combinations.
See: Clarinex-D 24 Hour.
•**deslorelin.** (DESS-low-REH-lin) USAN.
Use: Gonadotropin inhibitor; LHRH agonist. [Orphan Drug]
See: Somagard (as acetate).

Desma. (Tablicaps) Diethylstilbestrol 25 mg. Tab. Patient dispenser 10s. *Rx.*
Use: Estrogen.
•**desmopressin acetate.** (DESS-moe-PRESS-in) USAN.
Use: Posterior pituitary hormone.
See: DDAVP.
Stimate.
W/Chlorobutanol.
See: Minirin.
desmopressin acetate. (Bausch & Lomb) Desmopressin acetate 0.1 mg/mL (10 mcg/spray), chlorobutanol 0.5%. Nasal Soln. Nasal pump dispenser. *Rx.*
Use: Posterior pituitary hormone.
desmopressin acetate. (Various Mfr.) Desmopressin acetate 4 mcg/mL. Inj. Single-dose Amp. 1 mL, multidose vial 10 mL. *Rx.*
Use: Posterior pituitary hormone.
•**desmoteplase.** (des-moe-TE-plase) USAN.
Use: Cardiovascular agent.
Desogen. (Organon) Desogestrel 0.15 mg, ethinyl estradiol 30 mcg, lactose. Tab. Pack. 28s. *Rx.*
Use: Sex hormone, contraceptive hormone.
•**desogestrel.** (DESS-oh-JESS-trell) *USP 28.*
Use: Hormone, progestin.
W/Ethinyl estradiol.
See: Apri.
Cesia.
Desogen.
Mircette.
Ortho-Cept.
Velivet.
•**desonide.** (DESS-oh-nide) USAN.
Use: Anti-inflammatory.
See: LoKara.
Tridesilon.
desonide. (Fougera) Desonide 0.05%, light mineral oil, cetyl alcohol, stearyl alcohol, parabens, EDTA. Lot. 59 mL, 118 mL. *Rx.*
Use: Anti-inflammatory; corticosteroid, topical.
desonide. (Various Mfr.) Desonide 0.05%. Oint. Cream. Tube 15 g, 60 g. *Rx.*
Use: Anti-inflammatory; corticosteroid, topical.
desonide cream. (Galderma) Desonide 0.05% in cream base. Tube 15 g, 60 g. *Rx.*
Use: Corticosteroid, topical.
DesOwen. (Galderma) Desonide 0.05%. Cream. Tube 15 g, 60 g. *Rx.*
Use: Corticosteroid, topical.

• **desoximetasone.** (dess-OX-ee-MET-ah-sone) *USP 28.*
Use: Anti-inflammatory; corticosteroid, topical.
See: Topicort.

• **desoxycorticosterone acetate.** (dess-OX-ee-core-tih-koe-STURR-ohn ASS-eh-tate) *USP 28.*
Use: Adrenocortical steroid (salt-regulating).

• **desoxycorticosterone pivalate.** (dess-OX-ee-core-tih-koe-STURR-ohn) *USP 28.*
Use: Adrenocortical steroid (salt-regulating).

• **desoxycorticosterone trimethylacetate.** (dess-OX-ee-core-tih-koe-STURR ohn) *USP 28.*
Use: Adrenocortical steroid (salt-regulating).

desoxyephedrine hydrochloride. (Various Mfr.) *c-II.*
Use: CNS stimulant.
See: Methamphetamine hydrochloride.

Desoxyn. (Abbott) Methamphetamine hydrochloride 5 mg, lactose. Tab. Bot. 100s. *c-II.*
Use: CNS stimulant, amphetamine.

desoxy norephedrine.
Use: CNS stimulant.
See: Amphetamine hydrochloride.

desoxyribonuclease.
Use: Enzyme, topical.
W/Fibrinolysin.
See: Elase.

Desquam-E 5 & 10. (Westwood Squibb) Benzoyl peroxide 5%, 10%, EDTA. Gel. Tube 10.5 g, 0n.
Use: Dermatologic, acne.

Desquam-X 5. (Westwood Squibb) Benzoyl peroxide 5%, EDTA. Gel. 42.5 g, 85 g. *Rx.*
Use: Dermatologic, acne.

Desquam-X 10. (Westwood Squibb) Benzoyl peroxide 10%. **Bar:** Lactic acid, EDTA, sorbitol. 106 g. **Gel:** EDTA. 42.5 g, 85 g. *Rx.*
Use: Dermatologic, acne.

de-Stat. (Sherman Pharmaceuticals, Inc.) Surfactant cleaner, benzalkonium Cl 0.01%, EDTA 0.25%. Soln. Bot. 118 mL. *OTC.*
Use: Contact lens care.

de-Stat 4. (Sherman Pharmaceuticals, Inc.) Benzyl alcohol 0.3%, EDTA 0.5%, lauryl sulfate, salt of imidazdinyl urea, octylphenoxy polyethoxyethanol, thimerosal free. Soln. Bot. 118 mL. *OTC.*
Use: Contact lens care.

de-Stat 3. (Sherman Pharmaceuticals, Inc.) Octylphenoxy polyethoxyethanol, benzyl alcohol 0.1%, EDTA 0.5%, lauryl sulfate salt of imidazodinyl urea. Soln. Bot. 118 mL. *OTC.*
Use: Contact lens care.

• **desvenlafaxine succinate.** (des-VEN-la-fax-een) USAN.
Use: Antidepressant.

Desyrel. (Apothecon) Trazodone hydrochloride 50 mg, 100 mg. Bot. 100s, 1000s, UD 100s. *Rx.*
Use: Antidepressant.

Desyrel Dividose. (Apothecon) Trazodone hydrochloride 150 mg, 300 mg. Dividose Tab. Bot. 100s, 500s (150 mg only). *Rx.*
Use: Antidepressant.

Detachol. (Ferndale) Bland, nonirritating liquid for removing adhesive tape. Pkg. 4 oz.
Use: Adhesive remover.

De Tal. (de Leon) Phenobarbital 0.25 g, hyoscyamine sulfate 0.1037 mg, atropine sulfate 0.0194 mg, hyoscine HBr 0.0065 mg. **Tab.:** Bot. 100s. **Elix.:** W/alcohol 20%. Bot. Pt. *Rx.*
Use: Anticholinergic; antispasmodic; hypnotic; sedative.

Detane. (Del) Benzocaine 7.5%. Tube 0.5 oz. *OTC.*
Use: Anesthetic, local.

• **deterenol hydrochloride.** (dee-TEER-eh-nahl) USAN.
Use: Adrenergic, ophthalmic.

detergents. Surface-active.
See: pHisoDerm.
pHisoHex.
Zephiran.

detigon hydrochloride.
See: Chlophedianol hydrochloride.

• **detirelix acetate.** (DEH-tih-RELL-ix) USAN.
Use: Antagonist (LHRH).

• **detomidine hydrochloride.** (deh-TOE-mih-deen) USAN.
Use: Hypnotic; sedative.

detoxification agents.
See: Antidotes.
Chelating Agents.
Deferoxamine Mesylate.
Dimercaprol.
Edetate Calcium Disodium.
Flumazenil.
Naltrexone Hydrochloride.
Pentetate Calcium Trisodium.
Pentetate Zinc Trisodium.
Sodium Nitrite.
Sodium Thiosulfate.
Succimer.

Trientine Hydrochloride.

Detrol. (Pharmacia) Tolterodine tartrate 1 mg, 2 mg. Tab. Bot. 60s, 500s, UD 140s. *Rx.*
Use: Anticholinergic.

Detrol LA. (Pharmacia) Tolterodine tartrate 2 mg, 4 mg, sucrose. ER Cap. Bot. 30s, 90s, 500s, UD blisters. *Rx.*
Use: Anticholinergic.

Detussin. (Alpharma) Pseudoephedrine hydrochloride 60 mg, hydrocodone bitartrate 5 mg/5 mL, alcohol 5%, corn syrup, saccharin, methylparaben, cherry flavor. Liq. Bot. 473 mL. *c-III.*
Use: Upper respiratory combination, antitussive, decongestant.

Detussin Expectorant. (Various Mfr.) Pseudoephedrine hydrochloride 60 mg, hydrocodone bitartrate 5 mg, guaifenesin 200 mg, alcohol. Liq. Bot. 480 mL. *c-III.*
Use: Antitussive, decongestant, expectorant.

•**deuterium oxide.** (doo-TEER-ee-uhm) USAN.
Use: Radiopharmaceutical.

•**devazepide.** (dev-AZE-eh-PIDE) USAN.
Use: Antagonist (cholecystokinin); antispasmodic, gastrointestinal.

Devrom. (Parthenon) Bismuth subgallate 200 mg, lactose, sugar. Chew. Tab. Bot. 100s.
Use: Deodorant, systemic.

Dexacort Phosphate Respihaler. (Medeva) Dexamethasone sodium phosphate equivalent to 0.1 mg dexamethasone phosphate ($\approx$ 0.084 mg dexamethasone) w/fluorochlorohydrocarbons as propellants, alcohol 2%. Aerosol for oral inhalation, 170 sprays in 12.6 g pressurized container.
Use: Bronchodilator.

Dexacort Phosphate Turbinaire. (Medeva) Dexamethasone sodium phosphate 0.1 mg equivalent to dexamethasone 0.084 mg w/fluorochlorohydrocarbons as propellants and alcohol 2%. Aerosol w/nasal applicator. Container 170 sprays; refill package without nasal applicator.
Use: Nasal corticosteroid.

Dexafed. (Roberts) Phenylephrine hydrochloride 5 mg, dextromethorphan HBr 10 mg, guaifenesin 100 mg/5 mL. Syr. Bot. 120 mL. *OTC.*
Use: Antitussive, decongestant, expectorant.

DexAlone. (DexGen) Dextromethorphan HBr 30 mg, sorbitol. Gelcap. Pkg. 30s. *OTC.*
Use: Antitussive.

•**dexamethasone.** (DEX-uh-METH-uh-sone) *USP 28.*
Use: Adrenocortical steroid, glucocorticoid; corticosteroid, topical.
See: Aeroseb-Dex.
  Decaderm in Estergel.
  Decadron.
  Decameth.
  Decameth L.A.
  Dexaport.
  Maxidex.
  TobraDex.
W/Ciprofloxacin.
See: Ciprodex.
W/Neomycin sulfate.
See: NeoDecadron
W/Neomycin sulfate, polymyxin B sulfate.
See: Dexacidin.
  Maxitrol.
  NeoDecaspray.
  Neomycin and Polymyxin B Sulfates and Dexamethasone.

dexamethasone. (Roxane) Dexamethasone 1 mg, 2 mg. Tab. 100s, UD 100s. *Rx.*
Use: Adrenocortical steroid, glucocorticoid.

dexamethasone. (Steris) Dexamethasone 0.1%. Susp. Bot. 5 mL. *Rx.*
Use: Corticosteroid, ophthalmic.

dexamethasone. (Various Mfr.) Dexamethasone. **Elix.:** 0.5 mg/5 mL. May contain alcohol. 100 mL, 237 mL. **Oral Soln.:** 0.5 mg/5 mL. May contain sorbitol. Sugar free. 500 mL, UD 5 mL, UD 20 mL, 237 mL. **Tab.:** 0.25 mg, 0.5 mg, 0.75 mg, 1.5 mg, 4 mg, 6 mg. 50s (1.5 mg, 4 mg, 6 mg only), 100s, 500s (0.75 mg, 1.5 mg, 4 mg only), 1,000s (except 6 mg), UD 100s (except 0.25 mg). *Rx.*
Use: Adrenocortical steroid, glucocorticoid.

•**dexamethasone acefurate.** (DEX-ah-METH-ah-sone ASS-eh-fer-ate) USAN.
Use: Anti-inflammatory; topical steroid.

•**dexamethasone acetate.** (DEX-ah-METH-ah-sone) *USP 28.*
Use: Adrenocortical steroid (anti-inflammatory).
See: Dalalone.
  Dexone LA.

•**dexamethasone beloxil.** (DEX-ah-METH-ah-sone bel-OX-il) USAN.
Use: Anti-inflammatory.

•**dexamethasone dipropionate.** (DEX-ah-METH-ah-sone die-PRO-pee-oh-nate) USAN.
Use: Anti-inflammatory; steroid.

Dexamethasone Intensol. (Roxane) Dexamethasone 1 mg/mL. Alcohol 30%. Concentrated oral soln. Bot. 30 mL w/dropper. *Rx.*
Use: Glucocorticoid, adrenocortical steroid.

dexamethasone ophthalmic. (Various Mfr.) Dexamethasone 0.1%. Susp. Bot. 5 mL. *Rx.*
Use: Corticosteroid.

●**dexamethasone sodium phosphate.** (DEX-ah-METH-ah-sone) *USP 28.*
Use: Adrenocortical steroid (anti-inflammatory); corticosteroid, topical.
See: Dalalone.
Decadron Phosphate.
Decaject.
Decameth.
Dexone.
Hexadrol Phosphate.
Maxidex.
Savacort D.
Solurex.
W/Neomycin sulfate.
See: NeoDecadron.
Neo-Dexameth.
W/Neomycin and polymyxin B sulfates.
See: Dexasporin.
Maxitrol.

dexamethasone sodium phosphate. (Various Mfr.) Dexamethasone sodium phosphate **Soln.:** 0.1%. Bot. 5 mL. **Oint.;** 0.05%. Tube 3.5 g. *Rx.*
Use: Adrenocortical steroid (anti-inflammatory); corticosteroid, topical.

●**dexamisole.** (DEX-AM-ih-sole) USAN.
Use: Antidepressant.

dexamphetamine.
300. Bolti vampi trinine

Dexaphen-S.A. Tablets. (Major) Pseudoephedrine sulfate 120 mg, dexbrompheniramine maleate 6 mg. Bot. 100s, 500s. *Rx.*
Use: Antihistamine, decongestant.

Dexaport. (Freeport) Dexamethasone 0.75 mg. Tab. Bot. 1000s. *Rx.*
Use: Corticosteroid.

Dexasone. (Various Mfr.) Dexamethasone sodium phosphate 4 mg/mL, parabens, sodium bisulfite. Vial 5 mL, 10 mL, 30 mL. *Rx.*
Use: Corticosteroid.

Dexasone Injection. (Roberts) Dexamethasone sodium phosphate 4 mg/mL. Vial 5 mL, 30 mL. *Rx.*
Use: Corticosteroid.

Dexasone L.A. Injection. (Roberts) Dexamethasone acetate 8 mg/mL. Vial 5 mL. *Rx.*
Use: Corticosteroid.

Dexasporin Ointment. (Bausch & Lomb) Dexamethasone 0.1%, neomycin sulfate equivalent to 0.35% neomycin base and 10,000 units polymyxin B sulfate. Ophth. Oint. Tube 3.5 g. *Rx.*
Use: Steroid; anti-infective, ophthalmic.

Dexasporin Suspension. (Various Mfr.) Dexamethasone 0.1%, neomycin sulfate equivalent to 0.35%, neomycin base and 10,000 units polymyxin B sulfate/mL, hydroxypropyl methylcellulose, polysorbate 20, benzalkonium chloride. Drops. Bot. 5 mL. *Rx.*
Use: Anti-infective; corticosteroid, ophthalmic.

Dexatrim Natural Caffeine Free Caplets. (Chattem) Chromium 250 mcg, heartleaf 120 mg, thermonutrient blend 100 mg, vanadium 100 mcg. Box. Blister pak 30s. *OTC*
Use: Dietary aid.

●**dexbrompheniramine maleate.** (dex-brome-fen-EER-ah-meen MAL-ee-ate) *USP 28.*
Use: Antihistamine.
W/Combinations.
See: DEKA.
DEKA Pediatric.
Notuss PD.
W/Pseudoephedrine sulfate.
See: Disophrol Chronotab.
Drixomed.
Drixoral Cold & Allergy.
Drixoral S.A.
W/Pseudoephedrine Sulfate, Acetaminophen.
See: Acetaminophen, dexbrompheniramine maleate, and pseudoephedrine sulfate combinations.

●**dexchlorpheniramine maleate.** *USP 28.*
Use: Antihistamine, nonselective alkylamine.
See: Polaramine.
Polaramine Repetabs.
W/Combinations.
See: Panatuss DX.
Polaramine Expectorant.

dexchlorpheniramine maleate. (Morton Grove) Dexchlorpheniramine maleate 2 mg/5 mL. Alcohol, orange flavor. Syrup. 473 mL. *Rx.*
Use: Antihistamine.

dexchlorpheniramine maleate. (Various Mfr.) Dexchlorpheniramine maleate 4 mg, 6 mg. ER Tab. Bot. 100s, 1000s. *Rx.*
Use: Antihistamine, non-selective alkylamine.

●**dexclamol hydrochloride.** (DEX-claymahl) USAN.
Use: Hypnotic; sedative.

Dexedrine. (GlaxoSmithKline) Dextroamphetamine sulfate. **Tab.**: 5 mg, tartrazine, lactose, sucrose. Bot. 100s. **Spansule:** 5 mg, 10 mg, 15 mg, sugar spheres. SR, Cap. Bot. 100s. *c-II.*
Use: CNS stimulant, amphetamine.
●**dexetimide.** (dex-ETT-ih-mid) USAN.
Use: Anticholinergic; antiparkinsonian.
DexFerrum. (American Regent) Iron 50 mg/mL (as dextran). Inj. Single-dose vial. 1 mL, 2 mL. *Rx.*
Use: Hematinic, trace element.
DexFol. (Rising) Vitamin B$_1$ 1.5 mg, vitamin B$_2$ 1.5 mg, vitamin B$_3$ 20 mg, vitamin B$_5$ 10 mg, vitamin B$_6$ 50 mg, vitamin B$_{12}$ 1 mg, C 60 mg, FA 5 mg, biotin 300 mcg. Tab. 90s. *Rx.*
Use: Nutritional product.
Dex4 Glucose. (Can-Am Care) Glucose, lemon, orange, raspberry, grape flavors. Chew. Tab. Bot. 10s, 50s. *OTC.*
Use: Glucose-elevating agent.
Dex GG. (Boca Pharmacal) Dextromethorphan HBr 60 mg, guaifenesin 1000 mg. ER Tab. Bot. 100s. *Rx.*
Use: Upper respiratory combination, antitussive, expectorant.
●**dexibuprofen.** (dex-EYE-byoo-PRO-fen) USAN.
Use: Analgesic; anti-inflammatory.
●**dexibuprofen lysine.** (dex-EYE-byoo-PRO-fen LIE-seen) USAN.
Use: Analgesic (cyclooxygenase inhibitor); anti-inflammatory.
●**deximafen.** (dex-IH-mah-fen) USAN.
Use: Antidepressant.
●**dexivacaine.** (dex-IH-vah-CANE) USAN.
Use: Anesthetic.
●**dexmedetomidine.** (DEX-meh-dih-TOE-mih-deen) USAN.
Use: Anxiolytic.
●**dexmedetomidine hydrochloride.** (DEX-meh-dih-TOE-mih-deen high-droe-KLOR-ide)
Use: Sedative/hypnotic, nonbarbiturate.
See: Precedex.
●**dexmethylphenidate hydrochloride.** (dex-meth-il-FEN-i-date) USAN.
Use: CNS stimulant.
See: Focalin.
  Focalin XR.
Dexone LA. (Keene Pharmaceuticals) Dexamethasone acetate suspension equivalent to dexamethasone 8 mg, polysorbate 80, carboxymethylcellulose, sodium bisulfite, EDTA, benzyl alcohol. Vial 5 mL. *Rx.*
Use: Corticosteroid.
●**dexormaplatin.** (DEX-ore-mah-PLAT-in) USAN.

Use: Antineoplastic.
●**dexoxadrol hydrochloride.** (dex-OX-ah-drole) USAN.
Use: Antidepressant; stimulant (central); analgesic.
●**dexpanthenol.** (DEX-PAN-theh-nahl) *USP 28.*
Use: Treatment of paralytic ileus and postoperative distention; cholinergic.
See: Ilopan.
  Panthoderm.
●**dexpemedolac.** (dex-peh-MED-oh-lack) USAN.
Use: Analgesic.
●**dexpropanolol hydrochloride.** (DEX-pro-PRAN-oh-lole) USAN.
Use: Antiadrenergic (β-receptor); cardiovascular agent (antiarrhythmic).
●**dexrazoxane.** (dex-ray-ZOX-ane) USAN.
Use: Cytoprotective agent.
See: Zinecard.
dexrazoxane. (Bedford) Dexrazoxane 250 mg, 500 mg. 10 mg/mL reconstituted. Pow. for Inj., lyophilized. Single-use vials with 25 mL sodium lactate injection (250 mg) or 50 mL sodium lactate injection (500 mg). *Rx.*
Use: Cytoprotective agent.
●**dexsotalol hydrochloride.** (DEX-ah-tah-lahl) USAN.
Use: Cardiovascular agent (antiarrhythmic).
●**dextofisopam.** (dex-toe-FIS-oh-pam) USAN.
Use: Crohn disease
dextran adjunct. *Rx.*
Use: Plasma expander.
See: Promit.
dextran and deferoxamine.
Use: Acute iron poisoning. [Orphan Drug]
See: Bio-Rescue.
●**dextran 40.** (DEX-tran 40) USAN. Polysaccharide (m.w. 40,000) produced by the action of *Leuconostoc mesenteroides* on sucrose.
Use: Blood flow adjuvant; plasma volume extender.
See: 10% LMD.
  Gentran 40.
  Rheomacrodex.
dextran 40. (McGaw) Dextran 40 10% with 0.9% sodium chloride or in 5% dextrose. Inj. 500 mL. *Rx.*
Use: Plasma expander.
dextran 45, 75. Polysaccharide (m.w. 45,000, 75,000) produced by the action of *Leuconostoc mesenteroides* on saccharose. Rheotran (45). *Rx.*
Use: Blood volume expander.

●**dextran 1.** (DEX-tran 1) *USP 28.*
Use: Plasma volume extender.
See: Promit.
●**dextran 70.** (DEX-tran 70) USAN. Polysaccharide (m.w. 70,000) produced by the action of *Levconostoc mesenteroides* on sucrose.
Use: Plasma volume extender.
See: Aquasite.
Gentran 70.
Hyskon.
Macrodex.
dextran 70. (McGaw) Dextran 70 6% in 0.9% sodium chloride. Inj. 500 mL. *Rx.*
Use: Plasma expander.
●**dextran 75.** (DEX-tran 75) USAN. Polysaccharide (m.w. 75,000) produced by the action of *Louuvnoui ion mesentemides* on sucrose.
Use: Plasma volume extender.
See: Macrodex.
dextran 75. (Abbott) Dextran 75 6% in 0.9% sodium chloride or 5% dextrose. Inj. Vial 500 mL. *Rx.*
Use: Plasma expander.
dextran 6%. (Abbott) *Rx.*
See: Dextran 75.
dextran sulfate, inhaled aerosolized.
Use: Antiviral. [Orphan Drug]
See: Uendex.
dextran sulfate sodium. (Ueno Fine Chemicals Industry)
Use: AIDS drug. [Orphan Drug]
●**dextrates.** (DEX-traytz) *NF 23.* Mixture of sugars (≈ 92% dextrose monohydrate and 8% higher saccharides; dextrose equivalent is 95% to 97%) resulting from the controlled enzymatic hydrolysis of starch.
Use: Pharmaceutic aid (tablet binder, diluent).
●**dextrin.** *NF 23.*
Use: Pharmaceutic aid (suspending, viscosity-increasing agent; tablet binder; tablet, capsule diluent).
●**dextroamphetamine.** (DEX-troe-am-FET-ah-meen) USAN.
Use: Stimulant (central).
dextroamphetamine phosphate. Monobasic d-a-methylphenethlyamine phosphate. (+)-α-Methylphenethylamine phosphate.
Use: CNS stimulant.
dextroamphetamine saccharate.
Use: CNS stimulant.
W/Combinations.
See: Adderall.
Adderall XR.
Amphetamine Salt Combo.

●**dextroamphetamine sulfate.** (DEX-troe-am-FET-uh-meen) *USP 28.*
Use: CNS stimulant, amphetamine.
See: Dexampex.
Dexedrine.
Dexedrine Spansules.
Dextrostat.
Tidex.
W/Combinations.
See: Adderall.
Adderall XR.
Amphetamine Salt Combo.
dextroamphetamine sulfate. (Various Mfr.) Dextroamphetamine sulfate. **Tab:** 5 mg, 10 mg. Bot. 100s. **SR Cap:** 5 mg, 10 mg, 15 mg. Bot. 100s. *c-ii.*
Use: CNS stimulant, amphetamine.
Dextro-Check Normal Control. (Bayer Corp. (Consumer Div.)) Clear liquid containing measured amount of glucose 0.1%.
Use: Glucometer calibration aid.
Dextro-Chek Calibrators. (Bayer Corp. (Consumer Div.)) Clear liquid soln. containing measured amounts of glucose. Low calibrator contains 0.05% w/v glucose. High calibrator contains 0.3% w/v glucose.
Use: Glucometer calibration aid.
Dextro-Chlorpheniramine Maleate.
Use: Antihistamine.
See: Polaramine.
●**dextromethorphan.** (DEX-troe-meth-OR-fan) *USP 28.*
Use: Cough suppressant; antitussive.
W/Combinations.
See: DMax Pediatric.
●**dextromethorphan hydrobromide.** (DEX-troe-meth-OR-fan HIGH-droe-BROE-mide) *USP 28.*
Use: Antitussive.
See: Benylin.
Creo-Terpin.
Delsym.
DexAlone.
ElixSure Children's Cough.
Hold DM.
Little Colds Cough Formula.
Mediquell.
PediaCare Infants' Long-Acting Cough.
Robitussin Cough Gels.
Robitussin Maximum Strength Cough.
Robitussin Pediatric Cough.
Scot-Tussin DM Cough Chasers.
Silphen DM.
Simply Cough.
TheraFlu Thin Strips Long Acting Cough.
Triaminic Thin Strips Long Acting Cough.
Vicks 44 Cough Relief.

W/Benzocaine.
See: Cough-X.
Spec-T.
Vicks Cough Silencers.
W/Combinations.
See: AccuHist DM Pediatric.
AccuHist PDX.
Alacol DM.
Alka-Seltzer Plus Cold & Cough.
Alka-Seltzer Plus Cold & Cough Medicine Effervescent.
Alka Seltzer Plus Cold & Flu.
Alka-Seltzer Plus Flu Medicine.
Alka-Seltzer Plus Liqui-Gels Flu Medicine.
Alka-Seltzer Plus Night-Time Cold Medicine.
Alka-Seltzer Plus Nose & Throat.
Allfen-DM.
All-Nite.
AMBI 1000/55.
AMBI 60/580/30.
Amerituss AD.
Anaplex-DM.
Andehist DM.
Andehist DM NR.
Andehist DM Oral.
Anti-Tuss D.M.
Anti-Tussive.
AquaTab C.
AquaTab DM.
Atuss DM.
Balamine DM.
Balamine DM Oral.
Benylin Expectorant.
Bromanate DM Cold & Cough.
Bromatane DX.
Bromfed DM Cough.
Bromhist-DM.
Bromhist PDX Drops.
Bromhist-PDX Syrup.
Carbodex DM.
Carbofed DM.
Carbofed DM Oral.
Cardec DM.
Cheracol D.
Cheracol D Cough Formula.
Cheracol Plus.
Children's Elixir DM Cough & Cold.
Codal-DM.
Codimal DM.
Cold & Cough Tussin.
Coldec DM.
Cold Symptoms Relief Maximum Strength.
Comtrex Cough and Cold Relief, Multi-Symptom Maximum Strength.
Comtrex Day & Night Cold & Cough Relief, Multi-Symptom Maximum Strength.
Comtrex Maximum Strength Night-time Cold & Cough.
Comtrex Multi-Symptom Deep Chest Cold & Congestion Relief.
Comtrex Multi-Symptom Maximum Strength Non-Drowsy Cold & Cough Relief.
Contac Day & Night Cold & Flu.
Contac Severe Cold & Flu Maximum Strength.
Coricidin HBP Chest Congestion & Cough.
Coricidin HBP Cough & Cold.
Coricidin HBP Maximum Strength Flu.
C.P.-DM.
Cydec-DM.
DEKA.
DEKA Pediatric.
Dex GG TR.
Diabetic Tussin.
Diabetic Tussin DM.
Diabetic Tussin Maximum Strength DM.
Dicomal-DM.
Dimaphen DM Cold & Cough.
Dimetapp Children's Nighttime Flu.
Dimetapp Children's Non-Drowsy Flu.
Dimetapp Decongestant Plus Cough Infant.
Dimetapp DM Children's Cold & Cough.
Dimetapp Long Acting Cough Plus Cold.
DMax.
Donatussin.
Duraflu.
Duratuss DM.
Extra Action Cough.
Father John's Medicine Plus.
Fenesin DM.
Gani-Tuss-DM NR.
Genacol Maximum Strength Cold & Flu Relief.
Genatuss DM.
GFN 550/PSE 60/DM 30.
GFN 1000/DM 60.
GFN 1200/DM 60.
GFN 1200/DM 60/PSE 120.
Guaifenesin DM.
Guaifenesin-DM NR.
Guaifenesin 1000 mg and Dextromethorphan HBr 60 mg LA.
Guaifenex DM.
Guiadrine DM.
Histacol DM.
Histenol-Forte.
Humibid DM.
Hydro-Tussin DM.
Iobid DM.
Kid Kare Children's Cough/Cold.
Kolephrin/DM.
Kolephrin GG/DM.

Lemotussin-DM.
Lortuss DM.
Mapap Cold Formula.
Maxifed DM.
Maxifed DMX.
MAXIPHEN DM.
Maxi-tuss DM.
Mucinex DM.
Muco-Fen-DM.
Mytussin DM.
Nil Tuss.
Nite Time Children's.
Nite Time Cold Formula for Adults.
Norel DM.
Nyquil.
Panatuss DX.
PanMist-DM.
PediaCare Children's Long-Lasting
  Cough Plus Cold.
PediaCare Children's Multi-Symptom
  Cold.
PediaCare Cough-Cold.
PediaCare Infants' Decongestant &
  Cough.
PediaCare Multi-Symptom Cold.
PediaCare NightRest Cough & Cold.
Pediahist DM.
Pediatex-DM.
Phanatuss DM Cough.
Phenergan.
Polytuss-DM.
Profen Forte DM.
Profen II DM.
Promethazine w/Dextromethrophan
  Cough.
Prometh w/Dextromethorphan.
Rescon-DM.
Robafen CF.
Robitussin Allergy & Cough.
Robitussin-CF.
Robitussin Cold & Cough.
Robitussin Cold, Cold & Congestion.
Robitussin Cold, Cold & Cough.
Robitussin Cold, Multi-Symptom Cold
  & Flu.
Robitussin Cough & Cold Infant.
Robitussin Cough & Congestion For-
  mula.
Robitussin-DM.
Robitussin DM Infant.
Robitussin Flu.
Robitussin Honey Cough & Cold.
Robitussin Honey Flu Multi-
  Symptom.
Robitussin Honey Flu Nighttime.
Robitussin Honey Flu Non-Drowsy.
Robitussin Maximum Strength Cough
  & Cold.
Robitussin Night Relief.
Robitussin Pediatric Cough & Cold
  Formula.

Robitussin Pediatric Night Relief
  Cough & Cold.
Robitussin PM Cough & Cold.
Robitussin Sugar Free Cough.
Rondamine DM.
Rondec-DM.
Rondec-DM Oral.
Safe Tussin.
Scot-Tussin DM.
Scot-Tussin Senior Clear.
Sildec-DM.
Sildec-DM Oral.
Siltussin DM Cough.
SINUtuss DM.
666 Cold Preparation Maximum
  Strength.
Sudafed Children's Non-Drowsy Cold
  & Cough.
Sudafed Multi-Symptom Cold &
  Cough.
Sudafed Non-Drowsy Severe Cold
  Formula Maximum Strength.
Sudal-DM.
SU-TUSS DM.
TheraFlu Cold & Cough Night Time.
TheraFlu Flu and Chest Congestion
  Non-Drowsy.
TheraFlu Flu & Cough Night Time,
  Maximum Strength.
TheraFlu Flu, Cold, & Cough and
  Sore Throat, Maximum Strength.
TheraFlu Flu, Cold & Cough Night-
  Time, Maximum Strength.
TheraFlu Maximum Strength Flu, Cold
  & Cough.
TheraFlu Maximum Strength Night
  Time Formula Flu, Cold, & Cough
  Medicine.
TheraFlu Non-Drowsy Flu, Cold &
  Cough Maximum Strength.
TheraFlu Non-Drowsy Formula Maxi-
  mum Strength.
TheraFlu Severe Cold & Congestion
  Night Time, Maximum Strength.
TheraFlu Severe Cold & Congestion
  Non-Drowsy, Maximum Strength.
Thera-Hist Cold & Cough.
Tolu-Sed DM.
Top Care LiquiCaps Nite Time Multi-
  Symptom Cold/Flu Relief.
Top Care Maximum Strength Flu,
  Cold, & Cough Medicine Night Time.
Top Care Maximum Strength Soothing
  Cough & Head Congestion Relief
  D.
Top Care Multi-Symptom Pain Relief
  Cold.
Touro CC.
Touro DM.
Tri-Acting Cold & Cough.
Triaminic AM Non-Drowsy Cough &
  Decongestant.

Triaminic Cold & Cough.
Triaminic Cough.
Triaminic Cough & Sore Throat.
Triaminic Flu, Cough & Fever.
Triaminic Night Time Cough & Cold.
Triaminic Softchews Cold & Sore Throat.
Triaminic Throat Pain & Cough Softchews.
Tricodene Sugar Free.
Tussafed.
Tussafed-EX.
Tussafed-LA.
Tuss-DM.
TUSSI-bid.
Tussi-Organidin DM NR.
TUSSI-PRES.
Tylenol.
Tylenol Children's Cold Plus Cough.
Tylenol Children's Flu.
Tylenol Cold Complete Formula.
Tylenol Cold Non-Drowsy Formula.
Tylenol Flu Maximum Strength Non-Drowsy.
Tylenol Flu NightTime, Maximum Strength.
Tylenol Infants' Cold Decongestant & Fever Reducer Plus Cough.
Tylenol Multi-Symptom Cold Severe Congestion.
Unproco.
Vicks Children's NyQuil Cold/Cough Relief.
Vicks Cough.
Vicks DayQuil LiquiCaps Multi-Symptom Cold/Flu Relief.
Vicks DayQuil Multi-Symptom Cold/Flu Relief.
Vicks 44D Cough & Head Congestion Relief.
Vicks 44E Cough & Chest Congestion Relief.
Vicks 44M Cough, Cold, & Flu Relief.
Vicks NyQuil Cough.
Vicks NyQuil Multi-Symptom Cold/Flu Relief.
Vicks Pediatric 44E Cough & Chest Congestion Relief.
Vicks Pediatric 44M Cough & Cold Relief.
Z-Cof DM.
Z-Cof LA.

dextromethorphan hydrobromide/ guaifenesin. (URL) Dextromethorphan HBr 30 mg, guaifenesin 500 mg. Dye-free. ER Tab. 100s. *Rx.*
Use: Antitussive, expectorant.

•**dextromethorphan polistirex.** (DEX-troe-meth-OR-fan pahl-ee-STIE-rex) USAN.
Use: Antitussive.

W/Combinations.
See: Atuss-12 DX.
dextromethorphan tannate.
Use: Antitussive.
W/Combinations.
See: Atuss-12 DM.
Viravan-DM.
dextromoramide tartrate.
Use: Analgesic; narcotic.
dextro-pantothenyl alcohol.
See: Ilopan.
Panthenol.
dextropropoxyphene hydrochloride.
c-iv.
Use: Analgesic.
See: Propoxyphene hydrochloride.
•**dextrorphan hydrochloride.** (DEX-trorefan) USAN.
Use: Treatment of cerebral ischemia; vasospastic therapy adjunct.
•**dextrose.** (DEX-trose) *USP 28.*
Use: Fluid and nutrient replenisher.
W/Calcium ascorbate and benzyl alcohol injection.
See: Calscorbate.
W/Psyllium mucilloid.
See: V-lax.
dextrose-alcohol injection. *Rx.*
Use: Nutritional supplement, parenteral.
See: 5% Alcohol and 5% Dextrose in Water.
dextrose and Isolyte combinations.
Use: Intravenous nutritional therapy, intravenous replenishment solution.
See: Isolyte M in 5% Dextrose.
Isolyte H in 5% Dextrose.
Isolyte P in 5% Dextrose.
Isolyte S with 5% Dextrose.
Isolyte R in 5% Dextrose.
dextrose and Normosol combinations.
Use: Intravenous nutritional therapy, intravenous replenishment solution.
See: Normosol-M and 5% Dextrose.
Normosol-R and 5% Dextrose.
dextrose and Plasmalyte combinations.
Use: Intravenous nutritional therapy, intravenous replenishment solution.
See: Plasma-Lyte 56 and 5% Dextrose.
Plasma-Lyte M and 5% Dextrose.
Plasma-Lyte 148 and 5% Dextrose.
Plasma-Lyte R and 5% Dextrose.
dextrose and Ringer's combinations.
Use: Intravenous nutritional therapy, intravenous replenishment solution.
See: Half-Strength Lactated Ringer's in 2.5% dextrose.
Lactated Ringer's in 5% Dextrose.
Ringer's in 5% Dextrose.
dextrose-electrolyte solutions. *Rx.*
Use: Intravenous nutritional therapy,

intravenous replenishment solutions.
See: Dextrose 2.5% with 0.45% Sodium
Chloride.
Dextrose 3.3% and 0.3% Sodium
Chloride.
Dextrose 5% and Electrolyte No. 48.
Dextrose 5% and Electrolyte No. 75.
Dextrose 5% with 0.2% Sodium
Chloride.
Dextrose 5% and 0.225% Sodium
Chloride.
Dextrose 5% with 0.3% Sodium
Chloride.
Dextrose 5% with 0.33% Sodium
Chloride.
Dextrose 5% with 0.45% Sodium
Chloride.
Dextrose 5% with 0.9% Sodium
Chloride.
Dextrose 10% and Fluidolyte No. 40.
Dextrose 10% with 0.2% Sodium
Chloride.
Dextrose 10% with 0.225% Sodium
Chloride.
Dextrose 10% with 0.45 Sodium
Chloride.
Dextrose 10% and 0.9% Sodium
Chloride.
Half-Strength Lactated Ringer's in
2.5% Dextrose.
Isolyte H in 5% Dextrose.
Isolyte M in 5% Dextrose.
Isolyte P in 5% Dextrose.
Isolyte R in 5% Dextrose.
Isolyte S with 5% Dextrose.
Lactated Ringer's in 5% Dextrose.
Normosol-M and 5% Dextrose.
Normosol-R and 5% Dextrose.
Plasma-Lyte 56 and 5% Dextrose.
Plasma-Lyte M and 5% Dextrose.
Plasma-Lyte 148 and 5% Dextrose.
Plasma-Lyte R and 5% Dextrose.
Potassium Chloride in 5% Dextrose
and Lactated Ringer's.
Potassium Chloride in 5% Dextrose.
Potassium Chloride in 3.3% Dextrose
and 0.3% Sodium Chloride.
Potassium Chloride in 5% Dextrose
and 0.2% Sodium Chloride.
Potassium Chloride in 5% Dextrose
and 0.33% Sodium Chloride.
Potassium Chloride in 5% Dextrose
and 0.45% Sodium Chloride.
Potassium Chloride in 5% Dextrose
and 0.9% Sodium Chloride.
Potassium Chloride in 10% Dextrose
and 0.2% Sodium Chloride.
Ringer's in 5% Dextrose.
•**dextrose excipient.** NF 23.
Use: Pharmaceutic aid (tablet
excipient).

dextrose 5% and electrolyte No. 48.
(Baxter PPI) Dextrose 50 g, calories
180/L with Na$^+$ 25 mEq, K$^+$ 20 mEq,
Mg^{++} 3 mEq, Cl$^-$ 24 mEq, phosphate
3 mEq, acetate 23 mEq with osmolarity
348 mOsm/L. Soln. Bot. 250 mL. Rx.
Use: Intravenous nutritional therapy,
intravenous replenishment.
dextrose 5% and electrolyte No. 75.
(Baxter PPI) Dextrose 50 g, calories
180/L with Na$^+$ 40 mEq, K$^+$ 35 mEq, Cl$^-$
48 mEq, phosphate 15 mEq, and lactate 20 mEq with osmolarity 402 mOsm/
L. Soln. Bot. 250 mL, 500 mL,
1000 mL. Rx.
Use: Intravenous nutritional therapy,
intravenous replenishment.
**dextrose 5% and lactated ringer's and
potassium chloride.**
Use: Intravenous nutritional therapy,
intravenous replenishment solution.
See: Potassium Chloride in 5% Dextrose and Lactated Ringer's.
dextrose 5% and potassium chloride.
Use: Intravenous nutritional therapy,
intravenous replenishment solution.
See: Potassium Chloride in 5% Dextrose.
**dextrose 5% and sodium chloride
0.45% and potassium chloride.**
Use: Intravenous nutritional therapy,
intravenous replenishment solution.
See: Potassium Chloride in 5% Dextrose and 0.45% Sodium Chloride.
•**dextrose 5% and sodium chloride 0.9%
and potassium chloride.**
Use: Intravenous nutritional therapy,
intravenous replenishment solution.
See: Potassium Chloride in 5% Dextrose and 0.9% Sodium Chloride.
**dextrose 5% and sodium chloride
0.33% and potassium chloride.**
Use: Intravenous nutritional therapy,
intravenous replenishment solution.
See: Potassium Chloride in 5% Dextrose and 0.33% Sodium Chloride.
**dextrose 5% and sodium chloride 0.2%
and potassium chloride.**
Use: Intravenous nutritional therapy,
intravenous replenishment solution.
See: Potassium Chloride in 5% Dextrose and 0.2% Sodium Chloride.
**dextrose 5% and 0.225% sodium chlor-
ide.** (Abbott) Dextrose 50 g, calories
170/L, Na$^+$ 38.5 mEq, Cl$^-$ 38.5 mEq,
osmolarity 329 mOsm/L. Soln. Bot.
250 mL, 500 mL, 1000 mL. Rx.
Use: Intravenous nutritional therapy,
intravenous replenishment solution.
**dextrose 5% with 0.45% sodium chlor-
ide.** (Various Mfr.) Dextrose 50 g, calo-

ries 170/L, Na$^+$ 77 mEq, Cl$^-$ 77 mEq, osmolarity ≈ 405 mOsm/L. Soln. Bot. 250 mL, 500 mL, 1000 mL. *Rx.*
Use: Intravenous nutritional therapy, intravenous replenishment solution.

dextrose 5% with 0.9% sodium chloride. (Various Mfr.) Dextrose 50 g, calories 170/L, Na$^+$ 154 mEq, Cl$^-$ 154 mEq, osmolarity ≈ 560 mOsm/L. Soln. Bot. 250 mL, 500 mL, 1000 mL. *Rx.*
Use: Intravenous nutritional therapy, intravenous replenishment solution.

dextrose 5% with 0.3% sodium chloride. (Abbott) Dextrose 50 g, calories 170/L, Na$^+$ 51 mEq, Cl$^-$ 51 mEq, osmolarity 355 mOsm/L. Soln. Bot. 250 mL, 500 mL, 1000 mL. *Rx.*
Use: Intravenous nutritional therapy, intravenous replenishment solution.

dextrose 5% with 0.33% sodium chloride. (Various Mfr.) Dextrose 50 g, calories 170/L, Na$^+$ 56 mEq, Cl$^-$ 56 mEq, osmolarity 365 mOsm/L. Soln. Bot. 250 mL, 500 mL, 1000 mL. *Rx.*
Use: Intravenous nutritional therapy, intravenous replenishment solution.

dextrose 5% with 0.2% sodium chloride. (Various Mfr.) Dextrose 50 g, calories 170/L, Na$^+$ 34 mEq, Cl$^-$ 34 mEq, osmolarity ≈ 320 mOsm/L. Soln. Bot. 250 mL, 500 mL, 1000 ML. *Rx.*
Use: Intravenous nutritional therapy, intravenous replenishment solution.

dextrose large volume parenterals. (Abbott Hospital Products) *Rx.*
Use: Nutritional supplement, parenteral.

dextrose small volume parenterals. (Abbott Hospital Products) **Dextrose 5%:** 50 mL, 100 mL pressurized pintop vial. **Dextrose 10%:** 5 mL amp. **Dextrose 25%:** 10 mL syringe. **Dextrose 50%:** 50 mL Abboject syringe (18 g × 1.5″), 50 mL Fliptop vial. **Dextrose 70%:** 70 mL pressurized pintop vial. *Rx.*
Use: Nutritional supplement, parenteral.

dextrose-sodium chloride injection. (Abbott) 10% dextrose and 0.225% sodium chloride. Inj. Single-dose container. 500 mL.
Use: Nutritional supplement, parenteral.

dextrose 10% and electrolyte no. 48. (Baxter Healthcare) Dextrose 100 g, calories 350/L, Na$^+$ 25 mEq, K$^+$ 20 mEq, Mg^{++} 3 mEq, Cl$^-$ 24 mEq, phosphate 3 mEq, lactate 23 mEq, osmolarity 600 mOsm/L, sodium bisulfite Soln. Bot. 250 mL. *Rx.*
Use: Intravenous nutritional therapy, intravenous replenishment solution.

dextrose 10% and 0.9% sodium chloride. (Various Mfr.) Dextrose 100 g, calories 340/L, Na$^+$ 154 mEq, Cl$^-$ 154 mEq, osmolarity 813–815 mOsm/ L. Soln. Bot. 500 mL, 1000 mL. *Rx.*
Use: Intravenous nutritional therapy, intravenous replenishment solution.

dextrose 10% and 0.2% sodium chloride and potassium chloride.
Use: Intravenous nutritional therapy, intravenous replenishment solution.
See: Potassium Chloride in 10% Dextrose and 0.2% Sodium Chloride.

dextrose 10% with 0.45% sodium chloride. (B. Braun) Dextrose 100 g, calories 340/L, Na$^+$ 77 mEq, Cl$^-$ 77 mEq, osmolarity 660 mOsm/L. Soln. Bot. 1000 mL. *Rx.*
Use: Intravenous nutritional therapy, intravenous replenishment solution.

dextrose 10% with 0.2% sodium chloride. Various Mfr. Dextrose 100 g, calories 340/L, Na$^+$ 34 mEq, Cl$^-$ 34 mEq, osmolarity 575 mOsm/L. Soln. Bot. 250 mL. *Rx.*
Use: Intravenous nutritional therapy, intravenous replenishment solution.

dextrose 10% with 0.225% sodium chloride. (Abbott) Dextrose 100 g, calories 340/L, Na$^+$ 38.5 mEq, Cl$^-$ 38.5 mEq, osmolarity 582 mOsm/L. Soln. Bot. 250 mL, 500 mL. *Rx.*
Use: Intravenous nutritional therapy, intravenous replenishment solution.

dextrose 3.3% and 0.3% sodium chloride. (B. Braun) Dextrose 33 g, calories 110/L, Na$^+$ 51 mEq, Cl$^-$ 51 mEq, osmolarity 270 mOsm/L. Soln. Bot. 250 mL, 500 mL, 1000 mL. *Rx.*
Use: Intravenous nutritional therapy, intravenous replenishment solution.

dextrose 3.3% dextrose and 0.3% sodium chloride and potassium chloride.
Use: Intravenous nutritional therapy, intravenous replenishment solution.
See: Potassium chloride in 3.3% Dextrose and 0.3% Sodium Chloride.

dextrose 2.5% with 0.45% sodium chloride. Various Mfr. Dextrose 25 g, calories 85/L, Na$^+$ 77 mEq, Cl$^-$ 77 mEq, osmolarity 280 mOsm/L. Soln. Bot. 500 mL, 1000 mL. *Rx.*
Use: Intravenous nutritional therapy, intravenous replenishment solution.

Dextrostat. (Shire Richwood) Dextroamphetamine sulfate 5 mg, 10 mg, sucrose, lactose, tartrazine. Tab. Bot. 100s, 500s; 1000s (5 mg only). *c-ii.*
Use: CNS stimulant, amphetamine.

Dexule. (Health for Life Brands) Vitamins A 1333 units, D 133 units, B$_1$

0.33 mg, B₂ 0.4 mg, C 10 mg, niacinamide 3.3 mg, iron 3.3 mg, calcium 29 mg, phosphorus 15 mg, methylcellulose 100 mg, benzocaine 3 mg. Cap. Bot. 21s, 90s. *OTC.*
Use: Mineral, vitamin supplement.
Dexyl. (Pinex) Dextromethorphan HBr 15 mg, vitamin C 20 mg. Tab. Box 20s. *OTC.*
Use: Antitussive; vitamin supplement.
●**dezaguanine.** (DEH-zah-GWAHN-een) USAN.
Use: Antineoplastic.
●**dezaguanine mesylate.** (DEE-zah-GWAHN-een MEH-sih-late) USAN.
Use: Antineoplastic.
●**dezinamide.** (deh-ZIN-ah-mide) USAN.
Use: Anticonvulsant.
D Film. (Ciba Vision) Polovamer 407, EDTA 0.25%, benzalkonium Cl 0.025%. Gel. Tube 25 g. *OTC.*
Use: Contact lens care.
DFMO. Eflornithine hydrochloride. *Rx.*
Use: Anti-infective.
See: Ornidyl.
d4T.
Use: Antiviral.
See: Stavudine.
DFP. Disopropyl fluorophosphate (Various Mfr.)
d-Glucose. Dextrose. *Rx.*
Use: Nutritional supplement, parenteral.
See: D-10-W.
D-2½-W.
DHC Plus. (Purdue) Dihydrocodeine bitartrate 16 mg, acetaminophen 356.4 mg, caffeine 30 mg. Cap. Bot. 100s. *c-III.*
Use: Analgesic combination; narcotic.
DHEA. (Athena Neurosciences) EL10. *Rx.*
Use: Antiviral; immunomodulator.
D.H.E. 45. (Xcel) Dihydroergotamine mesylate 1 mg/mL, alcohol 6.2%, glycerin 15%. Inj. Amp. 1 mL. *Rx.*
Use: Antimigraine.
DHPG. Ganciclovir sodium. *Rx.*
Use: Antiviral.
See: Cytovene.
DHS Conditioning Rinse. (Person and Covey) Conditioning ingredients. Bot. 8 oz. *OTC.*
Use: Dermatologic, hair.
DHS Shampoo. (Person and Covey) Blend of cleansing surfactants and emulsifiers. Plastic bot. w/dispenser 8 oz, 16 oz. *OTC.*
Use: Dermatologic, hair, and scalp.
DHS Tar Gel Shampoo. (Person and Covey) Coal tar 0.5% Bot. 240 g. *OTC.*

Use: Antipsoriatic; antiseborrheic.
DHS Tar Shampoo. (Person and Covey) Coal tar 0.5%. Liq. Bot. 120 mL, 240 mL, 480 mL. *OTC.*
Use: Antipsoriatic; antiseborrheic.
DHS Zinc. (Person and Covey) Zinc pyrithione 2%. Shampoo. Bot. 240 mL, 360 mL. *OTC.*
Use: Antiseborrheic.
DHT. (Roxane) Dihydrotachysterol. **Tab.:** 0.125 mg, 0.2 mg, 0.4 mg, lactose, sucrose. Bot. 50s, 100s (0.2 mg only), UD 100s (except 0.4 mg). **Intensol Soln.:** 0.2 mg/mL, alcohol 20%. Bot. 30 mL w/dropper. *Rx.*
Use: Antihypocalcemic.
DiaBeta. (Hoechst) Glyburide. **1.25 mg:** Bot. 50s. **2.5 mg:** Bot. 100s, 500s, UD 100s. **5 mg:** Bot. 100s, 500s, 1000s, UD 1000s. *Rx.*
Use: Antidiabetic.
Diabetic Tussin. (Health Care Products) Guaifenesin 100 mg/5 mL, aspartame, menthol, methylparaben, phenylalanine 8.4 mg/5 mL. Alcohol- and dye-free. Liq. Bot. 118 mL. *Rx.*
Use: Antitussive, decongestant, expectorant.
Diabetic Tussin DM. (Health Care Products) Dextromethorphan HBr 10 mg, guaifenesin 100 mg/5 mL, methylparaben, menthol, aspartame, phenylalanine 8.4 mg, alcohol and dye free. Liq. Bot. 118 mL. *OTC.*
Use: Upper respiratory combination, antitussive, expectorant.
Diabetic Tussin Maximum Strength DM. (Health Care Products) Dextromethorphan HBr 10 mg, guaifenesin 200 mg/5 mL, aspartame, phenylalanine 8.4 mg, menthol, methylparaben, alcohol and dye free. Liq. Bot. 118 mL, 237 mL. *OTC.*
Use: Upper respiratory combination, antitussive, expectorant.
Diabinese. (Pfizer) Chlorpropamide 100 mg, 250 mg. Tab. Bot. 100s, 250s (250 mg only), 500s (100 mg only), 1000s (250 mg only), UD 100s. *Rx.*
Use: Antidiabetic.
diacetic acid test.
See: Acetest.
Diaceto w/Codeine. (Archer-Taylor) Codeine 0.25 g, 0.5 g. Tab. or Cap. Bot. 500s, 1000s. *c-II.*
Use: Analgesic; narcotic.
Diaceto w/Gelsemium. (Archer-Taylor) Phenobarbital 0.5 g, gelsemium 3 min. Tab. Bot. 1000s. *c-IV.*
Use: Hypnotic; sedative.

•diacetolol hydrochloride. (DIE-ah-SEET-oh-lahl HIGH-droe-KLOR-ide) USAN.
Use: Antiadrenergic (β-receptor).
diacetrizoate, sodium.
See: Diatrizoate.
•diacetylated monoglycerides. *NF 23.*
Use: Pharmaceutic aid (plasticizer).
diacetylcholine chloride. Succinylcholine Cl.
See: Anectine Chloride.
diacetyl-dihydroxydiphenylisatin.
See: Oxyphenisatin acetate.
diacetyldioxyphenylisatin.
See: Oxyphenisatin acetate.
diacetylmorphine salts. Heroin. Illegal in USA by federal statute because of its addiction potential.
Di-Ademil.
See: Hydroflumethiazide.
diagniol.
See: Sodium Acetrizoate.
diagnostic agents.
See: Acholest.
Aplisol.
Aplitest.
Candida Skin Test Antigen.
Candin.
Cardio-Green.
Cardiografin.
Cea-Roche.
Cholecystography Agents.
Cholografin.
Coccidioidin.
Dextrostix.
Dey-Pak Sodium Chloride.
Evans Blue Dye.
EZ Detect Strep-A Test.
Fertility Tape.
First Choice.
Fluorescein Sodium.
Fluor-I-Strip.
Fluor-I-Strip A.T.
Fluress.
Hema-Combistix.
Hemastix.
Histalog.
Histolyn-CYL.
Histoplasmin.
HIVAB HIV-1/HIV-2 (rDNA) EIA.
Hymenoptera Venoms.
Immunex CRP.
Indigo Carmine.
Kidney Function Agents.
Liver Function Agents.
Mannitol.
Mono-Latex.
Mono-Plus.
MSTA.
Multitest-CMI.
Mumps Skin Test Antigen.
Persantine IV.
Pharmalgen.
Phentolamine Methanesulfonate.
Prepen.
Regitine.
Rheumanosticon Slide Test.
Rheumatrex.
Rheumaton.
Spherulin.
SureCell Chlamydia Test.
SureCell Herpes (HSV) Test.
SureCell Strep A Test.
Sodium Dehydrochol.
Tes-Tape.
Tine Test.
True Test.
Tubersol.
Urography Agents.
Venomil.
diagnostic agents for urine.
See: Acetest.
Albustix.
Biotel Diabetes.
Biotel Kidney.
Biotel U.T.I.
Chemstrip Micral.
Clinistix.
Clinitest.
Fortel Midstream.
Fortel Plus.
HCG-nostick.
Hema-Combistix.
Hemastix.
Hematest.
Ictotest.
Ketostix.
SureCell hCG-Urine Test.
Uristix.
Wampole One-Step hCG.
diallylamicol. Diallyl-diethylaminoethyl phenol di hydrochloride.
diallylbarbituric acid. Allobarbital, Allobarbitone, Curral.
dialminate. Mixture of magnesium carbonate and (aluminate) dihydroxyaluminum glycinate.
W/Aspirin.
See: Bufferin.
Dialyte Pattern LM w/4.25% Dextrose. (Gambro) Dextrose 42.5 g/L, Na^+ 131.5, Ca^{++} 3.5, Mg^{++} 0.5, Cl^- 94, and lactate 40 with osmolarity 485 mOsm/L. Soln. Bot. 1000 mL, 2000 mL, 4000 mL. *Rx.*
Use: Peritoneal dialysis solution.
Dialyte Pattern LM w/1.5% Dextrose. (Gambro) Dextrose 15 g/L, Na^+ 131 mEq, Ca^{++} 3.5 mEq, Mg^{++} 0.5 mEq, Cl^- 94 mEq, and lactate 40 mEq with osmolarity 345 mOsm/L. Soln. Bot. 1000 mL, 2000 mL, 4000 mL. *Rx.*

Use: Peritoneal dialysis solution.

Dialyte Pattern LM w/2.5% Dextrose.
(Gambro) Dextrose 25 g/L, Na⁺
131.5 mEq, Ca⁺⁺ 3.5 mEq, Mg⁺⁺
0.5 mEq, Cl⁻ 94 mEq, and lactate
40 mEq with osmolarity 395 mOsm/L.
Soln. Bot. 1000 mL, 2000 mL, 4000 mL.
Rx.
Use: Peritoneal dialysis solution.

Dialyvite 3000. (Hillestad) Vitamin C
100 mg, B_1 1.5 mg, B_2 1.7 mg, B_3
20 mg, B_5 10 mg, B_6 25 mg, B_{12} 1 mg,
FA 3 mg, biotin 300 mcg, E 30 units,
Se 70 mcg, Zn 15 mg. Tab. 90s. *OTC.*
Use: Nutritional combination product.

diamethine.
See: Dimethyl Tubocurarine.

**di-amino acetate complex w/calcium
aluminum carbonate.** Cap. units.
See: Ancid.

•**diaminodiphenylsulfone.** *USP 28.*
Use: Antimalarial.
See: Dapsone.

diaminopropyl tetramethylene.
See: Spermine.

3,4-diaminopyridine. (Jacobus)
Use: Lambert-Eaton myasthenic syndrome. [Orphan Drug]

•**diamocaine cyclamate.** (die-AM-oh-
CANE SIH-klah-mate) USAN.
Use: Anesthetic, local.

diamthazole dihydrochloride. Asterol.

Dianeal 137 w/4.25% Dextrose. (Baxter
PPI) Dextrose 42.5 g/L, Na⁺ 132 mEq,
Ca⁺⁺ 3.5 mEq, Mg⁺⁺ 1.5 mEq, Cl⁻
102 mEq, lactate 35 mEq with osmolar-
ity 486 mOsm/L. Soln. Bot. 2000 mL.
Rx.
Use: Peritoneal dialysis solution.

Dianeal 137 w/1.5% Dextrose. (Baxter
PPI) Dextrose 15 g/L, Na⁺ 132 mEq,
Ca⁺⁺ 3.5 mEq, Mg⁺⁺ 1.5 mEq, Cl⁻
102 mEq, lactate 35 mEq with osmolar-
ity 347 mOsm/L. Soln. Bot. 2000 mL.
Rx.
Use: Peritoneal dialysis solution.

**dianeal PD-2 peritoneal dialysis solu-
tion with 1.1% amino acid.**
Use: Nutritional supplement for dialysis
patients. [Orphan Drug]

Dianeal w/4.25% Dextrose. (Baxter PPI)
Dextrose 42.5 g/L, Na⁺ 141 mEq, Ca⁺⁺
3.5 mEq, Mg⁺⁺ 1.5 mEq, Cl⁻ 101 mEq,
lactate 45 mEq with osmolarity 503
mOsm/L. Soln. Bot. 2000 mL. *Rx.*
Use: Peritoneal dialysis solution.

Dianeal w/1.5% Dextrose. (Baxter PPI)
Dextrose 15 g/L, Na⁺ 141 mEq, Ca⁺⁺
3.5 mEq, Mg⁺⁺1.5 mEq, Cl⁻ 101 mEq,
lactate 45 mEq with osmolarity 364
mOsm/L. Soln. Bot. 1000 mL, 2000 mL.

Rx.
Use: Peritoneal dialysis solution.

•**diapamide.** (die-APP-am-ide) USAN.
Use: Antihypertensive; diuretic.

Diapantin. (Janssen) Isopropamide bromide. *Rx.*
Use: Anticholinergic.

Diaparene. (Bayer Corp. (Consumer
Div.)) Methylbenzethonium chloride.
Pow. Bot. 4 oz, 9 oz, 12.5 oz, 14 oz.
Use: Disinfectant; surface active agent.

Diaparene Ointment. (Bayer Corp. (Consumer Div.)) Methylbenzethonium chloride 0.1% w/petrolatum, glycerin. Tube
1 oz, 2 oz, 4 oz. *OTC.*
Use: Antimicrobial, topical.

Diaparene Peri-Anal Cream. (Bayer
Corp. (Consumer Div.)) Methylbenzethonium chloride 1:1000, zinc oxide,
starch, cod liver oil, white petrolatum,
lanolin, calcium caseinate. Cream. Tube
1 oz, 2 oz, 4 oz. *OTC.*
Use: Antimicrobial; astringent.

Diaper Guard. (Del) Dimethicone 1%,
white petrolatum 66%, cocoa butter,
parabens, vitamins A, D_3, E, zinc oxide. Oint. Tube 49.6 g, 99.2 g. *OTC.*
Use: Diaper rash preparation.

Diaper Rash. (Various Mfr.) Zinc oxide,
cod liver oil, lanolin, methylparaben,
petrolatum, talc. Oint. Tube 113 g. *OTC.*
Use: Diaper rash preparation.

diaphenylsulfone. Dapsone.
Use: Leprostatic.

Di-Ap-Trol. (Foy Laboratories) Phendimetrazine tartrate 35 mg. Tab. Bot.
100s, 1000s. *c-III.*
Use: Anorexiant.

Diarrest. (Dover Pharmaceuticals) Calcium carbonate, pectin. Tab. Sugar,
lactose, salt free. UD box 500s. *OTC.*
Use: Antidiarrheal.

diarrhea therapy.
See: Antidiarrheal.

Diaserp. (Major) Chlorothiazide 250 mg,
500 mg, w/reserpine. Tab. Bot. 100s.
Rx.
Use: Antihypertensive.

Diasorb. (Columbia) Activated nonfibrous
attapulgite. Liq.: 750 mg per 5 mL. Bot.
120 mL. Tab.: 750 mg. Pkg. 24s. *OTC.*
Use: Antidiarrheal.

Diasporal. (Doak Dermatologics) Formerly Sulfur Salicyl Diasporal. Sulfur
3%, salicylic acid 2%, isopropyl alcohol
in diasporal base. Cream. Jar 3¾ oz.
OTC.
Use: Antiseptic, topical.

Diastase.
See: Aspergillus oryzae enzyme.

Diastat. (Xcel) Diazapam. Benzyl alcohol 1.5%, ethyl alcohol 10%. **Pediatric:** 2.5 mg, 5 mg, 10 mg. **Adult:** 10 mg, 15 mg, 20 mg. Rectal gel. Twin pack. Includes lubricating jelly, plastic applicator with flexible, molded tip in two lengths.
Use: Anticonvulsant.
Diastix Reagent Strips. (Bayer Corp. (Consumer Div.)) Broad range test for glucose in urine. Containing glucose oxidase, peroxidase, potassium iodide w/blue background dye. Tab. Pkg. 50s, 100s.
Use: Diagnostic aid.
•**diatrizoate meglumine.** (die-ah-TRIH-zoe-ate meh-GLUE-meen) *USP 28.*
Use: Radiopaque agent, parenteral agent.
See: Angiovist 282.
Cardiografin.
Cystografin.
Cystografin Dilute.
Gastrografin.
Hypaque-Cysto.
Hypaque Meglumine 60%.
Hypaque-76.
MD-76 R.
RenoCal-76.
Renografin 60.
Reno-DIP.
Reno-60.
Reno-30.
Urovist.
W/Iodipamide methylglucamine.
See: Sinografin.
W/Sodium diatrizoate.
See: Renovist.
diatrizoate meglumine and diatrizoate sodium injection.
Use: Radiopaque agent, parenteral agent.
See: Angiovist 370.
Angiovist 292.
Hypaque-M.
Hypaque-76.
MD-76 R.
RenoCal-76.
Renografin-60.
diatrizoate meglumine and diatrizoate sodium solution.
Use: Radiopaque agent, iodinated GI contrast agent.
See: Gastrografin.
Renografin-76.
Renografin-60.
Renovist.
diatrizoate meglumine 52.7% and iodipamide meglumine 26.8% (38% iodine).
Use: Diagnostic aid (radiopaque agent).

See: Sinografin.
diatrizoate methylglucamine.
Use: Diagnostic aid (radiopaque medium).
See: Diatrizoate Meglumine.
diatrizoate methylglucamine sodium.
Use: Diagnostic aid (radiopaque medium).
•**diatrizoate sodium.** *USP 28.*
Use: Diagnostic aid (radiopaque medium).
See: Hypaque.
Urovist Sodium.
W/Meglumine diatrizoate.
See: Gastrografin.
Renografin-76.
Renografin-60.
Renovist II.
W/Methylglucamine diatrizoate, sodium citrate, disodium ethylenediamine tetraacetate dihydrate, methylparaben, propylparaben.
See: Renovist.
diatrizoate sodium (59.87% iodine).
Use: Radiopaque agent, iodinated GI contrast agent.
See: Hypaque Sodium.
diatrizoate sodium 50%.
Use: Radiopaque, parenteral.
See: Hypaque Sodium 50%.
•**diatrizoate sodium I-131.** USAN.
Use: Radiopharmaceutical.
•**diatrizoate sodium I-125.** USAN.
Use: Radiopharmaceutical.
•**diatrizoic acid.** (DIE-at-rih-ZOE-ik) *USP 28.*
Use: Diagnostic aid (radiopaque medium).
See: Hypaque Sodium Salt.
Diatx. (Pan American) Vitamin B_1 1.5 mg, B_2 1.5 mg, B_3 20 mg, B_5 10 mg, B_6 50 mg, B_{12} 1 mg, C 60 mg, folic acid 5 mg, D-biotin 300 mcg, dye free. Tab. Bot. 90s. *Rx.*
Use: Vitamin supplement.
DiatxFe. (Pan American) Fe (as ferrous fumarate) 100 mg, B_1 1.5 mg, B_2 1.5 mg, B_3 20 mg, B_5 10 mg, B_6 50 mg, B_{12} 1 mg, C 60 mg, folic acid 5 mg, D-biotin 300 mcg, dye free. Tab. Bot. 90s. *Rx.*
Use: Vitamin supplement.
•**diaveridine.** (DIE-ah-ver-ih-deen) USAN.
Use: Anti-infective.
•**diazepam.** (DIE-aze-uh-pam) *USP 28.*
Use: Agent for control of emotional disturbances; anxiolytic; hypnotic; sedative.
See: Diastat.
Diazepam Intensol.

Valium.
diazepam. (Various Mfr.) **Tab.:** 2 mg,
5 mg, 10 mg. May contain lactose. Bot.
100s, 500s, 1000s, 5000s. **Inj.:** 5 mg/
mL. Propylene glycol 40%, ethyl alcohol
10%, sodium benzoate 5%, benzoic
acid, benzyl alcohol 1.5%. 2 mL *Carpuject* cartridges. **Oral Soln.:** (Roxane)
5 mg/5 mL, sorbitol, wintergreen spice
flavor. 500 mL, 5 mg patient cups,
10 mg patient cups. *c-iv.*
Use: Agent for control of emotional disturbances; anxiolytic; hypnotic; sedative.
diazepam. (Various Mfr.) Diazepam.
Tab.: 2 mg, 5 mg, 10 mg. 100s, 500s,
1000s, 5000s, UD 100s. **Soln.:** 1 mg/
mL. Sorbitol, wintergreen spice flavor.
500 ml , UD 5 mL, UD 10 mL. **Inj.:**
5 mg/mL. Benzyl alcohol 1.5%, alcohol
10%. Cartridges 2 mL. *c-iv.*
Use: Anticonvulsant.
Diazepam Intensol. (Roxane) Diazepam
5 mg/mL. Alcohol 19%. Oral Soln.
30 mL with dropper. *c-iv.*
Use: Anxiolytic.
diazepam viscous rectal solution.
(Athena Neurosciences)
Use: To treat acute repetitive seizures.
[Orphan Drug]
•**diaziquone.** (DIE-azz-ih-kwone) USAN.
Use: Antineoplastic.
diazomycins a, b, and c. Antibiotic obtained from *Streptomyces ambofaciens.* Under study.
•**diazoxide.** (DIE-aze-OX-ide) *USP 28.*
Use: Antihypertensive.
See: Proglycem.
diazoxide, parenteral.
Use: Antihypertensive.
See: Hyperstat IV.
dibasic calcium phosphate dihydrate.
Use: Replenisher (calcium); pharma-
ceutic aid (tablet base).
See: Diostate D.
Dibatrol. (Lexis Laboratories) Chlor-
propamide 100 mg, 250 mg. Tab. Bot.
100s, 1000s. *Rx.*
Use: Antidiabetic.
Dibent. (Roberts) Dicyclomine 10 mg/mL
with chlorobutanol. Inj. Vial 10 mL. *Rx.*
Use: Gastrointestinal, anticholinergic.
dibenzapine derivatives.
Use: Antipsychotic.
See: Clozapine.
Loxapine.
Olanzapine.
Quetiapine Fumarate.
•**dibenzepin hydrochloride.** (die-BEN-
zeh-pin) USAN.

Use: Antidepressant.
•**dibenzothiophene.** (die-BEN-zoe-
THIGH-oh-feen) USAN.
Use: Keratolytic.
Dibenzyline. (Wellspring) Phenoxy-
benzamine hydrochloride 10 mg. Cap.
Bot. 100s. *Rx.*
Use: Pheochromocytoma agent; antihy-
pertensive.
•**dibotermin alfa.** (dye-BOE-ter-min)
USAN.
Use: Osteoinductive agent.
dibromodulcitol. (Biopharmaceutics)
Use: Antineoplastic. [Orphan Drug]
•**dibromsalan.** (die-BROME-sah-lan)
USAN.
Use: Antimicrobial; disinfectant.
•**dibucaine.** (DIE-byoo-cane) *USP 28.*
Use: Anesthetic, local.
See: D-Caine.
Nupercainal.
Nupercainal Heavy.
W/Dextrose.
See: Nupercaine Heavy.
W/Sodium bisulfite.
See: Nupercainal.
W/Zinc oxide, bismuth subgallate, ac-
etone sodium bisulfite.
See: Nupercainal.
•**dibucaine hydrochloride.** *USP 28.*
Use: Anesthetic, local.
See: Nupercaine hydrochloride.
W/Antipyrine, hydrocortisone, polymyxin
B sulfate, neomycin sulfate.
See: Otocort.
W/Colistin sodium methanesulfonate, cit-
ric acid, sodium citrate.
See: Coly-Mycin M.
dibutoline sulfate. Ethyl (2-hydroxy-
ethyl)-dimethylammonium sulfate (2:1)
bis (dibutyl-carbam-ate).
Use: Anticholinergic; antispasmodic.
•**dibutyl sebacate.** *NF 23.*
Use: Pharmaceutic aid (plasticizer).
Dical. (Rugby) Calcium 116 mg, vitamin
D 133 units, phosphorus 90 mg.
Captab. Bot. 1000s. *OTC.*
Use: Mineral, vitamin supplement.
dicalcium phosphate. (Various Mfr.) Di-
basic calcium phosphate, monocalcium
phosphate. **Cap.:** 7.5 g, 10 g. **Tab.:**
7.5 g, 10 g, 15 g. **Wafer:** 15 g. *OTC.*
Use: Mineral supplement.
W/Calcium gluconate and Vitamin D.
See: CalciCaps.
Dical-D. (Abbott) Calciuim 105 mg, vita-
min D 120 units, phosphorus 81 mg.
Tab. 100s. *OTC.*
Use: Mineral, vitamin supplement.

Dical-Dee. (Alpharma) Vitamin D 350 units, dibasic calcium phosphate 4.5 g, calcium gluconate 3 g. Cap. Bot. 100s, 1000s. *OTC.*
Use: Mineral, vitamin supplement.

Dicaldel. (Faraday) Dibasic calcium phosphate 300 mg, calcium gluconate 200 mg, vitamin D 33 units. Cap. Bot. 100s, 250s, 500s, 1000s. *OTC.*
Use: Mineral, vitamin supplement.

Dical-D with Vitamin C. (Abbott) Dibasic calcium phosphate containing calcium 116.7 mg, phosphorus 90 mg, vitamin D 133 units, ascorbic acid 15 mg. Cap. Bot. 100s.
Use: Mineral, vitamin supplement.

Dicaltabs. (Faraday) Dibasic calcium phosphate 108 mg, calcium gluconate 140 mg, vitamin D 35 units. Tab. Bot. 100s, 250s, 1000s. *OTC.*
Use: Mineral, vitamin supplement.

Dicarbosil. (BIRA) Calcium carbonate 500 mg. Chew. Tab. Roll 12s. *OTC.*
Use: Antacid.

Di-Cet. (Sanford & Son) Methylbenze-thonium Cl 24.4 g, sodium carbonate monohydrate 48.8 g, sodium nitrite 24.4 g, trisodium ethylenediamine tetra-acetate monohydrate 2.4 g. Pow. Pkg. 2.4 g. Box 24s.
Use: Disinfectant.

dichloralantipyrine. Dichloral-phenazone. Chloralpyrine. A complex of 2 mol. chloral hydrate with 1 mol. antipyrine. Sominat.
W/Isometheptene mucate, acetamino-phen.
See: Midrin.

•**dichloralphenazone.** (die-klor-al-FEN-ah-zone) *USP 28.*
Use: Hypnotic; sedative.
W/Combinations.
See: Duradrin.
Midrin.

Dichloramine T. (Various Mfr.) (1% to 5% in chlorinated paraffin). P-Toluene-sulfone-dichloramine.
Use: Antiseptic.

dichloren.
See: Mechlorethamine hydrochloride.

dichloroacetate sodium.
Use: Lactic acidosis; hypercholesterol-emia. [Orphan Drug]

dichloroacetic acid. *Rx.*
Use: Cauterizing agent.

•**dichlorodifluoromethane.** (die-KLOR-oh-die-flure-oh-METH-ane) *NF 23.*
Use: Pharmaceutic aid (aerosol propel-lant).

dichlorodiphenyl trichloroethane.
See: Chlorophenothane.

dichlorophenarsine hydrochloride. (Chlorarsen, Clorarsen, Fontarsol, Ha-larsol).

dichlorophene. Related to hexachloro-phene.
W/Undecylenic acid.
See: Onychomycetin.

•**dichlorotetrafluoroethane.** (die-KLOR-oh-teh-trah-flur-oh-ETH-ane) *NF 23.*
Use: Pharmaceutic aid (aerosol propel-lant).

•**dichlorvos.** (DIE-klor-vahs) USAN.
Use: Anthelmintic.

•**dicirenone.** (die-sigh-REN-ohn) USAN.
Use: Hypotensive; aldosterone antago-nist.

Dickey's Old Reliable Eye Wash. (Dickey Drug) Berberine sulfate, boric acid, parabens. Plastic dropper bot. 8 mL, 12 mL, 1 oz. *OTC.*
Use: Counterirritant, ophthalmic.

•**diclofenac potassium.** (die-KLOE-fen-ak) USAN.
Use: Analgesic; NSAID.
See: Cataflam.

diclofenac potassium. (Various Mfr.) Diclofenac potassium 50 mg. Tab. Bot. 100s, 500s. *Rx.*
Use: Analgesic; NSAID.

•**diclofenac sodium.** (die-KLOE-fen-ak) *USP 28.*
Use: Analgesic; NSAID.
See: Solaraze.
Voltaren.
Voltaren-XR.

diclofenac sodium. (Various Mfr.) Diclo-fenac sodium. **ER Tab.:** 100 mg. Bot. 100s. **DR Tab.:** 25 mg, 50 mg, 75 mg. Bot. 42s (except 25 mg), 60s, 100s, 500s (except 25 mg), 1000s (except 25 mg), UD 100s (50 mg only). *Rx.*
Use: Analgesic; NSAID.

diclofenac sodium and misoprostol.
Use: Arthritis treatment, antiulcerative.
See: Arthrotec.

diclofenac sodium ophthalmic solu-tion 0.1%. Diclofenac sodium 0.1%, mannitol. Soln. Bot. 5 mL. *Rx.*
Use: Analgesic; NSAID, ophthalmic.

Dicloxacil. (Ivax) Dicloxacillin sodium 250 mg, 500 mg. Cap. Bot. 100s. *Rx.*
Use: Anti-infective; penicillin.

•**dicloxacillin.** (DIE-klox-uh-SILL-in) USAN.
Use: Anti-infective.
See: Dynapen.
Pathocil.

•**dicloxacillin sodium.** (DIE-klox-uh-SILL-in) *USP 28.*
Use: Anti-infective.

dicloxacillin sodium. (Various Mfr.)
Dicloxacillin sodium 250 mg, 500 mg.
Cap. Bot. 30s (500 mg only), 40s, 50s
(500 mg only), 100s, 500s, UD 100s.
Rx.
Use: Anti-infective
Dicole. (Halsey Drug) Docusate sodium
100 mg. Cap. Bot. 100s. *OTC.*
Use: Laxative.
Dicomal-DH. (Econolab) Hydrocodone
bitartrate 1.66 mg, pyrilamine maleate
8.33 mg, phenylephrine hydrochloride
5 mg/5 mL. Syr. Bot. 473 mL. *c-iii.*
Use: Upper respiratory combination, antitussive, antihistamine, deconges-
tant.
Dicomal-DM. (Econolab) Dextromethor-
phan HBr 10 mg, pyrilamine maleate
8.33 mg, phenylephrine hydrochloride
5 mg/5 mL, menthol, saccharin, sorbitol,
alcohol and dye free. Syr. Bot. 473 mL.
OTC.
Use: Upper respiratory combination, an-
titussive, antihistamine, deconges-
tant.
dicophane.
Use: Pediculicide.
See: Chlorophenothane.
DDT.
•**dicyclomine hydrochloride.** (die-SIGH-
kloe-meen) *USP 28.*
Use: Anticholinergic; antispasmodic.
See: Antispas.
Bentyl.
Dysaps.
Nospaz.
Triactin.
W/Phenobarbital.
See: Bentyl with Phenobarbital.
Dicynene. (Baxter PPI) *Rx.*
Use: Hemostatic.
See: Ethamsylate.
dicysteine.
See: Cystine.
•**didanosine.** (die-DAN-oh-SEEN) USAN.
Use: Antiretroviral, nucleoside reverse
transcriptase inhibitor.
See: Videx.
Videx EC.
didanosine. (Barr) Didanosine 200 mg,
250 mg, 400 mg. Dextrose, talc. En-
teric-coated beadlets. DR Cap. UD 30s.
Rx.
Use: Antiretroviral agent.
didehydrodideoxythymidine.
Use: Antiviral.
See: Stavudine.
Di-Delamine. (Del) Tripelennamine hy-
drochloride 0.5%, diphenhydramine hydrochloride 1%, benzalkonium chloride
0.12%. **Gel:** In clear gel. Tube 1.25 oz.

Spray: Spray pump 4 oz. *OTC.*
Use: Antipruritic, topical.
dideoxycytidine. (Roche) *Rx.*
Use: Antiviral.
See: HIVID.
2,3 dideoxycytidine. (Roche; Bristol-
Myers Squibb) *Rx.*
Use: Antiviral (AIDS).
dideoxyinisine.
Use: Antiviral.
Didrex. (Pharmacia) Benzphetamine hy-
drochloride. 50 mg, lactose, sorbitol.
Tab. Bot. 100s, 500s. *c-iii.*
Use: CNS stimulant. anorexiant.
Didronel. (Procter & Gamble Pharm)
Etidronate disodium 200 mg, 400 mg.
Tab. Bot. 60s. *Rx.*
Use: Antihypercalcemia, bisphospho-
nate,
•**dienestrol.** (die-en-ESS-trole) *USP 28.*
Use: Estrogen therapy; atrophic vagi-
nitis.
See: D V.
Ortho Dienestrol.
dienestrol. (Ortho-McNeil) Dienestrol
0.01%. Tube 78 g w/applicator.
Use: Estrogen.
•**dienogest.** USAN.
Use: Oral contraceptive; hormone re-
placement therapy.
diet aids, nonprescription.
Use: Dietary aid.
See: Extra Strength Grapefruit Diet Plan
w/Diadax.
Maximum Strength Dexatrim Plus Vitamin C.
•**diethanolamine.** *NF 23.*
Use: Pharmaceutic acid (alkalizing
agent).
See: Diolamine.
diethazine hydrochloride.
Use: Antiparkinsonian.
diethoxin. Intracaine hydrochloride.
•**diethylcarbamazine citrate.** (die-ETH-ill-
car-BAM-ah-zeen SIH-trate) *USP 28.*
Use: Anthelmintic.
diethyldithiocarbamate.
Use: Trial drug for AIDS. [Orphan Drug]
See: Imuthiol.
diethylenediamine citrate. Piperazine
Citrate, Piperazine Hexahydrate.
diethylmalonylurea.
See: Barbital.
•**diethyl phthalate.** *NF 23.*
Use: Pharmaceutic aid (plasticizer).
diethylpropion. (Various Mfr.) **Tab.:**
Diethylpropion 25 mg. Bot. 100s, 500s,
1000s. **SR Tab.:** Diethylpropion 75 mg.
Bot. 100s, 250s, 500s, 1000s. *c-iv.*
Use: Anorexiant.

• **diethylpropion hydrochloride.** (die-ETH-uhl-PRO-pee-ahn) *USP 28.*
Use: Anorexic.
See: Tenuate.
　Tenuate Dospan.
　Tepanil.
　Tepanil Ten-Tab.
diethylpropion hydrochloride. (Various Mfr.) Diethlpropion hydrochloride. **Tab.:** 25 mg. Bot. 100s. **CR Tab.:** 75 mg. Bot. 100s. *c-iv.*
Use: CNS stimulant, anorexiant.
diethylstilbestrol dipropionate. (Various Mfr.) Diethylstilbestrol dipropionate. **Amp.:** In oil, 0.5 mg, 1 mg, 5 mg/mL. **Tab.:** 0.5 mg, 1 mg, 5 mg.
Use: Estrogen.
• **diethyltoluamide.** (die-ETH-ill-toe-LOO-ah-mide) *USP 28.*
Use: Repellent (arthropod).
See: RV Pellent.
n, n-diethylvanillamide.
See: Ethamivan.
Diet-Tuss. (Health for Life Brands) Dextromethorphan 30 mg, thenylpyramine hydrochloride, pyrilamine maleate 80 mg, sodium salicylate 200 mg, sodium citrate 600 mg, ammonium Cl 100 mg/fl oz. Sugar free. Bot. 4 oz. *OTC.*
Use: Analgesic, antihistamine, antitussive, expectorant.
• **difenoximide hydrochloride.** (DIE-fen-OX-ih-mid) USAN.
Use: Antiperistaltic.
• **difenoxin.** (DIE-fen-OX-in) USAN.
Use: Antidiarrheal; antiperistaltic.
W/Atropine sulfate.
See: Motofen.
Differin. (Galderma) Adapalene. **Gel:** 0.1%, EDTA, methylparaben. Tube. 45 g. **Cream:** 0.1%, EDTA, glycerin, parabens. Tube. 45 g. **Soln.:** 0.1%, alcohol 30%, PEG-400. 30 mL glass bottles with applicator and 60 unit-of-use pledgets. *Rx.*
Use: Dermatologic, acne; retinoid.
• **diflorasone diacetate.** (die-FLORE-ah-sone die-ASS-eh-tate) *USP 28.*
Use: Anti-inflammatory, topical; antipruritic.
See: ApexiCon.
　ApexiCon E.
　Florone.
　Maxiflor.
　Psorcon E.
diflorasone diacetate. (Various Mfr.) Diflorasone diacetate 0.05%. Cream. Oint. Tube. 15 g, 30 g, 60 g. *Rx.*
Use: Anti-inflammatory, topical; antipruritic.

• **difloxacin hydrochloride.** (die-FLOX-ah-SIN) USAN.
Use: Anti-infective (DNA gyrase inhibitor).
• **difluanine hydrochloride.** (die-FLEW-an-EEN) USAN.
Use: CNS stimulant.
Diflucan. (Pfizer) Fluconazole. **Tab.:** 50 mg, 100 mg, 150 mg, 200 mg. Bot. 30s (except 150 mg), UD 100s (100 mg, 200 mg only), UD 1s (150 mg only). **Inj.:** 2 mg/mL. Bot. or *Viaflex Plus* (sodium chloride 9 mg/mL or dextrose hydrous 56 mg/mL) 100 mL, 200 mL. **Pow. for Oral Susp.:** 10 mg/mL when reconstituted, sucrose, orange flavor. Bot. 350 mg; 40 mg/mL when reconstituted, sucrose, orange flavor. Bot. 1400 mg. *Rx.*
Use: Antifungal.
• **diflucortolone.** (die-flew-CORE-toe-lone) USAN.
Use: Corticosteroid, topical.
• **diflucortolone pivalate.** USAN.
Use: Corticosteroid, topical.
• **diflumidone sodium.** (die-FLEW-mih-DOHN) USAN.
Use: Anti-inflammatory.
• **diflunisal.** (die-FLOO-nih-sal) *USP 28.*
Use: Analgesic; NSAID.
See: Dolobid.
diflunisal. (Various Mfr.) Diflunisal 250 mg, 500 mg. Tab. Bot. 100s, 500s, unit-of-use 60s. *Rx.*
Use: Analgesic; NSAID.
• **difluprednate.** (DIE-flew-PRED-nate) USAN.
Use: Anti-inflammatory.
• **diftalone.** (DIFF-tah-lone) USAN.
Use: Anti-inflammatory; analgesic.
• **digalloyl trioleate.** USAN.
Di-Gel. (Schering-Plough) Aluminum hydroxide (equivalent to dried gel) 200 mg, magnesium hydroxide 200 mg, simethicone 20 mg/5 mL, saccharin, sorbitol. Liq. Bot. 180 mL, 360 mL. *OTC.*
Use: Antacid; antiflatulent.
Di-Gel, Advanced. (Schering-Plough) Magnesium hydroxide 128 mg, calcium carbonate 280 mg, simethicone 20 mg. Tab. Bot. 30s, 60s, 90s. *OTC.*
Use: Antacid; antiflatulent.
Digestamic. (Lexis Laboratories) Pancrelipase 300 mg, pepsin 100 mg. Tab. Bot. 50s. *Rx-OTC.*
Use: Digestive aid.
Digestamic Liquid. (Lexis Laboratories) Belladonna leaf fluid extract 0.64 min/ 5 mL. Bot. 8 oz. *Rx-OTC.*

Use: Anticholinergic; antispasmodic.
Digestant. (Canright) Pancreatin 5.25 g, ox bile extract 2 g, pepsin 5 g, betaine hydrochloride 1 g. Tab. Bot. 100s, 1000s. *Rx-OTC.*
Use: Digestive aid.
Digestive Compound. (Thurston) Betaine hydrochloride 3.25 g, pepsin 1 g, papain 2 g, mycozyme 2 g, ox bile 2 g. 2 Tab. Bot. 100s, 500s. *Rx-OTC.*
Use: Digestive aid.
digestive enzymes.
See: Kutrase.
　Ku-Zyme.
　Lipram.
　Pancrease.
　Pancrecarb.
　Pancrelipase.
　Panokase.
　Plaretase
　Ultrase.
　Viokase.
digestive products, miscellaneous.
Use: Digestive enzyme supplement.
See: Arco-Lase.
　Digestozyme.
　Enzobile Improved.
　Ku-Zyme
Digibind. (GlaxoSmithKline) Digoxin immune fab (ovine) 38 mg/vial, sodium chloride 28 mg, preservative free. Each vial will bind ≈ digoxin 0.5 mg. Pow. for Inj., lyophilized. Vial. *Rx.*
Use: Antidote.
Digidote. (Boehringer Mannheim)
Use: Antidote. [Orphan Drug]
DigiFab. (Savage) Digoxin immune fab (ovine) 40 mg/vial, sodium acetate 2 mg, preservative free. Each vial will bind ≈ 0.5 mg digoxin. Pow. for Inj., lyophilized. Vial. *Rx.*
Use: Antidote.
•**digitalis.** (dih-jih-TAL-iss) *USP 28.*
Use: Cardiovascular agent.
See: Crystodigin.
　Deslanoside.
　Digoxin.
　Lanoxin.
digitalis leaf, powdered.
Use: Cardiovascular agent.
digitalis tincture.
Use: Cardiovascular agent.
Digitek. (Bertek) Digoxin 0.125 mg, 0.25 mg, lactose. Tab. Bot. 100s, 1000s, 5000s. *Rx.*
Use: Inotropic agent; cardiac glycoside.
•**digoxin.** (dih-JOX-in) *USP 28.*
Use: Cardiovascular agent.
See: Digitek.
　Lanoxicaps.
　Lanoxin.

digoxin. (Various Mfr.) Digoxin. **Tab.:** 0.125 mg, 0.25 mg. Bot. 1000s **Ped. Elix.:** 0.05 mg/mL. Bot. 60 mL; UD 2.5 mL, 5 mL. **Inj.:** 0.25 mg/mL, alcohol 10%, proplyene glycol 40% per mL. *Tubex* or *Carpuject* 1 mL, 2 mL. *Rx.*
Use: Inotropic agent; cardiac glycoside.
digoxin. (Elkins-Sinn) Digoxin 0.25 mg/mL, alcohol 0.1 mL, propylene glycol 0.4 mL per mL. Inj. Amp. 2 mL. *Rx.*
Use: Inotropic agent; cardiac glycoside.
digoxin antibody.
See: Digibind.
digoxin immune fab (ovine).
Use: Antidote.
See: Digibind.
　Digidote.
　DigiFab.
digoxin injection, pediatric. (Abbott) Digoxin 0.1 mg/mL, propylene glycol 40%, alcohol 10%. Ped. Inj. Amp. 1 mL. *Rx.*
Use: Inotropic agent; cardiac glycoside.
digoxin I-125 immunoassay. (Abbott Diagnostics) Digoxin diagnostic kit for the quantitative determination of serum digoxin. 100s, 300s.
Use: Diagnostic aid.
Digoxin Riabead. (Abbott Diagnostics) Solid-phase radioimmunoassay for quantitative measurement of serum digoxin. Test kit 100s, 300s.
Use: Diagnostic aid.
dihematoporphyrin ethers.
Use: Photodynamic therapy of transitional cell carcinoma in situ of urinary bladder or primary or recurrent obstructing esophageal carcinoma. [Orphan Drug]
See: Photofrin.
•**dihexyverine hydrochloride.** (die-HEX-ih-ver-een) USAN.
Use: Anticholinergic.
Dihistine DH. (Alpharma) Pseudoephedrine hydrochloride 30 mg, chlorpheniramine maleate 2 mg, codeine phosphate 10 mg/5 mL, alcohol 5%. Elix. Bot. 118 mL, 473 mL, 3.8 L. *c-v.*
Use: Upper respiratory combination, antihistamine, antitussive, decongestant.
Dihistine Elixir. (Various Mfr.) Phenylephrine hydrochloride 5 mg, chlorpheniramine maleate 2 mg/5 mL. Bot. Pt, gal. *OTC.*
Use: Antihistamine, decongestant.
Dihistine Expectorant. (Alpharma) Pseudoephedrine hydrochloride 30 mg, codeine phosphate 10 mg, guaifenesin 100 mg/5 mL, alcohol 7.5%, saccharin, sorbitol, sucrose. Liq. Bot. 473 mL. *c-v.*

Use: Upper respiratory combination, antitussive, decongestant, expectorant.

dihydan soluble.
See: Phenytoin Sodium.

dihydrocodeine. Paracodin. Drocode.
Use: Analgesic, antitussive.

• **dihydrocodeine bitartrate.** (die-high-droe-KOE-deen bye-TAR-trate) *USP 28.*
Use: Analgesic.
See: Hydrocodone Bitartrate.
W/Caffeine, acetaminophen.
See: DHC Plus.
Panlor DC.
Panlor SS.
W/Caffeine, aspirin.
See: Synalgos-DC.
W/Caffeine, phenacetin, aspirin.
See: Drocogesic #3.
Duradyne DHC.
W/Combinations.
See: Pancof.
Pancof PD.

dihydrocodeinone resin complex.
W/Phenyltoloxamine resin complex.
See: Tussionex.

dihydroergocornine. Ergot alkaline component of hydergine.

dihydroergocristine. Ergot alkaloid component of hydergine.

dihydroergocryptine. Ergot alkaloid component of hydergine.

dihydroergotamine. (Sandoz) (D.H.E. 45) Dihydroergotamine mesylate. Amp.
Rx.
Use: Agent for migraine; antiadrenergic.

• **dihydroergotamine mesylate.** (DIE-high-droe-err-GOT-uh-meen) *USP 28.*
Dihydroergotamine methanesulfonate.
Use: Antiadrenergic; antimigraine.
See: D.H.E. 45.
Migranal.

dihydroergotamine mesylate. (Various Mfr.) Dihydroergotamine mesylate 1 mg/mL. Alcohol 6%. Inj. Vial 1 mL.
Rx.
Use: Migraine agent.

dihydroergotoxine. Ergoloid mesylate.
Rx.
Use: Psychotherapeutic agent.
See: Ergoloid Mesylates.
Gerimal.
Hydergine.
Hydergine LC.

5,6-dihydro-5-azacytidine. (Ilex Oncology)
Use: Antineoplastic. [Orphan Drug]

dihydrofollicular hormone.
See: Estradiol.

dihydrofolliculin.
See: Estradiol.

dihydrohydroxycodeinone. *C-II.*
Use: Analgesic; narcotic.
See: Oxycodone. (Ducodal, Eukodal, Eucodal).

dihydrohydroxycodeinone hydrochloride or bitartrate. Oxycodone hydrochloride or bitartrate.
W/Combinations.
See: Cophene-S.
Damason-P.
Percodan.

dihydroindolone derivatives.
Use: Antipsychotic.
See: Molindone Hydrochloride.

dihydromorphinone hydrochloride.
See: Dilaudid.

• **dihydrostreptomycin sulfate.** (die-HIGH-droe-strep-toe-MY-sin) *USP 28.*
Use: Anti-infective.

dihydrotachysterol. (die-HIGH-droe-tack-ISS-ter-ole)
Use: Antihypocalcemic.
See: DHT.

dihydrotestosterone.
Use: AIDS. [Orphan Drug]
See: Androgel-DHT.

dihydrotheelin.
See: Estradiol.

dihydroxyacetone.
See: Chromelin.

• **dihydroxyaluminum aminoacetate.** (die-high-DROX-ee-ah-LOO-min-uhm ah-MEE-no-ASS-eh-tate) *USP 28.*
Use: Antacid.
W/Methscopolamine bromide, sodium lauryl sulfate, magnesium hydroxide.
See: Alu-Scop.

• **dihydroxyaluminum sodium carbonate.** *USP 28.*
Use: Antacid.
See: Rolaids.

dihydroxycholecalciferol.
See: Rocaltrol.

24,25 dihydroxycholecalciferol. (Lemmon)
Use: Uremic osteodystrophy. [Orphan Drug]

dihydroxyestrin.
See: Estradiol.

dihydroxyfluorane. Fluorescein.

dihydroxyphenylisatin.
See: Oxyphenisatin.

dihydroxyphenyloxindol.
See: Oxyphenisatin.

dihydroxypropyl theophylline. Dyphylline.
See: Neothylline

dihydroxy (stearato) aluminum. *NF 23.*
Aluminum monostearate.

diiodohydroxyquin.
Use: Amebicide.
See: Iodoquinol.
diiodohydroxyquinoline.
See: Iodoquinol.
diisopromine hydrochloride. (Lab. for Pharmaceutical Development, Inc.)
See: Desquam-X.
diisopropyl phosphorofluoridate.
See: Floropryl.
diisopropyl sebacate.
Use: Moisturizing agent.
Dilacor XR. (Watson) Diltiazem hydrochloride 120 mg, 180 mg, 240 mg. ER Cap. Bot. 100s, 500s. *Rx.*
Use: Calcium channel blocker.
dilaminate. Mixture of magnesium carbide and dihydroxyaluminum glycinate. *OTC.*
Use: Antacid.
Dilantin. (Parke-Davis) Phenytoin. **30 Susp.:** 30 mg/5 mL. Bot. 8 oz, UD 5 mL. **125 Susp.:** 125 mg/5 mL. Bot. 8 oz, UD 5 mL. **Infatab:** 50 mg. Bot. 100s, UD 100s. *Rx.*
Use: Anticonvulsant.
Dilantin Sodium. (Parke-Davis) Extended phenytoin sodium. **Kapseal:** 30 mg, 100 mg. Bot. 100s, 1000s, UD 100s. **Amp.:** (w/propylene glycol 40%, alcohol 10%, sodium hydroxide) 100 mg/2 mL. UD 10s; 250 mg/5 mL. Amp. 10s, UD 10s. *Rx.*
Use: Anticonvulsant.
Dilantin Sodium w/Phenobarbital Kapseal. (Parke-Davis) Phenytoin sodium 100 mg, phenobarbital 16 mg, 32 mg. Cap. Bot. 100s, 1000s, UD 100s (32 mg only). *Rx.*
Use: Anticonvulsant; hypnotic; sedative.
Dilantin-30 Pediatric. (Parke-Davis) Phenytoin 30 mg/5 mL, alcohol 0.6%. Susp. Bot. 240 mL, 5 mL. *Rx.*
Use: Anticonvulsant.
Dilatrate-SR. (Schwarz Pharma) Isosorbide dinitrate 40 mg. SR Cap. Bot. 60s, 100s. *Rx.*
Use: Antianginal.
Dilaudid. (Abbott) Hydromorphone hydrochloride. **Inj.:** 1 mg/mL, 2 mg/mL, 4 mg/mL. Amp. 1 mL. Multidose vials (with EDTA and methyl- and propylparabens, vial stopper contains latex). 20 mL (2 mg/mL only). **Oral Soln.:** 1 mg/1 mL. Parabens, sucrose, glycerin. May contain sodium metabisulfite. 473 mL. **Supp.:** 3 mg. Cocoa butter. Box 6s. **Tab.:** 2 mg, 4 mg, 8 mg (sodium metabisulfite). Lactose. Bot. 100s, 500s (except 8 mg), UD 100s

(except 8 mg). *c-II.*
Use: Opioid analgesic.
Dilaudid HP. (Abbott) Hydromorphone hydrochloride. **Inj.:** 10 mg/mL. Amps. 1 mL, 5 mL. Single-dose vials. 50 mL. **Pow. for Inj. (lyophilized):** 250 mg (10 mg/mL after reconstitution). Single-dose vial. *c-II.*
Use: Opioid analgesic.
Dilaudid Syrup. (Abbott) Hydromorphone hydrochloride 1 mg, guaifenesin 100 mg/5 mL, alcohol 5%, peach flavor. Bot. 473 mL. *c-II.*
Use: Upper respiratory combination, antitussive, expectorant, analgesic; narcotic.
● **dilevalol hydrochloride.** (DIE-LEV-ah-lole) USAN.
Use: Antihypertensive; antiadrenergic (β-receptor).
dilithium carbonate. Lithium carbonate, *USP.*
Use: Antipsychotic.
Dilor. (Savage) Dyphylline 200 mg. Tab. Bot. 100s, 1,000s, UD 100s. *Rx.*
Use: Bronchodilator.
Dilor 400. (Savage) Dyphylline 400 mg. Bot. 100s, 1000s, UD 100s. *Rx.*
Use: Bronchodilator.
Dilotab. (Zee Medical) Acetaminophen 500 mg, pseudoephedrine hydrochloride 30 mg. Tab. 24s. *OTC.*
Use: Analgesic, decongestant.
● **diloxanide furoate.** *USP 28.*
Use: Anti-infective.
Diltia XT. (Andrx) Diltiazem hydrochloride 120 mg, 180 mg, 240 mg. ER Cap. Bot. 100s, 500s, 1000s. *Rx.*
Use: Antihypertensive.
● **diltiazem hydrochloride.** (dill-TIE-uh-zem) *USP 28.*
Use: Vasodilator (coronary), calcium channel blocker.
See: Cardizem.
Cardizem CD.
Cardizem LA.
Cartia XT.
Dilacor XR.
Diltia XT.
Dilt-XR.
Taztia XT.
Tiamate.
Tiazac.
Tiazac ER.
diltiazem hydrochloride extended-release capsules. (Various Mfr.) Diltiazem hydrochloride 60 mg, 90 mg, 120 mg, 180 mg, 240 mg, 300 mg, 360 mg. May contain sucrose or sugar spheres. ER Cap. Bot. 30s (except

60 mg, 90 mg, 360 mg), 90s (except 60 mg, 90 mg), 100s (except 300 mg, 360 mg), 500s (except 60 mg, 90 mg, 360 mg), 1000s (except 60 mg, 90 mg, 360 mg). *Rx.*
Use: Antihypertensive.

diltiazem hydrochloride injection. (Various Mfr.) Diltiazem 5 mg/mL. Vial 5 mL, 10 mL, 25 mL. *Rx.*
Use: Calcium channel blocker.

diltiazem hydrochloride tablets. (Various Mfr.) Diltiazem hydrochloride 30 mg, 60 mg, 90 mg, 120 mg. Bot. 100s, 500s, 1000s. *Rx.*
Use: Calcium channel blocker.

•**diltiazem maleate.** (dill-TIE-ah-zem MAL-ate) USAN.
Use: Calcium channel blocker; antihypertensive.
See: Tiamate.

diltiazem maleate and enalapril maleate.
Use: Antihypertensive.
See: Teczem.

Dilt-XR. (Apotex) Diltiazem hydrochloride 120 mg, 180 mg, 240 mg. ER Cap. 100s. *Rx.*
Use: Calcium channel blocker.

diluent.
See: Broncho Saline.
Sodium Chloride.
Sodium Chloride 0.45%.
Sodium Chloride 0.9%.

Dimaphen DM Cold & Cough. (Major) Pseudoephedrine hydrochloride 15 mg, brompheniramine maleate 1 mg, dextromethorphan HBr 5 mg/5mL, saccharin, sorbitol, grape flavor, alcohol free. Elix. Bot. 118 mL. *OTC.*
Use: Upper respiratory combination, decongestant, antihistamine, antitussive.

Dimaphen Elixir. (Major) Pseudoephedrine hydrochloride 15 mg, brompheniramine maleate 1 mg/5 mL, saccharin, sorbitol, grape flavor, alcohol free. Elix. Bot. 237 mL. *OTC.*
Use: Upper respiratory combination, antihistamine, decongestant.

•**dimefadane.** (DIE-meh-fah-dane) USAN.
Use: Analgesic.

•**dimefilcon a.** (DIE-meh-FILL-kahn A) USAN.
Use: Contact lens material (hydrophilic).

•**dimefline hydrochloride.** (DIE-meh-fleen) USAN.
Use: Respiratory.

•**dimefocon a.** (DIE-meh-FOE-kahn A) USAN.
Use: Contact lens material (hydrophobic).

Dimenest. (Forest) Dimenhydrinate 50 mg/mL. Vial 10 mL. *Rx.*
Use: Antiemetic; antivertigo.

•**dimenhydrinate.** (die-men-HIGH-drih-nate) *USP 28.*
Tall Man: DimenhyDRINATE
Use: Antiemetic; antihistamine.
See: Dimenest.
Dimentabs.
Dramamine.
Dymenate.
Hydrate.
Signate.
Traveltabs.

Dimentabs. (Jones Pharma) Dimenhydrinate 50 mg. Tab. Bot. 100s. *OTC.*
Use: Antiemetic; antivertigo.

•**dimepranol acedoben.** (DIE-MEH-prah-nahl ah-SEE-doe-BEN) USAN.
Use: Immunomodulator.

•**dimercaprol.** (die-mer-CAP-role) *USP 28.* Formerly BAL.
Use: Antidote to gold, arsenic, and mercury poisoning; metal complexing agent.
See: BAL in oil.

Dimetane Decongestant. (Wyeth) **Capl.:** Brompheniramine maleate 4 mg, phenylephrine hydrochloride 10 mg. Capl. Bot. 24s, 48s. **Elix.:** Brompheniramine maleate 2 mg, phenylephrine hydrochloride 5 mg/5 mL, alcohol 2.3%. Bot. 120 mL. *OTC.*
Use: Antihistamine, decongestant.

Dimetapp Children's ND Non-Drowsy Allergy. (Wyeth) Loratadine. **Orally Disintegrating Tab.:** 10 mg. Aspartame, corn syrup, mannitol, phenylalanine. 6s, 12. **Syrup:** 5 mg/5 mL. Sucrose. 118 mL. *OTC.*
Use: Antihistamine.

Dimetapp Children's Nighttime Flu. (Wyeth) Pseudoephedrine hydrochloride 15 mg, brompheniramine maleate 1 mg, dextromethorphan HBr 5 mg/5 mL, corn syrup, saccharin, sorbitol, bubble gum flavor, alcohol free. Syr. Bot. 118 mL. *OTC.*
Use: Upper respiratory combination, decongestant, antihistamine, antitussive, analgesic.

Dimetapp Children's Non-Drowsy Flu. (Wyeth) Pseudoephedrine hydrochloride 15 mg, dextromethorphan HBr 5 mg, acetaminophen 160 mg/5 mL, corn syrup, saccharin, sorbitol, fruit flavor, alcohol free. Syr. Bot. 118 mL. *OTC.*
Use: Upper respiratory combination, decongestant, antitussive, analgesic.

Dimetapp Cold & Allergy Elixir. (Wyeth) Pseudoephedrine hydrochloride 15 mg, brompheniramine maleate 1 mg/ 5 mL, corn syrup, saccharin, sorbitol, grape flavor, alcohol free. Elix. Bot. 118 mL, 237 mL. *OTC.*
Use: Upper respiratory combination, decongestant, antihistamine.

Dimetapp Decongestant Pediatric. (Wyeth) Pseudoephedrine hydrochloride 7.5 mg/0.8 mL, corn syrup, menthol, sorbitol, sucrose. Drops. Bot. 15 mL. *OTC.*
Use: Nasal decongestant, arylalkylamine.

Dimetapp Decongestant Plus Cough Infants. (Wyeth) Pseudoephedrine hydrochloride 9.375 mg, dextromethorphan HBr 3.125 mg/mL, corn syrup, menthol, sucrose, grape flavor, alcohol free. Drops. Bot. 15 mL w/dropper. *OTC.*
Use: Upper respiratory combination, decongestant, antitussive.

Dimetapp DM Children's Cold & Cough. (Wyeth) Pseudoephedrine hydrochloride 15 mg, brompheniramine maleate 1 mg, dextromethorphan HBr 5 mg/5 mL, sorbitol, saccharin, corn syrup, grape flavor, alcohol free. Elix. Bot. 118 mL, 237 mL. *OTC.*
Use: Upper respiratory combination, decongestant, antihistamine, antitussive.

Dimetapp Long Acting Cough Plus Cold. (Wyeth) Dextromethorphan HBr 7.5 mg, pseudoephedrine hydrochloride 15 mg/5 mL. Corn syrup, saccharin. Fruit punch flavor. Syrup. 118 mL. *OTC.*
Use: Antitussive combination.

Dimetapp, Maximum Strength, Non-Drowsy. (Wyeth) Pseudoephedrine hydrochloride 30 mg, mannitol, sorbitol. Softgel cap. Pkg. 12s. *OTC.*
Use: Nasal decongestant, arylalkylamine.

Dimetapp, Maximum Strength 12-Hour Non-Drowsy. (Wyeth) Pseudoephedrine hydrochloride 120 mg. ER Tab. Pkg. 10s. *OTC.*
Use: Nasal decongestant, arylalkylamine.

Dimetapp Sinus. (Wyeth) Pseudoephedrine hydrochloride 30 mg, ibuprofen 200 mg/ cap. Cap. Bot. 20s, 40s. *OTC.*
Use: Antihistamine, decongestant.

•**dimethadione.** (DIE-meth-ah-DIE-ohn) USAN.
Use: Anticonvulsant.

•**dimethicone.** (DIE-meth-ih-cone) *NF 23.*
Use: Prosthetic aid (soft tissue); compo-

nent of barrier creams; lubricant; hydrophobic agent.
See: Aloe Vesta.
Pro-Q.
Silicone.

•**dimethicone 350.** (DIE-meth-ih-cone 350) USAN.
Use: Prosthetic aid for soft tissue.

•**dimethindene maleate.** (DIE-METH-in-deen) *USP 28.*
Use: Antihistamine.

•**dimethisoquin hydrochloride.** (die-meh-THIGH-so-kwin) USAN.

•**dimethisterone.** (DIE-meth-ISS-ter-ohn) *NF 23.*
Use: Hormone, progestin.

dimethoxyphenyl penicillin sodium.
Use: Anti-infective.
See: Methicillin Sodium

dimethpyridene maleate. Dimethindene Maleate.

dimethylaminophenazone.
See: Aminopyrine.

dimethylamino pyrazine sulfate.
See: Ampyzine Sulfate.

dimethylcarbamate.
See: Mestinon.

dimethylhexestrol dipropionate. Promethestrol Dipropionate.

dimethyl polysiloxane.
See: Dimethicone.

•**dimethyl sulfoxide.** (die-METH-uhl sull-FOX-ide) *USP 28.*
Use: Anti-inflammatory, topical.
See: Rimso-50.

dimethyl sulfoxide. (Pharma 21)
Use: Increased intracranial pressure. [Orphan Drug]

dimethyl-tubocurarine iodide.
Use: Muscle relaxant.
See: Metocurine Iodide.

dimethylurethimine.
See: Meturedepa.

•**dimoxamine hydrochloride.** (die-MOX-AH-meen) USAN.
Use: Memory adjuvant.

Dimycor. (Standard Drug Co.) Pentaerythritol tetranitrate 10 mg, phenobarbital 15 mg. Tab. Bot. 1000s. *Rx.*
Use: Antianginal; hypnotic; sedative.

Dinacrin. (Sanofi-Synthelabo) Isonicotinic acid, hydrazide. *Rx.*
Use: Antituberculosal.

Dinate. (Blaine) Dimenhydrinate 50 mg/ mL. Vial 10 mL. *Rx.*
Use: Antiemetic; antivertigo.

•**dinoprost.** (DIE-no-proste) USAN.
Use: Oxytocic; prostaglandin.

•**dinoprostone.** (DIE-no-PROSTE-ohn) *USP 28.*

Use: Abortifacient; agent for cervical ripening; oxytocic; prostaglandin.
See: Cervidil.
  Prepidil.
  Prostin E₂.
•**dinoprost tromethamine.** (DIE-noproste troe-METH-ah-meen) *USP 28.*
Use: Oxytocic; prostaglandin.
Diocto. (Various Mfr.) Docusate sodium.
Syr.: 60 mg/15 mL. Bot. 480 mL. **Liq.:** 150 mg/15 mL. Bot. 480 mL. *OTC.*
Use: Laxative.
Dioctolose. (Ivax) Docusate potassium 100 mg. Cap. Bot. 100s, 1000s.
Use: Laxative.
dioctyl calcium sulfosuccinate. (die-OCK-till SULL-foe-SUCK-sih-nate) Docusate Calcium.
Use: Laxative.
dioctyl sodium sulfosuccinate.
Use: Non-laxative fecal softener.
See: Docusate Sodium.
diodone injection.
See: Iodopyracet injection.
•**diohippuric acid I 125.** (dye-oh-hip-YOOR-ik) USAN.
Use: Radiopharmaceutical.
•**diohippuric acid I 131.** USAN.
Use: Radiopharmaceutical.
Dio-Hist. (Health for Life Brands) Dextromethorphan 30 mg, thenylpyramine hydrochloride 80 mg, phenylephrine hydrochloride 20 mg, potassium tartrate ¹⁄₂₄ g/oz. Bot. 4 oz. *OTC.*
Use: Antihistamine.
diolamine. Diethanolamine.
diolostene.
See: Methandriol.
Dionex. (Henry Schein) Docusate sodium 100 mg, 250 mg. Cap. Bot. 100s, 250s, 1000s. *OTC.*
Use: Laxative.
dionin. Ethylmorphine hydrochloride.
Use: Cough depressant, oral; ocular lymphagogue.
Dionosil Oily. (GlaxoSmithKline) Propyliodone 60% in peanut oil. Inj. Vial 20 mL.
Use: Radiopaque agent.
diophyllin.
See: Aminophylline.
diopterin. Pteroylglutamic acid, PDGA, Pteroyl-alpha-glutamylglutamic acid.
Use: Antineoplastic.
Diorapin. (Standex) **Tab.:** Estrogenic conjugate 0.625 mg, methyltestosterone 5 mg. Bot. 100s. **Inj.:** Estrone 2 mg, testosterone 25 mg/mL. Vial 10 mL. *Rx.*
Use: Androgen, estrogen combination.

Diosmin. Buchu resin obtained from lvs. of barosma serratifolia and alliedrutaceae.
Dio-Soft. (Standex) Docusate sodium 100 mg, casanthranol 30 mg. Cap. Bot. 100s. *OTC.*
Use: Laxative.
Diostate D. (Pharmacia) Vitamin D 400 units, calcium 343 mg, phosphorus 265 mg. 3 Tab. Bot. 100s. *OTC.*
Use: Mineral, vitamin supplement.
•**diotyrosine I 125.** (die-oh-TIE-row-seen) USAN.
Use: Radiopharmaceutical.
•**diotyrosine I 131.** USAN.
Use: Radiopharmaceutical.
Diovan. (Novartis) Valsartan 40 mg, 80 mg, 160 mg, 320 mg. Tab. Bot. 30s (40 mg only), 100s (except 40 mg), UD 100s. *Rx.*
Use: Antihypertensive.
Diovan HCT. (Novartis) Valsartan 80 mg, hydrochlorothiazide 12.5 mg, 25 mg, valsartan 160 mg, hydrochlorothiazide 12.5 mg. Tab. Bot. 100s, 4000s, UD 100s. *Rx.*
Use: Antihypertensive.
Diovocylin. (Novartis)
See: Estradiol.
•**dioxadrol hydrochloride.** (die-OX-ah-drole) USAN.
Use: Antidepressant.
dioxindol. Diacetylhydroxyphenylisatin.
dioxyanthranol.
See: Anthralin.
•**dioxybenzone.** (die-ox-ee-BEN-zone) *USP 28.*
Use: Ultraviolet screen.
W/Oxybenzone, benzophene.
See: Solbar.
dipalmitoylphosphatidylcholine. Colfosceril palmitate.
Use: Synthetic lung surfactant.
See: Exosurf Neonatal.
dipalmitoylphosphatidylcholine/phosphatidylglycerol.
Use: Neonatal respiratory distress syndrome. [Orphan Drug]
See: ALEC.
diparcol hydrochloride. Diethazine.
Dipegyl.
See: Nicotinamide.
Dipentum. (Celltech) Osalazine sodium 250 mg. Cap. Bot. 100s, 500s. *Rx.*
Use: Gastrointestinal.
diperodon hydrochloride.
Use: Anesthetic.
See: Diothane.
  Proctodon.

W/Bacitracin, neomycin sulfate, poly-myxin.
See: Boro.
W/Furacin (nitrofurazone).
See: Furacin E.
Furacin H.C.
W/Furacin (nitrofurazone) and Microfur (nituroxime).
See: Furacin Otic.
W/Hydrocortisone, polymyxin B sulfate, neomycin.
See: My Cort Otic #1.
W/Hydroxyquinoline Benzoate.
See: Diothane.
W/Methapyrilene hydrochloride, pyril-amine maleate, allantoin, benzocaine, menthol.
See: Antihistamine.
diphenadione.
Use: Anticoagulant.
Diphen AF. (Morton Grove) Diphenhydra-mine hydrochloride 12.5 mg/5 mL, sac-charin, sugar, cherry flavor. Liq. Bot. 118 mL, 237 mL, 473 mL. OTC.
Use: Antihistamine, nonselective ethanolamine.
Diphenatol. (Rugby) Diphenoxylate hy-drochloride 2.5 mg, atropine sulfate 0.025 mg. Tab. Bot. 100s, 500s, 1000s.
Use: Antidiarrheal.
Diphenhist. (Rugby) Diphenhydramine hydrochloride 12.5 mg/5 mL, saccha-rin sucrose. Soln. Bot. 473 mL. OTC.
Use: Antihistamine.
Diphenhist Captabs. (Rugby) Diphen-hydramine hydrochloride 25 mg, lac-tose. Tab. Bot. 100s. OTC.
Use: Antihistamine, nonselective ethanolamine.
• **diphenhydramine.**
Use: Antihistamine.
See: AllerMax.
AllerMax Caplets, Maximum Strength.
Banophen.
Benadryl.
Benadryl Allergy.
Benadryl Children's Allergy.
Benadryl Children's Dye-Free Allergy.
Benadryl Dye-Free Allergy LiquiGels.
Children's Benadryl Allergy Fastmelt.
Diphen AF.
Diphenhist Captabs.
Genahist.
Scot-Tussin Allergy Relief Formula Clear.
Siladryl.
Tusstat.
diphenhydramine. (Various Mfr.) Diphenhydramine hydrochloride 25 mg. Tab. Bot. 24s, 100s. OTC.
Use: Antihistamine, nonselective ethanolamine.

diphenhydramine and pseudoephed-rine capsules.
Use: Antihistamine, decongestant.
• **diphenhydramine citrate.** (die-fen-HIGH-druh-meen SIH-trate) USP 28.
Tall Man: DiphenhydrAMINE
Use: Antihistamine.
diphenhydramine citrate and phenyl-alanine.
Use: Antihistamine.
See: Benadryl Children's Allergy Fast-melt.
diphenhydramine citrate and pseudo-ephedrine hydrochloride combina-tions.
Use: Upper respiratory combination, an-tihistamine, decongestant.
See: Benadryl Allergy & Sinus Fast-melt.
Benadryl Children's Allergy & Cold Fastmelt.
• **diphenhydramine hydrochloride.** (die-fen-HIGH-druh-meen) USP 28.
Tall Man: DiphenhydrAMINE
Use: Antihistamine, nonselective ethanolamine, antitussive.
See: Altaryl Children's Allergy.
Bax.
Benadryl Hydrochloride.
Benadryl Itch Stopping Spray, Extra Strength.
Benadryl Itch Stopping Spray, Origi-nal Strength.
Benahist.
Benylin Cough.
Clearly Cala-gel.
Dermamycin.
Dermarest.
Fenylhist.
40 Winks.
Histine.
Hydramine Cough.
Hyrexin.
Mouthkote P/R.
Nighttime Sleep Aid.
Scot-Tussin Allergy.
Scot-Tussin Allergy DM.
Silphen Cough.
Silphen DM.
Simply Sleep.
Span-Lanin.
Snooze Fast.
TheraFlu Thin Strips Multi Symptom.
Triaminic Thin Strips Long Acting Cough.
W/Combinations.
See: Anti-Itch.
Ardeben.
Bendylate.
Excedrin PM.
Fenylex.

Legatrin PM.
Midol PM.
Tusstat.
diphenhydramine hydrochloride.
(Various Mfr.) Diphenhydramine hydrochloride 25 mg, 50 mg. Cap. Bot. 24s (25 mg only), 100s, 1000s. *Rx-OTC.*
Use: Antihistamine.
diphenhydramine hydrochloride.
(Various Mfr.) Diphenhydramine hydrochloride 50 mg/mL. Inj. 1 mL fill in 2 mL cartridges. *Rx.*
Use: Antihistamine.
diphenhydramine hydrochloride.
(Various Mfr.) Diphenhydramine hydrochloride 50 mg/mL. Inj. 1 mL fill in 2 mL cartridges. *Rx.*
Use: Antihistamine.
diphenhydramine hydrochloride, acetaminophen, and pseudoephedrine hydrochloride combinations.
Use: Upper respiratory combination, antihistamine, analgesic, decongestant.
See: Acetaminophen, diphenhydramine hydrochloride, and pseudoephedrine hydrochloride combinations.
Tylenol Flu Maximum Strength.
diphenhydramine hydrochloride, acetaminophen, dextromethorphan HBr, pseudoephedrine hydrochloride combinations.
Use: Upper respiratory combination, antihistamine, analgesic, antitussive, decongestant.
See: Acetaminophen, dextromethorphan HBr, diphenhydramine hydrochloride, pseudoephedrine hydrochloride combinations.
diphenhydramine hydrochloride and acetaminophen combinations.
Use: Upper respiratory combination, antihistamine, analgesic.
See: Acetaminophen and diphenhydramine hydrochloride combinations.
diphenhydramine hydrochloride and pseudoephedrine hydrochloride combinations.
Use: Upper respiratory combination, antihistamine, decongestant.
See: Benadryl Allergy & Sinus.
Benadryl Children's Allergy & Sinus.
diphenhydramine tannate.
See: Ben-Tann.
Dytan.
W/Combinations.
See: Dytan-CS.
diphenhydramine w/combinations.
See: Banophen Decongestant.
Benadryl Itch.
Benadryl Itch Stopping Spray, Extra Strength.

Benadryl Itch Stopping Spray, Original Strength.
Dermarest.
Dermarest Plus.
Dermaycin.
Dytan-D.
Hydro-HP.
Maximum Strength Ivarest.
Pancof-EXP.
•**diphenidol hydrochloride.** (die-FEN-ih-dahl) USAN.
Use: Antiemetic
•**diphenidol pamoate.** (die-FEN-ih-dahl) USAN.
Use: Antiemetic.
•**diphenoxylate hydrochloride.** (die-fen-OX-ih-late) *USP 28.*
Use: Antiperistaltic to treat diarrhea. W/Atropine.
See: Lomotil.
diphenylhydantoin. Phenytoin.
Use: Anticonvulsant.
diphenylhydantoin sodium. Phenytoin sodium.
Use: Anticonvulsant.
diphenylhydroxycarbinol. Benzhydrol hydrochloride.
diphenylisatin.
See: Oxyphenisatin.
diphosphonic acid.
See: Etidronic acid.
diphosphopyridine (DPN).
Use: Antialcoholic. Under study.
diphosphothiamin. Cocarboxylase.
diphtheria, acellular pertussis, tetanus vaccine. (diff-THEER-ee-uh, ay-SELL-you-luhr per-TUSS-iss, TET-ah-nus)
Use: Immunization.
See: Certiva.
Infanrix.
TriHIBit.
Tripedia.
diphtheria and tetanus toxoid, adult.
(Massachusetts Public Health Biologic Labs) Diphtheria 2 Lf units, tetanus 2 Lf units/0.5 mL dose, aluminum potassium sulfate, thimerosal. Inj. Vial 5 mL, 10 mL. *Rx.*
Use: Active immunization, toxoid.
diphtheria and tetanus toxoids, acellular pertussis and haemophilus influenzae type B conjugate vaccines (DTaP-HIB).
Use: Active immunization, toxoid.
See: TriHIBit.
diphtheria and tetanus toxoids, adsorbed (for adult use).
Use: Active immunization, toxoid.
See: Decavac.
Diphtheria & Tetanus Toxoids, Adult.

diphtheria and tetanus toxoids, adsorbed (for pediatric use).
Use: Active immunization, toxoid.
See: Diphtheria & Tetanus Toxoids, Pediatric.
diphtheria and tetanus toxoids, adult. (Aventis Pasteur) Diphtheria 2 Lf units, tetanus 5 Lf units/0.5 mL dose, aluminum potassium sulfate, thimerosal. Inj. Vial 5 mL. Syr. 0.5 mL. *Rx.*
Use: Active immunization, toxoid.
diphtheria and tetanus toxoids and acellular pertussis adsorbed, hepatitis B (recombinant) and inactivated poliovirus vaccine combined.
Use: Active immunization, toxoid.
See: Pediarix.
diphtheria and tetanus toxoids and acellular pertussis vaccine, adsorbed.
Use: Prevention against diphtheria, tetanus, and pertussis; immunizing agent.
See: Daptacel.
  Infanrix.
  TriHIBit.
  Tripedia.
diphtheria and tetanus toxoids, pediatric. (Aventis Pasteur) Diphtheria 6.7 Lf units, tetanus 5 Lf units/0.5 mL dose, aluminum potassium sulfate, thimerosal. Inj. Multidose vial 5 mL. *Rx.*
Use: Active immunization, toxoid.
diphtheria equine antitoxin. *Rx.*
Use: Prophylaxis and treatment of diphtheria.
● **diphtheria toxin for Schick Test.** (diff-THEER-ee-uh) *USP 28.* Formerly Diphtheria Toxin, Diagnostic
Use: Diagnostic aid (dermal reactivity indicator).
Dipimol. (Everett) Dipyridamole 25 mg, 50 mg, 75 mg. Tab. Bot. 100s, 500s, 1000s.
Use: Antianginal.
dipivalyl epinephrine.
See: Propine.
● **dipivefrin.** (die-PIHV-eh-FRIN) USAN. Formerly Dipivalyl Epinephrine.
Use: Adrenergic, ophthalmic.
● **dipivefrin hydrochloride.** (die-PIHV-eh-FRIN) *USP 28.*
Use: Antiglaucoma agent.
See: AKPro.
  Propine.
dipivefrin hydrochloride. (Various Mfr.) Dipivefrin hydrochloride 0.1% Soln. 5 mL, 10 mL, 15 mL. *Rx.*
Use: Antiglaucoma agent.

Diprivan. (AstraZeneca) Propofol 10 mg/mL, soybean oil 100 mg, glycerol 22.5 mg, egg lecithin 12 mg, EDTA 0.005%, ph = 7 to 8.5. Inj. Single-use amp. 20 mL. Single-use infusion vial 50 mL, 100 mL. Prefilled single-use syr. 50 mL. *Rx.*
Use: Anesthetic, general.
Diprolene. (Schering-Plough) Betamethasone dipropionate 0.05%.
Cream: In cream base. Tube 15 g.
Oint.: In ointment base. Tube 15 g, 45 g. *Rx.*
Use: Anti-inflammatory; antipruritic, topical.
Diprolene AF Cream. (Schering-Plough) Betamethasone dipropionate cream equivalent to 0.05% betamethasone. Tube 15 g, 45 g. *Rx.*
Use: Corticosteroid, topical.
dipropylacetic acid.
See: Valproic Acid.
Diprosone. (Schering-Plough) Betamethasone dipropionate 0.64 mg (equiv. to 0.5 mg betamethasone).
Cream: W/mineral oil, white petrolatum, polyethylene glycol 1000 monocetyl ether, cetostearyl alcohol, phosphoric acid, monobasic sodium phosphate with 4-chloro-m-cresol as preservative. Tube 15 g, 45 g. **Lot.:** W/isopropyl alcohol (46.8%). Bot. 20 mL, 60 mL.
Oint.: In white petrolatum and mineral oil base. Tube 15 g, 45 g. *Rx.*
Use: Corticosteroid, topical.
Diprosone Aerosol 0.1%. (Schering-Plough) Betamethasone dipropionate 6.4 mg (equiv. to 5 mg betamethasone) in vehicle of mineral oil, caprylic-capric triglyceride w/isopropyl alcohol 10%, inert hydrocarbon propellants (propane and isobutane). Can 85 g. *Rx.*
Use: Corticosteroid, topical.
● **dipyridamole.** (DIE-pih-RID-uh-mole) *USP 28.*
Use: Coronary vasodilator; antiplatelet agent.
See: Persantine.
  Persantine IV.
W/Aspirin.
See: Aggrenox.
dipyridamole. (Various Mfr.) Tab. **25 mg:** Bot. 90s, 100s, 500s, 1000s, 5000s, UD 100s. **50 mg, 75 mg:** Bot. 100s, 500s, 1000s, UD 100s. *Rx.*
Use: Coronary vasodilator; antiplatelet agent.
● **dipyrithione.** (DIE-pihr-ih-THIGH-ohn) USAN.
Use: Antifungal; anti-infective.

•**dipyrone.** (DIE-pie-rone) USAN. Formerly Methampyrone.
Use: Analgesic; antipyretic.

•**diquafosol tetrasodium.** (dye-kwa-FOS-ol) USAN.
Use: Dry eye.

•**dirithromycin.** (die-RITH-row-MY-sin) USAN.
Use: Anti-infective, macrolide.
See: Dynabac.

disaccharide tripeptide glycerol dipalmitoyl.
Use: Antineoplastic. [Orphan Drug]
See: ImmTher.

Disalcid. (3M) Salsalate. **Tab.**: 500 mg, 750 mg. Bot. 100s, 500s, UD 100s. **Cap.:** 500 mg. Bot. 100s. *Rx.*
Use: Analgesic.

Discase. (Omnis Surgical) Chymopapain 5 units/2 mL. Vial 5 mL. *Rx.*
Use: Intradiscal injection for herniated lumbar intervertebral discs.

Disinfecting Solution. (Bausch & Lomb) Sodium Cl, sodium borate, boric acid, chlorhexidine 0.005%, EDTA 0.1%, thimerosal 0.001%. Bot. 355 mL. *OTC.*
Use: Contact lens care.

•**disiquonium chloride.** (die-SIH-CONE-ee-uhm) USAN.
Use: Antiseptic.

Dismiss Douche. (Schering-Plough) Sodium Cl, sodium citrate, citric acid, cetearyl octoate, ceteareth-27, fragrance. Pow. for dilution. Pkg. 2s.
Use: Vaginal agent.

Disobrom. (Geneva) Pseudoephedrine sulfate 120 mg, dexbrompheniramine maleate 6 mg. Tab. Bot 100s, 1000s. *Rx.*
Use: Antihistamine, decongestant.

•**disobutamide.** (DIE-so-BYOO-tam-ide) USAN.
Use: Cardiovascular agent (antiarrhythmic).

disodium carbonate.
See: Sodium Carbonate.

disodium chromate. Sodium Chromate Cr 51 Injection.

disodium chromoglycate.
See: Intal.
Nasalcrom.

disodium clodronate. (Discovery)
Use: Antihypercalcemic. [Orphan Drug]

disodium clodronate tetrahydrate.
Use: Increased bone resorption due to malignancy. [Orphan Drug]
See: Bonefos.

disodium edathamil.
See: Edathamil Disodium.

disodium edetate. Disodium ethylenediaminetetra acetate.

See: Edetate disodium.

disodium phosphate.
See: Sodium phosphate.

disodium phosphate heptahydrate.
See: Sodium phosphate.

disodium thiosulfate pentahydrate.
See: Sodium thiosulfate.

di-sodium versenate.
See: Edathamil Disodium.

•**disofenin.** (DIE-so-FEN-in) USAN.
Use: Diagnostic aid (carrier agent).

Disophrol. (Schering-Plough) Pseudoephedrine sulfate 60 mg, dexbrompheniramine maleate 2 mg. Tab. Bot. 100s. *OTC.*
Use: Antihistamine, decongestant.

Disophrol Chronotabs. (Schering-Plough) Dexbrompheniramine maleate 6 mg, pseudoephedrine sulfate 120 mg. SA Tab. Bot. 100s. *OTC.*
Use: Antihistamine, decongestant.

•**disopyramide.** (DIE-so-PIR-uh-mide) USAN.
Use: Cardiovascular agent (antiarrhythmic).

•**disopyramide phosphate.** (DIE-so-PIHR-ah-mid) *USP 28.*
Use: Cardiovascular agent; antiarrhythmic.
See: Norpace.
Norpace CR.

disopyramide phosphate. (Various Mfr.) Disopyramide phosphate. **Cap.:** 100 mg, 150 mg. Bot. 100s, 500s. **ER Cap.:** 150 mg. Bot. 100s. *Rx.*
Use: Antiarrhythmics.

•**disoxaril.** (die-SOX-ar-ILL) USAN.
Use: Antiviral.

Di-Spaz. (Vortech Pharmaceuticals) Dicyclomine hydrochloride. **Cap.:** 10 mg. Bot. 1000s. **Inj.:** 10 mg. Vial 10 mL. *Rx.*
Use: Gastrointestinal; anticholinergic.

DisperMox. (Ranbaxy) Amoxicillin 200 mg, 400 mg. Aspartame, phenylalanine 5.6 mg. Strawberry flavor. Tab. for Oral Susp. 20s, 60s, 500s (400 mg only), 1000s (200 mg only), UD 100s. *Rx.*
Use: Anti-infective.

Dispos-a-Med. (Parke-Davis) Isoetharine hydrochloride 0.5%, 1%. Can of prefilled sterile tubes 0.5 mL. 50s. *Rx.*
Use: Bronchodilator.

distaquaine.
See: Penicillin V.

distigmine bromide. Hexamarium bromide.

•**disufenton sodium.** (dye-soo-FEN-ton) USAN.

Use: Neuroprotectant.
●**disulfiram.** (die-SULL-fih-ram) *USP 28.*
Use: Alcohol deterrent.
See: Antabuse.
Ditate DS. (Savage) Testosterone enanthate 360 mg, estradiol valerate 16 mg, benzyl alcohol 2% in sesame oil. Syringe 2 mL. Box 10s. Vial 2 mL. *Rx.*
Use: Androgen, estrogen combination.
●**ditekiren.** (DIE-teh-KIE-ren) USAN.
Use: Antihypertensive.
dithranol.
See: Anthralin.
D.I.T.I. Creme. (Dunhall Pharmaceuticals, Inc.) Iodoquinol 100 mg, sulfanilamide 500 mg, diethylstilbestrol 0.1 mg/g. Jar. 4 oz. *Rx.*
Use: Anti-infective, vaginal.
D.I.T.I. 2 Creme. (Dunhall Pharmaceutical cals, Inc.) Sulfanilamide 15%, aminacrine hydrochloride 0.2%, allantoin 2%. Tube 142 g. *Rx.*
Use: Anti-infective, vaginal.
●**ditiocade sodium.** (DIT-ee-oh-kade) USAN.
Use: Radiopharmaceutical.
Ditropan. (ALZA) Oxybutynin chloride. **Syr.:** 5 mg/5 mL sorbitol, sucrose, methylparaben. Bot. 473 mL. **Tab.:** 5 mg, lactose. Bot. 100s, 1000s, UD 100s. *Rx.*
Use: Anticholinergic.
Ditropan XL. (ALZA) Oxybutynin chloride 5 mg, 10 mg, 15 mg, lactose. ER Tab. Bot. 100s *Rx.*
Use: Anticholinergic.
Diulo. (Pharmacia) Metolazone 2.5 mg, 5 mg, 10 mg. Tab. Bot. 100s. *Rx.*
Use: Antihypertensive, diuretic.
Diurese. (American Urologicals, Inc.) Trichlormethiazide 4 mg. Tab. Bot. 100s, 1000s. *Rx.*
Use: Diuretic.
diuretic combinations.
See: Alazide.
　Aldactazide.
　Dyazide.
　Maxzide.
　Maxzide-25 MG.
　Moduretic.
　Spironazide.
　Spironolactone w/Hydrochlorothiazide.
　Spirozide.
　Triamterene w/Hydrochlorothiazide.
diuretics, loop.
See: Bumex.
　Edecrin.
　Edecrin Sodium.
　Furosemide.

　Lasix.
　Luramide.
diuretics, osmotic.
See: Ismotic.
　Mannitol.
　Osmitrol.
　Osmoglyn.
　Ureaphil.
diuretics, potassium-sparing.
See: Alatone.
　Aldactone.
　Amiloride Hydrochloride.
　Dyrenium.
　Midamor.
　Spironolactone.
diuretics, thiazides.
See: Aquatensen.
　Chlorothiazide.
　Chlorthalidone.
　Diucardin.
　Diulo.
　Diurese.
　Diurigen.
　Diuril.
　Diuril Sodium.
　Enduron.
　Esidrix.
　Ethon.
　Exna.
　Hydrochlorothiazide.
　HydroDiuRIL.
　Hydroflumethiazide.
　Hydromal.
　Hydro-T.
　Hydro-Z-50.
　Hygroton.
　Hylidone.
　Lozol.
　Metahydrin.
　Methyclothiazide.
　Mictrin.
　Mykrox.
　Naqua.
　Naturetin.
　Niazide.
　Oretic.
　Renese.
　Saluron.
　Thalitone.
　Trichlormethiazide.
　Zaroxolyn.
Diuretic Tablets. (Faraday) Buchu leaves 150 mg, uva ursi leaves 150 mg, juniper berries 120 mg, bone meal, parsley, asparagus. Bot. 100s. *Rx.*
Use: Diuretic.
Diurigen Tablets. (Ivax) Chlorothiazide 500 mg. Bot. 100s, 1000s. *Rx.*
Use: Diuretic.
Diurigen w/Reserpine 500 Tablets. (Ivax) Chlorothiazide 500 mg, reser-

pine 0.125 mg. Bot. 100s, 1000s. *Rx.*
Use: Antihypertensive combination.
Diurigen w/Reserpine 250 Tablets.
(Ivax) Chlorothiazide 250 mg, reserpine
0.125 mg. Bot. 100s, 1000s. *Rx.*
Use: Antihypertensive combination.
Diuril. (Merck & Co.) Chlorothiazide,
USP. **Tab.:** 250 mg. Bot. 100s, 1000s.
500 mg. Bot. 100s, 1000s, UD 100s.
Oral Susp.: 250 mg/5 mL w/methyl-
paraben 0.12%, propylparaben 0.02%,
benzoic acid 0.1%, alcohol 0.5%. Bot.
237 mL. *Rx.*
Use: Antihypertensive; diuretic.
W/Methyldopa.
See: Aldoclor.
Diuril Sodium Intravenous. (Merck &
Co.) Chlorothiazide sodium equivalent
to 0.5 g chlorothiazide w/mannitol
0.25 g sodium hydroxide, thimerosal
0.4 mg. Vial 20 mL. *Rx.*
Use: Antihypertensive; diuretic.
Diutensen-R. (Wallace) Methyclothiazide
2.5 mg, reserpine 0.1 mg. Tab. Bot.
100s, 500s, 5000s. *Rx.*
Use: Antihypertensive combination.
•**divalproex sodium.** (die-VAL-pro-ex)
USAN.
Use: Anticonvulsant.
See: Depakote.
divinyl oxide. Vinyl ether, divinyl ether.
Use: Inhalation anesthetic.
Dizac. (Ohmeda) Diazepam 5 mg/mL,
preservative free. Inj. Vial 3 mL. *c-IV.*
Use: Anxiolytic; anticonvulsant; muscle
relaxant.
Dizmiss. (Jones Pharma) Meclizine hydrochloride 25 mg. Tab. Bot. 100s,
1000s. *OTC.*
Use: Antiemetic; antivertigo.
•**dizocilpine maleate.** (die-ZOE-sill-
PEEN) USAN.
Use: Neuroprotective.
dl-desoxyephedrine hydrochloride.
See: dl-Methamphetamine hydrochloride.
dl-methamphetamine hydrochloride.
dl-Desoxyephedrine hydrochloride.
See: Oxydess.
dl-norephedrine hydrochloride.
DMax. (Great Southern) Dextromethorphan HBr 15 mg, phenylephrine hydrochloride 8 mg, carbinoxamine
maleate 4 mg/5 mL. Berry flavor. Syrup.
30 mL, 473 mL. *Rx.*
Use: Antitussive, antihistamine, decongestant.
DMax Pediatric. (Great Southern) Dextromethorphan 4 mg, phenylephrine
2 mg, carbinoxamine maleate 2 mg/mL.
Purple, berry flavor. Drops. 30 mL bot.

with 1 mL dropper. *Rx.*
Use: Antitussive, antihistamine, decon-
gestant.
DM Cough. (Rosemont) Dextromethor-
phan HBr 10 mg/5 mL, alcohol 5%.
Syr. Bot. 120 mL, pt, gal. *OTC.*
Use: Antitussive.
DMCT. (Wyeth) Demethylchlortetracycline. *Rx.*
Use: Anti-infective; tetracycline.
See: Declomycin hydrochloride.
d-methorphan hydrobromide.
See: Dextromethorphan HBr.
d-methylphenylamine sulfate.
See: Dextroamphetamine Sulfate.
**DML Dermatological Moisturizing Lo-
tion.** (Person and Covey) Purified water, petrolatum, glycerin, methyl glucose sesquisterate, dimethicone,
methyl gluceth-20 sesquisterate, benzyl alcohol, volatile silicone, glyceryl
stearate, stearic acid, palmitic acid, cetyl alcohol, xanthan gum, magnesium
aluminum silicate carbomer 941, sodium hydroxide. Bot. 8 oz. *OTC.*
Use: Emollient.
DML Facial Moisturizer. (Person and
Covey) Octyl methoxycinnamate 8%,
oxybenzone 4%, benzyl alcohol, petrolatum, EDTA. SPF 15. Cream. Tube
45 g. *OTC.*
Use: Sunscreen.
DML Forte. (Person and Covey) Petrolatum, PPG-2 myristyl ether propionate,
glyceryl stearate, glycerin, stearic acid,
d-panthenol, DEA-cetyl phosphate, si-
methicone, PVP eicosene copolymer,
benzyl alcohol, cetyl alcohol, silica, di-
sodium EDTA, BHA, magnesium alumi-
num silicate, sodium carbomer 1342.
Tube 113 g. *OTC.*
Use: Emollient.
dmp 777. (DuPont)
Use: Cystic fibrosis. [Orphan Drug]
DMSO.
See: Dimethyl sulfoxide.
DNA demethylation agents.
See: Azacitidine.
DNA topoisomerase inhibitors.
See: Irinotecan hydrochloride.
Topotecan hydrochloride.
Doak Tar. (Doak) **Lot.:** Tar distillate 5%.
Bot. 118 mL. **Oil:** Tar distillate 2%. Min-
eral oil. Bot. 237 mL. **Shampoo:** Coal
tar 1.2%, isopropyl alcohol. Bot.
237 mL. *OTC.*
Use: Antiseborrheic.
Doak Tar Oil Forte. (Doak Dermatolog-
ics) Tar distillate 5%. Bot. 4 oz.
Use: Antiseborrheic.

Doak Tersaseptic. (Doak Dermatologics) Liquid cleanser, pH 6.8. Bot. 4 oz, pt, gal. *OTC.*
Use: Detergent.
Doan's Backache Spray. (DEP Corp.) Methyl salicylate 15%, menthol 8.4%, methyl nicotinate 0.6%. Aerosol Can 4 oz. *OTC.*
Use: Analgesic, topical.
Doan's Pills. (DEP Corp.) Magnesium salicylate 325 mg. Tab. Ctn. 24s, 48s. *OTC.*
Use: Analgesic.
Doan's PM, Extra Strength.
See: Extra Strength Doan's PM.
•**dobutamine hydrochloride.** (doe-BYOOT-ah-meen) *USP 28.*
Tall Man: DOBUTamine
Use: Cardiovascular agent.
See: Dobutrex.
dobutamine hydrochloride. (Various Mfr.) Dobutamine hydrochloride 12.5 mg/mL. May contain sulfites. Inj. Vial 20 mL.
Tall Man: DOBUTamine
Use: Cardiovascular agent.
•**dobutamine in dextrose for injection,** (doe-BYOOT-ah-meen) *USP 28.*
Tall Man: DOBUTamine
Use: Cardiovascular agent.
•**dobutamine lactobionate.** (doe-BYOOT-ah-meen) USAN.
Tall Man: DOBUTamine
Use: Cardiovascular agent.
•**dobutamine tartrate.** (doe-BYOOT-ah-meen) USAN.
Use: Cardiovascular agent.
Dobutrex Solution. (Eli Lilly) Dobutamine hydrochloride 250 mg. Inj. Vial 20 mL. *Rx.*
Use: Cardiovascular agent.
•**docebenone.** (dah-SEH-beh-nohn) USAN.
Use: Inhibitor (5-lipoxygenase).
•**docetaxel.** (doe-seh-TAX-ehl) USAN.
Use: Antineoplastic, antimitotic.
See: Taxotere.
•**doconazole.** (doe-KOE-nah-zole) USAN.
Use: Antifungal.
•**docosanol.** (doe-KOE-sah-nole) USAN.
Use: Antiviral.
See: Abreva.
Doctase. (Purepac) Docusate sodium 100 mg, casanthranol 30 mg. Cap. Bot. 100s. *OTC.*
Use: Laxative.
Doctyl. (Health for Life Brands) Docusate sodium 100 mg. Tab. Bot. 40s, 100s, 1000s. *OTC.*
Use: Laxative.

Doctylax. (Health for Life Brands) Docusate sodium 100 mg, acetophenolisatin 2 mg, prune conc. ¾ mg. Tab. Bot. 40s, 100s, 1000s. *OTC.*
Use: Laxative.
Docu. (Hi-Tech Pharmacal) Docusate sodium. **Syr.:** 20 mg/5 mL, alcohol 5%. Bot. 480 mL. **Liq.:** 150 mg/15 mL. Bot. 480 mL. *OTC.*
Use: Laxative.
•**docusate calcium.** (DOCK-you-sate) *USP 28.* Formerly Dioctyl Calcium Sulfosuccinate.
Use: Laxative; stool softener.
See: DC Softgels.
Doxidan.
Stool Softner.
Stool Softner DC.
Surfak.
docusate calcium. (Various Mfr.) Docusate calcium 240 mg. Cap. Bot. 100s, 500s, UD 100s, 300s. *OTC.*
Use: Laxative.
•**docusate potassium.** *USP 28.*
Use: Laxative; stool softener.
•**docusate sodium.** (DOCK-you-sate) *USP 28.* Formerly Dioctyl Sodium Sulfosuccinate.
Use: Pharmaceutical aid (surfactant); stool softener.
See: Colace.
Coloctyl.
Comfolax.
Correctol Extra Gentle.
Dialose.
Diocto.
Diomedicone.
Docu.
DOK.
D.O.S.
Doss, Super Doss.
Doxinate.
D-S-S.
Dulcolax Stool Softener.
Duosol.
Dynoctol.
Easy-Lax.
ex-lax Stool Softener.
Genasoft.
Konsto.
Laxatab.
Liqui-Doss.
Non-Habit Forming Stool Softner.
Phillips' Liqui-Gels.
Regul-Aid.
Regulax SS.
Silace.
Sof-lax.
Stool Softner.
Stulex.

Surfak.
W/Ascorbic acid, ferrous fumarate.
See: Hemaspan.
W/Betaine hydrochloride, zinc, manganese, molybdenum.
See: Hemaferrin.
W/Bisacodyl.
See: Laxadan.
W/Brewer's yeast.
See: Doss or Super Doss.
W/Casanthranol.
See: Calotabs.
Constiban.
Diolax.
Dio-Soft.
DOK-Plus.
Doxidan.
Easy-Lax Plus.
Genericace.
Laxative and Stool Softener.
Neo-Vadrin D-D-S.
Nuvac.
W/Casanthranol, sodium carboxymethylcellulose.
See: Dialose Plus.
Tri-Vac.
W/D-calcium pantothenate and acetaphenolisatin.
See: Peri-Pantyl.
W/Dehydrocholic acid.
See: Dubbalax-B.
Dubbalax-N.
Neolax.
W/Ferrous fumarate, betaine hydrochloride, desiccated liver, vitamins, minerals.
See: Hemaferrin.
W/Ferrous fumarate, vitamin C.
See: Hemaspan.
Recoup.
W/Ferrous fumarate, vitamins.
See: Bevitone.
W/Glycerin.
See: Barc.
W/Petrolatum.
See: Milkinol.
W/Phenolphthalein.
See: Correctol.
ex-lax.
Feen-A-Mint.
Phillips' LaxCaps.
W/Phenolphthalein, dehydrocholic acid.
See: Bolax.
Tripalax.
W/Polyoxyethylene-nonyl-phenol, sodium edetate, 9-aminoacridine hydrochloride.
See: Vagisec Plus.
W/Senna concentrate.
See: DSS 100 Plus.
Genasoft Plus.
Gentlax S.

PeriColace.
Peri-Dos.
Senna Plus.
Senokap-DDS.
Senokot S.
W/Sennosides.
See: ex-lax Gentle Strength.
docusate sodium. (Roxane) Docusate sodium 50 mg/15 mL, 100 mg/30 mL, saccharin, sucrose, parabens. Syr. UD 15 mL, 30 mL (100s). *OTC.*
Use: Laxative.
docusate sodium. (UDL) Docusate sodium 50 mg. Softgel cap. Bot. 100s, UD 100s *OTC.*
Use: Laxative.
docusate sodium. (Various Mfr.) Docusate sodium. **Cap.:** 250 mg. Bot. 100s, 1000s, UD 100s. **Softgel Cap.:** 100 mg, 250 mg. Bot. 100s, 1000s, UD 100s, 300s (100 mg only). *OTC.*
Use: Laxative.
docusate with casanthranol. (Various Mfr.) Docusate sodium 100 mg, casanthranol 30 mg. Cap. Bot. 100s, 1000s, UD 100s, 300s, 600s. *OTC.*
Use: Laxative; stool softener.
•**dofetilide.** (doe-FEH-till-ide) USAN.
Use: Cardiovascular agent; antiarrhythmic.
See: Tikosyn.
Dofus. (Miller Pharmacal Group) Freeze-dried *Lactobacillus acidophilus* minimum of 1 billion organisms. Cap. w/*Lactobacillus bifidus* organisms added. Bot. 60s. *OTC.*
Use: Nutritional supplement; antidiarrheal.
DOK. (Major) Docusate sodium 250 mg. Cap. 100s. *OTC.*
Use: Laxative.
DOK-Plus. (Major) Docusate sodium 60 mg, casanthrol 30 mg/15 mL, alcohol 10%, parabens, saccharin, sucrose. Syr. Bot. 473 mL. *OTC.*
Use: Laxative.
Doktors Spray. (Scherer) Phenylephrine hydrochloride 0.25%, chlorobutanol, sodium bisulfite, benzalkonium chloride. Soln. Bot. 30 mL. *OTC.*
Use: Decongestant.
Dolacet. (Roberts) Hydrocodone bitartrate 5 mg, acetaminophen 500 mg. Cap. Bot. 100s. *c-III.*
Use: Analgesic combination, narcotic.
Dolamide Tabs. (Major) Chlorpropamide 100 mg, 250 mg. Bot. 100s, 500s, 1000s. *Rx.*
Use: Antidiabetic.
Dolamin. (Harvey) Ammonium sulfate 0.75% with sodium chloride, benzyl al-

cohol. Amp. 10 mL. In 12s, 25s, 100s.
Rx.
Use: Antineuralgic.
dolantin.
See: Meperidine hydrochloride.
•**dolasetron mesylate.** (dahl-AH-set-rahn) *USP 28.*
Use: Antiemetic; antimigraine.
See: Anzemet.
Dolcin. (Dolcin) Aspirin 3.7 g, calcium succinate 2.8 g. Tab. Bot. 100s, 200s. *OTC.*
Use: Analgesic.
Doldram. (Dram) Salicylamide 7.5 g. Tab. Bot. 100s.
Use: Analgesic.
Dolene AP-65. (Wyeth) Propoxyphene hydrochloride 65 mg, acetaminophen 650 mg. Tab. Bot. 100s, 500s. *c-IV.*
Use: Analgesic combination; narcotic.
Dolene Compound-65. (Wyeth) Propoxyphene hydrochloride 65 mg, aspirin 389 mg, caffeine 32.4 mg. Cap. Bot. 100s, 500s. *c-IV.*
Use: Analgesic combination; narcotic.
Dolene Plain. (Wyeth) Propoxyphene hydrochloride 65 mg. Cap. Bot. 100s, 500s. *c-IV.*
Use: Analgesic; narcotic.
Dolgic. (Athlon) Acetaminophen 650 mg, butalbital 50 mg. Tab. Bot. 100s. *Rx.*
Use: Analgesic.
Dolgic LQ. (Athlon) Acetaminophen 108.3 mg, caffeine 13.3 mg, butlabital 16.6 mg/5 mL, alcohol 7.368%, orange, tropical fruit punch flavors. Soln. 473 mL. *Rx.*
Use: Analgesic, nonnarcotic.
Dolobid. (Merck & Co.) Diflunisal 250 mg, 500 mg. Tab. Unit-of-use 60s, UD 100s. *Rx.*
Use: Analgesic.
Dolomite. (NBTY) Magnesium 78 mg, calcium 130 mg. Tab. Bot. 100s, 250s. *OTC.*
Use: Mineral supplement.
Dolomite. (Halsey Drug) Calcium 426 mg, magnesium 246 mg. Tab. w/guar and acacia gum. Bot. 250s. *OTC.*
Use: Mineral supplement.
Dolomite Plus Capsules. (Barth's) Magnesium 37 mg, calcium 187 mg, phosphorus 50 mg, iodine 0.25 mg. Bot. 100s, 500s, 1000s. *OTC.*
Use: Mineral supplement.
Dolomite Tablets. (Faraday) Calcium 150 mg, magnesium 90 mg. Bot. 250s. *OTC.*
Use: Mineral supplement.
•**dolonil.** (Parke-Davis)
See: Pyridium Plus.

Dolono. (R.I.D.) Acetaminophen 160 mg/ 5 mL, sorbitol, sucrose, alcohol free, cherry flavor. Elixir. Bot. 120 mL. *OTC.*
Use: Analgesic.
Dolophine Hydrochloride. (Roxane) Methadone hydrochloride 5 mg, 10 mg. Tab. Bot. 100s. *c-II.*
Use: Opioid analgesic.
Dolopirona Tablets. (Sanofi-Synthelabo) Dipyrone with chlormezanone. *Rx.*
Use: Analgesic; anxiolytic; muscle relaxant.
Dolorac. (GenDerm) Capsaicin 0.25%, benzyl alcohol, cetyl alcohol. Cream. Tube 28 g. *OTC.*
Use: Analgesic, topical.
Doloral. (Progressive Enterprises) Colchicine salicylate 0.1 mg, phenobarbital 8 mg, sodium para-aminobenzoate 15 mg, vitamins B, 25 mg, aspirin 325 mg. Tab. Bot. 100s, 1000s. *Rx.*
Use: Antiarthritis, antigout.
dolosal.
See: Meperidine hydrochloride.
Dolsed. (American Urologicals, Inc.) Methenamine 40.8 mg, phenylsalicylate 18.1 mg, atropine sulfate 0.03 mg, hyoscyamine 0.03 mg, benzoic acid 4.5 mg, methylene blue 5.4 mg. Tab. Bot. 100s, 1000s. *Rx.*
Use: Anti-infective, urinary.
dolvanol.
Use: Analgesic; narcotic.
See: Meperidine hydrochloride.
•**domazoline fumarate.** (DOME-AZE-oh-leen) *USAN.*
Use: Anticholinergic.
Domeboro. (Bayer Corp. (Consumer Div.)) Aluminum sulfate and calcium acetate when added to water gives therapeutic effect of Burow's. One pkg. or Tab./pt water approximately equivalent to 1:40 dilution. **Pkg.:** 2.2 g, 12s, 100s. **Effervescent Tab.:** Box 12s, 100s, 1000s. *OTC.*
Use: Anti-inflammatory, topical.
Domeboro Otic. (Bayer Corp. (Consumer Div.)) Acetic acid 2% (in aluminum acetate solution). Soln. Bot. 60 mL with dropper. *Rx.*
Use: Otic.
Dome-Paste Bandage. (Bayer Corp. (Consumer Div.)) Zinc oxide, calamine and gelatin bandage. Pkg. 4" × 10 yd. and 3" × 10 yd. impregnated gauze bandage. *OTC.*
Use: Dermatologic, wound therapy.
domestrol.
See: Diethylstilbestrol.
D.O.M.F.
Use: Antimicrobial.

See: Merbromin (Mercurochrome).

●**domiodol.** (dome-EYE-oh-DOLE) USAN.
Use: Mucolytic.

●**domiphen bromide.** (DOE-mih-fen)
USAN.
Use: Antiseptic; anti-infective, topical.
See: Bradosol.

Domol Bath and Shower Oil. (Bayer
Corp. (Consumer Div.)) D₁-isopropyl sebacate, isopropyl myristate with mineral oil. Bot. 240 mL. *OTC.*
Use: Emollient.

●**domperidone.** (dome-PEH-rih-dohn)
USAN.
Use: Investigational antiemetic.

Donatussin. (Laser) Dextromethorphan
HBr 15 mg, guaifenesin 100 mg,
phenylephrine hydrochloride 10 mg,
chlorpheniramine maleate 2 mg/5 mL.
Syrup. 30 mL, 115 mL, 473 mL. *Rx.*
Use: Antitussive and expectorant combination.

Donatussin DC. (Laser) Hydrocodone bitartrate 2.5 mg, guaifenesin 50 mg,
phenylephrine hydrochloride 7.5 mg/
5 mL, alcohol free. Syr. Bot. 118 mL,
473 mL. *c-III.*
Use: Upper respiratory combination, antitussive, expectorant, decongestant.

Donatussin Drops. (Laser) Guaifenesin
20 mg, chlorpheniramine maleate
1 mg, phenylephrine hydrochloride
2 mg/mL, peach flavor. Bot. 30 mL
w/dropper. *Rx.*
Use: Upper respiratory combination, antihistamine, decongestant, expectorant.

Donatussin Syrup. (Laser) Phenylephrine 10 mg, chlorpheniramine
maleate 2 mg, dextromethorphan HBr
7.5 mg, guaifenesin 100 mg/5 mL, alcohol free. Liq. Bot. 473 mL. *Rx.*
Use: Upper respiratory combination, antihistamine, antitussive, decongestant, expectorant.

Dondril. (Whitehall-Robins) Dextomethorphan HBr 10 mg, phenylephrine hydrochloride 5 mg, chlorpheniramine
maleate 1 mg. Tab. Bot. 24s. *OTC.*
Use: Antihistamine; antitussive; decongestant.

●**donepezil hydrochloride.** (doe-NEPP-
eh-zill HIGH-droe-KLOR-ide) USAN.
Use: Treatment of mild to moderate de-
mentia of the Alzheimer type.
See: Aricept.
Aricept ODT.

●**donetidine.** (doe-NEH-tih-DEEN) USAN.
Use: Antiulcerative.

Donna. (Arcum) Menthol, thymol, eucalyptol, exsiccated alum, boric acid.
4 oz, 14 oz. *Rx.*
Use: Vaginal agent.

Donnamar. (H.L. Moore Drug Exchange)
Atropine sulfate 0.0194 mg, scopolamine HBr 0.0065 mg, hyoscyamine
HBr, or SO₄ 0.1037 mg, phenobarbital
16.2 mg/5 mL, alcohol 23%. Elix. Bot.
120 mL, pt, gal. *Rx.*
Use: Anticholinergic; antispasmodic.

Donnamar. (Marnel) Hyoscyamine sulfate 0.125 mg. Tab. Bot. 100s. *Rx.*
Use: Anticholinergic; antispasmodic.

Donnaphen. (Health for Life Brands)
Phenobarbital 16.2 mg, hyoscyamine
sulfate 0.1037 mg, atropine sulfate
0.0194 mg, hyoscine HBr 0.0065 mg/
5 mL. Elix. Bot. Pt, gal. *Rx.*
Use: Anticholinergic; antispasmodic.

Donna-Sed Elixir. (Vortech Pharmaceuticals) Atropine sulfate 0.0194 mg,
scopolamine HBr 0.0065, hyoscyamine
HBr, or SO₄ 0.1037 mg, phenobarbital 16.2 mg, alcohol 23%. Liq. Bot.
118 mL, gal. *Rx.*
Use: Gastrointestinal; anticholinergic.

Donnatal. (PBM Pharm) **Elix.:** Atropine
sulfate 0.0194 mg, scopolamine hydrobromide 0.0065 mg, hyoscyamine
hydrobromide 0.1037 mg, phenobarbital
16.2 mg per 5 mL. Ethyl alcohol 95%,
saccharin, sucrose, sorbitol. Grape flavor. 118 mL, 473 mL. **Tab.:** Atropine
sulfate 0.0194 mg, scopolamine hydrobromide 0.0065 mg, hyoscyamine hydrobromide 0.1037 mg, phenobarbital
16.2 mg. Lactose. 100s, 1,000s. *Rx.*
Use: Gastrointestinal anticholinergic.

Donnatal Extentabs. (PBM Pharm) Atropine sulfate 0.0582 mg, scopolamine
hydrobromide 0.0195 mg, hyoscyamine
sulfate 0.3111 mg, phenobarbital
48.6 mg. Lactose, polydextrose. Film
coated. ER Tab. 100s, 500s. *Rx.*
Use: Gastrointestinal anticholinergic.

Don't. (Del) Sucrose octa acetate 5%,
isopropyl alcohol 54%. Bot. 0.45 oz.
OTC.
Use: Nail-biting deterrent.

●**dopamantine.** (DOE-pah-MAN-teen)
USAN.
Use: Antiparkinsonian.

dopamine. (AstraZeneca) Dopamine.
Amp.: 200 mg/5 mL, Box 10s; 400 mg/
10 mL, Box 5s. **Additive Syringe:**
200 mg/5 mL, Box 1s; 400 mg/10 mL,
Box 1s. *Rx.*
Use: Inotropic agent.

●**dopamine hydrochloride.** (DOE-puh-
meen) *USP 28.*
Tall Man: DOPamine

Use: Adrenergic.
dopamine hydrochloride and dextrose injection.
Use: Adrenergic; emergency treatment of low blood pressure.
dopaminergics.
Use: Antiparkinson agents.
See: Apomorphine Hydrochloride.
   Pramipexole.
   Ropinirole Hydrochloride.
Dopar. (Procter & Gamble) Levodopa 100 mg, 250 mg, 500 mg. Cap. Bot. 100s, 1000s (500 mg only). *Rx.*
Use: Antiparkinsonian.
•**dopexamine.** (doe-PEX-ah-MEEN) USAN.
Use: Cardiovascular agent.
•**dopexamine hydrochloride.** (doe-PEX-al-MLLN) UUAN.
Use: Cardiovascular agent.
Dopram. (Baxter Healthcare Corp.) Doxapram hydrochloride 20 mg/mL, 0.9% benzyl alcohol. Inj. Multiple-dose vial 20 mL. *Rx.*
Use: CNS stimulant, analeptic.
Doral. (Wallace) Quazepam 7.5 mg, 15 mg. Tab. Bot. 100s, 500s, UD 100s. *c-iv.*
Use: Sedative/hypnotic, nonbarbiturate.
•**doramapimod.** (dore-a-MAP-i-mod) USAN.
Use: Crohn disease; RA; psoriasis.
•**dorastine hydrochloride.** (DAI in ass teen HIGH-droe-KLOR-ide) USAN.
Use: Antihistamine.
•**doretinel.** (DOE-REH-tin-ell) USAN.
Use: Antikeratinizing agent.
Doriglute Tabs DEA. (Major) Glutethimide 0.5 g. Tab. Bot. 100s, 250s, 1000s. *c-ii.*
Use: Hypnotic.
•**doripenem.** (dore-i-PEN-em) USAN.
Use: Antibiotic.
Dormeer. (Taylor Pharmaceuticals) Scopolamine aminoxide HBr 0.2 mg. Cap. Bot. 100s, 1000s. *Rx.*
Use: Hypnotic; sedative.
dormethan.
See: Dextromethorphan HBr.
Dormin Capsules. (Randob) Diphenhydramine hydrochloride 25 mg, lactose. Bot. 32s, 72s. *OTC.*
Use: Sleep aid.
Dormin Sleeping Caplets. (Randob) Diphenhydramine hydrochloride 25 mg. Bot. 32s. *OTC.*
Use: Sleep aid.
dormiral.
See: Phenobarbital.

dormonal.
See: Barbital.
Dormutol. (Health for Life Brands) Scopolamine aminoxide HBr 0.2 mg. Cap. Bot. 24s, 60s. *Rx.*
Use: Hypnotic; sedative.
dornase alfa. (DOR-nace AL-fuh)
Use: Cystic fibrosis. [Orphan Drug]
See: Pulmozyme.
Doryx. (Warner Chilcott) Doxycycline hyclate 75 mg, 100 mg. Cap., pellets. Bot. 50s (100 mg only), 60s (75 mg only). *Rx.*
Use: Anti-infective; tetracycline.
•**dorzolamide hydrochloride.** (dore-ZOLE-lah-mide) *USP 28.*
Use: Carbonic anhydrase inhibitor.
See: TruSopt.
dorzolamide hydrochloride and timolol maleate.
Use: Antiglaucoma.
See: Cosopt.
D.O.S. (Goldline Consumer) Docusate sodium 100 mg, 250 mg, parabens. Softgel Cap. Bot. 100s, 500s (250 mg only), 1000s (100 mg only). *OTC.*
Use: Laxative.
Dosaflex. (Richwood Pharmaceuticals) Senna fruit extract, parabens, sucrose, alcohol 7%. Syr. Bot. 237 mL. *OTC.*
Use: Laxative.
Doss Syrup. (Rosemont) Docusate sodium 20 mg/5 mL. Bot. Pt, gal. *OTC.*
Use: Laxative; stool softener.
Dostinex. (Pharmacia) Cabergoline 0.5 mg. Tab. Bot. 8s. *Rx.*
Use: Antihyperprolactinemic.
•**dothiepin hydrochloride.** (DOE-THIGH-eh-pin) USAN.
Use: Antidepressant.
Dotirol. (Sanofi-Synthelabo) Ampicillin trihydrate available in Cap, Susp., Inj. (IV, IM). *Rx.*
Use: Anti-infective; penicillin.
Double-Action Toothache Kit. (C.S. Dent & Co.) **Liq.:** Benzocaine, alcohol 74%, chlorobutanol anhydrous 0.09%. Bot. 3.7 mL. **Maronox Pain Relief Tablets:** Acetaminophen 325 mg. Tab. Box. 8s. *OTC.*
Use: Analgesic, topical.
Double Antibiotic. (E. Fougera) Polymyxin B sulfate 10,000 units, bacitracin zinc 500 units/g. Oint. Tube 15 g, 30 g, UD 0.9 g (144s). *OTC.*
Use: Topical anti-infective, antibiotic.
Double Sal. (Pal-Pak, Inc.) Sodium salicylate 648 mg. EC Tab. Bot. 1000s. *OTC.*
Use: Analgesic.
Double Strength Gaviscon-2. (Glaxo-SmithKline) Aluminum hydroxide

160 mg, magnesium trisilicate 40 mg, alginic acid, calcium stearate, sodium bicarbonate, sucrose. Tab. Bot. 48s. *OTC.*
Use: Antacid.

Dovacet Capsules. (Pal-Pak, Inc.) Dover's powder 24.3 mg, aspirin 324 mg, caffeine 32.4 mg. Bot. 1000s.
Use: Analgesic.

Dover's Powder. Ipecac 1 part, opium 1 part, lactose 8 parts.
Use: Analgesic; diaphoretic; sedative.
W/Acetophenetidin, atropine sulfate, aspirin, camphor, caffeine, sodium sulfate, dried.
See: Dovium.
W/Acetophenetidin, camphor, aspirin, caffeine, atropine sulfate.
See: Analgestine.
W/Acetophenetidin, sodium citrate, potassium guaiacolsulfonate.
See: Doverlyn.
W/A.P.C. camphor monobromated.
See: Coldate.
W/Aspirin, phenacetin, camphor monobromated, caffeine.
See: Coldate.
W/Atropine sulfate, A.P.C., camphor.
See: Dasin.

Dovonex. (Bristol-Myers Squibb) Calcipotreine 0.005% alcohols, EDTA, mineral oil. Oint. Tube 30 g, 60 g, 100 g. Soln. Menthol. Bot. 50 mL. Cream. Tube 30 g, 60 g, 100 g. *Rx.*
Use: Dermatologic; antipsoriatic.

Dowicil 200.
Use: Antibacterial.
See: Derma Soap.

Dow-Isoniazid. (Hoechst) Isoniazid 300 mg. Tab. Bot. 30s. *Rx.*
Use: Antituberculousal.

Doxamin. (Forest) Thiamine hydrochloride 100 mg, vitamin B_6 100 mg/mL. Vial 10 mL. *Rx.*
Use: Vitamin supplement.

Doxapap-N. (Major) Propoxyphene napsylate 100 mg, acetaminophen 650 mg. Tab. Bot. 100s, 500s. *c-iv.*
Use: Analgesic combination, narcotic.

Doxaphene Capsules. (Major) Propoxyphene hydrochloride 65 mg. Cap. Bot. 1000s. *c-iv.*
Use: Analgesic; narcotic.

Doxaphene Compound 65 Caps. (Major) Propoxyphene hydrochloride, acetaminophen. Cap. Bot. 1000s. *c-iv.*
Use: Analgesic combination, narcotic.

•**doxapram hydrochloride.** (DOX-uh-pram) *USP 28.*
Use: Respiratory and CNS stimulant, analeptic.

See: Dopram.
doxapram hydrochloride. (Bedford) Doxapram hydrochloride 20 mg/mL. Benzyl alcohol 0.9%. Inj. Multiple-dose vial. 20 mL.
Use: Respiratory and CNS stimulant.

•**doxaprost.** (DOX-ah-proste) USAN.
Use: Bronchodilator.

Doxate. Docusate sodium. *OTC.*
Use: Laxative.

•**doxazosin mesylate.** (DOX-uh-ZOE-sin) USAN.
Use: Antihypertensive, antiadrenergic.
See: Cardura.

doxazosin mesylate. (Various Mfr.) Doxazosin 1 mg, 2 mg, 4 mg, 8 mg, may contain lactose. Tab. Bot. 100s, 500s, 1000s, UD 100s. *Rx.*
Use: Antihypertensive, antiadrenergic.

•**doxepin hydrochloride.** (DOX-uh-pin) *USP 28.*
Use: Psychotherapeutic agent; antidepressant.
See: Sinequan.

doxepin hydrochloride. (Various Mfr.) Doxepin hydrochloride. **Cap.:** 10 mg, 25 mg, 50 mg, 75 mg, 100 mg, 150 mg. Bot. 50s (150 mg only), 100s, 500s, 1000s (except 150 mg), UD 100s (except 150 mg). **Oral Conc.:** 10 mg/mL. Bot. 120 mL. *Rx.*
Use: Antidepressant.

•**doxercalciferol.** (dox-ehr-kal-SIFF-eh-role) USAN.
Use: Secondary hyperparathyroidism associated with end-stage renal disease.
See: Hectorol.

Doxidan. (Pharmacia) Bisacodyl 5 mg. DR Tab. 10s, 30s, 90s. *OTC.*
Use: Laxative.

Doxil. (Sequus) Doxorubicin (liposomal) 20 mg, sucrose. Inj. Single-use vial 10 mL. *Rx.*
Use: Antibiotic.

•**doxofylline.** (DOX-oh-fill-een) USAN.
Use: Bronchodilator.

•**doxorubicin.** (DOX-oh-ROO-bih-sin) USAN.
Tall Man: DOXOrubicin
Use: Antineoplastic.
See: Doxil.

•**doxorubicin hydrochloride.** (DOX-oh-ROO-bih-sin) *USP 28.*
Tall Man: DOXOrubicin
Use: Antineoplastic; antibiotic.
See: Adriamycin PFS.
Adriamycin RDF.

doxorubicin hydrochloride. (Bedford Labs) Doxorubicin hydrochloride. **Pow.**

for Inj., lyophilized: 10 mg: w/lactose 50 mg. **20 mg:** w/lactose 100 mg. **50 mg:** w/lactose 250 mg. Single-dose flip-top Vial. **Inj., aqueous:** 2 mg/mL, sodium chloride 0.9%, hydrochloric acid. Vial 5 mL, 10 mL, 25 mL, 100 mL. *Rx.*
Use: Antibiotic.

•**doxpicomine hydrochloride.** (DOX-PIH-koe-meen) USAN. Formerly doxpicodin hydrochloride.
Use: Analgesic.

Doxy. (APP) **100:** Doxycycline hyclate 100 mg, mannitol 300 mg. Pow. for Inj., lyophilzed. Vial. **200:** Doxycycline hyclate 200 mg, mannitol 600 mg. Pow. for Inj. Vial. *Rx.*
Use: Anti-infective; tetracycline.

•**doxycycline.** (LMJX-ee-SIGH-kleen) *USP 28.*
Use: Anti-infective, tetracycline; mouth and throat product.
See: Adoxa.
Atridox.
Dorxy.
Doxy.
Monodox.
Periostat.
Vibramycin.
Vibra-Tabs.

doxycycline. (Various Mfr.) Doxycycline hyclate. **Tab.:** 100 mg. Bot. 50s, 100s, 200s, 500s, UD 100s. **Cap.:** 50 mg, 100 mg. Bot. 50s, 500s, UD 100s (100 mg only). **Pow. for Inj., lyophilized:** 100 mg. Vials. *Rx.*
Use: Anti-infective, tetracycline.

doxycycline monohydrate. (Watson) Doxycycline (as monohydrate) 50 mg, 100 mg. Cap. 50s (100 mg only), 100s (50 mg only), 250s (100 mg only). *Rx.*
Use: Tetracycline.

•**doxylamine succinate.** (dox-IL-a-meen) *USP 28.*
Use: Antihistamine.
See: Decapryn.
Unisom.

W/Acetominophen, ephedrine sulfate, dextromethorphan HBr, alcohol.
See: Nyquil.

W/Dextromethorphan HBr, alcohol.
See: Consotuss Antitussive.

W/Dextromethorphan HBr, sodium citrate, alcohol.
See: Vicks Formula 44 Cough Mixture.

W/Combinations.
See: Alka-Seltzer Plus Night-Time Cold Medicine.
All-Nite.
Nite Time Cold Formula for Adults.

Top Care LiquiCaps Nite Time Multi-Symptom Cold/Flu Relief.
Tylenol Flu NightTime, Maximum Strength.
Vicks NyQuil Cough.
Vicks NyQuil Multi-Symptom Cold/Flu Relief.

•**doxylamine succinate, acetaminophen, and pseudoephedrine hydrochloride combinations.**
Use: Upper respiratory combination, antihistamine, analgesic, decongestant.
See: Acetaminophen, Doxylamine Succinate, and Pseudoephedrine hydrochloride Combinations.

Doxy-Lemmon. (Teva) **Cap.:** Doxycycline hyclate equivalent to 100 mg of doxycycline base. Cap. Bot. 50s, 500s, UD 100s. **Tab.:** Doxycycline hyclate equivalent to 100 mg doxycycline base. Tab. Bot. 50s, 500s, UD 100s. *Rx.*
Use: Anti-infective; tetracycline.

Doxy-Tabs. (Houba) Doxycycline hyclate 100 mg. FC Tab. Bot. 50s, 500s. *Rx.*
Use: Anti-infective; tetracycline.

Doxy-Tabs-50. (Houba) Doxycycline hyclate 50 mg. Tab. Bot. 50s. *Rx.*
Use: Anti-infective; tetracycline.

DPPC. Colfosceril palmitate. *Rx.*
Use: Lung surfactant.
See: Exosurf Neonatal.

•**draflazine.** (DRAFF-lah-ZEEN) USAN.
Use: Cardioprotectant.

Dramamine. (Pharmacia) Dimenhydrinate. **Liq.:** 12.5 mg/4 mL. Bot. 90 mL, pt. **Tab.:** 50 mg. Bot. 36s, 100s, 1000s, Blister pkg. 12s, UD 100s. *OTC.*
Use: Antiemetic; antivertigo.

Dramamine, Children's. (Pharmacia) Dimenhydrinate 12.5 mg/5 mL, alcohol 5%, sucrose. Liq. Bot. 120 mL. *OTC.*
Use: Antiemetic; antivertigo.

Dramamine Less Drowsy Formula. (Pharmacia & Upjohn) Meclizine hydrochloride 25 mg, lactose. Tab. Pkg. 8s. *OTC.*
Use: Antiemetic/antivertigo agent.

Dramamine II. (Pharmacia) Meclizine hydrochloride 25 mg, lactose. Tab. Pkg. 8s. *OTC.*
Use: Antiemetic; antivertigo.

Dramanate. (Taylor Pharmaceuticals) Dimenhydrinate 50 mg/mL. Inj. Vial 10 mL. *Rx.*
Use: Antiemetic; antivertigo.

dramarin.
See: Dramamine.

dramyl.
See: Dramamine.

Drawing Salve. (Whiteworth Towne) Tube oz. *OTC.*
Use: Dermatologic, wound therapy.
Drawing Salve with Triquinodin. (Towne) Tube 2 oz. *OTC.*
Use: Dermatologic, wound therapy.
Dr. Berry's Skin Toner. (Last) Hydroquinone 2%. Jar oz. *Rx.*
Use: Dermatologic.
Dr. Brown's Home Drug Testing System. (Personal Health and Hygiene) 1 urine specimen collection kit for detecting drugs of abuse (marijuana, cocaine, amphetamine, methamphetamine, phencyclidine, codeine, morphine, heroin). Kit 1s. *OTC.*
Use: Diagnostic aid.
DRC Peri-Anal Cream. (Xttrium) Lassar's paste 37.5%, anhydrous lanolin, 37.5%, cold cream 25%. Tube 5 oz. *OTC.*
Use: Dermatologic protectant, perianal.
Dr. Dermi-Heal. (Quality Formulations, Inc.) Zinc oxide 25%, allantoin 1%, peruvian balsam, castor oil, white petrolatum. Oint. Tube 75 g. *OTC.*
Use: Astringent.
Dr. Drake's Cough Medicine. (Last) Dextromethorphan HBr 10 mg/5 mL. Bot. 2 oz. *OTC.*
Use: Antitussive.
Dri-A Caps. (Barth's) Vitamin A 10,000 units. Cap. Bot. 100s, 500s. *OTC.*
Use: Vitamin supplement.
Dri A & D Caps. (Barth's) Vitamins A 10,000 units, D 400 units. Cap. Bot. 100s, 500s. *OTC.*
Use: Vitamin supplement.
•**dribendazole.** (dry-BEN-dah-ZOLE) USAN.
Use: Anthelmintic.
Dri-E. (Barth's) Vitamin E. Cap.
100 units: Bot. 100s, 500s, 1000s.
200 units: Bot. 100s, 250s, 500s.
400 units: Bot. 100s, 250s. *OTC.*
Use: Vitamin supplement.
Dri/Ear. (Pfeiffer) Boric acid 2.75% in isopropyl alcohol. Soln. Dropper Bot. 30 mL. *OTC.*
Use: Otic.
dried aluminum hydroxide gel.
Use: Antacid.
See: Aluminum Hydroxide Gel, dried.
dried yeast.
See: Yeast, dried.
DriHist SR. (Prasco) Phenylephrine hydrochloride 20 mg, chlorpheniramine maleate 8 mg, methscopolamine nitrate 2.5 mg. SR Tab. 100s. *Rx.*
Use: Upper respiratory combination, de-

congestant, antihistamine, anticholinergic.
Driminate Tabs. (Major) Dimenhydrinate 50 mg. Tab. Bot. 100s, 1000s. *OTC.*
Use: Antiemetic; antivertigo.
•**drinidene.** (DRIH-nih-deen) USAN.
Use: Analgesic.
Drisdol. (Sanofi-Synthelabo) Ergocalciferol (Vitamin D_2). **Cap.:** 50,000 units, tartrazine. Bot. 50s. **Drops:** 8000 units/ mL in propylene glycol. Liq. Bot. 60 mL. *Rx.*
Use: Refractory rickets; hypophosphatemia; hypoparathyroidism.
Dristan Allergy. (Whitehall-Robins) Pseudoephedrine hydrochloride 60 mg, brompheniramine maleate 4 mg. Cap. Bot. 20s. *OTC.*
Use: Antihistamine, decongestant.
Dristan Capsules. (Whitehall-Robins) Phenylephrine hydrochloride 5 mg, chlorpheniramine maleate 2 mg, acetaminophen 325 mg. Bot. 16s, 36s, 75s. *OTC.*
Use: Analgesic, antihistamine, decongestant.
Dristan Cold. (Whitehall-Robins) Pseudoephedrine hydrochloride 30 mg, acetaminophen 500 mg. Capl. Bot. 20s, 40s. *OTC.*
Use: Analgesic, decongestant.
Dristan Cold & Flu. (Whitehall-Robins) Acetaminophen 500 mg, pseudoephedrine hydrochloride 60 mg, chlorpheniramine maleate 4 mg, dextromethorphan HBr 20 mg. Pow. Pkts. 6s. *OTC.*
Use: Analgesic, antihistamine, antitussive, decongestant.
Dristan Cold Multi-Symptom Formula. (Whitehall-Robins) Phenylephrine hydrochloride 5 mg, chlorpheniramine maleate 2 mg, acetaminophen 325 mg. Tab. Bot. 20s, 40s, 75s. *OTC.*
Use: Upper respiratory combination, analgesic, antihistamine, decongestant.
Dristan Cold Non-Drowsy Maximum Strength. (Whitehall-Robins) Pseudoephedrine hydrochloride 30 mg, acetaminophen 500 mg. Tab. Pkg. 20s. *OTC.*
Use: Upper respiratory combination, decongestant, analgesic.
Dristan Fast Acting Formula. (Whitehall-Robins) Phenylephrine hydrochloride 0.5%, pheniramine maleate 0.2%, mannitol, sorbitol, benzalkonium chloride, benzyl alcohol. Soln. Spray Bot. 15 mL. *OTC.*
Use: Nasal decogestant, imidazoline.
Dristan Juice Mix-In. (Whitehall-Robins) Acetaminophen 500 mg, pseudoephedrine hydrochloride 60 mg, dextrometh-

orphan 20 mg. Pow. Pkts. 5s. *OTC.*
Use: Upper respiratory combination, analgesic, antitussive, decongestant.
Dristan Maximum Strength. (Whitehall-Robins) Pseudoephedrine hydrochloride 30 mg, acetaminophen 500 mg. Capl. Bot. 24s. *OTC.*
Use: Analgesic, decongestant.
Dristan Menthol Nasal Mist. (Whitehall-Robins) Phenylephrine hydrochloride 0.5%, pheniramine maleate 0.2%. Bot. 0.5 oz, 1 oz. *OTC.*
Use: Antihistamine, decongestant.
Dristan Nasal Mist. (Whitehall-Robins) Phenylephrine hydrochloride 0.5%, pheniramine maleate 0.2%. Bot. 15 mL, 30 mL. *OTC.*
Use: Antihistamine, decongestant.
Dristan No Drowsiness Cold. (Whitehall-Robins) Pseudoephedrine hydrochloride 30 mg, acetaminophen 500 mg. Cap. Bot. 20s. *OTC.*
Use: Analgesic, decongestant.
Dristan Saline Spray. (Whitehall-Robins) Sodium chloride. Soln. Bot. 15 mL.
Use: Nasal product.
Dristan Sinus. (Whitehall-Robins) Pseudoephedrine hydrochloride 30 mg, ibuprofen 200 mg, parabens, sucrose. Tab. Pkg. 20s. *OTC.*
Use: Upper respiratory combination, analgesic, decongestant.
Dristan 12 Hour. (Whitehall-Robins) Chlorpheniramine maleate 4 mg, phenylephrine hydrochloride 20 mg. Cap. Bot. 6s, 10s, 15s. *OTC.*
Use: Antihistamine, decongestant.
Dristan 12-Hr Nasal. (Whitehall-Robins) Oxymetazoline hydrochloride 0.05%, benzalkonium chloride, thimerosal, hydroxypropylmethylcellulose, sodium chloride. Spray Bot. 15 mL. *OTC.*
Use: Nasal decongestant, imidazoline.
Dritho Creme. (Dermik) Anthralin 0.1%, 0.25%, 0.5%. Tube 50 g. *Rx.*
Use: Antipsoriatic.
Dritho Creme HP 1.0%. (Dermik) Anthralin 1%. Tube 50 g. *Rx.*
Use: Antipsoriatic.
Dritho-Scalp. (Dermik) Anthralin 0.25%, 0.5%. Tube 50 g. *Rx.*
Use: Antipsoriatic.
Drixomed. (Iopharm) Dexbrompheniramine maleate 6 mg, pseudoephedrine sulfate 120 mg. SR Tab. Bot. 100s, 500s. *Rx.*
Use: Upper respiratory combination, antihistamine, decongestant.
Drixoral. (Schering-Plough) Dexbrompheniramine maleate 6 mg,

pseudoephedrine sulfate 120 mg. SA Tab. Box 10s, 20s, 40s. Bot. 48s, 100s. *OTC.*
Use: Antihistamine, decongestant.
Drixoral. (Schering-Plough) Pseudoephedrine sulfate 30 mg, brompheniramine maleate 2 mg, sorbitol, sugar. Syrup. Bot. 118 mL. *OTC.*
Use: Antihistamine, decongestant.
Drixoral Allergy Sinus. (Schering-Plough Healthcare) Pseudoephedrine sulfate 60 mg, dexbrompheniramine maleate 3 mg, acetaminophen 500 mg, parabens. ER Tab. Pkg. 12s. *OTC.*
Use: Upper respiratory combination, decongestant, antihistamine, analgesic.
Drixoral Cold & Allergy. (Schering-Plough) Dexbrompheniramine maleate 6 mg, pseudoephedrine sulfate 120 mg, sugar, lactose, butylparaben. Tab. Pkg. 10s. *OTC.*
Use: Upper respiratory combination, antihistamine, decongestant.
Drixoral Cough & Congestion Liquid Caps. (Schering-Plough) Pseudoephedrine hydrochloride 60 mg, dextromethorphan HBr 30 mg. Cap. Pkg. 10s. *OTC.*
Use: Antihistamine, decongestant.
Drixoral Non-Drowsy Formula. (Schering-Plough) Pseudoephedrine sulfate 120 mg, sugar. Tab. Pkg. 10s, 20s. *OTC.*
Use: Decongestant.
Drixoral Plus. (Schering-Plough) Pseudoephedrine sulfate 60 mg, dexbrompheniramine maleate 3 mg, acetaminophen 500 mg. TR Tab. Bot. 12s, 24s. *OTC.*
Use: Analgesic, antihistamine, decongestant.
Drixoral Sustained-Action. (Schering-Plough) Pseudoephedrine sulfate 120 mg, dexbrompheniramine maleate 6 mg, sugar, lactose. Tab. Pkg. 10s. Bot. 20s, 40s. *OTC.*
Use: Antihistamine; decongestant.
Drixoral 12 Hour Non-Drowsy Formula. (Schering-Plough) Pseudoephedrine sulfate 120 mg, sugar, lactose, butylparabens. ER Tab. Pkg. 10s. *OTC.*
Use: Nasal decongestant, arylalkylamine.
●**drobuline.** (DROE-byoo-leen) USAN.
Use: Cardiovascular agent (antiarrhythmic).
●**drocinonide.** (droe-SIN-oh-nide) USAN.
Use: Anti-inflammatory.
drocode.
See: Dihydrocodeine.

•**droloxifene.** (drole-OX-ih-feen) USAN.
Use: Antineoplastic.

•**droloxifene citrate.** (drole-OX-ih-feen) USAN.
Use: Antineoplastic.

•**drometrizole.** (DROE-meh-TRY-zole) USAN.
Use: Ultraviolet screen.

•**dromostanolone propionate.** (DRAHM-oh-STAN-oh-lone) *USP 28.*
Use: Antineoplastic.

•**dronabinol.** (droe-NAB-ih-nahl) *USP 28.*
Use: Antiemetic.
See: Marinol.

drop chalk. (Various Mfr.) Calcium carbonate, prepared. Prepared chalk.

•**droperidol.** (dro-PER-i-dahl) *USP 28.*
Use: Antipsychotic; anxiolytic; general anesthetic.
See: Inapsine.

droperidol. (Various Mfr.) Droperidol 2.5 mg/mL. Inj. Vial 2 mL. *Rx.*
Use: Anesthetic, general.

•**droprenilamine.** (droe-preh-NILL-ah-meen) USAN.
Use: Vasodilator (coronary).

•**drospirenone.** (droe-SPYE-reh-nohn) USAN.
Use: Sex hormone, contraceptive, hormone.
See: Yasmin.

Drotic Sterile Otic Solution. (B.F. Ascher) Hydrocortisone 10 mg (1%), polymyxin B sulfate 10,000 units, neomycin 5 mg/mL, preservatives. Dropper bot. 10 mL. *Rx.*
Use: Otic.

drotrecogin alfa (activated).
Use: Thrombolytic agent, recombinant human activated protein C.
See: Xigris.

•**droxacin sodium.** (DROX-ah-sin) USAN.
Use: Anti-infective.

Droxia. (Bristol-Myers Squibb Oncology/Virology) Hydroxyurea 200 mg, 300 mg, 400 mg, lactose. Cap. Bot. 60s. *Rx.*
Use: Antisickling agent.

•**droxifilcon a.** (DROX-ih-fill-kahn A) USAN.
Use: Contact lens material (hydrophilic).

•**droxinavir hydrochloride.** (drox-IN-ah-veer HIGH-droe-KLOR-ide) USAN.
Use: Antiviral.

Dr. Scholl's Advanced Pain Relief Corn Removers. (Schering-Plough) Salicylic acid 40% in a rubber-based vehicle. Disc. 6s. *OTC.*
Use: Keratolytic.

Dr. Scholl's Athlete's Foot. (Schering-Plough) **Pow.:** Tolnaftate 1%. Talc. Bot. 63 g. **Spray Liq.:** Tolnaftate 1%, alcohol 36%. Bot. 113 mL. *OTC.*
Use: Antifungal, topical.

Dr. Scholl's Athlete's Foot Cream. (Schering-Plough) Tolnaftate 1%. Tube 0.5 oz. *OTC.*
Use: Antifungal, topical.

Dr. Scholl's Callus Removers. (Schering-Plough) Salicylic acid 40% in a rubber-based vehicle. 6 pads, 4 discs. Extra thick in 4 discs. *OTC.*
Use: Keratolytic.

Dr. Scholl's Clear Away. (Schering-Plough) Salicylic acid 40% in a rubber-based vehicle. Disc 18s. *OTC.*
Use: Keratolytic.

Dr. Scholl's Clear Away One Step. (Schering-Plough) Salicylic acid 40% in a rubber-based vehicle. Strip 14s. *OTC.*
Use: Keratolytic.

Dr. Scholl's Clear Away Plantar. (Schering-Plough) Salicylic acid 40% in a rubber-based vehicle. Disc 24s. *OTC.*
Use: Keratolytic.

Dr. Scholl's Corn/Callus Remover. (Schering-Plough) Salicylic acid 12.6% in a flexible collodion, alcohol 18%, ether 55%, hydrogenated vegetable oil. Liq. 10 mL with 3 cushions. *OTC.*
Use: Keratolytic.

Dr. Scholl's Corn/Callus Salve. (Schering-Plough) Salicylic acid 15%. Tube 0.4 oz. *OTC.*
Use: Keratolytic.

Dr. Scholl's Corn Remover. (Schering-Plough) Salicylic acid 40% in a rubber-based vehicle. Discs: 6s as wrap-arounds, 9s as ultra thin, small, waterproof, regular, soft, and extra-thick. *OTC.*
Use: Keratolytic.

Dr. Scholl's Corn Salve. (Schering-Plough) Salicylic acid 15%. Jar 0.4 oz. *OTC.*
Use: Keratolytic.

Dr. Scholl's Cracked Heel Relief. (Schering-Plough) Lidocaine 2%, benzalkonium chloride 0.13%. Cream. Tube 5.6 g. *OTC.*
Use: Anesthetic, local.

Dr. Scholl's Ingrown Toenail Reliever. (Schering-Plough) Sodium sulfide 1%. Bot. 0.33 oz. *OTC.*
Use: Foot preparation.

Dr. Scholl's Maximum Strength Tritan. (Schering-Plough) Tolnaftate 1%. **Pow.:** Talc. Bot. 56 g. **Spray Pow.:** SD alcohol 40 14%. Bot. 85 g. *OTC.*
Use: Antifungal, topical.

Dr. Scholl's Moisturizing Corn Remover Kit. (Schering-Plough) Salicylic acid 40% in a rubber-based vehicle, moisturizing cream, pain relief cushions. Disc 6s. *OTC.*
Use: Keratolytic.

Dr. Scholl's One Step Corn Removers. (Schering-Plough) Salicylic acid 40% in a rubber-based vehicle. Strips 6s. *OTC.*
Use: Keratolytic.

Dr. Scholl's Pro Comfort Jock Itch Spray. (Schering-Plough) Tolnaftate 1%. Aerosol Can 3.5 oz. *OTC.*
Use: Antifungal, topical.

Dr. Scholl's Wart Remover Kit. (Schering-Plough) Salicylic acid 17% in a flexible collodion, alcohol 17%, ether 52%. Liq. 10 mL with brush and 6 adhesive pads. *OTC.*
Use: Keratolytic.

Dr. Scholl's Zino Pads with Medicated Disks. (Schering-Plough) Salicylic acid 20%, 40%. Protective pads designed for use with and without salicylic acid-impregnated disks. *OTC.*
Use: Keratolytic.

Dr. Smith's Adult Care. (Beta Dermaceuticals) Zinc oxide 10%, petrolatum, lanolin, mineral oil, olive oil. Oint. Tube. 85 g. *OTC.*
Use: Topical protectant.

Dr. Smith's Diaper. (Beta Dermaceuticals) Zinc oxide 10%, petrolatum, lanolin, mineral oil, olive oil. Oint. Tube. 05 g. *OTC.*
Use: Topical protectant.

Drucon C R. (Standard Drug Co.) Phenylephrine hydrochloride 25 mg, chlorpheniramine maleate 4 mg. Tab. Bot. 100s. *OTC.*
Use: Antihistamine, decongestant.

Drucon with Codeine. (Standard Drug Co.) Codeine phosphate 10 mg, phenylephrine hydrochloride 10 mg, chlorpheniramine maleate 2 mg, menthol 1 mg, alcohol 5%/5 mL. Bot. Pt. *c-v.*
Use: Antihistamine, antitussive, decongestant.

Dry Eyes. (Bausch & Lomb) White petrolatum, mineral oil, lanolin. Oint. Tube 3.5 g. *OTC.*
Use: Lubricant, ophthalmic.

Dry Eyes Solution. (Bausch & Lomb) Polyvinyl alcohol 1.4%, benzalkonium Cl 0.01%, sodium phosphate, EDTA, NaCl. Ophth. Soln. Bot. 15 mL. *OTC.*
Use: Lubricant, ophthalmic.

Dry Eye Therapy. (Bausch & Lomb) Glycerin 0.3%, potassium chloride, sodium chloride, sodium citrate, sodium phosphate, zinc chloride. Drop. Single-use Bot. 0.3 mL (UD 32s). *OTC.*
Use: Ophthalmic.

drying agents.
See: Aluminum Chloride (Hexahydrate). Formaldehyde.

Dryphen, Multi-Symptom Formula. (Major) Phenylephrine hydrochloride 5 mg, chlorpheniramine maleate 2 mg, actaminophen 325 mg. Tab. Bot. 40s. *OTC.*
Use: Upper respiratory combination, decongestant, antihistamine, analgesic.

Dry Skin Creme. (Gordon Laboratories) Cetyl alcohol, lubricating oils in a water-soluble base. Jar 2 oz, 1 lb, 5 lb. *OTC.*
Use: Emollient.

Drysol. (Person & Covey) Aluminum chloride hexahydrate 20% in 93% SD alcohol 40. Bot. 37.5 mL; 35 mL, 60 mL w/*Dab-O-Matic* applicator. *Rx.*
Use: Drying agent.

Drysum Shampoo. (Summers) Alcohol 15%, acetone 6%. Plastic bot. 4 oz. *OTC.*
Use: Dermatologic, hair.

Drytergent. (C & M Pharmacal) TEA-dodecylbenzenesulfonate, boric acid, lauramide DEA, propylene glycol, tartrazine, purified water, color, fragrance. Liq. Bot. 240 mL, 480 mL. *OTC.*
Use: Dermatologic, acne.

Drytex. (C & M Pharmacal) Salicylic acid 2%, benzalkonium chloride 0.1%, acetone 10%, isopropyl alcohol 40%, tartrazine. Lot. Bot. 240 mL. *OTC.*
Use: Dermatologic, acne.

Dryvax. (Wyeth-Ayerst) Vaccinia virus ≈ 100 million infectious vaccinia viruses/mL, polymyxin B sulfate, dihydrostreptomycin sulfate, chlortetracycline hydrochloride, neomycin sulfate. Pow. for Inj. Vials with 1 diluent syringe (glycerin 50%, phenol 25%), 1 vented needle, 100 bifurcated needles. *Rx.*
Use: Immunization.

DSS. (Dioctyl sodium sulfosuccinate) Docusate sodium. *OTC.*
Use: Laxative.
See: Colace.
Docusate Sodium.
DOK.
DOS.
D-S-S.
Modane Soft.
Pro-Sof.

D-S-S. (Magno-Humphries) Docusate sodium 100 mg. Cap. Bot. 100s. *OTC.*
Use: Laxative; stool softener.

DST. Dihydrostreptomycin.
See: Dihydrostreptomycin.
D-10-W. (Various Mfr.) Dextrose in water injection 10% (amps 3 mL); vials 250 mL, 500 mL, 1000 mL; 17 mL fill in 20 mL, 500 mL fill in 1000 mL, 1000 mL fill in 2000 mL vials. *Rx.*
Use: Carbohydrate supplement.
D-Test 100. (Burgin-Arden) Testosterone cypionate 100 mg/mL. Vial 10 mL. *c-III.*
Use: Androgen.
D-Test 200. (Burgin-Arden) Testosterone cypionate 200 mg/mL. Vial 10 mL. *c-III.*
Use: Androgen.
D-3. D vitamin.
See: Cholecalciferol.
DTIC. Dacarbazine. *Rx.*
Use: Antineoplastic.
See: DTIC-Dome.
DTIC-Dome. (Bayer) Dacarbazine 100 mg, 200 mg. May contain mannitol. Inj. Vials. *Rx.*
Use: Antineoplastic.
DTP. Diphtheria and tetanus toxoids and pertussis vaccine, adsorbed. *Rx.*
Use: Immunization.
See: Acel-Imune.
  Diphtheria and Tetanus Toxoids and Whole-Cell Pertussis Vaccine
  DTwP.
  Infanarix.
  Tri-Immunol.
  Tripedia.
D-2. D vitamin.
See: Ergocalciferol.
Duac. (Steifel) Benzoyl peroxide 5%, clindamycin 1%, EDTA, glycerin, methylparaben. Gel 45 g. *Rx.*
Use: Anti-infective, topical.
Dual-Wet. (Alcon) Polyvinyl alcohol, duasorb water-soluble polymetric system, benzalkonium chloride 0.01%, disodium edetate 0.05%. Bot. 2 oz. *OTC.*
Use: Contact lens care.
●**duazomycin.** (doo-AZE-oh-MY-sin) USAN. Antibiotic isolated from broth filtrates of *Streptomyces ambofaciens.*
Use: Antineoplastic.
Duazomycin A. Name used for Duazomycin.
Use: Antineoplastic.
Duazomycin B. Name used for Azotomycin.
Use: Antineoplastic.
Duazomycin C. Name used for Ambomycin.
Use: Antineoplastic.
Duet. (Integrity) Vitamin A 3000 units, D 400 units, C 120 mg, folic acid 1 mg, B_1 1.8 mg, B_2 4 mg, niacinamide 20 mg, B_6 25 mg, B_{12} 12 mcg, calcium

200 mg, copper 2 mg, iron 29 mg, zinc 25 mg, magnesium 25 mg, sucrose. Tab. 100s. *Rx.*
Use: Vitamin, mineral supplement.
Dulcagen Suppositories. (Ivax) Bisacodyl 10 mg. Box 12s, 100s. *OTC.*
Use: Laxative.
Dulcolax. (Boehringer Ingelheim) **EC Tab.:** Bisacodyl 5 mg, lactose, sucrose, parabens. Bot. 10s, 25s, 50s, 100s. **Liq.:** Magnesia (magnesium hydroxide) 400 mg per 5 mL. Original flavor. Sugar free. 355 mL. **Supp.:** Bisacodyl 10 mg. Pkg. 4s, 8s, 16s, 50s. *OTC.*
Use: Laxative; antacid.
Dulcolax Stool Softener. (Boehringer Ingelheim Consumer) Docusate sodium 100 mg. Glycerin, sorbitol. Soft Gel Cap. 25s. *OTC.*
Use: Laxative.
Dull-C. (Freeda) Ascorbic acid 1060 mg/ ¼ tsp. Pow. Bot. 120 g, 1 lb. *OTC.*
Use: Vitamin supplement.
●**duloxetine.** (doo-LOX-eh-teen) USAN.
Use: Antidepressant.
●**duloxetine hydrochloride.** (doo-LOX-eh-teen)
Use: Antidepressant.
See: Cymbalta.
Dulphalac. (Solvay) Lactulose 10 g/ 5 mL. Syr. Bot. 240 mL, 480 mL, 960 mL, UD 30 mL. *Rx.*
Use: Laxative.
Duo. (GlaxoSmithKline) Tube 0.5 oz.
Use: Adhesive.
Duocaine. (Amphastar) Lidocaine hydrochloride 10 mg/mL, bupivacaine hydrochloride 3.75 mg/mL. Preservative free. Inj. 10 mL single-dose vials. Cartons of 25. *Rx.*
Use: Anesthetic, injectable local.
Duocet. (Mason) Hydrocodone bitartrate 5 mg, acetaminophen 500 mg. Tab. Bot. 100s. *c-III.*
Use: Analgesic combination; narcotic.
DuoDERM. (ConvaTec) **Sterile dressing:** 10 cm × 10 cm. Pack 5s. 20 cm × 20 cm. Pack 3s. **Sterile gran.:** Packet 4 g. Pack 5s. *OTC.*
Use: Dermatologic, wound therapy.
DuoDERM Extra Thin. (ConvaTec) Flexible hydroactive sterile dressings. 4" × 4", 6" × 6". Pck. 10s. *OTC.*
Use: Dressing, topical.
Duofilm. (Stiefel) Salicylic acid 16.7%, lactic acid 16.7% in flexible collodion. Bot. 15 mL w/applicator. *OTC.*
Use: Keratolytic.
Duo-Flow. (Ciba Vision) Poloxamer 188, benzalkonium Cl 0.013%, EDTA 0.25%. Soln. Bot. 120 mL. *OTC.*

Use: Contact lens care.
Duo-K. (Various Mfr.) Potassium 20 mEq, chloride 3.4 mEq/15 mL (from potassium gluconate and potassium chloride). Bot. Pt, gal. *Rx.*
Use: Mineral supplement.
Duolube. (Bausch & Lomb) White petrolatum, mineral oil. Sterile, preservative and lanolin free. Oint. Tube 3.5 g. *OTC.*
Use: Lubricant, ophthalmic.
duomycin.
See: Aureomycin.
Duonate-12. (URL) Phenylephrine tannate 5 mg, pyrilamine tannate 30 mg/5 mL. Susp. Unit of use 118 mL w/oral syr. *Rx.*
Use: Upper respiratory combination, decongestant, antihistamine.
DuoNeb. (Dey) Ipratropium bromide 0.5 mg, albuterol sulfate 3 mg (equivalent to albuterol base 2.5 mg). Inhalation soln. Unit-dose vial 3 mL. Box 30s, 60s. *Rx.*
Use: Bronchodialator, anticholinergic.
• **duoperone fumarate.** (DOO-oh-per-OHN) USAN.
Use: Neuroleptic.
DuoPlant. (Stiefel) Salicylic acid 27%, alcohol 50%, flexible collodion, hydroxypropyl cellulose, lactic acid. Liq. Bot. 14 g. *OTC.*
Use: Ketatolytic (wart removal).
Duosol. (Kirkman) Docusate sodium 100 mg, 250 mg. Cap. Bot. 100s, 1000s. *OTC.*
Use: Laxative.
Duotal. (Health for Life Brands) **1.5 g.:** Secobarbital sodium ¾ g, amobarbital g. Cap. **3 g.:** Secobarbital sodium 1.5 g, amobarbital 1.5 g. Cap. Bot. 100s, 500s, 1000s. *c-ii.*
Use: Hypnotic; sedative.
duotal.
See: Guaiacol Carbonate.
Duotrate 45. (Jones Pharma) Pentaerythritol tetranitrate 45 mg. SR Cap. Bot. 100s. *Rx.*
Use: Antianginal.
Duotrate 30. (Jones Pharma) Pentaerythritol tetranitrate 30 mg. SR Cap. Bot. 100s. *Rx.*
Use: Antianginal.
Duovin-S. (Spanner) Estrone 2.5 mg, progesterone 25 mg/mL. Vial 10 mL. *Rx.*
Use: Estrogen, progestin combination.
Duo-WR, No. 1 & No. 2. (Whorton Pharmaceuticals, Inc.) **No. 1:** Salicylic acid, compound tincture benzoin. **No. 2:** Compound tincture benzoin, formaldehyde. Bot. 0.25 oz. *OTC.*

Use: Keratolytic.
Duphalac. (Solvay) Lactulose 10 g/15 mL < 1.6 g galactose, 1.2 g lactose, 1.2 g or less of other sugars). Soln. Bot. 240 mL, 480 mL, 960 mL, UD 30 mL. *Rx.*
Use: Laxative.
Duplast. (Beiersdorf) Adhesive coated elastic cloth. 8" × 4" Strip. Box 10s. 10" × 5" Strip. Box 8s, 10s.
Duplex Shampoo. (C & M Pharmacal) Sodium lauryl sulfate 15%, lauramide DEA, purified water. Bot. Pt, gal. *OTC.*
Use: Dermatologic.
duponol.
See: Gardinol type detergents (Sodium Lauryl Sulfate).
DURAcare. (Blairex) Buffered hypertonic salt solution, non-ionic detergents with thimerosal 0.001%, EDTA 0.1%. Soln. Bot. 30 mL. *OTC.*
Use: Contact lens care.
DURAcare II. (Blairex) Buffered hypertonic, ethylene and propylene oxide, octylphenoxypolyethoxyethanol, lauryl sulfate salt of imidazoline, sodium bisulfite 0.1%, sorbic acid 0.1%, EDTA 0.25%. Soln. Bot. 30 mL. *OTC.*
Use: Contact lens care.
Duraclon. (aaiPharma) Clonidine hydrochloride 100 mcg, 500 mcg/mL, preservative free. Inj. Vials. 10 mL. *Rx.*
Use: Analgesic.
Duradrin. (Barr) Isometheptene mucate 65 mg, dichoralphenazone 100 mg, acetaminophen 325 mg. Cap. Bot. 100s, 250s, 1000s. *c-iv.*
Use: Agent for migraine.
Duradryl. (Breckenridge Pharm.) Phenylephrine hydrochloride 10 mg, chlorpheniramine maleate 2 mg, methscopolamine nitrate 1.25 mg/5mL, corn syrup. Syr. Bot. 473 mL. *Rx.*
Use: Upper respiratory combination, decongestant, antihistamine, anticholinergic.
Dura-Estrin. (Roberts) Estradiol cypionate in oil 5 mg/mL. Inj. Vial 10 mL. *Rx.*
Use: Estrogen.
Duraflu. (ProEthic) Dextomethorphan HBr 20 mg, guaifenesin 200 mg, pseudoephedrine hydrochloride 60 mg, acetaminophen 500 mg. Dye free. Tab. 100s. *Rx.*
Use: Upper respiratory combination, antitussive, expectorant, decongestant, analgesic.
Duragen. (Roberts) Estradiol valerate in oil 20 mg, 40 mg/mL. Inj. Vial 10 mL. *Rx.*

Use: Estrogen.
Duragesic-50. (Janssen) Fentanyl 5 mg (50 mcg/h). Transdermal System. Alcohol < 0.2 mL released during use. Cartons containing 5 individually packaged systems. *c-II.*
Use: Opioid analgesic.
Duragesic-100. (Janssen) Fentanyl 10 mg (100 mcg/h). Transdermal System. Alcohol < 0.2 mL released during use. Cartons containing 5 indivually packaged systems. *c-II.*
Use: Opioid analgesic.
Duragesic-75. (Janssen) Fentanyl 7.5 mg (75 mcg/h). Transdermal System. Alcohol < 0.2 mL released during use. Cartons containing 5 individually packaged systems. *c-II.*
Use: Opioid analgesic.
Duragesic-12. (Janssen) Fentanyl 1.25 mg (12.5 mcg/h). Transdermal System. Alcohol < 0.2 mL released during use. Cartons containing 5 individually packaged systems. *c-II.*
Use: Opioid analgesic.
Duragesic-25. (Janssen) Fentanyl 2.5 mg (25 mcg/h). Transdermal System. Alcohol < 0.2 mL released during use. Cartons containing 5 individually packaged systems. *c-II.*
Use: Opioid analgesic.
Durahist. (ProEthic) Pseudoephedrine hydrochloride 60 mg, chlorpheniramine maleate 8 mg, methscopolamine nitrate 1.25 mg, talc. SR Tab. 100s. *Rx.*
Use: Upper respiratory combination, decongestant, antihistamine, anticholinergic.
Duralex. (American Urologicals, Inc.) Pseudoephedrine hydrochloride 120 mg, chlorpheniramine maleate 8 mg. SR Cap. Bot. 100s, 1000s. *Rx.*
Use: Antihistamine, decongestant.
Dura-Meth. (Foy Laboratories) Methylprednisolone 40 mg/mL. Vial 5 mL, 10 mL. *Rx.*
Use: Corticosteroid.
Duramist Plus 12–Hr Decongestant. (Pfeiffer) Oxymetazoline hydrochloride 0.05%, benzalkonium chloride, EDTA, sodium chloride. Spray. Bot. 15 mL. *OTC.*
Use: Nasal decongestant, imidazoline.
Duramorph. (Baxter) Morphine sulfate 0.5 mg/mL, 1 mg/mL. Inj. Single-use amp. 10 mL. *c-II.*
Use: Opioid analgesic.
Durapam. (Major) Flurazepam hydrochloride 15 mg, 30 mg. Cap. Bot. 100s, 500s. *c-IV.*
Use: Hypnotic; sedative.

•**durapatite.** (der-APP-ah-tite) USAN.
Use: Prosthetic aid.
Duraphen II. (ProEthic) Phenylephrine hydrochloride 25 mg, guaifenesin 800 mg. ER Tab. 100s. *Rx.*
Use: Decongestant and expectorant.
Duraquin. (Parke-Davis) Quinidine gluconate 330 mg. SR Tab. Bot. 100s, UD 100s. *Rx.*
Use: Cardiovascular agent.
Durasal II. (Prasco) Pseudoephedrine hydrochloride 60 mg, guaifenesin 600 mg. SR Tab. 100s. *Rx.*
Use: Upper respiratory combination, decongestant, expectorant.
DuraScreen. (Schwarz Pharma) SPF 30. Octyl methoxycinnamate, octyl salicylate, oxybenzone, 2-phenylbenzimidazole-sulfonic acid, titanium dioxide, cetearyl alcohol, diazolidinyl urea, parabens, shea butter. Lot. Bot. 105 mL. *OTC.*
Use: Sunscreen.
DuraScreen SPF 15. (Schwarz Pharma) SPF 15. Ethylhexyl p-methoxycinnamate, 2-ethylhexyl salicylate, oxybenzone, parabens, titanium dioxide. Lot. Bot. 105 mL. *OTC.*
Use: Sunscreen.
Dura-Tap/PD. (Dura) Pseudoephedrine hydrochloride 60 mg, chlorpheniramine maleate 4 mg. Cap. Bot. 100s. *Rx.*
Use: Antihistamine, decongestant.
Duratears Naturale. (Alcon) White petroleum, anhydrous liquid lanolin, mineral oil. Oint. Tube 3.5 g. *OTC.*
Use: Lubricant, ophthalmic.
Durathate-200 Injection. (Roberts) Testosterone enanthate in oil 200 mg/mL. Vial 10 mL. *c-III.*
Use: Androgen.
Duration. (Schering-Plough Healthcare) Oxymetazoline hydrochloride 0.05%, benzalkonium chloride, EDTA. Soln. Spray Bot. 30 mL. *OTC.*
Use: Nasal decongestant, imidazoline.
Duration Mentholated Vapor Spray. (Schering-Plough) Oxymetazoline hydrochloride 0.05%, aromatics. Squeeze bot. 15 mL. *OTC.*
Use: Decongestant.
Duration Mild Nasal Spray. (Schering-Plough) Phenylephrine hydrochloride 0.5%. Bot. 15 mL. *OTC.*
Use: Decongestant.
Duratuss. (Victory Pharma) Phenylephrine hydrochloride 25 mg, guaifenesin 900 mg. Tab. 100s. *Rx.*
Use: Decongestant and expectorant.
Duratuss DM. (Victory Pharma) Dextromethorphan hydrobromide 25 mg,

guaifenesin 225 mg/5 mL. Saccharin, sorbitol. Grape flavor. Elix. 473 mL. *Rx.*
Use: Antitussive with expectorant.

Duratuss GP. (Victory Pharma) Phenylephrine hydrochloride 25 mg, guaifenesin 1,200 mg. ER Tab. 100s. *Rx.*
Use: Decongestant and expectorant.

Duratuss HD. (Victory Pharma) Hydrocodone bitartrate 2.5 mg, guaifenesin 225 mg, phenylephrine hydrochloride 10 mg/5 mL. Saccharin, sorbitol. Wild cherry flavor. Elix. 473 mL. *c-III.*
Use: Antitussive and expectorant.

Duraxin. (Portal) Phenyltoloxamine citrate 25 mg, acetaminophen 325 mg, salicylamide 200 mg. Cap. 30s. *Rx.*
Use: Antitussive combination.

Durazyme. (Blairex) Nonionic detergent preserved w/thimerosal 0.004%, EDTA 0.1% in sterile buffered hypertonic soln. Bot. 30 mL. *OTC.*
Use: Contact lens care.

Duricef. (Mead Johnson) Cefadroxil.
Tab.: 1 g. Bot. 50s, 100s, UD 100s.
Cap.: 500 mg. Bot. 50s, 100s, UD 100s.
Susp.: 125 mg/5 mL, 250 mg/5 mL, 500 mg/5 mL Bot. 50 mL, 75 mL (500 mg/5 mL), 100 mL. *Rx.*
Use: Anti-infective; cephalosporin.

Dusotal. (Harvey) Sodium amobarbital ¾ g, sodium secobarbital g. Cap. Bot. 1000s. (3 g) Bot. 1000s. *c-II.*
Use: Hypnotic; sedative.

•**dusting powder, absorbable.** *USP 28.*
Use: Lubricant.

dusting powder, surgical.
See: B-F-I.

•**dutasteride.** (doo-TASS-teer-ide) USAN.
Use: Benign prostatic hyperplasia, sex hormone, androgen hormone inhibitor.
See: Avodart.

dutch oil. Oil of turpentine, sulfurated.

D V Cream. (Hoechst) Dienestrol 0.01% w/lactose, propylene glycol, stearic acid, diglycol stearate, TEA, benzoic acid, butylated hydroxytoluene, disodium edetate, buffered w/lactic acid to an acid pH. Tube 3 oz, w/applicator. *Rx.*
Use: Estrogen.

Dwelle. (Dakryon Pharmaceuticals) EDTA 0.09%, sodium chloride, potassium chloride, boric acid, povidone, NPX 0.001%. Drop. Bot. 15 mL. *OTC.*
Use: Artificial tears.

DX 114 Foot Powder. (Amlab) Zinc undecylenate 1%, salicylic acid 1%, benzoic acid 1%, ammonium alum 5%, boric acid 10.5% w/zinc stearate, chlorophyll, talc, kaolin, starch, calcium silicate, oil of wormwood. Cont. 2 oz. *OTC.*
Use: Antifungal, topical.

Dyantoin Caps. (Major) Phenytoin sodium 100 mg. Cap. Bot. 100s, 1000s. *Rx.*
Use: Anticonvulsant.

Dyazide. (GlaxoSmithKline) Triamterene 37.5 mg, hydrochlorothiazide 25 mg. Cap. Bot. 1000s, UD 100s, Patient Pack 100s. *Rx.*
Use: Antihypertensive; diuretic.

Dycill. (GlaxoSmithKline) Dicloxacillin sodium 250 mg, 500 mg. Cap. Bot. 100s. *Rx.*
Use: Anti-infective; penicillin.

•**dyclonine hydrochloride.** (DIE-kloe-neen) *USP 28.*
Use: Anesthetic, topical.
W/Benzethonium chloride.
See: Skin Shield.

Dycomene. (Hance) Hydrocodone bitartrate ⅙ g, pyrilamine maleate 1 g/fl. oz. Bot. 3 oz, gal. *c-III.*
Use: Antitussive; sleep aid.

•**dydrogesterone.** (DIE-droe-JESS-ter-ohn) *USP 28.*
Use: Hormone, progestin.

dyes.
See: Antiseptic, Dyes.

Dyflex-G Tablets. (Econo Med Pharmaceuticals) Dyphylline 200 mg, guaifenesin 200 mg. Bot. 100s, 1000s. *Rx.*
Use: Bronchodilator; expectorant.

Dyflex-200 Tablets. (Econo Med Pharmaceuticals) Dyphylline 200 mg. Bot. 100s, 1000s. *Rx.*
Use: Bronchodilator.

Dy-G Liquid. (Cypress) Dyphylline 100 mg, guaifenesin 100 mg/5 mL. Bot. Pt. *Rx.*
Use: Bronchodilator; expectorant.

dylate. Clonitrate.
Use: Coronary vasodilator.

Dylix. (Lunsco) Dyphylline 100 mg per 15 mL. Alcohol 20%. Elix. 473 mL. *Rx.*
Use: Bronchodilator.

•**dymanthine hydrochloride.** (DIE-man-theen) USAN.
Use: Anthelmintic.

Dymelor. (Eli Lilly) Acetohexamide 250 mg, 500 mg. Tab. Bot. 50s (500 mg only), 200s. *Rx.*
Use: Antidiabetic.

Dymenate. (Keene Pharmaceuticals) Dimenhydrinate 50 mg/mL. Vial 10 mL. *Rx.*
Use: Antiemetic; antivertigo.

Dynabac. (Muro) Dirithromycin 250 mg. Enteric coated. DR Tab. Bot. 60s. *D5-*

Pak of 10. *Rx.*
Use: Anti-infective, macrolide.
Dynacin. (Medicis) Minocycline hydrochloride **Cap.:** 50 mg, 75 mg, 100 mg. Bot. 50s (100 mg only), 100s (except 100 mg), 500s, 1000s. **Tab.:** 50 mg, 75 mg, 100 mg. Lactose. 50s (100 mg only), 100s (except 100 mg), 1000s. *Rx.*
Use: Anti-Infective; tetracycline.
DynaCirc. (Reliant) Isradipine. 2.5 mg, 5 mg, lactose. May contain benzyl alcohol and parabens. Cap. Bot. 60s, 100s. *Rx.*
Use: Calcium channel blocker.
DynaCirc CR. (Reliant) Isradipine 5 mg, 10 mg. CR Tab. Bot. 30s, 100s. *Rx.*
Use: Calcium channel blocker.
Dynafed Asthma Relief. (BDI) Ephedrine hydrochloride 25 mg, guaifenesin 200 mg. Tab. Bot. 60s. *OTC.*
Use: Upper respiratory combination, decongestant, expectorant.
Dynafed Ex, Extra Strength. (BDI)
See: Extra Strength Dynafed.
Dynafed Jr., Children's. (BDI)
See: Children's Dynafed Jr.
Dynafed Plus, Maximum Strength. (BDI)
See: Maximum Strength Dynafed Plus.
Dyna-Hex Skin Cleanser. (Western Medical) Chlorhexidine gluconate 4%, isopropyl alcohol 4%. Liq. Bot. 120 mL, 240 mL, 480 mL, gal. *OTC.*
Use: Antimicrobial; antiseptic.
Dyna-Hex 2 Skin Cleanser. (Western Medical) Chlorhexidine gluconate 2%, isopropyl alcohol 4%. Liq. Bot. 120 mL, 240 mL, 480 mL, gal. *OTC.*
Use: Antimicrobial; antiseptic.
dynamine. (Mayo Foundation)
Use: Antispasmodic, Lambert-Eaton myasthenic syndrome, hereditary motor and sensory neuropathy type I (Charcot-Marie-Tooth Disease). [Orphan Drug]
Dynapen. (Apothecon) Dicloxacillin sodium. **Cap.:** 125 mg, 250 mg, 500 mg. Bot. 24s (except 500 mg), 50s (500 mg only), 100s (except 500 mg). **Pow. for Oral Susp.:** 62.5 mg/5 mL. Bot. 100 mL, 200 mL. *Rx.*
Use: Anti-infective; penicillin.
Dynaplex. (Alton) Vitamin B complex. Bot. 100s, 1000s. *OTC.*
Use: Vitamin supplement.
dynarsan.
See: Acetarsone
Dynex. (Athlon) Pseudoephedrine hydrochloride 90 mg, guaifenesin 1200 mg, dye free. SR Tab. Bot. 30s, 100s. *Rx.*

Use: Upper respiratory combination, decongestant, expectorant.
Dy-O-Derm. (Galderma) Purified water, isopropyl alcohol, acetone, dihydroxyacetone, FD&C yellow No. 6, FD&C blue No. 1, FD&C red No. 33. Bot. 4 oz.
Use: Dermatologic, vitiligo stain.
Dy-Phyl-Lin. (Foy Laboratories) Dyphylline 250 mg/mL with benzyl alcohol. Inj. Vial 10 mL. *Rx.*
Use: Bronchodilator.
•**dyphylline.** (DIE-fih-lin) *USP 28.*
Use: Vasodilator; bronchodilator.
See: Brophylline.
    Dilor.
    Dylix.
    Emfabid TD.
    Lardet.
    Neothylline.
    Prophyllin.
W/Chlorpheniramine maleate, guaifenesin, dextromethorphan HBr, phenylephrine hydrochloride.
See: Dilor G.
    Neothylline GG.
W/Guaifenesin.
See: Dy-G.
    Dyphylline and Guaifenesin.
    Panfil G.
•**dyphylline and guaifenesin.** (DIE-fih-lin and GWIE-fen-ah-sin) *USP 28.*
Use: Bronchodilator; expectorant.
dyphylline and guaifenesin. (Econolab) Dyphylline 200 mg, guaifenesin 200 mg. Tab. Bot. 100s. *Rx.*
Use: Bronchodilator; expectorant.
Dyphylline GG Elixir. (Various Mfr.) Dyphylline 100 mg, guaifenesin 100 mg/15 mL. Bot. 473 mL. *Rx.*
Use: Bronchodilator.
Dyprotex. (Blairex) Micronized zinc oxide 40%, petrolatum 37.6%, dimethicone 2.5%, cod liver oil, aloe extract, zinc stearate. Pad. Pkg. 3s (9 applications). *OTC.*
Use: Astringent.
Dyrenium. (GlaxoSmithKline) Triamterene. 50 mg, 100 mg. Cap. Bot. 100s, 1000s (100 mg only), UD 100s. *Rx.*
Use: Diuretic.
Dyretic. (Keene Pharmaceuticals) Furosemide 10 mg/mL. Vial 10 mL. *Rx.*
Use: Diuretic.
Dyrexan-OD. (Trimen Laboratories, Inc.) Phendimetrazine tartrate 105 mg. SR Cap. Bot. 100s. *c-III.*
Use: Anorexiant.
Dyspel. (Dover Pharmaceuticals) Acetaminophen, ephedrine sulfate, atropine sulfate. Sugar, lactose, salt free. Tab. UD Box 500s. *Rx.*

Use: Analgesic.

Dytan. (Hawthorn) Diphenhydramine tannate. **Chew. Tab.:** 25 mg. Phenylalanine. Strawberry flavor. 60s. **Susp.:** 25 mg per 5 mL. Phenylalanine. Strawberry flavor. 118 mL. *Rx.*
Use: Antihistamine.

Dytan-CS. (Hawthorn) Carbetapentane tannate 30 mg, diphenhydramine tannate 25 mg, phenylephrine tannate 10 mg. Tab. 60s. *Rx.*
Use: Antitussive.

Dytan-D. (Hawthorn) Phenylephrine tannate 10 mg, diphenhydramine tannate 25 mg, aspartame, sorbitol, phenylalanine 1.5 mg, berry flavor. Chew. Tab. 60s. *Rx.*
Use: Upper respiratory combination, decongestant, antihistamine.

E

EACA. (Wyeth) Epsilon aminocaproic acid. *Rx.*
Use: Antifibrinolytic.
See: Amicar.

Ear Drops. (Weeks & Leo) Carbamide peroxide 6.5% in an anhydrous glycerin base. Bot. oz. *OTC.*
Use: Otic.

Ear-Dry. (Scherer) Isopropyl alcohol, boric acid 2.75%. Dropper bot. 30 mL. *OTC.*
Use: Otic.

Earex Ear Drops. (Health for Life Brands) Benzocaine 0.15 g, antipyrine 0.7 g/0.5 oz. Bot. 0.5 oz. *Rx.*
Use: Otic.

Ear-Eze. (Hyrex) Hydrooorticono 1%, chloroxylenol 0.1%, pramoxine hydrochloride 1%. Dropper bot. 15 mL. *Rx.*
Use: Anesthetic, local; anti-infective; corticosteroid.

Earocol Ear Drops. (Roberts) Benzocaine 1.4%, antipyrine 5.4%, glycerin, oxyquinoline sulfate. Soln. Dropper bot. 15 mL. *Rx.*
Use: Otic.

earthnut oil. Peanut oil.

Ease. (NeuroGenesis/Matrix Tech.) D, L-phenylalanine 500 mg, L-glutamine 15 mg, L-tyrosine 25 mg, L-carnitine 10 mg, L-arginine pyroglutamate 10 mg, L-ornithine/L-aspartate 10 mg, OI 0.033 mg, Se 0.012 mg, B₁ 0.33 mg, B₂ 5 mg, B₃ 3.3 mg, B₅ 0.33 mg, B₆ 0.33 mg, B₁₂ 1 mcg, E 5 units, biotin 0.05 mg, FA 0.066 mg, Fe 1 mg, Zn 2.5 mg, Ca 35 mg, I 0.25 mg, Cu 0.33 mg, Mg 25 mg. Cap. Bot. 42s. *OTC.*
Use: Nutritional supplement.

Easprin. (Parke-Davis) Aspirin 15 g. EC Tab. Bot. 100s. *Rx.*
Use: Analgesic.

East-A. (Eastwood) Therapeutic lotion. Bot. 16 oz. *OTC.*
Use: Emollient.

Easy-Lax. (Walgreen) Docusate sodium 100 mg. Cap. Bot. 60s. *OTC.*
Use: Laxative; stool softener.

Easy-Lax Plus. (Walgreen) Docusate sodium 100 mg, casanthranol 30 mg. Cap. Bot. 60s. *OTC.*
Use: Laxative; stool softener.

Eazol. (Roberts) Fructose, dextrose, orthophosphoric acid with controlled hydrogen ion concentration. Bot. 473 mL. *OTC.*
Use: Antinauseant.

●**ebanicline tosylate.** (EE-ba-ni-kleen) USAN.
Use: Analgesic.

E-Base. (Barr) Erythromycin. **Cap.:** 333 mg. Bot. 100s, 500s, 1000s. **Tab.:** 333 mg, 500 mg. Bot. 100s, 500s. *Rx.*
Use: Anti-infective; erythromycin.

●**ebastine.** (EBB-ass-teen) USAN.
Use: Antihistamine.

EBV-VCA. (Wampole) Epstein-Barr virus, viral capsid antigen antibody test. Qualitative and semi-quantitative detection of EBV antibody in human serum. Test 100s.
Use: Diagnostic aid.

EBV-VCA Ig. (Wampole) Epstein-Barr virus, viral capsid antigen Ig antibody. Qualitative and semiqualitative detection of EBV VCA Ig antibody in human serum. Test 50s.
Use: Diagnostic aid.

●**ecadotril.** (ee-CAD-oh-trill) USAN.
Use: Antihypertensive.

●**ecalcidene.** (ee-KAL-si-deen) USAN.
Use: Psoriasis.

●**ecamsule.** (eh-KAM-sool) USAN.
Use: Sunscreen.

Ecee Plus. (Edwards) Vitamin E 165 mg, ascorbic acid 100 mg, magnesium sulfate 70 mg, zinc sulfate 80 mg. Tab. Bot. 100s. *OTC.*
Use: Mineral, vitamin supplement.

●**echinacea angustifolia.** *NF 23.*
Use: Dietary supplement.

●**echinacea pallida.** *NF 23.*
Use: Dietary supplement.

●**echinacea purpurea.** *NF 23.*
Use: Dietary supplement.

echinocandins.
Use: Antifungal.
See: Caspofungin Acetate.
Micafungin Sodium.

●**echothiophate iodide.** (eck-oh-THIGH-oh-fate EYE-oh-dide) *USP 28.*
Use: Glaucoma agent.
See: Phospholine Iodide.

●**eclanamine maleate.** (eh-KLAN-ah-MEEN) USAN.
Use: Antidepressant.

●**eclazolast.** (eh-CLAY-zole-AST) USAN.
Use: Antiallergic; inhibitor (mediator release).

Eclipse After Sun. (Novartis) Petrolatum, glycerin, oleth-3 phosphate, carbomer-934, imidazolidinyl urea, benzyl alcohol, cetyl esters wax. Lot. Bot. 180 mL. *OTC.*
Use: Emollient.

Eclipse Lip and Face Protectant. (Novartis) Padimate O, oxybenzone. Stick

4.5 g. *OTC.*
Use: Lip protectant.
Eclipse Original Sunscreen. (Novartis) Padimate O, glyceryl PABA. Lot. Bot. 120 mL. *OTC.*
Use: Sunscreen.
Eclipse Suntan, Partial. (Novartis) Padimate O. Lot. Bot. 120 mL. *OTC.*
Use: Sunscreen.
EC-Naprosyn. (Roche) Naproxen 375 mg, 500 mg. DR Tab. Bot. 100s. *Rx.*
Use: NSAID.
•**econazole.** (ee-CON-uh-zole) USAN.
Use: Antifungal.
•**econazole nitrate.** (ee-CON-uh-zole) *USP 28.*
Use: Antifungal.
See: Spectazole.
econazole nitrate. (Various Mfr.) Econazole nitrate 1%. Cream. 15 g, 30 g, 85 g. *Rx.*
Use: Antifungal.
Econo B & C. (Vangard Labs, Inc.) Vitamins B$_1$ 15 mg, B$_2$ 10.2 mg, B$_3$ 50 mg, B$_5$ 10 mg, B$_6$ 5 mg, C 300 mg. Cap. Bot. 100s, UD 100s. *OTC.*
Use: Vitamin supplement.
Econopred. (Alcon) Prednisolone acetate 0.125%. Susp. *Drop-Tainer* 5 mL, 10 mL. *Rx.*
Use: Corticosteroid, ophthalmic.
Econopred Plus. (Alcon) Prednisolone acetate 1%. Susp. *Drop-Tainer* 5 mL, 10 mL. *Rx.*
Use: Corticosteroid, ophthalmic.
•**ecopipam hydrochloride.** (E-koe-pi-pam) USAN.
Use: Addiction disorders.
•**ecopladib.** (ek-oh-PLA-dib) USAN.
Use: Analgesic.
Ecotrin Adult Low Strength. (Glaxo-SmithKline) Aspirin 81 mg, tartrazine. EC Tab. Bot. 36s. *OTC.*
Use: Analgesic.
Ecotrin Maximum Strength. (Glaxo-SmithKline) Acetylsalicylic acid 500 mg. **Tab.:** Bot. 60s, 150s. **Cap.:** Bot. 60s. *OTC.*
Use: Analgesic.
Ecotrin Regular Strength. (GlaxoSmith-Kline) Aspirin 325 mg. EC Tab. Bot. 100s, 250s, 1000s. *OTC.*
Use: Analgesic.
•**ecraprost.** (E-kra-prost) USAN.
Use: Peripheral arterial occlusive disease.
•**ecromeximab.** (e-KROE-mek-si-mab) USAN.
Use: Monoclonal antibody.

•**eculizumab.** (ek-yoo-LYE-zyoo-mab) USAN.
Use: Treatment of autoimmune diseases.
Ed A-Hist Liquid. (Edwards) **Liq.:** Phenylephrine hydrochloride 10 mg, chlorpheniramine maleate 4 mg/5 mL, alcohol 5%, grape flavor. Liq. Bot. 473 mL. **Tab.:** Chlorpheniramine maleate 8 mg, phenylephrine hydrochloride 20 mg. SR Tab. Bot. 100s. *Rx.*
Use: Upper respiratory combination, antihistamine, decongestant.
edathamil. Edetate ethylenediamine tetraacetic acid.
edathamil calcium-disodium. Calcium disodium ethylenediamine tetraacetate.
See: Calcium Disodium Versenate.
edathamil disodium. Disodium salt of ethylenediamine tetraacetic acid.
See: Endrate.
•**edatrexate.** (EE-dah-TREX-ate) USAN.
Use: Antineoplastic.
Ed-Chlor-Tan. (Edwards) Chlorpheniramine tannate 8 mg. Tab. 100s. *Rx.*
Use: Antihistamine.
Edecrin. (Merck & Co.) Ethacrynic acid 25 mg, 50 mg. Tab. Bot. 100s. *Rx.*
Use: Diuretic.
Edecrin Sodium Intravenous. (Merck & Co.) Ethacrynate sodium equivalent to 50 mg ethacrynic acid w/mannitol 62.5 mg, thimerosal 0.1 mg. Vial. 50 mL for reconstitution. *Rx.*
Use: Diuretic.
•**edetate calcium disodium.** (EH-duh-tate) *USP 28.* Formerly Edathamil.
Use: Chelating agent (metal).
See: Calcium Disodium Versenate.
•**edetate dipotassium.** (EH-deh-tate) USAN.
Use: Pharmaceutic aid (chelating agent).
•**edetate disodium.** (EH-duh-tate) *USP 28.*
Use: Chelating agent (metal); pharmaceutic aid (chelating agent).
See: Disotate.
Endrate.
W/Benzalkonium chloride, boric acid, potassium chloride, sodium carbonate anhydrous.
See: Swim-Eye.
W/Phenylephrine hydrochloride, benzalkonium chloride, sodium bisulfate.
See: Sinarest.
W/Phenylephrine hydrochloride, methapyrilene hydrochloride, benzalkonium chloride, sodium bisulfite.
See: Allerest.

W/Potassium chloride, benzalkonium chloride, isotonic boric acid.
See: Dacriose.
W/Prednisolone sodium phosphate, niacinamide, sodium bisulfite, phenol.
See: P.S.P. IV.
W/Sodium thiosulfate, salicylic acid, isopropyl alcohol, propylene glycol, menthol, colloidal alumina.
See: Tinver.
edetate disodium. (Various Mfr.) Edetate disodium 150 mg/mL. Inj. Vial 20 mL. *Rx.*
Use: Antihypercalcemia; cadiovascular agent.
●**edetate sodium.** (EH-deh-tate) USAN.
Use: Chelating agent.
See: Disodium Versenate.
Vagisec.
●**edetate trisodium.** (EH-deh-tate) USAN.
Use: Chelating agent.
●**edetic acid.** (ED-eh-tic) *NF 23.*
Use: Pharmaceutic aid (chelating agent).
●**edetol.** (eh-deh-TOLE) USAN.
Use: Pharmaceutic aid (alkalinizing agent).
Edex. (Schwarz Pharma) Alprostadil. **Inj.:** 10 mcg, 20 mcg, 40 mcg (after reconstitution), lactose. Inj. Single-dose vial or kit containing prefilled syringe (with 1.2 mL of 0.9% sodium chloride), plunger rod, 2 one-half inch needles (one 27-gauge and one 30-gauge), 2 alcohol swabs, tape. **Pow. for Inj., lyophilized:** 10 mcg, 20 mcg, 40 mcg. Lactose. Single-dose, dual-chamber cartridges for use with reusable injection device. *Rx.*
Use: Anti-impotence agent.
Ed-Flex. (Edwards) Phenyltoloxamine citrate 20 mg, acetaminophen 300 mg, salicylamide 200 mg. Cap. Bot. 30s, 100s. *Rx.*
Use: Upper respiratory combination, antihistamine, analgesic.
●**edifoligide sodium.** (e-dif-oh-LIG-ide) USAN.
Use: Graft-vs-host disease.
●**edifolone acetate.** (EH-DIH-fah-LONE) USAN.
Use: Cardiovascular agent (antiarrhythmic).
edithamil.
See: Edathamil.
●**edobacomab.** (eh-dah-BACK-ah-mab) USAN.
Use: Antiendotoxin monoclonal antibody.

●**edodekin alfa.** (e-DOE-de-kin AL-fa) USAN.
Use: Antiasthmatic.
●**edonetan.** (ed-ON-en-tan) USAN.
Use: Heart failure.
●**edotreotide.** (ed-oh-TREE-oh-tide) USAN.
Use: Tumor staging.
●**edratide.** (ED-ra-tide) USAN.
Use: Lupus erythematosus.
●**edoxudine.** (ee-DOX-you-DEEN) USAN.
Use: Antiviral.
●**edrecolomab.** (edd-reh-KOE-lah-mab) USAN.
Use: Monoclonal antibody (antineoplastic adjuvant).
edrofuradene. Name used for Nifurdazil.
●**edrophonium chloride.** (eh-droe-FOE-nee-uhm) *USP 28.*
Use: Antidote to curare principles; diagnostic aid, myasthenia gravis.
See: Enlon.
Reversol.
Tensilon Chloride.
edrophonium chloride/atropine sulfate.
See: Atropine sulfate/edrophonium chloride.
ED-SPAZ. (Edwards) Hyoscyamine sulfate 0.125 mg. Tab. Bot. 100s. *Rx.*
Use: Anticholinergic; antispasmodic.
EDTA.
See: Edathamil.
ED-TLC. (Edwards) Phenylephrine hydrochloride 5 mg, chlorpheniramine maleate 2 mg, hydrocodone bitartrate 1.67 mg/5 mL. Liq. Bot. 473 mL. *c-III.*
Use: Upper respiratory combination, antihistamine, antitussive, decongestant.
ED Tuss HC. (Edwards) Phenylephrine hydrochloride 10 mg, chlorpheniramine maleate 4 mg, hydrocodone bitartrate 2.5 mg, alcohol 5%/5 mL, saccharin, sorbitol, grape flavor. Liq. Bot. 473 mL. *c-III.*
Use: Upper respiratory combination, antihistamine, antitussive, decongestant.
E.E.S. 400. (Abbott) Erythromycin ethylsuccinate (as base). **Tab.:** 400 mg. Sugar. Film coated. Bot. 100s, 500s, UD 100s. **Susp.:** 400 mg/5 mL. Parabens, sucrose. Orange flavor. Bot. 100 mL, 473 mL. *Rx.*
Use: Anti-infective; erythromycin.
E.E.S. Granules. (Abbott) Erythromycin ethylsuccinate (as base) 200 mg/5 mL when reconstituted. Sucrose. Cherry flavor. Pow. for Oral Susp. Bot. 100 mL,

200 mL. *Rx.*
Use: Anti-infective; erythromycin.
E.E.S. 200. (Abbott) Erythromycin ethylsuccinate 200 mg/5 mL. Parabens, sucrose. Fruit flavor. Bot. 100 mL, 473 mL. *Rx.*
Use: Anti-infective; erythromycin.

•**efalizumab.** (e-fa-li-ZOO-mab) USAN.
Use: Humanized anti-CD11a monoclonal antibody; immunosuppressive.
See: Raptiva.

•**efaproxiral.** (ef-a-PROKS-ir-al) USAN.
Use: Investigational hemoglobin modifier.

efavirenz.
Use: Antiretroviral agent, nonnucleoside reverse transcriptase inhibitor.
See: Sustiva.

Efedron Nasal. (Hyrex) Ephedrine hydrochloride 0.6%, chlorobutanol 0.5% w/sodium Cl, menthol, and cinnamon oil in a water-soluble jelly base. Tube 20 g. *OTC.*
Use: Decongestant.

Efed-II. (Alto) Ephedrine sulfate 25 mg. Cap. Box 24s. *OTC.*
Use: Decongestant.

•**efegatran sulfate.** (EH-feh-GAT-ran) USAN.
Use: Antithrombotic.

E-Ferol. (Forest) **Spray:** Alpha tocopherol equivalent to 30 units vitamin E/mL. Can 6 oz. **Vanishing Cream:** Alpha tocopherol. Jar 2 oz. *OTC.*
Use: Emollient.

E-Ferol Succinate. (Forest) d-alpha tocopherol acid succinate, equivalent to Vitamin E. **Cap. 100 units, 400 units:** Bot. 100s, 500s, 1000s. **Cap. 200 units:** Bot. 50s, 100s, 500s, 1000s. **Tab. 50 units:** Bot. 100s, 500s, 1000s. *OTC.*
Use: Vitamin supplement.

Effectin Tablets. (Sanofi-Synthelabo) Bitolterol mesylate. *Rx.*
Use: Bronchodilator.

Effective Strength Cough Formula. (Alra) Chlorpheniramine maleate 2 mg, dextromethorphan HBr 15 mg, alcohol 10%. Liq. Bot. 240 mL. *OTC.*
Use: Antihistamine, antitussive.

Effective Strength Cough w/Decongestant. (Alra) Pseudoephedrine hydrochloride 20 mg, dextromethorphan HBr 10 mg, alcohol 10%. Liq. Bot. 240 mL. *OTC.*
Use: Antitussive, decongestant.

Effer-K. (Nomax) Potassium 25 mEq (as bicarbonate and citrate), saccharin. Effervescent tab. Box foil 30s, 250s. *Rx.*

Use: Mineral supplement.

Effervescent Potassium/Chloride. (Qualitest) Potassium and chloride 25 mEq (from potassium chloride and bicarbonate, l-lysine monohydrochloride, and citric acid). Saccharin. Fruit punch flavor. Tab., effervescent. 30s, 100s, 250s. *Rx.*
Use: Potassium replacement product.

Effexor. (Wyeth-Ayerst) Venlafaxine hydrochloride 25 mg, 37.5 mg, 50 mg, 75 mg, 100 mg, lactose. Tab. Bot. 100s, *Redipak* 100s. *Rx.*
Use: Antidepressant.

Effexor XR. (Wyeth-Ayerst) Venlafaxine hydrochloride 37.5 mg, 75 mg, 150 mg. ER Cap. Bot. 100s, *Redipak* 100s. *Rx.*
Use: Antidepressant.

Efidac 24. (Hogil) Chlorpheniramine maleate 16 mg, mannitol. ER Tab. Pkg. 6s. *OTC.*
Use: Antihistamine, nonselective alkylamine.

Efidac 24 Chlorpheniramine. (Hogil) Chlorpheniramine maleate 16 mg. ER Tab. Pkg. 6s. *OTC.*
Use: Antihistamine.

Efidac 24 Pseudoephedrine. (Hogil) Pseudoephedrine hydrochloride 240 mg (immediate-release 60 mg, controlled-release 180 mg). CR Tab. Pkg. 6s, 12s, UD 1s. *OTC.*
Use: Nasal decongestant, arylalkylamine.

•**efletirizine dihydrochloride.** (ef-le-TI-razeen) USAN.
Use: Antihistaminic.

•**eflornithine hydrochloride.** (ee-FLAHR-nih-THEEN) USAN.
Use: Antineoplastic; antiprotozoal.
See: Ornidyl.
Vaniqa.

Efudex. (ICN Pharmaceuticals) Fluorouracil. **Soln.:** Fluorouracil 2%, 5%, EDTA, parabens. Dropper Bot. 10 mL. **Cream:** Fluorouracil 5%, parabens in a white petrolatum base. Tube 25 g. *Rx.*
Use: Antineoplastic.

•**eglumegad.** (e-GLUE-me-gad) USAN.
Use: Anti-anxiety agent; smoking cessation.

egraine. A protein binder from oats.

•**egtazic acid.** (egg-TAY-zik) USAN.
Use: Pharmaceutic aid.

EHDP.
See: Etidronate Disodium.

8-MOP. (ICN Pharmaceuticals) Methoxsalen 10 mg. Cap. 50s. *Rx.*
Use: Pigmenting agent.

●**elacridar hydrochloride.** (eh-LACK-rih-dahr) USAN.
Use: Potentiation of chemotherapy in cancer (multidrug resistance inhibitor in cancer); antineoplastic (adjunct).

●**elantrine.** (EL-an-treen) USAN.
Use: Anticholinergic.

●**elarofiban.** (el-a-roe-FYE-ban) USAN.
Use: Thrombotic disorders.

●**elastofilcon a.** (ee-LASS-toe-FILL-kahn A) USAN.
Use: Contact lens material, hydrophilic.

elcatonin. (Innapharma, Inc.)
Use: Intrathecal treatment of intractable pain. [Orphan Drug]

●**eldacimibe.** (ell-DASS-ih-mibe) USAN.
Use: Antiatherosclerotic; antihyperlipidemic.

Eldoo Kapooala. (Parke-Davis) Elemental iron 3.3 mg, Vitamins A 1667 units, E 10 mg, B₁ 10 mg, B₂ 0.9 mg, B₃ 17 mg, B₅ 10 mg, B₆ 0.7 mg, B₁₂ 2 mcg, C 67 mg, folic acid 0.3 mg, calcium iodine. Cap. Bot. 100s. *OTC.*
Use: Mineral, vitamin supplement.

Eldecort. (AstraZeneca) Hydrocortisone 2.5%, light mineral oil, propylene glycol, allantoin. Cream. Tube 15 g, 30 g. *Rx.*
Use: Corticosteroid, topical.

Eldepryl. (Somerset) Selegiline hydrochloride 5 mg, lactose. Cap. Bot. 60s, 300s. *Rx.*
Use: Antiparkinsonian.

Eldercaps. (Merz) Vitamins A 4000 units, D 400 units, E 25 units, B₁ 10 mg, B₂ 5 mg, B₃ 25 mg, B₅ 10 mg, B₆ 2 mg, C 200 mg, folic acid 1 mg, Zn 15.8 mg, Mg, Mn. Cap. Bot. 100s. *Rx.*
Use: Mineral, vitamin supplement.

Eldertonic. (Merz) Vitamins B₁ 0.17 mg, B₂ 0.19 mg, B₃ 2.22 mg, B₅ 1.11 mg, B₆ 0.22 mg, B₁₂ 0.67 mcg, alcohol 13.5%, Mg, Mn, zinc 1.7 mg/5 mL. Bot. 473 mL. *OTC.*
Use: Mineral, vitamin supplement.

Eldisine. (Eli Lilly)
See: Vindesine sulfate.

Eldo-B & C. (Canright) Vitamins C 250 mg, B₁ 25 mg, B₂ 10 mg, B₆ 5 mg, niacinamide 150 mg, d-calcium pantothenate 20 mg. Tab. Bot. 100s, 1000s. *OTC.*
Use: Mineral, vitamin supplement.

Eldofe. (Canright) Ferrous fumarate 225 mg. Chew. Tab. Bot. 100s, 1000s. *OTC.*
Use: Mineral supplement.

Eldofe-C. (Canright) Ferrous fumarate 225 mg, ascorbic acid 50 mg. Tab. Bot. 100s. *OTC.*
Use: Mineral, vitamin supplement.

Eldopaque. (ICN) Hydroquinone 2% with sunblock. Cream. Tube. 14.2 g, 28.4 g. *OTC.*
Use: Dermatologic.

Eldopaque Forte. (ICN) Hydroquinone 4% in a sunblock base. Talc, light mineral oil, EDTA, sodium metabisulfite. Cream. Tube. 28.4 g. *Rx.*
Use: Dermatologic.

Eldoquin Forte. (ICN) Hydroquinone 4% in vanishing base. Light mineral oil, propylparaben, sodium metabisulfite. Cream. Tube. 28.4 g. *Rx.*
Use: Dermatologic.

Elecal. (Western Research) Calcium 250 mg, magnesium 15 mg. Tab. Bot. 1000s. *OTC.*
Use: Mineral supplement.

electrolyte and invert sugar solutions.
Use: Intravenous nutritional therapy, intravenous replenishment solution.
See: Invert Sugar-Electrolyte Solutions.

electrolyte concentrates, combined.
Use: Intravenous nutritional therapy, intravenous replenishment solution.
See: Hyperlyte CR.
Lypholyte.
Lypholyte-II.
Multilyte-40.
Multilyte-20.
Nutrilyte.
Nutrilyte II.
TPN Electrolytes.
TPN Electrolytes III.
TPN Electrolytes II.

electrolyte-dextrose solutions.
Use: Intravenous nutritional therapy, intravenous replenishment solution.
See: Dextrose-Electrolyte Solutions.

electrolyte No. 48 and dextrose 10%.
Use: Intravenous nutritional therapy, intravenous replenishment solution.
See: Dextrose 10% and Electrolyte No. 48.

electrolyte No. 48 injection.
Use: Intravenous nutritional therapy, intravenous replenishment solution.
See: Dextrose 5% and Electrolyte No. 48.

electrolyte No. 75 and 5% dextrose.
Use: Intravenous nutritional therapy, intravenous replenishment solution.
See: 5% Dextrose and Electrolyte No. 75.

electrolyte solutions, combined.
Use: Intravenous nutritional therapy, intravenous replenshment solution.
See: Isolyte S pH 7.4.
Lactated Ringer's.

Normosol-M.
Normosol-R.
Normosol-R pH 7.4.
Plasma-Lyte A pH 7.4.
Plasma-Lyte 148.
Plasma-Lyte R.
Potassium Chloride in 0.9% Sodium Chloride.
Ringer's.
Elegen-G. (Grafton) Amitriptyline 10 mg, 25 mg, 50 mg. Tab. Bot. 100s, 1000s. *Rx.*
Use: Antidepressant, tricyclic.
Elestat. (Allergan) Epinastine hydrochloride 0.05%. Benzalkonium chloride 0.01%, EDTA. Soln., Ophthalmic. 8 mL, 15 mL. *Rx.*
Use: Ophthalmic antihistamine.
• **eletriptan hydrobromide.** (all-eh-TRIP-tan HIGH-droe-BROE-mide)
Use: Antimigraine agent, serotonin 5-HT receptor agonist.
See: Relpax.
• **eleuthero.** *NF 23.*
Use: Dietary supplement.
Elevites. (Barth's) Vitamins A 6000 units, D 400 units, B_1 1.5 mg, B_2 3 mg, B_{12} 10 mcg, C 60 mg, niacin 1 mg, E 10 units, malt diastase 15 mg, iron 15 mg, calcium 381 mg, phosphorus 0.172 mg, citrus bioflavonoid complex 15 mg, rutin 15 mg, nucleic acid 3 mg, red bone marrow 30 mg, peppermint leaves 10 mg, wheat germ 30 mg. Tab. or Cap. Bot. 100s, 500s, 1000s. *Rx.*
Use: Mineral, vitamin supplement.
Elidel. (Novartis) Pimecrolimus 1%. Cream. Tube. 30 g, 100 g. *Rx.*
Use: Topical immunomodulator.
Eligard. (Sanofi-Synthelabo) Leuprolide acetate **7.5 mg:** Inj. Single-use kit w/2-syringe mixing system and 20-gauge, ½-inch needle. **22.5 mg:** Single-use kit with 2-syringe mixing system and 20-gauge, ½-inch needle. **30 mg:** Inj. Single-use kit w/2-syringe mixing system and syringe containing *Atrigel.* **45 mg:** Single-use kit with 2-syringe mixing system and syringe containing *Atrigel. Rx.*
Use: Antineoplastic.
Eligard 22.5 mg. (Sanofi-Synthelabo) Leuprolide acetate 22.5 mg. Inj. Single-use kit w/2-syringe mixing system and 20-gauge, ½-inch needle. *Rx.*
Use: Antineoplastic.
Elimite. (Allergan) Permethrin 5%. Lanolin alcohols, coconut oil, mineral oil. Cream. Tube 60 g. *Rx.*
Use: Scabicide; pediculicide.

Elitek. (Sanofi-Synthelabo) Rasburicase 1.5 mg/vial, mannitol 10.6 mg. Pow. for Inj., lyophilized. Single-use vials with 1 mL amps of diluent. *Rx.*
Use: Antimetabolite.
Elixicon. (Berlex) Theophylline 100 mg/5 mL with methylparabens and propylparabens. Susp. Bot. 237 mL. *Rx.*
Use: Bronchodilator.
Elixiral. (Vita Elixir) Phenobarbital 16.2 mg, hyoscyamine sulfate 0.1037 mg, atropine sulfate 0.194 mg, hyoscine HBr 0.0065 mg/5 mL. Liq. Pt, gal. *Rx.*
Use: Anticholinergic; antispasmodic; hypnotic; sedative.
Elixophyllin Capsules, Dye-Free. (Forest) Anhydrous theophylline. Cap. **100 mg:** Bot. 100s. **200 mg:** Bot. 100s, 500s, UD 100s. *Rx.*
Use: Bronchodilator.
Elixophyllin Elixir. (Forest) Anhydrous theophylline 80 mg, alcohol 20%/15 mL. Bot. Pt, qt, gal. *Rx.*
Use: Bronchodilator.
Elixophyllin GG Liquid. (Forest) Theophylline 100 mg, guaifenesin 100 mg/15 mL. Alcohol free. Bot. 237, 480 mL. *Rx.*
Use: Antiasthmatic combination.
Elixophyllin-KI Elixir. (Forest) Anhydrous theophylline 80 mg, potassium iodide 130 mg/15 mL. Bot. 237 mL. *Rx.*
Use: Antiasthmatic combination.
ElixSure Children's Congestion. (Taro Consumer) Pseudoephedrine 15 mg per 5 mL. Glycerin, propylparaben, sucralose. Bubble gum, cherry, and grape flavors. Syrup. 118 mL. *OTC.*
Use: Nasal decongestant.
ElixSure Children's Cough. (Taro Consumer) Dextromethorphan hydrobromide 7.5 mg per 5 mL. Propylparaben, sorbitol, sucralose. Cherry bubble gum flavor. Syrup. 118 mL. *OTC.*
Use: Nonnarcotic antitussive.
Ellence. (Pharmacia & Upjohn) Epirubicin hydrochloride 2 mg/mL, preservative free. Inj. Single-use vial 25 mL, 100 mL. *Rx.*
Use: Antibiotic.
Ellesdine. (Janssen) Pipenperone. *Rx.*
Use: Anxiolytic.
Elliot's B Solution. (Orphan Medical)
Use: Acute lymphatic leukemias and acute lymphoblastic lymphomas. [Orphan Drug]
• **elm.** *USP 28.* Dried inner bark of *Ulmus rubra* Muhlenberg (*Ulmus fulva* Michaux).
Use: Pharmaceutic aid (suspending agent); demulcent.

Elmiron. (Baker Norton) Pentosan polysulfate 100 mg. Cap. Bot. 100s. *Rx.*
Use: Relief of bladder pain associated with interstitial cystitis.
Elocon Cream. (Schering-Plough)
Cream: Mometasone furoate 0.1%, hexylene glycol, phosphoric acid, propylene glycol stearate, stearyl alcohol, ceteareth-20, titanium dioxide, aluminum starch octenyl succinate, white wax, white petrolatum. Tube 15 g, 45 g.
Lot.: Mometasone furoate 0.1%. Bot. 30 mL, 60 mL. **Oint.:** Mometasone furoate 0.1%, hexylene glycol, propylene glycol stearate, white wax, white petrolatum. Tube 15 g, 45 g. *Rx.*
Use: Corticosteroid, topical.
Elon Barrier Protectant. (Dartmouth)
Paraffinum, liquidum, isopropyl palmitate, cetearyl alcohol, polyglyceryl-2, dipolyhydroxystearate, propylene glycol, cetearyl glucoside, C12-15 alkyl benzoate, stearic acid, bisabalol, petrolatum, phenoxyethanol, PEG-30 dipolyhydroxystearate, PEG-40 stearate, parabens, *Hamamelis virginiana*, denatured alcohol. Liq. 28 g. *OTC.*
Use: Protectant.
Elon Dual Defense Antifungal Formula. (Dartmouth) Undecylenic acid 25%. Alcohol. Soln. 30 mL. *OTC.*
Use: Antifungal agent.
Eloxatin. (Sanofi-Synthelabo) Oxaliplatin. **Inj.:** 5 mg/mL. Preservative free. Single-use vials. 10 mL, 20 mL. **Pow. for Inj., lyophilized:** 50 mg, 100 mg, preservative free, lactose. Single-use vials. *Rx.*
Use: Antineoplastic.
Elphemet. (Canright) Phendimetrazine tartrate 35 mg. Tab. Bot. 100s, 1000s. *c-III.*
Use: Anorexiant.
Elprecal. (Canright) Vitamins A 5000 units, D 400 units, B₁ 3 mg, B₂ 2 mg, B₆ 0.1 mg, B₁₂ 1 mcg, C 50 mg, E 2 units, calcium pantothenate 2.5 mg, niacinamide 15 mg, inositol 5 mg, choline 5 mg, calcium lactate 500 mg, ferrous sulfate 50 mg, Cu 1 mg, Mn 1 mg, Mg 2 mg, K 2 mg, Zn 0.5 mg, sulfur 1 mg. Cap. Bot. 100s. *OTC.*
Use: Mineral, vitamin supplement.
•**elsamitrucin.** (els-AM-ih-TRUE-sin) USAN.
Use: Antineoplastic.
Elserpine. (Canright) Reserpine 0.25 mg. Tab. Bot. 100s, 1000s. *Rx.*
Use: Antihypertensive.

Elspar. (Merck & Co.) Asparaginase 10,000 units, mannitol 80 mg. Inj. Vial 10 mL. *Rx.*
Use: Antineoplastic.
EL 10. (Elan) *Rx.*
Use: Antiviral; immunomodulator.
•**elucaine.** (eh-LOO-cane) USAN.
Use: Anticholinergic, gastric.
Elvanol. (DuPont) Polyvinyl alcohol. *Rx.*
Use: Pharmaceutical aid.
•**elvucitabine.** (el-vue-SYE-ta-been) USAN.
Use: Hepatitis B; HIV.
•**elzasonan citrate.** (el-za-SONE-an) USAN.
Use: Antidepressant.
•**elzasonan hydrochloride.** (el-za-SONE-an) USAN.
Use: Antidepressant.
Emadine (Alcon) Emedastine difumarate 0.05% (0.5 mg/mL), benzalkonium chloride 0.01%. Ophth. Soln. Dispenser 5 mL. *Rx.*
Use: Antihistamine, ophthalmic.
embechine. Aliphatic chloroethylamine.
Use: Antineoplastic.
Embeline. (Healthpoint Medical) Clobetasol propionate 0.5%. **Cream:** White petrolatum, cetyl alcohol, stearyl alcohol, lanolin oil, parabens. 15 g, 30 g, 45 g, 60 g. **Oint.:** White petrolatum. 15 g, 30 g, 45 g, 60 g. **Gel:** 15 g, 30 g, 60 g. *Rx.*
Use: Anti-inflammatory.
Embeline E, 0.05%. (Healthpoint Medical) Clobetasol propionate 0.5 mg/g, cetostearyl alcohol. Cream. Tube 15 g, 30 g, 60 g. *Rx.*
Use: Anti-inflammatory.
Embrox 600 (Andrx) Ca 240 mg, Fe (as carbonyl iron) 90 mg, vitamin A 3500 units, D₃ 400 units, E (dl alpha tocopherol acetate) 30 units, B₁ 2 mg, B₂ 3 mg, B₆ 3 mg, B₁₂ 12 mg, C 60 mg, folic acid 1 mg, Zn 20 mg, Cu, Mg, dioctylsulfosuccinate sodium 50 mg. Chew. Tab. Blister pack 35s, 91s. *Rx.*
Use: Vitamin, mineral supplement.
Emcodeine Tabs. (Major) Aspirin with codeine as #2, #3, #4. Bot. 100s, 500s. *c-III.*
Use: Analgesic combination; narcotic.
Emcyt. (Pharmacia) Estramustine phosphate sodium equivalent to 140 mg estramustine phosphate. Cap. Bot. 100s. *Rx.*
Use: Antineoplastic; hormone, alkylating agent.
Emdol. (Health for Life Brands) Salicylamide, para-aminobenzoic acid, sodium calcium succinate, vitamin D-

1250. Bot. 100s, 1000s. *OTC.*
Use: Analgesic combination.

•**emedastine difumarate.** (eh-meh-DASS-teen die-FEW-mah-rate) *USP 28.*
Use: Management of allergic conjunctivitis; antiasthmatic; antiallergic; antihistamine (H_1-receptor).
See: Emadine.

Emend. (Merck) Aprepitant 80 mg, 125 mg, sucrose. Cap. Bot. 30s, UD 5s (tri-fold pack containing one 125 mg capsule and two 80 mg capsules). *Rx.*
Use: Antiemetic.

emergency contraceptives.
See: Plan B.
Preven.

emergency kits.
See: Cyanide Antidote Package.

Emeroid. (Delta Pharmaceutical Group) Zinc oxide 5%, diperodon hydrochloride 0.25%, bismuth subcarbonate 0.2%, pyrilamine maleate 0.1%, phenylephrine hydrochloride 0.25%, in a petrolatum base containing cod liver oil. Tube 1.25 oz. *OTC.*
Use: Anorectal preparation.

Emerson 1% Sodium Fluoride Dental Gel. (Emerson) Red and plain. Bot. 2 oz. *Rx.*
Use: Dental caries agent.

emetics.
See: Apomorphine hydrochloride.
Cupric sulfate.
Ipecac.

•**emetine hydrochloride.** (EM-eh-teen) *USP 28.*
Use: Antiamebic.

Emetrol. (Pharmacia) Dextrose 1.87 g, fructose 1.87 g, phosphoric acid 21.5 mg, methylparaben, lemon, mint, or cherry flavor. Soln. Bot. 118 mL, 236 mL, 473 mL. *OTC.*
Use: Antiemetic.

EMF. (Wesley Pharmacal) Alanine, arginine, aspartic acid, cysteine, glutamic acid, glycine, histidine, hydroxylysine, hydroxyproline, isoleucineline, leucine, lysine, methionine, phenylalanine, proline, serine, threonine, tyrosine, valine, protein 15 g, sorbitol, saccharin, cherry flavor. Liq. Bot. Qt. *OTC.*
Use: Amino acid.

Emgel. (GlaxoSmithKline) Erythromycin 2%. Alcohol 77%. Gel. Tube 27 g, 50 g. *Rx.*
Use: Dermatologic, acne.

EM-GG. (Econo Med Pharmaceuticals) Guaifenesin 100 mg/5 mL. Bot. Pt. *OTC.*
Use: Expectorant.

•**emilium tosylate.** (EE-MILL-ee-uhm TAH-sill-ate) USAN.
Use: Cardiovascular agent (antiarrhythmic).

Emitrip Tabs. (Major) Amitriptyline. Tab. **10 mg, 25 mg:** Bot. 100s, 250s, 1000s, UD 100s. **50 mg:** Bot. 100s, 250s, 1000s, UD 100s. **75 mg:** Bot. 100s, 250s, UD 100s. **100 mg:** Bot. 100s, 250s, 1000s, UD 100s. **150 mg:** Bot. 100s, 250s. *Rx.*
Use: Antidepressant, tricyclic.

•**emivirine.** (e-mi-VYE-rene) USAN.
Use: HIV-1 infection.

EMLA. (AstraZeneca) Lidocaine 2.5%, prilocaine 2.5%. Cream. Tube 5 g, 30 g. *Rx.*
Use: Anesthetic, local.

EMLA Anesthetic. (AstraZeneca) EMLA emulsion 1 g (lidocaine 2.5%, prilocaine 2.5%). Contact surface ≈ 10 cm^2. Disc. Box. 2s, 10s. *Rx.*
Use: Anesthetic, local.

Emollia-Creme. (Gordon Laboratories) Cetyl alcohol, lubricating oils in water-soluble base. Jar 4 oz, 5 lb. *OTC.*
Use: Emollient.

Emollia-Lotion. (Gordon Laboratories) Water-dispersable waxes, lubricating bland oils in a water-soluble lotion base. Bot. 1 oz, 4 oz, gal. *OTC.*
Use: Emollient.

Empirin Aspirin. (GlaxoSmithKline) Aspirin 325 mg. Tab. Bot. 50s, 100s, 250s. *OTC.*
Use: Analgesic.

Empirin w/Codeine. (GlaxoSmithKline) Aspirin 325 mg with codeine phosphate 15 mg, 30 mg, 60 mg. Tab. **No. 2:** Codeine phosphate 15 mg. Bot. 100s. **No. 3:** Codeine phosphate 30 mg. Bot. 100s, 500s, 1000s, *Dispenserpak* 25s. **No. 4:** Codeine phosphate 60 mg. Bot. 100s, 500s, *Dispenserpak* 25s. *c-III.*
Use: Analgesic combination; narcotic.

•**emtricitabine.** (em-try-SIGH-tah-bean) USAN.
Use: Antiviral.
See: Emtriva.
W/Tenofovir Disoproxil.
See: Truvada.

Emtriva. (Gilead) Emtricitabine 200 mg. Cap. 30s. *Rx.*
Use: Antiviral.

Emulave. (Rydelle)
See: Aveenobar Oilated.

Emulsoil. (Paddock) Castor oil 95% w/emulsifuing agents, butylparaben. Emulsion. Bot. 63 mL. *OTC.*
Use: Laxative.

E-Mycin. (Pharmacia) Erythromycin 250 mg, 333 mg. EC Tab. Bot. 40s (250 mg only), 100s, 500s, UD 100s. *Rx.*
Use: Anti-infective; erythromycin.

Enablex. (Novartis) Darifenacin 7.5 mg, 15 mg. Lactose. ER Tab. 30s, 90s, UD 100s. *Rx.*
Use: Treatment of overactive bladder.

• **enadoline hydrochloride.** (en-AHD-oleen) USAN.
Use: Analgesic; severe head injury. [Orphan Drug]

• **enalaprilat.** (EH-NAL-uh-prill-at) *USP 28.*
Use: Antihypertensive.
See: Vasotec.

enalaprilat. (Various Mfr.) Enalaprilat 1.25 mg/mL. Inj. Vial 1 mL, 2 mL. *Rx.*
Use: Antihypertensive.

• **enalapril maleate.** (EH-NAL-uh-prill) *USP 28.*
Use: Antihypertensive.
See: Enalaprilat.
Vasotec.
W/Diltiazem maleate.
See: Teczem.
W/Felodipine.
See: Lexxel.
W/Hydrochlorothiazide.
See: Enalapril Maleate/Hydrochlorothiazide.
Vaseretic.

enalapril maleate. (Various Mfr.) Enalapril maleate 2.5 mg, 5 mg, 10 mg, 20 mg. Tab. Bot. 100s, 1000s. *Rx.*
Use: Antihypertensive.

enalapril maleate/hydrochlorothiazide. (Eon) Hydrochlorothiazide 12.5 mg or 25 mg, enalapril maleate 5 mg or 10 mg, lactose. Tab. Bot. 100s, 1000s. *Rx.*
Use: Antihypertensive.

• **enalkiren.** (en-al-KIE-ren) USAN.
Use: Antihypertensive.

• **enazadrem phosphate.** (eh-NAZZ-ahdrem) USAN.
Use: Antipsoriatic; inhibitor (5-lipoxygenase).

Enbrel. (Amgen) Etanercept. **Inj.:** 50 mg/mL. In 0.98 mL prefilled single-use syringe with 27-gauge, ½-inch needle. Carton contains 4 prefilled syringes. Preservative free. Sucrose 10 mg/mL, sodium chloride 5.8 mg/mL, L-arginine hydrochloride 5.3 mg/mL, sodium phosphate monobasic, monohydrate 2.6 mg/mL, sodium phosphate, dibasic, anhydrous 0.9 mg/mL. **Pow. for Inj., lyophilized:** 25 mg, preservative free, mannitol 40 mg, sucrose 10 mg, tromethamine 1.2 mg. Multiple-use vial with syr., alcohol swabs, diluent (sterile bacteriostatic water for injection 1 mL contains benzyl alcohol 0.9%), plunger. Ctn. containing 4 dose trays. *Rx.*
Use: Antiarthritic; immunologic agent, immunomodulator.

encapsulated porcine islet preparation.
Use: Type 1 diabetes. [Orphan Drug]
See: BetaRx.

Encare. (Thompson Medical) Nonoxynol 9 (2.27%). Supp. 12s. *OTC.*
Use: Vaginal contraceptive.

• **enciprazine hydrochloride.** (en-SIH-PRAH-zeen) USAN.
Use: Anxiolytic.

• **enclomiphene.** (en-KLOE-mih-FEEN) USAN. *Formerly Clomiphene.*

• **encyprate.** (en-SIGH-prate) USAN.
Use: Antidepressant.

Endafed. (Forest) Pseudoephedrine hydrochloride 120 mg, brompheniramine maleate 12 mg. SR Cap. Bot. 100s. *Rx.*
Use: Antihistamine, decongestant.

Endagen-HD. (Jones Pharma) Phenylephrine hydrochloride 5 mg, chlorpheniramine maleate 2 mg, hydrocodone bitartrate 1.7 mg, cherry flavor. Liq. Bot. 473 mL. *c-III.*
Use: Upper respiratory combination, antihistamine, antitussive, decongestant.

Endal-HD Plus. (PediaMed) Hydrocodone bitartrate 3.5 mg, phenylephrine hydrochloride 7.5 mg, chlorpheniramine maleate 2 mg, saccharin, sorbitol, alcohol free, black raspberry flavor. Liq. Bot. 473 mL. *c-III.*
Use: Antihistamine, antitussive, decongestant.

Endal Nasal Decongestant. (PediaMed) Phenylephrine hydrochloride 20 mg, guaifenesin 300 mg. TR Tab. Bot. 100s. *Rx.*
Use: Decongestant, expectorant.

Endep. (Roche) Amitriptyline hydrochloride 10 mg, 25 mg, 50 mg, 75 mg, 100 mg, 150 mg. Tab. **10 mg:** Bot. 100s, *Tel-E-Dose* 100s. **25 mg:** Bot. 100s, 500s, *Tel-E-Dose* 100s. **50 mg:** Bot. 100s, 500s, *Tel-E-Dose* 100s. **75 mg:** Bot. 100s, *Tel-E-Dose* 100s. **100 mg:** Bot. 100s, *Tel-E-Dose* 100s. **150 mg:** Bot 100s. *Rx.*
Use: Antidepressant, tricyclic.

endobenziline bromide.
Use: Anticholinergic.

endocaine. Pyrrocaine.
Use: Anesthetic, local.

Endocet. (Endo) Oxycodone hydrochloride/acetaminophen 5 mg/325 mg, 7.5 mg/325 mg, 7.5 mg/500 mg, 10 mg/325 mg, 10 mg/650 mg. Tab. Bot. 100s, 500s. *c-II.*
Use: Analgesic; narcotic.

endojodin.
See: Entodon.

endomycin. A new antibiotic obtained from cultures of *Streptomyces endus.* Under study.

endophenolphthalein. (Roche) Diacetyldioxyphenylisatin-isacen-bisatin. *OTC.*
Use: Laxative.

endothelin receptor antagonists.
Use: Vasodilator.
See: Bosentan.

• **endralazine mesylate.** (en-DRAL-ahzeen MEH-sih-late) USAN.
Use: Antihypertensive.

Endrate. (Abbott Hospital Products) Edetate disodium 150 mg/mL. Inj. Amp. 20 mL. *Rx.*
Use: Antihypercalcemic; cardiovascular agent.

• **endrysone.** (EN-drih-sone) USAN.
Use: Anti-inflammatory, topical; ophthalmic.

Enduron. (Abbott) Methyclothiazide 5 mg. Tab. Bot. 100s, 1000s, UD 100s. *Rx.*
Use: Diuretic.

Enduronyl. (Abbott) Methyclothiazide 5 mg, deserpidine 0.25 mg. Lactose. Tab. 100s. *Rx.*
Use: Antihypertensive combination.

Enecat CT. (Mallinckrodt) Barium sulfate 5%, simethicone, sorbitol. Conc. Susp. Bot. 110 mL w/480 mL bot. for dilution w/flexible tubing, clamp, enema tip. *Rx.*
Use: Radiopaque agent, GI contrast agent.

Enemark. (Lafayette) Rectal marker. 85% w/v liquid barium. Case of 12 kits.
Use: Rectal marker during radiation therapy.

enemas.
See: Fleet.
    Fleet Bisacodyl.
    Fleet Mineral Oil.
    Therevac-SB.

Enerjets. (Chilton) Caffeine 75 mg, sugar, coffee, mocha mint, and "butterscotch" flavors. Loz. Pkg. 10s. *OTC.*
Use: CNS stimulant, analeptic.

Eneset 1. (Lafayette) Barium sulfate suspension 300 mL/air contrast examination kit. Unit-of-use kit. Case 12s.
Use: Radiopaque agent.

Eneset 600. (Lafayette) Barium sulfate suspension 600 mL/air contrast exami-

nation kit. Unit-of-use kit. Case 12s.
Use: Radiopaque agent.

Eneset 2. (Lafayette) Barium sulfate suspension 450 mL/contrast examination kit. Unit-of-use kit. Case 12s.
Use: Radiopaque agent.

EnfaCare. (Mead Johnson Nutritionals) Protein (nonfat milk, whey protein concentrate, taurine, L-carnitine) 2.8 g, carbohydrate (maltodextrin, lactose) 10.7 g, fat (high oleic sunflower oil, soy oil, medium chain triglycerides, coconut oil, monoglycerides and diglycerides, soy lecithin) 5.3 g/100 cal, vitamins A, B_1, B_2, B_3, B_5, B_6, B_{12}, C, D, E, K, folic acid 26 mcg/100 cal, biotin, choline, inositol, linoleic acid, Ca, chloride, Cu, Fe 1.8 mg, I, Mg, Mn, P, Se, Zn, Na 35 mg, K 105 mg/100 cal, 22 cal/oz. Liq. Pow. *Nursette* bot. 3 oz. (Liq. only). Can 14 oz (Pow. only). *OTC.*
Use: Enteral nutritional therapy.

Enfamil. (Mead Johnson Nutritionals) Vitamins A 2000 units, D 400 units, E 20 units, C 52 mg, B_1 0.5 mg, B_2 1 mg, B_6 0.4 mg, B_{12} 1.5 mcg, niacin 8 mg, Ca 440 mg, P 300 mg, folic acid 100 mcg, pantothenic acid 3 mg, inositol 30 mg, biotin 15 mcg, K-1 55 mcg, choline 100 mg, Fe 1.4 mg, K 650 mg, Cl 400 mg, Cu 0.6 mg, I 65 mcg, Na 175 mg, Mg 50 mg, Zn 5 mg, Mn 100 mg. Qt. Concentrated Liq. 13 fl oz, Instant Pow. lb. *OTC.*
Use: Nutritional supplement.

Enfamil Human Milk Fortifier. (Mead Johnson Nutritionals) Whey protein, casein, corn syrup solids, lactose, protein 0.7 g, carbohydrate 2.7 g, fat 0.04 g, calories 14. Pow. Packet 0.95 g, Box 100s. *OTC.*
Use: Nutritional supplement.

Enfamil with Iron. (Mead Johnson Nutritionals) Iron 12 mg. Qt. Pkg. Con. Liq. 13 fl oz. 24s. Pow. 1 lb. 6s. *OTC.*
Use: Nutritional supplement.

Enfamil with Iron Ready to Use. (Mead Johnson Nutritionals) Ready-to-use infant formula 20 kcal/fl oz. Can 8 fl oz, 6-can pack; 32 fl oz, 6 cans per case. *OTC.*
Use: Nutritional supplement.

Enfamil LactoFree. (Mead Johnson Nutritionals) Protein 2.1 g, fat 5.3 g, carbohydrate 10.9 g, calories 100/serving, linoleic acid 860 mg, A 300 units, D 60 units, E 2 units, K 8 mcg, B_1 80 mcg, B_2 140 mcg, B_3 1000 mcg, B_5 500 mcg, B_6 60 mcg, B_{12} 0.3 mcg, folic acid 16 mcg, biotin 3 mcg, C 12 mg, choline 12 mg, inositol (liquid only)

17 mg, inositol (powder only) 6 mg, Ca 82 mg, P 55 mg, Mg 8 mg, Fe 1.8 mg, Zn 1 mg, Mn 15 mcg, Cu 75 mcg, I 15 mcg, Se 2.8 mcg, Na 30 mg, K 110 mg, Cl 67 mg. Liq., Liq. Conc., Pow. Bot. 397 g (pow.), 384 mL (liq. conc.), 946 mL (liq.). *OTC.*
Use: Nutritional therapy, enteral.

Enfamil LIPIL with Iron. (Mead Johnson Nutritionals) Protein (reduced minerals, whey, nonfat milk, taurine) 2.1 g, fat (vegetable oil [palm olein, soy, coconut, and high-oleic sunflower oils], and less than 1% mortierella alpina oil, crypthecodinium cohnii oil, mono- and diglycerides, soy, lecithin) 5.3 g, carbohydrate (lactose) 10.9 g/100 cal, A, B_1, B_2, B_3, B_5, B_6, B_{12}, C, D, E, K, folic acid 16 mg/cal, biotin, chloride, choline, inositol, linoleic acid, Ca, Cu, Fe, I, Mg, Mn, P, Se, Zn, Na 27 mg and K 108 mg/100 cal. 20 cal/oz. **Liq.:** *Nursette* bottles 3 oz, 6 oz. **Liq. Conc.:** Cans 13 oz. **Pow.:** Cans. 12.9 oz, 25.7 oz. *OTC.*
Use: Nutritional therapy.

Enfamil Natalins Rx. (Mead Johnson Nutritionals) Ca 100 mg, Fe 27 mg, vitamin A 2000 units, D 200 units, E 7.5 units, B_1 0.75 mg, B_2 0.8 mg, B_3 8.5 mg, B_5 3.5 mg, B_6 2 mg, B_{12} 1.25 mcg, C 40 mg, folate 0.5 mg, biotin 15 mcg, Zn 12.5 mg, Cu, Mg. TR Tab, Bot. 200s. *Rx.*
Use: Vitamin, mineral supplement.

Enfamil Next Step. (Mead Johnson Nutritionals) Protein 17.3 g, carbohydrates 74 g, fat 33.3 g/liter, with appropriate vitamins and minerals. **Liq.:** 390 mL concentrate, 1 qt ready to use. **Pow.:** 360 g, 720 g. *OTC.*
Use: Nutritional supplement.

Enfamil Nursette. (Mead Johnson Nutritionals) Ready-to-feed *Enfamil* 20 kcal/fl oz, 4 fl oz, 6 fl oz and 8 fl oz. 4 bottles/sealed carton. W/Iron. Ready to use. Bot. 6 fl oz 4s, 24s. *OTC.*
Use: Nutritional supplement.

Enfamil Premature Formula. (Bristol-Myers Squibb) Nonfat milk, whey protein concentrate, corn syrup solids, lactose, coconut oil, corn oil, medium chain triglycerides, soy lecithin. Protein 2.8 g, carbohydrate 10.7 g, fat 4.9 g, calories 96. Pow. *Nursettes* 120 mL. *OTC.*
Use: Nutritional supplement.

Enfamil Ready To Use. (Mead Johnson Nutritionals) Ready-to-use *Enfamil* infant formula 20 kcal/fl oz. Can 8 fl oz, 6-can pack; 32 fl oz, 6 cans per case.

OTC.
Use: Nutritional supplement.

● **enflurane.** (EN-flew-rane) *USP 28.*
Use: Anesthetic, inhalation.
See: Compound 347.
Ethrane.

enflurane. (Abbott) Enflurane 125 mL and 250 mL/Inhalation. *Rx.*
Use: Anesthetic, inhalation.

● **enfuvirtide.** (en-FYOO-veer-tide) USAN.
Use: Antiretroviral.
See: Fuzeon.

Engerix-B. (GlaxoSmithKline) Hepatitis B vaccine (recombinant). **Adult:** 20 mcg/mL hepatitis B surface antigen, thimerosal (mercury < 1 mcg), preservative free. Inj. Single-dose vial, prefilled syr. **Pediatric:** 10 mcg/0.5 mL hepatitis B surface antigen, preservative free, thimerosal (mercury < 0.5 mcg). Inj. Single-dose vial, prefilled syr. *Rx.*
Use: Active immunization, viral vaccine.

● **englitazone sodium.** (EN-GLIH-tah-zone) USAN.
Use: Antidiabetic.

Enhancer. (Mallinckrodt) Barium sulfate 98%, simethicone, sorbitol, sucrose, lemon-vanilla flavor. Susp. Bot. 312 g. *Rx.*
Use: Radiopaque agent, GI contrast agent.

Enjuvia. (Duramed) Synthetic conjugated estrogens D 0.0 mg, 0.16 mg, 0.625 mg, 1.25 mg. EDTA, lactose. Film-coated. Tab. 100s. *Rx.*
Use: Sex hormone.

● **enilconazole.** (EE-nill-KOE-nah-zole) USAN.
Use: Antifungal.

● **eniluracil.** (en-ill-YOUR-ah-sill) USAN.
Use: Potentiator of antineoplastic activity of fluorouracil (uracil reductase inhibitor); antineoplastic (adjunct).

● **enisoprost.** (en-EYE-so-prahst) USAN.
Use: Antiulcerative.

Enisyl. (Person and Covey) L-Lysine monohydrochloride 334 mg, 500 mg. Tab. Bot. 100s, 250s. *OTC.*
Use: Nutritional supplement.

● **enlimomab.** (en-LIE-moe-mab) USAN.
Use: Anti-inflammatory; monoclonal antibody.

Enlive!. (Abbott) Protein (whey protein isolate) 10 g, carbohydrates (maltodextrin, sucrose) 65 g, fat 0 g, Na 65 mg, K 40 mg/L. H_2O 840 mOsm/kg, 1.25 cal/mL. Vitamin A, B_1, B_2, B_3, B_5, B_6, B_{12}, C, D, E, K, biotin, chlorine, Ca, Cl, Cu, Cr, Fe, I, Mg, Mo, P, Se, Zn.

Gluten-free. Apple and peach flavors. Liq. 240 mL. *OTC.*
Use: Enteral nutrition therapy.

Enlon Injection. (Ohmeda) Edrophonium Cl 10 mg/mL, phenol 0.45%, sodium sulfite 0.2%. Vial 15 mL. *Rx.*
Use: Cholinergic muscle stimulant.

Enlon-Plus. (Ohmeda) Edrophonium chloride 10 mg, atropine sulfate 0.14 mg. Inj. Amp. 5 mL, Multi-dose vial 15 mL. *Rx.*
Use: Muscle stimulant.

•**enloplatin.** (en-LOW-PLAT-in) USAN.
Use: Antineoplastic.

Ennex Ointment. (Ennex) Aloe vera extract 37.5%. **Skin Oint.:** Zinc oxide 12.5%, coal tar 1.5%, alcohol 4.5%. Tube oz. **Hemorrhoidal Oint.:** Tube oz. *OTC.*
Use: Anti-inflammatory; astringent; antipruritic.

•**enofelast.** (EE-no-fell-ast) USAN.
Use: Antiasthmatic.

•**enolicam sodium.** (ee-NO-lih-kam) USAN.
Use: Anti-inflammatory; antirheumatic.

Enovid-E 21. (Pharmacia) Norethynodrel 2.5 mg, mestranol 0.1 mg. Tab. Compack disp. 21s, 6 × 21. Refill 21s, 12 × 21. *Rx.*
Use: Estrogen, progestin combination.

Enovil. (Roberts) Amtriptyline hydrochloride 10 mg/mL. Vial 10 mL. *Rx.*
Use: Antidepressant.

•**enoxacin.** (en-OX-ah-SIN) USAN.
Use: Anti-infective.

•**enoxaparin sodium.** (ee-NOX-ah-PAR-in) USAN.
Use: Anticoagulant.
See: Lovenox.

•**enoximone.** (EN-ox-ih-MONE) USAN.
Use: Cardiovascular agent.

•**enpiroline phosphate.** (en-PIHR-oh-LEEN) USAN.
Use: Antimalarial.

Enpresse. (Barr) Levonorgestrel 0.05 mg, ethinyl estradiol 30 mcg. Pink tab. Levonorgestrel 0.075 mg, ethinyl estradiol 40 mcg. White tab. Levonorgestrel 0.125 mg, ethinyl estradiol 30 mcg. Orange tab. Lactose. Box. 28s. *Rx.*
Use: Sex hormone, contraceptive hormone.

•**enprofylline.** (en-PRO-fih-lin) USAN.
Use: Bronchodilator.

•**enpromate.** (EN-pro-mate) USAN.
Use: Antineoplastic.

•**enprostil.** (en-PRAHS-till) USAN.
Use: Antisecretory; antiulcerative.

Enrich. (Ross) Liquid food with fiber providing complete, balanced nutrition as a full liquid diet, liquid supplement, or tube feeding. One serving provides 5 g dietary fiber. 1100 calories/L. 1530 calories provides 100% US RDA for vitamins and minerals. Ready-to-Use: Can 8 fl oz (vanilla, chocolate). *OTC.*
Use: Nutritional supplement, enteral.

Ensidon. (Novartis) Opipramol hydrochloride. *Rx.*
Use: Antidepressant.

•**ensulizole.** (en-SUL-i-zole) *USP 28.* Formerly phenylbenzimidazole sulfonic acid.
Use: Sunscreen.

Ensure. (Ross) Liquid food providing 1.06 calories/mL. Can be used as a full liquid diet, liquid supplement or tube feeding. Two quarts (2000 calories) provides 100% US RDA for vitamins and minerals for adults and children over 4 yrs. **Ready-to-Use:** Bot. 8 fl oz (vanilla). Can 8 fl oz (chocolate, black walnut, coffee, strawberry, eggnog, vanilla), 32 fl oz (vanilla, chocolate). **Pow.:** Can 14 oz (400 g) (vanilla). *OTC.*
Use: Nutritional supplement.

Ensure High Protein. (Ross) Protein 50.4 g, carbohydrate 129.4 g, fat 25.2 g, < 21 mg cholesterol, Na 1218 mg, K 2100 mg, vitamin A 5250 units, D 420 units, E 47.5 units, K 84 mcg, C 125 mg, folic acid 420 mg, B_1 1.6 mg, B_2 1.8 mg, B_3 21 mg, B_5 10.5 mg, B_6 2.1 mg, B_{12} 6.3 mcg, biotin 315 mcg, Ca 1050 mg, Cl, P, Mg, I, Mn, Cu, Zn 24 mg, Fe 19 mg, Se, Cr, Mo, 945 calories/237 mL. Liq. Bot. 237 mL. *OTC.*
Use: Nutritional supplement.

Ensure HN. (Ross) High nitrogen low residue liquid food providing complete, balanced nutrition as tube feeding or oral supplement with 1.06 calories/mL. Provides 100% US RDA for vitamins and minerals for adults and children over 4 yrs. 1400 calories (1321 mL). Ready-to-Use: Can 8 fl oz (vanilla). *OTC.*
Use: Nutritional supplement.

Ensure Osmolite. (Ross)
See: Osmolite.

Ensure Plus. (Ross) High-calorie liquid food w/caloric density of 1500 calories/L. Six servings (8 oz and 2130 calories each) provides 100% US RDA for vitamins and minerals for adults and children. Ready-to-Use: Bot. 8 fl oz (vanilla). Can 8 fl oz (chocolate, vanilla, eggnog, coffee, strawberry). *OTC.*

Use: Nutritional supplement.

Ensure Plus HN. (Ross) High-calorie, high-nitrogen liquid food providing 1.5 calories/mL; 1420 calories provides 100% US RDA for vitamins and minerals for adults and children. Calorie/nitrogen ratio is 150:1. Can 8 fl oz (vanilla). *OTC.*
Use: Nutritional supplement.

Ensure Pudding. (Ross) Protein 6.8 g (nonfat milk), carbohydrate 34 g (sucrose, modified food starch), fat 9.7 g (partially hydrogenated soybean oil), vitamin A 850 units, D 68 units, E 7.7 units, K 12 mcg, C 15.4 mg, folic acid 68 mcg, B_1 0.25 mg, B_2 0.29 mg, B_3 3.4 mg, B_5 1.7 mg, B_6 0.34 mg, B_{12} 1.1 mcg, choline, biotin, Na 240 mg, K 330 mg, Cl 220 mg, Ca 200 mg, P, Mg, I, Mn, Cu, Zn 3.83 mg, Fe 3.06 mg, 250 calories/Can. Pudding. 150 g. *OTC.*
Use: Nutritional supplement.

Entab 650. (Merz) Aspirin 650 mg. EC tab. Bot. 100s. *OTC.*
Use: Analgesic.

•**entacapone.** (en-TACK-ah-pone) USAN.
Use: Antidyskinetic; antiparkinsonian.
See: Comtan.
W/Carbidopa and Levodopa.
See: Stalevo.

•**entecavir.** (en-TE-ka-vihr) USAN.
Use: Antiviral.
See: Baraclude.

Entero-Test. (HDC) Cap. to identify duodenal parasites; to diagnose and locate upper GI bleeding, pH disorders, achlorhydria, and esophageal reflux. Bot. 10s, 25s.
Use: Diagnostic aid.

Entero-Test Pediatric. (HDC) To identify duodenal parasites; to diagnose and locate upper GI bleeding, pH disorders, achlorhydria, and esophageal reflux. Cap. Bot. 10s, 25s.
Use: Diagnostic aid.

Enterotube. (Roche) Culture-identification method for Enterobacteriaceae ACA. Test kit 25s.
Use: Diagnostic aid.

Entertainer's Secret. (KLI Corp.) Sodium carboxymethylcellulose, potassium chloride, dibasic sodium phosphate, aloe vera gel, glycerin, parabens. Soln. Bot. 60 mL spray. *OTC.*
Use: Saliva substitute.

Entex HC. (Andrx Laboratories) Hydrocodone bitartrate 5 mg, guaifenesin 100 mg, phenylephrine hydrochloride 7.5 mg/5 mL, cherry flavor, alcohol and dye free. Liq. Bot. 15 mL, 473 mL. *c-III.*
Use: Upper respiratory combination, antitussive, expectorant, decongestant.

Entex LA. (Andrx) Phenylephrine hydrochloride (extended release) 30 mg, guaifenesin (immediate release) 400 mg. Maltodextrin, sucrose. Cap. Bot. 100s. *Rx.*
Use: Upper respiratory combination, decongestant, expectorant.

Entex Liquid. (Andrx) Phenylephrine hydrochloride 7.5 mg, guaifenesin 100 mg/5 mL, alcohol and dye free, punch flavor. Liq. Bot. 15 mL, 473 mL. *Rx.*
Use: Upper respiratory combination, decongestant, expectorant.

Entex PSE. (Andrx) Pseudoephedrine hydrochloride (extended release) 120 mg, guaifenesin (immediate release) 400 mg. Maltodextrin, sucrose. Cap. Bot. 100s. *Rx.*
Use: Upper respiratory combination, decongestant, expectorant.

Entocort EC. (Prometheus) Budesonide 3 mg (micronized), sugar spheres. Cap. Bot. 100s. *Rx.*
Use: Adrenocortical steroid, glucocorticoid.

entoidoin.
See: Entodon.

Entolase HP. (Wyeth) Lipase 8000 units, protease 50,000 units, amylase 40,000 units. Cap. (enteric coated microbeads). Bot. 100s, 250s. *Rx.*
Use: Digestive enzyme.

Entrition Half Strength. (Biosearch Medical Products) Calcium and sodium caseinates, maltodextrin, corn oil, soy lecithin, monoglycerides and diglycerides, protein 17.5 g, carbohydrate 68 g, fat 17.5 g, Na 350 mg, K 600 mg, calories 0.5/mL, osmolarity 120 mOsm/kg, water, vitamins A, B_1, B_2, B_3, B_5, B_6, B_{12}, C, D, E, K, Ca, P, Mg, I, Fe, Zn, Mn, Cu, Cl, biotin, choline, folic acid. Pouch 1 liter. *OTC.*
Use: Nutritional supplement.

Entrition HN Entri-Pak. (Biosearch Medical Products) Sodium and calcium caseinates, soy protein isolate, maltodextrin, corn oil, soy lecithin, monoglycerides and diglycerides, vitamins A, B_1, B_2, B_3, B_5, B_6, B_{12}, C, D, E, K, folic acid, biotin, choline, Ca, Cl, Cu, Fe, I, Mg, Mn, P, Zn. Pouch 1 liter. *OTC.*
Use: Nutritional supplement.

Entrobag Set. (Lafayette) Enteroclysis set. Case 6 sets.
Use: Enteroclysis of the small intestine.

Entrobar. (Mallinckrodt) Barium sulfate 50%, simethicone. Susp. Bot. 500 mL

w/ or w/out kit. *Rx.*
Use: Radiopaque agent, GI contrast agent.
EntroEase. (Mallinckrodt) Barium sulfate 13%, simethicone. Susp. Bot. 600 mL. *Rx.*
Use: Radiopaque agent, GI contrast agent.
EntroEase Dry. (Mallinckrodt) Barium sulfate 92%. Pow. for Susp. Can. 90 g. *Rx.*
Use: Radiopaque agent, GI contrast agent.
Entrokit. (Lafayette) Barium sulfate susp. (*Entrobar*), methylcellulose (*Entrolcel*). Case 4 kits.
Use: Radiopaque agent.
Entrolcel. (Lafayette) Methylcellulose 1.8% w/w concentrate for dilution at time of use. Bot. 500 mL, case 24 Bot.
Use: Diagnostic aid.
•**entsufon sodium.** (ENT-sue-fahn) USAN.
Use: Detergent.
Entuss. (Roberts) **Tab.:** Hydrocodone bitartrate 5 mg, guaifenesin 300 mg. Bot. 100s. **Syr.:** Hydrocodone bitartrate 5 mg, potassium guaiacolsulfonate 300 mg/5 mL, alcohol free. Bot. 120 mL, 480 mL. *c-III.*
Use: Antitussive, expectorant.
Entuss-D Junior. (Roberts) Pseudoephedrine hydrochloride 30 mg, hydrocodone bitartrate 2.5 mg, guaifenesin 100 mg w/alcohol 5%, saccharin, sorbitol, sucrose. Liq. Bot. 120 mL, pt. *c-III.*
Use: Antitussive, expectorant combination.
Entuss-D Liquid. (Roberts) Hydrocodone bitartrate 5 mg, pseudoephedrine 30 mg/5 mL. 473 mL. *c-III.*
Use: Antitussive, decongestant.
Entuss-D Tablets (Roberts) Pseudoephedrine 30 mg, hydrocodone bitartrate 5 mg, guaifenesin 300 mg. Tab. Bot. 100s. *c-III.*
Use: Antitussive, decongestant, expectorant.
Enuclene. (Alcon) Tyloxapol 0.25%. Soln. *Drop-tainer* 15 mL. *OTC.*
Use: Artificial eye care.
Enulose. (Alra) Lactulose 10 g, (< galactose 1.6 g, lactose 1.2 g, other sugars 1.2 g). Soln. Bot. 473 mL, 1.89 L. *Rx.*
Use: Laxative.
•**enviradene.** (en-VIE-rah-DEEN) USAN.
Use: Antiviral.
Enviro-Stress. (Vitaline) Vitamins B$_1$ 50 mg, B$_2$ 50 mg, B$_3$ 100 mg, B$_5$ 50 mg, B$_6$ 50 mg, B$_{12}$ 25 mcg, C 600 mg, E 30 units, folic acid 0.4 mg, zinc 30 mg,

Mg, Se, PABA. SR Tab. Bot. 90s, 1000s. *OTC.*
Use: Mineral, vitamin supplement.
•**enviroxime.** (en-VIE-rox-eem) USAN.
Use: Antiviral.
Envisan Treatment Multipack. (Hoechst) Dextranomer with PEG 3000 and PEG 600. Paste 10 g packets with nylon net and semi-occlusive film. *OTC.*
Use: Dermatologic, wound therapy.
•**enzacamene.** (en-za-KAM-een) USAN.
Use: Sunscreen.
•**enzastaurin hydrochloride.** (en-za-STORE-in) USAN.
Use: Antineoplastic.
Enzest. (Barth's) Seven natural enzymes, calcium carbonate 250 mg. Tab. Bot. 100s, 250s, 500s. *OTC.*
Use: Digestive enzymes, antacid.
Enzobile Improved. (Roberts) Pancreatic enzyme concentrate 100 mg, ox bile extract 100 mg, cellulase 10 mg in inner core and pepsin 150 mg in outer layer. EC Tab. Bot. 100s. *Rx-OTC.*
Use: Digestive enzymes.
Enzone. (Forest) Hydrocortisone acetate 1%, pramoxine hydrochloride 1% in hydrophilic base w/stearic acid, aquaphor, isopropyl palmitate, polyoxyl 40, stearate, triethanolamine lauryl sulfate. Cream. Tube 30 g w/rectal applicator. *Rx.*
Use: Corticosteroid combination.
Enzymatic Cleaner for Extended Wear. (Alcon) Highly purified pork pancreatin to dilute in saline solution. Tab. Pkg. 12s. *OTC.*
Use: Contact lens care.
enzyme combinations, topical.
See: Accuzyme.
    Ethezyme.
    Ethezyme 830.
    Gladase.
    GranulDerm.
    Granulex.
    Panafil.
    Papain-Urea-Chlorophyllin.
Enzyme Formula #E-2. (Barth's) Amylase 30 mg, lipase 25 mg, bile salts 1 g, wilzyme 10 mg, pepsin 2 g, pancreatin 0.5 g, calcium carbonate 4 g. Tab. Bot. 100s, 250s. *Rx-OTC.*
Use: Digestive aid.
enzyme preparations.
See: Collagenase.
    Enzyme Combinations, Topical.
enzymes.
See: Alpha Chymar.
    Cholinesterase.
    Chymotrypsin.

Cotazym.
Creon.
Diastase.
Pancreatin.
Papain.
Pepsin.
EPA. (NBTY) N-3 fat content (mg) EPA 180 mg, DHA 120 mg, vitamin E 1 units. Cap. Bot. 50s, 100s. *OTC.*
Use: Nutritional supplement.
●**eperezolid.** (eh-per-EH-zoe-lid) USAN.
Use: Anti-infective.
●**ephedrine.** (eh-FED-rin) *USP 28.*
Use: Adrenergic (bronchodilator).
See: Bofedrol Inhalant.
Racephedrine hydrochloride.
W/Procaine.
See: Ephedrine and Procaine.
●**ephedrine hydrochloride.** (eh-FED-rin) *USP 28.*
Use: Bronchodilator.
W/Combinations.
See: Broncholate.
Bronkaid Dual Action.
Ceepa.
Co-Xan.
Derma Medicone.
Derma Medicone HC.
Dynafed Asthma Relief.
Golacol.
Kie.
Lardet.
Lardet Expectorant.
Mini Two Way Action.
Mudrane.
Mudrane GG.
Primatene.
Quelidrine.
Quibron Plus.
ephedrine hydrochloride. (Various Mfr.)
Ephedrine hydrochloride. Cryst. Box 0.25 oz, 4 oz.
Use: Bronchodilator.
ephedrine hydrochloride nasal jelly.
See: Efedron Nasal.
●**ephedrine sulfate.** (eh-FED-rin) *USP 28.*
Use: Bronchodilator, sympathomimetic.
See: Pretz-D.
W/Combinations.
See: Bronkaid.
Marax.
Marax DF.
Pazo.
Wyanoids.
ephedrine sulfate. (West-Ward) Ephedrine sulfate 25 mg. Cap. Bot. 100s. *OTC.*
Use: Bronchodilator, sympathomimetic.
ephedrine sulfate. (Various Mfr.) Ephedrine sulfate 50 mg. Inj. Amp. 1 mL. *Rx.*

Use: Bronchodilator, sympathomimetic.
ephedrine sulfate and phenobarbital.
Use: Bronchodilator; hypnotic; sedative.
ephedrine tannate w/combinations.
See: Quad Tann.
Rynatuss.
Rynatuss Pediatric.
Tuss-Tan.
Tuss-Tan Pediatric.
Ephenyllin. (CMC) Theophylline 130 mg, ephedrine hydrochloride 24 mg, phenobarbital 8 mg. Tab. Bot. 100s, 500s, 1000s. *Rx.*
Use: Bronchodilator; decongestant; hypnotic; sedative.
Epi-C. (Mallinckrodt) Barium sulfate 150%, simethicone, spearmint flavor. Susp. Bot. 450 mL. *Rx.*
Use: Radiopaque agent, GI contrast agent.
●**epicillin.** (EH-pih-SILL-in) USAN.
Use: Anti-infective.
epidermal growth factor (human). (Chiron Therapeutics)
Use: Accelerate corneal healing.
[Orphan Drug]
epidermal growth factor receptor inhibitors.
See: Erlotinib.
Geftinib.
Epi-Derm Balm. (Pedinol Pharmacal) Methyl salicylate, menthol, propylene glycol, alcohol. Bot. Gal. *OTC.*
Use: Analgesic, topical.
Epifoam. (Schwarz Pharma) Hydrocortisone acetate 1%, pramoxine hydrochloride 1% in base of propylene glycol, cetyl alcohol, PEG-100 stearate, glyceryl stearate, laureth-23, polyoxyl 40 stearate, methylparaben, propylparaben, trolamine, or hydrochloric acid to adjust pH, purified water, butane, propane inert propellant. Aerosol container 10 g. *Rx.*
Use: Corticosteroid, topical.
Epiform-HC. (Delta Pharmaceutical Group) Hydrocortisone 1%, iodohydroxyquin 3% in cream base. Tube 20 g. *Rx.*
Use: Antifungal; corticosteroid, topical.
Epilyt. (Stiefel) Propylene glycol, glycerin, oleic acid, quaternium-26, lactic acid, BHT. Lotion. Bot. 118 mL. *OTC.*
Use: Emollient.
●**epimestrol.** (EH-pih-MESS-trole) USAN.
Use: Anterior pituitary activator.
Epinal. (Alcon) Epinephrine borate 0.5%, 1%. Dropper Bot. 7.5 mL. *Rx.*
Use: Antiglaucoma.
epinastine hydrochloride. (epp-ih-NASteen) USAN.

Use: Ophthalmic antihistamine.
See: Elestat.
epinephran.
See: Epinephrine.
●**epinephrine.** (epp-ih-NEFF-rin) *USP 28.*
Use: Bronchodilator, sympathomimetic, vasopressor.
See: Adrenalin Chloride.
  Asmolin.
  Asthma Meter.
  Emergency Ana-Kit.
  Epinephrine Mist.
  EpiPen.
  EpiPen Jr.
  microNefrin.
  Nephron.
  Primatene Mist.
  S2.
W/Combinations.
See: Septocaine.
W/Lidocaine hydrochloride.
See: Ardecaine.
  Lidocaine and Epinephrine.
  Lidocaine hydrochloride.
  Lidocaine hydrochloride and Epinephrine.
  Lidosite Topical System.
  Octocaine.
  Xylocaine.
  Xylocaine MPF.
epinephrine. (Abbott) Epinephrine 1:1000 (1 mg/mL), sodium metabisulfite 0.9 mg, sodium chloride 9 mg/mL. 1 mL amp. Epinephrine 1:10,000 (0.01 mg/mL), sodium metabisulfite 0.46 mg, sodium chloride 8.16 mg/mL. Soln. Single-dose *Abboject* (prefilled) syringe 10 mL as either 18–G/3½ inch needle or 21–G1½ needle, single-dose *Abboject* (prefilled) 10 mL *LifeShield* syringe 10 mL vials. *Rx.*
Use: Asthma, hayfever, acute allergic states, cardiac arrest, acute hypersensitivity reactions, adrenergic (vasoconstrictor).
epinephrine. (Various Mfr.) Epinephrine 1:1000 (1 mg/mL as hydrochloride), 1:10,000 (0.1 mg/mL). Soln. Inj. Amp. 1 mL (1:1000 only) (may contain sodium metabisulfite). Prefilled Syr. 10 mL (1:10,000 only), sodium bisulfite. *Rx.*
Use: Bronchodilator, sympathomimetic.
●**epinephrine bitartrate.** (epp-ih-NEFF-rin) *USP 28.*
Use: Adrenergic, ophthalmic.
epinephrine borate.
Use: Adrenergic, ophthalmic.
See: Epinal.
epinephrine hydrochloride.
See: Adrenalin Cl.
  Ana-Guard Epinephrine.

  EpiEZPen.
  EpiEZPen Jr.
  Epinal.
  EpiPen.
  EpiPen Jr.
  Sus-Phrine.
  Vaponefrin.
epinephrine hydrochloride. (Ciba Vision) Epinephrine hydrochloride 0.1%. Soln. 1 mL Dropperettes (12s). *Rx.*
Use: Adrenergic, ophthalmic. Emergency kit, anaphylaxis.
epinephrine hydrochloride. (Various Mfr.) Epinephrine hydrochloride 1 mg/mL (1:1000 solution). Inj. Amp 1 mL. 0.1 mg/mL (1:10,000 solution). Inj. Vial 10 mL. *Rx.*
Use: Bronchodilator.
Epinephrine Mist. (Various Mfr.) Epinephrine 0.22 mg/spray, may contain alcohol. Aer. Kit 15 mL. *OTC.*
Use: Bronchodilator, sympathomimetic.
epinephrine, racemic.
See: AsthmaNefrin.
epinephrine-related compounds.
See: Sympathomimetic agents.
●**epinephryl borate ophthalmic solution.** (EPP-ih-NEFF-rill) *USP 28.*
Use: Adrenergic.
epinephryl borate ophthalmic solution.
Use: Adrenergic, ophthalmic.
See: Epinal.
  Eppy.
EpiPen. (Dey) Epinephrine injection 1:1000 (1 mg/mL), sodium metabisulfite 0.5 mg, sodium chloride 1.8 mg. Single-dose auto-injector 0.3 mL. *Rx.*
Use: Emergency kit.
EpiPen Jr. (Dey) Epinephrine injection 1:2000 (0.5 mg/mL), sodium chloride 1.8 mg, sodium metabisulfite 0.5 mg. Single-dose auto-injectors 0.3 mL. *Rx.*
Use: Emergency kit.
●**epipropidine.** (EPP-ih-PRO-pih-deen) USAN.
Use: Antineoplastic.
EpiQuin Micro. (SkinMedica) Hydroquinone 4%, vitamin A, E, and C, cetyl alcohol, benzyl alcohol, EDTA, glycerin, methylparaben, sodium metabisulfite. Cream. 30 g. *Rx.*
Use: Dermatologic, pigment agent.
epirenan.
See: Epinephrine.
●**epirizole.** (eh-PEER-IH-zole) USAN.
Use: Analgesic; anti-inflammatory.
●**epirubicin hydrochloride.** (EH-pih-ROO-bih-sin) USAN.
Use: Antineoplastic; antibiotic.

See: Ellence.

•**epitetracycline hydrochloride.** (epp-ih-TEH-trah-SIGH-kleen HIGH-droe-KLOR-ide) *USP 28.*
Use: Anti-infective.

•**epithiazide.** (EH-pih-THIGH-azz-ide) USAN.
Use: Antihypertensive; diuretic.

Epitol. (Teva) Carbamazepine 200 mg. Lactose. Tab. Bot. 100s. *Rx.*
Use: Anticonvulsant.

Epivir. (GlaxoSmithKline) Lamivudine. **Tab.:** 150 mg, 300 mg. Bot. 30s (300 mg only), 60s (150 mg only). **Oral Soln.:** 10 mg/mL, parabens, sucrose, strawberry-banana flavor. Bot. 240 mL. *Rx.*
Use: Antiretroviral agent, nucleoside reverse transcriptase inhibitor.

Epivir-HBV. (GlaxoSmithKline) Lamivudine. **Tab.:** 100 mg. Bot. 60s. **Oral Soln.:** 5 mg/mL, sucrose, parabens, strawberry-banana flavor. Bot. 240 mL. *Rx.*
Use: Antiretroviral agent, nucleoside reverse transcriptase inhibitor.

•**eplerenone.** (eh-PLER-en-ohn) USAN.
Use: Antihypertensive, aldosterone antagonist, renin angiotensin system antagonist.
See: Inspra.

EPO.
See: Epogen.
Procrit.

•**epoetin alfa, recombinant.** (eh-POE-eh-tin) USAN.
Use: Antianemic; hematinic; hematopoietic.
See: Epogen.
Procrit.

•**epoetin beta.** (eh-POE-eh-tin) USAN.
Use: Hematopoietic; hematinic; antianemic. [Orphan Drug]

•**epoetin delta.** (eh-POE-eh-tin) USAN.
Use: Antianemic.

Epogen. (Amgen) Epoetin alfa (Erythropoietin; EPO) 2,000 units/mL, 3,000 units/mL, 4,000 units/mL, 10,000 units/mL, 20,000 units/mL, 40,000 units/mL. Preservative free w/2.5 mg albumin (human) per mL. Single-dose vials. 1 mL (except 20,000 units/mL and 40,000 units/mL). Multidose vials. 1 mL (20,000 units/mL, 40,000 units/mL only), 2 mL (10,000 units/mL only) (benzyl alcohol 1%). *Rx.*
Use: Hematopoietic.

•**epoprostenol.** (EH-poe-PROSTE-eh-nole) USAN. *Formerly Prostacyclin,*

PGI_2, *Prostagland in* I_2, *Prostaglandin X, PGX.*
Use: Inhibitor (platelet). Primary pulmonary hypertension.
See: Flolan.

•**epoprostenol sodium.** (EH-poe-PROSTE-eh-nole) USAN.
Use: Inhibitor (platelet).
See: Flolan.

•**epostane.** (EH-poe-stain) USAN.
Use: Interceptive.

epoxytropine tropate methylbromide.
See: Methscopolamine Bromide.

Eppy/N. (PBH Wesley Jessen) Epinephryl borate ophthalmic soln. 0.5%, 1%, 2%. Bot. 7.5 mL. *Rx.*
Use: Antiglaucoma.

•**epristeride.** (eh-PRISS-the-ride) USAN.
Use: Inhibitor (alpha reductase.)

Epromate. (Major) Aspirin 325 mg, meprobamate 200 mg Tab. Bot. 100s, 500s. *c-iv.*
Use: Analgesic; anxiolytic.

•**eprosartan.** (eh-pro-SAHR-tan) USAN.
Use: Antihypertensive.

eprosartan and hydrochlorothiazide.
Use: Antihypertensive.
See: Teveten HCT.

•**eprosartan mesylate.** (eh-pro-SAHR-tan) USAN.
Use: Antihypertensive.
See: Teveten.

Epsal. (Press Chem. & Pharm Labs) Saturated soln. of epsom salts 80% in ointment form. Jar 0.5 oz, 2 oz. *OTC.*
Use: Drawing ointment.

Epsivite Forte. (Standex) Vitamin E 1000 units. Cap. Bot. 100s. *OTC.*
Use: Vitamin supplement.

Epsivite 400. (Standex) Vitamin E 400 units. Cap. Bot. 100s. *OTC.*
Use: Vitamin supplement.

Epsivite 100. (Standex) Vitamin E 100 units. Cap. Bot. 100s. *OTC.*
Use: Vitamin supplement.

Epsivite 200. (Standex) Vitamin E 200 units. Cap. Bot. 100s. *OTC.*
Use: Vitamin supplement.

Epsom salt. (Various Mfr.) Magnesium sulfate. Gran. Bot. 120 g, 1 lb., 4 lb. *OTC.*
Use: Laxative.
See: Magnesium Sulfate.

eptifibatide.
Use: Antiplatelet agent, glycoprotein IIb/IIIa inhibitor.
See: Integrilin.

eptoin.
See: Phenytoin Sodium.

e.p.t. Stick Test. (Parke-Davis) Reagent in-home kit for urine testing. Pregnancy test. Kit 1s. *OTC.*
Use: Diagnostic aid.

Epulor. (VistaPharm) **Liq.:** Fat 31 g, carbohydrate 5 g, protein 4 g, calories 315/serving, biotin 100 mcg, Ca 333 mg, chloride 12 mg, Cr 40 mcg, Cu 200 mcg, folic acid 133 mcg, I 50 mcg, Fe 6 mg, Mg 133 mg, Mn 667 mcg, Mo 25 mcg, P 333 mg, K 35 mg, Se 23 mcg, Si 667 mcg, Na 7 mg, Sn 3 mcg, V 3 mcg, vitamin A 1667 units, B_1 500 mcg, B_2 567 mcg, B_3 7 mg, B_5 3 mg, B_6 667 mcg, B_{12} 2 mcg, Ni 2 mcg, C 20 mg, D 133 units, E 58 units, K 8 mcg, Zn 5 mg. Pkg. 24s. **Pow.:** Protein (milk protein, isoleucine, leucine, lysine, methionine/cystine, phenylalanine/tyrosine, threonine, trytophan, valine) 89 g, fat (soybean oil) 755 g/L, vitamin A, B_1, B_2, B_3, B_5, B_6, B_{12}, C, D, E, K, biotin, folate, B, Ca, chloride, Cr, Cu, Fe, I, Mg, Mn, Mo, Ni, P, Se, Si, Sn, V, Zn, lemon flavor, 7.1 cal/mL. Pouch. 1.5 oz. *OTC.*
Use: Nutritional therapy, enteral.

Epzicom. (GlaxoSmithKline) Abacavir (as sulfate) 600 mg/lamivudine 300 mg. Film coated. Tab. 30s. *Rx.*
Use: Antiretroviral agent.

Equal. (Nutrasweet) Aspartame. **Packet:** 0.035 oz. (1 g). Box 50s, 100s, 200s. **Tab.:** Bot. 100s. *OTC.*
Use: Artificial sweetener.

Equalactin. (Numark) Calcium polycarbophil 625 mg (equivalent to 500 mg polycarbophil), citrus acid flavor. Chew. Tab. Bot. 24s, 48s. *OTC.*
Use: Antidiarrheal; laxative.

Equazine M. (Rugby) Aspirin 325 mg, meprobamate 200 mg, tartrazine. Tab. Bot. 100s, 500s. *c-iv.*
Use: Analgesic; anxiolytic.

Equetro. (Shire) Carbamazepine 100 mg, 200 mg, 300 mg. Lactose. ER Cap. 120s. *Rx.*
Use: Anticonvulsant.

•**equilin.** *USP 28.*
Use: Estrogen.

Equipertine. (Sanofi-Synthelabo) Oxypertine. Cap. *Rx.*
Use: Anxiolytic.

Eradacil. (Sanofi-Synthelabo) Rosoxacin. Cap. *Rx.*
Use: Antigonococcal agent.

Eramycin. (Wesley) Erythromycin FC Tab. Bot. 100s, 500s. *Rx.*
Use: Anti-infective; erythromycin.

Erbitux. (Bristol-Myers Squibb) Cetuximab 2 mg/mL. Preservative-free. So-dium phosphate dibasic heptahydrate 1.88 mg/mL, sodium phosphate monobasic monohydrate 0.42 mg/mL. Inj. Single-use 50 mL vial. *Rx.*
Use: Monoclonal antibody.

•**erbulozole.** (ehr-BYOO-low-zole) USAN.
Use: Radiosensitizer; antineoplastic (adjunct).

Ercaf. (Geneva) Ergotamine tartrate 1 mg, caffeine 100 mg. Tab. Bot. 100s, 1000s. *Rx.*
Use: Antimigraine.

Ergamisol. (Janssen) Levamisole (base) 50 mg. Tab. Blister pack 36s. *Rx.*
Use: Antineoplastic.

Ergo Caff. (Rugby) Ergotamine tartrate 1 mg, caffeine 100 mg. Tab. Bot. 100s. *Rx.*
Use: Antimigraine.

•**ergocalciferol.** (ehr-go-kal-SIFF-eh-role) *USP 28. Formerly Oleovitamin D, Synthetic; Calciferol.*
Use: Treatment of refractory ricket; familial hypophosphatemia; hypoparathyroidism, vitamin (antirachitic).
See: Calciferol.
Drisdol.

ergocornine. (Various Mfr.) Ergot alkaloid. *Rx.*
Use: Peripheral vascular disorders.

ergocristine. (Various Mfr.) Ergot alkaloid. *Rx.*
Use: Vascular disorders.

ergocryptine. (Various Mfr.) Ergot alkaloid. *Rx.*
Use: Peripheral vascular disorders.

•**ergoloid mesylates.** (err-GO-loyd) *USP 28. Formerly Dihydroergotoxine Mesylate; Dihydroergotoxine Methanesulfonate; Dihydrogenated Ergot Alkaloids, Hydrogenated Ergot Alkaloids.*
Use: Psychotherapeutic; cognition adjuvant.
See: Hydergine.

Ergomar. (Lotus Biochemical) Ergotamine tartrate 2 mg, lactose, saccharin. Sublingual Tab. Pkg. 20s. *Rx.*
Use: Antimigraine.

ergometrine maleate.
See: Ergonovine.

Ergonal. (Vita Elixir) Ergot powder 259.2 mg, aloin 8.1 mg, apiol fluid green 290 mg, oil pennyroyal 28 mg. Cap. Bot. 24s. *Rx.*
Use: Oxytocic.

ergonovine. (Various Mfr.) Ergobasine, ergometrine, ergostetrine, ergotocine. *Rx.*
Use: Oxytocic.
See: Ergonovine Maleate.

• **ergonovine maleate.** (ehr-go-NO-veen)
USP 28.
Use: Oxytocic.
See: Ergotrate.
ergosterol, activated, or irradiated.
USP 28.
See: Ergocalciferol.
ergostetrine.
See: Ergonovine.
Ergot Alkalside Dihydrogenated.
See: Ergoloid mesylates.
ergotamine derivatives.
See: Dihydroergotamine Mesylate.
Ergotamine Tartrate.
• **ergotamine tartrate.** (ehr-GOT-ah-
mean) *USP 28.*
Use: Analgesic (specific in migraine).
See: Ergomar.
W/Belladonna alkaloids, phenobarbital.
See: Bellamine.
Cafergot P-B.
W/Caffeine, homatropine methylbromide.
See: Cafergot.
W/Cyclizine hydrochloride, caffeine.
See: Ergotatropin.
W/Combinations.
See: Folergot-DF.
ergotamine tartrate and caffeine.
(West-Ward) Ergotamine tartrate 1 mg,
caffeine 100 mg. Sugar, mannitol. Tab.
30s, 100s, 500s. *Rx.*
Use: Migraine combination.
**ergotamine tartrate and caffeine sup-
positories.**
Use: Vascular headache; analgesic
(specific in migraine).
See: Cafergot.
**ergotamine tartrate and caffeine
tablets.**
Use: Vascular headache; analgesic
(specific in migraine).
ergot, fluid extract. (Various Mfr.) Ergot
1 g/mL Bot. 4 oz, pt.
ergotidine.
See: Histamine.
ergotocine.
See: Ergonovine.
Ergotrate. (HPS Rx Enterprises) Ergono-
vine maleate 0.2 mg. Mannitol. Tab.
100s, 500s, 1,000s. *Rx.*
Use: Oxytocic.
ergot-related products.
See: Cafergot.
Cafergot P-B.
D.H.E. 45.
Ergonovine.
Ergotamine.
Ergotrate.
Hydergine.
Hydro-Ergot.

Methergine.
Wigraine.
eriodictin.
See: Vitamin P & Rutin.
eriodictyon. Flext., aromatic syrup.
Use: Pharmaceutic aid (flavor).
See: Vitamin P & Rutin.
• **eritoran tetrasodium.** (ER-i-TORE-an)
USAN.
Use: Endotoxin antagonist.
• **erlotinib.** (er-LOE-tye-nib) USAN.
Use: Epidermal growth factor receptor
inhibitor.
See: Tarceva.
E-R-O. (Scherer) Propylene glycol, gly-
cerol. Bot. w/dropper tip 15 mL. *OTC.*
Use: Otic.
Errin. (Barr) Norethindrone 0.35 mg, lac-
tose. Tab. Box. 28s. *Rx.*
Use: Sex hormone, contraceptive hor-
mone.
• **ersofermin.** (EER-so-FEER-min) USAN.
Use: Dermatologic, wound therapy.
Ertaczo. (OrthoNeutrogena) Sertacona-
zole nitrate 2%. Light mineral oil, meth-
ylparaben. Cream. Tubes. 15 g, 30 g.
Rx.
Use: Antifungal.
• **ertapenem sodium.** (er-ta-PEN-em)
USAN.
Use: Antibacterial; carbapenem.
See: Invanz.
Ertine. (Health for Life Brands) Hexa-
chlorophene, benzocaine, cod liver oil,
allantoin, boric acid, lanolin. Tube
1.5 oz. *Rx.*
Use: Burn and first aid remedy.
• **ertiprotafib.** (er-ti-PROE-ta-fib) USAN.
Use: Antidiabetic.
erwina L-asparaginase.
Use: Acute lymphocytic leukemia.
See: Erwinase.
Erwinase. (Porton Product Limited) Er-
winia L-asparaginase.
Use: Acute lymphocytic leukemia.
[Orphan Drug]
Eryc. (FH Faulding & Co. Ltd.) Erythro-
mycin 250 mg. Enteric-coated pellets.
DR Cap. Bot. 100s. *Rx.*
Use: Anti-infective; erythromycin.
Erycette. (Ortho-McNeil) Erythromycin
2%. Pkg. 60 pledgets. *Rx.*
Use: Dermatologic, acne.
Erymax. (Allergan) Erythromycin 2%.
Soln. 59 mL, 118 mL. *Rx.*
Use: Dermatologic, acne.
Ery Pads. (Glades) Erythromycin 2%, al-
cohol 60.5%. Pledgets. 60s. *Rx.*
Use: Anti-infective, topical.

Erypar. (Parke-Davis) Erythromycin stearate. Filmseal. **250 mg:** Bot. 100s, 500s. **500 mg:** Bot. 100s. *Rx.*
Use: Anti-infective; erythromycin.
EryPed Drops. (Abbott) Erythromycin ethylsuccinate (as base) 100 mg/ 2.5 mL. Sucrose, fruit flavor. Susp. Bot. 50 mL. *Rx.*
Use: Anti-infective; erythromycin.
EryPed 400. (Abbott) Erythromycin ethylsuccinate (as base) 400 mg/5 mL when reconstituted. Sucrose, banana flavor. Pow. for Oral Susp. Bot. 60 mL, 100 mL, 200 mL, UD 5 mL (100s). *Rx.*
Use: Anti-infective; erythromycin.
EryPed 200. (Abbott) Erythromycin ethylsuccinate (as base) 200 mg/5 mL when reconstituted. Sucrose, fruit flavor. Pow. for Oral Susp. Bot. 100 mL, 200 mL, UD 5 mL (100s). *Rx.*
Use: Anti-infective; erythromycin.
Ery-Tab. (Abbott) Erythromycin enteric coated 250 mg, 333 mg, 500 mg. DR Tab. Bot. 100s, 500s (except 500 mg), UD 100s. *Rx.*
Use: Anti-infective; erythromycin.
•**erythrityl tetranitrate, diluted.** (eh-RITH-rih-till TEH-trah-NYE-trate) *USP 28. Formerly Erythrol Tetranitrate.*
Use: Coronary vasodilator.
See: Cardilate.
erythrityl tetranitrate tablets. (Various Mfr.) Erythritol, erythrol tetranitrate, nitroerythrite, tetranitrin, tetranitrol.
Use: Coronary vasodilator.
See: Anginar.
W/Phenobarbital.
See: Cardilate.
Erythrocin Lactobionate. (Hospira) Erythromycin lactobionate (as base) 500 mg, 1 g. May contain benzyl alcohol. Pow. for Inj., lyophilized. Vials. *Rx.*
Use: Anti-infective; erythromycin.
•**erythromycin.** (eh-RITH-row-MY-sin) *USP 28.*
Use: Anti-infective.
See: Akne-Mycin.
A/T/S.
Del-Mycin.
E-Base.
Emgel.
E-Mycin.
Erymax.
Ery Pads.
Erythrocin.
Erythromycin.
Erythromycin Base.
Erythromycin Estolate.
Erythromycin Ethylsuccinate.
Erythromycin Lactobionate.
Erythromycin Stearate.
Ilotycin.
Robimycin.
erythromycin. (Various Mfr.) Erythromycin base 250 mg. Enteric-coated pellets. DR Cap. 100s, 500s. *Rx.*
Use: Anti-infective.
•**erythromycin acistrate.** (eh-RITH-row-MY-sin ass-IH-strate) USAN.
Use: Anti-infective.
erythromycin base.
Use: Anti-infective.
See: Eryc.
Ery-Tab.
Erythromycin Filmtabs.
PCE Dispertab.
erythromycin-benzoyl peroxide.
(Various Mfr.) Erythromycin 3%, benzoyl peroxide 5%. Gel. 23 g, 46 g. *Rx.*
Use: Anti-infective.
•**erythromycin estolate.** (eh-RITH-row-MY-sin ESS-toe-late) *USP 28. Formerly Erythromycin Propionate Lauryl Sulfate.*
Use: Anti-infective; erythromycin.
erythromycin estolate. (Alpharma) Erythromycin estolate (as base) 125 mg/5 mL, 250 mg/5 mL. May contain EDTA, parabens, saccharin, sucrose. Susp. Bot. 473 mL. *Rx.*
Use: Anti-infective.
•**erythromycin ethylsuccinate.** (eh-RITH-row-MY-sin ETH-il-SUX-i-nate) *USP 28.*
Use: Anti-infective; erythromycin.
See: E.E.S.
EryPed.
erythromycin ethylsuccinate. (Various Mfr.) Erythromycin ethylsuccinate (as base). **Tab.:** 400 mg. Bot. 100s, 500s. **Susp.:** 200 mg/5 mL, 400 mg/5 mL. Bot. 473 mL. *Rx.*
Use: Anti-infective.
erythromycin ethylsuccinate and sulfisoxazole acetyl for oral suspension. (eh-RITH-row-MY-sin Eth-ill-SUCK-sih-nate and sull-fih-SOX-ah-zole ASS-eh-till)
Use: Anti-infective.
See: Pediazole.
erythromycin filmtabs. (Abbott) Erythromycin base 250 mg, 500 mg. Film coated. Tab. Bot. 100s; 500s, UD 100s (except 500 mg). *Rx.*
Use: Anti-infective; erythromycin.
erythromycin gel. (Glades) Erythromycin 2%, alcohol 95%. Gel. Tube 30 g, 60 g. *Rx.*
Use: Dermatologic, acne.

- **erythromycin gluceptate, sterile.** (eh-RITH-row-MY-sin glue-SEP-tate) *USP 28.*
  Use: Anti-infective; erythromycin.
  See: Ilotycin Gluceptate.
- **erythromycin glucoheptonate.**
  See: Erythromycin Gluceptate, Ilotycin Glucoheptonate.
- **erythromycin lactobionate.** (eh-RITH-row-MY-sin lack-toe-BYE-oh-nate) *USP 28.*
  Use: Anti-infective; erythromycin.
  See: Erythrocin Lactobionate.
- **erythromycin ointment.** (Various Mfr.) Erythromycin 0.5%. Oint. Tube 3.5 g. *Rx.*
  Use: Anti-infective, topical.
- **erythromycin pledgets.** (eh-RITH-row-MY-sin)
  Use: Anti-infective; erythromycin.
- **Erythromycin Pledgets.** (Glades) Erythromycin 2%, alcohol 68.5%. Pledgets. Bot. 60s. *Rx.*
  Use: Anti-infective; erythromycin.
- **erythromycin propionate.** (eh-RITH-row-MY-sin) USAN.
  Use: Anti-infective.
- **erythromycin propionate lauryl sulfate.**
  Use: Anti-infective; erythromycin.
  See: Erythromycin Estolate. Ilosone.
- **erythromycin salnacedin.** (eh-RITH-row-MY-sin sal-NAH-seh-din) USAN.
  Use: Dermatologic, acne.
- **erythromycin stearate.** (eh-RITH-row-MY-sin STEE-ah-rate) *USP 28.*
  Use: Anti-infective; erythromycin.
- **erythromycin stearate.** (Abbott) Erythromycin stearate (as base) 250 mg, 500 mg. Film coated. Tab. Bot. 100s, 500s (250 mg only). *Rx.*
  Use: Anti-infective.
- **erythromycin sulfate.**
  Use: Anti-infective; erythromycin.
- **erythromycin tablets.** (Various Mfr.) Erythromycin 100 mg, 250 mg. Tab. Bot. 25s (250 mg only,) 100s. *Rx.*
  Use: Anti-infective.
- **erythromycin topical.** (Various Mfr.) Erythromycin. **Gel:** 2%. Contains alcohol. Tube 30 g, 60 g. **Soln.:** 2%. Contains alcohol. Bot. 60 mL. *Rx.*
  Use: Dermatologic, acne.
- **erythromycin 2-propionate dodecyl sulfate.** *USP 28.* Erythromycin Estolate
  Use: Anti-infective; erythromycin.
- **erythrosine sodium.** *USP 28.*
  Use: Diagnostic aid (dental disclosing agent).

- **Eryzole.** (Alra) Erythromycin ethylsuccinate 200 mg, acetyl sulfisoxazole 600 mg/5 mL when reconstituted. Gran. for Susp. 100 mL, 150 mL, 200 mL. *Rx.*
  Use: Anti-infective.
- **escitalopram oxalate.** (ESS-sigh-TAL-oh-pram)
  Use: Antidepressant, serotonin reuptake inhibitor.
  See: Lexapro.
- **esclabron.** Guaithylline.
  Use: Antiasthmatic.
- **Esclim.** (Women First Healthcare) Estradiol 5 mg (0.025 mg/day), 7.5 mg (0.0375 mg/day), 10 mg (0.05 mg/day), 15 mg (0.075 mg/day), 20 mg (0.1 mg/day). Transdermal system. Patient pack 8s. *Rx.*
  Use: Estrogen.
- **Eserdine Forte Tabs.** (Major) Methyclothiazide, reserpine 0.5 mg. Bot. 100s. *Rx.*
  Use: Antihypertensive; diuretic.
- **Eserdine Tabs.** (Major) Methyclothiazide, reserpine 0.25 mg. Bot. 100s, 250s. *Rx.*
  Use: Antihypertensive; diuretic.
- **Eserine.** Physostigmine as alkaloid, salicylate or sulfate salt. *Rx.*
  Use: Antiglaucoma.
- **Eserine Salicylate.** (Alcon) Physostigmine 0.5%. Soln. 2 mL. *Rx.*
  Use: Antiglaucoma.
- **Eserine Sulfate Sterile Ophthalmic Ointment.** (Ciba Vision) Physostigmine sulfate 0.25%. Tube 3.5 g. *Rx.*
  Use: Antiglaucoma.
- **Esgic.** (Gilbert Laboratories.) Butalbital 50 mg, caffeine 40 mg, acetaminophen 325 mg. Cap. Tab. Bot. 100s. *Rx.*
  Use: Analgesic; hypnotic; sedative.
- **Esgic-Plus.** (Forest) Acetaminophen 500 mg, butalbital 50 mg, caffeine 40 mg. Tab. Bot. 100s, 500s. Cap. Bot. 20s, 100s, 500s. *Rx.*
  Use: Analgesic; hypnotic; sedative.
- **Esidrix.** (Novartis) Hydrochlorothiazide 25 mg, 50 mg. Tab. **25 mg:** Bot. 100s, 1000s, UD 100s. **50 mg:** Bot. 100s, 360s, 720s, 1000s, UD 100s. *Rx.*
  Use: Antihypertensive; diuretic.
  W/Apresoline.
  See: Apresoline-Esidrix.
- **Esimil.** (Novartis) Hydrochlorothiazide 25 mg, guanethidine monosulfate 10 mg. Tab. Bot. 100s. *Rx.*
  Use: Antihypertensive; diuretic.
- **Eskalith.** (GlaxoSmithKline) Lithium carbonate 300 mg. Cap. Bot. 100s, 500s. *Rx.*
  Use: Antipsychotic.

Eskalith CR. (GlaxoSmithKline) Lithium carbonate 450 mg. CR Tab. Bot. 100s. *Rx.*
Use: Antipsychotic.

•**esmolol hydrochloride.** (ESS-moe-lahl) USAN.
Use: Antiadrenergic/sympatholytic, beta-adrenergic blocking agent.
See: Brevibloc.
    Brevibloc Double Strength.

esmolol hydrochloride. (Baxter) Esmolol hydrochloride 10 mg/mL. Preservative-free. Inj. Vials. 10 mL. *Rx.*
Use: Antiadrenergic/sympatholytic, beta-adrenergic blocking agent.

•**esomeprazole magnesium.** (es-oh-ME-pray-zole) USAN.
Use: Proton pump inhibitor.
See: Nexium.

•**esomeprazole sodium.** (es-oh-ME-pray-zole) USAN.
Use: Proton pump inhibitor.
See: Nexium.

•**esorubicin hydrochloride.** (ESS-oh-ROO-bih-sin) USAN.
Use: Antineoplastic.

Esoterica Dry Skin Treatment Lotion. (GlaxoSmithKline) Bot. 13 fl oz. *OTC.*
Use: Emollient.

Esoterica Facial. (Medicis) Hydroquinone 2%, octyldimethyl PABA, benzophone, stearyl alcohol, sodium bisulfite, parabens, EDTA. Cream. Tube 90 g. *OTC.*
Use: Dermatologic.

Esoterica Regular. (Medicis) Hydroquinone 2%, light mineral oil, stearyl alcohol, parabens, sodium bisulfite, EDTA. Cream. Jar 90 g. *OTC.*
Use: Dermatologic.

Esoterica Sunscreen. (Medicis) Hydroquinone 2%, padimate O 3.3%, oxybenzone 2.5%, mineral oil, parabens, sodium bisulfite, EDTA. Cream. Jar 85 g. *OTC.*
Use: Dermatologic.

•**esoxybutynin chloride.** (es-ox-i-BUE-ti-nin) USAN.
Use: Antispasmodic, anticholinergic.

•**esproquin hydrochloride.** (ESS-pro-kwin) USAN.
Use: Adrenergic.

Essential-8. Liquid amino acid protein supplement.
Use: Protein supplement.
See: Vivonex Diets.

Essential ProPlus. (NutriSoy) Protein 16.3 g, fat 0.2 g, carbohydrates 6.4 g, Na 242.5 mg, K 112.5 mg, Ca 70 mg, Mg 31.3 mg, Fe 3 mg, P 187.5 mg, Cu 0.4 mg, Zn 0.5 mg, I 12.9 mcg, B_1 0.1 mg, B_3 0.2 mg, folic acid 0.1 mg/ 25 g. Pow. Cont. 2 lb. *OTC.*
Use: Nutritional supplement.

Essential Protein. (NutriSoy) Protein 16 g, fat 0.3 g, carbohydrates 5.6 g, sodium 5 mg, K 750 mg, Ca 97.5 mg, Mg 80 mg, Fe 2.5 mg, P 202.5 g, Cu 0.4 mg, Zn 0.8 mg, I 10 mcg, B_1 0.1 mg, B_3 0.2 mg, B_6 0.1 mg, folic acid 0.1 mg/25 g. Pow. Cont. 2 lb. *OTC.*
Use: Nutritional supplement.

•**estazolam.** (ess-TAZZ-OH-lam) USAN.
Use: Sedative/hypnotic, nonbarbiturate.
See: ProSom.

estazolam. (Zenith-Goldline) Estazolam 1 mg, 2 mg Tab. Bot. 30s, 100s, 500s, 1000s. *Rx.*
Use: Sedative/hypnotic, nonbarbiturate.

Ester-C Plus 500 mg Vitamin C. (Solgar) Vitamin C 500 mg, citrus bioflavonoids 25 mg, acerola 10 mg, rutin 5 mg, rose hips 10 mg, calcium 62 mg, sodium free. Cap. Bot. 250s. *OTC.*
Use: Mineral, vitamin supplement.

Ester-C Plus Multi-Mineral. (Solgar) Vitamin C 425 mg, citrus bioflavonoid complex 50 mg, acerola 12.5 mg, rose hips 12.5 mg, rutin 5 mg, calcium 25 mg, magnesium 13 mg, potassium 12.5 mg, zinc 2.5 mg, sodium free. Cap. Bot. 60s, 90s. *OTC.*
Use: Mineral, vitamin supplement.

Ester-C Plus 1000 mg Vitamin C. (Solgar) Vitamin C 1000 mg, citrus bioflavonoid complex 200 mg, acerola 25 mg, rutin 25 mg, rose hips 25 mg, calcium 125 mg, sodium free. Tab. Bot. 90s. *OTC.*
Use: Mineral, vitamin supplement.

esterified estrogens.
See: Estrogens, esterified.

•**esterifilcon a.** (ess-TER-ih-FILL-kahn A) USAN.
Use: Contact lens material, hydrophilic.

ester local anesthetics.
Use: Injectable local anesthetic.
See: Chloroprocaine Hydrochloride.
    Procaine Hydrochloride.
    Tetracaine Hydrochloride.

Estilben.
See: Diethylstilbestrol Dipropionate.

Estinyl. (Schering-Plough) Ethinyl estradiol. **Tab., coated. 0.02 mg, 0.05 mg:** Bot. 100s, 250s; **Tab. 0.5 mg:** Bot. 100s. *Rx.*
Use: Estrogen.

estopen.
See: Benzylpenicillin 2-diethylamino-ethyl ester HI.

Estrace. (Warner Chilcott) Estradiol micronized 0.5 mg, 1 mg, 2 mg, lactose, tartrazine (2 mg only). Tab. Bot. 100s, 500s (except 0.5 mg). *Rx.*
Use: Estrogen.
Estrace Vaginal. (Warner Chilcott) Estradiol 0.1 mg/g in a nonliquefying base, EDTA, methylparaben, steryl alcohol. Cream. Tube w/calibrated applicator 42.5 g. *Rx.*
Use: Estrogen.
Estracon. (Freeport) Conjugated estrogens 1.25 mg. Tab. Bot. 1000s. *Rx.*
Use: Estrogen.
Estraderm. (Novartis) Estradiol 4 mg (0.05 mg/day), 8 mg (0.1 mg/day). Calendar packs of 8 and 24 systems. *Rx.*
Use: Estrogen.
estradiol (ESS-trah-DIE-ole) *USP 29.* The form now known to be physiologically active is the β form rather than the α.
Use: Estrogen.
See: Alora.
　Aquagen.
　Climara.
　Esclim.
　Estrace.
　Estraderm.
　Estring.
　Estrogel.
　Femogen.
　FemPatch.
　Gynodial.
　Progynon.
　Vivelle.
　Vivelle-Dot.
W/Estriol, estrone.
See: Hormonin No. 1 and 2.
W/Estrone, estriol.
See: Sanestro.
W/Estrone, potassium estrone sulfate.
See: Tri-Estrin.
W/Norethindrone acetate.
See: CombiPatch.
W/Norgestimate.
See: Prefest.
W/Progesterone, testosterone, procaine hydrochloride, procaine base.
See: Horm-Triad.
W/Testosterone and chlorobutanol in cottonseed oil.
See: Climara.
　Depo-Testadiol.
　Estraderm.
estradiol. (Various Mfr.) Micronized estradiol 0.5 mg, 1 mg, 2 mg. May contain lactose. Tab. Bot. 100s, 500s (except 0.5 mg). *Rx.*
Use: Estrogen.

• **estradiol acetate.** (ESS-trah-DIE-ole) USAN.
Use: Estrogen.
estradiol cyclopentylpropionate.
W/Testosterone cypionate.
See: Depo-Testadiol.
• **estradiol cypionate.** (ESS-trah-DIE-ole SIP-ee-oh-nate) *USP 28.*
Use: Estrogen.
See: Depo-Estradiol.
W/Estradiol cyclopentylpropionate.
See: depGynogen.
　DepoGen.
　Estroject-L.A.
　Hormogen Depot.
　Span-A.
W/Testosterone cypionate.
See: Dep-Testestro.
　Menoject, L.A.
W/Testosterone cypionate, chlorobutanol.
See: Depo-Testadiol.
　Span FM.
　TE Ionate P.A.
estradiol cypionate. (Various Mfr.) Estradiol cypionate 5 mg/mL, cottonseed oil w/chlorobutanol. Inj. Vial. 10 mL. *Rx.*
Use: Estrogen.
estradiol dipropionate.
Use: Estrogen.
• **estradiol enanthate.** (ESS-trah-DIE-ole eh-NAN-thate) USAN.
Use: Estrogen.
estradiol, ethinyl.
See: Ethinyl Estradiol.
estradiol hemihydrate.
Use: Estrogen.
See: Vagifem.
estradiol, micronized.
Use: Estrogen.
See: Estrace.
　Gynodial.
estradiol monobenzoate
See: Estradiol benzoate.
estradiol, oral. (Teva) Micronized estradiol 0.5 mg, 1 mg, 2 mg. Tab. Bot. 100s. *Rx.*
Use: Estrogen.
estradiol, topical emulsion.
Use: Sex hormone.
See: Estrasorb.
estradiol transdermal system.
Use: Estrogen.
See: Alora.
　Climara.
　ClimaraPro.
　CombiPatch.
　Esclim.
　Estraderm.
　Menostar.
　Vivelle.
　Vivelle-Dot.

estradiol transdermal system. (Mylan)
Estradiol 1.94 mg (0.05 mg/day),
3.88 mg (0.1 mg/day). Patch. 4s. *Rx.*
Use: Estrogen.
• **estradiol undecylate.** (ESS-trah-DIE-ole
UHN-DEH-sill-ate) USAN.
See: Delestrec.
estradiol vaginal cream. (ESS-trah-DIE-
ole)
Use: Estrogen.
• **estradiol valerate.** (ESS-trah-DIE-ole
VAL-eh-rate) *USP 28.*
Use: Estrogen.
See: Ardefem 10, 20.
Deladiol.
Delestrogen.
Depogen.
Dioval.
Duragen.
Duratrad.
Estate.
Estra-L.
Gyneticsogen L.A.
Span-Est.
Valergen.
W/Benzyl alcohol.
See: Estate.
W/Hydroxyprogesterone caproate.
See: Depo-Testadiol.
W/Testosterone enanthate.
See: Ardiol 90/4, 180/8.
Deladumone.
Delatestadiol.
Duoval-P.A.
Estra-Testrin.
Span-Est-Test 4.
Teev.
Tesogen LA.
Valertest.
estradiol valerate. (Various Mfr.) Estra-
diol valerate 20 mg/mL, 40 mg/mL. Inj.
Vial 10 mL. 40 mg/mL. Vial 10 mL. *Rx.*
Use: Estrogen.
Estra-L. (Taylor Pharmaceuticals) Estra-
diol valerate in oil 40 mg/mL. Vial
10 mL. *Rx.*
Use: Estrogen.
• **estramustine.** (ESS-truh-muss-TEEN)
USAN.
Use: Antineoplastic.
• **estramustine phosphate sodium.** (Ess-
truh-muss-TEEN) USAN.
Use: Antineoplastic, alkylating agent.
See: Emcyt.
Estrasorb. (Novavax) Estradiol hemihy-
drate 2.5 mg/g. Soybean oil, ethanol.
Top. Emulsion. 1.74 g pouches (each
pouch contains estradiol hemihydrate
4.35 mg). *Rx.*
Use: Sex hormone; estrogen.

Estratab. (Solvay) Esterified estrogens
0.3 mg, 0.625 mg, 2.5 mg. Tab. Bot.
100s, 1000s (0.625 mg only). *Rx.*
Use: Estrogen.
Estratest. (Solvay) Esterified estrogens
1.25 mg, methyltestosterone 2.5 mg,
lactose, sucrose, parabens. Tab. Bot.
100s, 1000s. *Rx.*
Use: Estrogen, androgen combination.
Estratest H.S. (Solvay) Esterified estro-
gens 0.625 mg, methyltestosterone
1.25 mg, lactose, sucrose, parabens.
Tab. Bot. 100s. *Rx.*
Use: Estrogen, androgen combination.
• **estrazinol hydrobromide.** (ESS-trazz-
ih-nahl) USAN.
Use: Estrogen.
estrin.
See: Estrone.
Estrinex. (Pharmacia)
See: Toremifene.
Estring. (Pharmacia) Estradiol 2 mg.
Vaginal ring. Single packs. *Rx.*
Use: Estrogen.
• **estriol.** (ESS-tree-ole) *USP 28.*
Use: Estrogen.
Estrobene DP.
See: Diethylstilbestrol Dipropionate.
Estrofem. (Taylor Pharmaceuticals)
Estradiol cypionate 5 mg/mL in oil. Inj.
Vial 10 mL.
Use: Estrogen.
• **estrofurate.** (ESS-troe-FYOOR-ate)
USAN.
Use: Estrogen.
Estrogel. (Unimed) Estradiol 0.06%
(estradiol 0.75 mg/1.25 g unit dose). Al-
cohol. Gel. Pump. 93 g. Tube. 80 g.
Rx.
Use: Sex hormone.
estrogen and androgen combinations.
Use: Sex hormone.
See: Estratest.
Estratest H.S.
estrogen-androgen therapy.
See: Androgen-estrogen therapy.
estrogenic substance aqueous.
(Various Mfr.) Estrogenic substance or
estrogens (mainly estrone) 2 mg/mL.
Inj. Vial 10 mL, 30 mL. *Rx.*
Use: Estrogen.
estrogenic substances, conjugated.
(Water-soluble) A mixture containing
the sodium salts of the sulfate esters of
the estrogenic substances, principally
estrone and equilin that are of the type
excreted by pregnant mares. *Rx.*
See: Aquagen.
Ces.
Estroject, I.V.

Estroquin.
Estrosan.
Evestrone.
Orapin.
Prelestrin.
Premarin.
W/Ethinyl estradiol.
See: Demulen.
W/Meprobamate.
See: Milprem.
PMB 400.
PMB 200.
W/Methyltestosterone.
See: Estratest.
Estratest HS.
Premarin with Methyltestosterone.
estrogenic substances in aqueous suspension. (Wyeth) Sterile estrone suspension 2 mg/mL. Vial 10 mL. Rx.
Use: Estrogen.
estrogenic substances mixed. May be a crystalline or an amorphous mixture of the naturally occurring estrogens obtained from the urine of pregnant mares. **Aqueous Susp.:** Inj. **Cap.:** W/Androgen therapy, vitamins, iron, d-desoxyephedrine hydrochloride.
See: Gravigen, Inj. Aqueous Susp.
Premarin w/methyltestosterone, Cap.
estrogen/nitrogen mustard.
Use: Alkylating agent.
See: Estramustine Phosphate Sodium.
estrogens.
Use: Sex hormones.
See: Conjugated Estrogens.
Esterified Estrogens.
Estradiol.
Estradiol Cypionate in Oil.
Estradiol Topical Emulsion.
Estradiol Transdermal System
Estradiol Valerate in Oil.
Estropipate.
Synthetic Conjugated Estrogens, A.
Synthetic Conjugated Estrogens, B.
Topical Estrogens, Miscellaneous.
•**estrogens, conjugated.** (ESS-truh-janz KAHN-juh-gay-tuhd) USP 28.
Use: Estrogen.
See: Conest.
Ganeake.
PMB.
Premarin.
Premarin Intravenous.
Premarin with Methyltestosterone.
estrogens, conjugated and medroxy-progesterone acetate.
Use: Sex hormone.
See: Premphase.
Prempro.
estrogens equine.
See: Estrogen.

PMB.
Premarin.
Premarin with Methyltestosterone.
•**estrogens, esterified.** (ESS-troe-jenz, ess-TER-ih-fide) USP 28.
Use: Estrogen.
See: Estratab.
Menest.
Menogen.
Menogen HS.
estrogens, esterified & androgens.
Use: Estrogen, androgen supplement.
See: Estratab.
Estratest.
Menest.
estrogens, miscellaneous topical.
Use: Sex hormone, estrogen.
See: Estrogel.
•**estrogens, miscellaneous, vaginal.**
Use: Estrogen, sex hormone
See: Estrace Vaginal.
Estring.
Femring.
Ogen Vaginal.
Premarin Vaginal.
Vagifem.
estrogens, natural.
Use: Estrogen.
See: Depogen.
Estradiol.
Estrogenic Substance.
Estrone.
PMB.
Premarin.
Premarin with Methyltestosterone.
estrogens and progestins combined.
Use: Sex hormone.
See: Activella.
Alesse.
Anri.
Aviane.
Brevicon.
ClimaraPro.
CombiPatch.
Demulen 1/50.
Demulen 1/35.
Desogen.
Estrostep Fe.
Estrostep 21.
Femhrt.
Jenest-28.
Levlen.
Levlite.
Levora.
Loestrin Fe 1/20.
Loestrin Fe 1.5/30.
Loestrin 21 1/20.
Loestrin 21 1.5/30.
Lo/Ovral.
Low-Ogestrel.
Microgestin Fe 1/20.

Microgestin Fe 1.5/30.
Mircette.
Modicon.
MonoNessa.
Necon 1/50.
Necon 1/35.
Necon 10/11.
Necon 0.5/35.
Nordette.
Norinyl 1 + 50.
Norinyl 1 + 35.
Nortrel 1/35.
Nortrel 0.5/35.
Ogestrel.
Ortho-Cept.
Ortho-Cyclen.
Ortho-Novum 1/50.
Ortho-Novum 1/35.
Ortho-Novum 7/7/7.
Ortho-Novum 10/11.
Ortho-Prefest.
Ortho Tri-Cyclen.
Ovcon-50.
Ovcon-35.
Ovral-28.
Prefest.
Premphase.
Prempro.
Tri-Levlen.
Tri-Norinyl.
Triphasil.
Trivora-28.
Yasmin.
Zovia 1/50E.
Zovia 1/35E.
estrogens, synthetic.
See: Cenestin.
Dienestrol.
Diethylstilbestrol.
Enjuvia.
Stilphostrol.
Estrogestin A. (Harvey) Estrogenic sub-
stance 1 mg, progesterone 10 mg/mL
in peanut oil. Vial 10 mL. Rx.
Use: Estrogen, progestin combination.
Estrogestin C. (Harvey) Estrogenic sub-
stance 1 mg, progesterone 12.5 mg/mL
in peanut oil. Vial 10 mL. Rx.
Use: Estrogen, progestin combination.
•**estrone.** (ESS-trone) USP 28.
Use: Estrogen.
See: Bestrone Suspension.
Estrogenic Substances in Aqueous
Susp.
Foygen.
Kestrone 5.
Menagen.
Menformon (A).
Par-Supp.
Propagon-S.
Theelin.

W/Estriol, estradiol.
See: Hormonin.
W/Estrogens.
See: Estrogenic Mixtures.
Estrogenic Substances.
W/Hydrocortisone acetate.
See: Ovulin.
W/Lactose.
See: Estrovag.
W/Potassium estrone sulfate.
See: Mer-Estrone.
Sodestrin.
W/Progesterone.
See: Duovin-S.
W/Testosterone.
See: Andesterone.
Anestro.
Di-Hormone.
Di-Met.
Diorapin.
DI-Steroid.
Estratest
W/Testosterone, sodium carboxymethyl-
cellulose, sodium chloride.
See: Android-G.
Geratic Forte.
Geriamic.
Geritag.
estrone aqueous. (Various Mfr.) Estrone
aqueous 5 mg/mL. Inj. Vial 10 mL. Rx.
Use: Estrogen.
estrone sulfate, piperazine.
See: Ogen.
estrone sulfate, potassium.
See: Estrogen.
•**estropipate.** (ESS-troe-PIH-pate)
USP 28. Formerly Piperazine Estrone
Sulfate.
Use: Estrogen.
See: Ogen.
Ortho-Est.
estropipate. (Various Mfr.) Estropipate
0.75 mg, 1.5 mg, 3 mg, 6 mg. Tab. Bot.
30s, 100s, 500s. Rx.
Use: Estrogen.
Estroquin. (Sheryl) Purified conjugated
estrogens 1.25 mg. Tab. Bot. 100s. Rx.
Use: Estrogen.
Estrostep Fe. (Warner Chilcott) Norethin-
drone acetate 1 mg, ethinyl estradiol
20 mcg. Triangular Tab. Norethindrone
acetate 1 mg, ethinyl estradiol 30 mcg.
Square Tab. Norethindrone acetate
1 mg, ethinyl estradiol 35 mcg. Round
Tab. Ferrous fumarate 75 mg, lactose,
sucrose. Box. 28s. Rx.
Use: Sex hormone, contraceptive hormone.
Estrostep 21. (Pfizer) Norethindrone
acetate 1 mg, ethinyl estradiol 20 mcg.
Triangular Tab. Norethindrone acetate

1 mg, ethinyl estradiol 30 mcg. Square Tab. Norethindrone acetate 1 mg, ethinyl estradiol 35 mcg. Round Tab. Lactose. Box. 21s. *Rx.*
Use: Sex hormone, contraceptive hormone.

•**eszopiclone.** (es-zoe-PIK-lone) USAN.
Use: Insomnia.
See: Lunesta.

•**etafedrine hydrochloride.** (EH-tah-FED-rin) USAN.
Use: Bronchodilator; adrenergic.
See: Nethamine.

•**etafilcon a.** (EH-tah-FILL-kahn A) USAN.
Use: Contact lens material, hydrophilic.

Etalent. (Roger) Ethaverine hydrochloride 100 mg. Cap. Bot. 50s, 500s. *Rx.*
Use: Vasodilator.

•**etalocib.** (e-TAL-oh-kib) USAN.
Use: Antineoplastic.

•**etanercept.** (et-a-NER-sept) UCAN.
Use: Antiarthritic; immunologic agent, immunomodulator.
See: Enbrel.

•**etanidazole.** (ETT-ah-NIDE-ah-zole) USAN.
Use: Antineoplastic (hypoxic cell radiosensitizer).

•**etarotene.** (ett-AHR-oh-teen) USAN.
Use: Keratolytic.

•**etazolate hydrochloride.** (eh-TAY-zoe-late) USAN.
Use: Antipsychotic.

Eterna 27. (Revlon) Pregnenolone acetate 0.5% in cream base. *OTC.*
Use: Emollient.

•**eterobarb.** (ee-TEER-oh-barb) USAN.
Use: Anticonvulsant.

•**ethacrynate sodium for injection.** (ETH-ah-KRIN-ate) *USP 28.*
Use: Diuretic.
See: Edecrin Sodium I.V.

•**ethacrynic acid.** (eth-uh-KRIN-ik) *USP 28.*
Use: Diuretic.
See: Edecrin.

•**ethambutol hydrochloride.** (eth-AM-byoo-tahl) *USP 28.*
Use: Anti-infective (tuberculostatic).
See: Myambutol.

Ethamicort.
See: Hydrocortamate.

•**ethamivan.** (eth-AM-ih-van) USAN.
Use: Stimulant (central and respiratory).

Ethamolin. (Questcor) Ethanolamine oleate 5%. Inj. Amp. 2 mL. *Rx.*
Use: Sclerosing agent.

•**ethamsylate.** (ETH-AM-sill-ate) USAN.
Use: Hemostatic.

ethanol. (Various Mfr.) Alcohol, anhydrous.

ethanolamine. Olamine.

•**ethanolamine oleate.** (ETH-ah-nahl-ah-MEEN OH-lee-ate) USAN.
Use: Sclerosing agent.
See: Ethamolin.

ethanolamines, nonselective.
Use: Antihistamine.
See: Carbinoxamine Maleate.
Clemastine Fumarate.
Diphenhydramine Hydrochloride.

EtheDent. (Ethex) Fluoride 0.25 mg, 0.5 mg, 1 mg. Chew. Tab. 120s, 1000s (0.5 mg, 1 mg). *Rx.*
Use: Dental caries agent.

ethenol, homopolymer. *USP 28.* Polyvinyl alcohol.

•**ether.** (EE-ther) *USP 28.*
Use: Anesthetic, general; inhalation.

Ethezyme. (Ethex) Papain 1.1 × 10^6 units and urea 100 mg per g. Hydrophilic base. EDTA, glycerin, parabens. Oint. 30 g. *Rx.*
Use: Enzyme preparation.

Ethezyme 830. (Ethex) Papain 8.3 × 10^5 units, urea 100 mg/g in a hydrophilic ointment base, EDTA, glycerin, parabens. Oint. Tube. 30 g. *Rx.*
Use: Enzyme preparation.

•**ethinyl estradiol.** (ETH-in-ill ess-trah-DIE-ole) *USP 28.*
Use: Estrogen.
See: Estinyl.
Feminone.
Menolyn.

ethinyl estradiol. (Bio-Technology General)
Use: Turner syndrome. [Orphan Drug]

ethinyl estradiol and dimethisterone tablets.
Use: Estrogen, progestin combination.

ethinyl estradiol w/combinations.
See: Alesse.
Apri.
Aranelle.
Aviane.
Brevicon.
Cesia.
Demulen 1/50.
Demulen 1/35.
Desogen.
Estrostep Fe.
Estrostep 21.
Femhrt.
GenCept.
Jenest-28.
Junel Fe 1/20.
Junel Fe 1.5/30.
Leena.

Levlen.
Levlite.
Levora.
Loestrin 21 1/20.
Loestrin 21 1.5/30.
Loestrin Fe 1/20.
Loestrin Fe 1.5/30.
Lo/Ovral.
Low-Ogestrel.
Lutera.
Microgestin Fe 1/20.
Microgestin Fe 1.5/30.
Mircette.
Modicon.
MonoNessa.
Nelova 1/35E.
Nelova 10/11.
Nelova 0.5/35E.
Nelulen.
Nordette.
Norinyl 1 + 35.
Norlestrin.
Norlestrin Fe.
NuvaRing.
Ortho-Cept.
Ortho-Cyclen.
Ortho-Evra.
Ortho-Novum 1/35, 7/7/7, 10/11.
Ortho Tri-Cyclen.
Ovcon-50.
Ovcon-35.
Ovlin.
Ovral-28.
Preven.
Seasonale.
Solia.
Tri-Levlen.
Tri-Norinyl.
Triphasil.
Tri-Previfem.
Trivora-28.
Velivet.
Yasmin.
Zovia 1/50E.
Zovia 1/35E.
ethinyl estrenol.
See: Lynestrenol.
•**ethiodized oil injection.** (eth-EYE-oh-dized) *USP 28.*
Use: Radiopaque agent.
See: Ethiodol.
•**ethiodized oil I 131.** (eth-EYE-oh-dized OIL I 131) USAN.
Use: Antineoplastic; radiopharmaceutical.
Ethiodol. (Savage) Ethiodized oil (iodine 37%). Iodine 475 mg/mL, poppyseed oil 1%. Inj. Amp. 10 mL. *Rx.*
Use: Radiopaque agent.
•**ethionamide.** (eh-THIGH-ohn-ah-mide) *USP 28.*

Use: Anti-infective (tuberculostatic).
See: Trecator-SC.
ethisterone.
See: Anhydrohydroxyprogesterone.
Ethmozine. (Shire) Moricizine hydrochloride 200 mg, 250 mg, 300 mg. Lactose. Tab. 100s, UD 100s. *Rx.*
Use: Antiarrhythmic.
Ethocaine.
See: Procaine hydrochloride.
ethocylorvynol. *USP 28.*
ethodryl.
See: Diethylcarbamazine citrate.
ethohexadiol. Used in Comp. dimethyl phthalate.
Use: Insect repellent.
•**ethonam nitrate.** (ETH-oh-nam NYE-trate) USAN.
Use: Antifungal.
•**ethosuximide.** (ETH-oh-SUX-ih-mide) *USP 28.*
Use: Anticonvulsant.
See: Zarontin.
ethosuximide. (Copley) Ethosuximide 250 mg/5 mL, saccharin, sucrose, raspberry flavor. Syr. Bot. 483 mL. *Rx.*
Use: Anticonvulsant.
ethosuximide. (Sidmark) Ethosuximide 250 mg. Cap. 100s. *Rx.*
Use: Anticonvulsant.
•**ethotoin.** (ETH-oh-toyn) *USP 28.*
Use: Anticonvulsant.
See: Peganone.
ethovan. Ethyl Vanillin.
•**ethoxazene hydrochloride.** (eth-OX-ah-zeen) USAN.
Use: Analgesic.
ethoxzolamide.
Use: Carbonic anhydrase inhibitor.
Ethrane. (Ohmeda) Enflurane. Volatile Liq. Bot. 125 mL, 250 mL. *Rx.*
Use: Anesthetic, general.
•**ethybenztropine.** (ETH-ih-BENZ-troe-peen) USAN.
Use: Anticholinergic.
•**ethyl acetate.** (ETH-ill) *NF 23.*
Use: Pharmaceutic aid, flavoring; solvent.
ethyl aminobenzoate. Anesthesin, anesthrone, benzocaine, parathesin.
Use: Anesthetic, local.
See: Benzocaine.
ethyl bromide. (Various Mfr.) Bromoethane. *Rx.*
Use: Anesthetic, general.
ethyl carbamate.
See: Urethan.
•**ethylcellulose.** (eth-il-SEL-yoo-lose) *NF 23.*

Use: Tablet binder; pharmaceutic aid.
ethylcellulose aqueous dispersion.
Use: Tablet binder; pharmaceutic aid.
ethyl chaulmoograte.
Use: Hansen disease; sarcoidosis.
● **ethyl chloride.** (ETH-ill) *USP 28.*
Use: Anesthetic, topical.
ethyl chloride. (Various Mfr.) Ethyl chloride 100 g chloroethane. Spray. Bot. 105 mL, 120 mL. *Rx.*
Use: Anesthetic, local.
● **ethyl dibunate.** (ETH-ill DIE-byoo-nate) USAN.
Use: Cough suppressant; antitussive.
ethyl diiodobrassidate. Iodobrassid. Lipoiodine.
ethyldimethylammonium bromide.
See: Ambutonium bromide.
ethylene. (Various Mfr.) Ethene. *Rx.*
Use: Anesthetic, general.
● **ethylenediamine** (eth-ih-leen-DIF-ah-meen) *USP 28.*
Use: Component of aminophylline injection.
ethylenediamine solution. (67% w/v).
Use: Solvent (Aminophylline Inj.).
ethylenediamine tetraacetic acid disodium salt.
See: Endrate Disodium.
ethylenediaminetetraacetic acid.
See: Edathamil.
EDTA.
ethylenimines/methylmelamines.
Use: Alkylating agents.
See: Altretamine.
Thiotepa.
● **ethylestrenol.** (ETH-ill-ESS-tree-nahl) USAN.
Use: Anabolic.
ethylhydrocupreine hydrochloride.
Use: Antiseptic.
ethylmorphine hydrochloride.
Use: Narcotic.
ethyl nitrite spirit. Ethyl nitrite. Sweet Spirit of Niter. Spirit of Nitrous Ether.
● **ethyl oleate.** (ETH-ill) *NF 23.*
Use: Pharmaceutic aid (vehicle).
ethyl oxide; ethyl ether.
Use: Solvent.
● **ethylparaben.** (eth-ill-PAR-ah-ben) *NF 23.*
Use: Pharmaceutic aid (antifungal preservative).
ethylstibamine. Astaril, neostibosan.
Use: Antimony therapy.
● **ethyl vanillin.** (ETH-ill) *NF 23.*
Use: Pharmaceutic aid (flavor).
● **ethynerone.** (eth-EYE-ner-ohn) USAN.
Use: Hormone, progestin.

● **ethynodiol diacetate.** (eh-THIN-oh-die-ole die-ASS-eh-tate) *USP 28.*
Use: Progesterone, progestin.
W/Ethinyl estradiol.
See: Demulen.
Estrostep Fe.
Estrostep 21.
Nelulen.
Ovulen.
Zovia.
W/Mestranol.
See: Ovulen.
ethynodiol diacetate and ethinyl estradiol tablets.
Use: Contraceptive.
ethynodiol diacetate and mestranol tablets.
Use: Contraceptive.
ethynylestradiol.
See: Ethinyl Estradiol.
Mestranol.
ethynylestradiol 3-methyl ether.
See: Enovid.
Ethyol. (MedImmune Oncology) Amifostine 500 mg (anhydrous basis). Pow. for Inj., lyophilized. Single-use vial 10 mL. *Rx.*
Use: Antineoplastic; cytoprotective agent.
● **etibendazole.** (eh-tie-BEN-dah-ZOLE) USAN.
Use: Anthelmintic.
Eticylol. (Novartis) Ethinyl estradiol. *Rx.*
Use: Estrogen.
● **etidocaine.** (eh-TIE-doe-cane) USAN.
Use: Anesthetic, local.
● **etidronate disodium.** (eh-TIH-DROE-nate) *USP 28.*
Use: Bisphosphonate.
See: Didronel.
Didronel IV.
● **etidronic acid.** (eh-tih-DRAH-nik) USAN.
Use: Calcium regulator.
● **etifenin.** (EH-tih-FEN-in) USAN.
Use: Diagnostic aid.
● **etilevodopa.** (et-il-ee-voe-DOE-a) USAN.
Use: Parkinson disease.
● **etintidine hydrochloride.** (ett-IN-tih-DEEN) USAN.
Use: Antiulcerative.
etiocholanedoine. (SuperGen)
Use: Aplastic anemia; Prader-Willi syndrome. [Orphan Drug]
● **etiprednol dicloacetate.** (e-ti-PRED-nole dye-KLOE-a-se-tate) USAN.
Use: Anti-inflammatory; corticosteroid.
● **etocrylene.** (EH-toe-KRIH-leen) USAN.
Use: Ultraviolet screen.

●**etodolac.** (EE-toe-DOE-lak) *USP 28.*
Use: Analgesic; NSAID.
See: Lodine.
Lodine XL.
etodolac. (Various Mfr.) Etodolac **Tab.:**
400 mg, 500 mg. Bot. 100s, 500s,
1000s (400 mg only). **Cap.:** 200 mg,
300 mg. Bot. 100s, 500s, 1000s. **ER**
Tab.: 400 mg, 500 mg, 600 mg. Bot.
100s, 500s (400 mg only). *Rx.*
Use: Analgesic; NSAID.
●**etofenamate.** (EH-toe-FEN-am-ate)
USAN.
Use: Analgesic; anti-inflammatory.
●**etoformin hydrochloride.** (EH-toe-
FORE-min) USAN.
Use: Antidiabetic.
●**etomidate.** (eh-TAHM-ih-date) USAN.
Use: Hypnotic; sedative.
See: Amidate.
etomide hydrochloride. (ETT-oh-mide)
Bandol. carbiphene hydrochloride.
●**etonogestrel.** (ETT-oh-no-JESS-trell)
USAN.
Use: Hormone, progestin.
W/Ethinyl estradiol.
See: NuvaRing.
●**etoperidone hydrochloride.** (EH-toe-
PURR-ih-dohn) USAN.
Use: Antidepressant.
See: Vepesid.
Etopophos. (Bristol-Myers Squibb On-
cology/Virology) Etoposide phosphate
diethanolate 119.3 mg (100 mg etopo-
side), dextran 40 300 mg. Pow. for Inj.
Vial. Single dose. *Rx.*
Use: Antineoplastic.
●**etoposide.** (EH-toe-POE-side) *USP 28.*
Use: Antineoplastic.
See: Etopophos.
Toposar.
Vepesid.
etoposide. (Various Mfr.) Etoposide
20 mg/mL, alcohol 30.5%, benzyl alco-
hol 30 mg, polysorbate 80 80 mg, PEG
300 650 mg, citric acid 2 mg/mL. Inj.
Vial 5 mL, 12.5 mL, 25 mL. *Rx.*
Use: Antineoplastic.
●**etoposide phosphate.** (ee-toe-POE-
side) USAN.
Use: Antineoplastic.
See: Etopophos.
●**etoprine.** (ETT-oh-preen) USAN.
Use: Antineoplastic.
etoval.
See: Butethal.
●**etoxadrol hydrochloride.** (eh-TOX-ah-
drole) USAN.
Use: Anesthetic.

●**etozolin.** (EAT-oh-zoe-lin) USAN.
Use: Diuretic.
Etrafon-A (4-10). (Schering-Plough) Per-
phenazine 4 mg, amitriptyline hydro-
chloride 10 mg. Tab. Bot. 100s, UD
100s. *Rx.*
Use: Psychotherapeutic combination.
Etrafon Forte (4-25). (Schering-Plough)
Perphenazine 4 mg, amitriptyline hy-
drochloride 25 mg. Tab. Bot. 100s,
500s, UD 100s. *Rx.*
Use: Psychotherapeutic combination.
Etrafon (2-10). (Schering-Plough) Per-
phenazine 2 mg, amitriptyline hydro-
chloride 10 mg. Tab. Bot. 100s, 500s,
UD 100s. *Rx.*
Use: Psychotherapeutic combination.
Etrafon (2-25). (Schering-Plough) Per-
phenazine 2 mg, amitriptyline hydro-
chloride 25 mg. Tab. Bot. 100s, 500s,
UD 100s. *Rx.*
Use: Psychotherapeutic combination.
●**etretinate.** (eh-TRETT-ih-nate) USAN.
Use: Antipsoriatic.
etrynit. Propatyl nitrate.
Use: Cardiovascular agent.
●**etryptamine acetate.** (ee-TRIP-tah-
meen) USAN.
Use: Central stimulant.
E.T.S.-2%. (Paddock) Erythromycin topi-
cal 2%. Soln. Bot. 60 mL. *Rx.*
Use: Dermatologic, acne.
ettriol trinitrate.
See: Propatyl nitrate.
etybenzatropine. Ethybenztropine.
etynodiol acetate. Ethynodiol diacetate.
eubasin.
See: Sulfapyridine.
eucaine hydrochloride. (Novartis) Men-
thol 8%, eucalyptus oil, SD 3A alcohol.
Gel. Tube 60 g. *OTC.*
Use: Liniment.
Eucalyptamint. (Novartis) Menthol 8%,
eucalyptus oil, SD 3A alcohol. Gel
60 g. *OTC.*
Use: Liniment.
Eucalyptamint Maximum Strength.
(Novartis) Menthol 16%, lanolin, euca-
lyptus oil. Oint. Tube 60 mL. *OTC.*
Use: Liniment.
●**eucalyptol.** (yoo-ka-LIP-tol) USAN.
Use: Pharmaceutic aid (flavor); antitus-
sive; decongestant, nasal.
See: Vicks.
Vicks Sinex.
Vicks Va-Tro-Nol.
eucalyptus oil.
Use: Flavor; antitussive; decongestant,
nasal; expectorant; analgesic,
topical.

See: Vicks.
Victors Regular.
•**eucatropine hydrochloride.** (you-CAT-troe-peen) *USP 28.*
Use: Pharmaceutical necessity for ophthalmic dosage form; anticholinergic, ophthalmic.
eucatropine hydrochloride. (Glogau) Crystal, Bot. g.
Use: Pharmaceutical necessity for ophthalmic dosage form; anticholinergic, ophthalmic.
Eucerin. (Beiersdorf) Unscented moisturizing formula. **Creme:** Jar 120 g, lb. **Lot.:** Bot. 240 mL, 480 mL. *OTC.*
Use: Emollient.
Eucerin Cleansing. (Beiersdorf) Sodium laureth sulfate, cocoamphocarboxyglycinate, cocamidopropyl betaine, cocamide MEA, PEG 7 glyceryl cocoate, PEG-5 lanolate, PEG-120 methyl glucose dioleate, lanolin alcohol, imidazolidinyl urea. Soap free. Lot. Bot. 240 mL. *OTC.*
Use: Dermatologic, cleanser.
Eucerin Dry Skin Care Daily Facial. (Beiersdorf) Ethylhexyl p-methoxycinnamate, titanium dioxide, 2-phenylbenzimidazole-5-sulfonic acid, 2-ethylhexyl salicylate, mineral oil, cetearyl alcohol, castor oil, lanolin alcohol, EDTA. SPF 20. Lot. Bot. 120 mL. *OTC.*
Use: Sunscreen.
Eucerin Itch-Relief Moisturizing. (Beiersdorf) Menthol 0.15%, glycerin, mineral oil, cetyl alcohol, *Oenothera biennis* (evening primrose oil). Spray. 200 mL. *OTC.*
Use: Emollient.
Eucerin Plus. (Beiersdorf) Mineral oil, hydrogenated castor oil, sodium lactate 5%, urea 5%, glycerin, lanolin alcohol. Lot. Bot. 177 mL. *OTC.*
Use: Emollient.
eucodal.
See: Oxycodone.
eucupin dihydrochloride. Isoamylhydrocupreine dihydrochloride.
Eudal-SR. (Forest) Pseudoephedrine 120 mg, guaifenesin 400 mg. SR Tab. Bot. 100s. *Rx.*
Use: Decongestant, expectorant.
euflavine.
See: Acriflavine.
•**eugenol.** (you-jeh-nole) *USP 28.*
Use: Dental analgesic; oral anesthetic.
See: Benzodent.
eukadol.
See: Dihydrohydroxycodeinone.
Eulcin. (Leeds) Methscopolamine bromide 2.5 mg, butabarbital sodium

10 mg, aluminum hydroxide gel, dried, 250 mg, magnesium trisilicate 250 mg. Tab. Bot. 100s. *Rx.*
Use: Antacid; anticholinergic; antispasmodic; hypnotic; sedative.
Eulexin. (Schering-Plough) Flutamide 125 mg, lactose, parabens, EDTA. Cap. Bot. 180s, 500s, UD 100s. *Rx.*
Use: Antineoplastic; hormone, antiandrogen.
Eumydrin Drops. (Sanofi-Synthelabo) Atropine methonitrate. *Rx.*
Use: Anticholinergic; antispasmodic.
euneryl.
See: Phenobarbital.
Euphorbia Compound. (Sherwood Davis & Geck) Euphorbia pilulifera fluid extract 1.5 mL, lobelia tincture 2.2 mL, nitroglycerin spirit 0.29 mL, sodium iodide 1.04 g, sodium bromide 1.04 g, alcohol 24%/30 mL. Bot. Pt, gal. *Rx.*
Use: Expectorant; hypnotic; sedative.
euphorbia pilulifera.
W/Cocillana, squill, antimony potassium tartrate, senega.
See: Cylana.
W/Phenyl salicylate and various oils.
See: Rayderm.
Eupractone. (Baxter PPI) Dimethadione.
•**euprocin hydrochloride.** (YOU-pro-sin) USAN.
Use: Anesthetic, local.
See: Eucupin hydrochloride.
euquinine. Quinine ethyl carbonate.
Use: Antimalarial; antipyretic.
Eurax. (Bristol-Myers Squibb) Crotamiton. **Cream:** 10% in vanishing base. Cetyl alcohol. Tube 60 g. **Lotion:** 10% in emollient base. Cetyl alcohol. Bot. 60 g, 454 g. *Rx.*
Use: Scabicide; pediculicide.
Evac. (Burgin-Arden) **Supp.:** Sodium bicarbonate, sodium biphosphate, dioctyl sodium sulfosuccinate 50 mg. Supp. **Tab.:** Guar gum 300 mg, danthron 50 mg, sodium 100 mg. Tab. *OTC.*
Use: Laxative.
Evactol. (Delta Pharmaceutical Group) Docusate sodium 100 mg, sodium carboxymethyl cellulose 200 mg. Cap. Pkg. 10s. Bot. 10s, 30s, 100s. *OTC.*
Use: Laxative.
Evac-U-Gen. (Lee Pharmaceuticals) Sennosides 10 mg. Sugar. Chew. Tab. 35s. *OTC.*
Use: Laxative.
Evans Blue. *USP 28.*
Use: Diagnostic aid (blood volume determination).
Evans Blue Dye. (New World Trading Corp.) Evans blue dye 5 mL. Inj. *Rx.*

Use: Diagnostic aid.
- **evernimicin.** USAN.
  Use: Antibacterial.
- **everolimus.** (e-ver-OH-li-mus) USAN.
  Use: Immunosuppressant.
Evicyl Tablets. (Sanofi-Synthelabo) Inositol hexanicotinate. *Rx.*
  Use: Hypolipidemic; peripheral vasodilator.
Eviron. (Delta Pharmaceutical Group) Ferrous fumarate 160 mg, copper 1 mg, ascorbic acid 75 mg. Tab. *OTC.*
  Use: Mineral, vitamin supplement.
Evista. (Eli Lilly) Raloxifene 60 mg, lactose. Tab. Unit-of-use. 30s, 100s, 2000s. *Rx.*
  Use: Osteoporosis prevention; sex hormone, selective estrogen receptor modulator.
E-Vital Creme. (Taylor Pharmaceuticals) Vitamins E 100 units, A 250 units, D 100 units, d-panthenol 0.2%, allantoin 0.1%/g. Jar 2 oz, lb. *OTC.*
  Use: Emollient.
Evoclin. (Connetics) Clindamycin 1%. Cetyl alcohol, dehydrated alcohol (ethanol 58%), stearyl alcohol. Foam. 50 g. *Rx.*
  Use: Anti-infective, topical.
Evoxac. (Daiichi) Cevimeline hydrochloride 30 mg, lactose. Cap. Bot. 100s, 500s. *Rx.*
  Use: Sjögran syndrome; dry mouth.
Ewin Ninos Tablets. (Sanofi-Synthelabo) Aspirin. *OTC.*
  Use: Analgesic.
- **exametazime.** (EX-ah-MET-ah-zeen) USAN.
  Use: Diagnostic aid (regional cerebral perfusion imaging).
- **exaprolol hydrochloride.** (EX-ah-PRO-lahl) USAN.
  Use: Antiadrenergic (β-receptor).
- **exatecan mesylate.** (ex-a-TE-can) USAN.
  Use: Antineoplastic.
Ex-Caloric Wafers. (Eastern Research) Carboxymethylcellulose 181 mg, methylcellulose 272 mg. Bot. 100s, 500s, 5000s. *OTC.*
  Use: Dietary aid.
Excedrin Aspirin Free. (Bristol-Myers Squibb) Acetaminophen 500 mg, caffeine 65 mg, saccharin, parabens (Cap. only). Cap. Geltab. Bot. 24s; 50s, 100s. *OTC.*
  Use: Analgesic combination.
Excedrin Extra Strength. (Bristol-Myers Squibb) Acetaminophen 250 mg, aspirin 250 mg, caffeine 65 mg, saccha-

rin. **Cap.:** Bot. 24s, 50s, 100s, 175s, 275s. **Tab.:** Bot. 24s, 50s, 100s, 175s, 275s. **Geltab.:** Bot. 24s, 40s, 80s. *OTC.*
  Use: Analgesic combination.
Excedrin Migraine. (Bristol-Myers Squibb) Acetaminophen 250 mg, aspirin 250 mg, caffeine 65 mg. Tab. Bot. 50s, 100s. *OTC.*
  Use: Analgesic combination.
Excedrin P.M. (Bristol-Myers Squibb) **Tab.:** Acetaminophen 500 mg, diphenhydramine citrate 38 mg, parabens, mineral oil. Bot. 50s. **Capl.:** Acetaminophen 500 mg, diphenhydramine citrate 38 mg. Bot. 30s, 50s. **Liquigels:** Acetaminophen 500 mg, diphenhydramine hydrochloride 25 mg. Bot. 20s, 40s. **Liq.:** Acetaminophen 1000 mg, diphenhydramine hydrochloride 50 mg/30 mL, alcohol 10%, sucrose. Bot. 180 mL. **Geltab:** Acetaminophen 500 mg, diphenhydramine citrate 38 mg, EDTA, parabens. Bot. 100s. *OTC.*
  Use: Analgesic; sleep aid.
Excedrin QuickTabs. (Bristol-Myers Squibb) Acetaminophen 500 mg, caffeine 65 mg, mannitol, sucralose, spearmint and peppermint flavors. Quick-dissolving Tab. 16s, 32s. *OTC.*
  Use: Analgesic; CNS stimulant.
Excedrin Tension Headache. (Bristol-Myers Squibb) Acetaminophen 500 mg, caffeine 65 mg. Parabens. Caplets, Geltabs. 50s, 100s. *OTC.*
  Use: Nonnarcotic analgesic combination.
Excita Extra. (Durex) Nonoxynol-9 8% Ribbed Condom. Box 3s, 12s, 36s. *OTC.*
  Use: Condom with spermicide.
ExeFen-PD. (Larken) Phenylephrine hydrochloride 10 mg, guaifenesin 600 mg. ER Tab. 100s. *Rx.*
  Use: Decongestant and expectorant.
Exelon. (Novartis) Rivastigmine tartrate. **Cap.:** 1.5 mg, 3 mg, 4.5 mg, 6 mg. Bot. 60s, 500s, UD 100s. **Soln.:** 2 mg/mL. Bot. 120 mL. *Rx.*
  Use: Cholinesterase inhibitor.
- **exemestane.** (ex-e-MES-tane) USAN.
  Use: Antineoplastic.
exemestane.
  Use: Hormonal therapy of metastatic breast carcinoma. [Orphan Drug]
  See: Aromasin.
- **exenatide.** (ex-EN-a-tide) USAN.
  Use: Antidiabetic agent.
  See: Byetta.
Ex-Histine. (WE Pharmaceuticals) Phenylephrine hydrochloride 10 mg, chlorpheniramine maleate 2 mg, meth-

scopolamine nitrate 1.25 mg/5 mL, root beer flavor. Syr. Bot. 473 mL. *Rx.*
Use: Upper respiratory combination, anticholinergic, antihistamine, decongestant.
Exidine-4 Scrub. (Baxter PPI) Chlorhexidine gluconate 4%, isopropyl alcohol 4%. Soln. Bot. 120 mL, 240 mL, 480 mL, 887 mL, gal. *OTC.*
Use: Antiseptic; antimicrobial.
Exidine Skin Cleanser. (Xttrium) Chlorhexidine gluconate 4%, isopropyl alcohol 4%. Bot. 120 mL, 240 mL, 16 oz, 32 oz, gal. *OTC.*
Use: Antiseptic; antimicrobial.
Exidine-2 Scrub. (Baxter PPI) Chlorhexidine gluconate 2%, isopropyl alcohol 4%. Soln. Bot. 120 mL. *OTC.*
Use: Antiseptic; antimicrobial.
exisulind.
Use: Investigational apoptotic antineoplastic drug.
ex-lax. (Novartis) Sennosodes 15 mg, sucrose. Tab. Pkg. 8s, 30s, 60s. *OTC.*
Use: Laxative.
ex-lax Chocolated. (Novartis) Sennosides 15 mg, sugar, oil, dry milk, chocolated. Tab. Pkg. 6s, 18s, 48s. *OTC.*
Use: Laxative.
ex-lax Gentle Strength. (Novartis) Docusate sodium 65 mg, sennosides 10 mg, lactose, methylparaben, polydextrose. Tab. Box. 24s. *OTC.*
Use: Laxative.
ex-lax, Maximum Relief. (Novartis) Sennosides 25 mg, sucrose. Tab. Pkg. 24s, 48s. *OTC.*
Use: Laxative.
ex-lax Stool Softener. (Novartis) Docusate sodium 100 mg, methylparabens. Tab. Bot. 40s. *OTC.*
Use: Laxative.
Exocaine Plus. (Del) Methyl salicylate 30%. Jar 4 oz, Tube 1.3 oz. *OTC.*
Use: Analgesic, topical.
exol. Di-isobutyl ethoxy ethyl dimethyl benzyl ammonium chloride.
exonic ot. Dioctyl sodium sulphosuccinate.
Use: Laxative.
expectorant and antitussive combinations.
Use: Upper respiratory combination.
See: Antitussive and expectorant combinations.
expectorant and decongestant combinations.
Use: Upper respiratory combination.
See: Decongestant and expectorant combinations.

expectorant, antihistamine, and decongestant combinations.
Use: Upper respiratory combination.
See: Antihistamine, decongestant, and expectorant combinations.
expectorant, antitussive, and decongestant combinations.
Use: Upper respiratory combination.
See: Antitussive, decongestant, and expectorant combinations.
Expectorant DM Cough Syrup. (Weeks & Leo) Dextromethorphan HBr 15 mg, guaifenesin 100 mg/5 mL, alcohol 7.125%. Bot. 6 oz. *OTC.*
Use: Antitussive, expectorant.
expectorants.
See: Guaifenesin.
Expendable Blood Collection Unit ACD. (Baxter PPI) Citric acid 540 mg, sodium citrate 1.49 g, dextrose 1.65 g/ 67.5 mL. *Rx.*
Use: Anticoagulant.
Exratuss. (Midlothian) Carbetapentane tannate 30 mg, chlorpheniramine tannate 4 mg, phenylephrine tannate 12.5 mg/5 mL. Methylparaben, saccharin, sucrose. Strawberry flavor. Susp. 118 mL. *Rx.*
Use: Antitussive.
extended-spectrum penicillins.
Use: Anti-infective.
See: Mezlin.
Mezlocillin sodium.
Extendryl Chewable Tablets. (Cornerstone Biopharma) Chlorpheniramine maleate 2 mg, phenylephrine hydrochloride 10 mg, methscopolamine nitrate 1.25 mg, root beer flavor. Chew. Tab. Bot. 100s, 1000s. *Rx.*
Use: Upper respiratory combination, anticholinergic, antihistamine, antispasmodic, decongestant.
Extendryl JR. (Fleming & Co.) Chlorpheniramine maleate 4 mg, phenylephrine hydrochloride 10 mg, methscopolamine nitrate 1.25 mg. Cap. Bot. 100s, 1000s. *Rx.*
Use: Upper respiratory combination, anticholinergic, antihistamine, decongestant.
Extendryl SR. (Fleming & Co.) Chlorpheniramine maleate 8 mg, phenylephrine hydrochloride 20 mg, methscopolamine nitrate 2.5 mg. SR Cap. Bot. 100s, 1000s. *Rx.*
Use: Upper respiratory combination, anticholinergic, antihistamine, decongestant.
Extendryl Syrup. (Cornerstone Biopharma) Chlorpheniramine maleate 2 mg, phenylephrine hydrochloride

10 mg, methscopolamine nitrate 1.25 mg/5 mL, root beer flavor. Syr. Bot. 473 mL, 3.8 L. *Rx.*
Use: Upper respiratory combination, anticholinergic, antihistamine, decongestant.

Exten Strone 10. (Schlicksup) Estradiol valerate 10 mg/mL. Vial 10 mL. *Rx.*
Use: Estrogen.

Extenzyme Soflens Protein Cleaner. (Allergan) Papain, sodium chloride, sodium carbonate, sodium borate, edetate disodium. Vial w/Tab. 24s. Refill 36s. *OTC.*
Use: Contact lens care.

Extra Action Cough. (Rugby) Dextromethorphan HBr 10 mg, guaifenesin 100 mg/5 mL corn syrup, saccharin, glucose. Syr. Bot. 118 mL. *OTC.*
Use: Upper respiratory combination, antitussive, expectorant.

Extraneal. (Baxter) Icodextrin 75 g, Na 132 mEq, Ca 3.5 mEq, Mg 0.5 mEq, Cl 96 mEq, lactate 40 mEq/L. Soln. *Ultrabag* and *Ambu-Flex* 1.5, 2, 2.5 L. *Rx.*
Use: Peritoneal dialysis solution.

Extra Strength Adprin-B. (Pfeiffer) Aspirin 500 mg, calcium carbonate, magnesium carbonate, magnesium oxide. Tab, coated. Bot. 130s. *OTC.*
Use: Analgesic.

Extra Strength Alka-Seltzer Effervescent. (Bayer Corp. (Consumer Div.)) Sodium bicarbonate (heat-treated) 1985 mg, aspirin 500 mg, citric acid 1000 mg, sodium 588 mg. Tab. Bot. 12s and 24s. *OTC.*
Use: Antacid.

Extra Strength Aspirin Capsules. (Walgreen) Aspirin 500 mg. Bot. 80s. *OTC.*
Use: Analgesic.

Extra Strength Bayer Enteric 500 Aspirin. (Bayer Corp. (Consumer Div.)) Aspirin 500 mg. Tab. Enteric coated. Bot. 60s. *OTC.*
Use: Analgesic.

Extra Strength Bayer Plus. (Bayer Corp. (Consumer Div.)) Aspirin 500 mg buffered with calcium carbonate, magnesium carbonate, magnesium oxide. Cap. Bot. 30s, 60s. *OTC.*
Use: Analgesic.

Extra Strength Doan's PM. (Novartis) Magnesium salicylate 500 mg, diphenhydramine hydrochloride 25 mg. Capl. Pkg. 20s. *OTC.*
Use: Sleep aid.

Extra Strength Dynafed EX. (BDI) Acetaminophen 500 mg, fruit favor. Tab. Bot. 36s. *OTC.*

Use: Analgesic.

Extra Strength Excedrin Capsules and Tablets. (Bristol-Myers Squibb) Acetaminophen 250 mg, aspirin 250 mg, caffeine 65 mg. Cap. Bot. 24s, 50s, 80s. Tab. Bot. 30s, 60s, 100s, 165s, 225s, Pkg. 12s. *OTC.*
Use: Analgesic combination.

Extra Strength 5 mg Biotin Forte. (Vitaline) Vitamins B_1 10 mg, B_2 10 mg, B_3 40 mg, B_5 10 mg, B_6 25 mg, B_{12} 10 mcg, C 100 mg, biotin 5 mg, FA 800 mcg. Tab. Bot. 60s, 1000s. *OTC.*
Use: Mineral, vitamin supplement.

Extra Strength Gas-X. (Novartis) Simethicone 125 mg. Tab. Pkg. 18s. *OTC.*
Use: Antiflatulent.

Extra Strength Tylenol PM. (McNeil Consumer) Diphenhydramine 25 mg, acetaminophen 500 mg. **Tab.:** 24s, 50s. **Capl.:** 24s, 50s. **Gelcap:** 20s, 40s. *OTC.*
Use: Sleep aid.

Extra Strength Vicks Cough Drops. (Procter & Gamble) Menthol 8.4 mg (menthol flavor) or menthol 10 mg (cherry and honey lemon flavors), corn syrup, sucrose. Loz. Pkg. 9s, 30s. *OTC.*
Use: Mouth and throat preparation.

Extreme Cold Formula. (Major) Pseudoephedrine hydrochloride 30 mg, chlorpheniramine maleate 1 mg, dextromethorphan HBr 15 mg, acetaminophen 500 mg. Cap. Bot. 10s. *OTC.*
Use: Analgesic, antihistamine, antitussive, decongestant.

Eye Drops. (Bausch & Lomb) Tetrahydrozoline hydrochloride 0.05%. Drop. Bot. 15 mL. *OTC.*
Use: Ophthalmic vasoconstrictor; mydriatic.

Eye, Face, and Body Wash Station. (Lavoptik) Sodium chloride 0.49 g, sodium biphosphate 0.4 g, sodium phosphate 0.45 g/100 mL, benzalkonium chloride 0.005%. Bot. 32 oz. *OTC.*
Use: Emergency wash.

Eye Irrigating Solution. (Rugby) Sodium chloride, sodium phosphate mono- and dibasic, benzalkonium chloride, EDTA. Soln. Bot. 118 mL. *OTC.*
Use: Irrigant, ophthalmic.

Eye Irrigating Wash. (Roberts) Boric acid, potassium chloride, sodium carbonate anhydrous, EDTA 0.01%, benzalkonium chloride. Soln. Bot. 120 mL. *OTC.*
Use: Irrigant, ophthalmic.

Eye-Lube-A. (Optopics) Glycerin 0.25%, EDTA, NaCl, benzalkonium chloride. Soln. Bot. 15 mL. *OTC.*

Use: Lubricant, ophthalmic.

Eye Mo. (Sanofi-Synthelabo) Boric acid, benzalkonium chloride, phenylephrine hydrochloride, zinc sulfate. *OTC.*
Use: Astringent, ophthalmic.

Eye Scrub. (Novartis Ophthalmics) PEG-200 glyceryl monotallawate, disodium laureth sulfosuccinate, cocoamidopropylamineoxide, PEG-78 glyceryl monococoate, benzyl alcohol, EDTA. Soln. Bot. 240 mL. *OTC.*
Use: Cleanser, ophthalmic.

Eye-Stream. (Alcon) Sodium Cl 0.64%, potassium chloride 0.075%, magnesium chloride hexahydrate 0.03%, calcium chloride dihydrate 0.048%, sodium acetate trihydrate 0.39%, sodium citrate dihydrate 0.17%, benzalkonium chloride 0.013%. Bot. 30 ml, 118 mL. *OTC.*
Use: Irrigant, ophthalmic.

Eye Wash. (Bausch & Lomb) Boric acid, potassium chloride, EDTA, sodium carbonate, benzalkonium chloride 0.01%. Soln. Bot. 118 mL. *OTC.*
Use: Irrigant, ophthalmic.

Eye Wash. (Ivax) Boric acid, potassium chloride, EDTA, anhydrous sodium carbonate, benzalkonium chloride 0.1%. Soln. Bot. 118 mL. *OTC.*
Use: Irrigant, ophthalmic.

Eye Wash. (Lavoptik) Sodium chloride 0.49%, sodium biphosphate 0.4%, sodium phosphate 0.45%, benzalkonium chloride 0.005%. Soln. Bot. 180 mL with eye cup. *OTC.*
Use: Irrigant, ophthalmic.

EZ-Detect. (Biomerica) Occult blood screening test. Kit 3s.
Use: Diagnostic aid.

EZ Detect Strep-A Test. (Biomerica) Coated stick test for detection of group A streptococci taken directly from a throat swab.
Use: Diagnostic aid.

Eze Pain. (Halsey Drug) Acetaminophen 2.5 g, salicylamide, caffeine. Cap. Bot. 21s. *OTC.*
Use: Analgesic combination.

●**ezetimibe.** (ezz-ET-ih-mibe) USAN.
Use: Antihyperlipidemic.
See: Zetia.
W/Simvastatin
See: Vytorin.

Ezide. (Econo Med Pharmaceuticals) Hydrochlorothiazide 50 mg. Tab. Bot. 100s, 1000s. *Rx.*
Use: Diuretic.

●**ezlopitant.** (ez-LOE-pi-tant) USAN.
Use: Emesis; pain; inflammation.

Ezol. (Stewart-Jackson Pharmacal) Butalbital 50 mg, caffeine 40 mg, acetaminophen 325 mg. Bot. 100s. *Rx.*
Use: Analgesic; hypnotic; sedative.

Ezol #3. (Stewart-Jackson Pharmacal) Acetaminophen 650 mg, codeine 30 mg. Bot. 100s. *c-III.*
Use: Analgesic combination; narcotic.

F

Fabrase.
Use: Fabry disease. [Orphan Drug]
Fabrazyme. (Genzyme) Agalsidase beta.
5.5 mg: 5 mg/mL when reconstituted.
Mannitol 33 mg, sodium phosphate
monobasic monohydrate 3 mg, sodium
phosphate dibasic heptahydrate
8.8 mg. Preservative free. Pow. for Inj.,
lyophilized. Single-use vials. 5 mL.
37 mg (5 mg/mL when reconstituted):
Mannitol 222 mg, sodium phosphate
monobasic monohydrate 20.4 mg, sodium phosphate dibasic heptahydrate
59.2 mg/vial. Preservative free. Pow. for
Inj., lyophilized. Single-use vials.
20 mL. *Rx.*
Use: Fabry disease.

**Faces Only Moisturizing Sunblock by
Coppertone.** (Schering-Plough) Ethylhexyl p-methoxycinnamate, oxybenzone. SPF 15. Lot. Bot. 55.5 mL. *OTC.*
Use: Sunscreen.

Fact Home Pregnancy Test. (Johnson
& Johnson) Accurate test for pregnancy in 45 minutes, for use as early
as 3 days after a missed period. Test kit
1s.
Use: Diagnostic aid.

Factive. (Oscient) Gemifloxacin mesylate 320 mg, film coated. Tab. Unit of
use 5s, 7s, hospital pack 30s. *Rx.*
Use: Fluoroquinolone.

factor VIIa recombinant, DNA orgin.
(Novo/Nordisk)
Use: Antihemophilic; von Willebrand
disease. [Orphan Drug]

factor VIII.
See: Antihemophilic factor.

factor IX, coagulation.
See: Coagulation factor ix.

• **factor IX complex.** (FAK-tuhr-[IX] KAHM-
plex) *USP 28.*
Use: Hemostatic.
See: Alpha Nine SD.
Konyne 80.
Mononine.
Profilnine SD.
Proplex T.

**factor IX complex, vapor heated Bebu-
lin VH immuno.** (Immuno U.S.) Purified sterile, stable freeze-dried concentrate of coagulation Factor IX (Christ-
mas Factor), Factors II (prothrombin)
and X (Stuart Prower), low amounts of
Factor VII, ≤ 0.15 International Units
(units) heparin/units Factor IX. Pow. for
Inj. Single-dose vial w/Sterile Water
for Injection, double-ended needle, filter needle. *Rx.*

Use: Hemostatic.
factor IX concentrates.
Use: Antihemophilic.
See: AlphaNine SD.
Bebulin VH.
BeneFix.
Mononine.
Profilnine SD.
Proplex T.

factor XIII (plasma-derived).
Use: Congenital Factor XIII deficiency.
[Orphan Drug]
See: Fibrogammin P.

Fact Plus. (Johnson & Johnson) Reagent
in-home kit for urine testing. Pregnancy
test. Kit 1s, 2s.
Use: Diagnostic aid.

Factrel. (Wyeth) Gonadorelin hydrochloride, 100 mcg, 500 mcg, lactose
100 mg. Pow. for Inj., lyophilized. Vial.
2 mL sterile diluent, benzyl alcohol 2%.
Rx.
Use: In vivo diagnostic aid.

• **fadolmidine hydrochloride.** (fa-DOL-
mid-ine) USAN.
Use: Analgesic (spinal).

• **fadrozole hydrochloride.** (FAHD-rah-
ZOLE) USAN.
Use: Antineoplastic.

Falgos. (Sanofi-Synthelabo) Acetylsalicylic acid. Tab. *OTC.*
Use: Analgesic.

Falmonox. (Sanofi-Synthelabo) Teclozan
Susp., Tab. *Rx.*
Use: Amebicide.

• **famciclovir.** (fam-SIGH-kloe-veer)
USAN.
Use: Antiviral.
See: Famvir.

• **famotidine.** (fah-MOE-tih-den) *USP 28.*
Use: Histamine H$_2$ antagonist.
See: Pepcid.
Pepcid AC.
Pepcid AC Maximum Strength.
Pepcid RPD.

famotidine. (Ivax) Famotidine 10 mg.
Tab. Bot. 18s, 30s, 50s, 70s. *OTC.*
Use: Histamine H$_2$ antagonist.

famotidine. (Various Mfr.) Famotidine.
Tab.: 20 mg, 40 mg. May contain lactose. Bot. 30s, 100s, 500s, 1000s, UD
100s; *Robot–Ready* 25s (20 mg only).
Inj.: 10 mg/mL. May contain mannitol
or benzyl alcohol. Single-dose vial
1 mL, 2 mL. Multiple-dose vial 4 mL,
20 mL, 50 mL. *Rx.*
Use: Histamine H$_2$ antagonist.

**famotidine, calcium carbonate, and
magnesium hydroxide combinations.**
Use: Histamine H$_2$ antagonist.

See: Pepcid Complete.

●**famotine hydrochloride.** (FAM-oh-teen) USAN.
Use: Antiviral.

●**fampridine.** (FAHM-prih-DEEN) USAN.
Use: Symptomatic treatment of multiple sclerosis.

Famvir. (Novartis) Famciclovir 125 mg, 250 mg, 500 mg, lactose. Tab. Bot. 30s, UD 50s (500 mg only). *Rx.*
Use: Management of acute herpes zoster (shingles).

●**fananserin.** (fan-AN-ser-in) USAN.
Use: Antipsychotic; antischizophrenic (dual dopamine D_4 and serotonin 5-HT_2 receptor antagonist).

●**fandosentan potassium.** (fan-doe-SEN-tan) USAN.
Use: Pulmonary hypertension.

●**fanetizole mesylate.** (fan-EH-tih-zole) USAN.
Use: Immunoregulator.

Fansidar. (Roche) Sulfadoxine 500 mg, pyrimethamine 25 mg, lactose, talc. Tab. UD 25s. *Rx.*
Use: Antimalarial.

●**fantridone hydrochloride.** (FAN-trih-dohn) USAN.
Use: Antidepressant.

Faramals. (Faraday) Vitamins A 10,000 units, D 2000 units, B_1 6 mg, B_2 4 mg, B_6 0.5 mg, folic acid 0.1 mg, C 100 mg, calcium pantothenate 5 mg, niacinamide 30 mg, E 5 units, B_{12} 3 mcg. Tab. Bot. 100s, 250s, 500s, 1000s. *OTC.*
Use: Mineral, vitamin supplement.

Faramals-M. (Faraday) Faramals plus calcium 103 mg, cobalt 0.1 mg, Cu 1 mg, I 0.15 mg, Fe 10 mg, Mg 6 mg, Mo 0.2 mg, P 80 mg, K 5 mg, Zn 1.2 mg. Tab. Bot. 100s, 250s, 500s, 1000s. *OTC.*
Use: Mineral, vitamin supplement.

Faramins. (Faraday) Vitamins B_1 20 mg, B_2 6 mg, C 40 mg, niacinamide 20 mg, calcium pantothenate 3 mg, B_6 0.5 mg, powdered whole dried liver 125 mg, dried debittered yeast 125 mg, choline dihydrogen citrate 20 mg, inositol 20 mg, dl-methionine 20 mg, folic acid 0.1 mg, B_{12} 10 mcg, ferrous gluconate 30 mg, dicalcium phosphate 250 mg, copper sulfate 5 mg, magnesium sulfate 10 mg, manganese sulfate 5 mg, cobalt sulfate 0.2 mg, potassium Cl 2 mg, potassium iodide 0.15 mg. Tab. Bot. 100s, 250s, 500s, 1000s. *OTC.*
Use: Mineral, vitamin supplement.

Faratol. (Faraday) Vitamins A 12,500 units, D 1000 units, B_1 20 mg, B_2 6 mg, B_6 0.5 mg, B_{12} 15 mcg, folic acid 0.1 mg, niacinamide 10 mg, calcium pantothenate 3 mg, C 60 mg, E 5 units, choline dihydrogen citrate 20 mg, inositol 20 mg, dl-methionine 20 mg, whole dried liver 100 mg, dried debittered yeast 100 mg, dicalcium phosphate 200 mg, ferrous gluconate 30 mg, potassium iodide 0.2 mg, magnesium sulfate 7.2 mg, copper sulfate 5 mg, manganese sulfate 3.4 mg, cobalt sulfate 0.2 mg, potassium Cl 1.3 mg, zinc sulfate 2 mg, molybdenum 0.2 mg in a base of alfalfa. Tab. Bot. 100s, 250s, 500s, 1000s. *OTC.*
Use: Mineral, vitamin supplement.

Farbee with Vitamin C. (Major) Vitamins B_1 15 mg, B_2 10.2 mg, B_3 50 mg, B_5 10 mg, B_6 5 mg, C 300 mg. Capl. Bot. 100s, 130s, 1000s. *OTC.*
Use: Vitamin supplement.

Farbital. (Major) Butalbital. Tab. Bot. 100s. *c-III.*
Use: Hypnotic; sedative.

Farbital Compound. (Major) Butalbital, caffeine, aspirin. Cap. Bot. 100s. *c-III.*
Use: Analgesic; hypnotic; sedative.

Farbital Compound with Codeine #3. (Major) Butalbital, caffeine, aspirin, codeine 30 mg. Bot. 1000s. *c-III.*
Use: Analgesic; hypnotic; sedative.

Fareston. (Shire) Toremifene citrate 60 mg, lactose. Tab. Bot. 30s, 100s. *Rx.*
Use: Antiestrogen; hormone.

Faslodex. (AstraZeneca) Fulvestrant 50 mg/mL, alcohol, benzyl alcohol, castor oil. Inj. Prefilled Syr. 2.5 mL (2s), 5 mL. *Rx.*
Use: Hormone, antiestrogen.

Fastlene. (BDI) Caffeine 200 mg. Cap. Bot. 100s, 500s. *OTC.*
Use: CNS stimulant, analeptic.

fat emulsion, intravenous.
See: Intralipid 10%.
Intralipid 20%.
Liposyn 10%.
Liposyn 20%.
Liposyn II 10%.
Liposyn II 20%.
Travamulsion 10%.
Travamulsion 20%.

●**fat, hard.** *NF 23.*
Use: Pharmaceutic aid (suppository base).

Father John's Medicine Plus. (Oakhurst) Phenylephrine hydrochloride 1.66 mg, chlorpheniramine maleate 0.66 mg, dextromethorphan HBr 1.66 mg/5 mL, alcohol free. Liq. Bot. 118 mL. *OTC.*

Use: Upper respiratory combination, antihistamine, antitussive, decongestant.
fat soluble vitamins.
See: AquaMEPHYTON.
Aquasol A.
Aquavit-E.
Beta-carotene.
Calcifediol.
Calciferol.
Calcijex.
Calcitriol.
Calderol.
Cholecalciferol.
d' ALPHA E 400 Softgels.
d' ALPHA E 1000 Softgels.
Delta-D.
DHT.
Dihydrotachysterol (DHT).
Doxorualolfurul.
Drisdol.
Dry E 400.
Ergocalciferol.
Hectorol.
Hytakerol.
Mephyton.
Mixed E 400 Softgels.
Mixed E 1000 Softgels.
Palmitate-A 5000.
Paricalcitol.
Phytonadione.
Rocaltrol.
Vita-Plus E.
Vitamin A,
Vitamin D_3.
Vitamin E.
Vitamin E with Mixed Tocopherols.
Vitamin K.
Zemplar.
Fattibase. (Paddock) Preblended fatty acid suppository base composed of triglycerides of coconut oil and palm kernel oil. Jar 1 lb, 5 lb.
Use: Pharmaceutical aid; suppository base.
FazaClo. (Alamo) Clozapine 25 mg (phenylalanine 1.74 mg), 100 mg (phenylalanine 6.96 mg). Aspartame. Orally Disintegrating Tab. 48s. *Rx.*
Use: Antipsychotic.
fazadinium bromide.
Use: Neuromuscular blocking agent.
•**fazarabine.** (fah-ZAY-rah-BEAN) USAN.
Use: Antineoplastic.
Feberin. (Arcum) Ferrous gluconate 3 g, vitamins C 25 mg, B_1 2 mg, B_6 1 mg, B_2 1 mg, niacinamide 5 mg. Tab. Bot. 100s, 1000s. *OTC.*
Use: Mineral, vitamin supplement.
febrile antigens. (Laboratory Diagnostics) Group O antigens (somatic) are

dyed blue and group H antigens (flagellars) are dyed red for clear identification for detection of bacterial agglutinins, bacterial infections. Vial 5 mL.
Use: Diagnostic aid.
Febrinol. (Eon Labs) Acetaminophen 325 mg. Tab. Bot. 100s, 1000s. *OTC.*
Use: Analgesic.
Fe-Brone. (Forest) Vitamins B_{12} 1 units, folic acid 1 mg, ferrous sulfate exsiccated (powdered) 200 mg, ferrous sulfate exsiccated (timed) 200 mg, C acid 100 mg, B_6 0.5 mg, B_1 2 mg, B_2 1 mg, copper 0.9 mg, zinc 0.5 mg, manganese 0.3 mg. Cap. Bot. 30s, 100s, 1000s. *Rx.*
Use: Mineral, vitamin supplement.
•**febuxostat.** (feb-UX-oh-stat) USAN.
Use: Investigational drug for hyperuricemia; xanthine oxidase/dehydrogenase inhibitor.
fecal softeners/surfactants.
See: Colace.
DC Softgels.
Diocto.
Docu.
Docusate Calcium).
Docusate Sodium.
D.O.S..
D-S-S.
ex-lax Stool Softener
Genasoft.
Modane Soft.
Non-Habit Forming Stool Softener.
Phillips Liqui-Gels.
Regulax SS.
Silace.
Stool Softener.
Stool Softener DC.
Surfak Liquigels.
Fedahist Expectorant. (Schwarz Pharma) Guaifenesin 200 mg, pseudoephedrine hydrochloride 20 mg/5 mL, sorbitol, alcohol free. *OTC.*
Use: Antihistamine; decongestant.
Fedahist Gyrocaps. (Schwarz Pharma) Pseudoephedrine hydrochloride 65 mg, chlorpheniramine maleate 10 mg. SR Cap. Bot. 100s. *Rx.*
Use: Antihistamine; decongestant.
Fedahist Tablets. (Schwarz Pharma) Pseudoephedrine hydrochloride 60 mg, chlorpheniramine maleate 4 mg, sorbitol (alcohol and sugar free). Tab. Bot. 100s. *Rx.*
Use: Antihistamine; decongestant.
Fedahist Timecaps. (Schwarz Pharma) Pseudoephedrine hydrochloride 120 mg, chlorpheniramine maleate 8 mg. SR Cap. Bot. 100s. *Rx.*
Use: Antihistamine; decongestant.

Feen-a-Mint. (Schering-Plough) Bisacodyl 5 mg, talc, lactose, sugar. EC Tab. Pkg. 30s. *OTC.*
Use: Laxative.

Feen-a-Mint Dual Formula. (Schering-Plough) Docusate sodium 100 mg, yellow phenolphthalein 65 mg. Tab. Box 15s, 30s, 60s. *OTC.*
Use: Laxative.

Feen-a-Mint Gum. (Schering-Plough) Yellow phenolphthalein 97.2 mg. Chewing gum. Tab. Box 5s, 16s, 40s. *OTC.*
Use: Laxative.

Feg-I. (Western Research) Ferrous gluconate 300 mg. Tab. Handicount 28s (36 bags of 28 tab.). *OTC.*
Use: Mineral supplement.

Feiba VH Immuno. (Immuno US) Freeze-dried anti-inhibitor coagulant complex. Heparin free. Vapor heated, sodium ≈ 8 mg/mL. Inj. Vial with diluent and needle. Each bottle is labeled with the units of Factor VIIII inhibitor bypassing activity it contains. *Rx.*
Use: Antihemophilic agent.

• **felbamate.** (FELL-buh-MATE) USAN.
Use: Antiepileptic; treatment of Lennox-Gastaut syndrome [Orphan Drug]
See: Felbatol.

Felbatol. (Wallace) Felbamate. **Tab.:** 400 mg, 600 mg, lactose. Bot. 100s, UD 100s. **Susp.:** 600 mg/5 mL, sorbitol, parabens, saccharin. Bot. 240 mL, 960 mL. *Rx.*
Use: Antiepileptic. It has been recommended that use of this drug be discontinued if aplastic anemia or hepatic failure occurs unless, in the judgement of the physician, continued therapy is warranted. For further information contact Wallace Labs at 609-655-6000.

• **felbinac.** (FELL-bih-nak) USAN.
Use: Anti-inflammatory.

Feldene. (Pfizer) Piroxicam 10 mg, 20 mg, lactose. Cap. Bot. 100s; 500s, UD 100s (20 mg only). *Rx.*
Use: Analgesic; NSAID.

Fellobolic. (Forest) Methandriol dipropionate 50 mg/mL. Inj. Vial 10 mL. *Rx.*

• **felodipine.** (feh-LOW-dih-peen) *USP 28.*
Use: Vasodilator, calcium channel blocker.
See: Plendil.

felodipine and enalapril maleate.
Use: Antihypertensive.
See: Lexxel.

• **felvizumab.** (fell-VYE-zoo-mab) USAN.
Use: Antiviral (systemic); monoclonal antibody.

• **felypressin.** (fell-ih-PRESS-in) USAN.
Use: Vasoconstrictor.

Femagene. (Tennessee Pharmaceutic) Boric acid, sodium borate, lactic acid, menthol, methylbenzethonium Cl, parachlorometaxylenol, lactose, surface-active agents. Pow. 6 oz. *OTC.*
Use: Feminine hygiene.

Femara. (Novartis) Letrozole 2.5 mg, lactose. Tab. Bot. 30s. *Rx.*
Use: Hormone; aromatase inhibitor.

Femazole. (Major) Metronidazole 250 mg, 500 mg. Tab. **250 mg:** Bot. 100s, 250s, 500s. **500 mg:** Bot. 50s, 100s. *Rx.*
Use: Anti-infective.

FemBack. (CCA Inducstries) Acetaminophen 150 mg, salicylamide 150 mg, phenyltoloxamine citrate 44 mg. Capl. Bot. 24s. *OTC.*
Use: Analgesic.

Femcaps. (Buffington) Acetaminophen, caffeine, ephedrine sulfate, atropine sulfate. Tab. Sugar, lactose, and salt free Dispens-a-Kit 500s, Aidpaks 100s. *Rx.*
Use: Analgesic; anticholinergic; antispasmodic; bronchodilator.

femergin.
See: Ergotamine Tartrate.

Femhrt. (Warner Chilcott) Ethinyl estradiol/norethindrone acetate 2.5 mcg/0.5 mg, 5 mcg/1 mg, lactose. Tab. Bot. 90s, blister card 28s. *Rx.*
Use: Sex hormone, estrogens and progestins combined.

Femidyn.
See: Estrone.

Feminique Disposable Douche. (Durex) Sodium benzoate, sorbic acid, lactic acid, octoxynol-9. Twin-pack Bot. 120 mL. *OTC.*
Use: Douche.

Feminique Disposable Douche. (Durex) Vinegar and water. Soln. Twin-packs. Bot. 180 mL. *OTC.*
Use: Douche.

Feminone. (Pharmacia) Ethinyl estradiol 0.05 mg. Tab. Bot. 100s. *Rx.*
Use: Estrogen.

Femiron. (Menley & James Labs, Inc.) Ferrous fumarate 63 mg (iron 20 mg). Tab. Bot. 40s, 120s. *OTC.*
Use: Mineral supplement.

Femizol-M. (Lake Consumer) Miconazole nitrate 2%. Vaginal cream. Tube with applicator 45 g. *OTC.*
Use: Antifungal; vaginal.

Femizol-M. (Lake Consumer) Miconazole nitrate 2%, mineral oil. Vag. Cream. Tube 45 g with applicator. *OTC.*

Use: Vaginal preparation.

Fem-1. (BDI) Acetaminophen 500 mg, pamabrom 25 mg. Tab. Pkg. 16s. *OTC.*
Use: Analgesic.

Femotrone. (Bluco) Progesterone in oil 50 mg/mL. Vial 10 mL. *Rx.*
Use: Hormone; progestin.

FemPatch. (Parke-Davis) Estradiol 10.3 mg (0.025 mg/day). Patch. Box. 4s. *Rx.*
Use: Estrogen.

Fem ph. (Pharmics) Glacial acetic acid 0.9%, oxyquinoline sulfate 0.025%, glycerin, PEG 4500. Vaginal jelly. 50 g w/applicator. *OTC.*
Use: Vaginal preparation.

Femring. (Galen) Estradiol acetate 0.05 mg/day, 0.1 mg/day. Vaginal Ring. Single packs. *Rx.*
Use: Estrogen.

Femtrace. (Warner Chilcott) Estradiol acetate 0.45 mg, 0.9 mg, 1.8 mg. Lactose. Tab. 100s. *Rx.*
Use: Sex hormone, estrogen.

•**fenalamide.** (fen-AL-am-IDE) USAN.
Use: Muscle relaxant.

fenamisal. Phenyl aminosalicylate.

•**fenamole.** (FEN-ah-mole) USAN.
Use: Anti-inflammatory.

Fenaprin. (Sanofi-Synthelabo) Aspirin, chlormezanone. Tab. *Rx.*
Use: Analgesic; anxiolytic.

Fenarol. (Sanofi-Synthelabo) Chlormezanone 100 mg, 200 mg. Tab. Bot. 100s.
Use: Anxiolytic.

fenarsone.
See: Carbarsone.

•**fenbendazole.** (FEN-BEND-ah-zole) USAN.
Use: Anthelmintic.

•**fenbufen.** (FEN-byoo-fen) USAN.
Use: Anti-inflammatory.

•**fencibutirol.** (fen-sih-BYOO-tih-role) USAN.
Use: Choleretic.

•**fenclofenac.** (FEN-kloe-fen-ACK) USAN.
Use: Anti-inflammatory.

•**fenclonine.** (fen-KLOE-neen) USAN. Under study by Pfizer.
Use: Serotonin inhibitor.

•**fenclorac.** (FEN-kloe-rack) USAN.
Use: Anti-inflammatory.

Fend. (Mine Safety Appliances) **A-2:** Water-soluble cream which forms a physical barrier to water-insoluble irritants. Tube 3 oz, Jar lb. **E-2:** This cream combines the functions of the water-soluble **Fend A-2. and water-insoluble Fend I-2. creams. Tube 3 oz, Jar lb. I-2:** Water-insoluble cream which forms a physical barrier to water-soluble irritants. Tube 3 oz, Jar lb. **S-2:** A silicone cream which forms a barrier against a combination of water-soluble and water-insoluble irritants Tube 3 oz, Jar lb. **X:** Industrial cold cream which rubs well into the skin and serves as a skin conditioner. Tube 3 oz, Jar lb. *OTC.*
Use: Skin protectant.

Fendol. (Buffington) Salicylamide, caffeine, acetaminophen, phenylephrine hydrochloride. Sugar, lactose and salt free. Tab. Dispens-A-Kit 500s. Bot., 100s. *OTC.*
Use: Analgesic combination.

•**fendosal.** (FEN-doe-sal) USAN.
Use: Anti-inflammatory.

Fenesin. (Biovail) Guaifenesin 600 mg. SR Tab. Bot. 100s, 600s. *Rx.*
Use: Expectorant.

Fenesin DM. (Biovail) Dextromethorphan HBr 30 mg, guaifenesin 600 mg. SR Tab. Bot. 100s. *Rx.*
Use: Upper respiratory combination, antitussive, expectorant.

•**fenestrel.** (feh-NESS-trell) USAN. Under study.
Use: Estrogen.

•**fenethylline hydrochloride.** (FEN-ETH-ill-in) USAN.
Use: Stimulant (central).

•**fengabine.** (FEN-GAH-bean) USAN.
Use: Mood regulator.

•**fenimide.** (FEN-ih-mid) USAN.
Use: Anxiolytic; antipsychotic.

•**fenisorex.** (fen-EYE-so-rex) USAN.
Use: Anorexigenic; anorexic.

•**fenmetozole hydrochloride.** (FEN-MET-oh-zole) USAN.
Use: Antidepressant; antagonist (to narcotics).

•**fenmetramide.** (fen-MEH-trah-mide) USAN.
Use: Antidepressant.

•**fennel oil.** (FEN-el) *NF 23.*
Use: Pharmaceutic aid (flavor).

•**fenobam.** (FEN-oh-bam) USAN.
Use: Hypnotic; sedative.

•**fenoctimine sulfate.** (fen-OCK-tih-MEEN) USAN.
Use: Gastric antisecretory.

fenofibrate.
Use: Antihyperlipidemic.
See: Antara.
 Lofibra.
 Tricor.
 Triglide.

fenofibrate. (Teva) Fenofibrate (micronized) 134 mg, lactose. Cap. 100s. *Rx.*

Use: Antihyperlipidemic.

●**fenoldopam mesylate.** (feh-NAHL-doe-pam) *USP 28.*
Use: Antihypertensive; dopamine agonist.
See: Corlopam.

fenoldopam mesylate. (Baxter) Fenoldopam mesylate 10 mg/mL. Sodium metabisulfite. Inj. Single-dose amps. 1 mL, 2 mL. *Rx.*
Use: Antihypertensive.

●**fenoprofen.** (FEN-oh-PRO-fen) USAN.
Use: Anti-inflammatory; analgesic.

fenoprofen. (Qualitest) Fenoprofen 200 mg, 300 mg. Cap. Bot. 100s. *Rx.*
Use: Anti-inflammatory; analgesic.

fenoprofen. (Various Mfr.) Fenoprofen. **Cap.:** 200 mg, 300 mg. Bot. 100s. **Tab.:** 600 mg. Bot. 100s, 500s, 1000s; UD 100s; unit-of-use 30s, 60s, 90s, 120s. *Rx.*
Use: Anti-inflammatory; analgesic, NSAID.

●**fenoprofen calcium.** (FEN-oh-PRO-fen) *USP 28.*
Use: Anti-inflammatory; analgesic.
See: Nalfon.

●**fenoterol HBr.** (FEN-oh-TER-ahl) USAN.
Use: Investigational bronchodilator.

●**fenpipalone.** (FEN-PIP-ah-lone) USAN.
Use: Anti-inflammatory.

●**fenprinast hydrochloride.** (fen-PRIH-nast) USAN.
Use: Bronchodilator, antiallergic.

●**fenprostalene.** (FEN-PRAHST-ah-leen) USAN.
Use: Luteolysin.

●**fenquizone.** (FEN-kwih-zone) USAN.
Use: Diuretic.

●**fenretinide.** (fen-RET-ih-nide) USAN.
Use: Investigational antineoplastic.

●**fenspiride hydrochloride.** (fen-SPIH-rid) USAN.
Use: Bronchodilator; antiadrenergic (α-receptor).

fentanyl.
Use: Analgesic, narcotic.
See: Duragesic.

fentanyl. (Various Mfr.) Fentanyl citrate (as base) 50 mcg/mL. Inj. Amp. 2 mL, 5 mL, 10 mL, 20 mL. Single-dose vials. 30 mL, 50 mL. *c-ıı.*
Use: Opioid analgesic.

●**fentanyl citrate.** (FEN-tuh-nill) *USP 28.*
Use: Opioid analgesic.
See: Sublimaze.

fentanyl citrate transmucosal system.
Use: Opioid analgesic.
See: Actiq.

fentanyl transdermal system.
Use: Opioid analgesic.
See: Duragesic-12.
Duragesic-50.
Duragesic-100.
Duragesic-75.
Duragesic-25.

fentanyl transdermal system. (Various Mfr.) Fentanyl 2.5 to 2.75 mg (25 mcg/h), 5 to 5.5 mg (50 mcg/h), 7.5 to 8.25 mg (75 mcg/h), 10 to 11 mg (100 mcg/h). Transdermal system. Cartons containing 5 individually packaged systems. *c-ıı.*
Use: Opioid analgesic.

●**fentiazac.** (fen-TIE-azz-ACK) USAN.
Use: Anti-inflammatory.

●**fenticlor.** (FEN-tih-Klor) USAN.
Use: Antifungal; antiseptic, topical.

●**fenticonazole nitrate.** (FEN-tih-KOE-nah-zole) USAN.
Use: Antifungal.

Fenton. (Sanofi-Synthelabo) Ferrous gluconate. Elix. *OTC.*
Use: Mineral supplement.

Fenylhist. (Roberts) Diphenhydramine hydrochloride 25 mg, 50 mg. Cap. Bot. 1000s. *OTC.*
Use: Antihistamine.

fenyramidol hydrochloride. Phenyramidol hydrochloride.

●**fenyripol hydrochloride.** (FEH-nee-rih-pahl) USAN.
Use: Muscle relaxant.

Feocyte Injectable. (Oxypure) Peptonized iron 15 mg, vitamin B_{12} 200 mcg, liver injection, beef 10 units, sodium citrate 10 mg, benzyl alcohol 2%/mL. Inj. Vial 10 mL. *Rx.*
Use: Mineral, vitamin supplement.

Feocyte Tablets. (Oxypure) Iron 110 mg, vitamins C 100 mg, B_6 2 mg, B_{12} 50 mcg, copper sulfate, folic acid 0.8 mg, desiccated liver 15 mg. Prolonged Action Tab. Bot. 100s. *Rx.*
Use: Mineral, vitamin supplement.

FeoGen. (Rising) Fe 66 mg (as elemental iron), vitamin B_{12} 10 mcg, desiccated stomach substance 100 mg, C 250 mg. Cap. UD 100s. *Rx.*
Use: Vitamin, mineral supplement.

FeoGen FA. (Rising) Fe 66 mg (as elemental iron), vitamin B_{12} 10 mcg, C 250 mg, folic acid 1 mg. Cap. UD 100s. *Rx.*
Use: Vitamin, mineral supplement.

FeoGen Forte. (Rising Pharmaceuticals) Fe 15 mg, B_{12} 10 mcg, C 60 mg, folic acid 1 mg. Softgel Cap. 100s. *Rx.*
Use: Vitamin, mineral supplement.

Feosol. (GlaxoSmithKline) Carbonyl iron 45 mg. Tab. Bot. 30s, 60s. *OTC.*
Use: Mineral supplement.

Feosol. (GlaxoSmithKline) Ferrous sulfate exsiccated (dried) 200 mg (iron 65 mg), 325 mg (65 mg). Glucose (200 mg only). Tab. Bot. 100s. *OTC.*
Use: Mineral supplement.

Feosol Elixir. (GlaxoSmithKline) Ferrous sulfate (44 mg iron) 220 mg/5 mL, alcohol 5%. Elix. Bot. 16 oz. *OTC.*
Use: Mineral supplement.

Feostat. (Forest) Ferrous fumarate 100 mg (33 mg iron). Dextrose, saccharin, chocolate flavor. Chew. Tab. Bot. UD 100s. *OTC.*
Use: Mineral supplement.

FE-Plus Protein. (Miller Pharmacal Group) Iron (as an iron-protein complex) 50 mg. Tab. Bot. 100s. *OTC.*
Use: Mineral supplement.

Feratab. (Upsher-Smith) Ferrous sulfate exsiccated (dried) 300 mg (iron 60 mg-Tab. Bot. UD 100s. *OTC.*
Use: Mineral supplement.

Ferate-C. (Pal-Pak, Inc.) Ferrous fumarate 150 mg, ascorbic acid 200 mg, docusate sodium 25 mg. Tab. Bot. 100s, 1000s. *OTC.*
Use: Mineral, vitamin supplement; stool softener.

Fer-Gen-Sol. (Goldline) Ferrous sulfate 75 mg/0.6 mL (iron 15 mg/0.6 mL), alcohol 0.2%, sodium bisulfite, sorbitol, sugar, potassium sorbate, lemon flavor. Drops. Bot. 50 mL. *OTC.*
Use: Mineral supplement.

Fergon. (Bayer) Ferrous gluconate 225 mg (iron 27 mg). Tab. Bot. 100s. *OTC.*
Use: Mineral supplement.

Feridex I.V. (Berlex) Iron 11.2 mg (iron 56 mg/vial). Soln. Inj. Single dose vial w/administration filter 5 mL. *Rx.*
Use: Radiopaque agent, parenteral.

Fer-In-Sol. (Mead Johnson Nutritionals) Ferrous sulfate 75 mg per 0.6 mL (iron 15 mg per 0.6 mL). Alcohol 0.2%, sodium bisulfite, sorbitol, sugar. Drops. Dropper Bot. 50 mL. *OTC.*
Use: Mineral supplement.

Ferocyl. (Arco) Ferrous fumarate 150 mg (iron 50 mg), docusate sodium 100 mg. TR Cap. Bot. 100s. *OTC.*
Use: Mineral supplement; stool softener.

Fero-Folic 500. (Abbott) Ferrous sulfate controlled-release (equivalent to 105 mg iron), vitamin C 500 mg, folic acid 0.8 mg. Filmtab. Bot. 100s, 500s. *Rx.*

Use: Mineral, vitamin supplement.

Fero-Grad-500. (Abbott) Sodium ascorbate 500 mg, ferrous sulfate equivalent to 105 mg iron. Castor oil. CR Tab. Blisterpack 30s. *OTC.*
Use: Mineral supplement.

Ferolix. (Century) Ferrous sulfate 5 g, alcohol 5%/10 mL Elix. Bot. 8 oz, pt, gal. *OTC.*
Use: Mineral supplement.

Ferosan. (Sandia) Ferrous fumarate 91.2 mg, B_1 10 mg, B_6 3 mg, B_{12} 25 mcg/5 mL. Syr. Bot. 16 oz, gal. *OTC.*
Use: Mineral, vitamin supplement.

Ferosan Forte. (Sandia) Ferrous fumarate 300 mg, liver-stomach concentrate 150 mg, vitamin B_{12} w/intrinsic factor concentrate 7.5 mcg, intrinsic factor concentrate 150 mg, B_{12} 7.5 mcg, ascorbic acid 75 mg, folic acid 1 mg, sorbitol 50 mg. Tab. Bot. 100s. *Rx.*
Use: Mineral, vitamin supplement.

Ferospace. (Hudson Corp.) Ferrous sulfate 250 mg (iron 50 mg). TR Cap. Bot. 100s. *OTC.*
Use: Mineral supplement.

FeroSul. (Major) Ferrous sulfate 325 mg (iron 65 mg). Tab. 100s, 1,000s. *OTC.*
Use: Mineral supplement.

Ferotrinsic. (Rugby) Iron 110 mg (from ferrous fumarate), vitamins B_{12} 15 mcg, C 75 mg, intrinsic factor (as concentrate or from stomach preparations) 240 mg, folic acid 0.5 mg. Cap. 100s, 500s, 1000s. *Rx.*
Use: Mineral, vitamin supplement.

Feroweet. (Barth's) Vitamins B_1 6 mg, B_2 12 mg, niacin 4 mg, iron 30 mg, B_{12} 10 mcg, B_6 95 mcg, pantothenic acid 50 mcg. 3 Cap. Bot. 100s, 500s, 1000s. *OTC.*
Use: Mineral, vitamin supplement.

Ferracomp. (Roberts) Liver 2 mcg, vitamins B_{12} 15 mcg, B_1 10 mg, B_2 5 mg, B_6 1 mg, calcium pantothenate 1 mg, niacinamide 10 mg, iron 31.3 mg/mL. Vial 30 mL. *OTC.*
Use: Mineral, vitamin supplement.

Ferralet Plus. (Mission Pharmacal) Ferrous gluconate equivalent to 46 mg iron, C 400 mg, folic acid 0.8 mg, vitamin B_{12} 25 mcg. Tab. Bot. 60s. *OTC.*
Use: Mineral, vitamin supplement.

Ferrets. (Pharmics) Ferrous fumarate 325 mg, iron 106 mg. Polydextrose. Film coated. Tab. Bot. 60s. *OTC.*
Use: Mineral supplement.

Ferrex 150. (Breckenridge) Iron (as polysaccharide-iron complex) 150 mg. Cap. UD 100s. *OTC.*
Use: Mineral supplement.

Ferrex 150 Forte. (Breckenridge) Iron 150 mg (as polysaccharide-iron complex), folic acid 1 mg, B_{12} 25 mcg. Cap. UD 100s. *Rx.*
Use: Vitamin, mineral supplement.

Ferrex 150 Forte Plus. (Breckenridge) Fe (from ferrous sulfate) 150 mg, vitamin B_{12} 25, C 60 mg, folic acid 1 mg. Cap. UD 100s. *Rx.*
Use: Mineral, vitamin supplement.

Ferrex 150 Plus. (Breckenridge) Fe (from polysaccharide iron and ferrous bisglycinate) 150 mg, ascorbic acid 50 mg. Cap. UD 100s. *OTC.*
Use: Mineral, vitamin supplement.

Ferrex PC. (Breckenridge) Iron 60 mg (as polysaccharide-iron complex), folic acid 1 mg, C 50 mg, B_{12} 3 mcg, A 4000 units, D 400 units, B_1 3 mg, B_2 3 mg, B_6 2 mg, niacinamide 10 mg, Ca 25 mg, Zn 18 mg. Tab. UD 100s. *Rx.*
Use: Vitamin, mineral supplement.

Ferrex PC Forte. (Breckenridge) Vitamins A 5000 units, C 80 mg, Ca 250 mg, iron 60 mg (as polysaccharide-iron complex), D 400 units, E (as dl–alpha–tocopheryl acetate) 30 units, B_1 3 mg, B_2 3.4 mg, niacinamide 20 mg, B_6 4 mg, folic acid 1 mg, B_{12} 12 mcg, I, Mg, Zn 25 mg, Cu. Tab. UD 100s. *Rx.*
Use: Vitamin, mineral supplement.

•**ferric ammonium citrate.** (FER-ik) *USP 28.* Ammonium iron (Fe^{+++}) citrate.
Use: Mineral supplement.

•**ferric ammonium citrate for oral solution.** (FER-ik) *USP 28.*
Use: Mineral supplement.

ferric ammonium sulfate. (Various Mfr.)
Use: Astringent.

ferric ammonium tartrate. (Various Mfr.)
Use: Mineral supplement.

ferric cacodylate. (Various Mfr.)
Use: Leukemias; hematinic.

ferric chloride. (Various Mfr.)
Use: Astringent.

•**ferric chloride Fe 59.** (FER-ik) USAN.
Use: Radiopharmaceutical.

ferric citrochloride tincture. Iron (Fe^{+++}) chloride citrate.
Use: Hematinic.

•**ferric fructose.** (FER-ik FRUKE-tose) USAN.
Use: Hematinic.

ferric glycerophosphate. Glycerol phosphate iron (Fe^{+++}) salt.
Use: Pharmaceutic necessity.

ferric hypophosphate. Iron (Fe^{+++}) phosphinate.

Use: Pharmaceutic necessity.

•**ferriclate calcium sodium.** (fer-ih-KLATE) USAN.
Use: Hematinic.

•**ferric oxide.** (FER-ik) *NF 23.*
Use: Pharmaceutic aid (color).

ferric oxide, yellow.
Use: Pharmaceutic aid (color).

ferric "peptonate". (Various Mfr.)
See: Iron Peptonized.

ferric pyrophosphate, soluble. Iron (Fe^{+++}) citrate pyrophosphate.

ferric quinine citrate, "green". (Various Mfr.)
Use: Mineral supplement.

•**ferric subsulfate solution.** (FER-ik) *USP 28.*
Use: Local use on the skin.

•**ferric sulfate.** (FER-ik) *USP 28.*

•**ferristene.** (FER-ih-steen) USAN.
Use: Diagnostic aid, paramagnetic.

Ferrizyme. (Abbott Diagnostics) Enzyme immunoassay for qualitative determination of ferritin in human serum or plasma. Test kit 100s.
Use: Diagnostic aid, paramagnetic.

Ferrlecit. (Watson Pharma) Sodium ferric gluconate complex 62.5 mg/5 mL (12.5 mg/mL of elemental iron), benzyl alcohol 9 mg/mL, sucrose 20%. Inj. Amp. 5 mL. *Rx.*
Use: Iron-containing product.

ferrocholate.
See: Ferrocholinate.

ferrocholinate. Ferrocholate. Ferrocholine. A chelate prepared by reacting equimolar quantities of freshly precipitated ferric hydroxide with choline dihydrogen citrate.
Use: Mineral supplement.

ferrocholine.
See: Ferrocholinate.

Ferro-Cyte. (Spanner) Iron peptonate 20 mg, liver injection (20 mg/mL) 0.25 mL, vitamins B_1 22 mg, B_2 0.5 mg, B_6 2.5 mg, B_{12} 30 mcg, niacinamide 25 mg, panthenol 1 mg/mL. Inj. Multiple-dose vial 10 mL. *Rx.*
Use: Mineral, vitamin supplement.

Ferro-Docusate TR. (Parmed Pharmaceuticals, Inc.) Ferrous fumarate 150 mg (iron 50 mg), docusate sodium 100 mg. TR Cap. Bot. 100s. *OTC.*
Use: Mineral supplement; stool softener.

Ferro-Dok TR. (Major) Ferrous fumarate 150 mg (iron 50 mg), docusate sodium 100 mg. TR Cap. Bot. 100s. *OTC.*
Use: Mineral supplement; stool softener.

Ferrodyl Chewable Tablets. (Arcum) Ferrous fumarate 320 mg, vitamin C 200 mg. Bot. 100s, 1000s. *OTC.*
Use: Mineral, vitamin supplement.

Ferromar. (Marnel) Ferrous fumarate 201.5 mg (iron 65 mg), vitamin C 200 mg. SR Capl. Bot. 100s. *OTC.*
Use: Mineral supplement.

Ferroneed. (Hanlon) Ferrous gluconate 300 mg, ascorbic acid 60 mg. Cap. Bot. 100s. *OTC.*
Use: Mineral, vitamin supplement.

Ferroneed T-Caps. (Hanlon) Ferrous fumarate 250 mg, thiamine hydrochloride 5 mg, ascorbic acid 50 mg. TD Cap. Bot. 100s. *OTC.*
Use: Mineral, vitamin supplement.

Ferronex. (Taylor Pharmaceuticals) Iron from ferrous gluconate 2.9 mg, vitamins B_{12} equivalent 1 mcg, B_2 0.75 mg, B_3 60 mg, B_5 1.25 mg, B_{12} 18 mcg, procaine 2%/mL. Inj. Vial 30 mL. *Rx.*
Use: Mineral, vitamin supplement.

Ferro-Sequels. (Inverness) Ferrous fumarate 150 mg (iron 50 mg), sodium docusate 100 mg, lactose. TR Tab. Bot. 30s, 90s. *OTC.*
Use: Mineral supplement.

Ferrospan. (Imperial Lab) Ferrous fumarate 200 mg, ascorbic acid 100 mg. Tab. Bot. 100s, 1000s. *OTC.*
Use: Mineral, vitamin supplement.

Ferrosyn Injection. (Standex) Cyanocobalamin 30 mcg, liver 2 mcg, ferrous gluconate 100 mg, riboflavin 1.5 mg, panthenol 2.5 mg, niacinamide 100 mg, procaine 2%. Inj. Vial 30 mL. *Rx.*
Use: Mineral, vitamin supplement.

Ferrosyn S.C. (Standex) Iron 60 mg, vitamin B_{12} 5 mcg, magnesium 0.6 mg, copper 0.3 mg, manganese 0.1 mg, potassium 0.5 mg, zinc 0.15 mg. Tab. Bot. 100s, 1000s. *OTC.*
Use: Mineral, vitamin supplement.

Ferrosyn See. (Standex) Iron 34 mg, ascorbic acid 60 mg. Tab. Bot. 100s, 1000s. *OTC.*
Use: Mineral, vitamin supplement.

Ferrosyn Tablets. (Standex) Fe 60 mg, vitamin B_{12} 5 mcg, Mg 0.6 mg, Cu 0.3 mg, Mn 0.1 mg, K 0.5 mg, Zn 0.15 mg. Tab. Bot. 100s. *OTC.*
Use: Mineral, vitamin supplement.

ferrous bromide. (FER-uhs) (Various Mfr.)
Use: In chorea & tuberculous cervical adenitis.

ferrous carbonate mass. Vallet's mass. (Various Mfr.)
Use: Mineral supplement.

ferrous carbonate, saccharated. (Various Mfr.)

Use: Mineral supplement.

● **ferrous citrate Fe 59.** (FER-uhs) USAN.
Use: Radiopharmaceutical.

● **ferrous fumarate.** (FER-uhs) *USP 28.*
Use: Hematinic.
See: Feostat.
  Ferro-Sequels.
  Ferretts.
  Hemocyte.
  Nephro-Fer.
W/Ascorbic Acid.
See: C-Ron.
  Cytoferin.
  Eldofe-C.
  Ferancee.
  Ferancee-HP.
  Ferrodyl.
  Ferromar.
  Mili-Hema.
W/Ascorbic Acid and Folic Acid.
See: Fer-Regules.
  Ferro-Docusate TR.
  Ferro Dok TR.
  Ferro-DSS SR.
  Ferro-Sequels.
W/Norethindrone, Mestranol.
See: Ortho Novum Fe-28.
W/Vitamins and Minerals.
See: Stuart Formula.
  Stuartnatal 1 + 1.
  Stuart Prenatal.

ferrous fumarate. (Mission) Ferrous fumarate 90 mg (iron 29.5 mg). Sugar. Tab. Bot. 100s. *OTC.*
Use: Mineral supplement.

ferrous fumarate. (Various Mfr.) Ferrous fumarate 324 mg (iron 106 mg). Tab. 100s. *OTC.*
Use: Mineral supplement.

ferrous fumarate and docusate sodium.
Use: Mineral supplement.

● **ferrous gluconate.** (FER-uhs) *USP 28.*
Use: Hematinic.
See: Fergon.
W/Ascorbic Acid, Desiccated Liver, Vitamin B Complex.
See: I.L.X. w/B_{12}.
  Stuart Hematinic.
W/Polyoxyethylene Glucitan Monolaurate.
See: Simron.

ferrous gluconate. (Various Mfr.) Ferrous gluconate 225 mg (iron 27 mg), 300 mg (iron 35 mg), 324 mg (iron 38 mg), 325 mg (iron 36 mg). Tab. Bot. 100s (except 325 mg), 1,000s (325 mg only). *OTC.*
Use: Mineral supplement.

ferrous iodide. (Various Mfr.)
Use: In chronic tuberculosis.
ferrous iodide syrup. (Various Mfr.)
Use: In chronic tuberculosis.
ferrous lactate. (Various Mfr.)
Use: Mineral supplement.
•**ferrous sulfate.** (FER-uhs) *USP 28.*
Use: Hematinic.
See: Feosol.
  Fer-Gen-Sol.
  Fer-In-Sol.
  Fero-Gradumet.
  Ferolix.
  FeroSul.
  Fesotyme SR.
  Irospan.
  Mol-Iron.
W/Ascorbic Acid.
See: Fero-Grad-500.
  Mol-Iron w/Vitamin C.
W/Ascorbic Acid, Folic Acid.
See: Fero-Folic-500.
W/Cyanocobalamin, Ascorbic Acid, Folic
  Acid.
See: Intrin.
W/Folic Acid.
See: Folvron.
•**ferrous sulfate.** (Rugby) Ferrous sulfate
exsiccated (dried) 160 mg (iron 50 mg).
SR Tab. Blisterpack 60s. *OTC.*
Use: Mineral supplement.
ferrous sulfate. (Various Mfr.) Ferrous
sulfate. **Tab.:** 325 mg (iron 65 mg).
100s, 1,000s, UD 100s. **Elix.:** 220 mg/
5 mL (iron 44 mg/5 mL). May contain
alcohol. Bot. 473 mL. **Drops:** 75 mg/
0.6 mL (iron 15 mg/0.6 mL). May con-
tain alcohol. Bot. 50 mL. *OTC.*
Use: Mineral supplement.
ferrous sulfate. (Ivax) Ferrous sulfate
325 mg (elemental iron 65 mg). Tab.
Bot. 100s. *OTC.*
Use: Mineral supplement.
•**ferrous sulfate, dried.** (FER-uhs)
USP 28.
Use: Antianemic.
See: Feosol.
  Fer-In-Sol.
  Ferrous Sulfate.
  Slow Fe.
ferrous sulfate exsiccated (dried).
Use: Mineral supplement.
See: Feosol.
  Feratab.
  Slow FE.
  Slow Release Iron.
•**ferrous sulfate Fe 59.** (FER-uhs) USAN.
Use: Radiopharmaceutical.
Fertility Tape. (Weston Labs.) Regular,
extrasensitive, less-sensitive. W/Fertil-

ity Testor, cervical glucose test. Pkg.
test 60s.
Use: Diagnostic aid.
•**ferucarbotran.** (fur-you-CAR-boe-tran)
USAN.
Use: Diagnostic aid (paramagnetic).
•**ferumoxides.** (feh-roo-MOX-ides) USAN.
Use: Diagnostic aid (paramagnetic),
parenteral.
See: Feridex I.V.
ferumoxtran-10. (fur-you-MOX-tran 10)
Use: Diagnostic aid (paramagnetic).
•**ferumoxytol.** (fer-yoo-MOX-i-tole)
USAN.
Use: Diagnostic aid (MRI); iron deficiency.
Ferusal. (Eon Labs) Ferrous sulfate
325 mg. Tab. *OTC.*
Use: Mineral supplement.
Festalan. (Hoechst) Lipase 6000 units,
amylase 30,000 units, protease
20,000 units, atropine methylnitrate
1 mg. EC Tab. Bot. 100s, 1000s. *Rx.*
Use: Digestive enzyme.
Fetinic. (Roberts) Iron 3.6 mg, vitamins
B_{12} equivalent to 2 mcg, B_1 10 mg, B_2
0.5 mg, B_3 10 mg, B_5 1 mg, B_6 1 mg,
B_{12} 15 mcg, chlorobutanol 0.5%, ben-
zyl alcohol 2%/mL. Vial 30 mL. *Rx.*
Use: Mineral, vitamin supplement.
Fetinic-MW. (Roberts) Iron 66 mg (from
ferrous fumarate), vitamins B_{12} 5 mcg,
C 60 mg. SR Cap. Bot. 100s. *OTC.*
Use: Mineral, vitamin supplement.
Fe-Tinic 150. (Ethex Corp.) Iron 150 mg
(as polysaccharide-iron complex). Cap.
1,000s, UD 100s. *Rx.*
Use: Mineral supplement.
Fe-Tinic 150 Forte. (Ethex) Iron 150 mg
(as polysaccharide-iron complex), folic
acid 1 mg, B_{12} 25 mcg. Cap. UD 100s.
Rx.
Use: Vitamin, mineral supplement.
•**fetoxylate hydrochloride.** (fee-TOX-ih-
LATE) USAN.
Use: Muscle relaxant.
Feverall Children's. (Alpharma) Aceta-
minophen 120 mg. Supp. Pkg. 6s. *OTC.*
Use: Analgesic.
Feverall, Infants'. (Alpharma) Aceta-
minophen 80 mg. Supp. Pkg. 6s. *OTC.*
Use: Analgesic.
Feverall, Junior Strength. (Alpharma)
Acetaminophen 325 mg. Supp. Pkg.
6s. *OTC.*
Use: Analgesic.
Feverall Sprinkle. (Alpharma) Aceta-
minophen 80 mg, 160 mg. Cap. Bot.
20s. *OTC.*
Use: Analgesic.

FeverAll Suppositories. (Alpharma) Acetaminophen 120 mg, 325 mg, 650 mg. Supp. Ctn. 12s, 50s, 500s (650 mg). *OTC.*
Use: Analgesic.

•**feverfew.** (FEE-ver-fyoo) *NF 23.*
Use: Dietary supplement.

•**fexofenadine.** (fex-oh-FEN-ah-deen) USAN.
Use: Antihistamine, peripherally-selective piperidine.
See: Allegra.
W/Combinations.
See: Allegra-D 12 Hour Tablets.
Allegra-D 24 Hour.

•**fezolamine fumarate.** (feh-ZOLE-ah-MEEN) USAN.
Use: Antidepressant.

fgn-1. (Cell Pathways, Inc.)
Use: Treatment of adenomatous polyposis coli. [Orphan Drug]

•**fiacitabine.** (fih-AH-sit-ah-BEEN) USAN.
Use: Antiviral.

•**fialuridine.** (fie-al-YOUR-ih-deen) USAN.
Use: Antiviral.

FIAU. (Oclassen)
Use: Antiviral, hepatitis B. [Orphan Drug]

Fiberall Natural Flavor. (Novartis) **Pow.:**
Psyllium hydrophilic mucilloid 3.4 g, wheat bran, sodium < 10 mg, potassium 60 mg, calories 6/5.9 g, saccharin. Can 150 g, 300 g, 450 g. **Wafer:** Psyllium hydrophilic mucilloid 3.4 g, wheat bran, oats, sucrose. Box 14s. *OTC.*
Use: Laxative.

Fiberall Orange Flavor. (Heritage Consumer) Psyllium hydrophilic mucilloid 3.5 g/dose, aspartame. Pow. Can 480 g. *OTC.*
Use: Laxative.

Fiberall Tropical Fruit Flavor. (Heritage Consumer) Psyllium hydrophilic mucilloid 3.5 g/dose, aspartame. Pow. Can. 454 g, UD 10 g packets. *OTC.*
Use: Laxative.

FiberCon. (Wyeth) Calcium polycarbophil 625 mg (equiv. to 500 mg polycarbophil). Tab. Bot. 36s, 60s, 90s. *OTC.*
Use: Laxative.

Fiber Guard. (Wyeth) All natural high-fiber supplement 530 mg. Tab. Bot. 100s, 200s. *OTC.*
Use: Fiber supplement.

Fiberlan. (Elan) Protein 50 g, fat 40 g, carbohydrates 160 g, Na 920 mg, K 1.56 g, fiber 14 g/per L. With vitamins A, C, B, B_2, B_3, D, E, B_5, B_6, B_{12}, K, Ca, Fe, folic acid, P, I, Mg, Zn, Cu, biotin,

Mn, choline, Cl, Se, Cr, Mo. Liq. Bot. 237 mL. *OTC.*
Use: Nutritional supplement.

Fiber-Lax. (Rugby) Calcium polycarbophil 625 mg (equiv. to 500 mg polycarbophil). Tab. Bot. 60s, 90s, 500s. *OTC.*
Use: Laxative.

Fibermed High-Fiber Snacks. (Purdue) One serving (15 snacks) contains 5 g dietary fiber. Box 8 oz. Packs of 24 × 1.3 oz. *OTC.*
Use: Fiber supplement.

Fibermed High-Fiber Supplement. (Purdue) Each supplement contains 5 g dietary fiber. Box 14s. Institutional pack, Box 144s of two supplements. *OTC.*
Use: Fiber supplement.

FiberNorm. (G & W) Polycarbophil 625 mg. Tab. Bot. 60s, 90s. *OTC.*
Use: Laxative.

Fibre Trim. (Schering-Plough) Grain and citrus fruit concentrated dietary fiber. Tab. Bot. 100s, 250s. *OTC.*
Use: Dietary aid.

Fibre Trim w/Calcium. (Schering-Plough) Grain and citrus fruit concentrated dietary fiber w/calcium. Tab. Bot. 90s, 225s. *OTC.*
Use: Dietary aid.

fibric acid derivatives.
Use: Antihyperlipidemic.
See: Fenofibrate.
Gemfibrozil.

fibrinogen (human). (Alpha Therapeutic) Partially purified fibrinogen prepared by fractionation from normal human plasma.
Use: Coagulant, clotting factor. [Orphan Drug]

•**fibrinogen I 125.** (FIE-BRIN-oh-jen I 125) USAN.
Use: Diagnostic aid (vascular patency); radiopharmaceutical.

fibrinolysis inhibitor.
See: Amicar.

Fibrogammin P. (Aventis Behring)
Use: Congenital Factor XIII deficiency. [Orphan Drug]

•**fidexaban.** (fye-DEX-a-ban) USAN.
Use: Anticoagulant.

•**fiduxosin hydrochloride.** (fi-DUX-oe-sin) USAN.
Use: Benign prostatic hyperplasia.

•**filaminast.** (fih-LAM-in-ast) USAN.
Use: Antiasthmatic (selective phosphodiesterase IV inhibitor).

Filaxis. (Amlab) Vitamins A 25,000 units, D 1250 units, C 150 mg, E 5 units, B_1

12 mg, B_2 5 mg, B_6 0.5 mg, B_{12} 5 mcg, calcium pantothenate 5 mg, niacinamide 100 mg, Fe 15 mg, I 0.15 mg, Mg 10 mg, K 5 mg, Ca 75 mg, P 60 mg. Tab. Bot. 30s, 100s. Available w/B_{12}. Bot. 30s, 60s, 100s. *OTC.*
Use: Mineral, vitamin supplement.

•**filgrastim.** (fill-GRAH-stim) USAN. *Use:* Biological response modifier; antineoplastic adjunct; antineutropenic; hematopoietic stimulant. [Orphan Drug]
See: Neupogen.

•**filipin.** (FIH-lih-pin) USAN. *Use:* Antifungal.

Finac. (C & M Pharmacal) Salicylic acid 2%, isopropyl alcohol 22.5%, propylene glycol, acetone in lotion base. Bot. 60 mL. *OTC.*
Use: Dermatologic, acne.

Finacea. (Berlex Labs) Azelaic acid 15%, EDTA, benzoic acid. Gel. 30 g. *Rx.*
Use: Anti-inflammatory.

•**finasteride.** (fih-NASS-teer-ide) *USP 28.*
Use: Benign prostatic hypertrophy therapy; antineoplastic; antineutropenic; inhibitor (alpha-reductase); androgen hormone inhibitor.
See: Propecia.
Proscar.

Finevin. (Berlex) Azelaic acid 20%, glycerin, cetearyl alchol. Cream. Tube. 30 g. *Rx.*
Use: Anti-infective, antibiotic, topical.

Fioricet. (Novartis) Acetaminophen 325 mg, butalbital 50 mg, caffeine 40 mg. Tab. Bot. 100s, 500s, UD 100s. *Rx.*
Use: Analgesic; hypnotic; sedative.

Fioricet with Codeine. (Novartis) Codeine phosphate 30 mg, acetaminophen 325 mg, caffeine 40 mg, butalbital 50 mg. Cap. Bot. 100s, *ControlPak* 25s. *c-III.*
Use: Narcotic analgesic combination.

Fiorinal. (Novartis) Butalbital 50 mg, caffeine 40 mg, aspirin 325 mg, benzyl alcohol, parabens, EDTA. Cap. Bot. 100s, 500s, UD 25s. *c-III.*
Use: Analgesic; hypnotic; sedative.

Fiorinal with Codeine No. 3. (Novartis) Butalbital 50 mg, caffeine 40 mg, aspirin 325 mg, codeine phosphate 30 mg. Cap. Bot. 100s. *Control Pak* 25s. *c-III.*
Use: Analgesic combination; hypnotic; sedative.

fire ant venom, allergenic extract, imported.
Use: Dermatologic aid-skin test; immunotherapy. [Orphan Drug]

Firmdent. (Moyco Union Broach Division) *Formerly Moy.* Karaya gum 94.6%, sodium borate 5.36% Pkg. 3 oz. *OTC.*
Use: Denture adhesive.

•**firocoxib.** (fir-oh-KOX-ib) USAN. *Use:* Analgesic, anti-inflammatory.

First Aid Cream. (Johnson & Johnson) Cetyl alcohol, glyceryl stearate, isopropyl palmitate, stearyl alcohol, synthetic beeswax. Tube 0.8 oz, 1.5 oz, 2.5 oz. *OTC.*
Use: Antiseptic; dermatologic, protectant.

First Aid Cream. (Walgreen) Benzocaine 3%, allantoin 0.2%, benzyl alcohol 4%, phenol 0.25%. Tube 1.5 oz. *OTC.*
Use: Anesthetic; antiseptic.

First Choice. (Polymer Technology) 50s.
Use: Diagnostic aid.

First Response Ovulation Predictor. (Tambrands, Inc.) Monoclonal antibody-based enzyme immunoassay test for hLH in urine. Test kit 1s. *OTC.*
Use: Diagnostic aid.

First Response Pregnancy Test. (Tambrands, Inc.) Reagent in-home kit for urine testing. Test kit 1s.
Use: Diagnostic aid.

fish oil concentrate, natural. Natural fish oil concentrate containing EPA (Eicosanoic acid) and DHA (Docosahexaenoic acid).
Use: Nutritional supplement.

FIV-ASA. (Paddock) 5-aminosalicylic acid 500 mg. Supp. Bot. 30s. *Rx.*
Use: Gastrointestinal agent.

5-FC.
See: Flucytosine.

5-FU.
See: Fluorouracil.

523. (Enzyme Process) Pancreatin 200 mg, tryspin, chymotrypsin, amylase, lipase enzymes from pancreatin, raw beef pancreas. Tab. Bot. 100s, 250s.
Use: Digestive enzyme.

Fixodent. (Procter & Gamble) Calcium sodium poly (vinyl methyl ether-maleate), carboxymethylcellulose sodium in a petrolatum base. Tube 0.75 oz, 1.5 oz, 2.5 oz. *OTC.*
Use: Denture adhesive.

FK506.
See: Prograf.

FK-565.
Use: Immunomodulator.

Flagyl. (Pharmacia) Metronidazole 250 mg, 500 mg. Bot. 50s, 100s, 500s (500 mg only), 2500s (250 mg only). *Rx.*

Use: Anti-infective.

Flagyl ER. (Pharmacia) Metronidazole 750 mg, lactose. ER Tab. Bot. 30s. Rx.
Use: Anti-infective.

Flagyl IV. (Pharmacia) Metronidazole 500 mg, mannitol 415 mg (per vial). Pow. for Inj., lyophilized. Single-dose vial. Rx.
Use: Anti-infective.

Flagyl IV RTU. (Pharmacia) Metronidazole 5 mg/mL, sodium 14 mEq (per vial). Inj. Single-dose plastic container 100 mL. Rx.
Use: Anti-infective.

Flagyl 375. (Pharmacia) Metronidazole 375 mg. Cap. Bot. 50s, UD 100s. Rx.
Use: Anti-infective.

Flanders Buttocks Ointment. (Flanders) Zinc oxide, castor oil, balsam peru, boric acid in an emollient base. Tube. 60 g. OTC.
Use: Dermatologic, counterirritant.

Flarex. (Alcon) Fluorometholone acetate 0.1%. Susp. Bot. 2.5 mL, 5 mL, 10 mL Drop-Tainers. Rx.
Use: Corticosteroid, ophthalmic; anti-inflammatory.

Flatulence. (Pal-Pak, Inc.) Nux vomica 16.2 mg, cascara sagrada extract 64.8 mg, ginger 48.6 mg, capsicum 16.2 mg, asafetida. Tab. Bot. OTC.
Use: Antiflatulent; laxative.

Flatulex. (Dayton) **Tab.:** Simethicone 80 mg, activated charcoal 250 mg. Bot. 100s. **Drops:** Simethicone 40 mg/0.6 mL. Bot. 30 mL with calibrated dropper. OTC.
Use: Antiflatulent.

Flatus. (Foy Laboratories) Nux vomica extract 0.25 g, cascara extract 1 g, ginger ¾ g, capsicum g, w/asafetida qs. Tab. Bot. 1000s. OTC.
Use: Antiflatulent; laxative.

Flav-A-D. (Kirkman) Vitamins A 5000 units, D 1000 units, C 100 mg. Tab. Bot. 100s, 1000s. Also w/fluoride. Bot. 100s, 1000s. Rx-OTC.
Use: Vitamin supplement.

flavine.
See: Acriflavine Hydrochloride.

Flavinoid-C. (Barth's) **Tab.:** Vitamin C 150 mg, hesperidin complex 10 mg, citrus bioflavonoid 50 mg, rutin 20 mg. Bot. 100s, 500s, 1000s. **Liq.:** Vitamin C 100 mg, bioflavonoid complex 100 mg/5 mL. Bot. 4 oz. OTC.
Use: Vitamin supplement.

flavocoxid.
Use: Oral nutritional supplement.
See: Limbrel.

•**flavodilol maleate.** (FLAY-voe-DILL-ole) USAN.
Use: Antihypertensive.

flavolutan.
See: Progesterone.

flavonoid compounds.
See: Bio-Flavonoid Compounds; Vitamin P.

Flavons. (Freeda) Bioflavonoids 500 mg, calcium carbonate, calcium stearate. Tab. Bot. 100s, 250s. OTC.
Use: Vitamin supplement.

Flavons-500. (Freeda) Citrus bioflavonoids 500 mg. Tab. Bot. 100s, 250s. OTC.
Use: Vitamin supplement.

flavored diluent. (Roxane) Flavored vehicle for the immediate administration of crushed tablet or capsule product. Bot. 500 mL, UD 15 mL × 100.
Use: Flavored vehicle.

•**flavoxate hydrochloride.** (flay-VOKES-ate) USAN.
Use: Antispasmodic, urinary; muscle relaxant; anticholinergic.
See: Urispas.

flavoxate hydrochloride. (Global) Flavoxate hydrochloride 100 mg. Tab. 100s. Rx.
Use: Anticholinergic.

flavurol. Merbromin.
Use: Antiseptic.

•**flazalone.** (FLAY-zah-lone) USAN.
Use: Anti-inflammatory.

Flebogamma 5%. (Grifols) Immune globulin (human) 5% (50 mg/mL). Sorbitol 50 mg, polyethylene glycol ≤ 6 mg/mL, preservative-free. Inj. Vials. 10 mL, 50 mL, 100 mL, 200 mL. Rx.
Use: Immune globulin.

•**flecainide acetate.** (fleh-CANE-ide) USP 28.
Use: Antiarrhythmic agent.
See: Tambocor.

flecainide acetate. (Various Mfr.) Flecainide acetate 50 mg, 100 mg, 150 mg. Tab. 100s. Rx.
Use: Antiarrhythmic agent.

Fleet. (Fleet) Dibasic sodium phosphate 7 g, monobasic sodium phosphate 19 g/118 mL delivered dose (sodium 4.4 g/dose). Disp. enema. Squeeze bot. Pediatric 66 mL, Adult 133 mL. OTC.
Use: Laxative, enema.

Fleet Babylax. (Fleet) Glycerin 4 mL per applicator. Liq. Pkg. App. 6s. OTC.
Use: Laxative.

Fleet Bagenema. (Fleet) Castile soap or Fleets bisacodyl prep. OTC.
Use: Laxative.

Fleet Bisacodyl. (Fleet) Bisacodyl 10 mg/30 mL delivered dose. Disp. enema. Squeeze bot. 37 mL. *OTC.*
Use: Laxative, enema.

Fleet Enema. (Fleet) Sodium biphosphate 19 g, sodium phosphate 7 g/118 mL. Bot. w/rectal tube 4.5 oz. Pediatric size 67.5 mL, 135 mL. *OTC.*
Use: Laxative.

Fleet Glycerin Suppositories. (Fleet) Adult: Jar 12s, 24s, 50s. Child Size: Jar 12s. *OTC.*
Use: Laxative.

Fleet Laxative. (Fleet) Bisacodyl. **EC Tab.:** 5 mg, sucrose. Bot. 25s, 100s. **Supp.:** 10 mg. Box 4s, 12s, 50s, 100s. *OTC.*
Use: Laxative.

Fleet Medicated Wipes. (Fleet) Hamamelis water 50%, alcohol 7%, glycerin 10%, benzalkonium Cl, methylparaben. Rectal pads. 100s. *OTC.*
Use: Perianal hygiene.

Fleet Mineral Oil. (Fleet) Mineral oil. Squeeze bot. 133 mL. *OTC.*
Use: Laxative, enema.

Fleet Pain Relief. (Fleet) Pramoxine hydrochloride 1%, glycerin 12%. Pads. 100s. *OTC.*
Use: Anorectal preparation.

Fleet Phospho-Soda. (Fleet) Monobasic sodium phosphate 2.4 g, dibasic sodium phosphate 0.9 g/5 mL (sodium 556 mg/5 mL), saccharin, regular and ginger-lemon flavor. Soln. Bot. 45 mL, 90 mL, 240 mL. *OTC.*
Use: Laxative.

Fleet Prep Kit 1. (Fleet) *Phospho-Soda* 45 mL (monobasic sodium phosphate 21.6 g, dibasic sodium phosphate 8.1 g), 4 bisacodyl tablets (5 mg each), 1 bisacodyl suppository (10 mg). *OTC.*
Use: Laxative, enema.

Fleet Prep Kit 3. (Fleet) *Phospho-Soda* 45 mL (monobasic sodium phosphate 21.6 g, dibasic sodium phosphate 8.1 g), 4 bisacodyl tablets (5 mg each), bisacodyl enema 30 mL (10 mg). *OTC.*
Use: Laxative, enema.

Fleet Prep Kit 2. (Fleet) *Phospho-Soda* 45 mL (monobasic sodium phosphate 21.6 g, dibasic sodium phosphate 8.1 g), 4 bisacodyl tablets (5 mg each), 1 bag enema. *OTC.*
Use: Laxative, enema.

•**fleroxacin.** (fler-OX-ah-SIN) USAN.
Use: Anti-infective.

•**flestolol sulfate.** (FLESS-toe-lahl) USAN.
Use: Antiadrenergic (β-receptor).

•**fletazepam.** (FLET-AZE-eh-pam) USAN.
Use: Muscle relaxant.

Fletcher's Castoria. (Mentholatum Co.) Senna concentrate 33.3 mg/mL, alcohol free, sucrose, parabens. Liq. Bot. 74 mL, 150 mL. *OTC.*
Use: Laxative.

Fletcher's Castoria for Children. (Mentholatum Co.) Senna 6.5%, alcohol 3.5%. Liq. Bot. 74 mL, 150 mL. *OTC.*
Use: Laxative.

Flexall 454. (Chattem) Menthol 7%, alcohol, allantoin, aloe vera gel, boric acid, carbomer 940, diazolidinyl urea, eucalyptus oil, glycerin, iodine, parabens, methyl salicylate, peppermint oil, polysorbate 60, potassium iodide, propylene glycol, thyme oil, triethanolamine. Gel. Tube. 240 g. *OTC.*
Use: Analgesic, topical.

Flexall 454, Maximum Strength. (Chattem) Menthol 16%, aloe vera gel, eucalyptus oil, methylsalicylate, SD alcohol 38-B, thyme oil. Gel. Tube. 90 mg. *OTC.*
Use: Analgesic, topical.

Flex Anti-Dandruff Shampoo. (Revlon) Zinc pyrithione 1% in liquid shampoo. *OTC.*
Use: Antiseborrheic.

Flex Anti-Dandruff Styling Mousse. (Revlon) Zinc pyrithione 0.1%. Aerosol foam. *OTC.*
Use: Antiseborrheic.

Flexaphen. (Trimen Laboratories, Inc.) Chlorzoxazone 250 mg, acetaminophen 300 mg. Cap. Bot 100s. *Rx.*
Use: Muscle relaxant.

Flex-Care Especially for Sensitive Eyes. (Alcon) EDTA 0.1%, chlorhexidine gluconate 0.005%, sodium Cl, sodium borate, boric acid. Soln. Bot. 118 mL, 237 mL, 355 mL, 360 mL. *OTC.*
Use: Contact lens care.

Flexeril. (McNeil) Cyclobenzaprine hydrochloride 5 mg, 10 mg. Tab. Bot. 100s, UD 100s. *Rx.*
Use: Muscle relaxant.

flexible hydroactive dressings/granules.
See: DuoDerm.
  Intra Site.
  Shur-Clens.
  Sorbsan.

FlexiGel Strands. (Smith-Nephew) Single-use absorbent matrix. 6 g unit. Absorbent wound dressing. 10s. *OTC.*
Use: Dressing.

Flexoject. (Merz) Orphenadrine citrate 30 mg/mL. Inj. Vial 10 mL, Amp 2 mL.

Rx.
Use: Muscle relaxant.
Flexon. (Keene Pharmaceuticals)
Orphenadrine citrate 30 mg/mL. Inj. Vial
10 mL. *Rx.*
Use: Muscle relaxant.
Flex-Power Performance Sports. (Flex-Power) Trolamine salicylate 10%. Cetyl
alcohol, EDTA, parabens, glycerols,
stearyl alcohol, sodium metabisulfite.
Cream. Citrus light and clean scents.
120 g. *OTC.*
Use: Rub and liniment.
Flexsol. (Alcon) Sterile, buffered, isotonic aqueous soln. of sodium Cl, sodium borate, boric acid, adsorbobase.
Bot. 6 oz. *OTC.*
Use: Contact lens care.
Flextra-DS. (Poly Pharmaceuticals)
Acetaminophen 500 mg, phenyltoloxamine citrate 50 mg. Tab. Bot. 100s.
OTC.
Use: Analgesic.
●**flibanserin.** (flib-AN-ser-in) USAN.
Use: Antidepressant.
●**flindokalner.** (flin-doe-KAL-ner) USAN.
Use: Neuroprotectant.
Flintstones Children's. (Bayer Corp.
(Consumer Div.)) Vitamin A 2500 units,
E 15 mg, C 60 mg, folic acid 0.3 mg,
B_1 1.05 mg, B_2 1.2 mg, B_3 13.5 mg, B_6
1.05 mg, B_{12} 4.5 mcg, D 400 units.
Chew. Tab. Bot. 60s, 100s. *OTC.*
Use: Vitamin supplement.
Flintstones Complete. (Bayer Corp.
(Consumer Div.)) Elemental iron 18 mg,
vitamins A 5000 units, D 400 units, E
30 mg, B_1 1.5 mg, B_2 1.7 mg, B_3 20 mg,
B_5 10 mg, B_6 2 mg, B_{12} 6 mcg, C
60 mg, folic acid 0.4 mg, biotin 40 mcg,
Ca, Cu, I, Mg, P, zinc 15 mg. Chew.
Tab. Bot. 60s, 120s. *OTC.*
Use: Mineral, vitamin supplement.
Flintstones Plus Calcium. (Bayer Corp.
(Consumer Div.)) Vitamin A 2500 units,
D units 400, E 15 units, C 60 mg, folic acid 0.3 mg, B_1 1.05 mg, B_2 1.2 mg,
B_3 13.5 mg, B_6 1.05 mg, B_{12} 4.5 mcg,
Ca 200 mg. Chew. Tab. Bot. 60s. *OTC.*
Use: Mineral, vitamin supplement.
Flintstones Plus Extra C Children's.
(Bayer Corp. (Consumer Div.)) Vitamins A 2500 units, D 400 units, E
15 mg, C 250 mg, folic acid 0.3 mg, B_1
1.05 mg, B_2 1.2 mg, niacin 13.5 mg,
B_6 1.05 mg, B_{12} 4.5 mcg. Tab. Bot. 60s,
100s. *OTC.*
Use: Vitamin supplement.
Flintstones Plus Iron Multivitamins.
(Bayer Corp. (Consumer Div.)) Vitamins
A 2500 units, E 15 mg, C 60 mg,

folic acid 0.3 mg, B_1 1.05 mg, B_2 1.2 mg,
niacin 13.5 mg, B_6 1.05 mg, B_{12}
4.5 mcg, D 400 units, iron 15 mg. Chew.
Tab. Bot. 60s, 100s. *OTC.*
Use: Mineral, vitamin supplement.
Flo-Coat. (Mallinckrodt) Barium sulfate
100%, simethicone. Susp. Bot.
1850 mL. *Rx.*
Use: Radiopaque agent, GI contrast
agent.
●**floctafenine.** (FLOCK-tah-FEN-een)
USAN.
Use: Analgesic.
Flolan. (GlaxoSmithKline) Epoprostenol
sodium 0.5 mg, 1.5 mg, mannitol,
NaCl. Vial. Pow. for Inj. 17 mL. *Rx.*
Use: Antihypertensive.
Flomax. (Abbott) Tamsulosin hydrochloride 0.4 mg. Cap. Bot. 100s, 1000s.
Rx.
Use: Benign prostatic hyperplasia treatment, antiadrenergic.
Flonase. (GlaxoSmithKline) Fluticasone
propionate 50 mcg/actuation, dextrose,
polysorbate 80, benzalkonium chloride
w/w 0.02%, phenylethyl alcohol w/w
0.25%. Spray. Amber glass. Bot. w/metering atomizer pump and nasal
adapter. 16 g (120 actuations). *Rx.*
Use: Respiratory inhalant product, intranasal steroid.
Floranex. (Rising) Mixed culture of *Lactobacillus acidophilus* and *L. bulgaricus*
1 million CFU. Lactose, non-fat dried
milk, sucrose. Chew. Tab. 50s. *OTC.*
Use: Nutritional supplement.
Flor-D Chewable Tab. (Derm Pharm.)
Fluoride 1 mg, vitamins A 4000 units,
D 400 units, C 75 mg, B_1 1.5 mg, B_2
1.8 mg, niacinamide 15 mg, B_6 1 mg,
B_{12} 3 mcg, calcium pantothenate 10 mg.
Chew. Tab. Bot. 100s. *Rx.*
Use: Mineral, vitamin supplement.
Flor-D Drops. (Derm Pharm.) Fluoride
0.5 mg, vitamins A 3000 units, D
400 units, C 60 mg, B_1 1 mg, B_2 1.2 mg,
niacinamide 8 mg/0.6 mL. Drops. Bot.
60 mL. *Rx.*
Use: Mineral, vitamin supplement.
●**flordipine.** (FLORE-dih-peen) USAN.
Use: Antihypertensive.
Florical. (Mericon) Sodium fluoride
8.3 mg, calcium carbonate 364 mg
(equivalent to 145.6 mg calcium). Cap.
Tab. Bot. 100s, 500s. *OTC.*
Use: Mineral supplement, calcium.
Florida Foam. (Hill Dermaceuticals)
Benzalkonium Cl, aluminum subacetate, boric acid 2%. Bot. 8 oz. *OTC.*
Use: Soap substitute; antiseborrheic;
antifungal; dermatologic-acne.

Florida Sunburn Relief. (Pharmacel Laboratory, Inc.) Benzyl alcohol 3%, phenol 0.4%, camphor 0.2%, menthol 0.15%. Lot. Bot. 60 mL. *OTC.*
Use: Sunburn relief.

Florinef Acetate. (Monarch) Fludrocortisone acetate, 0.1 mg, lactose. Tab. Bot. 100s. *Rx.*
Use: Corticosteroid.

Florone Cream. (Dermik) Diflorasone diacetate 0.5 mg/g (0.05%) w/stearic acid, sorbitan mono-oleate, polysorbate 60, sorbic acid, citric acid, propylene glycol, purified water. Cream. Tube 15 g, 30 g, 60 g. *Rx.*
Use: Corticosteroid, topical.

Florone E. (Dermik) Diflorasone diacetate 0.5 mg. Tube 15 g, 30 g, 60 g. *Rx.*
Use: Corticosteroid, topical.

Florone Ointment. (Dermik) Diflorasone diacetate 0.5 mg/g (0.05%), polyoxypropylene 15-stearyl ether, stearic acid, lanolin alcohol, white petrolatum. Oint. Tube 15 g, 30 g, 60 g. *Rx.*
Use: Corticosteroid, topical.

Floropryl. (Merck & Co.) Isoflurophate 0.025% in sterile ophthalmic ointment in polyethylene-mineral oil gel. Tube 3.5 g. *Rx.*
Use: Agent for glaucoma.

Florvite. (Everett) Vitamins, fluoride 0.5 mg. Chew. Tab. Bot 100s. *Rx.*
Use: Dental caries agent.

Florvite Drops. (Everett) Fluoride 0.25 mg, 0.5 mg, A 1500 units, D 400 units, E 5 units, B_1 0.5 mg, B_2 0.6 mg, B_3 8 mg, B_6 0.4 mg, B_{12} 2 mcg, C 35 mg. Bot. 50 mL. *Rx.*
Use: Mineral, vitamin supplement; dental caries agent.

Florvite Half Strength. (Everett) Elemental fluoride 0.5 mg, vitamins A 2500 units, D 400 units, E 15 mg, B_1 1.05 mg, B_2 1.2 mg, B_3 13.5 mg, B_6 1.05 mg, B_{12} 4.5 mcg, C 60 mg, folic acid 0.3 mg. Chew. Tab. Bot. 100s. *Rx.*
Use: Mineral, vitamin supplement; dental caries agent.

Florvite Pediatric Drops. (Everett) Elemental fluorine, 0.25 mg/mL, 0.5 mg/mL, Vitamins A 1500 units, D 400 units, E 5 mg, B_1 0.5 mg, B_2 0.6 mg, B_3 8 mg, B_6 0.4 mg, B_{12} 2 mcg, C 35 mg/mL. Bot. 50 mL *Rx.*
Use: Mineral, vitamin supplement; dental caries agent.

Florvite + Iron Chewable. (Everett) Fluoride 1 mg, iron 12 mg, vitamins A 2500 units, D 400 units, E 15 mg, B_1 1.05 mg, B_2 1.2 mg, B_3 13.5 mg, B_6 1.05 mg, B_{12} 4.5 mcg, C 60 mg, folic acid 0.3 mg, Cu, Zn 10 mg, sucrose. Chew. Tab. Bot. 100s. *Rx.*
Use: Mineral, vitamin supplement; dental caries agent.

Florvite + Iron Drops. (Everett) Elemental fluorine 0.25 mg, 0.5 mg, Vitamins A 1500 units, D 400 units, E 5 mg, B_1 0.5 mg, B_2 0.6 mg, B_3 8 mg, B_6 0.4 mg, C 35 mg, iron 10 mg/mL. Liq. Bot. 50 mL. *Rx.*
Use: Mineral, vitamin supplement; dental caries agent.

Florvite Tablets. (Everett) Fluoride 1 mg, vitamins A 2500 units, D 400 units, E 15 mg, B_1 1.05 mg, B_2 1.2 mg, B_3 13.5 mg, B_6 1.05 mg, B_{12} 4.5 mcg, C 60 mg, folic acid 0.3 mg. Chew. Tab. Bot. 100s, 1000s. *Rx.*
Use: Mineral, vitamin supplement; dental caries agent.

•**flosequinan.** (flow-SEH-kwih-NAHN) USAN.
Use: Antihypertensive (vasodilator).

Flovent Diskus. (GlaxoSmithKline) Fluticasone propionate 50 mcg, 100 mcg, 250 mcg. Pow. for Inh. Inhalation device containing 28 or 60 blisters. *Rx.*
Use: Respiratory inhalant, corticosteroid.

Flovent HFA. (GlaxoSmithKline) Fluticasone propionate/actuation 44 mcg, 110 mcg, 220 mcg. Aerosol. Canister with actuator. 10.6 g (120 metered inhalations) (44 mcg only), 12 g (120 metered inhalations) (110 mcg and 220 mcg only). *Rx.*
Use: Respiratory inhalant, corticosteroid.

Flovent Rotadisk. (GlaxoSmithKline) Fluticasone propionate 50 mcg, 100 mcg, 250 mcg, lactose. Pow. for Inh. 4 Blisters containing 15 *Rotodisks* w/inhalation device. *Rx.*
Use: Respiratory inhalant, corticosteroid.

•**floxacillin.** (FLOX-ah-SILL-in) USAN.
Use: Anti-infective.

Floxin. (Ortho-McNeil) **Tab.:** Ofloxacin, 200 mg, 300 mg, 400 mg, lactose. Bot. 50s (except 400 mg), 100s (400 mg only); UD 6s (200 mg only), 100s. **Otic Soln.:** 3 mg/mL, benzalkonium chloride. Bot. 5 mL w/dropper. *Rx.*
Use: Anti-infective, fluoroquinolone.

•**floxuridine.** (flox-YOUR-ih-deen) *USP 28.*
Use: Antiviral; antineoplastic.
See: FUDR.

floxuridine. (Various Mfr.) Floxuridine 500 mg. Pow. for Inj., lyophilized. Vial

5 mL. *Rx.*
Use: Antiviral; antineoplastic.
●**fluazacort.** (flew-AZE-ah-kort) USAN.
Use: Anti-inflammatory.
●**flubanilate hydrochloride.** (flew-BAN-ill-ate) USAN.
Use: Antidepressant; CNS stimulant.
●**flubendazole.** (FLEW-BEN-dah-zole) USAN.
Use: Antiprotozoal.
flucarbril.
Use: Muscle relaxant; analgesic.
●**flucindole.** (flew-SIN-dole) USAN.
Use: Antipsychotic.
●**flucloronide.** (flew-KLOR-oh-nide) USAN.
Use: Corticosteroid, topical.
Flu, Cold & Cough Medicine. (Major) Pseudoephedrine hydrochloride 60 mg, chlorpheniramine 4 mg, dextromethorphan HBr 20 mg, acetaminophen 500 mg. Pow. Pck. 6s. *OTC.*
Use: Analgesic; antihistamine; antitussive; decongestant.
●**fluconazole.** (flew-KOE-nuh-sole) *USP 28.*
Use: Antifungal.
See: Diflucan.
fluconazole. (Mayne) Fluconazole 2 mg/mL. Inj. 100 mL, 200 mL. *Rx.*
Use: Antifungal.
fluconazole. (Various Mfr.) Fluconazole 50 mg, 100 mg, 150 mg, 200 mg. May contain lactose. Tab. 30s, 100s, UD 100s (except 150 mg); unit-of-use cards (150 mg only). *Rx.*
Use: Antifungal agent.
●**flucrylate.** (FLEW-krih-late) USAN.
Use: Surgical aid (tissue adhesive).
●**flucytosine.** (flew-SITE-oh-seen) *USP 28.*
Use: Antifungal.
See: Ancobon.
●**fludalanine.** (flew-DAL-AH-neen) USAN.
Use: Anti-infective.
Fludara. (Berlex) Fludarabine 50 mg. Mannitol 50 mg, sodium hydroxide. Pow. for Inj., lyophilized. Single-dose vial. *Rx.*
Use: Antineoplastic.
●**fludarabine phosphate.** (flew-DAR-uh-BEAN) USAN.
Use: Antineoplastic. [Orphan Drug]
See: Fludara.
fludarabine phosphate. (Sicor) Fludarabine phosphate 25 mg/mL. Preservative free. Mannitol 25 mg/mL, sodium hydroxide. Inj. Single-dose vials. *Rx.*
Use: Antimetabolite.

●**fludazonium chloride.** (FLEW-dazz-OH-nee-uhm) USAN.
Use: Anti-infective, topical.
●**fludeoxyglucose F 18 injection.** (FLEW-dee-OX-ee-GLUE-kose F 18) *USP 28.*
Use: Diagnostic aid (brain disorders, thyroid disorders, liver disorders, cardiac disease, and neoplastic disease); radiopharmaceutical.
●**fludorex.** (FLEW-doe-rex) USAN.
Use: Anorexic; antiemetic.
●**fludrocortisone acetate.** (flew-droe-CORE-tih-sone) *USP 28.*
Use: Adrenocortical steroid (salt-regulating).
See: Florinef Acetate.
fludrocortisone acetate. (Various Mfr.) Fludrocortisone acetate 0.1 mg. Tab. Bot. 100s. *Rx.*
Use: Adrenocortical steroid.
●**flufenamic acid.** (FLEW-fen-AM-ik) USAN.
Use: Anti-inflammatory.
●**flufenisal.** (flew-FEN-ih-sal) USAN.
Use: Analgesic.
Fluidex. (Columbia) Natural botanical ingredients. Tab. Bot. 36s, 72s.
Use: Diuretic.
Flu-Imune. (Wyeth) Influenza virus vaccine. Vial 5 mL (10 doses). (Purified surface antigen). *Rx.*
Use: Immunization.
fluitran. Trichlormethiazide.
Flumadine. (Forest) **Tab.:** Rimantadine hydrochloride 100 mg. Bot. 100s. **Syr.:** Rimantadine hydrochloride 50 mg/5 mL, saccharin, sorbitol, parabens, raspberry flavor. Bot. 240 mL. *Rx.*
Use: Antiviral.
●**flumazenil.** (flew-MAZ-ah-nil) USAN.
Use: Antagonist (to benzodiazepine); antidote.
See: Romazicon.
flumazenil. (Various Mfr.) Flumazenil 0.1 mg/mL. May contain EDTA, parabens, sodium chloride. Inj. Multidose vials. 5 mL, 10 mL. *Rx.*
Use: Antidote.
●**flumequine.** (FLEW-meh-kwin) USAN.
Use: Anti-infective.
●**flumeridone.** (FLEW-MER-ih-dohn) USAN.
Use: Antiemetic.
●**flumethasone.** (FLEW-meth-ah-zone) USAN.
Use: Corticosteroid, topical.
See: Locorten.
●**flumethasone pivalate.** (FLEW-meth-ah-zone PIH-vah-late) *USP 28.*
Use: Corticosteroid, topical.

flumethiazide.
Use: Diuretic.

•**flumetramide.** (flew-MEH-trah-mide)
USAN.
Use: Muscle relaxant.

•**flumezapine.** (FLEW-MEZZ-ah-peen)
USAN.
Use: Antipsychotic; neuroleptic.

•**fluminorex.** (flew-MEE-no-rex) USAN.
Use: Anorexic.

FluMist. (MedImmune Vaccines/Wyeth)
Influenza virus vaccine. A/New Cale-
donia/20/99 (H1N1), A/Wyoming
(H3N2), B (Jilin/20/2003). Preservative-
free. Intranasal spray. Prefilled single-
use sprayers. 0.5 mL. Rx.
Use: Active immunization agent, viral
vaccine.

•**flumizole.** (FLEW-mih-zole) USAN.
Use: Anti-inflammatory.

•**flumoxonide.** (flew-MOX-OH-nide)
USAN.
Use: Adrenocortical steroid.

flunarizine.
Use: Alternating hemiplegia. [Orphan
Drug]
See: Sibelium.

•**flunarizine hydrochloride.** (flew-NAR-
ih-zeen) USAN.
Use: Vasodilator.

•**flunidazole.** (FLEW-nih-dah-ZOLE)
USAN.
Use: Antiprotozoal.

•**flunisolide.** (flew-NIH-sole-ide) USP 28.
  Use: Corticosteroid, topical, respiratory
inhalant.
See: AeroBid.
  AeroBid-M.
  Nasarel.

flunisolide. (Bausch & Lomb) Flunisolide 0.025% (25 mcg/actuation), propylene glycol, polyethylene glycol 3350,
EDTA, benzalkonium chloride. Soln.
Bot. 25 mL nasal pump dispenser (200
sprays/bot). Rx.
Use: Corticosteroid, topical; intranasal
steroid.

•**flunisolide acetate.** (flew-NIH-sole-ide)
USAN.
Use: Anti-inflammatory.

•**flunitrazepam.** (flew-NYE-TRAY-zeh-
pam) USAN.
Use: Hynoptic; sedative.

•**flunixin.** (flew-NIX-in) USAN.
Use: Analgesic; anti-inflammatory.

•**flunixin meglumine.** (flew-NIX-in meh-
GLUE-meen) USP 28.
Use: Analgesic; anti-inflammatory.

Fluocet. (Alra) Fluocinolone acetonide
0.025%, 0.01%. Cream. Tube 15 g,
60 g. Rx.
Use: Corticosteroid, topical.

fluocinolide.
See: Fluocinonide.

•**fluocinolone acetonide.** (flew-oh-SIN-
oh-lone ah-SEE-toe-nide) USP 28.
Use: Corticosteroid, topical; corticoste-
roid, ophthalmic.
See: Fluonid.
  Retisert.
  Synalar.
W/Combinations.
See: Tri-Luma.

•**fluocinonide.** (FLEW-oh-SIN-oh-nide)
USP 28. Formerly Fluocinolide.
Use: Corticosteroid, topical.
See: Lidex.
  Lidex-E.
  Vanos.

fluocinonide. (E. Fougera) Fluocinonide
0.05%. Tube 15 g, 60 g.
Use: Corticosteroid, topical.

fluocinonide topical solution. (E. Fougera) Fluocinonide 0.05%. Soln. Bot.
60 mL.
Use: Corticosteroid, topical.

•**fluocortin butyl.** (FLEW-oh-CORE-tin
BYOO-tuhl) USAN.
Use: Anti-inflammatory.

•**fluocortolone.** (FLEW-oh-CORE-toe-
lone) USAN.
Use: Corticosteroid, topical.

•**fluocortolone caproate.** (FLEW-oh-
CORE-toe-lone) USAN.
Use: Corticosteroid, topical.

Fluonex. (AstraZeneca) Fluocinonide
0.05%. Cream. Tube. 15 g, 30 g. Rx.
Use: Corticosteroid, topical.

Fluonid. (Allergan) Fluocinolone aceto-
nide 0.01%. Soln. Bot. 20 mL, 60 mL.
Rx.
Use: Corticosteroid, topical.

Fluoracaine. (Akorn) Proparacaine hydrochloride 0.5%, fluorescein sodium
0.25%. Dropper Bot. 5 mL. Rx.
Use: Anesthetic, local; ophthalmic.

•**fluorescein.** (FLURE-eh-seen) USP 28.
Use: Diagnostic aid (corneal trauma in-
dicator).
See: Fluorescite.

•**fluorescein sodium.** (FLURE-eh-seen)
USP 28. Formerly Fluorescein, soluble.
Use: Diagnostic aid (corneal trauma
indicator).
See: AK-Fluor.
  Fluorets.
  Fluor-I-Strips.
  Ful-Glo.
  Funduscein.

fluorescein sodium. (Various Mfr.) Fluorescein sodium 2%. Ophth. Soln. Bot. 1 mL, 2 mL, 15 mL.
Use: Diagnostic aid (corneal trauma indicator).

fluorescein sodium intravenous.
See: Fluorescite.

fluorescein sodium/sodium hyaluronate.
See: Sodium Hyaluronate and Fluorescein Sodium Healon Yellow.

fluorescein sodium 2%. (Ciba Vision) Sterile aqueous solution containing fluorescein sodium 2%. *Dropperette* 1 mL, Box 12s.
Use: Diagnostic aid, ophthalmic.

fluorescein sodium 2% solution. (Alcon) *Drop-Tainer* 15 mL, *Steri-Unit* 2 mL 12s.
Use: Diagnostic aid, ophthalmic.

fluorescein sodium w/combinations.
See: Flurate.

fluorescein sodium w/proparacaine hydrochloride. (Taylor Pharmaceuticals) Proparacaine hydrochloride 0.5%, fluorescein sodium 0.25%. Ophthalmic soln. Bot. 5 mL. *Rx.*
Use: Anesthetic, local; diagnostic aid, ophthalmic.

Fluorescite. (Alcon) Fluorescein as sodium salt. Inj. Soln. **10%:** Amp. 5 mL with syringes. **25%:** Amp 2 mL. *Rx.*
Use: Diagnostic aid, ophthalmic.

Fluoresoft 0.35%. (Various Mfr.) Fluorexon 0.35%. Preservative-free. Soln. 0.35 mL ampules. 20s. *OTC.*
Use: Diagnostic aid, ophthalmic.

Fluorets. (Akorn) Fluorescein sodium 1 mg. Strip. Box 100s. *OTC.*
Use: Diagnostic aid, ophthalmic.

fluorexon.
Use: Ophthalmic diagnostic product.
See: Fluoresoft 0.35%.

fluoride. (Kirkman) Fluoride 1 mg (sodium fluoride 2.21 mg). Tab. Bot. 1000s. *Rx.*
Use: Dental caries agent.

Fluoride Loz. (Kirkman) Fluoride 1 mg (sodium fluoride 2.21 mg). Bot. 1000s. *Rx.*
Use: Dental caries agent.

fluoride sodium.
See: Sodium Fluoride.

fluoride therapy.
See: Adeflor.
Cari-Tab.
ControlRx.
Coral.
Fluora.
Fluorineed.
Fluorinse.

Luride.
Monocal.
Mulvidren-F.
OrthoWash.
PerioMed.
Point Two.
Poly-Vi-Flor.
Soluvite-F.
Tri-Vi-Flor.

Fluorigard. (Colgate Oral) Fluoride 0.02% (from sodium fluoride 0.05%), alcohol 6%, tartrazine. Bot. 180 mL, 300 mL, 480 mL. *Rx.*
Use: Dental caries agent.

Fluorineed. (Hanlon) Fluoride 1 mg. Chew. Tab. Bot. 100s, 1000s. *Rx.*
Use: Dental caries agent.

Fluorinse. (Oral-B) Fluoride 0.09% from sodium fluoride 0.2%. Bot. 480 mL. *Rx.*
Use: Dental caries agent.

Fluorinse. (Pacemaker) Fluoride mouthwash. Pack. Fluoride ion level 0.05%, 0.2%. UD Bot. 32 oz. Concentrate 1 oz, 4 oz, gal. *Rx.*
Use: Dental caries agent.

Fluor-I-Strip. (Wyeth) Fluorescein sodium 9 mg. Ophthalmic strip. Box. 300s. *Rx.*
Use: Diagnostic aid, ophthalmic.

Fluor-I-Strip-A.T. (Wyeth) Fluorescein sodium 1 mg. Ophthalmic strip. Box 300s. *Rx.*
Use: Diagnostic aid, ophthalmic.

Fluoritab. (Fluoritab) Sodium fluoride 2.2 mg equivalent to 1 mg of fluorine (as fluoride ion) w/inert organic filler 75.8 mg. Tab. Bot. 100s; Liq. Dropper Bot. Fluorine 0.25 mg from 0.55 mg sodium fluoride. Drop 19 mL. *Rx.*
Use: Dental caries agent.

5-fluorocytosine.
See: Ancobon.

•fluorodopa F 18 injection. (FLEW-roe-DOE-pah) *USP 28.*
Use: Diagnostic aid (brain imaging); radiopharmaceutical.

fluorogestone acetate.
Use: Hormone, progestin.

fluorohydrocortisone acetate. 9-α-Fluorohydrocortisone.
See: Fludrocortisone Acetate.

•fluorometholone. (flure-oh-METH-oh-lone) *USP 28.*
Use: Corticosteroid, ophthalmic.
See: Fluor-Op.
FML.

fluorometholone. (Various Mfr.) Fluorometholone 0.1%, benzalkonium chloride 0.004%, EDTA, polysorbate 80, polyvinyl alcohol 1.4%. Ophth. Susp. Bot. 5 mL, 10 mL, 15 mL. *Rx.*

Use: Corticosteroid, ophthalmic; anti-inflammatory.

•**fluorometholone acetate.** (flure-oh-METH-oh-LONE) USAN.
Use: Corticosteroid, ophthalmic; anti-inflammatory.

Fluor-Op. (Novartis Ophthalmics) Fluro-metholone 0.1%, benzalkonium chloride 0.004%, EDTA, polysorbate 80, polyvinyl alcohol 1.4%. Susp. 3 mL, 5 mL, 10 mL, 15 mL. *Rx.*
Use: Corticosteroid, ophthalmic.

fluorophene.
Use: Antiseptic.

Fluoroplex. (Allergan) Fluorouracil. **Soln.:** 1%. Bot. w/dropper 30 mL. **Cream:** 1%, benzyl alcohol, emulsifying wax, mineral oil. Tube 30 g. *Rx.*
Use: Topical treatment of multiple actinic (solar) keratoses.

fluoroquinolones.
Use: Anti-infective.
See: Ciprofloxacin.
Enoxacin.
Gatifloxacin.
Gemifloxacin Mesylate.
Grepafloxacin.
Levofloxacin.
Lomefloxacin hydrochloride.
Moxifloxacin hydrochloride.
Norfloxacin.
Ofloxacin.
Sparfloxacin.

•**fluorosalan.** (FLEW-oh-row-SAH-lan) USAN.
Use: Antiseptic; disinfectant.

fluorothyl.
See: Flurothyl.

•**fluorouracil.** (FLURE-oh-YOUR-uh-sill) *USP 28.*
Use: Antineoplastic. [Orphan Drug]
See: Adrucil.
Carac.
Efudex.
Fluoroplex.

fluorouracil. (Taro) Fluorouracil 2%, 5%. Soln. 10 mL. *Rx.*
Use: Antineoplastic.

fluorouracil. (Various Mfr.) Fluorouracil 50 mg/mL. Vial 10 mL, 20 mL, 100 mL. Amp. 10 mL. *Rx.*
Use: Antineoplastic; antimetabolite.

Fluothane. (Wyeth) Halothane. Bot. 125 mL, 250 mL. *Rx.*
Use: Anesthetic, general.

•**fluotracen hydrochloride.** (FLEW-oh-TRAY-sen) USAN.
Use: Antipsychotic; antidepressant.

•**fluoxetine hydrochloride.** (flew-OX-eh-teen) *USP 28.*

Use: Antidepressant.
See: Prozac.
Prozac Weekly.
Sarafem.
W/Olanzapine.
See: Symbyax.

fluoxetine hydrochloride. (Various Mfr.) Fluoxetine hydrochloride. **Cap.:** 10 mg, 20 mg, 40 mg (may contain parabens, EDTA, lactose [except 40 mg]). Bot. 30s (except 10 mg), 100s; 1000s, 2000s, unit-of-use 30s (except 40 mg); UD 100s (10 mg only). **Tab.:** 10 mg, 20 mg. Bot. 30s, 100s, 500s (10 mg only), 1000s, 5000s (10 mg only), UD 100s (10 mg only). **Oral Soln.:** 20 mg/5 mL, may contain alcohol, sucrose. Bot. 120 mL, 473 mL. *Rx.*
Use: Antidepressant.

Flu-Oxinate. (Taylor Pharmaceuticals) Benoxinate hydrochloride 0.4%, fluorescein sodium 0.25%. Ophthalmic Soln. Bot. 5 mL. *Rx.*
Use: Local anesthetic; diagnostic aid; ophthalmic.

•**fluoxymesterone.** (flew-ox-ee-MESS-teh-rone) *USP 28.*
Use: Androgen.

fluoxymestrone. (Various Mfr.) Fluoxymesterone 10 mg. Tab. Bot. 100s. *c-iii.*
Use: Sex hormone, androgen.

•**fluparoxan hydrochloride.** (flew-pah-ROX-an) USAN.
Use: Antidepressant.

•**fluperamide.** (flew-purr-ah-mide) USAN.
Use: Antiperistaltic.

•**fluperolone acetate.** (FLEW-per-oh-lone) USAN.
Use: Corticosteroid, topical.

•**fluphenazine decanoate.** (flew-FEN-uh-zeen) *USP 28.*
Use: Antipsychotic.
See: Prolixin Decanoate.

fluphenazine decanoate. (Various Mfr.) Fluphenazine decanoate 25 mg/mL, may contain sesame oil and benzyl alcohol. Inj. Multidose vials 5 mL. *Rx.*
Use: Antipsychotic.

•**fluphenazine enanthate.** (flew-FEN-uh-zeen) *USP 28.*
Use: Antipsychotic; anxiolytic.
See: Prolixin Enanthate.

•**fluphenazine hydrochloride.** (flew-FEN-uh-zeen) *USP 28.*
Use: Antipsychotic; anxiolytic.
See: Prolixin.

fluphenazine hydrochloride. (American Pharmaceutical Partners) Fluphenazine hydrochloride. **Elix.:** 2.5 mg/mL. May contain alcohol 14% and sucrose.

60 mL, 473 mL. **Inj.:** 2.5 mg/mL. Parabens. Vial. 10 mL. *Rx.*
Use: Antipsychotic.
fluphenazine hydrochloride. (Various Mfr.) Fluphenazine hydrochloride. **Tab.:** 1 mg, 2.5 mg, 5 mg, 10 mg. Bot. 50s, 100s, 500s, 1000s, UD 100s. **Elixir:** 2.5 mg/mL. May contain alcohol 14% and sucrose. 60 mL, 473 mL. *Rx.*
Use: Antipsychotic.
•**flupirtine maleate.** (flew-PIHR-teen) USAN.
Use: Investigational analgesic.
•**fluprednisolone.** (FLEW-pred-NIH-solone) USAN.
Use: Corticosteroid, topical.
•**fluprednisolone valerate.** (FLEW-pred-NIH-so-lone VAL-eh-rate) USAN.
Use: Corticosteroid, topical.
•**fluproquazone.** (FLEW-PRO-kwah-zone) USAN.
Use: Analgesic.
•**fluprostenol sodium.** (flew-PROSTE-een-ole) USAN.
Use: Prostaglandin.
•**fluquazone.** (FLEW-kwah-zone) USAN.
Use: Anti-inflammatory.
•**fluradoline hydrochloride.** (FLURE-ade-OLE-een) USAN.
Use: Analgesic.
Flura-Drops. (Kirkman) Fluoride. **Drops:** 0.25 mg (from 0.55 mg sodium fluoride). Bot. 30 mL. **Rinse:** 0.02% (from 0.05% sodium fluoride). Bot. 480 mL. *Rx.*
Use: Dental caries agent.
Flura-Loz. (Kirkman) Sodium fluoride 2.2 mg providing 1 mg fluoride. Loz. Bot. 100s, 1000s. *Rx.*
Use: Dental caries agent.
•**flurandrenolide.** (FLURE-an-DREEN-oh-lide) *USP 28.* Cream; Ointment, USP. *Formerly Flurandrenolone.*
Use: Corticosteroid, topical.
See: Cordran.
flurandrenolone. (FLURE-an-DREE-nahl-ohn)
Use: Corticosteroid, topical.
Flura-Tablets. (Kirkman) Sodium fluoride 2.21 mg, equivalent to 1 mg fluoride ion. Tab. Bot. 100s, 1000s. *Rx.*
Use: Dental caries agent.
Flurate. (Bausch & Lomb) Benoxinate hydrochloride 0.4%, fluorescein sodium 0.25%, chlorobutanol 1%, povidone. Soln. Bot. 5 mL. *Rx.*
Use: Diagnostic aid, ophthalmic.
•**flurazepam hydrochloride.** (flure-AZE-uh-pam) *USP 28.*
Use: Anticonvulsant; hypnotic; muscle

relaxant; sedative/hypnotic, nonbarbiturate.
See: Dalmane.
flurazepam hydrochloride. (Various Mfr.) Flurazepam hydrochloride 15 mg, 30 mg. Cap. 100s. *c-iv.*
Use: Sedative/hypnotic, nonbarbiturate.
•**flurbiprofen.** (FLURE-bih-PRO-fen) *USP 28.*
Use: Analgesic; anti-inflammatory.
flurbiprofen. (Various Mfr.) Flurbiprofen 50 mg, 100 mg. Tab. 100s, 500s (100 mg only). *Rx.*
Use: Analgesic, NSAID.
•**flurbiprofen sodium.** (FLURE-bih-PRO-fen) *USP 28.*
Use: Analgesic, NSAID; prostaglandin synthesis inhibitor.
See: Ocufen
flurbiprofen sodium ophthalmic. (FLURE-bih-PRO-fen) (Various Mfr.) Flurbiprofen sodium 0.03%, polyvinyl alcohol 1.4%, thimerosal 0.005%, EDTA. Soln. Bot. 2.5 mL. *Rx.*
Use: Analgesic, NSAID.
Fluress. (PBH Wesley Jessen) Fluorescein sodium 0.25%. Bot. 5 mL. *Rx.*
Use: Anesthetic; diagnostic aid.
•**fluretofen.** (flure-EH-TOE-fen) USAN.
Use: Anti-inflammatory; antithrombotic.
flurfamide. (FLURE-fah-MIDE)
See: Flurofamide.
•**flurocitabine.** (FLEW-row-SIGH-tah-been) USAN.
Use: Antineoplastic.
Fluro-Ethyl. (Gebauer) Ethyl Cl 25%, dichlorotetrafluoroethane 75%. Spray. Can 270 g. *Rx.*
Use: Anesthetic, topical.
•**flurofamide.** (FLEW-row-fah-MIDE) USAN. *Formerly Flurfamide.*
Use: Enzyme inhibitor (urease).
•**flurogestone acetate.** (FLEW-row-JEST-ohn) USAN.
Use: Hormone, progestin.
Flurosyn. (Rugby) **Cream:** Fluocinolone acetonide 0.01%, 0.025%. Tube 15 g, 60 g, 425 g. **Oint.:** Fluocinolone acetonide 0.025% in a white petrolatum base. Tube 15 g, 60 g. *Rx.*
Use: Corticosteroid, topical.
•**flurothyl.** (FLURE-oh-thill) USAN.
Use: Stimulant (central).
•**fluroxene.** (flure-OX-een) USAN.
Use: General inhalation anesthetic.
•**fluspiperone.** (FLEW-spih-per-OHN) USAN.
Use: Antipsychotic.
•**fluspirilene.** (flew-SPIRE-ih-leen) USAN.
Use: Antipsychotic; anxiolytic.

•**flutamide.** (FLEW-tuh-mide) *USP 28.*
Use: Hormone, antiandrogen.
See: Eulexin.

flutamide. (Various Mfr.) Flutamide
125 mg, may contain lactose. Cap. Bot.
100s, 180s, 500s, UD 100s. *Rx.*
Use: Hormone, antiandrogen.

•**fluticasone propionate.** (flew-TICK-ah-
SONE) USAN.
Use: Anti-inflammatory, respiratory in-
halant, intranasal steroid, corticoste-
roid.
See: Cutivate.
Flonase.
Flovent Diskus.
Flovent HFA.
Flovent Rotadisk.
W/Salmeterol.
See: Advair Diskus.

fluticasone propionate. (Fougera) Fluti-
casone propionate 0.005%. Oint.
Tubes. 15 g, 30 g, 60 g. *Rx.*
Use: Anti-inflammatory agent.

fluticasone propionate. (Sandoz) Fluticasone propionate 0.05%. Cetostearyl
alcohol, mineral oil. Cream. Tubes.
15 g, 30 g, 60 g. *Rx.*
Use: Anti-inflammatory agent.

fluticasone propionate. (Various Mfr.)
Fluticasone propionate 0.05%. Cetostearyl alcohol, mineral oil. Cream.
15 g, 30 g, 60 g. *Rx.*
Use: Anti-inflammatory agent.

Flutra. Trichlormethiazide.
Use: Diuretic.

•**flutroline.** (FLEW-troe-LEEN) USAN.
Use: Antipsychotic.

•**fluvastatin sodium.** (FLEW-vah-STAT-
in) USAN.
Use: Antihyperlipidemic inhibitor, HMG-
CoA reductase inhibitor.
See: Lescol.
Lescol XL.

Fluvirin. (Evans Vaccine Ltd.) Influenza
virus vaccine. A/Wyoming/3/2003/X-
147 (A/Fujian/411/2003 [H3N2]-like),
A/New Caledonia/20/99 IVR-116, and
B/Jiangsu/10/2003 (B/Shanghai/361/
2002-like) 15 mcg each per 0.5 mL, thimerosal. Purified split-virus. Inj. Prefilled Syr. 0.5 mL (mercury 0.98 mcg/
0.5 mL dose). *Rx.*
Use: Active immunization agent, viral
vaccine.

•**fluvoxamine maleate.** (flew-VOX-ah-
meen) USAN.
Use: Antidepressant; anti-obsessional
agent, selective serotonin reuptake
inhibitor.

fluvoxamine maleate. (Various Mfr.) Fluvoxamine maleate 25 mg, 50 mg,
100 mg. Tab. Bot. 100s, 500s (except
100 mg), 1000s (except 25 mg). *Rx.*
Use: Antidepressant, SSRI.

•**fluzinamide.** (flew-ZIN-ah-mide) USAN.
Use: Anticonvulsant.

Fluzone. (Aventis Pasteur) Influenza virus vaccine. A/Wyoming/03/2003
(H3N2) (A/Fujian/411/2002-like)
15 mcg, A/New Caledonia/20/99
(H1N1) 15 mcg, B/Jiangsu/10/2003
(B/Shanghai/361/2002-like) 15 mcg per
0.5 mL, thimerosal. Inj. (Purified split-
virus). Vial 5 mL (mercury 25 mcg/
0.5 mL dose), Prefilled Syr. 0.25 mL
(mercury 0.5 mcg or less per 0.25 mL
dose), 0.5 mL (mercury 0.98 mcg or
less per 0.5 mL dose). *Rx.*
Use: Active immunization agent, viral
vaccine.

FML. (Allergan) Fluorometholone 0.1%,
benzalkonium chloride 0.004%, EDTA,
polysorbate 80, polyvinyl alcohol.
Ophth. Susp. Bot. 5 mL, 10 mL. *Rx.*
Use: Corticosteroid, ophthalmic; anti-
inflammatory.

FML Forte. (Allergan) Fluorometholone
0.25%, benzalkonium chloride 0.005%,
EDTA, polysorbate 80, polyvinyl alcohol 1.4%. Ophth. Susp. Bot. 2 mL,
5 mL, 10 mL, 15 mL. *Rx.*
Use: Corticosteroid, ophthalmic; anti-
inflammatory.

FML-S. (Allergan) Fluorometholone
0.1%, sulfacetamide sodium 10%.
Susp. Dropper Bot. 5 mL, 10 mL. *Rx.*
Use: Corticosteroid, ophthalmic.

FML S.O.P. (Allergan) Fluorometholone
0.1%, phenylmercuric acetate
0.0008%, white petrolatum, mineral oil,
lanolin alcohol. Oint. Tube 3.5 g. *Rx.*
Use: Corticosteroid, ophthalmic; anti-
inflammatory.

Foamicon. (Invamed) Aluminum hydroxide 80 mg, magnesium trisilicate 20 mg,
alginic acid, calcium stearate, compressible sugar, sodium bicarbonate,
sucrose. Chew. Tab. Bot. 100s. *OTC.*
Use: Antacid.

Focalin. (Novartis) Dexmethylphenidate
hydrochloride 2.5 mg, 5 mg, 10 mg,
lactose. Tab. Bot. 100s. *c-II.*
Use: CNS stimulant.

Focalin XR. (Novartis) Dexmethylphenidate hydrochloride 5 mg, 10 mg,
20 mg. Sugar spheres. ER Cap. 100s.
c-II.
Use: Central nervous system stimulant.

•**focofilcon a.** (FOE-koe-FILL-kahn A)
USAN.
Use: Contact lens material (hydrophilic).

•**fodipir.** (FO-di-pir) USAN.
Use: Excipient.

Foille. (Blairex) Benzocaine 2%, benzyl alcohol 4% in a bland vegetable oil base. Oint. Tube 30 g. *OTC.*
Use: Anesthetic, local.

Foillecort. (Blairex) Hydrocortisone acetate 0.5%. Cream. Tube 3.5 g. *OTC.*
Use: Corticosteroid, topical.

Foille Medicated First Aid. (Blairex) **Aerosol:** Benzocaine 5% with chloroxylenol 0.1% in a bland vegetable oil base with benzyl alcohol. Spray 92 g. **Oint.:** Benzocaine 5%, chloroxylenol 0.1% in a bland vegetable oil base. Tube 30 g. **Lot.:** Benzocaine 5%, chloroxylenol 0.1% in a bland vegetable oil base with benzyl alcohol 30 mL. **Oint.:** Benzocaine 5%, chloroxylenol, benzyl alcohol, EDTA, corn oil 3.5 g, 28 g. **Spray:** Benzocaine 5%, chloroxylenol, benzyl alcohol, corn oil. 92 mL. *OTC.*
Use: Anesthetic, local.

Foille Plus. (Blairex) **Cream:** Benzocaine 5%, benzyl alcohol 4% in a nonstaining washable base. Tube 3.5 g. **Soln.:** Benzocaine 5%, benzyl alcohol, alcohol 77.8%. Aerosol spray 105 g. **Spray:** Benzocaine 5%, chloroxylenol, alcohol. 105 mL. *OTC.*
Use: Anesthetic, local.

Folabee. (Vortech Pharmaceuticals) Liver inj. B_{12} equivalent to 10 mcg, crystalline B_{12} 100 mcg, folic acid 0.4 mg. Inj. Vial 10 mL. *Rx.*
Use: Anemia.

folacin.
See: Folic acid.

Folergot-DF. (Marnel) Phenobarbital 40 mg, ergotamine tartrate 0.6 mg, levorotatory alkaloids of belladonna 0.2 mg, dye-free. Tab. Bot. 100s. *Rx.*
Use: Anticholinergic, gastrointestinal.

Folgard. (Upsher-Smith) B_6 10 mg, B_{12} 115 mcg, folic acid 0.8 mg. Tab. Bot. 60s. *OTC.*
Use: Vitamin, mineral supplement.

Folgard Rx. (Upsher-Smith) B_6 25 mg, B_{12} 500 mcg, folic acid 2.2 mg. Tab. Bot. 100s. *Rx.*
Use: Vitamin, mineral supplement.

•**folic acid.** (FOLE-ik) *USP 28.*
Use: Anemia; vitamin (hematopoietic).

folic acid. (Various Mfr.) Folic acid. Tab. **0.4 mg, 0.8 mg:** Bot. 100s. **1 mg:** Bot. 30s, 100s, 1000s, UD 100s. *Rx.*
Use: Vitamin supplement.

folic acid. (Fujisawa Healthcare) Folic acid 5 mg/mL w/benzyl alcohol 1.5%, EDTA. Inj. Vials 10 mL. *Rx.*

Use: Vitamin supplement.

folic acid antagonists.
See: Daraprim.
Methotrexate.
Pemetrexed.
Pyrimethamine.

folinic acid. Leucovorin Calcium, USP.

Fol-Li-Bee. (Foy Laboratories) Liver inj. equivalent to cyanocobalamin 10 mcg, folic acid 1 mg, cyanocobalamin 100 mcg/mL, phenol 0.5% pH adjusted w/sodium hydroxide and/or hydrochloride. Vial 10 mL multi-dose, Monovials. *Rx.*
Use: Anemia.

follicle-stimulating hormone, human. Menotropins, Pergonal.

follicormon.
Use: Estradiol Benzoate

follicular hormones.
See: Estrone.

folliculin.
See: Estrone .

Follistim. (Organon) FSH activity 75 units (as follitropin beta), sucrose 25 mg. Pow. for Inj., lyophilized. Vial w/5 mL Sterile Water for Injection as diluent. *Rx.*
Use: Sex hormone, ovulation stimulant.

follitropin alfa.
Use: Sex hormone, ovulation stimulant.
See: Gonal-F.
Gonal-f RFF Pen

follitropin beta.
Use: Sex hormone, ovulation stimulant.
See: Follistim.

Folpace. (Alaven) Vitamin B_6 25 mg, vitamin B_{12} 425 mcg, FA 2.05 mg, E 100 units, Mg 100 mg. Tab. 90s. *Rx.*
Use: Nutritional product.

Foltrin. (Eon Labs) Liver and stomach concentrate 240 mg, B_{12} 15 mcg, iron 110 mg, C 75 mg, folic acid 0.5 mg. Cap. Bot. 100s, 1000s. *Rx.*
Use: Mineral, vitamin supplement.

FOLTX. (PAMLAB) B_{12} 2,000 mcg, B_6 25 mg, folic acid 2.5 mg, sugar free, dye free. Tab. Bot. 90s. *Rx.*
Use: Vitamin, mineral supplement.

•**fomepizole.** (foe-MEH-pih-ZOLE) USAN.
Use: Antidote (alcohol dehydrogenase inhibitor).
See: Antizol.

•**fomivirsen sodium.** (foe-MIH-vihr-sen) USAN.
USAN: Antiviral (CMV retinitis).
See: Vitravene.

fonatol.
See: Diethylstilbestrol.

• **fonazine mesylate.** (FAH-nazz-een) USAN.
Use: Serotonin inhibitor.

• **fondaparinux sodium.** (fon-da-PAR-in-ux) USAN.
Use: Anticoagulant, selective factor Xa inhibitor.
See: Arixtra.

fontarsol.
See: Dichlorophenarsine Hydrochloride.

• **fontolizumab.** (fon-toe-LIZ-oo-mab) USAN.
Use: Immunoregulator.

Foradil Aerolizer. (Schering) Formoterol fumarate 12 mcg, lactose 25 mg (as carrier). Inh. Pow. in Cap. Blister Pack 18s, 60s w/*Aerolizer Inhaler. Rx.*
Use: Bronchodilator, sympathomimetic.

Foralicon Plus. (Forbes) Vitamins B_{12} 16.7 mcg, B_6 4 mg, iron 200 mg (equivalent to elemental iron 24 mg), niacinamide 40 mg, folic acid 0.8 mg, sorbitol soln. q.s./15 mL. Elix. Bot. 8 oz, 16 oz. *Rx.*
Use: Mineral, vitamin supplement.

Forane. (Ohmeda) Isoflurane. Gas. Volume 100 mL. *Rx.*
Use: Anesthetic, general.

• **forasartan.** (far-ah-SAHR-tan) USAN.
Use: Antihypertensive.

Fordustin. (Sween) Cornstarch based powder with deodorizing action. Bot. 3 oz, 8 oz. *OTC.*
Use: Powder, topical.

Formadon. (Gordon Laboratories) Formalin 3.7% to 4% (10% of USP strength) in an aqueous perfumed base. Soln. Bot. 1 oz, 4 oz, 0.5 gal, gal. *Rx.*
Use: Bromhidrosis, hyperhidrosis agent.

formaldehyde. (for-MAL-deh-hide)
Use: Drying agent.
See: Formalyde 10.
Lazer Formalyde.

formalin.
See: Formaldehyde

Formalyde-10. (Pedinol) Formaldehyde 10%, SD-40 alcohol. Spray. Bot. 60 mL. *Rx.*
Use: Drying agent.

Forma-Ray. (Gordon Laboratories) Formalin 7.4% to 8% (20% of USP strength) in aqueous, scented, tinted solution. Soln. Bot. 1.5 oz, 4 oz. *OTC.*
Use: Drying.

• **formocortal.** (FORE-moe-CORE-tal) USAN.
Use: Corticosteroid, topical.

• **formoterol fumarate.** (fore-MOE-ter-ole) USAN.

Use: Bronchodilator, sympathomimetic.
See: Foradil Aerolizer.

Formula B. (Major) Vitamins B_1 15 mg, B_2 15 mg, B_3 100 mg, B_5 18 mg, B_6 4 mg, B_{12} 5 mcg, C 500 mg, folic acid 0.5 mg. Tab. Bot 250 g. *Rx.*
Use: Vitamin supplement.

Formula B Plus. (Major) Iron 27 mg, A 5000 units, E 30 units, B_1 20 mg, B_2 20 mg, B_3 100 mg, B_5 25 mg, B_6 25 mg, B_{12} 50 mcg, C 500 mg, folic acid 0.8 mg, biotin 0.15 mg, Cr, Cu, Mg, Mn, Zn. Tab. Bot 100s, 500s. *Rx.*
Use: Mineral, vitamin supplement.

Formula EM. (Major) Dextrose 1.87 g, fructose 1.87 g, phosphoric acid 21.5 mg/5 mL, methylparaben, cherry-flavor. Soln. Bot. 118 mL. *OTC.*
Use: Antiemetic, antivertigo agent.

Formula 44 Cough Control Discs.
See: Vicks Formula 44 Cough Discs.

Formula 44 Cough Mixture. (Procter & Gamble) Chlorpheniramine maleate 2 mg, dextromethorphan HBr 15 mg, alcohol 10%/5 mL. Liq. Bot. 120 mL, 240 mL. *OTC.*
Use: Antihistamine; antitussive.

Formula 44D Decongestant Cough Mixture. (Procter & Gamble) Pseudoephedrine hydrochloride 20 mg, dextromethorphan HBr 10 mg, guaifenesin 67 mg, alcohol 10%/5 mL. Liq. Bot. 120 mL, 240 mL. *OTC.*
Use: Antitussive; decongestant; expectorant.

Formula 44M Cough and Cold. (Procter & Gamble) Pseudoephedrine hydrochloride 15 mg, dextromethorphan HBr 7.5 mg, chlorpheniramine maleate 1 mg, acetaminophen 125 mg/5 mL, alcohol 20%, saccharin, sucrose. Liq. Bot. 120 mL, 240 mL. *OTC.*
Use: Analgesic; antihistamine; antitussive; decongestant.

Formula 405. (Doak Dermatologics) Sodium tallowate, sodium cocoate, Doak Additive A, PPF-20 methyl glucose ether, titanium dioxide, trochlorocarbanilide, pentasodium pentatate, EDTA. Bar 100 g. *OTC.*
Use: Dermatologic, cleanser.

Formula No. 81. (Fellows) Liver (beef) 1 mcg, ferrous gluconate 100 mg, niacinamide 100 mg, B_2 1.5 mg, panthenol 2.5 mg, B_{12} 3 mcg, procaine hydrochloride 25 mg/2 mL. Inj. Vial 30 mL. *OTC.*
Use: Mineral, vitamin supplement.

Formula 1207. (Thurston) Iodine, liver fraction No. 2, caseinates. Tab. Bot. 100s, 250s. *OTC.*
Use: Mineral supplement.

Formulation R. (G & W Labs) **Cream:** Glycerin 12%, petrolatum 18%, phenylephrine hydrochloride 0.025%. Tube. 52 g. **Oint.:** Petrolatum 71.9%, mineral oil 14%, phenylephrine hydrochloride 0.25%, parabens. Tube. 28.4 g, 56.8 g. *OTC.*
Use: Anorectal preparation.

Formula VM-2000. (Solgar) Iron 5 mg, A 12,500 units, D 200 units, E 100 units, B_1 50 mg, B_2 50 mg, B_3 50 mg, B_5 50 mg, B_6 50 mg, B_{12} 50 mcg, C 150 mg, folic acid 0.2 mg, B, Ca, Cr, Cu, I, K, Mg, Mn, Mo, Se, Zn 7.5 mg, betaine, biotin 50 mcg, choline, bioflavonoids, amino acids, hesperidin, inositol, l-glutethione, PABA, rutin. Tab. Bot. 30s, 60s, 90s, 180s. *OTC.*
Use: Mineral, vitamin supplement.

formyl tetrahydropteroylglutamic acid. Leucovorin Calcium.

•**forodesine hydrochloride.** (fore-OH-deseen) USAN.
Use: Antineoplastic.

Forta Drink. (Ross) Whey protein concentrate, sucrose, vitamins A, B_1, B_2, B_3, B_5, B_6, B_{12}, C, D, E, folic acid, biotin, Ca, Cu, Fe, I, Mg, Mn, P, Zn. Pow. Can. 482 g. *OTC.*
Use: Nutritional supplement.

Forta-Flora. (Barth's) Whey-lactose 90%, pectin. Pow. Jar lb. Wafer. Bot. 100s. *OTC.*

Forta Instant Cereal. (Ross) Lactose-free oat or bran cereal provides 6.25 g dietary fiber/serving. Can 1 lb 1 oz. *OTC.*
Use: Nutritional supplement.

Forta Instant Pudding. (Ross) Lactose-free in pudding base. Can 1 lb 12 oz. Vanilla, chocolate, butterscotch flavors. *OTC.*
Use: Nutritional supplement.

Fortamet. (Andrx) Metformin hydrochloride 500 mg, 1000 mg. Film-coated. ER Tab. 60s. *Rx.*
Use: Antidiabetic agent.

Forta Pudding Mix. (Ross) Milk protein isolate, sucrose, hydrolyzed cornstarch, modified tapioca starch, partially hydrogenated soybean oil, vitamins A, B_1, B_2, B_3, B_5, B_6, B_{12}, C, D, E, folic acid, biotin, Ca, Fe, P, I, Mg, Zn, Cu, Mn, tartrazine. Can 794 g. *OTC.*
Use: Nutritional supplement.

Forta Shake Powder. (Ross) Nonfat dry milk, sucrose, vitamins A, B_1, B_2, B_3, B_5, B_6, B_{12}, C, D, E, folic acid, biotin, Ca, Cu, Fe, I, Mg, Mn, P, Zn, tartrazine. Can lb, pkt. 1.4 oz. Can 1 lb 2.7 oz, pkt. 1.6 oz. *OTC.*

Use: Nutritional supplement.

Forta Soup Mix. (Ross) Milk protein isolate, sodium and calcium caseinate, hydrolyzed cornstarch, modified tapioca starch, powdered shortening (partially hydrogenated coconut oil), vitamins A, B_1, B_2, B_3, B_5, B_6, B_{12}, C, D, E, folic acid, biotin, Ca, Cu, Fe, I, Mg, Mn, P, Zn. Chicken flavor. Can. 454 g. *OTC.*
Use: Nutritional supplement.

Fortaz. (GlaxoSmithKline) Ceftazidime Pow. for Inj. **500 mg:** Vial. **1 g:** Vial, *ADD-Vantage* vial, Infusion Pack. **2 g:** Vial, *ADD-Vantage* vial, Infusion Pack. **6 g:** Bulk Pkg. **Inj.:** 1 g. Vial 50 mL, premixed, frozen. *Rx.*
Use: Anti-infective, cephalosporin.

Forte L.I.V. (Foy Laboratories) Cyanocobalamin 15 mcg liver injection equivalent to vitamin B_{12} activity 1 mcg, ferrous gluconate 60 mg, B_2 0.75 mg, panthenol 25 mg, niacinamide 50 mg, citric acid 8.2 mg, sodium citrate 118 mg/mL, procaine hydrochloride 2%. Bot. 30 mL. *OTC.*
Use: Mineral, vitamin supplement.

Fortel Midstream. (Biomerica) Reagent in-home urine test for pregnancy. 1 test stick per kit.
Use: Diagnostic aid, pregnancy.

Fortel Ovulation. (Biomerica) Monoclonal antibody-based home test to predict ovulation. Kit 1s.
Use: Diagnostic aid.

Fortel Plus. (Biomerica) Reagent in-home urine pregnancy test. Kit contains urine collection cup, dropper, test device.
Use: Diagnostic aid, pregnancy.

Forteo. (Lilly) Teriparatide 250 mcg/mL, mannitol 45.4 mg. Inj. Prefilled pen delivery device 3 mL. *Rx.*
Use: Parathyroid hormone.

Fortovase. (Roche) Saquinavir 200 mg. Softgel Cap. Bot. 180s. *Rx.*
Use: Antiviral.

Fortral. (Sanofi-Synthelabo) Pentazocine as solution and tablets. *c-iv.*
Use: Analgesic, narcotic.

Fortramin. (Thurston) Vitamins E 200 units, A 6000 units, D 600 units, B_1 4.5 mg, B_2 4.5 mg, B_6 4.5 mg, B_{12} 5 mcg, C 2.75 mg, rutin 8 mg, hesperidin complex 10 mg, lemon bioflavonoids 15 mg, d-calcium pantothenate 50 mg, para-aminobenzoic acid 7.5 mg, biotin 10 mg, folic acid 24 mcg, niacinamide 20 mg, desiccated liver 25 mg, iron 3 mg, calcium 75 mg, phosphorus 34 mg, manganese 10 mg, copper 0.5 mg, zinc 0.5 mg, iodine 0.375 mg,

potassium 500 mg, magnesium 5 mg.
Tab. Bot. 100s, 250s. *OTC.*
Use: Mineral, vitamin supplement.
.44 Magnum. (BDI) Caffeine 200 mg.
Cap. Bot. 100s, 500s. *OTC.*
Use: CNS stimulant, analeptic.
40 Winks. (Roberts) Diphenhydramine
hydrochloride 50 mg. Cap. Bot. 30s.
OTC.
Use: Nonprescription sleep aid.
Fosamax. (Merck) Alendronate sodium
(as base). **Oral Soln.:** 70 mg. Parabens, saccharin. Raspberry flavor.
75 mL. **Tab.:** 5 mg, 10 mg, 35 mg,
40 mg, 70 mg, lactose. Unit-of-use 30s
(5 mg, 10 mg, 40 mg), 100s (5 mg,
10 mg); unit-of-use 4s and UD 20s
(35 mg, 70 mg); Bot. 1000s, *Uniblister*
cards of 31, UD 100s (10 mg). *Rx.*
Use: Bone resorption inhibitor.
Fosamax Plus D. (Merck) Alendronate
sodium 70 mg/cholecalciferol
2,800 units. Lactose, sucrose. Tab.
Unit-of-use blisters of 4, unit-of-use
bottles of 4 and 12, and UD 20s. *Rx.*
Use: Bisphosphonate.
•**fosamprenavir calcium.** (FOSS-am-
PREN-ah-veer) USAN.
Use: Antiretroviral agents.
See: Lexiva.
•**fosamprenavir sodium.** (FOSS-am-
PREN-ah-veer) USAN.
Use: Antiviral.
•**fosarilate.** (FOSS-ah-RILL-ate) USAN.
Use: Antiviral.
•**fosazepam.** (foss-AZZ-eh-pam) USAN.
Use: Hypnotic; sedative.
•**foscarnet sodium.** (foss-CAR-net)
USAN.
Use: Antiviral.
See: Foscavir.
Foscavir. (AstraZeneca) Foscarnet so-
dium 24 mg/mL. Inj. Bot. 250 mL,
500 mL. *Rx.*
Use: Anti-infective, antiviral.
•**fosfomycin.** (foss-foe-MY-sin) USAN.
Use: Anti-infective.
See: Monurol.
•**fosfomycin tromethamine.** (foss-foe-
MY-sin troe-METH-ah-meen) USAN.
Use: Anti-infective.
See: Monurol.
•**fosfonet sodium.** (FOSS-foe-net) USAN.
Use: Antiviral.
Fosfree. (Mission Pharmacal) Iron
14.5 mg, A 1500 units, D_3 150 units, B_1
4.5 mg, B_2 2 mg, B_3 10.5 mg, B_5 1 mg,
B_6 2.5 mg, B_{12} 2 mcg, C 50 mg, Ca
175.5 mg, sugar. Tab. Bot. 120s. *OTC.*
Use: Mineral, vitamin supplement.

fosinopril. (FAH-sen-oh-PRIL)
Use: Angiotensin-converting enzyme inhibitor; antihypertensive.
See: Monopril.
•**fosinoprilat.** (fah-SIN-oh-prill-at) USAN.
Use: Antihypertensive.
•**fosinopril sodium.** (FAH-sen-oh-PRIL)
USAN.
Use: Antihypertensive; enzyme inhibitor
(angiotensin-converting).
See: Monopril.
W/Hydrochlorothiazide.
See: Monopril-HCT.
fosinopril sodium. (Teva) Fosinopril sodium 10 mg, 20 mg, 40 mg. Isopropyl
alcohol, lactose. Tab. 90s, 1,000s. *Rx.*
Use: Antihypertensive.
**fosinopril sodium/hydrochlorothia-
zide.** (Ranbaxy) Hydrochlorothiazide/
fosinopril sodium 12.5 mg/10 mg,
12.5 mg/20 mg. Lactose. Tab. 30s,
100s, 1,000s. *Rx.*
Use: Antihypertensive combination.
•**fosphenytoin sodium.** (FOSS-FEN-ih-
toe-in) USAN.
Use: Anticonvulsant.
See: Cerebyx.
•**fosquidone.** (FOSS-kwih-dohn) USAN.
Use: Antineoplastic.
Fosrenol. (Shire) Lanthanum carbonate
250 mg, 500 mg. Chew. Tab. 100s. *Rx.*
Use: Phosphate reduction.
•**fostedil.** (FOSS-teh-dill) USAN.
Use: Vasodilator, calcium channel
blocker.
Fostex. (Bristol-Myers Squibb) Benzoyl
peroxide 10%, EDTA, urea. Bar. 106 g.
OTC.
Use: Dermatologic, acne.
Fostex Acne Cleansing Cream. (Bristol-
Myers Squibb) Salicylic acid 2%, EDTA,
stearyl alcohol. Cream. Bot. 118 g.
OTC.
Use: Dermatologic, acne.
**Fostex Acne Medication Cleansing
Bar.** (Bristol-Myers Squibb) Salicylic
acid 2%, EDTA. Bar. 106 g. *OTC.*
Use: Dermatologic, acne.
•**fostriecin sodium.** (FOSS-try-eh-SIN)
USAN.
Use: Antineoplastic.
•**fosveset.** (FOS-ve-set) USAN.
Use: Ligant excipient.
Fototar. (ICN Pharm) Coal tar extract
(equiv. to 2% coal tar) in emollient mois-
turizing cream base. Cream. Tube
85 g, 454 g. *OTC.*
Use: Dermatologic.
4 Hair Softgel. (Marlyn Nutraceuticals)
Iron 2.5 mg, A 1250 units, E 10 units,

B_3 5 mg, B_5 2.5 mg, B_6 1.5 mg, B_{12} 44 mcg, C 25 mg, folic acid 33.3 mg, biotin 250 mcg, I, Mg, Cu, Zn 7.5 mg, choline bitartrate, inositol, Mn, methionine, PABA, B_1, L-cysteine, tyrosine, Si. Cap. Bot 60s. *OTC.*
Use: Mineral, vitamin supplement.

4 Nails Softgel. (Marlyn Nutraceuticals) Ca 167 mg, iron 3 mg, A 833 units, D 67, E 10 mg, B_1 3.3 mg, B_2 1.7 mg, B_3 8.3 mg, B_5 8.3 mg, B_6 8.3 mg, B_{12} 8.3 mcg, C 10 mg, folic acid 33.3 mg, biotin 8.3 mcg, P, I, Mg, Cu, Zn 3.3 mg, Cr, Mn, methionine, inositol, choline bitartrate, Se, PABA, protein isolate, gelatin, lecithin, unsaturated fatty acid, predigested protein L-cysteine, B mucopolysaccharides, silicon amino acid chelate, Si. Cap. Bot. 60s. *OTC.*
Use: Mineral, vitamin supplement.

4 Trace Elements. (Hospira) Chromium (as chloride) 6 mcg, copper (as chloride) 0.42 mg, manganese (as chloride) 0.37 mg, zinc (as chloride) 1.67 mg. Vials. 5 mL, 10 mL, 50 mL. Syringes 5 mL. *Rx.*
Use: Intravenous nutritional therapy.

4 Way Fast Acting Nasal Spray. (Bristol-Myers) Phenylephrine hydrochloride 1%, benzalkonium chloride, boric acid, sodium borate. Soln. Spray Bot. 30 mL. *OTC.*
Use: Nasal decongestant, arylalkylamine.

4-Way Long Acting Nasal Spray. (Bristol-Myers Squibb) Oxymetazoline hydrochloride 0.05% in isotonic buffered soln. Spray Bot. 15 mL. *OTC.*
Use: Decongestant.

Fowler's Solution. Potassium Arsenite Solution (Various Mfr.).

Foxalin. (Standex) Digitoxin 0.1 mg, sodium carboxymethylcellulose. Cap. Bot. 100s. *Rx.*
Use: Cardiovascular agent.

foxglove.
See: Digitalis.

Foygen Aqueous. (Foy Laboratories) Estrogenic substance or estrogens 2 mg/mL with sodium carboxymethylcellulose, povidone, benzyl alcohol, methyl and propyl parabens. Inj. Vial 10 mL. *Rx.*
Use: Estrogen.

Foyplex. (Foy Laboratories) Sterile injectable soln. of nine water-soluble vitamins. Packaged as 2 separate solutions for extemporaneous combination. Inj. *Rx.*
Use: Nutritional supplement, parenteral.

Fragmin. (Pfizer) Dalteparin sodium 2,500 units/0.2 mL (16 mg/0.2 mL), 5,000 units/0.2 mL (32 mg/0.2 mL), 7,500 units/0.3 mL (48 mg/0.3 mL), 10,000 units/mL (64 mg/mL), 25,000 units/mL (160 mg/mL). Preservative free (except 25,000 units/mL). Anti-Factor Xa International Units. Inj. Single-dose prefilled syringe 0.2 mL with 27-gauge × ½-inch needle (2,500 units/0.2 mL, 5,000 units/0.2 mL only), single-dose prefilled syringe 0.3 mL with 27-gauge × ½-inch needle (7,500 units/0.3 mL only), single-dose graduated syringes with 27-gauge × ½-inch needle, multidose vials 9.5 mL with benzyl alcohol 14 mg/mL (10,000 units/mL only), multidose vials 3.8 mL (25,000 units/mL only). *Rx.*
Use: Anticoagulant.

FreAmine HBC 0.9%. (B. Braun) High branched 6.9% amino acid formulation for hypercatabolic patients. Bot. 1000 mL. *Rx.*
Use: Nutritional supplement, parenteral.

FreAmine III. (B. Braun) Amino acid 8.5%, 10%. Bot. 500 mL, 1000 mL. *Rx.*
Use: Nutritional supplement, parenteral.

FreAmine III 8.5% w/Electrolytes. (B. Braun) Sodium 60 mEq/L, potassium 60 mEq/L, magnesium 10 mEq/L, Cl 60 mEq/L, phosphate 40 mEq/L, acetate 125 mEq/L. Soln. Bot. 500 mL, 1000 mL. *Rx.*
Use: Nutritional supplement, parenteral.

FreAmine III 3% w/Electrolytes. (B. Braun) Amino acid 3% with electrolytes. Bot. 1000 mL. *Rx.*
Use: Nutritional supplement, parenteral.

Free & Clear. (Pharmaceutical Specialties) Ammonium laureth sulfate, disodium cocamide MEA sulfosuccinate, cocamidopropyl hydroxysultaine, cocamide DEA, PEG-120 methyl glucose dioleate, EDTA, potassium sorbate, citric acid. Shampoo. Bot. 240 mL. *OTC.*
Use: Dermatologic, cleanser.

Freedavite. (Freeda) Iron 10 mg (from ferrous fumarate), vitamins A 5000 units, D 400 units, E 3 units, B_1 5 mg, B_2 3 mg, B_3 25 mg, B_5 5 mg, B_6 2 mg, B_{12} 2 mcg, C 60 mg, choline, inositol, potassium iodide, Ca, Cu, K, Mg, Mn, Se, Zn 0.2 mg. Bot. 100s, 250s. *OTC.*
Use: Mineral, vitamin supplement.

Freedox. (Pharmacia) Tirilazad.
Use: A 21 aminosteroid antioxidant.

• **frentizole.** (FREN-tih-zole) USAN.
Use: Immunoregulator.

FreshBurst Listerine. (Warner Lambert) Thymol 0.064%, eucalyptol 0.092%, methyl salicylate 0.06%, menthol 0.042%, alcohol 21.6%. Rinse. Bot. 250 mL. *OTC.*
Use: Mouthwash.

Fresh n' Feminine. (Walgreen) Benzethonium Cl 0.2% Bot. 8 oz. *OTC.*
Use: Vaginal agent.

Frova. (Elan) Frovatriptan succinate 2.5 mg, lactose. Tab. Blister card 9s. *Rx.*
Use: Agent for migraine, serotonin 5-HT$_1$ receptor agonist.

• **frovatriptan succinate.** (froe-va-TRIP-tan) USAN.
Use: Antimigraine, serotonin 5-HT$_1$ receptor agonist.
See: Frova.

• **fructose.** (FRUK-tose) *USP 28.*
Use: Nutritional supplement.
See: Frutabs.

fructose. (Various Mfr.) Fructose 10%. Soln. Bot. 1000 mL.
Use: Nutritional supplement.

fructose and sodium chloride injection.
Use: Electrolyte, fluid, nutrient replacement.

Fruit C 500. (Freeda) Vitamin C 500 mg (as calcium ascorbate and ascorbic acid), rose hips. Chew. Tab. Bot. 100s, 250s. *OTC.*
Use: Vitamin supplement.

Fruit C 100. (Freeda) Vitamin C 100 mg (as calcium ascorbate and ascorbic acid). Chew. Tab. Bot. 250s. *OTC.*
Use: Vitamin supplement.

Fruit C 200. (Freeda) Vitamin C 200 mg (as calcium ascorbate and ascorbic acid), rose hips. Chew. Tab. Bot. 100s, 250s. *OTC.*
Use: Vitamin supplement.

Fruity Chews. (Ivax) Vitamins A 2500 units, D 400 units, E 15 mg, B$_1$ 1.05 mg, B$_2$ 1.2 mg, B$_3$ 13.5 mg, B$_6$ 1.05 mg, B$_{12}$ 4.5 mcg, C (as sodium ascorbate and ascorbic acid) 60 mg, folic acid 0.3 mg. Chew. Tab. Bot. 100s. *OTC.*
Use: Mineral, vitamin supplement.

Fruity Chews w/Iron. (Ivax) Elemental iron 12 mg, vitamins A 2500 units, D 400 units, E 15 mg, B$_1$ 1.05 mg, B$_2$ 1.2 mg, B$_3$ 13.5 mg, B$_6$ 1.05 mg, B$_{12}$ 4.5 mcg, C (as sodium ascorbate and ascorbic acid) 60 mg, folic acid 0.3 mg, zinc 8 mg. Chew. Tab. Bot. 100s. *OTC.*
Use: Mineral, vitamin supplement.

frusemide.
See: Lasix.

Frutabs. (Pfanstiehl) Fructose 2 g. Tab. Bot. 100s. *OTC.*
Use: Carbohydrate supplement.

FS Shampoo. (Hill Dermaceuticals) *OTC.*
See: Capex.

FTA-ABS. (Wampole) Fluorescent treponemal antibody-absorbed test in vitro for confirming a positive reagent test for syphillis. Test 100s.
Use: Diagnostic aid.

FTA-ABS/DS. (Wampole) Fluorescent treponemal antibody-absorbed test in vitro for confirming a positive reagent test for syphilis. Test 100s.
Use: Diagnostic aid.

• **fuchsin, basic.** (FYOO-sin) *USP 28.*
Use: Anti-infective, topical.

FUDR. (Roche) Floxuridine 500 mg. Pow. for Inj. Vial 5 mL. *Rx.*
Use: Antineoplastic; antimetabolite.

Ful-Glo. (PBH Wesley Jessen) Fluorescein sodium 0.6 mg. Strip. Box 300s. *OTC.*
Use: Diagnostic aid, ophthalmic.

Fuller. (Birchwood) Pkg. 1 shield.
Use: Anorectal preparation.

Full Spectrum B. (National Vitamin) Vitamin B$_1$ 1.5 mg, B$_2$ 1.7 mg, B$_3$ 20 mg, B$_5$ 10 mg, B$_6$ 10 mg, B$_{12}$ 6 mcg, C 60 mg, FA 800 mcg, biotin 3 mg. Preservative-free. Tab. 100s. *OTC.*
Use: Nutrition combination product.

fulvestrant.
Use: Hormone, antiestrogen.
See: Faslodex.

• **fumaric acid.** (fyoo-MAR-ik) *NF 23.*
Use: Acidifier.

Fumatinic. (Laser) Iron 90 mg (from ferrous fumarate equivalent to elemental iron 66 mg), vitamins C 60 mg, B$_{12}$ 5 mcg. ER Cap. Bot. 100s. *Rx.*
Use: Mineral, vitamin supplement.

• **fumoxicillin.** (fyoo-MOX-ih-SILL-in) USAN.
Use: Antibacterial.

Funduscein. (Ciba Vision) Fluorescein sodium. Inj. **10%:** Amp. 5 mL. **25%:** Amp. 3 mL. *Rx.*
Use: Diagnostic aid, ophthalmic.

Fungacetin. (Blair) Triacetin (glyceryl triacetate) 25% in a water-miscible ointment base. Tube 30 g. *Rx.*
Use: Antifungal, topical.

Fungatin. (Major) Tolnaftate 1%. Cream. Tube 15 g. *OTC.*
Use: Antifungal, topical.

fungicides.
See: Amphotericin B.
Ancobon.
Arcum.

Asterol.
Basic Fuchsin.
Desenex.
Dichlorophene.
Diflucan.
Fluconazole.
Fungizone Intravenous.
Grifulvin V.
Grisactin.
Griseofulvin Ultramicrosize.
Gris-PEG.
Itraconazole.
Miconazole Nitrate.
Monistat IV.
Mycostatin.
Nifuroxime.
Nilstat.
Nizoral.
Nyntntin
Phenylmercuric.
Sporanox.
Undecylenic Acid.
●**fungimycin.** (FUN-jih-MY-sin) USAN.
Use: Antifungal.
Fungi-Nail. (Kramer) Resorcinol 1%, salicylic acid 2%, parachlorometaxylenol 2%, benzocaine 0.5%, acetic acid 2.5%, propylene glycol, hydroxypropyl methylcellulose, alcohol 0.5%. Bot. 30 mL. *OTC.*
Use: Antifungal, topical.
Fungizone for Laboratory Use in Tissue Culture. (Bristol-Myers Squibb) Amphotericin B 50 mg, sodium desoxycholate 41 mg. Vial 20 mL.
Use: Diagnostic aid.
Fungizone Intravenous. (Apothecon) Amphotericin B 50 mg, as desoxycholate. Pow for Inj. Vial. *Rx.*
Use: Antifungal.
Fungoid-HC Creme. (Pedinol Pharmacal) Miconazole nitrate 2%, hydrocortisone 1%. Cream. In 56.7 g, 1 g dual packets. *Rx.*
Use: Antifungal, topical.
Fungoid Tincture. (Pedinol Pharmacal) Miconazole nitrate 2%, alcohol. Soln. Bot. with brush applicator 7.39 mL, 29.57 mL. *Rx.*
Use: Antifungal, topical.
Furacin Soluble Dressing. (Roberts) Nitrofurazone 0.2%, polyethylene glycol base. Oint. (soluble) Jar 454 g, Tube 28 g, 56 g. *Rx.*
Use: Burn therapy.
Furacin Topical Cream. (Roberts) Nitrofurazone 0.2% in a water-miscible base, cetyl alcohol, mineral oil, parabens. Cream. Tube 28 g. *Rx.*
Use: Burn therapy.

Furacin Topical Solution. (Roberts) Nitrofurazone 0.2%. Top. Soln. Bot. 480 mL. *Rx.*
Use: Burn therapy.
Furadantin. (First Horizon) Nitrofurantoin 25 mg per 5 mL. Glycerin, parabens, saccharin, sorbitol. Oral Susp. Bot. 60 mL, 470 mL. *Rx.*
Use: Anti-infective, urinary.
furalazine hydrochloride.
Use: Antimicrobial compound.
Furanite. (Major) Nitrofurantoin 50 mg, 100 mg. Tab. Bot. 100s. *Rx.*
Use: Anti-infective, urinary.
●**furaprofen.** (FYOOR-ah-PRO-fen) USAN. *Formerly Enprofen.*
Use: Anti-inflammatory.
●**furazolidone.** (fyoor-ah-ZOE-lih-dohn) *USP 28.*
Use: Antiprotozoal.
See: Furoxone.
●**furazolium chloride.** (FYOOR-ah-zoe-lee-uhm) USAN.
Use: Anti-infective.
●**furazolium tartrate.** (FYOOR-ah-ZOE-lee-uhm) USAN.
Use: Anti-infective.
furazosin hydrochloride. (FYOOR-ah-zoe-sin) Under study.
Use: Antihypertensive.
●**furegrelate sodium.** (fyoor-eh-GRELL-ate) USAN.
Use: Inhibitor (thromboxane synthetase).
●**furobufen.** (FER-oh-BYOO-fen) USAN.
Use: Anti-inflammatory.
●**furodazole.** (fyoor-OH-dah-zole) USAN.
Use: Anthelmintic.
Furonatal FA. (Lexis Laboratories) Vitamins A 8000 units, D 400 units, E 30 units, C 60 mg, folic acid 1 mg, B_1 2 mg, B_2 2.8 mg, B_6 2.5 mg, B_{12} 8 mcg, niacinamide 20 mg, iron 65 mg, calcium 125 mg. Tab. Bot. 100s, 1000s. *Rx.*
Use: Mineral, vitamin supplement.
●**furosemide.** (fyu-ROH-se-mide) *USP 28.* Oral Solution, USP.
Use: Diuretic.
See: Lasix.
furosemide. (Roxane) Furosemide. **10 mg/mL:** Soln. Dropper bot. 60 mL. **40 mg/5 mL:** Soln. Bot. 5 mL, 10 mL, 500 mL. *Rx.*
Use: Diuretic.
furosemide. (Various Mfr.) **Tab.:** 20 mg, 40 mg, 80 mg. Bot. 60s (40 mg only), 100s, 500s, 1000s, UD 100s. **Oral Soln.:** 10 mg/mL Bot. 60 mL, 120 mL. **Inj.:** 10 mg/mL Vial 10 mL; single-dose vial 2 mL, 10 mL; partial fill single-dose

vial 4 mL. *Rx.*
Use: Diuretic.
Furoxone. (Procter & Gamble Pharm) Furazolidone 100 mg. Sucrose. Tab. Bot. 20s, 100s. *Rx.*
Use: Antiprotozoal.
•**fursalan.** (FYOOR-sal-an) USAN. Under study.
Use: Disinfectant.

•**fusidate sodium.** (FEW-sih-DATE) USAN.
Use: Anti-infective.
•**fusidic acid.** (few-SIH-dik) USAN.
Use: Anti-infective.
Fuzeon. (Hoffman-LaRoche) Enfuvirtide 108 mg. Pow. for Inj., lyophilized. Convenience Kit with single-use vials, syringes, diluent, alcohol wipes. *Rx.*
Use: Anti-infective, tetracycline.

G

●**gabapentin.** (GAB-uh-PEN-tin) USAN.
Use: Anticonvulsant; amyotrophic lateral sclerosis agent.
See: Gabarone.
Neurontin.

gabapentin. (Various Mfr.) Gabapentin 100 mg, 300 mg, 400 mg. Cap. 100s, 500s. *Rx.*
Use: Anticonvulsant.

Gabarone. (Ivax) Gabapentin 100 mg, 300 mg, 400 mg. Lactose. Tab. 100s, 500s, 1,000s (400 mg only), 2,000s (300 mg only), 5,000s (100 mg only), UD 100s. *Rx.*
Use: Anticonvulsant.

gabbromicina. Aminosidine.
Use: Anti-infective. [Orphan Drug]

Gabitril. (Cephalon) Tiagabine hydrochloride 2 mg, 4 mg, 12 mg, 16 mg, 20 mg, lactose. Tab. Bot. 100s, 500s, *Abbo-Pac* 100s. *Rx.*
Use: Partial seizure treatment.

Gacid. (Arcum) Magnesium trisilicate 500 mg, aluminum hydroxide 250 mg. Tab. Bot. 100s, 1000s. *OTC.*
Use: Antacid.

●**gadobenate dimeglumine.** (gad-oh-BEN-ate die-meh-GLUE-meen) USAN.
Use: Diagnostic aid (paramagnetic), brain tumors, spine disorders.

●**gadodiamide.** (GAD-oh-DIE-ah-mide) *USP 28.*
Use: Radiopaque agent, parenteral.
See: Omniscan.

gadodiamide/caldiamide.
Use: Radiopaque agent.
See: Omniscan.

●**gadofosveset trisodium.** (gad-oh-FOS-ve-set) USAN.
Use: Diagnostic contrast agent.

●**gadopentetate dimeglumine.** (GAD-oh-PEN-teh-tate die-meh-GLUE-meen) *USP 28.*
Use: Radiopaque agent, parenteral.
See: Magnevist.

●**gadoteridol.** (GAD-oh-TER-ih-dahl) *USP 28.*
Use: Radiopaque agent, parenteral.
See: ProHance.

●**gadoversetamide.** (gad-oh-ver-SET-ah-mide) *USP 28.*
Use: Radiopaque agent, parenteral.
See: OptiMARK.

●**gadoxanum.** (gad-oh-ZAN-uhm) USAN.
Use: Diagnostic aid.

●**gadoxetate disodium.** (gad-OX-e-tate) USAN.
Use: Contrast agent.

●**gadozelite.** (gad-oh-ZEH-lite) USAN.
Use: Diagnostic aid.

●**galantamine.** (ga-LAN-ta-meen) USAN.
Use: Alzheimer disease; cholinesterase inhibitor.

galantamine hydrobromide.
Use: Cholinesterase inhibitor; Alzheimer disease.
See: Razadyne.
Razadyne ER.

Galardin. (Glycomed, Inc.) Matrix metalloproteinase inhibitor.
Use: Corneal ulcers. [Orphan Drug]

●**galasomite.** (GAL-ah-som-ite) USAN.
Use: Verocytotoxogenic *E. coli* infections.

●**galdansetron hydrochloride.** (gahl-DAN-seh-trahn) USAN.
Use: Antiemetic.

●**galiximab.** (gal-IX-i-mab) USAN.
Use: Psoriasis.

●**gallamine triethiodide.** (GAL-ah-meen try-eth-EYE-oh-dide) *USP 28.*
Use: Neuromuscular blocker.

●**gallium citrate Ga 67 injection.** (GAL-ee-uhm SIH-trate) *USP 28.*
Use: Diagnostic aid (radiopaque medium); radiopharmaceutical.

●**gallium nitrate.** (GAL-ee-uhm NYE-trate) USAN.
Use: Calcium regulator; antihypercalcemic.
See: Ganite

gallochrome.
See: Merbromin.

gallotannic acid.
See: Tannic Acid.

gallstone solubilizing agents.
See: Ursodiol.

●**galsulfase.** (gal-SUL-fase) USAN.
Use: Mucopolysaccharidosis VI.
See: Naglazyme.

Galzin. (Lemmon) Zinc acetate.
Use: Wilson disease. [Orphan Drug]

Gamazole Tabs. (Major) Sulfamethoxazole 500 mg. Tab. Bot. 100s, 500s, 1000s. *Rx.*
Use: Anti-infective; sulfonamide.

●**gamfexine.** (gam-FEX-ine) USAN.
Use: Antidepressant.

gamma benzene hexachloride.
See: Lindane.

gamma globulin.
See: Immune Globulin Intramuscular.
Immune Globulin Intravenous.

gamma-hydroxybutyrate. (Biocraft)
Use: Narcolepsy. [Orphan Drug]

gamma interferon.
See: Actimmune.

gammalinolenic acid.
Use: Juvenile rheumatoid arthritis.
[Orphan Drug]
Gammar-P I.V. (Aventis) Immune globulin intravenous (IGIV) 5% IgG, human albumin 3%, sucrose 5%, sodium chloride 0.5%, preservative free, heat-treated. Pow. for Inj., lyophilized. Single-dose vial 1 g, 2.5 g, 5 g w/diluent; 10 g w/administration set and diluent. W/vented transfer spike. Bulk pack 6s, diluent not supplied. *Rx.*
Use: Immunization.
Gamunex. (Bayer) Immune globulin (human) 10%, glycine 0.16 to 0.24 M. Caprylate/chromatography purified. Inj. 10 mL, 25 mL, 50 mL, 100 mL, 200 mL. *Rx.*
Use: Immune globulin.
ganaxolone. (Cocensys, Inc.)
Use: Infantile spasms; epilepsy; migraine. [Orphan Drug]
•**ganciclovir.** (gan-SIGH-kloe-VIHR) *USP 28.*
Use: Antiviral.
See: Cytovene.
ganciclovir. (Ranbaxy) Ganciclovir 250 mg, 500 mg. Cap. 100s. *Rx.*
Use: Antiviral.
ganciclovir intravitreal free implant.
Use: Cytomegalovirus retinitis. [Orphan Drug]
See: Vitrasert.
•**ganciclovir sodium.** (gah-SIGH-kloe-VIHR) *USAN.*
Use: Antiviral.
See: Cytovene.
Ganeake. (Geneva) Conjugated Estrogens, 0.625 mg, 1.25 mg, 2.5 mg. Tab. Bot. 100s, 1000s. *Rx.*
Use: Estrogen.
ganglionic blocking agents.
See: Dibenzyline Hydrochloride.
Hexamethonium Chloride and Bromide.
Hydergine.
Priscoline Hydrochloride.
Regitine.
Ganidin NR. (Cypress) Guaifenesin 100 mg/5 mL. Liq. 473 mL. *Rx.*
Use: Expectorant.
•**ganirelix acetate.** (ga-ni-REL-ix) *USAN.*
Use: Sex hormone.
ganirelix acetate. (Organon) Ganirelix acetate 250 mcg/0.5 mL. Inj. Prefilled disp. syr. 1 mL. Box 1s, 5s, 50s. *Rx.*
Use: Sex hormone.
Ganite. (Genta) Gallium nitrate 25 mg/mL. Preservative free. Inj. Single-dose vials. 20 mL. *Rx.*

Use: Calcium regulator; antihypercalcemic.
Gani-Tuss-DM NR. (Cypress) Dextromethorphan HBr 10 mg, guaifenesin 100 mg/5 mL, raspberry flavor, alcohol free. Liq. Bot. 118 mL, 473 mL. *Rx.*
Use: Upper respiratory combination, antitussive, expectorant.
Gani-Tuss NR. Various Mfr. Codeine phosphate 10 mg, guaifenesin 100 mg/5 mL, raspberry flavor, alcohol free. Liq. Bot. 120 mL, 473 mL. *c-v.*
Use: Upper respiratory combination, antitussive, expectorant.
Gantrisin. (Roche) Sulfisoxazole as acetyl sulfisoxazole 0.5 g/5 mL, alcohol 0.3%, parabens, sugar, sucrose, raspberry flavor. Ped. Susp. Bot. 473 mL. *Rx.*
Use: Anti-infective.
Garamycin. (Schering) Gentamicin sulfate. **Inj.:** 40 mg/mL. Parabens, EDTA, sodium bisulfite. Vials. 2 mL, 20 mL. **Oint.:** 3 mg/g. White petrolatum, parabens. Tube 3.5 g. **Soln.:** 3 mg/mL. Benzalkonium chloride 0.1 mg/mL, sodium phosphate, NaCl. Dropper Bot. 5 mL. *Rx.*
Use: Anti-infective, ophthalmic; aminoglycoside.
gardinol type detergents. Aurinol, cyclopon, dreft, drene, duponol, lissapol, maprofix, modinal, orvus, sandopan, sadipan.
Use: Detergent.
gardol. Sodium lauryl sarcosinate.
•**garenoxacin mesylate.** (gar-en-OX-a-sin) *USAN.*
Use: Antibacterial.
Garfield. (Menley & James Labs, Inc.) Vitamin A 2500 units, D 400 units, E 15 units, C 60 mg, folic acid 0.3 mg, B_1 1.05 mg, B_2 1.2 mg, B_3 13.5 mg, B_6 1.05 mg, B_{12} 4.5 mcg, sucrose, lactose. Chew. Tab. Bot. 60s. *OTC.*
Use: Vitamin supplement.
Garfield Complete w/Minerals. (Menley & James Labs, Inc.) Vitamin A 5000 units, D 400 units, E 30 units, C 60 mg, folic acid 0.4 mg, B_1 1.5 mg, B_2 1.7 mg, B_3 20 mg, B_5 10 mg, B_6 2 mg, B_{12} 6 mcg, biotin 40 mcg, iron 18 mg, Ca, Cu, P, I, Mg, zinc 15 mg, aspartame, phenylalanine, sorbitol. Chew. Tab. Bot. 60s. *OTC.*
Use: Mineral, vitamin supplement.
Garfield Plus Extra C. (Menley & James Labs, Inc.) Vitamin A 2500 units, D 400 units, E 15 units, C 250 mg, folic acid 0.3 mg, B_1 1.05 mg, B_2 1.2 mg, B_3 13.5 mg, B_6 1.05 mg, B_{12} 4.5 mcg, su-

crose, lactose. Chew. Tab. Bot. 60s. OTC.
Use: Vitamin supplement.

Garfield Plus Iron. (Menley & James Labs, Inc.) Vitamins A 2500 units, D 400 units, E 15 units, C 60 mg, folic acid 0.3 mg, B_1 1.05 mg, B_2 1.2 mg, B_3 13.5 mg, B_6 1.05 mg, B_{12} 4.5 mcg, iron 15 mcg, sucrose, lactose. Chew. Tab. Bot. 60s. OTC.
Use: Mineral, vitamin supplement.

Garfield's Tea. (Last) Senna leaf powder 68.3%. Bot. 2 oz. OTC.
Use: Laxative.

Garitabs. (Halsey Drug) Iron 50 mg, vitamins B_1 5 mg, B_2 5 mg, B_5 2 mg, B_6 0.5 mg, B_{12} 3 mcg, C 75 mg, niacinamide 30 mg. Bot. 1000s. OTC.
Use: Mineral, vitamin supplement.

Garl Tonic Hematinic. (Halsey Drug) Vitamins B_1 5 mg, B_2 5 mg, B_6 1 mg, B_{12} 6 mcg, pantothenic acid 4 mg, niacinamide 100 mg, choline bitartrate 100 mg, iron 100 mg/30 mL Bot. 16 oz. OTC.
Use: Mineral, vitamin supplement.

• **garlic.** NF 23. Allium.
Use: Antispasmodic.

garlic capsules. (Miller Pharmacal Group) Garlic 166 mg. Cap. Bot. 100s. OTC.
Use: Antispasmodic.

garlic oil.
See: Natural Garlic Oil.

garlic oil capsules. (Kirkman) Bot. 100s. OTC.

• **garnocestim.** (gar-no-SES-tim) USAN.
Use: Chemotherapeutic aid.

Gas Ban. (Roberts) Calcium carbonate 300 mg, simethicone 40 mg. Tab. Bot. UD 8s, 1000s. OTC.
Use: Antacid.

Gas Ban DS. (Roberts) Aluminum hydroxide 400 mg, magnesium hydroxide 400 mg, simethicone 40 mg/5 mL. Liq. Bot. 150 mL. OTC.
Use: Antacid.

Gas Permeable Daily Cleaner. (PBH Wesley Jessen) Potassium sorbate 0.13%, EDTA 2%, ethoxylated polyoxypropylene glycol, tris (hydroxymethyl) amino methane, hydroxymethylcellulose, thimerosal free. Soln. Bot. 30 mL. OTC.
Use: Contact lens care.

Gas Permeable Lens Starter System. (PBH Wesley Jessen) Daily cleanser, Bot. 3 mL, Wetting and soaking soln., Bot. 60 mL, Hydra-Mat II spin cleansing unit. Kit. OTC.
Use: Contact lens care.

Gas Permeable Wetting & Soaking Solution. (PBH Wesley Jessen) Sterile aqueous, isotonic soln. of low viscosity, buffered to physiological pH. Bot. 60 mL, 120 mL. OTC.
Use: Contact lens care.

Gas Relief. (Rugby) Simethicone 80 mg, 125 mg. Chew Tab. Bot. 60s (125 mg only), 100s (80 mg only). OTC.
Use: Antiflatulant.

gastric acidifiers.
See: Glutamic Acid hydrochloride.

Gastroccult. (SmithKline Diagnostics) Occult blood screening test. In 40s.
Use: Diagnostic aid.

Gastrocrom. (Celltech) Cromolyn sodium 100 mg/5 mL. Oral Conc. 8 UD Amps/foil pouch. Rx.
Use: Antiasthmatic.

Gastrografin. (Bracco Diagnostics) Diatrizoate meglumine 660 mg, diatrizoate sodium 100 mg, iodine 367 mg/mL, EDTA, polysorbate 80, saccharin, simethicone, lemon flavor. Soln. Bot. 120 mL. Rx.
Use: Radiopaque agent.

gastrointestinal function tests.
See: Secretin.
Simethicone-coated Cellulose Suspension.
Sincalide.

gastrointestinal tests.
See: Entero-Test.
Gastro-Test.

Gastrosed. (Roberts) Hyoscyamine sulfate. Soln.: 0.125 mg/mL. Dropper Bot. 5 mL. Alcohol free. Tab.: 0.125 mg. Bot. 100s. Rx.
Use: Anticholinergic; antispasmodic.

Gastro-Test. (HDC) To determine stomach pH and to diagnose and locate gastric bleeding. Test 25s.
Use: Diagnostic aid.

Gas-X. (Novartis) Simethicone 80 mg. Softgel Cap. Pkg. 12s, 30s. OTC.
Use: Antiflatulent.

Gas-X, Extra Strength. (Novartis) Simethicone 125 mg, sorbitol. Softgel Cap. Box 30s, 100s. OTC.
Use: Antiflatulent.

Gas-X with Maalox. (Novartis) Calcium carbonate 500 mg, simethicone 125 mg. Dextrose, mannitol. Orange and wild berry flavors. Chew. Tab. 8s, 24s. OTC.
Use: Antacid.

• **gatifloxacin.** (gat-ih-FLOX-ah-sin) USAN.
Use: Fluoroquinolone, antibiotic.
See: Tequin.
Zymar.

●**gauze, absorbent.** *USP 28.*
Use: Surgical aid.
●**gauze, petrolatum.** *USP 28.*
Use: Surgical aid.
●**gavestinel.** (ga-VE-sti-nel) USAN.
Use: Stroke.
Gaviscon. (GlaxoSmithKline) Aluminum
hydroxide 80 mg, magnesium trisilicate
20 mg, alginic acid, sodium bicarbonate, sucrose, calcium stearate. Chew.
Tab. Bot. 30s, 100s. *OTC.*
Use: Antacid.
**Gaviscon Extra Strength Relief For-
mula Liquid.** (GlaxoSmithKline) **Liq.:**
Aluminum hydroxide 254 mg, magnesium carbonate 237.5 mg, parabens,
EDTA, saccharin, sorbitol, simethicone,
sodium alginate/5 mL. Bot. 355 mL.
Tab.: Aluminum hydroxide 160 mg,
magnesium carbonate 105 mg, alginic
acid, sodium bicarbonate, sucrose, calcium stearate. Chew. Tab. Bot. 30s,
100s. *OTC.*
Use: Antacid.
Gaviscon Liquid. (GlaxoSmithKline) Alu-
minum hydroxide 31.7 mg, magnesium
carbonate 119.3 mg/5 mL. Bot.
177 mL, 355 mL. *OTC.*
Use: Antacid.
Gaviscon-2, Double Strength Tablets.
(GlaxoSmithKline) Aluminum hydrox-
ide 160 mg, magnesium trisilicate
40 mg, alginic acid, sodium bicarbo-
nate, sucrose. Chew. Tab. Bot. 48s.
OTC.
Use: Antacid.
GBA.
See: Gamma hydroxybutyrate.
G.B.H. Lotion. (Century) Gamma benz-
ene hexachloride 1%. Bot. 2 oz, pt, gal.
Use: Scabicide; pediculicide.
G.B.S. (Forest) Dehydrocholic acid
125 mg, phenobarbital 8 mg, homatro-
pine methylbromide 2.5 mg. Tab. 100s,
1000s. *Rx.*
Use: Hydrocholeretic.
G-CSF.
See: Neupogen.
Gebauer's 114. (Gebauer) Dichlorotetra-
fluoroethane 100%. Can 8 oz.
Use: Anesthetic, local.
Gebauer's Spray and Stretch. (Ge-
bauer) Tetrafluoroethane and pentaf-
luoropropane. Spray. 103.5 mL. *Rx.*
Use: Local anesthetic, topical.
●**gefitinib.** (ge-FI-tye-nib) USAN.
Use: Antineoplastic.
See: Iressa.
Geladine. (Barth's) Gelatin, protein, vita-
min D. Cap. Bot. 100s, 500s. *OTC.*

Gelamal. (Halsey Drug) Magnesium-
aluminum hydroxide gel. Bot. 12 oz.
OTC.
Use: Antacid.
●**gelatin.** *NF 23.*
Use: Pharmaceutic aid (encapsulating,
suspending agent, tablet binder, tab-
let coating agent).
●**gelatin film, absorbable.** *USP 28.*
Use: Local hemostatic.
See: Gelfilm.
gelatin film, sterile.
See: Neupogen.
gelatin powder, sterile.
See: Gelfoam.
gelatin sponge.
See: Gelfilm.
●**gelatin sponge, absorbable.** *USP 28.*
Use: Hemostatic, local.
See: Gelfoam.
gelatin, zinc.
See: Zinc gelatin.
Gel-Clean. (PBH Wesley Jessen) Gel for-
mulated with nonionic surfactant. Tube
30 g. *OTC.*
Use: Contact lens care.
G-11. (Givaudan) Hexachlorophene Pow.
for Mfg.
See: Hexachlorophene.
Gelfilm. (Pharmacia) Sterile, absorbable
gelatin film. Envelope 1s. 100 mm ×
125 mm. Also available as Ophth. Ster-
ile 25 × 50 mm. Box 6s. *Rx.*
Use: Hemostatic, topical.
Gelfoam Dental Pack. (Pharmacia) Size
4, 20 mm × 20 mm × 7 mm. Jar
15 sponges. *Rx.*
Use: Hemostatic, topical.
Gelfoam Powder. (Pharmacia) Sterile
Jar 1 g. *Rx.*
Use: Hemostatic, topical.
Gelfoam Prostatectomy Cones. (Phar-
macia) Prostatectomy cones (for use
with Foley catheter) 13 cm, 18 cm in diameter. Box 6s. *Rx.*
Use: Hemostatic.
Gelhist Pediatric Suspension. (Econolab) Phenylephrine tannate 5 mg,
chlorpheniramine tannate 2 mg, pyrilamine tannate 12.5 mg/5 mL, methylparaben, saccharin, sucrose. Susp. Bot.
118 mL, 473 mL. *Rx.*
Use: Antihistamine, decongestant.
Gel Jet Gelatin Capsules. (Kirkman)
Bot. 100s, 250s.
Gel-Kam. (Colgate-Palmolive) Fluoride
0.1% (stannous fluoride 0.4%). Mint,
fruit, berry, bubble gum, cinnamon flavors. Gel. Bot. w/applicator tip. 4.3 oz,
7 oz. *OTC.*
Use: Dental caries agent.

Gelocast. (Beiersdorf) Unna's Boot medicated bandage: Semi-rigid cast impregnated with zinc oxide mixtures. Box 4 inches × 10 yd, 3 inches × 10 yd.
Use: Unna's cast dressing.

gelsemium. (Various Mfr.) Pkg. oz.
Use: Neuralgia.
W/A.P.C.
See: APC Combinations.
W/Combinations
See: UB.
Urisan-P.

gelsolin, recombinant human. (Biogen)
Use: Cystic fibrosis. [Orphan Drug]

Gel-Tin. (Young Dental) Fluoride 0.1% (from stannous fluoride 0.4%). Gel Bot. 57 g, 623 g. *Rx.*
Use: Dental caries agent.

•**gemcabene calcium.** (JLM-ka been) USAN.
Use: Atherosclerosis.

•**gemcadiol.** (JEM-kah-DIE-ole) USAN.
Use: Antihyperlipoproteinemic.

•**gemcitabine.** (JEM-sit-ah-BEAN) USAN.
Use: Antineoplastic.

•**gemcitabine hydrochloride.** (JEM-sit-ah-BEAN) *USP 28.*
Use: Antineoplastic.
See: Gemzar.

•**gemeprost.** (JEH-meh-PRAHST) USAN.
Use: Prostaglandin.

•**gemfibrozil.** (gem-FIE-broe-ZILL) *USP 28.*
Use: Antihyperlipidemic.
See: Lopid.

gemfibrozil. (Various Mfr.) Gemfibrozil 600 mg. Tab., Bot. 60s, 500s; blisterpack 25s; UD 100s. *Rx.*
Use: Antihyperlipidemic.

•**gemifloxacin mesylate.** (jeh-mih-FLOKS-ah-sin MEH-sih-LATE) USAN.
Use: Fluoroquinolone.
See: Factive.

gemopatrilat. (ge-moe-PA-tril-at) USAN.
Use: Hypertension; congestive heart failure.

gemtuzumab ozogamicin.
Use: Monoclonal antibody.
See: Mylotarg.

Gemzar. (Eli Lilly) Gemcitabine hydrochloride 20 mg/mL. Pow for Inj. Vial 10 mL, 50 mL. *Rx.*
Use: Antineoplastic.

Genac. (Ivax) Triprolidine hydrochloride 2.5 mg, pseudoephedrine hydrochloride 60 mg, lactose. Tab. Bot. 48s. *OTC.*
Use: Upper respiratory combination, antihistamine, decongestant.

Genacol. (Ivax) Pseudoephedrine hydrochloride 30 mg, chlorpheniramine maleate 2 mg, dextromethorphan HBr 10 mg, acetaminophen 325 mg. Tab. Bot. 50s. *OTC.*
Use: Analgesic, antihistamine, antitussive, decongestant.

Genacol Maximum Strength Cold & Flu Relief. (Ivax) Dextromethorphan HBr 15 mg, chlorpheniramine maleate 2 mg, pseudoephedrine hydrochloride 30 mg, acetaminophen 500 mg. Tab. Bot. 50s. *OTC.*
Use: Upper respiratory combination, antitussive, antihistamine, decongestant, analgesic.

Genagesic. (Ivax) Propoxyphene hydrochloride 165 mg, acetaminophen 650 mg. Tab. Bot. 100s, 500s. *c-iv.*
Use: Analgesic combination, narcotic.

Genahist. (Goldline) Diphenhydramine hydrochloride. Liq.: 12.5 mg/5 mL, cherry flavor. Bot. 118 mL. **Tab.:** 25 mg. 24s. **Cap.:** 25 mg, lactose, parabens. 100s. *OTC.*
Use: Antihistamine.

Genallerate. (Ivax) Chlorpheniramine maleate 4 mg, lactose. Tab. Bot. 24s. *OTC.*
Use: Antihistamine.

Genapap. (Ivax) Acetaminophen 325 mg. Tab. Bot. 100s. *OTC.*
Use: Analgesic.

Genapap, Children's Chewable Tabs. (Ivax) Acetaminophen 80 mg. Bot. 30s. *OTC.*
Use: Analgesic.

Genapap, Children's Elixir. (Ivax) Acetaminophen 160 mg/5 mL. Cherry flavor. Bot. 120 mL. *OTC.*
Use: Analgesic.

Genapap, Infants Drops. (Ivax) Acetaminophen 100 mg/mL, alcohol 7%. Coln. Dropper Bot. 15 mL. *OTC.*
Use: Analgesic.

Genapax. (Key) Gentian violet 5 mg. Tampon. Box 12s.
Use: Antifungal, vaginal.

Genaphed. (Goldline) Pseudoephedrine hydrochloride 30 mg, lactose. Tab. Bot. 24s. *OTC.*
Use: Nasal decongestant, arylalkylamine.

Genasal. (Goldline) Oxymetazoline hydrochloride 0.05%, benzalkonium chloride, phenylmercuric acetate, sorbitol. Soln. Spray Bot. 15 mL, 30 mL. *OTC.*
Use: Nasal decongestant, arylalkylamine.

Genasoft. (Goldline Consumer) Docusate sodium 100 mg, methylparaben Softgel Cap. Bot. 60s. *OTC.*

Use: Laxative, stool softener.

Genaspor Antifungal. (Ivax) Tolnaftate 1%. Cream. Bot. 15 g. *OTC.*
Use: Antifungal, topical.

Genasyme. (Ivax) Simethicone 80 mg. Tab. Bot. 100s. *OTC.*
Use: Antiflatulent.

Genaton. (Ivax) Aluminum hydroxide 80 mg, magnesium trisilicate 20 mg, alginic acid, sodium bicarbonate, sodium 18.4 mg, sucrose, sugar. Chew. Tab. Bot. 100s. *OTC.*
Use: Antacid.

Genaton, Extra Strength. (Ivax) Aluminum hydroxide 160 mg, magnesium carbonate 105 mg, alginic acid, sodium bicarbonate, sodium 29.9 mg, sucrose, calcium stearate. Chew. Tab. Bot. 100s. *OTC.*
Use: Antacid.

Genaton Liquid. (Ivax) Aluminum hydroxide 31.7 mg, magnesium carbonate 137.3 mg, sodium alginate, sodium 13 mg, EDTA, saccharin, sorbitol/ 5 mL. Bot. 355 mL. *OTC.*
Use: Antacid.

genatropine hydrochloride. (jen-AT-row-peen) Atropine-N-oxide hydrochloride. Aminoxytropine tropate hydrochloride.
See: X-tro.

Genatuss DM. (Ivax) Dextromethorphan HBr 10 mg, guaifenesin 100 mg/5 mL, corn syrup, menthol, saccharin, alcohol free. Syr. Bot. Bot. 118 mL. *OTC.*
Use: Upper respiratory combination, antitussive, expectorant.

Gen-bee with C. (Ivax) Vitamins B_1 15 mg, B_2 10.2 mg, B_3 50 mg, B_5 10 mg, B_6 5 mg, C 300 mg. Cap. Bot. 130s, 1000s. *OTC.*
Use: Vitamin supplement.

Gencept. (Gencon) **0.5/35:** Norethindrone 0.5 mg, ethinyl estradiol, 35 mcg. Tab (with 7 inert tabs). Pkgs 21s and 28s. **1/35:** Norethindrone 1 mg, ethinyl estradiol 35 mcg. Tab (with 7 inert tabs). Pkgs 21s and 28s. **10/11:** Norethindrone 0.5 mg and 1 mg, ethinyl estradiol 35 mcg. Tab (with 7 inert tabs). Pkg 21s and 28s. *Rx.*
Use: Contraceptive.

Gendecon. (Ivax) Phenylephrine hydrochloride 5 mg, chlorpheniramine maleate 2 mg, acetaminophen 325 mg. Tab. Bot. 50s. *OTC.*
Use: Analgesic, antihistamine, decongestant.

Genebs Extra Strength. (Ivax) Acetaminophen 500 mg. Cap. Bot. 100s, 1000s. *OTC.*
Use: Analgesic.

Genebs Extra Strength Tablets. (Ivax) Acetaminophen 500 mg. Tab. Bot. 100s, 1000s. *OTC.*
Use: Analgesic.

Genebs Tablets. (Ivax) Acetaminophen 325 mg. Bot. 100s, 1000s. *OTC.*
Use: Analgesic.

• **general anesthetics.**
Use: Anesthetics, general.

Generet-500. (Ivax) Iron 105 mg, Vitamins B_1 6 mg, B_2 6 mg, B_3 30 mg, B_5 10 mg, B_6 5 mg, B_{12} 25 mcg, C (as sodium ascorbate) 500 mg. TR Tab. Bot. 60s. *OTC.*
Use: Mineral, vitamin supplement.

Generix-T. (Ivax) Iron 15 mg, vitamins A 10,000 units, D 400 units, E 5.5 mg, B_1 15 mg, B_2 10 mg, B_3 100 mg, B_5 10 mg, B_6 2 mg, B_{12} 7.5 mcg, C 150 mg, Cu, I, Mg, Mn, zinc 1.5 mg. Tab. Bot. 100s. *OTC.*
Use: Mineral, vitamin supplement.

GenESA. (Gensia Sicor) Arbutamine hydrochloride 0.05 mg/mL. Inj. Syringe 20 mg (containing 1 mg arbutamine). *Rx.*
Use: Diagnostic aid.

Geneye. (Ivax) Tetrahydrozoline hydrochloride 0.05%. Drop. Bot. 15 mL. *OTC.*
Use: Mydriatic, vasoconstrictor.

Geneye Extra. (Ivax) Tetrahydrozoline hydrochloride 0.05%, PEG 400 1%, benzalkonium chloride, EDTA. Drops. Bot. 15 mL. *OTC.*
Use: Ophthalmic vasoconstrictor.

Genfiber. (Goldline Consumer) Psyllium hydrophilic mucilloid fiber 3.4 g, 14 cal/ dose, dextrose. Pow. Can 595 g. *OTC.*
Use: Laxative.

Genfiber, Orange Flavor. (Goldline Consumer) Psyllium hydrophilic mucilloid fiber 3.4 g/dose, sucrose, orange flavor. Pow. Can 397 g. *OTC.*
Use: Laxative.

Gengraf. (Abbott) Cyclosporine. **Cap:** 25 mg, 100 mg, alcohol 12.8%, castor oil. UD 30s. **Oral Soln:** 100 mg/mL. Castor oil. 50 mL. *Rx.*
Use: Immunosuppressant.

genital herpes treatment.
See: Acyclovir.
Zovirax.

Genite. (Ivax) Pseudoephedrine hydrochloride 10 mg, doxylamine succinate 1.25 mg, dextromethorphan HBr 5 mg, acetaminophen 167 mg, alcohol 25%/ 5 mL. Bot. 177 mL. *OTC.*
Use: Analgesic, antihistamine, antitussive, decongestant.

genitourinary irrigants.
See: Acetic Acid for Irrigation.
Glycine (Aminoacetic Acid) for Irrigation.
Neosporin G.U. Irrigant.
Renacidin.
Resectisol.
Sodium Chloride for Irrigation.
Sorbitol.
Sorbitol-Mannitol.
Sterile Water for Irrigation.
Suby's Solution G.
Gen-K. (Ivax) **Pow.:** Potassium chloride. Bot. 20 mEq. Pkt. Box 30s. **Tab.:** Effervescent potassium. Bot. 30s. *Rx.*
Use: Electrolyte supplement.
Genna Tablets. (Ivax) Senna concentrate 217 mg. Bot. 100s, 1000s. *OTC.*
Use: Laxative
Gennin. (Ivax) Buffered aspirin 5 g. Tab. Bot. 100s. *OTC.*
Use: Analgesic.
genophyllin.
See: Aminophylline.
Genoptic Liquifilm Sterile Ophthalmic Solution. (Allergan) Gentamicin sulfate 3 mg/mL. Bot. 1 mL, 5 mL. *Rx.*
Use: Anti-infective, ophthalmic.
Genoptic S.O.P. Sterile Ophthalmic Ointment. (Allergan) Gentamicin sulfate 3 mg/g. Tube 3.5 g. *Rx.*
Use: Anti-infective, ophthalmic.
Genotropin (Pharmacia) Somatropin 1.5 mg (≈ 4.5 units/vial), preservative free. In 1.5 mg *Intra-Mix* 2-chamber cartridge with pressure-release needle. Box 5s. Somatropin 5.8 mg (≈17.4 units/vial), mannitol 46.8 mg. In 5.8 *Intra-Mix* 2-chamber cartridge with pressure-release needle and 2–chamber cartridge. Box 1s, 5s. Somatriptan 13.8 mg (≈ 41.4 units/vial), mannitol 46 mg. In *Intra-Mix* 2–chamber cartridge of 1s, 5s. Pow. for Inj. *Rx.*
Use: Growth hormone.
Genotropin MiniQuick. (Pharmacia) Somatropin 0.2 mg, 0.4 mg, 0.6 mg, 0.8 mg, 1 mg, 1.2 mg, 1.4 mg, 1.6 mg, 1.8 mg, 2 mg/vial, glycine 0.23 mg, mannitol 13.74 mg, preservative free. Pow. for Inj., lyophilized. Single-use syringe w/2-chamber cartridge. Box 7s. *Rx.*
Use: Growth hormone.
Genprep Ointment. (Ivax) Live yeast cell derivative supplying 2000 units skin respiratory factor/oz of ointment w/shark liver oil 3%, phenylmercuric nitrate 1:10,000. Tube 2 oz. *OTC.*
Use: Anorectal preparation.

Genpril. (Ivax) Ibuprofen 200 mg, lactose. Tab. Bot. 100s. *OTC.*
Use: Analgesic, NSAID.
Genprin. (Ivax) Aspirin 325 mg. Tab. 100s. *OTC.*
Use: Analgesic.
gensalate sodium.
Use: Analgesic.
Gentacidin Ophthalmic. (Novartis Ophthalmics) **Oint.:** Gentamicin 3 mg/g. Tube 3.5 g. **Soln.:** Gentamicin sulfate 3 mg/mL. Bot. 5 mL. *Rx.*
Use: Anti-infective, ophthalmic.
Gentafair. (Bausch & Lomb) **Oint.:** Gentamicin 3 mg/g with liquid lanolin, white petrolatum, mineral oil, parabens. Tube 3.75 g, 15 g. **Soln.:** Gentamicin 3 mg/mL, polyoxyl 40 stearate, polyethylene glycol. Dropper bot. 5 mL, 16 mL. *Rx.*
Use: Anti-infective, ophthalmic.
Gentak. (Akorn) **Oint.:** Gentamicin 3 mg/g. Tube 3.5 g. **Soln.:** Gentamicin 3 mg/mL. Bot. 5 mL, 15 mL. *Rx.*
Use: Anti-infective, ophthalmic.
gentamicin. (Various Mfr.) Gentamicin sulfate. **Oint.:** 0.1% (as base), may contain white petrolatum, parabens. 15 g. **Cream:** 0.1% (as base), may contain propylene glycol, parabens. 15 g. *Rx.*
Use: Anti-infective, topical.
gentamicin and prednisolone acetate ophthalmic suspension.
Use: Anti-infective; anti-inflammatory.
gentamicin impregnated PMMA beads on surgical wire.
Use: Chronic osteomyelitis. [Orphan Drug]
gentamicin liposome injection.
Use: Mycobacterium avium-intracellulare infection. [Orphan Drug]
• **gentamicin sulfate.** (JEN-tuh-MY-sin) *USP 28.*
Use: Anti-infective.
See: Genoptic.
Gentacidin.
Gentak.
W/Prednisolone acetate.
See: Pred-G ophthalmic suspension.
gentamicin sulfate. (Schering-Plough) Produced by *Micromonospora purpurea.* (Various Mfr.). **Ophthalmic Oint.:** 3 mg/g Tube 3.5 g. **Ophthalmic Soln.:** 3 mg/mL Bot. 5 mL, 15 mL. **Inj.:** 40 mg/mL. Vial 2 mL, 20 mL. Cartridge-needle units 1.5 mL, 2 mL. **Ped. Inj.:** 10 mg/mL. Vial 2 mL. *Rx.*
Use: Anti-infective.
gentamicin sulfate ophthalmic. (E. Fougera) Gentamicin sulfate 3 mg/g.

Mineral oil, white petrolatum base. Oint. 3.5 g. *Rx.*
Use: Antibiotic.

GenTeal. (Novartis Ophthalmics) Hydroxypropyl methylcellulose 0.3%, boric acid, phosphone acid, sodium chloride, sodium perborate. Drops. 15, 25 mL. *OTC.*
Use: Lubricant, ophthalmic.

•**gentian violet.** (JEN-shun) *USP 28. Formerly Methylrosaniline Chloride.*
Use: Anti-infective, topical.

gentian violet. (Various Mfr.) Gentian violet 1%, 2%. Top. Soln. Bot. 30 mL. *OTC.*
Use: Anti-infective; antifungal, topical.

•**gentisic acid ethanolamide.** *NF 23.*
Use: Pharmaceutic aid, complexing agent.

Gentle Cream. (Geritrex) Mineral oil, cetearyl alcohol, petrolatum, castor oil, lanolin, triethanolamine, propylene glycol, EDTA, zinc oxide, vitamins A, D, & E, aloe vera oil. Cream. 120 g. *OTC.*
Use: Emollient.

Gentle Iron. (Nature's Bounty) Fe 28 mg (as ferrous bisglycinate), vitamin B_{12} 8 mcg, C 60 mg, FA 0.4 mg. Cap. 90s. *OTC.*
Use: Vitamin.

Gentle Nature Natural Vegetable Laxative. (Novartis) Sennosides A and B as calcium salts. 20 mg. Tab. Box 16s, 32s. *OTC.*
Use: Laxative.

Gentle Shampoo. (Ulmer Pharmacal) Bot. 4 oz, gal. *OTC.*
Use: Dermatologic, hair.

Gentran 40. (Baxter PPI) Dextran 40 10% w/sodium chloride 0.9% or Dextran 40 10% w/dextrose 5%. Inj. Plastic Bot. 500 mL. *Rx.*
Use: Plasma expander.

Gentran 70. (Baxter PPI) Dextran 70 6% w/sodium chloride 0.9%. Inj. Plastic Bot. 500 mL. *Rx.*
Use: Plasma expander.

Gentran 75. (Baxter PPI) Dextran 75 6% in sodium chloride 0.9%. Inj. Bot. 500 mL. *Rx.*
Use: Plasma expander.

Gentrasul. (Bausch & Lomb) Gentamicin. **Oint.:** 3 mg. **Soln.:** 3.5 g. Dropper bot. 5 mL. *Rx.*
Use: Anti-infective, ophthalmic.

Gentz Rectal Wipes. (Roxane) Pramoxine hydrochloride 1%, alcloxa 0.2%, witch hazel 50%, propylene glycol 10%. Box 100s, 120s (individually wrapped disposable wipes). *OTC.*
Use: Anorectal preparation.

Genuine Bayer Aspirin. (Bayer Corp. (Consumer Div.)) Aspirin 325 mg. FC Tab. Bot. 12s, 24s, 50s, 200s, 300s. *OTC.*
Use: Analgesic.

Geocillin. (Roerig) Carbenicillin indanyl sodium 382 mg (indanyl sodium ester 118 mg). Film coated. Tab. Bot. 100s, UD 100s. *Rx.*
Use: Anti-infective, penicillin.

Geodon. (Pfizer) **Cap.:** Ziprasidone hydrochloride 20 mg, 40 mg, 60 mg, 80 mg, lactose. Bot. 60s, UD 80s. **Pow. for Inj.:** 20 mg (as mesylate). Vials. Single use. *Rx.*
Use: Antipsychotic; benzisoxazole derivative.

Geopen. (Roerig) Carbenicillin disodium. Inj. **Vial:** 1 g, 2 g, 5 g. Pkg. 10s. **Piggyback Vial:** 2 g, 5 g, 10 g. **Bulk Pharmacy Pack:** 30 g. *Rx.*
Use: Anti-infective, penicillin.

•**gepirone hydrochloride.** (jeh-PIE-rone) USAN.
Use: Anxiolytic; antidepressant.

Gera Plus. (Towne) Iron 50 mg, vitamins B_1 5 mg, B_2 5 mg, B_6 0.5 mg, B_{12} 3 mcg, C 75 mg, niacinamide 30 mg, calcium pantothenate 2 mg. Tab. Bot. 100s. *OTC.*
Use: Mineral, vitamin supplement.

Geravim. (Major) Vitamins B_1 0.83 mg, B_2 0.42 mg, B_3 8.3 mg, B_5 1.67 mg, B_6 0.17 mg, B_{12} 0.17 mg, I, Fe 2.5 mg, Zn 0.3 mg, choline, Mn, alcohol 18%. Liq. Bot. Pt, gal. *OTC.*
Use: Mineral, vitamin supplement.

Geravite. (Roberts) Vitamins B_1 0.3 mg, B_2 0.4 mg, B_3 33.3 mg, B_{12} 3.3 mcg, L-lysine, alcohol 15%, parabens, sorbitol, sucrose. Elix. Bot. 480 mL. *OTC.*
Use: Mineral, vitamin supplement.

Gerber Baby Formula Low Iron Formula. (Bristol-Myers Squibb) Protein (from non-fat milk) 14.7 g, carbohydrate (from lactose) 71.3 g, fat (from palm olein, soy, coconut, and high oleic sunflower oils) 36 g, linoleic acid 5.9 g, vitamins A, D, E, K, C, B_1, B_2, B_3, B_5, B_6, B_{12}, folic acid, biotin, choline, inositol, Ca, P, Mg, Fe 3.4 mg, Zn, Mn, Cu, I, Na 220 mg, K 720 mg, Cl, taurine, calories per L 666.7. **Ready to use liq.:** Bot. 943 mL. **Concentrated liq.:** Bot. 433 mL. **Pow.:** Can 457 g and 914 g. *OTC.*
Use: Nutritional supplement.

Geref. (Serono) Sermorelin acetate 50 mcg (lyophilized). Pow. for Inj. Amp. 2 mL w/sodium chloride 0.9%.
Use: Diagnostic aid.

Geri-All-D. (Barth's) Vitamins A 10,000 units, D 400 units, B_1 7 mg, B_2 14 mg, B_6 0.35 mg, B_{12} 25 mcg, C 200 mg, niacin 4.17 mg, E 50 units, pantothenic acid 0.63 mg, trace minerals, and other factors. 2 Cap. Bot. 1 mo., 3 mo., and 6 mo. supply of *Geri-All* regular and *Geri-All-D* *OTC*.
Use: Mineral, vitamin supplement.
geriatric supplements with multivitamins/minerals.
See: Geravite.
Gerimed.
Gerineed.
Geriot.
Geri-Plus.
Geritol Complete.
Gerivite.
Glorix.
Hep-Forte.
Mega VM-80.
Optivite P.M.T.
Strovite Plus.
Ultra Freeda.
Ultra Freeda Iron Free.
Vigortol.
Viminate.
Vita-Plus G.
Geriatroplex. (Morton Grove) Cyanocobalamin 30 mcg, liver inj. 0.1 mL, vitamins B_2 1.5 mg, B_{12} activity 2 mcg, ferrous gluconate 50 mg, calcium pantothenate 2.5 mg, niacinamide 100 mg, citric acid 16.4 mg, sodium citrate 23.6 mg/2 mL. Vial 30 mL. *OTC.*
Use: Mineral, vitamin supplement.
Geri-Derm. (Barth's) Vitamins A 400,000 units, D 40,000 units, E 800 units, panthenol 800 mg/4 oz. Jar 4 oz. *OTC.*
Use: Skin supplement.
Geridium Tablets. (Ivax) Phenazopyridine hydrochloride 100 mg, 200 mg. Tab. Bot. 100s, 1000s. *Rx.*
Use: Analgesic; anti-infective, urinary.
Geri-Hydrolac. (Geritrex) Ammonium lactate (equiv. to 12% lactic acid), light mineral oil, petrolatum, propylene glycol, glycerin, cetyl alcohol, parabens. Cream. 140 g. *OTC.*
Use: Emollient.
Gerilets. (Abbott) Vitamins A 5000 units, D 400 units, E 45 units, C 90 mg (from sodium ascorbate), folic acid 0.4 mg, B_1 2.25 mg, B_2 2.6 mg, niacin 30 mg, B_6 3 mg, B_{12} 9 mcg, biotin 0.45 mg, pantothenic acid 15 mg, iron 27 mg (from ferrous sulfate). Tab. Bot. 100s. *OTC.*
Use: Mineral, vitamin supplement.

Gerimal. (Rugby) Ergoloid mesylates. **Sublingual Tab.:** 0.5 mg, 1 mg. Bot. 100s, 500s, 1000s. **Oral Tab.:** 1 mg. Bot. 100s, 500s, 1000s. *Rx.*
Use: Psychotherapeutic agent.
Gerimed. (Fielding) Vitamins A 5000 units, D 400 units, E 30 mg, B_1 3 mg, B_2 3 mg, B_3 25 mg, B_6 2 mg, B_{12} 6 mcg, C 120 mg, calcium 370 mg, zinc 15 mg, Mg, P. Tab. Bot. 60s. *OTC.*
Use: Mineral, vitamin supplement.
Gerineed. (Hanlon) Vitamins A 5000 units, B_1 20 mg, B_2 5 mg, B_6 0.5 mg, B_{12} 5 mcg, niacinamide 20 mg, calcium pantothenate 5 mg, rutin 25 mg, C 50 mg, E 10 units, choline 50 mg, inositol 50 mg, calcium lactate 1.64 mg, iron sulfate 10 mg, Cu 1 mg, iodine 0.5 mg, Mn 1 mg, magnesium sulfate 1 mg, potassium sulfate 5 mg, zinc sulfate 0.5 mg. Cap. Bot. 100s. *OTC.*
Use: Mineral, vitamin supplement.
Geriot. (Ivax) Vitamins A 6000 units, D 400 units, E 30 units, B_1 1.5 mg, B_2 1.7 mg, B_3 20 mg, B_5 10 mg, B_6 2 mg, B_{12} 6 mcg, C 60 mg, folic acid 0.4 mg, iron 50 mg (from ferrous sulfate), biotin 45 mcg, Ca, Cl, Cr, Cu, I, K, Mg, Mn, Mo, Ni, P, Se, Si, Sn, V, Zn, vitamin K. Tab. Bot. 100s. *OTC.*
Use: Mineral, vitamin supplement.
Geri-Plus. (Health for Life Brands) **Cap.:** Vitamins A 12,500 units, D 1200 units, B_1 15 mg, B_2 10 mg, B_6 0.5 mg, B_{12} 15 mcg, C 75 mg, niacinamide 30 mg, calcium pantothenate 2 mg, E 5 units, Brewer's yeast 10 mg, iron 11.58 mg, desiccated liver 15 mg, choline bitartrate 99 mg, inositol 30 mg, Co 50 mg, P 45 mg, Zn 0.68 mg, francium dicalcium phosphate 200 mg, Mn, enzymatic factors, amino acids. Cap. Bot. 50s, 100s, 1000s. **Elix.:** Vitamins B_1 25 mg, B_2 10 mg, B_6 1 mg, B_{12} 20 mcg, niacinamide 100 mg, calcium pantothenate 5 mg, iron ammonium citrate 100 mg, choline 200 mg, inositol 100 mg, magnesium chloride 2 mg, manganese citrate 2 mg, zinc acetate 2 mg, amino acids/fl oz. Bot. Pt. *OTC.*
Use: Mineral, vitamin supplement.
Geri-Soft. (Geritrex) Mineral oil, propylene glycol, cetearyl alcohol, sorbitol, petrolatum, dimethicone, lanolin, castor oil, stearic acid, parabens, stearyl alcohol, EDTA, lemon oil. Lot. 240 g. *OTC.*
Use: Emollient.
Geri SS. (Geritrex) Mineral oil, propylene glycol, cetearyl alcohol, petrolatum, gly-

cerin, dimethicone, colloidal oatmeal, hydrogenated castor oil, parabens, stearyl alcohol, EDTA, lemon oil, tocopheryl acetate. Lot. 240 g. *OTC.*
Use: Emollient.

Geritol Complete. (GlaxoSmithKline) **Complete:** Vitamins A 6000 units, E 30 units, C 60 mg, folic acid 400 mcg, B_1 1.5 mg, B_2 1.7 mg, B_3 20 mg, B_5 10 mg, B_6 2 mg, B_{12} 6 mcg, D 400 units, K, biotin 45 mcg, iron 18 mg, Ca, Cl, Cr, Cu, I, K, Mg, Mn, Mo, Ni, P, Se, Si, Sn, V, Zn, vitamin K. Tab. Bot. 14s, 40s, 100s, 180s. **Extended:** Iron 10 mg, vitamins A 3333 units, D 200 units, E 15 units, B_1 1.2 mg, B_2 1.4 mg, B_3 15 mg, B_6 2 mg, B_{12} 2 mg, C 60 mg, folic acid 0.2 mg, vitamin K, Ca, I, Mg, Se, Zn 15 mg. Capl. Bot. 40s, 100s. **Tonic Liq.:** Iron 18 mg, vitamins B_1 2.5 mg, B_2 2.5 mg, B_3 50 mg, B_5 2 mg, B_6 0.5 mg, methionine 25 mg, choline bitartrate 50 mg/15 mL, alcohol 12%. Bot. 120 mL, 360 mL. *OTC.*
Use: Mineral, vitamin supplement.

Gerivite. (Ivax) Vitamins B_1 0.8 mg, B_2 0.4 mg, B_3 8.3 mg, B_5 1.7 mg, B_6 0.2 mg, B_{12} 0.2 mcg, iron 0.3 mg, Zn 0.3 mg, choline, I Mg, Mn, alcohol 18%, methylparaben, sorbitol. Liq. Bot. 473 mL. *OTC.*
Use: Mineral, vitamin supplement.

Gerix. (Abbott) Vitamins B_1 6 mg, B_2 6 mg, B_6 1.6 mg, niacin 100 mg, iron 15 mg, cyanocobalamin 6 mcg, alcohol 20%/30 mL. Elix. Bot. 480 mL. *OTC.*
Use: Mineral, vitamin supplement.

germanin. (Centers for Disease Control & Prevention) *Rx.*
Use: Anti-infective.
See: Suramin Sodium (Naphuride sodium).

Germicin. (CMC) Benzalkonium chloride 50%. Bot. Pt, gal. *OTC.*
Use: Antiseptic; antimicrobial.

Ger-O-Foam. (Roberts) Methyl salicylate 30%, benzocaine 3%, volatile oils. Aerosol Can 4 oz. *OTC.*
Use: Analgesic; anesthetic.

Geroton Forte. (Kenwood) Vitamin B_1 1.7 mg, B_2 1.9 mg, B_3 2.22 mg, B_5 1.11 mg, B_6 0.22 mg, B_{12} 0.67 mcg, Zn 1.7 mg, Mg, Mn, alcohol 13%. Liq. Bot. 473 mL. *OTC.*
Use: Mineral, vitamin supplement.

Gerterol Depo. (Fellows) Medroxyprogesterone acetate 50 mg, 100 mg/mL. Vial 5 mL. *Rx.*
Use: Hormone, progestin.

Gesic. (Lexalabs) Aspirin 226.8 mg, caffeine 32.4 mg, codeine 32.4 mg. Tab.

Bot. 100s. *c-III.*
Use: Analgesic combination, narcotic.

• **gestaclone.** (JEST-ah-klone) USAN.
Use: Hormone, progestin.

• **gestodene.** (JEST-oh-deen) USAN.
Use: Hormone, progestin.

Gestoneed. (Hanlon) Calcium lactate 1069 mg, vitamins C 100 mg, nicotinic acid 18 mg, B_1 1.8 mg, B_2 2.4 mg, B_6 9 mg, D 500 units, A 6000 units. Cap. Bot. 100s. *OTC.*
Use: Mineral, vitamin supplement.

• **gestonorone caproate.** (jess-TOE-noreohn CAP-row-ate) USAN.
Use: Hormone, progestin.

• **gestrinone.** (JESS-trih-nohn) USAN.
Use: Hormone, progestin.

Get Better Bear Sore Throat Pops. (Whitehall-Robins) Pectin 19 mg, corn syrup, sucrose, parabens. Loz. on a stick. Pkg. 10s. *OTC.*
Use: Mouth and throat product.

Gets-It. (Oakhurst) Salicylic acid, zinc chloride, collodion in ether ≈ 35%, alcohol ≈ 28%. Liq. Bot. 12 mL. *OTC.*
Use: Keratolytic.

• **gevotroline hydrochloride.** (jeh-VOE-troe-LEEN) USAN.
Use: Antipsychotic.

Gevrabon. (Wyeth) Vitamins B_1 0.83 mg, B_2 0.42 mg, B_3 8.3 mg, B_5 1.67 mg, B_6 0.17 mg, B_{12} 0.17 mcg, Fe 2.5 mg, choline, I, Mg, Mn, Zn 0.3 mg, alcohol 18%. Liq. Bot. 480 mL. *OTC.*
Use: Mineral, vitamin supplement.

Gevral. (Wyeth) Vitamins A 5000 units, B_1 1.5 mg, B_2 1.7 mg, B_3 20 mg, B_6 2 mg, B_{12} 6 mcg, folic acid 0.4 mg, C 60 mg, E 30 mg, Ca, P, iron 18 mg, Mg, I, lactose, parabens, sucrose. Tab. Bot. 100s. *OTC.*
Use: Mineral, vitamin supplement.

Gevral Protein. (Wyeth) Calcium caseinate, sucrose, protein 15.6 g, carbohydrate 7.05 g, fat 0.52 g, Na 50 mg, K 13 mg, calories 95.3/26 g. Pow. Can 8 oz, 5 lb. *OTC.*
Use: Nutritional supplement.

GFN 550/PSE 60/DM 30. (Cypress) Pseudoephedrine hydrochloride 60 mg, dextromethorphan HBr 30 mg, guaifenesin 550 mg. Dye-free. ER Tab. 100s. *Rx.*
Use: Antitussive, expectorant, decongestant.

GFN 1000/DM 50. (Cypress) Dextromethorphan HBr 50 mg, guaifenesin 1000 mg. ER Tab. 100s. *Rx.*
Use: Antitussive, expectorant.

GFN 1000/DM 60. (Cypress) Dextromethorphan HBr 60 mg, guaifenesin 1000 mg. SR Tab. Bot. 100s. *Rx.*
Use: Upper respiratory combination, antitussive, expectorant.

GFN/PSE. (Cypress) Pseudoephedrine hydrochloride 120 mg, guaifenesin 1200 mg. SR Tab. Bot. 100s. *Rx.*
Use: Upper respiratory combination, decongestant, expectorant.

GFN 600/Phenylephrine 20. (Cypress) Phenylephrine hydrochloride 20 mg, guaifenesin 600 mg, dye free, Tab. Bot. 100s. *Rx.*
Use: Upper respiratory combination, decongestant, expectorant.

GFN 600/PSE 60/DM 30. (Cypress) Dextromethorphan HBr 30 mg, guaifenesin 600 mg, pseudoephedrine hydrochloride 60 mg, dye free. SR Tab. 100s. *Rx.*
Use: Upper respiratory combination, decongestant, expectorant.

GFN 1200/DM 60. (Cypress) Dextromethorphan HBr 60 mg, guaifenesin 1200 mg. SR Tab. Bot. 100s. *Rx.*
Use: Upper respiratory combination, antitussive, expectorant.

GFN 1200/DM 60/PSE 120. (Cypress) Dextromethorphan HBr 60 mg, guaifenesin 1200 mg, pseudoephedrine hydrochloride 120 mg, dye free. SR. Tab. Bot. 100s. *Rx.*
Use: Upper respiratory combination, antitussive, expectorant, decongestant.

G-4.
See: Dichlorophene.

GI contrast agents (iodinated).
Use: Radiopaque agent.
See: Diatrizoate meglumine and diatrizoate sodium.
Diatrizoate sodium.
Gastrografin.
Hypaque Sodium.
MD-Gastroview.

GI contrast agents (miscellaneous).
Use: Radiopaque agent.
See: Anatrast.
Baricon.
Barium sulfate.
Barobag.
Baro-cat.
Baros.
Barosperse.
Bear•E•Yum CT.
Bear•E•Yum GI.
Cheetah.
Enecat CT.
Enhancer.
Entrobar.
Entroease.
Entroease Dry.

Epi-C.
Flo-coat.
HD 85.
HD 200 Plus.
Imager ac.
Intropaste.
Liqui-Coat HD.
Liquid Barosperse.
Medebar Plus.
Medescan.
Pediatric Bear•E•Bag.
Prepcat.
Radiopaque polyvinyl chloride.
Sitzmarks.
Sodium bicarbonate and tartaric acid.
Tomocat.
Tonopaque.

• **ginger.** *NF 23.*
Use: Dietary supplement.

• **ginseng, american.** *NF 23.*
Use: Dietary supplement.

• **ginseng, asian.** *NF 23.*
Use: Dietary supplement.

• **ginseng extract.** *NF 23.*
Use: Dietary supplement.

GI stimulants.
See: Maxolon.
Metoclopramide.
Metoclopramide hydrochloride.
Octamide.
Reclomide.
Reglan.

Gladase. (Smith & Nephew) Papain 8.3 × 10⁵ units, urea 100 mg per g. Glycerin, parabens. Oint. 30 g. *Rx.*
Use: Enzyme preparation.

Gladase-C. (Smith & Nephew) Papain ≥ 521,700 units, urea 10%, chlorophyllin copper complex sodium 0.5%/g. Boric acid, glycerin, gyceryl stearate, parabens, stearyl alcohol. Oint. 6 g, 30 g. *Rx.*
Use: Enzyme preparation.

glandubolin.
See: Estrone.

• **glatiramer acetate.** (glah-TEER-ah-mer ASS-eh-tate) USAN.
Use: Multiple sclerosis; immunosuppressant.
See: Copaxone.

glauber's salt.
See: Sodium Sulfate.

glaucoma, agents for.
See: Brinzolamide.
Carbonic Anhydrase Inhibitors.
Dorzolamide Hydrochloride.
Echothiophate Iodide.
Latanoprost.
Miotics, Cholinesterase Inhibitors.
Prostaglandin Agonist.

•**glaze, pharmaceutical.** *NF 23.*
Use: Pharmaceutic aid (tablet coating agent).
Gleevec. (Novartis) Imatinib (as mesylate) 100 mg, 400 mg. Film-coated. Tab. Bot. 30s (400 mg), 1000s (100 mg). *Rx.*
Use: Protein-tyrosine kinase inhibitor.
•**glemanserin.** (gleh-MAN-ser-in) USAN.
Use: Anxiolytic.
Gliadel. (Guilford Pharm) Carmustine (BCNU) 7.7 mg, preservative free. Wafer. Single-dose treatment box with 8 individually pouched wafers. *Rx.*
Use: Alkylating agent.
•**gliamilide.** (glie-AM-ih-lide) USAN.
Use: Antidiabetic.
glibenclamide.
See: Glyburide.
•**glibornuride.** (glie-BORN-you-ride) USAN.
Use: Oral hypoglycemic agent; antidiabetic.
•**glicetanile sodium.** (glie-SET-AH-nile) USAN. *Formerly Glydanile Sodium.*
Use: Antidiabetic.
•**gliflumide.** (GLIH-flew-mide) USAN.
Use: Antidiabetic.
glim.
See: Gardinol Type Detergents.
•**glimepiride.** (GLIE-meh-pie-ride) USAN.
Use: Hypoglycemic.
See: Amaryl.
•**glipizide.** (GLIP-ih-zide) *USP 28.*
Tall Man: GlipiZIDE
Use: Antidiabetic.
See: Glucotrol.
  Glucotrol XL.
glipizide. (Various Mfr.) Glipizide 5 mg, 10 mg. Tab. 100s, 500s, 1000s, UD 100s. *Rx.*
Use: Antidiabetic.
glipizide and metformin hydrochloride.
Use: Antidiabetic.
See: Metaglip.
glipizide ER. (Watson) Glipizide 5 mg, 10 mg. Film-coated. ER Tab. 100s. *Rx.*
Use: Antidiabetic.
glipizide extended-release. (Andrx) Glipizide 2.5 mg, 5 mg, 10 mg. ER Tab. 30s (2.5 mg only); 100s, 500s (except 2.5 mg). *Rx.*
Use: Antidiabetic.
globulin, cytomegalovirus immune.
See: CytoGam.
globulin, gamma.
See: Immune Globulin Intramuscular.
  Immune Globulin Intravenous.

globulin, hepatitis b immune.
See: BayHep B.
  H-BIG.
•**globulin, immune.** (GLAH-byoo-lin) *USP 28. Formerly Globulin, Immune Human Serum.*
Use: IM, measles prophylactic and polio; immunization.
globulin, immune, intravenous.
Use: Immunodeficiency; immune thrombocytopenia purpura; Kawasaki syndrome.
See: Gamimune N.
  Gammagard S/D.
  Gammar-P IV.
  Iveegam.
  Polygam S/D.
  Sandoglobulin.
  Venoglobulin-I.
  Venoglobulin-S.
globulin, rabies immune.
Use: Immunization.
See: Bayrab.
  Imogam Rabies.
globulin, Rh$_o$(D) immune.
Use: Prevention of Rh isoimmunization; immune thrombocytopenic purpura.
See: BayRho D.
  Gamulin Rh.
  MICRhoGAM.
  Mini-Gamulin Rh.
  RhoGAM.
  WinRho SD.
•**globulin serum, anti-human.** *USP 28.*
Use: Immunization.
globulin, tetanus immune.
Use: Immunization.
See: Baytet.
globulin, vaccinia immune.
Use: Immunization.
globulin, varicella-zoster immune.
Use: Immunization.
See: Varicella-zoster Immune Globulin (VZIG).
•**gloximonam.** (GLOX-ih-MOE-nam) USAN.
Use: Anti-infective.
GL-7 Skin Adherent. (Gordon Laboratories) Plastic material which may be used full strength or diluted with 3 to 10 parts 99% isopropyl alcohol, acetone or naphtha. Pkg. Pt, qt, gal. *OTC.*
GL-2 Skin Adherent. (Gordon Laboratories) Ready-to-use. Bot. Pt, qt, gal. *OTC.*
GlucaGen. (Bedford Laboratories) Glucagon 1 mg (1 unit), lactose 107 mg. Pow. for Inj. Vials with 1 mL diluent. *Rx.*
Use: Glucose-elevating agent, diagnostic aid, emergency kit.

- **glucagon.** (GLUE-kuh-gahn) *USP 28.*
  Use: Emergency treatment of hypo-
  glycemia; antidiabetic.
  See: GlucaGen.
    Glucagon Diagnostic Kit.
    Glucagon Emergency Kit.
- **glucagon.** (Eli Lilly) 1 unit/mL w/diluent.
  10 units w/10 mL diluent. Glucagon hydrochloride 1 mg, 10 mg w/diluent;
  soln. contains lactose, glycerin 1.6%
  w/phenol 0.2% as a preservative. Vial.
  Use: Hypoglycemic shock; antidiabetic.
- **Glucagon Diagnostic Kit.** (Eli Lilly) Glucagon 1 mg (1 unit), lactose 49 mg, glycerin 12 mg/mL. Pow. for Inj. Vial
  w/1 mL syringe diluent. *Rx.*
  Use: Glucose-elevating agent.
- **Glucagon Emergency Kit.** (Eli Lilly) Glucagon 1 mg (1 unit), lactose 49 mg, glycerin 12 mg/mL. Pow. for Inj. Vial
  w/1 mL syr. diluent. 1 mL, 10 mL. *Rx.*
  Use: Glucose-elevating agent.
- **Glucamide.** (Teva) Chlorpropamide
  100 mg, 250 mg. Tab. Bot. 100s, 250s,
  500s, 1000s, UD 100s. *Rx.*
  Use: Antidiabetic.
- **gluceptate sodium.** (GLUE-sep-tate)
  USAN.
  Use: Pharmaceutic aid.
- **Glucerna.** (Ross) Protein 41 g (amino acids), carbohydrate 93 g (hydrolyzed
  cornstarch, fructose, soy fiber), fat 55 g
  (high oleic safflower oil, soy oil, soy
  lecithin), sodium 917 mg (40 mEq), potassium 1542 mg (40 mEq), vitamins
  A, B_1, B_2, B_3, B_5, B_6, B_{12}, C, D, E, K, folic acid, Cl, Ca, P, Mg, I, Mn, Cu, Zn,
  Fe, Se, Cr, Mo, biotin, choline. Liq. Can
  240 mL, Cont. 1 L. Ready-to-use. *OTC.*
  Use: Nutritional supplement.
- **Glucerna Select.** (Abbott) Protein (sodium and calcium caseinates, soy protein isolate) 50 g, carbohydrates (fructose, fructooligosaccharides, maltodextrin, soy fiber, sugar alcohols) 95.7 g,
  fat (canola oil, high oleic safflower oil,
  soy lecithin) 54.4 g, Na 940 mg,
  1810 mg K/L. H_2O 470 mOsm/kg,
  1 cal/mL. Vitamin A, B_1, B_2, B_3, B_5, B_6,
  B_7, B_9, B_{12}, C, D, E, K, choline, Ca,
  Cl, Cu, Cr, Fe, I, Mg, Mn, Mo, P, Se, Zn.
  Gluten-free. Vanilla flavor. Liq. 240 mL,
  1000 mL, 1500 mL. *OTC.*
  Use: Enteral nutrition therapy.
- **Glucerna Weight Loss Shake.** (Abbott)
  Protein (sodium and calcium caseinates, soy protein isolate) 54.6 g, carbohydrates (fructose, fructooligosaccharides, maltodextrin, soy fiber, sugar alcohols) 163.8 g, fat (canola oil, high
  oleic safflower oil, soy lecithin) 46.2 g,

Na 1176 mg, K 2100 mg. 0.89 cal/mL.
Vitamin A, B_1, B_2, B_3, B_5, B_6, B_{12}, FA,
C, D, E, K, biotin, choline, Ca, Cl, Cu,
Cr, Fe, I, Mg, Mn, Mo, P, Se, Zn. Glu-
ten-free. Vanilla, chocolate, banana,
peach, dulce de leche flavors. Liq.
325 mL. *OTC.*
Use: Enteral nutrition therapy.
glucocerebrosidase-beta-glucosidase.
  Use: Treatment of Gaucher disease.
  See: Ceredase.
glucocerebrosidase (PEG).
  See: PEG-glucocerebrosidase.
**glucocerebrosidase, recombinant ret-
roviral vector.** (Genetic Therapy)
  Use: Treatment for Gaucher disease.
  [Orphan Drug]
glucocorticoids.
  See: Betamethasone.
    Betamethasone Sodium Phosphate.
    Betamethasone Sodium Phosphate
      and Betamethasone Acetate.
    Budesonide.
    Cortical Hormone Products.
    Cortisone.
    Dexamethasone.
    Dexamethasone Acetate.
    Dexamethasone Sodium Phosphate.
    Dexamethasone Sodium Phosphate
      with Lidocaine Hydrochloride.
    Hydrocortisone.
    Hydrocortisone Acetate.
    Hydrocortisone Cypionate.
    Hydrocortisone Sodium Phosphate.
    Hydrocortisone Sodium Succinate.
    Methylprednisolone.
    Methylprednisolone Acetate.
    Methylprednisolone Sodium Succi-
      nate.
    Prednisolone.
    Prednisolone Acetate.
    Prednisolone Sodium Phosphate.
    Prednisolone Tebutate.
    Prednisone.
    Triamcinolone.
    Triamcinolone Acetonide.
    Triamcinolone Diacetate.
    Triamcinolone Hexacetonide.
Glucolet Automatic Lancing Device.
  (Bayer Corp. (Consumer Div.)) To ob-
  tain sample for blood glucose testing.
  Automatic spring-loaded lancing de-
  vice.
  Use: Diagnostic aid.
Glucolet Endcaps. (Bayer Corp. (Con-
  sumer Div.)) To obtain sample for
  blood glucose testing. Controls depth
  of lancet penetration. Regular or super
  puncture.
  Use: Diagnostic aid.
Glucometer II Blood Glucose Meter.
  (Bayer Corp. (Consumer Div.)) Elec-

tronic meter for blood glucose testing. *OTC.*
Use: Diagnostic aid.

d-gluconic acid, calcium salt. Calcium gluconate.

gluconic acid salts.
See: Calcium gluconate.
Ferrous gluconate.
Magnesium gluconate.
Potassium gluconate.

•**gluconolactone.** (glue-koe-no-LACK-tone) *USP 28.*
Use: Chelating agent.

Glucophage. (Bristol-Myers Squibb) Metformin hydrochloride 500 mg, 850 mg, 1000 mg. Film coated. Tab. Bot. 100s, 500s (500 mg only). *Rx.*
Use: Antidiabetic, biguanide.

Glucophage XR. (Bristol-Myers Squibb) Metformin hydrochloride 500 mg, 750 mg. ER Tab. Bot. 100s. *Rx.*
Use: Antidiabetic, biguanide.

•**glucosamine.** (glue-KOSE-ah-meen) USAN.
Use: Pharmaceutic aid.
W/Oxytetracycline.
See: Terramycin.
W/Tetracycline.
See: Tetracyn.

glucose.
See: Glutose.
Insta-Glucose.

glucose-elevating agents.
See: B-D Glucose.
Glucagon.
Glutose.
Insta-Glucose.
Insulin Reaction.
Proglycem.

glucose enzymatic test strip.
Use: Diagnostic aid (in vitro, reducing sugars in urine).

glucose (hk) reagent strips. Reagent strip test for detection of glucose in serum or plasma. Bot. 50s.
Use: Diagnostic aid.

Glucose & Ketone Urine Test. (Major) Reagent test for glucose and ketones in urine. Bot. 100s.
Use: Diagnostic aid.

•**glucose, liquid.** (GLUE-kose) *NF 23.*
Use: As a 5% to 50% solution as nutrient; for acute hepatitis and dehydration; to increase blood volume; pharmaceutic aid (tablet binder, tablet-coating agent).

d-glucose, monohydrate. Dextrose.

glucose oxidase.
W/Peroxidase, potassium iodide.
See: Diastix.

glucose polymers.
See: Polycose.

Glucose Reagent Strips. (Bayer Corp. (Consumer Div.)) A quantitative strip test for glucose in serum or plasma. Seralyzer reagent strips. Bot. 50s.
Use: Diagnostic aid.

glucose test.
See: Combistix.
First Choice.
Glucose Reagent.

Glucostix Reagent Strips. (Bayer Corp. (Consumer Div.)) Cellulose strip containing glucose oxidase and indicator system. Bot. 50s, 100s, UD 25s. *OTC.*
Use: Diagnostic aid.

glucosulfone sodium, injection.
See: Sodium Glucosulfone.

Gluco System Lancets. (Bayer Corp. (Consumer Div.)) Disposable lancets for use in Miles diagnostic autolet or glucolet.
Use: Diagnostic aid.

Glucotrol. (Pfizer) Glipizide 5 mg, 10 mg, lactose. Tab. Bot. 100s, 500s, UD 100s. *Rx.*
Use: Antidiabetic.

Glucotrol XL. (Pfizer) Glipizide 2.5 mg, 5 mg, 10 mg. ER Tab. Bot. 30s, 100s, 500s. *Rx.*
Use: Antidiabetic.

Glucovance. (Bristol-Myers Squibb) Glyburide 1.25 mg, 2.5 mg, 5 mg. Metformin hydrochloride 250 mg, 500 mg. Tab. Bot. 100s, 500s (except 5 mg/ 500 mg). *Rx.*
Use: Antidiabetic combination.

Glucovite. (Pal-Pak, Inc.) Ferrous gluconate 260 mg, vitamins B_1 1 mg, B_2 0.5 mg, C 10 mg. Tab. Bot. 1000s, 5000s. *OTC.*
Use: Mineral, vitamin supplement.

glucurolactone. Gamma lactone of glucofuranuronic acid.

glufanide disodium. (GLOO-fa-nide)
See Oglufanide disodium.

Glu-K. (Western Research) Potassium gluconate 486 mg. Tab. Bot. 1000s. *OTC.*
Use: Electrolyte supplement.

gluside.
See: Saccharin.

•**glutamic acid.** *USP 28.*
Use: Nutritional supplement.
See: Glutamic acid.

glutamic acid. (Various Mfr.) Glutamic acid 500 mg. Tab. Bot. 100s, 500s. *OTC.*
Use: Nutritional supplement.

glutamic acid. (J. R. Carlson Laboratories) Glutamic acid. Pow. Bot. 100 g.

OTC.
Use: Nutritional supplement.
glutamic acid hydrochloride. Acidogen, aciglumin, glutasin. *OTC.*
Use: Gastric acidifier.
glutamic acid salts.
See: Calcium Glutamate.
•**glutamine.** (GLOO-ta-meen) *USP 28.*
Use: Dietary supplement; treatment of short bowel syndrome. [Orphan Drug]
•**glutaral concentrate.** (GLUE-tah-ral) *USP 28.*
Use: Disinfectant.
See: Cidex.
glutaraldehyde.
Use: Sterilizing, disinfecting agent.
See: Cidex.
Cidex Plus.
Cidex-7
Glutarex-1. (Ross) Protein 15 g, fat 23.9 g, carbohydrates 46.3 g, linoleic acid 1800 mg, Fe 9 mg, Na 190 mg, K 675 mg, Ca, vitamins A, B_1, B_2, B_3, B_5, B_6, B_{12}, C, D, E, K, biotin, choline, folic acid, inositol, Cl, Cu, I, Mg, Mn, P, Se, Zn, and 480 Cal per 100 g, lysine and tryptophan free. Pow. Can 350 g. *OTC.*
Use: Nutritional supplement.
Glutarex-2. (Ross) Protein 30 g, fat 15.5 g, carbohydrates 30 g, Fe 13 mg, Na 880 mg, K 1370 mg, Ca, vitamins A, B_1, B_2, B_3, B_5, B_6, B_{12}, C, D, E, K, biotin, choline, folic acid, inositol, Cl, Cu, I, Mg, Mn, P, Se, Zn, and 410 Cal per 100 g, lysine and tryptophan free. Pow. Can 325 g. *OTC.*
Use: Nutritional supplement.
l-glutathione.
Use: Treatment of AIDS-associated cachexia. [Orphan Drug]
See: Cachexon.
Glutofac. (Kenwood) Vitamins A 500 units, E 30 units, B_1 15 mg, B_2 10 mg, B_3 50 mg, B_5 20 mg, B_6 50 mg, C 300 mg, Zn 5 mg, Ca, Cr, Cu, Fe, K, Mg, Mn, P, Se. Capl. Bot. 90s. *OTC.*
Use: Mineral, vitamin supplement.
Glutofac-ZX. (Kenwood) Vitamin A 5000 units, D 400 units, E (succinate) 50 units, B 20 mg, B_2 20 mg, B_3 100 mg, B_5 25 mg, B_6 25 mg, B_{12} 50 mcg, C 500 mg, folic acid 1 mg, Zn, Ca, Cr, Cu, Mg, Mn, Se 20 mg, biotin 200 mg. Parabens, sorbitol. Capl. 60s. *Rx.*
Use: Mineral, vitamin supplement.
Glutol. (Paddock) Dextrose 100 g/180 mL. Bot. 180 mL.
Use: Diagnostic aid.

Glutose. (Paddock) Liquid glucose (40% dextrose). Concentrated glucose for insulin reactions. Gel. Bot. 60 g. *OTC.*
Use: Hyperglycemic.
•**glyburide.** (glie-BYOO-ride) *USP 28.*
Tall Man: GlyBURIDE
Use: Antidiabetic.
See: DiaBeta.
Glynase.
Micronase.
glyburide. (Various Mfr.) Glyburide. Tab., micronized. **1.25 mg:** Bot. 50s, 100s, 500s. **1.5 mg:** Bot. 100s, UD 100s. **2.5 mg & 5 mg:** Bot. 90s, 100s, 500s, 1000s, UD 100s; Blister pack 25s, 100s, 600s. **3 mg:** Bot. 100s, 500s, 1000s, UD 100s. **4.5 mg:** Bot. 100s, 500s, UD 100s. **6 mg:** 100s. *Rx.*
Use: Antidiabetic.
glyburide and metformin hydrochloride.
Use: Antidiabetic combination.
See: Glucovance.
glyburide/metformin hydrochloride. (PAR) Glyburide/metformin hydrochloride 1.25 mg/250 mg, 2.5 mg/500 mg, 5 mg/500 mg. Film-coated. Tab. 100s. *Rx.*
Use: Antidiabetic combination.
glyburide, micronized. (Various Mfr.) Micronized glyburide 1.5 mg, 3 mg, 4.5 mg, 6 mg. Tab. Bot. 100s, 500s (except 4.5 mg), 1000s, UD 100s (1.5 mg and 3 mg only). *Rx.*
Use: Antidiabetic.
Glycate Chewables. (Forest) Glycine 150 mg, calcium carbonate 300 mg. Chew. Tab. Bot. 1000s. *OTC.*
Use: Antacid.
•**glycerin.** (GLIH-suh-rin) *USP 28.*
Use: Pharmaceutic aid (humectant, solvent).
See: Colace.
Corn Huskers.
Fleet Babylax.
Ophthalgan Ophthalmic.
Osmoglyn.
Sani-Supp.
W/Dimethicone.
See: Dermasil.
glycerin. (Various Mfr.) Various concentrations of glycerin from 10% to > 95% for use as sterile allergen-extract diluents.
glycerin suppositories. (Various Mfr.) Glycerin. **Aduts:** Box 10s, 12s, 25s, 50s, 100s. **Pediatric:** 10s, 12s, 25s. *OTC.*
Use: Rectal evacuant, cathartic.
glycerol.
See: Glycerin.

•**glycerol, iodinated.** (GLIH-ser-ole EYE-oh-dih-nay-tehd) USAN.
Use: Expectorant.

•**glyceryl behenate.** *NF 23.*
Use: Pharmaceutic aid (tablet/capsule lubricant).

glyceryl guaiacolate.
Use: Expectorant.
See: Guaifenesin.

glyceryl guaiacolate carbamate. Methocarbamol.
See: Robaxin.
Robaxin 750.

glyceryl guaiacolether.
See: Guaifenesin.

•**glyceryl monostearate.** *NF 23.*
Use: Pharmaceutic aid (emulsifying agent).

Glyceryl-T. (Rugby) **Cap.:** Theophylline 150 mg, guaifenesin 90 mg. Bot. 100s.
Liq.: Theophylline 150 mg, guaifenesin 90 mg/15 mL. Bot. 480 mL. *Rx.*
Use: Bronchodilator; expectorant.

glyceryl triacetate.
See: Triacetin.

glyceryl triacetin. (Various Mfr.) Triacetin.
See: Fungacetin.

glyceryl trierucate.
Use: Adrenoleukodystrophy. [Orphan Drug]

glyceryl trinitrate ointment.
See: Nitrol.

glyceryl trinitrate tablets.
See: Nitroglycerin.
Nitroglyn.

glyceryl trioleate.
Use: Adrenoleukodystrophy. [Orphan Drug]

Glycets-Antacid Tablets. (Weeks & Leo) Calcium carbonate 350 mg, simethicone 25 mg. Chew. Tab. Bot. 100s. *OTC.*
Use: Antacid; antiflatulent.

glycinato dihydroxyaluminum hydrate.
See: Dihydroxyaluminum aminoacetate.

•**glycine.** (GLIE-seen) *USP 28.* Formerly *Aminoacetic Acid.*
Use: Myasthenia gravis treatment, irrigating solution.
W/Aluminum hydroxide-magnesium carbonate coprecipitated gel.
See: Glycogel.
W/Calcium carbonate.
See: Antacid No. 6.
Glycate Chewables.
Titralac.
W/Calcium carbonate, amylolytic, proteolytic cellulolytic enzymes.

See: Co-gel.
W/Chlor-Trimeton, sodium salicylate.
See: Corilin.
W/Glutamic acid, alanine.
See: Prostall.

glycine, aluminum salt.
See: Dihydroxyaluminum Aminoacetate.

glycine hydrochloride. (Various Mfr.)
Use: Gastric acidifier.

glycobiarsol.
Use: Amebiasis, *Trichomonas vaginalis, Monilia albicans.*

glycocoll. Glycine.
See: Aminoacetic Acid.

glycocyamine. Guanidoacetic acid.

Glycofed. (Pal-Pak, Inc.) Pseudoephedrine 30 mg, guaifenesin 100 mg. Tab. Bot. 1000s. *OTC.*
Use: Decongestant, expectorant.

GlycoLax. (Kremers Urban) PEG 3350 17 g in 14 single-dose packets, 255 g in 16 oz with dosing cup, 527 g in 24 oz with dosing cup. Pow. for Oral Soln. *Rx.*
Use: Laxative.

•**glycol distearate.** (GLIE-kole dih-STEE-ah-rate) USAN.
Use: Pharmaceutic aid (thickening agent).

glycol monosalicylate.
W/Oil of mustard, camphor, menthol, methyl salicylate.
See: Musterole.

glycophenylate bromide.
See: Mepenzolate methylbromide.

glycoprotein.
Use: Antiplatelet agent.
See: Kogenate FS.

•**glycoprotein IIb/IIIa inhibitors.**
Use: Antiplatelet agent.
See: Abciximab.
Eptifibatide.
Tirofiban.

•**glycopyrrolate.** (glie-koe-PIE-row-late) *USP 28.*
Use: Anticholinergic.
See: Robinul.
Robinul Forte.

glycopyrrolate. (Rising) Glycopyrrolate 1 mg, 2 mg. Lactose. Tab. 100s, 1,000s. *Rx.*
Use: Gastrointestinal anticholinergic/ antispasmodic.

glycopyrrolate. (Various Mfr.) Glycopyrrolate 0.2 mg/mL. Inj. Vials. 1 mL, 2 mL, 5 mL, 20 mL. *Rx.*
Use: Anticholinergic.

Glycotuss. (Pal-Pak, Inc.) Guaifenesin 100 mg. Tab. Bot. 100s, 1000s. *OTC.*

Use: Expectorant.
Glycotuss-dM. (Pal-Pak, Inc.) Guaifenesin 100 mg, dextromethorphan HBr 10 mg. Tab. Bot. 100s, 1000s. *OTC.*
Use: Antitussive, expectorant.
glycyrrhiza. Pure extract, fluid extract. Licorice root.
Use: Flavoring agent.
glycyrrhiza extract, pure.
Use: Flavoring agent.
glycyrrhiza fluid extract.
Use: Flavoring agent.
glydanile sodium. (GLIE-dah-neel SO-dee-uhm) See Glicetanile Sodium.
•**glyhexamide.** (glie-HEX-ah-mid) USAN.
Use: Antidiabetic.
Glylorin. (Cellegy) Monolaurin.
Use: Congenital primary ichthyosis.
[Orphan Drug]
•**glymidine sodium.** (GLIE-mih-deen) USAN.
Use: Oral hypoglycemic agent; antidiabetic.
glymol.
See: Petrolatum Liquid.
Glynase PresTab. (Pharmacia) Glyburide (micronized) **1.5 mg:** Tab. Bot. 100s, UD 100s. **3 mg:** Tab. Bot. 100s, 500s, 1000s, UD 100s. **6 mg:** Tab. Bot. 100s, 500s. *Rx.*
Use: Antidiabetic.
•**glyoctamide.** (glie-OCKT-am-id) USAN.
Use: Hypoglycemic agent; antidiabetic.
Gly-Oxide Liquid. (GlaxoSmithKline) Carbamide peroxide 10%. Soln. Bot. 15 mL, 60 mL. *OTC.*
Use: Mouth and throat product.
glyoxyldiureide.
See: Allantoin.
•**glyparamide.** (glie-PAR-am-ide) USAN.
Use: Oral hypoglycemic agent; antidiabetic.
Glypressin. (Ferring) Terlipressin.
Use: Bleeding esophageal varicies.
[Orphan Drug]
Glyquin. (ICN) Hydroquinone 4%, padimate O, oxybenzone, octyl methoxycinnamate, methylparaben. SPF 15. In a vanishing base. Cream. Tube. 28 g. *Rx.*
Use: Pigment agent.
Glyquin-XM. (ICN) Hydroquinone 4%. Octocrylene, oxybenzone, avobenzone, vitamin E, methylparaben, EDTA, SPF 15. In a vanishing base. Cream. 28 g. *Rx.*
Use: Pigment agent.
Glyset. (Bayer Corp. (Consumer Div.)) Miglitol 25 mg, 50 mg, 100 mg. Tab. Bot. 100s, 1000s (except 25 mg), UD

100. *Rx.*
Use: Antidiabetic.
GM-CSF. Granulocyte macrophage colony-stimulating factor.
See: Leukine.
gododiamide.
Use: Diagnostic aid.
Golacol. (Arcum) Codeine sulfate 30 mg, papaverine hydrochloride 30 mg, emetine hydrochloride 2 mg, ephedrine hydrochloride 15 mg, q.s./30 mL, alcohol 6.25%. Syr. Bot. 4 oz, 16 oz, gal. Orange flavor. *c-iii.*
Use: Antitussive; bronchodilator.
Gold Alka-Seltzer Effervescent. (Bayer Corp. (Consumer Div.)) Sodium bicarbonate (heat treated) 958 mg, citric acid 832 mg, potassium bicarbonate 312 mg. Tab. Bot. 20s, 36s. *OTC.*
Use: Antacid.
gold compounds.
See: Gold Sodium Thiosulfate.
Ridaura.
Solganal.
•**goldenseal.** (GOLD-n-seal) *NF 23.*
Use: Dietary supplement.
Golden-West Compound. (Golden-West) Gentian root, licorice root, cascara sagrada, damiana leaves, senna leaves, psyllium seed, buchu leaves, crude pepsin. Box 1.5 oz. *OTC.*
Use: Laxative.
Goldicide Concentrate. (Pedinol Pharmacal) Bot. oz. Ctn. 10s.
Use: Disinfectant.
Gold Seal Calcium 600. (Walgreen) Calcium 1200 mg. Tab. Bot. 60s. *OTC.*
Use: Mineral supplement.
Gold Seal Calcium 600 with Vitamin D. (Walgreen) Calcium 1200 mg, vitamin D. Tab. Bot. 60s. *OTC.*
Use: Mineral supplement.
Gold Seal Chewable Vitamin C. (Walgreen) Ascorbic acid 250 mg, 500 mg. Tab. Bot. 100s. *OTC.*
Use: Vitamin supplement.
Gold Seal Ferrous Gluconate. (Walgreen) Iron 37 mg. Tab. Bot. 100s. *OTC.*
Use: Mineral supplement.
Gold Seal Ferrous Sulfate. (Walgreen) Ferrous sulfate 325 mg. Tab. Bot. 100s, 1000s. *OTC.*
Use: Mineral supplement.
Gold Seal Time Release Ferrous Sulfate. (Walgreen) Iron 50 mg. Tab. Bot. 100s. *OTC.*
Use: Mineral supplement.
•**gold sodium thiomalate.** (gold SO-dee-uhm thigh-oh-MAL-ate) *USP 28.*
Use: Antirheumatic.
See: Aurolate.

Myochrisine.

gold sodium thiomalate. (Parenta) Gold sodium thiomalate 50 mg/mL. Benzyl alcohol 0.5%. Inj. 1 mL single-dose and 10 mL multidose vials. *Rx.*
Use: Antirheumatic agent.

gold sodium thiosulfate. Sterile, auricidine, aurocidin, aurolin, auropin, aurosan, novacrysin, solfocrisol, thiochrysine.
Use: Antirheumatic.

gold thioglucose.
See: Aurothioglucose.

•**golimumab.** (goe-li-MUE-mab) USAN.
Use: Monoclonal antibody.

GoLYTELY. (Braintree) **Disp. Jug:** PEG 3350 236 g, sodium sulfate 22.74 g, sodium bicarbonate 6.74 g, sodium chloride 5.86 g, potassium chloride 2.97 g. Pow. for Oral Soln. **Packet:** PEG 3350 227.1 g, sodium sulfate 21.5 g, sodium bicarbonate 6.36 g, sodium chloride 5.53 g, potassium chloride 2.82 g. *Rx.*
Use: Bowel evacuant.

•**gomiliximab.** (goe-mi-LIX-i-mab) USAN.
Use: Allergic asthma.

gonacrine.
See: Acriflavine.

•**gonadorelin hydrochloride.** (go-NAD-oh-RELL-in) USAN. *Formerly Luteinizing Hormone-releasing Factor Dihydrochloride.*
Use: Gonad-stimulating principle; in vivo diagnostic aid.
See: Factrel.

gonadotropic substance.
See: Gonadotropin chorionic.

•**gonadotropin, chorionic.** (go-NAD-oh-TROE-pin, core-ee-AHN-ik) *USP 28.*
Use: Gonad-stimulating principle. In women: Chronic cystic mastitis, functional sterility, dysmenorrhea, premenstrual tension, threatened abortion. In men: Cryptorchidism, hypogenitalism, dwarfism, impotency, enuresis.
See: A.P.L.
Chorex-5.
Chorex-10.
Choron 10.
Gonic.
Pregnyl.
Profasi.

gonadotropin, pituitary anterior lobe.
Extracted from anterior lobe of equine pituitaries (not pregnant mare urine) (rat unit = 1 Fevold-Hisaw unit).

gonadotropin-releasing hormone analog.
See: Goserelin Acetate.
Histrelin Acetate.
Leuprolide Acetate.
Triptorelin Pamoate.

gonadotropin-releasing hormone antagonists.
Use: Sex hormone.
See: Abarelix.
Cetrorelix Acetate.
Ganirelix Acetate.

gonadotropin-releasing hormones.
Use: Sex hormone.
See: Gonadorelin Acetate.
Histrelin Acetate.
Nafarelin Acetate.

gonadotropins.
Use: Ovulation stimulant.
See: Menotropins.
Lutropin Alfa.
Pergonal.

gonadotropin serum. Pregnant mare's serum.

gonadotropins, follitropin alfa.
Use: Sex hormone, ovulation stimulant.
See: Gonal-f.
Gonal-f RFF Pen.

gonadotropins, follitropin beta.
Use: Sex hormone, ovulation stimulant.
See: Follistim.

gonadotropins, menotropins.
Use: Sex hormone, ovulation stimulant.
See: Pergonal.
Repronex.

gonadotropins, urofollitropin.
Use: Sex hormone, ovulation stimulant.
See: Bravelle.

Gonak. (Akorn) Hydroxypropyl methylcellulose 2.5%. Soln. Bot. 15 mL. *OTC.*
Use: Ophthalmic.

Gonal-f. (Serono) Follitropin alfa 82 units (to deliver 75 units), 600 units (to deliver 450 units), 1, 200 units (to deliver 1,050 units) FSH activity, sucrose 30 mg. Pow. for Inj., lyophilized. Single-dose vials with sterile water for injection as diluent. 1, 10 (82 units only). Multi-dose vials with prefilled syringes of bacteriostatic water (with 0.9% benzyl alcohol) for injection as diluent. 1 (600 units and 1,200 units only), 5 (1,200 units only), 10 (1,200 units only). *Rx.*
Use: Sex hormone, ovulation stimulant.

Gonal-f RFF Pen. (Serono) Follitropin alfa 415 units (to deliver ≥ 300 units/ 0.5 mL), 568 units (to deliver ≥ 450 units/0.75 mL), 1,026 units (to deliver ≥ 900 units/1.5 mL) FSH activity. Inj. Prefilled pens with needles with ben-

zyl alcohol 0.9%. *Rx.*
Use: Ovulation stimulant.
Gonic. (Hauck) Chorionic gonadotropin 10,000 units vial with 10 mL diluent (1,000 units/mL), mannitol, benzyl alcohol 0.9%. Pow. for Inj. Vial 10 mL. *Rx.*
Use: Ovulation stimulant.
gonioscopic hydroxypropyl methylcellulose.
See: Goniosol.
Gonioscopic Solution. (Alcon) Hydroxyethyl cellulose. *Drop-Tainer* 15 mL. *Rx.*
Use: Ophthalmic.
Goniosol. (Novartis Ophthalmics) Gonioscopic hydroxypropyl methylcellulose 2.5%. Bot. 15 mL. *OTC.*
Use: Ophthalmic.
Gonodecten Test Kit. (United States Pooknging) Tube tort for urethral discharge from males, for detection of *Neisseria gonorrhoeae.* Test kit 10s, 25s.
Use: Diagnostic aid.
gonorrhea tests.
See: Biocult-GC.
Gonodecten Test Kit.
Gonozyme Diagnostic Kit.
Isocult for *Neisseria gonorrhoeae.*
MicroTrak *Neisseria gonorrhoeae* Culture Test.
Gonozyme. (Abbott Diagnostics) Enzyme immunoassay for detection of *Neisseria gonorrhoeae* in urogenital swab specimens. Test kit 100s.
Use: Diagnostic aid.
Good Samaritan Ointment. (Good Samaritan) Tube 1.25 oz. *OTC.*
Use: Counterirritant.
Good Sense Maximum Strength Dose Sinus. (Perrigo) Pseudoephedrine hydrochloride 30 mg, chlorpheniramine maleate 2 mg, acetaminophen 500 mg. Tab. Pkg. 24s. *OTC.*
Use: Upper respiratory combination, decongestant, antihistamine, analgesic.
Good Sense Maximum Strength Pain Relief Allergy Sinus. (Perrigo) Pseudoephedrine hydrochloride 30 mg, chlorpheniramine maleate 2 mg, acetaminophen 500 mg. Gelcap. Pkg. 24s. *OTC.*
Use: Upper respiratory combination, decongestant, antihistamine, analgesic.
Goody's Body Pain Powder. (GlaxoSmithKline) Acetaminophen 325 mg, aspirin 500 mg, lactose. Pow. Pkg. 6s, 24s. *OTC.*
Use: Analgesic.
Goody's Extra Strength Headache Powder. (GlaxoSmithKline) Acetaminophen 260 mg, aspirin 520 mg, caffeine 32.5 mg, lactose. Pow. Pkg. 2s, 6s, 24s, 50s. *OTC.*
Use: Analgesic.
Goody's Headache Powders. (GlaxoSmithKline) Aspirin 520 mg, acetaminophen 260 mg, caffeine 32.5 mg/dose. Pow. Pkg. 2s, 6s, 24s, 50s. *OTC.*
Use: Analgesic.
Gordobalm. (Gordon Laboratories) Chloroxylenol, methyl salicylate, menthol, camphor, thymol, eucalyptus oil, isopropyl alcohol 16%, fast-drying gum base. Bot. 4 oz, gal. *OTC.*
Use: Analgesic, topical.
Gordochom. (Gordon Laboratories) Undecylenic acid 25%, chloroxylenol in an oily base. Soln. Bot. 30 mL. *OTC.*
Use: Antifungal, topical.
Gordofilm. (Gordon Laboratories) Salicylic acid 16.7%, lactic acid 16.7% in flexible colloidan. Bot. 15 mL. *OTC.*
Use: Keratolytic.
Gordogesic Cream. (Gordon Laboratories) Methyl salicylate 10% in absorption base. Jar 2.5 oz, 1 lb. *OTC.*
Use: Analgesic, topical.
Gordomatic. (Gordon Laboratories) **Crystals:** Sodium borate, sodium bicarbonate, sodium chloride, thymol, menthol, eucalyptus oil. Jar 8 oz, 7 lb. **Lot.:** Menthol, camphor, propylene glycol, isopropyl alcohol. Bot. 1 oz, 4 oz, gal. **Pow.:** Menthol, thymol camphor, eucalyptus oil, salicylic acid, alum bentonite, talc. Shaker can 3.5 oz. Can 1 lb, 5 lb. *OTC.*
Use: Counterirritant.
Gordon's Urea. (Gordon Laboratories) Urea 40% in petrolatum base. Jar oz. *Rx.*
Use: Emollient.
Gordophene. (Gordon Laboratories) Neutral coconut oil soap 15%, glycerin with Septi-Chlor (trichlorohydroxy diphenyl ether) broad-spectrum antimicrobial and bacteriostatic agent. Bot. 4 oz, gal.
Use: Dermatologic, cleanser.
Gordo-Vite A. (Gordon Laboratories) **Creme:** Vitamin A 100,000 units/oz. in water-soluble base. Jar 0.5 oz, 2.5 oz, 4 oz, lb, 5 lb. **Lot.:** Vitamin A 100,000 units/oz. Plastic bot. 4 oz, gal. *OTC.*
Use: Emollient.
Gordo-Vite E Creme. (Gordon Laboratories) Vitamin E 1500 units/oz in water-soluble base. Jar 2.5 oz, lb. *OTC.*
Use: Emollient.
Gormel Cream. (Gordon Laboratories) Urea 20% in emollient base. Jar

0.5 oz, 2.5 oz, 4 oz, 1 lb, 5 lb. *OTC.*
Use: Emollient.
•**goserelin.** (GO-suh-REH-lin) USAN.
Use: LHRH agonist.
See: Zoladex.
goserelin acetate.
Use: Gonadotropin-releasing hormone analog.
See: Zoladex.
gossypol.
Use: Antineoplastic. [Orphan Drug]
gotamine. (Vita Elixir) Ergotamine tartrate 1 mg, caffeine 100 mg. Tab. *Rx.*
Use: Antimigraine.
gout, agents for.
See: Allopurinol.
 Colchicine.
 Probenecid.
 Probenecid with Colchicine.
 Sulfinpyrazone.
•**govafilcon a.** (GO-vaff-ILL-kahn A) USAN.
Use: Contact lens material, hydrophilic.
GP-500. (Marnel) Pseudoephedrine hydrochloride 120 mg, guaifenesin 500 mg, dye free. SR Tab. Bot. 100s. *Rx.*
Use: Upper respiratory combination, decongestant, expectorant.
gp 100 adenoviral gene therapy. (Genzyme)
Use: Antineoplastic. [Orphan Drug]
G/P 1200/60. (Cypress) Pseudoephedrine hydrochloride 60 mg, guaifenesin 1200 mg. SR Tab. Bot. 100s. *Rx.*
Use: Upper respiratory combination, decongestant, expectorant.
•**gramicidin.** (gram-ih-SIH-din) *USP 28.*
Use: Anti-infective.
W/Neomycin.
See: Spectrocin.
W/Neomycin sulfate, polymyxin B sulfate, thimerosal.
See: AK-Spore Ophthalmic Solution.
 Neo-Polycin.
 Neosporin Ophthalmic Solution.
W/Neomycin sulfate, polymyxin B sulfate, benzocaine.
See: Mycolog Cream.
W/Polymyxin B sulfate, neomycin sulfate.
See: AK-Spore.
 Neosporin.
 Neosporin-G.
 Ocutricin.
W/Polymyxin B sulfate, neomycin sulfate, hydrocortisone acetate.
See: Cortisporin.
•**granisetron.** (gran-IH-SEH-trahn) USAN.
Use: Antiemetic.
See: Kytril.

•**granisetron hydrochloride.** (gran-IH-SEH-trahn) USAN.
Use: Antiemetic.
See: Kytril.
GranulDerm. (Qualitest) Trypsin 0.1 mg, balsam peru 72.5 mg, castor oil 650 mg/0.82 mL. Aerosol. 113.4 g. *Rx.*
Use: Enzyme preparation, topical.
Granulex. (Bertek) Trypsin 0.12 mg, balsam peru 87 mg, castor oil 788 mg/g. Aerosol. 113.4 g. *Rx.*
Use: Enzyme preparation, topical.
granulocyte colony-stimulating factor.
See: Neupogen.
granulocyte macrophage colony-stimulating factor.
See: Leukine.
gratus strophanthin. Ouabain.
Gravineed. (Hanlon) Vitamins C 100 mg, E 10 units, B_1 3 mg, B_2 2 mg, B_6 10 mg, B_{12} 5 mcg, A 4000 units, D 400 units, niacin 10 mg, folic acid 0.1 mg, iron fumarate 40 mg, calcium 67 mg. Cap. Bot. 100s. *OTC.*
Use: Mineral, vitamin supplement.
Green mint. (Block Drug) Urea, glycine, polysorbate 60, sorbitol, alcohol 12.2%, peppermint oil, menthol, chlorophyllin-copper complex. Bot. 7 oz, 12 oz. *OTC.*
Use: Mouth and throat preparation.
green soap.
Use: Detergent.
Green Throat Spray. (Clay-Park Labs) Phenol 1.4%. Glycerin, saccharin. Alcohol-free. Throat spray. 473 mL. *OTC.*
Use: Mouth and throat product.
•**grepafloxacin hydrochloride.** (grep-ah-FLOX-ah-sin) USAN.
Use: Antibacterial.
•**griseofulvin.** (griss-ee-oh-FULL-vin) *USP 28.*
Use: Antifungal.
See: Fulvicin P/G.
 Fulvicin U/F.
 Grifulvin V.
 Griseofulvin Ultramicrosize.
 Gris-PEG.
griseofulvin. (Various Mfr.) Griseofulvin 165 mg, 330 mg. Tab. Bot. 100s.
Use: Antifungal.
griseofulvin microsize. (Glades) Griseofulvin microsize 125 mL per 5 mL. Alcohol 0.2%, menthol, parabens, saccharin, sucrose. Orange-cream flavors. Oral Susp. 120 mL. *Rx.*
Use: Antifungal agent.
griseofulvin, ultramicrosize. (Various Mfr.) Griseofulvin ultramicrosize 165 mg. Tab. Bot. 100s. *Rx.*
Use: Antifungal.
See: Fulvicin P/G.

Grisactin Ultra.
Gris-PEG.
Gris-PEG. (Pedinol) Griseofulvin ultramicrosize 125 mg, 250 mg, lactose (125 mg only), parabens. Tab. Bot. 100s, 500s (250 mg only). *Rx.*
Use: Antifungal.
growth hormone. Extract of human pituitaries containing predominantly growth hormone.
See: Crescormon.
growth hormone releasing factor. (ICN)
Use: Long-term treatment of growth failure. [Orphan Drug]
g-strophanthin. Ouabain.
guaiacol carbonate. (Various Mfr.) Duotal.
Use: Expectorant.
guaiacol glyceryl ether.
See: Guaifenesin.
guaiacol potassium sulfonate.
See: Bronchial.
W/Ammonium chloride, sodium citrate, benzyl alcohol, carbinoxamine maleate.
See: Clistin Expectorant.
W/Dextromethorphan HBr.
See: Bronchial DM.
W/Pheniramine maleate, pyrilamine maleate, codeine phosphate.
See: Tritussin.
guaianesin.
Use: Expectorant.
See: Guaifenesin.
•**guaiapate.** (GWIE-ah-pate) USAN.
Use: Antitussive.
Guaifed Capsules. (Verum Pharm) Guaifenesin 400 mg, phenylephrine 15 mg. Sucrose, parabens, maltodextrin. ER Cap. Bot. 30s, 100s. *Rx.*
Use: Upper respiratory combination, decongestant, expectorant.
Guaifed-PD Capsules. (Verum Pharm) Guaifenesin 200 mg, phenylephrine 7.5 mg. Maltodextrin, parabens, sucrose. ER. Cap. Bot. 30s, 100s. *Rx.*
Use: Upper respiratory combination, decongestant, expectorant.
Guaifed Syrup. (Muro) Pseudoephedrine hydrochloride 30 mg, guaifenesin 200 mg/5 mL, EDTA, menthol, saccharin, sorbitol, sucrose, cherry flavor, alcohol free. Syr. Bot. 473 mL. *OTC.*
Use: Upper respiratory combination, decongestant, expectorant.
•**guaifenesin.** (GWIE-fen-ah-sin) *USP 28.*
Formerly Glyceryl Guaiacolate. Synonyms: Glyceryl guaiacolate, glyceryl guaiacol ether, guaianesin, guaifylline, guayanesin.
Use: Expectorant.
See: Allfen Jr.

AMBI.
Consin-GG.
Diabetic Tussin EX.
Duratuss-G.
GG-Cen.
Glycotuss.
G-100.
G-Tussin.
Guiatuss.
Hytuss.
Liquibid.
Monafed.
Mucinex.
Muco-Fen-LA.
Organidin NR.
Pheunomist.
Robitussin.
Scot-Tussin Expectorant.
Siltussin.
Tusibron.
2/G.
W/Combinations.
See: AccuHist DM Pediatric.
AccuHist PDX
Actifed C Expectorant.
Airet G.G.
Allfen-DM.
AMBI 1000/55.
AMBI 60/580.
AMBI 60/580/30.
Anti-tuss D.M.
Antitussive Guaiacolate.
AquaTab C.
AquaTab D.
AquaTab DM.
Aspirin-Free Bayer Select Head & Chest Cold.
Atuss EX.
Atuss G.
Atuss-12 DX.
Benylin Expectorant.
Broxin.
Bromhist-DM.
Bromhist-PDX Syrup.
Broncholate.
Bronkaid Dual Action.
Brontex.
Bur-Tuss Expectorant.
Cheracol Cough.
Cheracol D.
Cheracol D Cough Formula.
Cheracol Plus.
Chlor-Trimeton.
Codeine Phosphate and Guaifenesin.
Codiclear DH.
Cold & Cough Tussin.
Coldloc.
Coldloc-LA.
Coldmist JR.
Coldmist LA.

Comtrex Multi-Symptom Deep Chest
Cold & Congestion Relief.
Congestac.
Coricidin Children's Cough.
Coricidin HBP Chest Congestion &
Cough.
Cortane D.C.
Crantex ER.
Cycofed Pediatric.
Decolate.
Deconamine CX.
Deconsal Pediatric.
Deconsal II.
DEKA.
DEKA Pediatric.
Dex GG TR.
Diabetic Tussin.
Diabetic Tussin DM.
Diabetic Tussin Maximum Strength
DM.
Dihistine Expectorant.
Dilaudid.
Dilaudid Cough.
Dimetane Expectorant.
Dimetane Expectorant-DC.
DM Plus.
Donatussin.
Donatussin DC.
Duraflu.
Dura-Gest.
Duraphen II.
Durasal II.
Duratuss.
Duratuss DM.
Duratuss GP.
Duratuss HD.
Dura-Vent.
Dy-G.
Dynafed Asthma Relief.
Dynex.
Dyphylline & Guaifenesin.
Endal.
Endal Expectorant.
Entex.
Entex HC.
Entex LA.
Entex PSE.
ExeFen-PD.
Extra Action Cough.
Fenesin.
Fenesin DM.
Formula 44D Decongestant Cough
Mixture.
Gani-Tuss-DM NR.
Gani-Tuss NR.
Genatuss DM.
GFN/PSE.
GFN 550/PSE 60/DM 30.
GFN 1000/DM 50.
GFN 1000/DM 60.
GFN 600/Phenylephrine 20.

GFN 1200/DM 60.
GFN 1200/DM 60/PSE 120.
Glycotuss-DM.
GP-500.
G/P 1200/60.
Guaifed.
Guaifed-PD.
Guaifenesin DAC.
Guaifenesin DM.
Guaifenesin-DM NR.
Guaifenesin 1000 mg and Dextro-
methorphan HBr 60 mg LA.
Guaifenesin/Pseudoephedrine hydro-
chloride.
Guaifenex DM.
Guaifenex GP.
Guaifenex PSE 120.
Guaifenex PSE 60.
Guaimax-D.
Guaipax PSE.
Guaitab.
Guaitex PSE.
Guaivent.
Guaivent PD.
Guai-Vent/PSE.
Guiadrine DM.
Guiatex LA.
Guiatuss AC.
Guiatuss DAC.
Guiatussin/Codeine.
Guistrey Fortis.
Histacol DM.
H 9600 SR.
Humibid DM.
Humibid L.A.
Hycoclear Tuss.
Hycotuss Expectorant.
Hycosin Expectorant.
Hydrocodone Bitartrate and Guaifen-
esin.
Hydrocodone GF.
Hydro-Tussin DM.
Hydro-Tussin HD.
Iobid DM.
Iosal II.
Isoclor Expectorant.
Kolephrin GG/DM.
Kwelcof.
Lardet Expectorant.
Lemotussin-DM.
Levall.
Levall 5.0.
Liquibid-D.
Liquibid-D 1200.
Liquibid-PD.
Maxifed.
Maxifed DM.
Maxifed DMX.
Maxifed-G.
MAXIPHEN DM.
Maxi-Tuss DM.

Maxi-Tuss HCG.
Med-Rx.
Mini Two-Way Action.
Miraphen PSE.
Mucinex DM.
Muco-Fen-DM.
Mudrane GG.
Mytussin AC Cough.
Mytussin DAC.
Mytussin DM.
Nalex Expectorant.
Nasabid.
Nasabid SR.
Nasatab LA.
Novagest Expectorant with Codeine.
Novahistine.
Novahistine Cough Formula.
Norel.
Nucofed Expectorant.
Nucofed Pediatric Expectorant.
Nucotuss Expectorant.
Nucotuss Pediatric Expectorant.
Panatuss DX.
Pancof-EXP.
Pancof-XP.
Panfil G.
PanMist-DM.
PanMist JR.
PanMist LA.
PanMist-S.
Partuss AC.
Pediacon DX Children's.
Pediacon DX Pediatric.
Pediacon EX.
Pediahist DM.
Phanatuss DM Cough.
PhenaVent D.
PhenaVent LA.
Phenylfenesin LA.
PMP Expectorant.
Pneumotussin.
Pneumotussin 2.5 Cough.
Polaramine Expectorant.
Poly-Histine Expectorant.
Polytuss-DM.
Primatene.
Profen Forte.
Profen Forte DM.
Profen LA.
Profen II.
Profen II DM.
Pseudovent.
Pseudovent-PED.
Quibron.
Quibron Plus.
Quibron-300.
Refenesen Plus Severe Strength
   Cough & Cold Medicine.
Rescon-GG.
Respaire-120 SR.
Respaire-60 SR.

Robafen CF.
Robafen PE.
Robitussin AC, CF, DAC, DM, PE.
Robitussin Cold & Cough.
Robitussin Cold, Cold & Congestion.
Robitussin Cold, Cold & Cough.
Robitussin Cold, Multi-Symptom Cold
   & Flu.
Robitussin Cold Sinus & Congestion.
Robitussin Cough and Cold Infant.
Robitussin Cough & Congestion
   Formula.
Robitussin-DM.
Robitussin-DM Cough Calmers.
Robitussin DM Infant.
Robitussin Severe Congestion.
Robitussin Sugar Free Cough.
Romilar AC.
Rondec-DM.
Rymed.
Safe Tussin.
Scot-Tussin Senior Clear.
Severe Congestion Tussin.
Silaminic Expectorant.
Sildicon-E.
Sil-Tex.
Siltussin-CF.
Siltussin DM.
Siltussin DM Cough.
Sinutab Non-Drying.
SINUtuss DM.
SINUvent PE.
Sorbase II Cough.
Stamoist E.
Sudafed Multi-Symptom Cold &
   Cough.
Sudafed Non-Drowsy Non-Drying
   Sinus.
Sudal-DM.
Sudal 120/600.
Sudal 60/500.
Su-Tuss DM.
Su-Tuss HD.
Syn-Rx.
TheraFlu Maximum Strength Flu &
   Congestion Non-Drowsy.
TheraFlu Maximum Strength Flu, Cold
   & Cough.
Thera-Hist Expectorant Chest Con-
   gestion.
Tolu-Sed.
Tolu-Sed DM.
Touro CC.
Touro DM.
Touro LA.
Triacting.
Triaminic Chest & Nasal Congestion
   Liquid.
Triaminic Expectorant.
Tri-Histin Expectorant.
Trind.

Tussafed.
Tussafed EX.
Tussafed HC.
Tussafed-LA.
Tussar SF.
Tussar-2.
Tuss-DM.
Tussend.
TUSSI-bid.
Tussi-Organidin DM NR.
Tussi-Organidin DM-S.
Tussi-Organidin NR.
TUSSI-PRES.
Tylenol Multi-Symptom Cold Severe Congestion.
Tylenol Sinus Severe Congestion.
V-Dec-M.
Versacaps.
Vicks Cough.
Vicks Formula 44D Decongestant Cough Mixture.
Vicks 44E.
Vicks 44E Cough & Chest Congestion Relief.
Vicks Pediatric 44e Cough & Chest Congestion Relief.
Vitussin.
Z-Cof DM.
Z-Cof LA.
Zephrex.
Zephrex LA.
ZTuss Expectorant.

guaifenesin. (URL) Guaifenesin 400 mg. Dye-free. Tab. 50s, 100s. *OTC.*
Use: Expectorant.

guaifenesin. (Various Mfr.) Guaifenesin. **ER Tab.:** 600 mg. Bot. 100s, **SR Tab.:** 1000 mg. Bot. 100s. **Syr.:** 100 mg/5 mL. Bot. 473 mL. **Tab.:** 200 mg. 100s. *Rx-OTC.*
Use: Expectorant.

• **guaifenesin and codeine phosphate oral solution.** *USP 28.*
Use: Antitussive, expectorant.

Guaifenesin DAC. (Cypress) Codeine phosphate 10 mg, pseudoephedrine hydrochloride 30 mg, guaifenesin 100 mg/5 mL, alcohol 1.9%, saccharin, sorbitol. Liq. Bot. 480 mL. *OTC.*
Use: Antitussive, decongestant, expectorant.

Guaifenesin DM. (UDL) Dextromethorphan HBr 10 mg, guaifenesin 100 mg/5 mL, saccharin, sorbitol, alcohol free. Syr. UD 5 mL, 10 mL. *OTC.*
Use: Upper respiratory combination, antitussive, expectorant.

Guaifenesin DM. (Prasco) Dextromethorphan HBr 30 mg, guaifenesin 600 mg. ER Tab. 100s. *Rx.*
Use: Upper respiratory combination, antitussive, expectorant.

Guaifenesin-DM NR. (Silarx) Dextromethorphan HBr 10 mg, guaifenesin 100 mg/5 mL, methylparaben, saccharin, sorbitol, raspberry flavor, alcohol free. Liq. Bot. 118 mL, 473 mL, 3.8 L. *Rx.*
Use: Upper respiratory combination, antitussive, expectorant.

Guaifenesin NR. (Silarx) Guaifenesin 100 mg/5 mL. Raspberry flavor. Liq. 473 mL. *Rx.*
Use: Expectorant.

guaifenesin 1000 mg and dextromethorphan HBr 60 mg. (URL Laboratories) Dextromethorphan HBr 60 mg, guaifenesin 1000 mg. LA Tab. Bot. 100s. *Rx.*
Use: Upper respiratory combination, antitussive, expectorant.

guaifenesin/pseudoephedrine hydrochloride. (Major) Pseudoephedrine hydrochloride 60 mg, guaifenesin 600 mg. SR Tab. Bot. 100s. *Rx.*
Use: Upper respiratory combination, decongestant, expectorant.

guaifenesin/pseudoephedrine hydrochloride/codeine phosphate syrup. (Schein) Pseudoephedrine hydrochloride 30 mg, codeine phosphate 10 mg, guaifenesin 100 mg, alcohol 1.4%/5 mL. Bot. 473 mL. *c-v.*
Use: Antitussive, decongestant, expectorant.
See: Guaifenesin DAC.

Guaifenex DM. (Ethex) Guaifenesin 600 mg, dextromethorphan HBr 30 mg. ER Tab. Bot. 100s. *Rx.*
Use: Upper respiratory combination, antitussive, expectorant.

Guaifenex GP. (Ethex) Pseudoephedrine hydrochloride 120 mg, guaifenesin 1200 mg, lactose, dye free. ER Tab. Bot. 100s. *Rx.*
Use: Upper respiratory combination, decongestant, expectorant.

Guaifenex PSE 120. (Ethex) Guaifenesin 600 mg, pseudoephedrine hydrochloride 120 mg, dye free. ER Tab. Bot. 100s. *Rx.*
Use: Upper respiratory combination, decongestant, expectorant.

Guaifenex PSE 60. (Ethex) Guaifenesin 600 mg, pseudoephedrine hydrochloride 60 mg, lactose. ER Tab. Bot. 100s. *Rx.*
Use: Upper respiratory combination, decongestant, expectorant.

Guaimax-D. (Schwarz Pharma) Pseudoephedrine hydrochloride 120 mg, guaifenesin 600 mg. ER Tab. Bot. 100s.

Rx.
Use: Upper respiratory combination, decongestant, expectorant.
Guaipax PSE. (Eon) Pseudoephedrine hydrochloride 120 mg, guaifenesin 600 mg. SR Tab. Bot. 100s, 250s, 500s. *Rx.*
Use: Upper respiratory combination, decongestant, expectorant.
Guaiphotol. (Foy Laboratories) Iodine 1/30 g, calcium creosote 4 g. Tab. Bot. 1000s. *Rx.*
Use: Expectorant.
Guaitab. (Muro) Pseudoephedrine hydrochloride 60 mg, guaifenesin 400 mg, lactose. Tab. Bot. 100s. *OTC.*
Use: Decongestant; expectorant.
Guaitex PSE. (Rugby) Pseudoephedrine hydrochloride 120 mg, guaifenesin 500 mg. Tab. Bot. 100s. *Rx.*
Use: Decongestant, expectorant.
•**guaithylline.** (GWIE-thill-in) USAN.
Use: Bronchodilator; expectorant.
Guaivent. (Ethex) Guaifenesin 250 mg, pseudoephedrine hydrochloride 120 mg, parabens, EDTA, sucrose. Cap. Bot. 100s, 500s. *Rx.*
Use: Decongestant, expectorant.
Guaivent PD. (Ethex) **300:** Guaifenesin 300 mg, pseudoephedrine hydrochloride 60 mg, parabens, sucrose. Cap. Bot. 100s, 500s. **600:** Guaifenesin 600 mg, pseudoephedrine hydrochloride 00 mg, parabens, EDTA, sucrose. Cap. Bot. 100s, 500s. *Rx.*
Use: Decongestant, expectorant.
Guai-Vent/PSE. (Biovail) Pseudoephedrine hydrochloride 120 mg, guaifenesin 600 mg. SR Tab. Bot. 100s. *Rx.*
Use: Upper respiratory combination, decongestant, expectorant.
guamide.
See: Sulfaguanidine.
•**guanabenz.** (GWAHN-uh-benz) USAN.
Use: Antihypertensive.
See: Wytensin.
•**guanabenz acetate.** (GWAHN-uh-benz) *USP 28.*
Use: Antihypertensive.
guanabenz acetate. (Various Mfr.) Guanabenz acetate 4 mg, 8 mg. Tab. Bot. 30s, 100s, 500s.
Use: Antihypertensive.
•**guanacline sulfate.** (GWAHN-ah-kleen) USAN.
Use: Antihypertensive.
•**guanadrel sulfate.** (GWAHN-uh-drell) *USP 28.*
Use: Antihypertensive.
See: Hylorel.

•**guancydine.** (GWAHN-sigh-deen) USAN.
Use: Antihypertensive.
•**guanethidine monosulfate.** (gwahn-ETH-ih-deen MAH-no-SULL-fate) *USP 28.*
Use: Antihypertensive. Reflex sympathetic dystrophy and causalgia.
[Orphan Drug]
W/Hydrochlorothiazide.
See: Ismelin.
See: Esimil.
•**guanethidine sulfate.** (gwahn-ETH-ih-deen) USAN.
Use: Antihypertensive.
See: Ismelin.
W/Hydrochlorothiazide.
See: Esimil.
-**guanfacine hydrochloride.** (GWAHN-fay-seen) *USP 28.*
Use: Antihypertensive.
See: Tenex.
guanidine hydrochloride. (Key) Guanidine hydrochloride 125 mg. Mannitol. Tab. Bot. 100s. *Rx.*
Use: Muscle stimulant.
guanisoquin. (GWAN-eye-so-KWIN)
Use: Antihypertensive.
•**guanisoquin sulfate.** (GWAHN-eye-so-kwin) USAN.
Use: Antihypertensive.
•**guanoclor sulfate.** (GWAHN-oh-klahr) USAN.
Use: Antihypertensive.
•**guanoctine hydrochloride.** (GWAHN-ock-teen) USAN.
Use: Antihypertensive.
•**guanoxabenz.** (gwahn-OX-ah-benz) USAN.
Use: Antihypertensive.
•**guanoxan sulfate.** (GWAHN-ox-an) USAN.
Use: Antihypertensive.
•**guanoxyfen sulfate.** (GWAHN-OX-eh-fen) USAN.
Use: Antihypertensive; antidepressant.
Guardal. (Morton Grove) Vitamins A 10,000 units, B_1 20 mg, B_2 8 mg, B_6 0.5 mg, B_{12} 8 mcg, C 50 mg, niacinamide 10 mg, calcium d-pantothenate 5 mg, iron 10 mg, dried whole liver 100 mg, yeast 100 mg, choline bitartrate 30 mg, mixed tocopherols 5 mg, dicalcium phosphate anhydrous 150 mg, magnesium sulfate dried 7.2 mg, sodium 1 mg, potassium chloride 1.3 mg. Tab. Bot. 100s. *OTC.*
Use: Mineral, vitamin supplement.
Guardex. (Archer-Taylor) Tube 4 oz, 1 lb, 4.5 lb. *OTC.*

Use: Emollient.

•**guar gum.** *NF 23.*
Use: Pharmaceutic aid (tablet binder; tablet disintegrant).
See: Benefiber.
W/Danthron, docusate sodium.
See: Guarsol.
W/Standardized senna concentrate.
See: Gentlax B.

guayanesin.
Use: Expectorant.
See: Guaifenesin.

Guiadrine DM. (Breckenridge Pharmaceutical) Dextromethorphan HBr 30 mg, guaifenesin 600 mg. SR Tab. Bot. 100s, 250s. *Rx.*
Use: Upper respiratory combination, antitussive, expectorant.

Guiamid Expectorant. (Vangard Labs, Inc.) Guaifenesin 100 mg/5 mL, alcohol 3.5%. Bot. Pt, gal. *OTC.*
Use: Expectorant.

Guiaphed. (Various Mfr.) Theophylline 45 mg, ephedrine sulfate 36 mg, guaifenesin 150 mg, phenobarbital 12 mg, alcohol 19%/15 mL. Elix. Bot. 480 mL. *Rx.*
Use: Antiasthmatic combination.

Guiatex PSE. (Rugby) Pseudoephedrine hydrochloride, guaifenesin 500 mg. Tab. Bot. 100s. *Rx.*
Use: Decongestant, expectorant.

Guiatuss. (Various Mfr.) Guaifenesin 100 mg/5 mL, may contain saccharin, menthol, corn syrup. Syr. Bot. 118 mL. *OTC.*
Use: Expectorant.

Guiatuss AC. (Various Mfr.) Codeine phosphate 10 mg, guaifenesin 100 mg, alcohol 3.5%/5 mL. Syr. Bot. 118 mL, 473 mL. *c-v.*
Use: Upper respiratory combination, antitussive, expectorant.

Guiatuss DAC. (Various Mfr.) Pseudoephedrine hydrochloride 30 mg, codeine phosphate 10 mg, guaifenesin 100 mg/5 mL, may contain alcohol. Liq. Bot. 473 mL. *c-v.*
Use: Upper respiratory combination, antitussive, decongestant, expectorant.

Guiatussin/Codeine Expectorant. (Rugby) Codeine phosphate 10 mg, guaifenesin 100 mg/5 mL, alcohol 3.5%. Syr. Bot. 120 mL, pt, gal. *c-v.*
Use: Antitussive, expectorant.

Guiatussin/Dextromethorphan. (Rugby) Dextromethorphan HBr 15 mg, guaifenesin 100 mg, alcohol 1.4%/5 mL. Liq. Bot. 480 mL. *OTC.*
Use: Antitussive, expectorant.

Guiatuss Syrup. (Various Mfr.) Guaifenesin 100 mg/5 mL. Syr. Bot. 120 mL, 240 mL, pt, gal. *OTC.*
Use: Expectorant.

Guistrey Fortis. (Jones Pharma) Guaifenesin 100 mg, phenylephrine hydrochloride 10 mg, chlorpheniramine maleate 1 mg. Tab. Bot. 1000s. *OTC.*
Use: Antihistamine, decongestant, expectorant.

Gulfasin. (Major) Sulfisoxazole 500 mg. Tab. Bot. 100s, 250s, 1000s.
Use: Anti-infective, sulfonamide.

guncotton, soluble. Pyroxylin.

gusperimus.
Use: Acute renal graft-rejection episodes.

•**gusperimus trihydrochloride.** (guss-PURR-ih-muss try-HIGH-droe-KLOR-ide) USAN.
Use: Immunosuppressant.

Gustalac. (Roberts) Calcium carbonate 300 mg, defatted skim milk pow. 200 mg. Tab. Bot. 100s, 250s, 1000s. *OTC.*
Use: Antacid; calcium supplement.

•**gutta percha.** *USP 28.*
Use: Dental restoration agent.

G-vitamin.
See: Riboflavin.

Gynazole-1. (Ther-Rx) Butoconazole nitrate 2%, EDTA, parabens, mineral oil. Vag. Cream. Prefilled, single-dose applicator 5 g (1s). *Rx.*
Use: Antifungal, vaginal.

Gynecort 10, Extra Strength. (Combe) Hydrocortisone acetate 1%, parabens, zinc pyrithione. Cream. Tube 15 g. *OTC.*
Use: Corticosteroid, topical.

Gyne-Lotrimin 3. (Schering-Plough) Clotrimazole. **Vag. Supp.:** 200 mg. Pkg. 3s w/applicator. **Vag. Cream:** 2%, benzyl alcohol. Tube 21 g w/3 disp. applicators. *OTC.*
Use: Antifungal, vaginal.

Gyne-Lotrimin 3 Combination Pack. (Schering-Plough) **Vaginal Supp.:** Clotrimazole 200 mg, lactose. Pkg. 3s w/applicator. **Topical Cream:** Clotrimazole 1%, benzyl alcohol, cetyl stearyl alcohol. Tube 7 g. *OTC.*
Use: Antifungal, vaginal.

gynergon.
See: Estradiol.

Gynodiol. (Fielding) Estradiol, micronized 0.5 mg, 1 mg, 1.5 mg, 2 mg, lactose. Tab. Bot. 30s, 100s. *Rx.*
Use: Estrogen.

Gynogen L.A. (Forest) **10:** Estradiol valerate in sesame oil 10 mg/mL. Vial

10 mL. **20:** Estradiol valerate in castor oil 20 mg/mL. Inj. Multi-dose Vial 10 mL. **40:** Estradiol valerate in castor oil 40 mg/mL. Inj. Vial 10 mL. *Rx.*
Use: Estrogen.

Gynol II Contraceptive. (Johnson & Johnson) Nonoxynol-9 in 2% concentration. Starter 75 g tube w/applicator. Refill 75 g, 114 g. Tube. *OTC.*
Use: Contraceptive.

Gynol II Extra Strength Contraceptive. (Johnson & Johnson) Nonoxynol-9 3%. Jelly. 75 g, 114 g. *OTC.*
Use: Contraceptive, spermicide.

Gyno-Petraryl. (Janssen) Econazole nitrate. *Rx.*
Use: Antifungal, vaginal.

Gynovite Plus. (Optimox) Vitamins A 833 units, D 67 units, E 67 mg (as d-alpha tocopheryl acid succinate), B_1 1.7 mg, B_2 1.7 mg, B_3 3.3 mg, B_5 1.7 mg, B_6 3.3 mg, B_{12} 21 mcg, C 30 mg, calcium 83 mg, iron 3 mg, folic acid 0.07 mg, boron, betaine, biotin, Cr, Cu, hesperidin, I, inositol, Mg, Mn, PABA, pancreatin, rutin, Se, Zn 2.5 mg. Tab. Bot. 100s. *OTC.*
Use: Mineral, vitamin supplement.

H

Habitrol. (Basel Pharm.) Nicotine transdermal system. Dose absorbed in 24 hours. Patch 21 mg, 14 mg, 7 mg. Box 30 systems. *OTC.*
Use: Smoking deterrent, nicotine.
haemophilus b conjugate vaccine.
Use: Vaccine, bacterial.
See: ActHIB.
  HibTITER.
  Liquid Pedvax HIB.
  OmniHIB.
  ProHIBiT.
  W/DTP vaccine.
See: ActHIB/DTP, set of DTwP vial plus Hib.
haemophilus conjugate vaccine with hepatitis B vaccine.
Use: Vaccine, bacterial.
See: Comvax.
haemophilus influenzae type b conjugate vaccines (DTaP-HIB).
Use: Active immunization, toxoid.
See: Diphtheria and tetanus toxoids, acellular pertussis and *Haemophilus influenzae* type b conjugate vaccines (DTaP-HIB).
Hair Booster Vitamin. (NBTY) Vitamin B_3 35 mg, B_5 100 mg, B_{12} 6 mcg, folic acid 0.4 mg, zinc 15 mg, Cu, iron 18 mg, I, Mn, choline bitartrate, inositol, PABA, protein. Tab. Bot. 60s. *OTC.*
Use: Mineral, vitamin supplement.
•**halazone.** (HAL ah zone) *USP 20.*
Use: Disinfectant.
•**halcinonide.** (hal-SIN-oh-nide) *USP 28.*
Use: Corticosteroid, topical; anti-inflammatory.
See: Halog.
Halcion. (Upjohn) Triazolam. Tab. **0.125 mg:** Bot. 100s, 500s, UD 100s, Visipak 100s. **0.25 mg.** Bot. 500s. c-iv.
Use: Sedative/hypnotic, nonbarbiturate.
Haldol. (McNeil-CPC) Haloperidol 5 mg/mL, parabens. Inj. Amp. 1 mL. Multidose vial 10 mL. *Rx.*
Use: Antipsychotic.
Haldol Decanoate 50. (McNeil, Bedford) Haloperidol 50 mg/mL (70.5 mg decanoate), sesame oil, benzyl alcohol 1.2%. Amp. 1 mL. Vial 5 mL. *Rx.*
Use: Antipsychotic.
Haldol Decanoate 100. (McNeil) Haloperidol 100 mg/mL (141.04 mg decanoate), sesame oil, benzyl alcohol 1.2%. Amp. 1 mL. Vial 5 mL. *Rx.*
Use: Antipsychotic.
Haldrone. (Eli Lilly) Paramethasone acetate 1 mg, 2 mg. Tab. Bot. 100s. *Rx.*
Use: Corticosteroid.

Halenol Children's. (Halsey Drug) Acetaminophen 160 mg/5 mL. Elix. Bot. 120 mL, 240 mL, pt, gal. *OTC.*
Use: Analgesic.
Halercol. (Roberts) Vitamins A 5000 units, D 400 units, E 1.36 mg, B_1 1.5 mg, B_2 2 mg, B_3 20 mg, B_5 1 mg, B_6 0.1 mg, B_{12} 1 mcg, C 37.5 mg. Cap. Bot. 100s. *OTC.*
Use: Vitamin supplement.
Haley's M-O. (Bayer Corp. (Consumer Div.)) Magnesium hydroxide $\approx$ 900 mg, mineral oil 3.75 mL/15 mL, saccharin (vanilla creme only). Regular or vanilla creme. Liq. Bot. 360 mL, 780 mL (vanilla creme only). *OTC.*
Use: Laxative.
HalfLytely. (Braintree) **DR Tab.:** Bisacodyl 5 mg. Lactose, sucrose, sugar. Enteric-coated, 4s. **Kit, Pow. for Oral Soln.:** PEG 3350 210 g, sodium chloride 5.6 g, sodium bicarbonate 2.86 g, potassium chloride 0.74 g. Lemon-lime flavor. Bot. 2 L. *Rx.*
Use: Bowel evacuant.
Halfort-T. (Halsey Drug) Vitamins C 300 mg, B_1 15 mg, B_2 10 mg, niacin 100 mg, B_6 5 mg, B_{12} 4 mcg, pantothenic acid 20 mg. Tab. Bot. 100s. *OTC.*
Use: Vitamin supplement.
Halfprin 81. (Kramer) Aspirin 81 mg. EC Tab. Bot. 90s. *OTC.*
Use: Analgesic.
Half Strength Entrition Entri-Pak. (Biosearch Medical Products) Protein 17.5 g (Na and Ca caseinates), carbohydrate 68 g (maltodextrin), fat 17.5 g (corn oil, soy lecithin, monoglycerides and diglycerides), sodium 350 mg, potassium 600 mg, mOsm/120 kg H_2O, calories 0.5/mL, vitamins A, B_1, B_2, B_3, B_5, B_6, B_{12}, C, D, E, K, P, Ca, Mg, I, Fe, Zn, Mn, Cu, Cl, biotin, choline, folic acid. Liq. Pouch 1 L. *OTC.*
Use: Nutritional supplement.
Half Strength Florvite with Iron. (Everett) Fluoride 0.5 mg, Vitamins A 2500 units, D 400 units, E 15 units, B_1 1.05 mg, B_2 1.2 mg, B_3 13.5 mg, B_6 1.05 mg, B_{12} 4.5 mcg, C 60 mg, folic acid 0.3 mg, Cu, iron 12 mg, Zn 10 mg, sucrose. Tab. Bot. 100s. *Rx.*
Use: Mineral, vitamin supplement; dental caries agent.
Half Strength Introlan. (Elan) Protein 22.5 g, fat 18 g, carbohydrates 70 g, Na 345 mg, K 585 mg/L. Vitamins A, C, B_1, B_2, B_3, B_5, B_6, B_{12}, D, E, K, Ca, Fe, folic acid, P, I, Mg, Zn, Cu, biotin, Mn, choline, Cl, Se, Cr, Mo. Liq. In 1,000 mL *New Pak* closed systems with and

without color check. *OTC.*
Use: Nutritional supplement.

Half-Strength Lactated Ringer's in 2.5% Dextrose. (Various Mfr.) Dextrose 25 g/L, calories 85 to 89/L, Na$^+$ $\approx$ 65.5 mEq, K$^+$ 2 mEq, Ca^{++} $\approx$ 1.5 mEq, Cl$^-$ $\approx$ 55 mEq, lactate 14 mEq/L, osmolarity $\approx$ 264 mOsm/L. Soln. Bot. 250 mL, 500 mL, 1,000 mL. *Rx.*
Use: Intravenous nutritional therapy, intravenous replenishment solution.

Hali-Best. (Barth's) Vitamins A 10,000 units, D 400 units. Cap. Bot. 100s, 500s. *OTC.*
Use: Vitamin supplement.

halibut liver oil.
Use: Vitamin supplement.

haliver oil.
See: Halibut liver oil.

Hall's Mentho-Lyptus Cough Lozenges. (Warner Lambert) Menthol and eucalyptus oil in varying amounts and flavors. *Stick-Pack* 9s. Bag 30s. *OTC.*
Use: Mouth and throat preparation.

Hall's Mentho-Lyptus Sugar Free. (Warner Lambert) Menthol 5 mg, 6 mg, eucalyptus oil 2.8 mg. Tab. Pkg. 25s. *OTC.*
Use: Mouth and throat preparation.

Hall's-Plus Maximum Strength. (Warner Lambert) Menthol 10 mg, corn syrup, sugar. Cherry, honey-lemon, and regular flavors. Tab. Pkg. 10s, 25s. *OTC.*
Use: Mouth and throat preparation.

Hall's Zinc Defense. (Warner Lambert) Zinc acetate 5 mg, sugar, cherry, or peppermint flavor. Loz. 24s. *OTC.*
Use: Mineral supplement.

• **halobetasol propionate.** (hal-oh-BEH-tah-sahl PRO-pee-oh-nate) USAN.
Use: Anti-inflammatory; corticosteroid, topical.
See: Ultravate.

halobetasol propionate. (Various Mfr.) Halobetasol propionate. **Cream:** 0.05%. May contain cetyl alcohol, glycerin, diazolidinyl urea. 15 g, 50 g. **Oint.:** 0.05%. May contain petrolatum. 15 g, 50 g. *Rx.*
Use: Anti-inflammatory.

Halofed. (Halsey Drug) **Tab.:** Pseudoephedrine hydrochloride 30 mg, 60 mg. Bot. 100s, 1000s. **Syr.:** Pseudoephedrine hydrochloride 30 mg/5 mL. Bot. 120 mL, 240 mL, pt, gal. *OTC.*
Use: Decongestant.

• **halofenate.** (HAY-low-FEN-ate) USAN.
Use: Antihyperlipoproteinemic; uricosuric.

• **halofuginone hydrobromide.** (HAY-low-FOO-jin-ohn HIGH-droe-BROE-mide) USAN.
Use: Antiprotozoal.

Halog. (Westwood-Squibb) Halcinonide. **Cream:** 0.1%, in specially formulated cream base consisting of glyceryl monostearate, cetyl alcohol, myristyl stearate, isopropyl palmitate, polysorbate 60, propylene glycol, purified water. Tube 15 g, 30 g, 60 g. Jar 240 g. **Oint.:** Halcinonide 0.1%, in *Plastibase* (plasicized hydrocarbon gel), PEG 400, PEG 6000 distearate, PEG 300, PEG 1540, butylated hydroxy toluene. Tube 15 g, 30 g, 60 g. Jar 240 g. **Sol.:** 0.1%, EDTA, PEG 300, purified water, butylated hydroxy toluene as preservative. Bot. 20 mL, 60 mL. *Rx.*
Use: Corticosteroid, topical.

Halog-E Cream. (Westwood-Squibb) Halcinonide 0.1% in hydrophilic vanishing cream base consisting of propylene glycol dimethicone 350, castor oil, cetearyl alcohol, ceteareth-20, propylene glycol stearate, white petrolatum, water. Tube 15 g, 30 g, 60 g. *Rx.*
Use: Corticosteroid, topical.

• **halopemide.** (hay-LOW-PEH-mid) USAN.
Use: Antipsychotic.

• **haloperidol.** (HAY-low-PURR-ih-dahl) *USP 28.*
Use: Antipsychotic; tranquilizer; antidyskinetic (in Gilles de la Tourette disease).
See: Haldol.

haloperidol. (Various Mfr.) Haloperidol. **Tab.:** 0.5 mg, 1 mg, 2 mg, 5 mg, 10 mg, 20 mg. Tab. Bot. 100s, 1000s (except 20 mg), UD 100s. **Conc.:** 2 mg/mL. Bot. 15 mL, 120 mL, UD 100s 5 mL, and 10 mL. **Inj.:** 5 mg/mL. May contain parabens. Vial 1 mL, multidose 10 mL. *Rx.*
Use: Antipsychotic.

• **haloperidol decanoate.** (HAY-low-PURR-ih-dahl deh-KAN-oh-ate) USAN.
Use: Antipsychotic.

haloperidol decanoate. (Various Mfr.) Haloperidol 50 mg/mL (70.5 mg decanoate), 100 mg/mL (141.04 mg decanoate), may contain sesame oil, benzyl alcohol 1.2%. Inj. Multidose vial 1 mL, 5 mL. *Rx.*
Use: Antipsychotic.

• **halopredone acetate.** (HAY-low-PREH-dohn) USAN.
Use: Anti-inflammatory, topical.

• **haloprogesterone.** (HAL-oh-pro-jeh-STEE-rone) USAN.

Use: Hormone, progestin.
• **halothane.** (HAL-oh-thane) *USP 28.*
Use: General anesthetic, inhalation.
See: Fluothane.
Halothane.
Halotussin. (Halsey Drug) Guaifenesin 100 mg/5 mL. Bot. 4 oz, 8 oz, pt, gal. *OTC.*
Use: Expectorant.
• **halquinols.** (HAL-kwin-oles) USAN.
Use: Anti-infective, topical; antimicrobial.
HAMA. Hydroxyaluminum magnesium aminoacetate.
hamamelis water.
See: Succus Cineraria maritima.
Witch hazel.
Tucks.
• **hamycin.** (HAY MY sin) USAN.
Use: Antifungal.
Hang-Over-Cure. (Silvers) Calcium carbonate, glycine, thiamine hydrochloride, pyridoxine hydrochloride, aspirin. Cont. Tab. 6 g. *OTC.*
Use: Antacid; analgesic combination.
Haniform. (Hanlon) Vitamins A 25,000 units, D 1000 units, B_1 10 mg, B_2 5 mg, C 150 mg, niacinamide 150 mg. Cap. Bot. 100s. *OTC.*
Use: Vitamin supplement.
Haniplex. (Hanlon) Vitamins B_1 20 mg, B_2 10 mg, B_6 1 mg, B_{12} 5 mcg, calcium pantothenate 10 mg, niacin 20 mg, liver concentrate 50 mg, C 150 mg. Cap. Bot. 100s. *OTC.*
Use: Mineral, vitamin supplement.
Harbolin. (Arcum) Hydralazine hydrochloride 25 mg, hydrochlorothiazide 15 mg, reserpine 0.1 mg. Tab. Bot. 100s, 1000s. *Rx.*
Use: Antihypertensive combination.
hard fat.
Use: Pharmaceutic necessity.
hartshorn. Ammonium carbonate.
Haugase. (Madland) Trypsin, chymotrypsin. Bot. 50s, 250s.
Use: Enzyme preparation.
Havab. (Abbott Diagnostics) Radioimmunoassay or enzyme immunoassay for detection of antibody to hepatitis A virus. Test kit 100s.
Use: Diagnostic aid.
Havab EIA. (Abbott Diagnostics) Enzyme immunoassay for the detection of antibody to hepatitis A virus.
Use: Diagnostic aid.
Havab-M. (Abbott Diagnostics) Radioimmunoassay for the detection of specific Ig antibody to hepatitis A virus. Test kit 100s.

Use: Diagnostic aid.
Havab-M EIA. (Abbott Diagnostics) Enzyme immunoassay for the detection of Ig antibody to hepatitis A virus.
Use: Diagnostic aid.
Havrix. (GlaxoSmithKline) Hepatitis A vaccine, inactivated. **Adult:** 1440 ELU units/mL. Single-dose vial, prefilled syringe. **Pediatric:** 360 ELU/0.5 mL, 720 ELU/0.5 mL. Single-dose vial; prefilled syringe (720 ELU only). *Rx.*
Use: Immunization, viral vaccine.
Hawaiian Tropic Aloe Paba Sunscreen. (Tanning Research Labs) Padimate O, oxybenzone. Cream. Bot. 120 g. *OTC.*
Use: Sunscreen.
Hawaiian Tropic Baby Faces. (Tanning Research Labs) SPF 20. Octyl methoxycinnamate, octocrylene, benzophenone-3, menthyl anthranilate, PABA free, waterproof. Gel. Tube 120 g. *OTC.*
Use: Sunscreen.
Hawaiian Tropic Baby Faces Sunblock. (Tanning Research Labs) Octyl methoxycinnamate, benzophenone-3, octyl salicylate, titanium dioxide, octocrylene, PABA free, waterproof. **SPF 35:** Lot. Bot. 60 mL, 120 mL, 300 mL. **SPF 50:** Lot. Bot. 120 mL. *OTC.*
Use: Sunscreen.
Hawaiian Tropic Cool Aloe with I.C.E. (Tanning Research Labs) Lidocaine, menthol, aloe, SD alcohol 40, diazolidinyl urea, EDTA, vitamins A and E, tartrazine. Gel. Jar 360 g. *OTC.*
Use: Emollient.
Hawaiian Tropic Dark Tanning. (Tanning Research Labs) **Gel:** Phenylbenzimidazole sulfonic acid. SPF 2. Bot. 240 mL. **Oil:** 2-ethylhexyl methoxycinnamate, octyl dimethyl, PABA, waterproof. Bot. 240 mL. *OTC.*
Use: Sunscreen.
Hawaiian Tropic Dark Tanning with Sunscreen. (Tanning Research Labs) **Oil:** Ethylhexyl p-methoxycinnamate, octyl dimethyl, PABA, waterproof. SPF 4. Bot. 240 mL. **Gel:** Phenylbenzimidazole, sulfonic acid. PABA free. SPF 4. Tube 240 g. *OTC.*
Use: Sunscreen.
Hawaiian Tropic 8 Plus. (Tanning Research Labs) Octyl methoxycinnamate, benzophenone-3, menthyl anthranilate, PABA free, waterproof. SPF 8+. Gel. Tube 120 g. *OTC.*
Use: Sunscreen.
Hawaiian Tropic 15 Plus. (Tanning Research Labs) Octyl methoxycinnamate, octocrylene, benzophenone-3, menthyl anthranilate, PABA free, waterproof.

Gel. Tube 120 g. *OTC.*
Use: Sunscreen.

Hawaiian Tropic 15 Plus Sunblock.
(Tanning Research Labs) Menthyl anthranilate, octyl methoxycinnamate, benzophenone-3, PABA free, waterproof. Lot. Bot. 7.5 mL, 15 mL, 60 mL, 120 mL, 240 mL, 300 mL. *OTC.*
Use: Sunscreen.

Hawaiian Tropic 15 Plus Sunblock Lip Balm. (Tanning Research Labs) Padimate O, oxybenzone. SPF 15, waterproof. Stick 4.2 g. *OTC.*
Use: Sunscreen.

Hawaiian Tropic 45 Plus Sunblock Lip Balm. (Tanning Research Labs) Octyl methoxycinnamate, benzophenone-3, octyl salicylate, titanium dioxide, menthyl anthranilate, PABA free, waterproof. SPF 45+. Lip balm 4.2 g. *OTC.*
Use: Sunscreen.

Hawaiian Tropic Just for Kids Sunblock. (Tanning Research Labs) **SPF 30:** Homosalate, octyl methoxycinnamate, benzophenone-3, menthyl anthranilate, octyl salicylate, PABA free, waterproof. Lot. Bot. 88.7 mL. **SPF 45:** Octyl methoxycinnamate, benzophenone-3, octyl salicylate, octocrylene, titanium dioxide, PABA free, waterproof. Lot. Bot. 88.7 mL. *OTC.*
Use: Sunscreen.

Hawaiian Tropic Lip Balm Sunblock. (Tanning Research Labs) Padimate O, oxybenzone. Stick 4 g. *OTC.*
Use: Sunscreen.

Hawaiian Tropic Protective Tanning. (Tanning Research Labs) Titanium dioxide, PABA free, waterproof. SPF 6. Lot. Bot. 240 mL. *OTC.*
Use: Sunscreen.

Hawaiian Tropic Protective Tanning Dry. (Tanning Research Labs) SPF 6. **Oil:** 2-ethylhexyl p-methoxycinnamate, homosalate, menthyl anthranilate, waterproof. Bot. 180 mL. **Gel:** Phenylbenzimidazole, sulfonic acid, benzophenone-4. Tube 180 g. *OTC.*
Use: Sunscreen.

Hawaiian Tropic Self Tanning Sunblock. (Tanning Research Labs) Octyl methoxycinnamate, benzophenone-3, aloe, cetyl alcohol, stearyl alcohol, cocoa butter, parabens, vitamin E, PABA free. SPF 15. Cream. Tube 93.75 mL. *OTC.*
Use: Sunscreen.

Hawaiian Tropic Sport Sunblock. (Tanning Research Labs) SPF 15, SPF 30. Methoxycinnamate, octocrylene, benzophenone-3, octyl salicylate, titanium

dioxide, PABA free, waterproof. Lot. Bot. 88.7 mL. *OTC.*
Use: Sunscreen.

Hawaiian Tropic Sunblock. (Tanning Research Labs) Titanium dioxide, octyl methoxycinnamate, benzophenone-3, octyl salicylate, octocrylene, PABA free, waterproof. **SPF 30+:** Lot. Bot. 120 mL. **SPF 45+:** Lot. Bot. 120 mL, 300 mL. *OTC.*
Use: Sunscreen.

Hawaiian Tropic Swim n Sun. (Tanning Research Labs) Padimate O, oxybenzone. Lot. Bot. 120 mL. *OTC.*
Use: Sunscreen.

Hawaiian Tropic 10 Plus. (Tanning Research Labs) Octyl methoxycinnamate, benzophenone-3, menthyl anthranilate, PABA free, waterproof. SPF 10+. Gel. Tube 120 g. *OTC.*
Use: Sunscreen.

• **hawthorne leaf with flower.** *NF 23.*
Use: Dietary supplement.

Hayfebrol Liquid. (Scot-Tussin) Pseudoephedrine hydrochloride 30 mg, chlorpheniramine 2 mg. Syr. Bot. 118 mL. *OTC.*
Use: Antihistamine; decongestant.

Hazogel Body and Foot Rub. (Vortech Pharmaceuticals) Witch hazel 70%, isopropanol 20% in a neutralized resin vehicle. Bot. 4 oz. *OTC.*
Use: Astringent; antipruritic.

1% HC. (C & M Pharmacal) Hydrocortisone 1%, petrolatum base. Oint. Tube 15, 20, 30, 60, 120, 240 g, lb. *OTC.*
Use: Corticosteroid, topical.

HC Derma-Pax. (Recsei) Hydrocortisone 0.5% in liquid base. Dropper Bot. 2 oz. *OTC.*
Use: Corticosteroid, topical.

HCG.
See: Chorionic gonadotropin.

HCG-Nostick. (Organon Teknika) Sol Particle Immunoassay (SPIA) for detection of hCG in urine. Stick 30s.
Use: Diagnostic aid, pregnancy.

HC Pramoxine. (Veracity) Hydrocortisone acetate 2.5%, pramoxine hydrochloride 1%. Cetyl alcohol. Cream. 28 g. *Rx.*
Use: Anorectal preparations.

HD 85. (Mallinckrodt) Barium sulfate 85%, raspberry flavor. Susp. Kit 150 mL, 450 mL. Bot. 1900 mL. *Rx.*
Use: Radiopaque agent, GI contrast agent.

HD 200 Plus. (Mallinckrodt) Barium sulfate 98%, strawberry flavor. Pow. for Susp. UD 312 g. *Rx.*
Use: Radiopaque agent, GI contrast agent.

Head & Shoulders. (Procter & Gamble) Pyrithione zinc 1%. **Cream:** Tube 51 g, 75 g, 120 g, 210 g. **Lot.:** Bot. 120 mL, 210 mL, 330 mL, 450 mL. **Shampoo:** Cetyl and benzyl alcohol. Normal to oily and normal to dry formulas. 200 mL, 400 mL, 750 mL. *OTC.*
Use: Antiseborrheic.

Head & Shoulders Conditioner. (Procter & Gamble) Pyrithione zinc 0.3%. Bot. 4 oz, 11 oz. *OTC.*
Use: Antiseborrheic.

Head & Shoulders Dry Scalp. (Procter & Gamble) Pyrithione zinc 1%, cetyl and benzyl alcohol, regular and conditioning formulas. Shampoo. Bot. 200 mL, 400 mL, 750 mL, 1000 mL. *OTC.*
Use: Antiseborrheic.

Head & Shoulders Intensive Treatment. (Procter & Gamble) Selenium sulfide 1%. Lotion/Shampoo. Bot. 400 mL. *OTC.*
Use: Antiseborrheic.

Healon. (Pharmacia) Sodium hyaluronate 10 mg/mL. Inj. Syringe 0.4 mL, 0.55 mL, 0.85 mL, 2 mL. *Rx.*
Use: Surgical aid, ophthalmic.

Healon GV. (Pharmacia) Sodium hyaluronate 14 mg/mL. Inj. Syringe 0.55 mL, 0.85 mL. *Rx.*
Use: Surgical aid, ophthalmic.

Healon Yellow. (Pharmacia) Sodium hyaluronate 10 mg, fluorescein sodium 0.005 mg/mL. Inj. Syringe 0.55 mL, 0.85 mL. *Rx.*
Use: Surgical and diagnostic aid, ophthalmic.

Healthbreak. (Lemar Labs) Silver acetate 6 mg. Chewing gum. Pack 24s. *OTC.*
Use: Smoking deterrent.

Heartburn Antacid. (Walgreen) Aluminum hydroxide dried gel 80 mg, magnesium trisilicate 60 mg. Tab. Bot. 100s. *OTC.*
Use: Antacid.

Heartline. (BDI) Aspirin 81 mg. EC Tab. Bot. 36s. *OTC.*
Use: Anti-inflammatory.

heavy metal poisoning, antidote.
See: BAL.
Calcium disodium versenate.

Hectorol. (Bone Care International) Doxercalciferol 2.5 mcg, BHA, ethanol. Cap. Bot. 50s. *Rx.*
Use: Hyperparathyroidism.

Heet Liniment. (Whitehall-Robins Laboratories) Methyl salicylate 15%, camphor 3.6%, oleoresin capsicum 0.025%, alcohol 70%. Bot. 2⅓ oz, 5 oz. *OTC.*

Use: Analgesic-topical.

•**hefilcon A.** (heh-FILL-kahn A) USAN.
Use: Contact lens material (hydrophilic).

•**hefilcon B.** (heh-FILL-kahn B) USAN.
Use: Contact lens material (hydrophilic).

•**hefilcon C.** (heh-FILL-kahn C) USAN.
Use: Contact lens material (hydrophilic).

Helidac. (Procter & Gamble) Bismuth subsalicylate 264.4 mg. Tab. Metronidazole 250 mg. Tab. Tetracycline 500 mg. Cap. Box. 4s, 8s (bismuth subsalicylate only). *Rx.*
Use: Antiulcerative.

Helistat. (Hoechst) Absorbable collagen hemostatic sponge. 1" × 2" and 3" × 4" in 10s, 9" × 10" in 5s. *Rx.*
Use: Hemostatic.

•**helium.** (HEE-lee-uhm) *USP 28.*
Use: Diluent for gases.

Helixate. (Aventis) Concentrated recombinant hemophilic factor. After reconstitution, also contains glycine 10 to 30 mg, imidazole ≤ 500 mcg/1000 units, polysorbate 80 H 600 mcg/1000 units, Calcium Cl 2 to 5 mM, sodium 100 to 130 mEq/L, chloride 100 to 130 mEq/L, albumin (human) 4 to 10 mg/mL. units 250, 500, 1000. *Rx.*
Use: Antihemophilic.

Helixate FS. (Aventis) Concentrate of antihemophilic factor (recombinant). When reconstituted contains glycine 21 to 25 mg/mL, imidazole ≤ 20 mcg/1,000 IU, CaCl 2 to 3 mM, chloride 32 to 40 mEq/L, histidine 18 to 23 mM, Cu < 0.6 mcg/1,000 IU, Na 27 to 36 mEq/L, tri-n-butyl-phosphate < 5 mcg/1,000 IU, sucrose 28 mg, solvent/detergent treated, preservative and albumin free. Inj., lyophilized. Vial 250, 500, 1,000 IU w/diluent, double-ended needle, filter needle, administration set. Actual number of antihemophilic factor units are indicated on vials. *Rx.*
Use: Antihemophilic agent.

Hemabate. (Pharmacia) Carboprost tromethamine equivalent to 250 mcg carboprost, tromethamine 83 mcg/mL. Inj. Amp. 1 mL. *Rx.*
Use: Abortifacient.

Hema-Chek Slides. (Bayer Corp. (Consumer Div.)) Fecal occult blood test containing slide tests, developer, and applicators. Pkg. 100s, 300s, 1000s.
Use: Diagnostic aid.

Hema-Combistix Reagent Strips. (Bayer Corp. (Consumer Div.)) Four-way strip test for urinary pH, glucose, protein, and occult blood. Strip. Bot. 100s.

Use: Diagnostic aid.

Hemaferrin. (Western Research) Ferrous fumarate 150 mg, desiccated liver 50 mg, docusate sodium 25 mg, betaine hydrochloride 100 mg, folic acid 0.4 mg, vitamins C 50 mg, B_6 2 mg, B_{12} 5 mcg, Mn 2 mg, Cu 1 mg, Zn 2 mg, Mo 0.4 mg. Tab. 28s. Pack 1000s. *OTC.*
Use: Mineral, vitamin supplement; stool softener.

Hemafolate. (Canright) Ferrous gluconate 293 mg, liver fraction II 250 mg, gastric substance 100 mg, vitamins C 50 mg, B_{12} 10 mcg. Tab. Bot. 100s, 1000s. *OTC.*
Use: Mineral, vitamin supplement.

Hemalive. (Barth's) **Liq.:** Vitamins B_1 3.15 mg, B_2 3.33 mg, B_6 0.81 mg, B_{12} 6 mcg, biotin 3.6 mcg, iron 60 mg, choline, inositol, liver fraction No. 1, niacin 22.5 mg, pantothenic acid/15 mL. Bot. 8 oz, 24 oz. **Tab.:** Vitamins B_1 2.5 mg, B_2 5 mg, B_6, B_{12} 25 mcg, iron 75 mg, niacin 1.4 mg, C 30 mg, liver 240 mg, pantothenic acid, aminobenzoic acid, choline, inositol, biotin, Mg, Mn, Cu. Tab. Bot. 100s, 500s, 1000s. *OTC.*
Use: Mineral, vitamin supplement.

Hemaneed. (Hanlon) Hematinic B_{12}, intrinsic factor, Fe. Cap. Bot. 100s. *OTC.*
Use: Mineral, vitamin supplement.

Hemastix Reagent Strips. (Bayer Corp. (Consumer Div.)) Cellulose strip, impregnated with a peroxide and orthotolidine for detection of hematuria and hemoglobinuria. Strip Bot. 50s.
Use: Diagnostic aid.

Hematest Reagent Tablets. (Bayer Corp. (Consumer Div.)) Reagent Tab. for blood in the feces. Bot. 100s.
Use: Diagnostic aid.

hematin.
Use: Porphyria.
See: Panhematin.

Hematinic. (Cypress) Ferrous fumarate 106 mg, folic acid 1 mg. Tab. Bot. 100s. *Rx.*
Use: Mineral, vitamin supplement.

Hematinic Plus. (Cypress) Ferrous fumarate 106 mg, vitamin B_1 10 mg, B_2 6 mg, B_3 30 mg, B_6 5 mg, B_{12} 15 mcg, C 200 mg, folic acid 1 mg, pantothenic acid, Cu, Mg, Mn, Zn 18.2 mg. Tab. 100s. *Rx.*
Use: Mineral, vitamin supplement.

hematinics.
See: Iron products.
  Ferric compounds.
  Ferrous compounds.
  Liver products.

Vitamin B_{12}.
  Vitamin products.

hematopoietic agents.
See: Colony Stimulating Factors.
  Darbepoetin Alfa.
  Epoetin Alfa, Recombinant.
  Filgrastim.
  Interleukins.
  Oprelvekin.
  Pegfilgrastim.
  Recombinant Human Erythropoietin.
  Sargramostim.

Hematrin. (Towne) Iron 50 mg, vitamins B_1 10 mg, B_2 10 mg, B_6 2 mg, B_{12} 10 mcg, C 150 mg, copper 2 mg, niacinamide 50 mg, calcium pantothenate 5 mg, desiccated liver 200 mg. Captab. Bot. 60s, 100s. *OTC.*
Use: Mineral, vitamin supplement.

heme arginate.
Use: Acute porphyria; myelodysplastic syndromes. [Orphan Drug]

HemeSelect. (SmithKline Diagnostics) Occult blood screening test. Box 40 test kits.
Use: Diagnostic aid, fecal.

Hemex. Hemin and zinc mesoporphyrin.
Use: Acute porphyric syndromes. [Orphan Drug]

Hemex. (Vogarell) Oint. Tube 1.25 oz. Supp. Box 12s.
Use: Anorectal preparation.

Hemiacidrin. Citric acid, glucono-delta-lactone, magnesium carbonate.
Use: Genitourinary irrigant.
See: Renacidin.

hemin.
Use: Acute intermittent porphyria. [Orphan Drug]
See: Panhematin.

hemin and zinc mesoporphyrin.
Use: Acute porphyric syndromes. [Orphan Drug]
See: Hemex.

hemisine.
See: Epinephrine.

Hemoccult SENSA. (SmithKline Diagnostics) Occult blood screening tests.
Use: Diagnostic aid, fecal.

Hemoccult Slides. (SmithKline Diagnostics) Occult blood detection (fecal). In 100s, 1000s, and tape dispensers (test 100s).
Use: Diagnostic aid.

Hemoccult II. (SmithKline Diagnostics) Occult blood detection (fecal). In 102s, kit 100s.
Use: Diagnostic aid.

Hemocitrate. (Hemotec Medical Products) Trisodium citrate concentrate.
Use: Leukapheresis procedures.

[Orphan Drug]
Hemocyte. (US Pharmaceutical Corp.) Ferrous fumarate 324 mg (iron 106 mg). Tab. Bot. 30s, 100s. *OTC.*
Use: Mineral supplement.
Hemocyte-F. (US Pharmaceutical Corp.) **Elix.:** Fe (as polysaccharide-iron complex) 100 mg, B_{12} 25 mcg, folic acid 1 mg/5 mL, alcohol 10%, parabens, saccharin, sorbitol, sherry wine flavor. 473 mL. **Tab.:** Iron 106 mg (from ferrous fumarate), folic acid 1 mg. 100s. *Rx.*
Use: Mineral supplement.
Hemocyte Plus. (US Pharmaceutical Corp.) Iron 106 mg (from ferrous fumarate), sodium ascorbate 200 mg, vitamins B_1 10 mg, B_2 6 mg, B_3 30 mg, B_5 10 mg, B_6 5 mg, B_{12} 15 mcg, folic acid 1 mg, zinc 18 mg, Mg, Mn sulfate, Cu Tabule. Bot. 100s. *Rx.*
Use: Mineral, vitamin supplement.
Hemocyte Plus Elixir. (US Pharmaceutical Corp.) Polysaccharide iron complex 12 mg, vitamin B_3 13.3 mg, B_5 3.3 mg, B_6 1.3 mg, B_{12} 4 mcg, folic acid 0.33 mg, zinc 5 mg, Mn 1.3 mg/15 mL. Bot. 473 mL. *Rx.*
Use: Mineral, vitamin supplement.
Hemofil M. (Baxter Healthcare) Preparation of human antihemophilic factor in concentrated form. When reconstituted, contains human albumin ≤ 12.5 mg/mL, PEG 3350 0.07 mg/mL, histidine 0.39 mg, glycine 0.1 mg, mouse protein ≤ 1 ng, tri-n-butyl-phosphate 18 ng. Solvent/detergent-treated. Monoclonal purified. Inj. Single-dose bot. w/diluent, double-ended needle, filter needle. Actual number of antihemophilic factor units indicated on vials. *Rx.*
Use: Antihemophilic agent.
Hemofil T. (Baxter PPI) Antihemophilic factor (human), method four, dried, heat-treated 225 to 375 units/10 mL; 450 to 650 units/20 mL; 675 to 999 units/30 mL; 1000 to 1600 units/30 mL. *Rx.*
Use: Antihemophilic.
●**hemoglobin crosfumaril.** (HEE-moe-GLOBE-in CROSS-FEW-mah-ril) USAN.
Use: Red cell substitute; treatment of prefusion deficit disorders.
●**hemoglobin raffimer.** (HEE-moe-GLOBE-in RAF-fi-mer) USAN.
Use: Blood substitute.
Hemoglobin Reagent Strips. (Bayer Corp. (Consumer Div.)) Seralyzer reagent strips. Bot. 50s. Quantitive strip test for hemoglobin in whole blood.

Use: Diagnostic aid.
Hemopad. (AstraZeneca) Fibrous absorbable collagen hemostat. 2.5 cm × 5 cm, 5 cm × 8 cm, 8 cm × 10 cm. *Rx.*
Use: Hemostatic.
hemorheologic agent. Pentoxifylline.
See: Trental.
Hemorid for Women. (Thompson Medical) **Lotion:** Mineral oil, petrolatum, diazolidinyl urea, cetyl alcohol, glycerin, parabens. Bot. 118 mL. **Cream:** White petrolatum 30%, mineral oil 20%, pramoxine hydrochloride 1%, phenylephrine hydrochloride 0.25%, aloe vera gel, parabens, cetyl and stearyl alcohols. Tube 28.3 g. **Supp.:** Zinc oxide 11%, phenylephrine hydrochloride 0.25%, hard fat 88.25%, aloe vera. Box 12s. *OTC.*
Use: Perianal hygiene.
Hemorrhoidal HC. (Various Mfr.) Hydrocortisone acetate 25 mg. Supp. Box 12s, 24s, 50s, 100s, UD 12s. *Rx.*
Use: Anorectal preparation.
Hemorrhoidal Ointment. (Ivax) Live yeast cell derivative supplying skin respiratory factor 2000 units/oz of ointment w/shark liver oil 3%, phenyl mercuric nitrate 1:10,000. *OTC.*
Use: Anorectal preparation.
Hemorrhoidal Suppositories. (Ivax) Bismuth subgallate 2.25%, bismuth resorcin compound 1.75%, benzyl benzoate 1.2%, balsam Peru 1.8%, zinc oxide 11%. Supp. Box 12s. *OTC.*
Use: Anorectal preparation.
Hemorrhoidal Uniserts. (Upsher-Smith) Bismuth subgallate 2.25%, bismuth resorcin compound 1.75%, benzyl benzoate 1.2%, balsam Peru 1.8%, zinc oxide 11%. Supp. Carton 12s, 50s. *OTC.*
Use: Anorectal preparation.
hemostatics, local.
See: Absorbable Gelatin Sponge.
Gelfilm.
Helistat.
Hemotene.
Oxidized cellulose.
Thrombin.
hemostatics, systemic.
See: Amicar.
Aminocaproic acid.
hemostatics, topical. Thrombin.
See: Thrombinar.
Thrombostat.
hemostatin.
See: Epinephrine.
Hemotene. (AstraZeneca) Absorbable collagen hemostat. 1 g. Pkg. 5s. *Rx.*
Use: Hemostatic, topical.

Hemovit. (Dayton) Vitamin B_1 1.5 mg, B_2 1.7 mg, B_3 20 mg, B_5 10 mg, B_6 10 mg, B_{12} 6 mcg, C 60 mg, folic acid 1 mg, d-biotin 300 mcg, dye free. Tab. Blister 100s. *Rx.*
Use: Nutritional product.

Hemozyme Elixir. (Barrows) Vitamins B_1 5 mg, B_2 5 mg, B_6 1 mg, panthenol 4 mg, niacinamide 100 mg, B_{12} 3 mcg, iron 100 mg, choline bitartrate 100 mg, dl-methionine 100 mg, yeast extract, alcohol 12%/fl oz. Bot. 12 oz. *OTC.*
Use: Mineral, vitamin supplement.

Hem-Prep. (G & W) Phenylephrine hydrochloride 0.25%, zinc oxide 11%. Supp. Bot. 12s. *OTC.*
Use: Anorectal preparation.

Hem-Prep Ointment. (G & W) Phenylephrine hydrochloride 0.025%, zinc oxide 11%, white petrolatum. Oint. 42.5 g. *OTC.*
Use: Anorectal preparation.

Hemril-HC Uniserts. (Upsher-Smith) Hydrocortisone acetate 25 mg. Supp. 12s. *Rx.*
Use: Anorectal preparation.

Hemril Uniserts. (Upsher-Smith) Bismuth subgallate 2.25%, bismuth resorcin compound 1.75%, benzyl benzoate 1.2%, balsam Peru 1.8%, zinc oxide 11%. Supp. Box 12s, 50s. *OTC.*
Use: Anorectal preparation.

henbane.
See: Hyoscyamus.

Henydin-M. (Arcum) Thyroid desiccated pow. 0.5 g, vitamins B_1 1 mg, B_2 0.5 mg, B_6 0.5 mg, niacinamide 2.5 mg. Tab. Bot. 100s, 1000s. *Rx.*
Use: Vitamin supplement.

Henydin-R. (Arcum) Thyroid desiccated pow. 1 g, vitamins B_1 2 mg, B_2 1 mg, B_6 1 mg, niacinamide 5 mg. Tab. Bot. 100s, 1000s. *Rx.*
Use: Vitamin supplement.

heparin.
Use: Anticoagulant.
See: Heparin Sodium and Sodium Chloride.
Heparin Sodium Injection.
Heparain Sodium Lock Flush Solution.

heparin antagonist.
See: Protamine sulfate.

•**heparin calcium.** (HEP-uh-rin KAL-see-uhm) *USP 28.*
Use: Anticoagulant.

heparin I.V. flush syringe. (Medefil) Heparin sodium 1 unit/mL. Inj. Syringe 1 mL, 2 mL, 2.5 mL, 5 mL, 10 mL. *Rx.*
Use: Anticoagulant.

heparin lock flush solution. (Sanofi-Synthelabo) **10 USP units/1 mL:** Cartridge 2 mL *HEP-PAK* containing 1 cartridge heparin lock flush soln. (1 mL) and 2 cartridges sodium Cl Inj. *HEP-PAK-2* containing 1 cartridge heparin lock flush soln. (1 mL) and 1 cartridge sodium Cl Inj. **10 USP units/2 mL:** Cartridge 2 mL. **100 USP units/1 mL:** Cartridge 2 mL *HEP-PAK* containing 1 cartridge heparin lock flush soln. (1 mL) and 2 cartridges sodium Cl Inj. *HEP-PAK-2* containing 1 cartridge of heparin lock flush soln. (1 mL) and 1 cartridge sodium Cl Inj. **100 USP units/2 mL:** Cartridge 2 mL. *Rx.*
Use: Catheter patency agent.

heparin lock flush solution. (Wyeth) Heparin sodium 10 units/mL, 100 units/mL vial. Pkg. 50 *Tubex* 1 mL, 2 mL. *Rx.*
Use: Infusion set patency agent.

•**heparin sodium.** (HEP-uh-rin) *USP 28.*
Use: Anticoagulant. Note: Protamine sulfate is antidote.
See: Hepathrom.
Hepflush-10.
Heprinar.
Lipo-Hepin.
Lipo-Hepin/BL.
Liquaemin.

heparin sodium. (Pharmacia) Heparin sodium 1000 units/mL. Vial 10 mL, 30 mL. 5000 units/mL. Vial 1 mL, 10 mL. 10,000 units/mL. Vial 1 mL, 4 mL. (Sanofi Winthrop Pharmaceuticals) 5000 USP units/1 mL. *Carpuject* 1 mL fill in 2 mL cartridge.
Use: Anticoagulant. Note: Protamine sulfate is antidote.

heparin sodium and 0.45% sodium chloride. (Abbott) Heparin sodium 12,500, 25,000 units in 250 mL Inj. *Rx.*
Use: Anticoagulant.

heparin sodium and 0.9% sodium chloride. (Baxter PPI) Heparin sodium 1000 units in 500 mL *Viaflex.* 2000 units in 1000 mL *Viaflex.* Inj. *Rx.*
Use: Anticoagulant.

heparin sodium lock flush solution. *Rx.*
Use: Anticoagulant.
See: Heparin Lock Flush.
Hepflush-10.
Hep-Lock.
Hep-Lock U/P.

heparin, 2-0-desulfated.
Use: Cystic fibrosis. [Orphan Drug]
See: Aeropin.

HepatAmine. (McGaw) Amino acid 8%. Inj. Bot. 500 mL. *Rx.*

Use: Nutritional supplement, parenteral.

Hepatic-Aid II Instant Drink Powder.
(McGaw) Amino acids (high BCAA, low AAA), maltodextrin, sucrose, partially hydrogenated soybean oil, lecithin, monoglycerides and diglycerides. In 3 oz packet of 12s. *OTC.*
Use: Nutritional supplement.

hepatitis A, inactivated and hepatitis B, recombinant vaccine.
Use: Active immunization, viral vaccine.
See: Twinrix.

hepatitis A vaccine, inactivated. (hep-uh-TIGHT-iss) *Rx.*
Use: Immunization.
See: Havrix.
Vaqta.

hepatitis B and haemophilus type b vaccines, combined.
See: Comvax.

●**hepatitis B immune globulin.** (hep-uh-TIGHT-iss B ih-myoon GLAH-byoo-lin) *USP 28.*
Use: Immunization.
See: BayHep B.
H-BIG.
Nabi-HB.

hepatitis B immune globulin IV.
Use: Prophylaxis against hepatitis B virus reinfection in liver transplant patients. [Orphan Drug]
See: H-BIGIV.

hepatitis B vaccine, recombinant. *Rx.*
Use: Immunization.
See: Engerix-B.
Recombivax HB.

hepatitis B vaccine (recombinant) and inactivated poliovirus vaccine combined, diphtheria and tetanus toxoids and acellular pertussis adsorbed.
Use: Active immunization, toxoid.
See: Diphtheria and tetanus toxoids and acellular vaccine adsorbed and hepatitis B vaccine (recombinant) and inactivated poliovirus vaccine combined.

●**hepatitis B virus vaccine inactivated.** (hep-uh-TIGHT-iss B vak-SEEN) *USP 28.*
Use: Immunization.

Hepflush-10. (American Pharmaceutical Partners) Heparin sodium 100 units/ 10 mL, preservative free. Inj. Single-dose vial 10 mL (25s). *Rx.*
Use: Catheter patency agent.

Hepfomin R Injection. (Keene Pharmaceuticals) Liver inj. equivalent to cyanocobalamin 10 mcg, folic acid 0.4 mg, cyanocobalamin 100 mcg. Vial 10 mL. *Rx.*

Use: Nutritional supplement, parenteral.

Hep-Forte. (Marlyn Nutraceuticals) Vitamins A 1200 units, E 10 mg, B$_1$ 1 mg, B$_2$ 1 mg, B$_3$ 10 mg, B$_5$ 2 mg, B$_6$ 0.5 mg, B$_{12}$ 1 mcg, C 10 mg, folic acid 0.06 mg, zinc 0.5 mg, choline, inositol, biotin, dl-methionine, desiccated liver, liver concentrate, liver fraction No. 2. Cap. Bot. 100s, 300s, 500s. *OTC.*
Use: Vitamin, liver supplement.

Hep-Lock. (Wyeth) Sterile heparin sodium soln. in saline 10 units/mL, 100 units/mL. Dosette 1 mL, 2 mL, multiple-dose vial 10 mL, 30 mL. *Rx.*
Use: Catheter patency agent.

Hep-Lock PF. (Wyeth) Preservative-free heparin flush soln. 10 units/mL, 100 units/mL. Vial 1 mL. *Rx.*
Use: Catheter patency agent.

Hepsera. (Gilead Sciences) Adefovir dipivoxil 10 mg, lactose. Tab. Bot. 30s. *Rx.*
Use: Antiviral.

Herbal Cellulex. (NBTY) Vitamin C 83 mg, K 33 mg, iron 9 mg. Tab. Bot. 90s. *OTC.*
Use: Vitamin supplement.

Herceptin. (Genentech) Trastuzumab 440 mg. Pow. for Inj., lyophilized. Vial. Preservative free. Diluent: 20 mL vial of Bacteriostatic Water for Inj. w/1.1% benzyl alcohol. *Rx.*
Use: Antineoplastic; monoclonal antibody.

Herbal Bath Oil. (Healthpoint Medical) Soybean oil-based bath oil. Bot. 8 oz, 32 oz. *OTC.*
Use: Emollient.

Herpecin-L. (Campbell Laboratories) Allantoin, octyl-p-(dimethylamino)-benzoate (Padimate O), titanium dioxide, pyridoxine hydrochloride in a balanced, acidic lipid system. Lip balm. Tube 2.5 g. *OTC.*
Use: Cold sores.

herpes simplex virus gene. (Genetic Therapy)
Use: Antineoplastic. [Orphan Drug]

Herrick Lacrimal Plug. (Lacrimedics) Silicone plug 0.3 mm, 0.5 mm Pkg. 2 plugs. *Rx.*
Use: Punctal plug.

HES. Hetastarch.
Use: Plasma expander.
See: Hespan.

Hespan Injection. (DuPont) Hetastarch 6 g, sodium Cl 0.9%/100 mL. Bot. 500 mL. *Rx.*
Use: Plasma volume expander.

hesperidin.
Use: Capillary fragility and permeability; hemorrhage.

See: Vitamin P; also Rutin.
W/Combinations.
See: A.C.N.
   Hesper Bitabs.
   Nialex.
   Vita Cebus.
hesperidin methyl chalcone.
   Use: Vitamin P supplement.
Hesperidin w/C. (Various Mfr.)
   Use: Vitamin supplement.
•**hetacillin.** (HET-ah-SILL-in) USAN.
   Use: Anti-infective.
•**hetacillin potassium.** (HET-ah-SILL-in
   poe-TASS-ee-uhm) *USP 28.*
   Use: Anti-infective.
•**hetaflur.** (HEH-tah-flure) USAN.
   Use: Dental caries prophylactic.
•**hetastarch.** (HET-uh-starch) USAN.
   Use: Plasma volume extender.
   See: Hespan.
•**heteronium bromide.** (HET-er-oh-nee-
   uhm) USAN.
   Use: Anticholinergic.
Hexabamate #1. (Rugby) Tridihexethyl
   Cl 25 mg, meprobamate 200 mg. Tab.
   Bot. 100s, 500s. *Rx.*
   Use: Anticholinergic combination.
Hexabamate #2. (Rugby) Tridihexethyl
   Cl 25 mg, meprobamate 400 mg. Tab.
   Bot. 100s, 500s. *Rx.*
   Use: Anticholinergic combination.
Hexa-Betalin. (Eli Lilly) Pyridoxine hydro-
   chloride. Inj. Vial 100 mg/mL. Ctn. 10s,
   vial 10 mL. *Rx.*
   Use: Vitamin supplement.
Hexabrix. (Mallinckrodt) Ioxaglate meglu-
   mine 393 mg, ioxaglate sodium 196 mg,
   iodine 320 mg/mL, EDTA. Inj. Vial
   20 mL, 30 mL, 50 mL. Bot. 150 mL,
   75 mL fill in 150 mL, 100 mL fill in
   150 mL, 200 mL fill in 250 mL. Power
   Inj. Syr. 125 mL, 50 mL fill in 125 mL,
   100 mL fill in 125 mL. *Rx.*
   Use: Radiopaque agent, parenteral.
•**hexachlorophene.** (hex-ah-KLOR-oh-
   feen) *USP 28.*
   Use: Anti-infective, topical; antiseptic;
   detergent.
   See: Derl.
   Gamophen, Leaves.
   pHisoHex.
hexachlorophene cleansing emulsion.
   Use: Anti-infective, topical detergent.
**hexachlorophene liquid soap, deter-
   gent liquid.**
   Use: Anti-infective, topical detergent.
   See: pHisoHex.
hexacose. Mixture of C-6 alcohols derived from oxidation of tetracosane
   $C_{24}H_{50}$.

hexadecadrol.
   See: Dexamethasone.
hexadienol. Hexacose.
Hexadrol Phosphate. (Organon Teknika)
   Dexamethasone sodium phosphate
   4 mg/mL, 10 mg/mL, 20 mg/mL, benzyl
   alcohol. **4 mg/mL:** Vial 1 mL, 5 mL,
   disposable syringe 1 mL. **10 mg/mL:**
   Vial 10 mL, disposable syringe 1 mL.
   20 mg/mL: Vial 5 mL, disposable syringe 5 mL. *Rx.*
   Use: Corticosteroid.
•**hexafluorenium bromide.** (HEK-sah-
   flure-EE-nee-uhm) USAN.
   Use: Muscle relaxant, synergist (succi-
   nycholine).
hexafluorodiethyl ether. Name used for
   Flurothyl.
hexahydroxycyclohexane.
   See: Inositol.
hexakose. Mixture of tetracosanes and
   oxidation products.
Hexalen. (MGI Pharma) Altretamine
   50 mg, lactose. Cap. Bot. 100s. *Rx.*
   Use: Antineoplastic.
hexamethonium chloride. (Various Mfr.)
   Hexamethylene (bistrimethylammo-
   nium) chloride.
hexamethylamine.
   Use: Hypotensive.
   See: Hexastat.
hexamethylenamine.
   See: Methenamine.
hexamethylenetetramine.
   See: Methenamine.
hexamethylmelamine. Altretamine.
   Use: Antineoplastic.
   See: Hexalen.
hexamethylpararosaniline chloride.
   See: Bismuth violet.
hexamethylrosaniline chloride.
   See: Gentian violet.
hexamine.
   See: Methenamine.
•**hexaminolevulinate hydrochloride.**
   (hex-a-MIN-oh-le-VUE-lin-ate) USAN.
   Use: Diagnostic agent, bladder cancer.
hexapradol hydrochloride.
   Use: CNS stimulant.
Hexate. (Davis & Sly) Atropine sulfate
   $\frac{1}{2000}$ g, extract of hyoscyamus 0.25 g,
   methylene blue g, methanamine 0.5 g,
   benzoic acid 0.5 g, salol 0.5 g. Tab. Bot.
   1000s. *Rx.*
   Use: Anti-infective, urinary.
Hexavitamin SC. (Halsey Drug)
   Use: Vitamin supplement.
Hexavitamin Tablets. (Various Mfr.) Vitamins A 5000 units, B_1 2 mg, B_2 3 mg,
   B_3 20 mg, C 75 mg, D 400 units. Bot.
   100s, 1000s, UD 100s. *OTC.*

Use: Vitamin supplement.
hexcarbacholine bromide.
•**hexedine.** (HEX-eh-deen) USAN.
Use: Anti-infective.
hexene-ol. Hexacose.
hexenol. Hexacose.
hexitol irrigants.
Use: Irrigant, genitourinary.
See: Resectisol.
Sorbitol.
Sorbitol-mannitol.
hexobarbital. *Name previously used*
Hexobarbitone.
•**hexobendine.** (HEX-oh-BEN-deen)
USAN.
Use: Vasodilator.
Hexopal. (Bayer Corp. (Consumer Div.))
Inositol hexanicotinate. *Rx.*
Use: Hypolipidemic; peripheral vasodi-
lator.
•**hexoprenaline sulfate.** (hex-oh-PREN-
ah-leen) USAN.
Use: Tocolytic.
•**hexylene glycol.** *NF 23.*
Use: Pharmaceutic aid (humectant, sol-
vent).
•**hexylresorcinol.** (hex-ill-reh-SORE-sih-
nole) *USP 28.*
Use: Anthelmintic (intestinal round-
worms and trematodes); throat
preparation.
See: Sucrets Sore Throat.
H-F Gel. (Paddock) Calcium gluconate
gel 2.5%.
Use: Emergency burn treatment.
[Orphan Drug]
H.H.R. (Geneva) Hydralazine hydrochlo-
ride 25 mg, hydrochlorothiazide 15 mg,
reserpine 0.1 mg. Tab. Bot. 100s,
1000s. *Rx.*
Use: Antihypertensive.
Hibiclens. (J & J Merck Consumer
Pharm.) Chlorhexidine gluconate 4%,
isopropyl alcohol 4%, in a nonalkaline
base. Bot. 4 oz, 8 oz, 16 oz, 32 oz, gal.
Packette 15 mL. *OTC.*
Use: Antimicrobial; antiseptic.
Hibiclens Sponge Brush. (J & J Merck
Consumer Pharm.) Chlorhexidine glu-
conate impregnated sponge brush.
Unit-of-use 22 mL sponge brushes.
OTC.
Use: Antimicrobial; antiseptic.
Hibistat. (J & J Merck Consumer Pharm.)
Chlorhexidine gluconate 0.5%. **Liq.:**
Isopropyl alcohol 70%, emollients. Bot.
4 oz, 8 oz. **Towelettes:** Unit-of-use
pocket-size towelette impregnated with
5 mL. *OTC.*
Use: Antimicrobial; antiseptic.

Hibplex. (Standex) Vitamins B_1 100 mg,
B_2 2 mg, B_3 100 mg, panthenol 2 mg/
mL. Vial 30 mL. *Rx.*
Use: Vitamin supplement.
HibTITER. (Wyeth-Lederle) Purified *Hae-*
mophilus b saccharide capsular oligo-
saccharide 10 mcg, diphtheria CRM_{197}
protein ≈ 25 mcg per 0.5 mL; thimerosal 1:10,000 (multidose vial). Inj.
Vials 1, 10 dose. *Rx.*
Use: Immunization.
Hi B with C. (Towne) Vitamin C 300 mg,
B_1 15 mg, B_2 10.2 mg, B_6 5 mg, niacin
50 mg, pantothenic acid 10 mg. Cap.
Bot. 100s. *Rx.*
Use: Vitamin supplement.
Hi-Cor 1.0. (C & M Pharmacal) Hydro-
cortisone 1% in a nonionic, ester-free,
salt-free, paraben-free washable base.
Tube 30 g, Jar 60 g. *Rx.*
Use: Corticosteroid, topical.
Hi-Cor 2.5. (C & M Pharmacal) Hydro-
cortisone 2.5% in a nonionic, ester-
free, salt-free, paraben-free washable
base. Tube 30 g. Jar 60 g. *Rx.*
Use: Corticosteroid, topical.
hiestrone.
See: Estrone.
High B12. (Barth's) Vitamin B_{12}, desic-
cated liver. Cap. Bot. 100s, 500s. *OTC.*
Use: Vitamin supplement.
High Potency Cold Cap. (Weeks & Leo)
Salicylamide 325 mg, chlorpheniramine
maleate 4 mg, dextromethorphan HBr
15 mg, caffeine 16.2 mg. Tab. Bot. 18s.
OTC.
Use: Analgesic; antihistamine; antitus-
sive.
high potency insulin.
Use: Antidiabetic.
See: Humulin R Regular U-500 (Con-
centrated).
Insulin Injection Concentrated.
High Potency N-Vites. (Nion Corp.) Vita-
mins B_1 15 mg, B_2 10 mg, B_3 100 mg,
B_5 20 mg, B_{12} 10 mcg, C 500 mg. Tab.
Bot. 100s. *OTC.*
Use: Vitamin supplement.
High Potency Pain Relievers. (Weeks
& Leo) Acetaminophen 300 mg, sali-
cylamide 300 mg. Cap. Bot. 20s, 40s.
OTC.
Use: Analgesic.
High Potency Vitamins and Minerals.
(Burgin-Arden) Vitamins A 25,000 units,
D 400 units, B_1 10 mg, B_2 5 mg, B_6
1 mg, B_{12} 5 mcg, C 150 mg, niacin-
amide 100 mg, calcium 103 mg, phos-
phorus 80 mg, iron 10 mg, magnesium
5.5 mg, manganese 1 mg, potassium
5 mg, zinc 1.4 mg. Tab. Bot.

100s. *OTC.*
Use: Mineral, vitamin supplement.
• **hilafilcon A.** (high-lah-FILL-kahn A) USAN.
Use: Contact lens material (hydrophilic).
• **hilafilcon B.** (high-lah-FILL-kahn B) USAN.
Use: Contact lens material (hydrophilic).
Hill-Shade Lotion. (Hill Dermaceuticals) Para-aminobenzoic acid, alcohol 65%. SPF 22. *OTC.*
Use: Sunscreen.
• **hioxifilcon A.** (high-ock-sih-FILL-kahn A) USAN.
Use: Contact lens material (hydrophilic).
Hipotest. (Marlop) Ca 53.5 mg, iron 50 mg, vitamins A 10,000 units, D 400 units, E 2.5 mg, B_1 25 mg, B_2 25 mg, B_3 50 mg, B_5 13 mg, B_6 15 mg, B_{12} 50 mcg, C 150 mg, choline, betaine, PABA, rutin, bioflavonoids, biotin 1 mg, desiccated liver, bone meal, Cu, Mg, Mn, Zn 2.2 mg, I, P, lecithin. Tab. Bot. 100s. *OTC.*
Use: Mineral, vitamin supplement.
Hi-Po-Vites Tablets. (Hudson Corp.) Iron 6 mg, vitamins A 10,000 units, D 400 units, E 13 mg, B_1 25 mg, B_2 25 mg, B_3 50 mg, B_5 12.5 mg, B_6 15 mg, B_{12} 50 mcg, C 150 mg, folic acid 0.4 mg, Ca, Cr, Cu, I, K, Mg, Mn, Mo, P, Se, Zn 5 mg, biotin 1 mg, bioflavonoids, bone meal, PABA, choline bitartrate, betaine, inositol, lecithin, desiccated liver, rutin. Tab. Bot. 100s. *OTC.*
Use: Mineral, vitamin supplement.
hippramine.
See: Methenamine hippurate.
hipputope. (Bristol-Myers Squibb) Radioiodinated sodium iodohippurate (^{131}I) Inj. Bot. 1 m Ci, 2 m Ci.
Use: Diagnostic aid.
Hiprex. (Hoechst) Methenamine hippurate 1 g. Tab. Bot. 100s. *Rx.*
Use: Anti-infective, urinary.
Histacol DM. (Breckenridge) Pseudoephedrine hydrochloride 30 mg, brompheniramine maleate 2 mg, dextromethorphan hydrobromide 5 mg, guaifenesin 50 mg per 5 mL. Alcohol free. Corn syrup, sorbitol. Grape flavor. Syrup. 473 mL. *Rx.*
Use: Antitussive and expectorant.
Histade. (Breckenridge) Pseudoephedrine hydrochloride 120 mg, chlorpheniramine maleate 12 mg, sucrose. SR Cap. Tab. Bot. 100s. *Rx.*
Use: Upper respiratory combination, antihistamine, decongestant.

Histagesic Modified Tablets. (Jones Pharma) Phenylephrine hydrochloride 10 mg, chlorpheniramine maleate 4 mg, acetaminophen 324 mg. Tab. Bot. 1000s. *OTC.*
Use: Analgesic, antihistamine, decongestant.
Histalet. (Solvay) Pseudoephedrine hydrochloride 45 mg, chlorpheniramine maleate 3 mg/5 mL. Syr. Bot. 473 mL. *Rx.*
Use: Antihistamine, decongestant.
Histalet X. (Solvay) **Syr.:** Pseudoephedrine hydrochloride 45 mg, guaifenesin 200 mg/5 mL, alcohol 15%. Bot. 480 mL. **Tab.:** Pseudoephedrine hydrochloride 120 mg, guaifenesin 400 mg. Tab. Bot. 100s. *Rx.*
Use: Decongestant, expectorant.
• **histamine dihydrochloride.** (HISS-tah-meen die-HIGH-droe-KLOR-ide) *USP 28.*
Use: Analgesic, topical.
histamine H$_2$ antagonists.
See: Cimetidine.
Famotidine.
Nizatidine.
Ranitidine Hydrochloride.
W/Combinations.
See: Pepcid Complete.
Histatab Plus. (Century) Phenylephrine hydrochloride 5 mg, chlorpheniramine maleate 2 mg. Tab. Bot. 30s, 100s, 1000s. *OTC.*
Use: Upper respiratory combination, decongestant, antihistamine.
Histatrol. (Center) 2.75 mg/mL histamine phosphate, equivalent to 1 mg/mL histamine base, in 50% glycerin w/v, 5 mL vial; available in a Multitest dosage form or dropper bottle; 0.275 mg/mL histamine phosphate, equivalent to 0.1 mg/mL histamine base, 5 mL vial.
Use: Diagnostic aid, skin test control.
Hista-Vent DA. (Ethex) Phenylephrine hydrochloride 20 mg, chlorpheniramine maleate 8 mg, methscopolamine nitrate 2.5 mg. SR Tab. Bot. 100s. *Rx.*
Use: Upper respiratory combination, decongestant, antihistamine, anticholinergic.
Histenol-Forte. (Zee Medical) Acetaminophen 325 mg, pseudoephedrine hydrochloride 30 mg, dextromethorphan HBr 10 mg. Tab. 24s. *OTC.*
Use: Antitussive combination.
Histex CT. (Teamm Pharm) Carbinoxamine maleate 8 mg. Film coated. TR Tab. Bot. 30s, 100s. *Rx.*
Use: Antihistamine, nonselective ethanolamine.

Histex HC. (Teamm Pharm) Pseudo-ephedrine hydrochloride 30 mg, hydro-codone bitartrate 5 mg, carbinoxamine maleate 2 mg/5 mL, saccharin, sorbitol, alcohol free, peach flavor. Liq. Bot. 473 mL. *c-III.*
Use: Decongestant, antitussive, antihis-tamine.

Histex I/E. (Teamm Pharm) Carbinox-amine maleate 10 mg. ER Cap. 60s. *Rx.*
Use: Antihistamine.

Histex Pd. (Teamm Pharm) Carbinox-amine maleate 4 mg/5 mL. Dye, alco-hol, and sugar free. Saccharin, sorbitol, gum fruit flavor. Liq. Bot. 473 mL. *Rx.*
Use: Antihistamine.

Histex SR. (Teamm Pharm) Pseudo-ephedrine hydrochloride 120 mg, brom-pheniramine maleate 10 mg. ER Cap. Bot. 30s, 100s. *Rx.*
Use: Upper respiratory combination, an-tihistamine, decongestant.

•**histidine.** (HISS-tih-deen) *USP 28.*
Use: Amino acid.
W/Combinations.
See: Monarc-M.

histidine monohydrochloride.
Use: I.M., peptic and jejunal ulcers.

Histine-8. (Freeport) Chlorpheniramine maleate 8 mg. TR Tab. Bot. 1000s. *OTC.*
Use: Antihistamine.

Histine-50. (Freeport) Diphenhydramine hydrochloride 50 mg. Cap. Bot. 1000s. *OTC.*
Use: Antihistamine, antitussive; anticho-linergic; antiemetic; sedative.

Histine-4. (Freeport) Chlorpheniramine maleate 4 mg. Tab. Bot. 1000s. *OTC.*
Use: Antihistamine.

Histine-1. (Freeport) Diphenhydramine hydrochloride 10 mg, alcohol 12% to 14%/4 mL. Bot. 4 oz. *OTC.*
Use: Antihistamine, antitussive; anticho-linergic; antiemetic; sedative.

Histine-12. (Freeport) Chlorpheniramine maleate 12 mg. TR Tab. Bot. 1000s. *OTC.*
Use: Antihistamine.

Histine-25. (Freeport) Diphenhydramine hydrochloride 25 mg. Cap. Bot. 1000s. *OTC.*
Use: Antihistamine, antitussive; anticho-linergic; antiemetic; sedative.

Histine-2. (Freeport) Diphenhydramine hydrochloride 12.5 mg/5 mL w/alcohol 5%. Bot. 4 oz. *OTC.*
Use: Antihistamine, antitussive; anticho-linergic; antiemetic; sedative.

Histinex-D. (Ethex) Hydrocodone bitar-trate 5 mg, pseudoephedrine hydro-chloride 60 mg/5 mL. Liq. Bot. 480 mL, 960 mL. *c-III.*
Use: Antitussive, decongestant.

Histinex HC. (Ethex) Hydrocodone bitar-trate 2.5 mg, phenylephrine hydrochlo-ride 5 mg, chlorpheniramine maleate 2 mg/5 mL, sorbitol, saccharin, fruit fla-vor, alcohol free. Syr. Bot. 473 mL, 946 mL. *c-III.*
Use: Upper respiratory combination, an-titussive, decongestant, antihistamine.

Histinex PV. (Ethex) Hydrocodone bitar-trate 2.5 mg, pseudoephedrine hydro-chloride 30 mg, chlorpheniramine maleate 2 mg/5 mL, parabens, saccha-rin, sorbitol, alcohol free. Syr. Bot. 473 mL. *c-III.*
Use: Upper respiratory combination, an-tihistamine, antitussive, deconges-tant.

Histolyn-CYL. (ALK) Histoplasmin sterile filtrate from yeast cells of *Histoplasma capsulatum.* Vial 1.3 mL. *Rx.*
Use: Diagnostic aid, skin test.

•**histoplasmin.** (hiss-toe-PLAZZ-min) *USP 28.* (Parke-Davis) An aqueous so-lution containing standardized sterile culture filtrate of *Histoplasma capsula-tum* grown on liquid synthetic medium.
Use: Diagnostic aid (dermal reactivity indicator).
See: Histolyn-CYL.

Histoplasmin, diluted.

histoplasmin, diluted. (Parke-Davis) 1:100 w/v. Standardized sterile filtrate from cultures of *Histoplasma capsula-tum,* 0.5% phenol, polysorbate 80. 1 mL. Inj. *Rx.*
Use: Diagnostic aid.

•**histrelin.** (hiss-TRELL-in) USAN.
Use: LHRH agonist; treatment of por-phyria. [Orphan Drug]
See: Supprelin.

histrelin acetate.
Use: Treatment of advanced prostate cancer.
See: Vantas.

Histussin D. (Sanofi-Synthelabo) Hydro-codone bitartrate 5 mg, pseudoephed-rine hydrochloride 60 mg/5 mL. Liq. Bot. 473 mL. *c-III.*
Use: Upper respiratory combination, an-titussive, decongestant.

Histussin HC. (Sanofi-Synthelabo) Phenylephrine hydrochloride 5 mg, chlorpheniramine maleate 2 mg, hydro-codone bitartrate 2.5 mg/5 mL, orange/ pineapple flavor, alcohol free. Syr. Bot. 473 mL. *c-III.*

Use: Upper respiratory combination, antihistamine, decongestant, antitussive.

Hitone. (Lafayette) Barium sulfate suspension 125% w/v. Bot. 2000 mL. Case 4s.
Use: Radiopaque agent.

Hi-Tor. (Barth's) B_1 6 mg, B_2 12 mg, B_6 54 mcg, Vitamins B_{12} 15 mcg, niacin 1.5 mg, pantothenic acid 150 mcg, choline 3.75 mg, inositol 5.25 mg. Tab. Bot. 100s, 500s, 1000s. *OTC.*
Use: Vitamin supplement.

Hi-Tor 900. (Barth's) Vitamins B_1 13.5 mg, B_2 5.2 mg, B_6 0.6 mg, B_{12} 2.5 mcg, niacin 15 mg, pantothenic acid 1.2 mg, biotin, iron 0.9 mg, protein 7.5 g, inositol 50 mg, choline 40 mg, aminobenzoic acid 0.15 to 2.4 mg/15 g. Bot. 1 lb, 3 lb. *OTC.*
Use: Mineral, vitamin supplement.

HIVAG HIV-1/HIV-2 (rDNA) EIA. (Abbott) Enzyme immunoassay for qualitative detection of antibodies to human immunodeficiency virus type 1 or type 2 in human serum or plasma. Test kits 100s, 1000s, 5000s.
Use: Diagnostic aid.

Hi-Vegi-Lip Tablets. (Freeda) Pancreatin 2400 mg, lipase 12,000 units, protease 60,000 units, amylase 60,000 units. Tab. Bot. 100s, 250s. *OTC.*
Use: Digestive aid.

Hivid. (Roche) Zalcitabine 0.375 mg, 0.75 mg, lactose. Tab. Bot. 100s. *Rx.*
Use: Antiretroviral, nucleoside reverse transcriptase inhibitor.

Hivig. (NABI) Human immunodeficiency virus immune globulin.
Use: Antiviral, HIV. [Orphan Drug]

Hiwolfia. (Jones Pharma) Rauwolfia 25 mg, 50 mg, 100 mg. Tab. Bot. 100s, 1000s.
Use: Antihypertensive.

HMG-CoA reductase inhibitors.
Use: Antihyperlipidemic.
See: Atorvastatin calcium.
Fluvastatin sodium.
Lovastatin.
Pravastatin sodium.
Rosuvastatin calcium.
Simvastatin.

HMM.
See: Hexamethylmelamine.

HMS. (Allergan) Medrysone 1%. Ophth. Susp. Bot. 5 mL, 10 mL. *Rx.*
Use: Anti-inflammatory, ophthalmic.

HN₂. Mechlorethamine hydrochloride.
Use: Antineoplastic.
See: Mustargen.

H 9600. (Cypress) Pseudoephedrine hydrochloride 90 mg, guaifenesin 600 mg, dye free. SR Tab. Bot. 100s. *Rx.*
Use: Upper respiratory combination, decongestant, expectorant.

•**hofocon A.** (hoe-FOE-kon) USAN.
Use: Hydrophobic.

H₂ OEX. (Fellows) Benzthiazide 50 mg. Tab. Bot. 100s, 1000s. *Rx.*
Use: Diuretic.

Hold. (GlaxoSmithKline) Dextromethorphan HBr 5 mg. Loz. Plastic tube 10 oz. *OTC.*
Use: Antitussive.

Hold DM. (B.F. Ascher) Dextromethorphan HBr 5 mg, corn syrup, sucrose, cherry flavor. Loz. Pkg. 10s. *OTC.*
Use: Antitussive.

holocaine hydrochloride. (Various Mfr.) Phenacaine hydrochloride.
Use: Anesthetic, local.

homarylamine hydrochloride. N-Methyl-3,4-methylenedioxyphenethylamine hydrochloride.

•**homatropine hydrobromide.** (hoe-MA-troe-peen) *USP 28.*
Use: Anticholinergic, ophthalmic; mydriatic, cycloplegic.
See: Homatropine HBr.
Isopto Homatropine.
Murocoll.

homatropine hydrobromide. (Various Mfr.) Homatropine HBr 5% Soln. Bot. 1 mL, 2 mL, 5 mL. *Rx.*
Use: Mydriatic, cycloplegic.

homatropine hydrochloride.
Use: Anticholinergic, topical; mydriatic, cycloplegic.

•**homatropine methylbromide.** (hoe-MA-troe-peen) *USP 28.*
Use: Anticholinergic.
W/Combinations.
See: Hycodan.
Hydromet.
Hydromide.
Hydropane.
Panitol H.M.B.
Spasmatol.
Tapuline.
Tussigon.

homatropine methylbromide and phenobarbital combinations.
Use: Anticholinergic.
See: Gustase Plus.

Hominex-1. (Ross) Protein 15 g, fat 23.9 g, carbohydrate 46.3 g, linoleic acid 1800 mg, Fe 9 mg, Na 190 mg, K 675 mg, Ca, vitamins A, B_1, B_2, B_3, B_5, B_6, B_{12}, C, D, E, K, biotin, choline, folic acid, inositol, Cl, Cu, I, Mg, Mn, P, Se, Zn and 480 Cal per 100 g.

Methionine free. Pow. Can 350 g. *OTC.*
Use: Nutritional supplement.
Hominex-2. (Ross) Protein 30 g, fat
15.5 g, carbohydrate 30 g, Fe 13 mg,
Na 880 mg, K 1370 mg, Ca, vitamins A,
B_1, B_2, B_3, B_5, B_6, B_{12}, C, D, E, K, bio-
tin, choline, folic acid, inositol, Cl, Cu,
I, Mg, Mn, P, Se, Zn and 410 Cal per
100 g. Methionine free. Pow. Can
325 g. *OTC.*
Use: Nutritional supplement.
Homogene-S. (Spanner) Testosterone
25 mg/mL, 50 mg/mL, 100 mg/mL. Vial
10 mL. *c-III.*
Use: Androgen.
•**homosalate.** (hoe-moe-SAL-ate) USAN.
Formerly Homomenthyl Salicylate.
Use: Ultraviolet screen.
W/Combinations.
See: Coppertone.
honey bee venom.
See: Albay.
Pharmalgen.
Venomil.
•**hoquizil hydrochloride.** (HOE-kwih-zill)
USAN.
Use: Bronchodilator.
hormofollin.
See: Estrone.
hormones.
See: Anastrozole.
Androgens.
Antiandrogens.
Antioestrogens.
Bicalutamide.
Cetrorelix Acetate.
Choriogonadotropin Alfa.
Clomiphene Citrate.
Diethylstilbestrol Dipropionate.
Estramustine Phosphate Sodium.
Estrogen/Nitrogen Mustard.
Flutamide.
Fulvestrant.
Ganirelix Acetate.
Gonadotropin-Releasing Hormone
Analog.
Goserelin Acetate.
Histrelin Acetate.
Intrauterine Progesterone Contracep-
tive System.
Letrozole.
Leuprolide Acetate.
Lovonorgestrel-Releasing Intrauterine
System.
Medroxyprogesterone Acetate.
Medroxyprogesterone Acetate/Estra-
diol Cypionate.
Medroxyprogesterone Contraceptive
Injection.
Megestrol Acetate.
Nilutamide.

Raloxifene.
Tamoxifen Citrate.
Testolactone.
Toremifene Citrate.
Triptorelin Pamoate.
hormones, contraceptive.
Use: Contraceptive hormones.
hormones, growth.
Use: Growth hormones.
hormones, posterior pituitary.
Use: Posterior pituitary hormones.
hormones, sex.
Use: Sex hormones.
hornet venom.
See: Albay.
Pharmalgen.
Venomil.
•**horse chestnut.** *NF 23.*
Use: Anti-inflammatory.
Hospital Foam Cleaner. (Health & Medi-
cal Techniques) 0-phenylphenol 0.1%,
4-chloro-2-cyclopentyl-phenol 0.08%,
lauric diethanolamide 0.2%, triethanol-
amine dodecylbenzenesulfonate 0.3%.
Aerosol spray 19 oz.
Use: Antimicrobial; disinfectant.
Hospital Lotion. (Paddock) Diisobutyl-
cresoxyethoxy-ethyl dimethyl benzyl
ammonium chloride, menthol, lanolin,
mineral and vegetable oils. Bot. 4 oz,
8 oz, gal. *OTC.*
Use: Emollient.
H.P. Acthar Gel. (Aventis) Repository
corticotropin injection 80 units/ml, gelatin 16%. Multidose vial 5 mL. *Rx.*
Use: Corticosteroid.
HRC-Tylaprin. (Cenci, H.R. Labs, Inc.)
Acetaminophen 120 mg, alcohol 7%/
5 mL. Elix. Bot. 2 oz, 4 oz. *OTC.*
Use: Analgesic.
H-R Lubricating Jelly. (Wallace)
Hydroxypropyl methycellulose, para-
bens. Jelly 150 g. *OTC.*
Use: Lubricant.
H.S. Need. (Hanlon) Chloral hydrate
3¾ g, 7.5 g. Cap. Bot. 100s. *Rx.*
Use: Sedative.
HSV-1. (Wampole) Herpes simplex virus
type 1 test system. For the qualitative
and semi-quantitative detection of HSV-
1 antibody in human serum. Test 100s.
Use: Diagnostic aid.
HSV-2. (Wampole) Herpes simplex virus
type 2 antibody test. For the qualita-
tive and semi-quantitative detection of
HSV-2 antibody in human serum. Test
100s.
Use: Diagnostic aid.
H.T. Factorate. (Centeon) Antihemophilic
factor (human) dried, heat treated for
IV administration only. Single-dose vial

w/diluent and needles. *Rx.*
Use: Antihemophilic.
H.T. Factorate Generation II. (Centeon)
Antihemophilic factor (human) dried,
heat treated for IV administration only.
Single-dose vial w/diluent and needles.
Rx.
Use: Antihemophilic.
HTSH EIA. (Abbott Diagnostics) Enzyme
immunoassay for the quantitative deter-
mination of human thyroid-stimulating
hormone (TSH) in human serum or
plasma.
Use: Diagnostic aid.
HTSH RIAbead. (Abbott Diagnostics) Im-
munoradiometric assay for the quantita-
tive measurement of human thyroid-
stimulating hormone (TSH) in serum.
Use: Diagnostic aid.
5-HT$_3$ receptor antagonists.
See: Alosetron hydrochloride.
Dolasetron mesylate.
Granisetron hydrochloride.
Ondansetron hydrochloride.
Palonosetron hydrochloride.
H-Tuss-D. (Cypress) Hydrocodone bitar-
trate 5 mg, pseudoephedrine hydro-
chloride 60 mg/5 mL, Liq. Bot. 473 mL.
Rx.
Use: Expectorant.
**Hulk Hogan Multi-Vitamins Plus Extra
C.** (S.G. Labs, Inc.) Vitamins A
2500 units, E 15 units, D$_3$ 400 units, B$_1$
1.05 mg, B$_2$ 1.2 mg, B$_3$ 13.5 mg, B$_6$
1.05 mg, B$_{12}$ 4.5 mcg, C 300 mg, folic
acid 300 mcg, sucrose. Chew. Tab. Bot.
60s. *OTC.*
Use: Mineral, vitamin supplement.
Humalog. (Lilly) Human insulin lispro
(rDNA) 100 units/mL. Inj. Vials. 10 mL.
Cartridges. 5 × 1.5 mL, 5 × 3 mL.
Disp. pen insulin delivery devices.
5 × 3 mL. *Rx.*
Use: Antidiabetic, insulin.
Humalog Mix 50/50. (Eli Lilly) Human insulin lispro (rDNA) 100 units/mL, protamine sulfate 0.19 mg. Inj. Vial 10 mL,
Cartridge 5 × 3 mL, Disp. insulin delivery device 5 × 3 mL. *Rx.*
Use: Antidiabetic.
Humalog Mix 75/25. (Lilly) Human insulin lispro (rDNA) 100 units/mL, protamine sulfate 0.28 mg. Contains 75% insulin lispro protamine suspension and
25% insulin lispro injection (rDNA). Inj.
Disp. pen insulin delivery devices. 5 ×
3 mL. Vials. 10 mL. *Rx.*
Use: Antidiabetic, insulin.
human acid alphaglucosidase. (Phar-
main BV)
Use: Glycogen storage disease type II.

[Orphan Drug]
human albumin grifols. (Grifols) Hu-
man albumin 25%. Inj. 50 mL, 100 mL.
Rx.
Use: Plasma expander.
human albumin microspheres.
Use: Radiopaque agent, parenteral.
See: Optison.
human antihemophilic factor.
See: Antihemophilic.
human B-type natriuretic peptide.
Use: Vasodilator.
See: Nesiritide.
human growth hormone. (Nutritional
Restart)
Use: With glutamine in the treatment of
short bowel syndrome. [Orphan Drug]
human growth hormone function test.
See: R-Gene 10.
•**human insulin.** *USP 28.* Insulin Human.
Use: Hypoglycemic.
See: Humulin.
humanized anti-tac.
Use: Immunosuppressant. [Orphan
Drug]
See: Zenapax.
human serum albumin.
See: Albumotope.
**human thyroid-stimulating hormone
(THS).**
Use: Diagnostic aid. [Orphan Drug]
**human t-lymphotropic virus type III gp
160 antigens.**
Use: AIDS. [Orphan Drug]
See: Vaxsyn HIV-1.
Humate-P. (Aventis Behring) Antihemophilic factor and von Willebrand factor: Ristocetin cofactor (vWF/RCo)
250 units/500 units per vial, 500 units/
1,000 units per vial, 1,000 units/
2,000 units per vial. When reconstituted, each milliliter contains Factor VIII
activity 20 to 40 units, vWF/RCo activity 50 to 100 units, glycine 15 to
33 mg, sodium citrate 3.5 to 9.3 mg,
sodium chloride 2 to 5.3 mg, albumin
(human) 4 to 8 mg, other proteins 1 to
7 mg, total proteins 5 to 15 mg. Contains anti-A and anti-B blood group iso-
agglutinins. Heat-treated. Pow. for Inj.,
lyophilized. Single-dose vials with
10 mL (250 units/500 units), 20 mL
(500 units/1,000 units), 30 mL
(1,000 units/2,000 units) diluent, sterile
tranfer set for reconstitution, and a
sterile filter spike for withdrawal. *Rx.*
Use: Antihemophilic agent.
Humatin. (Parke-Davis) Paromomycin
sulfate 250 mg. Cap. Bot. 16s. *Rx.*
Use: Amebicide.

Humatrope. (Eli Lilly) Somatropin. 5 mg (≈ 15 units/vial). Vial. Mannitol 25 mg, glycine 5 mg with 5 mL diluent (Water for Injection with metacresol 0.3%, glycerin 1.7%). 6 mg (18 units/cartridge). Cartridge w/prefilled syr. of diluent (mannitol 18 mg, glycine 6 mg, Water for Injection with metacresol 0.3%). 12 mg (36 units/cartridge). Cartridge w/prefilled syr. of diluent (mannitol 36 mg, glycine 12 mg, Water for Injection with metacresol 0.3%). 24 mg (72 units/cartridge). Cartridge w/prefilled syr. of diluent (mannitol 72 mg, glycine 24 mg, Water for Injection with metacresol 0.3%). Pow. for Inj. (lyophilized). *Rx.*
Use: Hormone, growth.

Humibid DM. (Carolina Pharmaceuticals) Dextromethorphan HBr 50 mg, guaifenesin 400 mg, potassium guaiacolsulfonate 200 mg. Sucrose. ER Cap. Bot. 30s, 100s. *Rx.*
Use: Upper respiratory combination, antitussive, expectorant.

Humira. (Abbott) Adalimumab 40 mg/ 0.8 mL, preservative free. Inj. In prefilled syringes and alcohol preps. *Rx.*
Use: Immunomodulator.

HuMist. (Scherer) Sodium Cl 0.65%, chlorobutanol. Soln. Bot. 45 mL. *OTC.*
Use: Nasal decongestant.

Humulin 50/50. (Lilly) Human insulin (rDNA) 100 units/mL. Inj. Vials. 10 mL. *OTC.*
Use: Antidiabetic, insulin.

Humulin L. (Lilly) Human insulin (rDNA) 100 units/mL. Inj. Vials. 10 mL. *OTC.*
Use: Antidiabetic, insulin.

Humulin N. (Lilly) Human insulin (rDNA) 100 units/mL. Inj. Disp. pen insulin delivery device 5 × 3 mL, Vials. 10 mL. *OTC.*
Use: Antidiabetic, insulin.

Humulin R. (Lilly) Regular insulin (rDNA) 100 units/mL. Inj. Vials. 10 mL. *OTC.*
Use: Antidiabetic, insulin.

Humulin R Regular U-500 (Concentrated). (Eli Lilly) Human insulin (rDNA) 500 units/mL, m-cresol 2.5 mg, glycerin 16 mg/mL. Inj. Vial 20 mL. *Rx.*
Use: Antidiabetic, insulin.

Humulin 70/30. (Lilly) Human insulin (rDNA) 100 units/mL. Inj. Disp. pen insulin delivery devices. 5 × 3 mL. Vials. 10 mL. *OTC.*
Use: Antidiabetic, insulin.

Humulin U. (Lilly) Human insulin (rDNA) 100 units/mL. Inj. Vials. 10 mL. *OTC.*
Use: Antidiabetic, insulin.

Hurricaine. (Beutlich) Benzocaine 20%. **Liq.:** 0.25 mL, 3.75 mL, 30 mL. **Gel:** 3.75 mL, 30 g. **Spray:** 60 mL. *OTC.*
Use: Anesthetic, topical.

Hurricaine Topical Anesthetic Spray Kit. (Beutlich) Benzocaine 20%. Kit: Aerosol 60 g plus 200 disposable extension tubes. *OTC.*
Use: Anesthetic, topical.

HVS 1 & 2. (Chemi-Tech Laboratories) Benzalkonium Cl in a specially formulated base. Soln. Bot. 15 mL. *OTC.*
Use: Cold sores, fever blisters, herpes virus.

Hyacide. (Niltig) Benzethonium chloride 0.1%, sodium nitrite 0.55%. Soln. Bot. oz. *OTC.*
Use: Antiseptic.

Hyalex. (Miller Pharmacal Group) Magnesium salicylate 260 mg, magnesium p-aminobenzoate 163 mg, vitamins A 1500 units, C 30 mg, D 100 units, E 3 units, B$_{12}$ 2 mcg, pantothenic acid 5 mg, zinc 0.7 mg. Tab. Bot. 100s. *OTC.*
Use: Mineral, vitamin supplement.

Hyalgan. (Sanofi-Synthelabo) Sodium hyaluronate 20 mg/2 mL. Vial 2 mL, Prefilled Syr. *Rx.*
Use: Antiarthritic.

hyalidase.
See: Hyaluronidase.

hyaluronic acid.
Use: Physical adjunct, correction of facial wrinkles and folds.
See: Restylane.

hyaluronic acid derivatives.
See: Hyalgan.
Orthovisc.
Supartz.
Synvisc.

●**hyaluronidase.** (hyo al ur ON i dase)
Use: Physical adjunct.
See: Amphadase
Vitrase.

●**hyaluronidase injection.** (high-uhl-yur-AHN-ih-dase) *USP 28.* Hyalidase, Hydase Enzymes which depolymerize hyaluronic acid. Hyalase, Rondase.
Use: Hypodermoclyses, promotion of diffusion, spreading agent.
See: Wydase.

hyamagnate. Hydroxy-Aluminum-Magnesium-Aminoacetate, Sodium-free.

Hyate:C (Porcine). (IPSEN) Concentrate of antihemophilic factor (VIII):C. Each vial contains 400 to 700 porcine units, citrate ions 10 to 30 mmol/L, sodium ions 110 to 135 mmol/L, preservative free. Pow. for Inj., lyophilized. Vial with filter needle. Actual number of AHF units indicated on vial. *Rx.*
Use: Antihemophilic agent.

Hybec Forte. (Amlab) Vitamins B₁
100 mg, B₂ 20 mg, B₆ 2.5 mg, B₁₂
10 mcg, niacinamide 25 mg, C 200 mg,
calcium pantothenate 5 mg, iron
10 mg, choline bitartrate 24 mg, inositol
10 mg, biotin 5 mcg, liver 50 mg, yeast
100 mg. Tab. Bot. 30s, 100s. *OTC.*
Use: Mineral, vitamin supplement.

Hycamtin. (GlaxoSmithKline) Topotecan
hydrochloride 4 mg (free base), mannitol 48 mg. Pow. for Inj., lyophilized.
Vial. Single-dose. *Rx.*
Use: Antineoplastic; DNA topoisomerase inhibitor.

•**hycanthone.** (HIGH-kan-thone) USAN.
Use: Antischistosomal.

Hyclorite. *USP 28.* Sodium hypochlorite
soln.

Hycet. (Xanodyne) Hydrocodone bitartrate 2.5 mg/acetaminophen 108 mg
per 5 mL. Alcohol 7%, glycerin, parabens, saccharin, sorbitol, sucrose. Oral
Soln. 473 mL. *c-III.*
Use: Analgesic, narcotic.

HycoClear Tuss. (Ethex) Hydrocodone
bitartrate 5 mg, guaifenesin 100 mg/
5 mL. Alcohol, dye, sugar free. Syr. Bot.
118 mL, 473 mL. *c-III.*
Use: Antitussive, expectorant.

Hycodan. (Endo) Hydrocodone bitartrate
5 mg, homatropine methylbromide
1.5 mg/5 mL or Tab. **Syr.:** Sorbitol,
sugar, parabens, cherry flavor. Bot.
473 mL. **Tab.:** Lactose. Bot. 100s, 500s.
c-III.
Use: Upper respiratory combination, antitussive, anticholinergic.

Hycort. (Everett) **Cream:** Hydrocortisone
1% in a cream base. Tube oz. **Oint.:**
Hydrocortisone 1% in ointment base.
Tube oz. *Rx.*
Use: Corticosteroid, topical.

Hycortole. (Teva) Hydrocortisone.
Cream: 0.5%: 5 g, 20 g; 1%: 5 g, 20 g,
4 oz; 2.5%: Tube 5 g, 20 g. **Oint.:** 1%,
2.5%. Tube 5 g, 20 g.
Use: Corticosteroid, topical.

Hycosin. (Alpharma) Hydrocodone bitartrate 5 mg, guaifenesin 100 mg/5 mL,
alcohol 10%, parabens, saccharin,
sorbitol, sucrose, butterscotch flavor.
Syr. Bot. 473 mL. *c-III.*
Use: Upper respiratory combination, antitussive, expectorant.

Hycotuss Expectorant. (Endo) Hydrocodone bitartrate 5 mg, guaifenesin
100 mg/5 mL alcohol 10%, saccharin,
sorbitol, sugar, parabens, butterscotch
flavor. Syr. Bot. 473 mL. *c-III.*
Use: Upper respiratory combination, antitussive, expectorant.

hydantoin derivatives.
Use: Anticonvulsant.
See: Dilantin.
Diphenylhydantoin sodium.
Ethotoin.
Mesantoin.
Phenantoin.

hydase.
Use: Hypodermoclyses, promotion of
diffusion.
See: Hyaluronidase.

Hydergine. (Novartis) **Liq.:** Equal parts
of dihydroergocornine, dihydroergocristine, dihydroergocryptine (Ergoloid
Mesylates). 1 mg/mL. Bot. 100 mL
w/dropper. **Oral:** Equal parts of dihydroergocornine, dihydroergocristine, dihydroergocryptine (Ergoloid Mesylates).
1 mg. Tab. Bot. 100s, 500s. *SandoPak*
(UD) 100s, 500s. **Sublingual:** Equal
parts of dihydroergocornine, dihydroergocristine, dihydroergocryptine (Ergoloid Mesylates). 0.5 mg, 1 mg. Tab. Bot.
100s, 1000s, *SandoPak* (UD) 100s.
Rx.
Use: Psychotherapeutic agent.

Hydoril. (Cenci, H.R. Labs, Inc.) Hydrochlorothiazide 25 mg, 50 mg. Tab. Bot.
100s, 1000s. *Rx.*
Use: Diuretic.

**hydrabamine phenoxymethyl peni-
cillin.**
See: Penicillin V hydrabamine.

hydracrylic acid beta lactone.
See: Propiolactone.

hydralazine. (Solopak Pharmaceuticals,
Inc.) Hydralazine hydrochloride 20 mg/
mL Inj. Vial 1 mL. *Rx.*
Use: Antihypertensive.

•**hydralazine hydrochloride.** (high-
DRAL-uh-zeen) *USP 28.*
Tall Man: HydrALAZINE
Use: Antihypertensive.
See: Apresoline.
W/Hydrochlorothiazide.
See: Apresazide.
Apresoline-Esidrix.
Hydralazide.
Hydroserpine Plus.
W/Reserpine.
See: Dralserp.
Serpasil-Apresoline.
W/Reserpine, hydrochlorothiazide.
See: Harbolin.
Ser-Ap-Es.

hydralazine hydrochloride. (Various
Mfr.) Hydralazine hydrochloride 10 mg,
25 mg, 50, mg 100 mg. Tab. Bot. 100s,
1000s, UD 100s (except 100 mg).
Use: Antihypertensive.

•**hydralazine polistirex.** (high-DRAL-ah-zeen pahl-ee-STIE-rex) USAN.
Tall Man: HydrALAZINE
Use: Antihypertensive.

Hydra Mag Tablets. (Pal-Pak, Inc.) Aluminum hydroxide gel, dried, 195 mg, magnesium trisilicate 195 mg, kaolin 162 mg. Tab. Bot. 1000s. *OTC.*
Use: Antacid.

Hydramine Cough. (Various Mfr.) Diphenhydramine hydrochloride 12.5 mg/mL, may contain alcohol. Syr. Bot. 473 mL. *Rx-OTC.*
Use: Antitussive.

Hydrap-ES. (Parmed Pharmaceuticals, Inc.) Hydrochlorothiazide 15 mg, reserpine 0.1 mg, hydralazine hydrochloride 25 mg. Tab. Bot. 100s, 500s, 1000s. *Rx.*
Use: Antihypertensive.

Hydraserp. (Geneva) Hydrochlorothiazide 25 mg, 50 mg, reserpine 0.1 mg. Tab. Bot. 100s, 1000s. *Rx.*
Use: Antihypertensive combination.

hydrastine hydrochloride. (Penick) Pow. Bot. oz.
Use: Hemostatic.

Hydrate. (Hyrex) Dimenhydrinate 50 mg/mL w/propylene glycol 50%, benzyl alcohol 5%. Amp. 1 mL. Box 25s, 100s; Vial 10 mL. *Rx.*
Use: Antiemetic; antihistamine; antivertigo.

Hydrazide. (Ivax) **25/25:** Hydrochlorothiazide 25 mg, hydralazine 25 mg. Cap. **50/50:** Hydrochlorothiazide 50 mg, hydralazine 50 mg. Cap. Bot. 100s. *Rx.*
Use: Antihypertensive.

Hydra-Zide. (Par Pharmaceuticals) Hydralazine hydrochloride 50 mg, hydrochlorothiazide 50 mg. Cap. Bot. 100s, 500s, 1000s. *Rx.*
Use: Antihypertensive.

hydrazone.
Use: Pulmonary tuberculosis.
See: Rimactane.

Hydrea. (Bristol-Myers Squibb) Hydroxyurea 500 mg, lactose. Cap. Bot. 100s. *Rx.*
Use: Antineoplastic.

hydriodic acid. (Various Mfr.)
Use: Expectorant.

hydriodic acid therapy.
See: Aminoacetic acid hydrochloride.

Hydrisinol Creme and Lotion. (Pedinol Pharmacal) Sulfonated hydrogenated castor oil. **Cream:** Spout Cap Jar 4 oz, lb. **Lot.:** Bot. 8 oz. *OTC.*
Use: Emollient.

Hydro-Ban. (Whiteworth Towne) Juniper oil 10 mg, uva ursi 50 mg, buchu extract 50 mg, parsley piert extract 50 mg, iron 6 mg. Cap. Bot. 42s. *OTC.*
Use: Diuretic.

Hydrocare Cleaning and Disinfecting. (Allergan) Tris (2-hydroxyethyl) tallow ammonium Cl, thimerosal 0.002%, bis (2-hydroxyethyl) tallow ammonium Cl, sodium bicarbonate, sodium phosphates, hydrochloric acid, propylene glycol, polysorbate 80, polyhema. Soln. Bot. 240 mL, 360 mL. *OTC.*
Use: Contact lens care, disinfective.

Hydrocare Preserved Saline. (Allergan) Isotonic, buffered, NaCl, sodium hexametaphosphate, boric acid, sodium borate, EDTA 0.01%, thimerosal 0.001%. Soln. Bot. 240 mL, 360 mL. *OTC.*
Use: Contact lens care, rinsing/storage solution.

Hydrocerin. (Geritrex) **Cream:** Petrolatum, mineral oil, mineral wax, ceresin, lanolin alcohol, parabens. 480 g. **Lotion:** EDTA, lanolin alcohol, parabens, PEG-40 sorbitan, peroleate, propylene glycol, sorbitol, water. 240 g. *OTC.*
Use: Emollient.

Hydrocet. (Carnrick) Hydrocodone bitartrate 5 mg, acetaminophen 500 mg. Cap. Bot. 100s. *c-III.*
Use: Narcotic analgesic combination.

hydrochlorate. Same as Hydrochloride.

•**hydrochloric acid.** *NF 23.*
Use: Well diluted, achlorhydria; pharmaceutic aid (acidifying agent).

hydrochloric acid. (Various Mfr.) Muriatic acid, Absolute 38%. Diluted 10%.

hydrochloric acid therapy.
Use: Well diluted, achlorhydria; pharmaceutic aid (acidifying agent); gastric acidifier.
See: Betaine hydrochloride.
Glutamic acid hydrochloride.
Glycine hydrochloride.

Hydrochloroserpine. (Freeport) Hydralazine hydrochloride 25 mg, hydrochlorothiazide 15 mg, reserpine 0.1 mg. Tab. Bot. 1000s.
Use: Antihypertensive combination.

•**hydrochlorothiazide.** (high-droe-klor-oh-THIGH-uh-zide) *USP 28.*
Use: Diuretic.
See: Chlorzide.
Delco-Retic.
Diu-Scrip.
Esidrix.
HydroDiuril.
Hydromal.
Microzide.
Oretic.
Zide.

W/Bisoprolol fumarate.
See: Bisoprolol fumarate and hydro-
chlorothiazide.
W/Candesartan cilexetil.
See: Atacand HCT.
W/Captopril.
See: Captopril and hydrochlorothiazide.
W/Deserpidine.
See: Oreticyl.
W/Enalapril.
See: Enalapril maleate/hydrochlorothia-
zide.
Vaseretic.
Vaseretic 50-12.5.
W/Fosinopril sodium.
See: Monopril-HCT.
W/Guanethidine monosulfate.
See: Esimil.
W/Hydralazine hydrochloride.
See: Apresazide.
Apresoline-Esidrix.
Hydralazide.
W/Lisinopril.
See: Prinzide.
Zestoretic.
W/Losartan potassium.
See: Hyzaar.
W/Methyldopa.
See: Aldoril.
W/Moexipril.
See: Uniretic.
W/Olmesartan medoxomil.
See: Benicar HCT.
W/Propranolol.
See: Inderide.
W/Quinapril hydrochloride.
See: Accuretic.
W/Reserpine.
See: Hydropres.
Hydroserp.
Hydroserpine.
Hydrotensin.
Serpasil-Esidrix.
W/Reserpine, Hydralazine hydrochloride.
See: Aldactazide.
Harbolin.
Hydroserpine Plus.
Ser-Ap-Es.
W/Telmisartan.
See: Micardis HCT.
W/Timolol maleate.
See: Timolide.
W/Triamterene.
See: Dyazide.
Triamterene/Hydrochlorothiazide.
hydrochlorothiazide. (Various Mfr.)
Hydrochlorothiazide 12.5 mg. Cap. Bot.
100s, 500s. Rx.
Use: Diuretic.
hydrochlorothiazide/amiloride.
See: Amiloride hydrochloride and

hydrochlorothiazide.
hydrochlorothiazide and benazepril
hydrochloride.
See: Benazepril hydrochloride and
hydrochlorothiazide.
hydrochlorothiazide/hydralazine.
(Various Mfr.) Hydrochlorothiazide
25 mg, hydralazine hydrochloride
25 mg. Cap. Hydrochlorothiazide
50 mg, hydralazine hydrochloride
50 mg. Cap. Bot. 100s, 500s, 1000s.
Rx.
Use: Antihypertensive.
hydrochlorothiazide/metoprolol tartrate.
See: Metoprolol Tartrate/Hydrochloro-
thiazide.
hydrocholeretic combinations.
See: G.B.S.
hydrocholeretics.
See: Bile salts.
Dehydrocholic acid.
Ox bile extract.
Hydrocil Instant. (Numark) Psyllium hy-
drophilic mucilloid 3.5 g/dose. Pow. Jar
250 g. OTC.
Use: Laxative.
Hydro Cobex. (Taylor Pharmaceuticals)
Hydroxocobalamin 1000 mcg. Vial
30 mL. Rx.
Use: Vitamin B$_{12}$ supplement.
•hydrocodone bitartrate. (HIGH-droe-
KOE-dohn by-TAR-TRATE) USP 28.
Dihydrocodeinone bitartrate.
Use: Antitussive, analgesic, narcotic.
W/Combinations.
See: Alor 5/500.
Anaplex HD.
Anexsia.
Anexsia 10/660.
Atuss G.
Atuss HC.
Atuss HD.
Atuss MS.
Codal-DH.
Codiclear DH.
Codimal DH.
Comtussin HC.
Cytuss HC.
Deconamine CX.
Detussin.
Dicomal-DH.
Donatussin DC.
Duratuss HD.
ED-TLC.
ED Tuss HC.
Endagen-HD.
Entex HC.
Histex HC.
Histinex-D.
Histinex HC.

Histinex PV.
Histussin D.
Histussin HC.
H-Tuss-D.
Hycet.
Hycoclear Tuss.
Hycodan.
Hycosin.
Hycotuss.
Hydrocet.
Hydrocodone w/acetaminophen.
Hydrocodone bitartrate and aceta-
minophen.
Hydrocodone bitartrate and guaifen-
esin.
Hydrocodone bitartrate and ibuprofen.
Hydrocodone CP.
Hydrocodone GF.
Hydrocodone HD.
Hydrocodone PA.
Hydro-DP.
Hydromet.
Hydromide.
Hydron CP.
Hydron EX.
Hydron KGS.
Hydron PSC.
Hydropanc.
Hydro-PC.
Hydro-PC II.
Hydro-Tussin HC.
Hydro-Tussin HD.
Hyphed.
Kwelcof
Levall 5.0.
Lortab.
Lortab 10/500.
Lortuss HC.
Marcof.
Maxidone.
Maxi-Tuss HC.
Maxi-Tuss HCG.
Maxi-Tuss HCX.
Nalex DH.
Nalex Expectorant.
Norco.
Norco 5/325.
Notuss PD.
Panacet 5/500.
Panasal 5/500.
Pancof-HC.
Pancof XP.
Pneumotussin.
Pneumotussin 2.5 Cough.
Poly-Tussin.
Prolex DH.
P-V-Tussin.
Statuss Green.
S-T Forte 2.
Su-Tuss HD.
Tussafed HC.

Tussend.
Tussigon.
Tyrodone.
Vanex HD.
Vetuss HC.
Vicodin.
Vicodin ES.
Vicodin HP.
Vicoprofen.
Vitussin.
Z-Cof HC.
Zydone.
ZTuss.

**hydrocodone bitartrate and aceta-
minophen.** (Qualitest) Hydrocodone bitartrate 2.5 mg, acetaminophen
500 mg. Sucrose. Tab. 100s, 500s,
1,000s. *c-III.*
Use: Narcotic analgesic.

**hydrocodone bitartrate and aceta-
minophen.** (Various Mfr.) **Caplets:**
Hydrocodone bitartrate 7.5 mg, acetaminophen 650 mg. Cap. Bot. 100s,
500s. **Capsules:** Hydrocodone bitartrate 5 mg, acetaminophen 500 mg.
Cap. Bot. 100s, 500s. **Elixir:** Hydrocodone bitartrate 2.5 mg, acetaminophen 167 mg/5 mL, alcohol 7%. Bot.
473 mL. **Tab.:** Hydrocodone bitartrate
5 mg, 7.5 mg, 10 mg, acetaminophen
325 mg, 500 mg, 650 mg, 660 mg,
750 mg. Tab. 30s, 60s, 90s, 120s
(10 mg/500 mg only); 100s; 500s;
1,000s (except 10 mg/500 mg and
10 mg/750 mg); UD 100s. *c-III.*
Use: Analgesic combination, narcotic.

**hydrocodone bitartrate and guaifene-
sin.** (Various Mfr.) Hydrocodone bitartrate 5 mg, guaifenesin 100 mg/5 mL,
may contain menthol, parabens, sorbitol, saccharin, alcohol and dye free.
Liq. Bot. 473 mL, 946 mL. *c-III.*
Use: Upper respiratory combination, antitussive, expectorant.

hydrocodone bitartrate and ibuprofen.
(Teva) Hydrocodone bitartrate 7.5 mg,
ibuprofen 200 mg, lactose. Tab. 100s.
c-III.
Use: Narcotic analgesic.

**hydrocodone bitartrate 5 mg/pseudo-
ephedrine hydrochloride 30 mg/car-
binoxamine maleate 2 mg.** (URL)
Hydrocodone bitartrate 5 mg, carbinoxamine maleate 2 mg, pseudoephedrine hydrochloride 30 mg/5 mL, alcohol
free. Liq. Bot. 473 mL. *c-III.*
Use: Upper respiratory combination, antitussive, antihistamine, decongest-
tant.

hydrocodone bitartrate, phenylephrine hydrochloride, chlorpheniramine maleate. (Cypress) Hydrocodone bitartrate 1.67 mg, phenylephrine hydrochloride 5 mg, chlorpheniramine maleate 2 mg/5 mL. Syr. Bot. Pt, gal. *c-III.*
Use: Decongestant, antihistamine, antitussive.
● **hydrocodone bitartrate tablets.**
USP 28.
Use: Analgesic, narcotic.
hydrocodone comp. syrup. (Various Mfr.) Hydrocodone bitartrate 5 mg, homatropine methylbromide 1.5 mg. Bot. 473 mL, gal. *c-III.*
Use: Antitussive.
Hydrocodone CP. (Morton Grove) Hydrocodone bitartrate 2.5 mg, phenylephrine hydrochloride 5 mg, chlorpheniramine maleate 2 mg/5 mL, saccharin, sorbitol, fruit flavor, alcohol free. Syr. Bot. 237 mL, 473 mL. *c-III.*
Use: Upper respiratory combination, antitussive, antihistamine, decongestant.
Hydrocodone GF. (Morton Grove) Hydrocodone bitartrate 5 mg, guaifenesin 100 mg/5 mL, saccharin, sorbitol, fruit flavor, alcohol and dye free. Syr. Bot. 237 mL, 473 mL. *c-III.*
Use: Upper respiratory combination, antitussive, expectorant.
Hydrocodone HD. (Morton Grove) Hydrocodone bitartrate 1.67 mg, phenylephrine hydrochloride 5 mg, chlorpheniramine maleate 2 mg/5 mL, sugar, menthol, parabens, cherry flavor, alcohol free. Liq. Bot. 236 mL, 473 mL. *c-III.*
Use: Upper respiratory combination, antihistamine, decongestant, antitussive.
● **hydrocodone polistirex.** (high-droe-KOE-dohn pahl-ee-STIE-rex) USAN.
Use: Antitussive.
See: Tussionex PennKinetic.
hydrocodone resin complex.
Use: Antitussive.
W/Phenyltoloxamine resin complex.
See: Tussionex.
hydrocodone w/acetaminophen.
Use: Analgesic combination, narcotic.
See: Alor 5/500.
  Anexsia 10/660.
  Lortab.
  Vicodin.
hydrocodone w/acetaminophen. (Pharmics) Hydrocodone bitartrate 7.5 mg, acetaminophen 500 mg. Tab. Bot. 100s, 500s. *c-III.*

Use: Analgesic combination, narcotic.
hydrocortamate hydrochloride. 17-Hydroxycorticosterone-21-diethylaminoacetate hydrochloride.
Use: Anti-inflammatory, topical.
● **hydrocortisone.** (HIGH-droe-CORE-tih-sone) *USP 28.*
Use: Anti-inflammatory, topical; corticosteroid, topical.
See: Acticort Lotion 100.
  Alcortin.
  Alphaderm.
  Caldecort.
  Cetacort.
  Cort-Dome.
  Cortef.
  Cortizone for Kids.
  Cortizone-10 Plus.
  Cortizone-10 Quickshot.
  Cortril.
  Delacort.
  Dermacort.
  Dermolate.
  Dermol HC.
  Eldecort.
  HC Derma-Pax.
  Hi-Cor 1.0.
  Hi-Cor 2.5.
  Hycort.
  Hycortole.
  Hydrocortone.
  Hydroskin.
  Hytone.
  Ivy Soothe.
  Ivy Stat.
  My Cort.
  Proctocort.
  proctoCream●HC 2.5%.
  Scalpicin.
  Signef.
  Synacort.
  Texacort 25, 50.
  T/Scalp.
W/Combinations.
See: Mediotic-HC.
hydrocortisone. (Pharmacia) Micronized nonsterile powder for prescription compounding.
Use: Anti-inflammatory, topical; corticosteroid, topical.
hydrocortisone. (Various Mfr.) Hydrocortisone 2.5%, may contain stearyl alcohol, cetyl alcohol, light mineral oil. Lot. Bot. 59 mL. Rx.
Use: Anti-infalmmatory, corticosteroid, topical.
● **hydrocortisone acetate.** *USP 28.*
Use: Glucocorticoid.
See: Anucort-HC.
  Anuprep HC.
  Anusol-HC.

Caldecort.
Caldecort Light.
Cortifoam.
Cortril Acetate.
Gynecort.
Hemril-HC Uniserts.
Hydrocort.
Hydrocortone acetate.
Hydrosone.
Maximum Strength Corticaine.
Maximum Strength Dermarest Dricort.
Novacort.
Pramosone Cream.
Proctocort.
U-cort.
W/Combinations.
See: Anusol-HC.
Carmol HC.
Coly-Mycin S Otic Drops w/Neomycin and Hydrocortisone.
Cortaid.
Cortic.
Cortisporin-TC.
Derma Medicone-HC.
Epifoam.
Furacin HC.
HC Pramoxine.
Lida-Mantle HC
Neo-Cortef.
Otomar-HC.
Proctofoam-HC.
Rectal Medicone-HC.
Wyanoids HC.

hydrocortisone acetate. (Pharmacia) Micronized nonsterile powder for prescription compounding.
Use: Anti-inflammatory, topical; corticosteroid, topical.

hydrocortisone acetate. (Various Mfr.) Hydrocortisone acetate 25 mg. Supp. 12s, 24s. *Rx.*
Use: Anorectal preparation.

hydrocortisone acetate maximum strength. (Clay-Park) Hydrocortisone acetate 1% (equiv. to hydrocortisone 10 mg/g), aloe extract, white petrolatum. Oint. Tube 28 g. *OTC.*
Use: Anti-inflammatory, corticosteroid, topical.

hydrocortisone and acetic acid. (Taro) Hydrocortisone 1%, acetic acid 2%, propylene glycol diacetate 3%, sodium acetate 0.015%, benzethonium chloride 0.02%. Citric acid 0.2%. Otic Soln. 10 mL dropper tip bottle. *Rx.*
Use: Otic preparation.

hydrocortisone and acetic acid otic solution.
Use: Anti-inflammatory, otic.

hydrocortisone and iodoquinol 1%. (Various Mfr.) Hydrocortisone 1%, iodoquinol 1%, may contain cetearyl alcohol, EDTA. Cream. Tube 30 g. *Rx.*
Use: Anti-inflammatory, corticosteroid, topical.

•**hydrocortisone butyrate.** (HIGH-droe-CORE-tih-sone BYOO-tih-rate) *USP 28.*
Use: Corticosteroid, topical.
See: Locoid.

hydrocortisone butyrate. (Taro) Hydrocortisone butyrate 0.1%. Isopropyl alcohol 50%, glycerin. Soln. 20 mL, 60 mL. *Rx.*
Use: Anti-inflammatory agent.

•**hydrocortisone cypionate.** *USP 28.*
Oral Susp. Hydrocortisone cypionate.
Use: Corticosteroid, topical.

hydrocortisone diethylaminoacetate hydrochloride.
See: Hydrocortamate.

•**hydrocortisone hemisuccinate.** (HIGH-droe-CORE-tih-sone hem-ih-SUCK-sih-nate) *USP 28.*
Use: Adrenocortical steroid.

hydrocortisone intravenous.
See: A-Hydro Cort.
Solu-Cortef.

hydrocortisone/iodochlorhydroxyquin. (Various Mfr.) **Cream:** Hydrocortisone 0.5%, 3%, iodochlorhydroxyquin 3%. 15 g, 30 g, 480 g. **Oint.:** Hydrocortisone 1%, iodochlorhydroxyquin 3%. 20 g, 30 g. *Rx-OTC.*
Use: Corticosteroid, topical.

hydrocortisone-neomycin. (Various Mfr.) Hydrocortisone 1%, neomycin sulfate 0.5%. Oint. 20 g. *Rx-OTC.*
Use: Corticosteroid, topical.

hydrocortisone phosphate.
See: Hydrocortone phosphate.

•**hydrocortisone probutate.** USAN.
Use: Atopic dermatitis (glucocorticoid).
See: Pandel.

•**hydrocortisone sodium phosphate.** (HIGH-droe-CORE-tih-sone) *USP 28.*
Use: Adrenocortical steroid (anti-inflammatory); corticosteroid, topical.

•**hydrocortisone sodium succinate.** (HIGH-droe-CORE-tih-sone) *USP 28.*
Use: Adrenocortical steroid (anti-inflammatory); corticosteroid, topical.
See: A-hydroCort.
Solu-Cortef.

•**hydrocortisone valerate.** (HIGH-droe-CORE-tih-sone VAL-eh-rate) *USP 28.*
Use: Corticosteroid, topical.
See: Westcort.

hydrocortisone valerate. (Copley) Hydrocortisone valerate 0.2% in hydrophilic base, white petrolatum, alcohol.

Cream. Tube 15 g, 45 g, 60 g. *Rx.*
Use: Corticosteroid, topical.
hydrocortisone valerate. (Taro) Hydrocortisone valerate 0.2% in hydrophilic base, white petrolatum, alcohol, mineral oil. Oint. Tube 15 g, 45 g, 60 g. *Rx.*
Use: Corticosteroid, topical.
hydrocortisone w/combinations.
See: AnaMantle HC.
Carmol HC.
Cipro HC.
Cortane-B.
Cortef.
Cortic.
Cortisporin.
Cortisporin-TC.
Doak Oil Forte.
Drotic No. 2.
Fostril HC.
Hysone.
Kleer.
Neo-Cort Dome.
Neo Cort Top.
Nutracort.
1 + 1.
1 + 1-F.
Oti-Med.
Oto.
Otobiotic.
Otocalm-H.
Otomar-HC.
Pyocidin-Otic.
Rectal Medicone-HC.
Terra-Cortril.
Tri-Otic.
Vanoxide-HC.
Vytone.
Zoto-HC.
Hydrocortone Acetate Saline Suspension. (Merck & Co.) Hydrocortisone acetate 25 mg, 50 mg/mL, sodium Cl 9 mg, polysorbate 80 4 mg, sodium carboxymethylcellulose 5 mg/mL, benzyl alcohol 9 mg q.s. water for injection to 1 mL. Vial 5 mL. *Rx.*
Use: Corticosteroid.
Hydrocortone Phosphate Injection. (Merck & Co.) Hydrocortisone sodium phosphate equivalent to hydrocortisone 50 mg/mL, creatinine 8 mg, sodium citrate 10 mg/mL, sodium hydroxide to adjust pH, sodium bisulfite 3.2 mg, methylparaben 1.5 mg, propylparaben 0.2 mg, water for injection q.s./mL. Vial 2 mL multiple dose, 10 mL multiple dose. Disposable syringe 2 mL single dose. *Rx.*
Use: Corticosteroid.
Hydrocortone Tablets. (Merck & Co.) Hydrocortisone 10 mg, 20 mg. Bot. 100s. *Rx.*

Use: Corticosteroid.
Hydrocream Base. (Paddock) Petrolatum, mineral oil, woolwax alcohol, imidazolidinyl urea, methyl- and propylparabens. Cream. Jar lb.
Use: Emollient.
Hydro-Crysti 12. (Roberts) Hydroxocobalamin, crystalline (vitamin B_{12}) 1000 mcg/mL. Inj. Vial 30 mL. *Rx.*
Use: Vitamin B_{12} supplement.
HydroDIURIL. (Merck & Co.) Hydrochlorothiazide 25 mg, 50 mg. Tab. Bot. 100s, 1000s, UD 100s. *Rx.*
Use: Diuretic.
Hydro-DP. (Cypress) Hydrocodone bitartrate 2 mg, diphenhydramine hydrochloride 12.5 mg, phenylephrine hydrochloride 7.5 mg/5 mL. Alcohol-free. Saccharin, sorbitol. Cherry flavor. Syr. 118 mL, 473 mL. *c-III.*
Use: Antitussive combination.
Hydro-D Tablets. (Halsey Drug) Hydrochlorothiazide. 25 mg, 50 mg. Bot. 1000s. *Rx.*
Use: Diuretic.
Hydro-Ergot. (Henry Schein) Hydrogenated ergot alkaloids 0.5 mg, 1 mg. Tab. Bot. 100s. *Rx.*
Use: Psychotherapeutic agent.
• **hydrofilcon a.** (HIGH-droe-FILL-kahn A) USAN.
Use: Contact lens material (hydrophilic).
• **hydroflumethiazide.** (HIGH-droe-flew-meth-EYE-ah-zide) *USP 28.*
Use: Antihypertensive; diuretic.
See: Saluron.
W/Reserpine.
See: Salutensin.
Salutensin-Demi.
hydrogen dioxide.
See: Hydrogen peroxide.
hydrogen iodide.
Use: Expectorant.
See: Hydriodic acid.
• **hydrogen peroxide concentrate.** (HIGH-droe-jen per-OX-ide) *USP 28.*
Use: Anti-infective, topical.
hydrogen peroxide solution 30%. Perhydrol, hydrogen peroxide. Bot. 0.25 lb, 0.5 lb, 1 lb.
Use: Dentistry, preparing the 3% solution.
hydrogen peroxide topical solution. (Various Mfr.) Hydrogen peroxide (3%). Bot. 4 oz, 8 oz, pt.
Use: Anti-infective, topical.
Hydrogesic. (Edwards) Hydrocodone bitartrate 5 mg, acetaminophen 500 mg. Cap. Bot. 100s. *c-III.*
Use: Analgesic combination, narcotic.

HYDROPHILIC OINTMENT 413

Hydroloid-G Sublingual. (Major) Ergoloid mesylates 0.5 mg, 1 mg. Tab. Bot. 100s, 250s, 500s (0.5 mg only), 1000s (1 mg only), UD 100s. *Rx.*
Use: Psychotherapeutic agent.
Hydroloid-G Tabs. (Major) Ergoloid mesylates 1 mg. Tab. Bot. 100s, 250s, 1000s, UD 100s. *Rx.*
Use: Psychotherapeutic agent.
Hydromal. (Roberts) Hydrochlorothiazide 50 mg. Tab. Bot. 1000s. *Rx.*
Use: Diuretic.
Hydromet. (Alra) Hydrocodone bitartrate 5 mg, homatropine MBr 1.5 mg/5 mL, saccharin, sucrose, methylparaben, cherry flavor. Syr. Bot. 473 mL, 3.8 L. *c-III.*
Use: Upper respiratory combination, antitussive, anticholinergic.
Hydromide. (Major) Hydrocodone bitartrate 5 mg, homatropine MBr 1.5 mg/5 mL, alcohol < 0.1%, cherry flavor. Syr. Bot. 473 mL. *c-III.*
Use: Upper respiratory combination, antitussive, anticholinergic.
hydromorphone. *c-II.*
Use: Analgesic, narcotic.
• **hydromorphone hydrochloride.** (HIGHdroe-MORE-phone) *USP 28.* Formerly *Dihydromorphinone Hydrochloride.*
Use: Opioid analgesic.
See: Dilaudid.
Dilaudid-HP.
Palladone.
W/Combinations.
See: Dilaudid Cough.
hydromorphone hydrochloride. (Paddock) Hydromorphone hydrochloride 3 mg. Supp. Box 6s. *c-II.*
Use: Opioid analgesic.
hydromorphone hydrochloride. (Various Mfr.) Hydromorphone hydrochloride. **Tab.:** 2 mg, 4 mg, 8 mg. Bot. 100s, UD 25s (except 8 mg), UD 100s (except 8 mg). **Inj.:** 1 mg/mL, 2 mg/mL, 4 mg/mL, 10 mg/mL. Prefilled syringes. 1 mL (except 10 mg/mL). Vials (2 mg/mL only). 1 mL, 20 mL. Single-dose vials (10 mg/mL only). 1 mL, 5 mL, 50 mL. **Oral Soln.:** 1 mg/1 mL. UD patient cups. 4 mL, 8 mL. Bot. 250 mL. *c-II.*
Use: Opioid analgesic.
hydromorphone sulfate.
Use: Analgesic, narcotic.
Hydron CP. (Cypress) Hydrocodone bitartrate 5 mg, chlorpheniramine maleate 2 mg, phenylephrine hydrochloride 10 mg/5 mL, saccharin, sorbitol, pineapple-orange flavor, alcohol free. Liq. 473 mL. *c-III.*

Use: Antitussive, antihistamine, decongestant combination.
Hydron EX. (Cypress) Hydrocodone bitartrate 2.5 mg, potassium guaiacolsulfonate 120 mg/5 mL, saccharin, sorbitol, alcohol free, cherry flavor. Liq. 473 mL. *c-III.*
Use: Antitussive and expectorant.
Hydron KGS. (Cypress) Hydrocodone bitartrate 5 mg, potassium guaiacolsulfonate 300 mg/5 mL, saccharin, sorbitol, wild cherry flavor, alcohol free. Liq. Bot. 473 mL. *c-III.*
Use: Upper respiratory combination, antitussive, expectorant.
Hydron PSC. (Cypress) Hydrocodone bitartrate 5 mg, chlorpheniramine maleate 2 mg, pseudoephedrine hydrochloride 30 mg/5 mL, menthol, saccharin, sorbitol, alcohol free, vanilla flavor. Liq. 473 mL. *c-III.*
Use: Antitussive, antihistamine, decongestant combination.
Hydropane. (Watson) Hydrocodone bitartrate 5 mg, homatropine methylbromide 1.5 mg/5 mL, parabens, sucrose, cherry flavor. Syr. Bot. 473 mL, 3.8 L. *c-III.*
Use: Upper respiratory combination, antitussive, anticholinergic.
Hydro-PC. (Cypress) Hydrocodone bitartrate 2 mg, chlorpheniramine maleate 2 mg, phenylephrine hydrochloride 5 mg/5 mL, strawberry flavor. Liq. Bot. 473 mL. *c-III.*
Use: Upper respiratory combination, antitussive, antihistamine, decongestant.
Hydro-PC II. (Cypress) Hydrocodone bitartrate 2 mg, chlorpheniramine maleate 2 mg, phenylephrine hydrochloride 7.5 mg/5 mL, strawberry flavor. Liq. Bot. 473 mL. *c-III.*
Use: Upper respiratory combination, antitussive, antihistamine, decongestant.
Hydropel. (C & M Pharmacal) Silicone 30%, hydrophobic starch derivative 10%, petrolatum. Jar 2 oz, lb. *OTC.*
Use: Emollient.
Hydrophed. (Rugby) Theophylline 130 mg, ephedrine sulfate 25 mg, hydroxyzine hydrochloride 10 mg. Tab. Bot. 100s, 1000s. *Rx.*
Use: Antiasthmatic combination.
hydrophilic ointment. (E. Fougera) Stearyl alcohol, white petrolatum, propylene glycol, sodium lauryl sulfate, water. Jar lb.
Use: Pharmaceutic aid, ointment base.

hydrophilic ointment base. (Emerson) Oil in water emulsion bases. 1 lb.
Use: Pharmaceutic aid, ointment base.
See: Aquaphilic.
Cetaphil.
Dermovan.
Lanaphilic.
Polysorb.
Unibase.
Hydropine. (Rugby) Hydroflumethiazide 25 mg, reserpine 0.125 mg. Tab. Bot. 100s. *Rx.*
Use: Antihypertensive combination.
Hydropine H.P. Tablets. (Rugby) Hydroflumethiazide 50 mg, reserpine 0.125 mg. Bot. 100s, 500s, 1000s. *Rx.*
Use: Antihypertensive combination.
Hydropres-50. (Merck & Co.) Hydrochlorothiazide 50 mg, reserpine 0.125 mg. Tab. Bot. 100s, 1000s. *Rx.*
Use: Antihypertensive combination.
• **hydroquinone.** (high-DROE-KWIN-ohn) *USP 28.*
Use: Depigmentor.
See: Aclaro.
Artra Skin Tone, Cream.
Black and White Bleaching.
Claripel.
Eldopaque.
Eldopaque Forte.
Eldoquin Forte.
EpiQuin Micro.
Esoterica.
Glyquin.
Lustra.
Lustra-AF.
Melpaque HP.
Melquin HP.
NeoStrata Skin Lightening.
Nuquin HP.
Solaquin.
W/Combinations.
See: Tri-Luma.
hydroquinone. (Glades) Hydroquinone.
Gel: 3%, 4%. Padimate O, dioxybenzone, EDTA, sodium metabisulfite, alcohol (4% only), hydroalcoholic base. 30 g (3% only), 28.35 g (4% only).
Soln.: 3%, SD Alcohol 40-B, isopropyl alcohol. 29 mL with applicator. *Rx.*
Use: Depigmentor.
hydroquinone. (Various Mfr.) Hydroquinone 4%. May contain EDTA, parabens, mineral oil, sodium metabisulfite. Cream 28.35 g. *Rx.*
Use: Depigmentor.
hydroquinone monobenzyl ether.
See: Benoquin.
hydroquinone with sunscreen. (Various Mfr.) Hydroquinone 4%. May contain padimate O, dioxybenzone, oxybenzone, octyl methoxycinnamate, octyl dimethyl-p-aminobenzoate, cetearyl alcohol, vitamin E, parabens, mineral oil, stearyl alcohol, lactic acid, EDTA, sodium metabisulfite. Cream 28.35 g. *Rx.*
Use: Depigmentor.
Hydrosal. (Hydrosal Co.) Aluminum acetate 5%. **Susp.:** Bot. 16 oz, gal. **Oint.:** 54 g, 113.4 g, Jar 54 g, 454 g. *OTC.*
Use: Astringent.
Hydro-Serp. (Ivax) Hydrochlorothiazide 25 mg, 50 mg, reserpine 0.125 mg, 0.1 mg. Tab. Bot. 100s, 1000s. *Rx.*
Use: Antihypertensive combination.
Hydroserpine #1. (Various Mfr.) Hydrochlorothiazide 25 mg, reserpine. Bot. 100s, 1000s. *Rx.*
Use: Antihypertensive combination.
Hydroserpine #2. (Various Mfr.) Hydrochlorothiazide 50 mg, reserpine. Bot. 100s, 250s, 400s, 1000s. *Rx.*
Use: Antihypertensive combination.
Hydrosine 50. (Major) Hydrochlorothiazide 50 mg, reserpine 0.125 mg. Tab. Bot. 100s. *Rx.*
Use: Antihypertensive combination.
Hydrosine 25. (Major) Hydrochlorothiazide 25 mg, reserpine 0.125 mg. Tab. Bot. 100s. Tartrazine. *Rx.*
Use: Antihypertensive combination.
HydroSKIN. (Rugby) Hydrocortisone 1%.
Cream: Mineral oil, lanolin alcohol, cetyl alcohol, parabens. Tube 113.4 g.
Oint.: Mineral oil, white petrolatum base. Tube 28.4 g. **Lot.:** Cetyl alcohol, parabens. Bot. 118 mL. *OTC.*
Use: Anti-inflammatory, corticosteroid, topical.
Hydrosone. (Sigma-Tau) Hydrocortisone acetate 25 mg, 50 mg, lactose/mL. Vial 5 mL. *Rx.*
Use: Corticosteroid.
HydroStat IR. (Richwood Pharmaceuticals) Hydromorphone hydrochloride 1 mg, 2 mg, 3 mg, 4 mg. Tab. Bot. 100s. *c-II.*
Use: Analgesic, narcotic.
Hydro-T. (Major) Hydrochlorothiazide 25 mg, 50 mg, 100 mg. Tab. Bot. 100s, 250s (100 mg only), 1000s, UD 100s. *Rx.*
Use: Diuretic.
Hydrotensin. (Merz) Hydrochlorothiazide 50 mg, reserpine 0.125 mg. Tab. Bot. 100s, 1000s. *Rx.*
Use: Antihypertensive combination.
Hydro-Tussin DM. (Ethex) Dextromethorphan HBr 20 mg, guaifenesin 200 mg/5 mL, saccharin, sorbitol. Liq. Bot. 473 mL. *Rx.*

Use: Upper respiratory combination, antitussive, expectorant.

Hydro-Tussin HC. (Ethex) Hydrocodone bitartrate 3 mg, chlorpheniramine maleate 2 mg, pseudoephedrine hydrochloride 15 mg/5 mL, alcohol and dye free. Syr. Bot. 473 mL. *c-III.*
Use: Upper respiratory combination. antitussive, antihistamine, decongestant.

Hydro-Tussin HD. (Ethex) Hydrocodone bitartrate 2.5 mg, guaifenesin 100 mg, pseudoephedrine hydrochloride 30 mg/ 5 mL, saccharin, sorbitol, alcohol free. Liq. Bot. 473 mL. *c-III.*
Use: Upper respiratory combination, antitussive, expectorant, decongestant.

Hydro-12. (Table Rock) Crystalline hydroxocobalamin 1000 mcg/mL. Pkg. 10 mL. *Rx.*
Use: Vitamin supplement.

•**hydroxocobalamin.** (high-DROX-oh-koe-BAL-ah-meen) *USP 28.*
Use: Treatment of megaloblastic anemia; vitamin (hematopoietic).

hydroxocobalamin, crystalline. (Various Mfr.) 1000 mcg/mL. Inj. 30 mL. *Rx.*
Use: Vitamin supplement.
See: Hydro Cobex.
Hydro-Crysti.
Hydroxocobalamin.
LA-12.

•**hydroxyamphetamine hydrobromide.** (high-DROX-ee-am-FET-uh-meen HIGH-droe-BROE-mide) *USP 28.*
Use: Adrenergic (ophthalmic); mydriatic.
See: Paredrine.

2-hydroxybenzamide.
See: Salicylamide.

hydroxy bis (acetato) aluminum. Aluminum Subacetate Topical Soln.

hydroxy bis (salicylato) aluminum diacetate.
See: Aluminum aspirin.

hydroxybutyrate, sodium/gamma.
See: Sodium gamma-hydroxybutyrate acid.

hydroxycholecalciferol. (D_3).
Use: Antihypocalcemia.
See: Calcifediol.

•**hydroxychloroquine sulfate.** (high-drox-ee-KLOR-oh-kwin) *USP 28.*
Use: Antimalarial; lupus erythematosus suppressant; antirheumatic agent.
See: Plaquenil.

hydroxychloroquine sulfate. (Various Mfr.) Hydroxychloroquine sulfate 200 mg (equiv. to 155 mg base). Tab.

Bot. 100s, 500s, 1000s. *Rx.*
Use: Antimalarial; lupus erythematosus suppressant; antirheumatic agent.

•**hydroxyethyl cellulose.** (high-drox-ee-ETH-ill SELL-you-lohs) *NF 23.*
Use: Pharmaceutic aid (suspending, viscosity-increasing agent).
See: Gonioscopic.

hydroxyethyl starch. (HES).
Use: Plasma volume expander.
See: Hespan.

hydroxyisoindolin. Under study.
Use: Antihypertensive.

hydroxymagnesium aluminate.
Use: Antacid.
See: Magaldrate.

hydroxymycin. An antibiotic substance obtained from cultures of *Streptomyces paucisporogenes.*

•**hydroxyphenamate.** (high-DROX-ee-FEN-ah-mate) USAN.
Use: Anxiolytic.

•**hydroxypropyl cellulose.** (high-drox-ee-PRO-pill SELL-you-lohs) *NF 23.*
Use: Topical protectant; pharmaceutic aid, emulsifying tablet-coating agent.

hydroxypropyl methylcellulose.
See: Hypromellose.

•**hydroxypropyl methylcellulose phthalate.** *NF 23.*
Use: Pharmaceutic aid (coating agent).
See: Hypromellose phthalate.

hydroxypropyl methylcellulose phthalate 200731.
Use: Pharmaceutic aid (coating agent).

hydroxypropyl methylcellulose phthalate 220824.
Use: Pharmaceutic aid (coating agent).

hydroxystearin sulfate. Sulfonate hydrogenated castor oil.

L-5 Hydroxytryptophan (L-5HTP). (Circa)
Use: Postanoxic intention myoclonus. [Orphan Drug]

•**hydroxyurea.** (high-DROX-ee-you-REE-uh) *USP 28.*
Use: Antineoplastic; sickle cell disease.
See: Droxia.
Hydrea.
Mylocel.

hydroxyurea. (Various Mfr.) Hydroxyurea 500 mg. Cap. Bot. 100s, UD 100s. *Rx.*
Use: Antineoplastic.

•**hydroxyzine.** (high-DROX-ih-zeen) *USP 28.*
Tall Man: HydrOXYzine
Use: Anxiolytic; antihistamine.
See: Vistaril.
W/Ephedrine sulfate, theophylline.

See: Marax.
Marax DF.
Theo-Drox.
hydroxyzine. (Various Mfr.) Hydroxyzine. **Tab.:** 10 mg, 25 mg, 50 mg. Bot. 20s (except 50 mg), 30s (except 50 mg), 40s (25 mg only), 50s (except 50 mg), 60s (25 mg only), 100s, 250s (except 50 mg), 500s (except 50 mg), 1000s (except 50 mg), UD 32s (10 mg only), UD 100s (except 50 mg). **Syrup:** 10 mg/5 mL. Bot. 16 mL, 120 mL, 473 mL, gal, UD 5 mL, UD 12.5 mL, UD 25 mL. *Rx.*
Use: Antihistamine, nonselective piperazine; anxiolytic.
hydroxyzine hydrochloride. (Various Mfr.) Hydroxyzine hydrochloride 25 mg/mL, 50 mg/mL. Vials. 1 mL, 2 mL, 10 mL. *Rx.*
Use: Antihistamine.
• **hydroxyzine pamoate.** *USP 28.*
Tall Man: HydrOXYzine
Use: Tranquilizer (minor); antihistamine.
See: Vistaril.
hydroxyzine pamoate. (Various Mfr.) Hydroxyzine pamoate 25 mg, 50 mg, 100 mg (equivalent to hydrochloride). Cap. Bot. 12s (except 100 mg), 20s (except 100 mg), 50s (25 mg only), 100s, 500s, 1000s, UD 32s (except 100 mg), UD 100s. *Rx.*
Use: Antihistamine, nonselective piperazine; anxiolytic.
Hydro-Z-50. (Merz) Hydrochlorothiazide 50 mg. Tab. Bot. 100s, 1000s. *Rx.*
Use: Diuretic.
Hyflex-650. (Breckenridge) Acetaminophen 650 mg, phenyltoloxamine citrate 60 mg. Tab. 100s. *Rx.*
Use: Nonnarcotic analgesic.
Hy-Flow Solution. (Ciba Vision) Polyvinyl alcohol with hydroxyethylcellulose, benzalkonium Cl, EDTA. Bot. 60 mL. *OTC.*
Use: Contact lens care.
Hygienic Cleansing. (Rugby) Witch hazel 50%, glycerin, benzalkonium Cl, methylparaben. Pads 100s. *OTC.*
Use: Anorectal preparation.
Hygroton. (Aventis) Chlorthalidone 25 mg, 50 mg. Tab. Lactose (25 mg, 50 mg). Bot. 100s. *Rx.*
Use: Diuretic.
Hylaform. (Inamed Aesthetics) Hylan B 5.5 mg/mL. Gel for Inj. Single-use, prefilled syringes. *Rx.*
Use: Physical adjunct.
hylan.
Use: Physical adjunct.
See: Hylaform.

Hylidone. (Major) Chlorthalidone. Tab. **25 mg, 50 mg:** Bot. 100s, 250s, 1000s, UD 100s. **100 mg:** Bot. 100s, 250s, 500s, 1000s. *Rx.*
Use: Diuretic.
Hyliver Plus. (Hyrex) Folic acid 0.4 mg, liver 10 mcg, vitamin B_{12} 100 mcg/mL. Vial 10 mL with phenol. *Rx.*
Use: Vitamin supplement.
Hylorel Tablets. (Medeva) Guanadrel sulfate 10 mg, 25 mg. Tab. Bot. 100s. *Rx.*
Use: Antihypertensive.
• **hymecromone.** (HIGH-meh-KROE-mone) USAN.
Use: Choleretic.
hymenoptera venom/venom protein. Purified venoms of honeybee, wasp, white faced hornet, yellow hornet, yellow jacket, and mixed vespids (both hornets and yellow jackets). *Rx.*
Use: Allergenic extract.
See: Albay.
Venomil.
HY-N.B.P. Ointment. (Jones Pharma) Bacitracin zinc 400 units, neomycin sulfate 5 mg, polymixin B sulfate 10,000 units/g. Tube ⅛ oz. *Rx.*
Use: Anti-infective, topical.
hyoscine hydrobromide. *USP 28.*
Scopolamine HBr.
Use: Antispasmodic.
hyoscine-hyoscyamine-atropine.
Use: Anticholinergic.
See: Atropine w/hyoscyamine w/hyoscine.
• **hyoscyamine.** (high-oh-SIGH-ah-meen) *USP 28.*
Use: Anticholinergic.
See: Cystospaz.
hyoscyamine-atropine-hyoscine.
Use: Anticholinergic.
See: Atropine w/hyoscyamine w/hyoscine.
• **hyoscyamine hydrobromide.** *USP 28.*
Use: Anticholinergic.
See: Combinations.
Phenazopyridine Plus.
hyoscyamine hydrochloride. (Various Mfr.)
hyoscyamine salts.
Use: Anticholinergic.
W/Atropine salts.
See: Atropine w/hyoscyamine.
• **hyoscyamine sulfate.** *USP 28.*
Use: Anticholinergic.
See: Anaspaz.
A-Spas S/L.
Cystospaz.
ED-SPAZ.

IB-Stat.
Levbid.
Levsin.
Levsinex Timecaps.
Levsin/SL.
Neosol.
NuLev.
Symax-SL.
Symax-SR.
W/Combinations.
See: Belladonna.
Bellahist-D LA.
Cystospaz-SR.
DeTal.
Donnatal.
Donnatal Extentabs.
Peece.
Sedamine.
Spasaid.
Stahist.
Urimax.
Uritact DS.
hyoscyamine sulfate. (Ethex) Hyoscyamine sulfate 0.375 mg. ER Cap. Bot.
100s. *Rx.*
Use: Anticholinergic.
hyoscyamine sulfate. (Goldline) Hyoscyamine sulfate 0.125 mg/mL, alcohol 5%. Soln. Bot. with dropper. 15 mL.
Rx.
Use: Anticholinergic.
hyoscyamine sulfate. (Various Mfr.)
Hyoscyamine sulfate. **ER Tab.:**
0.075 mg. Dot. 100s, 1,000s. **TR Cap.:**
0.375 mg. Bot. 100s. *Rx.*
Use: Anticholinergic.
hyoscyamus extract.
W/A.P.C.
See: Valacet Junior.
W/A.P.C., gelsemium extract.
See: Valacet.
hyoscyamus products and phenobarbital combinations.
Use: Anticholinergic, sedative.
See: Anaspaz PB.
Donnatal.
Elixiral.
Hyosophen Elixir. (Rugby) Atropine sulfate 0.0194 mg, scopolamine HBr 0.0065 mg, hyoscyamine HBr or sulfate 0.1037 mg, phenobarbital 16.2 mg, alcohol 23%, sugar, sorbitol. Bot.
120 mL, pt, gal. *Rx.*
Use: Gastrointestinal, anticholinergic.
Hyosophen Tablets. (Rugby) Atropine sulfate 0.0194 mg, scopolamine HBr 0.0065 mg, hyoscyamine HBr or SO$_4$ 0.1037 mg, phenobarbital 16.2 mg. Bot.
1000s. *Rx.*
Use: Anticholinergic combination.

Hypaque-Cysto. (Nycomed Amersham) Diatrizoate meglumine 300 mg, iodine 141 mg/mL, EDTA, preservative free. Inj. Pediatric Bot. 100 mL in 300 mL, 250 mL in 500 mL. *Rx.*
Use: Radiopaque agent.
Hypaque Meglumine 60%. (Nycomed Amersham) Diatrizoate meglumine 600 mg, iodine 282 mg/mL, EDTA. Inj. Vial 50 mL, 100 mL. Bot. 150 mL fill in 200 mL bot., 200 mL fill in 200 mL bot. *Rx.*
Use: Radiopaque agent, parenteral.
Hypaque-M 90%. (Sanofi-Synthelabo) Diatrizoate meglumine 60%, diatrizoate sodium 30%, EDTA. Vial 50 mL.
Use: Radiopaque agent.
Hypaque-M 75%. (Sanofi-Synthelabo) Diatrizoate meglumine 50%, diatrizoate sodium 25%, iodine 38.5%, EDTA.
Vial 20 mL, 50 mL.
Use: Radiopaque agent.
Hypaque Oral. (Sanofi-Synthelabo)
Pow.: Diatrizoate sodium oral pow. containing iodine 600 mg/g. Can 250 g, Bot. 10 g. **Liq.:** Soln. 41.66%. Bot.
120 mL.
Use: Radiopaque agent.
Hypaque-76. (Nycomed Amersham) Diatrizoate meglumine 660 mg, diatrizoate sodium 100 mg, iodine 370 mg/mL, EDTA. Inj. Vial 50 mL. Bot. 100 mL, 150 mL, 200 mL. Power injector Syr. 125 mL. *Rx.*
Use: Radiopaque agent, parenteral.
Hypaque Sodium. (Nycomed Amersham) **Soln.:** Diatrizoate sodium 416.7 mg, iodine 249 mg/mL. Soln. Bot. 120 mL. **Pow.:** Diatrizoate sodium (59.87% iodine), iodine 600 mg/g, polysorbate 80. Bot. 10 g. Can 250 g with measuring spoon. *Rx.*
Use: Radiopaque agent, iodinated GI contrast agent.
Hypaque Sodium 50%. (Nycomed Amersham) Diatrizoate sodium 500 mg, iodine 300 mg/mL, EDTA. Inj. Vial 50 mL. *Rx.*
Use: Radiopaque agent, parenteral.
Hyperab.
See: Bayrab.
HyperHep.
See: BayHep B.
hypericin. (VIMRxyn Pharm/NIH) *Rx.*
Use: Antiviral.
hyperlipidemia, agents for.
See: Atromid-S.
Choloxin.
Clofibrate.
Colestid.
Lescol.
Lopid.

Lorelco.
Mevacor.
Pravachol.
Questran.
Questran Light.
Zocor.
Hyperlyte. (McGaw) Sodium 25 mEq, potassium 40.5 mEq, calcium 5 mEq, magnesium 8 mEq, chloride 33.5 mEq, acetate 40.6 mEq, gluconate 5 mEq, 6050 mOsm/L. Inj. Vial 25 mL fill in 50 mL. *Rx.*
Use: Nutritional supplement, parenteral.
Hyperlyte CR. (B. Braun) Sodium 25 mEq, potassium 20 mEq, calcium 5 mEq, magnesium 5 mEq, chloride 30 mEq, acetate 30 mEq, 5500 mOsm/L. Inj. Pharmacy bulk packaging. *Super-vial* 250 mL. *Rx.*
Use: Intravenous nutritional therapy, intravenous replenishment solution.
Hyperlyte R. (McGaw) Sodium 25 mEq, potassium 20 mEq, calcium 5 mEq, magnesium 5 mEq, chloride 30 mEq, acetate 25 mEq, 4200 mOsm/L. Inj. Vial 25 mL fill in 50 mL. *Rx.*
Use: Nutritional supplement, parenteral.
Hypermune RSV. (MedImmune) Respiratory syncytial virus immune globulin, human.
Use: Respiratory syncytial virus treatment. [Orphan Drug]
Hyperopto 5%. (Professional Pharmacal) Sodium Cl 5%. Oint. Tube 3.5 g. *OTC.*
Use: Ophthalmic.
Hyperopto Ointment. (Professional Pharmacal) Sodium hydrochloride 50 mg, D.I. water 150 mg, anhydrous lanolin 150 mg, liquid petrolatum 50 mg, white petrolatum 599 mg, methylparaben 7 mg, propylparaben 3 mg/g. Tube 3.5 g. *OTC.*
Use: Ophthalmic.
hyperosmotic agents.
Use: Laxative.
See: Cephulac.
Cholac.
Chronulac.
Colace.
Constilac.
Constulose.
Duphalac.
Enulose.
Fleet Babylax.
Glycerin.
Lactulose.
Sani-Supp.
Hyperstat IV Injection. (Schering-Plough) Diazoxide 15 mg/mL. Amp. 20 mL. *Rx.*

Use: Antihypertensive.
hypertension diagnosis.
See: Regitine.
hypertensive emergency drugs.
See: Diazoxide.
Hyperstat IV.
Nitropress.
Hyphed. (Cypress) Hydrocodone bitartrate 2.5 mg, pseudoephedrine hydrochloride 30 mg, chlorpheniramine maleate 2 mg/5 mL, alcohol 5%, raspberry flavor. Liq. Bot. 473 mL. *c-III.*
Use: Upper respiratory combination, antitussive, decongestant, antihistamine.
Hyphylline. Dyphylline. *Rx.*
See: Neothylline.
hypnogene.
See: Barbital.
Hypnomidate. (Janssen) Etomidate. *Rx.*
Use: Anesthetic, general.
hypnotics.
See: Sedative/hypnotic agents.
"hypo".
See: Sodium thiosulfate.
Hypo-Bee. (Towne) Vitamins B_1 50 mg, B_2 20 mg, B_6 5 mg, B_{12} 15 mcg, niacinamide 25 mg, calcium pantothenate 5 mg, C 300 mg, E 200 units, iron 10 mg. Tab. Bot. 30s, 100s. *OTC.*
Use: Mineral, vitamin supplement.
hypochlorite preps.
See: Antiformin.
Dakin's.
Hyclorite.
Hypoclear. (Bausch & Lomb) Isotonic soln. with sodium Cl 0.9%. Aerosol soln. 240 mL, 300 mL. *OTC.*
Use: Contact lens care.
hypoglycemic agents.
See: Chlorpropamide.
Diabeta.
Diabinese.
Dymelor.
Glucotrol.
Glynase.
Micronase.
Orinase.
Phenformin hydrochloride.
Tolbutamide.
Tolinase.
α-hypophamine. Oxytocin.
•**hypophosphorous acid.** (high-poe-FOSS-for-uhs) *NF 23.*
Use: Pharmaceutic aid (antioxidant).
HypoTears Ophthalmic Liquid. (Novartis Ophthalmics) Polyvinyl alcohol 1%, PEG-400, dextrose 1%, benzalkonium Cl 0.01%, EDTA. Bot. 15 mL, 30 mL. *OTC.*
Use: Lubricant, ophthalmic.

HypoTears Ophthalmic Ointment. (Novartis Ophthalmics) White petrolatum, light mineral oil. Tube 3.5 g. *OTC.*
Use: Lubricant, ophthalmic.

HypoTears PF. (Novartis Ophthalmics) Polyvinyl alcohol 1%, PEG 400, dextrose and EDTA. Soln. In 0.6 mL. *OTC.*
Use: Artificial tears.

hypotensive agents.
See: Antihypertensives.

•**hypromellose.** *USP 28. Formerly hydroxypropyl methylcellulose.*
Use: Pharmaceutical aid (suspending agent), tablet excipient, viscosity-increasing agent.
See: Bion Tears.
GenTeal.
Goniosol.
Gonak.
GouCuul.
Tears Naturale Free.
Tears Naturale II.
Tears Renewed.
W/Benzalkonium chloride.
See: Isopto Tears.
Tearisol.
Tears Naturale.
Ultra Tears.

Hyrexin-50. (Hyrex) Diphenhydramine hydrochloride 50 mg/mL, benzethonium chloride. Vial 10 mL. Amp. 1 mL. *Rx.*
Use: Antihistamine.

Hyscorbic Plus Tablets. (Sanofi-Synthelabo) Vitamins E 45 units, C 600 mg, folic acid 400 mcg, B₁ 20 mg, B₂ 10 mg, niacinamide 100 mg, B₆ 10 mg, B₁₂ 25 mcg, pantothenic acid 25 mg, copper 3 mg, zinc 23.9 mg. Tab. Bot. 60s. *OTC.*
Use: Mineral, vitamin supplement.

Hyserp. (Freeport) Reserpine alkaloid 0.25 mg. Tab. Bot. 1000s. *Rx.*
Use: Antihypertensive.

Hyskon. (Pharmacia) Dextran 70 32% in 10% w/v dextrose. Bot. 100 mL, 250 mL. *Rx.*
Use: Diagnostic aid. For distending the uterine cavity and irrigating and visualizing its surfaces.

Hysone. (Roberts) Clioquinol 30 mg, hydrocortisone 10 mg/g. Cream. Tube 20 g. *OTC.*
Use: Antifungal; corticosteroid, topical.

hysteroscopy fluid.
Use: Diagnostic aid.
See: Hyskon.

Hytinic. (Hyrex) Polysaccharide-iron complex 150 mg. Parabens, EDTA, castor oil. Cap. Bot. 50s, 500s. *OTC.*
Use: Mineral supplement.

Hytone Cream. (Dermik) Hydrocortisone in cream base. **1%:** 1 oz. Jar 4 oz. **2.5%:** Tube 1 oz, 2 oz. *Rx-OTC.*
Use: Corticosteroid, topical.

Hytone Lotion. (Dermik) Hydrocortisone. **1%:** (10 mg/mL). Bot. 120 mL. **2.5%:** (25 mg/mL) in lotion base. Bot. 60 mL. *Rx.*
Use: Corticosteroid, topical.

Hytone Ointment. (Dermik) Hydrocortisone in ointment base, mineral oil, white petrolatum. **1%:** Tube 28.3 g, 113.4 g. **2.5%:** Tube 28.3 g. *Rx.*
Use: Corticosteroid, topical.

Hytone Spray. (Dermik) Hydrocortisone 1%. 45 mL. *Rx.*
Use: Corticosteroid, topical.

Hytrin. (Abbott) Terazosin hydrochloride 1 mg, 2 mg, 5 mg, 10 mg, parabens. Cap. Bot. 100s, UD 100s. *Rx.*
Use: Antihypertensive, antiadrenergic.

Hytuss. (Hyrex) Guaifenesin 100 mg. Tab. Bot. 100s, 1000s. *OTC.*
Use: Expectorant.

Hytuss 2X. (Hyrex) Guaifenesin 200 mg, parabens, EDTA, benzyl alcohol. Cap. Bot. 100s. *OTC.*
Use: Expectorant.

Hyzaar. (Merck & Co.) Losartan potassium 50 mg, hydrochlorothiazide 12.5 mg, potassium 4.24 mg, lactose. Tab. Bot. 30s, 90s, 100s, UD 100s. Losartan potassium 100 mg, hydrochlorothiazide 25 mg, potassium 8.48 mg, lactose. Tab. Unit-of-use 30s, 100s, UD 100s. *Rx.*
Use: Antihypertensive.

Hyzine-50. (Hyrex) Hydroxyzine hydrochloride 50 mg as hydrochloride/mL. Vial 10 mL. *Rx.*
Use: Anxiolytic.

I

- **ibafloxacin.** (ih-BAH-FLOX-ah-sin) USAN.
  Use: Anti-infective.
- **ibandronate sodium.** (ih-BAN-droe-nate) USAN.
  Use: Bone resorption inhibitor; antihypercalcemic.
  See: Boniva.

ibenzmethyzin. Name used for Procarbazine Hydrochloride.

Iberet. (Abbott) Ferrous sulfate 105 mg, ascorbic acid 150 mg, vitamins B_1 6 mg, B_2 6 mg, niacinamide 30 mg, B_5 10 mg, B_6 5 mg, B_{12} 25 mcg. CR Filmtab. Bot. 60s. *Rx.*
Use: Mineral, vitamin supplement.

Iberet-500 Filmtab. (Abbott) Ascorbic acid 500 mg, ferrous sulfate 105 mg, vitamins B_1 6 mg, B_2 6 mg, B_3 30 mg, B_5 10 mg, B_6 5 mg, B_{12} 25 mcg. CR Filmtab. Bot. 60s, 100s, *Abbo-Pac* 100s. *Rx.*
Use: Mineral, vitamin supplement.

Iberet-Folic-500 Filmtab. (Abbott) Ferrous sulfate 105 mg, vitamin C 500 mg, B_1 6 mg, B_2 6 mg, B_3 30 mg, B_5 10 mg, B_6 5 mg, B_{12} 25 mcg, folic acid 0.8 mg. CR Filmtab. Bot. 60s. *Rx.*
Use: Mineral, vitamin supplement.

- **iboctadekin.** (ib-OK-ta-DE-kin) USAN.
  Use: Immunologic mediator.
- **ibopamine.** (EYE-BOE-pah-meen) USAN.
  Use: Dopaminergic (peripheral).
- **ibritumomab tiuxetan.** (ib-ri-TYOO-mo-mab tye-UX-e-tan) USAN.
  Use: Monoclonal antibody.
  See: Zevalin.
- **ibrolipim.** (ib-ROE-li-pim) USAN.
  Use: Antiatherogenic; anti-obesity; antidyslipidemia; anticachexia; antidiabetes agent.

IB-Stat. (InKine) L-hyoscyamine sulfate 0.125 mg/mL. Alcohol 5.3%, liquid sugar, methylparaben, sorbitol. Oral Spray. 30 mL. *Rx.*
Use: Anticholinergic/antispasmodic, belladonna alkaloid.

- **ibufenac.** (eye-BYOO-feh-nak) USAN.
  Use: Antirheumatic; anti-inflammatory; analgesic; antipyretic.
- **ibuprofen.** (eye-BYOO-pro-fen) *USP 28.*
  Use: Anti-inflammatory; analgesic.
  See: Advil.
    Advil Liqui-Gels.
    Advil Migraine.
    Children's Advil.
    Dynafed IB.

Genpril.
Ibuprin.
Ibutab.
Infants' Motrin.
Junior Strength Advil.
Junior Strength Motrin.
Menadol.
Midol IB.
Midol Maximum Strength Cramp Formula.
Motrin.
Motrin, Children's
Motrin, Children's Cold
Motrin IB.
Motrin, Junior Strength.
Motrin Migraine Pain.
Nuprin.
PediaCare Fever.
Pediatric Advil Drops.
Caldto.
W/Combinations.
See: Advil Allergy Sinus.
    Advil Cold & Sinus.
    Advil Flu & Body.
    Children's Ibuprofen Cold.
    Combunox.
    Dristan Sinus.
    Motrin Children's Cold.
    Motrin Sinus Headache.
    Vicoprofen.

ibuprofen. (Various Mfr.) Ibuprofen. **Tab.:** 200 mg, 400 mg, 600 mg, 800 mg. Bot. **200 mg:** 24s, 50s, 100s, 250s, 1000s, UD 100s. **400 mg, 600 mg, 800 mg:** 100s, 270s (600 mg, 800 mg only), 360s (400 mg only), 500s, UD 100s, UD 300s, unit-of-use 100s, *Robot* ready 25s, *Emergi-script* 60s. **Susp.:** 100 mg/5 mL. Bot. 118 mL. *Rx-OTC.*
Use: Analgesic; NSAID.

ibuprofen. (Perrigo) Ibuprofen 40 mg/mL. Oral Drops. Bot. 15 mL. *OTC.*
Use: Analgesic; NSAID.

- **ibuprofen aluminum.** (eye-BYOO-profen ah-LOO-min-uhm) USAN.
  Use: Anti-inflammatory.
- **ibuprofen piconol.** (eye-BYOO-pro-fen PIK-oh-nahl) USAN.
  Use: Anti-inflammatory, topical.

ibuprofen suspension. (Various Mfr.) Ibuprofen 100 mg/5 mL. UD 50s. *Rx.*
Use: Analgesic; NSAID.

Ibutab. (Zee Medical) Ibuprofen 200 mg. Tab. 24s. *OTC.*
Use: Analgesic; NSAID.

- **ibutilide fumarate.** (ih-BYOO-tih-lide) USAN.
  Use: Cardiac depressant (antiarrhythmic).
  See: Corvert.

ICAPS Plus. (Ciba Vision) Vitamin A 6000 units, C 200 mg, E 60 units, B_2 20 mg, Zn 14.25 mg, Cu, Se, Mn. Sugar free. Tab. Bot. 60s, 120s. *OTC.*
Use: Mineral, vitamin supplement.
ICAPS Time Release. (Ciba Vision) Vitamin A 7000 units, C 200 mg, E 100 units, B_2 20 mg, Zn 14.25 mg, Cu, Se. Sugar free. Tab. Bot. 60s, 120s. *OTC.*
Use: Mineral, vitamin supplement.
Icar. (Hawthorn) Carbonyl iron. **Chew. Tab.:** 15 mg. Sorbitol, grape flavor. 60s. **Susp.:** 15 mg/1.25 mL. Fructose, parabens, grape and lemon flavors. Bot. 118 mL. *OTC.*
Use: Mineral supplement.
•**icatibant acetate.** (eye-CAT-ih-bant) USAN.
Use: Bradykinin antagonist.
Ice Mint. (Bristol-Myers Squibb) Stearic acid, synthetic cocoa butter, lanolin oil, camphor, menthol, beeswax, mineral oil, sodium borate, aromatic oils, emulsifiers. Jar 4 oz. *OTC.*
Use: Emollient; counterirritant.
IC-Green. (Akorn) Indocyanine green 25 mg. Pow. for Inj. Vials with 10 mL amps of aqueous solvent. 6s. *Rx.*
Use: Ophthalmic diagnostic product.
I-Chlor 0.5%. (Akorn) Chloramphenicol 5 mg/mL. Bot. 7.5 mL, 15 mL. *Rx.*
Use: Anti-infective, ophthalmic.
•**ichthammol.** (ICK-thah-mole) *USP 28.*
Use: Anti-infective, topical.
W/Aluminum hydroxide, phenol, zinc oxide, camphor, eucalyptol.
See: Boil-Ease Anesthetic Drawing Salve.
W/Hydrocortisone acetate, benzocaine, oxyquinoline sulfate, ephedrine hydrochloride.
See: Derma Medicone-HC.
W/Naftalan, calamine, amber pet.
See: Naftalan.
ichthammol. (Eli Lilly) Ichthammol 10%, 20% Oint. *OTC.*
Use: Antiseptic.
ichthammol. (Alra) Ichthammol 10%, 20% in a lanolin-petrolatum base. Oint. Tube 28.4 g. *OTC.*
Use: Antiseptic.
ichthynate.
See: Ichthammol.
•**icodextrin.** (eye-koe-DEX-trin) USAN.
Use: Osmotic.
•**icopezil maleate.** (eye-KOE-peh-zill) USAN.
Use: Alzheimer disease treatment (cognition enhancer); cognition adjuvant;

acetylcholinesterase inhibitor.
•**icotidine.** (eye-KOE-tih-DEEN) USAN.
Use: Antagonist (to histamine H_2 and H_1 receptors).
•**ictasol.** (IK-tah-sahl) USAN.
Use: Disinfectant.
Ictotest Reagent Tablets. (Bayer Corp. (Consumer Div.)) Reagent Tab. for urinary bilirubin. Bot. 100s.
Use: Diagnostic aid.
Icy Hot Balm. (Procter & Gamble) Methyl salicylate 29%, menthol 7.6%. Jar 3.5 oz, 7 oz. *OTC.*
Use: Analgesic, topical.
Icy Hot Cream. (Procter & Gamble) Methyl salicylate 30%, menthol 10%. Tube 0.25 oz, 1.25 oz, 3 oz. *OTC.*
Use: Analgesic, topical.
Icy Hot, Extra Strength. (Procter & Gamble) Methyl salicylate 30%, menthol 10%, ceresin, cyclomethicone, hydrogenated castor oil, PEG-150 distearate, propylene glycol, stearic acid, stearyl alcohol. Stick 52.5 g. *OTC.*
Use: Liniment.
Icy Hot Stick. (Procter & Gamble) Methyl salicylate 15%, menthol 8%. Stick 1.75 oz. *OTC.*
Use: Analgesic, topical.
I.D.A. Capsules. (Ivax) Isometheptene mucate 65 mg, dichloralphenazone 100 mg, acetaminophen 324 mg. Bot. 100s. *Rx.*
Use: Analgesic.
Idamycin PFS. (Pfizer) Idarubicin hydrochloride 1 mg/mL, preservative free. Inj. Single-use vial 5 mL, 10 mL, 20 mL. *Rx.*
Use: Anti-infective; anthracycline.
•**idarubicin hydrochloride.** (eye-DUH-RUE-bih-sin) *USP 28.*
Use: Antineoplastic; antibiotic, anthracycline.
See: Idamycin PFS.
idarubicin hydrochloride. (GensiaSicor) Idarubicin hydrochloride 1 mg/mL. Inj. Single-use vials. 5 mL, 10 mL, 20 mL. *Rx.*
Use: Antibiotic, anthracycline.
•**idoxifene.** (ih-dox-ih-feen) USAN.
Use: Antineoplastic; hormone replacement therapy (estrogen receptor antagonist); osteoporosis treatment and prevention.
I-Drops. (Akorn) Tetrahydrozoline hydrochloride 0.5%. Ophthalmic Soln. Bot. 0.5 oz. *Rx.*
Use: Mydriatic, vasoconstrictor.
•**idronoxil.** (id-roe-NOX-il) USAN.
Use: Antineoplastic agent.

•**idursulfase.** (eye-dur-SUL-fase) USAN.
Use: Hunter syndrome.

•**ifetroban.** (ih-FEH-troe-ban) USAN.
Use: Antithrombotic.

•**ifetroban sodium.** (ih-FEH-troe-ban)
USAN.
Use: Antithrombotic.

Ifex. (Bristol-Myers Squibb) Ifosfamide
1 g, 3 g. Pow. for Inj. Vial single dose.
Rx.
Use: Antineoplastic.

•**ifosfamide.** (eye-FOSS-fuh-MIDE)
USP 28.
Use: Antineoplastic.
See: Ifex.

ifosfamide. (American Pharmaceutical
Partners) Ifosfamide 1 g, 3 g. Pow. for
Inj., lyophilized. Vials. Single-dose. *Rx.*
Use: Antineoplastic.

I-Gent. (Akorn) Gentamicin sulfate 3 mg/
mL. Ophthalmic soln. Bot. 5 mL. *Rx.*
Use: Anti-infective, ophthalmic.

Igepal Co-880. (General Aniline & Film)
Nonoxynol-30. *OTC.*
Use: Contraceptive, spermicide.

Igepal Co-430. (General Aniline & Film)
Nonoxynol-4. *OTC.*
Use: Contraceptive, spermicide.

Igepal Co-730. (General Aniline & Film)
Nonoxynol-15. *OTC.*
Use: Contraceptive, spermicide.

IgG monoclonal anti-CD4.
See: Chimeric m t110 (human murine)
IgG monoclonal anti-cd4.

IGIV. (Various Mfr.) Immune globulin intravenous. *Rx.*
Use: Immunomodulator (Phase II/III pediatric HIV), immunization.
See: Immune globulin intravenous

•**igmesine hydrochloride.** (IGG-meh-
seen) USAN.
Use: Antidepressant.

I-Homatrine 5%. (Akorn) Homatropine
hydrobromide 5%. Ophth. Soln. Bot.
5 mL. *Rx.*
Use: Cycloplegic; mydriatic.

•**ilepcimide.** (eye-LEPP-sih-mide) USAN.
Formerly antiepilepsirine.
Use: Anticonvulsant.

Iletin I. (Eli Lilly) Regular and modified in-
sulin products from beef and pork.
Regular: 100 units/mL. Bot. 10 mL.
Lente: 100 units/mL. Bot. 10 mL. **NPH:**
100 units/mL. Bot 10 mL. *OTC.*
Use: Antidiabetic.

Iletin II Concentrated. (Eli Lilly) Purified
pork regular insulin 500 units/mL. Vial
20 mL. *Rx.*
Use: Antidiabetic.

Iletin II Regular. (Eli Lilly) Insulin
100 units/mL purified pork. Inj. Vial
10 mL. *OTC.*
Use: Antidiabetic.

•**ilmofosine.** (ill-MOE-fose-een) USAN.
Use: Antineoplastic.

•**ilomastat.** (eye-LOW-mah-stat) USAN.
Use: Corneal ulcers; inflammatory conditions; cancers.

•**ilonidap.** (ile-OHN-ih-dap) USAN.
Use: Anti-inflammatory.

Ilopan. (Pharmacia) Dexpanthenol
250 mg/mL. Disp. syringe 2 mL. *Rx.*
Use: Gastrointestinal stimulant.

•**iloperidone.** (ill-oh-PURR-ih-dohn)
USAN.
Use: Antipsychotic.

•**iloprost.** (EYE-loe-prost)
Use: Treatment of pulmonary arterial
hypertension.
See: Ventavis.

Ilosone. (Eli Lilly) Erythromycin estolate.
Tab.: 500 mg, Bot. 50s. **Susp.:** 125 mg,
250 mg/5 mL. Bot. 100 mL (250 mg
only), 480 mL. *Rx.*
Use: Anti-infective, erythromycin.

Ilosone Pulvules. (Eli Lilly) Erythromycin
estolate 250 mg. Cap. Bot. 100s. *Rx.*
Use: Anti-infective, erythromycin.

Ilotycin Gluceptate. (Eli Lilly) Erythro-
mycin gluceptate 1 g. Inj. Vial 30 mL.
Rx.
Use: Anti-infective, erythromycin.

Ilotycin Ointment. (Dista) Erythromycin
0.5%, white petrolatum, mineral oil.
Oint. Tube 3.5 g. *Rx.*
Use: Anti-infective, ophthalmic.

Ilozyme. (Pharmacia) Pancrelipase
equivalent to lipase 11,000 units, protease 30,000 units, amylase
30,000 units. Tab. Bot. 250s. *Rx.*
Use: Digestive enzymes.

IL-2. (Various Mfr.) Interleukin-2. *Rx.*
Use: Immunomodulator.
See: Proleukin.

I.L.X. B12 Elixir. (Kenwood) Liver fraction 98 mg, iron 102 mg, vitamins B_1
5 mg, B_2 2 mg, B_3 10 mg, B_{12} 10 mcg/
15 mL. Bot. 240 mL. *OTC.*
Use: Mineral, vitamin supplement.

I.L.X. B12 Tablets and Caplets. (Kenwood) Iron 37.5 mg, vitamins C
120 mg, desiccated liver 130 mg, B_1
2 mg, B_2 2 mg, B_3 20 mg, B_{12} 12 mcg.
Tab. Bot. 100s. *OTC.*
Use: Mineral, vitamin supplement.

I.L.X. Elixir. (Kenwood) Iron 70 mg, liver
concentrate 98 mg, vitamins B_1 5 mg,
B_2 2 mg, B_3 10 mg/15 mL. Bot. 240 mL.
OTC.

Use: Mineral, vitamin supplement.
• **imafen hydrochloride.** (IH-mah-fen)
USAN.
Use: Antidepressant.
Imager ac. (Mallinckrodt) Barium sulfate
100%, simethicone, sorbitol, sodium
benzoate. Susp. Bot. 650 mL w/enema
tip-tubing assemblies w/kit, 1900 mL
bot. *Rx.*
Use: Radiopaque agent.
imatinib mesylate.
Use: Protein-tyrosine kinase inhibitor.
See: Gleevec.
• **imazodan hydrochloride.** (ih-MAY-zoe-
DAN) USAN.
Use: Cardiovascular agent.
• **imciromab pentetate.** (im-SIHR-ah-
mab) USAN.
Use: Monoclonal antibody (antimyosin).
[Orphan Drug]
See: Myoscint.
Imdur. (Key) Isosorbide mononitrate
30 mg, 60 mg, 120 mg. ER Tab. Bot.
30s, 100s, UD 100s. *Rx.*
Use: Antianginal.
Imenol. (Sigma-Tau) Guaiacol 0.1 g, eu-
calyptol 0.08 g, iodoform 0.02 g, cam-
phor 0.05 g/mL. Vial 30 mL. *Rx.*
Use: Expectorant.
l-methorphinan levorphanol.
See: Levo-Dromoran.
Imexon. (Amplimed) DM 06.002.
Use: Multiple myeloma. [Orphan Drug]
Imferon. (Medeva) An iron-dextran com-
plex containing iron 50 mg/mL. Amp.
2 mL. Box 10s. Vial (w/phenol 0.5%)
10 mL. Box 2s. *Rx.*
Use: Mineral supplement.
imidazole antifungal.
Use: Antifungal agent.
See: Ketoconazole.
imidazole carboxamide.
Use: Antineoplastic.
See: Dacarbazine.
DTIC-Dome.
imidazolines.
Use: Nasal decongestant.
See: Afrin No-Drip Sinus with Vapor-
nase.
Afrin No-Drip 12-Hour.
Afrin No-Drip 12-Hour Extra Moistur-
izing.
Afrin No-Drip 12-Hour Severe Con-
gestion with Menthol.
Afrin Severe Congestion with Men-
thol.
Afrin Sinus with Vapornase.
Afrin 12-Hour Original.
Benzedrex.
Dristan Fast Acting Formula.

Dristan 12-Hr Nasal.
Duramist Plus 12-Hr Decongestant.
Duration.
Genasal.
Naphazoline Hydrochloride.
Nasal Decongestant Combinations.
Nasal Decongestant Inhalers.
Nasal Decongestant, Maximum
Strength.
Nasal Relief.
Natru-Vent.
Neo-Synephrine 12-Hour.
Neo-Synephrine 12-Hour Extra Mois-
turizing.
Nöstrilla 12-Hour.
Otrivin.
Otrivin Pediatric Nasal.
Oxymetazoline Hydrochloride.
Privine.
Tetrahydrozoline Hydrochloride.
12 Hour Nasal.
Twice-A-Day 12-Hour Nasal.
Tyzine.
Tyzine Pediatric.
Vicks Sinex 12-Hour Long-Acting.
Vicks Sinex 12-Hour Ultra Fine Mist
for Sinus Relief.
Vicks Vapor Inhaler.
Xylometazoline Hydrochloride.
imidazopyridines.
Use: Sedative/hypnotic nonbarbiturate.
See: Zolpidem Tartrate.
• **imidecyl iodine.** (IH-mih-DEH-sill EYE-
uh-dine) USAN.
Use: Anti-infective, topical.
• **imidocarb hydrochloride.** (ih-MIH-doe-
KARB) USAN.
Use: Antiprotozoal (Babesia).
• **imidoline hydrochloride.** (im-ID-oh-
leen) USAN.
Use: Anxiolytic; antipsychotic.
• **imidurea.** (ih-mid-your-EE-ah) *NF 23.*
Use: Antimicrobial.
• **imiglucerase.** (ih-mih-GLUE-ser-ACE)
USAN.
Use: Enzyme replenisher; treatment for
Gaucher disease (glucocerebrosi-
dase). [Orphan Drug]
See: Cerezyme.
• **imiloxan hydrochloride.** (ih-mill-OX-
ahn) USAN.
Use: Antidepressant.
imipemide.
Use: Anti-infective.
See: Imipenem.
• **imipenem.** (ih-mih-PEN-em) *USP 28.*
Formerly imipemide.
Use: Anti-infective.
W/Cilastatin for Injection.
See: Primaxin.

- **imipramine hydrochloride.** (im-IPP-ruh-meen) *USP 28.*
  Use: Antidepressant.
  See: Janimine.
     Tofranil.
imipramine hydrochloride. (Various Mfr.) Imipramine hydrochloride 10 mg, 25 mg, 50 mg. Tab. Bot. 50s (50 mg only), 100s, 250s, 500s, 1000s, UD 20s (50 mg only). *Rx.*
  Use: Antidepressant.
imipramine pamoate.
  Use: Antidepressant.
  See: Tofranil-PM.
- **imiquimod.** (ih-mih-KWIH-mahd) USAN.
  Use: Immunomodulator.
  See: Aldara.
Imitrex. (GlaxoSmithKline) Sumatriptan succinate. **Inj.:** 6 mg/0.5 mL, sodium chloride 7 mg/mL. Inj. Single-dose vial. 0.5 mL in 2 mL, *STATdose System* (2 pre-filled single dose syringes, 1 *STATdose Pen* and instructions for use). **Nasal Spray:** 5 mg, 20 mg. Nasal spray. Unit-dose spray device 100 mcL. Box 6s. **Tab.:** 25 mg, 50 mg, 100 mg. Tab. Blister pack 9s. *Rx.*
  Use: Antimigraine, serotonin 5-HI₁ receptor agonist.
ImmTher. (Immuno Therapeutics) Disaccharide tripeptide glycerol dipalmitoyl.
  Use: Antineoplastic. [Orphan Drug]
Immun-Aid. (McGaw) A custard flavored liquid containing 18.5 g protein, 60 g carbohydrate, 11 g fat, sodium 290 mg, potassium 530 mg per liter. 1 calorie/mL. With appropriate vitamins and minerals. Pow. Packets 123 g. 24s. *OTC.*
  Use: Nutritional supplement, enteral.
immune globulin. (ih-MYOON GLAH-byoo-lin) Immune Serum Globulin Human. Gamma-globulin fraction of normal human plasma. Vial 10 mL. Tubex 1 mL, 2 mL w/thimerosal 1:10,000. *Rx.*
  Use: Modification of active measles; prophylaxis of hepatitis A; treatment of immune deficiencies; prevention of infection associated with bone marrow transplantation (BMT); decrease frequency of certain pediatric HIV-related infections and conjunctive therapy for Kawasaki syndrome.
  See: Flebogamma 5%.
     Gamimune N.
     Gammar-P IV.
     Gamunex.
     Polygam S/D.
     Varicella-Zoster Immune Globulin (Human).
     Venoglobulin-S.

immune globulin, antithymocyte (rabbit).
  Use: Immunization.
  See: Thymoglobulin.
immune globulin, cytomegalovirus.
  See: CytoGam.
immune globulin, hepatitis B.
  See: BayHep B.
     H-BIG.
     Nabi-HB.
immune globulin intramuscular.
  Use: Immunization.
- **immune globulin intravenous pentetate.** (ih-MYOON GLAH-byoo-lin in-trah-VEE-nuhs) USAN.
  Use: Diagnostic aid.
immune globulin intravenous.
  Use: Immunization.
  See: BayGam.
     Carimune NF.
     Flebogamma 5%.
     Gamimune N.
     Gammagard S/D.
     Gammar-P IV.
     Gamunex.
     Iveegam.
     Octagam.
     Panglobulin.
     Panglobulin NF.
     Polygam S/D.
     RespiGam.
     Respiratory Syncytial Virus Immune Globulin Intravenous (Human) (RSV-IGIV).
     Rho₀(D) Immune Globulin IV (Human).
     Sandoglobulin.
     Venoglobulin-I.
     Venoglobulin-S.
     WinRho SDF.
immune globulin intravenous, botulism.
  Use: Infant botulism.
  See: BabyBIG.
immune globulin intravenous, vaccinia.
  Use: Immunization.
immune globulin, lymphocyte, antithymocyte (equine).
  Use: Immunization.
  See: Atgam.
immune globulin, rabies.
  Use: Immunization.
  See: Bayrab.
     Imogam Rabies-HT.
immune globulin, Rh₀(D).
  See: BayRho D Full Dose.
     BayRho D Mini Dose.
     MICRhoGAM.
     RhoGAM.
     WinRho SDF.

immune globulins.
See: Antithymocyte Globulin (Rabbit).
Botulism Immune Globulin IV.
Cytomegalovirus Immune Globulin
Intravenous, Human.
Hepatitis B Immune Globulin
(Human).
Immune Globulin Intravenous.
Lymphocyte Immune Globulin, Anti-
thymocyte Globulin (Equine).
Rabies Immune Globulin, Human.
$Rho_o(D)$ Immune Globulin.
$Rho_o(D)$ Immune Globulin IV Human.
$Rho_o(D)$ Immune Globulin Micro-
Dose.
Respiratory Syncytial Virus Immune
Globulin Intravenous (Human).
Tetanus Immune Globulin (Human).
Vaccinia Immune Globulin IV.
Varicella-Zoster Immune Globulin
(Human).
immune globulin, tetanus.
Use: Immunization.
See: BayTet.
immune globulin, varicella-zoster.
Use: Immunization.
See: Varicella-Zoster Immune Globulin
(Human).
immune serum (animal).
See: Botulism Antitoxin.
Diphtheria Antitoxin.
immune serums.
See: Cytomegalovirus Immune Glob-
ulin Intravenous (Human).
Hepatitis B Immune Globulin.
Immune Globulin Intramuscular.
Immune Globulin Intravenous.
Immune Serum Globulin (Human).
Rabies Immune Globulin.
$Rho_o(D)$ Immune Globulin.
Tetanus Immune Globulin.
Vaccinia Immune Globulin.
Varicella-Zoster Immune Globulin.
Immunex C-RP. (Wampole) Two-minute
latex agglutination slide test for the
qualitative detection of C-Reactive pro-
tein in serum. Kit 100s.
Use: Diagnostic aid.
immunization, active.
See: BCG Vaccine.
Diphtheria and Tetanus Toxoids, Acel-
lular Pertussis and Haemophilus In-
fluenzae Type B Conjugate Vac-
cines (DTaP-HIB).
Diphtheria and Tetanus Toxoids, Ad-
sorbed.
Diphtheria & Tetanus Toxoids, Adult.
Diphtheria and Tetanus Toxoids and
Acellular Pertussis Vaccine, Adsorbed (DTaP).
Diphtheria & Tetanus Toxoids, Pediatric.

Haemophilus b Conjugate Vaccine.
Haemophilus b Conjugate Vaccine
with Hepatitis B Vaccine.
Hepatitis A, Inactivated.
Hepatitis A, Inactivated and Hepatitis
B, Recombinant Vaccine.
Hepatitis B, Recombinant.
Influenza Virus Vaccine.
Measles Virus Vaccine, Live, Attenu-
ated.
Meningococcal Polysaccharide Vac-
cine.
Pneumococcal 7-Valent Conjugate
Vaccine.
Pneumococcal Vaccine, Polyvalent.
Typhoid Vaccine.
Varicella Virus Vaccine.
Immuno-C. (Biomune Systems, Inc.) Bo-
vine Whey Protein Concentrate.
Use: Cryptosporidiosis treatment.
[Orphan Drug]
Immunocal. (Immunotech Research)
Protein (from milk protein isolate) 9 g/
10 g, vitamin A, Ca, chloride, Fe, MG, P,
Na 25 mg, K 30 mg/10 g, 37 cal/10 g.
Pow. Pouch. 10 g. OTC.
Use: Enteral nutritional therapy.
Immunocal. (Immunotech Research)
Protein (from milk protein isolate) 9 g/
10 g, sodium 25 mg, potassium 30 mg,
calcium 60 mg, magnesium 9 mg, P
21 mg, calories 37/pkt. Pow. Pkt. 10 g
(30s). OTC.
Use: Nutritional supplement.
immunologic agents.
See: Adalimumab.
Alefacept.
Anakinra.
Basiliximab.
Cyclosporine Ophthalmic Emulsion.
Efalizumab.
Entanercept.
Immunomodulators.
Immunostimulants.
Immunosuppressives.
Infliximab.
Interferon alfacon-1.
Interferon alfa-n3 (human leukocyte
derived).
Interferon alfa-2a.
Interferon alfa-2b.
Interferon alfa-2b and Ribavirin.
Interferon beta-1a.
Interferon beta-1b.
Mitoxantrone Hydrochloride.
Mycophenolate.
Natalizumab.
Pegademase Bovine.
Peginterferon alfa-2a.
Peginterferon alfa-2b.
Sirolimus.

Tacrolimus.
Thalidomide.
immunomodulators.
See: Adalimumab.
Anakinra.
Etanercept.
Imiquimod.
Infliximab.
Interferon alfacon-1.
Interferon alfa-n3 (human leukocyte derived).
Interferon alfa-2a.
Interferon alfa-2b.
Interferon alfa-2b and Ribavirin.
Interferon beta-1a.
Interferon beta-1b.
Interferon gamma-1b.
Mitoxantrone Hydrochloride.
Natalizumab.
Peginterferon alfa-2a.
Peginterferon alfa-2b.
Pimecrolimus.
Thalidomide.
Immunorex. (Antigen Laboratories) Allergenic extracts, various. Vial. *Rx.*
Use: Allergen desensitization.
immunostimulants.
See: Pegademase Bovine.
immunosuppressives.
See: Alefacept.
Azathioprine.
Basiliximab.
Cylcosporine.
Daclizumab.
Efalizumab.
Glatiramer Acetate.
Muromonab-CD3.
Mycophenolate.
Sirolimus.
Tacrolimus.
Immuno Therapeutics. Immune globulin IV (human).
Use: Immunosuppressant. [Orphan Drug]
Immuraid. (Immunomedics) Technetium Tc-99M murine monoclonal antibody to hCG and human AFP.
Use: Diagnostic aid. [Orphan Drug]
ImmuRAIT. (Immunomedics) Iodine I[131] murine monoclonal antibody IgG2a to B cell.
Use: Antineoplastic.
Imodium A-D Liquid. (Ortho-McNeil) Loperamide 1 mg/5 mL, alcohol 5.25%. Bot. 60 mL, 90 mL, 120 mL. *OTC.*
Use: Antidiarrheal.
Imodium Capsules. (Janssen) Loperamide 2 mg. Cap. Bot. 100s, 500s, UD 100s. *Rx.*
Use: Antidiarrheal.

Imogam Rabies-HT. (Aventis Pasteur) Rabies immune globulin (human) (RIG) 150 IU/mL, preservative free, glycine 0.3 M, heat treated. Vials 2 mL, 10 mL. *Rx.*
Use: Immunization, rabies.
Imovax Rabies I.D. (Aventis Pasteur) Rabies vaccine 0.25 units/0.1 mL for intradermal administration for preexposure treatment only. Wistar rabies virus strain PM-1503-3M grown in human diploid cell culture. Pow. for Inj. in single-dose syringe w/1 vial diluent. *Rx.*
Use: Immunization, rabies.
Imovax Rabies Vaccine. (Aventis Pasteur) Merieux rabies vaccine, Wistar rabies virus strain PM-1503-3M grown in human diploid cell cultures. Rabies Vaccine G 2.5 units/mL. Pow. for Inj. In single-dose vial with disposable needle and syringe containing diluent and disposable needle for administration. *Rx.*
Use: Immunization, rabies.
imported fire ant venom, allergenic extract. (ALK)
Use: Allergy testing. [Orphan Drug]
impotence agents.
See: Alprostadil.
Sildenafil Citrate.
Vardenafil Hydrochloride.
Yohimbine Hydrochloride.
Impromen. (Janssen) Bromperidol decanoate. *Rx.*
Use: Antipsychotic.
Impromen Decanoate. (Janssen) Bromperidol decanoate. *Rx.*
Use: Antipsychotic.
•**impromidine hydrochloride.** (im-PRAH-mid-deen) USAN.
Use: Diagnostic aid (gastric secretion indicator).
Improved Congestant Tablets. (Rugby) Chlorpheniramine maleate 2 mg, acetaminophen 325 mg. Tab. Bot. 100s, 1000s. *OTC.*
Use: Antihistamine, analgesic.
Imreg-1. (Imreg) *Rx.*
Use: Immunomodulator.
Imreg-2. (Imreg) *Rx.*
Use: Immunomodulator.
Imuran. (Prometheus) Azathioprine 50 mg. Tab. Bot. 100s, UD 100s. *Rx.*
Use: Immunosuppressant.
Imuthiol. (Aventis Pasteur) Diethyldithiocarbamate. *Rx.*
Use: Immunomodulator.
Imuvert. (Celltech) *Serratia marcescens* extract (polyribosomes).
Use: Primary brain malignancies. [Orphan Drug]
inamrinone. *USP 28.* Formerly Amrinone.

Use: Cardiovascular agent.
- **inamrinone lactate.** *USP 28. Formerly Amrinone Lactate.*
Use: Cardiovascular agent.
inamrinone lactate. (Abbott Hospital Products) Inamrinone lactate 5 mg/mL, sodium metabisulfate 0.25 mg/mL. Inj. Amp. 20 mL. *Rx.*
Use: Inotropic agent.
Inapsine. (Akorn) Droperidol 2.5 mg/mL. Inj. Amp. or vial 1 mL, 2 mL. *Rx.*
Use: Anesthetic, general.
W/Fentanyl citrate.
See: Innovar.
incretin mimetic agents.
Use: Antidiabetic agent.
See: Exenatide.
- **indacrinone.** (IN-dah-KRIH-nohn) USAN.
Use: Antihypertensive, diuretic.
indalone.
See: Butopyronoxyl.
indandione derivative.
Use: Anticoagulant.
See: Anisindione.
- **indapamide.** (IN-DAP-uh-mide) *USP 28.*
Use: Antihypertensive, diuretic.
See: Lozol.
indapamide. (Various Mfr.) Indapamide 1.25 mg, 2.5 mg, lactose (2.5 mg only). Tab. Bot. 100s, 500s (1.25 mg only), 1000s. *Rx.*
Use: Antihypertensive, diuretic.
- **indeloxazine hydrochloride.** (in-DELL-OX-ah-zeen) USAN.
Use: Antidepressant.
Inderal. (Wyeth-Ayerst) Propranolol hydrochloride. **Tab.:** 10 mg, 20 mg, 40 mg, 60 mg, 80 mg. Bot. 100s, 1000s, 5000s (except 60 mg), UD 100s (except 60 mg, 80 mg). **Inj.:** 1 mg/mL. Amp. 1 mL. *Rx.*
Use: Antiadrenergic/sympatholytic; beta-adrenergic blocker.
Inderal LA. (Wyeth-Ayerst) Propranolol hydrochloride 60 mg, 80 mg, 120 mg, 160 mg. ER Cap. Bot. 100s, 1000s, UD 100s (except 60 mg). *Rx.*
Use: Antiadrenergic/sympatholytic; beta-adrenergic blocker.
Inderide. (Wyeth) Propranolol hydrochloride 40 mg, hydrochlorothiazide 25 mg. Tab. Bot. 100s, 1000s, UD 100s. Propranolol hydrochloride 80 mg, hydrochlorothiazide 25 mg. Tab. Bot. 100s. *Rx.*
Use: Antihypertensive combination.
indian gum.
See: Karaya Gum.

indigo carmine. (Becton Dickinson & Co.) Sodium indigotindisulfonate 8 mg/mL. Amp. 5 mL. Box 10s, 100s.
Use: Diagnostic aid.
See: Sodium indigotindisulfonate.
indigo carmine solution. (Becton Dickinson & Co.) Indigotindisulfonate sodium (0.8% aqueous soln. sodium salt of indigotindisulfonic acid) 40 mg/5 mL. Inj. Amp. 5 mL, 10s.
Use: Diagnostic aid.
- **indigotindisulfonate sodium.** (IN-dih-go-tin-die-SULL-foe-nate) *USP 28.* Indigo Carmine.
Use: Diagnostic aid (cystoscopy).
See: Sodium Indigotindisulfonate.
- **indinavir.** (in-DIN-ah-veer) USAN.
Use: Antiviral (HIV-protease inhibitor).
- **indinavir sulfate.** (in-DIN-ah-veer) USAN.
Use: Antiretroviral, protease inhibitor.
See: Crixivan.
- **indiplon.** (IN-di-plon) USAN.
Use: Sedative, hypnotic.
- **indium chlorides In 113m.** (IN-dee-uhm) USAN.
Use: Radiopharmaceutical.
- **indium In 111 chloride solution.** (IN-dee-uhm) *USP 28.*
Use: Radiopharmaceutical.
- **indium In 111 ibritumomab tiuxetan injection.** (IN-dee-uhm) *USP 28.*
Use: Radiopharmaceutical.
indium In 111 murine monoclonal antibody fab to myosin.
Use: Diagnostic aid in myocarditis. [Orphan Drug]
See: Myoscint.
- **indium In 111 oxyquinoline solution.** (IN-dee-uhm OX-ee-KWIN-oh-lin) *USP 28.*
Use: Radiopharmaceutical, diagnostic aid.
- **indium In 111 pentetate injection.** (IN-dee-uhm) *USP 28.*
Use: Diagnostic aid (radionuclide cisternography), radiopharmaceutical.
- **indium In 111 pentetreotide.** (IN-dee-uhm In 111 pen-teh-TREE-oh-tide) *USP 28.*
Use: Diagnostic aid, radiopharmaceutical.
- **indium In 111 satumomab pendetide.** (IN-dee-uhm sat-YOU-mah-mab PEN-deh-TIDE) USAN.
Use: Radiodiagnostic monoclonal antibody (ovarian and colorectal carcinoma), radiopharmaceutical.
Indocin. (Merck & Co.) Indomethacin. **Cap.:** 25 mg, 50 mg, lactose, lecithin.

Bot. 100s, 1000s (25 mg only). **Supp.:**
50 mg. Pkg. 30s. **Oral Susp.:** 25 mg/
5 mL, alcohol 1%, sorbitol, pineapple,
coconut, and mint flavor. Bot. 237 mL.
Rx.
Use: Analgesic; NSAID.
Indocin I.V. (Merck & Co.) Indomethacin
sodium trihydrate equivalent to 1 mg
indomethacin/Vial. Vial single-dose. *Rx.*
Use: Arterial patency agent.
Indocin SR. (Forte Pharma) Indomethacin 75 mg. SR Cap. Unit-of-use 60s.
Rx.
Use: Analgesic; NSAID.
• **indocyanine green.** (in-doe-SIGH-ah-
neen) *USP 28.*
Use: Diagnostic aid (cardiac output de-
termination, hepatic function determi-
nation); ophthalmic diagnostic prod-
uct.
See: Cardio-Green.
IC-Green.
Indogesic. (Century) Acetaminophen
32.5 mg, butalbital 50 mg. Tab. Bot.
100s, 1000s. *Rx.*
Use: Analgesic; hypnotic, sedative.
Indoklon. Hexafluorodiethyl ether. Flurothyl. Bis-(2,2,2-trifluorethyl) ether. *Rx.*
Use: Shock-inducing agent (convul-
sant).
• **indolapril hydrochloride.** (in-DAHL-ah-
PRILL) USAN.
Use: Antihypertensive.
Indo-Lemmon. (Teva) Indomethacin
25 mg, 50 mg. Cap. Bot. 100s, 500s,
1000s. *Rx.*
Use: Analgesic; NSAID.
• **indolidan.** (in-DOE-lih-DAN) USAN.
Use: Cardiovascular agent.
Indometh. (Major) Indomethacin. Cap.
25 mg: Bot. 100s, 1000s. **50 mg:** Bot.
100s, 500s. *Rx.*
Use: Analgesic; NSAID.
• **indomethacin.** (in-doe-METH-ah-sin)
USP 28.
Use: Anti-inflammatory; analgesic.
See: Indochron E-R.
Indocin.
Indocin SR.
Indo-Lemmon.
indomethacin. (Various Mfr.) Indometha-
cin 25 mg, 50 mg. Cap. Bot. 50s (25 mg
only), 100s, 500s, 1000s, UD 100s,
Robot ready 25s. *Rx.*
Use: Anti-inflammatory; analgesic.
indomethacin extended-release. (In-
wood) Indomethacin 75 mg, sucrose,
parabens. SR Cap. Bot. 60s, 100s. *Rx.*
Use: Analgesic; NSAID.

• **indomethacin sodium.** (in-doe-METH-
ah-sin) *USP 28.*
Use: Anti-inflammatory; analgesic.
indomethacin sodium trihydrate. *Rx.*
Use: Arterial patency agent.
See: Indocin IV.
indomethacin sustained release.
(Various Mfr.) Indomethacin 75 mg.
SR Cap. Bot. 60s, 100s, 500s. *Rx.*
Use: Anti-inflammatory; analgesic.
• **indoprofen.** (in-doe-PRO-fen) USAN.
Use: Analgesic; anti-inflammatory.
• **indoramin.** (in-DAHR-ah-min) USAN.
Use: Antihypertensive.
• **indoramin hydrochloride.** (in-DAHR-ah-
min) USAN.
Use: Antihypertensive.
• **indorenate hydrochloride.** (in-DAHR-
en-ATE) USAN.
Use: Antihypertensive.
• **indoxole.** (IN-dox-OLE) USAN.
Use: Antipyretic; anti-inflammatory.
• **indriline hydrochloride.** (IN-drih-leen)
USAN.
Use: Stimulant, central.
I-Neocort. (American Pharmaceutical)
Neomycin sulfate 5 mg, hydrocortisone
acetate 15 mg/5 mL. Ophth. Susp. Bot.
5 mL. *Rx.*
Use: Anti-infective; corticosteroid.
I-Neospor. (American Pharmaceutical)
Polymyxin B sulfate, gramicidin, neomycin sulfate. Ophth. Soln. Bot. 10 mL.
Rx.
Use: Anti-infective, ophthalmic.
Infalyte Oral Solution. (Bristol-Myers
Squibb) Electrolyte mixture with 30 g/L
rice syrup solids containing 4.2 calo-
ries/fl. oz. In 1 liter. *OTC.*
Use: Nutritional supplement.
Infanrix. (GlaxoSmithKline) Diphtheria
toxoid 25 Lf units, tetanus toxoid 10 Lf
units, pertussis toxin 25 mcg, filamentous hemagglutinin 25 mcg, pertactin
8 mcg/0.5 mL. Inj. Single-dose Vials
(2-phenoxyethanol 2.5 mg, sodium
chloride 4.5 mg, not more than
0.625 mg aluminum by assay, not more
than 100 mcg of residual formaldehyde, and not more than 100 mcg of
polysorbate 80) and disposable *Tip-Lok*
syringes. *Rx.*
Use: Immunization, active toxoid.
Infantaire. (Altaire) Acetaminophen
80 mg/0.8 mL. Drops. 15 mL, 30 mL.
OTC.
Use: Analgesic.
infant foods.
Use: Nutritional supplement.
See: Enfamil.
Enfamil Human Milk Fortifier.

Enfamil Premature 20 Formula. RCF. Similac. Similac PM 60/40.

infant foods, hypoallergenic.
Use: Nutritional supplement.
See: Isomil.
Isomil SF.
I-Soyalac.
Nutramigen.
Pregestimil.
ProSobee.
Soyalac.

Infant's Feverall. (Upsher-Smith) Acetaminophen 80 mg. Supp. 6s. *OTC.*
Use: Analgesic.

Infants' Motrin. (McNeil) Ibuprofen 40 mg/mL, sorbitol, sucrose, berry flavor. Oral drops. Bot. 15 mL w/dropper. *OTC.*
Use: Anti-inflammatory; analgesic.

Infants' No-Aspirin Drops. (Walgreen) Acetaminophen 80 mg/0.8 mL. Nonalcoholic. Bot. 15 mL. *OTC.*
Use: Analgesic.

Infants' Silapap. (Silarx) Acetaminophen 80 mg/0.8 mL. Drops. Bot. 15 mL. Alcohol free. *OTC.*
Use: Analgesic; antipyretic.

Infarub Cream. (Whitehall-Robins Laboratories) Methyl salicylate 35%, menthol 10% in vanishing cream base. Tube 1.25 oz, 3.5 oz. *OTC.*
Use: Analgesic, topical.

Infasurf. (Forest) Phospholipids 35 mg/mL suspended in 0.9% sodium chloride solution, 0.65 mg proteins. Intratracheal Susp. Single-use vial 6 mL. *Rx.*
Use: Lung surfactant.

Infectrol Ointment. (Bausch & Lomb) Dexamethasone 0.1%, neomycin sulfate equivalent to 0.35% neomycin base, 10,000 units polymyxin B sulfate/g. White petrolatum, lanolin, mineral oil, parabens. Tube 3.5, 3.75 g. *Rx.*
Use: Anti-infective, corticosteroid, topical.

Infectrol Suspension. (Bausch & Lomb) Dexamethasone 0.1%, neomycin sulfate equivalent to 0.35% neomycin base, 10,000 units polymyxin B sulfate/mL. Hydroxypropyl methylcellulose, polysorbate 20, benzalkonium chloride. Drop. Bot. 5 mL. *Rx.*
Use: Anti-infective; corticosteroid, ophthalmic.

InFeD. (Schein) Iron 50 mg/mL (as dextran), sodium chloride approximately 0.9%. Inj. Single-dose Vial 2 mL. *Rx.*
Use: Mineral supplement.

Infergen. (InterMune) Interferon alfacon-1 9 mcg, 15 mcg, preservative free. Inj. Single-dose vial. 0.3 mL (9 mcg), 0.5 mL (15 mcg). *Rx.*
Use: Immunologic, immunomodulator.

Inflamase Forte. (Novartis Ophthalmic) Prednisolone sodium phosphate 1%. Bot. 5 mL, 10 mL, 15 mL. *Rx.*
Use: Corticosteroid, ophthalmic.

Inflamase Mild. (Novartis Ophthalmic) Prednisolone sodium phosphate 0.125%. Bot. 3 mL, 5 mL, 10 mL. *Rx.*
Use: Corticosteroid, ophthalmic.

infliximab.
Use: Crohn disease; rheumatoid arthritis; immunologic agent; immunomodulator; ankylosing spondylitis.
See: Remicade.

• **influenza virus vaccine.** (in-flew-EN-zuh) *USP 28.*
Use: Immunization.
See: FluMist.
Fluvirin.
Fluzone.

Infumorph 500. (Baxter) Morphine sulfate 25 mg/mL, preservative free. Soln. for Inj. Amp. 20 mL (500 mg). *c-II.*
Use: Opioid analgesic.

Infumorph 200. (Baxter) Morphine sulfate 10 mg/mL, preservative free. Inj. Amp. 20 mL (200 mg). *c-II.*
Use: Opioid analgesic.

Infuvite Adult. (Baxter) Vitamin A 2300 units, D_3 200 units, E (dl-alpha tocopheryl acetate) 10 units, B_1 6 mg, B_2 3.6 mg, B_3 40 mg, B_5 15 mg, B_6 6 mg, B_{12} 5 mcg, C 200 mg, K 150 mcg, biotin 60 mcg, folic acid 600 mcg/10 mL (after combining vials), polysorbate 80. Inj. Vials. 2.5 mL. *Rx.*
Use: Nutritional supplement.

Infuvite Pediatric. (Baxter) Vitamin A 2300 units, D_3 400 units, E (dl-alpha tocopheryl acetate) 7 units, B_1 1.2 mg, B_2 14 mg, B_3 17 mg, B_5 15 mg, B_6 1 mg, B_{12} 1 mcg, C 80 mg, K 0.2 mg, biotin 20 mcg, folic acid 140 mcg/5 mL (after combining vials), polysorbate 80. Inj. 2 vials (4 mL and 1 mL). *Rx.*
Use: Nutritional supplement.

Ingadine Tabs. (Major) Guanethidine sulfate 10 mg, 25 mg. Bot. 100s, 1000s. *Rx.*
Use: Antihypertensive.

• **ingliforib.** (in-gli-FOE-rib) USAN.
Use: Antidiabetic.

INH. (Novartis) Isoniazid 300 mg. Tab. *Rx.*
Use: Antituberculosal.

Inhal-Aid. (Key)
Use: Respiratory drug delivery system.

Inhibace. (Roche) Cilazapril. *Rx.*
Use: Antihypertensive.
injectable local anesthetics.
See: Anesthetics, Injectable Local.
Innerclean Herbal Laxative. (Last)
Senna leaf powder, psyllium seed,
buckthorne, anise seed, fennel seed.
Bot. 1 oz, 2 oz. *OTC.*
Use: Laxative.
Innertabs. (Last) Senna leaf powder and
psyllium seed tablets. Bot. 80s, 200s.
OTC.
Use: Laxative.
Innohep. (Pharmion Corp.) Tinzaparin
sodium 20,000 units/mL (Anti-Factor
Xa International Units), sodium metabi-
sulfite 3.1 mg/mL, benzyl alcohol
10 mg/mL. Inj. Multidose vial 2 mL. *Rx.*
Use: Anticoagulant; low molecular
weight heparin.
InnoPran XL. (Reliant) Propranolol hy-
drochloride 80 mg, 120 mg, sugar
spheres. ER Cap. 30s, 100s, 500s, UD
100s. *Rx.*
Use: Antiadrenergic/sympatholytic,
beta-adrenergic blocking agent.
Inocor Lactate. (Sanofi-Synthelabo)
Amrinone lactate (base equivalent)
5 mg/mL, sodium metabisulfite 0.25 mg.
Inj. Amp. 20 mL. Box 5s. *Rx.*
Use: Inotropic.
•**inocoterone acetate.** (ih-NO-koe-ter-
ohn) USAN.
Use: Dermatologic, acne.
INOmax. (INO Therapeutics) Nitric oxide
100 ppm, 800 ppm. Gas. Can. 353 L
(delivered volume 344 L), 1963 L (deliv-
ered volume 1918 L). *Rx.*
Use: Respiratory gas.
In-111 murine mab. (2B8-MX-DTPA).
Use: B-cell non-Hodgkin lymphoma.
[Orphan Drug]
inophylline.
See: Aminophylline.
inosine pranobex. Isoprinosine.
Use: Antiviral. [Orphan Drug]
See: Isoprinosine.
Inosiplex. (Newport Pharmaceuticals)
Isoprinosine. *Rx.*
Use: Antiviral.
inosit.
See: Inositol.
Inositech. (Bio-tech) Inositol 324 mg.
Cap. 100s. *OTC.*
Use: Lipotropic product.
inositol.
Use: Lipotropic.
See: Inositech.
•**inositol niacinate.** (in-OH-sih-tole NIE-
ah-sin-ate) USAN.
Use: Vasodilator.

inositol nicotinate.
See: Inositol Niacinate.
inotropic agents.
See: Digitek.
Digoxin.
Digoxin Injection, Pediatric.
Inamrinone Lactate.
Lanoxicaps.
Lanoxin.
Milrinone Lactate.
Primacor.
InspirEase. (Key) *Rx.*
Use: Respiratory drug delivery system.
Inspra. (Searle) Eplerenone 25 mg,
50 mg, lactose. Tab. Bot. 30s, 90s, unit
doses (25 mg only). *Rx.*
Use: Renin angiotensin system antago-
nist.
Insta-Char. (Kerr Drug) **Regular:** Aque-
ous suspension activated charcoal
50 g/8 oz. **Pediatric:** Aqueous suspen-
sion activated charcoal 15 g/4 oz. *OTC.*
Use: Antidote.
Insta-Glucose. (ICN) Undiluted USP glu-
cose. UD tube containing liquid glu-
cose 31 g. *OTC.*
Use: Hyperglycemic.
Inst-E-Vite. (Barth's) Vitamin E 100 units,
200 units. Cap. **100 units:** Bot 100s,
500s, 1000s. **200 units:** Bot. 100s,
250s, 500s. *OTC.*
Use: Vitamin supplement.
•**insulin.** (IN-suh-lin) *USP 28.*
Use: Antidiabetic.
See: Insulin Analog Injection.
Insulin Detemir.
Insulin Glargine.
Insulin Glulisine.
Insulin Injection Concentrated.
Insulin Injection (Regular).
Insulin Zinc Suspension, Extended
(Ultralente).
Insulin Zinc Suspension (Lente).
Isophane Insulin Suspension (NPH).
Isophane Insulin Suspension (NPH)
and Insulin Injection (Regular).
insulin analog injection.
Use: Antidiabetic.
See: Humalog.
Humalog Mix 75/25.
NovoLog.
NovoLog Mix 70/30.
•**insulin aspart.** (IN-suh-lin ASS-part)
USAN.
Use: Antidiabetic.
•**insulin, dalanated.** (IN-suh-lin dah-
LAHN-ate-ed) USAN.
Use: Antidiabetic.
•**insulin detemir.** (IN-suh-lin DEHT-ih-
meer) USAN.

Use: Antidiabetic.
See: Levemir.
•**insulin glargine.** (IN-suh-lin GLAHR-gine) USAN.
Use: Antidiabetic.
See: Lantus.
•**insulin glulisine.** (IN-suh-lin gloo-LIS-een) USAN.
Use: Antidiabetic.
See: Apidra.
•**insulin human.** (IN-suh-lin) *USP 28.*
Use: Antidiabetic.
See: Humulin.
•**insulin human, isophane, suspension.**
(IN-suh-lin hue-man EYE-so-fane)
USP 28.
Use: Antidiabetic.
•**insulin human zinc, extended, suspension.** (IN-suh-lin) *USP 28.*
Use: Antidiabetic.
•**insulin human zinc suspension.** (IN-suh-lin) *USP 28.*
Use: Antidiabetic.
insulin inhaled.
Use: Investigational antidiabetic agent.
insulin injection, concentrated.
Use: Antidiabetic.
See: Humulin R Regular U-500 (Concentrated).
insulin injection (regular).
Use: Antidiabetic.
See: Humulin R.
Novolin R.
Novolin R PenFill.
Novolin R Prefilled.
Regular Iletin II.
•**insulin, isophane, suspension.** (IN-suh-lin EYE-so-fane) *USP 28.*
Use: Antidiabetic.
See: NPH.
•**insulin I-131.** (IN-suh-lin) USAN.
Use: Radiopharmaceutical.
•**insulin I-125.** (IN-suh-lin) USAN.
Use: Radiopharmaceutical.
insulin-like growth factor-1.
Use: Amyotrophic lateral sclerosis.
[Orphan Drug]
•**insulin lispro.** (IN-suh-lin LICE-pro)
USP 28.
Use: Antidiabetic.
See: Humalog.
Humalog Mix 50/50.
Humalog Mix 75/25.
•**insulin, neutral.** (IN-suh-lin) USAN.
Use: Antidiabetic.
insulin Novo rapitard. Biphasic Insulin.
•**insulin, protamine zinc suspension.**
(IN-suh-lin PRO-tah-meen zingk)
USP 28. 40 units, 100 units/mL. Vials
10 mL.

Use: Antidiabetic.
insulin, regular.
Use: Antidiabetic.
See: Humulin BR.
Humulin R.
Novolin R.
Novolin R PenFill.
Pork Regular Iletin II (Pork).
Regular Insulin (Pork).
Velosulin.
Velosulin (Pork).
insulin, regular concentrate.
Use: Antidiabetic.
insulin suspension, isophane.
Use: Antidiabetic.
See: Humulin 50/50.
Humulin 70/30.
Novolin 70/30.
Novolin 70/30 PenFill.
insulin suspension, lente.
Use: Antidiabetic.
See: Humulin L.
Lente Insulin.
Lente Insulin (Beef).
Lente L.
Lente Iletin II (Beef).
Lente Iletin II (Pork).
Lente Purified Pork Insulin.
Novolin L.
insulin suspension, NPH.
Use: Antidiabetic.
See: Beef NPH Iletin II.
Humulin N.
Novolin N.
Novolin N PenFill.
NPH Iletin I (Beef and Pork).
NPH Insulin (Beef).
NPH-N Purified (Pork).
Pork NPH Iletin II.
insulin suspension, PZI. *OTC.*
Use: Antidiabetic.
See: Humulin U Ultralente.
insulin suspension semilente. *OTC.*
Use: Antidiabetic.
insulin suspension, ultralente. *OTC.*
Use: Antidiabetic.
See: Humulin U Ultralente.
Ultralente Insulin (Beef).
•**insulin zinc, prompt, suspension.** (IN-suh-lin) *USP 28.*
Use: Antidiabetic.
•**insulin zinc, suspension, extended (ultralente).** (IN-suh-lin) *USP 28.*
Use: Antidiabetic.
See: Humulin U.
•**insulin zinc suspension (lente).** (IN-suh-lin) *USP 28.*
Use: Antidiabetic.
See: Humulin L.
Lente Iletin II.

Intal. (Aventis) Cromolyn sodium.
Soln.: 20 mg/2 mL. UD Amps. 60, 120.
Aerosol: 800 mcg/actuation. 8.1 g
(≥ 112 metered sprays), 14.2 g
(≥ 200 metered sprays). *Rx.*
Use: Antiasthmatic.
Integrilin. (COR Therapeutics) Eptifibatide 0.75 mg/mL, 2 mg/mL. Inj. for
Soln. Vial 10 mL (2 mg/mL only),
100 mL. *Rx.*
Use: Antiplatelet, glycoprotein IIb/IIIa inhibitor.
Integrin Caps. (Sanofi-Synthelabo)
Oxypertine. *Rx.*
Use: Anxiolytic.
Intensol. (Roxane) A system of concentrated solutions of drugs w/calibrated
dropper: Chlorpromazine hydrochloride
30 mg/mL, 100 mg/mL; dexamethasone 1 mg/mL; dihydrotachysterol
0.2 mg/mL; hydrochlorothiazide
100 mg/mL; prednisone 5 mg/mL; thioridazine hydrochloride 30 mg/mL,
100 mg/mL.
interferon. A family of naturally occurring, small protein molecules with molecular weights of approximately
15,000 to 21,000 daltons. They are
formed by the interaction of animal cells
with viruses capable of conferring on
animal cells' resistance to virus infection. Three major classes of interferons have been identified: alpha, beta,
and gamma. Interferon was first derived
from human white blood cells and
originally used in Finland.
Use: Antineoplastic, antiviral; treatment
of breast cancer lymphoma, multiple
melanoma, and malignant melanoma.
See: Actimmune.
Avonex.
Betaseron.
Intron A.
Roferon-A.
interferon alfacon-1.
Use: Immunologic, immunomodulator.
See: Infergen.
•**interferon alfa-n1.** (IN-ter-FEER-ahn AL-fuh) USAN.
Use: Antineoplastic, antiviral; biological
response modifier. [Orphan Drug]
**interferon alfa-n3 (human leukocyte
derived).**
Use: Immunologic agent, immunomodulator.
See: Alferon N.
•**interferon alfa-2a, recombinant.** (IN-ter-FEER-ahn AL-fuh-2a ree-KAHM-bih-nent) USAN.
Use: Antineoplastic, antiviral; biological

response modifier; immunomodulator.
[Orphan Drug]
See: Roferon-A.
•**interferon alfa-2b.** (IN-ter-FEER-ahn AL-fuh-2b) USAN.
Use: Antineoplastic, antiviral; biological
response modifier; immunomodulator.
See: Intron A.
**interferon alfa-2b, recombinant and
ribavirin.**
Use: Antineoplastic; immunologic; immunomodulator.
See: Rebetron.
interferon, beta.
Use: Immunomodulator; treatment of
multiple sclerosis.
See: Avonex.
Betaseron.
•**interferon beta-1a.** (in-ter-FEER-ohn BAY-tuh-1a) USAN.
Use: Antineoplastic; biological response
modifier; immunologic agent, immunomodulator; antineoblast.
See: Avonex.
Rebif.
•**interferon beta-1b.** (IN-ter-FEER-ahn BAY-tuh-1b) USAN.
Use: Immunologic agent, immunomodulator.
See: Betaseron.
•**interferon gamma-1b.** (IN-ter-FEER-ahn GAM-uh-1b) USAN.
Use: Antineoplastic, antiviral; immunoregulator, biological response modifier. [Orphan Drug]
See: Actimmune.
interleukin-1 receptor antagonist, human recombinant.
Use: Juvenile rheumatoid arthritis; graft-vs-host disease in transplant patients.
[Orphan Drug]
See: Antril.
interleukins.
Use: Hematopoietic.
See: Oprelvekin.
interleukin-3, recombinant human.
(Novartis) *Rx.*
Use: Immunomodulator. [Orphan Drug]
interleukin-2.
Use: Immunomodulator; antineoplastic.
[Orphan Drug]
See: Proleukin.
Teceleukin.
interleukin-2 PEG. (Cetus) *Rx.*
Use: Immunomodulator.
**interleukin-2, recombinant liposome
encapsulated.**
Use: Antineoplastic. [Orphan Drug]

Intralipid 10% I.V. Fat Emulsion. (Pharmacia) IV fat emulsion containing soybean oil 10%, egg yolk phospholipids 1.2%, glycerin 2.25%, water for injection. I.V. Flask 50 mL, 100 mL, 250 mL, 500 mL. *Rx.*
Use: Nutritional supplement, parenteral.
Intralipid 20% I.V. Fat Emulsion. (Pharmacia) IV fat emulsion containing soybean oil 20%, egg yolk phospholipids 1.2%, glycerin 2.25%, water for injection. I.V. Flask 50 mL, 100 mL, 250 mL, 500 mL. *Rx.*
Use: Nutritional supplement, parenteral.
intranasal steroids.
See: Beclomethasone Dipropionate.
Budesonide.
Flunisolide.
Fluticasone Propionate.
Mometasone Furoate Monohydrate.
Triamcinolone Acetonide.
IntraSite. (Smith & Nephew) Graft T starch copolymer 2%, water 8%, propylene glycol 20%. Sterile amorphous interactive hydrogel dressing. 25 g. *Rx.*
Use: Dermatologic, wound therapy.
intrauterine progesterone system. *Rx.*
Use: Contraceptive.
See: Progestasert.
intraval sodium.
See: Pentothal Sodium.
intravenous nutritional therapy.
See: Combined Electrolyte Concentrates.
Combined Electrolyte Solutions.
Dextrose 2.5% with 0.45% Sodium Chloride.
Dextrose 3.3% and 0.3% Sodium Chloride.
Dextrose 5% and Electrolyte No. 48.
Dextrose 5% and Electrolyte No. 75.
Dextrose 5% with 0.2% Sodium Chloride.
Dextrose 5% and 0.225% Sodium Chloride.
Dextrose 5% with 0.3% Sodium Chloride.
Dextrose 5% with 0.33% Sodium Chloride.
Dextrose 5% with 0.45% Sodium Chloride.
Dextrose 5% with 0.9% Sodium Chloride.
Dextrose 10% and Electrolyte No. 48.
Dextrose 10% with 0.2% Sodium Chloride.
Dextrose 10% with 0.225% Sodium Chloride.
Dextrose 10% with 0.45% Sodium Chloride.
Dextrose 10% and 0.9% Sodium Chloride.
Half-Strength Lactated Ringer's in 2.5% Dextrose.
Hyperlyte CR.
Invert Sugar-Electrolyte Solutions.
Isolyte H in 5% Dextrose.
Isolyte M in 5% Dextrose.
Isolyte P in 5% Dextrose.
Isolyte R in 5% Dextrose.
Isolyte S pH 7.4.
Isolyte S with 5% Dextrose.
Lactated Ringer's.
Lactated Ringer's in 5% Dextrose.
Lypholyte.
Lypholyte-II.
Multilyte-20.
Multilyte-40.
Multiple Electrolytes and 5% Travert.
Multiple Electrolytes and 10% Travert.
Normosol-M.
Normosol-M and 5% Dextrose.
Normosol-R.
Normosol-R and 5% Dextrose.
Normosol-R pH 7.4.
Nutrilyte.
Nutrilyte II.
Plasma-Lyte A pH 7.4.
Plasma-Lyte 56 and 5% Dextrose.
Plasma-Lyte 148.
Plasma-Lyte 148 and 5% Dextrose.
Plasma-Lyte R.
Plasma-Lyte R and 5% Dextrose.
Potassium Chloride in 0.9% Sodium Chloride.
Potassium Chloride in 3.3% Dextrose and 0.3% Sodium Chloride.
Potassium Chloride in 5% Dextrose.
Potassium Chloride in 5% Dextrose and Lactated Ringer's.
Potassium Chloride in 5% Dextrose and 0.2% Sodium Chloride.
Potassium Chloride in 5% Dextrose and 0.33% Sodium Chloride.
Potassium Chloride in 5% Dextrose and 0.45% Sodium Chloride.
Potassium Chloride in 5% Dextrose and 0.9% Sodium Chloride.
Potassium Chloride in 10% Dextrose and 0.2% Sodium Chloride.
Ringer's.
Ringer's in 5% Dextrose.
TPN Electrolytes.
TPN Electrolytes II.
TPN Electrolytes III.
intravenous replenishment solutions.
Use: Intravenous nutritional therapy.
See: Intravenous Nutritional Therapy.
•**intrazole.** (IN-trah-zole) USAN.
Use: Anti-inflammatory.
•**intriptyline hydrochloride.** (in-TRIP-tih-leen) USAN.

Use: Antidepressant.

Introlite. (Ross) Protein 22.2 g, carbohydrate 70.5 g, fat 18.4 g, Na 930 mg, K 1570 mg/L with 200 mOsm/kg water, with appropriate vitamins and minerals, 0.53 Cal/mL. Liq. *OTC.*
Use: Nutritional supplement.

Intron A. (Schering-Plough) Interferon alfa-2b. **Pow. for Inj.:** 5 million, 10 million, 18 million, 25 million, 50 million units/vial. Each mL contains human albumin 1 mg, glycine 20 mg, sodium phosphate dibasic 2.3, sodium phosphate monobasic 0.55 mg. Vial w/1 mL diluent vial (5 million, 18 million, 50 million); vial w/2 mL diluent vial (10 million); vial w/5 mL diluent vial (25 million). **Soln. for Inj.:** 3 million, 5 million, 10 million, 18 million, 25 million units/vial. Each mL contains sodium chloride 7.5 mg, sodium phosphate dibasic 1.8 mg, sodium phosphate monobasic 1.3 mg, EDTA 0.1 mg, polysorbate 80 0.1 mg, m-cresol 1.5 mg. Vial Pak-3 (6 vials, 6 syr.) (3 million); Pak-5 (6 vials, 6 syr.) (5 million); Pak-10 (6 vials, 6 syr.) (10 million); multidose vial (22.8 million units/ 3.8 mL) (18 million units); multidose vial (32 million units/3.2 mL) (25 million). **Inj.:** 3 million, 5 million, 10 million units/dose. Each mL contains sodium chloride 7.5 mg, sodium phosphate dibasic 1.8 mg, sodium phosphate monobasic 1.3 mg, EDTA 0.1 mg, polysorbate 80 0.1 mg, m-cresol 1.5 mg. Multidose pens 6 doses (22.5 million units/1.5 mL per pen) (3 million); (37.5 million units/1.5 mL per pen) (5 million); (75 million units/1.5 mL per pen) (10 million) w/needles. *Rx.*
Use: Antineoplastic; immunologic, immunomodulator.

Intropaque Liquid. (Lafayette) Barium sulfate 60% w/v suspension. Bot. Gal. Case 4s.
Use: Radiopaque agent.

Intropaste. (Mallinckrodt) Barium sulfate 70%, simethicone, sorbitol, saccharin, parabens. Paste. Tube 454 g. *Rx.*
Use: Radiopaque agent, GI contrast agent.

Intropin. (Faulding USA) Dopamine 40 mg/mL, sodium metabisulfite 1%. Inj. 5 mL. *Rx.*
Use: Vasoconstrictor.

•**inulin.** (IN-you-lin) *USP 28.*
Use: Diagnostic aid (renal function determination).

inulin. (DuPont) Purified inulin 5 g/50 mL sodium Cl 0.9%, sodium hydroxide to adjust pH. Amp. 50 mL.
Use: Diagnostic aid.

Invanz. (Merck & Co.) Ertapenem sodium 1.046 g (equivalent to ertapenem 1 g), sodium bicarbonate 175 mg, sodium hydroxide. Pow., lyophilized. Vial. *Rx.*
Use: Anti-infective.

Inversine. (Targacept) Mecamylamine hydrochloride 2.5 mg, lactose, talc. Tab. Bot. 100s. *Rx.*
Use: Antiadrenergic/sympatholytic.

invert sugar. (Abbott) 10%. Soln. Bot. 1000 mL. *Rx-OTC.*
Use: Nutritional supplement, parenteral.
See: Travert.

invert sugar-electrolyte solutions. *Rx.*
Use: Nutritional supplement, parenteral.
See: 5% Travert and Electrolyte No. 2.
10% Travert and Electrolyte No. 2.
Ionosol B and 10% Invert Sugar.
Ionosol D and 10% Invert Sugar.
Ionosol G and 10% Invert Sugar.
Multiple Electrolytes and 5% Travert.
Multiple Electrolytes and 10% Travert.
Multiple Electrolyte 2 w/5% Invert Sugar.
Multiple Electrolyte 2 w/10% Invert Sugar.

invert sugar injection.
Use: Fluid, nutrient replacement.

Invirase. (Roche) Saquinavir mesylate 200 mg, lactose. Cap. Bot. 270s. *Rx.*
Use: Antiviral.

in vivo diagnostic aids.
See: Gonadorelin Hydrochloride.
Methacholine Chloride.
Secretin.
Simethicone-coated Cellulose Suspension.
Sincalide.
Sodium Iodide I¹²³.
Tolbutamide Sodium.
Thyroid Function Tests.
Thyrotropin Alfa.
Tuberculin Purified Protein Derivative.

•**iobenguane I 131.** (EYE-oh-BEN-gwane) USAN.
Use: Diagnostic aid; radiopharmaceutical.

•**iobenguane I 123 injection.** (EYE-oh-BEN-gwane) *USP 28.*
Use: Radiopharmaceutical.

•**iobenguane sulfate I 131.** (EYE-oh-BEN-gwane) USAN.
Use: Diagnostic aid; radiopharmaceutical.

• **iobenguane sulfate I 123.** (EYE-oh-BEN-gwane) USAN.
Use: Diagnostic aid, radioactive, adrenomedullary disorders, and neuroendocrine tumors; radiopharmaceutical.

• **iobenzamic acid.** (EYE-oh-ben-ZAM-ik) USAN.
Use: Diagnostic aid (radiopaque medium, cholecystographic).

Iobid DM. (Iopharm) Dextromethorphan HBr 30 mg, guaifenesin 600 mg. SR Tab. Bot. 100s. *Rx.*
Use: Upper respiratory combination, antitussive, expectorant.

• **iocanlidic acid I 123.** (eye-oh-kan-LIH-dik) USAN.
Use: Diagnostic aid (radioactive, cardiac disease) for assessment of viable myocardium.

Iocare Balanced Salt Solution. (Novartis Ophthalmic) Sodium Cl 0.64%, potassium Cl 0.075%, magnesium Cl 0.03%, calcium Cl 0.048%, sodium acetate 0.39%, sodium citrate 0.17%, sodium hydroxide or hydrochloric acid. Soln. Bot. 15 mL. *Rx.*
Use: Irrigant, ophthalmic.

• **iocarmate meglumine.** (EYE-oh-KAR-mate meh-GLUE-meen) USAN.
Use: Diagnostic aid (radiopaque medium).

• **iocarmic acid.** (EYE-oh-KAR-mik) USAN.
Use: Diagnostic aid (radiopaque medium).

• **iocetamic acid.** (eye-oh-seh-TAM-ik) *USP 28.*
Use: Diagnostic aid (radiopaque medium).

i-octadecanol. *NF 23.*
See: Stearyl Alcohol.

• **iodamide.** (EYE-oh-dah-MIDE) USAN.
Use: Diagnostic aid (radiopaque medium).

• **iodamide meglumine.** (EYE-oh-dah-MIDE meh-GLUE-meen) USAN.
Use: Diagnostic aid (radiopaque medium).
W/Combinations.
See: Renovue-Dip.
Renovue-65.

Iodex. (KM Lee) Iodine 4.7% in petrolatum ointment base. Jar 1 oz, 14 oz. *OTC.*
Use: Antimicrobial; antiseptic.

Iodex with Methyl Salicylate. (Lee) Iodine 4.7%, methyl salicylate 4.8%. Petrolatum. Oint. 28 g. *OTC.*
Use: Antiseptic; analgesic, topical.

iodide, sodium, I-131 capsules.
Use: Antineoplastic; diagnostic aid (thyroid function determination); radiopharmaceutical.
See: Iodotope.

iodide, sodium, I-131 solution.
Use: Antineoplastic; diagnostic aid (thyroid function determination); radiopharmaceutical.
See: Iodotope.

iodide, sodium, I-125 capsules.
Use: Diagnostic aid (thyroid function determination); radiopharmaceutical.

iodide, sodium, I-125 solution.
Use: Diagnostic aid (thyroid function determination), radiopharmaceutical.

iodide, sodium, I-123 capsules.
Use: Diagnostic aid (thyroid function determination).

iodide, sodium, I-123 tablets.
Use: Diagnostic aid (thyroid function determination).

iodinated glycerol and codeine phosphate liquid. (Various Mfr.) Codeine phosphate 10 mg, iodinated glycerol 30 mg. Liq. Bot. Pt, gal. *c-v.*
Use: Antitussive, expectorant, narcotic.

iodinated glycerol/theophylline.
See: Iophylline.

iodinated human serum albumin.
See: Albumotope.

iodinated I-131 albumin aggregated injection.
Use: Radiopharmaceutical.
See: Albumin, Aggregated Iodinated I-131 serum.

iodinated I-131 albumin injection.
Use: Diagnostic aid (blood volume determination and intrathecal imaging); radiopharmaceutical.
See: Albumin, Iodinated I-131.

iodinated I-125 albumin injection.
Use: Diagnostic aid (blood volume determination); radiopharmaceutical.
See: Albumin, Iodinated I-125.

• **iodine.** (EYE-uh-dine) *USP 28.*
Use: Anti-infective, topical; source of iodine.
See: Kelp.
W/Methyl Salicylate
See: Iodex with Methyl Salicylate.

iodine cacodylate, colloidal. Cacodyne Iodine.

iodine combination.
See: Calcidrine.

iodine-iodophor.
See: Betadine.

iodine I^{131} metaiodobenzylguanidine sulfate.
Use: Diagnostic aid. [Orphan Drug]

iodine I¹³¹ murine monoclonal antibody IgG2a to B cell.
Use: Antineoplastic. [Orphan Drug]
See: Immurait.

iodine I¹³¹ murine monoclonal antibody to alpha-fetoprotein. (Immunomedics)
Use: Antineoplastic. [Orphan Drug]

iodine I¹³¹ murine monoclonal antibody to hCG. (Immunomedics)
Use: Antineoplastic. [Orphan Drug]

iodine I¹³¹ 6b-iodomethyl-19-norcholesterol.
Use: Diagnostic aid. [Orphan Drug]

iodine I¹²³ murine monoclonal antibody to alpha-fetoprotein. (Immunomedics)
Use: Diagnostic aid. [Orphan Drug]

iodine I¹²³ murine monoclonal antibody to hCG. (Immunomedics)
Use: Diagnostic aid. [Orphan Drug]

iodine 131: capsules diagnostic-capsules therapeutic-solution therapeutic oral.
See: Iodotope.

iodine ¹³¹I-tositumomab and tositumomab.
Use: Antineoplastic.
See: Bexxar.

iodine povidone.
See: Iodophor.
Mallisol.

iodine products, anti-infective.
See: Anayodin.
Betadine.
Chiniofon.
Diiodohydroxyquinoline.
Prepodyne.
Quinoxyl.
Surgidine.
Vioform.

iodine products, diagnostic.
See: Chloriodized Oil.
Ethyl Iodophenylundecylate.
Iodized Oil.
Iodoalphionic Acid.
Iodobrassid.
Iodohippurate Sodium.
Iodopanoic Acid.
Iodophthalein Sodium.
Iodopyracet.
Methiodal Sodium.
Optiray 350.
Pantopaque.
Sodium Acetrizoate.
Sodium Iodomethamate.
Telepaque.

iodine products, nutritional.
See: Calcium Iodobehenate.
Entodon.
Hydriodic Acid.

Iodobrassid.
Potassium Iodide.

iodine ration. (Barth's) Iodine (from kelp) 0.15 mg, trace minerals. Tab. Bot. 90s, 180s, 360s. *OTC.*
Use: Mineral supplement.

iodine ration. (Nion Corp.) Iodine (from kelp) 0.15 mg. 3 Tab. Bot. 175s, 500s. *OTC.*
Use: Mineral supplement.

iodine surface active complex.
See: Ioprep.

iodine tincture, strong.
Use: Anti-infective, topical.

• iodipamide. (eye-oh-DIH-pah-mide) *USP 28.*
Use: Pharmaceutic necessity for Iodipamide Meglumine Injection.

• iodipamide meglumine. (eye-oh-DIH-pah-mide meh-GLUE-meen) *USP 28.*
Use: Radiopaque agent, parenteral.
See: Cholografin Meglumine.

iodipamide methylglucamine. Also sodium salt injection.
W/Diatrizoate Methylglucamine.
See: Sinografin.

iodipamide sodium injection.
See: Cholografin Sodium.

• iodipamide sodium I-131. (eye-oh-DIH-pah-mide) USAN.
Use: Radiopharmaceutical.

iodipamide 26.8% and diatrizoate meglumine 52.7%.
Use: Radiopaque agent.
See: Diatrizoate Meglumine 52.7% and Iodipamide Meglumine 26.8% (38% Iodine).

• iodixanol. (EYE-oh-DIX-an-ole) *USP 28.*
Use: Radiopaque agent, parenteral.
See: Visipaque 270.
Visipaque 320.

iodized oil. A vegetable oil containing not less than 38% and not more than 42% of organically combined iodine.
Use: Diagnostic aid.

iodoalphionic acid. Biliselectan dikol, pheniodol.

• iodoantipyrine I-131. (EYE-oh-doe-ANN-tee-PI-reen) USAN.
Use: Radiopharmaceutical.

iodobehenate calcium. Calcium iododocosanoate.
Use: Antigoitrogenic.

iodobrassid. Ethyl Diiodobrassidate. Lipoiodine.

• iodocetylic acid I-123. (eye-OH-doe-SEE-till-ik) USAN.
Use: Diagnostic aid; radiopharmaceutical.

•**iodocholesterol I-131.** (EYE-oh-DOE-koe-LESS-teh-role) USAN.
Use: Radiopharmaceutical.

iodochlorhydroxyquin.
Use: Antiamebic; anti-infective, topical.
See: Clioquinol.

Iodo Cream. (Day-Baldwin) Clioquinol 3%. Tube 1 oz, Jar 1 lb. *OTC.*
Use: Antifungal, topical.

•**iodoform.** (EYE-oh-doe-form) *USP 28.*

Iodo H-C. (Day-Baldwin) Clioquinol 3%, hydrocortisone 1%. **Oint.:** Tube 20 g, Jar 1 lb. **Cream:** Tube 20 g, Jar 1 lb. *Rx.*
Use: Antifungal; corticosteroid.

•**iodohippurate, sodium I-131 injection.** (EYE-oh-doe-HIP-you-rate) *USP 28.*
Use: Diagnostic aid (renal function determination); radiopharmaceutical.
See: Hipputope.

•**iodohippurate sodium I-123 injection.** (EYE-oh-doe-HIP-you-rate) *USP 28.*
Use: Radiopharmaceutical; diagnostic aid (renal function determination).

•**iodohippurate sodium I-125.** (EYE-oh-doe-HIP-you-rate) USAN.
Use: Radiopharmaceutical.
See: Hipputope I-125.

iodohippuric acid.
See: Hipputope.

Iodo Ointment. (Day-Baldwin) Clioquinol 3%. Tube 1 oz, Jar 1 lb. *Rx.*
Use: Antifungal, topical.

Iodo-Pak. (SoloPak Pharmaceuticals, Inc.) Iodine 100 mcg/mL. Inj. Vial 10 mL. *Rx.*
Use: Nutritional supplement, parenteral.

iodopanoic acid.
Use: Diagnostic aid (radiopaque medium).

Iodopen. (American Pharmaceutical Partners) Sodium iodide 118 mcg/mL. Inj. 10 mL. *Rx.*
Use: Nutritional supplement, parenteral.

iodophene. Iodophthalein.

iodophene sodium.
See: Iodophthalein Sodium.

iodophor.
See: Betadine.

iodophthalein sodium. Tetraiodophenolphthalein Sodium, Tetraiodophthalein Sodium, Tetiothalein Sodium (Antinosin, Cholepulvis, Cholumbin, Foriod, Iodophene, Iodorayoral, Nosophene Sodium, Opacin, Photobiline, Piliophen, Radiotetrane).
Use: Radiopaque agent.

iodopropylidene glycerol.
See: Organidin.

iodopyracet compound. Diodrast.

iodopyracet concentrated. Diodrast.

iodopyracet injection. Diatrast, Diodone, Iopyracil, Neo-Methiodal, NeoSkiodan.
Use: Radiopaque medium.

•**iodopyracet I 131.** (EYE-oh-doe-peer-ah-set) USAN.
Use: Radiopharmaceutical.

•**iodopyracet I 125.** (EYE-oh-doe-peer-ah-set) USAN.
Use: Radiopharmaceutical.

iodopyrine. Antipyrine iodide.
Use: Iodides, analgesic.

•**iodoquinol.** (EYE-oh-doe-KWIH-nole) *USP 28.* Formerly Diiodohydroxyquin.
Use: Antiamebic.
See: Floraquin.
  Sebaquin.
  Yodoxin.
W/9-Aminoacridine hydrochloride.
See: Vagitric.
  Yodoxin.
W/Hydrocortisone alcohol.
See: Hydrocortisone and Iodoquinol 1%.
  Vytone.
W/Hydrocortisone, coal tar solution.
See: Gynben.
  Gynben Insufflate.
W/Surfactants.
See: Lycinate.
W/Sulfanilamide, diethylstilbestrol.
See: Amide V/S.
  D.I.T.I.

Iodotope (Diagnostic). (Bristol-Myers Squibb) Sodium iodide I-131 for oral use. 7, 14, 28, 70, 106 units Ci. Vial of 5, 10, 15, 20 Cap.
Use: Diagnostic aid.

Iodotope (Therapeutic Antibodies). (Bracco Diagnostics) Sodium iodide I-131. 1 to 50 mCi Cap. Sodium iodide I-151 7.05 m Ci/mL. Vial 7, 14, 28, 70, 106 mCi, EDTA 1 mg. Soln. *Rx.*
Use: Antithyroid agent.

•**iodoxamate meglumine.** (EYE-oh-DOX-ah-mate meh-GLUE-meen) USAN.
Use: Diagnostic aid (radiopaque medium).

•**iodoxamic acid.** (EYE-oh-dox-AM-ik) USAN.
Use: Diagnostic aid (radiopaque medium).

iodoxyl.
See: Sodium Iodomethamate.

Iofed. (Iomed) Brompheniramine maleate 12 mg, pseudoephedrine hydrochloride 120 mg. ER Cap. Bot. 100s. *Rx.*
Use: Antihistamine, decongestant.

Iofed PD. (Iomed) Brompheniramine maleate 6 mg, pseudoephedrine hydrochloride 60 mg. ER Cap. Bot. 100s. *Rx.*
Use: Antihistamine, decongestant.

•**iofetamine hydrochloride I 123.** (EYE-oh-FET-ah-meen) USAN.
Use: Diagnostic aid; radiopharmaceutical.

•**ioglicic acid.** (eye-oh-GLIH-sick) USAN.
Use: Diagnostic aid (radiopaque medium).

•**ioglucol.** (EYE-oh-GLUE-kahl) USAN.
Use: Diagnostic aid (radiopaque medium).

•**ioglucomide.** (EYE-oh-GLUE-koe-mide) USAN.
Use: Diagnostic aid (radiopaque medium).

•**ioglycamic acid.** (EYE-oh-glie-KAM-ik) USAN.
Use: Diagnostic aid (radiopaque medium, cholecystographic).

•**iogulamide.** (EYE-oh-GULL-ah-mide) USAN.
Use: Diagnostic aid (radiopaque medium).

•**iohexol.** (EYE-oh-HEX-ole) *USP 28.*
Use: Radiopaque agent, parenteral.
See: Omnipaque 140.
Omnipaque 180.
Omnipaque 240.
Omnipaque 300.
Omnipaque 350.

•**iomeprol.** (EYE-oh-MEH-prole) USAN.
Use: Diagnostic aid (radiopaque medium).

•**iomethin I-131.** (EYE-oh-METH-in) USAN.
Use: Diagnostic aid (neoplasm); radiopharmaceutical.

•**iomethin I-125.** (EYE-oh-METH-in) USAN.
Use: Diagnostic aid (neoplasm); radiopharmaceutical.

•**iometopane I-123.** (eye-oh-meh-TOE-pane) USAN.
Use: Diagnostic aid.

Ionamin. (Celltech) Phentermine resin 15 mg, 30 mg, lactose. Cap. Bot. 100s, 400s. *c-iv.*
Use: CNS stimulant, anorexiant.

Ionax Astringent Cleanser. (Galderma) Isopropyl alcohol 48%, acetone, salicylic acid. Bot. 240 mL. *OTC.*
Use: Dermatologic, acne.

Ionax Foam. (Galderma) Benzalkonium Cl, propylene glycol. Aerosol Can 150 mL. *OTC.*

Use: Dermatologic, acne.

Ionax Scrub. (Galderma) SD alcohol 40, benzalkonium Cl. Tube 60 g, 120 g. *OTC.*
Use: Dermatologic, acne.

I-131 radiolabeled b1 monoclonal antibody. (Coulter)
Use: Treatment for non-Hodgkin B-cell lymphoma. [Orphan Drug]

ion-exchange resins.
See: Polyamine Methylene Resin.
Resins, Sodium-Removing.

Ionil Plus Shampoo. (Galderma) Salicylic acid 2%, sodium laureth sulfate, lauramide DEA, quaternium-22, talloweth-60 myristyl glycol, laureth-23, TEA lauryl sulfate, glycol disterate, laureth-4, TEA-abietoyl hydrolyzed collagen, DMDM hydantoin, tetrasodium EDTA, sodium hydroxide, FD&C blue No. 1. Bot. 4 oz, 8 oz. *OTC.*
Use: Antiseborrheic.

Ionil Rinse. (Galderma) Conditioners with benzalkonium Cl in water base. Bot. 16 oz. *OTC.*
Use: Dermatologic, hair.

Ionil Shampoo. (Galderma) Salicylic acid, benzalkonium Cl, alcohol 12%, polyoxyethylene ethers. Plastic bot. w/dispenser cap 4 oz, 8 oz, 16 oz, 32 oz. *OTC.*
Use: Antiseborrheic.

Ionil T. (Galderma) A nonionic/cationic foaming shampoo w/coal tar, salicylic acid, benzalkonium Cl, alcohol 12%, polyoxyethylene ethers. Plastic bot. 4 oz, 8 oz, 16 oz, 32 oz. *OTC.*
Use: Antiseborrheic.

Ionil-T Plus Shampoo. (Healthpoint) Coal tar 2%. Shampoo. 120 mL, 240 mL. *OTC.*
Use: Antiseborrheic.

Ionosol D-CM. (Abbott Hospital Products) Sodium Cl 516 mg, potassium Cl 89.4 mg, calcium Cl anhydrous 27.8 mg, magnesium Cl anhydrous 14.2 mg, sodium lactate 560 mg/100 mL. Bot. 1000 mL. *Rx.*
Use: Nutritional supplement, parenteral.

•**iopamidol 51%.** (EYE-oh-PAM-ih-dahl) *USP 28.*
Use: Radiopaque agent, parenteral.
See: Isovue-250.

•**iopamidol 41%.** (EYE-oh-PAM-ih-dahl) *USP 28.*
Use: Radiopaque agent, parenteral.
See: Isovue-200.
Isovue-M 200.

•**iopamidol 76%.** (EYE-oh-PAM-ih-dahl) *USP 28.*

Use: Radiopaque agent, parenteral.
See: Isovue-370.
● **iopamidol 61%.** (EYE-oh-PAM-ih-dahl)
Use: Radiopaque agent, parenteral.
See: Isovue-300.
Isovue-M 300.
● **iopanoic acid.** (eye-oh-pan-OH-ik)
USP 28.
Use: Diagnostic aid (radiopaque medium).
See: Telepaque.
● **iopentol.** (EYE-oh-PEN-tole) USAN.
Use: Diagnostic aid (radiopaque medium).
Iophen-C. (Various Mfr.) Codeine phosphate 10 mg, iodinated glycerol 30 mg/5 mL. Liq. Bot. Pt, gal. *c-v.*
Use: Antitussive, expectorant.
Iophen-DM. (Various Mfr.) Dextromethorphan HBr, iodinated glycerol 30 mg/5 mL. Liq. Bot. 120 mL, pt, gal. *Rx.*
Use: Antitussive, expectorant.
● **iophendylate.** (eye-oh-FEN-dih-late)
USP 28. Benzenedecanoic acid, iodo-t-methyl, ethyl ester.
Use: Diagnostic aid (radiopaque medium).
iophendylate injection. Ethiodan, Myodil. Ethyl Iodophenylundecylate.
Use: Diagnostic aid (radiopaque medium).
See: Pantopaque.
Iophylline. (Various Mfr.) Theophylline 120 mg, iodinated glycerol 30 mg/15 mL. Elix. Bot. 480 mL. *Rx.*
Use: Antiasthmatic combination.
Iopidine. (Alcon) Apraclonidine 0.5%, 1%, benzalkonium Cl 0.01%. Dispenser Bot. 0.25 mL (1%), *Drop-Tainer* 5 mL (0.5%). *Rx.*
Use: Antiglaucoma agent.
iopodate sodium.
See: Ipodate Sodium.
Ioprep. (Johnson & Johnson) Nonyl-phenoxypolyethyleneoxy (4) ethanol and nonylphenoxypolyethyleneoxy (15) ethanol iodine complex 5.5%, nonyl-phenoxypolyethyleneoxy (30) ethanol 10%. Solution provides 1% available iodine. Plastic bot. Gal.
Use: Antiseptic.
● **ioprocemic acid.** (EYE-oh-pro-SEH-mik acid) USAN.
Use: Diagnostic aid (radiopaque medium).
● **iopromide.** (eye-oh-PRO-mide) *USP 28.*
Use: Radiopaque agent, parenteral.
See: Ultravist 150.
Ultravist 240.
Ultravist 300.

Ultravist 370.
● **iopronic acid.** (eye-oh-PRO-nik acid) USAN.
Use: Diagnostic aid (radiopaque medium, cholecystographic).
● **iopydol.** (eye-oh-PIE-dahl) USAN.
Use: Diagnostic aid (radiopaque medium, bronchographic).
● **iopydone.** (eye-oh-PIE-dohn) USAN.
Use: Diagnostic aid (radiopaque medium, bronchographic).
Iosal II. (Iopharm) Pseudoephedrine hydrochloride 60 mg, guaifenesin 600 mg. SR Tab. Bot. 100s. *Rx.*
Use: Upper respiratory combination, decongestant, expectorant.
● **iosefamic acid.** (EYE-oh-seh-FAM-ik) USAN.
Use: Diagnostic aid; radiopaque medium.
● **ioseric acid.** (eye-oh-SEH-rik) USAN.
Use: Diagnostic aid (radiopaque medium).
Iosopan. (Ivax) Magaldrate 540 mg/5 mL. Liq. Bot. 355 mL. *OTC.*
Use: Antacid.
Iosopan Plus. (Ivax) Magaldrate 540 mg, simethicone 40 mg/5 mL. Liq. Bot. 355 mL. *OTC.*
Use: Antacid.
● **iosulamide meglumine.** (eye-oh-SULL-ah-mide meh-GLUE-meen) USAN.
Use: Diagnostic aid (radiopaque medium).
● **iosumetic acid.** (eye-oh-sue-MEH-tick) USAN.
Use: Diagnostic aid (radiopaque medium).
● **iotasul.** (EYE-oh-tah-sull) USAN.
Use: Diagnostic aid (radiopaque medium).
● **iotetric acid.** (eye-oh-TEH-trick) USAN.
Use: Diagnostic aid (radiopaque medium).
iothalamate meglumide and iothalmate sodium injection.
Use: Diagnostic aid (radiopaque medium).
● **iothalamate sodium injection.** (eye-oh-THAL-am-ate) *USP 28.*
Use: Diagnostic aid (radiopaque medium).
See: Conray.
● **iothalamate sodium I-131.** (eye-oh-THAL-am-ate) USAN.
Use: Radiopharmaceutical.
● **iothalamate sodium I-125 injection.** (eye-oh-THAL-am-ate) *USP 28.*
Use: Radiopharmaceutical.

●**iothalamic acid.** (eye-oh-THAL-am-ik)
USP 28.
Use: Diagnostic aid (radiopaque medium).

iothiouracil sodium. Sodium salt of
5-iodo-2-thiouracil.

●**iotrolan.** (EYE-oh-TRAHL-an) USAN.
Formerly Iotrol.
Use: Diagnostic aid (radiopaque medium).

●**iotroxic acid.** (EYE-oh-TRAHK-sick)
USAN.
Use: Diagnostic aid (radiopaque medium).

●**iotyrosine I-131.** (eye-oh-TYE-roe-seen)
USAN.
Use: Radiopharmaceutical.

●**ioversol.** (EYE-oh-ver-sole) *USP 28.*
Use: Diagnostic aid (radiopaque medium).
See: Optiray.

ioversol 51%.
Use: Radiopaque agent, parenteral.
See: Optiray 240.

ioversol 74%.
Use: Radiopaque agent, parenteral.
See: Optiray 350.

ioversol 68%.
Use: Radiopaque agent, parenteral.
See: Optiray 320.

ioversol 64%.
Use: Radiopaque agent, parenteral.
See: Optiray 300.

ioversol 34%.
Use: Radiopaque agent, parenteral.
See: Optiray 160.

●**ioxaglate meglumine.** (eye-ox-AGG-late
meh-GLUE-meen) USAN.
Use: Diagnostic aid (radiopaque medium).
See: Hexabrix.

ioxaglate meglumine and ioxaglate sodium.
Use: Radiopaque agent, parenteral.
See: Hexabrix.

●**ioxaglate sodium.** (eye-ox-AGG-late)
USAN.
Use: Diagnostic aid (radiopaque medium).

●**ioxaglic acid.** (eye-ox-AGG-lick)
USP 28.
Use: Diagnostic aid (radiopaque medium).

●**ioxilan.** (eye-OX-ee-lan) USAN.
Use: Diagnostic aid.

●**ioxotrizoic acid.** (eye-OX-oh-TRY-zoe-ik) USAN.
Use: Diagnostic aid (radiopaque medium).

●**ipazilide fumarate.** (ih-PAZZ-ih-LIDE)
USAN.
Use: Cardiovascular agent.

●**ipecac.** (IPP-uh-kak) *USP 28.*
Use: Emetic.
W/Combinations.
See: Ipsatol.
Mallergan.

ipecac. (Various Mfr.) Ipecac alcohol
1.5% to 1.75%, 2%. Syr. Bot. 15 mL,
30 mL. *OTC.*
Use: Antidote.

●**ipexidine mesylate.** (eye-PEX-ih-DEEN)
USAN.
Use: Dental caries agent.

I-Pilopine. (Akorn) Pilocarpine hydrochloride 1%. Ophthalmic soln. Bot. 15 mL.
Rx.
Use: Antiglaucoma agent

●**ipodate calcium.** (EYE-poe-date)
USP 28.
Use: Diagnostic aid (radiopaque medium).
See: Oragrafin Calcium.

●**ipodate sodium.** (EYE-poe-date)
USP 28.
Use: Diagnostic aid (radiopaque medium).

IPOL. (Aventis Pasteur) Suspension of
3 types of poliovirus (Types 1, 2, and
3) grown in monkey kidney cell cultures,
2-phenoxyethanol 0.5%, formaldehyde
0.02% (maximum), $\leq$ streptomycin
200 ng, polymyxin B 25 ng, neomycin
5 ng. Inj. Single-dose syringe 0.5 mL.
Rx.
Use: Immunization.

Ipran. (Major) Propranolol hydrochloride
10 mg, 20 mg, 40 mg, 60 mg, 80 mg,
90 mg. Tab. **10 mg, 20 mg, 40 mg:** Bot.
100s, 250s, 1000s, UD 100s. **60 mg:**
Bot. 100s, 500s. **80 mg:** Bot. 100s,
500s, 1000s, UD 100s. **90 mg:** Bot.
100s, 500s. *Rx.*
Use: Beta-adrenergic blocker.

●**ipratropium bromide.** (IH-pruh-TROE-pee-uhm) USAN.
Use: Bronchodilator.
See: Atrovent.
Atrovent HFA.

ipratropium bromide. (Dey) Ipratropium
bromide 0.02% (500 mcg/vial) Soln. for
Inh. Vial 2.5 mL each. 25, 30, 60 unit-
dose. *Rx.*
Use: Anticholinergic.

ipratropium bromide. (Various Mfr.)
Ipratropium bromide 0.03% (21 mcg/
spray), 0.06% (42 mcg/spray). Nasal
Spray. 30 mL (345 sprays) (0.03%
only), 15 mL (165 sprays) (0.06% only).

Rx.
Use: Anticholinergic.
ipratropium bromide/albuterol sulfate.
Use: Bronchodilator, anticholinergic.
See: Combivent.
DuoNeb.
I-Pred. (Akorn) Prednisolone sodium
phosphate 0.5%, 1%. Ophth. Soln. Bot.
5 mL. *Rx.*
Use: Corticosteroid, ophthalmic.
• **iprindole.** (IH-prin-dole) USAN.
Use: Antidepressant.
Iprivask. (Aventis) Desirudin 15 mg, pre-
servative free. Pow. for Inj., lyophilized.
Single-use vials with diluent (manni-
tol 0.6 mL [3%] in water for injection).
Rx.
Use: Anticoagulant, antithrombin agent.
• **iprofenin.** (IH-pro-FEN-in) USAN.
Use: Diagnostic aid (hepatic function
determination).
• **ipronidazole.** (ih-pro-NIH-dah-zole)
USAN.
Use: Antiprotozoal *Histomonas.*
• **iproplatin.** (IH-pro-PLAT-in) USAN.
Use: Antineoplastic.
iproveratril. Name used for verapamil.
• **iproxamine hydrochloride.** (IH-PROX-
ah-meen) USAN.
Use: Vasodilator.
• **ipsapirone hydrochloride.** (ipp-sah-PIE-
rone) USAN.
Use: Anxiolytic.
IPV.
Use: Immunization.
See: IPOL.
Polio Virus Vaccine, Inactivated.
Iquix. (Santen) Levofloxacin 1.5%
(15 mg/mL). Soln. 5 mL. *Rx.*
Use: Ophthalmic antibiotic.
• **irbesartan.** (ihr-beh-SAHR-tan) *USP 28.*
Use: Antihypertensive (angiotensin II
receptor antagonist).
See: Avalide.
Avapro.
Ircon. (Kenwood) Iron (as carbonyl iron)
66 mg. Tab. Blister Pack 100s. *OTC.*
Use: Mineral supplement.
Ircon-FA. (Kenwood) Iron (as carbonyl
iron) 82 mg, folic acid 0.8 mg. Tab.
Blister pack 100s. *OTC.*
Use: Mineral supplement.
Iressa. (AstraZeneca) Gefitinib 250 mg,
lactose. Film-coated Tab. 30s. *Rx.*
Use: Antineoplastic.
Irgasan CF3. Cloflucarban.
Use: Antiseptic, topical.
• **iridium Ir 192.** (ih-RID-ee-uhm) USAN.
Use: Radioactive agent.

• **irinotecan hydrochloride.** (eye-rih-no-
TEE-can) USAN.
Use: Antineoplastic (DNA topoisomerase I inhibitor).
See: Camptosar.
irisin. A polysaccharide found in several
species of iris.
irocaine.
See: Procaine Hydrochloride.
Irodex. (Keene Pharmaceuticals) Iron
dextran complex 50 mg/mL. Vial 10 mL.
Rx.
Use: Mineral supplement.
Iromin-G. (Mission Pharmacal) Ferrous
gluconate 260 mg (iron 30 mg), vita-
mins B_{12} (crystalline on resin) 2 mcg,
C 100 mg, A acetate 4000 units, D
400 units, B_1 5 mg, B_2 2 mg, B_3 10 mg,
B_5 1 mg, B_6 20.6 mg, folic acid 0.8 mg,
Ca. Tab. Bot. 100s. *OTC.*
Use: Mineral, vitamin supplement.
iron.
See: Carbonyl Iron.
Ferrous Fumarate.
Ferrous Gluconate.
Ferrous Sulfate.
Ferrous Sulfate Exsiccated (Dried).
Iron Dextran.
Iron Sucrose.
Iron with Vitamin C.
Polysaccharide-Iron Complex.
Sodium Ferric Gluconate Complex.
iron carbonate complex.
See: Polyferose.
Ironco-B. (Pal-Pak, Inc.) Ferrous sulfate
120.4 mg, manganese sulfate 21.6 mg,
dicalcium phosphate 129.6 mg, vita-
mins B_1 1 mg, B_2 1 mg, niacin 6 mg, D
100 units. Tab. Bot. 100s, 1000s. *OTC.*
Use: Mineral, vitamin supplement.
• **iron dextran.** (iron DEX-tran) *USP 28.*
Use: Hematinic.
See: DexFerrum.
InFeD.
Iron-Folic 500. (Major) Ferrous sulfate
105 mg, B_1 6 mg, B_2 6 mg, B_3 30 mg,
B_5 10 mg, B_{12} 25 mcg, C 500 mg, folic
acid 0.8 mg. Tab. Bot. 100s, 500s. *OTC.*
Use: Mineral, vitamin supplement.
iron (2+) fumarate. Ferrous Fumarate,
USP.
iron (2+) gluconate.
See: Ferrous Gluconate.
iron/liver combinations, injection.
See: Hemocyte.
Hytinic.
Liver-Iron B Complex w/Vitamin B_{12}.
iron/liver combination, oral.
See: Feocyte.
I-L-X.
I-L-X B_{12}.

Liquid Geritonic.
iron oxide mixture with zinc oxide.
Calamine, *USP.*
iron, parenteral.
See: DexFerrum.
INFeD.
iron products, injection.
See: INFeD.
•**iron sorbitex injection.** (SORE-bih-tex)
USP 28.
Use: Hematinic.
•**iron sucrose.** *USP 28.*
Use: Trace element.
See: Venofer.
iron with vitamin B$_{12}$ and IFC.
See: Contrin.
Chromagen.
Fergon Plus.
Ferotrinsic.
Livitrinsic I.
Pronemia Hematinic.
TriHEMIC 600.
Trinsicon.
iron with vitamin C.
See: Fero-Grad-500.
Ferrex 150 Plus.
Niferex-150.
Vitelle Irospan.
Vitron-C.
iron with vitamins.
See: Gentle Iron.
Irospan. (Fielding) Ferrous sulfate
65 mg, vitamin C 150 mg. Cap. Bot.
60s, Tab, Bot, 100s, *OTC.*
Use: Mineral, vitamin supplement.
irradiated ergosterol.
See: Calciferol.
Irrigate Eye Wash. (Optopics) Sodium
Cl, monobasic and dibasic sodium
phosphate, benzalkonium Cl, EDTA.
Soln. Bot. 118 mL. *OTC.*
Use: Irrigant, ophthalmic.
irrigating solutions, physiological.
Use: Irrigant.
See: Lactated Ringer's Irrigation.
Physiolyte.
PhysioSol.
Tis-U-Sol.
irrigating solutions, urinary.
Use: Irrigant.
See: Acetic Acid.
Glycine (Aminoacetic acid).
Neosporin G.U. Irrigant.
Renacidin.
Resectisol.
Sodium Chloride.
Sorbitol-Mannitol.
Sterile Water.
irritant or stimulant laxatives.
See: Agoral.
Aromatic Cascara Fluid extract.

Bisac-Evac.
Bisacodyl.
Bisacodyl Uniserts.
Black-Draught.
Caroid.
Cascara Aromatic.
Cascara Sagrada.
Correctol.
Dulcolax.
ex-lax.
ex-lax chocolated.
Feen-a-mint.
Fleet Laxative.
Fletcher's Castoria.
Maximum Relief ex-lax.
Modane.
Reliable Gentle Laxative.
Senexon.
Senna Gen.
Sennosides.
Senokot.
Senokot XTRA.
Women's Gentle Laxative.
•**irtemazole.** (ihr-TEH-mah-zole) USAN.
Use: Uricosuric.
isacen.
See: Oxyphenisatin.
•**isamoxole.** (eye-SAH-MOX-ole) USAN.
Use: Antiasthmatic.
•**isatoribine.** (eye-sah-TORE-ih-been)
USAN.
Use: Immunomodulator.
iscador. (Weleda) Mistletoe.
Use: Cancer (not FDA-approved).
•**iseganan hydrochloride.** (eye-se-GAN-
an) USAN.
Use: Antimicrobial.
•**isepamicin.** (eye-SEP-ah-MY-sin) USAN.
Use: Antibacterial (aminoglycoside).
ISG. Immune globulin intramuscular. *Rx.*
Use: Immunization.
Ismelin. (Novartis) Guanethidine mono-
sulfate 10 mg, 25 mg. Tab. Bot. 100s.
Rx.
Use: Antihypertensive.
Ismo. (Wyeth) Isosorbide mononitrate
20 mg. Tab. Bot. 100s, UD 100s. *Rx.*
Use: Antianginal.
•**ismomultin alpha.** (IZ-moe-MUL-tin)
USAN.
Use: Rheumatoid arthritis.
Ismotic. (Alcon) Isosorbide solution.
W/sodium 4.6 mEq, potassium
0.9 mEq/220 mL, alcohol, saccharin,
sorbitol. In 220 mL. *Rx.*
Use: Diuretic.
iso-alcoholic elixir.
Use: Vehicle.

isoamylhydrocupreine dihydro-chloride.
See: Eucupin Dihydrochloride.
isoamyl methoxycinnamate.
See: Amiloxate.
isoamyl nitrate.
See: Amyl Nitrite.
isoamyne.
See: Amphetamine.
Iso-B. (Tyson) Vitamins B_1 25 mg, B_2 25 mg, B_3 75 mg, B_5 125 mg, B_6 50 mg, B_{12} 100 mcg, FA 0.2 mg, pyridoxal 5 phosphate 2.5 mg, PABA 50 mg, inositol 50 mg, choline bitartrate 125 mg, biotin 100 mcg. Cap. Bot. 120s. *OTC*.
Use: Mineral, vitamin supplement.
isobornyl thiocyanoacetate, technical.
Use: Pediculicide.
See: Barc.
W/Docusate sodium and related terpenes.
See: Barc.
●**isobucaine hydrochloride.** (eye-so-BYOO-kane) *USP 28*.
Use: Anesthetic, local.
●**isobucaine hydrochloride and epinephrine injection.** (eye-so-BYOO-kane HIGH-droe-KLOR-ide & epp-ih-NEFF-rin) *USP 28*.
Use: Anesthetic, local.
●**isobutamben.** (EYE-so-BYOO-tam-ben) USAN.
Use: Anesthetic, local.
●**isobutane.** (eye-so-BYOO-tane) *NF 23*.
Use: Aerosol propellant.
isobutylallylbarbituric acid.
W/Aspirin, phenacetin, caffeine.
See: Buff-A-Comp.
　Fiorinal.
　Palgesic.
　Tenstan.
W/Codeine phosphate.
See: Fiorinal w/Codeine.
isobutyl p-aminobenzoate.
See: Isobutamben, USAN.
isobutyramide. (Vertex)
Use: Sickle cell disease; beta-thalassemia. [Orphan Drug]
isobutyramide oral solution. (Alpha Therapeutic)
Use: Sickle call disease; beta-thalassemia. [Orphan Drug]
isocaine. Isobutamben, *USP*.
Isocal. (Bristol-Myers Squibb) Lactose-free isotonic liquid containing as a percentage of the calories protein 13% as caseinate and soy protein; fat 37% as soy oil and medium chain triglycerides; carbohydrate 50% as corn syrup solids w/vitamins and minerals for the tube-

fed patient. Bot. 8 fl oz, 12 fl oz, 32 fl oz. *OTC*.
Use: Nutritional supplement.
Isocal HCN. (Bristol-Myers Squibb) High calorie nitrogen nutritionally complete food. Protein 15%, fat 45%, carbohydrate 40%. Can 8 fl oz. *OTC*.
Use: Nutritional supplement.
Isocal HN. (Bristol-Myers Squibb) ≈ 1 Kcal/mL with protein 44 g, fat 45 g, carbohydrates 124 g/L. In 237 mL. *OTC*.
Use: Nutritional supplement.
●**isocarboxazid.** (eye-so-car-BOX-ah-zid) *USP 28*.
Use: Antidepressant.
See: Marplan.
Isochron. (Forest) Isosorbide dinitrate 40 mg. ER Tab. 100s. *Rx*.
Use: Vasodilator.
Isoclor Expectorant. (Medeva) Codeine phosphate 10 mg, pseudoephedrine hydrochloride 30 mg, guaifenesin 100 mg/5 mL, alcohol 5%. Bot. Pt. *c-v*.
Use: Antitussive, decongestant, expectorant.
isococaine. Pseudococaine.
Isocom. (Nutripharm Laboratories, Inc.) Isometheptene mucate 65 mg, dichloralphenazone 100 mg, acetaminophen 325 mg. Cap. Bot. 50s, 100s, 250s. *Rx*.
Use: Antimigraine.
●**isoconazole.** (EYE-so-CONE-ah-zole) USAN.
Use: Anti-infective; antifungal.
isoephedrine hydrochloride. d-Isoephedrine hydrochloride.
See: Pseudoephedrine Hydrochloride.
W/Chlorpheniramine maleate.
See: Isoclor.
W/Chlorprophenpyridamine maleate.
See: Isoclor.
d-isoephedrine sulfate.
See: Pseudoephedrine sulfate.
●**isoetharine.** (EYE-so-ETH-uh-reen) USAN.
Use: Bronchodilator.
●**isoetharine hydrochloride.** (EYE-so-ETH-uh-reen) *USP 28*.
Use: Bronchodilator, sympathomimetic.
isoetharine hydrochloride. (Roxane) Isoetharine hydrochloride 1%, EDTA, parabens, sulfites. Soln. for Inh. Bot. 10 mL, 30 mL, w/dropper. *Rx*.
Use: Bronchodilator, sympathomimetic.
●**isoetharine mesylate.** (EYE-so-ETH-uh-reen) *USP 28*.
Use: Bronchodilator.
See: Bronkometer.

●**isoflupredone acetate.** (eye-so-FLEW-PREH-dohn) USAN.
Use: Anti-inflammatory.

●**isoflurane.** (EYE-so-FLEW-rane) *USP 28.*
Use: Anesthetic, general.
See: Terrell.

●**isoflurophate.** (eye-so-FLURE-oh-fate) *USP 28.*
Use: Cholinergic, ophthalmic.
See: Floropryl.

iso-iodeikon.
See: Phentetiothalein Sodium.

Isoject. (Roerig) A purified, sterile, disposable injection system.
Use: Injection system.
See: Permapen (benzathine penicillin G) aqueous soln. 1,200,000 units/2 ml. I0n
Terramycin (oxytetracycline) Intramuscular.

Isolan. (Elan) Protein 40 g, fat 36 g, carbohydrates 144 g, Na 690 g, K 1.17 g/L, with appropriate vitamins and minerals. Lactose free. Liq. In 237 mL Tetra Pak containers and 1000 mL New Pak closed systems with and without Color Check. *OTC.*
Use: Nutritional supplement.

Isolate Compound Elixir. (Various Mfr.) Theophylline 45 mg, ephedrine sulfate 12 mg, isoproterenol hydrochloride 2.5 mg, potassium iodide 150 mg, phenobarbital 6 mg/15 mL, alcohol 19%. Elix. Bot. Pt, gal. *Rx.*
Use: Antiasthmatic combination.

●**isoleucine.** (EYE-so-LOO-seen) *USP 28.*
Use: Amino acid.

isoleucine. (Pfaltz & Bauer) Pow. 10 g.
Use: Amino acid.

Isolyte G with Dextrose. (McGaw) Sodium 65 mEq, potassium 17 mEq, chloride 150 mEq, NH_4 70 mEq, dextrose 50 g, 170 Cal, 555 mOsm/L. Bot. 1000 mL. *Rx.*
Use: Nutritional supplement, parenteral.

Isolyte H in 5% Dextrose. (B. Braun) Dextrose 50 g/L, calories 170 Cal/L, Na^+ 39 mEq, K^+ 13 mEq, Mg^{++} 3 mEq, Cl⁻ 44 mEq, acetate 16 mEq/L, osmolarity 360 mOsm/L. Inj. Soln. 1000 mL. *Rx.*
Use: Intravenous nutritional therapy, intravenous replenishment solution.

Isolyte M in 5% Dextrose. (B. Braun) Dextrose 50 g/L, calories 170 cal/L, Na^+ 36 mEq, K^+ 35 mEq, Cl⁻ 49 mEq, phosphate 15 mEq, acetate 20 mEq/L, osmolarity 390 mOsm/L. Inj. Soln. 500 mL, 1000 mL. *Rx.*

Use: Intravenous nutritional therapy, intravenous replenishment solution.

Isolyte P in 5% Dextrose. (B. Braun) Dextrose 50 g/L, calories 170 Cal/L, Na^+ 23 mEq, K^+ 20 mEq, Mg^{++} 3 mEq, Cl⁻ 29 mEq, phosphate 3 mEq, acetate 23 mEq/L, osmolarity 340 mOsm/L. Inj. Soln. 250 mL, 500 mL, 1000 mL. *Rx.*
Use: Intravenous nutritional therapy, intravenous replenishment solution.

Isolyte R in 5% Dextrose. (B. Braun) Sodium 39 mEq, potassium 16 mEq, calcium 5 mEq, magnesium 3 mEq, chloride 46 mEq, acetate 24 mEq, dextrose 50 g, 170 Cal, 375 mOsm/L. Inj. Soln. 1000 mL. *Rx.*
Use: Intravenous nutritional therapy, intravenous replenishment solution.

Isolyte S pH 7.4. (B. Braun) Sodium 141 mEq, potassium 5 mEq, magnesium 3 mEq, chloride 98 mEq, acetate 27 mEq, gluconate 23 mEq, phosphate 1 mEq, 295 mOsm/L, preservative free. Inj. Bot. Soln. 500 mL, 1000 mL. *Rx.*
Use: Intravenous nutritional therapy, intravenous replenishment solution.

Isolyte S with 5% Dextrose. (B. Braun) Sodium 140 mEq, potassium 5 mEq, magnesium 3 mEq, chloride 106 mEq, acetate 27 mEq, gluconate 23 mEq, dextrose 50 g, Cal 170, 550 mOsm/L. Inj. Soln. 1000 mL. *Rx.*
Use: Intravenous nutritional therapy, intravenous replenishment solution.

●**isomazole hydrochloride.** (eye-SO-mah-ZOLE) USAN.
Use: Cardiovascular agent.

isomeprobamate.
See: Carisoprodol.

●**isomerol.** (EYE-so-MER-ole) USAN. *Formerly Parahydrecin.*
Use: Antiseptic.

●**isometheptene/dichloralphenazone/acetaminophen.** (eye-so-meth-EPP-teen/die-klor-uhl-FEN-uh-zone/ASS-et-ah-MEE-noe-fen) *USP 28.*
Use: Antimigraine.
See: Duradrin.
Midrin.
Migratine.

isometheptene/dichloralphenazone/acetaminophen. (Various Mfr.) Isometheptene 65 mg, dichloralphenazone 100 mg, acetaminophen 325 mg. Cap. Bot. 50s, 100s, 250s, 500s. *c-iv.*
Use: Antimigraine.

●**isometheptene mucate.** (eye-so-meth-EPP-teen MYOO-kate) *USP 28.*
See: Midrin.

Isomil. (Ross) Soy protein isolate infant formula containing 20 calories/fl oz. **Pow.:** Can 14 oz. **Concentrated Liq.:** Can 13 fl oz. **Ready-to-feed:** Can 32 fl oz. **Nursing Bottles:** Hospital use. Bot. 8 fl oz. *OTC.*
Use: Nutritional supplement.

Isomil DF. (Ross) Protein 17.9 g, carbohydrates 67.3 g, fat 36.7 g, Fe 12 mg, Na 293 mg, K 720 mg, with appropriate vitamins and minerals. 676 cal/L. Lactose free. Liq. 960 mL prediluted, ready-to-use cans. *OTC.*
Use: Nutritional supplement.

Isomil SF. (Ross) Low osmolar sucrose-free soy protein isolate infant formula containing 20 calories/fl oz. **Concentrated Liq.:** Can 13 fl oz. **Ready-to-feed:** Can 32 fl oz. **Nursing Bottles:** Hospital use. Bot. 8 fl oz. *OTC.*
Use: Nutritional supplement, enteral.

Isomune-CK. (Roche) Rapid immunochemical separation method of the heart specific CK-MB isoenzyme for quantitating when used with an appropriate CK substrate reagent. Test kit 100s, 250s.
Use: Diagnostic aid.

Isomune-LD. (Roche) Rapid immunochemical separation method of the heart specific LD-1 isoenzyme for quantitating when used with an appropriate LD substrate reagent. Test kit 40s, 100s.
Use: Diagnostic aid.

• **isomylamine hydrochloride.** (EYE-so-MILL-ah-meen) USAN.
Use: Muscle relaxant.

isomyn.
See: Amphetamine.

Isonate Sublingual. (Major) Isosorbide 2.5 mg, 5 mg. Sublingual Tab. Bot. 100s, 1000s, UD 100s. *Rx.*
Use: Antianginal.

Isonate Tablets. (Major) Isosorbide. **5 mg, 10 mg:** Bot. 100s, 1000s, UD 100s. **20 mg, 30 mg:** Bot. 100s, 1000s. *Rx.*
Use: Antianginal.

Isonate TD-Caps. (Major) Isosorbide 40 mg. Bot. 100s, 1000s. *Rx.*
Use: Antianginal.

Isonate T.R. Tabs. (Major) Isosorbide 40 mg. Bot. 100s, 1000s. *Rx.*
Use: Antianginal.

• **isoniazid.** (eye-so-NYE-uh-zid) *USP 28.*
Use: Anti-infective (tuberculostatic).
See: Calpas-INH.
Dow-Isoniazid.
INH.
Laniazid.

Nydrazid.
W/Calcium p-aminosalicylate, vitamin B_6.
See: Calpas-INAH-6.
Calpas Isoxine.
W/Pyridoxine Hydrochloride (vitamin B_6).
See: Niadox.
Pasna, Tri-Pack 300.
Teebaconin w/B_6.
W/Rifampin.
See: Rifater.

isoniazid. (Carolina Medical Products) Isoniazid 50 mg/5 mL, sorbitol, orange flavor. Syr. Bot. Pt. *Rx.*
Use: Anti-infective (tuberculostatic).

isoniazid. (Various Mfr.) Isoniazid 100 mg, 300 mg. Tab. Bot. 30s, 60s (300 mg only), 100s, 200s (300 mg only), 1000s. *Rx.*
Use: Anti-infective (tuberculostatic).

isoniazid combinations.
Use: Antituberculous agent.
See: Rifamate.
Rifater.

isonicotinic acid hydrazide.
See: Isoniazid.

isonicotinyl hydrazide.
See: Isoniazid.

isonipecaine hydrochloride.
See: Meperidine Hydrochloride.

isopentaquine.
Use: Antimalarial.

isophane insulin suspension (NPH).
Use: Antidiabetic.
See: Humulin N.
Novolin N.
Novolin N PenFill.
Novolin N Prefilled.
NPH Iletin II.

isophane insulin suspension (NPH)/ insulin injection (regular).
Use: Antidiabetic.
See: Humulin 50/50.
Humulin 70/30.
Novolin 70/30.
Novolin 70/30 Penfill.
Novolin 70/30 Prefilled.

isopregnenone.
See: Dydrogesterone.

Isoprinosine. (Newport Pharmaceuticals) Inosine pranobex.
Use: Antiviral; immunomodulator.

isopropanol.
Use: Antiseptic.
W/Combinations.
See: Ivy-Dry.
Ivy Super Dry.

isoprophenamine hydrochloride. Name used for Clorprenaline hydrochloride.

isopropicillin potassium.
Use: Anti-infective.

• **isopropyl alcohol.** (eye-so-PRO-pill AL-koe-hahl) *USP 28.*
Use: Topical anti-infective; pharmaceutic aid (solvent).
isopropyl alcohol spray. (Morton Grove) Isopropyl alcohol w/propellant. Aer. Can 6 oz. *OTC.*
Use: Anti-infective.
isopropylarterenol hydrochloride.
Use: Asthma; vasoconstrictor, allergic states.
isopropylarterenol sulfate.
See: Isoproterenol Sulfate.
• **isopropyl myristate.** (eye-so-PRO-pill mih-RIST-ate) *NF 23.*
Use: Pharmaceutic aid (emollient).
isonoradrenaline.
See: Isoproterenol.
isopropyl-noradrenaline hydrochloride.
See: Isoproterenol Hydrochloride.
• **isopropyl palmitate.** (eye-so-PRO-pill pal-mih-tate) *NF 23.*
Use: Pharmaceutic aid (oleaginous vehicle).
isopropyl phenazone. 4-Isopropyl antipyrine. Larodon.
isopropyl rubbing alcohol.
Use: Rubefacient, solvent.
isoproterenol.
See: Norisodrine.
W/Butabarbital, theophylline, ephedrine hydrochloride.
See: Medihaler-Iso.
• **isoproterenol hydrochloride.** (eye-so-pro-TER-uh-nahl) *USP 28.*
Use: Bronchodilator; vasoconstrictor.
See: Isuprel.
Medihaler-ISO.
Norisodrine.
W/Aminophylline, ephedrine sulfate, phenobarbital.
See: Asminorel.
W/Clopane (clopentamine) hydrochloride, propylene glycol, ascorbic acid.
See: Aerolone Compound.
isoproterenol hydrochloride. (Abbott) Isoproterenol hydrochloride 0.02 mg/mL (1:50,000), sodium metabisulfite. Inj. Prefilled syr. 10 mL. *Rx.*
Use: Bronchodilator, sympathomimetic.
isoproterenol hydrochloride. (ESI Lederle) Isoproterenol hydrochloride 0.2 mg/mL (1:5000 solution), sodium bisulfite. Inj. Amp. 5 mL. *Rx.*
Use: Bronchodilator, sympathomimetic.
• **isoproterenol sulfate.** (eye-so-pro-TER-uh-nahl) *USP 28.*
Use: Bronchodilator.
See: Medihaler-Iso.

W/Calcium iodide (anhydrous), alcohol.
See: Norisodrine.
Isoptin SR. (Abbott) Verapamil hydrochloride 120 mg, 180 mg, 240 mg. Film-coated. Tab. Bot. 100s, 500s (240 mg only). *Rx.*
Use: Calcium channel blocker.
Isopto Alkaline. (Alcon) Hydroxypropyl methylcellulose 1%, benzalkonium Cl 0.01%. Sterile ophthalmic soln. Dropper bot. 15 mL. *OTC.*
Use: Artificial tears.
Isopto Atropine. (Alcon) Atropine sulfate 0.5%, 1%. **0.5%:** *Drop-Tainer* 5 mL. **1%:** *Drop-Tainer* 5 mL, 15 mL. *Rx.*
Use: Cycloplegic; mydriatic.
Isopto Carbachol. (Alcon) Carbachol 0.75%, 1.5%, 3%. Benzalkonium chloride 0.005%, hydroxypropyl methylcellulose 1%, sodium chloride, boric acid, sodium borate. Soln. *Drop-Tainer* 15 mL, 30 mL. *Rx.*
Use: Antiglaucoma agent.
Isopto Carpine. (Alcon) Pilocarpine hydrochloride 0.5%, 1%, 2%, 4%, 5%, 6%, 8%. Soln. Bot. 15 mL, 30 mL (except 5%). *Rx.*
Use: Antiglaucoma agent.
Isopto Cetamide. (Alcon) Sodium sulfacetamide 15%. Soln. *Drop-Tainer* 5 mL, 15 mL. *Rx.*
Use: Anti-infective, ophthalmic.
Isopto Frin. (Alcon) Phenylephrine hydrochloride 0.12% in a methylcellulose Soln. *Drop-Tainer* 15 mL. *Rx.*
Use: Mydriatic; vasoconstrictor.
Isopto Homatropine. (Alcon) Homatropine HBr 2%, 5%. Soln. *Drop-Tainer* 5 mL, 15 mL. *Rx.*
Use: Cycloplegic; mydriatic.
Isopto Hyoscine. (Alcon) Hyoscine HBr 0.25%. Soln. *Drop-Tainer* 5 mL, 15 mL. *Rx.*
Use: Cycloplegic; mydriatic.
Isopto Plain. (Alcon) Hydroxypropyl methylcellulose 2910 0.5%, benzalkonium Cl 0.01%, sodium Cl, sodium phosphate, sodium citrate. *Drop-Tainer* 15 mL. *OTC.*
Use: Artificial tears.
Isopto Tears. (Alcon) Hydroxypropyl methylcellulose 0.5%, benzalkonium Cl 0.01%, sodium Cl, sodium phosphate, sodium citrate. Bot. *Drop-Tainer* 15 mL, 30 mL. *OTC.*
Use: Artificial tears.
Isordil Sublingual. (Wyeth) Isosorbide dinitrate. Tab. **2.5 mg, 5 mg:** Bot. 100s, 500s, *Redi-pak* 100s. **10 mg:** Bot. 100s. *Rx.*
Use: Antianginal.

Isordil Titradose Tablets. (Biovail) Isosorbide dinitrate 5 mg, 10 mg, 20 mg, 30 mg, 40 mg. **5 mg, 10 mg:** Bot. 100s, 500s, 1000s, *Redi-pak* 100s. **20 mg, 30 mg:** Bot. 100s, 500s, *Redi-pak* 100s. **40 mg:** Bot. 100s, *Redi-pak* 100s. *Rx.*
Use: Antianginal.

Isorgen-G. (Grafton) Isosorbide 5 mg, 10 mg. Tab. Bot. 1000s. *Rx.*
Use: Antianginal.

•**isosorbide concentrate.** (EYE-sos-ORE-bide) *USP 28.*
Use: Diuretic.

isosorbide dinitrate. (Various Mfr.) Isosorbide dinitrate. **Sublingual:** 2.5 mg, 5 mg, 10 mg. **2.5 mg:** Bot. 100s, 500s, 1000s, UD 100s. **5 mg:** Bot. 100s, 1000s, UD 100s. **10 mg:** Bot. 100s, 1000s. **Oral:** 5 mg, 10 mg, 20 mg, 30 mg. Tab. 40 mg. SR Tab. **5 mg:** Bot. 100s, 1000s, UD 100s. **10 mg:** Bot. 100s, 500s, 1000s, UD 100s. **20 mg:** Bot. 90s, 100s, 120s, 180s, 240s, 360s, 500s, 1000s, UD 100s. **30 mg:** Bot. 100s, 500s, 1000s, UD 100s. **40 mg:** Bot. 90s, 100s, 250s, 1000s, UD 100s. *Rx.*
Use: Coronary vasodilator.

•**isosorbide dinitrate diluted.** (EYE-sos-ORE-bide die-NYE-trate dye-LOOT-ed) *USP 28.*
Use: Coronary vasodilator.
See: Dilatrate-SR.
  Iso-Bid
  Isochron.
  Isordil.
  Nitromed.
  Onset.
  W/Phenobarbital.
  See: Sorbitrate w/Phenobarbital.

•**isosorbide mononitrate.** (EYE-sos-ORE-bide MAH-no-NYE-trate) USAN.
Use: Coronary vasodilator.
See: Imdur.
  ISMO.
  Isotrate ER.
  Monoket.

isosorbide mononitrate. (Teva) Isosorbide mononitrate 20 mg, lactose. Tab. Bot. 100s, 500s. *Rx.*
Use: Coronary vasodilator.

isosorbide mononitrate. (Various Mfr.) Isosorbide mononitrate 10 mg, 30 mg, 60 mg, 120 mg, lactose. ER Tab. Bot. 100s, UD 100s (except 10 mg, 120 mg). *Rx.*
Use: Coronary vasodilator.

isosorbide oral solution.
Use: Diuretic.

Isosource. (Novartis) Protein (Ca and Na caseinate, soy protein isolate) 43.2 g, carbohydrate (maltodextrin) 1755 g, fat (MCT, canola oil, lecithin) 443.9 g, Na 760 mg, K 1182 mg, mOsm/kg H_2O 390, Cal/mL 1.2, vitamins A, B_1, B_2, B_3, B_5, B_6, B_{12}, C, D, E, K, FA, biotin, choline, Ca, Cl, Cu, Fe, I, Mg, Mn, P, Zn, Se, Cr, Mo. Liq. Bot. 250 mL, 1000 mL. *OTC.*
Use: Nutritional supplement.

Isosource HN. (Novartis) Protein (Ca and Na caseinate, soy protein isolate) 56.1 g, carbohydrate (maltodextrin) 165 g, fat (MCT, canola oil, lecithin) 43.9 g, Na 760 mg, K 1772 mg, mOsm/kg H_2O 390, Cal/mL 1.2, vitamins B_1, B_2, B_3, B_5, B_6, B_{12}, C, D, E, K, FA, biotin, choline, Ca, P, I, Fe, Mg, Cu, Zn, Cl, Mn, Se, Cr, Mo. Liq. Bot. 250 mL, 1000 mL. *OTC.*
Use: Nutritional supplement.

•**isostearyl alcohol.** (EYE-so-STEE-rill AL-koe-hahl) USAN.
Use: Pharmaceutic aid (emollient, solvent).

•**isosulfan blue.** (EYE-so-SULL-fan) USAN.
Use: Radiopaque agent, parenteral.
See: Lymphazurin 1%.

Isotein HN. (Novartis) Vanilla Flavor. Maltodextrin, delactosed lactalbumin, partially hydrogenated soy oil with BHA, fructose, medium chain triglycerides, artificial flavor, sodium caseinate, monoglycerides and diglycerides, sodium Cl, vitamins, minerals. Pow. Packet 2.75 oz. *OTC.*
Use: Nutritional supplement.

•**isotiquimide.** (eye-so-TIH-kwih-MIDE) USAN.
Use: Antiulcerative.

Isotrate ER. (Apothecon) Isosoribide mononitrate 60 mg, lactose. ER Tab. Bot. 100s, 500s. *Rx.*
Use: Coronary vasodilator.

•**isotretinoin.** (EYE-so-TREH-tin-NO-in) *USP 28.*
Use: Retinoid.
See: Accutane.
  Amnesteem.
  Claravis.
  Sotret.

•**isotretinoin anisatil.** (eye-so-TRETT-ih-noyn ah-NIH-sah-till) USAN.
Use: Dermatologic, acne.

isovorin. (Wyeth) L-leucovorin.
Use: Antineoplastic. [Orphan Drug]

Isovue-M 300. (Bracco Diagnostics) Iopamidol 612 mg, iodine 300 mg/mL,

EDTA. Inj. Vial 15 mL. For intrathecal use *Rx.*
Use: Radiopaque agent, parenteral.

Isovue-M 200. (Bracco Diagnostics) Iopamidol 408 mg, iodine 200 mg/mL, EDTA. Inj. Vial 10 mL, 20 mL. For intrathecal use. *Rx.*
Use: Radiopaque agent, parenteral.

Isovue-300. (Bracco Diagnostics) Iopamidol 612 mg, iodine 300 mg/mL, EDTA. Inj. Vial 30 mL, 50 mL. Bot. 75 mL, 100 mL, 150 mL w/wo administration sets. Power Injector Syr. 100 mL, 150 mL. *Rx.*
Use: Radiopaque agent, parenteral.

Isovue-370. (Bracco Diagnostics) Iopamidol 755 mg, iodine 370 mg/mL, EDTA. Inj. Vial 20 mL, 30 mL, 50 mL. Bot. 50 mL, 75 mL, 100 mL, 125 mL, 150 mL, 175 mL, 200 mL. Power Injector Syr. 75 mL, 100 mL. *Rx.*
Use: Radiopaque agent, parenteral.

Isovue-200. (Bracco Diagnostics) Iopamidol 408 mg, iodine 200 mg/mL, EDTA. Inj. Vial 50 mL. Bot. 100 mL, 200 mL w/infusion set. *Rx.*
Use: Radiopaque agent, parenteral.

Isovue-250. (Bracco Diagnostics) Iopamidol 510 mg, iodine 250 mg/mL, EDTA. Inj. Vial 50 mL. Bot. 100 mL, 150 mL, 200 mL. Power Injector Syr. 150 mL. *Rx.*
Use: Radiopaque agent, parenteral.

•**isoxepac.** (EYE-SOX-ee-pack) USAN.
Use: Anti-inflammatory.

•**isoxicam.** (eye-SOX-ih-kam) USAN.
Use: Anti-inflammatory.

•**isoxsuprine hydrochloride.** (eye-SOX-you-preen) *USP 28.*
Use: Vasodilator.
See: Vasodilan.

I-Soyalac. (Mt. Vernon Foods, Inc.) I-soy protein isolate, I-methionine, CHO-sucrose, tapioca dextrin. F-soy oil, soy lecithin. Corn free. Protein 20.2 g, carbohydrate 63.4 g, fat 35.5 g, iron 12 mg, 640 Cal/serving (1 qt). Concentrate 390 mL, ready-to-use 1 qt. *OTC.*
Use: Nutritional supplement.

•**isradipine.** (iss-RAHD-ih-peen) *USP 28.*
Use: Calcium channel blocker; antagonist (calcium channel).
See: DynaCirc.
     DynaCirc CR.

Istalol. (Ista) Timolol maleate 0.5%, benzalkonium chloride 0.005%, monobasic sodium phosphate monohydrate, potassium sorbate 0.47%, sodium hydroxide. Soln. 5 mL. *Rx.*
Use: Agents for glaucoma.

•**istradefylline.** (iz-TRA-de-fye-leen) USAN.
Use: Parkinson disease.

I-Sulfacet. (American Pharmaceutical) Sulfacetamide sodium 10%, 15%, 30% ophthalmic soln. Bot. 2 mL, 5 mL, 15 mL. *Rx.*
Use: Anti-infective, ophthalmic.

Isuprel Inhalation Solution. (Sanofi-Synthelabo) Isoproterenol hydrochloride 0.5% (1:200), 1% (1:100). Soln. for Inh. Bot. 10 mL. *Rx.*
Use: Bronchodilator; sympathomimetic.

Isuprel Mistometer. (Sanofi-Synthelabo) Isoproterenol hydrochloride 103 mcg/dose. Aer. Bot. 15 mL. Refill 15 mL. *Rx.*
Use: Bronchodilator; sympathomimetic.

Isuprel Sterile Injection. (Abbott) Isoproterenol hydrochloride 0.2 mg/mL (1:5000), sodium metabisulfite. Inj. Amp. 1 mL, 5 mL. *Rx.*
Use: Bronchodilator; sympathomimetic.

isuprene.
See: Isoproterenol.

•**itasetron.** (eye-tah-SEH-trahn) USAN.
Use: Antidepressant; antiemetic; anxiolytic.

•**itazigrel.** (ih-TAY-zih-GRELL) USAN.
Use: Platelet aggregation inhibitor.

Itchaway. (Moyco Union Broach Division) Zinc undecylenate 20%, undecylenic acid 2%. Pow. Can 1.5 oz. *OTC.*
Use: Antifungal, topical.

Itch Relief Gel Spritz. (Band-Aid) Camphor 0.5%, benzyl alcohol, glycerin SD alcohol 40 B (43%). Spray. 56 g. *OTC.*
Use: Poison ivy treatment.

Itch-X. (B.F. Ascher) Pramoxine hydrochloride 1%. **Gel:** Benzyl alcohol, aloe vera gel, diazolidinyl urea, SD alcohol 40, parabens. 35.4 g. **Spray:** Benzyl alcohol, aloe vera gel, SD alcohol 40. In 60 mL. *OTC.*
Use: Anesthetic, local.

itobarbital.
W/Acetaminophen.
See: Panitol.

•**itraconazole.** (ih-truh-KAHN-uh-zole) USAN.
Use: Antifungal, triazole.
See: Sporanox.

itraconazole. (Various Mfr.) Itraconazole 100 mg. Cap. 28s, 30s, 100s, 500s, UD 28s, UD 30s. *Rx.*
Use: Antifungal agent.

I-Valex-1. (Ross) Protein 15 g, fat 23.9 g, carbohydrates 46.3 g, linoleic acid 1800 mg, Fe 9 mg, Na 190 mg, K 675 mg, with appropriate vitamins and minerals. 480 Cal/100 g. Leucine free.

Pow. Can 350 g. *OTC.*
Use: Nutritional supplement.
I-Valex-2. (Ross) Protein 30 g, fat 15.5 g, carbohyrates 30 g, Na 880 mg, K 1370 mg, with appropriate vitamins and minerals. 410 Cal/100 g. Leucine free. Pow. Can 325 g. *OTC.*
Use: Nutritional supplement.
Ivarest Maximum Strength. (Blistex) Calamine 14%, diphenhydramine hydrochloride 2%, lanolin oil, petrolatum, propylene glycol. Cream. Tube. 56 g. *OTC.*
Use: Poison ivy product, topical.
•**ivermectin.** (eye-VER-MEK-tin) *USP 28.*
Use: Anthelmintic.
See: Stromectol.
Ivocort. (Roberts) Micronized hydrocortisone alcohol 0.5%, 1%. Bot. 4 oz. *OTC.*
Use: Corticosteroid, topical.
Ivy Block. (EnviroDerm) Bentoquatam 5%, benzyl alcohol, methylparaben, SDA 40 denatured alcohol. Lot. 118 mL. *OTC.*
Use: Poison ivy treatment.
Ivy Cleanse. (EnviroDerm) Isopropyl alcohol, cetyl alcohol. Wipes. Packets of 12 individually wrapped towelettes. *OTC.*

Use: Poison ivy treatment.
Ivy-Dry. (Ivy Corp.) Zinc acetate 2%, glycerin, methylparaben, isopropanol 12.5%. Lot. Bot. 118 mL. *OTC.*
Use: Poison ivy product, topical.
Ivy Soothe. (Enviroderm) Hydrocortisone 1%, parabens, cetyl alcohol, glycerin, white petrolatum. Cream. 28 g. *OTC.*
Use: Poison ivy treatment.
Ivy Stat. (Tec Labs) Hydrocortisone 1%, propylene glycol, menthol, SD alcohol 40–B. Gel. 89 mL. *OTC.*
Use: Poison ivy treatment.
Ivy Super Dry. (Ivy Corp.) Zinc acetate 2%, benzyl alcohol 10%, menthol, camphor, glycerin, parabens, isopropanol 35%. Lot. Bot. 177 mL. *OTC.*
Use: Poison ivy product, topical.
I-Wash. (Akorn) Phosphate buffered saline soln. Bot. 4 oz, 8 oz. *OTC.*
Use: Irrigant, ophthalmic.
I-White. (Akorn) Phenylephrine 0.12%, polyvinyl alcohol, hydroxyethyl cellulose. Soln. Bot. 15 mL. *OTC.*
Use: Mydriatic; vasoconstrictor.
•**ixabepilone.** (ix-ab-EP-i-lone) USAN.
Use: Antineoplastic; antimitotic.
Izonid. (Major) Isoniazid 300 mg. Tab. Bot. 100s. *Rx.*
Use: Antituberculosal.

J

jalovis.
See: Hyaluronidase.
Janimine. (Abbott) Imipramine hydrochloride 10 mg, 25 mg, 50 mg. Tab. Bot. 100s, 1000s. *Rx.*
Use: Antidepressant.
Jantoven. (Upsher-Smith) Warfarin sodium 1 mg, 2 mg, 2.5 mg, 3 mg, 4 mg, 5 mg, 6 mg, 7.5 mg, 10 mg. Lactose, povidone. Tab. 100s, 500s (7.5 mg, 10 mg only), 1000s (except 7.5 mg, 10 mg). *Rx.*
Use: Anticoagulant.
japan agar.
See: Agar.
japanese encephalitis virus vaccine.
Use: Immunization.
See: JE VAX.
japan gelatin.
See: Agar.
japan isinglass.
See: Agar.
Jenest-28. (Organon) 7 white tablets norethindrone 0.5 mg, ethinyl estradiol 35 mcg; 14 peach tablets norethindrone 1 mg, ethinyl estradiol 35 mcg; 7 inert tablets. Lactose. *Cyclic Tablet dispenser* 28s. *Rx.*
Use: Sex hormone, contraceptive hormone.
Jeri-Bath. (Dermik) Concentrated moisturizing bath oil. Plastic Bot. 8 oz. *OTC.*
Use: Dermatologic.
Jets. (Freeda) L-lysine 300 mg, vitamins C 25 mg, B_{12} 25 mcg, B_6 5 mg, B_1 10 mg. Chew. Tab. Bot. 100s. *OTC.*
Use: Vitamin supplement; amino acid.
JE-VAX. (Aventis Pasteur) Japanese encephalitis virus vaccine 2 to 3 mcg nitrogen content per mL. Pow. for Inj. Single-dose vial with 1.3 mL diluent; 10-dose vial with 11 mL diluent. *Rx.*
Use: Immunization.
Jevity. (Ross) Calcium and sodium caseinates, soy fiber, hydrolyzed cornstarch, MCT (fractionated coconut oil), soy oil, corn oil, soy lecithin, vitamins A, B_1, B_2, B_3, B_5, B_6, B_{12}, C, D, E, K, folic acid, biotin, choline, Ca, P, Mg, Fe, Mn, Cu, Zn, I, Cl. Liq. Bot. 240 mL. *OTC.*
Use: Nutritional supplement.
Jevity 1.5 Cal. (Ross) Protein 63.4 g, carbohydrate 214.2 g, fat 49.6 g/L. Na 1386 mg/L, K 1848 mg/L, cal 1.5/mL. Vitamins A, B_1, B_2, B_3, B_5, B_6, B_{12}, C, D, E, K, Ca, Cu, Fe, I, Mg, Mn, Mo, P, Se, Zn, biotin, chloride, choline, folic acid. Liq. Can. 237 mL. Ready-to-hang containers 1 L, 1.5 L. *OTC.*
Use: Enteral nutrition therapy.
Jiffy. (Block Drug) Benzocaine, menthol, eugenol in glycerin-water base with SD alcohol 38-B 76%. Bot. 0.125 oz. *OTC.*
Use: Anesthetic, local.
J-Liberty. (J Pharmacal) Chlordiazepoxide hydrochloride 5 mg, 10 mg, 25 mg. Cap. *c-iv.*
Use: Anxiolytic.
Johnson's Baby. (Johnson & Johnson) Dimethicone 2%. Cream. Jar 4 oz, 6 oz; Tube 2 oz. *OTC.*
Use: Dermatologic protectant.
Johnson's Baby Sunblock Extra Protection. (Johnson & Johnson) Octyl methoxycinnamate, octyl salicylate, titanium dioxide, oxybenzone, C12-15 alcohols benzoate, cetyl alcohol, EDTA, vitamin E. Lot. Bot. 120 mL. *OTC.*
Use: Sunscreen.
Johnson's Baby Sunblock SPF 15. (Johnson & Johnson) Octyl methoxycinnamate, octyl salicylate, oxybenzone, titanium dioxide, benzyl alcohol, cetyl alcohol. PABA free. Waterproof. **Cream:** Tube. 60 g. **Lot.:** Bot. 60 g. *OTC.*
Use: Sunscreen.
Johnson's Baby Sunblock SPF 30. (Johnson & Johnson) Benzophenone-3, octyl methoxycinnamate, octyl salicylate, titanium dioxide. PABA free. Waterproof. Lot. Bot. 120 mL.
Johnson's Medicated. (Johnson & Johnson) Bentonite, kaolin, talc, zinc oxide. Pow. Bot. Small, Medium, Large. *OTC.*
Use: Diaper rash preparation.
Jolivette. (Watson) Norethindrone 0.35 mg, lactose. Tab. 28s. *Rx.*
Use: Contraceptive hormone.
•josamycin. (JOE-sah-MY-sin) USAN.
Use: Anti-infective.
Junel Fe 1/20. (Barr) Norethindrone acetate 1 mg, ethinyl estradiol 20 mcg. Tab. 28s with 7 brown tablets (ferrous fumarate 75 mg/tab). *Rx.*
Use: Contraceptive hormone.
Junel Fe 1.5/30. (Barr) Norethindrone acetate 1.5 mg, ethinyl estradiol 30 mcg. Tab. 28s with 7 brown tablets (ferrous fumarate 75 mg/tab). *Rx.*
Use: Contraceptive hormone.
Junior Strength Advil. (Whitehall-Robins) Ibuprofen 100 mg, aspartame, phenylalanine 4.2 mg, grape and fruit flavor. Chew. Tab. Bot. 24s. *OTC.*
Use: Analgesic, NSAID.
Junior-Strength Feverall. (Upsher-Smith) Acetaminophen 120 mg,

325 mg. Supp. Pkg 6s. *OTC.*
Use: Analgesic.

Junior Strength Motrin. (Ortho-McNeil) Ibuprofen 100 mg. Tab. Bot. 24s. *OTC.*
Use: Analgesic, NSAID.

Junior Strength Panadol. (Bayer Consumer Care) Acetaminophen 160 mg. Capl. Bot. 30s. *OTC.*
Use: Analgesic.

•**juniper tar.** (JOO-nih-per tar) *USP 28.*
Use: Local antieczematic, pharmaceutic necessity.

Junyer-All. (Barth's) Vitamins A 6000 units, D 400 units, B$_1$ 3 mg, B$_2$ 6 mg, C 120 mg, niacin 1 mg, E 12 units, B$_{12}$ 10 mcg, calcium 217 mg, phosphorus 97.5 mg, red bone marrow 10 mg, organic iron 15 mg, iodine 0.1 mg, beef peptone 20 mg/2 Cap. Bot. 10 month, 3 month, 6 month supply. *OTC.*
Use: Vitamin, mineral supplement.

Just Tears. (Blairex) Benzalkonium chloride, EDTA, NaCl, polyvinyl alcohol 1.4%. Soln. Bot. 15 mL. *OTC.*
Use: Lubricant, ophthalmic.

juvocaine.
See: Procaine hydrochloride.

K

Kadian. (Alpharma) Morphine sulfate 20 mg, 30 mg, 50 mg, 60 mg, 100 mg, sucrose. SR Pellet Cap. Bot. 30s, 60s, 100s. *c-II.*
Use: Opioid analgesic.

Kaergona.
See: Menadione.

Kala. (Freeda) Soy-based acidophilus 2 million units. Tab. Bot. 100s, 250s, 500s. *OTC.*
Use: Nutritional supplement.

•**kalafungin.** (kal-ah-FUN-jin) USAN.
Use: Antifungal.

Kaletra. (Abbott) **Cap.:** Lopinavir 133.3 mg, ritonavir 33.3 mg, sorbitol. Soft gelatin Cap. Bot. 180s. **Oral Soln.:** Lopinavir 80 mg, ritonavir 20 mg/mL, alcohol 42.4%, menthol, corn syrup, saccharin, peppermint oil, cotton candy or vanilla flavor. Bot. with dosing cup 160 mL. *Rx.*
Use: Antiretroviral, protease inhibitor combination.

Kaltostat. (GlaxoSmithKline) Calcium-sodium alginate fiber, 3" × 4¾" sterile dressing. In 1s. *OTC.*
Use: Dressing, hydroactive.

Kaltostat Forte. (GlaxoSmithKline) Calcium-sodium alginate fiber, 4" × 4" sterile dressing. In 1s. *OTC.*
Use: Dressing, hydroactive.

Kamfolene. (Wade) Camphor, menthol, methyl salicylate, turpentine and eucalyptus oils, carbolic acid 2%, calamine, zinc oxide in lanolin base. Jar 2 oz, lb. *OTC.*
Use: Antiseptic.

•**kanamycin sulfate.** (kan-uh-MY-sin) *USP 28.*
Use: Anti-infective.
See: Kantrex.

Kank-A. (Blairex) Benzocaine 5%, cetylpyridinium chloride, castor oil, benzoin compound. Liq. Bot. 3.75 mL. *OTC.*
Use: Anesthetic, local.

Kantrex. (Bristol-Myers Squibb) Kanamycin sulfate. **Cap.:** 0.5 g. Bot. 20s, 100s. **Vial.:** 0.5 g/2 mL or 1 g/3 mL. **Pediatric Inj.:** 75 mg/2 mL. **Disposable Syringe:** 500 mg/2 mL. *Rx.*
Use: Anti-infective aminoglycoside.

Kaochlor-Eff. (Pharmacia) Elemental potassium 20 mEq, chloride 20 mEq. Tab. Supplied by: Potassium Cl 0.6 g, potassium citrate 0.22 g, potassium bicarbonate 1 g, betaine hydrochloride 1.84 g, saccharin 20 mg, artificial fruit flavor, tartrazine (color). Tab. Sugar free. Carton 60s. *Rx.*

Use: Electrolyte supplement.

Kaodene Non-Narcotic. (Pfeiffer) Kaolin 3.9 g, pectin 194.4 mg/30 mL, bismuth subsalicylate. Alcohol free. Liq. Bot. 120 mL. *OTC.*
Use: Antidiarrheal.

Kaodene with Codeine. (Pfeiffer) Codeine phosphate 32.4 mg, kaolin 3.9 g, pectin 194.4 mg, sodium carboxymethylcellulose, bismuth subsalicylate/ 30 mL. Susp. Bot. 120 mL. *OTC.*
Use: Antidiarrheal.

•**kaolin.** (KAY-oh-lin) *USP 28.*
Use: Adsorbent.
W/Belladonna, phenobarbital.
See: Bellkata.
W/Bismuth compound.
See: Kaomine.
W/Bismuth subgallate.
See: Diastop.
W/Bismuth subgallate, pectin, zinc phenolsulfonate, opium powder.
See: Diastay.
W/Cornstarch, camphor, zinc oxide, eucalyptus oil.
See: Mexsana.
W/Furazolidone, pectin.
See: Furoxone.
W/Hyoscyamine sulfate, sodium benzoate, atropine sulfate, hyoscine HBr, pectin.
See: Donnagel.
W/Neomycin sulfate, pectin.
See: Pecto-Kalin.
W/Pectin.
See: B-K-P Mixture.
Kapectin.
Pecto-Kalin.
W/Pectin, bismuth subcarbonate, belladonna.
See: Kay-Pec.
W/Pectin, bismuth subcarbonate, opium.
See: Palsorb Improved.
W/Pectin, opium, bismuth subgallate, zinc phenolsulfonate.
See: B.P.P.
Cholactabs.
W/Pectin, opium extract.
See: Pecto-Kalin.
W/Pectin, paregoric (equivalent).
See: Duosorb.
Kaoparin.
Kapectin.
Ka-Pek w/Paregoric.
W/Pectin, zinc phenolsulfonate.
See: Pectocel.
W/Phenobarbital, atropine sulfate, aluminum hydroxide gel.
See: Kao-Lumin.

kaolin colloidal.
W/Bismuth subcarbonate.

See: Bisilad.
W/Magnesium trisilicate, aluminum hydroxide dried gel.
See: Kamadrox.
Kathmagel.
W/Pectin, aromatics.
See: Paocin.
kaolin w/pectin. (Various Mfr.) Kaolin 90 g, pectin 2 g/30 mL. Susp. Bot. 180 mL, pt, UD 30 mL. *OTC.*
Use: Antidiarrheal combination.
Kaon Cl. (Pharmacia) Potassium Cl 500 mg, FD&C Yellow No. 5. CR Tab. Bot. 100s, 250s, 1000s. *Rx.*
Use: Electrolyte supplement.
Kaon Cl-10. (Pharmacia) Potassium Cl 750 mg. CR Tab. Bot. 100s, 500s, 1000s. Stat-Pak 100s. *Rx.*
Use: Electrolyte supplement.
Kaon Cl 20%. (Pharmacia) Potassium and chloride 40 mEq (to potassium Cl 3 g)/15 mL, saccharin, flavoring, alcohol 5%. Bot. Pt. *Rx.*
Use: Electrolyte supplement.
Kaon Elixir. (Pharmacia) Elemental potassium 20 mEq (as potassium gluconate 4.68 g)/15 mL, aromatics, grape and lemon-lime flavors, alcohol 5%, saccharin. Elix. Unit pkg. Pt, gal. *Rx.*
Use: Electrolyte supplement.
Kaon Tablets. (Pharmacia) Elemental potassium 5 mEq obtained from potassium gluconate 1.17 g. SC Tab. Bot. 100s, 500s. *Rx.*
Use: Electrolyte supplement.
Kaopectate. (Pharmacia) Bismuth subsalicylate 87.3 mg/5 mL, sucrose, regular and peppermint flavor. Liq. 236 mL, 355 mL. *OTC.*
Use: Antidiarrheal.
Kaopectate, Children's. (Pharmacia) Bismuth subsalicylate 87 mg/5 mL, sucrose, cherry flavor. Liq. 177 mL. *OTC.*
Use: Antidiarrheal combination.
Kaopectate Extra Strength. (Pharmacia) Bismuth subsalicylate 175 mg/5 mL, sucrose, peppermint flavor. Liq. 236 mL. *OTC.*
Use: Antidiarrheal.
Kaopectate, Maximum Strength. (Pharmacia) Attapulgite 750 mg, Capl. Pkg. 12s, 20s. *OTC.*
Use: Antidiarrheal combination.
Kaopectate Tablet Formula. (Pharmacia) Attapulgite 750 mg. Tab. Blister pak 12s, 20s. *OTC.*
Use: Antidiarrheal.
Kaophen. (Pal-Pak, Inc.) Phenobarbital 6.5 mg, belladonna extract 0.1 mg, kaolin 388.8 mg. Tab. Bot. 100s, 1000s. *OTC.*

Use: Antidiarrheal.
Kao-Spen. (Century) Kaolin 5.2 g, pectin 260 mg/30 mL. Susp. Bot. 120 mL, pt, gal. *OTC.*
Use: Antidiarrheal.
Kao-Tin. (Major) Kaolin 5.85 g, pectin 130 mg/30 mL. Susp. Bot. 120 mL, 240 mL, pt, gal. *OTC.*
Use: Antidiarrheal.
Kapectin. (Health for Life Brands) Kaolin 90 g, pectin 2 g/oz. Bot. Gal. *OTC.*
Use: Antidiarrheal.
Kapectolin. (United Research Laboratories) Bismuth subsalicylate 262 per 15 mL. Glycerin, saccharin, sorbitol. Mint flavor. Liq. 480 mL. *OTC.*
Use: Antidiarrheal.
Kapectolin. (Various Mfr.) Kaolin 90 g, pectin 2 g/30 mL. Susp. Bot. 360 mL. *OTC.*
Use: Antidiarrheal.
Ka-Pek. (A.P.C.) Kaolin 90 g, pectin 4.5 g/fl oz. Bot. 6 oz, gal. *OTC.*
Use: Antidiarrheal.
kapilin.
See: Menadione.
karaya gum. (Penick) Indian Gum. Sterculia Gum.
See: Tri-Costivin.
W/Psyllium seed, plantago ovata, brewers yeast.
See: Movicol.
W/Refined psyllium mucilloid.
See: Hydrocil Regular.
karaya powder. (Sween) Bot. 3 oz.
Use: Deodorant, ostomy.
Kareon.
See: Menadione.
Karidium. (Young Dental) **Tab.:** Sodium fluoride 2.21 mg, sodium Cl 94.49 mg, disintegrant 0.5 mg. Bot. 180s, 1000s. **Liq.:** Sodium fluoride 2.21 mg, sodium Cl 10 mg, purified water q.s./8 drops. Bot. 30 mL, 60 mL. *Rx.*
Use: Dental caries agent.
Karigel. (Young Dental) Fluoride ion 0.5%, pH 5.6. Gel. Bot. 30 mL, 130 mL, 250 mL. *Rx.*
Use: Dental caries agent.
Karigel-N. (Young Dental) Fluoride ion 0.5% in neutral pH gel. Bot. 24 mL, 125 mL. *Rx.*
Use: Dental caries agent.
Kariva. (Barr) **Phase 1:** Desogestrel 0.15 mg, ethinyl estradiol 20 mcg. **Phase 2:** Ethinyl estradiol 10 mcg, lactose. Tab. Blister card. 28s. *Rx.*
Use: Sex hormone, contraceptive update.

• **kasal.** (KAY-sal) USAN. Approximately
Na_8Al_2 $(OH)_2$ $(PO_4)_4$ with ≈ 30% of
dibasic sodium phosphate; sodium aluminum phosphate, basic.
Use: Food additive.

kasugamycin. Under study.
Use: Anti-infective.

Kaviton.
See: Menadione.

Kay Ciel. (Forest) Potassium chloride
1.5 g/Packette. (20 mEq/Packet), 4%
alcohol. Pow. Box 30s, 100s, 500s. *Rx.*
Use: Electrolyte supplement.

Kayexalate. (Sanofi-Synthelabo) Sodium
polystyrene sulfonate (sodium content
≈ 100 mg/g). Jar 1 lb. *Rx.*
Use: Potassium-removing resin.

K-C. (Century) **Susp.:** Kaolin 5.2 g, pectin 200 mg, bismuth subcarbonate
260 mg/30 mL. Bot. 120 mL, pt, gal.
Liq.: Kaolin 5.2 g, pectin 260 mg, bismuth subcarbonate 260 mg/oz. Bot.
4 oz, pt, gal. *OTC.*
Use: Antidiarrheal.

KCl-20. (Western Research) Potassium
Cl 1.5 g (potassium 20 mEq, chloride
20 mEq) Packet. Box 30s. *Rx.*
Use: Electrolyte supplement.

K-Dur 10 & 20. (Key) **10:** Potassium Cl
750 mg (10 mEq). SR Tab. **20:** Potassium Cl 1500 mg (20 mEq). SR Tab.
Bot. 100s. *Rx.*
Use: Electrolyte supplement.

KE.
See: Cortisone Acetate.

Keelamin. (Mericon Industries) Zinc
20 mg, manganese 5 mg, copper 3 mg.
Tab. Bot. 100s. *OTC.*
Use: Mineral supplement.

Keep Alert. (Magno-Humphries Labs.)
Caffeine 200 mg. Tab. Bot. 60s. *OTC.*
Use: CNS stimulant, analeptic.

Keep Going. (Block Drug) Caffeine
200 mg. Tab. Pkg. 4s. *OTC.*
Use: CNS stimulant, analeptic.

Keflex. (Advancis) **Capl.:** Cephalexin
250 mg, 500 mg. Bot. 20s, 100s
(250 mg only), UD 100s. **Pow. for Oral
Susp.:** Cephalexin 125 mg/5 mL,
250 mg/5 mL. Bot. 100 mL, 200 mL, UD
100 mL (250 mg/5 mL only). *Rx.*
Use: Anti-infective, cephalosporin.

Kell E. (Canright) dl-α Tocopheryl
100 units, 200 units, 400 units. Tab. Bot.
100s. *OTC.*
Use: Vitamin supplement.

Kellogg's Tasteless Castor Oil. (Glaxo-
SmithKline) Castor oil 100%. Bot. 2 oz.
OTC.
Use: Laxative.

Kelp. (Arcum) Tab. Bot. 100s, 1000s.
OTC.

Kelp. (Faraday) Iodine from kelp
0.15 mg. Tab. Bot. 100s. *OTC.*

Kelp Plus. (Barth's) Iodine from kelp plus
16 trace minerals. Tab. Bot. 100s, 500s,
1000s. *OTC.*

Kemadrin. (GlaxoSmithKline) Procyclidine hydrochloride 5 mg. Tab. Bot.
100s. *Rx.*
Use: Antiparkinsonian.

Kemstro. (Schwarz) Baclofen 10 mg
(with phenylalanine 3.7 mg), 20 mg
(phenylalanine 7.9 mg). Mannitol, aspartame. Orally Disintegrating Tab.
100s. *Rx.*
Use: Skeletal muscle relaxant.

Kenac. (Alra) Triamcinolone acetonide.
Cream: 0.025%, 0.1%. Tube 15 g,
60 g, 80 g; Jar 240 g. **Oint.:** 0.1%. Tube
15 g, 80 g. *Rx.*
Use: Corticosteroid, topical.

Kenaject-40. (Merz) Triamcinolone acetonide 40 mg/mL. Inj. Vial 5 mL. *Rx.*
Use: Corticosteroid.

Kenakion. (Harriett Lane Home of Johns
Hopkins Hospital) Vitamin K-1 oxide.
Rx.
Use: Vitamin K-induced kernicterus.

Kenalog. (Bristol-Myers Squibb) Triamcinolone acetonide. **0.1% Cream:**
Tube 15 g, 60 g, 80 g; Jar 240 g. In
aqueous lotion base w/propylene glycol, cetyl and stearyl alcohols, glyceryl
monostearate, sorbitan monopalmitate,
polyoxyethylene sorbitan monolaurate,
methylparaben, propylparaben, polyethylene glycol monostearate, simethicone, sorbic acid. **0.5% Cream:** Tube
20 g. **0.1% Oint.:** (w/base of polyethylene, mineral oil) Tube 15 g, 60 g, 80 g;
Jar 240 g. **0.5% Oint.:** Tube 20 g. **0.1%
Lot.:** Bot. 15 mL, 60 mL. **Spray:**
6.6 mg/100 g, alcohol 10.3%. Can 23 g,
63 g. *Rx.*
Use: Corticosteroid, topical.

Kenalog-40. (Bristol-Myers Squibb) Sterile triamcinolone acetonide suspension
40 mg/mL, sodium chloride for isotonicity, benzyl alcohol 0.9% (w/v) as a
preservative, sodium carboxymethylcellulose 0.75%, polysorbate 80 0.04%.
Sodium hydroxide or hydrochloride
acid may be present to adjust pH to 5
to 7.5. Nitrogen packed at the time of
manufacture. Inj. Vial 1 mL, 5 mL,
10 mL. *Rx.*
Use: Corticosteroid.

Kenalog-H. (Bristol-Myers Squibb) Triamcinolone acetonide cream USP
0.1%. Each g of cream provides 1 mg

of triamcinolone acetonide in a specially formulated hydrophilic vanishing cream base containing propylene glycol, dimethicone 350, castor oil, cetearyl alcohol and ceteareth-20, propylene glycol stearate, white petrolatum, purified water. Cream. Tube 15 g, 60 g. *Rx.*
Use: Corticosteroid, topical.

Kenalog in Orabase. (Apothecon) Triamcinolone acetonide 0.1% in Orabase. Triamcinolone acetonide 1 mg/g. Tube 5 g. *Rx.*
Use: Corticosteroid, topical.

Kenalog-10. (Bristol-Myers Squibb) Sterile triamcinolone acetonide suspension 10 mg/mL, sodium Cl for isotonicity, benzyl alcohol 0.9% (w/v) as a preservative, sodium carboxymethylcellulose 0.75%, polysorbate 80 0.04%. Sodium hydroxide or hydrochloric acid may be present to adjust pH to 5 to 7.5. Nitrogen packed at the time of manufacture. Inj. Vial 5 mL. *Rx.*
Use: Corticosteroid.

Kenalog 0.025%. (Bristol-Myers Squibb) Triamcinolone acetonide. **Cream:** Tube 15 g, 80 g; Jar 240 g. **Lot.:** In aqueous lotion base w/propylene glycol, cetyl and stearyl alcohols, glyceryl monostearate, sorbitan monopalmitate, polyoxyethylene sorbitan monolaurate, methylparaben, propylparaben, polyethylene glycol monostearate, simethicone, sorbic acid, tinted in an isopropyl palmitate vehicle with alcohol (4.7%). Bot. 60 mL. **Oint.:** Plastibase (w/base of polyethylene and mineral oil gel). Tube 15 g, 80 g, 240 g. *Rx.*
Use: Corticosteroid, topical.

Kendall's "Compound E".
See: Cortisone Acetate.

Kendall's "Desoxy Compound B".
See: Desoxycorticosterone Acetate.

Kenwood Therapeutic. (Kenwood) Vitamins A 3333 units, D 133 units, E 1.5 units, C 50 mg, B_1 2 mg, B_2 1 mg, B_3 20 mg, B_5 2 mg, B_6 0.33 mg, Ca, K, Mg, Mn, P/5 mL. Liq. Bot. 240 mL. *OTC.*
Use: Mineral, vitamin supplement.

Kepivance. (Amgen) Palifermin 6.25 mg. Sucrose. Preservative free. Pow. for Inj. Single-use vials. *Rx.*
Use: Keratinocyte growth factor.

Keppra. (UCB Pharma) Levetiracetam. **Oral Soln.:** 100 mg/mL. Dye-free. Parabens. Grape flavor. 480 mL. **Tab.:** 250 mg, 500 mg, 750 mg. Film-coated. Bot. 120s. *Rx.*
Use: Anticonvulsant.

Keralac. (Doak) Urea. **Cream:** 50%. EDTA. 18 mL. **Lot.:** 35%. Cetyl alcohol, EDTA. 207 mL, 325 mL. *Rx.*
Use: Emollient.

Keralac Nail Gel. (Doak) Urea 50%. EDTA. Gel. 18 mL. *Rx.*
Use: Emollient.

keratinocyte growth factors.
See: Palifermin.

keratolytics.
See: Condylox.
Diclofenac Sodium.
Solaraze.

Keri. (Bristol-Myers Squibb) Mineral oil, lanolin oil, water, propylene glycol, glyceryl stearate, PEG-100 stearate, PEG 40 stearate, PEG-4 dilaurate, laureth-4, parabens, docusate sodium, triethanolamine, quaternium 15, carbomer 934. Lot. Bot. 6.5 oz, 13 oz, 20 oz. *OTC.*
Use: Emollient.

Keri Facial Soap. (Bristol-Myers Squibb) Sodium tallowate, sodium cocoate, mineral oil, octyl hydroxystearate, fragrance, glycerin, titanium dioxide, PEG-75, lanolin oil, docusate sodium, PEG-4 dilaurate, propylparaben, PEG-40 stearate, glyceryl monostearate, PEG-100 stearate, sodium Cl, BHT, EDTA. Bar 3.25 oz. *OTC.*
Use: Dermatologic cleanser.

Keri Nourishing Shea Butter. (Bristol-Myers Squibb) Mineral oil, glycerin, shea butter, vitamin E acetate, parabens, sunflower seed oil, EDTA, aloe. Lot. 425 g. *OTC.*
Use: Emollient.

Keri Sensitive Skin. (Bristol-Myers Squibb) Glycerin, hydrogenated polyisobutane, petrolatum, cetyl alcohol, aloe, barbadensis gel, vitamin E acetate, EDTA, parabens. Lot. 241 g. *OTC.*
Use: Emollient.

Kerlone. (Sanofi) Betaxolol hydrochloride 10 mg, 20 mg, lactose. Tab. Bot. 100s. *Rx.*
Use: Antiadrenergic, sympatholytic, beta-adrenergic blocker.

Kerocaine.
See: Procaine hydrochloride.

Kerodex. (Wyeth) **No. 51:** Water-miscible. Tube 4 oz, Jar lb. **No. 71:** Water-repellent Tube 4 oz, Jar lb. *OTC.*
Use: Emollient.

kerohydric. A de-waxed, oil-soluble fraction of lanolin.
Use: Emollient, cleanser.
See: Alpha-Keri.
Keri.

W/Docusate sodium, sodium alkyl polyether sulfonate, sodium sulfoacetate, sulfur, salicylic acid, hexachlorophene.
See: Sebulex.
Kerr Insta-Char. (Kerr Drug) **Regular:** Aqueous suspension activated charcoal 50 g/8 oz. **Pediatric:** Aqueous suspension activated charcoal 15 g/4 oz. *OTC.*
Use: Antidote.
Kerr Triple Dye. (Kerr Drug) Gentian violet, proflavine hemisulfate, brilliant green in water. Dispensing bot. 15 mL. Single Use *Dispos-A-Swab* 0.65 mL, Box 10s, Case 10 × 50 Box. *OTC.*
Use: Antiseptic.
Kestrone 5. (Hyrex) Estrone 5 mg/mL, sodium carboxymethylcellulose, povidone, benzyl alcohol, propylparabens Inj. Multi-dose vial 10 mL. *Rx.*
Use: Estrogen.
Ketalar. (Monarch) Ketamine hydrochloride 10 mg, 50 mg, 100 mg/mL. Inj. Vial 20 mL (10 mg), 10 mL (50 mg), 5 mL (100 mg). Ctn. 10s. *c-III.*
Use: Anesthetic.
• **ketamine hydrochloride.** (KEET-uh-MEEN) *USP 28.*
Use: Anesthetic.
See: Ketalar.
• **ketanserin.** (KEET-AN-ser-in) USAN.
Use: Serotonin antagonist.
• **ketazocine.** (key-TAY-zoe-seen) USAN.
Use: Analgesic.
• **ketazolam.** (keet-AZE-oh-lam) USAN.
Use: Anxiolytic.
Ketek. (Aventis) Telithromycin 300 mg, 400 mg. Cornstarch (400 mg only) lactose. Film-coated. Tab. 60s; blister pack 10s, UD 100s (400 mg only). *Rx.*
Use: Anti-infective.
• **kethoxal.** (KEY-thox-al) USAN.
Use: Antiviral.
• **ketipramine fumarate.** (key-TIH-prah-MEEN) USAN.
Use: Antidepressant.
• **ketoconazole.** (KEY-toe-KOE-nuh-zole) *USP 28.*
Use: Antifungal.
See: Nizoral.
Nizoral A-D.
ketoconazole. (Clay-Park Labs) Ketoconazole 2%. Shampoo. 118 mL. *Rx.*
Use: Antifungal agent.
ketoconazole. (Teva) Ketoconazole 2% in aqueous vehicle, cetyl alcohol, stearyl alcohol, sodium sulfite. Cream. Tube. 15 g, 30 g, 60 g. *Rx.*
Use: Antifungal.

ketoconazole. (Various Mfr.) Ketoconazole 200 mg. Tab. Bot. 30s, 50s, 100s, 250s, 500s, 1000s; blister pack 10s; UD 30s, 50s, 100s. *Rx.*
Use: Antifungal.
Ketodestrin.
See: Estrone.
Keto-Diastix Reagent Strips. (Bayer Corp. (Consumer Div.)) Dip and read reagent strip test for glucose and ketones in urine. Two test areas: glucose levels from 30 mg to 5000 mg/dl; ketone test (acetoacetic acid) negative 5 mg, 40 mg, 80 mg, 160 mg/dL. Strip Bot. 50s, 100s.
Use: Diagnostic aid.
ketohexazine. (Wyeth)
Use: Hypnotic.
ketohydroxyestratriene
See: Estrone.
ketohydroxyestrin.
See: Estrone.
ketolides.
Use: Anti-infectives.
See: Telithromycin.
ketone tests.
Use: Diagnostic aid.
See: Acetest Reagent.
Chemstrip K.
Ketostix Strips.
Ketonex-1. (Ross) Protein 15 g, fat 23.9 g, carbohydrates 46.3 g, linoleic acid 1800 mg, Fe 9 mg, Na 190 mg, K 675 mg. With appropriate vitamins and minerals. 480 Cal/100 g. Isoleucine, leucine, and valine free. Pow. Can 350 g. *OTC.*
Use: Nutritional supplement.
Ketonex 2. (Ross) Protein 30 g, fat 15.5 g, carbohydrates 30 g, Fe 13 mg, Na 880 mg, K 1370 mg. With appropriate vitamins and minerals. 410 Cal/100 g. Isoleucine, leucine and valine free. Pow. Can 325 g. *OTC.*
Use: Nutritional supplement.
• **ketoprofen.** (KEY-to-pro-fen) *USP 28.*
Use: Anti-inflammatory, NSAID.
See: Orudis KT.
Oruvail.
ketoprofen. (Andrx) Ketoprofen 100 mg, 150 mg, 200 mg. ER Cap. Bot. 100s, 1000s. *Rx.*
Use: Anti-inflammatory, NSAID.
ketoprofen. (Various Mfr.) Ketoprofen 50 mg, 75 mg. Cap. Bot. 100s, 500s (75 mg only). *Rx.*
Use: Anti-inflammatory, NSAID.
• **ketorfanol.** (key-TAR-fan-AHL) USAN.
Use: Analgesic.

•**ketorolac tromethamine.** (KEY-TOR-oh-lak tro-METH-uh-meen) *USP 28.*
Use: Analgesic, NSAID, ophthalmic.
See: Acular.
Acular LS.
Toradol.
ketorolac tromethamine. (Bedford) Ketorolac tromethamine 15 mg/mL, 30 mg/mL. Inj. Vial 1 mL (15 mL only). Single dose Vial 1 mL, 2 mL; multiple-dose vial 10 mL. *Rx.*
Use: Analgesic, NSAID.
ketorolac tromethamine. (Various Mfr.) Ketorolac tromethamine 10 mg. Tab. Bot. 100s, 500s. *Rx.*
Use: Analgesic, NSAID.
Ketostix Reagent Strips. (Bayer Corp. (Consumer Div.)) Sodium nitroprusside, sodium phosphate, glycine. Stick test for ketones in urine (measures aceto-acetic acid). Bot. 50s, 100s, UD 20s.
Use: Diagnostic aid.
•**ketotifen fumarate.** (KEY-toe-TIE-fen) USAN.
Use: Antiasthmatic.
See: Zaditor.
Key-Plex. (Hyrex) Vitamins B_1 50 mg, B_2 5 mg, B_{12} 1000 mcg, pyridoxine hydrochloride 5 mg, d-panthenol 6 mg, niacinamide 125 mg, ascorbic acid 50 mg/mL. Inj. Vial 10 mL. *Rx.*
Use: Nutritional supplement, parenteral.
Key-Pred. (Hyrex) Prednisolone 25 mg/mL, 50 mg/mL. Inj. Vial 10 mL, 30 mL (50 mg/mL only). *Rx.*
Use: Corticosteroid.
Key-Pred-SP. (Hyrex) Prednisolone sodium phosphate 20 mg/mL. Inj. Vial 10 mL. *Rx.*
Use: Corticosteroid.
K-4. Menadiol sodium diphosphate.
Use: Vitamin K.
K-G Elixir. (Geneva) Potassium (as potassium gluconate) 20 mEq/15 mL, alcohol 5%. Elix. Bot. Pt. *Rx.*
Use: Electrolyte supplement.
kharophen.
See: Acetarsone.
khellin.
Use: Coronary vasodilator.
Kiddie Powder. (Gordon Laboratories) Pure fine Italian talc. Can. 3.5 oz. *OTC.*
Use: Antifungal.
Kiddi-Vites, Improved. (Geneva) Vitamins A 5000 units, D 500 units, B_1 1 mg, B_2 1.5 mg, B_{12} 2 mcg, C 50 mg, B_6 1 mg, pantothenate 2 mg, niacinamide 10 mg. Tab. Bot. 100s, 1000s. *OTC.*
Use: Vitamin supplement.
Kid Kare. (Rugby) Pseudoephedrine hydrochloride 7.5 mg/0.8 mL, sorbitol, sugar, cherry flavor, alcohol free. Drops. Bot. 30 mL w/dropper. *OTC.*
Use: Nasal decongestant, arylalkylamine.
Kid Kare Children's Cough/Cold. (Rugby) Pseudoephedrine hydrochloride 15 mg, chlorpheniramine maleate 1 mg, dextromethorphan HBr 5 mg/5 mL, sorbitol, corn syrup, cherry flavor, alcohol free. Liq. Bot. 118 mL. *OTC.*
Use: Upper respiratory combination, decongestant, antihistamine, antitussive.
kidney function agents.
See: Biotel Kidney.
Indigo Carmine.
Inulin.
Iodohippurate Sodium.
Methylene Blue.
KIE. (Laser) Potassium iodide 150 mg, ephedrine hydrochloride 8 mg/5 mL, saccharin, sorbitol, sucrose, cherry flavor. Syr. Bot. 473 mL. *Rx.*
Use: Upper respiratory combination, decongestant, expectorant.
kinate. Hexahydrotetra hydroxybenzoate salt, quinic acid salt.
Kindercal. (Mead Johnson Nutritionals) Protein 13%, carbohydrate 50%, fat 37%, 30 cal/oz, sucrose, vanilla flavor, lactose free, 30 cal/oz. Liq. Can. 8 oz. *OTC.*
Use: Nutritional supplement.
Kinerase Intensive Eye Cream. (Valeant) Kinetin 0.125%, safflower seed oil, cetyl alcohol, urea, parabens. Cream. 20 g. *OTC.*
Use: Emollient.
Kineret. (Amgen) Anakinra 100 mg/0.67 mL, sodium chloride, EDTA, preservative free. Inj. Single-use Prefilled syr 1 mL w/27-gauge needle. *Rx.*
Use: Immunologic, immunomodulator.
Kinevac. (Bracco Diagnostics) Sincalide 5 mcg/vial. Pow. for Inj., lyophilized. Vials. *Rx.*
Use: Diagnostic aid, gastrointestinal function test.
Kin White. (Whiteworth Towne) Triamcinolone acetonide. **Cream:** 0.025%, 1%. Tube 15 g, 80 g. **Oint.:** 1%. Tube 15 g, 80 g. *OTC.*
Use: Corticosteroid, topical.
Kionex. (Paddock) Finely ground sodium polystyrene sulfonate (4 level tsp ≈ 15 g), sodium content ≈ 100 mg (4.1 mEq)/g. Pow. Can. 454 g. *Rx.*
Use: Potassium-removing resin.
•**kitasamycin.** (kit-ah-sah-MY-sin) USAN. An antibiotic substance obtained from cultures of *Streptomyces kitasatoensis.* Under study.

Use: Anti-infective.

Klaron. (Dermik) Sodium sulfacetamide 10%, propylene glycol, polyethylene glycol 400, methylparaben, EDTA. Lot. Bot. 59 mL. *Rx.*
Use: Dermatologic.

Klavikordal. (US Ethicals) Nitroglycerin 2.6 mg. SR Tab. Bot. 100s, 1000s. *Rx.*
Use: Antianginal.

KLB6. (NBTY) Vitamin B_6 3.5 mg, soya lecithin 100 mg, kelp 25 mg, cider vinegar 80 mg Softgels. Bot. 100s. *OTC.*
Use: Vitamin supplement.

KLB6 Complete. (NBTY) Vitamins A 833.3 units, E 5 mg (as units), B_3 3.3 mg, C 10 mg, soya lecithin 200 mg, kelp 25 mg, cider vinegar 40 mg, wheat bran 83.3 mg, D 66.7 units, FA 0.067 mg, B_1 0.35 mg, B_6 0.20 mg, B_2 8.3 mg, B_{12} 1 mcg, biotin 0.05 mg. Tab. Bot. 100s. *OTC.*
Use: Vitamin supplement.

Kleen-Handz. (American Medical) Ethyl alcohol 62%, aloe vera. Soln. Bot. 60 mL. *OTC.*
Use: Antiseptic.

Kleer Improved. (Scrip) Atropine sulfate 0.2 mg, chlorpheniramine maleate 5 mg/mL. *Rx.*
Use: Anticholinergic; antihistamine.

Klerist-D. (Nutripharm Laboratories, Inc.) **Cap. SR:** Pseudoephedrine hydrochloride 120 mg, chlorpheniramine maleate 8 mg. Bot. 100s, 500s. **Tab.:** Pseudoephedrine hydrochloride 60 mg, chlorpheniramine maleate 4 mg. Bot. 24s, 100s. *Rx.*
Use: Antihistamine; decongestant.

Kler-Ro. (Ulmer Pharmacal) Surgical cleanser and laboratory detergent. **Liq.:** Bot. Gal. **Pow.:** Can 2 lb, Bot. 6 lb. *Rx.*
Use: Antiseptic.

KL4-Surfactant. (Acute Therapeutics) *Use:* Treatment of acute respiratory distress syndrome. [Orphan Drug]

Klonopin. (Roche) Clonazepam. **Orally Disintegrating Tab.:** 0.125 mg, 0.25 mg, 0.5 mg, 1 mg, 2 mg. Mannitol, parabens. Blister pack 60s. **Tab.:** 0.5 mg, 1 mg, 2 mg, lactose. 100s. *c-iv.*
Use: Anticonvulsant; antianxiety agent.

K-Lor. (Abbott) Potassium Cl equivalent to potassium 20 mEq and Cl 20 mEq/ 2.6 g for oral soln. w/saccharin. Pkg. 30s, 100s. 15 mEq/2 g Pkg. 100s. *Rx.*
Use: Electrolyte supplement.

Klor-Con 8. (Upsher-Smith) Potassium Cl 8 mEq. ER Tab. Bot. 100s, 500s. *Rx.*
Use: Electrolyte supplement.

Klor-Con M15. (Upsher-Smith) Potassium 15 mEq (from potassium chloride 1125 mg). ER Tab. Bot. 100s, 1000s, UD 100s. *Rx.*
Use: Electrolyte supplement.

Klor-Con M10. (Upsher-Smith) Potassium 10 mEq (from potassium chloride 750 mg). ER Tab. Bot. 90s, 100s, 1000s, UD 100s. *Rx.*
Use: Electrolyte supplement.

Klor-Con M20. (Upsher-Smith) Potassium 20 mEq (from potassium chloride 1500 mg). ER Tab. Bot. 90s, 100s, 500s, 1000s, UD 100s. *Rx.*
Use: Electrolyte supplement.

Klor-Con 10. (Upsher-Smith) Potassium Cl 10 mEq. ER Tab. Bot. 100s, 500s. *Rx.*
Use: Electrolyte supplement.

Klorvess. (Novartis) Liq.: Potassium Cl 1.5 g (20 mEq)/15 mL, alcohol 0.75%. Bot. pt. **Effervescent Granules:** Potassium 20 mEq, Cl 20 mEq supplied by potassium Cl 1.125 g, potassium bicarbonate 0.5 g, L-lysine monohydrochloride 0.913 g. Pkt. w/saccharin. Box 30s. **Effervescent Tablets:** Potassium Cl 1.125 g, potassium bicarbonate 0.5 g, L-lysine hydrochloride 0.913 g. Sodium and sugar free, saccharin. Pkg. 60s, 1000s. *Rx.*
Use: Electrolyte supplement.

Klotrix. (Bristol-Myers Squibb) Potassium Cl 10 mEq. SR Tab. Bot. 100s, 1000s, UD 100s. *Rx.*
Use: Electrolyte supplement.

K-Lyte. (Bristol-Myers Squibb) Potassium bicarbonate and citrate 25 mEq, saccharin. Lime and orange flavors. Effervescent Tab. Pkg. 30s, 100s, 250s. *Rx.*
Use: Electrolyte supplement.

K-Lyte/Cl. (Bristol-Myers Squibb) Potassium Cl 25 mEq, saccharin. Citrus and fruit punch flavor. Effervescent Tab. Pkg. 30s, 100s, 250s. Bulk powder 225 g Can. *Rx.*
Use: Electrolyte supplement.

K-Lyte/Cl 50. (Bristol-Myers Squibb) Potassium Cl 50 mEq, saccharin. Citrus and fruit punch flavors. Pkg. 30s, 100s. *Rx.*
Use: Electrolyte supplement.

K-Lyte DS. (Bristol-Myers Squibb) Potassium bicarbonate and citrate 50 mEq, saccharin. Lime and orange flavor. Effervescent Tab. Pkg. 30s, 100s. *Rx.*
Use: Electrolyte supplement.

Koate-DVI. (Bayer) Concentrate of antihemophilic factor (human). When reconstituted, contains PEG $\leq$ 1500 mcg/ mL, glycine $\leq$ 0.05 M, polysorbate 80

≤ 25 mcg/mL, calcium ≤ 3 mM, aluminum ≤ 1 mcg/mL, histidine ≤ 0.06 M, human albumin ≤ 10 mg/mL, tri-n-butylphosphate ≤ 5 mcg/g, solvent/detergent- and heat-treated. Inj., lyophilized. Vial ≈ 250 or 500 units Factor VIII activity and ≈ 1,000 IU Factor VIII activity with diluent (actual number of antihemophilic factor units indicated on vials), double-ended needle, filter needle, and administration set. *Rx.*
Use: Antihemophilic agent.

Kodonyl Expectorant. (Halsey Drug) Bromodiphenhydramine hydrochloride 3.75 mg, diphenhydramine hydrochloride 8.75 mg, ammonium Cl 80 mg, potassium guaiacolsulfonate 80 mg, menthol 0.5 mg/5 mL. Bot. 16 oz. *OTC.*
Use: Antihistamine; expectorant.

Kof-Eze. (Roberts) Menthol 6 mg. Loz. Pkg. 4s, Bot. 500s. *OTC.*
Use: Mouth and throat preparation.

Kogenate. (Bayer) Concentrate of AHF (recombinant). When reconstituted, contains glycine 10 to 30 mg/mL, imidazole ≤ 500 mcg/1000 units, CaCl 2 to 5 mM, chloride 100 to 130 mEq/L, human albumin 4 to 10 mg/mL, monoclonal purified, Na 100 to 130 mEq/L, preservative free. Inj., lyophilized. Single-dose bottles (actual number of AHF units indicated on bottles) with diluent, double-ended needle, filter needle, administration set. *Rx.*
Use: Antihemophilic.

Kogenate FS. (Bayer) Recombinant antihemophilic factor, glycine 21 to 25 mg/mL, histidine 18 to 23 mM, CaCl 2 to 3 mM, Na 27 to 36 mEq/L, Cl 32 to 40 mEq/L, polysorbate 80 ≤ 35 mcg/mL, imidazole ≤ 20 mcg/1,000 IU, tri-n-butyl phosphate ≤ 5 mcg/1,000 IU, Cu ≤ 0.6 mcg/1,000 IU, sucrose 28 mg/vial, preservative and albumin free, solvent/detergent-treated, monoclonal purified. Inj., lyophilized. Vial 250 units, 500 units, 1,000 IU w/diluent, double-ended transfer needle, filter needle, and administration set. *Rx.*
Use: Antihemophilic agent.

Kolephrin/DM. (Pfeiffer) Pseudoephedrine hydrochloride 30 mg, chlorpheniramine maleate 2 mg, dextromethorphan HBr 10 mg, acetaminophen 325 mg. Tab. Bot. 30s. *OTC.*
Use: Upper respiratpry combination, analgesic, antihistamine, antitussive, decongestant.

Kolephrin GG/DM. (Pfeiffer) Dextromethorphan HBr 10 mg, guaifenesin 150 mg/5 mL, glucose, saccharin, sucrose,

cherry flavor, alcohol free. Liq. Bot. 118 mL. *OTC.*
Use: Upper respiratory combination, antitussive, expectorant.

● **kolfocon a.** (KAHL-FOE-kahn A) USAN.
Use: Contact lens material (hydrophobic).

● **kolfocon b.** (KAHL-FOE-kahn B) USAN.
Use: Contact lens material (hydrophobic).

● **kolfocon c.** (KAHL-FOE-kahn C) USAN.
Use: Contact lens material (hydrophobic).

● **kolfocon d.** (KAHL-FOE-kahn D) USAN.
Use: Contact lens material (hydrophobic).

Kolyum. (Medeva) Potassium ion 20 mEq, chloride ion 3.4 mEq from potassium gluconate 3.9 g, potassium Cl 0.25 g/15 mL or 5 g/15 mL, saccharin, sorbitol. Liq. Bot. Pt, gal. *Rx.*
Use: Electrolyte supplement.

Kondon's Nasal Jelly. (Kondon) Tube 20 g w/ephedrine alkaloid. *OTC.*
Use: Decongestant.

Kondremul Plain. (Heritage Consumer) Mineral oil, Irish moss, acacia, glycerin. Emulsion Bot. 480 mL **W/Cascara:** 0.66 g/15 mL. Bot. 14 oz. *OTC.*
Use: Laxative.

K-1. Phytonadione.
Use: Vitamin K.
See: Aqua MEPHYTON.
Mephyton.

Konsto. (Freeport) Docusate sodium 100 mg. Cap. Bot. 1000s. *OTC.*
Use: Laxative.

Konsyl. (Konsyl) Psyllium 6 g. Pow. Canister 300 g, 450 g, UD Packet 6 g. *OTC.*
Use: Laxative.

Konsyl-D. (Konsyl) Psyllium 3.4 g, 14 cal/tsp, dextrose. Pow. Canister 325 g, 500 g, UD 6.5 g. *OTC.*
Use: Laxative.

Konsyl Easy Mix Formula. (Konsyl) Psyllium 6 g, Na 4.4 mg, Ca 48 mg, P 4 mg, Zn 0.06 mg, K 42 mg, carbohydrates 0.35 g, 4 cal/5 mL. Pow. Can. 200 g, Packets. *OTC.*
Use: Laxative

Konsyl Fiber. (Konsyl) Polycarbophil 500 mg Tab. Bot. 90s. *OTC.*
Use: Laxative.

Konsyl-Orange. (Konsyl) Psyllium fiber 3.4 g/tbsp., sucrose, orange flavor. Pow. Can. 538 g and Packets. *OTC.*
Use: Laxative.

Koro-Flex. (Holland-Rantos) Improved contouring-spring, natural latex diaphragm 60 mm to 95 mm. *OTC.*

Use: Contraceptive.

Korum. (Geneva) Acetaminophen 5 g.
Tab. Bot. 1000s. *OTC.*
Use: Analgesic.

Kotabarb. (Wesley) Phenobarbital ¼ g.
Tab. Bot. 1000s. *Rx.*
Use: Hypnotic, sedative.

Kovitonic. (Freeda) Iron 42 mg, vitamins
B_1 5 mg, B_6 10 mg, B_{12} 30 mcg, folic
acid 0.1 mg, l-lysine 10 mg/15 mL. Liq.
Bot. 120 mL, 240 mL. *OTC.*
Use: Mineral, vitamin supplement.

K-P. (Century) Kaolin 5.2 g, pectin
260 mg/oz. Susp. Bot. Gal. *OTC.*
Use: Antidiarrheal.

K-Pek. (Rugby) Bismuth subsalicylate
262 mg per 15 mL. Sugar. Peppermint
flavor. Susp. 237 mL, 473 mL. *OTC.*
Use: Antidiarrheal.

K Pek II. (Rugby) Loperamide hydrochloride 2 mg, lactose. Tab, Pkg. 12s. *OTC.*
Use: Antidiarrheal.

K-Phos M.F. (Beach) Potassium acid
phosphate 155 mg, sodium acid phosphate 350 mg Tab. Bot. 100s, 500s.
Rx.
Use: Acidifier, urinary.

K-Phos Neutral. (Beach) Phosphorus
250 mg, potassium 45 mg, sodium
298 mg. *Rx.*
Use: Mineral supplement.

K-Phos No. 2. (Beach) Potassium acid
phosphate 305 mg, sodium acid phosphate anhydrous 700 mg. Tab. Bot.
100s, 500s. *Rx.*
Use: Acidifier, urinary.

K-Phos Original. (Beach) Potassium
acid phosphate 500 mg. Tab. Bot. 100s,
500s. *Rx.*
Use: Urinary acidifier; electrolyte
supplement.

K + Care. (Alra) Potassium chloride, saccharin. Soln. Pkt. 15, 20, 25 mEq. 30s,
100s. *Rx.*
Use: Electrolyte supplement.

K + Care ET. (Alra) Potassium bicarbonate 25 mEq. Effervescent Tab. Bot.
30s, 100s, 1000s. *Rx.*
Use: Electrolyte supplement.

K+8. (Alra) Potassium chloride 8 mEq.
ER Tab. Bot. 100s, 500s. *Rx.*
Use: Electrolyte supplement.

K+10. (Alra) Potassium Cl 10 mEq. Tab.
Bot. 100s, 500s, 1000s. *Rx.*
Use: Electrolyte supplement.

K.P.N. (Freeda) Vitamins C 333 mg, Fe
11 mg, A 2667 units, D 133 units, E
10 mg, B_1 2 mg, B_2 2 mg, B_3 10 mg, B_5
3.3 mg, B_6 0.83 mg, B_{12} 2 mcg, C
33 mg, FA 0.27 mg, I, Cu, Mn, K, Mg,
Zn 6.7 mg, bioflavonoids. Tab. Bot.

100s, 250s, 500s. *OTC.*
Use: Mineral, vitamin supplement.

Kristalose. (Bertek) Lactulose (galactose and lactose < 0.3 g/10 g). Crystals
for reconstitution. Pack 10 g, 20 g.
Box. 30s. *Rx.*
Use: Laxative, hyperosmotic agent.

Kronofed-A. (Ferndale) Pseudoephedrine hydrochloride 120 mg, chlorpheni-
amine maleate 8 mg. SR Cap. Bot.
100s, 500s. *Rx.*
Use: Upper respiratory combination, antihistamine, decongestant.

Kronofed-A Jr. (Ferndale) Pseudoephedrine hydrochloride 60 mg, chlorpheniramine maleate 4 mg. SR Cap.
Bot. 100s, 500s. *Rx.*
Use: Upper respiratory combination, antihistamine, decongestant.

• **krypton clathrate Kr 85.** (KRIPP-tahn
KLATH-rate) USAN.
Use: Radiopharmaceutical.

• **krypton Kr 81m.** (KRIP-tahn Kr 81 m)
USP 28.
Use: Radiopharmaceutical.

K-Tab. (Abbott) Potassium Cl (10 mEq)
750 mg. ER Tab. Bot. 100s, 1000s, UD
100s. *Rx.*
Use: Electrolyte supplement.

K 34. Hexachlorophene.

K.T.V. (Knight) Vitamin B_{12}, minerals. Tab.
Bot. 50s. *OTC.*
Use: Mineral, vitamin supplement.

Kutrase Capsules. (Schwarz Pharma)
Lipase 2400 units, amylase
30,000 units, protease 30,000 units.
Cap. Bot. 100s. *Rx.*
Use: Digestive aid.

Ku-Zyme Capsules. (Schwarz Pharma)
Lipase 1200 units, amylase
15,000 units, protease 15,000 units.
Cap. Bot. 100s. *Rx.*
Use: Digestive aid.

Ku-Zyme HP Capsules. (Schwarz
Pharma) Lipase 8000 units, protease
30,000 units, amylase 30,000 units, lactose. Cap. Bot. 100s. *Rx.*
Use: Digestive aid.

K-Vescent Potassium Chloride. (Major)
Potassium and chloride 20 mEq from
potassium chloride 1.5 g, saccharin.
Pow. Pkt. 30s, 100s. *Rx.*
Use: Potassium replacement product.

Kwelcof. (B.F. Asher) Hydrocodone bitartrate 5 mg, guaifenesin 100 mg/5 mL,
menthol, saccharin, sorbitol, fruit flavor,
alcohol and dye free. Liq. Bot. 473 mL.
c-III.
Use: Upper respiratory combination, antitussive, expectorant.

Kwikderm. (Alra) Tolnaftate 1%. **Cream:** Tube. 15 g. **Soln.:** Bot. 10 mL. *OTC.*
Use: Antifungal, topical.

Kwildane. (Major) Gamma benzene hexachloride 1%. Shampoo. Bot. 60 mL, pt, gal. *OTC.*
Use: Pediculicide.

K-Y. (Johnson & Johnson) Glycerin, methylparaben, hydroxyethylcellulose. Sterile or regular. Jelly. Tube. 12 g, 60 g, 120 g. *OTC.*
Use: Lubricant.

Kyodex Reagent Strips. (Kyoto) A disposable plastic reagent strip for determination of glucose in whole blood. Vial 25s.
Use: Diagnostic aid.

Kyotest UGK Reagent Strip. (Kyoto) Disposable reagent strip for measurement of glucose and ketones in the urine. Vial 50s, 100s.
Use: Diagnostic aid.

Kyotest UG Reagent Strips. (Kyoto) Reagent strips for glucose and ketones in urine.
Use: Diagnostic aid.

Kyotest UK Reagent Strips. (Kyoto) Reagent strip for ketones in urine. Vial 50s.
Use: Diagnostic aid.

KY Plus. (Johnson & Johnson) Nonoxynol-9 2%, methylparaben. Nongreasy. 113 g. *OTC.*
Use: Lubricant.

Kytril. (Roche) Granisetron hydrochloride. **Inj.:** 1 mg per mL (1.12 mg/mL as hydochloride). Benzyl alcohol 10 mg, sodium chloride 9 mg/mL. Single-use vial 1 mL. Multidose vial 4 mL. **Tab.:** 1.12 mg, lactose. Pkg. SUP 20s, unit-of-use 2s. **Oral Soln.:** 1.12 mg/5 mL, sorbitol, orange flavor. Bot. 30 mL. *Rx.*
Use: Antiemetic (cancer therapy).

L

- **labetalol hydrochloride.** (la-BET-ul-lahl) *USP 28.*
  Use: Alpha/beta-adrenergic blocking agent; antiadrenergic/sympatholytic.
  See: Normodyne.
  Trandate.

labetalol hydrochloride. (Various Mfr.) Labetolol hydrochloride. **Inj.:** 5 mg/mL, EDTA 0.1 mg, methylparaben 0.8 mg, propylparaben 0.1 mg, dextrose. Multidose Vial 20 mL, 40 mL. **Tab.:** 100 mg, 200 mg, 300 mg. Bot. 30s, 100s, 250s, 500s, 1000s. *Rx.*
  Use: Antiandrenergic/sympatholytic; alpha/beta-adrenergic blocker.

- **labetuzumab.** (la-be-too-zoo-mab) UUAN.
  Use: Monoclonal antibody.

- **labradimil.** (la-BRAY-da-mil) USAN.
  Use: Adjuvant.

Labstix Reagent Strips. (Bayer Consumer Care) Urine screening test. Bot. 100s.
  Use: Diagnostic aid.

Lac-Hydrin. (Westwood-Squibb) Ammonium lactate 12%. Cetyl alcohol, glycerin, glyceryl stearate, light mineral oil, parabens. Cream. 280 g, 385 g. *Rx.*
  Use: Emollient.

Lac-Hydrin Lotion. (Bristol-Myers Squibb) Lactic acid 12% neutralized w/ammonium hydroxide, light mineral oil, cetyl alcohol, parabens. Tube 150 mL, 360 mL. *Rx.*
  Use: Emollient.

- **lacidipine.** (lah-SIH-dih-PEEN) USAN.
  Use: Antihypertensive.

Laclede Cleaner. (Laclede) Container. 2 lb. *OTC.*
  Use: Detergent.

Laclede Disclosing Swab. (Laclede) Swabs 6″. 100s, 500s, 1000s. *OTC.*
  Use: Dentrifice.

Laclede Topi-Fluor A.P.F. Topical Cream. (Laclede) Fluoride ion 1.23% (from sodium fluoride) in orthophosphoric acid 0.98%. Jar 50 mL, 500 mL, 1000 mL, 2000 mL. *Rx.*
  Use: Dental caries agent.

LAC-Lotion. (Paddock) Ammonium lactate 12% (12% lactic acid neutralized with ammonium hydroxide), mineral oil, cetyl alcohol, parabens, glycerin. Lotion. 225 g, 400 g. *Rx.*
  Use: Emollient.

Lacotein. (Christina) Protein digest 5% w/preservatives. Vial 30 mL (w/iodochin), Vial 30 mL. *Rx.*
  Use: Protein supplement.

Lacril. (Allergan) Hydroxypropyl methylcellulose 0.5%, gelatin A 0.01%, chlorobutanol 0.5%, polysorbate 80, dextrose, magnesium Cl, sodium borate, sodium chloride. Soln. Dropper bot. 15 mL. *OTC.*
  Use: Lubricant; ophthalmic.

Lacri-Lube NP. (Allergan) White petrolatum 55.5%, mineral oil 42.5%, petrolatum/lanolin alcohol 2%. Oint. 0.7 g. *OTC.*
  Use: Lubricant; ophthalmic.

Lacri-Lube S.O.P. (Allergan) White petrolatum 56.8%, mineral oil 41.5%, lanolin alcohols, chlorobutanol. Tube 3.5 g, 7 g. *OTC.*
  Use: Lubricant; ophthalmic.

Laurleurt. (Merck & Co.) Hydroxypropyl cellulose 5 mg/insert. Pkg. 60s w/applicators. *Rx.*
  Use: Artificial tears.

LactAid. (Ortho-McNeil) **Liq.:** Beta-D-galactosidase derived from *Kluyveromyces lactis* yeast (1000 Neutral Lactase units/5 drop dosage) in carrier of glycerol 50%, water 30%, inert yeast dry matter 20%. Units of 4, 12, 30, 75 one-quart dosages at 5 drops/dose. **Tab.:** Beta-D-galactosidase from *Aspergillus oryzae* (3300 FCC lactase units/Tab.) In 12s, 100s. *OTC.*
  Use: Digestive aid.

lactalbumin hydrolysate.
  See: Aminonat.

- **lactase.** (LAK-tase) USAN.
  Use: Digestive aid.
  See: Dairy Ease.
  LactAid.
  Lactrase.
  SureLac.

lactated Ringer's. (Various Mfr.) Na$^+$ 130 mEq, K$^+$ 4 mEq, Ca^{++} ≈ 3 mEq, Cl$^-$ ≈ 109 mEq, lactate 28 mEq, osmolarity ≈ 274 mOsm/L. Soln. Inj. Bot. 250 mL, 500 mL, 1000 mL. *Rx.*
  Use: Intravenous nutritional therapy, intravenous replenishment solution.

lactated Ringer's in 5% dextrose. (Various Mfr.) Dextrose 50 g, calories 170, Na$^+$ 130 mEq, K$^+$ 4 mEq, Ca^{++} ≈ 3 mEq, Cl$^-$ 109–112 mEq, lactate 28 mEq, osmolarity 525–530 mOsm/L. Soln. Bot. 250 mL, 500 mL, 1000 mL. *Rx.*
  Use: Intravenous nutritional therapy, intravenous replenishment solution.

- **lactic acid.** (LACK-tick) *USP 28.*
  Use: Pharmaceutic necessity for sodium lactate injection.

See: Lactrex 12%.
Penecare.
W/Sodium pyrrolidone carboxylate.
See: LactiCare.
Lactinol.
LactiCare. (Stiefel) Lactic acid 5%, sodium pyrrolidone carboxylate 2.5% in an emollient lotion base. Lot. Bot. 8 oz, 12 oz, w/pump dispenser. *OTC.*
Use: Emollient.
LactiCare-HC. (Stiefel) Hydrocortisone lotion 1%, 2.5%. **1%:** Bot 4 oz. **2.5%:** Bot. 2 oz. *Rx.*
Use: Corticosteroid, topical.
Lactinex. (Becton Dickinson & Co.) *Lactobacillus acidophilus* & *Lactobacillus bulgaricus* mixed culture. Tab. 250 mg, Bot. 50s. Gran. 1 g pkt. Box 12s. *OTC.*
Use: Antidiarrheal; nutritional supplement.
Lactinol. (Pedinol Pharmacal) Lactic acid 10%. Lot. Bot. 237 mL. *Rx.*
Use: Emollient.
Lactinol-E Creme. (Pedinol Pharmacal) Lactic acid 10%, vitamin E 3500 units/ 30 g. Cream 56.7 g, 113.4 g. *Rx.*
Use: Emollient.
Lactobacillus acidophilus. Preparation made from acid-producing bacterium.
Use: Antidiarrheal; nutritional supplement.
See: Bacid.
Dofus.
More Dophilus.
Pro-Bionate.
Superdophilus.
Lactobacillus acidophilus and bulgaricus mixed culture.
See: Floranex.
Lactinex.
Lactobacillus acidophilus, viable culture.
See: Dofus.
Lactinex Gran.
Lactobacillus bulgaricus. Antidiarrheal.
See: Bacid.
Lactinex B.
More Dophilus.
Lactocal-F. (Laser) Vitamin A 4000 units, D 400 units, E 30 units, C 100 mg, folic acid 1 mg, B_1 3 mg, B_2 3.4 mg, B_3 20 mg, B_6 5 mg, B_{12} 12 mcg, calcium 200 mg, I, Fe 65 mg, Mg, Cu, Zn 15 mg. Tab. Bot. 100s, 1000s. *Rx.*
Use: Mineral; vitamin supplement.
lactoflavin.
See: Riboflavin.
Lactofree. (Bristol-Myers Squibb) Protein 14.7 g, carbohydrates 69.3 g, fat 36.7 g, linoleic acid 6 g, Fe 12 mg, Na 200 mg, K 733.3 mg, with appropriate

vitamins and minerals. Lactose free. 666.7 cal/L. Pow. Can 400 g. *OTC.*
Use: Nutritional supplement; enteral.
lactose. Milk sugar.
Use: Pharmaceutic aid (tablet and capsule diluent).
See: Natur-Aid.
•**lactose anhydrous.** (LACK-tohs an-HIGH-druss) *NF 23.*
Use: Pharmaceutic aid (tablet and capsule diluent).
•**lactose monohydrate.** (LAK-tose) *NF 23.*
Use: Pharmaceutic aid (tablet and capsule diluent).
Lactrase. (Aventis) Standardized enzyme lactase (β-D-galactosidase) 125 mg dispersed in maltodextrins. Cap. Bot. 100s. *OTC.*
Use: Nutritional supplement.
Lactrex 12%. (SDR Pharmaceuticals) Lactic acid 12%, petrolatum, EDTA. Cream. Tube. 184 g. *OTC.*
Use: Emollient.
Lactrodectus Mactans Antivenin. (Merck & Co.) Antivenin 6000 units per vial (with 1:10,000 thimerosal), supplied with a 2.5 mL vial of Sterile Water for Injection and a 1 mg vial (with 1:10,000 thimerosal) of normal horse serum (1:10 dilution) for sensitivity testing. *Rx.*
Use: Antivenin (Black Widow spider).
See: antivenin *Lactrodectus Mactans.*
lactulose.
Use: Laxative.
See: Cephulac.
Cholac.
Chronulac.
Constilac.
Constulos.
Duphalac.
Enulose.
Kristalose.
lactulose. (Various Mfr.) Lactulose 10 g/ 15 mL (galactose < 1.6 g, lactose 1.2 g, other sugars 1.2 g). Soln. Bot. 237 mL, 473 mL, 960 mL, 1873 mL. *Rx.*
Use: Laxative.
•**lactulose concentrate.** (LAK-tyoo-lohs) *USP 28.*
Use: Laxative, treatment of hepatic coma and chronic constipation.
See: Cephulac.
Chronulac.
Evalose.
Heptalac.
ladakamycin.
Use: Refractory acute myelogenous leukemia (AML) agent.

See: Azacitidine.

Ladogal. (Sanofi-Synthelabo) Danazol. Rx.
Use: Androgen.

Ladogar. (Sanofi-Synthelabo) Danazol. Rx.
Use: Androgen.

•**ladostigil.** (LAD-oh-STIJ-il) USAN.
Use: Alzheimer disease.

Lady Esther. (Menley & James Labs, Inc.) Mineral oil. Cream. 120 g. OTC.
Use: Emollient.

L.A.E. 40. (Seatrace) Estradiol valerate 40 mg/mL. Inj. Vial 10 mL. Rx.
Use: Estrogen.

L.A.E. 20. (Seatrace) Estradiol valerate 20 mg/mL. Inj. Vial 10 mL. Rx.
Use: Estrogen.

Lamictal. (GlaxoSmithKline) Lamotrigine 25 mg, 100 mg, 150 mg, 200 mg, lactose. Tab. Bot. 60s (150 mg, 200 mg), 100s (25 mg, 100 mg). Rx.
Use: Anticonvulsant.

Lamictal Chewable Dispersible. (GlaxoSmithKline) Lamotrigine 2 mg, 5 mg, 25 mg, saccharin. Black currant flavor. Chew. Tab. Bot. 30s (2 mg only), 100s (except 2 mg). Rx.
Use: Anticonvulsant.

•**lamifiban.** (la-mih-FIE-ban) USAN.
Use: Antithrombotic; platelet aggregation inhibitor; fibrinogen receptor antagonist.

Lamisil. (Novartis) Terbinafine hydrochloride 250 mg. Tab. Bot. 30s, 100s. Rx.
Use: Antifungal, allyamine.

Lamisil AT. (Novartis) Terbinafine hydrochloride. **Spray:** 1%, ethanol, propylene glycol. Bot. 30 mL. OTC.
Use: Antifungal.

Lamisil Cream. (Novartis) Terbinafine. 1%, benzyl alcohol, cetyl alcohol, stearyl alcohol. Cream. Tube. 15 g, 30 g. OTC.
Use: Antifungal.

•**lamivudine.** (la-MIH-view-deen) USAN.
Use: Antiretroviral, nucleoside reverse transcriptase inhibitor.
See: Epivir.
Epivir-HBV.
W/Abacavir.
See: Epzicom.
W/Abacavir Sulfate and Zidovudine.
See: Trizivir.
W/Zidovudine.
See: Combivir.

lamivudine and zidovudine.
Use: Antiretroviral; AIDS.
See: Combivir.
W/Abacavir Sulfate.

See: Trizivir.

•**lamotrigine.** (lah-MOE-trih-JEEN) USAN.
Use: Anticonvulsant; Lennox-Gestaut syndrome. [Orphan Drug]
See: Lamictal.
Lamictal Chewable Dispersible.

Lampit. (Bayer Corp. (Biological and Pharmaceutical Div.)) Nifurtimox.
Use: Anti-infective.

Lamprene. (Novartis) Clofazimine 50 mg. Cap. Bot. 100s. Rx.
Use: Leprostatic, investigational. [Orphan Drug]

Lanabiotic. (Combe) Polymyxin B sulfate 10,000 units, neomycin (as sulfate) 3.5 mg, bacitracin zinc 500 units, lidocaine 40 mg, aloe, lanolin, mineral oil, petrolatum. Oint. Tube. 28 g. OTC.
Use: Anti-infective; antibiotic, topical; anesthetic, local.

Lanacane. (Combe) **Spray:** Benzocaine 20%, benzethonium Cl, ethanol, aloe extract. 113 mL. **Cream:** Benzocaine 6%, benzethonium Cl, aloe, parabens, castor oil, glycerin, isopropyl alcohol. 28 g, 56 g. OTC.
Use: Anesthetic, local.

Lanacort. (Combe) Hydrocortisone acetate 0.5%. Cream. Tube 0.5 oz, 1 oz. OTC.
Use: Corticosteroid, topical.

Lanacort 10. (Combe) Hydrocortisone acetate 1%. Cream. Tube 15, 00 g. **Oint.:** Tube 15 g. OTC.
Use: Corticosteroid, topical.

Lanaphilic. (Medco Lab) Sorbitol, isopropyl palmitate, stearyl alcohol, white petrolatum, lanolin oil, sodium lauryl sulfate, propylene glycol, methylparaben, propylparaben. Oint. Jar 16 oz. Also available w/urea 10% or 20%. OTC.
Use: Emollient.

Lanaphilic w/Urea 10%. (Medco Lab) Urea, stearyl alcohol, white petrolatum, isopropyl palmitate, propylene glycol, sorbitol, sodium lauryl sulfate, lactic acid, parabens. Oint. Jar 1 lb. OTC.
Use: Emollient.

•**lanimostim.** (LAN-i-MOE-stim) USAN.
Use: Antineoplastic agent.

•**lanolin.** (LAN-oh-lin) USP 28. Formerly Anhydrous lanolin.
Use: Pharmaceutic aid (ointment base, absorbent).
See: Kerohydric.
W/Coconut oil, pine oil, castor oil, cholesterols, lecithin, parachlorometaxylenol.
See: Sebacide.

W/Diiosbutylcresoxyethoxyethyl, dimethyl benzyl ammonium Cl, menthol.
See: Hospital Lot.
●**lanolin alcohols.** (LAN-oh-lin) *NF 23.*
Use: Pharmaceutic aid (emulsifying agent).
Lanoline. (GlaxoSmithKline) Perfumed emollient. Oint. Tube 1.75 oz. *OTC.*
Use: Pharmaceutic aid; ointment base; absorbent; emollient.
●**lanolin, modified.** (LAN-oh-lin) *USP 28.*
Use: Pharmaceutic aid (ointment base, absorbent).
Lano-Lo Bath Oil. (Whorton Pharmaceuticals, Inc.) 8 oz. *OTC.*
Lanolor. (Numark) Lanolin oil, glyceryl stearates, propylene glycol, sodium lauryl sulfate, simethicone, polyoxyl 40 stearate, cetyl esters wax, methylparaben. Cream Jar 60 g, 240 g. *OTC.*
Use: Emollient.
●**lanoteplase.** (lan-OH-teh-place) USAN.
Use: Thrombolytic; plasminogen activator.
Lanoxicaps. (Cardinal Health) Digoxin 0.05 mg, 0.1 mg, 0.2 mg, parabens, sorbitol. Cap. Bot. 100s. *Rx.*
Use: Inotropic agent; cardiac glycoside.
Lanoxin. (GlaxoSmithKline) Digoxin.
Tab.: 0.125 mg, 0.25 mg, lactose. Bot. 30s, 100s, 1000s, 5000s, UD 100s.
Pediatric Elix.: 0.05 mg/mL, alcohol 10%, methylparaben 0.1%, lime flavor. Bot. 60 mL w/calibrated dropper. **Inj.:** (w/propylene glycol 40%, alcohol 10%). Amp. 2 mL. **Pediatric Inj.:** 0.1 mg/mL (w/propylene glycol 40%, alcohol 10%). Amp. 1 mL. *Rx.*
Use: Inotropic agent; cardiac glycoside.
●**lanreotide acetate.** (lan-REE-oh-tide) USAN.
Use: Antineoplastic.
●**lansoprazole.** (lan-SO-pruh-zole) *USP 28.*
Use: Proton pump inhibitor.
See: Prevacid.
   Prevacid IV.
W/Amoxicillin and clarithromycin.
See: Prevpac.
W/Naproxen
See: Prevacid NapraPAC.
●**lanthanum carbonate.** (Lan-thah-num)
Use: Phosphate reduction.
See: Fosrenal.
Lanturil. (Sanofi-Synthelabo) Oxypertine. *Rx.*
Use: Anxiolytic.
Lantus. (Aventis) Insulin glargine 100 units/mL. Inj. Vial. 10 mL. *Rx.*
Use: Antidiabetic.

lanum. (Various Mfr.) Lanolin. *OTC.*
Use: Pharmaceutic aid.
●**lapatinib ditosylate.** (la-PA-tin-ib) USAN.
Use: Antineoplastic.
●**lapyrium chloride.** (LAH-pihr-ee-uhm KLOR-ide) USAN.
Use: Pharmaceutic aid (surfactant).
Lardet. (Standex) Phenobarbital 8 mg, theophylline 130 mg, ephedrine hydrochloride 24 mg. Tab. Bot. 100s. *Rx.*
Use: Antiasthmatic combination.
Lardet Expectorant. (Standex) Phenobarbital 8 mg, theophylline 130 mg, ephedrine hydrochloride 24 mg, guaifenesin 100 mg. Tab. Bot. 100s. *Rx.*
Use: Antiasthmatic combination.
Lariam. (Roche) Mefloquine hydrochloride 250 mg, lactose. Tab. UD 25s. *Rx.*
Use: Antimalarial.
Larodopa. (Roche) Levodopa. **Cap: 100 mg:** Bot. 100s. **250 mg, 500 mg:** Bot. 100s, 500s. **Tab: 100 mg:** Bot. 100s. **250 mg, 500 mg:** Bot. 100s, 500s. *Rx.*
Use: Antiparkinsonian.
●**laronidase.** (lare-AHN-ih-dase) USAN.
Use: Enzyme replacement in Mucopolysaccharidosis.
See: Aldurazyme.
Larotid. (GlaxoSmithKline) Amoxicillin. **Cap.: 250 mg:** Bot. 100s, 500s, UD 100s, unit-of-use 18s. **500 mg:** Bot. 50s, 500s. **Oral Susp.:** 125 mg, 250 mg (as trihydrate)/5 mL. Bot. 80 mL, 100 mL, 150 mL. **Pediatric drops:** 50 mg (as trihydrate)/mL. Bot. 15 mL. *Rx.*
Use: Anti-infective, penicillin.
Larynex. (Dover Pharmaceuticals) Benzocaine. Sugar, lactose and salt free. Loz. UD Box 500s. *OTC.*
Use: Anesthetic, local.
Lasix. (Aventis) Furosemide. **Tab.:** 20 mg, 40 mg. Tab. Bot. 100s, 500s, 1000s, UD 100s; 80 mg. Tab. Bot. 50s, 500s, UD 100s. **Inj.:** 10 mg/mL. 2 mL Amp. Box 5s, 50s, 4 mL Amp. Box 5s, 25s; 10 mL Amp. Box 5s, 25s; Syringe 2 mL, 4 mL, 10 mL. Box 5s. Single-use Vial 2 mL, 4 mL, 10 mL. *Rx.*
Use: Diuretic.
●**lasofoxifene tartrate.** (la-soe-FOX-i-feen) USAN.
Use: Osteoporosis; breast cancer.
lassar's paste.
See: Zinc Oxide Paste.
●**latanoprost.** (lah-TAN-oh-prahst) USAN.
Use: Antiglaucoma agent.
See: Xalatan.

Latest-CRP Kit. (Fischer) Measures C-reactive protein in serum. Kit 1s.
Use: Diagnostic aid.
LA-12. (Hyrex) Hydroxocobalamin 1000 mcg/mL. Inj. Vial 30 mL. *Rx.*
Use: Vitamin supplement.
•**laureth 4.** (LAH-reth 4) USAN.
Use: Pharmaceutic aid (surfacant).
•**laureth 9.** (LAH-reth 9) USAN.
Use: Pharmaceutical aid (surfactant); emulsifier; spermaticide.
•**laureth 10.** (LAH-reth 10s) USAN.
Use: Spermaticide.
•**laurocapram.** (LAHR-oh-KAH-pram) USAN.
Use: Pharmaceutic aid (excipient).
lauromacrogol 400. Laureth 9.
•**lauryl isoquinolinium bromide.** (LAH-rlll EYE uu KWIN-ul-lih-nee-uhm) USAN.
Use: Anti-infective.
lauryl sulfoacetate.
See: Lowila.
Lavacol. (Parke-Davis) Ethyl alcohol 70%. Bot. Pt.
Use: Anti-infective, topical.
Lavatar. (Doak Dermatologics) Coal tar distillate 25.5% in a bath oil base. Liq. Bot. 4 oz, pt. *OTC.*
Use: Antipsoriatic; antipruritic.
lavender oil.
Use: Perfume.
•**lavoltidine succinate.** (lahv-OLE-tih-DEEN) USAN. *Formerly Loxotidine.*
Use: Antiulcerative (histamine H_2-receptor blocker).
Lavoptik Emergency Wash. (Lavoptik) Eye, face, body wash. 32 oz/emergency station. *OTC.*
Use: Emergency wash.
Lavoptik Eye Wash. (Lavoptik) Sodium Cl 0.49%, sodium biphosphate 0.4%, sodium phosphate 0.45%/100 mL w/benzalkonium Cl 0.005%. Bot. 6 oz. *OTC.*
Use: Irrigant; ophthalmic.
Lavoris. (Procter & Gamble) Zinc Cl, glycerin, poloxamer 407, saccharin, polysorbate 80, flavors, clove oil, alcohol, citric acid, water. Bot. 6 oz, 12 oz, 18 oz, 24 oz. *OTC.*
Use: Mouthwash.
Laxative & Stool Softener. (Rugby) Docusate sodium 100 mg, casanthranol 30 mg, parabens, sorbitol. Softgel. Cap. Bot. 100s. *OTC.*
Use: Laxative.
Laxative Caps. (Weeks & Leo) Docusate sodium 100 mg, casanthranol 30 mg. Cap. Bot. 30s, 60s. *OTC.*

Use: Laxative.
laxatives.
See: Aloe.
   Aloin.
   Bile Salts.
   Bisacodyl.
   Bisacodyl Tannex.
   Bowel Evacuants.
   Carboxymethylcellulose Sodium.
   Casanthranol.
   Cascara.
   Cascara Sagrada.
   Castor Oil.
   Citrucel.
   Correctol.
   Docusate Sodium.
   Emulsoil.
   Enemas.
   Evac Q-Kwik.
   ex-lax.
   Feen-a-Mint.
   Fleet Prep Kit 1.
   Fleet Prep Kit 2.
   Fleet Prep Kit 3.
   Karaya Gum.
   Liquid Petrolatum.
   Magnesia Maga.
   Maltsupex.
   Methylcellulose.
   Mucilloid of Psyllium Seed W/Dextrose.
   Mylanta Natural Fiber Supplement.
   Nature's Remedy.
   Neoloid.
   Oxyphenisatin Acetate.
   Petrolatum.
   Phenolphthalein.
   Plantago Ovata, Coating.
   Poloxalkol.
   Prune Concentrate.
   Prune Preps.
   Purge.
   Restore.
   Senna, Alexandrian.
   Senna, Cassia angustifolia.
   Senna Conc, Standardized.
   Senna Fruit Extract.
   Sennosides A & B.
   Sodium Biphosphate.
   Sodium Phosphate.
   Tridrate Bowel Cleansing System.
   Unifiber.
   X-Prep Bowel Evacuant Kit-1.
   X-Prep Bowel Kit-2.
   X-Prep Liquid.
W/Choline base, cephalin, lipositol.
See: Alcolec.
W/CO_2-Releasing Suppositories.
See: Ceo-Two.
W/Coconut oil, pine oil, castor oil, lanolin, cholesterols, parachlorometaxylenol.

See: Sebacide.
W/Polycarbophil
  See: Bulk Forming Fiber Laxative.
  Cephulac.
  Cholac.
  Chronulac.
  Citrucel Sugar Free.
  Colace.
  Constilac.
  Constulose.
  DC Softgels.
  Diocto.
  Docu.
  Docusate Calcium.
  D.O.S.
  D-S-S.
  Duphalac.
  Enulose.
  Equalactin.
  ex-lax Stool Softener.
  FiberCon.
  Fiber-Lax.
  FiberNorm.
  Fleet.
  Fleet Babylax.
  Fleet Bisacodyl.
  Fleet Mineral Oil.
  Genasoft.
  Glycerin
  Kondremul Plain.
  Konsyl Fiber.
  Latulose.
  Milkinol.
  Mineral Oil.
  Mitrolan.
  Modane Soft.
  Non-Habit Forming Stool Softener.
  Phillips' Liqui-Gels.
  Regulax SS.
  Sani-Supp.
  Silace.
  Stool Softener.
  Stool Softener DC.
  Surfak Liquigels.
  Therevac-Plus.
  Therevac-SB.
W/Polyethylene Glycol-Electrolyte.
  See: CoLyte.
  Concentrated Milk of Magnesia-
    Cascara.
  Diocto C.
  DOK-Plus.
  Emulsoil.
  Evac-Q-Kwik.
  Fleet Prep Kit 1.
  Fleet Prep Kit 2.
  Fleet Prep Kit 3.
  GoLYTELY.
  Haley's M-O.
  Liqui-Doss.
  MiraLax.

  Neoloid.
  NuLYTELY.
  OCL.
  Perdiem Overnight Relief.
  Purge.
  Silace-C.
  Tridrate Bowel Cleansing System.
  X-Prep Bowel Evacuant Kit-1.
  X-Prep Bowel Kit-2.
  X-Prep Liquid.
W/Psyllium.
  See: Fiberall Orange Flavor.
  Fiberall Tropical Fruit Flavor.
  Genfiber.
  Genfiber, Orange Flavor.
  Hydrocil Instant.
  Konsyl.
  Konsyl-D.
  Konsyl Easy Mix Formula.
  Konsyl-Orange.
  Metamucil.
  Metamucil, Orange Flavor, Original
    Texture.
  Metamucil Orange Flavor, Smooth
    Texture.
  Metamucil, Original Texture.
  Metamucil, Sugar Free, Orange
    Flavor, Smooth Texture.
  Metamucil, Sugar Free, Smooth
    Texture.
  Modane Bulk.
  Natural Fiber Laxative.
  Perdiem Fiber Therapy.
  Reguloid.
  Reguloid, Orange.
  Reguloid, Sugar Free Orange.
  Reguloid, Sugar Free Regular.
  Serutan.
  Syllact.
W/Saline laxatives.
  See: Aromatic Cascara Fluid Extract.
  Cascara Aromatic.
  Epsom Salt.
  Fleet Phospho-soda.
  Magnesium Citrate.
  Milk of Magnesia.
  Milk of Magnesia-Concentrated.
  Phillips' Milk of Magnesia.
  Phillips' Milk of Magnesia, Concen-
    trated.
W/Sennosides.
  See: Agoral.
  Bisac-Evac.
  Bisacodyl Uniserts.
  Black Draught.
  Caroid.
  Docusate w/Casanthranol.
  Doxidan.
  DSS 100 Plus.
  Dulcolax.
  ex-lax Chocolated.

Fleet Laxative.
Fletcher's Castoria.
Genasoft Plus Softgels.
Maximum Relief ex•lax.
Modane.
Nature's Remedy.
Peri-Colace.
Reliable Gentle Laxative.
Senexon.
Senna-Gen.
Senokot.
Senokot-S.
SenokotxTRA.
Women's Gentle Laxative.
W/Vitamins.
See: Lec-E-Plex.
Laxinate 100. (Roberts) Dioctyl sodium
sulfosuccinate 100 mg. Cap. Bot. 100s,
1000s.
Use: Laxative.
Lax Pills. (G & W Labs) Sennosides
15 mg, 25 mg, EDTA, parabens, su-
crose. Tab. Blister pack 24s, 48s (25 mg
only); 30s, 60s (15 mg only). *OTC.*
Use: Laxative.
layor carang.
See: Agar.
•**lazabemide.** (la77-AH-bem-ide) USAN.
Use: Antiparkinsonian.
•**lazabemide hydrochloride.** (lazz-AH-
bem-ide) USAN.
Use: Antiparkinsonian.
Lazer Creme. (Pedinol Pharmacal) Vita-
mins E 3500 units. A 100,000 units/oz.
Cream. Jar 2 oz. *OTC.*
Use: Emollient.
Lazer Formalyde. (Pedinol) Formalde-
hyde 10%. Soln. Bot. 90 mL. *Rx.*
Use: Drying agent.
LazerSporin-C. (Pedinol Pharmacal)
Neomycin sulfate 3.5 mg, polymyxin B
sulfate 10,000 units, hydrocortisone
1%/mL. Soln. Bot. 10 mL. *Rx.*
Use: Anti-infective combination, topical.
L-baclofen.
Use: Antispasmodic. [Orphan Drug]
L-Caine E. (Century) Lidocaine hydro-
chloride 1%, 2%, epinephrine
1:100,000/mL. Inj. 20 mL, 50 mL. *Rx.*
Use: Anesthetic, local.
L-Caine Viscous. (Century) Lidocaine
hydrochloride 2% with sodium carboxy-
methylcellulose. Soln. Bot. 100 mL. *Rx.*
Use: Anesthetic, local.
l-carnitine. (Freeda Vitamins) Levocarnitine 500 mg. Tab. Bot. 50s, 100s. *OTC.*
Use: Amino acid.
l-carnitine. (Various Mfr.) Amino acid derivative 250 mg. Cap. Bot. 30s, 60s,
100s. *OTC.*
Use: Amino acid.

L.C.D. (Almay) Alcohol extractions of
crude coal tar. Cream, soln. Bot. 4 oz,
pt. *OTC.*
Use: Antipsoriatic; antipruritic; topical.
See: Coal Tar Topical Soln.
LCR. *Rx.*
Use: Antineoplastic.
See: Vincristine sulfate.
LC-65 Daily Contact Lens Cleaner.
(Allergan) Daily cleaning solution for all
hard, soft (hydrophilic), rigid gas per-
meable contact lenses. Bot. 15 mL,
60 mL. *OTC.*
Use: Contact lens care.
LCx Neisseria gonorrhoeae Assay. (Ab-
bott) Reagent kit for the detection of
Neisseria gonorrhoeae in female endo-
cervical, male urethral, and urine swab
specimens. Kit. 96s. *Rx.*
Use: Diagnostic aid.
L cycloserine.
Use: Gaucher disease. [Orphan Drug]
L-cysteine. (Tyson)
Use: Erythropoietic protoporphyria.
[Orphan Drug]
L-deprenyl.
See: Selegiline hydrochloride.
LDH Reagent Strip. (Bayer Consumer
Care) A quantitative strip test for LDH
in serum or plasma. Seralyzer reagent
strip. Bot. 25s. *Rx.*
Use: Diagnostic aid.
Leber Tabulae. (Paddock) Aloe 0.09 g,
extract of rhei 0.03 g, myrrh 0.01 g,
frangula 5 mg, galbanum 2 mg, oliba-
num 3 mg. Tab. Bot. 100s, 500s, 1000s.
OTC.
Lec-E-Plex. (Barth's) Vitamin E
100 units, 200 units, 400 units. Cap.
w/lecithin. Bot. 100s, 500s, 1000s.
OTC.
Use: Vitamin E supplement.
•**lecimibide.** (leh-SIM-ih-bide) USAN.
Use: Antihyperlipidemic.
•**lecithin.** (LESS-ih-thin) *NF 23.*
Use: Pharmaceutic aid (emulsifying
agent).
lecithin. (Various Mfr.) Lecithin. **Cap.:**
520 mg. Bot. 100s, 250s, 1000s;
650 mg. Bot. 90s, 100s, 250s, 500s.
Pow.: 120 g, kg, lb. *OTC.*
Use: Nutritional supplement.
lecithin. (Arcum) Lecithin 1200 mg. Cap.
Bot. 100s, 1000s; Gran. Bot. 8 oz; Pow.
Bot. 4 oz. (Barth's) 8 gr. Cap. Bot.
100s, 500s, 1000s; Gran. Can 8 oz,
16 oz; Pow. Can 10 oz. (Cavendish)
Tab. (0.5 g) Bot. 500s. (Quality Formulations, Inc.) 1200 mg, Cap. 100s. (De
Pree) Cap. Bot 100s. (Pfanstiehl) 25 g,
100 g, 500 g Pkg.
Use: Pharmaceutic aid (emulsifying
agent).

•**ledoxantrone trihydrochloride.** (led-OX-an-trone try-HIGH-droe-KLOR-ide) USAN.
Use: Antineoplastic.

Leena. (Watson) **Phase 1:** Norethindrone 0.5 mg, ethinyl estradiol 35 mcg. **Phase 2:** Norethindrone 1 mg, ethinyl estradiol 35 mcg. **Phase 3:** Norethindrone 0.5 mg, ethinyl estradiol 35 mcg. Lactose. Tab. 28s. *Rx.*
Use: Contraceptive hormone.

leflunomide.
Use: Antiarthritic.
See: Arava.

Legatrin PM. (Columbia) Acetaminophen 500 mg, diphenhydramine hydrochloride 50 mg. Capl. Bot. 30s, 50s. *OTC.*
Use: Sleep aid.

•**lemon oil.** *NF 23.*
Use: Pharmaceutic aid (flavor).

•**lemon tincture.** *NF 23.*
Use: Pharmaceutic aid (flavor).

Lemotussin-DM. (Seneca) Dextromethorphan HBr 7.5 mg, guaifenesin 50 mg, potassium guaiacolsulfonate 50 mg, pseudoephedrine hydrochloride 10 mg, chlorpheniramine maleate 2 mg/5 mL, parabens, saccharin, sorbitol, alcohol free. Liq. 473 mL. *Rx.*
Use: Antitussive and expectorant combination.

•**lenalidomide.** (le-na-LID-oh-mide) USAN.
Use: Immunomodulator.

•**lenefilcon A.** (len-e-FIL-kon) USAN.
Use: Hydrophilic.

•**lenercept.** (LEH-ner-sept) USAN.
Use: Treatment of septic shock, multiple sclerosis, inflammatory bowel disease, rheumatoid arthritis.

lenetran. Mephenoxalone.
Use: Anxiolytic.

lenicet.
See: Aluminum Acetate, Basic.

•**leniquinsin.** (LEN-ih-KWIN-sin) USAN. Under study.
Use: Antihypertensive.

Lenium Medicated Shampoo. (Sanofi-Synthelabo) Selenium sulfide. *OTC.*
Use: Antiseborrheic.

•**lenograstim.** (leh-no-GRAH-stim) USAN.
Use: Antineutropenic; hematopoietic stimulant; immunomodulator (granulocyte colony-stimulating factor).

•**lenperone.** (LEN-per-OHN) USAN.
Use: Antipsychotic.

Lens Clear. (Allergan) Sterile, isotonic solution surfactant cleaner w/sorbic acid 0.1%, edetate disodium 0.2%. Bot. 15 mL. *OTC.*

Use: Contact lens care.

Lens Drops. (Ciba Vision) Sodium chloride, borate buffer, carbamide, poloxamer 407, EDTA 0.2%, sorbic acid 0.15%. Soln. Bot. 15 mL. *OTC.*
Use: Contact lens care, rewetting.

Lensept Disinfecting Solution. (Ciba Vision) Micro-filtered hydrogen peroxide with sodium stannate 3%, sodium nitrate, phosphate buffers. Soln. Bot. 237, 355 mL. *OTC.*
Use: Disinfecting solution.

Lensept Rinse and Neutralizer. (Ciba Vision) Sodium chloride, sodium borate decahydrate, boric acid, bovine catalase, sorbic acid, EDTA. Soln. Bot. 237 mL. System includes lens cup and holder. *OTC.*
Use: Contact lens care, rinsing, neutralizing.

Lens Fresh. (Allergan) Sterile, buffered, isotonic aqueous soln., hydroxyethyl cellulose, sodium Cl, boric acid, sodium borate, sorbic acid 0.1%, edetate disodium 0.2%. Bot. 0.5 oz. *OTC.*
Use: Contact lens care.

Lensine Extra Strength. (Ciba Vision) Cleaning agent with benzalkonium Cl 0.01%, EDTA 0.1%. Soln. Bot. 45 mL. *OTC.*
Use: Contact lens care.

Lens Lubricant. (Bausch & Lomb) Povidone and polyoxyethylene with thimerosal 0.004%, EDTA 0.1% Soln. Bot. 15 mL. *OTC.*
Use: Contact lens care; lubricant.

Lens Plus. (Allergan) Isotonic soln. w/sodium Cl 0.9%. Aerosol 3 oz, 8 oz, 12 oz. Preservative free. *OTC.*
Use: Contact lens care.

Lens Plus Daily Cleaner. (Allergan) Buffered solution with cocoamphocarboxyglycinate, sodium lauryl sulfate, hexylene glycol, sodium chloride, sodium phosphate. Preservative free. Soln. Bot. 15 mL, 30 mL. *OTC.*
Use: Contact lens care, cleanser.

Lens Plus Oxysept Disinfecting Solution. (Allergan) Hydrogen peroxide with sodium stannate 3%, sodium nitrate, phosphate buffer. Soln. Bot. 240 mL. *OTC.*
Use: Contact lens care.

Lens Plus Oxysept Rinse and Neutralizer. (Allergan) Isotonic with sodium chloride, mono- and dibasic sodium phosphates, catalytic neutralizing agent, EDTA. Soln. Bot. 15 mL. *OTC.*
Use: Contact lens care.

Lens Plus Oxysept 2 Neutralizing. (Allergan) Catalase with buffering

agents used to neutralize the *Lens Plus Oxysept 1* disinfecting solution in a chemical lens care system. For soft contact lens. Tabs. Box 12s. Bot. 36s. *OTC.*
Use: Contact lens care.

Lens Plus Preservative Free. (Allergan) Isotonic sodium chloride 9%. Soln. Bot. 90 mL, 240 mL, 360 mL. *OTC.*
Use: Contact lens care.

Lens Plus Rewetting Drops. (Allergan) Isotonic solution with sodium chloride and boric acid. Thimerosal and preservative free. Soln. Bot. 0.3 mL (30s). *OTC.*
Use: Contact lens care.

Lens Plus Sterile Saline. (Allergan) Sodium Cl, boric acid, nitrogen. Soln. Bot. 90 mL, 240 mL, 360 mL. Aerosol. *OTC.*
Use: Contact lens care.

Lensrins. (Allergan) Sterile preserved saline for heat disinfection, rinsing and storage of soft (hydrophilic) contact lenses, rinsing solution for chemical disinfection. Soln. Bot. 8 oz. *OTC.*
Use: Contact lens care.

Lens-Wet. (Allergan) Isotonic, buffered soln. of polyvinyl alcohol, thimerosal 0.002%, EDTA 0.01%. Bot. 0.5 fl oz. *OTC.*
Use: Contact lens care.

Lente Iletin II. (Lilly) Insulin zinc suspension 100 units/mL. Purified pork. Inj. Vials. 10 mL. *OTC.*
Use: Antidiabetic.

lente insulin. Susp. of zinc insulin crystals. *OTC.*
See: Iletin Lente.

lente insulin. (Novo/Nordisk) Insulin zinc susp. 100 units/mL Beef. Inj. Vial 10 mL.
Use: Antidiabetic.

lentinan. (Lenti-Chemico Pharmaceuticals)
Use: Immunomodulator.

lepirudin. (LEP-ih-ru-din)
Use: Thrombin inhibitor. [Orphan Drug]
See: Refludan.

lepromin. (Louisiana State University) Lepromin, 30 to 40 million acid-fast bacilli/mL. Vial 5 mL, 10 mL, 20 mL, 50 mL.

leprostatics.
Use: Bactericidal.
See: Dapsone.

• **lercanidipine hydrochloride.** (ler-can-i-DIP-een) USAN.
Use: Antihypertensive; calcium channel blocker.

• **lergotrile.** (LER-go-trill) USAN.
Use: Enzyme inhibitor (prolactin).

• **lergotrile mesylate.** (LER-go-trill) USAN.
Use: Enzyme inhibitor (prolactin).

Lerton Ovules. (Vita Elixir) Caffeine 250 mg. Cap. *OTC.*
Use: CNS stimulant.

Lescol. (Novartis) Fluvastatin sodium (as base) 20 mg, 40 mg, benzyl alcohol, parabens, EDTA. Cap. Bot. 30s, 100s. *Rx.*
Use: Antihyperlipidemic, HMG-CoA reductase inhibitor.

Lescol XL. (Novartis) Fluvastatin sodium (as base) 80 mg. Film-coated. ER Tab. Bot. 30s, 100s. *Rx.*
Use: Antihyperlipidemic, HMG-CoA reductase inhibitor.

Lessina. (Barr) Levonorgestrel 0.1 mg, ethinyl estradiol 20 mcg, lactose. Tab. Packs. 21s, 28s. *Rx.*
Use: Sex hormone, contraceptive hormone.

• **lestaurtinib.** (le-STOR-tin-ib) USAN.
Use: Antineoplastic agent.

Lesterol. (Dram) Nicotinic acid 500 mg. Tab. Bot. 250s. *OTC.*
Use: Antihyperlipidemic.

• **leteprinim potassium.** (leh-TEPP-rin-nim) USAN.
Use: Central neurodegenerative disease; Alzheimer disease; spinal cord injury; stroke.

• **letimide hydrochloride.** (LET-ih-mide) USAN.
Use: Analgesic.

• **letrozole.** (let-ROW-zahl) *USP 28.*
Use: Antineoplastic, hormone, aromatase inhibitor.
See: Femara.

• **leucine.** (LOO-SEEN) *USP 28.*
Use: Amino acid.

• **leucovorin calcium.** (loo-koe-VORE-in) *USP 28.*
Use: Antianemic; folate-deficiency; antidote to folic acid antagonists.

leucovorin calcium. (American Regent) Leucovorin calcium 10 mg/mL. Inj. Single-dose vial 5 mL (25s). *Rx.*
Use: Antianemic; folate-deficiency; antidote to folic acid antagonists.

leucovorin calcium. (Various Mfr.) Leucovorin calcium 5 mg. Tab. Bot. 30s, 100s, UD 50s.
Use: Antagonist of amithopterin; antianemic (folate-deficiency); antidote to folic acid antagonists; antineoplastic.

leucovorin calcium. (Various Mfr.) Leucovorin calcium. **Tab.:** 15 mg, 25 mg as calcium. Pkg. 12s, 24s, 25s, UD 50s. **Inj.:** 3 mg/mL as calcium w/benzyl al-

cohol 0.9%. Amps 1 mL. **Pow. for Inj.:** 50 mg/vial, 100 mg/vial, 350 mg/vial. *Rx.*
Use: Folic acid antagonist overdosage.
Leukeran. (GlaxoSmithKline) Chlorambucil 2 mg. Film coated. Tab. Bot. 50s. *Rx.*
Use: Antineoplastic; alkylating agent.
Leukine. (Immunex) Sargramostim. **Pow. for Inj., lyophilized:** 250 mcg, mannitol 40 mg, sucrose 10 mg, tromethamine 1.2 mg/mL, preservative free. Vial. **Liq.:** 500 mcg/mL, benzyl alcohol 1.1%, mannitol 40 mg, sucrose 10 mg, tromethamine 1.2 mg/mL. Multipledose vial. *Rx.*
Use: Hematopoietic, colony stimulating factor.
leukocyte protease inhibitor, recombinant secretory.
Use: Alpha-1 antitrypsin deficiency; cystic fibrosis. [Orphan Drug]
leukocyte protease inhibitor, secretory.
Use: Bronchopulmonary dysplasia. [Orphan Drug]
leukocyte typing serum. (LOO-koe-site)
Use: Diagnostic aid, blood, in vitro.
leukotriene receptor antagonists.
Use: Antiasthmatic.
See: Montelukast Sodium.
Zafirlukast.
leupeptin. (Neuromuscular Agents)
Use: Adjunct to nerve repair. [Orphan Drug]
•**leuprolide acetate.** (loo-PRO-lide) USAN.
Use: Antineoplastic; LHRH agonist; central precocious puberty. [Orphan Drug]
See: Eligard.
Lupron.
Lupron Depot-4 Month.
Lupron Depot-Ped.
Lupron Depot-3 Month.
Lupron for Pediatric Use.
Viadur.
leuprolide acetate. (Various Mfr.) Leuprolide acetate 5 mg/mL, benzyl alcohol 9 mg/mL, sodium chloride. Inj. Multidose Vial 2.8 mL. *Rx.*
Use: Antineoplastic; hormone; gonadotropin-releasing hormone analog.
leurocristine.
See: Vincristine Sulfate.
leurocristine sulfate (1:1) (salt). Vincristine Sulfate, USP.
Use: Antineoplastic.
Leustatin. (Ortho Biotech) Cladribine. Soln. 1 mg/mL. Vial. 20 mL single-use. *Rx.*

Use: Antineoplastic.
leuteinizing hormone (recombinant) human.
Use: With recombinant human folliclestimulating hormone for chronic anovulation due to hypogonadotropic hypogonadism. [Orphan Drug]
Levacet. (Pharmakon) Phenyltoloxamine citrate 50 mg, acetaminophen 400 mg, salicylamide 150 mg, aspirin 400 mg, caffeine 40 mg. Tab. 50s. *Rx.*
Use: Narcotic analgesic.
•**levalbuterol hydrochloride.** (lev-al-BYOO-ter-ole) USAN.
Use: Bronchodilator, sympathomimetic; antiasthmatic.
See: Xopenex.
•**levalbuterol sulfate.** (lev-al-BYOO-terole) USAN.
Use: Bronchodilator, antiasthmatic.
•**levalbuterol tartrate.** (lev-al-BYOO-terole) USAN.
Use: Bronchodilator, antiasthmatic.
Levall. (Athlon Pharmaceuticals) Carbetapentane citrate 20 mg, guaifenesin 100 mg, phenylephrine hydrochloride 15 mg/5 mL, strawberry flavor, alcohol free. Liq. Bot. 15 mL, 473 mL. *Rx.*
Use: Upper respiratory combination, antitussive, expectorant, decongestant.
Levall 5.0. (Athlon Pharmaceuticals) Phenylephrine hydrochloride 15 mg, hydrocodone bitartrate 5 mg, guaifenesin 100 mg/5 mL, alcohol free, grape flavor. Liq. Bot. 15 mL, 473 mL. *c-III.*
Use: Upper respiratory combination, decongestant, antitussive, expectorant.
•**levamfetamine succinate.** (LEV-am-FET-ah-meen) USAN.
Use: Anorexic.
•**levamisole hydrochloride.** (lev-AM-ih-sole) *USP 28.*
Use: Biological response modifier; antineoplastic.
See: Ergamisol.
Levaquin. (Ortho-McNeil) Levofloxacin. **Tab.:** 250 mg, 500 mg, 750 mg. Film coated. Bot. 20s (750 mg only), 50s (except 750 mg), UD 100s, *Leva-Pak* 5s (750 mg only). **Inj. (conc.):** 500 mg (25 mg/mL), preservative free, singleuse vial 20 mL; 750 mg (25 mg/mL), preservative free, single-use vial 30 mL. **Inj. (premix):** 250 mg (5 mg/mL), 500 mg (5 mg/mL), 750 mg (5 mg/mL), preservative free. Flex. Cont 50 mL (250 mg only), 100 mL (500 mg only), 150 mL (750 mg only) w/dextrose solution 5%. **Oral Soln.:** 25 mg/mL. Benzyl alcohol, glycerin, sucrose. 480 mL.

Rx.
Use: Anti-infective, fluoroquinolone.
levarterenol.
See: Norepinephrine Bitartrate.
Levatol. (Schwarz Pharma) Penbutolol sulfate 20 mg. Tab. Bot. 100s. *Rx.*
Use: Antiadrenergic, sympatholytic, beta-adrenergic blocker.
Levbid. (Schwarz Pharma) L-hyoscyamine sulfate 0.375 mg. ER Tab. Bot. 100s. *Rx.*
Use: Anticholinergic; antispasmodic.
•**levcromakalim.** (lev-KROE-mah-KAY-lim) USAN.
Use: Antihypertensive; antiasthmatic.
•**levcycloserine.** (LEV-sigh-kloe-SER-een) USAN.
Use: Enzyme inhibitor (Gaucher disease).
•**levdobutamine lactobionate.** (LEV-dah-BYOOT-ah-meen LACK-toe-BYE-oh-nate) USAN.
Use: Cardiovascular agent.
Levemir. (Novo Nordisk) Insulin detemir (rDNA) 100 units/mL. Inj. Vial 10 mL, PenFill cartridge 3 mL, InnoLet 3 mL, FlexPen 3 mL. *Rx.*
Use: Antidiabetic, insulin.
•**levetiracetam.** (lee-ve-tye-RA-se-tam) USAN.
Use: Antiepileptic.
See: Keppra.
Leviron. (Health for Life Brands) Desiccated liver 7 gr, iron and ammonium citrate 3 gr, vitamins B_1 1 mg, B_2 0.5 mg, B_6 0.5 mg, calcium pantothenate 0.3 mg, niacinamide 2.5 mg, B_{12} 1 mcg. Cap. Bot. 100s, 1000s. *OTC.*
Use: Mineral, vitamin supplement.
Levitra. (Bayer) Vardenafil hydrochloride 2.5 mg, 5 mg, 10 mg, 20 mg. Tab. 6s (10 mg, 20 mg only), 30s. *Rx.*
Use: Impotence agents.
Levlen. (Berlex) Levonorgestrel 0.15 mg, ethinyl estradiol 30 mcg, lactose. Tab. Slidecase Dispenser 21s, 28s. *Rx.*
Use: Sex hormone, contraceptive hormone.
Levlite. (Berlex) Levonorgestrel 0.1 mg, ethinyl estradiol 20 mcg, lactose, sucrose. Tab. Slidecase 28s. *Rx.*
Use: Sex hormone, contraceptive hormone.
levmetamfetamine.
Use: Nasal decongestant.
See: Vicks Vapor Inhalant.
•**levoamphetamine.** (lee-voe-am-FET-uh-meen) *USP 28.*
Use: Nasal decongestant.

levo-amphetamine. Alginate (l-isomer) alpha-2-phenylaminopropane succinate.
•**levobetaxolol hydrochloride.** (LEE-voe-beh-TAX-oh-lahl) USAN.
Use: Antiadrenergic, β-receptor.
See: Betaxon.
•**levobunolol hydrochloride.** (LEE-voe-BYOO-no-lahl) *USP 28.*
Use: Antiadrenergic, β-receptor.
See: AKBeta.
Betagan Liquifilm.
levobunolol hydrochloride. (Various Mfr.) Levobunolol hydrochloride 0.25%, 0.5% Ophth. Soln. Bot. 5 mL, 10 mL, 15 mL (0.5% only). *Rx.*
Use: Antiglaucoma agent; beta-adrenergic blocker.
•**levobupivacaine hydrochloride.** (lee-voe-byoo-PIV-ah-caine) USAN.
Use: Local anesthetic, amide.
See: Chirocaine.
•**levocarnitine.** (LEE-voe-KAR-nih-teen) *USP 28.*
Use: Amino acid.
See: Carnitor.
L-Carnitine.
Vitacarn.
levocarnitine. (Rising) Levocarnitine. **Soln.:** 100 mg/mL. Sucrose, parabens. Cherry flavor. 118 mL. **Tab.:** 330 mg. Blisters of 90. *Rx.*
Use: Amino acid.
levocarnitine. (Various Mfr.) Levocarni tine 200 mg/mL. Inj. Single-dose vial. *Rx.*
Use: Amino acid.
•**levocarnitine propionate hydrochloride.** (lee-voe-KAR-ni-teen) USAN.
Use: Peripheral arterial disease.
•**levodopa.** (LEE-voe-DOE-puh) *USP 28.*
Use: Antiparkinsonian.
See: Bio Dopa.
Dopar.
Larodopa.
Levora.
W/Carbidopa.
See: Parcopa.
Sinemet CR.
Sinemet 10/100.
Sinemet 25/100.
Sinemet 25/250.
W/Carbidopa and Entacapone.
See: Stalevo.
Levo-Dromoran. (Valeant) Levorphanol tartrate. **Inj.:** 2 mg/mL. Amps (contains parabens). 1 mL. Multidose vials (phenol 14.5 mg/mL). 10 mL. **Tab.:** 2 mg, lactose. Bot. 100s. *c-II.*
Use: Opioid analgesic.

• **levofloxacin.** (lee-voe-FLOX-ah-sin) USAN.
Use: Anti-infective, fluoroquinolone.
See: Iquix.
  Levaquin.
  Quixin.

• **levofuraltadone.** (LEE-voe-fer-AL-tah-dohn) USAN.
Use: Anti-infective; antiprotozoal.

• **levoleucovorin calcium.** (LEE-voe-loo-koe-VORE-in) USAN.
Use: Antidote to folic acid antagonist.
See: Isovorin.

• **levomepromazine.** (LEE-voe-me-PROE-ma-zeen) USAN.
Use: Analgesic.

• **levomepromazine hydrochloride.** (LEE-voe-me-PROE-ma-zeen) USAN.
Use: Analgesic.

• **levomepromazine maleate.** (LEE-voe-me-PROE-ma-zeen) USAN.
Use: Analgesic.

• **levomethadyl acetate hydrochloride.** (LEE-voe-METH-uh-dill) USAN.
Use: Analgesic; narcotic. [Orphan Drug]

• **levonantradol hydrochloride.** (LEE-voe-NAN-trah-DAHL) USAN.
Use: Analgesic.

• **levonordefrin.** (lee-voe-nore-DEFF-rin) *USP 28.*
Use: Adrenergic, vasoconstrictor.
W/Combinations.
See: Mepivacaine hydrochloride and Levonordefrin.
  Polocaine with Levonordefrin.

• **levonorgestrel.** (LEE-voe-nor-JESS-truhl) *USP 28.*
Use: Hormone, progestin.
See: Alesse.
  Levora.
  Plan B.

levonorgestrel and ethinyl estradiol tablets.
Use: Contraceptive.
See: Alesse.
  Aviane.
  Levlen.
  Levlite.
  Levora.
  Levoral.
  Lutera.
  Nordette.
  Norplant System.
  Plan B.
  Preven.
  Seasonale.
  Tri-Levlen.
  Triphasil.
  Trivora-28.

levonorgestrel-releasing intrauterine system.
Use: Sex hormone, contraceptive system.
See: Mirena.

Levophed. (Abbott) Norepinephrine bitartrate 1 mg/mL, metabisulfite ≤ 2 mg. Amp. 4 mL. *Rx.*
Use: Vasoconstrictor.

Levophed Bitartrate. (Abbott) Norepinephrine bitartrate w/sodium Cl, sodium metabisulfite 1 mg, 2 mg/mL. Amp. 4 mL. Box 10s. *Rx.*
Use: Vasoconstrictor.

• **levopropoxyphene napsylate.** (lee-voe-pro-POX-ee-feen NAP-sih-late) *USP 28.*
Use: Antitussive.

• **levopropylcillin potassium.** (lee-voe-pro-pihl-SILL-in) USAN.
Use: Anti-infective.

Levora. (Watson) Ethinyl estradiol 30 mcg, levonorgestrel 0.15 mg, lactose. Tab. Pkt. 28s. *Rx.*
Use: Sex hormone, contraceptive hormone.

levorenine.
See: Epinephrine.

Levoroxine. (Bariatric) Sodium levothyroxine 0.05 mg, 0.1 mg, 0.2 mg, 0.3 mg. Tab. Bot. 100s, 500s. *Rx.*
Use: Hormone, thyroid.

• **levorphanol tartrate.** (lee-VORE-fah-nole TAR-trate) *USP 28.*
Use: Opioid analgesic.
See: Levo-Dromoran.

levorphanol tartrate. (Roxane) Levorphanol tartrate 2 mg, lactose. Tab. Bot. 100s. *c-II.*
Use: Opioid analgesic.

• **levosimendan.** (lee-voe-sih-MEN-dan) USAN.
Use: Investigational for congestive heart failure.

Levo-T. (Wyeth) Levothyroxine sodium 0.025 mg, 0.05 mg, 0.075 mg, 0.1 mg, 0.125 mg, 0.15 mg, 0.2 mg, 0.3 mg. Tab. Bot. 100s (all strengths), 1000s (0.05, 0.1, 0.15, 0.2 mg only). *Rx.*
Use: Hormone, thyroid.

Levothroid. (Forest) Levothyroxine sodium. **Tab.:** 0.025 mg, 0.05 mg, 0.075 mg, 0.088 mg, 0.1 mg, 0.112 mg, 0.125 mg, 0.150 mg, 0.175 mcg, 0.2 mg, 0.3 mg. Bot. 100s, 1000s. *Rx.*
Use: Hormone, thyroid.

• **levothyroxine sodium.** (lee-voe-thigh-ROX-een) *USP 28.*
Use: Hormone, thyroid.
See: Levothroid.

Levoxyl.
Synthroid.
Unithroid.
W/Mannitol.
See: Levoxine.
Synthroid.
W/Sodium liothyronine.
See: Thyrolar.
levothyroxine sodium. (Sandoz) Levothyroxine sodium (T_4, L-thyroxine) 0.137 mg. Tab. 100s. *Rx.*
Use: Hormone, thyroid.
levothyroxine sodium. (Various Mfr.) Levothyroxine sodium. **Pow. for Inj.:** 200 mcg, 500 mcg. Vial. 10 mL. **Tab.:** 0.025 mg, 0.05 mg, 0.075 mg, 0.088 mg, 0.1 mg, 0.112 mg, 0.125 mg, 0.15 mg, 0.175 mg, 0.2 mg, 0.3 mg. Bot. 100s. *Rx.*
Use: Hormone, thyroid.
• **levotofisopam.** (LEV-oh-toe-FIS-oh-pam) USAN.
Use: Anxiolytic agent.
• **levoxadrol hydrochloride.** (lev-OX-ah-drole) USAN.
Use: Anesthetic, local; muscle relaxant.
Levoxyl. (Jones Pharma) Levothyroxine sodium 0.025 mg, 0.05 mg, 0.075 mg, 0.088 mg, 0.1 mg, 0.112 mg, 0.125 mg, 0.137 mg, 0.15 mg, 0.175 mg, 0.2 mg, 0.3 mg. Tab. Bot. 100s, 1000s, UD 100s. *Rx.*
Use: Hormone, thyroid.
Levsin. (Schwarz Pharma) L-hyoscyamine sulfate. **Tab.:** 0.125 mg. Bot. 100s, 500s. **Elix.:** 0.125 mg/5 mL, alcohol 20%. Sorbitol, orange flavor. Bot. Pt. **Inj.:** 0.5 mg/mL. Amp. 1 mL, Vial 10 mL with benzyl alcohol 1.5%, sodium metabisulfite 0.1%. *Rx.*
Use: Anticholinergic; antispasmodic.
Levsin Drops. (Schwarz Pharma) L-hyoscyamine sulfate 0.125 mg/mL, alcohol 5%, sorbitol, orange flavor. Soln. Bot. 15 mL. *Rx.*
Use: Anticholinergic; antispasmodic.
Levsinex Timecaps. (Schwarz Pharma) L-hyoscyamine sulfate 0.375 mg. TR Cap. Bot. 100s, 500s. *Rx.*
Use: Anticholinergic; antispasmodic.
Levsin-PB Drops. (Schwarz Pharma) Hyoscyamine sulfate 0.125 mg, phenobarbital 15 mg/mL, alcohol 5%. Liq. Bot. 15 mL. *Rx.*
Use: Anticholinergic; antispasmodic; hypnotic; sedative.
Levsin/SL. (Schwarz Pharma) L-hyoscyamine sulfate 0.125 mg. Peppermint flavor. Tab. Sublingual. Bot. 100s, 500s. *Rx.*
Use: Anticholinergic; antispasmodic.

Levulan Kerastick. (DUSA) Aminolevulinic acid hydrochloride 20% (354 mg), ethanol v/v 48%, isopropyl alcohol. Top. Soln. Applicator (2 glass Amp, applicator tip. One amp 1.5 mL soln. vehicle, other amp aminolevulinic acid hydrochloride 354 mg). Box 4s, 6s, 12s. *Rx.*
Use: Photochemotherapy.
levulose. Fructose.
levulose-dextrose.
See: Invert Sugar.
Lexapro. (Forest) Escitalopram oxalate. **Tab.:** 5 mg, 10 mg, 20 mg. Talc, film-coated. Bot. 100s, UD 100s (except 5 mg). **Oral Soln.:** 5 mg/mL, sorbitol, parabens, peppermint flavor. Bot. 240 mL. *Rx.*
Use: Antidepressant, selective serotonin reuptake inhibitor.
• **lexipafant.** (lex-IH-pah-fant) USAN.
Use: Platelet-activating factor (PAP) antagonist.
• **lexithromycin.** (lex-ith-row-MY-sin) USAN.
Use: Anti-infective.
Lexiva. (GlaxoSmithKline) Fosamprenavir calcium 700 mg (equiv. to amprenavir 600 mg). Tab. 60s. *Rx.*
Use: Antiretroviral agent.
Lextron. (Eli Lilly) Liver-stomach concentrate 50 mg, iron 30 mg, vitamins B_1 1 mg, B_2 0.25 mg, B_{12} (activity equivalent) 2 mcg, other factors of vitamin D complex present in the liver-stomach concentrate. Pulv. Bot. 84s. *OTC.*
Use: Mineral; vitamin supplement.
Lexxel. (AstraZeneca) Enalapril maleate 5 mg, felodipine 2.5 mg, 5 mg. ER Tab. Bot. 30s, 100s, UD 100s. *Rx.*
Use: Antihypertensive combination.
L-5 hydroxytryptophan. (Circa)
Use: Postanoxic intention myoclonus. [Orphan Drug]
L'Homme. (Armenpharm Ltd.) Vitamins A 4000 units, D 400 units, B_1 1 mg, B_2 1.2 mg, B_3 10 mg, B_{12} 2 mcg, calcium pantothenate 5 mg, C 30 mg, Ca 100 mg, P 76 mg, Fe 10 mg, Mn 1 mg, Mg 1 mg, Zn 1 mg. Bot. 100s. *OTC.*
Use: Mineral, vitamin supplement.
• **liarozole fumarate.** (lie-AHR-oh-zole) USAN.
Use: Antipsoriatic.
• **liarozole hydrochloride.** (lie-AHR-oh-zole) USAN.
Use: Antineoplastic.
Li Ban. (Pfizer) Synthetic pyrethroid 0.5%, related compounds 0.065%, aromatic petroleum hydrocarbons 0.664%.

Spray. Bot. 5 oz, Box 6s. *OTC.*
Use: Pediculicide, inanimate objects.
(Not to be used on humans or animals).

•**libenzapril.** (lie-BENZ-ah-prill) USAN.
Use: ACE inhibitor.

Librax. (Victory Pharma) Methscopolamine nitrate 2.5 mg, chlordiazepoxide hydrochloride 5 mg. Lactose. Cap. Bot. 100s. *c-iv.*
Use: Anticholinergic combination.

Librium. (ICN) Chlordiazepoxide hydrochloride. **Cap.:** 5 mg, 10 mg, 25 mg. Lactose, parabens. Bot. 100s. **Pow. for Inj.:** 100 mg w/benzyl alcohol 1.5%, polysorbate 80, propylene glycol 20%. Amp. 5 mL w/2 mL diluent. *c-iv.*
Use: Anxiolytic.

Lice Treatment. (Goldline) Pyrethrins 0.33%, piperonyl butoxide. Benzyl alcohol. Shampoo. 59 mL, 118 mL with comb. *OTC.*
Use: Pediculicide.

•**licorice.** (LIK-o-ris) *NF 23.*
Use: Pharmaceutic aid (flavor).

•**licostinel.** (li-KOS-ti-nel) USAN.
Use: Treatment of stroke (NMDA receptor antagonist, glycine site).

•**licryfilcon a.** (lih-krih-FILL-kahn) USAN.
Use: Contact lens material (hydrophilic).

•**licryfilcon b.** (lih-krih-FILL-kahn) USAN.
Use: Contact lens material, hydrophilic.

LidaMantle. (Doak Dermatologics) Lidocaine hydrochloride 3%. Cetyl alcohol, stearyl alcohol, glycerin, petrolatum, parabens, light mineral oil. Cream. 28 g, 85 g. *Rx.*
Use: Anesthetic, topical.

LidaMantle HC. (Doak Dermatologics) Lidocaine hydrochloride 3%, hydrocortisone acetate 0.5%. Cetyl alcohol, mineral oil, methylparaben, petrolatum. Lot. 177 mL. *Rx.*
Use: Corticosteroid, topical.

LidaMantle HC Cream. (Doak Dermatologics) Lidocaine 3%, hydrocortisone acetate 0.5% in cream base. Tube 1 oz. *Rx.*
Use: Corticosteroid; anesthetic, local.

•**lidamidine hydrochloride.** (LIE-DAM-ih-deen) USAN.
Use: Antiperistaltic.

Lidex. (Roche) Fluocinonide 0.05%.
Cream: Tube 15 g, 30 g, 60 g, 120 g.
Oint.: Tube 15 g, 30 g, 60 g, 120 g.
Soln.: Bot. 20 mL, 60 mL. *Rx.*
Use: Corticosteroid, topical.

Lidex-E. (Roche) Fluocinonide 0.05% in aqueous emollient base. Tube 15 g,

30 g, 60 g, 120 g. *Rx.*
Use: Corticosteroid, topical.

•**lidocaine.** (LIE-doe-cane) *USP 28.*
Use: Anesthetic, local.
See: Dentipatch.
Dermaflex.
Lidosense 4.
L-M-X4.
Solarcaine Aloe Extra Burn Relief.
TheraPatch Cold Sore.
Xylocaine.
Zilactin-L.
W/Prilocaine.
See: EmLA Anesthetic.

lidocaine and epinephrine. (Abbott) Lidocaine 0.5%, epinephrine 1:200,000, methylparaben, sodium metabisulfite. Inj. Multidose vial 50 mL. Lidocaine 1%, epinephrine 1:100,000, methylparaben, sodium metabisulfite. Inj. Multidose vial 20 mL, 30 mL, 50 mL. Lidocaine 1%, epinephrine 1:200,000, sodium metabisulfite. Inj. Single-dose amp. 30 mL. Lidocaine 1.5%, epinephrine 1:200,000. Inj. Single-dose amp. 5 mL, 30 mL. Single-dose vial 30 mL (sodium metabisulfite). Lidocaine 2%, epinephrine 1:200,000, sodium metabisulfite. Inj. Single-dose vial 20 mL. *Rx.*
Use: Injectable local anesthetic, amide.

lidocaine and epinephrine. (Various Mfr.) Lidocaine 2%, epinephrine 1:100,000. Inj. Cart. 1.8 mL. Multidose vial 20 mL, 30 mL, 50 mL (may contain sodium metabisulfite and methylparaben) *Rx.*
Use: Injectable local anesthetic, amide.

lidocaine hydrochloride. (Abbott) Lidocaine hydrochloride. Inj. **1.5%:** With 1:200,000 epinephrine. Amp. 5 mL, 30 mL. Single-dose vial 30 mL (with sodium metabisulfite). With 7.5% dextrose. Amp. 2 mL **4%:** Single-dose amp. 5 mL. **5%:** With 7.5% dextrose. Single-dose amp. *Rx.*
Use: Injectable local anesthetic, amide.

lidocaine hydrochloride. (Various Mfr.) Lidocaine hydrochloride. Inj. **0.5%:** May contain methylparaben. Single-dose vial 50 mL; multidose vial 50 mL. **1%:** Amp. 2 mL, 5 mL. Vial 5 mL (preservative free). Single-dose vial 30 mL. Multidose vial 20 mL, 30 mL, 50 mL (may contain methylparaben). Syr. 5 mL. Cartridge. **1.5%:** Amp. 20 mL. **2%:** Amp. 2 mL, 10 mL. Vial 5 mL (preservative free). Single-dose vial 10 mL. Multidose vial 20 mL, 50 mL (may contain methylparaben). Syr. 5 mL *Rx.*
Use: Injectable local anesthetic, amide.

•**lidocaine hydrochloride.** (LIE-doe-cane) *USP 28.*
Use: Cardiovascular agent; antiarrhythmic agent; anesthetic, local.
See: Anestacon.
  Ardecaine 1%, 2%.
  Dolicaine.
  L-Caine.
  LidaMantle.
  LidoPen Auto-Injector.
  Norocaine.
  Octocaine hydrochloride.
  Xylocaine.
  Xylocaine 10% Oral.
  Xylocaine MPF.
  Xylocaine Viscous.
W/Benzalkonium Cl.
See: Bactine Pain Relieving Cleansing.
  Medi-Quik.
W/Benzalkonium Cl, phenol, menthol, eu-genol, thyme oil, eucalyptus oil.
See: Unguentine Spray.
W/Cetyltrimethylammonium bromide, hexachlorophene.
See: Hil-20.
W/Epinephrine.
See: Lidocaine and Epinephrine.
  Lidocaine hydrochloride.
  Lidosite Topical System.
  Otocaine.
  Xylocaine.
  Xylocaine MPF.
W/Hydrocortisone
See: AnaMantle HC.
  LidaMantle HC.
W/Methyl parasept.
See: L-Caine.
W/Methyl parasept, epinephrine.
See: L-Caine-E.
W/Orthohydroxyphenyl mercuric Cl, menthol, camphor, allantoin.
See: Unguentine Plus.
lidocaine hydrochloride and epineph-rine. (Eastman Kodak) Lidocaine 2%, epinephrine 1:50,000, sodium meta-bisulfite. Dental cart. 1.8 mL *Rx.*
Use: Injectable local anesthetic, amide.
lidocaine hydrochloride cream. (River's Edge) Lidocaine hydrochloride 3%. Alcohols, aluminum sulfate, glycerin, light mineral oil, parabens, petrolatum. Cream. 28.35 g, 85 g. *Rx.*
Use: Local anesthetic, topical.
lidocaine hydrochloride for cardiac ar-rhythmias. (Abbott) Lidocaine hydrochloride. **1%:** 10 mg/mL. Inj. (for direct IV administration). Amps. 5 mL. Vials. 20 mL, 30 mL, 50 mL. *Abboject* syringes. 5 mL. **10%:** 100 mg/mL. Inj. (for IV admixture). Additive vials. 10 mL. **20%:** 200 mg/mL. Inj. (for IV admixture).

Syringes. 5 mL, 10 mL. Vials. 10 mL. *Rx.*
Use: Antiarrhythmic agent.
lidocaine hydrochloride for cardiac ar-rhythmias. (Various Mfr.) Lidocaine hydrochloride. **2%:** 20 mg/mL. Inj. (for direct IV administration). Vials. 5 mL, 10 mL. 20 mL, 30 mL, 50 mL. Syringes. 5 mL. **4%:** 40 mg/mL. Inj. (for IV admixtures). Amps. 5 mL. Vials. 25 mL, 50 mL. *Rx.*
Use: Antiarrhythmic agent.
lidocaine hydrochloride in 5% dex-trose. (Various Mfr.) Lidocaine hydrochloride 0.2% (2 mg/mL), 0.4% (4 mg/mL), 0.8% (8 mg/mL). Inj. (for IV infusion). 250 mL (except 0.2%), 500 mL, 1,000 mL (0.2% only). *Rx.*
Use: Antiarrhythmic agent.
lidocaine hydrochloride lotion. (River's Edge) Lidocaine hydrochloride 3%. Alcohols, aluminum sulfate, glycerin, light mineral oil, parabens, petrolatum. Lot. 177 mL. *Rx.*
Use: Local anesthetic, topical.
lidocaine hydrochloride 2%. (IMS) Lidocaine hydrochloride 2%. Preservative-free. Jelly. UD 5, 10, and 20 mL single-use vials. 25s. *Rx.*
Use: Anesthetic, local.
lidocaine/hydrocortisone cream. (River's Edge) Hydrocortisone acetate 0.5%, lidocaine hydrochloride 3%. Aluminum sulfate, alcohols, glycerin, light mineral oil, parabens, petrolatum. Cream. 28.5 g, 85 g. *Rx.*
Use: Topical corticosteroid.
lidocaine/hydrocortisone rectal. (River's Edge) Hydrocortisone acetate 0.5%, lidocaine hydrochloride 3%. Aluminum sulfate, alcohols, glycerin, light mineral oil, parabens, petrolatum. Cream. Single-use units with applicator. 7 g. *Rx.*
Use: Anorectal preparation.
lidocaine patch 5%.
Use: Anesthetic, local topical.
See: EMLA Anesthetic.
  Lidoderm.
  TheraPatch Cold Sore.
lidocaine/prilocaine. (Hi-Tech) Lidocaine 2.5%, prilocaine 2.5%. Cream. 15 g, 30 g. *Rx.*
Use: Local anesthetic, topical.
lidocaine 2% viscous. (Various Mfr.) Lidocaine hydrochloride 2%. Soln. 100 mL, UD 20 mL. *Rx.*
Use: Anesthetic, local.
Lidoderm. (Endo) Lidocaine 5%, EDTA, glycerin, parabens, polyvinyl alcohol. Patch 10 × 14 cm. Box 5s. *Rx.*

Use: Anesthetic, local topical.

•**lidofenin.** (LIE-doe-FEN-in) USAN.
Use: Diagnostic aid (hepatic function determination).

•**lidofilcon a.** (lih-DAH-FILL-kahn A) USAN.
Use: Contact lens material (hydrophilic).

•**lidofilcon b.** (lih-DAH-FILL-kahn B) USAN.
Use: Contact lens material (hydrophilic).

•**lidoflazine.** (LIE-dah-FLAY-zeen) USAN.
Use: Coronary vasodilator.

Lidopen Auto-Injector. (Survival Technical) Lidocaine hydrochloride 300 mg/ 3 mL. EDTA, methylparaben. Inj. (for IM adminstration). Automatic-injection device. *Rx.*
Use: Antiarrhythmic.

•**lidorestat.** (lye-DOE-res-tat) USAN.
Use: Selective aldose reductase inhibitor.

Lidosense 4. (River's Edge) Lidocaine 4%. Benzyl alcohol. Cream. 5 g, 15 g, 30 g. *OTC.*
Use: Local anesthetic, topical.

Lidosite Topical System. (B. Braun) Lidocaine hydrochloride 10%/epinephrine 0.1%. EDTA. Patch. Single-use patches. *Rx.*
Use: Anesthetic, local, topical.

Lidox Caps. (Major) Chlordiazepoxide hydrochloride 10 mg, clidinium bromide 2.5 mg. Cap. Bot. 100s, 500s, 1000s, UD 100s. *Rx.*
Use: Anticholinergic combination.

Lidoxide. (Henry Schein) Chlordiazepoxide hydrochloride 5 mg, clidinium bromide 2.5 mg. Tab. Bot. 100s, 500s. *Rx.*
Use: Anticholinergic combination.

lid scrubs.
Use: Cleanser, ophthalmic.
See: OCuSOFT.

•**lifarizine.** (lih-FAR-ih-ZEEN) USAN.
Use: Cerebral anti-ischemic; platelet aggregation inhibitor.

Lifer-B. (Burgin-Arden) Cyanocobalamin 30 mcg, liver inj. 0.1 mL, ferrous gluconate 100 mg, riboflavin 1.5 mg, panthenol 2.5 mg, niacinamide 100 mg, citric acid 16.4 mg, sodium citrate 23.6 mg/mL. Vial 30 mL. *Rx.*
Use: Mineral; vitamin supplement.

Life Saver Kit. (Whiteworth Towne) Ipecac syrup two 1 oz bottles, activated charcoal pow. 1 oz, poison treatment instruction booklet. *OTC.*
Use: Antidote; poisons.

Life Spanner. (Spanner) Vitamins A 12,500 units, D 400 units, E 5 units, B_1

10 mg, B_2 5 mg, B_6 2 mg, B_{12} 5 mcg, niacinamide 50 mg, calcium pantothenate 10 mg, biotin 10 mcg, C 100 mg, hesperidin complex 10 mg, rutin 20 mg, choline bitartrate 40 mg, inositol 30 mg, betaine anhydrous 15 mg, l-lysine monohydrochloride 25 mg, Fe 30 mg, Cu 1 mg, Mn 1 mg, K 5 mg, Ca 105 mg, P 82 mg, Mg 5.56 mg, Zn 1 mg. Cap. Bot. 100s. *OTC.*
Use: Mineral; vitamin supplement.

•**lifibrate.** (lih-FIE-brate) USAN.
Use: Antihyperlipoproteinemic.

•**lifibrol.** (lie-FIB-rahl) USAN.
Use: Hypercholesterolemic.

Lifol-B. (Burgin-Arden) Liver inj. 10 mcg, folic acid 1 mg, cyanocobalamin 100 mcg, phenol 0.5%/mL. Inj. Vial 10 mL. *Rx.*
Use: Nutritional supplement.

Lifolex. (Taylor Pharmaceuticals) Liver 10 mcg, cyanocobalamin 100 mcg, folic acid 5 mg/mL. Inj. Vial 10 mL. *Rx.*
Use: Nutritional supplement.

Lilly Bulk Products. (Eli Lilly) The following products are supplied by Eli Lilly under the USP, NF, or chemical name as a service to the health professions:
See: Ammoniated Mercury Oint.
   Amyl Nitrite.
   Analgesic Balm.
   Apomorphine hydrochloride.
   Aromatic Ammonia.
   Aromatic Elix.
   Atropine Sulfate.
   Bacitracin.
   Belladonna Tincture.
   Benzoin.
   Boric Acid.
   Calcium Gluceptate.
   Calcium Gluconate.
   Calcium Gluconate with Vitamin D.
   Calcium Hydroxide.
   Calcium Lactate.
   Carbarsone.
   Cascara, Aromatic, Fluid Extract.
   Cascara Sagrada, Fluid Extract.
   Citrated Caffeine.
   Cocaine Hydrochloride.
   Codeine Phosphate.
   Codeine Sulfate.
   Colchicine.
   Compound Benzoin.
   Dibasic Calcium Phosphate.
   Diethylstilbestrol.
   Ephedrine Sulfate.
   Ferrous Gluconate.
   Ferrous Sulfate.
   Folic Acid.
   Glucagon for Inj.

Green Soap Tincture.
Heparin Sodium.
Histamine Phosphate.
Ipecac.
Isoniazid.
Isopropyl Alcohol, 91%.
Liver.
Magnesium Sulfate.
Mercuric Oxide, Yellow.
Methadone Hydrochloride.
Methenamine for Timed Burning.
Methyltestosterone.
Milk of Bismuth.
Morphine Sulfate.
Myrrh.
Neomycin Sulfate.
Niacin.
Niacinamide.
Nitroglycerin.
Opium (Deodorized)
Ox Bile Extract.
Pancreatin.
Papaverine hydrochloride.
Paregoric.
Penicillin G Potassium.
Phenobarbital.
Phenobarbital Sodium.
Potassium Cl.
Potassium Iodide.
Powder Papers (Glassine).
Progesterone.
Propylthiouracil.
Protamine Sulfate.
Pyridoxine Hydrochloride.
Quinidine Gluconate.
Quinidine Sulfate.
Quinine Sulfate.
Riboflavin.
Silver Nitrate.
Sodium Bicarbonate.
Sodium Chloride.
Sodium Salicylate.
Streptomycin Sulfate.
Sulfadiazine.
Sulfapyridine.
Sulfur.
Terpin Hydrate.
Terpin Hydrate and Codeine.
Testosterone Propionate.
Thiamine Hydrochloride.
Thyroid.
Tubocurarine Hydrochloride.
Tylosterone.
Whitfield's Oint.
Wild Cherry Syrup.
Zinc Oxide.
limarsol.
  See: Acetarsone.
Limbitrol. (Roche) Chlordiazepoxide
  5 mg, amitriptyline hydrochloride
  12.5 mg. Tab. Bot. 100s, 500s, *Tel-E-*

Dose 100s, Prescription pak 50s. *c-IV.*
  Use: Psychotherapeutic agent.
Limbitrol DS. (Roche) Chlordiazepoxide
  10 mg, amitriptyline hydrochloride
  25 mg. Tab. Bot. 100s, 500s, *Tel-E-*
  Dose 100s, Prescription pak 50s. *c-IV.*
  Use: Psychotherapeutic agent.
Limbrel. (Primus) Flavocoxid 250 mg.
  Dextrose, maltodextrin. Cap. 60s. *Rx.*
  Use: Nutrition supplement.
•**lime.** *USP 28.*
  Use: Pharmaceutical necessity.
•**lime solution, sulfurated.** *USP 28.*
  Use: Scabicide.
lime sulfur solution. Calcium poly-
  sulfide, calcium thiosulfate.
  Use: Wet dressing.
•**linarotene.** (lin-AHR-oh-teen) USAN.
  Use: Antikeratolytic.
Lincocin. (Pharmacia) Lincomycin hydro-
  chloride. Cap.: 500 mg. Bot. 100s.
  Soln.: 300 mg/mL. Benzyl alcohol
  9.45 mg/mL. Vial 2 mL, 10 mL. *Rx.*
  Use: Anti-infective.
•**lincomycin.** (LIN-koe-MY-sin) *USP 28.*
  Antibiotic produced by *Streptomyces
  lincolnensis* variant.
  Use: Anti-infective; infections due to
  gram-positive organisms.
•**lincomycin hydrochloride.** (LIN-koe-
  MY-sin) *USP 28.*
  Use: Anti-infective.
  See: Lincocin.
    Lincorex.
lincomycin hydrochloride. (Steris)
  Lincomycin hydrochloride 300 mg/mL.
  Inj. Vial 10 mL. *Rx.*
  Use: Anti-infective.
Lincorex. (Hyrex) Lincomycin hydrochlo-
  ride 300 mg/mL. Benzyl alcohol
  9.45 mg/mL. Inj. Vial 10 mL. *Rx.*
  Use: Anti-Infective.
•**lindane.** (LIN-dane) *USP 28.* Gamma-
  benzene-hexachloride; hexachlorocy-
  clohexane.
  Use: Pediculicide, scabicide.
lindane. (Various Mfr.) Lindane. Lot.: 1%.
  30 mL, 59 mL, pharmacy-size only pint.
  Shampoo: 1%. 30 mL, 59 mL, phar-
  macy-size only pint. *Rx.*
  Use: Pediculicide, scabicide.
Lindora. (Bristol-Myers Squibb) Sodium
  laureth sulfate, cocamide DEA, sodium
  Cl, lactic acid, tetra sodium EDTA,
  benzophenone-4, FD&C Blue No. 1.
  Bot. 8 oz. *OTC.*
  Use: Dermatologic, cleanser.
•**linezolid.** (lin-EH-zoe-lid) USAN.
  Use: Anti-infective, oxalodinone.
  See: Zyvox.

Linodil. (Sanofi-Synthelabo) Inositol hexanicotinate. Cap. *Rx.*
Use: Hyperlipidemic; peripheral vasodilator.

•**linogliride.** (lie-no-GLIE-ride) USAN.
Use: Antidiabetic.

•**linogliride fumarate.** (lih-no-GLIE-ride) USAN.
Use: Antidiabetic.

•**linopirdine.** (lih-no-PIHR-deen) USAN.
Use: Treatment of Alzheimer disease (cognition enhancer).

Lioresal. (Novartis) Baclofen 10 mg, 20 mg. Tab. Bot. 100s, UD 100s. *Rx.*
Use: Muscle relaxant.

Lioresal Intrathecal. (Medtronic) 0.05 mg/mL (50 mcg/mL), 10 mg/20 mL (500 mcg/mL), 10 mg/5 mL (2000 mcg/mL), preservative free. Single-use amps. 1 amp refill kit (10 mg/20 mL only), 2 and 4 amp refill kits (10 mg/5 mL only). *Rx.*
Use: Musle relaxant.

•**liothyronine I 131.** (lie-oh-THIGH-row-neen) USAN.
Use: Radiopharmaceutical.

•**liothyronine I 125.** (lie-oh-THIGH-row-neen) USAN.
Use: Radiopharmaceutical.

•**liothyronine sodium.** (lie-oh-THIGH-row-neen) *USP 28.*
Use: Hormone, thyroid.
See: Cytomel.
   Triostat.

liothyronine sodium injection.
Use: Myxedema coma/precoma. [Orphan Drug]

•**liotrix.** (LIE-oh-trix) *USP 28.*
Use: Hormone, thyroid.
See: Thyrolar.

lipase.
Use: Digestive enzyme.
W/Alpha-amylase W-100, proteinase W-300, cellase W-100, estrone, testosterone, vitamins, minerals.
See: Kutrase.
   Ku-Zyme.
W/Amylase, bile salts, wilzyme, pepsin, pancreatin, calcium.
See: Enzyme.
W/Amylase, protease.
See: Creon.
   Kutrase.
   Ku-Zyme.
   Lipram.
   Palcaps 10.
   Palcaps 20.
   Pancrelipase.
   Panocaps.
   Panocaps MT 16.

Panocaps MT 20.
PAN-2400.
Ultrase.
Ultrase MT 18.
Ultrase MT 12.
Ultrase MT 20.
Viokase.
W/Amylolytic, proteolytic, cellulolytic enzymes.
See: Arco-Lase.
W/Amylolytic, proteolytic, cellulolytic enzymes, phenobarbital, hyoscyamine sulfate, atropine sulfate.
See: Arco-Lase Plus.
W/Pancreatin, protease, amylase.
See: Dizymes.

lipid/DNA human cystic fibrosis gene. (Genzyme)
Use: Cystic fibrosis. [Orphan Drug]

lipids.
Use: Intravenous nutritional therapy.
See: Intralipid 10%.
   Intralipid 20%.
   Liposyn II 10%.
   Liposyn II 20%.
   Liposyn III 10%.
   Liposyn III 20%.

Lipisorb. (Bristol-Myers Squibb) Protein 35 g/L, fat 48 g/L, carbohydrates 115 g/L, Na 733.3 mg/L, K 1250 mg/L, H_2O 320 mOsm/kg. With appropriate vitamins and minerals. 1 calorie/mL. Vanilla flavored. Pow. Can 1 lb. *OTC.*
Use: Nutritional supplement.

Lipitor. (Pfizer) Atorvastatin calcium (as base) 10 mg, 20 mg, 40 mg, 80 mg, lactose. Film-coated. Tab. Bot. 90s, 500s (40 mg, 80 mg only), 5000s (10 mg, 20 mg only), UD 100s (except 40 mg, 80 mg). *Rx.*
Use: Antihyperlipidemic; HMG-CoA reductase inhibitor.

Lipkote by Coppertone. (Schering-Plough) Padimate O, oxybenzone. SPF 15. Lip balm 4.2 g. *OTC.*
Use: Sunscreen.

Lipkote SPF 15 Ultra Sunscreen Lipbalm. (Schering-Plough) Tube 0.15 oz. *OTC.*
Use: Sunscreen.

Lip Medex. (Blairex) Petrolatum, camphor 1%, phenol 0.54%, cocoa butter, lanolin. Oint. 210 g. *OTC.*
Use: Fever blisters; lip protectant.

lipocholine.
See: Choline dihydrogen citrate.

Lipoflavonoid. (Numark) Vitamins C 100 mg, B_1 0.33 mg, B_2 0.33 mg, B_3 3.33 mg, B_5 1.66 mg, B_6 0.33 mg, B_{12} 1.66 mcg, choline 111 mg, bioflavonoids 100 mg, inositol 111 mg. Capl. Bot.

100s, 500s. *OTC.*
Use: Vitamin supplement.
Lipoflavonoid. (Numark) Choline 111 mg, inositol 111 mg, vitamins B_1 0.3 mg, B_2 0.3 mg, B_3 3.3 mg, B_5 1.7 mg, B_6 0.3 mg, B_{12} 1.7 mcg, C 100 mg, lemon bioflavonoid complex. Cap. Bot. 100s, 500s. *OTC.*
Use: Vitamin supplement.
Lipogen. (Ivax) Choline 111 mg, inositol 111 mg, vitamins B_1 0.33 mg, B_2 0.33 mg, B_3 3.33 mg, B_5 1.7 mg, B_6 0.33 mg, B_{12} 1.7 mcg, C 20 mg, A 1667 units, E 10 units, Zn 30 mg, Cu, Se. Capl. Bot. 60s. *OTC.*
Use: Mineral, vitamin supplement.
Lipogen. (Various Mfr.) Choline 111 mg, inositol, vitamins B_1 0.33 mg, B_2 0.33 mg, B_3 3.33 mg, B_5 1.7 mg, B_6 0.33 mg, B_{12} 1.7 mcg, C 100 mg. Cap. Bot. 60s. *OTC.*
Use: Vitamin supplement.
• **lipoic acid, alpha.** (li-POE-ik) *NF 23.*
Use: Dietary supplement.
Lipomul. (Pharmacia) Corn oil 10 g/ 15 mL, d-alpha tocopheryl acetate, butylated hydroxyanisole, polysorbate 80, glyceride phosphates, sodium saccharin, sodium benzoate 0.05%, benzoic acid 0.05%, sorbic acid 0.07%. Bot. Pt. *OTC.*
Use: Nutritional supplement.
Lipo-Nicin/100 mg. (AstraZeneca) Nicotinic acid 100 mg, niacinamide 75 mg, vitamins C 150 mg, B_1 25 mg, B_2 2 mg, B_6 10 mg. Tab. Bot. 100s, 500s. *Rx.*
Use: Vasodilator combination.
Lipo-Nicin/300 mg. (AstraZeneca) Niacin 300 mg, vitamin C 150 mg, B_1 25 mg, B_2 2 mg, B_6 10 mg TR Cap. 100s. *Rx.*
Use: Vasodilator.
Liponol. (Rugby) Choline, inositol 83 mg, methionine 110 mg, vitamins B_1 3 mg, B_2 3 mg, B_3 10 mg, B_5 2 mg, B_6 2 mg, B_{12} 2 mcg, desiccated liver 56 mg, liver concentrate 30 mg, sorbitol, lecithin. Cap. Bot. 60s. *OTC.*
Use: Nutritional supplement.
lipopeptides.
Use: Anti-infectives.
See: Daptomycin.
liposomal amphotericin B.
Use: Antiviral. [Orphan Drug]
liposomal doxorubicin.
See: Doxorubicin hydrochloride.
liposome encapsulated recombinant interleukin-2. (Biomerica)
Use: Antineoplastic. [Orphan Drug]
Liposyn. (Abbott Hospital Products) Intravenous fat emulsion containing

safflower oil 10%, egg phosphatides 1.2%, glycerin 2.5% in water for inj. **10%:** Single-dose container 50 mL, 100 mL, 200 mL, 500 mL; Syringe Pump Unit 50 mL single-dose. **20%:** Single-dose container 200 mL, 500 mL Syringe Pump Unit 25 mL, 50 mL single-dose. *Rx.*
Use: Nutritional supplement, parenteral.
Liposyn III. (Hospira) Oil, soybean, egg yolk phospholipids. **10%:** 100, 200, 500 mL. **20%:** 100, 500 mL. *Rx.*
Use: Nutritional supplement, parenteral.
Liposyn II. (Hospira) Intravenous fat emulsion: **10%:** Safflower oil 5%, soybean oil 5%. Bot. 100 mL, 200 mL, 500 mL. **20%:** Safflower oil 10%, soybean oil 10%, egg phosphatides 1.2%, glycerin 2.5%. 200 mL, 500 mL. Bot. Syringe pump unit 25 mL, 50 ml. *Rx.*
Use: Nutritional supplement, parenteral.
Lipo-Tears. (Spectra Pharmaceuticals) Mineral oil, petrolatum, preservative free. Drops. Bot. 1 mL. 30s. *OTC.*
Use: Lubricant, ophthalmic.
Lipotriad. (Numark) Zn 30 mg, vitamin A 5000 units, C 60 mg, E 30 units, Cu, Se, B_3 20 mg, B_1 1.5 mg, B_2 1.7 mg, B_6 2 mg, B_{12} 6 mcg, B_5 10 mg, choline bitartrate, inositol. Capl. Bot. 60s. *OTC.*
Use: Mineral, vitamin supplement.
lipotropics with vitamins.
Use: Nutritional supplement.
See: Cholidase.
    Cholinoid.
    Lipoflavonoid.
    Lipogen.
    Liponol.
    Lipotriad.
    Methatropic.
Lipoxide. (Major) Chlordiazepoxide hydrochloride 5 mg, 10 mg, 25 mg. Cap. Bot. 100s, 500s, 1000s. *c-iv.*
Use: Anxiolytic.
Lipram. (Global) **Lipram-CR5:** Lipase 5000 U, amylase 16,600 U, protease 18,750 U. **Lipram-CR10:** Lipase 10,000 U, amylase 33,200 U, protease 37,500 U. **Lipram-CR20:** Lipase 20,000 U, amylase 66,400 U, protease 75,000 U. **Lipram-PN16:** Lipase 16,000 U, amylase 48,000 U, protease 48,000 U. **Lipram-PN10:** Lipase 10,000 U, amylase 30,000 U, protease 30,000 U. **Lipram-PN20:** Lipase 20,000 U, amylase 56,000 U, protease 44,000. **Lipram-UL12:** Lipase 12,000 U, amylase 39,000 U, protease 39,000 U. **Lipram-UL18:** Lipase 18,000 U, amylase 58,500 U, protease 58,500 U. **Lipram-UL20:** Lipase

20,000 U, amylase 65,000 U, protease 65,000 U. **Lipram 4500:** Lipase 4500 U, amylase 20,000 U, protease 25,000 U.DR Cap. Bot. 100s, 250s (4500, CR5, CR10, CR20 only), 500s (UL 20 only). *Rx.*
Use: Digestive enzyme.

Liqua-Gel. (Paddock) Boric acid, glycerine, propylene glycol, methylparaben, propylparaben, Irish moss extract, methylcellulose. Bot. 4 oz, 16 oz. *OTC.*

Liquibid. (Capellon) Guaifenesin 400 mg. Tab. 100s. *Rx.*
Use: Expectorant.

Liquibid-D. (Capellon) Guaifenesin 600 mg, phenylephrine hydrochloride 40 mg. Tab. Bot. 100s. *Rx.*
Use: Upper respiratory combination, decongestant, expectorant.

Liquibid-D 1200. (Capellon) Phenylephrine hydrochloride 40 mg, guaifenesin 1200 mg. SR Tab. 100s. *Rx.*
Use: Decongestant and expectorant.

Liquibid-PD. (Capellon) Phenylephrine hydrochloride 25 mg, guaifenesin 275 mg. SR Tab. 100s. *Rx.*
Use: Decongestant and expectorant.

Liqui-Char. (Jones Pharma) Activated charcoal. **Liq. Bot.:** 12.5 g/60 mL, 15 g/75 mL. **Squeeze container:** 25 g/120 mL, 50 g/240 mL, 30 g/120 mL. *OTC.*
Use: Antidote.

Liqui-Coat HD. (Mallinckrodt) Barium sulfate 210%, simethicone, sorbitol, saccharin, sodium benzoate, vanilla-raspberry flavor. Susp. UD Bot. 150 mL. *Rx.*
Use: Radiopaque agent, GI contrast agent.

Liquid Barosperse. (Mallinckrodt) Barium sulfate 60%, simethicone, vanilla flavor. Susp. Bot. 355 mL, 1900 mL. *Rx.*
Use: Radiopaque agent, GI contrast agent.

Liquid Geritonic. (Roberts) Fe 105 mg, liver fraction 1 375 mg, B_1 3 mg, B_2 3 mg, B_3 30 mg, B_6 0.3 mg, B_{12} 9 mcg, inositol 60 mg, glycine 180 mg, yeast concentrate 375 mg, Ca, I, K, Mg, Mn, P, alcohol 20%. Liq. Bot. 240 mL, gal. *OTC.*
Use: Nutritional supplement.

Liquid Lather. (Ulmer Pharmacal) Gentle wash for hands, body, face, hair. Bot. 8 oz, gal. *OTC.*
Use: Cleanser.

Liqui-Doss. (Ferndale) Mineral oil in emulsifying base, alcohol free. Emulsion. Bot. 60 mL, 480 mL. *OTC.*

Use: Laxative.

Liquid PedvaxHIB. (Merck) *Haemophilus* b PRP 7.5 mcg, *Neisseria meningitidis* OMPC 125 mcg, aluminum hydroxide 225 mcg/0.5 mL. Inj. Single-dose vial. *Rx.*
Use: Immunization, bacterial vaccine.

liquid petrolatum emulsion.
See: Mineral Oil Emulsion.

Liquid Pred. (Muro) Prednisone 5 mg/5 mL in syrup base. Alcohol 5%, saccharin, sorbitol. Syr. Bot. 120 mL, 240 mL. *Rx.*
Use: Corticosteroid.

Liquifilm Forte. (Allergan) Polyvinyl alcohol 3%, thimerosal 0.002%, EDTA, sodium Cl. Soln. Bot. 15 mL, 30 mL. *OTC.*
Use: Artificial tears.

Liquifilm Tears. (Allergan) Polyvinyl alcohol 1.4%, chlorobutanol 0.5%, sodium Cl. Bot. 15 mL, 30 mL. *OTC.*
Use: Artificial tears.

Liquifilm Wetting Solution. (Allergan) Polyvinyl alcohol, hydroxypropyl methylcellulose, edetate disodium, sodium Cl, potassium Cl, benzalkonium Cl 0.004%. Bot. 60 mL. *OTC.*
Use: Contact lens care.

Liquimat. (Galderma) Sulfur 5%, SD alcohol 40 22%, cetyl alcohol in drying makeup base. Plastic Bot. 45 mL. *OTC.*
Use: Dermatologic, acne.

Liquipake. (Lafayette) Barium sulfate suspension 100% w/v for dilution. Bot. 1850 mL, Case 4s.
Use: Radiopaque agent.

Liquiprin. (Menley & James Labs, Inc.) Acetaminophen 80 mg/1.66 mL, saccharin. Soln. Bot. 35 mL w/dropper. *OTC.*
Use: Analgesic.

liquor carbonis detergens.
See: Coal Tar Topical Soln.

• **lisadimate.** (liss-AD-ih-mate) USAN.
Use: Sunscreen.

• **lisinopril.** (lie-SIN-oh-pril) *USP 28.*
Use: Antihypertensive.
See: Prinivil.
Zestril.
W/Hydrochlorothiazide.
See: Prinzide.
Zestoretic.

lisinopril. (Various Mfr.) Lisinopril 2.5 mg, 5 mg, 10 mg, 20 mg, 30 mg, 40 mg. Tab. 100s, 500s (2.5 mg, 30 mg, 40 mg only), 1000s, UD 100s (40 mg only). *Rx.*
Use: Antihypertensive.

lisinopril/hydrochlorothiazide. (Various Mfr.) Lisinopril/hydrochlorothiazide 10 mg/12.5 mg, 20 mg/12.5 mg, 20 mg/

25 mg. Tab. 100s, 500s, 1000s, UD 100s. *Rx.*
Use: Antihypertensive combination.

•**lisofylline.** (lie-SO-fih-lin) USAN.
Use: Immunomodulator.

Listerine Antiseptic. (Warner Lambert) Thymol 0.06%, eucalyptol 0.09%, methyl salicylate 0.06%, menthol 0.04%. Alcohol 26.9% (regular flavor), 21.6% (cool mint flavor), sorbitol, saccharin. Bot. 90 mL, 180 mL, 360 mL, 540 mL, 720 mL, 960 mL, 1440 mL. *OTC.*
Use: Mouthwash, antiseptic.

Listerine, Natural Citrus. (Pfizer Consumer) Thymol 0.064%, eucalyptol 0.092%, methyl salicylate 0.06%, menthol 0.042%. Alcohol 21.6%, sorbitol, sucralose. Mouthwash. 250 mL, 500 mL, 1 L, 1.5 L. *OTC.*
Use: Mouth and throat product.

Listerine, Tartar Control. (Pfizer Consumer) Thymol 0.064%, eucalyptol 0.092%, methyl salicylate 0.06%, menthol 0.042%. Alcohol 21.6%, sorbitol, sucralose. Wintermint flavor. Mouthwash. 250 mL, 500 mL, 1 L, 1.5 L. *OTC.*
Use: Mouth and throat product.

Listermint Arctic Mint Mouthwash. (Warner Lambert) Glycerin, poloxamer 335, PEG 600, sodium lauryl sulfate, sodium benzoate, benzoic acid, zinc chloride, saccharin. Liq. 946 mL. *OTC.*
Use: Antiseptic, mouthwash.

Lite Pred. (Horizon) Prednisolone sodium phosphate 0.125%. Soln. Bot. 5 mL. *Rx.*
Use: Corticosteroid, ophthalmic.

lithium. (Various Mfr.) Lithium carbonate 300 mg (lithium 8.12 mEq). May contain sorbitol. ER Tab. 100s, 500s. *Rx.*
Use: Antipsychotic agent.

•**lithium carbonate.** (LITH-ee-uhm CARboe-nate) USP 28.
Use: Antipsychotic, manic-depressive state; antimanic; antidepressant.
See: Eskalith.
Lithonate.
Lithotabs.

lithium carbonate. (Roxane) Lithium carbonate. **ER Tab.:** 450 mg. 100s. **Tab.:** 300 mg. Bot. 100s, 1000s, UD 100s. **Cap.:** 150 mg, 300 mg, 600 mg. Bot. 100s, 1000s, UD 100s. *Rx.*
Use: Antipsychotic, manic-depressive state; antimanic; antidepressant.

•**lithium citrate.** (LITH-ee-uhm) USP 28.
Use: Antimanic.

lithium citrate. (Various Mfr.) Lithium citrate 8 mEq (equivalent to 300 mg lith-

ium carbonate)/5 mL. Syr. Bot. 480 mL, 500 mL, UD 5 mL, 10 mL. *Rx.*
Use: Antipsychotic.

•**lithium hydroxide.** (LITH-ee-uhm high-DROX-ide) USP 28.
Use: Antipsychotic, manic-depressive state; antimanic; antidepressant.

Lithonate. (Solvay) Lithium carbonate 300 mg. Cap. Bot. 100s, 1000s, UD 100s. *Rx.*
Use: Antipsychotic.

Lithostat. (Mission Pharmacal) Acetohydroxamic acid 250 mg. Tab. Bot. 100s. *Rx.*
Use: Anti-infective; urinary.

Lithotabs. (Solvay) Lithium carbonate 300 mg. Tab. Bot. 100s, 1000s, UD 100s. *Rx.*
Use: Antipsychotic.

Little Colds Cough Formula. (Vetco) Dextromethorphan hydrobromide 7.5 mg per mL. Glycerin, corn syrup. Natural grape flavor. Drops. 30 mL. *OTC.*
Use: Nonnarcotic antitussive.

Little Colds for Infants and Children. (Vetco) Phenylephrine hydrochloride 0.25%, sorbitol, sucralose, grape flavor, alcohol free. Soln. Oral Drops. Bot. 30 mL w/dropper. *OTC.*
Use: Nasal decongestant, arylalkylamine.

Little Noses Gentle Formula, Infants & Children. (Vetco) Phenylephrine hydrochloride 0.125%, EDTA, benzalkonuim chloride, alcohol free. Soln. Drops. Bot. 15 mL w/dropper. *OTC.*
Use: Nasal decongestant, arylalkylamine.

Livec. (Enzyme Process) Vitamins A 5000 units, B₁ 1.5 mg, B₂ 1.7 mg, niacin 20 mg, C 60 mg, B₆ 2 mg, pantothenic acid 10 mg, E 30 units, B₁₂ 6 mcg, Ca 250 mg, Fe 5 mg, D 400 units, folacin 0.075 mg/3 Tab. Bot. 100s, 300s. *OTC.*
Use: Mineral, vitamin supplement.

Liverbex. (Spanner) Liver 2 mcg, vitamins B₁, B₂, B₆, B₁₂, niacinamide, pantothenate/mL. Vial 30 mL. *OTC.*
Use: Nutritional supplement.

liver desiccated. Desiccated liver substance.

liver extract. Dry liver extract w/Vitamin B₁₂, folic acid.

liver function agents.
See: Iodophthalein.
Sulfobromophthalein Sodium.

Livergran. (Rawl) Desiccated whole liver 9 g, vitamins B₁ 18 mg, B₂ 36 mg, niacinamide 90 mg, choline bitartrate

216 mg, B_6 3.6 mg, calcium pantothenate 3.6 mg, inositol 90 mg, biotin 6 mcg, vitamins B_{12} 5.4 mcg, methionine 198 mg, arginine 242 mg, cysteine 72 mg, glutamic acid 675 mg, histidine 99 mg, isoleucine 333 mg, leucine 495 mg, lysine 297 mg, phenylalanine 189 mg, threonine 333 mg, tryptophan 45 mg, tyrosine 180 mg, valine 306 mg/3 Tsp. Bot. 15 oz. *OTC.*
Use: Nutritional supplement.

liver injection. (Various Mfr.) Liver extract for parenteral use. *Rx.*
Use: Parenteral liver supplement.

liver injection. (Arcum; Lederle Laboratories) Vitamin B_{12} 20 mcg/mL. Vial 10 mL. *Rx.*
Use: Nutritional supplement.

Liver Injection, Crude. (Eli Lilly and Co.) 2 mcg/mL. Vial 30 mL; (Medwick) 2 mcg/mL. Vial 30 mL. *Rx.*
Use: Liver supplement.

Liver Iron Vitamins. (Arcum) Liver inj. (10 mcg B_{12} activity/mL) 0.1 mL, crude liver inj. (2 mcg B_{12} activity/mL) 0.125 mL, green ferric ammonium citrate 20 mg, niacinamide 50 mg, vitamin B_6 0.3 mg, B_2 0.3 mg, procaine hydrochloride 0.5%, phenol 0.5%/2 mL. Inj. Vial 30 mL. *Rx.*
Use: Nutritional supplement.

Liver, Refined. (Medwick) 20 mcg/mL. Vial 10 mL, 30 mL. *Rx.*
Use: Nutritional supplement.

liver vasoconstrictor.
See: Kutapressin.

Livifol. (Oxypure) Vitamin B_{12} activity from liver inj. equivalent to cyanocobalamin 10 mcg, folic acid 1 mg, cyanocobalamin 100 mcg/mL. Vial 10 mL. *Rx.*
Use: Vitamin supplement.

Livitrinsic-f. (Ivax) Iron 110 mg, vitamins B_{12} 15 mcg, C 75 mg, intrinsic factor concentrate 240 mg, folic acid 0.5 mg. Cap. Bot. 100s, 1000s. *Rx.*
Use: Mineral, vitamin supplement.

•**lixazinone sulfate.** (lix-AZE-ih-NOHN) USAN.
Use: Cardiotonic (phosphodiesterase inhibitor).

•**lixivaptan.** (lix-i-VAP-tan) USAN.
Use: Nonhypovolemic hyponatremia.

Lixoil. (Lixoil Labs.) Sulfonated fatty oils and one or more esters of higher fatty acids. Bot. 16 oz. *OTC.*
Use: Dermatologic.

LKV-Drops. (Freeda) Vitamins A 5000 units, D 400 units, E 2 mg, B_1 1.5 mg, B_2 1.5 mg, B_3 10 mg, B_5 2 mg, B_6 2 mg, B_{12} 6 mcg, C 50 mg, biotin 50 mcg/0.6 mL. Bot. 60 mL. *OTC.*
Use: Vitamin supplement.

LKV Infant Drops. (Freeda) Vitamins A 2500 units, D 400 units, E 5 units, B_1 1 mg, B_2 1 mg, B_3 10 mg, B_5 3 mg, B_6 1 mg, B_{12} 4 mcg, C 50 mg, biotin 75 mcg/0.5 mL. Bot. 60 mL. *OTC.*
Use: Vitamin supplement.

lld factor.
See: Vitamin B_{12}.

L-leucovorin.
Use: Antineoplastic.
See: Isovorin.

L-Lysine. (Various Mfr.) L-lysine 312 mg, 500 mg. Tab. Bot. 100s. 1000 mg. Tab. Bot. 60s. 500 mg. Cap. Bot. 100s, 250s. *OTC.*
Use: Dietary supplement; amino acid.

LMD. (Abbott) Dextran 40 10%. 500 mL. With 0.9% sodium chloride or in 5% dextrose. *Rx.*
Use: Plasma volume expander.

lm-427. Ribabutin.
Use: CDC anti-infective agent.

LMWD-Dextran 40. (Pharmachemie USA, Inc.) Normal saline 0.9%, dextrose 10%. *Rx.*
Use: Plasma volume expander.

L-M-X4. (Ferndale) Lidocaine 4% (40 mg/g), benzyl alcohol. Cream. Tube 5 g, 30 g. *OTC.*
Use: Anesthetic, local.

Lobac. (Seatrace) Salicylamide 200 mg, phenyltoloxamine 20 mg, acetaminophen 300 mg. Cap. Bot. 100s. *Rx.*
Use: Analgesic, muscle relaxant.

Lobak. (Sanofi-Synthelabo) Chlormezanone 250 mg, acetaminophen 300 mg. Tab. 40s, 100s, 1000s. *Rx.*
Use: Anxiolytic; analgesic.

Lobana Body. (Ulmer Pharmacal) Mineral oil, triethanolamine stearate, stearic acid, lanolin, cetyl alcohol, potassium stearate, propylene glycol, parabens. Lot. Bot. 120, 240 mL, gal. *OTC.*
Use: Emollient.

Lobana Body Shampoo. (Ulmer Pharmacal) Chloroxylenol. Bot. 240 mL, gal. *OTC.*
Use: Dermatologic, hair and skin.

Lobana Conditioning Shampoo. (Ulmer Pharmacal) Bot. 8 oz, gal. *OTC.*
Use: Dermatologic, hair and scalp.

Lobana Derm-Ade. (Ulmer Pharmacal) Vitamin A, D, E. Cream Jar 2 oz, 8 oz. *OTC.*
Use: Dermatologic; counterirritant.

Lobana Liquid Lather. (Ulmer Pharmacal) Sodium laureth sulfate, sodium lauroyl sarcosinate, sodium myristyl

sarcosonate, lauramide DEA, linoleamide DEA, octyl hydroxystearate, polyquaternium 7, tetrasodium EDTA, quaternium 15, sodium chloride, citric acid. Liq. Bot. 240 mL, gal. *OTC.*
Use: Cleanser.

Lobana Peri-Gard. (Ulmer Pharmacal) Water-resistant ointment containing vitamins A & D. Oint. Jar 2 oz, 8 oz. *OTC.*
Use: Dermatologic, protectant.

Lobana Perineal Cleanser. (Ulmer Pharmacal) Sprayer 4 oz, 8 oz. Bot. Gal. *OTC.*
Use: Urine and fecal cleanser.

•**lobenzarit sodium.** (low-BENZ-ah-RIT) USAN.
Use: Antirheumatic.

Lobidram. (Dram) Lobeline sulfate 2 mg. Tab. Pkg. 15s, 30s. *OTC.*
Use: Smoking cessation aid.

•**lobucavir.** (lah-BYOO-kah-vihr) USAN.
Use: Antiviral.

LoCHOLEST. (Warner Chilcott) Cholestyramine resin 4 g/9 g, fructose, sorbitol, sucrose, strawberry flavor. Pow. for Susp. Pouch 9 g (60s), Can 378 g. *Rx.*
Use: Antihyperlipidemic; bile acid sequestrant.

LoCHOLEST Light. (Warner Chilcott) Cholestyramine resin 4 g/5.7 g, aspartame, fructose, mannitol, sorbitol, phenylalanine 3.93 mg/g, strawberry flavor. Pow. for Susp. Pouch 5.7 g (60s), Can 239.4 g. *Rx.*
Use: Antihyperlipidemic; bile acid sequestrant.

Locoid. (Ferndale) **Cream:** Hydrocortisone butyrate 0.1%. Tube 15 g, 45 g. **Oint.:** Hydrocortisone butyrate 0.1%. Tube 15 g, 45 g. **Soln.:** Hydrocortisone butyrate 0.1%, isopropyl alcohol 50%, glycerin, povidone. Bot. 20 mL, 60 mL. *Rx.*
Use: Corticosteroid, topical.

•**lodelaben.** (low-DELL-ah-ben) USAN.
Formerly Declaben.
Use: Antiarthritic; emphysema therapy adjunct.

•**lodenosine.** (loh-DEN-oh-seen) USAN.
Use: Antiviral (HIV reverse transcriptase inhibitor).

Lodine. (Wyeth-Ayerst) **Cap.:** Etodolac 200 mg, 300 mg, lactose. Bot. 100s, UD 100s. **Tab.:** Etodolac 400 mg, 500 mg, lactose. Bot. 100s, UD 100s. *Rx.*
Use: Analgesic, NSAID.

Lodine XL. (Wyeth-Ayerst) Etodolac 400 mg, 500 mg, 600 mg, lactose. ER Tab. Bot. 100s, UD 100s. *Rx.*

Use: Analgesic, NSAID.

Lodosyn. (Bristol-Myers Squibb Primary Care) Carbidopa 25 mg. Tab. Bot. 100s. *Rx.*
Use: Antiparkinsonian.

•**Iodoxamide ethyl.** (low-DOX-ah-mide ETH-uhl) USAN.
Use: Antiasthmatic, antiallergic, bronchodilator.

•**Iodoxamide tromethamine.** (low-DOX-ah-mide troe-METH-ah-meen) USAN.
Use: Antiasthmatic, antiallergic, bronchodilator; vernal keratoconjunctivitis.
See: Alomide.

Lodrane. (ECR) Pseudoephedrine hydrochloride 60 mg, brompheniramine maleate 4 mg/5 mL, cherry flavor, alcohol and dye free. Liq. Bot. 473 mL *Rx.*
Use: Upper respiratory combination, decongestant, antihistamine.

Lodrane D. (ECR) Pseudoephedrine tannate 90 mg, brompheniramine tannate 8 mg per 5 mL. Alcohol free, sugar free. Strawberry flavor. Susp. 473 mL. *Rx.*
Use: Decongestant and antihistamine.

Lodrane LD. (ECR) Brompheniramine maleate 6 mg, pseudoephedrine hydrochloride 60 mg, dye free. Cap. Bot. 100s. *Rx.*
Use: Upper respiratory combination, antihistamine, decongestant.

Lodrane 12 D. (ECR) Pseudoephedrine hydrochloride 45 mg, brompheniramine maleate 6 mg, dye free. ER Tab. 100s. *Rx.*
Use: Decongestant and antihistamine.

Lodrane 24. (ECR Pharmaceuticals) Brompheniramine maleate 12 mg. ER Cap. 100s. *Rx.*
Use: Antihistamine.

Lodrane XR. (ECR Pharmaceuticals) Brompheniramine tannate 8 mg/5 mL. Alcohol free, sugar free. Strawberry flavor. Oral Susp. Pints, 10 mL. *Rx.*
Use: Antihistamine.

Loestrin Fe 1/20. (Duramed) Norethindrone acetate 1 mg, ethinyl estradiol 20 mcg, lactose, sugar (active tablets), sucrose (inert tablets), ferrous fumarate 75 mg (brown tab. only). Tab. Pack 28s. *Rx.*
Use: Sex hormone, contraceptive hormone.

Loestrin Fe 1.5/30. (Duramed) Norethindrone acetate 1.5 mg, ethinyl estradiol 30 mcg, lactose, sugar (active tablets), sucrose (inert tablets), ferrous fumarate 75 mg (brown tab. only). Tab. Pack 28s. *Rx.*
Use: Sex hormone, contraceptive hormone.

Loestrin 21 1/20. (Duramed) Norethindrone acetate 1 mg, ethinyl estradiol 20 mcg, lactose, sugar. Tab. Packs 21s. *Rx.*
Use: Sex hormone, contraceptive hormone.

Loestrin 21 1.5/30. (Duramed) Norethindrone acetate 1.5 mg, ethinyl estradiol 30 mcg, lactose, sugar. Tab. Packs 21s. *Rx.*
Use: Sex hormone, contraceptive hormone.

•**lofemizole hydrochloride.** (low-FEM-ih-ZOLE) USAN.
Use: Anti-inflammatory; analgesic; antipyretic.

•**lofentanil oxalate.** (low-FEN-tah-NILL OX-ah-late) USAN.
Use: Analgesic, narcotic.

•**lofepramine hydrochloride.** (low-FEH-prah-MEEN) USAN.
Use: Antidepressant.

•**lofexidine hydrochloride.** (low-FEX-ih-DEEN) USAN.
Use: Treatment of opioid withdrawal symptoms.

Lofibra. (Gate) Fenofibrate (micronized) 67 mg, 134 mg, 200 mg, lactose. Cap. 100s. *Rx.*
Use: Antihyperlipidemic.

Logen. (Ivax) Diphenoxylate hydrochloride, atropine sulfate. **Liq.:** Bot. 2 oz. **Tab.:** Bot. 100s, 500s, 1000s. *c-v.*
Use: Antidiarrheal.

LoHist 12 Hour. (Larken) Brompheniramine tannate 6 mg. ER Tab. 100s. *Rx.*
Use: Antihistamine.

LoKara. (PharmaDerm) Desonide 0.05%. Light mineral oil, cetyl alcohol, stearyl alcohol, parabens, EDTA. Lot. 59 mL, 118 mL. *Rx.*
Use: Topical corticosteroid.

Lomanate. (Various Mfr.) Diphenoxylate hydrochloride 2.5 mg, atropine sulfate 0.025 mg/5 mL. Bot. 60 mL. *c-v.*
Use: Antidiarrheal.

•**lomefloxacin.** (low-MEH-FLOX-ah-sin) USAN.
Use: Anti-infective, fluoroquinolone.

•**lomefloxacin hydrochloride.** (low-MEH-FLOX-ah-sin) USAN.
Use: Anti-infective, fluoroquinolone.
See: Maxaquin.

•**lomefloxacin mesylate.** (low-MEH-FLOX-ah-sin) USAN.
Use: Anti-infective.

•**lometraline hydrochloride.** (low-MET-rah-LEEN) USAN.
Use: Antipsychotic; antiparkinsonian.

•**lometrexol sodium.** (LOW-meh-TREX-ole) USAN.
Use: Antineoplastic.

•**lomofungin.** (low-moe-FUN-jin) USAN.
Use: Antifungal.

Lomotil. (Pharmacia) Diphenoxylate hydrochloride 2.5 mg, atropine sulfate 0.025 mg. Tab. or 5 mL. **Tab.:** Bot. 100s, 500s, 1000s, 2500s, UD 100s. **Liq.:** Bot. w/dropper 2 oz. *c-v.*
Use: Antidiarrheal.

•**lomustine.** (LOW-muss-teen) USAN.
Use: Antineoplastic, alkylating agent.
See: CeeNu.

•**lonafarnib.** (loe-na-FAR-nib) USAN.
Use: Chemotherapeutic.

Lonalac. (Bristol-Myers Squibb) Protein as casein 21%, fat as coconut oil 49%, carbohydrate as lactose 30%, vitamins A 1440 units, B_1 0.6 mg, B_2 2.6 mg, niacin 1.2 mg, Ca 1.69 g, P 1.5 g, Cl 750 mg, K 1.88 g, Na 38 mg, Mg 135 mg/qt. Pow. Can 16 oz. *OTC.*
Use: Nutritional supplement.

•**lonapalene.** (low-NAP-ah-LEEN) USAN.
Use: Antipsoriatic.

Long Acting Nasal Spray. (Weeks & Leo) Oxymetazoline hydrochloride 0.05%. Soln. Bot. 0.75 oz. *OTC.*
Use: Decongestant.

Long Acting Neo-Synephrine II Nose Drops and Nasal Spray. (Sanofi-Synthelabo) Xylometazoline hydrochloride 0.1% (adult strength) or 0.05% (child strength). Bot. 1 oz, Spray 0.5 oz (adult strength). *OTC.*
Use: Decongestant.

Long Acting Neo-Synephrine II Vapor Spray. (Sanofi-Synthelabo) Xylometazoline hydrochloride 0.1%. Mentholated. Spray Bot. 0.5 fl oz. *OTC.*
Use: Decongestant.

Lonox. (Geneva) Diphenoxylate hydrochloride 2.5 mg, atropine sulfate 0.025 mg. Tab. Bot. 100s, 500s, 1000s, UD 100s. *c-v.*
Use: Antidiarrheal.

•**lontucirev.** (lon-TOO-si-rev) USAN.
Use: Antineoplastic agent.

Lo/Ovral. (Wyeth-Ayerst) Norgestrel 0.3 mg, ethinyl estradiol 30 mcg, lactose. Tab. *Pilpak* 21s, 28s. *Rx.*
Use: Sex hormone, contraceptive hormone.

•**loperamide hydrochloride.** (low-PURR-ah-mide) *USP 28.*
Use: Antiperistaltic.
See: Imodium.
  K-Pek II.
  Neo-Diaral.

Lopid. (Parke-Davis) Gemfibrozil 600 mg, parabens. Tab. Bot. 60s, 500s, UD 100s. *Rx.*
Use: Antihyperlipidemic; fibric acid derivative.

lopinavir and ritonavir.
Use: Antiretroviral; protease inhibitor combination.
See: Kaletra.

Lopressor HCT. (Novartis) Metoprolol tartrate/hydrochlorothiazide. 50/25 mg, 100/25 mg, 100/50 mg. Tab. Bot. 100s. *Rx.*
Use: Antihypertensive combination.

Loprox. (Medicis) Ciclopirox. **Cream:** 0.77%, water miscible base, benzyl alcohol 1%, cetyl alcohol, stearyl alcohol, myristyl alcohol, mineral oil. Tube. 15 g, 30 g, 90 g. **Gel:** 0.77%, isopropyl alcohol. 30 g, 45 g, 100 g. **Shampoo:** 1%. 120 mL. **Topical Susp.:** 0.77%, stearyl alcohol, cetyl alcohol, mineral oil, myristyl alcohol, benzyl alcohol, lactic acid. 30 mL, 60 mL. *Rx.*
Use: Antifungal, topical.

Lopurin. (Knoll) Allopurinol 100 mg, 300 mg. Tab. Bot. 100s, 1000s, UD 100s. *Rx.*
Use: Antigout agent.

Lorabid. (Monarch) Loracarbef. **Cap.:** 200 mg, 400 mg. Bot. 30s. **Pow. for Oral Susp.:** 100 mg/5 mL, 200 mg/5 mL, parabens, sucrose. Bot. 50 mL, 75 mL, 100 mL. *Rx.*
Use: Anti-infective, cephalosporin.

• **loracarbef.** (LOW-ra-CAR-beff) *USP 28.*
Use: Anti-infective.
See: Lorabid.

• **lorajmine hydrochloride.** (lahr-AZH-meen) USAN.
Use: Cardiovascular agent.

• **loratadine.** (lor-AT-uh-DEEN) *USP 28.*
Use: Antihistamine, peripherally-selective piperidine.
See: Alavert.
Alavert Children's.
Children's Loratadine.
Claritin.
Claritin Hives Relief.
Claritin RediTabs.
Claritin 24-Hour Allergy.
Clear-Atadine.
Dimetapp Children's ND Non-Drowsy Allergy.
Non-Drowsy Allergy Relief for Kids.
Tavist ND.
Triaminic Allerchews.
W/Pseudoephedrine sulfate.
See: Alavert Allergy & Sinus D-12 Hour.
Claritin-D 12 Hour.

Claritin-D 24 Hour.

loratadine. (Geneva) Loratadine 10 mg. Tab. 100s. *OTC.*
Use: Antihistamine, peripherally selective piperidine.

• **lorazepam.** (lore-AZE-uh-pam) *USP 28.*
Use: Anxiolytic; anticonvulsant.
See: Alzapam.
Ativan.

lorazepam. (Abbott) Lorazepam 2 mg/mL, 4 mg/mL. PEG 400, propylene glycol, benzyl alcohol 2%. Inj. Single and 10 mL multidose vials. *c-IV.*
Use: Anxiolytic; hypnotic; sedative.

lorazepam. (Various Mfr) Lorazepam 0.5 mg, 1 mg, 2 mg. Tab. Bot. 100s, 500s, 1000s. *c-IV.*
Use: Anxiolytic; hypnotic; sedative.

Lorazepam Intensol. (Roxane) Lorazepam 2 mg/mL, alcohol and dye free. Concentrated oral soln. Dropper Bot. 10 mL, 30 mL. *c-IV.*
Use: Anxiolytic; hypnotic; sedative.

• **lorbamate.** (lore-BAM-ate) USAN.
Use: Muscle relaxant.

• **lorcainide hydrochloride.** (lahr-CANE-ide) USAN.
Use: Cardiovascular agent; antiarrhythmic.

Lorcet-HD. (Forest) Hydrocodone bitartrate 5 mg, acetaminophen 500 mg. Cap. Bot. 500s. *c-III.*
Use: Analgesic combination, narcotic.

Lorcet Plus. (Forest) Hydrocodone bitartrate 7.5 mg, acetaminophen 650 mg. Tab. Bot. 100s, 500s, UD 100s. *c-III.*
Use: Analgesic combination, narcotic.

Lorcet 10/650. (Forest) Hydrocodone bitartrate 10 mg, acetaminophen 650 mg. Tab. Bot. 20s, 100s, UD 100s. *c-III.*
Use: Analgesic combination, narcotic.

• **lorcinadol.** (LORE-sin-ah-dole) USAN.
Use: Analgesic.

• **loreclezole.** (lahr-EH-kleh-zole) USAN.
Use: Antiepileptic.

Lorelco. (Hoechst) Probucol 250 mg. Tab. Bot. 120s. *Rx.*
Use: Antihyperlipidemic.

• **lormetazepam.** (LORE-met-AZE-eh-pam) USAN.
Use: Hypnotic, sedative.

• **lornoxicam.** (lore-NOX-ih-kam) USAN.
Use: Anti-inflammatory; analgesic.

Lortab. (UCB) Hydrocodone bitartrate 2.5 mg, acetaminophen 167 mg/5 mL, alcohol 7%, parabens, saccharin, sorbitol, sucrose. Elix. Bot. pt. *c-III.*
Use: Analgesic combination, narcotic.

Lortab ASA. (UCB) Hydrocodone bitartrate 5 mg, aspirin 500 mg. Tab. Bot.

100s. *c-III.*
Use: Analgesic combination, narcotic.
Lortab 5/500. (UCB) Hydrocodone 5 mg, acetaminophen 500 mg. Tab. Bot. 100s, 500s, UD 100s. *c-III.*
Use: Analgesic combination, narcotic.
Lortab 7/500. (UCB) Hydrocodone 7.5 mg, acetaminophen 500 mg. Tab. Bot. 100s, 500s, UD 100s. *c-III.*
Use: Analgesic combination, narcotic.
Lortab 10/500. (UCB) Hydrocodone bitartrate 10 mg, acetaminophen 500 mg. Tab. Bot. 100s, 500s. *c-III.*
Use: Analgesic combination, narcotic.
Lortab 2.5/500. (UCB) Hydrocodone 2.5 mg, acetaminophen 500 mg. Tab. Bot. 100s, 500s. *c-III.*
Use: Analgesic combination, narcotic.
• **lortalamine.** (lahr-TAHL-ah-MEEN) USAN.
Use: Antidepressant.
Lortuss DM. (ProEthic) Brompheniramine maleate 2 mg, phenylephrine hydrochloride 7.5 mg, dextromethorphan 15 mg/5 mL. Alcohol-free. Saccharin, sorbitol. Tutti-frutti flavor. Liq. 20 mL, 473 mL. *Rx.*
Use: Decongestant, antihistamine, antitussive.
Lortuss HC. (ProEthic) Hydrocodone bitartrate 3.75 mg, phenylephrine hydrochloride 7.5 mg/5 mL. Saccharin, sorbitol, grape flavor. Liq. 20 mL, 473 mL. *c-III.*
Use: Upper respiratory combination.
• **lorzafone.** (LAHR-zah-FONE) USAN.
Use: Anxiolytic.
• **losartan potassium.** (low-SAHR-tan) *USP 28.*
Use: Antihypertensive; treatment of CHF (angiotensin II receptor antagonist).
See: Cozaar.
W/Hydrochlorothiazide and potassium.
See: Hyzaar.
Losec.
See: Prilosec.
Losopan. (Ivax) Magaldrate 540 mg/5 mL. Liq. Bot. 12 oz. *OTC.*
Use: Antacid.
Losopan Plus. (Ivax) Magaldrate 540 mg, simethicone 20 mg/5 mL. Liq. Bot. 12 oz. *OTC.*
Use: Antacid; antiflatulent.
Losotron Plus. (Various Mfr.) Magaldrate 540 mg, simethicone 20 mg/5 mL. Liq. Bot. 360 mL. *OTC.*
Use: Antacid; antiflatulent.
• **losoxantrone hydrochloride.** (low-SOX-an-trone) USAN.

Use: Antineoplastic.
• **losulazine hydrochloride.** (low-SULL-ah-zeen) USAN.
Use: Antihypertensive.
Lotawin. (Sanofi-Synthelabo) Oxypertine. Cap. *Rx.*
Use: Anxiolytic.
Lotemax. (Bausch & Lomb) Loteprednol etabonate 0.5%, EDTA, benzalkonium chloride 0.01%. Ophth. Susp. Bot. 2.5 mL, 5 mL, 10 mL, 15 mL. *Rx.*
Use: Anti-inflammatory, topical.
Lotensin. (Novartis) Benazepril hydrochloride 5 mg, 10 mg, 20 mg, 40 mg, lactose, castor oil (except 40 mg). Tab. Bot. 90s, 100s, UD 100s. *Rx.*
Use: Antihypertensive.
• **loteprednol etabonate.** (low-TEH-PRED-nole ett-AB-ohn-ate) USAN.
Use: Anti-inflammatory, topical.
See: Alrex.
Lotemax.
lotio alba. White lotion. *OTC.*
Use: Antiseborrheic; dermatologic, acne.
lotio alsulfa. (Doak Dermatologics) Colloidal sulfur 5%. Bot. 4 oz. *OTC.*
Use: Antiseborrheic; dermatologic, acne.
Lotion-Jel. (C.S. Dent & Co.) Benzocaine in gel base. Tube 0.2 oz. *OTC.*
Use: Anesthetic, local.
• **lotrafiban hydrochloride.** (low-TRAFF-ih-ban) USAN.
Use: Antiplatelet.
Lotrel. (Novartis) Amlodipine 2.5 mg, 5 mg, benazepril hydrochloride 10 mg. Cap. Amlodipine 5 mg, benazepril hydrochloride 20 mg. Cap. Bot. 100s. Amlodipine 10 mg, benazepril 20 mg, lactose. Cap. Bot. 100s. *Rx.*
Use: Antihypertensive combination.
Lotrimin AF. (Schering-Plough) Clotrimazole 1%. **Cream:** Benzyl alcohol, cetearyl alcohol. Tube. 12 g, 24 g. **Top. Soln.:** PEG. Bot. 10 mL. **Lot.:** Benzyl alcohol, cetearyl alcohol. Bot. 20 mL. *OTC.*
Use: Antifungal, topical.
Lotrimin Ultra. (Schering Plough) Butenafine hydrochloride 1%, benzyl alcohol, cetyl alcohol, glycerin, white petrolatum. Cream. 12 g, 24 g. *OTC.*
Use: Antifungal.
Lotrisone. (Schering) **Cream.:** Clotrimazole 1%, betamethasone dipropionate 0.05%/g. Tube 15 g, 45 g. **Lot.:** Betamethasone (as dipropionate) 0.05%, clotrimazole 1%. Alcohols, hydrophilic, minieral oil, white petrolatum. 30 mL.

Rx.
Use: Antifungal, topical.
Lotronex. (GlaxoSmithKline) Alosetron hydrochloride 0.562 mg (equiv. to 0.5 mg alosetron base), 1.124 mg (equiv. to 1 mg alosetron), lactose. Tab. Bot. 30s. *Rx.*
Use: Antiemetic; antivertigo.
Lo-Trop. (Vangard Labs, Inc.) Diphenoxylate hydrochloride 2.5 mg, atropine sulfate 0.025 mg. Tab. Bot. 100s, 1000s. *c-v.*
Use: Antidiarrheal.
• **lovastatin.** (LOW-vuh-STAT-in) *USP 28.* Formerly Mevinolin.
Use: Antihypercholesterolemic; antihyperlipidemic, HMG-CoA reductase inhibitor.
See: Mevacor.
W/Niacin
See: Advicor.
lovastatin. (Various Mfr.) Lovastatin 10 mg, 20 mg, 40 mg, may contain lactose. Tab. Bot. 30s, 60s, 90s (except 10 mg), 100s, 500s, 1000s. *Rx.*
Use: Antihypercholesterolemic; antihyperlipidemic; HMG-COA reductase inhibitor.
Love Longer. (Durex) Benzocaine 7.5% in water-soluble lubricant base. Tube 0.5 oz. *OTC.*
Use: Anesthetic, local.
Lovenox. (Aventis) Enoxaparin sodium. 30 mg/0.3 mL, 40 mg/0.4 mL, 60 mg/ 0.6 mL, 80 mg/0.8 mL, 100 mg/1 mL, 120 mg/0.8 mL, 150 mg/1 mL, 300 mg/ 3 mL (benzyl alcohol 15 mg/15 mL). Preservative free (except 300 mg/ 3 mL). Approximate anti-factor Xa activity of 100 units/1 mg (with reference to the WHO First International Low Molecular Weight Heparin Reference Standard). Inj. **30 mg/0.3 mL:** Amps and single-dose prefilled syringes w/27-gauge × ½ inch needle. **40 mg/ 0.4 mL:** Single-dose prefilled syringes with a 27-gauge × ½ inch needle. **60 mg/0.6 mL, 80 mg/0.8 mL, 100 mg/ 1 mL, 120 mg/0.8 mL, 150 mg/mL:** Graduated single-dose prefilled syringes with a 27-gauge × ½ inch needle. **300 mg/3 mL:** 3 mL multidose vial. *Rx.*
Use: Anticoagulant, low molecular weight heparin (LMWH).
• **loviride.** (LOW-vihr-ide) USAN.
Use: Antiviral for chronic oral treatment of HIV-seropositive patients (nonnucleoside reverse transcriptase inhibitor).
Lowila Cake. (Bristol-Myers Squibb) Sodium lauryl sulfoacetate, dextrin, boric acid, urea, sorbitol, mineral oil, PEG 14 M, lactic acid, cellulose gum, docusate sodium. Cake 112.5 g. *OTC.*
Use: Dermatologic, cleanser.
low molecular weight heparins. LMWH.
Use: Anticoagulant.
See: Dalteparin Sodium.
Enoxaparin Sodium.
Tinzaparin Sodium.
Low-Ogestrel. (Watson) Ethinyl estradiol 30 mcg, norgestrel 0.3 mg, lactose. Tab. Pack 28s. *Rx.*
Use: Sex hormone, contraceptive hormone.
Low-Quel. (Halsey Drug) Diphenoxylate hydrochloride 2.5 mg, atropine sulfate 0.025 mg. Tab. Bot. 100s. *c-v.*
Use: Antidiarrheal.
Lowsium. (Rugby) Magaldrate 540 mg/ 5 mL. Susp. Bot. 360 mL. *OTC.*
Use: Antacid.
Lowsium Plus. (Rugby) **Tab.:** Magaldrate 480 mg, simethicone 20 mg. Bot. 60s. **Susp.:** Magaldrate 540 mg, simethicone 40 mg/5 mL. Bot. 360 mL. *OTC.*
Use: Antacid; antiflatulent.
• **loxapine.** (LOX-ah-peen) USAN.
Use: Anxiolytic; antipsychotic, dibenzapine derivative.
See: Loxapine Succinate.
Loxitane.
Loxitane IM.
loxapine hydrochloride.
Use: Anxiolytic.
See: Loxitane.
Loxitane-C Oral Concentrate.
• **loxapine succinate.** (LOX-ah-peen) *USP 28.*
Use: Anxiolytic; antipsychotic, dibenzapine derivative.
See: Loxitane.
loxapine succinate. (Various Mfr.) Loxapine succinate 5 mg, 10 mg, 25 mg, 50 mg. Cap. Bot. 100s, 1000s (5 mg only). *Rx.*
Use: Antipsychotic, dibenzapine derivative.
Loxitane. (Watson) Loxapine succinate 5 mg, 10 mg, 25 mg, 50 mg, lactose. Cap. Bot. 100s, 1000s. *Rx.*
Use: Antipsychotic, dibenzapine derivative.
• **loxoribine.** (LOX-ore-ih-BEAN) USAN.
Use: Immunostimulant; vaccine adjuvant.
L₂-oxothiazolidine₄-carboxylic acid.
Use: Treatment of adult respiratory distress syndrome. [Orphan Drug]
See: Procysteine.

Lozol. (Aventis) Indapamide 2.5 mg. Tab. Bot. 100s, 1000s, 2500s, Strip dispenser 100s. *Rx.*
Use: Diuretic; antihypertensive.

L-PAM.
See: Alkeran.

Lubafax. (GlaxoSmithKline) Surgical lubricant, sterile, water-soluble, nonstaining. Foil wrapper 2.7 g, 5 g. Box 144s.
Use: Lubricant.

Lubath. (Warner Lambert) Mineral oil, PPG-15, stearyl ether, oleth-2, nonoxynol 5, fragrance, FD&C Green No. 6. Bot. 4 oz, 8 oz, 16 oz. *OTC.*
Use: Emollient.

•**lubazodone hydrochloride.** (LOO-bazoe-done) USAN.
Use: Antidepressant; SSRI.

•**lubeluzole.** (loo-BELL-you-zole) USAN.
Use: Stroke treatment.

Lubinol. (Purepac) Light, heavy, and extra heavy mineral oil. Bot. Pt, qt, gal. (Extra heavy Bot.) 8 oz, pt, qt, gal. *OTC.*
Use: Emollient.

•**lubiprostone.** (loo-bi-PROS-tone) USAN.
Use: Bowel prep.

Lubraseptic Jelly. (Guardian Laboratories) Water-soluble amyl phenyl phenol complex 0.12%, phenylmercuric nitrate, 0.007%. Bellows-type tube 10 g, 24s.
Use: Genitourinary aid.

Lubricating Jelly. (Taro) Glycerin, propylene glycol. Tube. 60 g, 125 g. *OTC.*
Use: Vaginal agent.

Lubriderm. (Warner Lambert) Mineral oil, petrolatum, sorbitol, lanolin, lanolin alcohol, stearic acid, TEA, cetyl alcohol, fragrance (if scented), butylparaben, methylparaben, propylparaben, sodium Cl. Lot. Bot. (scented), 4 oz, 8 oz, 16 oz; (unscented) 8 oz, 16 oz. *OTC.*
Use: Emollient.

Lubrin. (Kenwood) Glycerin, caprylic/capric triglyceride. Inserts. Pkg. 5s, 12s. *OTC.*
Use: Lubricant.

Lubriskin. (Geritrex) Mineral oil, petrolatum, lanolin, lanolin alcohol, cetearyl alcohol, castor oil, triethanolamine, stearyl alcohol, propylene glycol, parabens, EDTA. Lot. 240 g. *OTC.*
Use: Emollient.

LubriTears. (Bausch & Lomb) White petrolatum, mineral oil, lanolin, chlorobutanol 0.5%. Oint. Tube 3.5 g. *OTC.*
Use: Lubricant, ophthalmic.

LubriTears Solution. (Bausch & Lomb) Hydroxypropyl methylcellulose 2906 0.3%, dextran 70 0.1%, EDTA, KCl, NaCl, benzalkonium chloride 0.01%. Bot. 15 mL. *OTC.*
Use: Artificial tears.

•**lucanthone hydrochloride.** (LOO-kanthone) USAN.
Use: Antischistosomal.

Lucidex. (Xanodyne) Caffeine 100 mg, enteric coated. Tab. 24s. *OTC.*
Use: Stimulant, analeptic.

•**lucinactant.** (loo-sin-AK-tant) USAN.
Use: Respiratory distress syndrome.

•**lufironil.** (loo-FIHR-ah-nill) USAN.
Use: Collagen inhibitor.

Lufyllin. (Medpointe) Dyphylline 200 mg. Tab. Bot. 100s, 1,000s, UD 100s. *Rx.*
Use: Bronchodilator.

Lufyllin-400. (Medpointe) Dyphylline 400 mg. Tab. Bot. 100s, 1000s. *Rx.*
Use: Bronchodilator.

Lufyllin-GG. (Medpointe) **Tab.:** Dyphylline 200 mg, guaifenesin 200 mg. Tab. Bot. 100s, 3000s, UD 100s. **Elix.:** Dyphylline 100 mg, guaifenesin 100 mg, alcohol 17%/15 mL. Elix. Bot. Pt, gal. *Rx.*
Use: Bronchodilator, expectorant.

Lugol's Solution. (Lyne) Iodine 5 g, potassium iodide 10 g, in purified water to make 100 mL. Soln. Bot. 15 mL. (Wisconsin Pharmacal Co.) Bot. Pt. *Rx-OTC.*
Use: Antithyroid; antiseptic, topical.

Lumigan. (Allergan) Bimatoprost 0.03%, benzalkonium chloride 0.05 mg/mL. Soln. Bot. 2.5 mL, 5 mL. *Rx.*
Use: Antiglaucoma; prostaglandin agonist.

•**lumiliximab.** (loo-mil-IX-i-mab) USAN.
Use: Monoclonal antibody.

Luminal Injection. (Sanofi-Synthelabo) Phenobarbital 130 mg/mL. Amp 1 mL. Box 100s. *Rx.*
Use: Hypnotic, sedative.

•**lumiracoxib.** (lue-mye-ra-KOX-ib) USAN.
Use: Rheumatoid arthritis; osteoarthritis.

Lumopaque Capsules. (Sanofi-Synthelabo) Tyropanoate sodium.
Use: Radiopaque agent.

Lunesta. (Sepracor) Eszopiclone 1 mg, 2 mg, 3 mg. Lactose. Film coated. Tab. 100s, cartons of 90s (except 1 mg). *c-IV.*
Use: Sedative/hypnotic, nonbarbiturate.

lung surfactants.
Use: Surfactant replacement therapy in neonatal respiratory distress syndrome.

See: Beractant.
Calfactant.
Poractant Alfa.
Lupron. (TAP) Leuprolide acetate 5 mg/ mL, benzyl alcohol 9 mg/mL, sodium chloride. Inj. Multiple-dose vial 2.8 mL. *Rx.*
Use: Hormone, gonadotropin-releasing hormone analog.
Lupron Depot. (TAP) Leuprolide acetate 3.75, 7.5 mg, mannitol, preservative free. Lyophilized microspheres for injection. Single-use kit, multi-pack, prefilled dual-chamber syringe. *Rx.*
Use: Hormone, gonadotropin-releasing hormone analog.
Lupron Depot-4 Month. (TAP) Leuprolide acetate 30 mg, mannitol, preservative free. Microspheres for injection, lyophilized. Single use kit w/diluent 1.5 mL and in prefilled dual-chamber syringe. *Rx.*
Use: Hormone, gonadotropin-releasing hormone analog.
Lupron Depot-Ped. (TAP) Leuprolide acetate 7.5 mg, 11.25 mg, 15 mg, mannitol. Preservative free. Microspheres for Inj. Single-dose kit, prefilled dual-chamber syringe. *Rx.*
Use: Hormone, gonadotropin-releasing hormone analog.
Lupron Depot-3 Month. (TAP) Leuprolide acetate 11.25 mg, 22.5 mg, mannitol, preservative free. Microspheres for injection. Single-use Kit, w/diluent 1.5 mL and in prefilled dual-chamber syringe. *Rx.*
Use: Hormone, gonadotropin-releasing hormone analog.
Lupron for Pediatric Use. (TAP) Leuprolide acetate 5 mg/mL, benzyl alcohol 9 mg/mL, sodium chloride. Inj. Multiple-dose vial 2.8 mL. *Rx.*
Use: Hormone, gonadotropoin-releasing hormone analog.
Lupron Injection. (TAP) Leuprolide acetate 1 mg/0.2 mL. Vial 2.8 mL. *Rx.*
Use: Antineoplastic.
Luramide. (Major) Furosemide 20 mg, 40 mg, 80 mg. Tab. Bot. 100s, 1000s. *Rx.*
Use: Diuretic.
Luride Drops. (Colgate Oral) Sodium fluoride equivalent to 0.5 mg of fluoride. Plastic dropper bot. 50 mL. *Rx.*
Use: Dental caries agent.
Luride-F Lozi Tablets. (Colgate Oral) Sodium fluoride in Lozi base tab. available as fluoride. **0.25 mg:** Bot. 120s; **0.5 mg:** Bot. 120s, 1200s; **1 mg:** Bot. 120s, 1000s, 5000s. *Rx.*

Use: Dental caries agent.
Luride Gel. (Colgate Oral) Fluoride (from sodium fluoride and hydrogen fluoride) 1.2%. Tube 7 g. *Rx.*
Use: Dental caries agent.
Luride Lozi-Tabs. (Colgate Oral) Sodium fluoride 0.25 mg Chew. Tab. Sugar free. Bot. 120s. *Rx.*
Use: Dental caries agent.
Luride Prophylaxis Paste. (Colgate Oral) Acidulated phosphate sodium fluoride containing 0.4% fluoride ion w/silicon dioxide abrasive. UD 3 g, Jar 50 g. *OTC.*
Use: Dentrifice.
Luride-SF Lozi Tablets. (Colgate Oral) Sodium fluoride equivalent to 1 mg. Bot. 120s. *Rx.*
Use: Dental caries agent.
Luride Topical Gel. (Colgate Oral) Fluoride 1.2%. Tube 7 g. *Rx.*
Use: Dental caries agent.
Luride Topical Solution. (Colgate Oral) Acidulated phosphate sodium fluoride w/pH 3.2. Bot. 250 mL. *OTC.*
Use: Dental caries agent.
Lurline PMS. (Fielding) Acetaminophen 500 mg, pamabrom 25 mg, pyridoxine 50 mg. Tab. Bot. 24s, 50s. *OTC.*
Use: Analgesic combination.
•**lurosetron mesylate.** (loo-ROW-set-rahn) USAN.
Use: Antiemetic.
Lurotin Caps. (BASF) Beta-carotene 25 mg. Cap. Bot. 100s. *OTC.*
Use: Nutritional supplement.
•**lurtotecan dihyrdochloride.** (lure-toe-TEE-kan die-HIGH-droe-KLOR-ide) USAN.
Use: Antineoplastic (DNA topoisomerase I inhibitor).
Lusonal. (WraSer) Phenylephrine hydrochloride 7.5 mg per 5 mL. Aspartame, parabens, phenylalanine. Strawberry flavor. Oral Liq. 473 mL. *Rx.*
Use: Nasal decongestant.
Lustra. (Medicis) Hydroquinone 4%, glycerin, alcohol, cetyl alcohol, cetearyl alcohol, benzyl alcohol, sodium metabisulfite, EDTA. Cream. Tube. 28.4 g. *Rx.*
Use: Depigmentor.
Lustra-AF. (Medicis) Hydroquinone 4%, glycerin, alcohol, cetyl alcohol, cetearyl alcohol, benzyl alcohol, sodium metabisulfite, EDTA, octyl methoxycinnamate, arobenzone. Cream. Tube. 28.4 g. *Rx.*
Use: Depigmentor.
luteogan.
See: Progesterone.
luteosan.
See: Progesterone.

Lutera. (Watson) Ethinyl estradiol 20 mcg, levonorgestrel 0.1 mg. Lactose. Tab. 28s. 7 peach inert tablets. *Rx.*
Use: Contraceptive hormone.

lutocylol. (Novartis) Ethisterone.

Lutolin-F. (Spanner) Progesterone 25 mg, 50 mg/mL. Vial 10 mL. *Rx.*
Use: Hormone, progestin.

Lutolin-S. (Spanner) Progesterone 25 mg/mL. Vial 10 mL. *Rx.*
Use: Hormone, progestin.

• **lutrelin acetate.** (loo-TRELL-in ASS-eh-tate) USAN.
Use: LHRH agonist.

lutren.
See: Progesterone.

• **lutropin alfa.** (LOO-troe-pin alfa) USAN.
Use: Ovulation stimulant.
See: Luveris.

Luveris. (Serono) Lutropin alfa 82.5 units/vial. Sucrose 48 mg. Pow. for Inj., lyophilized. Single-dose vials. Delivers 75 units lutropin alfa after reconstitution. *Rx.*
Use: Ovulation stimulant.

Luxiq. (Connetics) Betamethasone valerate 1.2 mg/g, cetyl alcohol, stearyl alcohol. Foam. Can. 100 g. *Rx.*
Use: Anti-inflammatory.

• **lyapolate sodium.** (lie-APP-oh-late) USAN.
Use: Anticoagulant.
See: Peson.

• **lycetamine.** (lie-SEET-ah-meen) USAN.
Use: Antimicrobial, topical.

lycine hydrochloride.
See: Betaine hydrochloride.

Lydia E. Pinkham Herbal Compound. (Numark) Vitamin C, iron. Liq. Bot. 8 fl oz, 16 fl oz.

Lydia E. Pinkham Tablets. (Numark) Vitamin C, iron, calcium. Bot. 72s, 150s. *OTC.*

• **lydimycin.** (lie-dih-MY-sin) USAN.
Use: Antifungal.

Lymphazurin 1%. (US Surgical) Isosulfan blue 10 mg/mL, preservative free. Inj. Vial 5 mL. *Rx.*
Use: Radiopaque agent, parenteral.

lymphocyte immune globulin antithymocyte globulin (equine).
Use: Immune globulin.
See: Atgam.

LymphoScan. (Immunomedics) Technetium TC-99M murine monoclonal antibody (IgG2a) to B-cell.
Use: Diagnostic aid. [Orphan Drug]

• **lynestrenol.** (lin-ESS-tree-nahl) *USP 28.*
Use: Hormone, progestin.

lynoestrenol. Lynestrenol.

lyophilized vitamin B complex and vitamin C with B$_{12}$. (McGuff) B$_1$ 50 mg, B$_2$ 5 mg, B$_3$ 125 mg, B$_5$ 6 mg, B$_6$ 5 mg, B$_{12}$ 1000 mcg, C 50 mg/mL. Inj. Vial 10 mL. *Rx.*
Use: Vitamin supplement; parenteral.

Lyphocin P. (Fujisawa Healthcare) Vancomycin hydrochloride 500 mg. Vial 10 mL. *Rx.*
Use: Anti-infective.

Lypholyte. (American Pharmaceutical Partners) Na$^+$ 25 mEq, K$^+$ ≈ 40 mEq, Ca^{++} 5 mEq, Mg^{++} 8 mEq, Cl$^-$ ≈ 33 mEq, acetate ≈ 41 mEq, gluconate 5 mEq, osmolarity ≈ 7562/20 mL or 25 mL after dilution. Conc. Single-dose vial 20 mL, 40 mL, *Maxivial* (pharmacy bulk packaging) 100 mL, 200 mL. *Rx.*
Use: Intravenous nutritional therapy, intravenous replenishment solution.

Lypholyte II. (American Pharmaceutical Partners) Na$^+$ 35 mEq, K$^+$ 20 mEq, Ca^{++} 4.5 mEq, Mg^{++} 5 mEq, Cl 35 mEq, acetate 29.5 mEq, osmolarity ≈ 6200/20 mL or 25 mL after dilution. Single-dose vial 20 mL, 40 mL; *Maxivial* (pharmacy bulk packaging) 100 mL, 200 mL. *Rx.*
Use: Intravenous nutritional therapy, intravenous replenishment solution.

• **lypressin nasal solution.** (LIE-PRESS-in) *USP 28.*
Use: Antidiuretic; vasoconstrictor.

lysidin. Methyl glyoxalidin.

• **lysine.** (LIE-SEEN) USAN.
Use: Nutrient; rapid weight gain; amino acid.

• **lysine acetate.** (LIE-SEEN) *USP 28.*
Use: Amino acid.

• **lysine hydrochloride.** (LIE-SEEN) *USP 28.*
Use: Amino acid.
See: Enisyl.

Lysodase. (Enzon) PEG-glucocerebrosidase.
Use: Gaucher disease. [Orphan Drug]

Lysodren. (Bristol-Myers Squibb Oncology) Mitotane 500 mg. Tab. Bot. 100s. *Rx.*
Use: Antineoplastic.

• **lysostaphin.** (LIE-so-STAFF-in) USAN. Enzyme produced by *Staphylococcus staphylolyticus.*
Use: Antibiotic; antibacterial enzyme.

Lytren. (Bristol-Myers Squibb) Dextrose, sodium citrate, citric acid, sodium Cl, potassium citrate. Ready-to-use Bot. 8 fl. oz. *OTC.*
Use: Electrolyte, fluid replacement.

M

Maagel. (Health for Life Brands) Aluminum and magnesium hydroxide. Bot. 12 oz, gal. *OTC.*
Use: Antacid.

Maalox Antacid/Calcium Supplement. (Novartis) Calcium carbonate 600 mg, aspartame, phenylalanine 0.5 mg, dextrose, mannitol, lemon flavor. Chew. Tab. Bot. 85s. *OTC.*
Use: Antacid; calcium supplement.

Maalox Anti-Gas. (Novartis) Simethicone 80 mg, sucrose. Chew. Tab. Bot. 12s. *OTC.*
Use: Antiflatulent.

Maalox Anti-Gas Extra Strength. (Novartis) Aluminum hydroxide 500 mg, magnesium hydroxide 450 mg, simethicone 40 mg/5 mL, calcium, saccharin, sorbitol, parabens, cherry and mint flavors. Liq. Bot. 769 mL. *OTC.*
Use: Antacid.

Maalox Extra Strength Anti-Gas. (Novartis) Simethicone 150 mg, mannitol, sucrose, lemon and peppermint flavors. Chew. Tab. Pkg. 10s. *OTC.*
Use: Antiflatulent.

Maalox Maximum Strength Quick Dissolve. (Novartis) Calcium carbonate 1000 mg, aspartame, phenylalanine 0.9 mg, dextrose, mannitol, wild berry and wintergreen flavors. Chew. Tab. Bot. 35s, 65s. *OTC.*
Use: Antacid.

Maalox Quick Dissolve. (Novartis) Calcium carbonate 600 mg, aspartame, phenylalanine, mannitol, dextrose, wild berry, lemon, and wintergreen flavors. Chew. Tab. Bot. 30s, 45s, 85s. *OTC.*
Use: Antacid.

Maalox Suspension. (Novartis) Magnesium hydroxide 200 mg, aluminum hydroxide 225 mg/5 mL. Bot. 148 mL, 355 mL, 769 mL. *OTC.*
Use: Antacid.

Maalox TC. (Novartis) Magnesium hydroxide 300 mg, aluminum hydroxide 600 mg/5 mL. Bot. 355 mL. *OTC.*
Use: Antacid.

Maalox Therapeutic Concentrate. (Novartis) Magnesium hydroxide 300 mg, aluminum hydroxide 600 mg. Tab. Bot. 48s. *OTC.*
Use: Antacid.

MacPac. (Procter & Gamble) Nitrofurantoin macrocrystals 50 mg, 100 mg. Cap. UD 28s. *Rx.*
Use: Anti-infective, urinary.

macroaggregated albumin. (Bristol-Myers Squibb) Albumotope I-131.

Macrobid. (Procter & Gamble) Nitrofurantoin (as monohydrate/macrocrytals) 100 mg. Lactose, talc. Cap. Bot. 100s. *Rx.*
Use: Anti-infective, urinary.

Macrodantin. (Procter & Gamble) Nitrofurantoin macrocrystals 25 mg, 50 mg, 100 mg. Lactose, talc. Cap. Bot. 100s, 1,000s. *Rx.*
Use: Anti-infective; urinary.

Macrodex. (Pharmacia) Dextran 6% w/v in normal saline, 6% w/v in Dextrose 5% in water. Bot. 500 mL. *Rx.*
Use: Plasma volume expander.

macrogol stearate 2000. Polyoxyl 40 Stearate.

macrolides.
Use: Anti-infective.
See: Azithromycin.
    Clarithromycin.
    Erythromycin.
    Dirithromycin.

Macrotec. (Bristol-Myers Squibb) Technetium Tc 99m Medronate kit. Vial Kit 10s.
Use: Radiopaque agent.

Macugen. (Eyetech) Pegaptanib sodium 0.3 mg (equiv. to 1.6 mg or 3.2 mg when expressed as the sodium salt form). Inj. Glass syringes. 1 mL with 27-gauge needle and shield. *Rx.*
Use: Treatment of age-related macular degeneration.

• **maduramicin.** (mau-UHR-ah-MY-sin) USAN.
Use: Anticoccidal.

• **mafenide.** (MAY-feh-NIDE) USAN.
Use: Anti-infective.

• **mafenide acetate.** (MAY-feh-NIDE) *USP 28.*
Use: Anti-infective, topical.
See: Sulfamylon Cream.

mafenide acetate solution.
Use: Prevent graft loss on burn wounds. [Orphan Drug]

• **mafilcon a.** (MAY-fill-kahn A) USAN.
Use: Contact lens material (hydrophilic).

Mafylon Cream. (Sanofi-Synthelabo) Mafenide acetate.
Use: Burn therapy.

• **magaldrate.** (MAG-al-drate) *USP 28.* (Wyeth) Monalium Hydrate. Aluminum Magnesium Hydroxide.
Use: Antacid.
See: Iosopan.
    Monalium Hydrate.
    Riopan.

magaldrate and simethicone.
Use: Antacid, antiflatulent.
See: Lowsium.

Lowsium Plus.
Riopan Plus.
magaldrate plus suspension. (Various Mfr.) Magaldrate 540 mg, simethicone 40 mg/5 mL. Susp. Bot. 360 mL. *OTC.*
Use: Antacid; antiflatulent.
Magan. (Pharmacia) Magnesium salicylate (anhydrous) 545 mg. Tab. Bot. 100s, 500s. *Rx.*
Use: Analgesic.
Mag-Cal Mega. (Freeda) Mg 800 mg, Ca 400 mg, kosher, sugar free. Tab. Bot. 100s, 250s. *OTC.*
Use: Mineral, vitamin supplement.
Mag-Cal Tablets. (Fibertone) Calcium 416.7 mg (as carbonate), calcium 166.7 mg (as elemental), vitamin D 66.7 units, Mg 83.3 mg, Cu 0.167 mg, Mn 0.83 mg, K 1.67 mg, Zn 0.167 mg. Tab. Bot. 90s, 180s. *OTC.*
Use: Mineral, vitamin supplement.
Mag-Caps. (Genesis) Magnesium oxide ≈ 140 mg (elemental magnesium 85 mg). Cap. 100s. *OTC.*
Use: Dietary supplement.
Magdrox. (Vita Elixir) Magnesium hydroxide, aluminum hydroxide. *OTC.*
Use: Antacid.
Mag-G. (Cypress) Magnesium gluconate dihydrate 500 mg (elemental magnesium 27 mg). Tab. Bot. 100s. *OTC.*
Use: Mineral supplement.
Magmalin. (Pal-Pak, Inc.) Magnesium hydroxide 0.2 g, aluminum hydroxide gel, dried 0.2 g/Loz. Bot. 1000s. *OTC.*
Use: Antacid.
Magnacal Liquid. (Biosearch Medical Products) Protein (from calcium, sodium caseinate), carbohydrate (from maltodextrin, sucrose), fat (partially hydrogenated from soy oil, lecithin, mono- and diglycerides). 1.5 Cal/mL, 590 mOsm/kg H₂O. Protein 70 g, CHO 250 g, fat 80 g, Na 1000 mg, K 1250 mg/L. Can 120 mL, 240 mL. *OTC.*
Use: Nutritional supplement.
Magnalum. (Global Source) Magnesium hydroxide 3.75 g, aluminum hydroxide 2 g. Tab. Bot. 1000s. *OTC.*
Use: Antacid.
Magnaprin. (Rugby) Aspirin 325 mg, dried aluminum hydroxide gel 75 mg, magnesium hydroxide 75 mg. Tab. Bot. 100s, 500s. *OTC.*
Use: Analgesic.
Magnaprin Arthritis Strength. (Rugby) Aspirin 325 mg, dried aluminum hydroxide gel 150 mg, magnesium hydroxide 150 mg. Tab. Bot. 100s, 500s. *OTC.*
Use: Analgesic.

MagneBind 400 Rx. (Nephro-Tech) Magnesium carbonate 400 mg, calcium carbonate 200 mg, folic acid 1 mg. Tab. Bot. 150s. *Rx.*
Use: Mineral supplement.
MagneBind 300. (Nephro-Tech) Magnesium carbonate 300 mg, calcium carbonate 250 mg. Tab. Bot. 150s. *OTC.*
Use: Mineral supplement.
MagneBind 200. (Nephro-Tech) Magnesium carbonate 200 mg, calcium carbonate 400 mg. Tab. Bot. 150s. *OTC.*
Use: Mineral supplement.
magnesia tablets.
Use: Antacid.
magnesia & alumina oral suspension. (Roxane) Oral Susp. 6 fl oz. 25s.
Use: Antacid.
See: Maalox.
magnesia & alumina tablets.
Use: Antacid.
See: Maalox.
magnesia magma. Milk of Magnesia.
Use: Antacid; cathartic; laxative.
See: Magnesium Hydroxide
•**magnesia, milk of.** (mag-NEE-zee-uh) *USP 28.*
Use: Antacid; laxative.
magnesium.
Use: Mineral.
See: Magnesium Citrate.
Magnesium Gluconate.
Magonate Natal.
Mag-Tab SR.
Mag-200.
Slow-Mag.
magnesium. (Various Mfr.) Elemental magnesium 30 mg. Tab. Bot. 100s. *OTC.*
Use: Mineral.
magnesium acetylsalicylate. Apyron, Magnespirin, Magisal, Novacetyl.
Use: Analgesic.
magnesium aluminate hydrated.
Use: Antacid.
See: Riopan.
•**magnesium aluminometasilicate.** (mag-NEE-zee-uhm ah-LOO-mihn-oh-met-uh-sill-ih-CATE) *NF 23.*
•**magnesium aluminosilicate.** (mag-NEE-zee-uhm ah-LOO-mihn-oh-sill-ih-CATE) *NF 23.*
magnesium aluminum hydroxide.
Use: Antacid.
See: Maalox.
Malogel.
Medalox.
W/A.P.C.
See: Buffadyne.
W/Calcium carbonate.

See: Maalox Plus.
• **magnesium aluminum silicate.** (mag-NEE-zee-uhm ah-LOO-mihn-num sill-ih-CATE) *NF 23.*
Use: Pharmaceutic aid; suspending agent.
• **magnesium carbonate.** (mag-NEE-zee-uhm kar-BAHN-ate) *USP 28.*
Use: Antacid.
magnesium carbonate and sodium bicarbonate for oral suspension.
Use: Antacid.
magnesium carbonate w/combinations.
Use: Antacid.
See: Alkets.
Antacid No. 2.
Bufferin.
Urocit.
MagneBind 400 Rx.
MagneBind 300.
MagneBind 200.
Marblen.
• **magnesium chloride.** (mag-NEE-zee-uhm) *USP 28.*
Use: Electrolyte replacement; pharmaceutical necessity for hemodialysis and peritoneal dialysis.
• **magnesium citrate.** (mag-NEE-zee-uhm) *USP 28.*
Use: Cathartic; laxative.
magnesium citrate. (Various Mfr.) Elemental magnesium 100 mg. Tab. Bot. 100s, 250s. *OTC.*
Use: Mineral.
magnesium citrate solution. (Humco Holding Group) Magnesium citrate 1.75 g/30 mL, saccharine, cherry, lemon flavors. Soln. Bot. 2% mL. *OTC.*
Use: Laxative.
• **magnesium gluconate.** *USP 28.*
Use: Vitamin supplement, replacement.
See: Mag-G.
Magonate.
Magtrate.
magnesium gluconate. (Various Mfr.) Elemental magnesium 27.5 mg. Tab. Bot. 100s, 500s. *OTC.*
Use: Mineral.
magnesium hydroxide. *USP 28.*
Use: Antacid; cathartic; laxative.
See: Dulcolax.
Magnesia Magma.
Milk of Magnesia.
Phillips' Chewable.
Phillips' Milk of Magnesia.
magnesium hydroxide w/combinations.
See: Aludrox.
Ascriptin.

Ascriptin A/D.
Ascriptin Extra Strength.
Ascriptin w/Codeine.
Banacid.
Delcid.
Gas Ban DS.
Maalox.
Maalox Anti-Gas Extra Strength.
Maalox TC.
Mylanta.
Mylanta Supreme.
Pepcid Complete.
Rolaids.
Rolaids Extra Strength.
Rolaids Multi-Symptom.
Trial AG.
magnesium-L-aspartate.
Use: Mineral.
• **magnesium oxide.** (mag-NEE-zee-uhm OX-ide) *USP 28.*
Use: Pharmaceutic aid (sorbent).
See: Mag-Caps.
Mag-Ox.
Mag-Ox 400.
Niko-Mag.
Par-Mag.
Uro-Mag.
W/Calcium, Vitamin D.
See: Elekap.
W/Magnesium carbonate, calcium carbonate.
See: Alkets.
W/Ox bile (desiccated), hog bile (desiccated).
See: Hyper-Cholate.
magnesium oxide. (Cypress) Magnesium oxide 400 mg (elemental magnesium 241.3 mg). Tab. Bot. 120s. *OTC.*
Use: Mineral.
magnesium oxide. (Manne) Magnesium oxide 420 mg. Tab. Bot. 250s, 1000s. (Stanlabs) 10 g. Tab. Bot. 100s, 1000s. (Cypress) 400 mg. Tab. Bot. 120s. *OTC.*
Use: Mineral.
• **magnesium phosphate.** (mag-NEE-zee-uhm) *USP 28.*
Use: Antacid.
• **magnesium salicylate.** (mag-NEE-zee-uhm suh-LIH-sih-late) *USP 28.*
Use: Analgesic; antipyretic; antirheumatic.
See: Analate.
Backache Maximum Strength Relief.
Bayer Select Maximum Strength Backache.
Efficin.
Magan.
Momentum Muscular Backache Formula.

Nuprin Backache.
W/Diphenhydramine HCl.
See: Extra Strength Doan's PM.
W/Phenyltoloxamine citrate.
See: Mobigesic.
Novasal.

magnesium salicylate tetrahydrate.
Use: Nonnarcotic analgesic.
See: Painaid BRF Back Relief Formula.

• **magnesium silicate.** (mag-NEE-zee-uhm sill-IH-cate) NF 23.
Use: Pharmaceutic aid (tablet excipient).

• **magnesium stearate.** (mag-NEE-zee-uhm STEER-ate) NF 23.
Use: Pharmaceutic aid (tablet and capsule lubricant).

• **magnesium sulfate.** (mag-NEE-zee-uhm) USP 28.
Use: Anticonvulsant; electrolyte replacement; laxative.

magnesium sulfate. (Abbott) Magnesium sulfate (as heptahydrate) 4% (0.325 mEq/mL), 8% (0.65 mEq/mL). Inj. Single-dose flexible containers. 50 mL (8% only); 100 mL, 500 mL, 1000 mL (except 8%). Rx.
Use: Anticonvulsant.

magnesium sulfate. (Various Mfr.) Magnesium sulfate (as heptahydrate). Inj. **12.5%:** (1 mEq/mL). Preservative-free. Single-dose vials. 8 mL. **50%:** (4 mEq/mL). Preservative-free. Single-dose amps. 2 mL, 10 mL. Single-dose vials. 2 mL, 10 mL, 20 mL. Multidose vials. 50 mL. Syringes. 5 mL, 10 mL. Rx.
Use: Anticonvulsant; electrolyte replacement; laxative.

• **magnesium trisilicate.** (mag-NEE-zee-uhm try-SILL-ih-cate) USP 28.
Use: Antacid.
See: Banacid.

magnesium trisilicate w/combinations.
See: Alsorb Gel C.T.
Arcodex Antacid.
Gacid.
Gaviscon.
Maracid 2.

Magnevist. (Hospira) Gadopentetate dimeglumine 469.01 mg/mL, preservative free. Inj. Single-dose vial 5 mL, 10 mL, 15 mL, 20 mL. Prefilled Disp. Syr. 10 mL, 15 mL, 20 mL. Pharmacy bulk pkg. 100 mL. Rx.
Use: Radiopaque agent, parenteral.

Magonate. (Fleming) **Tab.:** Magnesium gluconate dihydrate 500 mg (elemental magnesium 27 mg), Ca 87.5 mg, P 66 mg (dibasic calcium phosphate dihydrate 376 mg). Bot. 1000s. **Liq.:**

Magnesium gluconate dihydrate 1000 mg/5 mL (elemental magnesium 54 mg/5 mL), sorbitol, magnesium carbonate, melon flavored. Bot. 473 mL. OTC.
Use: Mineral supplement.

Magonate Natal. (Fleming) Elemental magnesium 3.52 mg (as gluconate)/mL. Liq. Bot. 480 mL. OTC.
Use: Mineral.

Mag-Ox 400. (Blaine) Magnesium oxide 400 mg (elemental magnesium 241.3 mg). Tab. Bot. 120s, 1000s, UD 100s. OTC.
Use: Antacid; vitamin supplement; mineral.

Magsal. (US Pharmaceutical Corp.) Magnesium salicylate tetrahydrate 600 mg, phenyltoloxamine dihydrogen citrate 25 mg. Tab. Bot. 100s. Rx.
Use: Analgesic combination.

Mag-Tab SR. (Niche) Elemental magnesium (as L-lactate dihydrate) 84 mg. SR Tab. 60s, 100s, 1000s. OTC.
Use: Mineral supplement.

Magtrate. (Mission) Magnesium gluconate 500 mg (elemental magnesium 29 mg). Tab. Bot. 100s. OTC.
Use: Mineral.

Mag-200. (Optimox) Elemental magnesium (as oxide) 200 mg, PABA 300 mg. Tab. Bot. 120s. OTC.
Use: Mineral.

Maintenance Vitamin Formula w/Minerals. (Towne) Vitamins A palmitate 10,000 units, D 400 units, B_1 5 mg, B_2 2.5 mg, C 75 mg, niacinamide 40 mg, B_6 1 mg, calcium pantothenate 4 mg, B_{12} 2 mcg, E 2 units, choline bitartrate 31.4 mg, inositol 15 mg, Ca 75 mg, P 58 mg, Fe 30 mg, Mg 3 mg, Mn 0.5 mg, K 2 mg, Zn 0.5 mg. Cap. Bot. 100s. OTC.
Use: Mineral; vitamin supplement.

majeptil. Thioproperazine. Psychopharmacologic agent; pending release.

Major-gesic. (Major) Phenyltoloxamine citrate 30 mg, acetaminophen 325 mg. Tab. Bot. 100s, 1000s. OTC.
Use: Upper respiratory combination, antihistamine, analgesic.

malagride. Acetarsone.

Malaraquin. (Sanofi-Synthelabo) Chloroquine phosphate. Rx.
Use: Antimalarial.

Malarone. (GlaxoSmithKline) Atovaquone 250 mg, proguanil HCl 100 mg. Film-coated. Tab. Bot. 100s, UD 24s. Rx.
Use: Antimalarial.

Malarone Pediatric. (GlaxoSmithKline) Atovaquone 62.5 mg, proguanil HCl 25 mg. Film-coated. Tab. Bot. 100s. *Rx.*
Use: Antimalarial.

●**malathion.** (mal-ah-THIGH-ahn) *USP 28.*
Use: Pediculicide.

●**malic acid.** (MAL-ik) *NF 23.*
Use: Pharmaceutic aid (acidifying agent).

Mallamint. (Roberts) Calcium carbonate 420 mg. Tab. Bot. 100s. *OTC.*
Use: Antacid.

Mallazine Drops. (Roberts) Tetra-hydrozoline 0.05%. Soln. 15 mL. *OTC.*
Use: Mydriatic; vasoconstrictor.

Mallergan-VC w/Codeine Syrup. (Roberts) Phenylephrine HCl 5 mg, pro-methazine HCl 6.25 mg, codeine phos-phate 10 mg/5 mL, alcohol 7%. Syr. Bot. 120 mL. *c-v.*
Use: Antihistamine, antitussive, decon-gestant.

Malogen Cyp. (Forest) Testosterone cypionate in oil 100 mg, 200 mg/mL. Inj. Vial 10 mL. *c-III.*
Use: Androgen.

Malogen Injection Aqueous. (Forest) Testosterone. **25 mg/mL:** 10 mL, 30 mL. **50 mg/mL:** 10 mL. **100 mg/mL:** 10 mL. *c-III.*
Use: Androgen.

Malogen 100 L.A. in Oil. (Forest) Testo-sterone enanthate 100 mg/mL. Inj. 10 mL. *c-III.*
Use: Androgen.

Malogen 200 L.A. in Oil. (Forest) Testo-sterone enanthate 200 mg/mL. Inj. 10 mL. *c-III.*
Use: Androgen.

malonal. (Various Mfr.) Barbital.

●**malotilate.** (mal-OH-tih-LATE) USAN.
Use: Liver disorder treatment.

Malotrone Aqueous Injection. (Bluco) Testosterone, USP 25 mg, 50 mg/mL in aqueous susp. Vial 10 mL. *c-III.*
Use: Androgen.

●**maltitol solution.** (MAL-tih-tahl) *NF 23.*
Use: Sweetener.

●**maltodextrin.** (mawl-toe-dex-trin) *NF 23.*
Use: Pharmaceutic aid (coating agent, tablet binder, tablet and capsule dilu-ent, viscosity-increasing agent).

●**maltose.** (mawl-toes) *NF 23.*
Use: Pharmaceutic aid.

Maltsupex. (Wallace) Malt soup extract 8 g/level scoop. Pow. Can. 227 g, 454 g. *OTC.*
Use: Laxative.

Mammol Ointment. (Abbott) Bismuth subnitrate 40%, castor oil 30%, an-hydrous lanolin 22%, ceresin wax 7%, balsam Peru 1%. Tube ⅞ oz. Ctn. 12s. *OTC.*
Use: Dermatologic; protectant; emol-lient.

mandameth. (Major) Methenamine man-delate 0.5 g. EC Tab. Bot. 1000s. *Rx.*
Use: Anti-infective; urinary.

Mandelamine. (Warner Chilcott) Methen-amine mandalate 0.5 g, 1 g. Tab. Bot. 100s. *Rx.*
Use: Anti-infective, urinary.

mandelic acid.
Use: Anti-infective; urinary.

mandelic acid salts. (Various Mfr.) Cal-cium mandelate.

mandelyltropeine. (Various Mfr.) Hom-atropine Salts.

●**mangafodipir trisodium.** (man-gah-FOE-dih-pihr try-SO-dee-uhm) *USP 28.*
Use: Radiopaque agent, parenteral.
See: Teslascan.

Manganese.
Use: Dietary supplement.
See: Chelated Manganese.

●**manganese chloride.** (MANG-ah-neese) *USP 28.* For Oral Solution.
Use: Manganese deficiency treatment; trace mineral supplement.

●**manganese gluconate.** (MANG-ah-neese GLOO-kahn-ate) *USP 28.*
Use: Manganese deficiency; trace min-eral supplement.

manganese glycerophosphate. Gly-cerol phosphate manganese salt.
Use: Pharmaceutical necessity.

manganese hypophosphite. Manga-nese⁺⁺ phosphinate.
Use: Pharmaceutical necessity.

●**manganese sulfate.** (MANG-ah-neese) *USP 28.*
Use: Trace mineral supplement.

Manga-Pak. (SoloPak Pharmaceuticals, Inc.) Manganese 0.1 mg/mL. Inj. Vial 10 mL, 30 mL. *Rx.*
Use: Nutritional supplement; parenteral.

mangofodopir trisodium.
Use: Diagnostic aid.
See: Teslascan.

Maniron. (Jones Pharma) Ferrous fuma-rate 3 mg. Tab. Bot. 100s, 1000s, 5000s. *OTC.*
Use: Mineral supplement.

Mannan. (Rugby) Purified glucomannan 500 mg. Cap. Bot. 90s. *OTC.*
Use: Nutritional supplement.

Mann Astringent Mouth Wash Concen-trate. (Manne) Bot. 4 oz, qt, 0.5 gal, gal. Mint flavored. Bot. 4 oz, qt, 0.5 gal, gal. *OTC.*

Use: Mouthwash.

manna sugar. (Various Mfr.) Mannitol.

Mann Body Deodorant. (Manne) Bot. 4 oz, 8 oz, pt, qt. *OTC.*
Use: Deodorant.

Mann Breath Deodorant. (Manne) Bot. 1 oz, 4 oz, 8 oz, pt, qt, 0.5 gal. *OTC.*
Use: Mouthwash.

Mann Emollient. (Manne) Jar. 100 g. *OTC.*
Use: Emollient.

Mannest. (Manne) Conjugated estrogens 0.625 mg, 1.25 mg, or 2.5 mg. Tab. Bot. 100s, 200s. *Rx.*
Use: Estrogen.

Mann Eugenol U.S.P. Extra. (Manne) 0.06 lb, 0.13 lb, 0.25 lb, 0.5 lb, 1 lb. *OTC.*
Use: Dermatologic, protectant.

Mann Germicidal Solution. (Manne) **Regular:** Bot. Gal, 4 gal. **Conc.:** 12.8%. Bot. Pt, qt, 0.5 gal, gal. *OTC.*
Use: Antimicrobial.

Mann Hand Lotion. (Manne) Twin pack, gal. *OTC.*
Use: Emollient.

Mann Hemostatic. (Manne) Bot. 1 oz, 4 oz, 8 oz, pt, qt. *OTC.*
Use: Hemostatic.

mannite.
See: Mannitol.

• **mannitol.** (MAN-ih-tole) *USP 28.*
Use: Diagnostic aid.
See: Osmitrol.

mannitol hexanitrate.
Use: Coronary vasodilator.
See: Vascunitol.

mannitol hexanitrate & phenobarbital tablets. (Jones Pharma) Mannitol hexanitrate 0.5 g, phenobarbital 0.25 g. Tab. Bot. 1000s. *c-iv.*
Use: Vasodilator.

mannitol hexanitrate with phenobarbital combinations.
See: Manotensin.
Vascused.

mannitol injection. (Abbott) Mannitol 15%, 20%. *Abbo-Vac* single-dose container 500 mL.
Use: Diagnostic aid (renal function determination); diuretic.
See: Mannitol Solution.

mannitol in sodium chloride injection.
Use: Diuretic.

Mann Liquid Soap. (Manne) Concentrated cococastile. Bot. Qt, 0.5 gal, gal. *OTC.*
Use: Emollient.

Mann Lubricant and Cleanser. (Manne) Bot. Pt, qt. *OTC.*
Use: Emollient.

Mann Superfatted Bar Soap. (Manne) Rich in lanolin. Cake. 12s. *OTC.*
Use: Emollient.

Mann Talbot's Iodine. (Manne) Glycerin base. Bot. 1 oz, 4 oz, 8 oz, pt, qt. *OTC.*
Use: Antiseptic.

Mann Topical Anesthetic. (Manne) Bot. 1 oz, 4 oz, 8 oz, pt. W/stain to indicate area treated. Bot. 1oz, 4 oz, 8 oz. *OTC.*
Use: Anesthetic, local.

Manotensin. (Oxypure) Mannitol hexanitrate 32 mg, phenobarbital 16 mg. Tab. Bot. 100s, 1000s. *c-iv.*
Use: Vasodilator.

Mantoux Test.
Use: Tuberculin test.

manvene.
Use: Antineoplastic.

MAOI.
See: Monoamine Oxidase Inhibitors.

Maolate. (Pharmacia) Chlorphenesin carbamate 400 mg. Tab. Bot. 50s, 500s. *Rx.*
Use: Muscle relaxant; anxiolytic.

Maox 420. (Manne) Magnesium oxide 420 mg. Tab. Bot. 250s, 1000s. *OTC.*
Use: Antacid.

Mapap Cold Formula. (Major) Acetaminophen 325 mg, pseudoephedrine HCl 30 mg, dextromethorphan HBr 15 mg, chlorpheniramine maleate 2 mg. Tab. Pkg. 24s. *OTC.*
Use: Upper respiratory combination, analgesic, decongestant, antitussive, antihistamine.

Mapap Extra Strength. (Major) Acetaminophen 500 mg. Tab. Bot. 30s, 60s, 100s, 200s, 1000s and UD 100s. *OTC.*
Use: Analgesic.

Mapap Infant Drops. (Major) Acetaminophen 100 mg/mL, alcohol free. Bot. 15 mL, 30 mL. *OTC.*
Use: Analgesic.

Mapap Regular Strength. (Major) Acetaminophen 325 mg. Scored Tab. Bot. 100s, 1000s, UD 100s. *OTC.*
Use: Analgesic.

Mapap Sinus Maximum Strength. (Major) Pseudoephedrine HCl 30 mg, acetaminophen 500 mg. Geltab. Pkg. 24s. *OTC.*
Use: Upper respiratory combination, decongestant, analgesic.

Maprofix.
See: Gardinol Type Detergents.

• **maprotiline.** (map-ROW-tih-leen) USAN.
Use: Antidepressant.

• **maprotiline hydrochloride.** (map-ROW-tih-leen) *USP 28.*
Use: Antidepressant, tetracyclic compound.

maprotiline hydrochloride. (Various Mfr.) Maprotiline HCl 25 mg, 50 mg, 75 mg. Tab. Bot. 30s, 100s, 500s. *Rx.*
Use: Antidepressant, tetracyclic compound.

Maracid 2. (Marlin Industries) Magnesium trisilicate 150 mg, aluminum hydroxide dried gel 90 mg, aminoacetic acid 75 mg. Tab. Bot. *OTC.*
Use: Antacid; adsorbent.

Maranox. (C.S. Dent & Co.) Acetaminophen 325 mg. Tab. Bot. 8s. *OTC.*
Use: Analgesic.

Marax-DF Syrup. (Roerig) Hydroxyzine HCl 7.5 mg, ephedrine sulfate 18.75 mg, theophylline 97.5 mg/15 mL. Color free, dye free. Bot. Pt, gal. *Rx.*
Use: Antiasthmatic combination.

Marax Tab. (Roerig) Hydroxyzine HCl 10 mg, ephedrine sulfate 25 mg, theophylline 130 mg. Tab. Bot. 100s, 500s. *Rx.*
Use: Antiasthmatic combination.

Marbaxin 750. (Vortech Pharmaceuticals) Methocarbamol 750 mg. Tab. Bot. 500s. *Rx.*
Use: Muscle relaxant.

Marblen Liquid. (Fleming & Co.) Magnesium carbonate 400 mg, calcium carbonate 520 mg/5 mL. Bot. 473 mL. *OTC.*
Use: Antacid.

Marblen Tablets. (Fleming & Co.) Calcium carbonate 520 mg, magnesium carbonate 400 mg. Tab. Bot. 100s, 1000s. *OTC.*
Use: Antacid.

Marcaine. (Abbott) Bupivacaine HCl. Multiple-dose vial also contains methylparaben 1 mg/mL as preservative. **0.25%:** Single-dose amp. 50 mL. Single-dose vial 10 mL, 30 mL. Multiple-dose vial 50 mL. **0.5%:** Single-dose amp. 30 mL. Single-dose vial 10 mL, 30 mL. Multiple-dose vial 50 mL. **0.75%:** Single-dose amp. 30 mL. Single-dose vial 10 mL, 30 mL. **0.25% with epinephrine 1:200,000:** Sodium metabisulfite 0.5 mg, edetate calcium disodium 0.1 mg. Amp. 50 mL, 5s. Vial 10 mL, 30 mL, 50 mL (methylparaben 1 mg/mL). **0.5% with epinephrine 1:200,000:** Sodium metabisulfite 0.5 mg, edetate calcium disodium 0.1 mg. Single-dose amp. 3 mL, 30 mL. Single-dose vial 10 mL, 30 mL. **0.75% with epinephrine 1:200,000:** Sodium metabisulfite 0.5 mg, edetate calcium disodium 0.1 mg. Amp. 30 mL. Inj. *Rx.*
Use: Anesthetic, local amide.

Marcaine. (Eastman-Kodak) Bupivacaine 0.5%, epinephrine 1:200,000, sodium metabisulfite, EDTA 0.1 mg/mL. Inj. Dental Cart. 1.8 mL. *Rx.*
Use: Anesthetic, local amide.

Marcillin. (Marnel) Ampicillin trihydrate 500 mg. Cap. Bot. 100s. *Rx.*
Use: Anti-infective; penicillin.

Marcof Expectorant. (Marnel) Hydrocodone bitartrate 5 mg, potassium guaiacolsulfonate 350 mg/5 mL, menthol, saccharin, sorbitol, alcohol and dye free. Syr. Bot. 473 mL. *c-III.*
Use: Upper respiratory combination, antitussive, expectorant, narcotic.

Mardon. (Armenpharm Ltd.) Propoxyphene HCl. **Cap.:** 32 mg Bot. 100s, 1000s. **65 mg:** Bot. 100s, 500s, 1000s. *c-IV.*
Use: Analgesic; narcotic.

Mardon Compound. (Armenpharm Ltd.) Propoxyphene compound 65 mg, aspirin 3.5 g, phenacetin 2.5 g, caffeine 0.5 g. Cap. Bot. 100s, 500s, 1000s. *c-IV.*
Use: Analgesic combination; narcotic.

Marezine. (Himmel) Cyclizine HCl 50 mg. Tab. Bot. 100s. Box 12s. *OTC.*
Use: Anticholinergic.

Margesic. (Marnel) Butalbital 50 mg, acetaminophen 325 mg, caffeine 40 mg. Cap. Bot. 100s. *Rx.*
Use: Analgesic; hypnotic; sedative.

Margesic H. (Marnel) Hydrocodone bitartrate 5 mg, acetaminophen 500 mg. Cap. Bot. 100s. *c-III.*
Use: Analgesic combination; narcotic.

Margesic No. 3. (Marnel) Codeine phosphate 30 mg, acetaminophen 300 mg. Tab. Bot. 100s. *c-III.*
Use: Analgesic combination; narcotic.

• **marimastat.** (mah-RIH-mah-stat) USAN.
Use: Antineoplastic (matrix metalloproteinase inhibitor).

Marine Lipid Concentrate. (Vitaline) Omega-3 1200 mg, EPA 360 mg, DHA 240 mg, E 5 units/Cap., sodium free. Bot. 90s. *OTC.*
Use: Nutritional supplement.

Marinol. (Solvay) Dronabinol 2.5 mg, 5 mg, 10 mg, in sesame oil, parabens. Gelatin Cap. Bot. 25s, 60s (except 5 mg), 100s (except 10 mg). *c-III.*
Use: Antiemetic, antivertigo agent.

• **maritime pine.** (mair-ih-time) *NF 23.*
Use: Pharmaceutic aid.

Marlin Salt System. (Marlin Industries) Sodium Cl 250 mg. Tab. Bot. 200s with bot. 27.7 mL. *OTC.*
Use: Contact lens care.

Marlyn Formula 50. (Marlyn Nutraceuticals) Vitamin B_6 w/18 amino acids. Cap. Bot. 100s, 250s, 1000s. *OTC.*

Use: Nutritional supplement.

Marnatal-F. (Marnel) Ca 250 mg, Fe 60 mg, vitamins A 4000 units, D 400 units, E 30 mg, B_1 3 mg, B_2 3.4 mg, B_3 20 mg, B_6 5 mg, B_{12} 12 mcg, C 100 mg, folic acid 1 mg, Mg, Zn 25 mg, Cu, I. Tab. Bot. 30s, 100s. *Rx.*
Use: Mineral; vitamin supplement; dental caries agent.

• **maropitant citrate.** (mar-oh-PIT-ant) USAN.
Use: Antiemetic.

Marplan. (Roche) Isocarboxazid 10 mg. Tab. Bot. 100s. *Rx.*
Use: Antidepressant.

Marten-Tab. (Marnel) Butalbital 50 mg, acetaminophen 325 mg. Tab. Bot. 100s. *Rx.*
Use: Analgesic.

Marthritic. (Marnel) Salsalate 750 mg. Tab. Bot. 100s. *Rx.*
Use: Analgesic.

Masse Breast Cream. (Johnson & Johnson) Glyceryl monostearate, glycerin, cetyl alcohol, lanolin, peanut oil, Span-60, stearic acid, Tween-60, sodium benzoate, propylparaben, methylparaben, potassium hydroxide. Tube 2 oz. *OTC.*
Use: Emollient.

Massengill Baking Soda Freshness. (GlaxoSmithKline) Sanitized water, sodium bicarbonate. Soln. Bot. 180 mL. *OTC.*
Use: Vaginal agent.

Massengill Disposable Douche. (GlaxoSmithKline) Water, SD alcohol 40, lactic acid, sodium lactate, octoxynol-9, cetylpyridinium Cl, propylene glycol, diazolidinyl urea, EDTA, parabens, fragrance, color. Bot. 180 mL. *OTC.*
Use: Vaginal agent.

Massengill Extra Cleansing w/Puraclean. (GlaxoSmithKline) Vinegar, water, cetylpyridinium chloride, diazolidinyl urea, EDTA. Soln. Bot. 180 mL. *OTC.*
Use: Vaginal agent.

Massengill Feminine Cleansing Wash. (GlaxoSmithKline) Sodium laureth sulfate, magnesium oleth sulfate, sodium oleth sulfate, magnesium oleth sulfate, PEG-120 methyl glucose dioleate, parabens. Liq. Bot. 240 mL. *OTC.*
Use: Vaginal agent.

Massengill Feminine Deodorant Spray. (GlaxoSmithKline) Aerosol Bot. 3 oz. *OTC.*
Use: Vaginal agent.

Massengill Liquid. (GlaxoSmithKline) Lactic acid, SD alcohol 40, octoxynol-9, water, sodium bicarbonate. Bot.

120 mL. *OTC.*
Use: Vaginal agent.

Massengill Medicated. (GlaxoSmithKline) Povidone-iodine 0.3% when added to sanitized fluid. Bot. 6 oz. *OTC.*
Use: Vaginal agent.

Massengill Medicated Disposable Douche w/Cepticin. (GlaxoSmithKline) Povidone-iodine 10%. Liq. Vial 5 mL w/180 mL bot. of sanitized water. *OTC.*
Use: Vaginal agent.

Massengill Medicated Douche w/Cepticin. (GlaxoSmithKline) Povidone-iodine 12%. Liq. concentrate. Bot. 120 mL, 240 mL. *OTC.*
Use: Vaginal agent.

Massengill Powder. (GlaxoSmithKline) Ammonium alum, PEG-8, methyl salicylate, eucalyptus oil, menthol, thymol, phenol. Jar 120 g, 240 g, 480 g, 660 g. UD Packette 10s, 12s. *OTC.*
Use: Vaginal agent.

Massengill Soft Cloth. (GlaxoSmithKline) Hydrocortisone 0.5%, diazolidinyl urea, DMDM hydantoin, isopropyl myristate, methylparaben, polysorbate 60, propylene glycol, propylparaben, sorbitan stearate, steareth-2, steareth-21. Towelettes 10s. *OTC.*
Use: Vaginal agent.

Massengill Unscented. (GlaxoSmithKline) Water, SD alcohol 40, lactic acid, sodium lactate, octoxynol-9, cetylpyridinium chloride, propylene glycol, diazolidinyl urea, parabens, EDTA. Soln. Bot. 180 mL. *OTC.*
Use: Vaginal agent.

Massengill Vinegar & Water Extra Cleansing with Puraclean. (GlaxoSmithKline) Vinegar, water, cetylpyridinium chloride, diazolidinyl urea, EDTA. Soln. Bot. 180 mL. *OTC.*
Use: Vaginal agent.

Massengill Vinegar & Water Extra Mild. (GlaxoSmithKline) Vinegar, water, preservative free. Soln. Bot. 180 mL. *OTC.*
Use: Vaginal agent.

Massengill Vinegar-Water Disposable Douche. (GlaxoSmithKline) Water and vinegar solution. Bot. 180 mL. *OTC.*
Use: Vaginal agent.

mast cell stabilizer.
Use: Ophthalmic agent.
See: Cromolyn Sodium.
  Nedocromil Sodium.
  Pemirolast Potassium.

Master Formula. (Barth's) Vitamins A 10,000 units, D 400 units, C 180 mg, B_1 7 mg, B_2 14 mg, niacin 4.6 mg, B_6 292 mcg, pantothenic acid 210 mcg, B_{12} 25 mcg, biotin 2.9 mcg, E 50 units,

Ca 800 mg, P 387 mg, Fe 10 mg, I 0.1 mg, Cl 7.78 mg, inositol 11.6 mg, aminobenzoic acid 35 mcg, rutin 30 mg, citrus bioflavonoid complex 30 mg/ 4 Tab. Bot. 120s, 600s, 1200s. *OTC. Use:* Mineral; vitamin supplement.

Mastisol. (Ferndale) Nonirritating medical adhesive. Bot. 4 oz.
Use: Adhesive.

matrix metalloproteinase inhibitor.
Use: Corneal ulcers. [Orphan Drug]

Matulane. (Sigma-Tau) Procarbazine HCl 50 mg. Talc, mannitol, parabens. Cap. Bot. 100s. *Rx.*
Use: Antineoplastic.

Mavik. (Abbott) Trandolapril 1 mg, 2 mg, 4 mg, lactose. Tab. Bot. 100s, UD 100s. *Rx.*
Use: Antihypertensive; renin angiotensin system antagonist; angiotensin-converting enzyme inhibitor.

Maxair Inhaler. (3M) Pirbuterol acetate 0.2 mg/actuation. Aer. Metered dose inhaler 25.6 g (300 inhalations). *Rx.*
Use: Bronchodilator sympathomimetic.

Maxalt. (Merck) Rizatriptan benzoate 5 mg, 10 mg, lactose. Tab. Unit-of-use carrying case 6s. *Rx.*
Use: Antimigraine, serotonin 5-HT$_1$ receptor agonist.

Maxalt-MLT. (Merck) Rizatriptan benzoate 5 mg, 10 mg, lyophilized, mannitol, aspartame, phenylalanine 1.05 mg (5 mg only), 2.1 mg (10 mg only). Orally disintegrating Tab. 2 unit of use carrying cases of 3 tabs (6 tabs total). *Rx.*
Use: Antimigraine, serotonin, 5-HT$_1$ receptor agonist.

Maxaquin. (Searle) Lomefloxacin HCl 400 mg, lactose. Tab. Bot. 20s. *Rx.*
Use: Anti-infective, fluoroquinolone.

Max EPA. (Various Mfr.) Omega 0 poly unsaturated fatty acids 1000 mg. Cap. containing EPA 180 mg, DHA 60 mg. Cap. Bot. 50s, 60s, 100s. *OTC.*
Use: Nutritional supplement.

Maxidex. (Alcon) Dexamethasone 0.1%. Susp. *Drop-Tainers* 5 mL, 15 mL. *Rx.*
Use: Corticosteroid; ophthalmic.

Maxidone. (Watson) Hydrocodone bitartrate 10 mg, acetaminophen 750 mg, lactose. Tab. Bot. 100s, 500s. *c-III.*
Use: Narcotic analgesic combination.

Maxifed. (MCR American) Guaifenesin 780 mg, pseudoephedrine HCl 80 mg. Tab. Bot. 100s. *Rx.*
Use: Upper respiratory combination, decongestant, expectorant.

Maxifed DM. (MCR American) Guaifenesin 580 mg, pseudoephedrine HCl 60 mg, dextromethorphan HBr 30 mg, dye free. ER Tab. Bot. 100s. *Rx.*
Use: Upper respiratory combination, decongestant, expectorant, antitussive.

Maxifed-DMX. (MCR American) Dextromethorphan HBr 40 mg, guaifenesin 780 mg, pseudoephedrine HCl 80 mg. Dye free. SR Tab. 100s. *Rx.*
Use: Upper respiratory combination, decongestant, expectorant, antitussive.

Maxifed-G. (MCR American) Guaifenesin 580 mg, pseudoephedrine HCl 60 mg. Tab. Bot. 100s. *Rx.*
Use: Upper respiratory combination, decongestant, expectorant.

Maxiflor. (Allergan) Diflorasone diacetate 0.05%. Cream, Oint. Tubes 15 g, 30 g, 60 g. *Rx.*
Use: Corticosteroid, topical.

Maxilube. (Mission Pharmacal) Water, silicone oil, glycerin, carbomer 934, triethanolamine, sodium lauryl sulfate, parabens. Jelly 90 g, 150 g. *OTC.*
Use: Vaginal agent.

Maximum Bayer Aspirin Tablets and Capsules. (Bayer Corp. (Consumer Div.)) Aspirin (Acetylsalicylic Acid; ASA) 500 mg. **Tab.:** 10s, 30s, 60s, 100s. **Capl.:** 60s. *OTC.*
Use: Analgesic.

Maximum Blue Label. (Vitaline) Vitamins A 2500 units, D 16.7 units, E 66.7 mg, B$_1$ 16.7 mg, B$_2$ 8.3 mg, B$_3$ 31.7 mg, B$_5$ 66.7 mg, B$_6$16.7 mg, B$_{12}$ 16.7 mcg, C 200 mg, folic acid 0.13 mg, Zn 5 mg, Ca, Cr, Cu, I, K, Mg, Mn, Mo, Se, Si, V, biotin 50 mcg, SOD, l-lysine. Tab. Bot. 180s. *OTC.*
Use: Mineral; vitamin supplement.

Maximum Green Label. (Vitaline) Vitamins A 2500 units, D 16.7 units, E 66.7 mg, B$_1$ 16.7 mg, B$_2$ 8.3 mg, B$_3$ 31.7 mg, B$_5$ 66.7 mg, B$_6$16.7 mg, B$_{12}$ 16.7 mcg, C 200 mg, folic acid 0.13 mg, Zn 5 mg, Ca, Cr, I, K, Mg, Mn, Mo, Se, Si, V, biotin 50 mcg, SOD, l-lysine. Tab. Bot. 180s. *OTC.*
Use: Mineral; vitamin supplement.

Maximum Pain Relief Pamprin. (Chattem) Acetaminophen 250 mg, magnesium salicylate 250 mg, pamabrom 25 mg. Capl. Bot. 16s, 32s. *OTC.*
Use: Analgesic combination.

Maximum Red Label. (Vitaline) Iron 3.3 mg, vitamins A 2500 units, D 67 units, E 66.7 mg, B$_1$ 16.7 mg, B$_2$ 8.3 mg, B$_3$ 31.7 mg, B$_5$ 66.7 mg, B$_6$ 16.7 mg, B$_{12}$ 16.7 mcg, C 200 mg, folic acid 0.13 mg, Zn 5 mg, Ca, Cr, Su, I, K, Mg, Mo, Se, Si, V, biotin 50 mcg, choline, inositol, bioflavonoids, l-lysine,

PABA. Tab. Bot. 180s. *OTC.*
Use: Mineral; vitamin supplement.
Maximum Relief ex•lax. (Novartis) Sennosides 25 mg, sucrose. Tab. Bot. 24s, 48s. *OTC.*
Use: Laxative.
Maximum Strength Allergy Drops. (Bausch & Lomb) Naphazoline HCl 0.03%. Soln. Bot. 15 mL. *OTC.*
Use: Mydriatic; vasoconstrictor.
Maximum Strength Anbesol. (Whitehall-Robins) **Gel:** Benzocaine 20%, alcohol 60%, saccharin. Tube 7.2 g. **Liq.:** Benzocaine 20%, alcohol 60%, saccharin. Bot. 9 mL. *OTC.*
Use: Anesthetic, local.
Maximum Strength Aqua-Ban. (Thompson Medical) Pamabrom 50 mg, lactose. Tab. Bot. 30s. *OTC.*
Use: Diuretic.
Maximum Strength Benadryl. (Parke-Davis) **Cream:** Diphenhydramine HCl 2%, parabens in a greaseless base. Jar 15 g. **Spray, non-aerosol:** Diphenhydramine HCl 2%, alcohol 85%. Bot. 60 mL. *OTC.*
Use: Antihistamine, topical.
Maximum Strength Benadryl Itch Relief. (Warner Lambert) Diphenhydramine HCl. **Cream:** 2%, zinc acetate 1%, parabens, aloe vera. 14.2 g. **Stick:** 2%, zinc acetate 1%. Alcohol 73.5%, aloe vera. 14 mL. *OTC.*
Use: Antihistamine.
Maximum Strength Clearasil Clearstick.
See: Clearasil.
Maximum Strength Clearasil Clearstick for Sensitive Skin.
See: Clearasil.
Maximum Strength Comtrex.
See: Comtrex.
Maximum Strength Cortaid. (Pharmacia) Hydrocortisone 1% in parabens, mineral oil, white petrolatum. Oint. Tube 15 g, 30 g. *OTC.*
Use: Corticosteroid, topical.
Maximum Strength Cortaid Faststick. (Pharmacia) Hydrocortisone 1%, alcohol 55%, methylparaben. Stick, roll-on. 14 g. *OTC.*
Use: Corticosteroid, topical.
Maximum Strength Corticaine. (UCB) Hydrocortisone acetate 1%, glycerin, menthol, EDTA, parabens. Cream Tube 30 g. *OTC.*
Use: Corticosteroid, topical.
Maximum Strength Dermarest Dricort Creme. (Del) Hydrocortisone (as acetate) 1%, white petrolatum. Cream Tube 14 g. *OTC.*

Use: Corticosteroid, topical.
Maximum Strength Desenex Antifungal. (Novartis) Miconazole nitrate 2%, EDTA. Cream Tube 14 g. *OTC.*
Use: Antifungal, topical.
Maximum Strength Dristan. (Whitehall-Robins) Pseudoephedrine HCl 30 mg, acetaminophen 500 mg. Cap. Bot. 24s, 48s, 100s. *OTC.*
Use: Decongestant, analgesic.
Maximum Strength Dristan Cold. (Whitehall-Robins) Pseudoephedrine HCl 30 mg, brompheniramine maleate 2 mg, acetaminophen 500 mg. Capl. Pkg. 16s, Bot. 36s. *OTC.*
Use: Decongestant, analgesic, antihistamine.
Maximum Strength Dynafed Plus. (BDI) Acetaminophen 500 mg, pseudoephedrine 30 mg. Tab. Bot. 30s. *OTC.*
Use: Analgesic, decongestant.
Maximum Strength Flexall 454. (Chattem) Menthol 16%, aloe vera gel, eucalyptus oil, methyl salicylate, SD alcohol 38-B, thyme oil. Gel Tube 90 g. *OTC.*
Use: Liniment.
Maximum Strength Halls-Plus. (Warner Lambert) Menthol 10 mg, corn syrup, sucrose. Loz. Pkg. 10s, 20s. *OTC.*
Use: Anesthetic.
Maximum Strength Ivarest. (Blistex) Calamine 14%, diphenhydramine HCl 2%. Lanolin oil, petrolatum, propylene glycol. Cream. 56 g. *OTC.*
Use: Poison ivy treatment.
Maximum Strength KeriCort-10. (Bristol-Myers Squibb) Hydrocortisone 1%, parabens, cetyl alcohol, stearyl alcohol. Cream Tube 56.7 g. *OTC.*
Use: Corticosteroid, topical.
Maximum Strength Meted. (Medicis) Sulfur 5%, salicylic acid 3%. Shampoo. Bot. 118 mL. *OTC.*
Use: Antiseborrheic combination.
Maximum Strength Midol. (Bayer Corp. (Consumer Div.)) Ibuprofen 200 mg. Tab. Bot. 24s *OTC.*
Use: Analgesic; NSAID.
Maximum Strength, Midol Multi-Symptom. (Bayer Corp. (Consumer Div.)) Acetaminophen 325 mg, pyrilamine maleate 12.5 mg. Tab. Bot. 30s. *OTC.*
Use: Analgesic combination.
Maximum Strength Midol PMS. (Bayer Corp. (Consumer Div.)) Acetaminophen 500 mg, pamabrom 25 mg, pyrilamine maleate 15 mg. Capl. Pkg. 8s, 16s. Bot. 32s. Gelcaps. Pkg. 12s, 24s. *OTC.*
Use: Analgesic combination.

Maximum Strength Nasal Decongestant. (Taro) Oxymetazoline HCl 0.05%, 0.002% phenylmercuric acetate, benzalkonium chloride. Spray Bot. 15 mL, 30 mL. *OTC.*
Use: Decongestant.

Maximum Strength No-Aspirin Sinus Medication. (Walgreen) Acetaminophen 500 mg, pseudoephedrine HCl 30 mg. Tab. Bot. 50s. *OTC.*
Use: Analgesic, decongestant.

Maximum Strength NoDoz. (Bristol-Myers) Caffeine 200 mg, sucrose. Tab. Pkg. 36s. *OTC.*
Use: CNS stimulant, analeptic.

Maximum Strength Nytol. (Block Drug) Diphenhydramine HCl 50 mg. Tab., lactose. Pkg. 8s, 16s. *OTC.*
Use: Sleep aid.

Maximum Strength Orajel Gel. (Del) Benzocaine 20%, saccharin. Tube 9.45 mL. *OTC.*
Use: Anesthetic, local.

Maximum Strength Orajel Liquid. (Del) Benzocaine 20%, ethyl alcohol 44.2%, phenol, tartrazine, saccharin. Liq. Bot. 13.3 mL. *OTC.*
Use: Anesthetic, local.

Maximum Strength Ornex. (Menley & James Labs, Inc.) Pseudoephedrine HCl 30 mg, acetaminophen 500 mg. Cap. Bot. 24s, 48s. *OTC.*
Use: Analgesic, decongestant.

Maximum Strength Oinc Aid. (McNeil Consumer) Pseudoephedrine HCl 30 mg, acetaminophen 500 mg. Cap., Tab., or Gelcap. **Cap. & Tab.:** Bot. 50s. **Gelcaps:** Bot. 40s. *OTC.*
Use: Analgesic, decongestant.

Maximum Strength Sinutab Nighttime. (Warner Lambert) Pseudoephedrine HCl 10 mg, diphenhydramine HCl 8.33 mg, acetaminophen 167 mg/5 mL. Liq. Alcohol free. 120 mL. *OTC.*
Use: Analgesic, antihistamine, decongestant.

Maximum Strength Sinutab Without Drowsiness. (Warner Lambert) Pseudoephedrine HCl 30 mg, acetaminophen 500 mg. Tab. or Capl. Bot. 24s, 48s (tab. only). *OTC.*
Use: Analgesic, decongestant.

Maximum Strength Sleepinal. (Thompson Medical) **Cap.:** Diphenhydramine HCl 50 mg, lactose. Pkg. 16s. **Soft gel:** Diphenhydramine HCl 50 mg, sorbitol. Pkg. 16s. *OTC.*
Use: Sleep aid.

Maximum Strength Sudafed Severe Cold Formula. (GlaxoSmithKline) Dextromethorphan HBr 15 mg, pseudoephedrine HCl 30 mg, acetaminophen 500 mg. Tab. 10s. *OTC.*
Use: Analgesic, antitussive, decongestant.

Maximum Strength Sudafed Sinus. (Warner Lambert) Pseudoephedrine HCl 30 mg, acetaminophen 500 mg. Tab. or Capl. Bot. 24s, 48s. *OTC.*
Use: Analgesic, decongestant.

Maximum Strength Thera-Flu Non-Drowsy.
See: Thera-Flu.

Maximum Strength Tylenol Allergy Sinus. (McNeil Consumer) Pseudoephedrine HCl 30 mg, chlorpheniramine maleate 2 mg, acetaminophen 500 mg. Tab. Bot. 24s, 60s. *OTC.*
Use: Analgesic, antihistamine, decongestant.

Maximum Strength Tylenol Cough. (McNeil Consumer) Dextromethorphan HBr 7.5 mg, acetaminophen 250 mg/5 mL, alcohol 10%. Liq. Bot. 120 mL. *OTC.*
Use: Analgesic, antitussive.

Maximum Strength Tylenol Cough w/Decongestant. (McNeil Consumer) Pseudoephedrine HCl 15 mg, dextromethorphan HBr 7.5 mg, acetaminophen 250 mg/5 mL, alcohol 10%. Liq. Bot. 120 mL. *OTC.*
Use: Analgesic, antitussive, decongestant.

Maximum Strength Tylenol Flu Night-Time Gelcaps. (McNeil Consumer) Pseudoephedrine HCl 30 mg, chlorpheniramine maleate 2 mg, acetaminophen 500 mg. Gelcap. Pkg. 12s, 20s. *OTC.*
Use: Analgesic, antihistamine, decongestant.

Maximum Strength Tylenol Flu Night-Time Powder. (McNeil Consumer) Pseudoephedrine HCl 60 mg, diphenhydramine HCl 50 mg, acetaminophen 1000 mg. Powd. Pkt. 6s. *OTC.*
Use: Analgesic, antihistamine, decongestant.

Maximum Strength Tylenol Select Allergy Sinus. (McNeil Consumer) Pseudoephedrine HCl 30 mg, diphenhydramine HCl 25 mg, acetaminophen 500 mg. Cap. Bot. 24s. *OTC.*
Use: Analgesic, antihistamine, decongestant.

Maximum Strength Tylenol Sinus. (McNeil Consumer) Pseudoephedrine HCl 30 mg, acetaminophen 500 mg. Tab., Capl., or Gelcap. **Tab. and Capl.:** Bot. 24s, 50s. **Gelcap:** Bot. 24s, 60s. *OTC.*
Use: Analgesic, decongestant.

Maximum Strength Unisom SleepGels.
(Pfizer) Diphenhydramine HCl 50 mg,
sorbitol. Cap. Pkg. 8s. *OTC.*
Use: Sleep aid.

Maximum Strength Wart Remover.
(Stiefel) Salicylic acid 17%, alcohol
29%, castor oil, flexible collodion. Liq.
13.3 mL. *OTC.*
Use: Keratolytic.

MAXIPHEN DM. (AMBI) Dextromethorphan HBr 60 mg, guaifenesin 1000 mg,
phenylephrine HCl 40 mg. Dye-free.
ER Tab. 100s. *Rx.*
Use: Antitussive, expectorant.

Maxipime. (Dura) Cefepime HCl 500 mg,
1 g, 2 g. Pow. for Inj. Vial 15 mL
(500 mg, 1 g), 20 mL (2 g), *ADD-Vantage* Vial (1 g, 2 g), piggyback bottle
100 mL (1 g, 2 g). *Rx.*
Use: Antibiotic; cephalosporin.

maxiton.
See: Amphetamine.

Maxitrol Ointment. (Alcon) Dexamethasone 0.1%, neomycin 0.35%, polymyxin B sulfate 10,000 units/g. Tube
3.5 g. *Rx.*
Use: Anti-infective; ophthalmic.

Maxitrol Ophthalmic Suspension. (Alcon) Dexamethasone 0.1%, neomycin
(as sulfate) 0.35%, polymyxin B sulfate 10,000 units/mL, benzalkonium
chloride 0.004%, hydroxypropyl methylcellulose 0.5%, hydrochloric acid, sodium chloride, polysorbate 20, sodium
hydroxide. *Drop-Tainer* 5 mL. *Rx.*
Use: Anti-infective; ophthalmic; steroid
antibiotic combination.

Maxi-Tuss DM. (MCR American Pharmaceuticals) Dextromethorphan HBr
20 mg, guaifenesin 200 mg/5 mL, glucose, menthol, parabens, saccharin,
black cherry flavor. Liq. Bot. 473 mL.
Rx.
Use: Upper respiratory combination, antitussive, expectorant.

Maxi-Tuss HC. (MCR American Pharmaceuticals.) Hydrocodone bitartrate
2.5 mg, chlorpheniramine maleate
4 mg, phenylephrine HCl 10 mg/5 mL.
Liq. Bot. 473 mL. *c-III.*
Use: Upper respiratory combination, antitussive, antihistamine, decongestant.

Maxi-Tuss HCG. (MCR American) Hydrocodone bitartrate 6 mg, guaifenesin
200 mg/5 mL. Alcohol-free. Aspartame,
parabens. Liq. *c-III.*
Use: Antitussive, expectorant.

Maxi-Tuss HCX. (MCR American) Hydrocodone bitartrate 6 mg, chlorpheni-
amine maleate 2 mg, phenylephrine

HCl 12 mg/5 mL. Alcohol-free. Liq. *c-III.*
Use: Antitussive combination.

Maxi-Vite. (Ivax) Vitamins A 10,000 units,
D 400 units, E 15 mg, B_1 10 mg, B_2
10 mg, B_3 100 mg, B_5 20 mg, B_6 5 mg,
B_{12} 5 mcg, C 200 mcg, Ca 53.5 mg, Fe
1.5 mg, folic acid 0.4 mg, biotin 1 mcg,
I, P, Cu, Mg, Mn, Zn 1.5 mg, PABA,
rutin, glutamic acid, inositol, choline bitartrate, bioflavonoids, l-lysine, betaine, lecithin. Tab. Bot. 60s. *OTC.*
Use: Mineral; vitamin supplement.

Maxolon Tablets. (GlaxoSmithKline)
Metoclopramide HCl 10 mg. Bot. 100s.
Rx.
Use: Antiemetic; gastrointestinal stimu-
lant.

Maxovite. (Tyson) Vitamins A 2083 units,
D 16.7 units, E 16.7 mg, B_1 5 mg, B_2
4.2 mg, B_3 4.2 mg, B_5 4.2 mg, B_6
54.2 mg, B_{12} 10.8 mcg, C 250 mg, folic
acid 0.33 mg, Zn 5 mg, Ca, Cr, Cu,
Fe, I, K, Mg, Mn, Se, biotin 11.7 mcg.
Tab. Bot. 120s, 240s. *OTC.*
Use: Mineral; vitamin supplement.

Maxzide. (Wyeth) Hydrochlorothiazide
50 mg, triamterene 75 mg. Tab. Bot.
100s, 500s, UD 10 × 10s. *Rx.*
Use: Antihypertensive; diuretic.

Maxzide-25MG. (Wyeth) Triamterene
37.5 mg, hydrochlorothiazide 25 mg.
Tab. Bot. 100s, UD 100s. *Rx.*
Use: Diuretic combination.

Mayotic. (Merz) Hydrocortisone 1%, neomycin sulfate 5 mg, polymyxin B sulfate 10,000 units/mL, thimerosal 0.01%.
Susp. Bot. 10 mL w/dropper. *Rx.*
Use: Otic.

• **maytansine.** (MAY-tan-SEEN) USAN.
Use: Antineoplastic.

• **mazapertine succinate.** (mazz-ah-
PURR-teen) USAN.
Use: Antipsychotic.

Mazicon. (Roche) Flumazenil 0.1 mg/
mL. Inj. Vial 5 mL, 10 mL. *Rx.*
Use: Antidote.

• **mazindol.** (MAZE-in-dole) *USP 28.*
Use: Anorexic; appetite suppressant;
Duchenne muscular dystrophy.
[Orphan Drug]

M-Caps. (Mill-Mark) Methionine 200 mg.
Cap. Bot. 50s, 1000s. *Rx.*
Use: Diaper rash preparation.

MCT Oil. (Bristol-Myers Squibb) Triglycerides of medium chain fatty acids.
Lipid fraction of coconut oil; fatty acid
shorter than C_8 < 6%, C_8 (octanoic)
67%, C_{10} (decanoic) 23%, longer than
C_{10} 4%. Bot. Qt. *OTC.*
Use: Nutritional supplement, enteral.

MDP-Squibb. (Bristol-Myers Squibb) Technetium Tc 99 medronate. Reaction vial pkg. 10s.
Use: Radiopaque agent.

MD-76 R. (Mallinckrodt) Diatrizoate meglumine 660 mg, diatrizoate sodium 100 mg, iodine 370 mg/mL. Inj. Vial 50 mL. Bot. 100 mL, 150 mL, 200 mL. Power injector syr. 125 mL. *Rx.*
Use: Radiopaque agent; parenteral.

MD-60. (Mallinckrodt) Diatrizoate meglumine 52%, diatrizoate sodium 8% (29.2% iodine). Inj. Vial 30 mL, 50 mL.
Use: Radiopaque agent.

meadinin. Mixture of Amoidin & Amidin alk. of Ammi Majus Linn.

measles, mumps, and rubella virus vaccine live. (MEE-zuhls, mumps, and ru-BELL-uh vaccine)
Use: Immunization.
See: M-M-R II.

measles prophylactic serum.
See: Immune Globulin (Intramuscular).

• **measles virus vaccine, live.** (MEE-zuhls) *USP 28.* Modified live-virus measles vaccine.
Use: Immunization.
See: Attenuvax.
W/Mumps virus vaccine, rubella virus vaccine.
See: M-M-R II.

measles virus vaccine, live attenuated. Moratonline derived from Enders' attenuated Edmonston strain grown in cell cultures of chick embryos.
See: Attenuvax.
W/Mumps virus vaccine, rubella virus vaccine.
See: M-M-R II.

Mebaral. (Ovation) Mephobarbital 0.5 gr, 0.75 gr, 1.5 gr. Tab. Bot. 250s. *c-iv.*
Use: Anticonvulsant; sedative.

• **mebendazole.** (meh-BEND-uh-zole) *USP 28.*
Use: Anthelmintic.
See: Vermox.

mebendazole. (Copley) Mebendazole 100 mg. Chew. Tab. Pkg. 12s, 36s. *Rx.*
Use: Anthelmintic.

• **mebeverine hydrochloride.** (MEH-BEH-ver-een) USAN.
Use: Spasmolytic agent; muscle relaxant.

• **mebrofenin.** (MEH-broe-FEN-in) *USP 28.*
Use: Diagnostic aid (hepatobiliary function determination).

• **mebutamate.** (MEH-byoo-TAM-at) USAN.
Use: Antihypertensive.

• **mecamylamine hydrochloride.** (mek-ah-MILL-ah-meen) *USP 28.*
Use: Antihypertensive, antiadrenergic.
See: Inversine.

• **mecasermin.** (mek-a-SER-min) USAN.
Use: Antidiabetic.

• **mecetronium ethylsulfate.** (MEH-seh-TROE-nee-uhm ETH-ill-SULL-fate) USAN.
Use: Antiseptic.

• **mechlorethamine hydrochloride.** (meh-klor-ETH-ah-meen) *USP 28.*
Use: Antineoplastic, alkylating agent.
See: Mustargen.

mecholin hydrochloride.
See: Methacholine Chloride.

Mecholyl Ointment. (Gordon Laboratories) Methacholine Cl 0.25%, methyl salicylate 10% in ointment base. Jar 4 oz, 1 lb, 5 lb. *OTC.*
Use: Analgesic, topical.

meclastine. Clemastine.

• **meclizine hydrochloride.** (MEK-lih-zeen) *USP 28.*
Use: Antinauseant; antiemetic.
See: Antivert.
Antivert/50.
Antivert/25.
Antrizine.
Dizmiss.
Dramamine II.
Dramamine Less Drowsy Formula.
Meclizine HCl.
Meni-D.

Meclizine HCl. (Various Mfr.) Meclizine HCl. **Tab.: 12.5 mg:** Bot. 30s, 60s, 100s, 500s, 1000s, UD 100s. **25 mg:** Bot. 12s, 20s, 30s, 60s, 100s, 500s, 1000s, UD 32s, 100s. **50 mg:** Bot. 100s. **Chew Tab.: 25 mg:** Bot. 20s, 30s, 60s, 100s, 1000s, UD 100s. *Rx-OTC.*
Use: Antiemetic/antivertigo agent.

• **meclocycline.** (meh-kloe-SIGH-kleen) USAN.
Use: Anti-infective.

• **meclofenamate sodium.** (mek-loe-FEN-uh-mate) *USP 28.*
Use: Anti-inflammatory.

meclofenamate sodium. (Various Mfr.) Meclofenamate sodium 50 mg, 100 mg. Cap. Bot. 100s, 500s, 1000s. *Rx.*
Use: Anti-inflammatory; NSAID.

• **meclofenamic acid.** (MEH-kloe-fen-AM-ik) USAN.
Use: Anti-inflammatory.

• **mecloqualone.** (MEH-kloe-KWAH-lone) USAN.
Use: Sedative, hypnotic.

- **meclorisone dibutyrate.** (MEH-KLAHR-ih-sone die-BYOO-tih-rate) USAN.
Use: Anti-inflammatory, topical.
- **mecobalamin.** (MEH-koe-BAHL-ah-min) USAN.
Use: Vitamin (hematopoietic).
mecodrin.
See: Amphetamine.
- **mecrylate.** (MEH-krih-late) USAN.
Use: Surgical aid (tissue adhesive).
mecysteine. Methyl Cysteine.
Meda Cap. (Circle) Acetaminophen 500 mg. Cap. Bot. 25s, 60s, 100s. *OTC.*
Use: Analgesic.
Medacote. (Dal-Med Pharmaceuticals) Pyrilamine maleate 1%, dimethyl polysiloxane, zinc oxide, menthol, camphor in a greaseless base. Lot. Bot. 120 mL. *OTC.*
Use: Antihistamine, topical.
Medadyne. (Dal-Med Pharmaceuticals) **Liq.:** Methyl benzethonium chloride, benzocaine, tannic acid, camphor, chlorothymol, menthol, benzyl alcohol, alcohol 61%. Bot. 15 mL, 30 mL. **Throat Spray:** Lidocaine, cetyl dimethyl ammonium chloride, ethyl alcohol. Bot. 30 mL. *OTC.*
Use: Mouth and throat preparation.
Meda-Hist Expectorant. (Medwick) Bot. 4 oz, pt, gal.
Use: Decongestant, antitussive.
Medalox Gel. (Davol) Magnesium aluminum hydroxide gel. Bot. 12 oz, pt, gal. *OTC.*
Use: Antacid.
Medamint. (Dal-Med Pharmaceuticals) Benzocaine 10 mg/Loz. Pkg. 12s, 24s. *OTC.*
Use: Mouth and throat preparation.
Meda Tab. (Circle) Acetaminophen 325 mg. Bot. 100s. *OTC.*
Use: Analgesic.
Medatussin Pediatric. (Dal-Med Pharmaceuticals) Dextromethorphan HBr 5 mg, guaifenesin 50 mg, potassium citrate, citric acid, sorbitol, saccharin. Syr. Bot. 120 mL. *OTC.*
Use: Antitussive, expectorant.
- **medazepam hydrochloride.** (med-AZE-eh-pam) USAN. Under study.
Use: Anxiolytic.
Medebar Plus. (Mallinckrodt) Barium sulfate 100%, simethicone. Susp. Bot. 1900 mL. Kit w/enema tip-tubing assemblies 650 mL. *Rx.*
Use: Radiopaque agent; GI contrast agent.
Medent. (Stewart-Jackson Pharmacal) Pseudoephedrine HCl 120 mg, guai-

fenesin 500 mg. Tab. Bot. 100s.
Use: Decongestant, expectorant.
Mederma. (Merz) PEG-4, onion (allium cepa) extract, xanthan gum, allantoin, fragrance, methylparaben. Gel. Tube. 50 g. *OTC.*
Use: Helps scars appear softer and smoother.
Medescan. (Mallinckrodt) Barium sulfate 2.3%, sorbitol, saccharin, sodium benzoate. Susp. Bot. 250 mL, 450 mL, 1900 mL. *Rx.*
Use: Radiopaque agent; GI contrast agent.
Medicaine Cream. (Walgreen) Benzocaine 3%, resorcinol 2%. Tube 1.25 oz. *OTC.*
Use: Antipruritic.
Medicated Acne Cleanser. (C & M Pharmacal) Sulfur 4%, resorcinol 2%, SD alcohol 40 11.65%, methylparaben. Lot. Bot. 120 mL. *OTC.*
Use: Dermatologic, acne.
Medicated Healer. (Walgreen) Strong ammonia soln. 10%, camphor 2.6%. Bot. 6 oz. *OTC.*
Use: Emollient.
Medicated Powder. (Johnson & Johnson) Zinc oxide, talc, fragrance, menthol. Plastic container 3 oz, 6 oz, 11 oz. *OTC.*
Use: Antipruritic.
Medicone Ointment. (Lee Pharma) Benzocaine 20%. 30 g. *OTC.*
Use: Anorectal preparation.
Medi-First Sinus Decongestant. (Textilease Medique) Pseudoephedrine HCl 30 mg. Tab. Bot. 100s, 250s. *OTC.*
Use: Nasal decongestant; arylalkylamine.
Medigesic. (US Pharmaceutical Corp.) Acetaminophen 325 mg, caffeine 40 mg, butalbital 50 mg. Cap. Bot. 100s. *Rx.*
Use: Analgesic; hypnotic, sedative.
Medihaler-Iso. (3M) Isoproterenol sulfate 80 mcg/actuation. Aer. Inhaler 15 mL ($\geq$ 300 doses) w/adapter and 15 mL refill. *Rx.*
Use: Sympathomimetic bronchodilator.
Mediotic-HC. (Dayton) Hydrocortisone 1%, pramoxine hydrochloride 1%, chloroxylenol 0.1%, benzalkonium chloride 0.01%. Drops. Vial. 15 mL with dropper. *Rx.*
Use: Miscellaneous otic preparation.
Medipak. (Armenpharm Ltd.) First-aid kit.
Medi-Phite. (Davol) Vitamins B_1 and B_{12}. Syr. Bot. 4 oz, pt, gal. *OTC.*
Use: Vitamin supplement.

Mediplast. (Beiersdorf) Salicylic acid plaster 40%. Box 25s. *OTC.*
Use: Keratolytic.
Mediplex Plus. (US Pharm) Vitamins E (dl-alpha tocopheryl) 50 units, B_1 25 mg, B_2 10 mg, B_3 100 mg, B_5 25 mg, B_6 10 mg, B_{12} 25 mcg, C 300 mg, folic acid 0.4 mg, Zn 18 mg, Cu, Mg, Mn. Bot. Tab. 100s. *OTC.*
Use: Multivitamin.
Mediplex Tabules. (US Pharmaceutical Corp.) Vitamins E 60 units, B_1 25 mg, B_2 10 mg, B_3 100 mg, B_5 25 mg, B_6 10 mg, B_{12} 25 mcg, C 300 mg, Zn 4 mg, Cu, Mg, Mn. Bot. 100s. *OTC.*
Use: Mineral; vitamin supplement.
Mediquell. (Parke-Davis) Dextromethorphan HBr 15 mg. Chewy Square. Pkg. 12s, 24s. *OTC.*
Use: Antitussive.
Medi-Quik Aerosol. (Mentholatum Co.) Lidocaine 2.5%, benzalkonium Cl 0.1%, ethanol 38%. Aerosol 3 oz. *OTC.*
Use: Antiseptic; anesthetic, local.
• **medorinone.** (MEH-doe-RIH-nohn) USAN.
Use: Cardiovascular agent.
Medotar. (Medco) Coal tar 1%, octoxynol-5, zinc oxide, white petrolatum. Oint. 454 g. *OTC.*
Use: Antipsoriatic; antipruritic.
• **medrogestone.** (MEH-droe-JEST-ohn) USAN.
Use: Hormone, progestin.
Medrol. (Pharmacia) Methylprednisolone. **Tab.:** 2 mg. Bot. 100s; 4 mg Bot. 30s, 100s, 500s, UD 100s; 8 mg Bot. 25s; 16 mg Bot. 50s; 24 mg Bot. 25s; 32 mg Bot. 25s. **Dosepak:** 4 mg Pkg. 21s. **Alternate Daypak:** 16 mg Pkg. 14s. *Rx.*
Use: Corticosteroid.
• **medronate disodium.** (MEH-droe-nate) USAN. *Formerly Disodium Methylene Diphosphonate; MDP.*
Use: Pharmaceutic aid.
• **medronic acid.** (meh-DRAH-nik) USAN.
Use: Pharmaceutic aid.
Medrosphol Hg-197. Merprane.
• **medroxalol.** (meh-DROX-ah-LAHL) USAN.
Use: Antihypertensive.
• **medroxalol hydrochloride.** (meh-DROX-ah-LAHL) USAN.
Use: Antihypertensive.
• **medroxyprogesterone acetate.** (meh-DROX-ee-pro-JESS-tuh-rone) *USP 28.*
Tall Man: MedroxyPROGESTERone
Use: Hormone, progestin.
See: Depo-Provera.

Depo-Sub Q Provera 104.
Provera.
W/Conjugated Estrogens.
See: Premphase.
Prempro.
medroxyprogesterone acetate. (CMC) Medroxyprogesterone acetate 50 mg, 100 mg/mL. Vial 5 mL.
Use: Hormone, progestin.
medroxyprogesterone acetate. (Sicor) Medroxyprogesterone acetate 150 mg/mL. PEG 28.9 mg, sodium chloride 8.68 mg, 2.41 mg, sodium chloride 8.68 mg, methylparaben 1.37 mg, propylparaben 0.15 mg. Inj. Vials. 1 mL. *Rx.*
Use: Contraceptive.
medroxyprogesterone acetate. (Wyeth) Medroxyprogesterone acetate 10 mg. Tab. Bot. 50s, 250s. *Rx.*
Use: Hormone, progestin.
medroxyprogesterone acetate. (Various Mfr.) Medroxyprogesterone acetate 2.5 mg, 5 mg, 10 mg. Tab. Bot. 30s, 40s (10 mg only), 50s (10 mg only), 90s (2.5 mg only), 100s, 250s (10 mg only), 500s, 1000s (2.5 and 5 mg only). *Rx.*
Use: Hormone, progestin.
MED-Rx. (Ionpharm) Pseudoephedrine HCl 60 mg, guaifenesin 600 mg. CR Tab. Box 28s. Guaifenesin 600 mg. CR Tab. Box 28s. *Rx.*
Use: Decongestant, expectorant.
• **medrysone.** (MEH-drih-sone) USAN.
Use: Ophthalmic corticosteroid, topical.
See: HMS.
• **mefenamic acid.** (MEH-fen-AM-ik) *USP 28.*
Use: Anti-inflammatory; analgesic.
See: Ponstel.
• **mefenidil.** (meh-FEN-ih-dill) USAN.
Use: Cerebral vasodilator.
• **mefenidil fumarate.** (meh-FEN-ih-dill) USAN.
Use: Cerebral vasodilator.
• **mefenorex hydrochloride.** (meh-FEN-oh-rex) USAN. Under study.
Use: Anorexic.
• **mefexamide.** (meh-FEX-am-IDE) USAN.
Use: Stimulant (central).
• **mefloquine hydrochloride.** (MEH-flow-kwin) USAN.
Use: Antimalarial. [Orphan Drug]
See: Lariam.
• **mefloquine hydrochloride.** (MEH-flow-kwin) (Geneva) Mefloquine HCl 250 mg. Tab. Bot. 25s. *Rx.*
Use: Antimalarial.
Mefoxin. (Merck & Co.) Sterile cefoxitin sodium. **Pow. for Inj.:** 1 g, 2 g, 10 g.

Vial and Infusion Bot. (1 g, 2 g), Bulk Bot. (10 g). **Inj.:** 1 g, 2 g, dextrose. Premixed, frozen in 50 mL plastic containers. *Rx.*
Use: Anti-infective; cephalosporin.

Mefoxin in 5% Dextrose. (Merck & Co.) Cefoxitin sodium 1 g, 2 g in Dextrose in Water 5%. Inj. Containers 50 mL. *Rx.*
Use: Anti-infective; cephalosporin.

•**mefruside.** (MEFF-ruh-side) USAN.
Use: Diuretic.

Mega B. (Arco) Vitamins B_1 100 mg, B_2 100 mg, B_3 100 mg, B_5 100 mg, B_6 100 mg, B_{12} 100 mcg, folic acid 100 mcg, d-biotin 100 mcg, PABA 100 mg. Tab. Bot. 100s. *OTC.*
Use: Vitamin supplement.

Megace. (Bristol-Myers Oncology) Megestrol acetate. **Tab.:** 40 mg, lactose. Bot. 250s, 500s. **Susp.:** 40 mg/mL, alcohol ≤ 0.06%, sucrose, lemon-lime flavor. Bot. 240 mL. *Rx.*
Use: Sex hormone, progestin.

•**megalomicin potassium phosphate.** (meh-GAL-OH-my-sin) USAN.
Use: Anti-infective.

Megaton. (Hyrex) Vitamins B_3 4.4 mg, B_5 1.1 mg, B_6 0.44 mg, B_{12} 1.33 mcg, FA 0.1 mg, Fe 4 mg, Mn, Zn 1.7 mg, alcohol 13%. Liq. Bot. 473 mL. *Rx.*
Use: Mineral; vitamin supplement.

Mega VM-80. (NBTY) Vitamins A 10,000 units, D 1000 units, E 100 mg, B_1 80 mg, B_2 80 mg, B_3 80 mg, B_5 80 mg, B_6 80 mg, B_{12} 80 mcg, C 250 mg, Fe 1.2 mg, folic acid 0.4 mg, Ca 4.5 mg, Zn 3.58 mg, choline, inositol, biotin 80 mcg, PABA, bioflavonoids, betaine, hesperidin, Cu, I, K, Mg, Mn. Tab. Bot. 60s, 100s. *OTC.*
Use: Mineral; vitamin supplement.

•**megestrol acetate.** (meh-JESS-trole) *USP 28.*
Use: Sex hormone, progestin.
See: Megace.

megestrol acetate. (Various Mfr.) Megestrol acetate. **Susp.:** 40 mg/mL. Alcohol, sorbitol, sucrose. 240 mL. **Tab.:** 20 mg, 40 mg. Bot. 100s, 500s (40 mg only), UD 100s; blister pkg. 25s (40 mg only). *Rx.*
Use: Sex hormone, progestin.

meglitinides.
Use: Antidiabetic.
See: Nateglinide.
Repaglinide.

•**meglumine.** (meh-GLUE-meen) *USP 28.*
Use: Diagnostic aid (radiopaque medium).

meglumine, diatrizoate injection.
Use: Diagnostic aid (radiopaque medium).
See: Cardiografin.
Cystografin.
Gastrografin.
Hypaque-M 90%.
Hypaque-M 75%.
Hypaque Meglumine.
Hypaque-76.
Reno-M-Dip.
Reno-M-60.
Reno-M-30.
W/Meglumine iodipamide.
See: Sinografin.
W/Sodium diatrizoate.
See: Gastrografin.
Renografin-76.
Renografin-60.
Renovist II.

meglumine, iodipamide inj.
Use: Diagnostic aid; radiopaque medium.
See: Cholografin.
W/Meglumine diatrizoate.
See: Sinografin.

meglumine, iothalamate inj.
Use: Diagnostic aid; radiopaque medium.

•**meglutol.** (MEH-glue-tahl) USAN.
Use: Antihyperlipoproteinemic.

•**melafocon a.** (MEH-lah-FOE-kahn) USAN.
Use: Contact lens material (hydrophobic).

melanoma cell vaccine.
Use: Invasive melanoma. [Orphan Drug]

melanoma vaccine.
Use: Stage III to IV melanoma. [Orphan Drug]

melarsoprol. (Mel B)
Use: Anti-infective.
See: Arsobal.

melatonin.
Use: Treatment of circadian rhythm sleep disorders in blind patients. [Orphan Drug]

Mel B.
See: Melarsoprol.

•**melengestrol acetate.** (meh-len-JESS-trole) USAN.
Use: Antineoplastic; hormone, progestin.

Melfiat-105 Unicelles. (Numark) Phendimetrazine tartrate 105 mg, sucrose. SR Cap. Bot. 100s. *c-III.*
Use: CNS stimulant, anorexiant.

Melhoral Child Tablet. (Sanofi-Synthelabo) Acetylsalicylic acid. *OTC.*
Use: Analgesic.

melitoxin.
See: Dicumarol.
- **melitracen hydrochloride.** (meh-lih-TRAY-sen) USAN.
Use: Antidepressant.
- **melizame.** (MEH-lih-zame) USAN.
Use: Sweetener.
mellose. Methylcellulose.
Melonex. Metahexamide.
Use: Oral antidiabetic.
- **meloxicam.** (mell-OX-ih-kam) USAN.
Use: Anti-inflammatory.
See: Mobic.
Melpaque HP. (Stratus) Hydroquinone 4% in a sunblocking base of mineral oil, parabens, talc, EDTA, sodium metabisulfite. Cream. Tinted. Tube 14.2 g, 28.4 g. Rx.
Use: Dermatologic.
- **melphalan.** (MELL-fuh-lan) USP 28.
Use: Antineoplastic.
See: Alkeran.
- **melphalan.**
Use: Antineoplastic. [Orphan Drug]
Melquin HP. (Stratus) Hydroquinone 4%, mineral oil, petrolatum, cetostearyl alcohol, glycerin, sodium metabisulfite. Vanishing base. Cream. Tube 14.2 g, 28.4 g. Rx.
Use: Dermatologic.
- **memantine hydrochloride.** (me-MAN-teen) USAN.
Use: Alzheimer disease.
See: Namenda.
- **memotine hydrochloride.** (MEH-moe-teen) USAN.
Use: Antiviral.
- **menabitan hydrochloride.** (meh-NAB-ih-tan) USAN.
Use: Analgesic.
Menactra (Groups A, C, Y, and W-135). (Aventis Pasteur) 4 mcg each of groups A, C, Y, and W-135. Inj. Single-dose vials (conjugated to approximately 48 mcg of diphtheria toxoid protein carrier). Stopper to the vial contains dry, natural latex rubber. Rx.
Use: Meningococcal vaccine.
- **menadiol sodium diphosphate.** (men-ah-DIE-ole) USP 28.
Use: Vitamin (prothrombogenic).
- **menadione.** (men-ah-DIE-ohn) USP 28.
Use: Oral & IM; Vitamin K therapy; vitamin (prothrombogenic).
W/Ascorbic acid, hesperidin.
See: Hescor-K.
menadione diphosphate sodium.
See: Menadiol sodium diphosphate.
Menadol. (Rugby) Ibuprofen 200 mg. Captab. Bot. 100s. OTC.

Use: Analgesic, NSAID.
menaphthene or menaphthone.
See: Menadione.
menaquinone.
See: Menadione.
Menest. (Monarch) Esterified estrogens. 0.3 mg, 0.625 mg, 1.25 mg, 2.5 mg, lactose. Film-coated. Tab. Bot. 50s. (2.5 mg only), 100s (except 2.5 mg). Rx.
Use: Estrogen, sex hormone.
Meni-D. (Seatrace) Meclizine hydrochloride 25 mg. Cap. Bot. 100s. Rx.
Use: Antiemetic/antivertigo agent.
meningococcal vaccine.
Use: Immunization.
See: Menactra (Groups A, C, Y, and W-135).
Menomune A/C/Y/W-135.
- **menoctone.** (meh-NOCK-tone) USAN.
Under study.
Use: Antimalarial.
- **menogaril.** (MEN-oh-gar-ILL) USAN.
Use: Antineoplastic.
Menoject L.A. (Merz) Testosterone cypionate, estradiol cypionate. Vial 10 mL. Rx.
Use: Androgen; estrogen combination.
Menolyn. (Arcum) Ethinyl estradiol 0.05 mg. Tab. Bot. 100s, 1000s. Rx.
Use: Estrogen.
Menomune-A/C/Y/W-135. (Aventis Pasteur) When reconstituted, each 0.5 mL contains 50 mcg isolated product from each of groups A, C, Y, and W-135. Freeze-dried. Lactose 2.5 to 5 mg per dose. Pow. for Inj. Single-dose vial w/preservative-free distilled water diluent 0.78 mL. 10-dose vial w/diluent 6 mL w/thimerosal 1:10,000 (stopper to vial contains dry, natural latex rubber). Rx.
Use: Immunization.
Menopur. (Ferring) FSH activity 75 units, LH activity (menotropin) 75 units. Pow. or Pellets for Inj., lyophilized. In vials with diluent. Rx.
Use: Ovulation stimulant.
Menostar. (Berlex) Estradiol 1 mg (0.014 mg/day). Patch 3.25 cm^2 surface area. 4s. Rx.
Use: Sex hormone, estradiol transdermal system.
- **menotropins.** (MEN-oh-trope-inz) USAN. Formerly Human Follicle-Stimulating Hormone.
Use: Sex hormone; ovulation stimulant; gonadotropin; gonad-stimulating principle.
See: Menopur.
Pergonal.

Repronex.

Men-Phor. (Geritrex) Camphor 0.5%, menthol 0.5%, carbopol, cetearyl alcohol, cetyl alcohol, hydantoin, castor oil, petrolatum. Lot. 222 mL. *OTC.*
Use: Topical combination.

Mentane. (Hoechst) Velnacrine.
Use: Cholinesterase inhibitor for Alzheimer disease.

Mentax. (Bertek) Butenafine HCl 1%, benzyl and cetyl alcohol, glycerin, white petrolatum. Cream. Tube. 15 g, 30 g. *Rx.*
Use: Anti-infective, antifungal, topical.

•**menthol.** (MEN-thole) *USP 28.*
Use: Topical antipruritic; local analgesic; nasal decongestant; antitussive.
See: BENGAY Patch.
  Blue Gel Muscular Pain Reliever.
  Menthol Cough Drops.
  Robitussin Liquid Center Cough Drops.
  Vicks Cough Silencers.
  Vicks Formula 44 Cough Control Discs.
  Vicks Inhaler.
  Vicks Medicated Cough Drops.
  Vicks Oracin Regular and Cherry.
  Vicks Sinex.
  Vicks Vaporub.
  Vicks Vaposteam.
  Vicks Va-Tro-Nol.
  Victors Regular and Cherry.
W/Combinations.
See: ArthriCare Bayer Muscle & Joint Cream.
  Eucalyptamint.
  Eucalyptamint Maximum Strength.
  Hall's Mentho-Lyptus Sugar Free.
  Listerine Antiseptic.

Mentholatum. (Mentholatum Co.) Menthol 1.3%, camphor 9%, petrolatum. Oint. Tube 28 g. *OTC.*
Use: Upper respiratory combination, analgesic, topical.

Mentholatum Cherry Chest Rub for Kids. (Mentholatum Co.) Camphor 4.7%, menthol 2.6%, eucalyptus oil 1.2%, petrolatum. Oint. Tube 28 g. *OTC.*
Use: Upper respiratory combination, topical.

Mentholatum Deep Heating Lotion. (Mentholatum Co.) Menthol 6%, methyl salicylate 20%, lanolin derivative in lotion base. Bot. 2 oz, 4 oz. *OTC.*
Use: Analgesic, topical.

Mentholatum Deep Heating Rub. (Mentholatum Co.) Menthol 5.8%, methyl salicylate 12.7%, eucalyptus oil, turpentine oil, anhydrous lanolin, vehicle and

fragrance. Tube 1.25 oz, 3.33 oz, 5 oz. *OTC.*
Use: Analgesic, topical.

Menthol Cough Drops. (Major) Menthol 6.5 mg. Eucalyptus oil, glucose syrup, sucrose. Lozenges. 30s. *OTC.*
Use: Mouth and throat product.

Mentholin. (Apco) Methyl salicylate 30%, chloroform 20%, hard soap 3%, camphor gum 2.2%, menthol 0.8%, alcohol 35%. Bot. 2 oz. *OTC.*
Use: Analgesic, topical.

•**menthyl anthranilate.**
See: Meradimate

•**meobentine sulfate.** (meh-OH-BEN-teen) USAN.
Use: Cardiovascular agent (antiarrhythmic).

mepacrine hydrochloride.
Use: Anthelmintic; antimalarial.

•**mepartricin.** (meh-PAR-trih-sin) USAN.
Use: Antifungal; antiprotozoal.

mepavlon. Meprobamate.

•**mepenzolate bromide.** (meh-PEN-zoe-late) *USP 28.*
Use: Anticholinergic.
See: Cantil.
W/Phenobarbital.
See: Cantil w/phenobarbital.

mepenzolate methyl bromide. Mepenzolate bromide.
Use: Anticholinergic.

•**meperidine hydrochloride.** (meh-PEHR-ih-deen) *USP 28.*
Use: Opioid analgesic.
See: Demerol.
W/Acetaminophen.
See: Demerol APAP.

meperidine hydrochloride. (Roxane) Meperidine HCl 50 mg/5 mL. Syr. Bot. 500 mL. *c-ii.*
Use: Opioid analgesic.

meperidine hydrochloride. (Various Mfr.) Meperidine HCl **Tab.:** 50 mg, 100 mg. Bot. 100s, 500s, 1000s, UD 25s. **Inj.:** 25 mg/mL, 50 mg/mL, 75 mg/mL, 100 mg/mL. Vials. 1 mL. Amps. 1 mL. *c-ii.*
Use: Opioid analgesic.

mephenesin.
Use: Muscle relaxant.
See: Myanesin.
W/Acetaminophen, Vitamin C, butabarbital.
See: T-Caps.
W/Pentobarbital.
See: Nebralin.
W/Salicylamide, butabarbital sodium.
See: Metrogesic.

mephenesin carbamate. Methoxydone.

●**mephobarbital.** (meh-foe-BAR-bih-tahl) *USP 28.*
Use: Anticonvulsant; hypnotic; sedative.
See: Mebaral.

mephone. Mephentermine.

Mephyton. (Merck & Co.) Phytonadione (vitamin K) 5 mg, lactose. Tab. Bot. 100s. *Rx.*
Use: Vitamin, prothrombogenic.

Mepiben. (Schein) Methylpiperidyl benzhydryl ether.
Use: Antihistamine.

mepiperphenidol bromide.
Use: Anticholinergic.

mepivacaine HCl and levonordefrin.
(Septodont) Mepivacaine HCl 2%, levonordefrin 1:20,000, sodium bisulfite. Inj. Dental Cart. 1.8 mL. *Rx.*
Use. Anesthetic, local amide.

●**mepivacaine hydrochloride.** (meh-PIHV-ah-cane) *USP 28.*
Use: Anesthetic, local amide.
See: Carbocaine.
　　Carbocaine Dental.
　　Polocaine.
　　Polocaine MPF.

mepivacaine hydrochloride. (Septodont) Mepivacaine HCl 3%. Inj. Dental Cart. 1.8 mL. *Rx.*
Use: Anesthetic, local amide.

mepivacaine hydrochloride and levonordefrin.
Use: Anesthetic, local amide.
See: Carbocaine with Neo-Cobefrin.
　　Polocaine with Levonordefrin.

●**meprednisone.** (meh-PRED-nih-sone) *USP 28.*
Use: Corticosteroid, topical.

●**meprobamate.** (meh-pro-BAM-ate) USP 28.
Use: Anxiolytic; hypnotic; sedative; antianxiety agent.
See: Arcoban.
　　Bamate.
　　Miltown.
　　Tranmep.
　　W/Benactyzine HCl.
See: Milprem.
　　W/Pentaerythritol tetranitrate.
See: Miltrate.
　　W/Premarin.
See: PMB 200.

meprobamate. (meh-pro-BAM-ate) (Various Mfr.) Meprobamate 200 mg, 400 mg. Tab. Bot. 20s, 100s, 500s (400 mg only), 1000s, UD 100s (400 mg only). *c-iv.*
Use: Antianxiety agent.

meprobamate/aspirin. (Various Mfr.) Aspirin 325 mg, meprobamate 200 mg. Tab. Bot. 100s, 500s. *Rx.*
Use: Analgesic combination.

meprobamate/benactyzine.
Use: Miscellaneous psychotherapeutic agent.

meprobamate, n-isopropyl.
See: Carisoprodol.

Meprogesic Q. (Various Mfr.) Aspirin 325 mg, meprobamate 200 mg. Tab. Bot. 100s, 500s. *Rx.*
Use: Analgesic combination.

Meprolone Tabs. (Major) Methylprednisolone 4 mg. Bot. 25s, 100s. *Rx.*
Use: Corticosteroid.

Mepron. (GlaxoSmithKline) Atovaquone 750 mg/5 mL. Susp. Bot. 210 mL. *Rx.*
Use: Anti-infective.

meprylcaine hydrochloride.
Use: Anesthetic, local.

●**meptazinol hydrochloride.** (mep-TAZE-ih-nahl) USAN.
Use: Analgesic.

mepyrapone.
See: Metopirone.

●**mequidox.** (MEH-kwih-dox) USAN.
Under study.
Use: Anti-infective.

●**mequinol.** (MEH-kwih-noll) USAN.
Use: Hyperpigmentation.
See: Solagé.

mequinolate. Name used for Proquinolate.

●**meradimate.** (mer-ADD-ih-mate) USAN.
Formerly menthyl anthranilate.
Use: Sunscreen.

●**meralein sodium.** (MER-ah-leen) USAN.
Use: Anti-infective, topical.
See: Sodium Meralein.

merbromin. *OTC.*
Use: Antiseptic, topical.

●**mercaptopurine.** (mer-cap-toe-PURE-een) *USP 28.*
Use: Antineoplastic.
See: Purinethol.

mercaptopurine. (PAR) Mercaptopurine 50 mg. Lactose. Tab. 60s. *Rx.*
Use: Antineoplastic.

mercazole.
See: Methimazole.

●**mercufenol chloride.** (MER-cue-FEEN-ole) USAN.
Use: Anti-infective, topical.

mercuranine.
See: Merbromin.

mercurial, antisyphilitics. Mercuric Oleate, Mercuric Salicylate.

mercuric oleate. Oleate of mercury.
Use: Parasitic and fungal skin diseases.

mercuric oxide ophthalmic ointment, yellow.
Use: Local anti-infective; ophthalmic.

mercuric salicylate. Mercury subsalicylate.
Use: Parasitic and fungal skin diseases.

mercuric succinimide. Bis-Succinimidato-mercury.

mercurocal.
See: Merbromin Soln.

mercurome.
See: Merbromin Soln.

•**mercury, ammoniated.** (mer-cue-REE, ah-MOHN-ee-ated) *USP 28.*
Use: Anti-infective, topical.

mercury compounds.
See: Antiseptics, Mercurials.

mercury oleate. Mercury++ oleate. Pharmaceutic aid.

mercury-197-203.
See: Chlormerodrin.

Merdex. (Faraday) Docusate sodium 100 mg. Tab. Vial 60 mL. *Rx-OTC.*
Use: Laxative.

Meridia. (Abbott) Sibutramine 5 mg, 10 mg, 15 mg, lactose. Cap. Bot. 100s. *c-IV.*
Use: CNS stimulant, anorexiant.

•**merimepodib.** (me-ri-ME-poe-dib) USAN.
Use: Inosine monophosphate dehydrogenase inhibitor.

•**merisoprol acetate Hg 197.** (mer-EYE-so-prole) USAN.
Use: Radiopharmaceutical.

•**merisoprol acetate Hg 203.** (mer-EYE-so-prole) USAN.
Use: Radiopharmaceutical.

Meritene Powder. (Novartis) Vanilla flavor: Specially processed nonfat dry milk, corn syrup solids, sucrose, fructose, calcium caseinate, sodium Cl, natural and artificial flavors, lecithin, vitamins and minerals. Can 1 lb, 4.5 lb, 25 lb. Packet 1.14 oz. Vanilla, chocolate, eggnog, milk chocolate, plain flavors. *OTC.*
Use: Nutritional supplement.

merodicein. Sodium meralein.

•**meropenem.** (meh-row-PEN-em) USAN.
Use: Anti-infective.
See: Merrem IV.

meroxapol 105.
Use: Irrigating solution.
See: Saf-Clens.

merprane.
Use: Diagnostic aid.

Merrem IV. (AstraZeneca) Meropenem 500 mg, 1 g. Pow. for Inj. Vial 20 mL (500 mg only), 30 mL (1 g only),

100 mL, *ADD-Vantage* Vial 15 mL. *Rx.*
Use: Anti-infective.

mersol. (Century) Thimerosal tincture 1/1000. 1 oz, 4 oz, pt, gal. *OTC.*
Use: Antiseptic.

Merthiolate. (Eli Lilly) Thimerosal. **Soln.:** 1:1000: 4 fl. oz, 16 fl oz, gal. **Tincture:** 1:1000: alcohol 50%, 0.75 oz, 4 fl oz, 16 fl oz, gal. *OTC.*
Use: Antiseptic.

Meruvax II. (Merck & Co.) Lyophilized, live attenuated rubella virus of the Wistar Institute RA 27/3 strain. Each dose contains ≈ 25 mcg of neomycin. Single-dose vial w/diluent. Pkg. 1s, 10s.
Use: Immunization.
W/Attenuvax.
See: M-R-Vax II.
W/Attenuvax, Mumpsvax.
See: M-M-R II.
W/Mumpsvax.
See: Biavax II.

Mervan. (Continental Pharma, Belgium) Alclofenac.
Use: Anti-inflammatory.

•**mesalamine.** (me-SAL-uh-MEEN) *USP 28.*
Use: Anti-inflammatory.
See: Asacol.
Canasa.
Pentasa.
Rowasa.

mesalamine. (Clay Park) Mesalamine 4 g/60 mL. EDTA, potassium acetate, potassium metabisulfite, sodium benzoate, white petrolatum. Enemas. 7s with lubricated applicator tip. *Rx.*
Use: Treatment of inflammatory bowel disease.

mescomine.
See: Methscopolamine Bromide.

•**meseclazone.** (meh-SAK-lah-zone) USAN.
Use: Anti-inflammatory.

•**mesifilcon a.** (MEH-sih-FILL-kahn A) USAN.
Use: Contact lens material; hydrophilic.

•**mesna.** (MESS-nah) USAN.
Use: Cytoprotective agent.
See: Mesnex.

mesna. (American Pharmaceutical Partners) Mesna 100 mg/mL, benzyl alcohol 10.4 mg, EDTA 0.25 mg/mL. Inj. Vial. 10 mL multidose. *Rx.*
Use: Cytoprotective agent.

mesna. (Baxter) Mesna 400 mg. May contain lactose. Tab. 10 blisters. *Rx.*
Use: Cytoprotective agent.

Mesnex. (Bristol-Myers Squibb) Mesna. **Inj.:** 100 mg/mL, EDTA 0.25 mg/mL, benzyl alcohol 10.4 mg. Multidose Vial 10 mL. **Tab.:** 400 mg, lactose, simethicone. Blisters. 10. *Rx.*
Use: Antidote; cytoprotective agent.

•**mespiperone c 11.** (meh-SPIH-peh-rone c 11) USAN.
Use: Radiopharmaceutical.

•**mesterolone.** (MESS-TER-oh-lone) USAN.
Use: Androgen.

mestibol. Monomestrol.

Mestinon. (ICN) Pyridostigmine bromide. **ER Tab.:** 180 mg. Bot. 30s. **Inj:** 5 mg/mL, parabens 0.2%, sodium citrate 0.02%. Amp. 2 mL. **Syr.:** 60 mg/5 mL, sucrose, sorbitol, alcohol 5%, raspberry flavor. Bot 480 mL. **Tab.:** 60 mg, lactose. Bot. 100s, 500s. *Rx.*
Use: Muscle stimulant.

•**mestranol.** (MESS-trah-nole) *USP 28.*
Use: Contraceptive; estrogen.
W/Ethynodiol Diacetate.
See: Ovulen.
Ovulen-28.
Ovulen-21.
W/Norethindrone.
See: Necon 1/50.
Nelova 1/50M.
Norinyl.
Norinyl-1 Fe 28.
Norinyl 1+50.
Ortho-Novum.
Ortho-Novum 1/50.
W/Norethindrone, ferrous fumarate.
See: Ortho-Novum Fe-28, Fe-28, 1 mg Fe-28.
W/Norethynodrel.
See: Enovid.
Enovid-E.
Enovid-E 21.

•**mesuprine hydrochloride.** (MEH-suh-PREEN) USAN.
Use: Vasodilator; muscle relaxant.

Metabolin. (Thurston) Vitamins A 833 units, D 66 units, B_1 833 mcg, B_2 500 mcg, B_6 0.083 mcg, calcium pantothenate 833 mcg, niacinamide 5 mg, folic acid 0.066 mcg, p-aminobenzoic acid 0.416 mcg, inositol 833 mcg, B_{12} 500 mcg, C 5 mg, Ca 33.1 mg, P 14.6 mg, Fe 2.5 mg, I 0.15 mg. Tab. Bot. 100s, 500s, 1000s. *OTC.*
Use: Mineral; vitamin supplement.

•**metabromsalan.** (MET-ah-BROME-sahlan) USAN.
Use: Antimicrobial; disinfectant.

metabutethamine hydrochloride.
Use: Anesthetic, local.

metabutoxycaine hydrochloride.
Use: Anesthetic, local.

metacaraphen hydrochloride. Netrin.

metacordralone.
See: Prednisolone.

metacortandracin.
See: Prednisone.

metacortin.
See: Meticorten.

•**metacresol.** (met-ah-KREE-sole) *USP 28.*
Use: Antiseptic, topical; antifungal.

Metadate CD. (Celltech) Methylphenidate HCl 10 mg, 20 mg, 30 mg, sugar spheres. ER Cap. Bot. 30s (20 mg only), 100s (except 20 mg), UD 100s (20 mg only). *c-II.*
Use: CNS stimulant.

Metadate ER. (Celltech) Methylphenidate HCl 10 mg, 20 mg, lactose, color-additive free. ER Tab. Bot. 100s. *c-II.*
Use: CNS stimulant.

meta-delphene. Diethyltoluamide.

Metaglip. (Bristol-Myers Squibb) Glipizide 2.5 mg, 5 mg. Metformin HCl 250 mg, 500 mg. Tab. Bot. 100s. *Rx.*
Use: Antidiabetic.

metaglycodol.
Use: Central nervous system depressant.

Metahydrin. (Hoechst) Trichlormethiazide 2 mg, 4 mg. Tab. Bot. 100s. *Rx.*
Use: Diuretic.

•**metalol hydrochloride.** (MEH-ta-lahl) USAN. Under study.
Use: Antiadrenergic beta-receptor.

Metalone T.B.A. (Foy Laboratories) Prednisolone tertiary butylacetate 20 mg, sodium citrate 1 mg, polysorbate 80 1 mg, d-sorbitol 450 mg/mL, benzyl alcohol 0.9%, water for inj. Vial 10 mL. *Rx.*
Use: Corticosteroid.

Metamucil. (Procter & Gamble) **Cap.:** Psyllium husk 0.52 g. 100s, 160s. **Pow.:** Psyllium hydrophilic mucilloid, sodium 1 mg, potassium 31 mg/Dose. **Regular Flavor:** w/dextrose. Jar 7 oz, 14 oz, 21 oz. Packette 5.4 g. Box 100s. **Orange and Strawberry Flavors:** w/flavoring, sucrose and coloring. Jar 7 oz, 14 oz, 21 oz. **Wafer:** Psyllium husk 3.4 g, carbohydrates 17 g, sodium 20 mg, fat 5 g, 120 cal/dose, sugar, fructose, molasses, sucrose, cinnamon spice, apple crisp flavors. Ctn. 24s. *OTC.*
Use: Laxative.

Metamucil Instant Mix. (Procter & Gamble) Psyllium hydrophilic mucilloid

with citric acid, sucrose, potassium bicarbonate, sodium bicarbonate. Powder when combined with water forms an effervescent, flavored liquid. **Lemon Lime Flavor:** w/calcium carbonate. Cartons of 16, 30, or 100 packets of 3.4 g. **Orange Flavor:** w/flavoring and coloring. Ctn. 16 or 30 packets of 3.4 g. *OTC.*
Use: Laxative.

Metamucil Orange Flavor, Original Texture. (Procter & Gamble) Approximately psyllium husk 3.4 g, carbohydrates 10 g, sodium 5 mg, 40 cal/dose, sucrose. Pow. Can. 210 g, 420 g, 538 g, 630 g. *OTC.*
Use: Laxative.

Metamucil Orange Flavor, Smooth Texture. (Procter & Gamble) Approximately psyllium husk 3.4 g, sodium 5 mg, carbohydrates 12 g, 45 cal/dose, sucrose. Pow. Can. 420 g, 630 g, 1368 g, 100 UD single-dose packs (100s). *OTC.*
Use: Laxative.

Metamucil Original Texture. (Procter & Gamble) Approximately psyllium husk 3.4 g, carbohydrates 6 g, sodium 3 mg, 25 cal/dose, sucrose. Pow. Can. 822 g, Pack. 30. *OTC.*
Use: Laxative.

Metamucil, Sugar Free. (Procter & Gamble) Psyllium hydrophilic mucilloidin sugar-free formula. **Regular Flavor:** Jar 3.7 oz, 7.4 oz, 11.1 oz. Packet 3.4 g. Box 100s. **Orange Flavor:** Jar 3.7 oz, 7.4 oz, 11.1 oz. *OTC.*
Use: Laxative.

Metamucil Sugar Free, Orange Flavor, Smooth Texture. (Procter & Gamble) Approximately psyllium husk 3.4 g, carbohydrates 5 g, sodium 5 mg, 20 cal/dose, aspartame, phenylalanine 25 mg. Pow. Can. 210 g, 420 g, 630 g, 660 g. *OTC.*
Use: Laxative.

Metamucil, Sugar Free, Smooth Texture. (Procter & Gamble) Approximately psyllium husk 3.4 g, carbohydrates 5 g, sodium 4 mg, 20 cal/dose. Pow. Can. 425 g, Pack. 30s, 100s. *OTC.*
Use: Laxative.

Metandren. (Novartis) Methyltestosterone. **Linguet:** 5 mg, 10 mg Bot. 100s. **Tab.:** 10 mg, 25 mg Bot. 100s. *Rx.*
Use: Androgen.

metaphenylbarbituric acid.
See: Mephobarbital.

metaphyllin.
See: Aminophylline.

Metaprel Syrup. (Novartis) Metaproterenol sulfate 10 mg/5 mL. Bot. Pt. *Rx.*
Use: Bronchodilator.

•**metaproterenol polistirex.** (MEH-tuh-pro-TEHR-uh-nahl pahl-ee-STIE-rex) USAN.
Use: Bronchodilator.

•**metaproterenol sulfate.** (MEH-tuh-pro-TEHR-uh-nahl) *USP 28.*
Use: Bronchodilator, sympathomimetic.
See: Alupent.

metaproterenol sulfate. (Various Mfr.) Metaproterenol sulfate. **Soln. for Inh.:** 0.4%, 0.6%, may contain EDTA. UD. Vial 2.5 mL. 5%, may contain EDTA, benzalkonium chloride. Vial 10 mL, 30 mL with dropper. **Tab.:** 10 mg, 20 mg, lactose. 100s, 1000s. *Rx.*
Use: Bronchodilator, sympathomimetic.

•**metaraminol bitartrate.** (met-uh-RAM-in-ole) *USP 28.*
Use: Adrenergic.
See: Aramine.

Metastron. (Medi-Physics, Inc., Amersham Healthcare) Strontium-89 Cl 10.9 to 22.6 mg/mL. Preservative free. Inj. Vial 10 mL.
Use: Radiopharmaceutical.

Metatensin #2 & #4. (Hoechst) Trichlormethiazide 2 mg, 4 mg, each containing reserpine 0.1 mg. Tab. Bot. 100s. *Rx.*
Use: Antihypertensive.

•**metaxalone.** (meh-TAX-ah-lone) USAN.
Use: Muscle relaxant.
See: Skelaxin.

Meted, Maximum Strength. (Medicis) Sulfur 5%, salicylic acid 3%. Shampoo. Bot. 118 mL. *OTC.*
Use: Antiseborrheic combination.

•**meteneprost.** (meh-TEN-eh-PRAHST) USAN.
Use: Oxytocic; prostaglandin.

•**metesind glucuronate.** (MEH-teh-sind glue-CURE-oh-nate) USAN.
Use: Antineoplastic (specific thymidylate synthase inhibitor).

metethoheptazine.
Use: Analgesic.

•**metformin.** (MET-fore-min) USAN.
Use: Oral hypoglycemic; antidiabetic.
See: Riomet.

•**metformin hydrochloride.** (MET-fore-min) *USP 28.*
Use: Antidiabetic.
See: Fortamet.
  Glucophage.
  Glucophage XR.
  Riomet.
W/Glyburide.

See: Glucovance.

metformin hydrochloride. (Barr) Metformin hydrochloride 750 mg. ER Tab. 100s. *Rx.*
Use: Antidiabetic.

metformin hydrochloride. (Various Mfr.) Metformin HCl 500 mg, 850 mg, 1,000 mg. Tab. Bot. 100s, 500s, 1,000s, 2,000s (500 mg only), UD 100s. *Rx.*
Use: Antidiabetic.

metformin hydrochloride ER. (PAR) Metformin HCl 500 mg. ER Tab. 100s. *Rx.*
Use: Antidiabetic.

methacholine bromide. Mecholin bromide.
Use: Cholinergic.

•**methacholine chloride.** (METH-uh-KOH Inrn) *USP 28.*
Use: Cholinergic.
See: Mecholyl Cl.
  Provocholine.

methacholine chloride.
Use: Diagnostic aid.
See: Provocholine.

•**methacrylic acid copolymer.** (meth-ah-KRILL-ik ASS-id koe-PAHL-ih-mer) *NF 23.*
Use: Pharmaceutic aid (tablet coating agent).

•**methacycline.** (meth-ah-SIGH-kleen) USAN.
Use: Anti-infective.

•**methadone hydrochloride.** (METH-uh-dohn) *USP 28.*
Use: Opioid analgesic; narcotic abstinence syndrome suppressant.
See: Dolophine Hydrochloride.
  Methadose.

•**methadone hydrochloride.** (aaiPharma) Methadone hydrochloride 10 mg/mL. Chlorobutanol 0.5%. Inj. Multidose vial 20 mL. *c-II.*
Use: Opioid analgesic.

methadone hydrochloride. (Roxane) Methadone hydrochoride. **Tab.:** 5 mg, 10 mg. Bot. 100s, UD 100s. **Oral Soln.:** 5 mg/5 mL, 10 mg/5 mL, alcohol 8%, sorbitol, citrus flavor. Bot. 500 mL. *c-II.*
Use: Opioid analgesic.

methadone hydrochloride. (Various Mfr.) Methadone hydrochloride. **Oral Conc.:** 10 mg/mL. 946 mL, 1 L. **Tab.:** 5 mg, 10 mg. 100s, UD 100s. *c-II.*
Use: Opioid analgesic.

methadone hydrochloride diskets. (Various Mfr.) Methadone hydrochloride 40 mg. Dispersible Tab. Bot. 100s. *c-II.*
Use: Opioid analgesic.

methadone hydrochloride intensol. (METH-uh-dohn HIGH-droe-KLOR-ide ihn-TEN-sahl) (Roxane) Methadone hydrohcloride 10 mg/mL. Oral Conc. Bot. 30 mg with calibrated dropper. *c-II.*
Use: Opioid analgesic.

Methadose. (Mallinckrodt) Methadone hydrochloride. **Tab.:** 5 mg, 10 mg. Bot. 100s. **Disp. Tab.:** 40 mg. Bot. 100s. **Oral Conc.:** 10 mg/mL. Sucrose, cherry flavor. Also available sugar free, dye free, unflavored. Bot. 1 L. *c-II.*
Use: Opioid analgesic.

•**methadyl acetate.** (METH-ah-dill) USAN.
Use: Analgesic, narcotic.

•**methafilcon b.** (METH-ah-FILL-kahn) USAN.
Use: Contact lens material (hydrophilic).

Methagual. (Gordon Laboratories) Guaiacol 8%, methyl salicylate 8% in petrolatum. Oint. 2 oz, lb. *OTC.*
Use: Analgesic, topical.

methalamic acid. Name used for lothalamic acid.

methalgen. (Alra) Camphor, menthol, mustard oil, methyl salicylate in nongreasy cream base. Bot. 2 oz, Jar 4 oz, lb.
Use: Analgesic, topical.

•**methalthiazide.** (METH-al-THIGH-ah-zide) USAN.
Use: Antihypertensive; diuretic.

methaminodiazepoxide.
See: Librium.

methamoctol.
Use: Adrenergic.

methamphetamine-dl hydrochloride.
See: dl-Methamphetamine HCl.

methamphetamine hydrochloride. (Able) Methamphetamine HCl 5 mg. Corn starch, lactose. Tab. 30s, 100s, 500s, 1000s. *c-II.*
Use: Central nervous system stimulant.

•**methamphetamine hydrochloride.** (meth-am-FET-uh-meen) *USP 28.*
Use: CNS stimulant.
See: Desoxyn.
W/Pamabrom, pyrilamine maleate, homatropine methylbromide, hyoscyamine-sulfate, scopolamine HBr.
See: Aridol.

methampyrone.
See: Dipyrone.

methandriol. (Various Mfr.) Methylandrostenediol.
See: Anabol.

methandriol dipropionate.
See: Arbolic.

Methaphor. (Borden) Protein hydrolysate (l-leucine, l-isoleucine, l-methionine, l-phenylalanine, l-tyrosine); methionine,

camphor, benzethonium Cl, in Dermabase vehicle. Oint. Tube 1.5 oz. *OTC.*
Use: Dermatologic, amino acid supplement.

•**methaqualone.** (METH-ah-kwan-lone) USAN.
Use: Hypnotic, sedative.

Methatropic Capsules. (Ivax) Choline 115 mg, inositol 83 mg, methionine 110 mg, vitamins B_1 3 mg, B_2 3 mg, B_3 10 mg, B_5 2 mg, B_6 2 mg, B_{12} 2 mcg, desiccated liver 86 mg. Bot. 100s. *OTC.*
Use: Vitamin supplement.

•**methazolamide.** (meth-ah-ZOLE-ahmide) *USP 28.*
Use: Carbonic anhydrase inhibitor.

methazolamide. (Various Mfr.) Methazolamide 25 mg or 50 mg. Tab. Bot. 100s. *Rx.*
Use: Carbonic anhydrase inhibitor.

Methblue 65. (Manne) Methylene blue 65 mg. Tab. Bot. 100s, 1000s. *Rx.*
Use: Antidote, cyanide.

Meth-Choline. (Schein) Choline 115 mg, inositol 83 mg, methionine 110 mg, vitamins B_1 3 mg, B_2 3 mg, B_3 10 mg, B_5 2 mg, B_6 2 mg, B_{12} 2 mcg, desiccated liver 56 mg, liver concentrate 30 mg. Cap. Bot. 100s, 250s, 1000s. *OTC.*
Use: Vitamin supplement.

Meth-Dia-Mer Sulfa. Trisulfapyrimidines. Tab.
Use: Triple sulfonamide therapy.
See: Chemozine.
Triple Sulfa.

Meth-Dia-Mer Sulfonamides.
Use: Triple sulfonamide therapy.
W/Sulfacetamide.
See: Sulfa-Plex.

Meth-Dia-Mer Sulfonamides Suspension. Trisulfapyrimidines Oral Suspension.
Use: Triple sulfonamide therapy.
See: Chemozine.
Triple Sulfa.

•**methdilazine hydrochloride.** (METHdill-ah-ZEEN) *USP 28.*
Use: Antipruritic.

•**methenamine.** (meh-THEN-uh-meen) *USP 28. Formerly Hexamethylenamine.*
Use: Anti-infective, urinary.

methenamine and monobasic sodium phosphate tablets.
Use: Anti-infective, urinary.

methenamine anhydromethylene citrate. Formanol, Uropurgol, Urotropin.

•**methenamine hippurate.** (meth-EE-nahmeen HIP-you-rate) *USP 28.*
Use: Anti-infective, urinary.
See: Hipre.

Urex.

•**methenamine mandelate.** (meth-EEnah-meen MAN-deh-late) *USP 28.*
Use: Anti-infective, urinary.
See: Mandelamine.

methenamine mandelate. (Various Mfr.)
Tab.: 0.5 g, 1 g. Tab. 100s, 1000s.
Susp.: 0.5 g/5 mL. Susp. Bot. 480 mL.
Use: Anti-infective, urinary.

methenamine mandelate w/combinations.
Use: Anti-infective, urinary.
See: Urisedamine.

methenamine w/combinations.
Use: Anti-infective, urinary.
See: Cystamine.
Cystex.
Cysto.
MHP-A.
Prosed/DS.
Urelle.
Uretron D/S.
Urimar-T.
Urimax.
Urisan-P.
Urised.
Uriseptic.
UriSym.
Uro Blue.
Urogesic Blue.
Uro Phosphate.
U-Tran.

•**methenolone acetate.** (meth-EEN-ohlone) USAN.
Use: Anabolic.

•**methenolone enanthate.** (meth-EENoh-lone eh-NAN-thate) USAN.
Use: Anabolic.

Metheponex. (Rawl) Choline 0.54 g, dlmethionine 1.80 g, inositol 0.27 g, whole desiccated liver 8.10 g, vitamins B_1 18 mg, B_2 36 mg, niacinamide 90 mg, B_6 3.6 mg, calcium pantothenate 3.6 mg, biotin 10.8 mcg, B_{12} 5.4 mcg and amino acid/daily therapeutic dose. Cap. Bot. 100s, 500s. *Rx.*
Use: Antidiabetic; nutritional supplement.

metheptazine.
Use: Analgesic.

Methergine. (Sandoz) Methylergonovine maleate. **Inj.:** 0.2 mg/mL. Ampuls. 1 mL. **Tab.:** 0.2 mg. Lactose, FD&C BLue No. 1, parabens, sucrose, coated. Bot. 100s. *Rx.*
Use: Oxytocic.

methestrol.
See: Promethestrol.

methetharimide bemegride. USAN.
Use: Anticonvulsant.

Methibon. (Barrows) Choline dihydrogen citrate 278 mg, dl-methionine 111 mg, inositol 83.3 mg, vitamin B$_{12}$ 2 mcg, liver concentrate, desiccated liver 86.6 mg. Cap. Bot. 100s. *Rx.*
Use: Antidiabetic; nutritional supplement.

methicillin sodium. (meth-ih-SILL-in)
Use: Anti-infective.

• **methimazole.** (meth-IMM-uh-zole) *USP 28.*
Use: Thyroid inhibitor.
See: Tapazole.

methimazole. Various Mfr. Methimazole 5 mg, 10 mg, may contain lactose. Tab. Bot. 100s. *Rx.*
Use: Thyroid inhibitor.

Methiokaps. (Pal-Pak, Inc.) dl-methionine 200 mg. Cap. Bot. 1000s. *Rx.*
Use: Diaper rash product.

methiomeprazine hydrochloride. (GlaxoSmithKline)
Use: Antiemetic.

• **methionine.** (meh-THIGH-oh-NEEN) *USP 28.*
Note: Also see Racemethionine.
Use: Amino acid.
See: M-Caps.

• **methionine C 11 injection.** (meh-THIGH-oh-NEEN) *USP 28.*
Use: Radiopharmaceutical.

methionyl human stem cell factor (recombinant).
Use: Combination w/filgrastim to decrease the number of phereses required to collect blood progenitor cells following myelosuppressive/myeloblative therapy. [Orphan Drug]

methionyl neurotrophic (brain-derived, recombinant) factor.
Use: Amyotrophic lateral sclerosis agent. [Orphan Drug]

Methioplex. (Lincoln Diagnostics) Methionine 25 mg, vitamins B$_1$ 50 mg, niacinamide 100 mg, B$_2$ 2 mg, choline 50 mg, B$_6$ 2 mg, panthenol 2 mg, benzyl alcohol 1%, distilled water q.s./mL. Vial 30 mL. *Rx.*
Use: Nutritional supplement.

• **methisazone.** (METH-eye-SAH-zone) USAN.
Use: Antiviral.

Methitest. (Global) Methyltestosterone 10 mg, 25 mg, lactose, sugar. Tab. Bot. 100s, 1000s (25 mg only). *c-III.*
Use: Sex hormone, androgen.

methitural sodium.
Use: Hypnotic, sedative.

• **methixene hydrochloride.** (meh-THIX-een) USAN.

Use: Muscle relaxant.

• **methocarbamol.** (meth-oh-CAR-buh-mahl) *USP 28.*
Use: Muscle relaxant.
See: Delaxin.
Robaxin Injection.
Robaxin-750.
Robaxin Tablets.

methocarbamol. (Various Mfr.) Methocarbamol. **Tab.:** 500 mg, 750 mg. Bot. 60s (750 mg only), 100s, 500s, UD 100s.
Use: Muscle relaxant.

Methocarbamol/ASA. (Various Mfr.) Methocarbamol 400 mg, aspirin 325 mg. Tab. Bot. 15s, 30s, 40s, 100s, 500s, 1000.
Use: Muscle relaxant.

methocel, Methylcellulose.

• **methohexital.** (meth-oh-HEX-ih-tahl) *USP 28.*
Use: Pharmaceutic necessity for Methohexital Sodium for Injection.

• **methohexital sodium for injection.** (METH-oh-HEX-ih-tahl) *USP 28.*
Use: Anesthetic, general; anesthetic (intravenous).
See: Brevital.

• **methoin.** (METH-eh-toe-in) USAN.
Use: Anticonvulsant.

• **methopholine.** (METH-oh-foe-leen) USAN.
Use: Analgesic.
See: Versidyne.

Methopto Forte 1%. (Professional Pharmacal) Methylcellulose pow. 10 mg (1% soln.), boric acid 12 mg, potassium Cl 7.3 mg, benzalkonium Cl 0.04 mg, glycerin 12 mg/mL w/sodium carbonate to adjust pH and purified water. Bot. 15 mL. *OTC.*
Use: Artificial tears.

Methopto Forte 0.5%. (Professional Pharmacal) Methylcellulose pow. 5 mg (0.5% soln.), boric acid 12 mg, potassium Cl 7.3 mg, benzalkonium Cl 0.4 mg, glycerin 12 mg/mL w/sodium carbonate to adjust pH and purified water. Bot. 15 mL. *OTC.*
Use: Artificial tears.

Methopto 0.25%. (Professional Pharmacal) Methylcellulose pow. 2.5 mg (0.25% soln.), boric acid 12 mg, potassium Cl 7.3 mg, benzalkonium Cl 0.04 mg, glycerin 12 mg/mL w/sodium carbonate to adjust pH and purified water. Bot. 15 mL, 30 mL. *OTC.*
Use: Artificial tears.

methopyraphone.
See: Metopirone.

methorate.
See: Dextromethorphan HBr.
Methorbate S.C. (Standex) Methenamine 40.8 mg, atropine sulfate 0.03 mg, hyoscyamine sulfate 0.03 mg, salol 18.1 mg, benzoic acid 4.5 mg, methylene blue 5.4 mg. Tab. Bot. 100s. Rx.
Use: Anti-infective, urinary.
d-methorphan hydrobromide.
See: Dextromethorphan HBr.
methorphinan. Racemorphan HBr.
Dromoran.
• **methotrexate.** (meth-oh-TREK-sate) USP 28. Formerly Amethopterin.
Use: Leukemia in children; antineoplastic; antipsoriatic; juvenile rheumatoid arthritis; folic acid antagonist.
See: Rheumatrex Dose Pack.
Trexall.
methotrexate. (Immunex) **Inj.:** 25 mg/mL as sodium, benzyl alcohol 0.9%, sodium Cl 0.26% and water for inj. Vials 2 mL, 10 mL. **Pow. for Inj.:** 20 mg or 1 g/vial as sodium. Single-use vials. Rx.
Use: Antipsoriatic.
methotrexate. (Various Mfr.) Methotrexate 2.5 mg (as sodium). Tab. Bot. 36s, 100s. Rx.
Use: Antineoplastic; antirheumatic.
methotrexate LPF sodium. (Xanodyne) Methotrexate sodium 25 mg/mL (as base). Preservative-free. Single-use vials. 2 mL (sodium 0.43 mEq/vial), 4 mL (sodium 0.86 mEq/vial), 10 mL (sodium 2.15 mEq/vial). Rx.
Use: Antimetabolite.
methotrexate sodium. (Various Mfr.) Methotrexate sodium. **Inj.:** 25 mg/mL (as base). Preservative-free. Single-use vials. 2 mL, 4 mL, 8 mL, 10 mL, 20 mL, 40 mL. **Pow. for Inj., lyophilized:** 20 mg (as base) (sodium 0.14 mEq/vial), 1 g (as base) (sodium 7 mEq/vial). Preservative-free. Single-use vials. Rx.
Use: Antimetabolite.
methotrexate sodium. (Various Mfr.) Methotrexate sodium 25 mg/mL (as base). Benzyl alcohol 0.9%. Must not be used for intrathecal or high-dose therapy. Vials. 2 mL, 10 mL. Rx.
Use: Antimetabolite.
methotrexate sodium for injection. (Wyeth) Methotrexate sodium 2.5 mg/mL Vial 2 mL; 25 mg/mL. Vial 2 mL w/preservatives; 20 mg, 50 mg, 100 mg Vial cryodesiccated, preservative free; 50 mg, 100 mg, 200 mg Vial; 25 mg/mL solution preservative free.
Use: Leukemia therapy; psoriasis; os-

teogenic sarcoma. [Orphan Drug]
See: Folex.
Folex PFS.
Methotrexate.
Mexate.
methotrexate USP with laurocapram.
Use: Topical treatment of Mycosis fungoides. [Orphan Drug]
• **methoxsalen.** (meth-OX-ah-len) USP 28.
Use: Pigmenting agent.
See: 8-MOP.
Oxsoralen.
Oxsoralen Ultra.
Uvadex.
8-methoxsalen.
Use: Treatment of diffuse systemic sclerosis, rejection of cardiac allografts. [Orphan Drug]
See: Uvadex.
methoxydone.
See: Mephenoxalone.
• **methoxyflurane.** (meth-OCK-sih-FLEW-rane) USP 28.
Use: Anesthetic, general.
See: Penthrane.
methoxyphenamine hydrochloride. USP 28.
Use: Adrenergic (bronchodilator).
W/Chlorpheniramine maleate, acetophenetidin, acetylsalicylic acid, caffeine.
See: Pyrroxate.
W/Dextromethorphan HCl, orthoxine, sodium citrate.
See: Orthoxicol.
W/Dextromethorphan HBr, phenylephrine HCl, chlorpheniramine maleate.
See: Statuss.
W/Medrol.
See: Medrol.
methoxypromazine maleate.
Use: CNS depressant.
methoxypsoralen, oral.
Use: Psoralen.
See: Oxsoralen.
Oxsoralen Ultra.
methscopolamine bromide.
Use: Anticholinergic.
See: Pamine.
Pamine Forte.
W/Amobarbital.
See: Scoline-Amobarbital.
W/Butabarbital sodium, dried aluminum hydroxide gel and magnesium trisilicate.
See: Eulcin.
W/Phenobarbital.
See: Pamine PB.
W/Chlorpheniramine maleate.
See: Bobid.
methscopolamine nitrate. (Various Mfr.) Scopolamine Methyl Nitrate, Preps.
Mescomine.

See: AlleRx.
Dallergy.
Extendryl.
Sanhist T.D. 12.
W/Combinations.
See: AeroHist Plus.
AeroKid.
AH-chew.
AlleRx.
AlleRx.
CPM 8/PSE 90/MSC 2.5.
D.A.
D.A. II.
Dallergy.
Dehistine.
DriHist-SR.
Duradryl.
Durahist.
Ex-Histine.
Extendryl.
Extendryl JR.
Hista-Vent DA.
Librax.
OMNIhist L.A.
Pannaz.
Pannaz S.
Pre-Hist-D.
PSE 120/MSC 2.5.
Rescon-MX.
•**methsuximide.** (meth-SUCK-sih-mide) *USP 28.*
Use: Anticonvulsant.
See: Celontin.
Methyclodine. (Rugby) Methyclothiazide 5 mg, deserpidine 0.25 mg. Tab. Bot. 100s. *Rx.*
Use: Antihypertensive; diuretic.
•**methyclothiazide.** (METH-ee-kloe-THIGH-ah-zide) *USP 28.*
Use: Antihypertensive; diuretic.
See: Enduron.
Methyclodine.
W/Deserpidine.
See: Enduronyl.
methylacetylcholine.
See: Methacholine.
•**methyl alcohol.** (METH-ill) *NF 23.*
Use: Pharmaceutic acid (solvent).
•**methyl aminolevulinate hydrochloride.** (METH-ill a-MEE-noe-lev-yoo-lin-ate) USAN.
Use: Antineoplastic.
methylamphetamine hydrochloride & sulfate.
See: Desoxyephedrine HCl.
methylandrostenediol. Methandriol.
See: Hybolin.
W/Adrenal cortex extract, Vitamin B_{12}.
See: Geri-Ace.
W/Carboxymethylcellulose sodium, thimerosal.

See: Cenabolic.
•**methylatropine nitrate.** (METH-ill-AT-row-peen) USAN.
Use: Anticholinergic.
•**methylbenzethonium chloride.** (meth-ill-benz-eth-OH-nee-uhm) *USP 28.*
Use: Bactericide, local anti-infective (topical).
See: Ammorid.
Benephen.
Cuticura Acne.
Cuticura Medicated First Aid.
Diaparene.
Fordustin.
Surgi-Kleen.
W/Cod liver oil.
See: Benephen.
Sween.
W/Magnesium stearate.
See: Mennen Baby.
methylbenztropine.
See: Ethybenztropine.
methylbromtropin mandelate. Homatropine Methylbromide.
•**methylcellulose.** (METH-ill-SELL-you-lohs) *USP 28.*
Use: Pharmaceutic aid (suspending agent).
See: Cellothyl, Tab.
Cologel.
Isopto-Plain.
Melozets.
W/Boric acid, glycerin, propylene glycol, methylparaben, propylparaben, Irish moss extract.
See: Canfield Lubricating Jelly.
W/Carboxymethylcellulose.
See: Ex-Caloric.
W/Dicyclomine HCl, magnesium trisilicate, aluminum hydroxide-magnesium carbonate, dried.
See: Triactin.
W/Dicyclomine HCl, aluminum hydroxide, and magnesium hydroxide.
See: Triactin.
W/Phenylephrine HCl, benzalkonium Cl.
See: Efricel.
W/Polysorbate 80, boric acid.
See: Lacril Artificial Tears.
methyl cysteine hydrochloride. Cysteine methyl ester hydrochloride.
Use: Mucolytic agent.
•**methyldopa.** (meth-ill-DOE-puh) *USP 28. Formerly Alpha-Methyldopa.*
Use: Antihypertensive.
•**methyldopa.** (Various Mfr.) Methyldopa 250 mg, 500 mg. Tab. Bot. 100s, 500s, 1000s (250 mg only), UD 100s. *Rx.*
Use: Antihypertensive.

methyldopa and chlorothiazide tablets.
Use: Antihypertensive.
See: Aldoclor.
methyldopa/hydrochlorothiazide.
(Various Mfr.) Methyldopa 250 mg, hydrochlorothiazide 15 mg, 25 mg. Tab. Bot. 100s, 500s, 1000s, UD 100s. *Rx.*
Use: Antihypertensive combination.
methyldopa/hydrochlorothiazide.
(Various Mfr.) Methyldopa 500 mg, hydrochlorothiazide 30 mg, 50 mg. Tab. Bot. 100s, 250s, 500s. *Rx.*
Use: Antihypertensive combination.
methyldopa/hydrochlorothiazide tablets.
Use: Antihypertensive.
See: Aldoril.
•**methyldopate hydrochloride.** (meth-ill-DOE-pate) *USP 28.*
Use: Antihypertensive.
methyldopate hydrochloride. (Various Mfr.) Methyldopate HCl 50 mg/mL. Inj. Single-dose vials, *ADD-vantage* vials. *Rx.*
Use: Antihypertensive.
•**methylene blue.** (METH-ih-leen) *USP 28.*
Use: Antidote; cyanide.
See: Methblue 65.
    Urolene Blue.
methylene blue. (Various Mfr.) Methylene blue 10 mg/mL. Inj. Vial 1 mL, 10 mL. *Rx.*
Use: GU antiseptic; antidote; cyanide.
methylene blue w/combinations.
See: Urised.
•**methylene chloride.** (METH-ih-leen) *NF 23.*
Use: Pharmaceutic aid (solvent).
•**methylergonovine maleate.** (METH-ill-err-go-NO-veen) *USP 28.*
Use: Oxytocic.
See: Methergine.
methylglucamine diatrizoate, injection.
A water-soluble radiopaque iodine cpd. N-methylglucamine salt of Diatrizoate.
See: Diatrizoate Inj.
    Diatrizoate Meglumine Inj.
methylglucamine iodipamide, inj.
See: Meglumine Iodipamide, Inj.
W/Diatrizoate methylglucamine.
See: Sinografin.
methylglyoxal-bis-guanylhydrazone.
Methyl GAG.
Methylin. (Alliant) Methylphenidate hydrochloride. **Chew. Tab.:** 2.5 mg, phenylalanine 0.42 mg; 5 mg, phenylalanine 0.84 mg; 10 mg, phenylalanine 1.68 mg. Aspartame, grape flavor. 30s,

100s, 1000s (except 2.5 mg). **Oral Soln.:** 5 mg per 5 mL. Grape flavor. 10 mg per 5 mL. 500 mL. *c-II.*
Use: CNS stimulant.
Methylin. (Mallinckrodt) Methylphenidate hydrochloride 5 mg, 10 mg, 20 mg. Lactose, talc. Tab. Bot. 100s, 1,000s. *c-II.*
Use: CNS stimulant.
Methylin ER. (Mallinckrodt) Methylphenidate HCl 10 mg, 20 mg, color-additive free. ER Tab. Bot. 100s. *c-II.*
Use: CNS stimulant.
•**methyl isobutyl ketone.** (METH-ill eye-so-BYOO-till KEE-tone) *NF 23.*
Use: Pharmaceutic aid (alcohol denaturant).
methyliso-octenylamine.
See: Isometheptene HCl.
methylmercadone. Name used for Nifuratel.
•**methyl nicotinate.** (METH-ill NIK-oh-TIN-ate) USAN.
W/Histamine dihydrochloride, oleoresin capsicum, glycomonosalicylate.
See: Akes-N-Pain Rub.
W/Methyl salicylate, menthol.
See: Musterole Deep Strength Oint.
Methylone. (Paddock) Methylprednisolone acetate 40 mg/mL. Vial 5 mL. *Rx.*
Use: Corticosteroid.
•**methyl palmoxirate.** (METH-ill pal-MOX-ihr-ate) USAN.
Use: Antidiabetic.
•**methylparaben.** (meth-ill-PAR-ah-ben) *NF 23.*
Use: Pharmaceutic aid (antifungal agent).
•**methylparaben sodium.** (meth-ill-PAR-ah-ben) *NF 23.*
Use: Pharmaceutic aid (antimicrobial preservative).
methylphenethylamine.
See: Amphetamine HCl.
•**methylphenidate.** (meth-ill-FEN-ih-date) USAN.
Use: CNS stimulant.
•**methylphenidate hydrochloride.** (meth-ill-FEN-ih-date) *USP 28.*
Use: CNS stimulant.
See: Concerta.
    Metadate CD.
    Metadate ER.
    Methylin.
    Methylin ER.
    Ritalin.
    Ritalin LA.
    Ritalin-SR.
methylphenidate hydrochloride. (Various Mfr.) Methylphenidate HCl.
Tab.: 5 mg, 10 mg, 20 mg. Bot. 100s,

1000s. **ER Tab.:** 20 mg, Bot. 30s, 100s. *c-II.*
Use: CNS stimulant.
methylphenidylacetate hydrochloride.
See: Methylphenidate HCl.
methylphenobarbital.
See: Mephobarbital.
d-methylphenylamine sulfate.
See: Dextroamphetamine Sulfate.
methyl phenylethylhydantoin.
See: Mesantoin.
methylphenylsuccinimide.
See: Milontin.
methylphytyl naphthoquinone.
Use: Vitamin supplement.
See: Phytonadione.
methyl polysiloxane.
See: Mylicon.
Simethicone.
methylprod-10. (Seatrace) Methylpred-
nisolone acetate 40 mg/mL. Vial 5 mL,
10 mL. *Rx.*
Use: Corticosteroid.
• **methylprednisolone.** (METH-ill-pred-
NIH-suh-lone) *USP 28.*
Tall Man: MethylPREDNISolone
Use: Corticosteroid, topical.
See: A-Methapred.
Dura-Meth.
Medrol.
W/Neomycin sulfate
See: Solu-Medrol.
methylprednisolone. (Prasco) Methyl-
prednisolone 8 mg. Lactose. Tab. 25s.
Rx.
Use: Adrenocortical steroid.
• **methylprednisolone acetate.** (METH-ill-
pred-NIH-suh-lone) *USP 28.*
Tall Man: MethylPREDNISolone
Use: Corticosteroid.
See: Depo-Medrol.
Depopred-40
• **methylprednisolone hemisuccinate.**
(METH-ill-pred-NIH-suh-lone hem-ih-
SUCK-sih-nate) *USP 28.*
Tall Man: MethylPREDNISolone
Use: Adrenocortical steroid.
• **methylprednisolone sodium phos-
phate.** (METH-ill-pred-NIH-suh-lone)
USAN.
Tall Man: MethylPREDNISolone
Use: Corticosteroid, topical.
• **methylprednisolone sodium succinate.**
(METH-ill-pred-NIH-suh-lone) *USP 28.*
Use: Adrenocorticoid steroid; cortico-
steroid, topical.
See: Solu-Medrol, Mix-O-Vial.
• **methylprednisolone suleptanate.**
(METH-ill-pred-NIH-suh-lone sull-EPP-
tah-NATE) USAN.

Tall Man: MethylPREDNISolone
Use: Adrenocortical steroid; anti-inflam-
matory.
4-methylpyrazole.
Use: Methanol or ethylene glycol poi-
soning. [Orphan Drug]
methylpyrimal.
See: Sulfamerazine.
methylrosaniline chloride.
Use: Anthelmintic; anti-infective.
See: Gentian Violet.
• **methyl salicylate.** (METH-ill sal-ISS-ih-
late) *NF 23.*
Use: Pharmaceutic aid (flavor).
methyl salicylate w/combinations.
Use: Rubefacient rub (topical).
See: Analbalm.
Analgesic Balm.
Banalg, Liniment.
Bayer Muscle & Joint Rub.
Cydonol.
Emul-o-balm.
Gordobalm.
Listerine Antiseptic.
Musterole.
Pain Bust-R II.
Sloan's Liniment.
Ziks.
methyl sulfanil amidoisoxazole. Sulfa-
methoxazole
See: Gantanol.
• **methyltestosterone.** (METH-ill-tess-
TAHS-ter-ohn) *USP 28.*
Tall Man: MethylTESTOSTERone
Use: Sex hormone, androgen.
See: Android
Methitest.
Testred.
Virilon.
Virilon IM.
methyltestosterone. (Various Mfr.)
Methyltestosterone. **Tab.:** 10 mg,
25 mg. Bot. 100s. **Tab., bucccal:**
10 mg. Bot. 100s. *c-III*
Use: Sex hormone, androgen.
methyltestosterone w/combinations.
Use: Androgen.
See: Android.
Menogen.
Premarin w/Methyltestosterone.
Virilon.
methylthionine chloride. Name used
for Methylene Blue.
methylthionine hydrochloride. Name
used for Methylene Blue.
methylthiouracil. *USP 28.*
Use: Antithyroid agent.
methyl violet.
See: Gentian Violet, Crystal Violet,
Methylrosaniline Cl.
methyndamine. Name used for Tetrydamine.

•**metiamide.** (meh-TIE-aim-id) USAN.
Histamine H_2 antagonist.
Use: Treatment for peptic ulcer; antiulcerative.

•**metiapine.** (meh-TIE-ah-PEEN) USAN.
Use: Antipsychotic.

meticlopindol. Name used for Clopidol.

Meticorten. (Schering-Plough) Prednisone 1 mg. Tab. Bot. 100s. *Rx.*
Use: Corticosteroid.

Metimyd Ophthalmic Oint. Sterile.
(Schering-Plough) Prednisolone acetate
0.5% (5 mg), sulfacetamide sodium
10%. Tube 3.5 g. *Rx.*
Use: Corticosteroid; sulfonamide,
topical.

Metimyd Ophthalmic Susp. Sterile.
(Schering-Plough) Prednisolone acetate
0.5%, sulfacetamide sodium 10%. Bot.
dropper 5 mL. *Rx.*
Use: Corticosteroid; sulfonamide,
topical.

•**metioprim.** (meh-TIE-oh-PRIM) USAN.
Use: Anti-infective.

•**metipranolol.** (meh-tih-PRAN-oh-lahl)
USAN.
Use: Antihypertensive (beta-blocker,
ophthalmic).

metipranolol. (Falcon Ophthalmics)
Metipranolol 0.3%, povidone, hydrochloric acid, NaCl, EDTA, benzalkonium
chloride 0.004%. Ophth. Soln. Bot.
5 mL, 10 mL. *Rx.*
Use: Antihypertensive, beta-blocker,
ophthalmic.

metipranolol hydrochloride.
Use: Antihypertensive (beta-blocker,
ophthalmic).
See: OptiPranolol.

metizoline.
Use: Decongestant.

•**metizoline hydrochloride.** (meh-TIH-
zoe-leen) USAN.
Use: Adrenergic vasoconstrictor.

•**metkephamid acetate.** (MET-KEFF-am-
id) USAN.
Use: Analgesic.

•**metoclopramide hydrochloride.** (MET-
oh-kloe-PRA-mide) *USP 28.*
Use: Antiemetic; gastrointestinal stimulant.
See: Reclomide.
Reglan.
Reglan Tablets.

metofurone. Name used for Nifurmerone.

•**metogest.** (MET-oh-JEST) USAN.
Use: Hormone.

•**metolazone.** (meh-TOLE-uh-ZONE)
USP 28.
Use: Antihypertensive; diuretic.
See: Mykrox.
Zaroxolyn.

•**metolazaone.** (Eon Labs) Metolazone
5 mg, 10 mg. Tab. 100s. *Rx.*
Use: Diuretic.

metolazone. (Various Mfr.) Metolazone
2.5 mg. Tab. 100s, 1000s. *Rx.*
Use: Diuretic.

•**metopimazine.** (meh-toe-PIH-mazz-
EEN) USAN.
Use: Antiemetic.

Metopirone. (Novartis) Metyrapone
250 mg. Softgel Cap. Pkg. 18s. *Rx.*
Use: Diagnostic aid.

•**metoprine.** (MET-oh-preen) USAN.
Use: Antineoplastic.

•**metoprolol.** (meh-TOE-pro-lahl) USAN.
Use: Antiadrenergic/sympatholytic,
beta-adrenergic blocker.
See: Lopressor.

•**metoprolol fumarate.** (meh-TOE-pro-
lahl) *USP 28.*
Use: Antihypertensive.

•**metoprolol succinate.** (meh-TOE-pro-
lahl) USAN.
Use: Antihypertensive; antianginal;
treatment of myocardial infarction.
See: Toprol XL.

•**metoprolol tartrate.** (meh-TOE-pro-lahl)
USP 28.
Use: Antiadrenergic (beta-receptor).
See: Lopressor.

metoprolol tartrate. (Abbott) Metoprolol
tartrate 1 mg/mL. Inj. Amp. *Carpuject*
sterile cartridge units with Interlink System Cannula, *Carpuject* sterile cartridge units with *Luer-Lock. Rx.*
Use: Antiadrenergic/sympatholytic,
beta-adrenergic blocker.

metoprolol tartrate. (Purepac) Metoprolol tartrate. **Tab.:** 50 mg, 100 mg,
lactose. Bot. 100s, 1000s, UD 100s.
Inj.: 1 mg/mL. Amp. 5 mL. *Rx.*
Use: Antiadrenergic/sympatholytic;
beta-adrenergic blocker.

metoprolol tartrate. (Various Mfr.) Metoprolol tartrate 25 mg. Tab. 30s, 90s,
100s, 1000s. *Rx.*
Use: Antiadrenergic, sympatholytic.

metoprolol tartrate. (Various Mfr.) Metoprolol tartrate 50 mg, 100 mg. Tab.
100s, 1000s. *Rx.*
Use: Antiadrenergic/sympatholytic,
beta-adrenergic blocker.

metoprolol tartrate and hydrochlorothiazide.
Use: Antihypertensive combination.
See: Lopressor HCT 50/25.
Lopressor HCT 100/25.

Lopressor HCT 100/50.

metoprolol tartrate/hydrochlorothia-zide. (Mylan) Hydrochlorothiazide/ metoprolol tartrate 25 mg/50 mg, 25 mg/100 mg, 50 mg/100 mg. Lactose. Tab. 100s, 500s. *Rx.*
Use: Antihypertensive.

metoquine.
Use: Antimalarial.

•**metoquizine.** (MET-oh-kwih-zeen) USAN.
Use: Anticholinergic; antiulcerative.

•**metreleptin.** (MEH-trah-lep-tihn) USAN.
Use: Obesity and related disorders.

Metreton Ophthalmic Solution. (Scher-ing-Plough) Prednisolone sodium phos-phate 5.5 mg/mL. Bot. 5 mL. *Rx.*
Use: Corticosteroid; ophthalmic.

Metric 21. (Fielding) Metronidazole 250 mg. Tab. Bot. 100s. *Rx.*
Use: Anti-infective.

•**metrifonate.** (meh-TRIH-foe-nate) *USP 28.* Formerly trichlorfon.
Use: Cholinesterase inhibitor.

•**metrizamide.** (meh-TRIH-zam-ide) USAN.
Use: Myelography, diagnostic aid (radi-opaque medium).
See: Amipaque.

•**metrizoate sodium.** (meh-trih-ZOE-ate) USAN.
Use: Diagnostic aid (radiopaque medium).

MetroCream. (Galderma) Metronidazole 0.75%, glycerin, benzyl alcohol. Cream. Tube. 45 g. *Rx.*
Use: Anti-infective.

MetroGel. (Galderma) Metronidazole 0.75%, parabens, EDTA. Gel Tube 28.4 g, 45 g. *Rx.*
Use: Dermatologic, acne.

MetroGel-Vaginal. (3M) Metronidazole 0.75%, EDTA, parabens. Gel Tube (with 5 applicators) 70 g. *Rx.*
Use: Anti-infective, vaginal.

Metrogesic. (Lexis Laboratories) Salicyl-amide 325 mg, acetaminophen 162 mg, phenacetin 65 mg. Tab. Bot. 100s.
Use: Analgesic.

metrogestone.
Use: Hormone, progestin.

MetroLotion. (Galderma) Metronidazole 0.75%, benzyl alcohol, stearyl alcohol, glycerin, mineral oil. Lot. Bot. 59 mL. *Rx.*
Use: Antiacne.

•**metronidazole.** (meh-troe-NID-uh-zole) *USP 28.*
Use: Antiprotozoal (trichomonas); anti-trichomonal.

See: Flagyl.
Flagyl ER.
Flagyl IV.
Flagyl IV RTU.
Flagyl 375.
MetroCream.
MetroGel.
MetroGel-Vaginal.
MetroLotion.
Metronid.
Metryl.
Noritate.
Rozex.

metronidazole. (Able) Metronidazole. **Cap.:** 375 mg. 30s, 50s, 100s, 500s, 1000s. **ER Tab.:** 750 mg, lactose, poly-dextrose. 30s, 100s, 500s, 1000s. *Rx.*
Use: Anti-infective.

metronidazole. (B. Braun) Metronida-zole 5 mg/mL. Inj. Vial 100 mL. *Rx.*
Use: Anti-infective.

metronidazole. (Fougera) Metronidazole 0.75%. Benzyl alcohol, glycerin. Cream. 45 g. *Rx.*
Use: Anti-infective, topical.

metronidazole. (Various Mfr.) Metronida-zole 250 mg, 500 mg. Tab. Bot. 25s, 50s (500 mg only), 100s, 250s, (250 mg only), 500s. *Rx.*
Use: Anti-infective.

•**metronidazole benzoate.** (meh-troe-NIH-dah-zole) *USP 28.*
Use: Anti-infective.

•**metronidazole hydrochloride.** (meh-troe-NIH-dah-zole) USAN.
Use: Anti-infective.
See: Flagyl IV.

•**metronidazole phosphate.** (meh-troe-NIH-dah-zole) USAN.
Use: Antibacterial; anti-infective; anti-protozoal.

Metrozole. (Lexis Laboratories) Metro-nidazole 250 mg, 500 mg. Tab. **250 mg:** Bot. 100s, 250s. **500 mg:** Bot. 100s. *Rx.*
Use: Amebicide; anti-infective.

MET-RX. (Met-Rx USA) **Pow. for Drink:** Fat 2 g, Na 37 mg, K 900 mg, carbohy-drate 22 g, protein, < 1 g dietary fiber, sugar, vitamins A, D, C, E, B_1, B_5, B_6, B_{12}, biotin, Mg, Zn, Ca, folate, P, Cu, Fe, riboflavin, iodine. 72 g. **Food Bar:** Fat 4 g, Na 110 mg, K 700 mg, car-bohydrate 50 g, protein 27 g, sugar, Ca, vitamins A, D, B_1, B_2, B_3, B_5, B_6, B_{12}, C, E, folate, biotin, P, Mg, Cu, Fe, I, Zn. 100 g. *OTC.*
Use: Nutritional therapy.

Metryl. (Teva) Metronidazole 250 mg. Tab. Bot. 100s, 250s, 500s, UD 100s.

Rx.
Use: Amebicide, anti-infective.
Metryl 500. (Teva) Metronidazole
500 mg. Tab. Bot. 100s, 500s. *Rx.*
Use: Amebicide; anti-infective.
• **meturedepa.** (meh-TOO-ree-DEH-pah)
USAN.
Use: Antineoplastic.
Metussin. (Faraday) Dextromethorphan.
Bot. 4 oz. *OTC.*
Use: Antitussive.
Metussin Jr. (Faraday) Dextromethor-
phan. Bot. 4 oz. *OTC.*
Use: Antitussive.
• **metyrapone.** (meh-TEER-ah-pone)
USP 28.
Use: Diagnostic aid (pituitary function
determination); adrenocortical en-
zyme inhibitor.
See: Metopirone.
• **metyrapone tartrate.** (meh-TEER-ah-
pone) USAN.
Use: Diagnostic aid (pituitary function
determination).
metyrapone tartrate injection.
Use: Diagnostic aid.
• **metyrosine.** (meh-TIE-roe-seen)
USP 28.
Use: Antihypertensive.
See: Demser.
Mevacor. (Merck) Lovastatin 10 mg,
20 mg, 40 mg, lactose. Tab. Bot. 1000s,
10,000s (except 10 mg); UD 100s
(20 mg only); unit-of-use 60s, 90s (except 10 mg). *Rx.*
Use: Antihyperlipidemic; HMG-CoA reductase inhibitor.
mevinolin.
See: Lovastatin.
Mexate-AQ. (Bristol-Myers Squibb On-
cology/Virology) Methotrexate 50 mg,
100 mg, 250 mg/preservative-free liquid
vial. *Rx.*
Use: Antineoplastic.
• **mexiletine hydrochloride.** (MEX-ih-leh-
teen) *USP 28.*
Use: Antiarrhythmic agent.
See: Mexitil.
Mexitil. (Boehringer Ingelheim) Mexiletine HCl 150 mg, 200 mg, 250 mg.
Cap. Bot. 100s, UD 100s. *Rx.*
Use: Antiarrhythmic.
• **mexrenoate potassium.** (mex-REN-oh-
ate) USAN.
Use: Aldosterone antagonist.
Mexsana Medicated Powder. (Schering-
Plough) Corn starch, kaolin, triclosan,
zinc oxide. Can 3 oz, 6.25 oz, 11 oz.
OTC.
Use: Diaper rash preparation.

Meyenberg Goat Milk. (Jackson-
Mitchell) Evaporated and powdered
cans of goat milk. Foil pack 4 oz.
(makes 1 quart). *OTC.*
Use: Cows' milk allergies.
MG Cold Sore Formula. (Outdoor Rec-
reation) Menthol 1%, lidocaine, propyl-
ene glycol in alcohol base. Soln. Bot.
7.5 mL. *OTC.*
Use: Cold sores; fever blisters.
MG400. (Triton) Colloidal sulfur in Guy-
Base II 5%, salicylic acid 3%. Sham-
poo. Bot. 240 mL, pt. *OTC.*
Use: Antiseborrheic.
MG-Oroate. (Miller Pharmacal Group)
Magnesium (as magnesium orotate)
33 mg. Tab. Bot. 100s. *OTC.*
Use: Vitamin supplement.
MG-Plus Protein. (Miller Pharmacal
Group) Magnesium-protein complex
made w/specially isolated soy protein
133 mg. Tab. Bot. 100s. *OTC.*
Use: Vitamin supplement.
MG217 Medicated Tar. (Triton) **Sham-
poo:** Coal tar solution 15%. Bot.
120 mL, 240 mL. **Oint.:** Coal tar solu-
tion 10%, petrolatum, cetyl alcohol.
107 g. **Lot.:** Coal tar solution 5%,
moisturizing base, cetyl alcohol, mineral oil. 120 mL. *OTC.*
Use: Antipruritic; antieczematic; keratolytic.
MG217 Medicated Tar-Free. (Triton) Colloidal sulfur 5%, salicylic acid 3%.
Shampoo. Bot. 120 mL, 240 mL. *OTC.*
Use: Antiseborrheic; antipruritic.
MG217 Sal-Acid. (Triton) Salicylic acid
3%, vitamin E. Oint. Tube. 60 g. *OTC.*
Use: Keratolytic.
MHP-A. (Cypress) Methenamine
40.8 mg, phenyl salicylate 18.1 mg,
atropine sulfate 0.03, hyoscyamine sulfate 0.03 mg, benzoic acid 4.5 mg,
methylene blue 5.4 mg. Tab. 100s. *Rx.*
Use: Anti-infective, urinary.
Miacalcin. (Novartis) Calcitonin-salmon
200 units, acetic acid 2.25 mg, phenol
5 mg, sodium acetate trihydrate 2 mg,
sodium chloride 7.5 mg/mL. Inj. Vial
2 mL. *Rx.*
Use: Hormone.
Mi-Acid Gelcaps. (Major) Calcium carbonate 311 mg, magnesium carbonate
232 mg, parabens, EDTA. Bot. 50s.
OTC.
Use: Antacid.
Mi-Acid Liquid. (Major) Aluminum
hydroxide 200 mg, magnesium hydroxide 200 mg, simethicone 20 mg/5 mL.
Bot. 355 mL, 780 mL. *OTC.*
Use: Antacid; antiflatulent.

Mi-Acid II Liquid. (Major) Aluminum hydroxide 400 mg, magnesium hydroxide 400 mg, simethicone 40 mg/5 mL. Bot. 355 mL. *OTC.*
Use: Antacid; antiflatulent.

miadone.
See: Methadone HCl.

• **mianserin hydrochloride.** (my-AN-ser-in) USAN. Under study.
Use: Serotonin inhibitor; antihistamine.

• **mibolerone.** (my-BOLE-ehr-ohn) USAN.
Use: Anabolic; androgen.

• **micafungin sodium.** (mi-ka-FUN-gin) USAN.
Use: Antifungal.
See: Mycamine.

Micardis. (Boehringer Ingelheim) Telmisartan 20 mg, 40 mg, 80 mg, sorbitol. Tab. Blister Pack 28s. *Rx.*
Use: Antihypertensive.

Micardis HCT. (Boehringer Ingelheim) Telmisartan/hydrochlorothiazide 40 mg/ 12.5 mg, 80 mg/12.5 mg, 80 mg/25 mg, sorbitol, lactose. Tab. Blister pack 28s (except 80 mg/25 mg), blister pack 30s (80 mg/25 mg only). *Rx.*
Use: Antihypertensive.

micasorb.
W/Red Veterinary Petrolatum.
See: RV Plus.

Micatin. (Johnson & Johnson) Miconazole nitrate 2%. **Cream:** Tube 0.5 oz, 1 oz. **Spray powder:** Aerosol 3 oz. **Spray Liquid Aerosol:** Bot. 3.5 oz. *OTC.*
Use: Antifungal, topical.

Mi-Cebrin. (Eli Lilly) Vitamins B_1 10 mg, B_2 5 mg, B_6 1.7 mg, pantothenic acid 10 mg, niacinamide 30 mg, B_{12} (activity equivalent) 3 mcg, C 100 mg, E 5.5 units, A 10,000 units, D 400 units, Fe 15 mg, Cu 1 mg, I 0.15 mg, Mn 1 mg, Mg 5 mg, Zn 1.5 mg. Tab. Pkg. 60s, 100s, 1000s, Blister pkg. 10 × 10s. *OTC.*
Use: Mineral; vitamin supplement.

Mi-Cebrin T. (Eli Lilly) Vitamins B_1 15 mg, B_2 10 mg, B_6 2 mg, pantothenic acid 10 mg, niacinamide 100 mg, B_{12} 7.5 mcg, C 150 mg, E 5.5 units, A 10,000 units, D 400 units, Fe 15 mg, Cu 1 mg, I 0.15 mg, Mn 1 mg, Mg 5 mg, Zn 1.5 mg. Tab. Bot. 30s, 100s, 1000s, Blister pkg. 10 × 10s. *OTC.*
Use: Mineral; vitamin supplement.

micofur.
Use: Antifungal; anti-infective, topical.

Miconal. (Bioglan Pharma) Anthralin 1%. Cream. Tube 50 g. *Rx.*
Use: Antipsoriatic.

• **miconazole.** (my-KAHN-uh-zole) *USP 28.*
Use: Antifungal.
See: Monistat IV.

• **miconazole nitrate.** (my-CONE-ah-zole) *USP 28.*
Use: Antifungal.
See: Breezee Mist Antifungal.
Femizol-M.
Fungoid Tincture.
Lotrimin AF.
Maximum Strength Desenex Antifungal.
Miconazole 7.
Monistat.
Monistat 3.
Monistat 3 Combination Pack.
Monistat 7.
Monistat 7 Combination Pack.
Monistat Derm.
Monistat Dual-Pak.
M-Zole 3 Combination Pack.
M-Zole 7 Dual Pack.
Neosporin AF.
Ting.
Zeasorb-AF.

miconazole nitrate. (Various Mfr.) Miconazole nitrate 2%. Vag. Cream. Tube 15 g, 30 g, 45 g. *OTC.*
Use: Antifungal, vaginal.

miconazole nitrate. (Taro) Miconazole nitrate 2%, benzoic acid, mineral oil, apricot kernel oil. Cream. Tube 15 g, 30 g. *OTC.*
Use: Antifungal, topical.

Miconazole 7. (Rugby) Miconazole nitrate 100 mg, hydrogenated vegetable oil base. Vag. Supp. Box 7s w/applicator. *OTC.*
Use: Antifungal.

micoren. (Novartis) A respiratory stimulant; pending release.

Micrainin. (Wallace) Meprobamate 200 mg, aspirin 325 mg. Tab. Bot. 100s. *c-iv.*
Use: Analgesic combination.

MICRhoGAM. (Ortho Diagnostics) Rh_0 (D) immune globulin micro-dose ≈ 5% ± 1% gamma globulin, sodium chloride 2.9 mg/mL, polysorbate 80 0.01%, glycine 15 mg/mL, preservative free. Soln. for Inj. Pkg. containing single-dose prefilled syringes, injection control form, patient ID card 5s, 25s. *Rx.*
Use: Immune globulin.

microbubble contrast agent.
Use: Aid in ID of intracranial tumors. [Orphan Drug]

Microcult-GC Test. (Bayer Corp. (Consumer Div.)) Miniaturized culture test for the detection of *Neisseria Gonor-*

rhoeae. Test Kit 25s.
Use: Diagnostic aid.
microfibrillar collagen hemostat.
Use: Hemostatic, topical.
See: Avitene.
Hemopad.
Hemotene.
Microgestin Fe 1/20. (Watson) Ethinyl estradiol 20 mcg, norethindrone acetate 1 mg, lactose. Tab. Pack 28s. *Rx.*
Use: Sex hormone, contraceptive hormone.
Microgestin Fe 1.5/30. (Watson) Ethinyl estradiol 30 mcg, norethindrone acetate 1.5 mg, lactose. Tab. Pack 28s. *Rx.*
Use: Sex hormone, contraceptive hormone.
Micro-Guard. (Sween) Antimicrobial skin cream. Tube 0.5 oz, Jar 2 oz. *OTC.*
Use: Antifungal, topical.
Micro-K Extencaps. (Wyeth) Potassium Cl (8 mEq) 600 mg. Cap. Bot. 100s, 500s, *Dis-Co* pack 100s. *Rx.*
Use: Electrolyte supplement.
Micro-K LS. (Wyeth) Potassium Cl 20 mEq (1500 mg). Extended release Susp. Packet 30s, 100s. *Rx.*
Use: Electrolyte supplement.
Micro-K 10 Extencaps. (Wyeth) Potassium Cl 750 mg (10 mEq). Cap. Bot. 100s, 500s, *Dis-co* UD 100s. *Rx.*
Use: Electrolyte supplement.
Microlipid. (Biosearch Medical Products) Fat emulsion 50%, safflower oil, polyglycerol esters of fatty acids, soy lecithin, xanthan gum, ascorbic acid. Cal 4500, fat 500 g/L, 80 mOsm/Kg. H_2O. 120 mL. *Rx.*
Use: Nutritional supplement.
Micronase. (Pharmacia) Glyburide 1.25, 2.5, 5 mg. Tab. **1.25 mg:** Bot. 100s.
2.5 mg: Bot. 100s, 1000s, UD 100s.
5 mg: Bot. 30s, 60s, 100s, 500s, 1000s, UD 100s. *Rx.*
Use: Antidiabetic.
microNefrin. (Bird Products) Racepinephrine HCl 2.25% (epinephrine base 1.125%), sodium bisulfite, potassium metabisulfite, chlorobutanol, benzoic acid, propylene glycol. Soln. for Inh. Bot 15 mL, 30 mL. *OTC.*
Use: Bronchodilator; sympathomimetic.
Micronor.
See: Ortho Micronor.
Microsol. (Star) Sulfamethizole 0.5 g, 1 g. Tab. Bot. 100s, 1000s. *Rx.*
Use: Anti-infective; urinary.
Microsol-A. (Star) Phenazopyridine 50 mg, sulfamethizole 0.5 g. Tab. Bot. 100s, 1000s. *Rx.*
Use: Anti-infective; urinary.

Microstix Candida. (Bayer Corp. (Consumer Div.)) Test for *Candida* species in vaginal specimens. Box 25s.
Use: Diagnostic aid.
Microstix-3 Reagent Strips. (Bayer Corp. (Consumer Div.)) For recognition of nitrite in urine and for semiquantitation of bacterial growth. Bot. 25s w/25 incubation pouches.
Use: Diagnostic aid.
MicroTrak Chlamydia Trachomatis Direct Specimen Test. (Syva) To detect and identify chlamydia trachomatis. Slide test 60s.
Use: Diagnostic aid.
MicroTrak HSV 1/HSV 2 Culture Confirmation/Typing Test. (Syva) For identification and typing of herpes simplex in tissue culture. Test kit 1s.
Use: Diagnostic aid.
MicroTrak Neisseria Gonorrhea Culture Test. (Syva) For endocervical, urethral, rectal, and pharyngeal cultures. Test kit 85s.
Use: Diagnostic aid.
Microzide. (Watson) Hydrochlorothiazide 12.5 mg, lactose. Cap. Bot. 100s. *Rx.*
Use: Diuretic.
micrurus fulvius antivenin. (Wyeth) Inj. Combination package: One vial antivenin, one vial diluent (Bacteriostatic Water for Injection 10 mL.).
Use: Antivenin.
Mictrin Plus. (Johnson & Johnson) Water, SD alcohol 38-B, glycerin, poloxamer 407, flavor, sodium saccharin, glutamic acid buffer, cetylpyridinium Cl, FD & C Yellow #5, Blue #1. Bot. 12 oz, 24 oz. *OTC.*
Use: Mouth preparation.
• **midaflur.** (MY-dah-flure) USAN.
Use: Hypnotic, sedative.
midamaline hydrochloride.
Use: Anesthetic, local.
Midamor. (Merck & Co.) Amiloride 5 mg. Tab. Bot. 100s. *Rx.*
Use: Diuretic; antihypertensive.
Midaneed. (Hanlon) Vitamins A 5000 units, D 500 units, B_1 5 mg, B_2 3 mg, B_6 0.5 mcg, B_{12} 5 mcg, C 100 mg, niacinamide 10 mg, calcium pantothenate 5 mg. Cap. Bot. 100s. *OTC.*
Use: Mineral; vitamin supplement.
• **midazolam hydrochloride.** (meh-DAZE-oh-lam) USAN.
Use: Anesthetic (injectable).
midazolam hydrochloride. (Various Mfr.) Midazolam HCl 1 mg/mL, 5 mg/mL. Inj. Vial 1 mL (5 mg only), 2 mL, 5 mL. *Carpuject* Vial 10 mL. Syr. 2 mL

(5 mg only). *c-iv.*
Use: Anesthetic.
● **midazolam maleate.** (meh-DAZE-oh-lam) USAN.
Use: Anesthetic, intravenous.
● **midodrine hydrochloride.** (MIH-doe-DREEN) USAN.
Use: Antihypotensive; vasoconstrictor.
See: ProAmatine.
midodrine hydrochloride. (Global) Midodrine hydrochloride 2.5 mg, 5 mg. Tab. 100s, 500s, 1,000s. *Rx.*
Use: Vasopressor used in shock.
midodrine hydrochloride. (Mylan) Midodrine hydrochloride 10 mg. Tab. 100s. *Rx.*
Use: Vasopressor used in shock.
midodrine hydrochloride. (Various Mfr.) Midodrine hydrochloride 2.5 mg, 5 mg. Tab. 100s, 500s (except 2.5 mg). *Rx.*
Use: Vasopressor used in shock.
Midol Extended Relief. (Bayer) Naproxen 200 mg (naproxen sodium 220 mg). Sodium 20 mg. Tab. 24s. *OTC.*
Use: Nonsteroidal anti-inflammatory drug.
Midol for Cramps. (Bayer Corp. (Consumer Div.)) Aspirin 500 mg, caffeine 32.4 mg, cinnamedrine HCl 14.9 mg. Capl. In 8s, 16s, 32s. *OTC.*
Use: Analgesic combination.
Midol Maximum Strength Cramp Formula. (Bayer Corp. (Consumer Div.)) Ibuprofen 200 mg. Tab. Bot. 24s. *OTC.*
Use: Analgesic; NSAID.
Midol Maximum Strength Menstrual. (Bayer Corp. (Consumer Div.)) Acetaminophen 500 mg, caffeine 60 mg, pyrilamine maleate 15 mg. Capl. Bot. 8s, 24s. Gelcap: EDTA. Bot. 24s. *OTC.*
Use: Analgesic.
Midol Maximum Strength Multi-Symptom Menstrual. (Bayer Corp. (Consumer Div.)) Acetaminophen 500 mg, caffeine 60 mg, pyrilamine maleate 15 mg. Capl. Pkg. 8s, 16s, 32s. Gelcaps. Pkg. 12s, 24s. *OTC.*
Use: Analgesic combination.
Midol Maximum Strength PMS. (Bayer Corp. (Consumer Div.)) Acetaminophen 500 mg, pamabrom 25 mg, pyrilamine maleate 15 mg. Capl. Bot. 24s. Gelcap: EDTA. Bot. 24s. *OTC.*
Use: Analgesic.
Midol Multi-Symptom, Maximum Strength. (Bayer Corp. (Consumer Div.)) Acetaminophen 500 mg, pyrilamine maleate 15 mg. Capl. Bot. 32s. *OTC.*
Use: Analgesic combination.

Midol Original Formula. (Bayer Corp. (Consumer Div.)) Cinnamedrine HCl 14.9 mg, aspirin 454 mg, caffeine 32.4 mg. Tab. Bot. 30s, 60s. Strip pack 12s. *OTC.*
Use: Analgesic combination.
Midol PM. (Bayer Corp. (Consumer Div.)) Acetaminophen 500 mg, diphenhydramine 25 mg. Capl. Pkg. 16s. *OTC.*
Use: Analgesic combination.
Midol Teen Maximum Strength. (Bayer Corp. (Consumer Div.)) Acetaminophen 500 mg, pamabrom 25 mg. Capl. Bot. 24s. *OTC.*
Use: Analgesic.
● **midostaurin.** (mi-doe-STOR-in) USAN.
Use: Antineoplastic.
Midrin. (Women First Healthcare) Isometheptene mucate 65 mg, acetaminophen 325 mg, dichloralphenazone 100 mg. Cap. Bot. 50s, 100s, 250s. *c-iv.*
Use: Antimigraine.
Midstream Pregnancy Test Kit. (Ivax) Stick for urine test. Kit 1s. *OTC.*
Use: Pregnancy test.
Mifeprex. (Danco Labs) Mifepristone 200 mg. Tab. Single-dose blister pack containing 3 tabs. *Rx.*
Use: Uterine-active agent; abortifacient.
mifepristone.
Use: Uterine-active agent; abortifacient.
See: Mifeprex.
● **mifobate.** (mih-FOE-bate) USAN.
Use: Antiatherosclerotic.
● **miglitol.** (mih-GLIH-tole) USAN.
Use: Antidiabetic.
See: Glyset.
● **miglustat.** (MIG-loo-stat)
Use: Gaucher disease.
See: Zavesca.
migraine agents.
See: Almotriptan Maleate.
Dihydroergotamine Mesylate.
Eletriptan HBr.
Ergotamine Derivatives.
Ergotamine Tartrate.
Frovatriptan Succinate.
Naratriptan Hydrochloride.
Rizatriptan Benzoate.
Sumatriptan Succinate.
Zolmitriptan.
migraine combinations.
See: Isometheptene/Dichloralphenazone/Acetaminophen.
Migranal. (Xcel) Dihydroergotamine mesylate 4 mg/mL, caffeine 10 mg, dextrose 50 mg. Nasal spray. Bot. 1 mL ampules. Kit with 4 unit-dose trays. *Rx.*

Use: Antimigraine.

Migratine. (Major) Isometheptene mucate 65 mg, dichloralphenazone 100 mg, acetaminophen 325 mg. Cap. Bot. 100s, 250s. *c-iv.*
Use: Antimigraine.

MIH.
Use: Antineoplastic.
See: Matulane.

• **milacemide hydrochloride.** (mill-ASS-eh-mide) USAN.
Use: Anticonvulsant; antidepressant.

• **milameline hydrochloride.** (mill-AM-eh-leen) USAN.
Use: Antidementia (partial muscarinic agonist).

mild silver protein.
See: Silver Protein, Mild.

• **milenperone.** (mih-LEN-per-OHN) USAN.
Use: Antipsychotic.

Miles Nervine. (Bayer Corp. (Consumer Div.)) Diphenhydramine HCl 25 mg. Tab. Pkg. 12s, Bot. 30s.
Use: Nonprescription sleep aid.

• **milipertine.** (MIH-lih-PURR-teen) USAN.
Use: Antipsychotic.

milk of bismuth. (Various Mfr.) Bismuth hydroxide, bismuth subcarbonate.
Use: Orally; intestinal disturbances.

• **milk of magnesia.** (mag-NEE-zhuh) *USP 28. Formerly Magnesia Magma.*
Use: Antacid; laxative.
See: Magnesium Hydroxide.

Milk of Magnesia. (Various Mfr.). Magnesium hydroxide 325 mg, 390 mg. **Tab.:** 250s, 1000s. **Liq.:** 120 mL, 360 mL, 720 mL, pt, qt, gal, UD 10 mL, 15 mL, 20 mL, 30 mL, 100 mL, 180 mL, 400 mL. **Susp.:** 400 mg/5 mL. Bot. 180 mL, 360 mL, 480 mL, UD 30 mL, gal. *OTC.*
Use: Antacid; laxative.

Milk of Magnesia-Concentrated.
(Roxane) Equivalent to milk of magnesia 30 mL susp. Bot. 100 mL, 400 mL, UD 10 mL. *OTC.*
Use: Antacid; laxative.

• **milk thistle extract.** *NF 23.*
Use: Anti-inflammatory.

Millazine. (Major) Thioridazine. **10 mg, 15 mg/Tab.:** Bot. 100s. **25 mg/Tab.:** Bot. 100s, 1000s. **100 mg, 150 mg, 200 mg/Tab.:** Bot. 100s, 500s. *Rx.*
Use: Antipsychotic.

milnacipran.
Use: Investigational serotonin norepinephrine reuptake inhibitor.

• **milodistim.** (my-low-DIH-stim) USAN.
Use: Immunomodulator (antineutropenic).

Milophene. (Milex) Clomiphene citrate 50 mg. Tab. Bot. 30s. *Rx.*
Use: Sex hormone; ovulation stimulant.

Milpar. (Sanofi-Synthelabo) Magnesium hydroxide, mineral oil. *OTC.*
Use: Antacid; laxative.

• **milrinone.** (MILL-rih-nohn) *USP 28.*
Use: Cardiovascular agent; congestive heart failure.
See: Primacor.

milrinone lactate. (Bedford) Milrinone lactate (as base) 1 mg/mL, dextrose 47 mg/mL. Single-dose vials. 10 mL, 20 mL, 50 mL. *Rx.*
Use: Cardiovascular agent; congestive heart failure.

Milroy Artificial Tears. (Milton Roy) Bot. 22 mL.
Use: Artificial tears.

Miltown. (Wallace) Meprobamate 200 mg, 400 mg. Tab. Bot. 100s; 500s, 1000s (400 mg only). *c-iv.*
Use: Anxiolytic; antianxiety agent.

Miltown 600. (Wallace) Meprobamate 600 mg. Tab. Bot. 100s. *c-iv.*
Use: Anxiolytic.

• **mimbane hydrochloride.** (MIM-bane) USAN.
Use: Analgesic.

• **minalrestat.** (min-AL-reh-stat) USAN.
Use: Aldose reductase inhibitor.

• **minaprine.** (MIN-ah-preen) USAN.
Use: Psychotherapeutic agent.

• **minaprine hydrochloride.** (MIN-ah-preen) USAN.
Use: Antidepressant.

• **minaxolone.** (min-AX-oh-lone) USAN.
Use: Anesthetic.

mincard.
Use: Diuretic.

Mineral Ice, Therapeutic. (Bristol-Myers Squibb) Menthol 2%, ammonium hydroxide, carbomer 934, cupric sulfate, isopropyl alcohol, magnesium sulfate, thymol. Gel Tube 105 g, 240 g, 480 g. *OTC.*
Use: Liniment.

mineralocorticoids.
Use: Adrenalocortical steroids.
See: Fludrocortisone Acetate.

• **mineral oil.** *USP 28.*
Use: Laxative; pharmaceutic aid (solvent, oleaginous vehicle).
See: Kondremul Plain.
Petrolatum.

mineral oil. (Various Mfr.) Mineral oil. Liq. Bot. 180 mL, 473 mL. *OTC.*
Use: Laxative.

• **mineral oil, light.** *NF 23.*
Use: Pharmaceutic aid (tablet and cap-

sule lubricant, vehicle).

minerals.
See: Calcium Acetate.
  Calcium Carbonate.
  Calcium Citrate.
  Calcium Glubionate.
  Calcium Gluconate.
  Calcium Lactate.
  Magnesium.
  Magnesium Citrate.
  Magnesium Gluconate.
  Magnesium Oxide.
  Phosphorus Replacement Products.
  Tricalcium Phosphate.

Minibex. (Faraday) Vitamins B_1 6 mg, B_2 3 mg, B_6 0.5 mg, C 50 mg, niacinamide 10 mg, calcium pantothenate 3 mg, B_{12} 2 mcg, folic acid 0.1 mg. Cap. Bot. 100s, 250s, 1000s. *OTC.*
Use: Mineral; vitamin supplement.

Minidyne 10%. (Pedinol Pharmacal) Povidone-iodine 10%, citric acid, sodium phosphate dibasic. Soln. Bot. 15 mL. *OTC.*
Use: Antimicrobial; antiseptic.

Minipress. (Pfizer) Prazosin HCl 1 mg, 2 mg, 5 mg. Cap. Bot. 250s. *Rx.*
Use: Antihypertensive, antiadrenergic.

Minirin. (Ferring) Desmopressin acetate 0.1 mg, chlorobutanol 5 mg/mL. Nasal spray. 5 mL (50 doses of 10 mcg). *Rx.*
Use: Posterior pituitary hormones.

Minitec. (Bristol-Myers Squibb) Sodium pertechnetate Tc 99 m generator.
Use: Radiopaque agent.

Minitec Generator (Complete with Components). (Bristol-Myers Squibb) Medotopes Kit.
Use: Diagnostic aid.

Minitran. (3M) Nitroglycerin 9 mg, 18 mg, 36 mg, 54 mg. Transdermal Patch 33s. *Rx.*
Use: Antianginal.

Minit-Rub. (Bristol-Myers Squibb) Methyl salicylate 15%, menthol 3.5%, camphor 2.3% in anhydrous base. Tube 1.5 oz, 3 oz. *OTC.*
Use: Analgesic, topical.

Mini Two Way Action. (BDI Pharm) Ephedrine HCl 12.5 mg, guaifenesin 200 mg; ephedrine HCl 25 mg, guaifenesin 200 mg. Tab. Bot. 6s, 24s (12.5 mg only), 48s (25 mg only), 60s. *OTC.*
Use: Upper respiratory combination, decongestant, expectorant.

Minizide. (Pfizer) Prazosin HCl and polythiazide. **Minizide 1:** Prazosin 1 mg, polythiazide 0.5 mg. Cap. **Minizide 2:** Prazosin 2 mg, polythiazide 0.5 mg. Cap. **Minizide 5:** Prazosin 5 mg, poly-

thiazide 0.5 mg. Cap. Bot. 100s. *Rx.*
Use: Antihypertensive.

Minocin. (Lederle) **Cap., Pellet-filled:** Mincocyline HCl 50 mg, 100 mg. Bot. 50s (100 mg only), 100s (50 mg only). **Oral Susp.:** Minocycline HCl 50 mg/ 5 mL, alcohol 5%, parabens, EDTA, saccharin, custard flavor. Bot. 60 mL. **Pow. for Inj., cryodesiccated:** Minocycline 100 mg. Vials. *Rx.*
Use: Anti-infective, tetracycline.

• **minocromil.** (MIH-no-KROE-mill) USAN.
Use: Antiallergic (prophylactic).

• **minocycline.** (mihn-oh-SIGH-kleen) USAN.
Use: Anti-infective.
See: Dynacin.
  Minocin.
  Myrac.

• **minocycline hydrochloride.** (mihn-oh-SIGH-kleen) *USP 28.*
Use: Anti-infective, mouth and throat product.
See: Arestin.
  Vectrin.

minocycline hydrochloride. (Various Mfr.) Minocycline HCl 50 mg, 75 mg, 100 mg. Cap. Bot. 50s (100 mg only), 100s (except 100 mg). *Rx.*
Use: Anti-infective, tetracycline.

• **minoxidil.** (min-OX-ih-dill) *USP 28.*
Use: Antihypertensive; vasodilator; antialopecia agent.
See: Rogaine.
  Rogaine Extra Strength for Men.

minoxidil. (Schein) Minoxidil 2.5 mg. Tab. Bot. 100s, 500s, 1000s. *Rx.*
Use: Antihypertensive.

minoxidil. (Rugby) Minoxidil 10 mg. Tab. Bot. 500s. *Rx.*
Use: Antihypertensive.

Minoxidil Extra Strength for Men. (Apotex) Minoxidil 5%, alcohol 30%. Top. Soln. Bot. 60 mL (1s and 2s). *OTC.*
Use: Male pattern baldness.

Minoxidil for Men. (Lemmon) Minoxidil 2%, alcohol 60%. Soln (topical). Pouches. 60 mL single and twin. *OTC.*
Use: Male pattern baldness.

Mintezol. (Merck & Co.) Thiabendazole. **Susp.:** 500 mg/5 mL. Bot. 120 mL. **Chew. Tab.:** 500 mg. Pkg. 36s. *Rx.*
Use: Anthelmintic.

Minto-Chlor Syrup. (Pal-Pak, Inc.) Codeine sulfate 10 mg, potassium citrate 219 mg/5 mL, alcohol 2%. Gal. *c-v.*
Use: Antitussive, expectorant.

Mintox. (Major) Aluminum hydroxide 200 mg, magnesium hydroxide 200 mg. Tab. Bot. 100s. *OTC.*

Use: Antacid.

Mintox Plus Extra Strength Liquid.
(Major) Aluminum hydroxide 500 mg,
magnesium hydroxide 450 mg, simethicone 40 mg/5 mL. Bot. 355 mL. *OTC.*
Use: Antacid, antiflatulent.

Mintox Plus Tablets. (Major) Aluminum
hydroxide 200 mg, magnesium hydroxide 200 mg, simethicone 25 mg. Chew.
Tab. 100s. *OTC.*
Use: Antacid; antiflatulent.

Mintox Suspension. (Major) Aluminum
hydroxide 225 mg, magnesium hydroxide 200 mg, parabens, saccharin,
sorbitol/5 mL. Bot. 355 mL, 780 mL.
OTC.
Use: Antacid; antiflatulent.

Mint Sensodyne. (Block Drug) Potassium nitrate 5%, saccharin, sorbitol.
Toothpaste. Tube 28.3 g. *OTC.*
Use: Toothpaste for sensitive teeth.

Minute-Gel. (Oral-B) Acidulated phosphate fluoride 1.23% Gel. Bot. 16 oz.
Rx.
Use: Dental caries agent.

Miochol-E. (Novartis Ophthalmic) Acetylcholine Cl 1:100, mannitol 2.8% when
reconstituted. Soln. In 2 mL Univials.
Rx.
Use: Antiglaucoma agent.

• **mioflazine hydrochloride.** (MY-ah-
FLAY-zeen) USAN.
Use: Vasodilator (coronary).

Miostat Intraocular Solution. (Alcon)
Carbachol 0.01%. Vial 1.5 mL. Pkg.
12s.
Use: Antiglaucoma agent.

miotics, cholinesterase inhibitors.
Use: Glaucoma agents.
See: Echothiophate Iodide.
　Eserine Salicylate.
　Eserine Sulfate.
　Floropryl.
　Humorsol.
　Isopto Eserine.

• **mipafilcon a.** (mih-paff-ILL-kahn) USAN.
Use: Contact lens material (hydrophilic).

MiraFlow Extra Strength. (Ciba Vision)
Isopropyl alcohol 15.7%, poloxamer
407, amphoteric 10. Thimerosal free.
Soln. Bot. 12 mL. *OTC.*
Use: Contact lens care.

Miral. (Armenpharm Ltd.) Dexamethasone 0.75 mg. Tab. Bot. 100s, 1000s.
Use: Corticosteroid.

MiraLax. (Braintree) PEG 3350 255 g,
527 g. Pow. for Oral Soln. Bot. 14 oz
(255 g only), 26 oz (527 g only). *Rx.*
Use: Laxative; bowel evacuant.

Mirapex. (Boehringer Ingelheim) Pramipexole dihydrochloride 0.125 mg,

0.25 mg, 0.5 mg, 1 mg, 1.5 mg, mannitol. Tab. Bot. 63s (0.125 mg only), 90s,
UD 100s (0.5 mg only). *Rx.*
Use: Antiparkinson agent.

Miraphen PSE. (Major) Pseudoephedrine HCl 120 mg, guaifenesin 600 mg.
ER Tab. Bot. 500s. *Rx.*
Use: Upper respiratory combination, decongestant, expectorant.

MiraSept. (Alcon) **Disinfecting Solution:** Hydrogen peroxide 3%, sodium
stannate, sodium nitrate. Bot. 120 mL.
Rinse and neutralizer: Boric acid, sodium borate, sodium Cl, sodium pyruvate, EDTA. Bot. 120 mL (2s). *OTC.*
Use: Contact lens care.

MiraSept Step 2. (Alcon) Boric acid, sodium borate, sodium chloride, EDTA,
sodium pyruvate. Soln. Bot. 120 mL.
OTC.
Use: Contact lens product.

Mircette. (Organon) **Phase 1:** Desogestrel 0.15 mg, ethinyl estradiol
20 mcg. **Phase 2:** Ethinyl estradiol
10 mcg. Lactose. Tab. Blister Card 28s.
Rx.
Use: Sex hormone, contraceptive hormone.

Mirena. (Berlex) T-shaped unit containing a reservoir of levonorgestrel 52 mg
covered by a silicone membrane. Intrauterine system. Pkg. 1s w/inserter. *Rx.*
Use: Sex hormone; contraceptive.

• **mirfentanil hydrochloride.** (MIHR-FEN-
tan-ill) USAN.
Use: Analgesic.

• **mirincamycin hydrochloride.** (mihr-IN-
kah-MY-sin) USAN.
Use: Anti-infective; antimalarial.

• **mirisetron maleate.** (my-RIH-seh-trahn)
USAN.
Use: Antianxiety.

• **mirtazapine.** (mihr-TAZZ-ah-PEEN)
USAN.
Use: Antidepressant, tetracyclic compound.
See: Remeron.
　Remeron SolTab.

mirtazapine. (Various Mfr.) Mirtazapine
7.5 mg, 15 mg, 30 mg, 45 mg. Tab.
30s, 100s, 500s (7.5 mg only), 1000s.
Rx.
Use: Antidepressant, tetracyclic compound.

• **misonidazole.** (MY-so-NIH-dah-zole)
USAN.
Use: Antiprotozoal (trichomonas).

• **misoprostol.** (MY-so-PRAHST-ole)
USAN.
Use: Antiulcerative.

See: Cytotec.

misoprostol. (Various Mfr.) Misoprostol 100 mcg, 200 mcg. Tab. Unit-of-use 60s, 100s (200 mcg only), 120s (120 mcg only). *Rx.*
Use: Antiulcerative.

misoprostol and diclofenac sodium.
Use: Arthritis; antiulcerative.
See: Arthrotec.

Mission Prenatal. (Mission Pharmacal) Ferrous gluconate 260 mg (iron 30 mg), vitamins C 100 mg, B₁ 5 mg, B₆ 3 mg, B₂ 2 mg, B₃ 10 mg, B₅ 1 mg, B₁₂ 2 mcg, A 4000 units, D 400 units, Ca, zinc 15 mg. Tab. Bot. 100s. *OTC.*
Use: Mineral; vitamin supplement.

Mission Prenatal F.A. (Mission Pharmacal) Ferrous gluconate 260 mg (iron 30 mg), vitamins C 100 mg, B₁ 5 mg, B₆ 10 mg, B₂ 2 mg, B₃ 10 mg, B₁₂ 2 mcg, folic acid 0.8 mg, A acetate 4000 units, D 400 units, Ca, B₅ 1 mg. Tab. Bot. 100s. *OTC.*
Use: Mineral; vitamin supplement.

Mission Prenatal H.P. (Mission Pharmacal) Ferrous gluconate 260 mg (iron 30 mg), vitamins C 100 mg, B₁ 5 mg, B₆ 25 mg, B₂ 2 mg, B₃ 10 mg, D₅ 1 mg, B₁₂ 2 mcg, folic acid 0.8 mg, A 4000 units, D 400 units, Ca. Tab. Bot. 100s. *OTC.*
Use: Mineral; vitamin supplement.

Mission Prenatal Rx. (Mission Pharmacal) Vitamins A 8000 units, D 400 units, C 240 mg, B₁ 4 mg, B₂ 2 mg, B₃ 20 mg, B₅ 10 mg, B₆ 20 mg, B₁₂ 8 mcg, folic acid 1 mg, Fe 60 mg, Ca 175 mg, I, Zn 15 mg, Cu. Tab. Bot. 100s. *Rx.*
Use: Mineral; vitamin supplement.

Mission Surgical Supplement. (Mission Pharmacal) Vitamins C 500 mg, B₁ 2.5 mg, D₂ 2.0 mg, D₃ 30 mg, B₅ 16.3 mg, B₆ 3.6 mg, B₁₂ 9 mcg, A 5000 units, D 400 units, E 45 units, Fe 27 mg, Zn 22.5 mg. Tab. Bot. 100s. *OTC.*
Use: Mineral; vitamin supplement.

• **mitemcinal fumarate.** (mye-TEM-cin-al) USAN.
Use: GERD.

• **mitindomide.** (my-TIN-doe-MIDE) USAN.
Use: Antineoplastic.

• **mitocarcin.** (MY-toe-CAR-sin) USAN. Antibiotic derived from *Streptomyces* species.
Use: Antineoplastic.

• **mitocromin.** (MY-toe-KROE-min) USAN. Produced by *Streptomyces virdochromogenes.*

Use: Antineoplastic.

• **mitogillin.** (MY-toe-GIH-lin) USAN. An antibiotic obtained from a "unique strain" of *Aspergillus restrictus.*
Use: Antitumorigenic antibiotic; antineoplastic.

mitoguazone. (CTRC Research Foundation)
Use: Treatment of diffuse non-Hodgkin lymphoma. [Orphan Drug]

mitolactol.
Use: Adjuvant therapy in the treatment of primary brain tumors. [Orphan Drug]

• **mitomalcin.** (MY-toe-MAL-sin) USAN. Produced by *Streptomyces malayensis.* Under study.
Use: Antineoplastic.

• **mitomycin.** (MY-toe-MY-sin) *USP 28.* In literature as Mitomycin C. Antibiotic isolated from *Streptomyces caespitosis.*
Use: Anti-infective, antibiotic; antineoplastic.
See: Mutamycin.

mitomycin. (Various Mfr.) Mitomycin 5 mg (mannitol 10 mg), 20 mg (mannitol 40 mg), 40 mg (mannitol 80 mg). Pow. for Inj. Vials. *Rx.*
Use: Antibiotic.

• **mitosper.** (MY-toe-sper) USAN. Substance derived from *Aspergillus* of the glaucus group.
Use: Antineoplastic.

• **mitotane.** (MY-toe-TANE) *USP 28.* Formerly o,p'-DDD.
Use: Antineoplastic.
See: Lysodren.

• **mitoxantrone hydrochloride.** (MY-toe-ZAN-trone) *USP 28.*
Use: Antineoplastic; immunologic agent; anthracenedione.
See: Novantrone.

• **mitumomab.** (mih-TOO-moe-mab) USAN.
Use: Antitumor monoclonal antibody.

Mivacron. (Abbott Hospital Products) Mivacurium chloride 0.5 mg/mL, 2 mg/mL. Inj. **0.5 mg:** Premixed infusion in 5% Dextrose Injection, USP in flexible plastic container 50 mL (100 mL unit). **2 mg:** Single-use vial 5 mL, 10 mL in Water for Injection. *Rx.*
Use: Muscle relaxant, adjunct to anesthesia.

• **mivacurium chloride.** (mih-vah-CURE-ee-uhm) USAN.
Use: Neuromuscular blocker.
See: Mivacron.

• **mivobulin isethionate.** (mih-VOE-byoo-lin eye-seh-THIGH-oh-nate) USAN.
Use: Antineoplastic (microtubule inhibitor).

Mixed E 400 Softgels. (Naturally Vitamins) Vitamin E 400 units. Cap. Bot. 60s, 90s, 180s. *OTC.*
Use: Vitamin supplement.

Mixed E 1000 Softgels. (Naturally Vitamins) Vitamin E 1000 units. Cap. Bot. 30s, 60s *OTC.*
Use: Vitamin supplement.

Mixed Respiratory Vaccine. Each mL contains *Staphylococcus aureus* 1,200 million organisms, *Streptococcus* (both *viridans* and nonhemolytic) 200 million organisms, *Streptococcus (Diplococcus) pneumoniae* 150 million organisms, *Moraxella (Branhamella, Neisseria) catarrhalis* 150 million organisms, *Klebsiella pneumoniae* 150 million organisms, and *Haemophilus influenzae* types a and b 150 million organisms. Vial. 20 mL.
Use: Bacterial vaccine.
See: MRV.

mixed vespid Hymenoptera venom. *Rx.*
Use: Agent for immunization.
See: Albay.
  Pharmalgen.
  Venomil.

• **mixidine.** (MIX-ih-deen) USAN.
Use: Vasodilator (coronary).

mixture 612. Dimethyl Phthalate Solution, Compound.

M-M-R II. (Merck & Co.) Lyophilized preparation of live attenuated measles virus vaccine (*Attenuvax*), live attenuated mumps virus vaccine (*Mumpsvax*), live attenuated rubella virus vaccine (*Meruvax II*). See details under *Attenuvax, Mumpsvax* and *Meruvax II.* Single dose vial w/diluent. Pkg. 1s, 10s. *Rx.*
Use: Agent for immunization.

Moban. (Endo) Molindone HCl 5 mg, 10 mg, 25 mg, 50 mg, lactose. Tab. Bot. 100s. *Rx.*
Use: Antipsychotic.

Mobic. (Boehringer Ingelheim) Meloxicam. **Oral Susp.:** 7.5 mg/5 mL. Saccharin, sorbitol. Raspberry flavor. 100 mL. **Tab.:** 7.5 mg, 15 mg, lactose. Bot. 30s, UD 100s (7.5 mg only); 100s. *Rx.*
Use: Anti-inflammatory, NSAID.

Mobidin. (B.F. Ascher) Magnesium salicylate, anhydrous 600 mg. Tab. Bot. 100s, 500s. *Rx.*
Use: Antiarthritic.

Mobigesic. (B.F. Ascher) Magnesium salicylate anhydrous 325 mg, phenyltolox-

amine citrate 30 mg. Tab. Bot. 50s, 100s, Pkg. 18s. *OTC.*
Use: Analgesic combination.

Mobisyl Creme. (B.F. Ascher) Trolamine salicylate in vanishing creme base. Tube 100 g. *OTC.*
Use: Analgesic, topical.

moccasin bite.
See: Antivenin.

• **moclobemide.** (moe-KLOE-beh-mide) USAN.
Use: Antidepressant.

• **modafinil.** (moe-DAFF-ih-nill) USAN.
Use: CNS stimulant, analeptic.
See: Provigil.

• **modaline sulfate.** (MODE-al-een) USAN.
Use: Antidepressant.

Modane. (Savage) Bisacodyl 5 mg, lactose. EC Tab. Bot. 10s, 30s, 100s. *OTC.*
Use: Laxative.

Modane Mild. (Pharmacia) Phenolphthalein 60 mg. Tab. Bot. 10s, 30s, 100s. *OTC.*
Use: Laxative.

Modane Versabran. (Pharmacia) Psyllium hydrophilic mucilloid in wheat bran base. Dose 3.4 g, Bot. 10 oz. *OTC.*
Use: Laxative.

• **modecainide.** (moe-deh-CANE-ide) USAN.
Use: Cardiovascular (antiarrhythmic).

Modicon. (Ortho-McNeil) Norethindrone 0.5 mg, ethinyl estradiol 35 mcg, lactose. Tab. *Dialpak* and *Veridate* 28s. *Rx.*
Use: Sex hormone, contraceptive hormone.

modinal.
See: Gardinol Type Detergents.

Moducal. (Bristol-Myers Squibb) Maltodextrin. Pow. Can 13 oz. *OTC.*
Use: Nutritional supplement.

Moduretic. (Merck & Co.) Hydrochlorothiazide 50 mg, amiloride 5 mg. Tab. Bot. 100s, UD 100s. *Rx.*
Use: Antihypertensive; diuretic.

moenomycin. Phosphorus-containing glycolipide antibiotic. Active against gram-positive organisms. Under study.

• **moexipril hydrochloride.** (moe-EX-ah-prill) USAN.
Use: Antihypertensive; ACE inhibitor.
See: Univasc.

moexipril hydrochloride and hydrochlorothiazide.
Use: Antihypertensive.
See: Uniretic.

• **mofegiline hydrochloride.** (moe-FEH-jih-leen) USAN.
Use: Antiparkinsonian.

Moist Again. (Lake Consumer) Aloe vera, EDTA, methylparaben, glycerin. Gel. Tube 70.8 g. *OTC.*
Use: Vaginal agent.

Moi-Stir. (Kingswood) Dibasic sodium phosphate; Mg, Ca, Na, K chlorides; sorbitol; sodium carboxymethyl-cellulose; parabens. Soln. Bot. 120 mL spray. *OTC.*
Use: Saliva substitute.

Moi-Stir Swabsticks. (Kingswood) Dibasic sodium phosphate; Mg, Ca, Na, K chlorides; sorbitol; sodium carboxymethylcellulose; parabens. Swabsticks. Pkt. 3s. *OTC.*
Use: Saliva substitute.

Moisture Drops. (Bausch & Lomb) Hydroxypropyl methylcellulose 0.5%, povidone 0.1%, glycerin 0.2%, benzalkonium Cl 0.01%, EDTA, NaCl, boric acid, KCl, sodium borate. Soln. Bot. 0.5 oz, 1 oz. *OTC.*
Use: Artificial tears.

molar phosphate.
W/Fluoride ion.
See: Coral.
   Karigel.

molecusol-carbamazepine.
See: PR-320.

•**molgramostim.** (mahl-GRAH-moe-STIM) USAN.
Use: Hematopoietic stimulant; antineu-tropenic.

•**molinazone.** (moe-LEEN-ah-zone) USAN.
Use: Analgesic.

•**molindone hydrochloride.** (moe-LIN-dohn) *USP 28.*
Use: Antipsychotic.
See: Moban.

Mollifene Ear Drops. (Pfeiffer) Glycerin, camphor, cajaput oil, eucalyptus oil, thyme oil. Soln. Bot. 24 mL. *OTC.*
Use: Otic.

•**molsidomine.** (mole-SIH-doe-meen) USAN.
Use: Antianginal; vasodilator (coronary).

molybdenum solution. (American Quinine) Molybdenum 25 mcg/mL (as 46 mcg/mL ammonium molybdate tetrahydrate). Inj. Vial 10 mL. *Rx.*
Use: Nutritional supplement; parenteral.

Molycu. (Burns) Meprobamate 400 mg, copper 60 mg/mL. *Rx.*
Use: Antidote.

Moly-Pak. (SoloPak Pharmaceuticals, Inc.) Molybdenum 25 mcg. Inj. Vial 10 mL. *Rx.*
Use: Nutritional supplement; parenteral.

Molypen. (American Pharmaceutical Partners) Ammonium molybdate tetra-hydrate 46 mcg/mL. Vial 10 mL. *Rx.*
Use: Nutritional supplement; parenteral.

Momentum. (Whitehall-Robins) Aspirin 500 mg, phenyltoloxamine citrate 15 mg. Capl. Bot. 24s, 48s. *OTC.*
Use: Analgesic.

Momentum Muscular Backache Formula. (Whitehall-Robins) Magnesium salicylate tetrahydrate 580 mg (equivalent to 467 mg magnesium salicylate anhydrous). Capl. Box. 48s. *OTC.*
Use: Analgesic compound.

•**mometasone furoate.** (moe-MET-uh-SONE FEW-roh-ate) *USP 28.*
Use: Corticosteroid, topical; intranasal steroid.
See: Elocon.
   Nasonex.

mometasone furoate. (Clay Park) Mometasone furoate. **Cream:** 0.1%. White petrolatum, stearyl alcohol. 15 g, 45 g. **Top. Soln.:** 0.1%. Isopropyl alcohol 40%, glycerin. 30 mL, 60 mL. *Rx.*
Use: Topical corticosteroid.

mometasone furoate. (Various Mfr.) Mometasone furoate 0.1%. Oint. 15 g, 45 g. *Rx.*
Use: Topical corticosteroid.

mometasone furoate inhalation.
Use: Corticosteroid.
See: Asmanex Twisthaler.

monoöctyl pyrogallol. Eugallol Pyrogal-lol Monoacetate.
Use: Keratolytic.

Monafed. (Monarch) Guaifenesin 600 mg, lactose. SR Tab. Bot. 100s. *Rx.*
Use: Expectorant.

monalium hydrate. Hydrated magnesium aluminate. Magaldrate.
See: Riopan.

Monarc-M. (American Red Cross) A concentrated preparation of antihemophilic factor (AHF). AHF 2 to 15 units/mg total protein and a maximum of albumin (human) 12.5 mg/mL and PEG 3350 0.07 mg, histidine 0.39 mg, glycine 0.1 mg/AHF IU, mouse protein ≤ 0.1 ng/AHF IU, organic solvent (tri-n-butyl-phosphate) 18 ng, detergent (octoxynol 9) 50 ng, monoclonal purified. Pow. for Inj. Single-dose bot. w/10 mL Sterile Water for Injection, double-ended needle, filter needle. *Rx.*
Use: Antihemophilic agent.

•**monatepil maleate.** (moe-NAT-eh-pill) USAN.
Use: Antianginal; antihypertensive.

monensin. (mah-NEN-sin) *USP 28.*
Use: Antifungal; anti-infective; antiproto-zoal.

monensin sodium. (mah-NEN-sin) *USP 28.*
Use: Antifungal; anti-infective; antiproto-zoal.

Monistat. (Personal Products) Micona-zole nitrate 2%. Top. Cream. Tube 9 g. *OTC.*
Use: Antifungal, vaginal.

Monistat-Derm Cream. (Personal Prod-ucts) Miconazole nitrate 2%, pegoxol 7 stearate, peglicol 5 oleate, mineral oil, benzoic acid, butylated hydroxyanis-ole. Tube 15 g, 30 g, 90 g. *OTC.*
Use: Antifungal, topical.

Monistat-Derm Lotion. (Personal Prod-ucts) Miconazole nitrate 2%, pegoxol 7 stearate, peglicol 5 oleate, mineral oil, benzoic acid, butylated hydroxyanis-ole. Squeeze bot. 30 mL, 60 mL. *Rx.*
Use: Antifungal, topical.

Monistat 1. (Personal Products) Tiocona-zole 6.5%. Vag. Oint. Prefilled single-dose applicator 4.6 g. *OTC.*
Use: Antifungal, vaginal.

Monistat 1 Combination Pack. (Per-sonal Products) Miconazole nitrate.
Supp.: 1200 mg, petrolatum w/parafin. Pkg. 1s w/applicator. **Cream:** 2%, steryl and cetyl alcohol. Tube 9 g. *Rx.*
Use: Antifungal, vaginal.

Monistat 7. (Personal Products) Micona-zole nitrate. **Vag. Supp.:** 100 mg. Box 7s w/applicator. **Vag. Cream:** 2%. Tube 35 g, 45 g w/1 applicator or 7 *Ultraslim* disp. applicators, or 7 pre-filled applicators w/5 g cream. *OTC.*
Use: Antifungal, vaginal.

Monistat 7 Combination Pack. (Per-sonal Products) **Vaginal Supp.:** Miconazole nitrate 100 mg. In 7s with applicator. **Topical Cream:** Miconazole nitrate 2%. Tube. *OTC.*
Use: Antifungal, vaginal.

Monistat 3. (Personal Products) Micona-zole nitrate 2%. Vag. Cream. Pkg. Pre-filled applicator (3). *OTC.*
Use: Antifungal, vaginal.

Monistat 3 Combination Pack. (Per-sonal Products) Miconazole nitrate.
Vag. Supp.: 200 mg. 3s w/1 reusable applicator or 3 disp. applicators. **Top. Cream:** 2%. Tube. *OTC.*
Use: Antifungal, vaginal.

monoamine oxidase inhibitors.
Use: Antidepressant.
See: Isocarboxazid.
 Phenelzine Sulfate.
 Tranylcypromine Sulfate.

mono- and di-acetylated monoglycer-ides. (mahn-OH and di-ah-SEE-till-ated mahn-OH-GLIH-sir-ides) *NF 23.* A mix-ture of glycerin esterfied mono- and diesters of edible fatty acids followed by direct acetylation.
Use: Pharmaceutic aid (plasticizer).

mono- and di-glycerides. (mahn-OH and di-GLIH-sir-ides) *NF 23.* A mixture of mono- and diesters of fatty acids from edible oils.
Use: Fatty acids; pharmaceutic aid (emulsifying agent).

monobenzone.
Use: Pigment agent.
See: Benoquin.

monobenzyl ether of hydroquinone.
See: Benoquin.

Monocal. (Mericon) Fluoride 3 mg, Ca 250 mg. Tab. Bot. 100s. *OTC.*
Use: Mineral supplement.

Monocaps Tablets. (Freeda) Iron 14 mg, vitamins A 10,000 units, D 400 units, E 15 units, B_1 15 mg, B_2 15 mg, B_3 41 mg, B_5 15 mg, B_6 15 mcg, B_{12} 15 mcg, C 125 mg, folic acid 0.1 mg, biotin 15 mg, PABA, L-lysine, Ca, Cu, I, K, Mg, Mn, Se, Zn 12 mg, lecithin. Tab. Bot. 100s, 250s, 500s. *OTC.*
Use: Mineral; vitamin supplement.

Mono-Chlor. (Gordon Laboratories) Monochloroacetic acid 80%. Bot. 15 mL.
Use: Cauterizing agent.

monochloroacetic acid.
Use: Cauterizing agent.
See: Mono-Chlor.

monochlorophenol-para.
See: Camphorated para-chlorophenol.

Monoclate. (Centeon) Monoclonal anti-body derived stable lyophilized con-centrate of Factor VIII: R heat-treated. With albumin (human) 1% to 2%, man-nitol 0.8%, histidine 1.2 mM. Inj. Vial 1 mL single dose with diluent. *Rx.*
Use: Antihemophilic.

Monoclate-P. (Aventis) Concentrate of human factor VIII: C. When reconsti-tuted, contains calcium chloride ≈ 2 to 5 mM/L, human albumin ≈ 1% to 2%, mannitol 0.8%, histidine 1.2 mM, trace murine monoclonal antibody < 50 ng/ 100 IU, sodium ions ≈ 300 to 450 mM/ L, heat-treated, monoclonal purified. Pow. for Inj., lyophilized. Vial with dilu-ent, double-ended needle, vented fil-ter spike, winged infusion set, alcohol swabs. Actual number of AHF units indicated on vial. *Rx.*
Use: Antihemophilic agent.

monoclonal antibodies.
See: Alemtuzumab.
Bevacizumab.
Cetuximab.
Gemtuzumab Ozogamicin.
Ibritumomab Tiuxetan.
Omalizumab.
Palivizumab.
Rituximab.
Tositumomab and Iodine ^{131}I-Tositumomab.
Trastuzumab.
monoclonal antibodies (murine) anti-idiotype melanoma associated antigen.
Use: Invasive cutaneous melanoma. [Orphan Drug]
monoclonal antibodies PM-81.
Use: Adjunctive treatment for leukemia. [Orphan Drug]
monoclonal antibodies PM-81 and AmL-2-23.
Use: Leukemic bone marrow transplantation. [Orphan Drug]
monoclonal antibody (human) against hepatitis B virus.
Use: Prophylaxis in hepatitis B reinfection in liver transplants. [Orphan Drug]
monoclonal antibody to CD4, 5a8.
(Biogen)
Use: Postexposure prophylaxis for HIV. [Orphan Drug]
monoclonal antibody to lupus nephritis. (Medclone, Inc.)
Use: Immunization. [Orphan Drug]
•**monoctanoin.** (MAHN-ahk-tuh-NO-in) USAN.
monocycline hydrochloride.
See: Minocin IV.
Mono-Diff Test. (Wampole)
Use: Diagnostic aid; mononucleosis.
Monodox. (Oclassen) Doxycycline monohydrate 50 mg, 100 mg. Cap. Bot. 50s (100 mg only), 100s (50 mg only), 250s, (100 mg only) *Rx.*
Use: Anti-infective; tetracycline.
•**monoethanolamine.** (mahn-oh-eth-an-OLE-ah-meen) *NF 23.*
Use: Pharmaceutic aid (surfactant).
Monojel. (Sherwood Davis & Geck) Glucose 40%. UD 25 g. *OTC.*
Use: Hyperglycemic.
Monoket. (Schwarz Pharma) Isosorbide mononitrate 10 mg, 20 mg. Tab. Bot. 60s, 100s, 180s, UD 100s. *Rx.*
Use: Antianginal.
Mono-Latex. (Wampole) Two-minute latex agglutination slide test for the qualitative or semiquantitative detection of infectious mononucleosis heterophile

antibodies in serum or plasma. Test kit 20s, 50s, 1000s.
Use: Diagnostic aid.
monolaurin.
Use: Treatment of congenital primary ichthyosis. [Orphan Drug]
See: Glylorin.
monomercaptoundecahydrocloso-do-decaborate sodium.
Use: Treatment of glioblastoma multiforme. [Orphan Drug]
MonoNessa. (Watson) Norgestimate 0.25 mg, ethinyl estradiol 35 mcg. Tab. Pkg. 28s. *Rx.*
Use: Sex hormone, contraceptive hormone.
Mononine. (Aventis) Sterile, lyophilized concentrate of Factor IX, plasma derived; heparin. Pow. for Inj. Single-dose vial 250 units, 500 units, 1000 units with diluent, double-ended needle, vented filter spike, winged infusion set, alcohol swabs. *Rx.*
Use: Antihemophilic.
mononucleosis tests.
Use: Diagnostic aid.
See: Mono-Diff Test.
Mono-Latex.
Mono-Plus.
Monospot.
Monosticon.
Monosticon Dri-Dot.
Mono-Sure Test.
Monopar. Stilbazium Iodide.
Use: Anthelmintic.
monophen.
Use: Orally; cholecystography.
Mono-Plus. (Wampole) To diagnose infectious mononucleosis from serum, plasma, or fingertip blood. Test kits 24s.
Use: Diagnostic aid.
Monopril. (Bristol-Myers Squibb) Fosinopril sodium 10 mg, 20 mg, 40 mg, lactose. Tab. Bot. 90s, 1000s (except 40 mg), UD 100s (20 mg only). *Rx.*
Use: Antihypertensive; congestive heart failure.
Monopril-HCT. (Bristol-Myers Squibb) Fosinopril sodium 10 mg, 20 mg, hydrochlorothiazide 12.5 mg, lactose. Tab. Bot. 100s. *Rx.*
Use: Antihypertensive.
•**monosodium glutamate.** (mahn-oh-SO-dee-uhm GLUE-tah-mate) *NF 23.*
Use: Pharmaceutic aid (flavor, perfume).
monosodium phosphate.
See: Sodium Biphosphate.
Monospot. (Ortho-Clinical Diagnostics) Diagnosis of infectious mononucleosis. Test kit 20s.

Use: Diagnostic aid.

monostearin. (Various Mfr.) Glyceryl monostearate.

Monosticon Dri-Dot. (Organon Teknika) Diagnosis of infectious mononucleosis. Test kit 40s, 100s.
Use: Diagnostic aid.

Mono-Sure Test. (Wampole) One-minute hemagglutination slide test for the differential qualitative detection and quantitative determination of infectious mononucleosis heterophile antibodies in serum or plasma. Kit 20s.
Use: Diagnostic aid.

Monosyl. (Arcum) Secobarbital sodium 1 gr, butabarbital 0.5 gr. Tab. Bot. 100s, 1000s. *c-II.*
Use: Hypnotic; sedative.

Monotard Human Insulin. (Bristol-Myers Squibb; Novo/Nordisk) Human insulin zinc 100 units/mL. Susp. Vial 10 mL. *OTC.*
Use: Antidiabetic.

•**monothioglycerol.** (mahn-oh-thigh-oh-GLIS-er-ole) *NF 23.*
Use: Pharmaceutic aid (preservative).

Mono-Vacc Test O.T. (Aventis Pasteur) 5 tuberculin units by the mantoux method. Multiple puncture disposable device. Box 25s (tamper-proof). *Rx.*
Use: Diagnostic aid; tuberculosis.

monoxychlorosene. A stabilized, buffered, organichypochlorous acid derivative.
See: Oxychlorosene.

Monsel Solution. (Wade) Bot. 2 oz, 4 oz.
Use: Styptic solution.

•**montelukast sodium.** (mahn-teh-LOO-kast) USAN.
Use: Antiasthmatic (leukotriene receptor antagonist).
See: Singulair.

Monurol. (Forest) Fosfomycin tromethamine 3 g/Gran. Single-dose packet. *Rx.*
Use: Anti-infective; urinary.

•**morantel tartrate.** (moe-RAN-tell) USAN.
Use: Anthelmintic.

moranyl.
See: Suramin Sodium.

Morco. (Archer-Taylor) Cod liver oil ointment, zinc oxide, benzethonium Cl, benzocaine 1%. 1.5 oz, lb. *OTC.*
Use: Antiseptic; antipruritic, topical.

More Dophilus. (Freeda) Acidophilus-carrot derivative 4 billion units/g. Pow. Bot. 120 g. *OTC.*
Use: Antidiarrheal; nutritional supplement.

•**moricizine.** (MAHR-IH-sizz-een) USAN.
Use: Cardiovascular agent (antiarrhythmic).
See: Ethmozine.

•**morniflumate.** (MAR-nih-FLEW-mate) USAN.
Use: Anti-inflammatory.

Moroline. (Schering-Plough) Petrolatum. Jar 1.75 oz, 3.75 oz, 15 oz. *OTC.*
Use: Dermatologic; lubricant; protectant.

Morpen. (Major) Ibuprofen 400 mg, 600 mg. Tab. Bot. 500s. *Rx.*
Use: Analgesic; NSAID.

morphine hydrochloride. (Various Mfr.) Pow. Bot. 1 oz, 5 oz. *c-II.*
Use: Analgesic.

•**morphine sulfate.** (MORE-feen) *USP 28.*
Use: Opioid analgesic; sedative.
See: Astramorph PF.
Avinza.
DepoDur.
Duramorph.
Infumorph 500.
Infumorph 200.
Kadian.
MS Contin.
MSIR.
Oramorph SR.
RMS.
Roxanol.
Roxanol 100.
Roxanol T.
W/Tartar emetic, bloodroot, ipecac, squill, wild cherry.
See: Roxanol T.

morphine sulfate. (Abbott) Morphine sulfate 0.5 mg/mL. Inj. Amps and vials 10 mL. *c-II.*
Use: Analgesic, narcotic agonist.

morphine sulfate. (Eli Lilly) Morphine sulfate 10 mg, 15 mg, 30 mg, Soln. Tab. Bot. 100s. *c-II.*
Use: Analgesic, narcotic.

morphine sulfate. (Endo) Morphine sulfate 15 mg, 30 mg, 60 mg, 100 mg, lactose. ER Tab. Bot. 100s, 500s. *c-II.*
Use: Analgesic, narcotic agonist.

morphine sulfate. (Ethex) Morphine sulfate 20 mg/mL, alcohol free. Soln. Bot. 30 mL, 120 mL, 240 mL. *c-II.*
Use: Analgesic, narcotic agonist.

morphine sulfate. (Paddock) Morphine sulfate. Compounding Pow. Bot. 25 g. *c-II.*
Use: Analgesic, narcotic agonist.

morphine sulfate. (Ranbaxy) Morphine sulfate 10 mg, 15 mg, 30 mg, lactose, sucrose. Soluble Tab. for Inj. Bot. 100s. *c-II.*
Use: Opioid analgesic.

morphine sulfate. (Roxane) Morphine sulfate 10 mg/5 mL, 20 mg/5 mL. Oral Soln. Bot. 100 mL, 500 mL. UD 5 mL (10 mg only), 10 mL (10 mg only). *c-II.*
Use: Opioid analgesic.

morphine sulfate. (Various Mfr.) Morphine sulfate. **ER Tab.:** 15 mg, 30 mg, 60 mg, 100 mg, 200 mg (for use only in opioid-tolerant patients). 50s (30 mg only), 100s, 500s (except 200 mg), UD 100s (except 200 mg). 150 punch cards (15 mg, 30 mg, 60 mg only). **Inj.:** 0.5 mg/mL (Amps. and vials, 10 mL), 1 mg/mL (Vial 10 mL, 30 mL. Amp. 10 mL), 2 mg/mL (Vial 30 mL, syringe, *Carpujet, Tubex* 1 mL); 4 mg/mL (Disp. Syr. 1 mL, 2 mL. *Tubex* and *Carpuject* 1 mL), 5 mg/mL (Vial 1 mL), 8 mg/mL (Vial, Amp., *Carpuject*, 1 mL), 10 mg/mL (1 mL *Carpuject*, Vial, Amp. Multidose vial 10 mL), 15 mg/mL (Amp., *Carpuject*, Vial 1 mL, Multidose vial 20 mL). **Oral Soln. (concentrate):** 20 mg/mL. Alcohol free. 15 mL, 30 mL, 120 mL, 240 mL with calibrated dropper or spoon. **Rec. Supp.:** 5 mg, 10 mg, 20 mg, 30 mg. Box 12s. **Soln. for Inj.:** 25 mg/mL (Syr. 4 mL, 10 mL, 20 mL, 40 mL); 50 mg/mL (Syr. 10 mL, 20 mL, 40 mL, 50 mL; Single-use vials). **Tab.:** 15 mg, 30 mg. Bot. 100s, UD 100s. *c-II.*
Use: Opioid analgesic.

● **morrhuate sodium.** (MORE-you-ate) *USP 28.*
Use: Sclerosing agent.
See: Scleromate.

morrhuate sodium. (Pasadena Research Labs) Morrhuate sodium 50 mg/mL. Inj. Multiple use vials. 30 mL. *Rx.*
Use: Sclerosing agent.

Morton Salt Substitute. (Morton Grove) Potassium Cl, fumaric acid, tricalcium phosphate, monocalcium phosphate. Na < 0.5 mg/5 g (0.02 mEq/5 g), K 2800 mg/5 g (72 mEq/5 g) 88.6 g. *OTC.*
Use: Salt substitute.

Morton Seasoned Salt Substitute. (Morton Grove) Potassium chloride, spices, sugar, fumaric acid, tricalcium phosphate, monocalcium phosphate. Na < 1 mg/5 g (< 0.04 mEq/5 g), K 2165 mg/5 g (56 mEq/5 g). Bot. 85.1 g. *OTC.*
Use: Salt substitute.

Mosco. (Medtech) 17.6% Salicylic acid. Jar 10 mL. *OTC.*
Use: Keratolytic.

● **motexafin gadolinium.** (moe-TEX-a-fin gad-OH-lihn-ee-uhm) USAN.
Use: Antineoplastic.

● **motexafin lutetium.** USAN.
Use: Photoantineoplastic.

Motilium. (Janssen) Domperidone maleate. *Rx.*
Use: Antiemetic.

Motion Aid. (Vangard Labs, Inc.) Dimenhydrinate 50 mg. Tab. Bot. 100s, 1000s, UD 10 × 10s.
Use: Antiemetic; antivertigo.

Motion Cure. (Wisconsin Pharmacal Co.) Meclizine 25 mg. Chew. Tab. 12s.
Use: Antiemetic; antivertigo.

motion sickness agents.
See: Antinauseants.
Bucladin.
Dramamine.
Emetrol.
Marezine.
Scopolamine HBr.

Mototen. (Garnrick) Difunoxin HCl 1 mg, atropine sulfate 0.025 mg. Tab. Bot. 50s, 100s. *c-IV.*
Use: Antidiarrheal.

● **motretinide.** (MOE-TREH-tih-nide) USAN.
Use: Keratolytic.

Motrin, Children's. (McNeil Consumer) Ibuprofen 100 mg/5 mL, sucrose. Susp. Bot. 120 mL, 480 mL. *Rx-OTC.*
Use: Analgesic, NSAID.

Motrin Children's Cold. (McNeil Consumer) Pseudoephedrine HCl 15 mg, ibuprofen 100 mg/5 mL, acesulfame K, sucrose, berry or grape flavors, dye free. Susp. Bot. 118 mL. *OTC.*
Use: Upper respiratory combination, decongestant, analgesic.

Motrin, Junior Strength. (McNeil Consumer) Ibuprofen 100 mg, aspartame, phenylalanine 6 mg, orange flavor. Chew. Tab. Pkg. 24s *OTC.*
Use: Analgesic, NSAID.

Motrin IB. (McNeil Consumer) Ibuprofen 200 mg. Tab. Bot. 100s. Gelcap Pkg. 8s. *OTC.*
Use: Analgesic; NSAID.

Motrin Migraine Pain. (McNeil Consumer) Ibuprofen 200 mg. Capl. Bot. 24s, 50s, 100s. *OTC.*
Use: Analgesic, NSAID.

mouth and throat products.
See: Amlexanox.
Carbamide Peroxide.
Doxycycline.
Minocycline HCl.
Pilocarpine HCl.
Saliva Substitutes.
Sulfuric Acid/Sulfonated Phenolics.
Tetracycline HCl.

MouthKote. (Parnell) Xylitol, sorbitol, yerba santa, citric acid, ascorbic acid,

sodium benzoate, saccharin, lemon-lime flavor. Soln. Spray Bot. 60 mL, 240 mL. *OTC.*
Use: Saliva substitute.

MouthKote O/R Rinse. (Unimed) Benzyl alcohol, menthol, sorbitol. Rinse. Sugar free. Bot. 240 mL. *OTC.*
Use: Antiseptic.

MouthKote O/R Solution. (Unimed) Diphenhydramine HCl 1.25%, cetylpyridinium Cl, EDTA, saccharin. Soln. Bot. 40 mL. *OTC.*
Use: Antiseptic.

●**moxalactam disodium for injection.** (MOX-ah-LACK-tam) *USP 28.*
Use: Anti-infective.
See: Moxam.

Moxam. (Eli Lilly) Moxalactam disodium. Vial 1 g/10 mL Traypak 10s; Vial 2 g/20 mL Traypak 10s; Vial 10 g/100 mL Traypak 6s. *Rx.*
Use: Anti-infective; cephalosporin.

●**moxazocine.** (MOX-AZE-oh-seen) USAN.
Use: Analgesic; antitussive.

●**moxifloxacin hydrochloride.** (mox-ih-FLOX-ah-sin) USAN.
Use: Anti-infective; fluoroquinolone; antibiotic, ophthalmic.
See: Avelox.
    Avelox IV.
    Vigamox.

●**moxilubant maleate.** (MOX-ill-yoo-bahnt) USAN.
Use: Treatment of rheumatoid arthritis and psoriasis (leukotriene B_4 receptor antagonist).

●**moxnidazole.** (MOX-NIH-dazz-ole) USAN.
Use: Antiprotozoal (trichomonas).

M-Oxy. (Mallinckrodt) Oxycodone hydrochloride 5 mg. Tab. Bot. 100s. *c-II.*
Use: Opioid analgesic.

Moxy Compound. (Major) Theophylline 130 mg, ephedrine 25 mg, hydroxyzine HCl 10 mg. Tab. Bot. 100s. *Rx.*
Use: Antiasthmatic compound.

Moyco Fluoride Rinse. (Moyco Union Broach Division) Fluoride 2%. Flavor. Bot. 128 oz. with pump. *Rx-OTC.*
Use: Dental caries agent.

6-MP.
Use: Antimetabolite.
See: Purinethol.

MRV. (Bayer Corp. (Consumer Div.)) 2000 million organisms/mL from *Staphylococcus aureus* (1200 million), *Streptococcus,* viridans and nonhemolytic (200 million), *Streptococcus pneumoniae* (150 million), *Branhamella ca-*

tarrhalis (150 million), *Klebsiella pneumoniae* (150 million), *Haemophilus influenzae* (150 million). Inj. Vial 20 mL. *Rx.*
Use: Immunization.

MS Contin. (Purdue Frederick) Morphine sulfate 15 mg, 30 mg, 60 mg, 100 mg, 200 mg. Lactose (except 100 mg, 200 mg). CR Tab. Bot. 100s, 500s (except 200 mg), UD 25s (except 200 mg). *c-II.*
Use: Opioid analgesic.

MSIR. (Purdue Frederick) Morphine sulfate. **Oral Soln.:** 10 mg/5 mL, 20 mg/5 mL. EDTA. Bot. 120 mL. **Oral Soln. (concentrate):** 20 mg/mL. EDTA. 30 mL with calibrated dropper. *c-II.*
Use: Opioid analgesic.

MS/L-Concentrate. (Richwood Pharmaceuticals) Morphine sulfate 100 mg/5 mL. Oral Soln. Bot. 120 mL w/calibrated dropper. *c-II.*
Use: Analgesic; narcotic.

MSL-109. (Novartis) Monoclonal antibody.
Use: Antiviral. [Orphan Drug]

MS/S. (Richwood Pharmaceuticals) Morphine sulfate 5 mg, 10 mg, 20 mg, 30 mg. Supp. 12s. *c-II.*
Use: Analgesic; narcotic.

MSTA. (Aventis Pasteur) Mumps skin test antigen 40 complement-fixing units/mL, Inj. Vial 1 mL. *Rx.*
Use: Diagnostic aid.

MTC. Mitomycin. *Rx.*
Use: Anti-infective.
See: Mutamycin.

M.T.E.-5. (Fujisawa Healthcare) Zn 1 mg, Cu 0.4 mg, Cr 4 mcg, Mn 0.1 mg, Se 20 mcg/mL. Inj. Vial 10 mL. *Rx.*
Use: Mineral supplement.

M.T.E.-5 Concentrated. (Fujisawa Healthcare) Zn 5 mg, Cu 1 mg, Cr 10 mcg, Mn 0.5 mg, Se 60 mcg/mL. Inj. Vial 1 mL, MD vial 10 mL.
Use: Mineral supplement.

M.T.E.-4. (Fujisawa Healthcare) Zn 1 mg, Cu 0.4 mg, Cr 4 mcg, Mn 0.1 mg/mL. Inj. Vial 3 mL, 10 mL, MD Vial 30 mL. *Rx.*
Use: Mineral supplement.

M.T.E.-4 Concentrated. (Fujisawa Healthcare) Zn 5 mg, Cu 1 mg, Cr 10 mcg, Mn 0.5 mg/mL. Inj. Vial 1 mL, MD Vial 10 mL. *Rx.*
Use: Mineral supplement.

M.T.E.-7. (Fujisawa Healthcare) Zn 1 mg, Cu 0.4 mg, Mn 0.1 mg, Cr 4 mcg, Se 20 mcg, I 25 mcg, Mo 25 mcg/mL. Vial 10 mL. *Rx.*
Use: Mineral supplement.

M.T.E.-6. (Fujisawa Healthcare) Zn 1 mg, Cu 0.4 mg, Cr 4 mcg, Mn 0.1 mg, Se 20 mcg, I 25 mcg/mL. Inj. Vial 10 mL. *Rx.*
Use: Mineral supplement.

M.T.E.-6 Concentrate. (Fujisawa Healthcare) Zn 5 mg, Cu 1 mg, Cr 10 mcg, Mn 0.5 mg, Se 60 mcg, I 75 mcg/mL. Inj. Vial 1 mL. MD vial 10 mL. *Rx.*
Use: Mineral supplement.

MTP-PE. (Novartis) Muramyl-tripeptide.
Use: Immunomodulator.

MTX. *Rx.*
Use: Antineoplastic; antipsoriatic.
See: Methotrexate.

• **mubritinib.** (mue-bri-TYE-nib) USAN.
Use: Antineoplastic agent.

mucilloid of psyllium seed.
W/Dextrose.
See: Metamucil

mucin.
See: Gastric Mucin.

Mucinex. (Adams) Guaifenesin 600 mg (100 mg immediate-release, 500 mg extended-release). ER Tab. Bot. 20s, 40s, 500s. *OTC.*
Use: Expectorant.

Mucinex DM. (Adams) Dextromethorphan hydrobromide 30 mg, guaifenesin 600 mg. ER Tab. 20s, 40s. *OTC.*
Use: Antitussive with expectorant.

MUC 9 + 4 Pediatric. (Fujisawa Healthcare) Vitamin A 2300 units, D 400 units, E 7 mg, B_1 1.2 mg, B_2 1.4 mg, B_3 17 mg, B_5 5 mg, B_6 1 mg, B_{12} 1 mcg, C 80 mg, biotin 20 mcg, folic acid 0.14 mg, K 200 mcg/5 mL, mannitol 375 mg. Pow. Vial. 10 mL. *Rx.*
Use: Nutritional supplement; parenteral.

Muco-Fen DM. (IVAX) Guaifenesin 1000 mg, dextromethorphan HBr 30 mg, dye free. Long-acting Tab. Bot. 100s. *Rx.*
Use: Upper respiratory combination, antitussive, expectorant.

Muco-Fen-LA. (Ivax) Guaifenesin 600 mg, dye free. TR Tab. Bot. 100s. *Rx.*
Use: Expectorant.

mucolytics.
Use: Respiratory.
See: Mucomyst.

Mucomyst. (Sandoz) Acetylcysteine 10%, 20%. EDTA. Oral Soln. Vials. 4 mL, 10 mL, 30 mL. *Rx.*
Use: Respiratory agent; antidote.

Mucomyst 10. (Bristol-Myers Squibb) A sterile 10% solution of acetylcysteine for nebulization or direct instillation into the lung as a mucolytic agent. Approved as antidote for acetaminophen overdose. Vial. **4 mL:** Ctn. 12s; **10 mL:** Ctn. 3s with dropper; **30 mL:** Ctn. 3s. *Rx.*
Use: Respiratory.

Mudd. (Chattem) Natural hydrated magnesium aluminum silicate. Topical preparation. *OTC.*
Use: Cleanser.

Mudrane. (ECR) Aminophylline (anhydrous) 130 mg, phenobarbital 8 mg, ephedrine HCl 16 mg, potassium iodide 195 mg. Tab. Bot. 100s. *Rx.*
Use: Antiasthmatic combination.

Mudrane GG. (ECR) Aminophylline (anhydrous) 130 mg, ephedrine HCl 16 mg, guaifenesin 100 mg, phenobarbital 8 mg. Tab. Bot. 100s. *Rx.*
Use: Antiasthmatic combination.

Mudrane GG Liixir. (ECR) Theophylline 20 mg, ephedrine HCl 4 mg, guaifenesin 26 mg, phenobarbital 2.5 mg/5 mL, alcohol 20%. Bot. pt, 0.5 gal. *Rx.*
Use: Antiasthmatic combination.

Mudrane GG-2. (ECR) Guaifenesin 100 mg, theophylline 111 mg. Tab. Bot. 100s. *Rx.*
Use: Antiasthmatic combination.

Mudrane-2. (ECR) Potassium iodide 195 mg, aminophylline (anhydrous) 130 mg. Tab. Bot. 100s. *Rx.*
Use: Antiasthmatic combination.

Multa-Gen 12 + E. (Jones Pharma) Vitamin A 5000 units, D 400 units, B_1 2 mg, B_2 2 mg, B_6 0.5 mg, B_{12} 3 mcg, C 37.5 mg, E 15 units, folic acid 0.2 mg, nicotinamide 20 mg. Cap. Bot. 60s, 500s, 1000s. *OTC.*
Use: Vitamin supplement.

MulTE-PAK-5. (SoloPak Pharmaceuticals, Inc.) Zn 1 mg, Cu 0.4 mg, Mn 0.1 mg, Cr 4 mg, Se 20 mcg/mL. Inj. Vial 3 mL, 10 mL. *Rx.*
Use: Mineral supplement.

MulTE-PAK-4. (SoloPak Pharmaceuticals, Inc.) Zn 1 mg, Cu 0.4 mg, Mn 0.1 mg, Cr 4 mg/mL. Inj. Vial 3 mL, 10 mL, 30 mL. *Rx.*
Use: Mineral supplement.

Multi-B-Plex. (Forest) Vitamins B_1 100 mg, B_2 1 mg, nicotinamide 100 mg, pantothenic acid 10 mg, B_6 10 mg/mL. Inj. Vial 10 mL, 30 mL. *Rx.*
Use: Mineral; vitamin supplement.

Multi-B-Plex Capsules. (Forest) Vitamins B_1 50 mg, B_2 5 mg, niacinamide 50 mg, calcium pantothenate 5.4 mg, B_6 0.2 mg, C 150 mg, B_{12} 1 mcg. Cap. Bot. 100s, 1000s. *OTC.*
Use: Mineral; vitamin supplement.

Multi-Day. (NBTY) Vitamins A 5000 units, D 400 units, E 30 mg, B_1 1.5 mg, B_2 1.7 mg, B_3 20 mg, B_5 10 mg, B_6 2 mg, B_{12} 6 mcg, C 60 mg, FA 0.4 mL. Tab. Bot. 100s. *OTC.*
Use: Vitamin supplement.

Multi-Day Plus Iron. (NBTY) Fe 18 mg, A 5000 units, D 400 units, E 15 mg, B_1 1.5 mg, B_2 1.7 mg, B_3 20 mg, B_6 2 mg, B_{12} 6 mcg, C 60 mg, FA 0.4 mg. Tab. Bot. 100s. *OTC.*
Use: Vitamin supplement.

Multi-Day Plus Minerals. (NBTY) Fe 18 mg, A 6500 units, D 400 units, E 30 mg, B_1 1.5 mg, B_2 1.7 mg, B_3 20 mg, B_5 10 mg, B_6 2 mg, B_{12} 6 mcg, C 60 mg, FA 0.4 mg, Ca, Cl, Cr, Cu, I, K, Mg, Mn, Mo, P, Se, Zn 15 mg, biotin 30 mcg. Tab. Bot. 100s. *OTC.*
Use: Vitamin supplement.

Multi-Day with Calcium and Extra Iron Tablets. (NBTY) Fe 27 mg, A 5000 units, D 400 units, E 30 mg, B_1 1.5 mg, B_2 1.7 mg, B_3 20 mg, B_5 10 mg, B_6 2 mg, B_{12} 6 mcg, C 60 mg, FA 0.4 mg, Ca, Zn 15 mg, tartrazine. Tab. Bot. 100s. *OTC.*
Use: Mineral; vitamin supplement.

Multifol. (Breckenridge) Ca 125 mg, iron (as ferrous fumarate) 65 mg, vitamin A 6000 units, D 400 units, E 30 units, B_1 1.1 mg, $B_2$1.8 mg, B_3 15 mg, B_6 2.5 mg, B_{12} 5 mcg, C 60 mg, FA 1 mg. Tab. UD 100s. *Rx.*
Use: Multivitamin.

Multi-Germ Oil. (Viobin) Corn, sunflower and wheat germ oils. Bot. 4 oz, 8 oz, pt, qt. *OTC.*
Use: Nutritional supplement.

Multi-Jets. (Kirkman) Vitamins A 10,000 units, D_2 400 units, B_1 20 mg, B_2 8 mg, C 120 mg, niacinamide 10 mg, calcium pantothenate 5 mg, B_6 0.5 mg, E 50 units, desiccated liver 100 mg, dried debittered yeast 100 mg, choline bitartrate 62 mg, inositol 30 mg, dl-methionine 30 mg, B_{12} 7 mcg, Fe 2.6 mg, Ca (dical phosphate) 58 mg, P (dical phosphate) 45 mg, I (potassium iodide) 0.114 mg, Mg sulfate 1 mg, Cu sulfate 1.99 mg, Mn sulfate 1.11 mg, KCl iodide 79 mg. Tab. Bot. 100s. *OTC.*
Use: Mineral; vitamin supplement.

Multilex Tablets. (Rugby) Fe 15 mg, vitamins A 10,000 units, D 400 units, E 5.5 mg, B_1 10 mg, B_2 5 mg, B_3 30 mg, B_5 10 mg, B_6 1.7 mg, B_{12} 3 mcg, C 100 mg, Zn 1.5 mg, Cu, I, Mg, Mn. Tab. Bot. 100s. *OTC.*
Use: Mineral; vitamin supplement.

Multilex T & M Tablets. (Rugby) Fe 15 mg, vitamins A 10,000 units, D 400 units, E 5.5 mg, B_1 15 mg, B_2 10 mg, B_3 100 mg, B_5 10 mg, B_6 2 mg, B_{12} 7.5 mcg, C 150 mg, Cu, I, Mg, Mn, Zn 1.5 mg, sugar. Tab. Bot. 100s. *OTC.*
Use: Mineral; vitamin supplement.

Multilyte. (Fujisawa Healthcare) Vitamins A 5000 units, D 400 units, E 15 mg, B_1 3 mg, B_2 3.4 mg, B_3 36 mg, B_5 14 mg, B_6 4.4 mg, B_{12} 6 mcg, C 120 mg, FA 0.4 mg, Zn 10.5 mg, biotin 100 mcg, Ca, K, Mg, Mn, phenylalanine. Tab. Pkg. 12s. *OTC.*
Use: Mineral; vitamin supplement.

Multilyte-40. (American Pharmaceutical Partners) Na 25 mEq, K $\approx$ 40 mEq, Ca 5 mEq, Mg 8 mEq, Cl $\approx$ 33 mEq, acetate $\approx$ 40 mEq, gluconate 5 mEq/ 25 mL, osmolarity $\approx$ 6015 mOsm/L. Single-dose vial 25 mL. *Rx.*
Use: Intravenous nutritional therapy, intravenous replenishment solution.

Multilyte-20. (American Pharmaceutical Partners) Na 25 mEq, K 20 mEq, Ca 5 mEq, Mg 5 mEq, Cl 30 mEq, acetate 25 mEq/25 mL, osmolarity $\approx$ 4205 mOsm/L. Single-dose vial 25 mL. *Rx.*
Use: Intravenous nutritional therapy, intravenous replenishment solution.

Multi-Mineral Tablets. (NBTY) Ca 166.7 mg, P 75.7 mg, I 25 mcg, Fe 3 mg, Mg 66.7 mg, Cu 0.33 mg, Zn 2.5 mg, K 12.5 mg, Mn 8.3 mg. Tab. Bot. 100s. *OTC.*
Use: Mineral; vitamin supplement.

Multipals. (Faraday) Vitamins A 5000 units, D 400 units, C 50 mg, B_1 3 mg, B_6 0.5 mg, B_2 3 mg, calcium pantothenate 5 mg, niacinamide 20 mg, B_{12} 2 mcg. Tab. Bot. 100s, 250s, 1000s. *OTC.*
Use: Mineral; vitamin supplement.

Multipals-M. (Faraday) Vitamins A 6000 units, D 400 units, B_1 3 mg, B_2 3 mg, B_6 0.5 mg, B_{12} 5 mcg, C 60 mg, E 2 units, niacinamide 20 mg, calcium pantothenate 5 mg, Fe 10 mg, I 0.15 mg, Cu 1 mg, Mg 6 mg, Mn 1 mg, K 5 mg. Tab. Bot. 100s, 250s, 1000s. *OTC.*
Use: Mineral; vitamin supplement.

Multiple Electrolytes and 5% Travert. (Baxter Healthcare) Invert sugar 50 g/ L, calories 196 cal/L, Na^+ 56 mEq, K^+ 25 mEq, Mg^{++} 6 mEq, Cl^- 56 mEq, phosphate 12.5 mEq, lactate 25 mEq/ L, osmolarity 449 mOsm/L, sodium 5 mEq/L sodium bisulfite. Soln. Bot. 1000 mL. *Rx.*
Use: Intravenous nutritional therapy, intravenous replenishment solution.

Multiple Electrolytes and 10% Travert. (Baxter Healthcare) Invert sugar 100 g/L, calories 384 cal/L, Na$^+$ 56 mEq, K$^+$ 25 mEq, Mg^{++} 6 mEq, Cl$^-$ 56 mEq, phosphate 12.5 mEq, lactate 25 mEq/L, osmolarity 726 mOsm/L, sodium 5 mEq/L, sodium bisulfite. Soln. Bot. 1000 mL. *Rx.*
Use: Intravenous nutritional therapy, intravenous replenishment solution.

Multiple Trace Element Neonatal. (American Regent) Zn 1.5 mg, Cu 0.1 mg, Mn 25 mcg, Cr 0.85 mcg/mL. Inj. Vial 2 mL single dose. *Rx.*
Use: Mineral supplement.

Multiple Vitamin Mineral Formula. (Kirkman) Vitamins A 5000 units, D$_2$ 400 units, C 50 mg, B$_1$ 2.5 mg, B$_2$ 2.6 mg, B$_6$ 0.6 mg, B$_{12}$ 1 mcg, niacinamide 15 mg, calcium pantothenate 5 mg, E 0.1 units, Ca 100 mg, Fe 7.5 mg, Mg 2.5 mg, K 2.5 mg, Zn 0.15 mg, Mn 0.5 mg, I 0.07 mg. Tab. Bot. 100s. *OTC.*
Use: Mineral; vitamin supplement.

Multiple Vitamins Chewable. (Kirkman) Vitamins A 5000 units, D 400 units, C 50 mg, B$_1$ 3 mg, B$_2$ 2.5 mg, B$_6$ 1 mg, B$_{12}$ 1 mcg, niacinamide 20 mg. Tab. Bot. 100s. *OTC.*
Use: Vitamin supplement.

Multiple Vitamins w/Iron. (Kirkman) Vitamins A 5000 units, D 400 units, C 50 mg, B$_1$ 3 mg, B$_2$ 2.5 mg, B$_6$ 1 mg, B$_{12}$ 1 mcg, niacinamide 20 mg, Fe 10 mg. Tab. Bot. 100s. *OTC.*
Use: Mineral; vitamin supplement.

Multi 75. (Fibertone) Vitamins A 25,000 units, D 500 units, E 150 units, B$_1$ 75 mg, B$_2$ 75 mg, B$_3$ 75 mg, B$_5$ 75 mg, B$_6$ 75 mg, B$_{12}$ 75 mcg, C 250 mg, FA 0.4 mg, Ca 50 mg, Fe 10 mg, biotin, I, Mg, Zn 15 mg, Cu, PABA, K, Mn, Cr, Se, Mo, B, Si, choline bitartrate, inositol, rutin, lemon bioflavonoid complex, hesperidin, betaine, HCl. TR Tab. Bot. 60s, 90s. *OTC.*
Use: Mineral; vitamin supplement.

Multistix 8. (Bayer Corp. (Consumer Div.)) Urinalysis reagent strip test for detecting glucose, ketone, blood, pH, protein, nitrite, bilirubin, leukocytes. Strip Box. 100s.
Use: Diagnostic aid.

Multistix 8 SG Reagent Strips. (Bayer Corp. (Consumer Div.)) Urinalysis reagent strip test for glucose, ketone, specific gravity, blood, pH, protein nitrite, leukocytes. Strip Box 100s.
Use: Diagnostic aid.

Multistix-N. (Bayer Corp. (Consumer Div.)) Glucose, protein, pH, blood, ketones, bilirubin, urobilinogen, nitrate, leukocytes. Kit. 100s.
Use: Diagnostic aid.

Multistix 9 Reagent Strips. (Bayer Corp. (Consumer Div.)) Urinalysis reagent strip test for glucose, bilirubin, ketone, blood, pH, protein, urobilinogen, nitrite, leukocytes. Strip Box 100s.
Use: Diagnostic aid.

Multistix 9 SG Reagent Strips. (Bayer Corp. (Consumer Div.)) Urinalysis reagent strip test for glucose, bilirubin, ketone, specific gravity, blood, pH, protein, nitrite, leukocytes. Strip Box 100s.
Use: Diagnostic aid.

Multistix-N S.G. Reagent Strips. (Bayer Corp. (Consumer Div.)) Urinalysis reagent strip test for pH, protein, glucose, ketones, bilirubin, blood nitrite, urobilinogen, specific gravity. Strip Bot. 100s.
Use: Diagnostic aid.

Multistix Reagent Strips. (Bayer Corp. (Consumer Div.)) Urinalysis reagent strip test for pH, protein, glucose, ketone, bilirubin, blood. Strip Box 100s.
Use: Diagnostic aid.

Multistix 7. (Bayer Corp. (Consumer Div.)) Urinalysis reagent strip test for glucose ketone, blood, pH, protein, nitrite, leukocytes. Strip Box 100s.
Use: Diagnostic aid.

Multistix SG Reagent Strips. (Bayer Corp. (Consumer Div.)) Urinalysis reagent strip test for pH, glucose, protein, ketones, bilirubin, blood, urobilinogen. Strip Box. 100s.
Use: Diagnostic aid.

Multistix 10 SG Reagent Strips. (Bayer Corp. (Consumer Div.)) Reagent strip test for glucose, bilirubin, ketone, specific gravity, blood, pH, protein, urobilinogen, nitrite, leukocytes in urine. Strip Box 100s.
Use: Diagnostic aid.

Multistix 2 Reagent Strips. (Bayer Corp. (Consumer Div.)) Urinalysis reagent strip test for nitrite and leukocytes. Strip Bot. 100s.
Use: Diagnostic aid.

Multi-Symptom Tylenol Cold. (McNeil Consumer) Pseudoephedrine HCl 30 mg, chlorpheniramine maleate 2 mg, dextromethorphan HBr 15 mg, acetaminophen 325 mg. Capl. or Tab. Bot. 24s, 50s. *OTC.*
Use: Analgesic, antihistamine, antitussive, decongestant.

Multi-Thera-M. (NBTY) Iron 27 mg, vitamins A 5500 units, D 400 units, E 30 mg, B$_1$ 3 mg, B$_2$ 3.4 mg, B$_3$ 30 mg,

B_5 10 mg, B_6 3 mg, B_{12} 9 mcg, C 120 mg, folic acid 0.4 mg, biotin 15 mcg, Zn 15 mg, Ca, Cl, Cr, Cu, I, K, Mg, Mn, Mo, Se. Tab. Bot. 130s. *OTC.*
Use: Mineral; vitamin supplement.

Multi-Thera Tablets. (NBTY) Vitamins A 5500 units, D 400 units, E 30 mg, B_1 3 mg, B_2 3.4 mg, B_3 30 mg, B_5 10 mg, B_6 3 mg, B_{12} 9 mcg, C 120 mg, folic acid 0.4 mg, biotin 15 mcg. Tab. Bot. 100s. *OTC.*
Use: Vitamin supplement.

Multitrace-5 Concentrate. (American Regent) Zinc sulfate 5 mg, copper sulfate 1 mg, manganese sulfate 0.5 mg, chromium Cl 10 mcg, selenium 60 mcg, benzyl alcohol 0.9%. Inj. Soln. Vial 1 mL, 10 mL. *Rx.*
Use: Mineral supplement.

Multi-Vita. (Rosemont) Vitamins A 1500 units, D 400 units, E 5 mg, B_1 0.5 mg, B_2 0.6 mg, B_3 8 mg, B_6 0.4 mg, B_{12} 2 mcg, C 35 mg/mL. Alcohol free. Drop. Bot. 50 mL. *OTC.*
Use: Vitamin supplement.

Multi-Vita Drops. (Rosemont) Vitamins A 1500 units, D 400 units, E 5 mg, B_1 0.5 mg, B_2 0.6 mg, B_3 8 mg, B_6 0.4 mg, B_{12} 2 mcg, C 35 mg/mL. Alcohol free. Drop. Bot. 50 mL. *OTC.*
Use: Mineral; vitamin supplement.

Multi-Vita Drops w/Fluoride. (Rosemont) Fluoride 0.5 mg, vitamins A 1500 units, D 400 units, E 5 mg, B_1 0.5 mg, B_2 0.6 mg, B_3 8 mg, B_6 0.4 mg, B_{12} 2 mcg, C 35 mg/mL. Alcohol free. Drop. Bot. 50 mL. *Rx.*
Use: Vitamin supplement; dental caries agent.

Multi-Vita Drops w/Iron. (Rosemont) Iron 10 mg, vitamins A 1500 units, D 400 units, E 5 mg, B_1 0.5 mg, B_2 0.6 mg, B_3 8 mg, B_6 0.4 mg, C 35 mg/mL. Alcohol free. Drop. Bot. 50 mL. *OTC.*
Use: Mineral; vitamin supplement.

multivitamin concentrate injection. (Fujisawa Healthcare) Vitamins A 10,000 units, D 1000 units, E 5 units, B_1 50 mg, B_2 10 mg, B_3 100 mg, B_5 25 mg, B_6 15 mg, C 500 mg/Inj. Vial 5 mL. *Rx.*
Use: Vitamin supplement.

multivitamin infusion (neonatal formula).
Use: Nutritional supplement for low birth weight infants. [Orphan Drug]

Multi-Vitamin Mineral w/Beta Carotene. (Mission Pharmacal) Iron 27 mg, A 5000 units, D 400 units, E 30 units, B_1 2.25 mg, B_2 2.6 mg, B_3 20 mg, B_5

10 mg, B_6 3 mg, B_{12} 9 mcg, C 90 mg, folic acid 0.4 mg, biotin 0.45 mg, Ca, Cl, Cr, Cu, I, K, Mg, Mn, Mo, P, Se, Zn 15 mg, Vitamin K. Tab. Bot. 130s. *OTC.*
Use: Mineral; vitamin supplement.

Multi-Vitamins Capsules. (Forest) Vitamins A 5000 units, D 400 units, B_1 1.5 mg, B_2 2 mg, B_6 0.1 mg, C 37.5 mg, calcium pantothenate 1 mg, niacinamide 20 mg. Cap. Bot. 100s, 1000s, 5000s. *OTC.*
Use: Mineral; vitamin supplement.

Multivitamins Capsules. (Solvay) Vitamins A 5000 units, D 400 units, B_1 2.5 mg, B_2 2.5 mg, C 50 mg, B_3 20 mg, B_5 5 mg, B_6 0.5 mg, B_{12} 2 mcg, E 10 units. Cap. Bot. 100s, UD 100s. *OTC.*
Use: Mineral; vitamin supplement.

Multivitamin with Fluoride Drops. (Major) Fluoride 0.5 mg, vitamins A 1500 units, D 400 units, E 4.1 units, B_1 0.5 mg, B_2 0.6 mg, B_3 8 mg, B_6 0.4 mg, B_{12} 2 mg, C 35 mg. Drop. Bot. 50 mL.
Use: Vitamin supplement; dental caries agent.

Multivitamin with Fluoride Drops. (Major) Fluoride 0.5 mg, vitamins A 1500 units, D 400 units, E 5 units, B_1 0.5 mg, B_2 0.6 mg, B_3 8 mg, B_6 0.4 mg, B_{12} 2 mcg, C 35 mg, F 0.25 mg. Drop. Bot. 50 mL. *Rx.*
Use: Vitamin supplement; dental caries agent.

Multi-Vit Drops. (Alra) Vitamins A 500 units, D 400 units, E 5 mg, B_1 0.5 mg, B_2 0.6 mg, B_3 8 mg, B_6 0.4 mg, B_{12} 2 mcg, C 35 mg/mL. Bot. 50 mL. *OTC.*
Use: Vitamin supplement.

Multi-Vit Drops w/Iron. (Alra) Iron 10 mg, vitamins A 1500 units, D 400 units, E 5 units, B_1 0.5 mg, B_2 0.6 mg, B_3 8 mg, B_6 0.4 mg, C 35 mg/mL. Methylparaben. Drop. Bot. 50 mL. *OTC.*
Use: Mineral; vitamin supplement.

multizine.
See: Trisulfapyrimidines.

Multorex. (Health for Life Brands) Vitamins A 6000 units, D 1250 units, C 50 mg, E 5 units, B_1 3 mg, B_2 3 mg, B_6 0.5 mg, niacinamide 20 mg, calcium pantothenate 5 mg, B_{12} 5 mcg, Ca 59 mg, P 45 mg. Cap. Bot. 100s, 250s, 1000s.
Use: Mineral; vitamin supplement.

Mulvidren-F Softabs. (Wyeth) Fluoride 1 mg, vitamins A 4000 units, D 400 units, B_1 1.6 mg, B_2 2 mg, B_3

10 mg, B_5 2.8 mg, B_6 1 mg, B_{12} 3 mcg, C 75 mg, saccharin. Tab. Bot. 100s. *Rx.*
Use: Mineral; vitamin supplement; dental caries agent.

•**mumps skin test antigen.** *USP 28.*
Use: Diagnostic aid (dermal reactivity indicator).
See: MSTA.

Mumpsvax. (Merck & Co.) Live mumps virus vaccine, Jeryl Lynn strain. Single-dose vial w/diluent Pkg. 1s, 10s. *Rx.*
Use: Agent for immunization.
W/Meruvax II.
See: Biavax II.

•**mumps virus vaccine live.** *USP 28.*
Use: Immunization.
See: Mumpsvax.

mumps virus vaccine, live attenuated. Jeryl Lynn (B level) strain.
See: Mumpsvax.
W/Measles virus vaccine, rubella virus vaccine.
See: M-M-R.

•**mupirocin.** (myoo-PIHR-oh-sin) *USP 28.*
Use: Anti-infective (topical and nasal).
See: Bactroban.

•**mupirocin calcium.** (myoo-PIHR-oh-sin) USAN.
Use: Anti-infective, topical.
See: Bactroban.

mupirocin 2%. (Various Mfr.) Mupirocin 2% in a polyethylene glycol base. Oint. 15 g, 22 g, 30 g. *Rx.*
Use: Anti-infective.

•**muplestim.** (myoo-PLEH-stim) USAN.
Use: Hematopoietic stimulant; antineutropenic.

•**muraglitazar.** (myoo-ra-GLI-ta-zar) USAN.
Use: Antidiabetic.

muriatic acid.
See: Hydrochloric Acid.

Muri-Lube. (Fujisawa Healthcare) Mineral Oil "Light." Vial 2 mL, 10 mL. *Rx.*
Use: Lubricant.

Murine Ear Drops. (Ross) Carbamide peroxide 6.5% in anhydrous glycerin. Bot. 0.5 oz. *OTC.*
Use: Otic.

Murine Ear Wax Removal System. (Ross) Carbamide peroxide 6.5% in anhydrous glycerin w/ear washing syringe. Bot. 0.5 oz. and ear washer 1 oz. *OTC.*
Use: Otic.

Murine Eye Drops. (Ross) Polyvinyl alcohol 0.5%, povidone 0.6%, benzalkonium chloride, dextrose, EDTA, NaCl, sodium bicarbonate, sodium phos-

phate. Soln. Bot. 15 mL, 30 mL. *OTC.*
Use: Artificial tears.

Murine Plus Eye Drops. (Ross) Tetrahydrozoline HCl 0.05%. Drop. Bot. 15 mL, 30 mL. *OTC.*
Use: Vasoconstrictor; ophthalmic.

Murine Regular Formula. (Ross) Sodium chloride, potassium chloride, sodium phosphate, glycerin, benzalkonium chloride 0.01%, EDTA 0.05%. Drop. Bot. 15, 30 mL. *OTC.*
Use: Artificial tears.

Murocel Solution. (Bausch & Lomb) Methylcellulose 1%, propylene glycol, sodium Cl, methylparaben 0.046%, propylparaben 0.02%, boric acid, sodium borate. Soln. Bot. 15 mL. *OTC.*
Use: Artificial tears.

Murocoll-2. (Bausch & Lomb) Phenylephrine HCl 10%, scopolamine HBr 0.3%. Bot. 5 mL. *Rx.*
Use: Cycloplegic; mydriatic.

•**muromonab-CD3.** (MYOO-row-MOE-nab) USAN.
Use: Monoclonal antibody (immunosuppressant).
See: Orthoclone OKT3.

Muro 128 Ointment. (Bausch & Lomb) Sodium Cl 5% in sterile ointment base. Tube 3.5 g. *OTC.*
Use: Hyperosmolar.

Muro 128 Solution. (Bausch & Lomb) Sodium Cl 2%, 5%. Soln. Bot. 15 mL, 30 mL (5% only). *OTC.*
Use: Hyperosmolar.

Muroptic-5. (Optopics) Sodium Cl, hypertonic 5%. Soln. Bot. 15 mL. *OTC.*
Use: Hyperosmolar.

Muro's Opcon A Solution. (Bausch & Lomb) Naphazoline HCl 0.025%, pheniramine maleate 0.3%. Bot. 15 mL. *OTC.*
Use: Antihistamine (ophthalmic), decongestant.

Muro's Opcon Solution. (Bausch & Lomb) Naphazoline HCl 0.1%. Bot. 15 mL. *OTC.*
Use: Decongestant; ophthalmic.

Muro Tears Solution. (Bausch & Lomb) Hydroxypropyl methylcellulose, dextran 40. Soln. Bot. 15 mL. *OTC.*
Use: Artificial tears.

muscle adenylic acid. (Various Mfr.) Active form of adenosine 5-monophosphate.
See: Adenosine 5-monophosphate.

muscle relaxants.
See: Arduan.
Curare.
Flexeril.
Lioresal.

Mephenesin.
Meprobamate.
Metubine Iodine.
Neostig.
Neuromuscular Blockers, Nondepolarizing.
Norflex.
Nuromax.
Pancuronium Bromide.
Parafon Forte.
Rapacuronium Bromide.
Raplon.
Rela.
Robaxin.
Rocuronium Bromide.
Soma.
Succinylcholine Cl.
Muse. (Vivus) Alprostadil 125 mcg, 250 mcg, 500 mcg, 1000 mcg. Pellet. Individual foil pouches. *Rx.*
Use: Anti-impotence agent.
mustaral oil.
See: Allyl Isothiocyanate.
Mustargen. (Merck) Mechlorethamine HCl 10 mg. Pow. for Inj. Vial. Set of 4s. *Rx.*
Use: Antineoplastic, alkylating agent.
Musterole. (Schering-Plough) **Regular:** Camphor 4%, menthol 2%. Jar 0.9 oz. **Extra Strength:** Camphor 5%, menthol 3%. Jar 0.9 oz., Tube 1 oz, 2.25 oz. *OTC.*
Use: Analgesic, topical.
Musterole Deep Strength. (Schering-Plough) Methyl salicylate 30%, menthol 3%, methyl nicotinate 0.5%. Jar 1.25 oz, Tube 3 oz. *OTC.*
Use: Analgesic, topical.
Musterole Extra Strength. (Schering-Plough) Camphor 5%, menthol 3%, methyl salicylate, lanolin, oil of mustard, petrolatum. 27, 30, 67.5 g. *OTC.*
Use: Liniment.
mustin.
See: Mechlorethamine HCl, Sterile.
mutalin. (Spanner) Protein and iodine. Vial 30 mL.
Mutamycin. (Bristol-Myers Oncology) Mitomycin 5 mg (mannitol 10 mg), 20 mg (mannitol 40 mg), 40 mg (mannitol 80 mg). Vials. *Rx.*
Use: Antineoplastic; antibiotic.
●**muzolimine.** (MYOO-ZOLE-ih-meen) USAN.
Use: Antihypertensive; diuretic.
M.V.I. Pediatric. (AstraZeneca) Vitamin A 2300 units, D 400 units, E 7 units, B_1 1.2 mg, B_2 1.4 mg, B_3 17 mg, B_5 5 mg, B_6 1 mg, B_{12} 1 mcg, C 80 mg, biotin 20 mcg, FA 0.14 mg, vitamin K 200 mcg, mannitol 375 mg. Inj. Vial. *Rx.*

Use: Nutritional supplement; parenteral.
M.V.I.-12. (AstraZeneca) Vitamins A 3300 units, D 200 units, E 10 units, B_1 3 mg, B_2 3.6 mg, B_3 40 mg, B_5 15 mg, B_6 4 mg, B_{12} 5 mcg, C 100 mg, biotin 60 mcg, FA 0.4 mg. Inj. Vials. 5 mL single-dose, 50 mL multiple-dose; Unit vial: 10 mL two-chambered vials. *Rx.*
Use: Nutritional supplement; parenteral.
M.V.M. (Tyson) Iron 3.6 mg, vitamins A 400 units, E 60 units, B_1 20 mg, B_2 10 mg, B_3 10 mg, B_5 100 mg, B_6 31 mg, B_{12} 160 mcg, C 50 mg, folic acid 0.08 mg, Ca, Cr, Cu, I, K, Mg, Mo, Zn 6 mg, biotin 160 mcg, PABA, Mn, Se, tryptophan. Cap. Bot 150s. *OTC.*
Use: Mineral; vitamin supplement.
Myadec. (Parke-Davis) Iron 18 mg, A 5000 units, D 400 units, E 30 units, B_1 1.7 mg, B_2 2 mg, B_3 20 mg, B_5 10 mg, B_6 3 mg, B_{12} 6 mcg, C 60 mg, folic acid 0.4 mg, biotin 30 mcg, vitamin K, Ca, P, I, Mg, Cu, Zn 15 mg, Mn, K, Cl, Cr, Mo, Se, Ni, Si, V, B, Sn. Tab. Bot. 130s. *OTC.*
Use: Mineral; vitamin supplement.
myagen. Bolasterone.
Use: Anabolic agent.
Myambutol. (X-Gen) Ethambutol HCl. Tab. **100 mg:** Bot. 100s. **400 mg:** Bot. 100s, 1000s, UD 10s. *Rx.*
Use: Antituberculous.
myanesin.
See: Mephenesin.
Myapap Drops. (Rosemont) Acetaminophen 80 mg/0.8 mL. Bot. 15 mL w/dropper. *OTC.*
Use: Analgesic.
Myapap Elixir. (Rosemont) Acetaminophen 160 mg/5 mL. Bot. 4 oz, pt, gal. *OTC.*
Use: Analgesic.
Myapap with Codeine Elixir. (Rosemont) Acetaminophen 120 mg, codeine phosphate 12 mg/5 mL. Bot. 4 oz, pt, gal. *c-v.*
Use: Analgesic, antitussive.
Mybanil. (Rosemont) Codeine phosphate 10 mg, bromodiphenhydramine HCl 12.5 mg/5 mL, alcohol 5%. Bot. 4 oz, pt, gal. *c-v.*
Use: Antihistamine, antitussive.
Mycadec DM Drops. (Rosemont) Pseudoephedrine 25 mg, carbinoxamine maleate 2 mg, dextromethorphan HBr 4 mg/mL. Bot. 30 mL. *Rx.*
Use: Antihistamine, antitussive, decongestant.
Mycadec DM Syrup. (Rosemont) Carbinoxamine maleate 4 mg, pseudoephedrine HCl 60 mg, dextromethor-

phan HBr 15 mg/5 mL, alcohol 0.6%. Bot. 4 oz, pt, gal. *Rx.*
Use: Antihistamine, antitussive, decongestant.

Mycadec Drops. (Rosemont) Pseudoephedrine HCl 25 mg, dextromethorphan HBr 4 mg, carbinoxamine maleate 2 mg/mL. Bot. 30 mL. *Rx.*
Use: Antihistamine, antitussive, decongestant.

Mycamine. (Astellas Pharma, Inc.) Micafungin sodium 50 mg (must be diluted with 0.9% sodium chloride injection or 5% dextrose injection). Pow. for Inj. Single-use vials. *Rx.*
Use: Antifungal agent.

Mycartal. (Sanofi-Synthelabo) Pentaerythritol tetranitrate. *Rx.*
Use: Coronary vasodilator.

Mycelex. (Bayer Corp. (Consumer Div.)) Clotrimazole. **Cream:** 1%. Tube 15 g, 30 g, 90 g (2 × 45 g). **Topical Soln.:** 1%. Bot. 10 mL, 30 mL. *Rx-OTC.*
Use: Antifungal, topical.

Mycelex-G 500. (Bayer Corp. (Consumer Div.)) Clotrimazole 500 mg. Vaginal Tab. w/applicator. *Rx.*
Use: Antifungal; vaginal.

Mycelex-7. (Bayer Corp. (Consumer Div.)) Clotrimazole 1%, benzyl alcohol, cetostearyl alcohol. Vag. Cream. Tube 45 g w/1 applicator or 7 disp. applicators. *OTC.*
Use: Antifungal; vaginal.

Mycelex-7 Combination Pack. (Bayer Corp. (Consumer Div.)) Clotrimazole. **Cream:** 1%, benzyl alcohol, cetostearyl alcohol, polysorbate 80. Tube 7 g. **Supp.:** 100 mg, lactose, povidone. Pkg. 7s w/applicator. *OTC.*
Use: Antifungal; vaginal.

Mycelex-3. (Bayer) Butoconazole nitrate 2%, cetyl and stearyl alcohol, parabens, mineral oil. Vag. Cream. Prefilled single-dose applicators (3s), 3 disp. applicators 20 g. *OTC.*
Use: Antifungal; vaginal.

Mycelex Troches. (Bayer Corp. (Consumer Div.)) Clotrimazole 10 mg. Troche 70s, 140s. *Rx.*
Use: Antifungal.

Mychel-S. (Houba) Sterile chloramphenicol sodium succinate. Vial 1 g/15 mL. Box 5s. *Rx.*
Use: Anti-infective.

Mycifradin. (Pharmacia) Neomycin sulfate 125 mg/5 mL (equivalent to 87.5 mg neomycin). Oral soln. Bot. Pt. *Rx.*
Use: Anti-infective.

Mycinaire Saline Mist. (Pfeiffer) Sodium chloride 0.65%, benzalkonium chloride. Soln. Spray Bot. 45 mL. *OTC.*
Use: Nasal decongestant.

Mycinette. (Pfeiffer) Benzocaine 15 mg, sorbitol, saccharin, menthol. Loz. 12s. *OTC.*
Use: Anesthetic, local; antiseptic; expectorant.

Mycinette Sore Throat. (Pfeiffer) Phenol 1.4%, alum 0.3%, alcohol free, sugar free. Spray 180 mL. *OTC.*
Use: Mouth and throat preparation.

Myci-Spray. (Edwards) Phenylephrine HCl 0.25%, pyrilamine maleate 0.15%/mL. Bot. 20 mL. *OTC.*
Use: Antihistamine, decongestant.

Mycitracin. (Pharmacia) Bacitracin 500 units, neomycin sulfate 5 mg, polymyxin B sulfate 5000 units/g. Oint. Tube 0.5 oz, Box 30s, 1 oz, UD 1/32 oz Box 144s. *OTC.*
Use: Anti-infective, topical.

Mycitracin Triple Antibiotic, Maximum Strength. (Pharmacia) Polymyxin B sulfate 5000 units/g, neomycin 3.5 mg/g, bacitracin 500 units/g, parabens, mineral oil, white petrolatum. Oint. Tube 30 g, UD 0.94 g. *OTC.*
Use: Anti-infective, topical.

Mycobutin. (Pharmacia) Rifabutin. 150 mg. Cap. Bot. 100s. *Rx.*
Use: Antituberculosal.

Mycocide NS. (Woodward) Benzalkonium Cl, propylene glycol, methylparaben. Soln. Bot. 30 mL. *OTC.*
Use: Antimicrobial; antiseptic.

Mycodone Syrup. (Rosemont) Hydrocodone bitartrate 5 mg, homatropine HBr 1.5 mg/5 mL. Bot. 4 oz, pt, gal. *c-III.*
Use: Antitussive.

Mycogen-II Cream. (Ivax) Nystatin 100,000 units, triamcinolone acetonide 1 mg/g. Cream Tube 15 g, 30 g, 60 g, 120 g, lb. *Rx.*
Use: Antifungal; corticosteroid, topical.

Mycogen-II Ointment. (Ivax) Nystatin 100,000 units, triamcinolone acetonide 1 mg/g. Oint. Tube 15 g, 30 g, 60 g. *Rx.*
Use: Antifungal; corticosteroid, topical.

Mycolog-II Cream and Ointment. (Bristol-Myers Squibb) Triamcinolone acetonide 1 mg, nystatin 100,000 units/g. Ointment base w/Plastibase (polyethylene, mineral oil). Tube 15 g, 30 g, 60 g, Jar 120 g. *Rx.*
Use: Antifungal; corticosteroid, topical.

Mycomist. (Gordon Laboratories) Chlorophyll, formalin, benzalkonium Cl. Bot. 4 oz, plastic Bot. 1 oz. *OTC.*

Use: Antifungal for clothing.

• **mycophenolate.** (my-koe-FEN-oh-LATE MOE-feh-till) USAN.
Use: Immunosuppressant.
See: CellCept.
Myfortic.

• **mycophenolate mofetil hydrochloride.** (my-koe-FEN-oh-late MOE-fen-till) USAN.
Use: Transplantation (immunosuppressant).

• **mycophenolate sodium.** (mye-koe-FEN-oh-late) USAN.
Use: Immunosuppressant (transplantation).

• **mycophenolic acid.** (MY-koe-fen-AHL-ik) USAN.
Use: Antineoplastic.
See: Myfortic.

Mycoplasma Pneumonia IFA IgM Test. (Wampole) Indirect fluorescent assay for IgM antibodies to *Mycoplasma pneumoniae.* Box test 100s.
Use: Diagnostic aid.

Mycoplasma Pneumonia IFA Test. (Wampole) Indirect fluorescent assay for antibodies to *Mycoplasma pneumoniae* Box test 100s.
Use: Diagnostic aid.

Mycostatin. (Bristol-Myers Squibb) Nystatin. **Tab.:** 500,000 units, lactose. Bot. 100s. **Cream:** 100,000 units/g in aqueous base. Tube 15 g, 30 g. **Oint.:** 100,000 units/g in Plastibase (polyethylene and mineral oil). Tube 15 g, 30 g. **Troche:** 200,000 units. 30s. **Vaginal Tab:** 100,000 units, lactose 0.95 g, ethyl cellulose, stearic acid, starch. Pkg. 15s, 30s. **Pow.:** (topical) 100,000 units/g in talc. Shaker bot. 15 g. *Rx.*
Use: Antifungal.

Mycostatin Pastilles. (Bristol-Myers Squibb Oncology/Virology) Nystatin, 200,000 units. Troche. 30s. *Rx.*
Use: Antifungal.

Myco-Triacet. (Various Mfr.) Triamcinolone acetonide 0.1%, neomycin sulfate 0.25%, gramicidin 0.25 mg, nystatin 100,000 units/g. **Cream:** 15 g, 30 g, 60 g, 480 g. **Oint.:** 15 g, 30 g, 60 g. *Rx.*
Use: Antifungal, corticosteroid, topical.

Myco-Triacet II Cream & Ointment. (Teva) Nystatin 100,000 units, triamcinolone acetonide 1 mg/g. **Cream:** White petrolatum and mineral oil. Tube 15 g, 30 g, 60g. **Oint.:** Tube 15 g, 30 g, 60 g. *Rx.*
Use: Antifungal, corticosteroid, topical.

Mycotussin Expectorant. (Rosemont) Pseudoephedrine HCl 60 mg, hydrocodone bitartrate 5 mg, guaifenesin 200 mg/5 mL, alcohol 12.5%. Liq. Bot. 4 oz, pt, gal. *c-III.*
Use: Antitussive, decongestant, expectorant.

Mycotussin Liquid. (Rosemont) Pseudoephedrine HCl 60 mg, hydrocodone bitartrate 5 mg/5 mL, alcohol 5%. Bot. 4 oz, pt, gal. *c-III.*
Use: Antitussive, decongestant.

Mydacol. (Rosemont) Vitamins B_1 5 mg, B_2 2.5 mg, niacinamide 50 mg, B_6 1 mg, B_{12} 1 mcg, pantothenic acid 10 mg, I 100 mcg, Fe 15 mg, Mg 2 mg, Zn 2 mg, choline 100 mg, Mn 2 mg/30 mL. Liq. Bot. Pt, gal. *OTC.*
Use: Mineral; vitamin supplement.

Mydfrin Ophthalmic 2.5%. (Alcon) Phenylephrine HCl 2.5%. Soln. *Drop-Tainers.* 3 mL, 5 mL. *Rx.*
Use: Mydriatic.

Mydriacyl. (Alcon) Tropicamide 0.5%, 1%. Soln. 3 mL (1% only), 15 mL *Drop-Tainer. Rx.*
Use: Cycloplegic; mydriatic.

mydriatics, parasympatholytic types.
See: Atropine Salts.
Homatropine Hydrobromide.
Scopolamine Salts.

mydriatics, sympathomimetic types.
See: Amphetamine Sulfate 3%.
Clopane HCl.
Ephedrine Sulfate.
Epinephrine HCl.
Neo-Synephrine HCl.
Phenylephrine HCl.

Myelo-Kit. (Sanofi-Synthelabo) Omnipaque 180, 240 in various sizes and one sterile myelogram tray.
Use: Radiopaque agent.

Myfed. (Rosemont) Triprolidine HCl 1.25 mg, pseudoephedrine HCl 30 mg/5 mL. Syr. Bot. 4 oz, pt, gal. *OTC.*
Use: Antihistamine, decongestant.

Myfedrine. (Rosemont) Pseudoephedrine 30 mg/5 mL. Liq. Bot. 473 mL. *OTC.*
Use: Decongestant.

Myfedrine Plus. (Rosemont) Pseudoephedrine HCl 30 mg, chlorpheniramine maleate 2 mg/5 mL. Syr. Bot. 4 oz, pt, gal. *OTC.*
Use: Antitussive, decongestant.

Myfortic. (Novartis) Mycophenolate (as sodium) 180 mg, 360 mg. Lactose. Film coated. DR Tab. 120s. *Rx.*
Use: Immunosuppressant.

Mygel Liquid. (Geneva) Aluminum hydroxide 200 mg, magnesium hydroxide 200 mg, simethicone 20 mg, Na

1.38 mg/5 mL. Liq. Bot. 360 mL. *OTC.*
Use: Antacid; antiflatulent.

Mygel Suspension. (Geneva) Aluminum hydroxide 200 mg, magnesium hydroxide 200 mg, simethicone 20 mg/5 mL. Bot. 360 mL. *OTC.*
Use: Antacid; antiflatulent.

Mygel II Suspension. (Geneva) Aluminum hydroxide 400 mg, magnesium hydroxide 400 mg, simethicone 40 mg/ 5 mL. Bot. 360 mL. *OTC.*
Use: Antacid; antiflatulent.

Myhistine DH. (Rosemont) Codeine phosphate 10 mg, chlorpheniramine maleate 2 mg, pseudoephedrine HCl 30 mg/5 mL. Liq. Bot. 4 oz, pt, gal. *c-v.*
Use: Antihistamine, antitussive, decongestant.

Myhistine Elixir. (Rosemont) Chlorpheniramine maleate 2 mg, phenylephrine HCl 5 mg/5 mL, alcohol 5%. Liq. Bot. 4 oz, pt, gal. *OTC.*
Use: Antihistamine, decongestant.

Myhistine Expectorant. (Rosemont) Codeine phosphate 10 mg, guaifenesin 100 mg, pseudoephedrine HCl 30 mg/ 5 mL, alcohol 7.5%. Liq. Bot. 4 oz, pt, gal. *c-v.*
Use: Antitussive, decongestant, expectorant.

Myidone Tabs. (Major) Primidone 250 mg. Tab. Bot. 100s, 1000s. *Rx.*
Use: Anticonvulsant.

Mykacet Cream. (Alra) Nystatin 100,000 units, triamcinolone acetonide 0.1%/g. Tube 15 g, 30 g, 60 g. *Rx.*
Use: Antifungal; corticosteroid, topical.

My-K Elixir. (Rosemont) Potassium 20 mEq/15 mL, alcohol 5%, saccharin. Bot. Pt, gal. *Rx.*
Use: Electrolyte supplement.

My-K Formula 77 Liquid. (Rosemont) Doxylamine succinate 3.75 mg, dextromethorphan HBr 7.5 mg/5 mL, alcohol 10%. Liq. Bot. 180 mL. *OTC.*
Use: Antihistamine, antitussive.

Mykinac. (Alra) Nystatin 100,000 units/g in cream base. Cream Tube 15 g, 30 g. *OTC.*
Use: Antifungal, topical.

My-K Nasal Spray. (Rosemont) Oxymetazoline HCl 0.05%. Soln. Bot. 0.5 oz. *OTC.*
Use: Decongestant.

Mykrox. (Medeva) Metolazone 0.5 mg. Tab. Bot. 100s. *OTC.*
Use: Diuretic.

Mylagen Gelcaps. (Ivax) Calcium carbonate 311 mg, magnesium carbonate 232 mg. Pkg. 24s. *OTC.*
Use: Antacid.

Mylagen Liquid. (Ivax) Magnesium hydroxide 200 mg, aluminum hydroxide 200 mg, simethicone 20 mg/5 mL. Bot. 355 mL. *OTC.*
Use: Antacid; antiflatulent.

Mylagen II Liquid. (Ivax) Aluminum hydroxide 400 mg, magnesium hydroxide 400 mg, simethicone 40 mg/5 mL. Bot. 355 mL. *OTC.*
Use: Antacid; antiflatulent.

Mylanta Double Strength. (J & J/Merck Consumer Pharm.) **Chew. Tab.:** Magnesium hydroxide 400 mg, aluminum hydroxide dried gel 400 mg, simethicone 40 mg, Bot. 24s, 60s. **Liq.:** Magnesium hydroxide 400 mg, aluminum hydroxide dried gel 400 mg, simethicone 40 mg, sorbitol/5 mL. Bot. 150 mL, 360 mL. **Susp.:** Magnesium hydroxide 400 mg, aluminum hydroxide dried gel 400 mg, simethicone 40 mg, Na 0.05 mEq/5 mL. Bot. 150 mL, 360 mL, 720 mL, UD 30, 150 mL. *OTC.*
Use: Antacid.

Mylanta Gas. (J & J/Merck Consumer Pharm.) Simethicone. **40 mg:** Chew. Tab. Bot. 100s, UD 100s. **80 mg:** Chew. Tab. Pkg. 12s, Bot. 48s, 100s, UD 100s. *OTC.*
Use: Antiflatulent.

Mylanta Gas, Maximum Strength. (J & J/Merck Consumer Pharm.) Simethicone 125 mg. Chew. Tab. Pkg. 12s, Bot. 60s. *OTC.*
Use: Antiflatulent.

Mylanta Gelcaps. (J & J/Merck Consumer Pharm.) Calcium carbonate 311 mg, magnesium carbonate 232 mg. Bot. 24s, 50s. *OTC.*
Use: Antacid.

Mylanta Liquid. (J & J/Merck Consumer Pharm.) Magnesium hydroxide 200 mg, aluminum hydroxide 200 mg, simethicone 20 mg/5 mL, parabens, sorbitol, saccharin (lemon, mint, cherry only), original, lemon, mint, cherry flavors. Liq. Bot. 150 mL (original), 355 mL, 720 mL (original, cherry). *OTC.*
Use: Antacid; antiflatulent.

Mylanta Maximum Strength. (J & J Merck) Aluminum hydroxide 400 mg; magnesium hydroxide 400 mg, simethicone 40 mg/5 mL; parabens; saccharin; sorbitol; original, cherry, mint flavors. Liq. 360 mL, 720 mL (original only). *OTC.*
Use: Antacid.

Mylanta Natural Fiber Supplement. (J & J/Merck Consumer Pharm.) Psyllium hydrophilic mucilloid fiber 3.4 g/ dose, sucrose, orange flavor. Pow. Can

390 g. *OTC.*
Use: Laxative.

Mylanta Regular Strength. (J & J Merck) Aluminum hydroxide 200 mg; magnesium hydroxide 200 mg; simethicone 20 mg/5 mL; parabens; sorbitol; saccharin; original, mint, cherry flavors. Liq. Bot. 150 mL (original), 360 mL (all flavors), 720 mL (original, cherry). *OTC.*
Use: Antacid.

Mylanta Soothing Antacids. (J & J/ Merck Consumer Pharm.) Calcium carbonate 600 mg, corn syrup, sucrose. Loz. Pkg. 18s. Bot. 50s. *OTC.*
Use: Antacid.

Mylanta Supreme. (J & J/Merck Consumer Pharm.) Calcium carbonate 400 mg, magnesium hydroxide 135 mg/5 mL, saccharin, sorbitol, mint, lemon, cherry flavors. Liq. Bot. 355 mL. *OTC.*
Use: Antacid.

Mylanta Tablets. (J & J Merck Consumer Pharm.) Magnesium hydroxide 200 mg, aluminum hydroxide 200 mg, simethicone 20 mg, Na 0.77 mg, sorbitol. Chew. Tab. Bot. 12s, 40s, 48s, 100s, 180s. *OTC.*
Use: Antacid; antiflatulent.

Mylanta-II Liquid. (J & J/Merck Consumer Pharm.) Magnesium hydroxide 400 mg, aluminum hydroxide 400 mg, simethicone 40 mg, Na 1.14 mg, sorbitol/5 mL. Bot. 0.5 oz, 12 oz, UD 30 mL, 100s. *OTC.*
Use: Antacid; antiflatulent.

Mylanta-II Tablets. (J & J/Merck Consumer Pharm.) Magnesium hydroxide 400 mg, aluminum hydroxide 400 mg, simethicone 40 mg, Na 1.3 mg. Chew. Tab. Box 24s, 60s. *OTC.*
Use: Antacid; antiflatulent.

Mylase 100. Alpha-amylase.
See: Diastase.

Myleran. (GlaxoSmithKline) Busulfan 2 mg. Tab. Bot. 25s. *Rx.*
Use: Alkylating agent.

Mylicon. (AstraZeneca) Simethicone 40 mg. **Chew. Tab.:** Bot. 100s, 500s, UD 100s. **Drops:** 40 mg/0.6 mL. Bot. 30 mL. *OTC.*
Use: Antiflatulent.

Mylicon-80. (AstraZeneca) Simethicone 80 mg. Chew. Tab. Bot. 100s, Box 12s, 48s, UD 100s. *OTC.*
Use: Antiflatulent.

Mylicon-125. (AstraZeneca) Simethicone 125 mg. Chew. Tab. In 12s, 50s. *OTC.*
Use: Antiflatulent.

Mylocaine 4% Solution. (Rosemont) Lidocaine HCl 4%. Bot. 50 mL, 100 mL.
Rx.
Use: Anesthetic, local.

Mylocaine 2% Viscous Solution. (Rosemont) Lidocaine HCl 2%. Bot. 100 mL.
Rx.
Use: Anesthetic, local.

Mylocel. (MGI Pharma) Hydroxyurea 1000 mg, alcohol. Tab. Unit-of-use 60s.
Rx.
Use: Antineoplastic.

Mylotarg. (Wyeth) Gemtuzumab ozogamicin 5 mg, sodium chloride, mono/ dibasic sodium phosphate, preservative free. Pow. for Inj., lyophilized. Single Vial 20 mL. *Rx.*
Use: Monoclonal antibody.

Mymethasone. (Rosemont) Dexamethasone 0.5 mg/5 mL, alcohol 5%. Elix. Bot. 100 mL, 240 mL. *Rx.*
Use: Corticosteroid.

Mynatal. (ME Pharmaceuticals) Ca 300 mg, Fe 65 mg, vitamins A 5000 units, D 400 units, E 30 mg, B$_1$ 3 mg, B$_2$ 3.4 mg, B$_3$ 20 mg, B$_5$ 10 mg, B$_6$ 10 mg, B$_{12}$ 12 mcg, C 120 mg, folic acid 1 mg, biotin 30 mcg, Cr, Cu, I, Mg, Mn, Mo, Zn 25 mg. Cap. Bot. 100s, 500s. *Rx.*
Use: Mineral; vitamin supplement.

Mynatal FC. (ME Pharmaceuticals) Ca 250 mg, Fe 60 mg, vitamin A 5000 units, D 400 units, E 30 units, B$_1$ 3 mg, B$_2$ 3.4 mg, B$_3$ 20 mg, B$_5$ 10 mg, B$_6$ 10 mg, B$_{12}$ 12 mcg, C 100 mg, folic acid 1 mg, biotin 30 mcg, Zn 25 mg, I, Mg, Cr, Cu, Mo, Mn. Capl. Bot. 100s.
Rx.
Use: Mineral; vitamin supplement.

Mynatal P.N. Captabs. (ME Pharmaceuticals) Ca 125 mg, Fe 60 mg, vitamins A 4000 units, D 400 units, B$_1$ 3 mg, B$_2$ 3 mg, B$_3$ 10 mg, B$_6$ 2 mg, B$_{12}$ 3 mcg, C 50 mg, folic acid 1 mg, Zn 18 mg. Tab. Bot. 100s. *Rx.*
Use: Mineral; vitamin supplement.

Mynatal P.N. Forte. (ME Pharmaceuticals) Fe 60 mg, vitamin A 5000 units, D 400 units, E 30 units, C 80 mg, B$_1$ 3 mg, B$_2$ 3.4 mg, B$_3$ 20 mg, B$_6$ 4 mg, B$_{12}$ 12 mcg, folic acid 1 mg, Ca 250 mg, Zn 25 mg, I, Mg, Cu. Capl. Bot. 100s.
Rx.
Use: Mineral; vitamin supplement.

Mynatal Rx. (ME Pharmaceuticals) Ca 200 mg, Fe 60 mg, vitamin A 4000 units, D 400 units, E 15 mg, B$_1$ 1.5 mg, B$_2$ 1.6 mg, B$_3$ 17 mg, B$_5$ 7 mg, B$_6$ 4 mg, B$_{12}$ 2.5 mcg, C 80 mg, folic acid 1 mg, biotin 0.03 mg, Zn 25 mg, Mg, Cu. Capl. Bot. 100s. *Rx.*
Use: Mineral; vitamin supplement.

Mynate 90 Plus. (ME Pharmaceuticals) Ca 250 mg, Fe 90 mg, vitamin A 4000 units, D 400 units, E 30 units, B_1 3 mg, B_2 3.4 mg, B_3 20 mg, B_6 20 mg, B_{12} 12 mcg, C 120 mg, folic acid 1 mg, Zn 25 mg, DSS, I, Cu. Capl. Bot. 100s. *Rx.*
Use: Mineral; vitamin supplement.

Myo-B. (Sigma-Tau) Adenosine-5-monophosphoric acid, vitamin B_{12}. Inj. Vial 10 mL. *Rx.*

Myobloc. (Elan) Botulinum toxin type B 5000 units/mL, human serum albumin 0.05%, sodium succinate 0.01 M, sodium chloride 0.1 M, preservative free. (One unit corresponds to the calculated median lethal intraperitoneal dose (LD_{50}) in mice.) Inj. Soln. Single-use Vial 3.5 mL. *Rx.*
Use: Botulinum toxin.

Myochrysine. (Taylor) Gold sodium thio malate 50 mg/mL. Benzyl alcohol 0.5%. Inj. Vials. 2 mL, 10 mL. *Rx.*
Use: Antirheumatic agent.

Myocide NS. (Woodward) Benzalkonium chloride, propylene glycol, methylparaben. Soln. 30 mL. *OTC.*
Use: Antiseptic.

myodil.
See: Iophendylate Inj.

Myoflex Creme. (Aventis) Trolamine salicylate 10% in a vanishing cream base. Tube 2 oz, 4 oz, Jar 8 oz, lb, Pump dispenser 3 oz. *OTC.*
Use: Analgesic, topical.

Myolin. (Roberts) Orphenadrine citrate 30 mg/mL. Inj. Vial 10 mL. *Rx.*
Use: Muscle relaxant.

Myorgal. (Mysuran) Ambenonium Cl.
Use: Cholinergic.

Myoscint. (Centocor) Imciromab pentetate 0.5 mg for conjugation with indium-111. Kit. *Rx.*
Use: Radioimmunoscintigraphy agent.

Myotalis. (Vita Elixir) Digitalis 1.5 gr. EC Tab. *Rx.*
Use: Cardiovascular agent.

Myotonachol. (Glenwood) Bethanechol Cl 10 mg, 25 mg. Tab. Bot. 100s. *Rx.*
Use: Urinary tract product.

Myotoxin. (Vita Elixir) **#1:** Digitoxin 0.1 mg. Tab. **#2:** Digitoxin 0.2 mg. Tab. *Rx.*
Use: Cardiovascular agent.

Myphentol Elixir. (Rosemont) Phenobarbital 16.2 mg, hyoscyamine SO_4 or HBr 0.1037 mg, atropine sulfate 0.0194 mg, scopolamine HBr 0.0065 mg/5 mL, alcohol 23%. Bot. 4 oz, pt, gal. *Rx.*
Use: Anticholinergic; antispasmodic; hypnotic; sedative.

Myphetane. (Rosemont) Brompheniramine maleate 2 mg/5 mL, alcohol. Elix. Bot. *OTC.*
Use: Antihistamine.

Myphetane DX Cough. (Various Mfr.) Brompheniramine maleate 2 mg, pseudoephedrine HCl 30 mg, dextromethorphan HBr 10 mg/5 mL, alcohol 0.95%. Syr. Bot. 4 oz, pt, gal. *Rx.*
Use: Antihistamine, antitussive, decongestant.

Myproic Acid. (Rosemont) Valproic acid 250 mg (as sodium valproate)/5 mL. Syr. Bot. Pt. *Rx.*
Use: Anticonvulsant.

Myrac. (Glades) Minocycline (as hydrochloride) 50 mg, 75 mg, 100 mg. Lactose. Film coated. Tab. 50s (100 mg only), 100s (except 100 mg). *Rx.*
Use: Anti infective.

Myriatin Drops. (Sanofi-Synthelabo) Atropine methonitrate BP. *Rx.*
Use: Antispasmodic.

myristica oil.
Use: Flavor.

• **myristyl alcohol.** (mih-RIST-ill) *NF 23.*
Use: Pharmaceutic aid (stiffening agent).

myristyl-picolinium chloride.
See: Wet Tone.

Myrj 53. (AstraZeneca) Polyoxyl 50 stearate.
Use: Surface active agent.

Myrj 52 and M2s. (AstraZeneca) Polyoxyethylene 40 stearate. Mixture of free polyoxyethylene glycol and its mono- and di-stearates.
Use: Surface active agent.

Myrj 45. (AstraZeneca) Mixture of free polyoxyethylene glycol and its mono- and di-stearates. Polyoxyl 8 stearate.
Use: Surface active agent.

Mysoline. (Xcel Pharm) Primidone 50 mg, 250 mg. Lactose. Tab. 100s, 500s (50 mg only), 1000s, UD 100s (250 mg only). *Rx.*
Use: Anticonvulsant.

Mysuran. Ambenonium Cl.
Use: Muscle stimulant.
See: Mytelase Cl.

Mytelase. (Sanofi-Synthelabo) Ambenonium Cl 10 mg. Cap. Bot. 100s. *Rx.*
Use: Muscle stimulant.

Myticin G Creme and Ointment.
See: G-myticin creme and ointment.

Mytomycin-C. (IOP)
Use: Antiglaucoma agent. [Orphan Drug]

Mytussin. (Rosemont) Guaifenesin 100 mg/5 mL, alcohol 3.5%. Syr. Bot. 4 oz, pt, gal. *OTC.*

Use: Expectorant.

Mytussin AC Cough. (Morton Grove) Guaifenesin 100 mg, codeine phosphate 10 mg/5 mL, alcohol 3.5%, menthol, saccharin, sorbitol, fruit flavor. Syr. Bot. 118 mL, 237 mL, 473 mL. *c-v.*
Use: Upper respiratory combination, antitussive, expectorant.

Mytussin DAC. (Morton Grove) Guaifenesin 100 mg, pseudoephedrine HCl 30 mg, codeine phosphate 10 mg/ 5 mL, alcohol 1.7%, menthol, saccharin, sorbitol, strawberry-raspberry flavor. Liq. Bot. 118 mL, 473 mL. *c-v.*
Use: Upper respiratory combination, antitussive, decongestant, expectorant.

Mytussin DM. (Morton Grove) Guaifenesin 100 mg, dextromethorphan HBr 10 mg/5 mL, alcohol free, sugar, menthol, saccharin, cherry flavor. Syr. Bot. 118 mL, 3.8 L. *OTC.*
Use: Upper respiratory combination, antitussive, expectorant.

Myverol. (Eastman Kodak) Glyceryl monostearate.

My-Vitalife. (ME Pharmaceuticals) Ca 130 mg, Fe 27 mg, vitamins A 6500 units, D 400 units, E 30 mg, B_1 1.5 mg, B_2 1.7 mg, B_3 20 mg, B_5 10 mg, B_6 2 mg, B_{12} 6 mcg, C 60 mg, folic acid 0.4 mg, Cr, Cu, K, I, Mg, Mn, Mo, P, Se, Zn 15 mg, vitamin K, biotin 30 mcg. Cap. Bot. 60s. *OTC.*
Use: Mineral; vitamin supplement.

M-Zole 7 Dual Pack. (Alra) Miconazole nitrate. **Vag. Supp.:** 100 mg, mineral oil. 7s w/1 applicator. **Top. Cream:** 2%. Tube 9 g. *OTC.*
Use: Antifungal; vaginal.

M-Zole 3 Combination Pack. (Alpharma) Miconazole nitrate. **Vag. Supp.:** 200 mg, vegetable oil. Box 3s w/reusable applicator or 3 disp. applicators. **Top Cream:** 2%. Tube 9 g. *OTC.*
Use: Antifungal; vaginal.

N

Na-Ana-Tal. (Churchill) Phenobarbital 0.25 g, phenacetin 2 g, aspirin 3 g, nicotinic acid 50 mg. Tab. Bot. 100s, Liq. Bot. 16 oz. *c-IV*.
Use: Analgesic; hypnotic; sedative.

●**nabazenil.** (nab-AZE-eh-nill) USAN.
Use: Anticonvulsant.

Nabi-HB. (NABI) Hepatitis B immune globulin (human) 5% ± 1% protein, glycine 0.15 M, solvent/detergent treated. Preservative free. Soln. for Inj. Single-dose vial 1 mL, 5 mL. *Rx.*
Use: Hepatitis B vaccine.

●**nabilone.** (NAB-ih-lone) USAN.
Use: Anxiolytic.

●**nabitan hydrochloride.** (NAB-ih-tan) USAN. *Formerly Nabutan Hydrochloride.*
Use: Analgesic.

●**naboctate hydrochloride.** (NAB-ock-tate) USAN.
Use: Antiglaucoma agent; antinauseant.

●**nabumetone.** (nab-YOU-meh-TONE) *USP 28.*
Use: Anti-inflammatory.
See: Relafen.

nabumetone. (Various Mfr.) Nabumetone 500 mg, 750 mg. Tab. 100s, 500s, UD 100s (500 mg only). *Rx.*
Use: Anti-inflammatory.

n-acetylcysteine.
See: Acetylcysteine.

n-acetyl-p-aminophenol. Acetaminophen.

●**nadide.** (NAD-ide) USAN. *Formerly Diphosphopyridine Nucleotide, Nicotinamide Adenine Dinucleotide.*
Use: Antagonist to alcohol and narcotics.

Nadinola (Deluxe) for Oily Skin. (Strickland) Hydroquinone 2%. Bot. 1.25 oz, 2.25 oz. *Rx.*
Use: Dermatologic.

Nadinola for Dry Skin. (Strickland) Hydroquinone 2%. Bot. 1.25 oz, 2.25 oz. *Rx.*
Use: Dermatologic.

Nadinola (Ultra) for Normal Skin. (Strickland) Hydroquinone 2%. Bot. 1.25 oz, 3.75 oz, Tube 1.85 oz. *Rx.*
Use: Dermatologic.

●**nadolol.** (nay-DOE-lahl) *USP 28.*
Use: Antihypertensive; antianginal; beta-adrenergic blocker.
See: Corgard.

nadolol. (nay-DOE-lahl) (Various Mfr.) Nadolol 20 mg, 40 mg, 80 mg, 120 mg, 160 mg. Tab. Bot. 30s (80 mg only), 100s; 500s (80 mg, 120 mg, 160 mg only); 1000s (except 20 mg); UD 100s (20 mg, 40 mg, 80 mg only). *Rx.*
Use: Antiadrenergic/sympatholytic, beta-adrenergic blocker.

nadolol and bendroflumethiazide.
Use: Antihypertensive; antianginal beta blocker.
See: Corzide.

naepaine hydrochloride.
Use: Anesthetic, local.

●**nafamostat mesylate.** (naff-AM-oh-stat) USAN.
Use: Anticoagulant; antifibrinolytic.

●**nafarelin acetate.** (NAFF-uh-RELL-in) USAN.
Use: LHRH agonist; agonist; hormone. [Orphan Drug]
See: Synarel.

Nafazair. (Bausch & Lomb) Naphazoline hydrochloride 0.1%. Soln. Bot. 15 mL. *Rx.*
Use: Mydriatic, vasoconstrictor.

Nafazair A. (Bausch & Lomb) Naphazoline hydrochloride 0.025%, pheniramine maleate 0.3%, benzalkonium chloride 0.01%, EDTA, boric acid, sodium borate. Bot. 15 mL. *Rx.*
Use: Decongestant combination, ophthalmic.

Nafcillin Injection. (Baxter) Nafcillin sodium 1 g, 2 g (as base). Single-dose Galaxy bags, 50 ml (1 g only), 100 ml (2 g only). *Rx.*
Use: Anti-infective, penicillin.

●**nafcillin, sodium.** (naff-SILL-in) *USP 28.*
Use: Anti-infective.
See: Nafcillin Injection.

Na-Feen. (Pacemaker) Fluoride 1 mg/ Dose. Tab. Bot. 100s, 500s, 1000s; Liq. 2 oz. *Rx.*
Use: Dental caries agent.

●**nafenopin.** (naff-EN-oh-pin) USAN.
Use: Antihyperlipoproteinemic.

●**nafimidone hydrochloride.** (naff-IH-mih-DOHN) USAN.
Use: Anticonvulsant.

●**naflocort.** (NAFF-lah-cort) USAN.
Use: Adrenocortical steroid (topical).

●**nafoxidine hydrochloride.** (naff-OX-ih-deen) USAN.
Use: Antiestrogen.

●**nafronyl oxalate.** (NAFF-row-NILL OX-ah-late) USAN.
Use: Vasodilator.

●**naftifine hydrochloride.** (NAFF-tih-FEEN) USAN.
Use: Antifungal.
See: Naftin.

Naftin. (Allergan) Naftifine hydrochloride 1%. Cream. 2 g, 15 g, 30 g. *Rx.*
Use: Antifungal, topical.

naganol.
See: Suramin Sodium.
Naphuride Sodium.

Naglazyme. (BioMarin) Galsulfase 1 mg/mL. Soln. for Inj. Single-use vial 5 mL. *Rx.*
Use: Mucopolysaccharidosis VI.

•**nagrestipen.** (na-gres-ti-pen) USAN.
Use: Stem cell inhibitory protein.

Nailicure. (Purepac) Denatonium benzoate in a clear nail polish base. Liq. Bot. 0.33 oz. *OTC.*
Use: Nail-biting deterrent.

Nail Plus. (Faraday) Gelatin Cap. Bot. 100s, 200s.

•**nalbuphine hydrochloride.** (NAL-byoo-FEEN) USAN.
Use: Narcotic agonist-antagonist analgesic.
See: Nubain.

nalbuphine hydrochloride. (Various Mfr.) Nalbuphine hydrochloride 10 mg/mL, 20 mg/mL. Inj. Vials. 1 mL, 10 mL. *Rx.*
Use: Narcotic agonist-antagonist analgesic.

Naldecon Senior EX. (Sandoz) Guaifenesin 200 mg/5 mL, saccharin, sorbitol. Alcohol-free. Liq. Bot. 120 mL. *OTC.*
Use: Expectorant.

Nalex-A. (Blansett) **Liq.:** Phenylephrine hydrochloride 5 mg, chlorpheniramine maleate 2.5 mg, phenyltoloxamine citrate 7.5 mg/5 mL. Alcohol free, sugar free. Cotton-candy flavor. 473 mL. **Tab.:** Phenylephrine hydrochloride 20 mg, chlorpheniramine maleate 4 mg, phenyltoloxamine 40 mg. Lactose. 100s. *Rx.*
Use: Decongestant and antihistamine.

Nalex-A 12. (Blansett) Phenylephrine tannate 5 mg, chlorpheniramine tannate 2 mg, pyrilamine tannate 12.5 mg/5 mL. Methylparaben, saccharin, sucrose. Raspberry flavor. Susp. 118 mL. *Rx.*
Use: Decongestant and antihistamine.

Nalex DH. (Blansett) Hydrocodone bitartrate 2.5 mg, phenylephrine hydrochloride 5 mg/5 mL. Alcohol free, sugar free. Cherry flavor. Liq. 15 mL, 437 mL. *c-III.*
Use: Antitussive.

Nalex Expectorant. (Blansett) Hydrocodone bitartrate 5 mg, guaifenesin 200 mg, pseudoephedrine hydrochloride 60 mg/5 mL. Alcohol 12.5%. Liq. 25 mL, 473 mL. *c-III.*
Use: Antitussive and expectorant.

Nalfon Pulvules. (Pedinol) Fenoprofen calcium 200 mg, 300 mg. Cap. Bot. 100s. *Rx.*
Use: Analgesic; NSAID.

•**nalidixate sodium.** (nal-ih-DIK-sate) USAN. Under study.
Use: Anti-infective.

•**nalidixic acid.** (nal-ih-DIK-sik) *USP 28.*
Use: Anti-infective.
See: NegGram.

•**nalmefene hydrochloride.** (NAL-meh-FEEN) USAN. *Formerly Naletrene.*
Use: Antagonist to narcotics.
See: Revex.

nalmetrene. (NAL-meh-treen)
Use: Antagonist to narcotics.

•**nalmexone hydrochloride.** (NAL-mex-ohn) USAN.
Use: Analgesic; narcotic.

•**nalorphine hydrochloride.** (nal-or-feen) *USP 28.*

•**naloxone hydrochloride.** (NAL-ox-ohn) *USP 28.*
Use: Narcotic antagonist.
See: Narcan.

naloxone hydrochloride. (Various Mfr.) Naloxone hydrochloride. **0.02 mg/mL:** Amp 2 mL. **0.4 mg/mL:** Amp 1 mL, syringe 1 mL, vial 1 mL, 2 mL, 10 mL. *Rx.*
Use: Narcotic antagonist.

•**naltrexone hydrochloride.** (nal-TREX-ohn high-droe-KLOR-ide) USAN.
Use: Antidote, antagonist to narcotics. [Orphan Drug]
See: ReVia.

naltrexone hydrochloride. (Various Mfr.) Naltrexone hydrochloride 50 mg. Tab. Bot. 30s, 100s, 500s. *Rx.*
Use: Narcotic antagonist; antidote.

Namenda. (Forest Laboratories) Memantine hydrochloride. **Oral Soln.:** 2 mg/mL. Sorbitol, parabens. Alcohol free. Peppermint flavor. 360 mL. **Tab.:** 5 mg, 10 mg. Lactose. 60s, UD 100s, titration paks (blister pack containing 49 tabs). *Rx.*
Use: Alzheimers disease.

•**naminidil.** (nam-IN-i-dil) USAN.
Use: Alopecia.

namol xenyrate. (NAY-mahl ZEH-neh-rate)
See: Namoxyrate.

•**namoxyrate.** (nam-OX-ee-rate) USAN.
Use: Analgesic.
See: Namol Xenyrate.

namuron.
See: Cyclobarbital Calcium.

• **nandrolone cyclotate.** (NAN-drole-ohn SIH-kloe-tate) USAN.
Use: Anabolic.

• **nandrolone decanoate.** (NAN-drole-ohn deh-KAN-oh-ate) *USP 28.*
Use: Anabolic steroid.

nandrolone decanoate. (Watson) Nandrolone decanoate. **100 mg /mL:** Sesame oil, benzyl alcohol. Inj. (in oil). Multiple-dose vials. 2 mL. **200 mg/mL:** Sesame oil, benzyl alcohol. Single-dose vials. 1 mL. *c-III.*
Use: Androgen.

• **nantradol hydrochloride.** (NAN-trah-DAHL) USAN.
Use: Analgesic.

Naotin. (Drug Products) Sodium nicotinate. Amp. (equivalent to 10 mg nicotinic acid/mL) 10 mL, Box 25s, 100s. *Rx.*
Use: Vitamin B₃ supplement.

NAPA. (Medco Research; Parke-Davis) Acecainide hydrochloride.
Use: Cardiovascular agent.

• **napactadine hydrochloride.** (nap-ACK-tah-deen) USAN.
Use: Antidepressant.

• **napamezole hydrochloride.** (nap-am-EH-zole) USAN.
Use: Antidepressant.

NAPAmide Caps. (Major) Disopyramide phosphate 100 mg or 150 mg. Bot. 100s, 500s, UD 100s. *Rx.*
Use: Antiarrhythmic.

• **naphazoline hydrochloride.** (naff-AZZ-oh-leen) *USP 28.*
Use: Adrenergic, vasoconstrictor; nasal decongestant, arylalkylamine.
See: AK-Con.
 Albalon.
 All Clear AR.
 Allerest Eye Drops.
 Clear Eyes.
 Comfort Eye Drops.
 Degest 2.
 Maximum Strength Allergy Drops.
 Muro's Opcon.
 Nafazair.
 Naphcon.
 Privine.
 VasoClear.
 Vasocon Regular.
W/Antazoline phosphate, boric acid, phenylmercuric acetate, sodium Cl, sodium carbonate anhydrous.
See: Antazoline-V.
 Vasocon-A Ophthalmic.
W/Antazoline phosphate, polyvinyl alcohol.
See: AK-Con-A.

Nafazair A.
Naphazole-A.
Naphazoline Plus.
Naphcon A.
Naphoptic-A.
W/PEG 300, benzalkonium Cl.
See: Allergy Drops.
 All Clear.
W/Polyvinyl alcohol.
See: Albalon.
 Albalon Liquifilm.

naphazoline hydrochloride. (Various Mfr.) Naphazoline hydrochloride. 0.1% Soln. Bot. 15 mL. *Rx.*
Use: Adrenergic, vasoconstrictor.

naphazoline hydrochloride & antazoline phosphate. (Various Mfr.) Naphazoline hydrochloride 0.05%, antazoline phosphate 0.5%. Soln. 5 mL, 15 mL. *OTC.*
Use: Antihistamine; decongestant, ophthalmic.

• **naphazoline hydrochloride & pheniramine maleate.** *USP 28.* (Various Mfr.) Naphazoline hydrochloride 0.025%, pheniramine maleate 0.3%. Soln. Bot. 15 mL. *OTC.*
Use: Antihistamine; decongestant, ophthalmic.

naphazoline plus. (Parmed Pharmaceuticals, Inc.) Naphazoline hydrochloride 0.025%, pheniramine maleate 0.3%. Bot. 15 mL. *OTC.*
Use: Decongestant combination, ophthalmic.

Naphcon. (Alcon) Naphazoline hydrochloride 0.012%. Soln. Bot. 15 mL. *OTC.*
Use: Mydriatic; vasoconstrictor.

Naphcon-A. (Alcon) Naphazoline hydrochloride 0.025%, pheniramine maleate 0.3%. Soln. Bot. 15 mL. *OTC.*
Use: Decongestant combination, ophthalmic.

Naphcon Forte. (Alcon) Naphazoline hydrochloride 0.1%/mL. Soln. *Drop-Tainer* Bot. 15 mL. *Rx.*
Use: Mydriatic; vasoconstrictor.

Napholine. (Horizon) Naphazoline hydrochloride 0.1%. Soln. Bot. 15 mL. *Rx.*
Use: Mydriatic; vasoconstrictor.

Naphoptic-A. (Optopics) Naphazoline hydrochloride 0.025%, pheniramine maleate 0.3%. Soln. Bot. 15 mL. *Rx.*
Use: Decongestant combination, ophthalmic.

Naphthyl-B Salicylate. Betol, Naphthosalol, Salinaphthol.
Use: GI & GU, antiseptic.

naphuride sodium. Suramin Sodium.

•**napitane mesylate.** (NAP-ih-tane) USAN.
Use: Antidepressant.

•**napitane mesylate.** (NAP-ih-tane) USAN.
Use: Antidepressant.

Naprelan. (Blansett Pharmacal) Naproxen 375 mg, 500 mg. CR Tab. Bot. 100s (375 mg), 75s (500 mg). *Rx.*
Use: Analgesic.

Naprosyn. (Roche) Naproxen. **Tab.:** 250 mg, 375 mg, 500 mg. Bot. 100s, 500s. **Susp.:** 125 mg/5 mL, sorbitol, sucrose, parabens, orange-pineapple flavor. Bot. 473 mL. *Rx.*
Use: Analgesic; NSAID.

•**naproxen.** (nah-PROX-ehn) *USP 28.*
Use: Analgesic; anti-inflammatory; antipyretic.
See: EC-Naprosyn.
Midol Extended Relief.
Naprelan.
Naprosyn.
Naproxen Sodium.
W/Lansoprazole.
See: Prevacid NapraPAC.

naproxen. (Various Mfr.) Naproxen. **Tab.:** 250 mg, 375 mg, 500 mg. Bot. 30s, 100s, 500s, 1000s, UD 100s, UD 300s (500 mg only); unit-of-use 30s, 60s, 90s, 120s; *Robot ready* 25s (except 375 mg). **DR Tab.:** 375 mg, 500 mg. Bot. 100s, 500s. **Susp.:** 125 mg/5 mL, methylparaben, sorbitol, sucrose, pineapple-orange flavor. Bot. 15 mL, 20 mL, 500 mL. *Rx.*
Use: Analgesic; NSAID; antipyretic.

•**naproxen sodium.** (nah-PROX-ehn) *USP 28.*
Use: Analgesic; anti-inflammatory; antipyretic.
See: Aleve.
Anaprox.
Anaprox DS.
Naprosyn.

naproxen sodium. (Various Mfr.) Naproxen sodium 200 mg, 250 mg, 500 mg. Tab. Bot. 24s, 50s (200 mg only), 100s, 500s, 1000s, UD 100s. *Rx-OTC.*
Use: Analgesic; NSAID.

naproxen sodium. (Ivax) Naproxen sodium 200 mg (220 mg naproxen sodium). Tab. Bot. 24s. *OTC.*
Use: Anti-inflammatory.

naproxen sodium and pseudoephedrine hydrochloride.
Use: Upper respiratory combination, decongestant, analgesic.
See: Aleve Cold & Sinus.

Aleve Sinus & Headache.

•**naproxol.** (nay-PROX-ole) USAN.
Use: Analgesic; anti-inflammatory; antipyretic.

•**napsagatran.** (nap-sah-GAT-ran) USAN.
Use: Antithrombotic.

Naqua. (Schering-Plough) Trichlormethiazide 2 mg, 4 mg. Tab. Bot. 100s, 1000s. *Rx.*
Use: Diuretic.

•**naranol hydrochloride.** (NARE-ah-nahl) USAN.
Use: Antipsychotic.

•**naratriptan hydrochloride.** (NAHR-ah-trip-tan) *USP 28.*
Use: Antimigraine, serotonin 5-HT$_1$ receptor antagonist.
See: Amerge.

Narcan. (DuPont) Naloxone hydrochloride 0.4 mg/mL. Inj. Amp. 1 mL, Box 10s. Prefilled syringe 1 mL, Tray 10s; 1 mL, 2 mL, 10 mL Multiple-dose vials. *Rx.*
Use: Narcotic antagonist.

narcotic agonist-analgesic combinations.
See: Floricet with codeine.
Florinal with codeine.

narcotic agonist-antagonist analgesics.
See: Buprenorphine Hydrochloride.
Buprenorphine Hydrochloride Combinations.
Butorphanol Tartrate.
Nalbuphine Hydrochloride.
Pentazocine.
Pentazocine Combinations.

narcotic antitussive.
See: Codeine Sulfate.

Nardil. (Parke-Davis) Phenelzine sulfate 15 mg. Tab. Bot. 100s. *Rx.*
Use: Antidepressant.

Naropin. (AstraZeneca) Ropivacaine hydrochloride 0.2%, 0.5%, 0.75%, 1%, preservative free. Inj. *PolyAmp DuoFit Sterile Paks* 10 mL (0.2%, 1% only), 20 mL. Single-dose vial 30 mL (0.5% only). Single-dose infusion bot. 100 mL, 200 mL (0.2% only). *Rx.*
Use: Anesthetic, local injectable.

Nasabid. (Jones Pharma) Pseudoephedrine hydrochloride 90 mg, guaifenesin 250 mg, sucrose. Cap., prolonged-action. Bot. 100s. *Rx.*
Use: Decongestant; expectorant.

Nasabid SR. (Jones Medical) Pseudoephedrine hydrochloride 90 mg, guaifenesin 600 mg. SR Tab. Bot. 100s. *Rx.*
Use: Decongestant; expectorant.

Nasacort AQ. (Aventis) Triamcinolone acetonide 55 mcg per actuation, benzalkonium chloride, dextrose, EDTA, polysorbate 80. Spray. Bot. 6.5 g, 16.5 g (30 and 120 actuations) w/metered dose pump unit w/nasal adapter. *Rx.*
Use: Respiratory inhalant, intranasal steroid.

Nasadent. (Scherer) Sodium metaphosphate, glycerin, dicalcium phosphate dihydrate, sodium carboxymethylcellulose, oil of spearmint, sodium benzoate, saccharin. *OTC.*
Use: Ingestible dentifrice.

NaSal. (Bayer Corp. (Consumer Div.)) Sodium chloride 0.65%, benzalkonium chloride, thimerosal, alcohol free. Soln. Drop bot. 15 mL. Spray bot. 30 mL. *OTC.*
Use: Nasal decongestant.

NasalCrom. (Pharmacia) Cromolyn sodium 40 mg/mL, benzalkonium Cl, EDTA. Nasal Soln. Delivers 5.2 mg/spray. Metered spray device 13 mL or 26 mL. *OTC.*
Use: Antiasthmatic.

Nasal Decongestant, Children's Non-Drowsy. Various Mfr. Pseudoephedrine hydrochloride 15 mg/5 mL. Liq. Bot. 118 mL. *OTC.*
Use: Nasal decongestant, arylalkylamine.

Nasal Decongestant, Maximum Strength. (Taro) Oxymetazoline hydrochloride 0.05%. Soln. Spray bot. 15 mL, 30 mL. *OTC.*
Use: Nasal decongestant, imidazoline.

Nasal Decongestant Oral. Various Mfr. Pseudoephedrine hydrochloride 7.5 mg/0.8 mL. Drops. Bot. 15 mL, 30 mL w/dropper. *OTC.*
Use: Nasal decongestant, arylalkylamine.

nasal decongestants.
See: Adrenalin Chloride.
Afrin No-Drip 12-Hour.
Afrin No-Drip 12-Hour Extra Moisturizing.
Afrin No-Drip 12-Hour Severe Congestion with Menthol.
Afrin Saline, Extra Moisturizing.
Afrin Severe Congestion with Menthol.
Afrin Sinus with Vapornase.
Afrin 12-Hour Original.
Afrin 12-Hour Original Pump Mist.
Afrin No-Drip Sinus with Vapornase.
Afrin Children's Pump Mist.
AH-chew D.
Ayr Saline.

Benzedrex.
Breathe Free.
Cenafed.
Decofed.
Dimetapp Decongestant Pediatric.
Dimetapp, Maximum Strength, Non-Drowsy.
Dimetapp, Maximum Strength 12-Hour Non-Drowsy.
Dristan Fast Acting Formula.
Dristan 12-Hour Nasal.
Drixoral 12-Hour Non-Drowsy Formula.
Duramist Plus 12-Hour Decongestant.
Duration.
Efidac 24-Hour Relief.
Ephedrine Sulfate.
Epinephrine hydrochloride.
4 Way Fast Acting.
Genaphed.
Genasal.
HuMist Moisturizing Mist.
Kid Kare.
Little Colds for Infants & Children.
Little Noses Gentle Formula, Infants & Children.
Medi-First Sinus Decongestant.
Mycinaire Saline Mist.
Naphazoline hydrochloride.
NaSal.
Nasal Decongestant, Children's Non-Drowsy.
Nasal Decongestant, Maximum Strength.
Nasal Decongestant Oral.
Nasal Ease with Zinc.
Nasal Ease with Zinc Gluconate.
Nasal Moist.
Nasal Relief.
Nasal Spray.
Natru-Vent.
Neo-Synephrine 4-Hour Extra Strength.
Neo-Synephrine 4-Hour Mild Formula.
Neo-Synephrine 4-Hour Regular Strength.
Neo-Synephrine 12-Hour.
Neo-Synephrine 12-Hour Extra Moisturizing.
Nōstrilla 12-Hour.
Ocean.
Otrivin.
Otrivin Pediatric Nasal.
Oxymetazoline hydrochloride.
PediaCare Decongestant, Infants'.
Phenylephrine hydrochloride.
Pretz-D.
Pretz Irrigation.
Pretz Moisturizing.
Privine.

Pseudoephedrine hydrochloride.
Pseudoephedrine Sulfate.
Rhinall.
Rhinaris Lubricating Mist.
Salinex.
Silfedrine, Children's.
Simply Saline.
Simply Stuffy.
Sinustop.
Sudafed, Children's Non-Drowsy.
Sudafed Non-Drowsy, Maximum
Strength.
Sudafed Non-Drowsy 12 Hour Long-
Acting.
Sudafed Non-Drowsy 24 Hour Long-
Acting.
Sudodrin.
Tetrahydrozoline hydrochloride.
Triaminic Allergy Congestion.
12–Hour Nasal.
Twice-A-Day 12-Hour Nasal.
Tyzine.
Tyzine Pediatric.
Vicks Sinex 12-Hour Long-Acting.
Vicks Sinex 12-Hour Ultra Fine Mist
for Sinus Relief.
Vicks Sinex Ultra Fine Mist.
Vicks Vapor Inhaler.
Xylometazoline hydrochloride.
**Nasal Decongestant Sinus Non-
Drowsy.** (Topco) Pseudoephedrine hy-
drochloride 30 mg, acetaminophen
500 mg. Tab. Pkg. 24s. *OTC.*
Use: Upper respiratory combination, de-
congestant, analgesic.
Nasal•Ease with Zinc. (Health Care
Products) Zinc acetate, aloe vera, ca-
lendula extract, parabens, tocopherol
acetate, EDTA, glycerin. Soln. Gel.
Tube 14.1 g. *OTC.*
Use: Nasal decongestant.
Nasal•Ease with Zinc Gluconate.
(Health Care Products) Zinc gluconate,
sodium chloride, benzalkonium chlor-
ide, glycerin. Soln. Spray. Bot. 30 mL.
OTC.
Use: Nasal decongestant.
Nasal Jelly. (Kondon) Phenol, camphor,
menthol, eucalyptus oil, lavender oil.
Oint. Tube. 20 g. *OTC.*
Use: Decongestant.
Nasal Moist. (Blairex) Sodium chloride
0.65%, alcohol and dye free. Soln.
Spray bot. 45 mL. Mist pump bot.
15 mL. Gel bot. 28.5 g, unit-of-use
2 mL, aloe vera. *OTC.*
Use: Nasal decongestant.
Nasal Relief. (Rugby) Oxymetazoline hy-
drochloride 0.05%, EDTA, phenylmer-
curic acetate, sodium chloride. Soln.
Spray bot. 15 mL. *OTC.*

Use: Nasal decongestant, imidazoline.
Nasal Saline. (Sanofi-Synthelabo) Nasal
spray and drops. Sodium Cl 0.65% buf-
fered w/phosphates, preservatives.
Bot. 15 mL. Spray Bot. 15 mL. *OTC.*
Use: Moisturizer, nasal.
NaSal Saline Nasal. (Sanofi-Synthelabo)
Sodium Cl 0.65%. Drops, Spray. Bot.
15 mL. *OTC.*
Use: Moisturizer, nasal.
Nasal Spray. Various Mfr. Sodium chloride. Soln. Spray bot. 45 mL. *OTC.*
Use: Nasal decongestant.
Nasarel. (Ivax) Flunisolide 0.025%
(29 mcg/actuation), benzylkonium
chloride 0.01%, butylated hydroxytoluene, EDTA, polyethylene glycol 400,
sorbitol. Spray. 25 mL spray bot.
(200 sprays/bot.) with meter pump and
nasal adapter. *Rx.*
Use: Anti-inflammatory; intranasal
steroid.
• **nasaruplase beta.** (na-SA-rue-plase)
USAN.
Use: Ischemic stroke, acute.
Nasatab LA. (ECR) Guaifenesin 500 mg,
pseudoephedrine hydrochloride
120 mg. SR Tab. Bot. 100s. *Rx.*
Use: Upper respiratory combination, decongestant, expectorant.
Nascobal. (Questcor) Cyanocobalamin.
Intranasal Gel: 500 mcg/0.1 mL, benzalkonium chloride. 500 mcg/actuation.
Bot. 5 mL (≈ 8 doses). **Intranasal
Spray:** 500 mcg per 0.1 mL (500 mcg/
actuation). Benzalkonium chloride.
2.3 mL (≈ 8 doses/bottle). *Rx.*
Use: Vitamin supplement.
Nashville Rabbit Antithymocyte. (Applied Medical Research) Antithymocyte
serum. *Rx.*
Use: Immunosuppresant.
Nasonex. (Schering) Mometasone furoate monohydrate 0.05% (50 mcg/ac-
tuation), glycerin, 0.25% w/w phenyl-
ethylalcohol, citric acid, benzalkonium
chloride, polysorbate 80. Spray. Bot.
17 g (120 sprays) w/metered-dose
manual pump spray unit. *Rx.*
Use: Repiratory inhalant product, intranasal steroid.
Nasop. (Hawthorn) Phenylephrine hydrochloride 10 mg. Phenylalanine 4 mg,
aspartame, sorbitol. Bubble gum flavor.
Orally Disintegrating Tab. 100s. *Rx.*
Use: Nasal decongestant.
Nasophen. (Premo) Phenylephrine hydrochloride 0.25%, 1%. Bot. Pt. *OTC.*
Use: Decongestant.
Natabec. (Parke-Davis) Vitamins A
4000 units, D 400 units, B$_1$ 3 mg, B$_2$

2 mg, B_6 3 mg, C 50 mg, B_{12} 5 mcg, B_3 10 mg, elemental calcium 240 mg, elemental iron 30 mg. Kapseal. Bot. 100s. *OTC.*
Use: Mineral, vitamin supplement.

Natabec-F.A. (Parke-Davis) Vitamins A 4000 units, D 400 units, B_1 3 mg, B_2 2 mg, B_6 3 mg, C 50 mg, B_{12} 5 mcg, B_3 10 mg, elemental calcium 240 mg, elemental iron 30 mg, folic acid 0.1 mg. Kapseal, magnesium, bisulfites. Bot. 100s. *OTC.*
Use: Mineral, vitamin supplement.

Natabec with Fluoride. (Parke-Davis) Vitamins A 4000 units, D 400 units, B_1 3 mg, B_2 2 mg, B_6 3 mg, C 50 mg, B_{12} 5 mcg, B_3 10 mg, elemental calcium 240 mg, elemental iron 30 mg, elemental fluoride 1 mg. Kapseal. Bot. 100s. *Rx.*
Use: Vitamin supplement, dental caries agent.

NataChew. (Warner Chilcott) Vitamin A 1000 units, D_3 400 units, E (as dl-alpha tocopheryl acetate) 11 units, C 120 mg, folic acid 1 mg, B_1 2 mg, B_2 3 mg, niacinamide 20 mg, B_6 10 mg, B_{12} 12 mcg, Fe (as ferrous fumarate) 29 mg, wildberry flavor. Chew. Tab. Bot. 90s. *Rx.*
Use: Vitamin, mineral supplement.

Natacyn. (Alcon) Natamycin 5%. Bot. 15 mL. *Rx.*
Use: Antifungal agent, ophthalmic.

NataFort. (Warner Chilcott) Vitamin A (as acetate and beta carotene) 1000 units, D_3 400 units, E (as dl-alpha tocopheryl acetate) 11 units, C 120 mg, folic acid 1 mg, B_1 2 mg, B_2 3 mg, niacinamide 20 mg, B_6 10 mg, B_{12} 12 mcg, Fe (as carbonyl iron and ferrous sulfate) 60 mg, lactose. Tab. UD 90s. *Rx.*
Use: Vitamin, mineral supplement.

NatalCare Plus. (Ethex) Vitamin A 4000 units, C 120 mg, calcium sulfate 200 mg, Fe 27 mg, D 400 units, E 22 units, B_1 1.84 mg, B_2 3 mg, niacinamide 20 mg, B_6 10 mg, folic acid 1 mg, B_{12} 12 mcg, Zn 25 mg, Cu 2 mg.Tab. Bot. 100s. *Rx.*
Use: Mineral, vitamin supplement.

NatalCare Three. (Ethex) Ca 200 mg, Fe (as ferrous fumarate) 27 mg, vitamin A (as beta carotene) 3000 units, D 400 units, E (as dl-alpha tocopheryl acetate) 30 units, B_1 1.8 mg, B_2 4 mg, B_3 20 mg, B_6 25 mg, B_{12} 12 mcg, C 120 mg, folic acid 1 mg, Zn 25 mg, Cu, Mg. Tab. Bot. 100s. *Rx.*
Use: Vitamin, mineral supplement.

Natalins. (Bristol-Myers Squibb) Ca 200 mg, Fe 30 mg, vitamins A 4000 units, D 400 units, E 15 units, B_1 1.5 mg, B_2 1.6 mg, B_3 17 mg, B_6 2.6 mg, B_{12} 2.5 mcg, C 70 mg, folic acid 0.5 mg, Mg, Cu, Zn 15 mg. Tab. Bot. 100s. *OTC.*
Use: Mineral, vitamin supplement.

•**natamycin.** (NAT-uh-MY-sin) *USP 28.*
Use: Anti-infective, ophthalmic.
See: Natacyn.

Natarex Prenatal. (Major) Ca 200 mg, iron 60 mg, vitamins A 4000 units, D 400 units, E 15 mg, B_1 1.5 mg, B_2 1.6 mg, B_3 17 mg, B_5 7 mg, B_6 4 mg, B_{12} 2.5 mcg, C 80 mg, folic acid 1 mg, Cu, Mg, Zn 25 mg, biotin 30 mcg. Tab. Bot 100s. *Rx.*
Use: Mineral, vitamin supplement.

Nata-San. (Sandia) Vitamins A 4000 units, D 400 units, D_1, D_1 5 mg, B_2 4 mg, B_6 10 mg, nicotinic acid 10 mg, C 100 mg, B_{12} activity 5 mcg, ferrous fumarate 200 mg (elemental iron 65 mg), calcium carbonate 500 mg (Ca 196 mg), Cu (sulfate) 0.5 mg, Mg (sulfate) 0.1 mg, Mn (sulfate) 0.1 mg, K (sulfate) 0.1 mg, Zn (sulfate) 0.5 mg. Tab. Bot. 100s, 1000s. *OTC.*
Use: Mineral, vitamin supplement.

Nata-San F.A. (Sandia) Vitamins A 4000 units, D 400 units, B_1 5 mg, B_2 4 mg, B_6 10 mg, nicotinic acid 10 mg, C 100 mg, B_{12} activity 5 mcg, folic acid 1 mg, Fe 65 mg, Ca 200 mg, Cu (sulfate) 0.5 mg, Mg (sulfate) 0.1 mg, Mn (sulfate) 0.1 mg, K (sulfate) 0.1 mg, Zn (sulfate) 0.5 mg. Tab. Bot. 100s, 1000s. *Rx.*
Use: Mineral, vitamin supplement.

NataTab CFe. (Ethex) Vitamin A 4000 units, C 120 mg, Ca 200 mg, Fe 50 mg, D 400 units, E 30 units, B_1 3 mg, B_2 3 mg, niacin 20 mg, B_6 3 mg, folic acid 1 mg, B_{12} 8 mcg, iodine, zinc, lactose. Tab. UD 10s (100s). *Rx.*
Use: Vitamin, mineral supplement.

NataTab FA. (Ethex) Vitamin A 4000 units, C 120 mg, Ca 200 mg, Fe 29 mg, D 400 units, E 30 units, B_1 3 mg, B_2 3 mg, niacin 20 mg, B_6 3 mg, folic acid 1 mg, B_{12} 8 mcg, iodine, zinc 15 mg, lacotse. Tab. Bot. 100s. *Rx.*
Use: Vitamin, mineral supplement.

NataTab Rx. (Ethex) Ca 200 mg, Fe (as carbonyl iron) 29 mg, vitamin A (as beta carotene) 4000 units, D_3 400 units, E (as dl-alpha tocopheryl acetate) 30 units, B_1 3 mg, B_2 3 mg, B_3 20 mg, B_5 7 mg, B_6 3 mg, B_{12} 8 mcg, C 120 mg, folic acid 1 mg, biotin 30 mcg, Zn 15 mg, Cu, I, Mg. Tab. Bot. 90s.

Rx.
Use: Vitamin, mineral supplement.
nateglinide.
Use: Antidiabetic; meglitinide.
See: Starlix.
Natelle-EZ. (Pharmelle) Ca 100 mg, Fe 25 mg, vitamin A 2700 units, D 400 units, E 20 units, B_1 3 mg, B_2 3.5 mg, B_3 20 mg, B_5 8 mg, B_6 30 mg, B_{12} 12 mcg, C 120 mg, FA 1 mg, biotin 30 mcg, Cu, Mg, Se, Zn 15 mg, choline bitartrate. Tab. 90s. *Rx.*
Use: Multivitamin with calcium and iron.
Natodine. (Faraday) Iodine in organic form as found in kelp 1 mg. Tab. Bot. 100s, 250s. *OTC.*
Natrapel. (Tender) Citronella 10% in 15% Aloe vera base. *OTC.*
Use: Insect repellent.
Natrecor. (Scios Nova) Nesiritide 1.58 mg, mannitol. Pow. for Inj., lyophilized. Single-use vial 1.5 mg. *Rx.*
Use: Vasodilator, human B-type natriuretic peptide.
Natrico. (Drug Products) Potassium nitrate 2 g, sodium nitrite 1 g, nitroglycerin 0.25 g, cratageus oxycantha 0.25 g. Pulvoid. Bot. 100s, 1000s. *Rx.*
Use: Antihypertensive.
Natru-Vent. (Boehringer Ingelheim Consumer Health) Xylometazoline hydrochloride 0.05%, 0.1% sorbitol, preservative free. Soln. Spray bot. Metered-dose pump 100 sprays (0.05% only), 210 mL bot. (0.1% only). *OTC.*
Use: Nasal decongestant, imidazoline.
Naturacil. (Bristol-Myers Squibb) Psyllium seed husks 3.4 g, carbohydrate 9.6 g, Na 11 mg, 54 cal/2 pieces. Ctn. 24s, 40s. *OTC.*
Use: Laxative.
Natur-Aid. (Scot-Tussin) Lactose, pectin, and carob-lemon juice. Pow. 90%. Bot. 8 oz. *OTC.*
Use: Increase in normal intestinal flora.
Natural Diuretic Water Tablet. (AmLab) Buchu leaves 1 g, uva ursi 1 g, trilicum 1 g, parsley 1 g, juniper berries 1 g, asparagus 1 g, alfalfa powder 1 gr. Tab. Bot. 100s. *OTC.*
Use: Diuretic.
Natural Fiber Laxative. (Apothecary Prods.) Approx. psyllium hydrophillic mucilloid 3.4 g/7 g dose, 14 cal/dose, sodium free. Pow. Can. 390 g. *OTC.*
Use: Laxative.
natural lung surfactant.
See: Survanta.
natural penicillins.
Use: Anti-infective.
See: Penicillin G (Aqueous).

Penicillin G Potassium.
Pfizerpen.
natural vitamin a in oil.
See: Oleovitamin A.
Naturalyte. (Unico Holdings) Na 45 mEq, K 20 mEq, Cl 35 mEq, citrate 48 mEq, dextrose 25 g/L. Soln. Bot. 240 mL, 1 liter. *OTC.*
Use: Electrolyte, mineral supplement.
Naturalyte Oral Electrolyte Solution. (Unico Holdings) Dextrose 20 g, K 20 mEq, fructose 5 g, Cl 35 mEq, Na 45 mEq, citrate 30 mEq. Soln. Bot. 1 liter. *OTC.*
Use: Mineral, electrolyte supplement.
Nature's Aid Laxative Tabs. (Walgreen) Docusate sodium 100 mg, yellow phenolphthalein 65 mg. Tab. Bot. 60s. *OTC.*
Use: Laxative.
Nature's Remedy. (Block Drug) Aloe 100 mg, cascara sagrada 150 mg, lactose. Tab. Bot. 15s, 30s, 60s. *OTC.*
Use: Laxative.
Nature's Tears. (Rugby) Hydroxypropyl methylcellulose 2906 0.4%, KCl, NaCl, sodium phosphate, benzalkonium Cl 0.01%, EDTA. Soln. Bot. 15 mL. *OTC.*
Use: Artificial tears.
Nature-Throid. (Western Research Labs) Thyroid desiccated 32.4 mg (½ gr), 64.8 mg (1 gr), 129.6 mg (2 gr), 194.4 mg (3 gr). Tab. Bot. 100s. *Rx.*
Use: Thyroid hormone.
Naturetin. (Bristol-Myers Squibb) Bendroflumethiazide 5 mg. Tab. 100s, 1,000s. *Rx.*
Use: Diuretic.
Natur-Lax Tablets. (Faraday) Rhubarb root, cape aloes, cascara sagrada extract, mandrake root, parsley, carrot. Protein-coated tab. Bot. 100s. *OTC.*
Use: Laxative.
Naus-A-Tories. (Table Rock) Pyrilamine maleate 25 mg, secobarbital 30 mg. Supp. Box 12s. *c-II.*
Use: Antiemetic.
Nausea Relief. (Ivax) Dextrose 1.87 g, fructose 1.87 g, phosphoric acid 21.5 mg, methylparaben. Soln. Bot. 118 mL. *OTC.*
Use: Antiemetic; antivertigo.
Nausetrol. (Walsh Dohmen) Dextrose 1.87 g, fructose 1.87 g, phosphoric acid 21.5 mg per 5 mL. Glycerin, methylparaben. Cherry flavor. Soln. Bot. 118 mL. *OTC.*
Use: Antiemetic; antivertigo.
Navane. (Roerig) Thiothixene. **Cap.:** 1 mg, 2 mg, 5 mg, 10 mg, 20 mg. Lactose. Bot. 100s. *Rx.*

Use: Antipsychotic.

Navelbine. (GlaxoSmithKline) Vinorelbine tartrate 10 mg/mL, preservative free. Inj. Single-use Vial 1 mL, 5 mL. *Rx.*
Use: Antineoplastic; vinca alkaloid.

• **naxagolide hydrochloride.** (nax-A-go-LIDE) USAN.
Use: Antiparkinsonian; dopamine agonist.

• **naxifylline.** (na-xee-FYE-leen) USAN.
Use: Edema.

Nazafair. (Various Mfr.) Naphazoline hydrochloride 0.1%. Soln. Bot. 15 mL. *Rx.*
Use: Mydriatic; vasoconstrictor.

ND-Gesic. (Hyrex) Acetaminophen 300 mg, pyrilamine maleate 12.5 mg, chlorpheniramine maleate 2 mg, phenylephrine hydrochloride 5 mg. Tab. Bot. 100s, 1000s. *OTC.*
Use: Analgesic; antihistamine; decongestant.

n-diethyl meta-toluamide.
W/Red Veterinary Petrolatum.
See: RV Pellent.

n-diethylvanillamide.
See: Ethamivan.

NDNA. (Wampole) Anti-native DNA test by IFA. Confirmatory test for active SLE. Test 48s. *Rx.*
Use: Diagnostic aid.

• **nebacumab.** (neh-BACK-you-mab) USAN. *Formerly Septomonab.*
Use: Monoclonal antibody, antiendotoxin.

• **nebivolol.** (neh-BIV-oh-lole) USAN.
Use: Antihypertensive, beta blocker.

• **nebramycin.** (neh-brah-MY-sin) USAN. A complex of antibiotic substances produced by *Streptomyces tenebrarius.*
Use: Anti-infective.

NebuPent. (American Pharmaceutical Partners) Pentamidine isethionate 300 mg. Aer. single-dose vial. *Rx.*
Use: Anti-infective.

Nebu-Prel. (Mahon) Isoproterenol sulfate 0.4%, phenylephrine hydrochloride 2%, propylene glycol 10%. Liq. Vial 10 mL. *Rx.*
Use: Bronchodilator.

Necon 1/50. (Watson) Mestranol 50 mcg, norethindrone 1 mg, lactose. Tab. Pkt. 21s, 28s. *Rx.*
Use: Sex hormone, contraceptive hormone.

Necon 1/35. (Watson) Ethinyl estradiol 35 mcg, norethindrone 1 mg, lactose. Tab. Pkt. 21s, 28s. *Rx.*
Use: Sex hormone, contraceptive hormone.

Necon 7/7/7. (Watson) **Phase 1:** Norethindrone 0.5 mg, ethinyl estradiol 35 mcg. 7 tabs. **Phase 2:** Norethindrone 0.75 mg, ethinyl estradiol 35 mcg. 7 tabs.Tab. 28s. *Rx.*
Use: Sex hormone, contraceptive hormone.

Necon 10/11. (Watson) **Phase 1:** Norethindrone 0.5 mg, ethinyl estradiol 35 mcg. 10 tabs. **Phase 2:** Norethindrone 1 mg, ethinyl estradiol 35 mcg. 11 tabs. Lactose. Tab. Pkt. 28s. *Rx.*
Use: Sex hormone, contraceptive hormone.

Necon 0.5/35. (Watson) Ethinyl estradiol 35 mcg, norethindrone 0.5 mg, lactose. Tab. Pkt. 21s, 28s. *Rx.*
Use: Sex hormone, contraceptive hormone.

• **nedocromil.** (NEH-doe-KROE-mill) USAN.
Use: Antiallergic, prophylactic.

• **nedocromil calcium.** (NEH-doe-KROE-mill) USAN.
Use: Antiallergic, prophylactic.
See: Tilade.

• **nedocromil sodium.** (NEH-doe-KROE-mill) USAN.
Use: Mast cell stabilizer, antiasthmatic.
See: Alocril.
Tilade.

N.E.E. (Lexis Laboratories) Ethinyl estradiol 35 mcg, norethindrone 1 mg. Tab. 6 pcks. 21s, 28s. *Rx.*
Use: Contraceptive.

• **nefazodone hydrochloride.** (neff-AZE-oh-dohn) USAN.
Use: Antidepressant.

nefazodone hydrochloride. (Various Mfr.) Nefazodone hydrochloride 50 mg, 100 mg, 150 mg, 200 mg, 250 mg. Tab. 60s, 100s (50 mg only). *Rx.*
Use: Antidepressant.

• **neflumozide hydrochloride.** (neh-FLEW-moe-ZIDE) USAN.
Use: Antipsychotic.

• **nefocon a.** (NEE-FOE-kahn A) USAN.
Use: Contact lens material, hydrophilic.

• **nefopam hydrochloride.** (NEFF-oh-pam) USAN.
Use: Muscle relaxant; analgesic.

Negacide. (Sanofi-Synthelabo) Nalidixic acid. *Rx.*
Use: Anti-infective, urinary.

NegGram. (Sanofi-Synthelabo) Nalidixic acid 500 mg. Capl. Bot. 56s, 500s. *Rx.*
Use: Anti-infective, urinary.

• **nelarabine.** (neh-LAY-rah-bean) USAN.
Use: Antineoplastic.

•**nelezaprine maleate.** (neh-LEH-zah-PREEN) USAN.
Use: Muscle relaxant.

•**nelfilcon a.** (nell-FILL-kahn A) USAN.
Use: Contact lens material, hydrophilic.

•**nelfinavir mesylate.** (nell-FIN-ah-veer) USAN.
Use: Antiviral.
See: Viracept

Nelulen. (Watson) **1/35 E:** Ethynodiol diacetate 1 mg, ethinyl estradiol 35 mcg. Tab. Pack 21s, 28s. **1/50 E:** Ethynodiol diacetate 1 mg, ethinyl estradiol 50 mcg. Tab. Pack 21s, 28s. *Rx.*
Use: Contraceptive.

•**nelzarabine.** (nell-ZARE-ah-bean) USAN.
Use: Antineoplastic.

nemazine. Under study.
Use: Anti-inflammatory.

•**nemazoline hydrochloride.** (neh-MAZZ-oh-leen) USAN.
Use: Decongestant, nasal.

Nembutal. (Ovation) Pentobarbital 20 mg/5 mL, alcohol 18%. Elixir. Bot. Pt. *c-II.*
Use: Hypnotic; sedative.

Nembutal Sodium. (Ovation) Pentobarbital sodium. **Inj.:** 50 mg/mL. Amp 2 mL; Vial 20 mL, 50 mL. Box 5s. **Cap.:** 50 mg. Bot. 100s; 100 mg. Bot. 100s, 500s. Display pack 100s. **Supp.:** 30 mg, 60 mg, 120 mg, 200 mg. Box 12s. *c-II.*
Use: Hypnotic; sedative.

•**nemifitide ditriflutate.** (ne-MI-fi-tide) USAN.
Use: Antidepressant.

Neo-Benz-All. (Xttrium) Benzalkonium Cl 20.1%. Packet 25 mL 15s. To make gal of 1:750 soln. Also Aqueous Neo-Benz-All 1:750 soln. Packet 20 mL, 50s. *OTC.*
Use: Antiseptic; antimicrobial.

Neo Beserol. (Sanofi-Synthelabo) Aspirin, methocarbamol. *Rx.*
Use: Analgesic; muscle relaxant.

Neocalamine. (Various Mfr.) Red ferric oxide 30 g, yellow ferric oxide 40 g, zinc oxide 930 g. *OTC.*
Use: Astringent; antiseptic.

Neocate One +. (Scientific Hospital Supplies, Inc.) Protein 2.5 g (amino acids 3 g), carbohydrates 14.6 g, fat 3.5 g, vitamins A, D, E, K, B_1, B_2, B_3, B_5, B_6, B_{12}, folic acid, biotin, C, choline, inositol, Ca, P, Mg, Fe, Zn, Mn, Cu, I, Mo, Cr, Se, Cl, Na 20 mg (0.9 mEq), K 93 mg (2.4 mEq) per 100 mL, 100 cal/mL. Liq. Bot. 237 mL. *OTC.*

Use: Nutritional supplement, enteral.

Neo-Cholex. (Lafayette) Fat emulsion containing 40%/ w/v pure vegetable oil. Bot. 60 mL. *Rx.*
Use: Cholecystokinetic.

Neocidin. (Major) Polymyxin B sulfate 10,000 units, neomycin sulfate 1.75 mg, gramicidin 0.025 mg/mL. Soln. Bot. 10 mL. *Rx.*
Use: Anti-infective, ophthalmic.

neo-cobefrin.
Use: Vasoconstrictor.

Neocurb. (Taylor Pharmaceuticals) Phendimetrazine tartrate 35 mg. Tab. Bot. 100s, 1000s. *c-III.*
Use: Anorexiant.

Neocylate. (Schwarz Pharma) Potassium salicylate 280 mg, aminobenzoic acid 250 mg. Tab. Bot. 100s, 1000s. *OTC.*
Use: Analgesic.

Neocyten. (Schwarz Pharma) Orphenadrine citrate 30 mg/mL. Vial 10 mL. *Rx.*
Use: Muscle relaxant.

NeoDecadron Ophthalmic Solution. (Merck & Co.) Dexamethasone sodium phosphate 0.1%, neomycin sulfate 0.35%, benzalkonium chloride 0.02%, EDTA, hydrochloric acid, sodium bisulfite 0.1%, polysorbate 80, sodium borate, sodium citrate. *Ocumeter* 5 mL. *Rx.*
Use: Anti-infective; corticosteroid, ophthalmic.

Neo-Dexair. (Bausch & Lomb) Dexamethasone sodium phosphate 0.1%, neomycin sulfate 0.35%, polysorbate 80, EDTA, benzalkonium Cl 0.02%, sodium bisulfite 0.1%. Soln. Bot. 5 mL. *Rx.*
Use: Anti-infective; corticosteroid, ophthalmic.

Neo-Dexameth. (Major) Dexamethasone sodium phosphate 0.1%, neomycin sulfate 0.35%, benzalkonium chloride 0.01%, EDTA, hydrochloric acid, polysorbate 80, sodium bisulfite, sodium borate, sodium citrate. Ophth. Soln. Bot. 5 mL. *Rx.*
Use: Anti-infective; corticosteroid, ophthalmic.

Neo-Diaral. (Roberts) Loperamide 2 mg. Cap. Bot. UD 8s, 250s. *OTC.*
Use: Antidiarrheal.

neodrenal.
See: Isoproterenol.

Neo-Durabolic. (Roberts) Nandrolone decanoate injection. **50 mg/mL, 100 mg/mL:** Vial 2 mL. **200 mg/mL:** Vial 1 mL. *c-III.*
Use: Anabolic steroid.

Neo-fradin. (Pharma-Tek) Neomycin sulfate 125 mg/5 mL, parabens. Oral Soln. Bot. 480 mL. *Rx.*
Use: Amebicide.

Neogesic. (Pal-Pak, Inc.) Aspirin 194.4 mg, acetaminophen 129.6 mg, caffeine 32.4 mg. Tab. Bot. 1000s. *OTC.*
Use: Analgesic combination.

Neoloid. (Kenwood) Castor oil 36.4% (emulsified), sodium benzoate 0.1%, potassium sorbate 0.2%, mint flavor. Emulsion. Bot. 118 mL. *OTC.*
Use: Laxative.

Neo-Mist Nasal Spray. (A.P.C.) Phenylephrine hydrochloride 0.5%, cetalkonium Cl 0.02%. Spray Bot. 20 mL. *OTC.*
Use: Antiseptic; decongestant.

Neo-Mist Pediatric 0.25% Nasal Spray. (A.P.C.) Phenylephrine hydrochloride 0.25%, cetalkonium Cl 0.02%. Squeeze Bot. 20 mL. *OTC.*
Use: Antiseptic; decongestant.

•**neomycin and polymyxin B sulfates and bacitracin ointment.** *USP 28.*
Use: Anti-infective, antibiotic, topical.
See: Bacitracin Zinc w/Neomycin Sulfate, Polymyxin B Sulfate.
Bacitracin Zinc w/Polymyxin B Sulfate, Neomycin, Pramoxine hydrochloride.

•**neomycin and polymyxin B sulfates and bacitracin ophthalmic ointment.** *USP 28.*
Use: Anti-infective, topical.

•**neomycin and polymyxin B sulfates and bacitracin zinc ointment.** *USP 28.*
Use: Anti-infective, topical.

•**neomycin and polymyxin B sulfates and bacitracin zinc ophthalmic ointment.** *USP 28.*
Use: Anti-infective, ophthalmic.

neomycin and polymyxin B sulfates and bacitracin zinc ophthalmic ointment. (Various Mfr.) Polymyxin B sulfate 10,000 units, neomycin 3.5 mg, bacitracin zinc 400 units/g, white petrolatum, mineral oil. Tube. 3.5 g. *Rx.*

neomycin and polymyxin B sulfates and dexamethasone ophthalmic ointment. (Various Mfr.) Dexamethasone 0.1%, neomycin sulfate 0.35%, polymyxin B sulfate 10,000 units. Tube 3.5 g.

•**neomycin and polymyxin B sulfates and dexamethasone ophthalmic suspension.** *USP 28.*
Use: Anti-infective; corticosteroid, ophthalmic.

neomycin and polymyxin B sulfates and dexamethasone ophthalmic

suspension. (Various Mfr.) Dexamethasone 0.1%, neomycin sulfate 0.35%, polymyxin B sulfate 10,000 units/mL, benzalkonium chloride 0.004%, hydroxypropyl methylcellulose 0.5%, hydrochloric acid, sodium chloride, polysorbate 20, sodium hydroxide. Bot. 5 mL. *Rx.*

•**neomycin and polymyxin B sulfates and gramicidin cream.** *USP 28.*
Use: Anti-infective, topical.

•**neomycin and polymyxin B sulfates and gramicidin ophthalmic solution.** *USP 28.*
Use: Anti-infective, ophthalmic.

neomycin and polymyxin B sulfates and hydrocortisone. (Falcon) Hydrocortisone 1%, neomycin sulfate equiv. to 0.35% neomycin base/mL, polymyxin B sulfate 10,000 units/mL. Thimerosal 0.001%, cetyl alcohol, glyceryl monostearate, mineral oil, propylene glycol. Susp. 7.5 mL *Drop-Tainers. Rx.*
Use: Otic preparations.

•**neomycin and polymyxin B sulfates and hydrocortisone acetate ointment.** *USP 28.*
Use: Anti-infective; corticosteroid, topical.

•**neomycin and polymyxin B sulfates and hydrocortisone acetate ophthalmic ointment.** *USP 28.*
Use: Anti-infective; corticosteroid, ophthalmic.

neomycin and polymyxin B sulfates and hydrocortisone acetate ophthalmic suspension. (Various Mfr.) Hydrocortisone 1%, neomycin sulfate 0.35%, polymyxin B sulfate 10,000 units. Bot. 7.5 mL, 10 mL.
Use: Anti-infective; corticosteroid, ophthalmic.

•**neomycin and polymyxin B sulfates and hydrocortisone otic suspension.** *USP 28.*
Use: Anti-infective; corticosteroid, otic.

neomycin and polymyxin B sulfates and hydrocortisone otic suspension. (Steris) Polymyxin B sulfate equiv. to 10,000 polymyxin B units, neomycin sulfate equiv. to 3.5 mg neomycin base/mL. Hydrocortisone 1%, thimerosal 0.01%, cetyl alcohol, propylene glycol, polysorbate 80. Susp. Bot. 10 mL.

•**neomycin and polymyxin B sulfates and pramoxine hydrochloride cream.** *USP 28.*
Use: Anti-infective, topical anesthetic.

●**neomycin and polymyxin B sulfates and prednisolone acetate ophthalmic suspension.** *USP 28.*
Use: Anti-infective; corticosteroid, ophthalmic.

●**neomycin and polymyxin B sulfates, bacitracin, and hydrocortisone acetate ointment.** *USP 28.*
Use: Anti-infective; corticosteroid, topical.

neomycin and polymyxin B sulfates, bacitracin, and hydrocortisone acetate ointment.
Use: Anti-infective; antifungal; antiinflammatory, topical.

●**neomycin and polymyxin B sulfates, bacitracin, and hydrocortisone acetate ophthalmic ointment.** *USP 28.*
Use: Anti-infective; corticosteroid, topical.

●**neomycin and polymyxin B sulfates, bacitracin, and hydrocortisone ointment.** *USP 28.*
Use: Anti-infective, corticosteroid.

●**neomycin and polymyxin B sulfates, bacitracin, and lidocaine ointment.** *USP 28.*
Use: Anti-infective, topical.
See: Lanabiotic.

●**neomycin and polymyxin B sulfates, bacitracin zinc, and hydrocortisone acetate ophthalmic ointment.** *USP 28.*
Use: Anti-infective, antifungal; anti-inflammatory, topical.

●**neomycin and polymyxin B sulfates, bacitracin zinc, and hydrocortisone ophthalmic ointment.** *USP 28.*
Use: Anti-infective, corticosteroid.

neomycin and polymyxin B sulfates cream.
Use: Anti-infective, topical.

●**neomycin and polymyxin B sulfates, gramicidin, and hydrocortisone acetate cream.** *USP 28.*
Use: Anti-infective, corticosteroid.

neomycin and polymyxin B sulfates, gramicidin, and hydrocortisone acetate cream.
Use: Anti-infective; corticosteroid, topical.

neomycin and polymyxin B sulfates ophthalmic ointment.
Use: Anti-infective, ophthalmic.

neomycin and polymyxin B sulfates ophthalmic solution.
Use: Anti-infective, ophthalmic.

neomycin and polymyxin B sulfates solution for irrigation.
Use: Irrigant, ophthalmic; anti-infective, topical.

See: Neosporin G.U. Irrigant.
neomycin base.
Use: Anti-infective.
W/Combinations.
See: Maxitrol.
Neosporin Plus.
Neotal.

●**neomycin boluses.** *USP 28.*
Use: Anti-infective.

●**neomycin palmitate.** (NEE-oh-MY-sin PAL-mih-tate) USAN.
Use: Anti-infective.

●**neomycin sulfate.** (NEE-oh-MY-sin) *USP 28.* Cream; Ointment; Ophthalmic Ointment, Oral Solution; Tablets.
Use: Anti-infective.
See: Mycifradin Sulfate.
Neo-fradin.
Neo-Tabs.
W/Combinations.
See: AK-Spore.
Bacitracin Neomycin.
Coracin.
Cordran-N.
Cortisporin.
Maxitrol.
Mycifradin Sulfate Sterile.
Mycitracin.
Neo-Cort Dome.
Neo-Cortef.
NeoDecadron Ophthalmic Solution.
Neosporin.
Neotal.
Neo-Thrycex.
Ocutricin.
Tigo.
Trimixin.

neomycin sulfate. (Pharmacia) Neomycin sulfate. Pow. micronized for compounding. Bot. 100 g.
Use: Anti-infective.

●**neomycin sulfate and bacitracin ointment.** *USP 28.*
Use: Anti-infective, topical.

●**neomycin sulfate and bacitracin zinc ointment.** *USP 28.*
Use: Anti-infective, topical.

●**neomycin sulfate and dexamethasone sodium phosphate cream.** *USP 28.*
Use: Anti-infective; corticosteroid, topical.

●**neomycin sulfate and dexamethasone sodium phosphate ophthalmic ointment.** *USP 28.*
Use: Anti-infective; corticosteroid, ophthalmic.

●**neomycin sulfate and dexamethasone sodium phosphate ophthalmic solution.** *USP 28.* (Various Mfr.) Dexamethasone sodium phosphate 0.1%,

neomycin sulfate 0.35%. Bot. 5 mL.
Use: Anti-infective; corticosteroid, ophthalmic.

•**neomycin sulfate and fluocinolone acetonide cream.** *USP 28.*
Use: Anti-infective; corticosteroid, topical.

•**neomycin sulfate and fluorometholone ointment.** *USP 28.*
Use: Anti-infective, corticosteroid, topical.

•**neomycin sulfate and flurandrenolide cream.** *USP 28.*
Use: Anti-infective, corticosteroid, topical.
See: Cordran.

•**neomycin sulfate and gramicidin ointment.** *USP 28.*
Use: Anti-infective, topical.

•**neomycin sulfate and hydrocortisone.** *USP 28.* Cream; Ointment; Otic Suspension, *USP.*
Use: Anti-infective; corticosteroid, topical.

•**neomycin sulfate and hydrocortisone acetate.** *USP 28.* Cream; Lotion; Ointment; Opthalmic Ointment; Ophthalmis Suspension, *USP.*
Use: Anti-infective; corticosteroid.

•**neomycin sulfate and methylprednisolone acetate cream.** *USP 28.*
Use: Anti-infective, corticosteroid, topical.

•**neomycin sulfate and prednisolone acetate ointment.** *USP 28.*
Use: Anti-infective, corticosteroid, topical.

•**neomycin sulfate and prednisolone acetate ophthalmic ointment.** *USP 28.*
Use: Anti-infective, corticosteroid, topical.

•**neomycin sulfate and prednisolone acetate ophthalmic suspension.** *USP 28.*
Use: Anti-infective; corticosteroid, topical.

•**neomycin sulfate and prednisolone sodium phosphate ophthalmic ointment.** *USP 28.*
Use: Anti-infective; corticosteroid, topical.

•**neomycin sulfate and triamcinolone acetonide cream.** *USP 28.*
Use: Anti-infective; corticosteroid, topical.

•**neomycin sulfate and triamcinolone acetonide ophthalmic ointment.** *USP 28.*

Use: Anti-infective; corticosteroid, ophthalmic.

neomycin sulfate, polymyxin B sulfate, and gramicidin solution. (Various Mfr.) Polymyxin B sulfate 10,000 units/mL, neomycin sulfate 1.75 mg/mL, gramicidin 0.025 mg/mL, sodium chloride, alcohol 0.5%, propylene glycol, hydrochloric acid, thimerosal 0.001%, poloxamer 188, ammonium hydroxide. Bot. 10 mL. *Rx.*
Use: Anti-infective, ophthalmic.

neomycin sulfate, polymyxin B sulfate, and lidocaine.
Use: Anti-infective; anesthetic, local.
See: Clomycin.
Neosporin Plus.
Tribiotic Plus.

•**neomycin sulfate, sulfacetamide sodium, and prednisolone acetate ophthalmic ointment.** *USP 28.*
Use: Anti-infective; corticosteroid, topical.

•**neomycin undecylenate.** (NEE-oh-MY-sin UHN-de-sih-LEN-ate) USAN.
Use: Anti-infective; antifungal.

Neopap. (PolyMedica) Acetaminophen 125 mg/Supp. In 12s. *OTC.*
Use: Analgesic.

Neopham 6.4%. (Pharmacia) Essential and non-essential amino acids 6.4%. Inj. 250 mL, 500 mL. *Rx.*
Use: Nutritional supplement, parenteral.

Neo Picatyl. (Sanofi-Synthelabo) Glycobiarsol. *Rx.*
Use: Amebicide.

Neo Quipenyl. (Sanofi-Synthelabo) Primaquine phosphate. *Rx.*
Use: Antimalarial.

Neoral. (Novartis) Cyclosporine. **Soft Gelatin Cap.:** 25 mg, 100 mg, dehydrated alcohol 11.9%. UD 30s. **Oral Soln.:** 100 mg/mL, dehydrated alcohol 11.9%. Bot. 50 mL. *Rx.*
Use: Immunosuppressant.

Neosar. (Gensia Sicor) Cyclophosphamide. 100 mg, sodium bicarbonate 82 mg. Pow. for Inj. Vial 100 mg, 200 mg, 500 mg, 1 g, 2 g. *Rx.*
Use: Antineoplastic; alkylating agent.

neo-skiodan. Iodopyracet, Diodrast.

Neosol. (Breckenridge) L-hyoscyamine sulfate 0.125 mg, mint flavor. Orally Disintegrating Tab. 100s. *Rx.*
Use: Gastrointestinal anticholinegic/antispasmodic.

Neosporin AF. (Pfizer Consumer Health) Miconazole nitrate. **Cream:** 2%. Mineral oil. 14 g. **Spray Liq.:** 2%. Alcohol. 105 g. *OTC.*
Use: Anti-infective, topical.

Neosporin G.U. Irrigant. (GlaxoSmith-Kline) Neomycin sulfate 40 mg, polymyxin B sulfate 200,000 units/mL. Amp. 1 mL. Box 10s, 50s, Multiple-dose vial 20 mL. *Rx.*
Use: Irrigant, genitourinary.

Neosporin Maximum Strength. (Warner Lambert) Polymyxin B sulfate 10,000 units, neomycin 3.5 mg, bacitracin 500 units/g, white petrolatum. Oint. Tube 15 g. *OTC.*
Use: Anti-infective, topical.

Neosporin Ophthalmic Ointment. (Monarch) Polymyxin B sulfate 10,000 units, bacitracin zinc 400 units, neomycin sulfate 3.5 mg/g, white petrolatum. Tube 3.5 g. *Rx.*
Use: Anti-infective, ophthalmic.

Neosporin Ophthalmic Solution. (Monarch) Polymyxin B sulfate 10,000 units, neomycin 1.75 mg, gramicidin 0.025 mg/mL, thimerosal 0.5%, thimerosal 0.001%, propylene glycol, sodium chloride. Bot. 10 mL. *Drop-dose. Rx.*
Use: Anti-infective, ophthalmic.

Neosporin Original. (Pfizer) Polymyxin B sulfate 5000 units, neomycin 3.5 mg, bacitracin zinc 400 units, cocoa butter, cottonseed oil, olive oil, white petrolatum. Oint. Tube 14 g, 28 g; UD 0.9 g (10s). *OTC.*
Use: Anti-infective, antibiotic, topical.

Neosporin Plus Pain Relief. (Pfizer) **Oint.:** Polymyxin B sulfate 10,000 units, neomycin 3.5 mg, bactracin zinc 500 units, pramoxine hydrochloride 10 mg/g, white petrolatum. Tube 15 g, 30 g. **Cream:** Polymyxin B sulfate 10,000 units, neomycin 3.5 mg, pramoxine hydrochloride 10 mg/g, methylparaben, mineral oil, white petrolatum. Tube. 15 g. *OTC.*
Use: Anti-infective, antibiotic, topical.

neostibosan. Ethylstibamine.

neostigmine. (nee-oh-STIGG-meen)
Use: Cholinergic.
See: Neostigmine Bromide.
Neostigmine Methylsulfate.
Prostigmin.

neostigmine and atropine sulfate.
Use: Muscle stimulant.
See: Neostigmine Min-I-Mix.

•**neostigmine bromide.** (nee-oh-STIGG-meen BROE-mide) *USP 28.*
Use: Cholinergic.
See: Prostigmin Bromide.

neostigmine bromide. (Lannett) Neostigmine bromide. 15 mg. Tab. 100s and 1000s.
Use: Cholinergic.

•**neostigmine methylsulfate.** (nee-oh-STIGG-meen METH-ill-SULL-fate) *USP 28.*
Use: Cholinergic.
See: Prostigmin.

neostigmine methylsulfate. (Various Mfr.) Neostigmine methylsulfate 1:2000 (0.5 mg/mL), 1:1000 (1 mg/mL). Inj. Vials. 1 mL, 2 mL, 10 mL (1:2000 only). Multidose vials. 10 mL. *Rx.*
Use: Cholinergic; urinary cholinergic.

Neostigmine Min-I-Mix. (I.M.S., Ltd.) Atropine sulfate 1.2 mg, neostigmine methylsulfate 2.5 mg. Inj. Vial. Use: Cholinergic muscle stimulant. *Rx.*
Use: Mydriatic, vasoconstrictor.

Neostrate Skin Lightening. (NeoStrata) Hydroquinone 2%, denatured alcohol, sodium bisulfite, EDTA. Gel. 4.8 g. *OTC.*
Use: Dermatologic.

neo-strepsan.
See: Sulfathiazole.

Neo-Synephrine. (Sanofi-Synthelabo) Phenylephrine hydrochloride 2.5% or 10%. Soln. Bot. 5 mL (10%), 15 mL (2.5%). *Rx.*
Use: Mydriatic; vasoconstrictor.

Neo-Synephrine 4-Hour Extra Strength. (Bayer) Phenylephrine hydrochloride 1%, benzalkonium chloride, thimerosal. Drop. bot., Spray bot. 15 mL. *OTC.*
Use: Nasal decongestant, arylalkylamine.

Neo-Synephrine 4-Hour Mild Formula. (Bayer) Phenylephrine hydrochloride 0.25%, benzalkonium chloride, thimerosal. Soln. Spray bot. 15 mL. *OTC.*
Use: Nasal decongestant, arylalkylamine.

Neo-Synephrine 4-Hour Regular Strength. (Bayer) Phenylephrine hydrochloride 0.5%, benzalkonium chloride, thimerosal. Soln. Spray bot., Drop. bot. 15 mL. *OTC.*
Use: Nasal decongestant, arylalkylamine.

Neo-Synephrine Hydrochloride. (Sanofi-Synthelabo) Phenylephrine hydrochloride. **Spray:** 0.25% children and adult, 0.5% adult. **Regular:** Squeeze bot. 0.5 oz. **0.5% mentholated:** Squeeze bot. 0.5 oz. **Drops:** 0.125% infant; 0.25% children and adult; 0.5% adult; 1% adult extra strength. Bot. 1 oz; 0.25% and 1%, also bot. 16 oz. **Jelly:** 0.5%. Tube 18.75 g. *OTC.*
Use: Decongestant.

Neo-Synephrine Hydrochloride. (Sanofi-Synthelabo) Phenylephrine hy-

drochloride. **Amp.:** 1%, Carpuject sterile cartridge-needle unit 10 mg/mL. (1 mL fill in 2 mL cartridge) w/22-gauge, 1.25 inch needle. Dispensing Bin 50s; Vial 1 mL. Box 25s. *Rx.*
Use: Vasoconstrictor.

Neo-Synephrine 12-Hour. (Bayer) Oxymetazoline hydrochloride 0.05%, benzalkonium chloride, phenylmercuric acetate, glycine, sorbitol, sodium chloride. Soln. Spray Bot. 15 mL. *OTC.*
Use: Nasal decongestant, imidazoline.

Neo-Synephrine 12-Hour Extra Moisturizing. (Bayer) Oxymetazoline hydrochloride 0.05%, benzalkonium chloride, phenylmercuric acetate, glycine, sorbitol, sodium chloride. Soln. Spray Bot. 15 mL. *OTC.*
Use: Nasal decongestant, imidazoline.

Neo-Synephrine Viscous Ophthalmic. (Sanofi-Synthelabo) Phenylephrine hydrochloride 10%. Soln. Bot. 5 mL. *Rx.*
Use: Mydriatic; vasoconstrictor.

Neo-Tabs. (Pharma-Tek) Neomycin sulfate 500 mg (equivalent to 350 mg neomycin base). Tab. Bot. 100s. *Rx.*
Use: Amebicide.

Ncotal. (Roberts) Zinc bacitracin 400 units, polymyxin B sulfate 5000 units, neomycin sulfate 5 mg, petrolatum and mineral oil base/g. Tube 3.5 g. *Rx.*
Use: Anti-infective, ophthalmic.

Neo-Thrycex. (Del) Bacitracin, neomycin sulfate, polymyxin B sulfate. Oint. Tube 0.5 oz. *Rx.*
Use: Anti-infective, topical.

Neothylline. (Teva) Dyphylline. Tab. **200 mg:** Bot. 100s, 1000s. **400 mg:** Bot. 100s, 500s. *Rx.*
Use: Bronchodilator.

Neothylline-GG (Teva) Dyphylline 200 mg, guaifenesin 200 mg. Tab. Bot. 100s, 1000s. *Rx.*
Use: Bronchodilator; expectorant.

Neotrace-4. (APP) Zn 1.5 mg, Cu 0.1 mg, Cr 0.85 mcg, Mn 25 mcg/mL. Vial 2 mL. *Rx.*
Use: Mineral supplement.

Neotricin HC. (Bausch & Lomb) Hydrocortisone acetate 1%, neomycin sulfate 0.35%, bacitracin zinc 400 units, polymyxin B sulfate 10,000 units. Oint. Tube 3.5 g. *Rx.*
Use: Anti-infective; corticosteroid, ophthalmic.

Neotricin Ophthalmic Ointment. (Bausch & Lomb) Polymyxin B sulfate 10,000 units, neomycin sulfate 3.5 mg, bacitracin 400 units/g. In 3.5 g. *Rx.*
Use: Anti-infective, ophthalmic.

Neotricin Ophthalmic Solution. (Bausch & Lomb) Polymyxin B sulfate 10,000 units, neomycin sulfate 1.75 mg, gramicidin 0.025 mg/mL. Dropper bot. 10 mL. *Rx.*
Use: Anti-infective, ophthalmic.

Neo-Trobex Injection. (Forest) Vitamins B_1 150 mg, B_6 10 mg, riboflavin 5-phosphate sodium 2 mg, niacinamide 150 mg, panthenol 10 mg, choline Cl 20 mg, inositol 20 mg/mL. Vial 30 mL. *Rx.*
Use: Vitamin supplement.

Neotrol. (Horizon) Phenylephrine hydrochloride 0.25%, pyrilamine maleate 0.2%, cetalkonium Cl 0.05%, tyrothricin 0.03%, phenylmercuric acetate 1:50,000. Soln. Squeeze Bot. 20 mL. *OTC.*
Use: Antihistamine, decongestant.

Neoval. (Halsey Drug) Vitamins A 10,000 units, D 400 units, B_1 10 mg, B_2 5 mg, B_6 2 mg, B_{12} 3 mcg, C 100 mg, E 5 mg, pantothenic acid 10 mg, niacinamide 30 mg, Fe 15 mg, Cu 1 mg, Mg 5 mg, Mn 1 mg, Zn 1.5 mg, I 0.15 mg. Tab. Bot. 100s. *OTC.*
Use: Mineral, vitamin supplement.

Neoval T. (Halsey Drug) Vitamins A 10,000 units, D 400 units, B_1 15 mg, B_2 10 mg, B_6 2 mg, C 150 mg, B_{12} 7.5 mcg, E 5 mg, pantothenic acid 10 mg, E 5 mg, niacinamide 100 mg, Fe 18 mg, Mg 5 mg, Mn 1 mg, Zn 1.5 mg, Cu 1 mg. Tab. Bot. 1000s. *OTC.*
Use: Mineral, vitamin supplement.

• **nepafenac.** (neh-pah-FEN-ack) USAN.
Use: Topical ocular anti-inflammatory, analgesic.

NephPlex Rx. (Nephro-Tech) B_1 1.5 mg, B_2 1.7 mg, B_3 20 mg, B_5 10 mg, B_6 10 mg, B_{12} 6 mcg, C 60 mg, folic acid 1 mg, biotin 300 mcg, Zn 12.5 mg. Tab. Bot. 100s. *Rx.*
Use: Mineral, vitamin supplement.

5.4% NephrAmine. (McGaw) Amino acid concentration 5.4%, nitrogen 0.65 g/100 mL. **Essential amino acids:** Isoleucine 560 mg, leucine 880 mg, lysine 640 mg, methionine 880 mg, phenylalanine 880 mg, threonine 400 mg, tryptophan 200 mg, valine 640 mg, histidine 250 mg/100 mL. **Nonessential amino acids:** Cysteine < 20 mg/100 mL, sodium 5 mEq, acetate 44 mEq, chloride 3 mEq/L, sodium bisulfite. Inj. 250 mL. *Rx.*
Use: Nutritional supplement, parenteral.

nephridine.
See: Epinephrine.

Nephro-Calci. (R & D Laboratories, Inc.) Calcium carbonate 1.5 g. Chew. Tab. (600 mg calcium). Bot. 100s, 200s, 500s, 1000s. *OTC.*
Use: Mineral supplement.

Nephro-Calci. (Watson) Calcium carbonate 1500 mg (elemental calcium 600 mg). Tab. Bot. 100s. *OTC.*
Use: Mineral supplement, calcium.

Nephrocaps. (Fleming & Co.) Vitamins B₁ 1.5 mg, B₂ 1.7 mg, B₃ 20 mg, B₅ 5 mg, B₆ 10 mg, B₁₂ 6 mcg, C 100 mg, folic acid 1 mg, biotin 150 mcg. Cap. Bot. 100s. *Rx.*
Use: Vitamin supplement.

Nephro-Fer. (Watson) Ferrous fumarate 350 mg (iron 115 mg). Lactose, tartrazine, sugar free. Tab. Bot. 30s. *OTC.*
Use: Mineral supplement.

Nephron. (Nephron) Racepinephrine hydrochloride 2.25% (epinephrine base 1.125%), sodium bisulfate, potassium metabisulfite, chlorobutanol, benzoic acid, propylene glycol. Soln. for Inh. Bot. 15 mL. *OTC.*
Use: Bronchodilator, sympathomimetic.

Nephron FA. (Nephro-Tech) Fe 66.6 mg, C 40 mg, B₁ 1.5 mg, B₂ 1.7 mg, B₃ 20 mg, B₅ 10 mg, B₆ 10 mg, B₁₂ 6 mcg, biotin 300 mcg, FA 1 mg, docusate sodium 75 mg. Tab. Bot. 100s. *Rx.*
Use: Mineral, vitamin supplement.

Nephro-Vite Rx. (R & D Laboratories, Inc.) Vitamins B₁ 1.5 mg, B₂ 1.7 mg, B₃ 20 mg, B₅ 10 mg, B₆ 10 mg, B₁₂ 6 mcg, C 60 mg, folic acid 1 mg, d-biotin 300 mcg. Tab. Bot. 100s. *Rx.*
Use: Mineral, vitamin supplement.

Nephro-Vite Vitamin B Complex & C Supplement. (R & D Laboratories, Inc.) Vitamins B₁ 1.5 mg, B₂ 1.7 mg, B₃ 20 mg, B₅ 10 mg, B₆ 10 mg, B₁₂ 6 mcg, C 60 mg, folic acid 800 mcg, biotin 300 mcg. Tab. Bot. 100s. *OTC.*
Use: Mineral, vitamin supplement.

Nephrox. (Fleming & Co.) Aluminum hydroxide 320 mg, mineral oil 10%/ 5 mL. Bot. Pt. *OTC.*
Use: Antacid.

Nepro. (Ross) Protein 6.6 g (as Ca, Mg, and Na caseinates), fat 22.7 g (as 90% high-oleic safflower oil, 10% soy oil), carbohydrate 51.1 g (assucrose, hydrolyzed corn starch), vitamins A, D, E, K, C, B₁, B₂, B₅, B₆, B₁₂, biotin, FA, Na, K, Cl, Ca, P, Mg, I, Mn, Cu, Zn, Fe, Se/ 240 mL. 59.4 calories. Liq. Can. 240 mL. *OTC.*
Use: Nutritional supplement, enteral.

●**neramexane mesylate.** (ner-a-MEX-ane) USAN.

Use: Depression; Alzheimer disease; pain.

neraval.
Use: Anesthetic, general.

●**nerelimomab.** (neh-reh-LI-moe-mab) USAN.
Use: Monoclonal antibody.

Nervine Nighttime Sleep-Aid. (Bayer Corp. (Consumer Div.)) Diphenhydramine hydrochloride 25 mg. Tab. Bot. 12s, 30s, 50s. *OTC.*
Use: Sleep aid.

Nesacaine. (AstraZeneca) Chloroprocaine hydrochloride 1%, 2%, methylparaben, EDTA. Inj. Multidose vial. 30 mL. *Rx.*
Use: Anesthetic, local injectable.

Nesacaine-MPF. (AstraZeneca) Chloroprocaine hydrochloride 2%, 3%, preservative-free. Inj. Single-dose vials. 20 mL. *Rx.*
Use: Anesthetic, local injectable.

Nesa Nine Cap. (Standex) Vitamins A 5000 units, D 400 units, C 37.5 mg, B₁ 1.5 mg, B₂ 2 mg, niacinamide 20 mg, B₆ 0.1 mg, calcium pantothenate 1 mg, E 2 units. Cap. Bot. 100s. *OTC.*
Use: Mineral, vitamin supplement.

nesdonal sodium.
See: Pentothal Sodium.
Thiopental Sodium.

●**nesiritide.** (ni-sir-i-tide) USAN.
Use: Vasodilator, human B-type natriuretic peptide.
See: Natrecor.

●**nesiritide citrate.** USAN.
Use: Treatment of congestive heart failure.

Nestabs. (Fielding) See Vitelle Nestabs OTC.

Nestabs CBF. (Fielding) Vitamins A 4000 units, D 400 units, E 30 units, C 120 mg, folic acid 1 mg, B₁ 3 mg, B₂ 3 mg, niacinamide 20 mg, B₆ 3 mg, B₁₂ 8 mcg, Ca 200 mg, I, Zn 15 mg, Fe 50 mg. Tab. Bot. 100s. *Rx.*
Use: Mineral, vitamin supplement.

Nestabs FA. (Fielding) Vitamins A 4000 units, D 400 units, E 30 units, C 120 mg, B₁ 3 mg, B₂ 3 mg, B₃ 20 mg, B₆ 3 mg, B₁₂ 8 mcg, Ca 200 mg, Fe 29 mg, folic acid 1 mg, Zn 15 mg, I. Tab. Bot. 100s. *Rx.*
Use: Mineral, vitamin supplement.

Nestle VHC 2.25. (Nestle Clinical Nutrition) Protein 90 g, carbohydrate 196 g, fat 120 g, vitamins A, B₁, B₂, B₃, B₅, B₆, B₁₂, C, D, E, K, folic acid, biotin, chloride, choline, Ca, Cr, Cu, Fe, I, Mg, Mn, Mo, P, Se, Zn, Na 1200 mg, K

1732 mg/L. Liq. Can. 250 mL. *OTC.*
Use: Enteral nutrition.

●**netilmicin sulfate.** (ne-til-MYE-sin)
USAN.

●**netoglitazone.** (net-oh-GLIT-a-zone)
USAN.
Use: Antidiabetic.

●**netrafilcon a.** (NET-rah-FILL-kahn A)
USAN.
Use: Contact lens material, hydrophilic.

netrin. Under Study.
Use: Anticholinergic.
See: Metcaraphen hydrochloride.

Neulasta. (Amgen) Pegfilgrastim 10 mg/
mL, preservative free. Soln. for Inj. Dispensing pack containing single-dose
syr. w/needle. *Rx.*
Use: Hematopoietic, colony stimulating
factor.

Neumega. (Genetics Institute) Oprelvekin
5 mg, dibasic sodium phosphate heptahydrate 1.6 mg, monobasic sodium
phosphate monohydrate 0.55 mg, preservative free. Pow. for Inj. lyophilized.
Box. Single-dose Vial with diluent. *Rx.*
Use: Hematopoietic, interleukin.

Neupogen. (Amgen) Filgrastim (G-CSF)
300 mcg/0.5 mL. Acetate 0.295 mg,
sorbitol 25 mg, 0.004% Tween 80,
0.0175 mg Na/0.5 mL. Preservative-
free. Inj. Prefilled syringe. 0.5 mL,
0.8 mL. *Rx.*
Use: Immunomodulator.

NeuRecover-DA. (NeuroGenesis) DL-
phenylalanine 460 mg, L-glutamine
25 mg, vitamin A 333.3 units, B₁
1.65 mg, B₂ 0.85 mg, B₃ 33 mg, B₅
15 mg, B₆ 3 mg, B₁₂ 5 mcg, FA
0.065 mg, C 100 mg, E 5 units, biotin
0.05 mg, Ca 25 mg, Cr 0.01 mg, Fe
1.5 mg, Mg 25 mg, Zn 2.5 mg. Cap. Bot.
180s. *OTC.*
Use: Amino acid.

NeuRecover-SA. (NeuroGenesis) DL-
phenylalanine 250 mg, L-tyrosine
150 mg, L-glutamine 50 mg, vitamins
B₁ 1.65 mg, B₂ 2.5 mg, B₃ 16.6 mg, B₅
15 mg, B₆ 3.36 mg, B₁₂ 5 mcg, FA
0.067 mg, C 100 mg, Ca 25 mg, Fe
1.5 mg, Mg 25 mg, Zn 5 mg. Cap. Bot.
180s. *OTC.*
Use: Amino acid.

Neurodep-Caps. (Medical Products
Panamericana) Vitamins B₁ 125 mg, B₆
125 mg, B₁₂ 1000 mcg. Cap. Bot. 50s.
OTC.
Use: Vitamin supplement.

Neurodep Injection. (Medical Products
Panamericana) Vitamins B₁ 50 mg, B₂
5 mg, B₃ 125 mg, B₅ 6 mg, B₆ 5 mg,

B₁₂ 1000 mcg, C 50 mg/mL. Inj. Vial
10 mL. *Rx.*
Use: Vitamin supplement, parenteral.

**neuromuscular blockers, nondepolar-
izing.**
Use: Muscle relaxants; adjuncts to an-
esthesia.
See: Pancuronium Bromide.
Rocuronium Bromide.

Neurontin. (Pfizer) Gabapentin. **Cap.:**
100 mg, 300 mg, 400 mg, lactose, talc.
Bot. 100s, UD 50s. **Tab.:** 600 mg,
800 mg, talc. Bot. 100s, 500s, UD 50s.
Oral Soln.: 250 mg/5 mL, xylitol, cool
strawberry anise flavor. Bot. 480 mL.
Rx.
Use: Anticonvulsant.

neurosin.
See: Calcium Glycerophosphate.

Neurotim. (NeuroGenesis) DL-phenyl-
alanine 500 mg, L-glutamine 15 mg, L-
tyrosine 25 mg, L-carnitine 10 mg, L-
arginine pyroglutamate 10 mg, ornithine
aspartate 10 mg, Cr 0.033 mg, Se
0.012 mg, vitamins B₁ 0.33 mg, B₂
0.5 mg, B₃ 3.3 mg, B₅ 0.012 mg, B₆
0.333 mg, B₁₂ 1 mcg, E 5 units, biotin
0.05 mg, FA 0.066 mg, Fe 1 mg, Zn
2.5 mg, Ca 35 mg, I 0.025 mg, Cu
0.33 mg, Mg 25 mg. Cap. Bot. 180s.
OTC.
Use: Amino acid.

neurotrophin-1.
Use: Motor neuron disease/amyotro-
phic lateral sclerosis. [Orphan Drug]

Neut. (Abbott) Sodium bicarbonate 4%.
Vial (2.4 mEq each of sodium and bicarbonate), disodium edetate anhydrous 0.05% as stabilizer. Pintop Vial
5 mL, 10 mL. Box 25s, 100s. *Rx.*
Use: Nutritional supplement, parenteral.

NeutraGuard Advanced. (Pascal) Fluo-
ride sodium 1.1%, wintermint flavor.
Dental Gel. 60 g. *Rx.*
Use: Prevention of dental caries.

neutral acriflavine.
See: Acriflavine.

Neutralin. (Dover Pharmaceuticals) Cal-
cium carbonate, magnesium oxide.
Tab. Sugar, lactose, and salt free. UD
Box 500s. *OTC.*
Use: Antacid.

neutral protamine hagedorn-insulin.
See: Insulin, N.P.H. Iletin.

●**neutramycin.** (NEW-trah-MY-sin) USAN.
A neutral macrolide antibiotic produced
by avariant strain of *Streptomyces rimosus.*
Use: Anti-infective.

Neutra-Phos. (Ortho-McNeil) Phosphorus 250 mg, potassium 278 mg, so-

dium 164 mg, fruit flavor. Pow. Bot. 64 g. UD Pkt. 1.25 g. *OTC.*
Use: Mineral supplement.
Neutra-Phos-K. (Ortho-McNeil) Phosphorus 250 mg, potassium 556 mg. Pow. Bot. 71 g. UD Pkt. 1.45 g. *OTC.*
Use: Mineral supplement.
Neutrexin. (US Bioscience) Trimetrexate glucuronate 25 mg. Pow. for Inj. (lyophilized). Vial 5 mL w/wo 50 mg leucovorin. *Rx.*
Use: Anti-infective.
neutroflavin.
See: Acriflavine.
Neutrogena Antiseptic Cleanser for Acne-Prone Skin. (Neutrogena) Benzethonium Cl, butylene glycol, methylparaben, menthol, peppermint oil, eucalyptus, mint, rosemary oils, witch hazel extract, camphor. Liq. Bot. 135 mL. *OTC.*
Use: Dermatologic, acne.
Neutrogena Baby Cleansing Formula Soap. (Neutrogena) Triethanolamine, glycerin, stearic acid, tallow, coconut oil, castor oil, sodium hydroxide, oleic acid, laneth-10 acetate, cocamide DEA, nonoxynol-14, PEG-4 octoate. Bar 105 g. *OTC.*
Use: Dermatologic, cleanser.
Neutrogena Body Lotion. (Neutrogena) Glyceryl stearate, isopropyl myristate, PEG-100 stearate, butylene glycol, imidazolidinyl urea, carbomer 934, parabens, sodium lauryl sulfate, triethanolamine, cetyl alcohol. Lot. Bot. 240 mL. *OTC.*
Use: Emollient.
Neutrogena Body Oil. (Neutrogena) Isopropyl myristate, sesame oil, PEG-40 sorbitan peroleate, parabens. Bot. 240 mL. *OTC.*
Use: Emollient.
Neutrogena Chemical-Free Sunblocker. (Neutrogena) Titanium dioxide, parabens, diazolidinyl urea, shea butter. SPF 17. Lot. Bot. 120 mL. *OTC.*
Use: Sunscreen.
Neutrogena Cleansing for Acne-Prone Skin. (Neutrogena) TEA-stearate, triethanolamine, glycerin, sodium tallowate, sodium cocoate, TEA-oleate, sodium ricinoleate, acetylated lanolin alcohol, cocamide DEA, TEA lauryl sulfate, tocopherol. Bar 105 g. *OTC.*
Use: Dermatologic, cleanser.
Neutrogena Clear Pore. (Neutrogena) Benzoyl peroxide 3.5%, glycerin, titanium dioxide, EDTA, menthol. Cleanser/mask. 125 mL. *OTC.*
Use: Dermatologic, acne.

Neutrogena Drying. (Neutrogena) Witch hazel, isopropyl alcohol, EDTA, parabens, tartrazine. Gel. Tube 22.5 mL. *OTC.*
Use: Dermatologic, acne.
Neutrogena Dry Skin Soap. (Neutrogena) Triethanolamine, stearic acid, tallow, glycerin, coconut oil, castor oil, sodium hydroxide, oleic acid, laneth-10 acetate, cocamide DEA, nonoxynol-14, PEG-14 octoate, BHT, O-tolyl biguanide. Bar 105 g, 165 g. Scented or unscented. *OTC.*
Use: Dermatologic, cleanser.
Neutrogena Glow Sunless Tanning. (Neutrogena) Octyl methoxycinnamate, cetyl alcohol, diazolidinyl urea, parabens, EDTA. SPF 8. Lot. Bot. 120 mL. *OTC.*
Use: Sunscreen.
Neutrogena Intensified Day Moisture. (Neutrogena) Octyl methoxycinnamate, 2-phenylbenzimidazole sulfonic acid, titanium dioxide, cetyl alcohol, diazolidinyl urea, parabens, EDTA. SPF 15. Cream 67.5 g. *OTC.*
Use: Dermatologic, moisturizer.
Neutrogena Lip Moisturizer. (Neutrogena) Octyl methoxycinnamate, benzophenone-3, corn oil, castor oil, mineral oil, lanolin oil, petrolatum, lanolin, stearyl alcohol. SPF 15. Lip balm 4.5 g. *OTC.*
Use: Lip protectant.
Neutrogena Moisture SPF 15. (Neutrogena) Octyl methoxycinnamate, benzophenone-3, glycerin, PEG-100 stearate, dimethicone, PEG-6000 monostearate, triethanolamine, parabens, imidazolidinyl urea, carbomer 954, PABA free. Lot. Bot. 120 mL. *OTC.*
Use: Sunscreen.
Neutrogena Moisture SPF 5. (Neutrogena) Octyl methoxycinnamate, petrolatum, cetyl alcohol, parabens, diazolidinyl urea, EDTA, cetyl alcohol. Lot. Bot 60 mL, 120 mL. *OTC.*
Use: Dermatologic, moisturizer.
Neutrogena Non-Drying Cleansing. (Neutrogena) Glycerin, caprylic/capric triglyceride, PEG-20 almond glycerides, cetyl ricinoleate, isohexadecane, TEA-cocoyl glutamate, PEG-20 methyl glucose sesquistearate, stearyl alcohol, cetyl alcohol, EDTA, dipotassium glycyrrhizate, stearyl glycyrrhetinate, bisabolol, parabens, acrylates/C 10-30 alkyl acrylate crosspolymer, triethanolamine, diazolidinyl urea. Lot. Bot. 165 mL. *OTC.*
Use: Dermatologic, cleanser.

Neutrogena Norwegian Formula Emulsion. (Neutrogena) Glycerin base 2%. Pump dispenser 5.25 oz. *OTC.*
Use: Emollient.

Neutrogena Norwegian Formula Hand Cream. (Neutrogena) Glycerin base 41%. Tube 2 oz. *OTC.*
Use: Emollient.

Neutrogena No-Stick Sunscreen. (Neutrogena) SPF 30. Homosalate 15%, octyl methoxycinnamate 7.5%, benzophenone-36%, octyl salicylate 5%, EDTA, parabens, diazolidinyl urea/ Cream. Waterproof 118 g. *OTC.*
Use: Sunscreen.

Neutrogena Oil-Free Acne Wash. (Neutrogena) Salicylic acid 2%, EDTA, propylene glycol, tartrazine, aloe extract. Liq. Dot. 100 mL. *OTC.*
Use: Dermatologic, acne.

Neutrogena Oily Skin Formula Soap. (Neutrogena) Triethanolamine, glycerin, fatty acids. Bar 3.5 oz. *OTC.*
Use: Dermatologic, cleanser.

Neutrogena Original Formula Soap. (Neutrogena) Triethanolamine, glycerin, fatty acids. Bar 3.5 oz, 5.5 oz. *OTC.*
Use: Dermatologic, cleanser.

Neutrogena Soap. (Neutrogena) TEA-stearate, triethanolamine, glycerin, sodium tallowate, sodium cocoate, sodium ricinoleate, TEA-oleate, cocamide DEA, tocopherol. Bar 105 g, 165 g. *OTC.*
Use: Dermatologic, cleanser.

Neutrogena Sunblock. (Neutrogena) **SPF 8:** Octyl methoxycinnamate, menthyl anthranilate, titanium dioxide, mineral oil. Cream 67.5 g. **SPF 15:** Octyl methoxycinnamate, octyl salicylate, menthyl anthranilate, mineral oil, titanium dioxide, propylparaben. Cream 67.5 g. **SPF 25:** Octyl methoxycinnamate, benzophenone-3, octyl salicylate, castor oil, cetearyl alcohol, propylparaben, shea butter. Stick 12.6 g. **SPF 30:** Octocrylene, octyl methoxycinnamate, menthyl anthranilate, zinc oxide, mineral oil, vitamin E. Cream 67.5 g. *OTC.*
Use: Sunscreen.

Neutrogena Sunscreen. (Neutrogena) Ethylhexyl p-methoxycinnamate 7%, oxybenzone 4%, titanium dioxide 2%. Tube 3 oz. *OTC.*
Use: Sunscreen.

Neutrogena T/Gel Original. (Neutrogena Corp) Coal tar extract 2%. Shampoo. Bot. 132 mL, 255 mL, 480 mL. *OTC.*
Use: Dermatologic.

Neutrogena T/Sal. (Neutrogena) Salicylic acid 2%, solubilized coal tar extract 2%. Shampoo. Bot. 135 mL. *OTC.*
Use: Antiseborrheic.

●**nevirapine.** (neh-VIE-rah-peen) *USP 28.*
Use: Antiviral.
See: Viramune.

●**nexeridine hydrochloride.** (NEX-eh-RIH-deen) USAN.
Use: Analgesic.

Nexium. (AstraZeneca) Esomeprazole magnesium 20 mg, 40 mg, sugar spheres, talc. DR Cap. Bot. 90s, 1000s, unit-of-use 30s, UD 100s. *Rx.*
Use: Proton pump inhibitor.

N.G.T. (Geneva) Triamcinolone acetonide 0.1%, nystatin 100,000 units/g. Cream. Tube 15 g. *Rx.*
Use: Antifungal; corticosteroid, topical.

NG-29.
Use: Diagnostic aid. [Orphan Drug]

Niacal. (Jones Pharma) Calcium lactate 324 mg, niacin 25 mg. Tab. Peppermint flavor. Bot. 100s, 1000s. *OTC.*
Use: Vasodilator; vitamin supplement.

●**niacin.** (NYE-uh-sin) *USP 28.*
Use: Antihyperlipidemic; vitamin, enzyme co-factor.
See: Niacal.
　Ni Cord XL.
　Niacor.
　Nico-400.
　Nicotinic Acid.
　Slo-Niacin.
　Span Niacin 300.
W/Combinations.
See: Advicor.
　Lipo-Nicin.

●**niacinamide.** (nye-ah-SIN-ah-mide) *USP 28.*
Use: Vitamin, enzyme co-factor.
W/Pentylenetetrazol, thiamine hydrochloride, cyanocobalamin, alcohol.
See: Cenalene.
W/Potassium iodide.
See: Riboflavin and Niacinamide, Amp.

niacinamide (nicotinamide). (Various Mfr.) Niacinamide (nicotinamide) 100 mg, 500 mg. Tab. Bot. 100s, 250s. *Rx-OTC.*
Use: Vitamin supplement; pellagra.

Niacor. (Upsher-Smith) Niacin 500 mg, lactose. Tab. Bot. 100s. *Rx.*
Use: Vitamin supplement, antihyperlipidemic.

Nialexo-C. (Roberts) Niacin 50 mg, vitamin C 30 mg. Tab. Bot. 100s. *OTC.*
Use: Vitamin supplement.

Niarb Super. (Miller Pharmacal Group) Magnesium 100 mg, vitamin C 200 mg, niacinamide 200 mg (as ascorbate).

Tab. Bot. 100s. *OTC.*
Use: Mineral, vitamin supplement.
Niaspan. (Kos Pharmaceuticals) Niacin 500 mg, 750 mg, 1000 mg. ER Tab. Bot. 100s. *Rx.*
Use: Antihyperlipidemic.
Niazide. (Major) Trichlormethiazide 4 mg. Tab. Bot. 100s, 1000s. *Rx.*
Use: Diuretic.
niazo. Neotropin.
Use: Antiseptic, urinary.
•**nibroxane.** (nye-BROX-ane) USAN.
Use: Antimicrobial, topical.
nicamindon.
See: Nicotinamide.
•**nicardipine hydrochloride.** (NYE-CAR-dih-peen) USAN.
Tall Man: NiCARdipine
Use: Vasodilator, calcium channel blocker.
See: Cardene.
Cardene IV.
Cardene SR.
nicardipine hydrochloride. (Mylan) Nicardipine hydrochloride 20 mg, 30 mg. Cap. Bot. 90s, 500s. *Rx.*
Use: Vasodilator, calcium channel blocker.
N'ice. (GlaxoSmithKline) Menthol 5 mg. Loz. in sugarless sorbitol base, saccharin. Pkg. 16s. *OTC.*
Use: Anesthetic, local.
N'ice 'n Clear. (GlaxoSmithKline) Menthol 5 mg, sorbitol. Loz. Pkg. 16s. *OTC.*
Use: Anesthetic, local.
•**nicergoline.** (nice-ERR-go-leen) USAN.
Use: Vasodilator.
N'ice Throat Spray. (GlaxoSmithKline) Menthol 0.12%, glycerin 25%, alcohol 23%, glucose, saccharin, sorbitol. Spray. 180 mL. *OTC.*
Use: Mouth and throat preparation.
N'ice w/Vitamin C Drops. (Heritage Consumer) Ascorbic acid 60 mg, menthol, sorbitol, orange flavor. Loz. Pks. 16s. *OTC.*
Use: Vitamin supplement; anesthetic, local.
Nichols Syphon Powder. (Last) Sodium bicarbonate, sodium Cl, sodium borate. Pouch 12.2 g (add to 32 oz. water to yield isotonic soln.).
•**niclosamide.** (nye-CLOSE-ah-mide) USAN.
Use: Anti-helminthic.
nicobion.
See: Nicotinamide.
Nicoderm CQ. (GlaxoSmithKline Consumer) Nicotine 7 mg, 14 mg, 21 mg/day (dose absorbed in 24 hours). Trans-

dermal system. Box 7s (21 mg only), 14s, original and clear patches. *OTC.*
Use: Smoking deterrent.
nicoduozide. A mixture of nicothazone and isoniazid.
Nicomide. (Sirius) Nicotinamide 750 mg, zinc oxide 25 mg, cupric oxide 1.5 mg, folic acid 500 mg. Tab. 60s. Rx.
Use: Nutritional supplement.
•**nicorandil.** (NIH-CAR-an-dill) USAN.
Use: Coronary vasodilator.
Ni Cord XL Caps. (Scot-Tussin) Nicotinic acid 400 mg. Cap. Bot. 100s, 500s. *OTC.*
Use: Vitamin supplement.
Nicorette. (GlaxoSmithKline Consumer) Nicotine polacrilex 2 mg, 4 mg/square; orange, mint, and original flavors. Chewing gum. Box 48, 108, 168 pieces. *OTC.*
Use: Smoking deterrent.
nicotamide.
See: Nicotinamide.
nicothazone. Nicotinal dehydethiose micarbazone.
nicotilamide.
See: Nicotinamide.
nicotinamide. Niacinamide, *USP.* Vitamin B$_3$, aminicotin, dipegyl, nicamindon, nicotamide, nicotilamide, nicotinic acid amide.
nicotinamide adenine dinucleotide. Name used for Nadide.
nicotine. (NIK-oh-TEEN) *USP 28.*
Use: Smoking cessation adjunct.
See: Nicotene Inhalation System.
Nicotine Nasal Spray.
Nicotine Polacrilex.
Nicotine Transdermal System.
nicotine gum. Various Mfr. Nicotine polacrilex 2 mg, 4 mg/square. Chewing gum. Box 48, 108 pieces. *OTC.*
Use: Smoking deterrent.
nicotine inhalation system.
Use: Smoking deterrent.
See: Nicotrol Inhaler.
nicotine nasal spray.
Use: Smoking deterrent.
See: Nicotrol NS.
•**nicotine polacrilex.** (NIK-oh-TEEN PAHL-ah-KRILL-ex) *USP 28.*
Use: Smoking cessation adjunct.
See: Commit.
Nicorette.
Nicotine Gum.
nicotine resin complex.
See: Nicotine Polacrilex.
•**nicotine transdermal system.** *USP 28.*
Use: Smoking cessation adjunct.

nicotine transdermal system.
Use: Smoking deterrent.
See: Habitrol.
  Nicoderm CQ.
  Nicotrol.
  Prostep.
nicotine transdermal system. Various
  Mfr. Nicotine 7 mg, 14 mg, 21 mg/day
  (dose absorbed in 24 hours). Transdermal system. Box 7s, 30s. *OTC.*
  Use: Smoking deterrent.
nicotinic acid. Niacin, *USP.*
nicotinic acid. (Various Mfr.) Nicotinic
  acid. **Tab.:** 50 mg, 100 mg, 250 mg,
  500 mg. Bot. 100s, 250s (50 mg,
  100 mg only), 1000s (500 mg only). **TR
  Tab.:** 250 mg, 500 mg. Bot. 100s, 250s
  (250 mg only), 1000s (500 mg only).
  SR Tab.: 500 mg. Bot. 100s. **ER Cap.:**
  250 mg, 400 mg. Bot. 100s, 1000s
  (250 mg only). **SR Cap.:** 125 mg,
  500 mg. Bot. 100s. **TR Cap.:** 250 mg,
  500 mg. Bot. 100s, 1000s (500 mg
  only). *Rx-OTC.*
  Use: Vitamin supplement.
nicotinic acid amide. Niacinamide,
  USP.
  See: Niacinamide.
nicotinic acid w/combinations.
  See: Niacin w/Combinations.
• **nicotinyl alcohol.** (NIK-oh-TIN-ill AL-
  koe-hahl) USAN.
  Use: Vasodilator, peripheral.
nicotinyl tartrate. 3-Pyridinemethanol
  tartrate.
Nicotrol. (Pharmacia) Nicotine 5 mg,
  10 mg, 15 mg (released gradually over
  16 hours). Trans. system. Box 7s, 14s.
  OTC.
  Use: Smoking deterrent.
Nicotrol Inhaler. (Pharmacia) Nicotine
  4 mg delivered (10 mg/cartridge). Inhaler Kit contains mouthpiece, storage
  trays each containing 6 cartridges,
  1 plastic storage case, patient information leaflet. Box 42s, 168s. *Rx.*
  Use: Smoking deterrent.
Nicotrol NS. (Pharmacia) Nicotine
  0.5 mg per actuation (10 mg/mL), parabens, EDTA. Spray pump. Bot. 10 mL.
  (200 sprays). Each unit has a glass container mounted with metered spray
  pump. *Rx.*
  Use: Smoking deterrent.
nieraline.
  See: Epinephrine.
Nifediac CC. (Teva) Nifedipine 30 mg,
  60 mg, 90 mg. Lactose. ER Tab. 100s,
  300s (except 90 mg), 1000s (except
  90 mg). *Rx.*
  Use: Calcium channel blocker.

Nifedical XL. (Teva) Nifedipine 30 mg,
  60 mg, lactose. ER Tab. Bot. 100s,
  300s. *Rx.*
  Use: Calcium channel blocker.
• **nifedipine.** (nye-FED-ih-peen) *USP 28.*
  Tall Man: NIFEdipine
  Use: Coronary vasodilator; calcium
  channel blocker; urinary tract agent.
  [Orphan Drug]
  See: Adalat.
  Adalat CC.
  Afeditab CR.
  Nifediac CC.
  Nifedical XL.
  Procardia.
  Procardia XL.
nifedipine. (Mylan) Nifedipine 30 mg,
  60 mg, 90 mg. ER Tab. Bot. 100s, 300s
  (except 90 mg). *Rx.*
  Use: Calcium channel blocker.
nifedipine. (Various Mfr.) Nifedipine
  10 mg, 20 mg. Cap. In 100s, 300s. *Rx.*
  Use: Calcium channel blocker.
Niferex. (Schwarz Pharma) Polysaccha-
  ride iron complex. Iron 100 mg/5 mL,
  alcohol 10%, sorbitol. Dye free, sugar
  free. Elix. Bot. 237 mL. *OTC.*
  Use: Mineral supplement.
Niferex. (Ther-Rx) Polysaccharide-iron
  complex. Iron 60 mg, lactose. Cap. UD
  100s. *OTC.*
  Use: Mineral supplement.
Niferex 150. (Ther-Rx) Polysaccharide
  iron complex equivalent to iron
  150 mg, calcium ascorbate and calcium
  threonate 50 mg. Cap. UD 100s. *OTC.*
  Use: Mineral supplement.
Niferex-150 Forte Capsules. (Ther-Rx)
  Elemental iron as polysaccharide-iron
  complex 150 mg, folic acid 1 mg, vitamin B_{12} 25 mcg. Bot. 100s, 1000s. *Rx.*
  Use: Mineral, vitamin supplement.
Niferex-PN. (Ther-Rx) Iron 60 mg, folic
  acid 1 mg, vitamins C 50 mg, B_{12}
  3 mcg, A 4000 units, D 400 units, B_1
  3 mg, B_2 3 mg, B_6 2 mg, B_3 10 mg, Zn
  18 mg, Ca, sorbitol. Bot. 30s, 100s,
  1000s. *Rx.*
  Use: Mineral, vitamin supplement.
Niferex-PN Forte. (Ther-Rx) Calcium
  250 mg, iron 60 mg, vitamins A
  5000 units, D 400 units, E 30 mg, B_1
  3 mg, B_2 3.4 mg, B_3 20 mg, B_6 4 mg,
  B_{12} 12 mcg, C 80 mg, folic acid 1 mg,
  Cu, I, Mg, Zn 25 mg. Bot. 100s. *Rx.*
  Use: Mineral, vitamin supplement.
• **nifluridide.** (nye-FLURE-ih-DIDE) USAN.
  Use: Ectoparasiticide.
• **nifungin.** (nih-FUN-jin) USAN. Substance derived from *Aspergillus gigan-
  teus.*

●**nifuradene.** (NYE-fyoor-ad-EEN) USAN.
Use: Anti-infective.

●**nifuraldezone.** (NYE-fer-AL-dee-zone) USAN. (Eaton Medical)
Use: Anti-infective.

●**nifuratel.** (NYE-fyoor-at-ell) USAN.
Use: Anti-infective; antifungal; antiprotozoal, trichomonas.

●**nifuratrone.** (nye-FYOOR-ah-trone) USAN.
Use: Anti-infective.

●**nifurdazil.** (NYE-fyoor-dazz-ill) USAN.
Use: Anti-infective.

nifurethazone.
Use: Anti-infective.

●**nifurimide.** (nye-FYOOR-ih-MIDE) USAN.
Use: Anti-infective.

●**nifurmerone.** (NYE-fyoor-MER-ohn) USAN.
Use: Antifungal.

nifuroxime.
Use: Antifungal; anti-infective, topical; antiprotozoal.
See: Micofur.

●**nifurpirinol.** (nye-fer-PIHR-ih-nole) USAN.
Use: Anti-infective.

●**nifurquinazol.** (NYE-fyoor-KWIN-azz-ole) USAN.
Use: Anti-infective.

●**nifurthiazole.** (NYE-fyoor-THIGH-ah-zole) USAN.
Use: Anti-infective.

nifurtimox.
Use: CDC anti-infective agent.
See: Lampit.

Nighttime Pamprin. (Chattem) Diphenhydramine hydrochloride 50 mg, acetaminophen 650 mg. Pow. Pkg. 4s. *OTC.*
Use: Sleep aid.

Nighttime Sleep Aid. (Rugby) Diphenhydramine hydrochloride 50 mg. Tab. Bot. 50s. *OTC.*
Use: Antihistimine, non-selective ethanolamine.

NightTime TheraFlu. (Novartis) Pseudoephedrine hydrochloride 60 mg, chlorpheniramine maleate 4 mg, dextromethorphan HBr 30 mg, acetaminophen 1000 mg. Pow. 6s. *OTC.*
Use: Analgesic; antihistamine; antitussive; decongestant.

nigrin. Streptonigrin.
Use: Antineoplastic.

Niko-Mag. (Scruggs) Magnesium oxide 500 mg. Cap. Bot. 100s, 1000s. *OTC.*
Use: Antacid.

Nikotime TD Caps. (Major) Niacin 125 mg, 250 mg. TD Cap. Bot. 100s, 1000s. *OTC.*
Use: Vitamin supplement.

Nilandron. (Aventis) Nilutamide 50 mg, 150 mg, lactose. Tab. Bot. 90s (50 mg only), 30s (150 mg only). *Rx.*
Use: Antineoplastic; hormone, antiandrogen.

Nilspasm. (Parmed Pharmaceuticals, Inc.) Phenobarbital 50 mg, hyoscyamine sulfate 0.31 mg, atropine sulfate 0.06 mg, scopolamine hydrobromide 0.0195 mg. Tab. Bot. 100s, 1000s. *Rx.*
Use: Anticholinergic; antispasmodic; hypnotic; sedative.

Nilstat Ointment & Cream. (Wyeth) Nystatin 100,000 units/g. **Cream base:** w/Emulsifying wax, isopropyl myristate, glycerin, lactic acid, sodium hydroxide, sorbic acid 0.2%. Tube 15 g, Jar 240 g. **Oint. base:** w/light mineral oil, Plastibase 50 W. Tube 15 g. *Rx.*
Use: Antifungal, topical.

Nilstat Oral. (Wyeth) Nystatin 500,000 units. FC Tab. Bot. 100s, UD 10 × 10s. *Rx.*
Use: Antifungal.

Nilstat Oral Suspension. (Wyeth) Nystatin 100,000 units/mL, methylparaben 0.12%, propylparaben 0.03%, cherry flavor. Bot. 60 mL w/dropper, 16 fl oz. *Rx.*
Use: Antifungal.

Nilstat Powder. (Wyeth) Nystatin pow. 150 million, 1 billion, 2 billion units. Bot. *Rx.*
Use: Antifungal.

Nil Tuss. (Minnesota Pharm) Dextromethorphan HBr 10 mg, chlorpheniramine maleate 1.25 mg, phenylephrine hydrochloride 5 mg, ammonium Cl 83 mg/5 mL. Syr. Bot. Pt. *OTC.*
Use: Antihistamine; antitussive; decongestant; expectorant.

●**nilutamide.** (nye-LOO-tah-mide) USAN.
Use: Antineoplastic; hormone, antiandrogen.
See: Nilandron.

●**nilvadipine.** (NILL-vah-DIH-peen) USAN.
Use: Antagonist, calcium channel.

Nil Vaginal Cream. (Century) Sulfanilamide 15%, 9-aminoacridine hydrochloride 0.2%, allantoin 1.5%. Bot. 4 oz. w/applicator. *OTC.*
Use: Anti-infective, vaginal.

●**nimazone.** (nih-mah-ZONE) USAN.
Use: Anti-inflammatory.

Nimbex. (GlaxoSmithKline) Cisatracurium besylate 2 mg/mL, Vial 5 mL, 10 mL; 10 mg/mL, Vial 20 mL. Inj. *Rx.*

Use: Nondepolarizing neuromuscular blocker; muscle relaxant.

Nimbus. (Biomerica) Monoclonal antibody-based enzyme immunoassay. Screens for urinary chorionic gonadotropin. Pkg. 10s, 25s, 50s. *Rx.*
Use: Diagnostic aid.

•**nimodipine.** (NYE-MOE-dih-peen) *USP 28.*
Use: Vasodilator, calcium channel blocker
See: Nimotop.

Nimotop. (Bayer) Nimodipine 30 mg. Liq. Cap. Bot. UD 30s, 100s. *Rx.*
Use: Calcium channel blocker.

Nion B Plus C. (Nion Corp.) Vitamins B$_1$ 15 mg, B$_2$ 10.2 mg, B$_3$ 50 mg, B$_5$ 10 mg, C 300 mg. Capl. Bot 100s. *OTC.*
Use: Vitamin supplement.

Niong. (US Ethicals) Nitroglycerin 2.6 mg, 6.5 mg. CR Tab. Bot. 100s. *Rx.*
Use: Antianginal.

Nipent. (SuperGen) Pentostatin 10 mg/vial. Mannitol 50 mg/vial. Pow. for Inj. Vial. Single-dose. *Rx.*
Use: Antineoplastic.

Niratron. (Progress) Chlorpheniramine maleate 4 mg/5 mL. Bot. pt. *Rx.*
Use: Antihistamine.

Niravam. (Schwarz Pharma) Alprazolam 0.25 mg, 0.5 mg, 1 mg, 2 mg. Sucralose, sucrose. Orange flavor. Orally Disintegrating Tab. 100s. *Rx.*
Use: Antianxiety agent.

•**niridazole.** (nye-RIH-dah-ZOLE) USAN.
Use: Antischistosomal.

•**nisbuterol mesylate.** (NISS-BYOO-teh-role) USAN.
Use: Bronchodilator.

•**nisobamate.** (NYE-so-BAM-ate) USAN.
Use: Anxlolytic, hypnotic; sedative.

•**nisoldipine.** (nye-SOLE-dih-peen) USAN.
Use: Vasodilator, coronary; calcium channel blocker.
See: Sular.

•**nisoxetine.** (NISS-OX-eh-teen) USAN.
Use: Antidepressant.

•**nisterime acetate.** (nye-STEER-eem) USAN.
Use: Androgen.

•**nitarsone.** (NITE-AHR-sone) USAN.
Use: Antiprotozoal, histomonas.

•**nitazoxanide.** (nye-tah-ZOX-ah-nide)
Use: Antiprotozoals.
See: Alinia.

Nite Time Children's. (Topco) Pseudoephedrine hydrochloride 10 mg, chlorpheniramine maleate 0.67 mg, dextromethorphan HBr 5 mg/5 mL, sucrose,

cherry flavor, alcohol free. Liq. Bot. 118 mL. *OTC.*
Use: Upper respiratory combination, decongestant, antihistimine, antitussive.

Nite Time Cold Formula. (Alra) Pseudoephedrine hydrochloride 10 mg, doxylamine succinate 1.25 mg, dextromethorphan HBr 5 mg, acetaminophen 167 mg, alcohol 25%. Liq. Bot. 180 mL, 300 mL. *OTC.*
Use: Analgesic; antihistamine; antitussive; decongestant.

Nite Time Cold Formula for Adults. (Alpharma) Dextromethorphan HBr 5 mg, doxylamine succinate 2.1 mg, pseudoephedrine hydrochloride 10 mg, acetaminophen 167 mg/5 mL, alcohol 10%, saccharin, corn syrup, original and cherry flavors. Liq. Bot. 177 mL. *OTC.*
Use: Upper respiratory combination, antitussive, antihistimine, decongestant, analgesic.

•**nitisinone.** (nit-IS-i-none) USAN.
Use: Tyrosinemia.

•**nitralamine hydrochloride.** (nye-TRAL-ah-meen) USAN.
Use: Antifungal.

•**nitramisole hydrochloride.** (nye-TRAM-ih-sole) USAN.
Use: Anthelmintic.

nitrates.
Use: Vasodilator.
See: Amyl Nitrate.
   Isosorbide Dinitrate.
   Isosorbide Mononitrate.
   Nitroglycerin.

•**nitrazepam.** (nye-TRAY-zeh-pam) USAN.
Use: Anticonvulsant; hypnotic; sedative.

Nitrek. (Bertek) Nitroglycerin 22.4 mg, 44.8 mg, 67.2 mg. Patch. Box 30s. *Rx.*
Use: Antianginal.

•**nitrendipine.** (NIGH-TREN-dih-peen) USAN.
Use: Antihypertensive.

•**nitric acid.** (NYE-trick) *NF 23.*
Use: Pharmaceutic aid, acidifying agent.
See: INOmax.

nitric acid silver. Silver Nitrate.
nitric oxide. (Ohmeda)
Use: Primary pulmonary hypertension agent. [Orphan Drug]
See: INOmax.

Nitro-Bid IV. (Hoechst) Nitroglycerin 5 mg/mL. Inj. Vial 1 mL box 10s; 5 mL Box 10s; 10 mL Box 5s. *Rx.*
Use: Antianginal.

Nitro-Bid Ointment. (Hoechst) Nitroglycerin (glyceryl trinitrate) 2%, in lanolin and petrolatum base. Tube 20 g, 60 g, UD 1 g (100s). *Rx.*
Use: Antianginal.

Nitrocap. (Freeport) Nitroglycerin 2.5 mg. TR Cap. Bot. 100s. *Rx.*
Use: Antianginal.

•**nitrocycline.** (NYE-troe-SIGH-kleen) USAN.
Use: Anti-infective.

•**nitrodan.** (NYE-troe-dan) USAN.
Use: Anthelmintic.

Nitrodisc. (Roberts) Nitroglycerin. Transdermal nitroglycerin discs releasing 16 mg, 24 mg, 32 mg. Patch. Ctn. 30s, 100s. *Rx.*
Use: Antianginal.

Nitro-Dur. (Key) Nitroglycerin. Transdermal system releasing 20 mg, 40 mg, 60 mg, 80 mg, 120 mg, 160 mg. Patch. Ctn. 30s, 100s, UD 30s, 100s (except 120 mg). *Rx.*
Use: Antianginal.

Nitrofan Caps. (Major) Nitrofurantoin 50 mg, 100 mg. Cap. Bot. 100s, 500s. *Rx.*
Use: Anti-infective, urinary.

nitrofurans.
See: Furazolidone.
Nitrofurantoin.

•**nitrofurantoin.** (nye-troe-FYOOR-antoyn) *USP 28.*
Use: Anti-infective, urinary.
See: Furadantin.
Macrobid.
Macrodantin.

nitrofurantoin. (Various Mfr.) Nitrofurantoin as macrocrystals 50 mg, 100 mg. Cap. Bot. 100s, 500s, 1000s. *Rx.*
Use: Anti-infective, urinary.

nitrofurantoin. (Various Mfr.) Nitrofurantoin (as monohydrate/macrocrystals) 100 mg. Cap. 100s, 500s. *Rx.*
Use: Anti-infective, urinary.

•**nitrofurazone.** (nye-troe-FYOOR-azone) *USP 28.*
Use: Anti-infective, topical.
See: Furacin.

nitrofurazone. (Various Mfr.) Nitrofurazone. **Top. Soln.:** 0.2%. Bot. Pt., gal. **Oint.:** 0.2%. Tube 480 g. *Rx.*
Use: Anti-infective, topical.

Nitrogard. (Forest) Transmucosal nitroglycerin 2 mg, 3 mg. Buccal CR Tab. Bot. 100s, UD 100s. *Rx.*
Use: Vasodilator.

•**nitrogen.** (NYE-troe-jen) *NF 23.*
Use: Pharmaceutic aid, air displacement.

nitrogen monoxide. Laughing Gas, Nitrous Oxide.
Use: Anesthetic, general; analgesic.

nitrogen mustard.
See: Mustargen.

nitrogen mustard derivatives.
See: Leukeran.
Mustargen hydrochloride.
Triethylene Melamine.

nitrogen mustards.
Use: Alkylating agents.
See: Chlorambucil.
Cyclophosphamide.
Ifosfamide.
Mechlorethamine Hydrochloride.
Melphalan.

nitroglycerin.
Use: Vasodilator.
See: Minitran.
Niglycon.
Niong.
Nitrek.
Nitro.
Nitro-Bid.
Nitrocels.
Nitrodisk.
Nitro-Dur.
Nitrodyl.
Nitrogard.
Nitrolingual.
Nitro-Lyn.
NitroQuick.
Nitrospan.
Nitrostat.
NitroTab.
Nitro-Time.
Transderm-Nitro.

•**nitroglycerin.** (nye-troe-GLH-suh-rin) (Various Mfr.) Nitroglycerin 0.3 mg (1/200 gr), 0.4 mg (1/150 gr), 0.6 mg (1/100 gr). Sublingual Tab. 25s (0.4 mg only), 100s. *Rx.*
Use: Antianginal.

nitroglycerin. (Various Mfr.) Nitroglycerin 5 mg/mL. Inj. Vial 5 mL, 10 mL. *Rx.*
Use: Antianginal.

nitroglycerin. (Various Mfr.) Nitroglycerin 2.5 mg, 6.5 mg, 9 mg. SR Cap. Bot. 30s (9 mg only), 60s, 100s, UD 60s (2.5 mg only), 100s. *Rx.*
Use: Vasodilator.

•**nitroglycerin, diluted.** (nye-troe-GLIH-suh-rin) *USP 28. Formerly Glyceryl Trinitrate.*
Use: Vasodilator, coronary.

nitroglycerin in 5% dextrose. (Various Mfr.) Nitroglycerin. **25 mg, 100 mg:** Inj. Soln. 250 mL. **50 mg:** Inj. Soln. 250, 500 mL. **200 mg:** Inj. Soln. 500 mL. *Rx.*
Use: Antianginal.

nitroglycerin injection. (Abbott) Nitroglycerin 25 mg/mL. Vial 5 mL, 10 mL.
Use: Antianginal; vasodilator.
See: Tridil.

nitroglycerin, intravenous.
Use: Vasodilator.
See: Nitro-Bid IV.

nitroglycerin ointment. (Various Mfr.) Nitroglycerin 2% in lanolin-petrolatum base. Tube 30 g, 60 g. *Rx.*
Use: Vasodilator.

nitroglycerin patch.
Use: Antianginal.
See: Nitrek.

nitroglycerin transdermal. (Mylan) Nitroglycerin 0.1 mg. Patch (4 cm^2 area). 30s. *Rx.*
Use: Vasodilator.

nitroglycerin transdermal. (Various Mfr.) Nitroglycerin 18 mg to 02.5 mg, 32 mg to 125 mg, or 75 mg to 187.5 mg (some systems have different release rates). Transdermal system. Box 30s. *Rx.*
Use: Vasodilator.

nitroglycerin transdermal system. (Hercon Laboratories, Inc.) Nitroglycerin 37.3 mg, 74.6 mg, 111.9 mg. Patch Pkg. 30s. *Rx.*
Use: Vasodilator.

nitroglycerol.
See: Nitroglycerin.

Nitrolan. (Elan) Protein 60 g, fat 40 g, carbohydrates 160 g, Na 690 mg, K 1.17 g/L, lactose free. With appropriate vitamins and minerals. Liq. In 237 mL *Tetra Pak* containers and 1000 mL *New Pak* closed systems with and without *Color Check. OTC.*
Use: Nutritional supplement.

Nitrolin. (Schein) Nitroglycerin 2.5 mg, 9 mg. SR Cap. **2.5 mg:** Bot. 100s. **9 mg:** Bot. 60s. *Rx.*
Use: Antianginal.

Nitrolingual. (Horizon) Nitroglycerin translingual aerosol 0.4 mg/metered dose. Canister 14.48 g containing 200 metered doses. Box 1s. *Rx.*
Use: Vasodilator.

Nitro-Lyn. (Lynwood) Nitroglycerin 2.5 mg. Cap. Bot. 100s. *Rx.*
Use: Antianginal.

nitromannite.
See: Mannitol Hexanitrate.

nitromannitol.
See: Mannitol Hexanitrate.

Nitromed. (US Ethicals) Nitroglycerin 2.6 mg, 6.5 mg. CR Tab. Bot. 100s. *Rx.*
Use: Antianginal.

•**nitromersol.** (nye-troe-MER-sole) *USP 28.*

Use: Anti-infective, topical.

•**nitromide.** (NYE-troe-mid) USAN.
Use: Anti-infective.

•**nitromifene citrate.** (nye-TROE-mih-feen) USAN.
Use: Antiestrogen.

Nitronet. (US Ethicals) Nitroglycerin 2.6 mg, 6.5 mg. CR Tab. Bot. 100s. *Rx.*
Use: Antianginal.

Nitropress. (Abbott) Sodium nitroprusside 50 mg/2 mL. Vial. *Rx.*
Use: Antihypertensive.

nitroprusside sodium.
Use: Antihypertensive.
See: Nitropress (Abbott).
Sodium Nitroprusside.

NitroQuick. (Ethex) Nitroglycerin 0.3 mg (1/200 g), 0.4 mg (1/150 g), 0.6 mg (1/100 g), lactose. Subling. Tab. Bot. 25s (0.4 mg only), 100s. *Rx.*
Use: Vasodilator.

nitrosoureas.
Use: Alkylating agent; antineoplastic.
See: Carmustine.
Lomustine.
Streptozocin.

Nitrostat. (Parke-Davis) Nitroglycerin 0.3 mg (1/200 g), 0.4 mg (1/150 g), 0.6 mg (1/100 g), lactose, sucrose. Tab. Bot. 100s. *Rx.*
Use: Vasodilator.

Nitrostat IV. (Parke-Davis) Nitroglycerin for infusion. **0.8 mg/mL:** Amp. 10 mL. **5 mg/mL:** Amp. 10 mL, Vial 10 mL. **10 mg/mL:** Vial 10 mL. *Rx.*
Use: Antianginal.

NitroTab. (Able) Nitroglycerin 0.3 mg (1/200 gr), 0.4 mg (1/150 gr), 0.6 mg (1/100 gr), lactose. Sublingual Tab. Bot. 100s. *Rx.*
Use: Vasodilator.

Nitro Time. (Time Cap Labs) Nitroglycerin 2.5 mg, 6.5 mg, 9 mg, lactose, sucrose. SR Cap. Bot. 60s, 90s, 100s. *Rx.*
Use: Antianginal.

nitrous acid, sodium salt. Sodium Nitrite.

•**nitrous oxide.** *USP 28.* Laughing Gas. Nitrogen Monoxide.
Use: Anesthesia, inhalation.

•**nivazol.** (NIH-vah-ZOLE) USAN.
Use: Corticosteroid, topical.

Nivea Moisturizing. (Beiersdorf) **Cream:** Mineral oil, petrolatum, lanolin alcohol, glycerin, microcrystalline wax, paraffin, magnesium sulfate, decyloleate, octyl dodecanol, aluminum stearate, citric acid, magnesium stearate. 120 g, 180 g, 300 g, 480 g. **Lot.:** Mineral oil, lanolin, isopropyl myristate, cetearyl al-

cohol, glyceryl stearate, acrylamide/ sodium acrylate copolymer, simethicone, methychloroisothiazolinone, methylisothiazolinone. In 180 mL, 300 mL, 450 mL. *OTC.*
Use: Emollient.

Nivea Moisturizing Creme Soap. (Beiersdorf) Sodium tallowate, sodium cocoate, glycerin, petrolatum, titanium dioxide, NaCl, octyldodecanol, macadamia nut oil, aloe, sodium thiosulfate, lanolin alcohol, pentasodium pentetate, EDTA, BHT, beeswax. Bar 90 g, 150 g. *OTC.*
Use: Dermatologic, cleanser.

Nivea Oil. (Beiersdorf) Emulsion of neutral aliphatic hydrocarbons. **Liq.:** Bot. 2 oz, 4 fl oz, pt, qt. **Cream:** Tube 1 oz, 2⅓ oz, Jar 4 oz, 6 oz, 1 lb, 5 lb. tin. **Soap:** Bath or toilet size. *OTC.*
Use: Emollient.
See: Basic.

Nivea Sun. (Beiersdorf) Octyl methoxycinnamate, octyl salicylate, benzophenone-3, 2-phenylbenzimidazole-5-sulfonic acid. Lot. Bot. 120 mL. *OTC.*
Use: Sunscreen.

•**nivimedone sodium.** (nih-VIH-mehdohn) USAN.
Use: Antiallergic.

Nix Creme Rinse. (Pfizer) Permethrin 1%. Isopropyl alcohol 20%, cetyl alcohol, parabens. Liq. (cream rinse). 60 mL with comb. *OTC.*
Use: Pediculicide.

•**nizatidine.** (nye-ZAT-ih-deen) *USP 28.*
Use: Histamine H_2 antagonist.
See: Axid AR.
    Axid Pulvules.

nizatidine. (Various Mfr.) Nizatidine 150 mg, 300 mg. Cap. 30s (300 mg only), 60s (150 mg only), 100s, 500s, 1000s (150 mg only), UD 100s (150 mg only). *Rx.*
Use: Histamine H_2 antagonist.

Nizoral A-D. (McNeil Consumer) Ketoconazole 1%. Shampoo. Bot. 207 mL. *OTC.*
Use: Antifungal, topical.

Nizoral Tablets. (Janssen) Ketoconazole 200 mg. Tab. Bot. 100s. *Rx.*
Use: Antifungal.

nmda receptors.
Use: Treatment of Alzheimer dementia.
See: Memantine hydrochloride.

n-methylhydrazine.
Use: Antineoplastic.
See: Procarbazine.

n-methylisatin beta-thiosemicarbazone. Under study.
Use: Smallpox protection.

N-Multistix. (Bayer Corp. (Consumer Div.)) Glucose, protein, pH, blood, ketones, bilirubin, urobilinogen, nitrate, leukocytes. Kit 100s. *Rx.*
Use: Diagnostic aid.

N-Multistix S. G. Reagent Strips. (Bayer Corp. (Consumer Div.)) Urinalysis reagent strip test for pH, protein, glucose, ketones, bilirubin, blood, nitrite, urobilinogen and specific gravity. Bot. 100s. *Rx.*
Use: Diagnostic aid.

n, n-diethylvanillamide.
See: Ethamivan.

No-Aspirin. (Walgreen) Acetaminophen 325 mg. Tab. Bot. 100s. *OTC.*
Use: Analgesic.

No-Aspirin Extra Strength. (Walgreen) Acetaminophen 500 mg. Tab. **Tab.:** Bot. 60s, 100s. **Cap.:** Bot. 50s, 100s. *OTC.*
Use: Analgesic.

•**noberastine.** (no-BER-ast-een) USAN.
Use: Antihistamine.

•**nocodazole.** (no-KOE-DAH-zole) USAN.
Use: Antineoplastic.

No Drowsiness Allerest. (Novartis) Pseudoephedrine hydrochloride 30 mg, acetaminophen 500 mg. Tab. Bot. 20s. *OTC.*
Use: Analgesic; decongestant.

No Drowsiness Sinarest. (Medeva) Pseudoephedrine hydrochloride 30 mg, acetaminophen 500 mg. Tab. Bot. 24s. *OTC.*
Use: Analgesic; decongestant.

nofetumomab merpentan.
See: Verluma.

•**nogalamycin.** (no-GAL-ah-MY-sin) USAN.
Use: Antineoplastic.

Nokane. (Wren) Salicylamide 4 g, n-acetyl-p-aminophenol 4 g, caffeine 0.5 gr. Tab. Bot. 40s. *OTC.*
Use: Analgesic combination.

Nolahist. (Amarin) Phenindamine tartrate 25 mg. Alcohol and dye free. Tab. Bot. 24s, 100s. *OTC.*
Use: Antihistamine, nonselective piperdine.

•**nolinium bromide.** (no-LIN-ee-uhm) USAN.
Use: Antisecretory; antiulcerative.

Nolvadex. (AstraZeneca) Tamoxifen citrate 10 mg, 20 mg. Tab. Box 30s (20 mg only), 60s (10 mg only). *Rx.*
Use: Antineoplastic; hormone; antiestrogen.

Nometic. Diphenidol.
Use: Antiemetic.

•nomifensine maleate. (NO-mih-FEN-seen) USAN.
Uour Antidepressant

Nonamin. (Western Research) Ca 100 mg, Cl 90 mg, Mg 50 mg, Zn 3.75 mg, Fe 4.5 mg, Cu 0.5 mg, I 37.5 mcg, K 49 mg, P 100 mg. Tab. Bot. 1000s. *OTC.*
Use: Mineral supplement.

nonbarbiturate sedative/hypnotic agents.
See: Sedative/Hypnotic Agents (Nonbarbiturate).

Non-Drowsy Allergy Relief for Kids. (Major) Loratadine 5 mg per 5 mL. Glycerin, sucrose. Fruit flavor. Syrup. 120 mL. *OTC.*
Use: Antihistamine.

Non-Drowsy Contac Sinus. (Glaxo-SmithKline) Pseudoephedrine hydrochloride 30 mg, acetaminophen 500 mg. Cap. Bot. 24s. *OTC.*
Use: Analgesic; decongestant.

None. (Forest) Heparin sodium 1000 units/mL. No preservatives. Amps 5 mL. Box 25s. *Rx.*
Use: Anticoagulant.

Non-Habit Forming Stool Softener. (Rugby) Docusate sodium 100 mg, sorbitol, parabens. Cap. Bot. 100s, 1000s. *OTC.*
Use: Laxative.

nonnarcotic analgesic combinations.
See: Aceta-Gesic.
Anacin.
Anacin Aspirin Free Extra Strength.
Anacin Aspirin Free Maximum Strength.
Anacin Maximum Strength.
APAP Plus.
Arthrotec.
Bayer Plus Extra Strength.
Bayer PM Extra Strength Aspirin Plus Sleep Aid.
BC Powder Arthritis Strength.
BC Powder Original Formula.
Diclofenac Sodium and Misoprostol.
Equagesic.
Excedrin Aspirin Free.
Excedrin Extra Strength.
Excedrin Migraine.
FemBack.
Fem-1.
Flextra-DS.
Goody's Body Pain.
Goody's Extra Strength Headache.
Magsal.
Micrainin.
Midol Maximum Strength Menstrual.
Midol Maximum Strength PMS.
Midol Teen Maximum Strength.

Mobigesic.
Naproxen and Lansoprazole.
P-A-C Analgesic.
Pamprin Maximum Pain Relief.
Pamprin Multi-Symptom Maximum Strength.
Prēmsyn PMS.
Saleto.
Summit Extra Strength.
Vanquish.
Vitelle Lurline PMS.
W/Barbiturates.
See: Americet.
Axocet.
Bucet.
Bupap.
Butalbital, Acetaminophen, and Caffeine.
Butalbital Compound.
Butex Forte.
Dolgic.
Esgic.
Esgic-Plus.
Fioricet.
Fiorinal.
Fiortal.
Margesic.
Marten Tab.
Medigesic.
Phrenilin.
Phrenilin Forte.
Repan.
Repan CF.
Sedapap.
Tencon.
Triad.

nonnarcotic antitussives.
See: Benzonatate.
Dextromethorphan HBr.
Dextromethorphan HBr/Benzocaine.
Diphenhydramine hydrochloride.

•non nucleoside reverse transcriptase inhibitors. *Rx.*
Use: Antiretroviral.
See: Delavirdine Mesylate.
Efavirenz.
Nevirapine.
Rescriptor.
Sustiva.

nonoxynol. (nahn-OCK-sih-nahl) (Ortho-McNeil) *OTC.*
Use: Contraceptive, spermicide.
See: Emko.

•nonoxynol-15. (NAHN-ox-sih-nahl 15) USAN.
Use: Pharmaceutic aid, surfactant.

•nonoxynol-4. (NAHN-ox-sih-nahl 4) USAN.
Use: Pharmaceutic aid, surfactant.

• **nonoxynol-9.** (NAHN-ox-sih-nahl 9)
USP 28.
Use: Spermaticide; pharmaceutic aid,
wetting and solubilizing agent.
See: Conceptrol.
Delfen.
Encare.
Gynol II.
Ortho-Gynol.
• **nonoxynol-10.** (nahn-OCK-sih-nahl 10)
NF 23.
Use: Pharmaceutic aid, surfactant.
• **nonoxynol-30.** (NAHN-ox-sih-nahl 30)
USAN. Under study.
Use: Pharmaceutic aid, surfactant.
nonselective alkylamines.
Use: Antihistamine.
See: Alkylamines, nonselective.
nonselective ethanolamines.
Use: Antihistamine.
See: Ethanolamines, nonselective.
nonselective piperazines.
Use: Antihistamine.
See: Piperazines, nonselective.
nonselective piperidines.
Use: Antihistamine.
See: Piperidines, nonselective.
nonspecific protein therapy.
See: Protein, Nonspecific Therapy.
nonsteroidal anti-inflammatory agents.
See: Celecoxib.
Diclofenac Potassium.
Diclofenac Sodium.
Etodolac.
Fenoprofen Calcium.
Flurbiprofen.
Ibuprofen.
Indomethacin.
Ketoprofen.
Ketorolac Tromethamine.
Meclofenamate Sodium.
Mefenamic Acid.
Meloxicam.
Nabumetone.
Naproxen.
Oxaprozin.
Piroxicam.
Rofecoxib.
Sulindac.
Tolmetin Sodium.
**nonsteroidal anti-inflammatory agents,
ophthalmic.**
See: Bromfenac.
Diclofenac Sodium.
Flurbiprofen Sodium.
Ketorolac Tromethamine.
Suprofen.
nonylphenoxypolyethoxy ethanol.
Nonoxynol.
Use: Contraceptive, spermicide.
See: Delfen.

No Pain-HP. (Young Again Products)
Capsaicin 0.075%. Roll-on. 60 mL.
OTC.
Use: Analgesic, topical.
Nora-BE. (Watson) Norethindrone
0.35 mg, lactose. Tab. 28s. *Rx.*
Use: Sex hormone, contraceptive hor-
mone.
• **noracymethadol hydrochloride.** (nahr-
ASS-ih-METH-ah-dole) USAN.
Use: Analgesic.
• **norbolethone.** (nahr-BOLE-eth-ohn)
USAN.
Use: Anabolic.
Norcet Tablets. (Holloway) Hydrocodone
bitartrate 5 mg, acetaminophen 500 mg.
Tab. Bot. 100s. *c-III.*
Use: Analgesic combination; narcotic.
Norco. (Watson) Hydrocodone bitartrate
10 mg, acetaminophen 325 mg. Tab.
Bot. 100s, 500s. *c-III.*
Use: Analgesic; narcotic.
Norco 5/325. (Watson) Hydrocodone bitartrate 5 mg, acetaminophen 325 mg,
sucrose. Tab. Bot. 100s, 500s. *c-III.*
Use: Narcotic analgesic combination.
Norcuron. (Organon Teknika) Vecuronium bromide 10 mg/5 mL. **With diluent:** Vial 5 mL lyophilized powder and
5 mL Amp. of sterile water for injection. Box 10s. **Without diluent:** Vial
5 mL lyophilized powder. Box 10s. **Prefilled syringe:** Vial 10 mL lyophilized
powder and 10 mL syringe w/bacterio-
static water for injection. Box 10s. *Rx.*
Use: Muscle relaxant.
norcycline.
Use: Anti-infective.
Nordette. (Barr/Duramed) Levonorgestrel 0.15 mg, ethinyl estradiol
30 mcg, lactose. Tab. *Pilpak*, 21s, 28s.
Rx.
Use: Sex hormone, contraceptive hormone.
Norditropin. (Novo/Nordisk) Somatropin.
Pow. for Inj., lyophilized: 4 mg
($\approx$ 12 units), 8 mg ($\approx$ 24 units), glycine
8.8 mg, mannitol 44 mg, Water for In-
jection with benzyl alcohol 1.5%. Vial
w/diluent. **Inj.:** 5 mg, 10 mg, 15 mg/mL,
phenol 4.5 mg, mannitol 60 mg (5 mg,
10 mg only), 58 mg (15 mg only). Cartridge. *Rx.*
Use: Hormone, growth.
Norel DM. (US Pharm) Dextromethorphan HBr 15 mg, chlorpheniramine
maleate 4 mg, phenylephrine hydrochloride 10 mg/5 mL, sorbitol, alcohol,
dye free. Liq. 473 mL. *OTC.*
Use: Antitussive combination.

norelgestromin/ethinyl estradiol.
Use: Sex hormone, contraceptive hormonal.
See: Ortho Evra.
Norel LA. (US Pharmaceuticals) Phenylephrine hydrochloride 40 mg, carbinoxamine maleate 8 mg. ER Tab. 100s. *Rx.*
Use: Decongestant and antihistamine.
●**norepinephrine bitartrate.** (NOR-eh-pih-NEFF-reen bye-TAR-trate) *USP 28.*
Formerly levarterenol bitartrate.
Use: Adrenergic, vasoconstricto, vasopressor.
See: Levophed.
norepinephrine bitartrate. (Abbott) Norepinephrine bitartrate 1 mg/mL, sodium metabisulfite 0.46 mg, sodium chloride 8.2 mg. Inj. Amps. 4 mL. *Rx.*
Use: Vasopressor.
●**norethindrone.** (nore-ethIN-drone) *USP 28.*
Use: Progestin.
See: Jolivette.
　Micronor.
　Norlutin.
　Nor-Q.D.
　Ortho Micronor.
W/Ethinyl estradiol.
See: Aranelle.
　Brevicon.
　Estrostep Fe.
　Estrostep 21.
　GenCept.
　Jenest-28.
　Junel 1/20.
　Junel 1.5/30.
　Leena.
　Loestrin Fe.
　Loestrin Fe 1/20.
　Loestrin Fe 1.5/30.
　Loestrin 21 1/20.
　Loestrin 21 1.5/30.
　Microgestin Fe 1.5/30.
　Microgestin Fe 1/20.
　Modicon.
　Nelova 0.5/35E.
　Nelova 1/35E.
　Nelova 10/11.
　Norinyl 1+ 35.
　Nortrel 1/35.
　Nortrel 0.5/35.
　Ortho-Novum 1/35.
　Ortho-Novum 10/11.
　Ortho-Novum 7/7/7.
　Ovcon-35.
　Ovcon-50.
　Tri-Norinyl.
W/Mestranol.
See: Necon 1/50.
　Nelova 1/50M.

　Norinyl 1+ 50.
　Ortho-Novum 1/50.
●**norethindrone acetate.** *USP 28.*
Use: Sex hormone, progestin.
See: Aygestin.
W/Ethinyl Estradiol.
See: CombiPatch.
　Femhrt.
norethindrone acetate. (Barr) Norethindrone acetate 5 mg. Tab. Bot. 50s. *Rx.*
Use: Sex hormone, progestin.
●**norethynodrel.** (nahr-eh-THIGH-nodrell) *USP 28.*
Use: Hormone, progestin.
See: Enovid.
Norflex. (3M) Orphenadrine citrate 100 mg. SR Tab. Bot. 100s, 500s. *Rx.*
Use: Muscle relaxant.
Norflex Injectable. (3M) Orphenadrine citrate 30 mg, sodium bisulfite 2 mg, sodium Cl 5.8 mg, water for injection qs 2 mL. Amp. 2 mL 6s, 50s. *Rx.*
Use: Muscle relaxant.
●**norfloxacin.** (nor-FLOX-uh-SIN) *USP 28.*
Use: Anti-infective.
See: Noroxin.
●**norflurane.** (nahr-FLEW-rane) USAN.
Under study.
Use: Anesthetic, general.
Norgesic Forte Tablets. (3M) Orphenadrine citrate 50 mg, aspirin 770 mg, caffeine 60 mg, lactose. Bot. 100s, 500s, UD 100s. *Rx.*
Use: Muscle relaxant; analgesic.
Norgesic Tablets. (3M) Orphenadrine citrate 25 mg, aspirin 385 mg, caffeine 30 mg, lactose. Bot. 100s, 500s, UD 100s. *Rx.*
Use: Muscle relaxant; analgesic.
●**norgestimate.** (nore-JEST-ih-mate) USAN. *Formerly Dexnorgestrel Acetime.*
Use: Hormone, progestin.
W/Ethinyl Estradiol.
See: MonoNessa.
　Ortho-Cyclen.
　Ortho-Prefest.
　Ortho Tri-Cyclen.
　Tri-Previfem.
●**norgestomet.** (nore-JESS-toe-met) USAN.
Use: Hormone, progestin.
●**norgestrel.** (nahr-JESS-trell) *USP 28.*
Use: Contraceptive; hormone, progestin.
See: Ovrette.
W/Ethinyl Estradiol.
See: Lo/Ovral.
　Low-Ogestrel.
　Ogestrel.

Ovral-28.

•norgestrel and ethinyl estradiol tablets. *USP 28.*
Use: Contraceptive.
See: Norinyl 1+35.

Norinyl 1 + 50. (Watson) Norethindrone 1 mg, mestranol 50 mcg, lactose. Tab. *Wallette.* 28s. *Rx.*
Use: Sex hormone, contraceptive hormone.

Norinyl 1 + 35. (Watson) Norethindrone 1 mg, ethinyl estradiol 35 mcg, lactose. Tab. *Wallette,* 28s. *Rx.*
Use: Sex hormone, contraceptive hormone.

Norinyl 2 mg. (Roche) Norethindrone 2 mg, mestranol 0.1 mg. Tab. *Memorette* Disp. of 20s. Refill folders of 20s. *Rx.*
Use: Contraceptive.

Norisodrine Aerosol. (Abbott) Norisodrine hydrochloride (isoproterenol hydrochloride) 0.25% (2.8 mg/mL) in inert chlorofluorohydrocarbon propellants, alcohol 33%, ascorbic acid 0.1% as preservative. Aerosol 15 mL. Box 12s. *Rx.*
Use: Bronchodilator.

Norisodrine/Calcium Iodide Syrup. (Abbott) Isoproterenol sulfate 3 mg, calcium iodide, anhydrous 150 mg/5 mL, alcohol 6%. Bot. Pt. *Rx.*
Use: Bronchodilator.

Noritate. (Dermik Labs) Metronidazole 1%. Parabens, glycerin. Cream. Tube 30 g. *Rx.*
Use: Dermatologic, acne.

Norlestrin Fe 1/50 Tablets. (Parke-Davis) Norethindrone acetate 1 mg, ethinyl estradiol 50 mcg. Compact 21 yellow Tab., 7 brown 75 mg ferrous fumarate Tab. Pkg. 5 compacts. Pkg. 5 refills; Ctn. 10 × 5 refills. *Rx.*
Use: Contraceptive.

Norlestrin Fe 2.5/50 Tablets. (Parke-Davis) Norethindrone acetate 2.5 mg, ethinyl estradiol 50 mcg. Compact 21 Tab., 7 brown 75 mg ferrous fumarate Tab. Pkg. 5 compacts. Pkg. 5 refills; Ctn. 10 × 5 refills. *Rx.*
Use: Contraceptive.

Norlestrin-28 1/50 Tablet. (Parke-Davis) Norethindrone acetate 1 mg, ethinyl estradiol 50 mcg. Compact 21 yellow, 7 white (inert) tablets. Pkg. 5 compacts. Pkg. 5 refills; Ctn. 10× 5 refills. *Rx.*
Use: Contraceptive.

Norlestrin-21 1/50 Tablets. (Parke-Davis) Norethindrone acetate 1 mg, ethinyl estradiol 50 mcg. Compact 21s. Pkg. 5 compacts. Pkg. 5 refills; Ctn. 10 × 5 refills. *Rx.*

Use: Contraceptive.

Norlestrin-21 2.5/50 Tablets. (Parke-Davis) Norethindrone acetate 2.5 mg, ethinyl estradiol 50 mcg. Tab. Compact 21s. Pkg. 5 compacts. Pkg. 5 refills; Ctn. 10 × 5 refills. *Rx.*
Use: Contraceptive.

Normaderm Cream & Lotion. (Doak Dermatologics) Buffered lactic acid in vanishing bases. **Cream:** Jar 3 ¾ oz, 16 oz. **Lot.:** Bot. 4 oz, 16 oz, 128 oz. *OTC.*
Use: Dermatologic, emollient.

normal human serum albumin. Albumin Human.

normal human serum albumin. (Baxter Healthcare) Normal human serum albumin. **5% Inj.:** 50 mL, 250 mL, 500 mL **25% Inj.:** 20 mL, 50 mL, 100 mL. *Rx.*
Use: Blood volume supporter.

Normaline. (Apothecary Prods.) Sodium chloride 250 mg. Tab. Bot. 200s, 500s. *OTC.*
Use: Ophthalmic.

normal saline.
See: Sodium chloride 0.9%.

Normodyne. (Key) Labetalol hydrochloride 5 mg/mL, dextrose, EDTA 0.1 mg, methylparaben 0.8 mg, propylparaben 0.1 mg. Inj. Multidose vial 20 mL, prefilled syringe. 4 mL, 8 mL. *Rx.*
Use: Antiadrenergic/sympatholytic, alpha/beta-adrenergic blocker.

Normol. (Alcon) Sterile, isotonic solution of thimerosal 0.004%, chlorhexidine gluconate 0.005%, edetate disodium 0.1%. Bot. 8 oz. *OTC.*
Use: Contact lens care.

Normosol-M. (Abbott) Na$^+$ 40 mEq, K$^+$ 13 mEq, Mg^{++} 3 mEq, Cl$^-$ 40 mEq, acetate 16 mEq, osmolarity 10% mOsm/L, ph ≈ 6. Soln. Single-dose container 1000 mL. *Rx.*
Use: Intravenous nutritional therapy, intravenous replenishment therapy.

Normosol-M and 5% Dextrose. (Abbott) Dextrose 50 g, calories 170, Na$^+$ 40 mEq, K$^+$ 13 mEq, Mg^{++} 3 mEq, Cl$^-$ 40 mEq, acetate 16 mEq, osmolarity 363 mOsm/L. Soln. Bot. 500 mL, 1000 mL. *Rx.*
Use: Intravenous nutritional therapy, intravenous replenishment solution.

Normosol-R. (Abbott) Na$^+$ 140 mEq, K$^+$ 5 mEq, Mg^{++} 3 mEq, Cl$^-$ 98 mEq, acetate 27 mEq, gluconate 23 mEq, osmolarity 294 mOsm/L, preservative free, ph ≈ 6. Soln. Single-dose container 500 mL, 1000 mL. *Rx.*
Use: Intravenous nutritional therapy, intravenous replenishment solution.

Normosol-R and 5% Dextrose. (Abbott) Dextrose 50 g, calories 185, Na⁺ 140 mEq, K⁺ 5 mEq, Mg⁺⁺ 3 mEq, Cl⁻ 98 mEq, acetate 27 mEq, gluconate 23 mEq, osmolarity 547 mOsm/L. Soln. Bot. 500 mL, 1000 mL. *Rx.*
Use: Intravenous nutritional therapy, intravenous replenishment solution.

Normosol-R pH 7.4. (Abbott) Na⁺ 140 mEq, K⁺ 5 mEq, Mg⁺⁺ 3 mEq, Cl⁻ 98 mEq, acetate 27 mEq, gluconate 23 mEq, osmolarity 295 mOsm/L, preservative free. Soln. Single-dose container 500 mL, 1000 mL. *Rx.*
Use: Intravenous nutritional therapy, intravenous replenishment solution.

Normotensin. (Marcen) Mucopolysaccharide 20 mg, sodium nucleate 25 mg, epinephrine-neutralizing factor 25 units, sodium citrate 10 mg, inositol 5 mg, phenol 0.5%/mL. IM Soln. for Inj. Multi-dose vial 10 mL, 30 mL. *Rx.*
Use: Antihypertensive.

Norolon. (Sanofi-Synthelabo) Chloroquine phosphate. *Rx.*
Use: Antimalarial.

Noroxin. (Merck & Co.) Norfloxacin 400 mg. Tab. Bot. 100s, UD 20s, UD 100s. *Rx.*
Use: Urinary anti-infective, fluoroquinolone.

Norpace. (Pharmacia) Disopyramide phosphate 100 mg, 150 mg, lactose. Cap. Bot. 100s, 1000s. *Rx.*
Use: Antiarrhythmic.

Norpace CR. (Pharmacia) Disopyramide phosphate 100 mg, 150 mg, sucrose. ER Cap. Bot. 100s, 500s, UD 100s. *Rx.*
Use: Antiarrhythmic.

Norphyl. (Vita Elixir) Aminophylline 100 mg. Tab. *Rx.*
Use: Bronchodilator.

Norpramin. (Hoechst) Desipramine hydrochloride 10 mg, 25 mg, 50 mg, 75 mg, 100 mg, 150 mg. Tab. Bot. 50s (150 mg only), 100s (except 150 mg), UD 100s (25 mg, 50 mg only). *Rx.*
Use: Antidepressant.

Nor-QD. (Watson) Norethindrone 0.35 mg, lactose. Tab. 28s. *Rx.*
Use: Sex hormone, contraceptive hormone.

Nortrel 1/35. (Barr) Ethinyl estradiol 35 mcg, norethindrone 1 mg, lactose. Tab. Pkt. 21s, 28s. *Rx.*
Use: Sex hormone, contraceptive hormone.

Nortrel 0.5/35. (Barr) Ethinyl estradiol 35 mcg, norethindrone 0.5 mg, lactose. Tab. Pkt. 21s, 28s. *Rx.*
Use: Sex hormone, contraceptive hormone.

nortriptyline. (Various Mfr.) Nortriptyline 10 mg, 25 mg, 50 mg, 75 mg. Cap. 100s, 500s. *Rx.*
Use: Antidepressant.

• **nortriptyline hydrochloride.** (nor-TRIP-tih-leen) *USP 28.*
Use: Antidepressant.
See: Aventyl hydrochloride.
  Aventyl hydrochloride Pulvule.
  Pamelor.

nortriptyline hydrochloride. (Various Mfr.). **Soln.:** Nortriptyline base 10 mg/ 5 mL, may contain alcohol, sorbitol. Soln. Bot. 480 mL, UD 12.5 mL. **Cap.:** Nortriptyline hydrochloride 10 mg, 25 mg, 50 mg, 75 mg. Bot. 100s, 500s, 1,000s; blister pack 25s (except 75 mg), 100s, 600s; UD 100s (except 75 mg). *Rx.*
Use: Antidepressant.

Norval. Docusate sodium.
Use: Laxative.

Norvasc. (Pfizer) Amlodipine **2.5 mg:** Bot. 90s, 100s; **5 mg:** Bot. 90s, 100s, 300s, UD 100s; **10 mg:** Bot. 90s, 100s, UD 100s. *Rx.*
Use: Calcium channel blocker.

Norvir. (Abbott) Ritonavir. **Soft Gelatin Cap.:** 100 mg, ethanol. Bot. 120s. **Oral Soln.:** 80 mg/mL, saccharin, ethanol, peppermint, caramel flavors. Bot. 240 mL. *Rx.*
Use: Antiretroviral, protease inhibitor.

Norwich Extra Strength. (Procter & Gamble) Aspirin 500 mg. Tab. Bot. 150s. *OTC.*
Use: Analgesic.

Nosalt. (GlaxoSmithKline) Potassium Cl, potassium bitartrate, adipic acid, mineral oil, fumaric acid. Na < 10 mg/5 g (0.43 mEq/5 g), K 2502 mg/5 g (64 mEq/5 g). Pkg. 330 g. *OTC.*
Use: Salt substitute.

Nosalt Seasoned. (GlaxoSmithKline) Potassium Cl, dextrose, onion, and garlic, spices, lactose, cream of tartar, paprika, silica, disodium inosinate, disodium guanylate, turmeric. Na < 5 mg/5 g (0.2 mEq/5 g), K 1328 mg/ 5 g (34 mEq/5 g). Pkg. 240 g. *OTC.*
Use: Salt substitute.

• **noscapine.** (NAHS-kah-peen) *USP 28.*
Use: Antitussive.

noscapine hydrochloride. l-Narcotine-hydrochloride.
Use: Antitussive.
See: Noscaps.

Noscaps. (Table Rock) Noscapine 7.5 mg, chlorpheniramine maleate 1 mg, phenylephrine hydrochloride 5 mg, N-acetyl-p-aminophenol 150 mg,

salicylamide 150 mg, vitamin C 20 mg. Cap. Bot. 100s, 500s. *OTC.*
Use: Analgesic; antihistamine; decongestant; vitamin C.

Nose Better. (Lee Pharm.) Allentoin 0.5%, camphor 0.75%, menthol 0.5%, lanolin, methylparaben. Gel. Tube 12.9 g. *OTC.*
Use: Upper respiratory combination, topical.

Noskote. (Schering-Plough) Oxybenzone 3%, homosalate 8%. SPF 8. Cream 13.2 g, 30 g. *OTC.*
Use: Sunscreen.

Noskote Sunblock. (Schering-Plough) Padimate O 8%, oxybenzone 3%, benzyl alcohol. SPF 15. Cream. Tube 30 g. *OTC.*
Use: Sunscreen.

Nostril. (Boehringer Ingelheim) Phenylephrine hydrochloride 0.25%, 0.5%, benzalkonium Cl 0.004% in buffered aqueous soln. Bot. 15 mL, pump spray. *OTC.*
Use: Decongestant.

Nōstrilla 12-Hour. (Heritage) Oxymetazoline hydrochloride 0.05%, benzalkonium chloride, glycine, sorbitol. Soln. Spray bot. 15 mL. *OTC.*
Use: Nasal decongestant, imidazoline.

Notuss PD. (Stewart-Jackson) Hydrocodone bitartrate 4 mg, dexchlorpheniramine maleate 2 mg, phenylephrine hydrochloride 5 mg/5 mL. Menthol, sorbitol, sugar. Grape flavor. Liq. 473 mL. *c-III.*
Use: Antitussive combination.

Nouriva Repair. (Ferndale) Petrolatum, paraffin, mineral oil, sorbitan oleate, carnauba wax, ceramide 3, cholesterol, glycerin, oleic acid, palmitic acid, acrylates/C 10–30 albyl acrylate crosspolymer, tromethamine. Cream. 30 g. *OTC.*
Use: Emollient.

Novacet. (Medicis) Sodium sulfacetamide 100 mg, sulfur 50 mg, benzyl alcohol, cetyl alcohol, sodium thiosulfate, EDTA. Lot. Bot. 30 mL. *Rx.*
Use: Dermatologic, acne.

Novacort. (Primus) Hydrocortisone acetate 2%, pramoxine 1%. Alcohols, aloe, glycerin. Gel. Tubes. 29 g. *Rx.*
Use: Anti-inflammatory agent.

Nova-Dec. (Rugby) Iron 18 mg, vitamins A 5000 units, D 400 units, E 30 units, B_1 1.7 mg, B_2 2 mg, B_3 20 mg, B_5 10 mg, B_6 3 mg, B_{12} 6 mcg, C 60 mg, folic acid 0.4 mg, Ca, Cr, Cu, I, Mg, Mo, Mn, P, Se, K, Zn 15 mg, vitamin K, Cl, Ni, Sn, V, B, biotin 30 mcg. Tab. Bot. 130s. *OTC.*

Use: Mineral, vitamin supplement.

Novadyne Expectorant. (Various Mfr.) Pseudoephedrine 30 mg, codeine phosphate 10 mg, guaifenesin 100 mg/5 mL, alcohol 7.5%. Bot. 120 mL, pt, gal. *c-III.*
Use: Antitussive; decongestant; expectorant.

Novagest Expectorant w/Codeine. (Major) Pseudoephedrine hydrochloride 30 mg, codeine phosphate 10 mg, guaifenesin 100 mg/5 mL, alcohol 8.2%, sugar, menthol, parabens. Liq. Bot. 118 mL, 473 mL. *c-v.*
Use: Upper respiratory combination, antitussive, decongestant, expectorant.

novamidon.
See: Aminopyrine.

Novamine. (Clintec Nutrition) Amino acid concentration 11.4%, for infusion. Nitrogen 1.8 g/100 mL. Essential amino acids (mg/100 mL): Isoleucine 570, leucine 790, lysine 900, methionine 570, phenylalanine 790, threonine 570, tryptophan 190, valine 730. Nonessential amino acids (mg/100 mL): Alanine 1650, arginine 1120, histidine 680, proline 680, serine 450, tyrosine 30, glycine 790, glutamic acid 570, aspartic acid 330, acetate 114 mEq/L, sodium metabisulfite 30 mg/100 mL. In 250 mL, 500 mL, 1 liter. *Rx.*
Use: Parenteral nutritional supplement.

Novamine 15%. (Clintec Nutrition) Amino acids 15%: Lysine 1.18 g, leucine 1.04 g, phenylalanine 1.04 g, valine 960 mg, isoleucine 749 mg, methionine 749 mg, threonine 749 mg, tryptophan 250 mg, alanine 2.17 g, arginine 1.47 g, glycine 1.04 g, histidine 894 mg, proline 894 mg, glutamic acid 749 mg, serine 592 mg, aspartic acid 434 mg, tyrosine 39 mg, nitrogen 2.37 g/100 mL. Inj. 500 mL, 1000 mL. *Rx.*
Use: Nutritional supplement, parenteral.

Novamine Without Electrolytes. (Clintec Nutrition) Amino acid concentration 8.5%, for infusion. Nitrogen 1.35 g/100 mL. Essential amino acids (mg/100 mL): Isoleucine 420, leucine 590, lysine 673, methionine 420, phenylalanine 590, threonine 420, tryptophan 140, valine 550. Nonessential amino acids (mg/100 mL): Alanine 1240, arginine 840, histidine 500, proline 500, serine 340, tyrosine 20, glycine 590, glutamic acid 420, aspartic acid 250, acetate 88 mEq/L, sodium bisulfite 30 mg/100 mL. In 500 mL, 1 liter. *Rx.*
Use: Nutritional supplement, parenteral.

Novantrone. (Serono) Mitoxantrone hydrochloride 2 mg free base/mL, sodium chloride 0.8%, sodium acetate 0.005%, acetic acid 0.046%, preservative free. Inj. Multi-dose Vial 10 mL, 12.5 mL, 15 mL. *Rx.*
Use: Antineoplastic; immunologic agent, immunomodulator; anthracenedione.

Novarel. (Ferring) Chorionic gonadotropin 10,000 units per vial with 10 mL diluent (1,000 units per mL), mannitol, benzyl alcohol 0.9%. Pow. for Inj. Vials. 10 mL. *Rx.*
Use: Ovulation stimulant.

Novasal. (US Pharm) Magnesium salicylate tetrahydrate 600 mg. Tab. 100s. *Rx.*
Use: Nonnarcotic analgesic combination.

NovaSource Renal. (Novartis Nutrition) Protein (sodium and calcium caseinates, arginine, taurine, carnitine) 74 g, carbohyrates (corn syrup, fructose, hydrolyzed corn starch) 200 g, fat (high oleic sunflower oil, corn oil, medium chain triglycerides, soy lecithin) 100 g/L, vitamins A, B_1, B_2, B_3, B_5, B_6, B_{12}, C, D, E, K, folic acid, biotin, choline, Ca chloride, Cu, Fe, I, Mg, Mn, P, Se, Zn, Na 1000 mg (43.5 mEq)/L, Na 1600 mg/complete feeding *Brik* Paks) (70 mEq)/L (closed system), K 810 mg (20.8 mEq)/L, K 1100 mg/complete feeding *Brik* Paks (28.2 mEq)/L (closed system), H_2O 700 mOsm/kg (complete feeding *Brik* Paks), H_2O 960 mOsm/kg (closed system), 2 cal/mL, vanilla flavor. Liq. *Tetra Brik* Paks 237 mL (27s), closed system containers 1000 mL (6s). *OTC.*
Use: Enteral nutritional therapy.

novatropine.
See: Homatropine Methylbromide.

Novocain. (Abbott) Procaine hydrochloride 1%, 10%. Inj. *Uni-Amp* 2 mL. Single-dose amp. 6 mL w/acetone sodium bisulfite (1% only). Multidose vial 30 mL w/acetone sodium bisulfite, chlorobutanol (1% only). *Rx.*
Use: Anesthetic, local ester.

Novocain for Spinal Anesthesia. (Sanofi-Synthelabo) Procaine hydrochloride 10% soln. Amp. 2 mL. Box 25s. *Rx.*
Use: Anesthetic, spinal.

Novolin N. (Novo Nordisk) Human insulin (rDNA) 100 units/mL. Inj. Vials. 10 mL. *OTC.*
Use: Antidiabetic, insulin.

Novolin N PenFill. (Novo Nordisk) Human insulin (rDNA) 100 units/mL. Cartridges. 5 × 1.5, 5 × 3 mL. Use with *NovoPen* and *Novolin Pen.* *OTC.*
Use: Antidiabetic, insulin.

Novolin N Prefilled. (Novo Nordisk) Human insulin (rDNA) 100 units/mL. Inj. Prefilled syringes. 5 × 1.5 mL. *OTC.*
Use: Antidiabetic, insulin.

Novolin R. (Novo Nordisk) Human insulin (rDNA) 100 units/mL. Inj. Vials. 10 mL. *OTC.*
Use: Antidiabetic, insulin.

Novolin R PenFill. (Novo Nordisk) Human insulin (rDNA) 100 units/mL. Cartridges. 5 × 1.5, 5 × 3 mL. Use with *NovoPen* and *Novolin Pen.* *OTC.*
Use: Antidiabetic, insulin.

Novolin R Prefilled. (Novo Nordisk) Human insulin (rDNA) 100 units/mL. Inj. Prefilled syringes. 5 × 1.5 mL. *OTC.*
Use: Antidiabetic, insulin.

Novolin 70/30. (Novo Nordisk) Human insulin (rDNA) 100 units/mL. Inj. Vials. 10 mL. *OTC.*
Use: Antidiabetic, insulin.

Novolin 70/30 PenFill. (Novo Nordisk) Human insulin (rDNA) 100 units/mL. Cartridges. 5 × 1.5 mL, 5 × 3 mL. Use with *NovoPen* and *Novolin Pen.* *OTC.*
Use: Antidiabetic, insulin.

Novolin 70/30 Prefilled. (Novo Nordisk) Human insulin (rDNA) 100 units/mL. Inj. Prefilled syringes. 5 × 1.5 mL. *OTC.*
Use: Antidiabetic, insulin.

NovoLog. (Novo Nordisk) Human insulin aspart (rDNA) 100 units/mL. Inj. *PenFill* cartridges. 3 mL. Vials. 10 mL. *Rx.*
Use: Antidiabetic, insulin.

NovoLog Mix 70/30. (Novo Nordisk) Insulin aspart 100 units/mL. 70% insulin aspart (rDNA origin) protamine suspension and 30% insulin aspart (rDNA origin). Inj. 3 mL *PenFill* cartridges and 3 mL *FlexPen* prefilled syringes. *Rx.*
Use: Antidiabetic, insulin.

NovoSeven. (Novo/Nordisk) Human coagulation factor VIIa (recombinant) Vial 1.2 mg, 2.4 mg, 4.8 mg. *Rx.*
Use: Antihemophilic.

Noxzema Antiseptic Cleanser Sensitive Skin Formula. (Noxell Corp.) Benzalkonium Cl 0.13%. Bot. 4 oz, 8 oz. *OTC.*
Use: Dermatologic, cleanser.

Noxzema Antiseptic Skin Cleanser. (Noxell Corp.) SD 40 alcohol 63%. Bot. 4 oz, 8 oz. *OTC.*
Use: Dermatologic, cleanser.

Noxzema Antiseptic Skin Cleanser Extra Strength Formula. (Noxell Corp.) SD 40 alcohol 36%, isopropyl alcohol 34%. Bot. 4 oz, 8 oz. *OTC.*

Use: Dermatologic, cleanser.
Noxzema Clear Ups. (Noxell Corp.) Salicylic acid 0.5% on pads. Jar 50s. *OTC.*
Use: Dermatologic, acne.
Noxzema Clear Ups Acne Medicine Maximum Strength Lotion. (Noxell Corp.) Benzoyl peroxide 10%. Bot. 1 oz. Vanishing formula. *OTC.*
Use: Dermatologic, acne.
Noxzema Clear Ups Maximum Strength. (Noxell Corp.) Salicylic acid 2% on pads. Jar 50s. *OTC.*
Use: Dermatologic, acne.
Noxzema Medicated Skin Cream. (Noxell Corp.) Menthol, camphor, clove oil, eucalyptus oil, phenol. Jar 2.5 oz, 4 oz, 6 oz, 10 oz. Tube 4.5 oz. Bot. 6 oz., 14 oz. Pump Bottle 10.5 oz. *OTC.*
Use: Counterirritant.
Noxzema On-The-Spot. (Noxell Corp.) Benzoyl peroxide 10% in vanishing and tinted lotion. Bot. 0.25 oz. *OTC.*
Use: Dermatologic, acne.
NPH Iletin II. (Lilly) Isophane insulin (NPH) 100 units/mL purified pork. Inj. Vials. 10 mL. *OTC.*
Use: Antidiabetic, insulin.
NTBC.
Use: Tyrosinemia type 1. [Orphan Drug]
N-Trifluoroacetyladriamycin-14-valerate. (Anthra) *Rx.*
Use: Antineoplastic.
NTS Transdermal System. (Circa) Nitroglycerin transdermal system 5 mg/24 hours or 15 mg/24 hours. Box 30s. *Rx.*
Use: Antianginal.
NTZ Long-Acting. (Sanofi-Synthelabo) Oxymetazoline hydrochloride 0.05%, benzalkonium Cl, phenylmercuric acetate 0.002% as preservatives. Drops. Bot. 1 oz. Spray Bot. 1 oz. *OTC.*
Use: Decongestant.
Nubain. (Endo) Nalbuphine hydrochloride 10 mg/mL, 20 mg/mL. Parabens. Amp (available as sulfite/paraben-free) 1 mL. Vial 10 mL. *Rx.*
Use: Narcotic agonist-antagonist analgesic.
Nu-Bolic. (Seatrace) Nandrolone phenpropionate 25 mg/mL. Vial 5 mL. *c-iii.*
Use: Anabolic steroid.
nucite.
See: Inositol.
nucleoside reverse transcriptase inhibitors.
Use: Antiretroviral.
See: Abacavir.
Didanosine.
Emtricitabine.
Lamivudine.
Stavudine.

Zalcitabine.
Zidovudine.
nucleoside analog reverse transcriptase inhibitor combination.
Use: Antiretroviral.
See: Abacavir/Lamivudine.
Abacavir Sulfate/Lamivudine/Zidovudine.
Emtricitabine/Tenofovir Disoproxil Fumarate.
Lamivudine/Zidovudine.
nucleotide analog reverse transcriptase inhibitor.
Use: Antiretroviral.
See: Tenofovir Disoproxil Fumarate.
Nucofed. (Monarch) Codeine phosphate 20 mg, pseudoephedrine hydrochloride 60 mg/5 mL or Cap. **Syr.:** Sorbitol, sucrose, mint flavor, alcohol free. Bot. 473 mL. **Cap.:** Lactose. Bot. 60s. *c-iii.*
Use: Antitussive; decongestant.
Nucofed Expectorant. (Monarch) Codeine phosphate 20 mg, pseudoephedrine hydrochloride 60 mg, guaifenesin 200 mg/5 mL, alcohol 12.5%, saccharin, sucrose, cherry flavor. Syr. Bot. 473 mL. *c-iii.*
Use: Upper respiratory combination, antitussive, decongestant, expectorant.
Nucofed Pediatric Expectorant. (Monarch) Codeine phosphate 10 mg, pseudoephedrine hydrochloride 30 mg, guaifenesin 100 mg/5 mL, alcohol 6%, EDTA, saccharin, sucrose, strawberry flavor. Syr. Bot. 473 mL. *c-v.*
Use: Upper respiratory combination, antitussive, decongestant, expectorant.
Nucotuss Expectorant. (Alra) Pseudoephedrine hydrochloride 60 mg, codeine phosphate 20 mg, guaifenesin 200 mg/5 mL, alcohol 12.5%. Syr. Bot. 473 mL. *c-iii.*
Use: Upper respiratory combination, antitussive, decongestant, expectorant.
Nucotuss Pediatric Expectorant. (Alra) Pseudoephedrine hydrochloride 30 mg, codeine phosphate 10 mg, guaifenesin 100 mg/5 mL, alcohol 6%, strawberry flavor. Syr. Bot. 473 mL. *c-v.*
Use: Upper respiratory combination, antitussive, decongestant, expectorant.
•**nufenoxole.** (NEW-fen-OX-ole) USAN.
Use: Antiperistaltic.
Nuhist. (Dayton) Phenylephrine tannate 5 mg, chlorpheniramine tannate 4.5 mg/5 mL, methylparaben, saccharin, sucrose. Susp. 473 mL. *Rx.*
Use: Decongestant and antihistamine.
Nu-Iron 150. (Merz) Polysaccharide-iron complex equivalent to 150 mg iron. Parabens, EDTA, castor oil, sucrose.

Cap. Bot. 100s. *OTC.*
Use: Mineral supplement.

Nu-Iron Plus Elixir. (Merz) Polysaccharide iron complex 300 mg, folic acid 3 mg, vitamin B_{12} 75 mcg/15 mL. Bot. 237 mL. *Rx.*
Use: Mineral, vitamin supplement.

Nu-Iron-V. (Merz) Polysaccharide iron 60 mg, folic acid 1 mg, vitamins A 4000 units, C 50 mg, D 400 units, B_1 3 mg, B_2 3 mg, B_3 10 mg, B_6 2 mg, B_{12} 3 mcg, Ca. Tab. Bot. 100s. *Rx.*
Use: Mineral, vitamin supplement.

NuLev. (Schwarz Pharma) L-hyoscyamine sulfate 0.125 mg, aspartame, mannitol, phenylalanine 1.7 mg, mint flavor. Orally disintegrating tab. Bot. 100s. *Rx.*
Use: Anticholinergic/antispasmodic.

Nul T900. (Duvic & 'sly) Potassium 16 mg, magnesium 13 mg, ascorbic acid 250 mg. Tab. Bot. 100s. *Rx.*
Use: Antiarrythmic.

NuLYTELY. (Braintree) PEG 3350 420 g, sodium bicarbonate 5.72 g, sodium chloride 11.2 g, potassium chloride 1.48 g, cherry, lemon-lime, orange flavors. Pow. for Recon. Disp. Jugs. 4 L. *Rx.*
Use: Laxative.

Numorphan. (Endo Laboratories) Oxymorphone hydrochloride. **Inj. 1 mg/mL:** Amp. 1 mL. **1.5 mg/mL:** Parabens. Multidose vials. 10 mL. **Supp.:** 5 mg. Box 6s. *c-II.*
Use: Opioid analgesic.

Numotizine Cataplasm. (Hobart) Guaiacol 0.26 g, beechwood creosote 1.302 g, methyl salicylate 0.26 g/100 g. Jar 4 oz. *OTC.*
Use: Analgesic, topical.

Numotizine Cough Syrup. (Hobart) Guaifenesin 5 g, ammonium Cl 5 g, sodium citrate 20 g, menthol 0.04 g/fl oz. Bot. 3 oz, pt, gal. *OTC.*
Use: Expectorant.

Numzident. (Purepac) Benzocaine 10%, PEG-400 NF 47.86%, PEG-3350 NF 10%, saccharin. Gel. 15 g. *OTC.*
Use: Anesthetic, local.

Numzit. (Purepac) Benzocaine, menthol, glycerin, methylparaben, alcohol 12%. Liq. Bot. 22.5 mL. *OTC.*
Use: Anesthetic, local.

Numzit Gel. (Purepac) Benzocaine, menthol. Tube 10 g. *OTC.*
Use: Anesthetic, local.

Numzit Teething Gel. (GlaxoSmithKline) Benzocaine 7.5%, peppermint oil 0.018%, clove leaf oil 0.09%, PEG-400 66.2%, PEG-3350 26.1%, saccharin

0.036%. Tube. 14.1 g. *OTC.*
Use: Anesthetic, local.

Numzit Teething Lotion. (GlaxoSmithKline) Benzocaine 0.2%, alcohol 12.1%, saccharin 0.02%, glycerin 2%, kelgin MU 0.5%, methylparaben. Lot. Bot. 15 mL. *OTC.*
Use: Anesthetic, local.

Nu-Natal Advanced. (Rising) Ca 200 mg, Fe (as carbonyl iron) 90 mg, vitamin D 400 units, E 30 units, B_1 3 mg, B_2 3.4 mg, B_3 20 mg, B_6 20 mg, B_{12} 12 mcg, C 120 mg, FA 1 mg, CU 2 mg, Mg, dioctyl sodium sulfosuccinate 50 mg, Zn 25 mg. Mineral oil. Film coated. Tab. UD 90s. *Rx.*
Use: Multivitamin.

nunol.
See: Phenobarbital.

Nupercainal. (Novartis) **Oint.:** Dibucaine 1%, acetone, sodium bisulfite, lanolin, mineral oil, white petrolatum. 30 g, 60 g. **Supp.:** Cocoa butter, zinc oxide, sodium bisulfite. 12s, 24s. *OTC.*
Use: Anesthetic, local (Oint., Cream); anorectal preparation (Supp.).

Nuprin. (Bristol-Myers Squibb) Ibuprofen 200 mg. Tab. Cap. Bot. 36s, 75s, 150s. *OTC.*
Use: Analgesic; NSAID.

Nuprin Backache. (Bristol-Myers Squibb) Magnesium salicylate tetrahydrate 580 mg (equivalent to 467 mg anhydrous magnesium salicylate). Capl. Bot. 50s. *OTC.*
Use: Anti-inflammatory.

Nuquin HP. (Stratus) **Cream:** 4% hydroquinone, octyl methoxycinnamate, glycerin, cetyl alcohol, cetostearyl alcohol, stearyl alcohol, sodium metabisulfite. Tube 14.2 g, 28.4 g, 56.7 g. **Gel:** 4% hydroquinone, 30 mg dioxybenzone per g. Alcohol, sodium metabisulfite, EDTA. Tube 14.2 g, 28.4 g. *Rx.*
Use: Dermatologic.

Nu-Salt. (Cumberland Packing Corp.) Potassium Cl, potassium bitartrate, calcium silicate, natural flavor derived from yeast. Sodium 0.85 mg/5 g (< 0.04 mEq/ 5 g), potassium 2640 mg/5 g (68 mEq/ 5 g). Pkg. 90 g. *OTC.*
Use: Salt substitute.

Nu-Tears. (Optopics) Polyvinyl alcohol 1.4%, EDTA, NaCl, benzalkonium chloride, potassium chloride. Soln. Bot. 15 mL. *OTC.*
Use: Artificial tears.

Nu-Tears II. (Optopics) Polyvinyl alcohol 1%, PEG-400 1%, EDTA, benzalkonium chloride. Soln. Bot. 15 mL. *OTC.*

Use: Artificial tears.

Nu-Thera. (Kirkman) Vitamins A 10,000 units, D 400 units, B_1 10 mg, B_2 5 mg, niacinamide 100 mg, B_6 1 mg, B_{12} 5 mcg, C 150 mg, Ca 103 mg, P 80 mg, Fe 10 mg, Mg 5.5 mg, Mn 1 mg, K 5 mg, Zn 1.4 mg. Cap. Bot. 100s. *OTC.*
Use: Mineral, vitamin supplement.

nutmeg oil.
Use: Pharmaceutic aid, flavor.

Nutracort. (Galderma) Hydrocortisone 1%. Cream Jar 4 oz. Tube 30 g, 60 g. *Rx.*
Use: Corticosteroid, topical.

Nutraderm. (Galderma) Oil-in-water emulsion. **Lot.:** Plastic bot. 8 oz, 16 oz. **Cream:** Tube 1.5 oz, 3 oz, Jar lb. *OTC.*
Use: Emollient.

Nutraderm Bath Oil. (Galderma) Mineral oil, PEG-4 dilaurate, lanolin oil, butylparaben, benzophenone-3, fragrance, D & C Green No. 6. Bot. 8 oz. *OTC.*
Use: Emollient.

Nutraloric. (Nutraloric) A chocolate, vanilla, or strawberry flavored liquid containing, when mixed with whole milk to make 1 L, 91.7 g protein, 175 g carbohydrates, 125 g fat, 875 mg Na, 3166.7 mg, K 2.2 calories/mL. Pow. Can 480 g. *OTC.*
Use: Nutritional supplement.

Nutrament Drink Box. (Drackett) Protein 10 g, fat 7 g, carbohydrate 35 g, vitamins, minerals/240 calories/8 oz. Liq. Drink Box. *OTC.*
Use: Nutritional supplement.

Nutrament Liquid. (Mead Johnson Nutritionals) Protein (calcium and sodium caseinates, skim milk, soy protein isolates [in all flavors except chocolate]) 44.5 g, carbohydrate (sugar, corn syrup) 144.6 g, fat (canola oil, high oleic sunflower oil, corn oil, soy lecithin) 27.8 g/L, vitamins A, B_1, B_2, B_3, B_5, B_6, B_{12}, C, D, E, K, biotin, folate, Ca, Cr, Cu, Fe, I, Mg, Mn, Mo, P, Se, Zn, Na 695 mg, K 1390 mg/L, 1 cal/mL, vanilla, strawberry, chocolate, banana, coconut, and eggnog flavors. Liq. Can. 12 oz. *OTC.*
Use: Nutritional supplement.

Nutramigen. (Bristol-Myers Squibb) Hypoallergenic formula that supplies 640 calories/qt. Protein 18 g, fat 25 g, carbohydrates 86 g, vitamins A 2000 units, D 400 units, E 20 units, C 52 mg, folic acid 100 mcg, B_1 0.5 mg, B_2 0.6 mg, niacin 8 mg, B_6 0.4 mg, B_{12} 2 mcg, biotin 50 mcg, pantothenic acid 3 mg, K-1 100 mcg, Cl 85 mg, inositol

30 mg, Ca 600 mg, P 400 mg, I 45 mcg, Fe 12 mg, Mg 70 mg, Cu 0.6 mg, Zn 5 mg, Mn 200 mcg, Cl 550 mg, K 700 mg, Na 300 mg/qt of formula (4.9 oz pow.). Liq. Can 16 oz, 390 mL concentrate, 1 qt ready-to-use. *OTC.*
Use: Nutritional supplement.

Nutramin. (Thurston) Vitamins A 666 units, D 66 units, B_1 666 mcg, B_2 333 mcg, niacinamide 2 mg, folic acid 0.0444 mcg, Ca 16.6 mg, P 8.33 mg, Fe 1.33 mg, I 0.15 mg. Tab. Bot. 200s, 500s, 1000s. *OTC.*
Use: Mineral, vitamin supplement.

Nutramin Granular. (Thurston) Vitamins A 333 units, D 333 units, B_1 3.3 mg, B_2 1.6 mg, niacinamide 10 mg, folic acid 0.133 mg, Ca 250 mg, P 115 mg, Fe 6.6 mg, I 0.15 mg/5 g. Bot. 10 oz, 32 oz. *OTC.*
Use: Mineral, vitamin supplement.

Nutraplus. (Galderma) Urea 10% in emollient cream base or lotion base with preservatives. **Cream:** Tube 3 oz, Jar lb. **Lot.:** Bot. 8 oz, 16 oz. *OTC.*
Use: Emollient.

Nutra-Soothe. (Pertussin) Colloidal oatmeal, light mineral oil. Emollient bath preparation. Pow. Pkts. 9s. *OTC.*
Use: Dermatologic.

Nutravims. (Health for Life Brands) Vitamins A 6000 units, D 1250 units, C 50 mg, E 5 units, B_{12} 5 mcg, B_1 3 mg, B_2 3 mg, B_6 0.5 mg, niacinamide 20 mg, calcium pantothenate 5 mg, Zn 1.5 mg, Mn 1 mg, I 0.15 mg, K 5 mg, Mg 4 mg, Fe 15 mg, Ca 59 mg, P 45 mg. Cap. Bot. 100s, 250s, 1000s. *OTC.*
Use: Mineral, vitamin supplement.

Nutren 1.5 Liquid. (Clintec Nutrition) Casein, maltodextrin, corn syrup, sucrose, MCT, corn oil, vitamins A, B_1, B_2, B_3, B_5, B_6, B_{12}, C, D, E, K, folic acid, biotin, choline, Ca, Cl, Cu, Fe, I, Mg, Mn, P, Zn. 250 mL. *OTC.*
Use: Nutritional supplement.

Nutren 1.0 Liquid. (Clintec Nutrition) Potassium and sodium caseinate, maltodextrin, sucrose, MCT, corn oil, lecithin, vitamins A, B_1, B_2, B_3, B_5, B_6, B_{12}, C, D, E, K, folic acid, biotin, choline, Ca, Cl, Cu, Fe, I, Mg, Mn, P, Zn. Can 250 mL. *OTC.*
Use: Nutritional supplement.

Nutren 2.0 Liquid. (Clintec Nutrition) Casein, maltodextrin, corn syrup, sucrose, MCT, corn oil, vitamins A, B_1, B_2, B_3, B_5, B_6, B_{12}, C, D, E, K, folic acid, biotin, choline, Ca, Cl, Cu, Fe, I, Mg, Mn, P, Zn. 250 mL. *OTC.*
Use: Nutritional supplement.

Nutr-E-Sol. (Advanced Nutritional Therapy) Vitamin E 133 units/5 mL, dye free. Liq. 473 mL. *OTC.*
Use: Vitamin.

Nutrex. (Holloway) Ca 162 mg, Fe 27 mg, vitamins A 5000 units, D 400 units, E 30 mg, B_1 2.25 mg, B_2 2.6 mg, B_3 20 mg, B_5 10 mg, B_6 3 mg, B_{12} 9 mcg, C 90 mg, folic acid 0.4 mg, Cu, I, K, Mg, Mn, P, Zn 22.5 mg, biotin 45 mcg. Tab. Bot. 100s. *OTC.*
Use: Mineral, vitamin supplement.

Nutricon Tablets. (Taylor Pharmaceuticals) Ca 200 mg, Fe 20 mg, vitamins A 2500 units, D 200 units, E 15 mg, B_1 1.5 mg, B_2 1.5 mg, B_3 10 mg, B_5 5 mg, B_6 2 mg, B_{12} 5 mcg, C 50 mg, folic acid 0.4 mg, Cu, I, Mg, Zn 3.75 mg, biotin 100 mcg. Bot. 120s. *OTC.*
Use: Mineral, vitamin supplement.

Nutri-E. (Nutri Vention) Vitamin E.
Cream: 200 units/g. Jar 1 oz, 2 oz. **Oil:** 1 oz. **Oint.:** 200 units/g. Tube 1 oz, 1.5 oz. **Cap.:** 200 units. Bot. 80s; 400 units. Bot. 60s, 100s; 800 units. Bot. 55s. *OTC.*
Use: Vitamin supplement.

Nutrifac ZX. (Rising Pharmaceuticals) Vitamin A 5000 units, D_3 400 units, E (succinate) 50 units, B_1 20 mg, B_2 20 mg, B_3 100 mg, B_5 25 mg, B_6 25 mg, B_{12} 50 mcg, C 500 mg, folic acid 1 mg, Zn 20 mg, Ca, Cr, Cu, Mg, Mn, Se, biotin 200 mcg, tartrazine, mineral oil. Tab. 60s. *Rx.*
Use: Multivitamin.

NutriFocus. (Ross) Protein (Na caseinate, milk protein isolate, soy protein isolate, arginine) 61.7 g, carbohydrate (corn syrup, sugar, fructooligosaccharides) 212.3 g, fat (canola oil, high-oleic safflower oil, corn oil, lecithin) 48.8 g/L, vitamins A, B_1, B_2, B_3, B_5, B_6, B_{12}, C, D, E, K, folic acid 417 mcg/L, beta carotene, biotin, choline, Ca, chloride, Cr, Cu, Fe, I, Mg, Mn, Mo, P, Se, Zn, Na 917 mg, K 1668 mg/L, fiber 20.85 g/L, 1.5 cal/mL, lactose and gluten free, chocolate and vanilla flavors. Liq. Can. 240 mL. *OTC.*
Use: Enteral nutritional therapy.

NutriHeal. (Nestle) Protein 62.4 g, carbohydrate 112.8 g, fat 33.2 g, Na 876 mg/L, K 1248 mg/L, cal 1/mL. Vitamins A, B_1, B_2, B_3, B_5, B_6, B_{12}, C, D, E, K, beta carotene, biotin, chloride, choline, folic acid, Ca, Cr, Cu, Fe, I, Mg, Mn, Mo, P, Se, Zn. Vanilla flavor. Liq. Can. 250 mL. *OTC.*
Use: Nutritional supplement.

Nutrilan. (Elan) A vanilla, chocolate, or strawberry flavored liquid containing 38 g protein, 37 g fat, 143 g carbohydrates, 632.5 mg Na, 1.073 g K/L. With appropriate vitamins and minerals. In 237 mL *Tetra Pak* containers. *OTC.*
Use: Nutritional supplement.

Nutrilipid. (McGaw) Soybean oil intravenous fat emulsion. **10%:** Calories 1.1/mL. Bot. 250 mL, 500 mL. **20%:** Calories 2/mL. Bot. 250 mL, 500 mL. *Rx.*
Use: Nutritional supplement, parenteral.

Nutrilyte. (American Regent) Na^+ 25 mEq, K^+ ≈ 40 mEq, Ca^{++} 5 mEq, Mg^{++} 8 mEq, Cl^- ≈ 33 mEq, acetate ≈ 41 mEq, gluconate 5 mEq/20 mL, osmolarity ≈ 7562 mOsm/L. Conc. Soln. Single-dose vial 20 mL, pharmacy bulk pkg. 100 mL. *Rx.*
Use: Intravenous nutritional therapy, intravenous replenishment solution.

Nutrilyte II. (American Regent) Na^+ 35 mEq, K^+ 20 mEq, Ca^{++} 4.5 mEq, Mg^{++} 5 mEq, Cl^- 35 mEq, acetate 29.5 mEq/20 mL, osmolarity ≈ 6212 mOsm/L. Conc. Soln. Single-dose vial 20 mL, pharmacy bulk pkg. Vial 100 mL. *Rx.*
Use: Intravenous nutritional therapy, intravenous replenishment solution.

Nutri-Plex Tablets. (Faraday) Vitamins B_1 5 mg, B_2 5 mg, B_6 5 mg, pantothenic acid 25 mg, B_{12} 12.5 mcg, niacinamide 50 mg, iron gluconate 30 mg, choline bitartrate 50 mg, inositol 50 mg, PABA 15 mg, C 150 mg/2 Tab. Bot. 100s, 250s. *OTC.*
Use: Mineral, vitamin supplement.

Nutrisource Modular System. (Novartis) Individual Nutrisource modules available: protein, amino acids, amino acids (high branched chain), carbohydrate, lipid (medium chain triglycerides), lipid (long branched chain triglycerides), vitamins, minerals. Cans of liquid. Packets of powder. *OTC.*
Use: Nutritional supplement.

Nutri-Val. (Marcen) Vitamins A 5000 units, D 500 units, B_1 10 mg, B_2 5 mg, B_{12} activity 5 mcg, B_6 5 mcg, C 50 mg, hesperidin 5 mg, niacinamide 15 mg, folic acid 0.2 mg, calcium pantothenate 50 mg, choline bitartrate 50 mg, betaine hydrochloride 25 mg, lipo-K 0.4 mg, duodenum substance 50 mg, pancreas substance 50 mg, inositol 25 mg, Cy-yeast hydrolysates 50 mg, rutin 5 mg, l-lysine hydrochloride 5 mg, E 5 units, Ossonate (glucuronic complex) 8 mg, glutamic acid 30 mg, lecithin 5 mg, Fe 20 mg, I 0.15 mg, Ca

50 mg, P 40 mg, B 0.1 mg, Cu 1 mg, Mn 1 mg, Mg 1 mg, K 5 mg, Zn 0.5 mg, biotin 0.02 mg. Cap. Bot. 100s, 500s, 1000s. *OTC.*
Use: Mineral, vitamin supplement.

Nutri-Vite Natural Multiple Vitamin and Minerals. (Faraday) Vitamins A 15,000 units, D 400 units, B_1 1.5 mg, B_2 3 mg, B_{12} 15 mcg, niacin 500 mcg, B_6 20 mcg, choline 1.75 mg, folic acid 13 mcg, pantothenic acid 50 mcg, p-aminobenzoic acid 12 mcg, inositol 1.72 mg, C 60 mg, citrus bioflavonoids 15 mg, E 50 units, iron gluconate 15 mg, Ca 192 mg, P 85 mg, I 0.15 mg, red bone marrow 30 mg/3 Tab. Protein-coated Tab. Bot. 100s, 250s. *OTC.*
Use: Mineral, vitamin supplement.

Nutrizyme. (Enzyme Process) Vitamins A 5000 units, D 400 units, C 60 mg, B_1 1.5 mg, B_2 1.7 mg, niacinamide 20 mg, B_6 2 mg, pantothenate 10 mg, B_{12} 6 mcg, E 30 units, Fe 10 mg, Cu 1 mg, Zn 1 mg, Folac in 0.025 mg. Tab. Bot. 90s, 250s. *OTC.*
Use: Mineral, vitamin supplement.

Nutropin. (Genentech) Somatropin 5 mg ($\approx$ 15 units)/vial, 10 mg ($\approx$ 30 units)/vial. Pow. for Inj. (lyophilized). **5 mg:** Ctn. of 2 vials (mannitol 45 mg, glycine 1.7 mg) w/10 mL multiple-dose vial of diluent (Bacteriostatic Water for Injection w/benzyl alcohol 0.9%). **10 mg:** Ctn. of 2 vials (mannitol 90 mg, glycine 3.4 mg) w/2 10 mL multiple-dose vials of diluent (Bacteriostatic Water for Injection w/benzyl alcohol 0.9%). *Rx.*
Use: Hormone, growth.

Nutropin AQ. (Genentech) Somatropin 10 mg ($\approx$ 30 units)/Vial. Inj. Multiple dose vial 2 mL (6s). *Rx.*
Use: Hormone, growth.

Nutrox Capsules. (Tyson) Vitamins A 10,000 units, E 150 units, B_1 25 mg, B_2 25 mg, B_3 50 mg, B_5 22 mg, C 80 mg, l-cysteine, taurine, glutathione, zinc oxide 15 mg, Se. Cap. Bot. 90s. *OTC.*
Use: Mineral, vitamin supplement.

NuvaRing. (Organon) Etonogestrel 0.12 mg, ethinyl estradiol 2.7 mg/sachet. Box 1s, 3s. *Rx.*
Use: Sex hormone, contraceptive hormone.

Nuzine Ointment. (Hobart) Guaiacol 1.66 g, oxyquinoline sulfate 0.42 g, zinc oxide 2.5 g, glycerine 1.66 g, lanum (anhydrous) 43.76 g, petrolatum 50 g/100 g. Tube 1 oz. *OTC.*
Use: Anorectal preparation.

Nycoff. (Dover Pharmaceuticals) Dextromethorphan HBr. Tab. UD Box 500s.

Sugar, lactose, and salt free. *OTC.*
Use: Antitussive.

Nyco-White. (Whitworth Towne) Nystatin, neomycin, gramicidin, triamcinolone. Cream. Tube 15 g, 30 g, 60 g. *Rx.*
Use: Anti-infective, topical.

Nyco-Worth. (Whitworth Towne) Nystatin. Cream. Tube 15 g. *Rx.*
Use: Antifungal, topical.

Nydrazid. (Apothecon) Isoniazid 100 mg/mL, chlorobutanol 0.25%. Inj. Vial 10 mL. *Rx.*
Use: Antituberculosal.

•**nylestriol.** (NYE-less-TRY-ole) USAN.
Use: Estrogen.

NyQuil Cough/Cold, Children's. (Procter & Gamble) Pseudoephedrine hydrochloride 10 mg, chlorpheniramine maleate 0.67 mg, dextromethorphan HBr 5 mg/5 mL, sucrose, alcohol free, cherry flavor. Liq. 120 mL. *OTC.*
Use: Antihistamine; antitussive; decongestant.

NyQuil Hot Therapy. (Procter & Gamble) Pseudoephedrine hydrochloride 60 mg, doxylamine succinate 12.5 mg, dextromethorphan HBr 30 mg, acetaminophen 1000 mg/pkt. Pow. 6s. *OTC.*
Use: Analgesic; antihistamine; antitussive; decongestant.

NyQuil Liqui-Caps. (Procter & Gamble) Pseudoephedrine hydrochloride 30 mg, diphenhydramine hydrochloride 25 mg, dextromethorphan HBr 15 mg, acetaminophen 250 mg. Cap. Bot. 20s. *OTC.*
Use: Analgesic; antihistamine; antitussive; decongestant.

NyQuil Nighttime Cold/Flu Medicine. (Procter & Gamble) Pseudoephedrine hydrochloride 10 mg, doxylamine succinate 2.1 mg, dextromethorphan HBr 5 mg, acetaminophen 167 mg/5 mL, alcohol 10%, sucrose, saccharin (cherry flavor), tartrazine (regular flavor). Liq. Bot. 295 mL. *OTC.*
Use: Analgesic; antihistamine; antitussive; decongestant.

NyQuil Nighttime Cold Medicine Liquid. (Procter & Gamble) Dextromethorphan HBr 30 mg, pseudoephedrine hydrochloride 60 mg, doxylamine succinate 7.5 mg, acetaminophen 1000 mg/oz, alcohol 25%. Regular and cherry flavors. Regular flavor contains FDC Yellow #5 tartrazine. Bot. 6 oz, 10 oz, 14 oz. *OTC.*
Use: Analgesic; antihistamine; antitussive; decongestant.

NyQuil Nighttime Head Cold Allergy Formula, Children's. (Procter & Gamble) Pseudoephedrine hydrochloride, chlorpheniramine maleate, 0.67 mg/5 mL, alcohol free, sorbitol, sucrose, grape flavor. Liq. Bot. 120 mL. *OTC.*
Use: Antihistamine; decongestant.

Nyral. (Pal-Pak, Inc.) Cetylpyridinium Cl 0.5 mg, benzocaine 5 mg/Loz. w/parabens. Pkg. 100s, 1000s. *OTC.*
Use: Antiseptic.

•**nystatin.** (nye-STAT-in) *USP 28.*
Use: Antifungal.
See: Mycostatin.
　Nilstat.
　Nystop.
　O-V Statin.
　Pedi Dri.
　W/Clioquinol.
　See: Mycolog.
　W/Tetracycline phosphate buffered.
　See: Achrostatin-V.

nystatin. (PAR) Nystatin 100,000 units/g. Talc. Pow. 15 g, 60 g. *Rx.*
Use: Antifungal agent.

nystatin. (Various Mfr.) Nystatin. **Tab.:** 500,000 units. Bot. 100s. **Vaginal Tab.:** 100,000 units. Pkg. 15s, 30s w/applicator(s). *Rx.*
Use: Antifungal.

nystatin and triamcinolone acetonide cream.
Use: Antifungal; corticosteroid, topical.

nystatin and triamcinolone acetonide ointment.
Use: Antifungal; corticosteroid, topical.

nystatin, neomycin sulfate, gramicidin, and triamcinolone acetonide.
Use: Antifungal; anti-infective; corticosteroid, topical.
See: Mycolog.

Nystop. (Paddock) Nystatin 100,000 units/g. Dispersed in talc. Pow. 15 g, 30 g. *Rx.*
Use: Antifungal.

Nytcold Medicine. (Rugby) Pseudoephedrine hydrochloride 10 mg, doxylamine succinate 1.25 mg, dextromethorphan HBr 5 mg, acetaminophen 167 mg, alcohol 25%, glucose, saccharin, sucrose, cherry flavor. Liq. Bot. 177 mL. *OTC.*
Use: Analgesic; antihistamine; antitussive; decongestant.

Nytime Cold Medicine. (Rugby) Acetaminophen 1000 mg, doxylamine succinate 7.5 mg, pseudoephedrine hydrochloride 60 mg, dextromethorphan HBr 30 mg/30 mL, alcohol 25%. Bot. 6 oz, 10 oz. *OTC.*
Use: Analgesic; antihistamine; antitussive; decongestant.

Nytol. (Block Drug) Diphenhydramine hydrochloride 25 mg. Tab. Bot. 16s, 32s, 72s. *OTC.*
Use: Sleep aid.

Nytol, Maximum Strength. (Block Drug) Diphenhydramine hydrochloride 50 mg, lactose. Tab. Bot. 8s. *OTC.*
Use: Sleep aid.

O

O.A.D. (Sween) Ostomy. Bot. 1.25 oz, 4 oz, 8 oz. *OTC.*
Use: Deodorant; ostomy.

Oasis. (Zitar) Artificial saliva. Bot. 6 oz. *OTC.*
Use: Antixerostomia agent.

● **oatmeal, colloidal.** *USP 28.*
Use: Antipruritic, topical.

oatmeal, gum fraction.
See: Aveeno.

Obepar. (Tyler) Vitamins A 3000 units, D 300 units, B₁ 3 mg, B₂ 2 mg, nicotinamide 10 mg, B₆ 3 mg, calcium pantothenate 2 mg, B₁₂ 3 mcg, C 37.5 mg, Ca 150 mg, Fe 5 mg, Mg 1 mg, Mn 0.1 mg, K 1 mg, Zn 0.15 mg. Cap. Bot. 100s. *OTC.*
Use: Mineral, vitamin supplement.

Obe-Tite. (Scot-Tussin) Phendimetrazine tartrate 35 mg. Tab. Bot. 100s, 500s. *c-III.*
Use: Anorexiant.

Obezine. (Western Research) Phendimetrazine tartrate 35 mg. Tab. *Handi count* 28 (36 bags of 28s). *c-III.*
Use: Anorexiant.

● **obidoxime chloride.** (OH-bih-DOX-eem) USAN.
Use: Cholinesterase reactivator.

● **oblimersen sodium.** (ob-li-MER-sen) USAN.
Use: Anticancer therapy.

Obrical. (Canright) Calcium lactate 500 mg, vitamins D 400 units, ferrous sulfate exsiccated 35 mg, B₁ 1 mg, B₂ 1 mg, C 10 mg. Tab. Bot. 100s, 1000s. *OTC.*
Use: Mineral, vitamin supplement.

Obrical-F. (Canright) Ferrous sulfate 50 mg, calcium lactate 500 mg, vitamins D 400 units, B₁ 1 mg, B₂ 1 mg, C 10 mg, folic acid 0.67 mg. Tab. Bot. 100s, 1000s. *OTC.*
Use: Mineral, vitamin supplement.

Obrite. (Milton Roy) Contact lens and eye glass cleaner. Plastic spray Bot. 30 mL, 55 mL. *OTC.*
Use: Contact lens and eye glass care.

Obstetrix-100. (Seyer) Ca 250 mg, Fe 100 mg, vitamin A 2700 units, D₃ 400 units, E (as dl-alpha tocopheryl) 30 mg, B₁ 3 mg, B₂ 3.4 mg, B₃ 20 mg, B₆ 20 mg, B₁₂ 12 mcg, C 250 mg, folic acid 1 mg, Zn 25 mg, sodium docusate 50 mg. Tab. UD 30s. *Rx.*
Use: Vitamin, mineral supplement.

OB-Tinic. (Roberts) Fe 65 mg, vitamins A 6000 units, D 400 units, E 30 units,

B₁ 1.1 mg, B₂ 1.8 mg, B₃ 15 mg, B₆ 2.5 mg, B₁₂ 5 mcg, C 60 mg, folic acid 1 mg, Ca Tab. Bot. 100s. *Rx.*
Use: Mineral, vitamin supplement.

Obtrex. (Pronova) Vitamin A 2700 units, E 18 mg, C 120 mg, selenium 65 mcg, D₃ 400 units, folic acid 1 mg, zinc 25 mg, B₁ 3 mg, B₂ 3.4 mg, B₃ 20 mg, B₆ 40 mg, B₁₂ 2 mcg, magnesium 30 mg, sodium docusate 50 mg. Tab. 60s. *Rx.*
Use: Vitamin, mineral supplement.

O-Cal f.a. (Pharmics) Tab.: Ca 200 mg, Fe 66 mg, vitamins A 5000 units, D 400 units, E 30 mg, B₁ 3 mg, B₂ 3 mg, B₃ 20 mg, B₆ 4 mg, B₁₂ 12 mcg, C 90 mg, folic acid 1 mg, fluoride 1.1 mg, Mg, I, Cu, Zn 15 mg. Bot. 100s. *Rx.*
Use: Mineral, vitamin supplement.

O-Cal Prenatal. (Pharmics) Ca 200 mg, Fe 15 mg, vitamin A 2500 units, D 400 units, E 30 units, B₁ 1.5 mg, B₂ 1.6 mg, B₃ 17 mg, B₆ 12 mg, B₁₂ 12 mcg, C 70 mg, folic acid 1 mg, Zn 15 mg, Cu, I, Mg. Tab. Bot. 100s. *Rx.*
Use: Multivitamin.

● **ocaperidone.** (oke-ah-PURR-ih-dohn) USAN.
Use: Antipsychotic.

Occlusal HP. (Medicis) Salicylic acid 17%. Soln. Bot. 10 mL. *OTC.*
Use: Keratolytic.

Occucoat. (Bausch & Lomb) Hydroxypropyl methylcellulose 2%. Soln. Syringe 1 mL with cannula. *Rx.*
Use: Ophthalmic.

Ocean. (Fleming & Co.) Sodium Cl 0.65%, benzalkonium chloride. Soln. Spray Bot. 45 mL, 473 mL. *OTC.*
Use: Nasal decongestant.

Ocean for Kids. (Fleming) Sodium chloride 0.65%. Alcohol free. Benzalkonium chloride, EDTA, glycerin. Nasal spray. 37.5 mL. *OTC.*
Use: Nasal decongestant.

Ocean Plus. (Fleming & Co.) Caffeine 2.5%, benzyl alcohol. Soln. Bot. 15 mL. *OTC.*
Use: Moisturizer, nasal.

● **ocfentanil hydrochloride.** (ock-FEN-tah-NILL) USAN.
Use: Analgesic, narcotic.

● **ocinaplon.** (oh-SIN-ah-plahn) USAN.
Use: Anxiolytic.

OCL. (Abbott Hospital Products) Sodium Cl 146 mg, sodium bicarbonate 168 mg, sodium sulfate decahydrate 1.29 g, potassium Cl 75 mg, PEG 3350 6 g, polysorbate 80 30 mg/100 mL. Oral Soln. Bot. 1500 mL (3 pack). *Rx.*

Use: Laxative.

• **ocrylate.** (AH-krih-late) USAN.
Use: Surgical aid, tissue adhesive.

• **octabenzone.** (OCK-tah-BEN-zone) USAN.
Use: Ultraviolet screen.

octadecanoic acid.
See: Stearic Acid.

octadecanoic acid, sodium salt.
See: Sodium Stearate.

octadecanoic acid, zinc salt.
See: Zinc Stearate.

octadecanol-l.
See: Stearyl Alcohol.

• **octafluoropropane.**
Use: Radiopaque agent.
See: Definity.

Octagam. (Octapharma) Immune globulin (human) 5% (50 mg/mL). Maltose 100 mg. Inj. Single-use bot. 1 g, 2.5 g, 5 g, 10 g. *Rx.*
Use: Immune globulin.

Octamide. (Pharmacia) Metoclopramide 10 mg. Tab. Bot. 100s, 500s. *Rx.*
Use: Gastrointestinal stimulant; antiemetic.

Octamide PFS. (Pharmacia) Metoclopramide hydrochloride 5 mg/mL, preservative free. Vial. Single dose; 2, 10, 30 mL. *Rx.*
Use: Antiemetic; gastrointestinal stimulant.

• **octanoic acid.** (OCK-tah-NO-ik) USAN.
Use: Antifungal.

octapeptide sequence.
Use: Antiviral.
See: Flumadine.

Octarex. (Health for Life Brands) Vitamins A 5000 units, D 1000 units, B₁ 1.5 mg, B₂ 2 mg, B₆ 0.1 mg, calcium pantothenate 1 mg, niacinamide 20 mg, C 37.5 mg, E 1 unit, B₁₂ 1 mcg. Cap. Bot. 100s, 1000s. *OTC.*
Use: Mineral, vitamin supplement.

Octavims. (Health for Life Brands) Vitamins A 6000 units, D 1250 units, C 50 mg, E 5 units, B₁ 3 mg, B₂ 3 mg, B₆ 0.5 mg, niacinamide 20 mg, calcium pantothenate 5 mg, B₁₂ 5 mcg, Ca 59 mg, P 45 mg. Cap. Bot. 100s, 250s, 1000s. *OTC.*
Use: Mineral, vitamin supplement.

• **octazamide.** (OCK-TAY-zah-mide) USAN.
Use: Analgesic.

• **octenidine hydrochloride.** (OCK-TEN-ih-deen) USAN.
Use: Anti-infective, topical.

• **octenidine saccharin.** (OCK-TEN-ih-deen SACK-ah-rin) USAN.

Use: Dental plaque inhibitor.

• **octicizer.** (OCK-tih-SIGH-zer) USAN. Santicizer 141.
Use: Pharmaceutic aid, plasticizer.

• **octinoxate.** (ok-TIN-ox-ate) *USP 28.*
Formerly octylmethoxycinnamate.
Use: Sunscreen.

• **octisalate.** (ok-ti-SAL-ate) *USP 28.*
Formerly octyl salicylate.
Use: Sunscreen.
W/Combinations.
See: Scar Cream Maximum Strength.

Octocaine. (Septodont) Lidocaine hydrochloride 2%, epinephrine 1:50,000 or 1:100,000, sodium bisulfite. Inj. Cartridge 1.8 mL. *Rx.*
Use: Anesthetic, local.

• **octocrylene.** (OCK-toe-KRIH-leen) *USP 28.*
Use: Ultraviolet screen.

• **octodrine.** (OCK-toe-DREEN) USAN. Under study.
Use: Adrenergic, vasoconstrictor; anesthetic, local.

• **octoxynol 9.** (ock-TOXE-ih-nahl 9) *NF 23.*
Use: Pharmaceutic aid, surfactant.

OctreoScan. (Mallinckrodt) Pentetreotide 10 mcg, indium in 111 chloride sterile solution. Kit. Vial 10 mL. *Rx.*
Use: Radiopaque agent.

• **octreotide.** (ock-TREE-oh-tide) USAN.
Use: Antisecretory, gastric.

• **octreotide acetate.** (ock-TREE-oh-tide) USAN.
Use: Antidiarrheal, gastrointestinal tumor; antihypotensive, carcinoid crisis; growth hormone suppressant, acromegaly, antisecretory, gastric.

• **octreotide pamoate.** (ock-TREE-oh-tide PAM-oh-ate) USAN.
Use: Antineoplastic.

• **octriptyline phosphate.** (ock-TRIP-tih-leen FOSS-fate) USAN.
Use: Antidepressant.

• **octrizole.** (OCK-TRY-zole) USAN.
Use: Ultraviolet screen.

• **octyldodecanol.** *NF 23.*
Use: Pharmaceutic aid, oleaginous vehicle.

octyl methoxycinnamate.
See: Octinoxate.

octylphenoxy polyethoxyethanol. A mono-ether of a polyethylene glycol. Igepal CA 630 (Antara).

octyl salicylate.
See: Octisalate.

OcuClear. (Schering-Plough) Oxymetazoline hydrochloride 0.025%. Soln. Bot.

30 mL. *OTC.*
Use: Mydriatic; vasoconstrictor.
OcuCoat. (Bausch & Lomb) Hydroxy-
propyl methylcellulose 2%. Soln. Sy-
ringe 1 mL. *Rx.*
Use: Lubricant, ophthalmic.
OcuCoat PF. (Bausch & Lomb) Dextran
70 0.1%, hydroxypropyl methylcellu-
lose, NaCl, KCl, dextrose, sodium phos-
phate, preservative free. Drops. 0.5 mL
single-dose containers. *OTC.*
Use: Lubricant, ophthalmic.
Ocufen. (Allergan) Flurbiprofen sodium
0.03%. Drops. Bot. 2.5 mL w/dropper.
Rx.
Use: NSAID, ophthalmic.
• **ocufilcon a.** (OCK-you-FILL-kahn A)
USAN.
Use: Contact lens material, hydrophilic.
• **ocufilcon b.** (OCK-you-FILL-kahn B)
USAN.
Use: Contact lens material, hydrophilic.
• **ocufilcon c.** (OCK-you-FILL-kahn C)
USAN.
Use: Contact lens material, hydrophilic.
• **ocufilcon d.** (OCK-you-FILL-kahn D)
USAN.
Use: Contact lens material, hydrophilic.
• **ocufilcon e.** (OCK-you-FILL-kahn E)
USAN.
Use: Contact lens material, hydrophilic.
• **ocufilcon f.** (OCK-you-FILL-kahn F)
USAN.
Use: contact lens material, hydrophilic.
Ocuflox. (Allergan) Ofloxacin 3 mg/mL,
benzalkonium chloride 0.005%. Soln.
Bot. 1 mL, 5 mL, 10 mL. *Rx.*
Use: Anti-infective, ophthalmic.
ocular lubricants.
Use: Ophthalmic.
See: Akwa Tears.
Artificial Tears.
Dry Eyes.
Duolube.
Duratears Naturale.
Hypotears.
Lacri-Lube NP.
Lacri-Lube S.O.P.
Lipo-Tears.
LubriTears.
OcuCoat PF.
Puralube.
Refresh PM.
Tears Renewed.
Vit-A-Drops.
Ocu-Lube. (Bausch & Lomb) Petrolatum
sterile, preservative and lanolin free.
Oint. Tube 3.5 g. *OTC.*
Use: Lubricant, ophthalmic.

Ocumeter.
See: Decadron Phosphate, Preps.
Humorsol.
NeoDecadron Ophthalmic.
Ocusert. (Alza) Pilocarpine ocular thera-
peutic system. **Pilo-20:** Releases
20 mcg pilocarpine/hour for one week.
Pkg. 8s. **Pilo-40:** Releases 40 mcg
pilocarpine/hour for one week. Pkg. 8s.
Rx.
Use: Antiglaucoma agent.
OCuSOFT. (OCuSOFT) PEG-80 sorbitan
laurate, sodium trideceth sulfate, PEG-
150 distearate, cocoamido propyl hy-
droxysultaine, lauroamphocarboxyglyci-
nate, sodium laureth-13 carboxylate,
PEG-15 tallow polyamine, quaternium-
15. Alcohol and dye free. Soln. Pads
UD 30s, Bot. 30 mL, 120 mL, 240 mL,
Complinoo kit (120 mL and 100
pads). *OTC.*
Use: Cleanser, ophthalmic.
OCuSOFT VMS. (OCuSOFT) Vitamins A
5000 units, E 30 units, C 60 mg, Cu,
Se, Zn 40 mg. Tab. Bot. 60s. *OTC.*
Use: Mineral, vitamin supplement.
Ocusulf-10. (Optopics) Sodium sulfacet-
amide 10%. Soln. Bot. 2 mL, 5 mL,
15 mL. *Rx.*
Use: Anti-infective, ophthalmic.
Ocutricin. (Bausch & Lomb) Polymyxin
B sulfate 10,000 units, bacitracin zinc
400 units, neomycin sulfate 3.5 mg.
Oint. Tube 3.5 g. *Rx.*
Use: Antibiotic, ophthalmic.
Ocuvite. (Bausch & Lomb) Vitamins A
5000 units, E 30 units, C 60 mg, Zn
40 mg, Cu, Se 40 mcg. Tab. Bot. 120s.
OTC.
Use: Mineral, vitamin supplement.
Ocuvite Extra. (Bausch & Lomb) Vita-
min A 1000 units, C 300 mg, E
100 units, Zn 40 mg, B_3 40 mg, B_2
3 mg, Cu, Se, Mn, l-glutathione, lutein
2 mg. Tab. Bot. 50s. *OTC.*
Use: Vitamin supplement.
Ocuvite Lutein. (Bausch & Lomb) Vita-
min E 30 units, C 60 mg, Zn 15 mg,
Cu, lutein 6 mg. Lactose. Cap. 36s.
OTC.
Use: Mineral, vitamin supplement.
Ocuvite PreserVision. (Bausch & Lomb)
Vitamin A 7160 units, E 100 units, C
113 mg, Zn 17.4 mg, Cu. Lactose. Tab.
120s. *OTC.*
Use: Mineral, vitamin supplement.
Odara. (Young Dental) Alcohol 48%, car-
bolic acid < 2%, zinc Cl, potassium io-
dide, glycerin, methyl salicylate, eu-
calyptus oil, myrrh tincture. Concen-
trated Liq. Bot. 8 oz. *OTC.*
Use: Mouthwash.

oestergon.
See: Estradiol.
Oesto-Mins. (Tyson) Ascorbic acid
500 mg, Ca 250 mg, Mg 250 mg, K
45 mg, vitamin D 100 units/4.5 g. Pow.
Bot. 200 g. *OTC.*
Use: Vitamin supplement.
oestradiol.
See: Estradiol.
oestrasid.
See: Dienestrol.
oestrin.
See: Estrone.
oestroform.
See: Estrone.
oestromenin.
See: Diethylstilbestrol.
oestromon.
See: Diethylstilbestrol.
OFF-Ezy Corn & Callous Remover.
(Del) Salicylic acid 17% in a collodion-
like vehicle of 65% ether and 21% alcohol. Kit. 13.5 mL with callous
smoother and 3 corn cushions. *OTC.*
Use: Keratolytic.
OFF-Ezy Corn Remover. (Del) Salicylic
acid 13.57%, inflexible collodion base,
ether 65%, alcohol 21%. Liq. Bot.
0.45 oz. *OTC.*
Use: Keratolytic.
OFF-Ezy Wart Remover. (Del) Salicylic
acid 17% in flexible collodion base,
ether 65%, alcohol 21%. Liq. Bot.
13.5 mL. *OTC.*
Use: Keratolytic.
• **ofloxacin.** (oh-FLOX-uh-SIN) *USP 28.*
Use: Anti-infective.
See: Floxin.
Ocuflox.
ofloxacin. (Various Mfr.) Ofloxacin.
Soln.: 0.3% (3 mg/mL). Dropper bot.
5 mL, 10 mL. **Tab.:** 200 mg, 300 mg,
400 mg. 50s (except 400 mg), 100s. *Rx.*
Use: Otic preparation; anti-infective.
• **ofornine.** (ah-FAR-neen) USAN.
Use: Antihypertensive.
Ogen. (Pharmacia) Estropipate 0.75 mg,
1.5 mg, 3 mg, lactose. Tab. Bot. 100s.
Rx.
Use: Estrogen.
Ogen Vaginal Cream. (Pharmacia)
Estropipate 1.5 mg/g, cetyl alcohol,
parabens, mineral oil. Cream. Tube
42.5 g w/calibrated applicator. *Rx.*
Use: Estrogen.
Ogestrel 0.5/50. (Watson) Norgestrel
0.5 mg, ethinyl estradiol 50 mcg, lac-
tose. Tab. Pack 28s. *Rx.*
Use: Sex hormone, contraceptive
hormone.

• **oglufanide disodium.** (oh-GLOO-fa-
nide) USAN. Previously Glufanide disodium.
Use: Immunomodulator; angiogenesis
inhibitor (Kaposi sarcoma).
Oilatum Soap. (Stiefel) Polyunsaturated
vegetable oil 7.5%. Bar 120 g, 240 g.
OTC.
Use: Dermatologic, cleanser.
oil of camphor w/combinations.
See: Sloan's Liniment.
oil of cloves w/alcohol.
See: Buckley "Z.O."
Oil of Olay Daily UV Protectant. (Procter & Gamble) SPF 15. **Cream:** Titanium dioxide, ethylhexyl p-methoxycinnamate, 2-phenylbenzimidazole-5-
sulfonic acid, glycerin, triethanolamine,
imidazolidinyl urea, parabens, carbomer, PEG-10, EDTA, castor oil, tartrazine. Scented and unscented. 51 g.
Lot.: Ethylhexyl p-methoxycinnamate,
2-phenylbenzimidazole-5-sulfonic acid,
titanium dioxide, cetyl alcohol, imidazolidinyl urea, parabens, EDTA, castor oil, tartrazine. Bot. 105 g, 157.7 g.
OTC.
Use: Sunscreen.
Oil of Olay Foaming Face Wash. (Procter & Gamble) Potassium cocoyl hydrolyzed collagen, glycerin, EDTA. Liq.
Bot. 90 mL, 210 mL. *OTC.*
Use: Dermatologic, acne.
oil of pine w/combinations.
See: Sloan's Liniment.
• **ointment and lotion base.**
See: Hydrocerin.
ointment base, washable.
See: Absorbent Base.
Cetaphil.
Velvachol.
• **ointment, bland lubricating ophthalmic.** *USP 28.*
Use: Lubricant, ophthalmic.
• **ointment, hydrophilic.** *USP 28.*
Use: Pharmaceutic aid, oil-in-water
emulsion ointment base.
• **ointment, rose water.** *USP 28.*
Use: Pharmaceutic aid, emollient, ointment base.
• **ointment, white.** *USP 28.*
Use: Pharmaceutical aid, oleaginous
ointment base.
• **ointment, yellow.** *USP 28.*
Use: Pharmaceutic aid, ointment base.
• **olaflur.** (OH-lah-flure) USAN.
Use: Dental caries agent.
olamine.
See: Ethanolamine.

• **olanexidine hydrochloride.** USAN.
Use: Antimicrobial.

• **olanzapine.** (oh-LAN-zah-PEEN) USAN.
Use: Antipsychotic, dibenzapine derivative.
See: Zyprexa.
Zyprexa Zydis.
W/Fluoxetine hydrochloride.
See: Symbyax.

old tuberculin.
See: Mono-Vacc Test (OT).
Tuberculin, Old, Tine Test.

oleandomycin phosphate. Phosphate of an antibacterial substance produced by *Streptomyces antibioticus.*
Use: Anti-infective.

oleandomycin, triacetyl. Troleandomycin, *USP.*

• **oleic acid.** (oh LAY ik) *NF 23.*
Use: Pharmaceutic aid, emulsion adjunct.

• **oleic acid I 131.** USAN.
Use: Radiopharmaceutical.

• **oleic acid I 125.** USAN.
Use: Radiopharmaceutical.

oleovitamin a.
See: Vitamin A.

• **oleovitamin a & d.** *USP 28.*
Use: Vitamin supplement.
See: Super D.

oleovitamin d, synthetic.
Use: Vitamin supplement.
See: Viosterol in Oil.

• **oleyl alcohol.** (oh-LAY-il) *NF 23.*
Use: Pharmaceutic aid, emulsifying agent, emollient.
See: Patanol.

• **olive oil.** *NF 23.*
Use: Emollient, pharmaceutic aid, not ting retardant for dental cements.

• **olmesartan.** (ole-mih-SAR-tan) USAN.
Use: Antihypertensive.

• **olmesartan medoxomil.** (ole-mih-SAR-tan meh-DOX-oh-mill) USAN.
Use: Antihypertensive.
See: Benicar.
W/Hydrochlorothiazide
See: Benicar HCT.

• **olopatadine hydrochloride.** (oh-low-pat-AD-een) USAN.
Use: Antiallergic, allergic rhinitis, urticria, allergic conjunctivitis, asthma.
See: Patanol.

• **olsalazine sodium.** (OLE-SAL-uh-zeen) USAN. *Formerly Sodium azodisalicylate, azodisal sodium.*
Use: Maintenance of remission of ulcerative colitis in patients intolerant of sulfasalazine; anti-inflammatory, gastrointestinal.

See: Dipentum.

Olux. (Connetics) Clobetasol propionate 0.05%, ethanol 60%, cetyl alcohol, stearyl alcohol. Foam. Can. 50 g, 100 g. *Rx.*
Use: Anti-inflammatory.

• **olvanil.** (OLE-van-ill) USAN.
Use: Analgesic.

• **omalizumab.** (oh-mah-lie-ZOO-mab) USAN.
Use: Monoclonal antibody.
See: Xolair.

omapatrilat.
Use: Vasopeptidase inhibitor.

Omega Oil. (Block Drug) Methyl nicotinate, methyl salicylate, capsicum oleoresin, histamine dihydrochloride, isopropyl alcohol 44%. Bot. 2.5 oz, 4.85 oz. *OTC.*
Use: Analgesic, topical.

• **omega-3-acid ethyl esters.** USAN.
Use: Hypolipidemic.

omega-3 (n-3) polyunsaturated fatty acids. From cold water fish oils.
Use: Dietary supplement to reduce risk of coronary artery disease.
See: Animi-3.
Cardi-Omega 3.
Marine 500, 1000.
Max EPA.
Promega.
Sea-Omega 50.
SuperEPA.

• **omeprazole.** (oh-MEH-pray-ZAHL) *USP 28.*
Use: Depressant, gastric acid secretory; agent for gastroesophageal reflux disease; proton pump inhibitor.
See: Prilosec.
Prilosec OTC.
Zegerid.

omeprazole. (Various Mfr.) Omeprazole 10 mg, 20 mg. Enteric-coated granules. DR Cap. Bot. 30s, 100s. *Rx.*
Use: Proton pump inhibitor; gastric acid secretory depressant; agent for gastroesophageal reflux disease.

• **omeprazole sodium.** (oh-MEH-pray-ZOLE) USAN.
Use: Antisecretory, gastric.

OM 401.
Use: Sickle cell disease. [Orphan Drug]

• **omiganan pentahydrochloride.** (oh-me-GAN-an) USAN.
Use: Antimicrobial.

Omnicef. (Abbott) **Cap.:** Cefdinir 300 mg. Bot. 60s. **Oral Susp.:** 125 mg/5 mL, 250 mg/5 mL, sucrose, strawberry flavor. Bot. 60 mL, 100 mL. *Rx.*
Use: Anti-infective, cephalosporin.

Omnicol. (Delta Pharmaceutical Group) Dextromethorphan HBr 15 mg, chlorpheniramine maleate 4 mg, phenylephrine hydrochloride 5 mg, phenindamine tartrate 4 mg, salicylamide 227 mg, acetaminophen 100 mg, caffeine alkaloid 10 mg, ascorbic acid 25 mg. Tab. Bot. 100s. *OTC.*
Use: Antitussive, antihistamine, decongestant, analgesic.

Omnihemin. (Delta Pharmaceutical Group) Fe 110 mg, vitamins C 150 mg, B_{12} 7.5 mcg, folic acid 1 mg, Zn 1 mg, Cu 1 mg, Mn 1 mg, Mg 1 mg. Tab. or Soln. 5 mL. **Tab.:** Bot. 100s. **Soln.:** Bot. Pt. *Rx.*
Use: Mineral, vitamin supplement.

OmniHIB. (GlaxoSmithKline) Purified *Haemophilus influenzae* type b capsular polysaccharide 10 mcg, tetanus toxoid 24 mcg/0.5 mL, sucrose 8.5%. Pow. for Inj. (lyophilized). Vial w/0.6 mL syringe of diluent. *Rx.*
Use: Immunization.

OMNIhist L.A. (WE Pharmaceuticals) Phenylephrine 20 mg, chlorpheniramine maleate 8 mg, methscopolamine nitrate 2.5 mg. SR Tab. Bot. 100s. *Rx.*
Use: Upper respiratory combination, anticholinergic, antihistamine, decongestant.

Omninatal. (Delta Pharmaceutical Group) Fe 60 mg, Cu 2 mg, Zn 15 mg, vitamins A 8000 units, D 400 units, C 90 mg, Ca 200 mg, folic acid 1.5 mg, B_1 2.5 mg, B_2 3 mg, niacinamide 20 mg, pyridoxine hydrochloride 10 mg, pantothenic acid 15 mg, B_{12} 8 mcg. Tab. Bot. 100s. *Rx.*
Use: Mineral, vitamin supplement.

Omnipaque 180. (Nycomed Amersham) Iohexol 388 mg equivalent to iodine 180 mg/mL, EDTA. Inj. Vial 10 mL, 20 mL. *Rx.*
Use: Radiopaque agent, parenteral.

Omnipaque 140. (Nycomed Amersham) Iohexol 302 mg equivalent to iodine 140 mg/mL, EDTA. Inj. Vial 50 mL, Bot. *Rx.*
Use: Radiopaque agent, parenteral.

Omnipaque 300. (Nycomed Amersham) Iohexol 647 mg equivalent to iodine 300 mg/mL, EDTA. Inj. Vial 10 mL, 30 mL, 50 mL. Bot. 50 mL. Flex. Cont. 100 mL, 150 mL. Prefilled Syringe 50 mL. 75 mL fill in 100 mL Bot. 100 mL fill in 100 mL Bot. 125 mL fill in 200 mL Bot. 150 mL fill in 200 mL Bot. 125 mL fill in 150 mL Flex. Cont. *Rx.*
Use: Radiopaque agent, parenteral.

Omnipaque 350. (Nycomed Amersham) Iohexol 755 mg equivalent to iodine 350 mg/mL, EDTA. Inj. Vial 50 mL. Bot. 50 mL. Flex. Cont. 100 mL, 150 mL, 200 mL. Prefilled Syringe 50 mL. 75 mL fill in 100 mL Bot., 100 mL fill in 100 mL Bot., 125 mL fill in 200 mL Bot., 150 mL fill in 200 mL Bot., 200 mL fill in 200 mL Bot., 250 mL fill in 300 mL Bot., 125 mL fill in 150 mL Flex. Cont. *Rx.*
Use: Radiopaque agent, parenteral.

Omnipaque 240. (Nycomed Amersham) Iohexol 518 mg equivalent to iodine 240 mg/mL, EDTA. Inj. Vial 10 mL, 20 mL, 50 mL. Bot. 50 mL. Flex. Cont. 100 mL, 150 mL, 200 mL. Prefilled Syringe 50 mL. 100 mL fill in 100 mL Bot. 150 mL fill in 200 mL Bot. 200 mL fill in 200 mL Bot. *Rx.*
Use: Radiopaque agent, parenteral.

Omnipen. (Wyeth) **Cap.:** Ampicillin anhydrous 250 mg, 500 mg. Bot. 100s, 500s. **Pow. for Oral Susp.:** Ampicillin trihydrate 125 mg, 250 mg/5 mL when reconstituted. Pow. for Oral Susp. Bot. 100 mL, 150 mL, 200 mL. *Rx.*
Use: Anti-infective, penicillin.

Omnipen-N. (Wyeth) Ampicillin sodium 125 mg, 250 mg, 500 mg, 1 g, 2 g, 10 g. Pow. for Inj. Vial, Piggyback and *ADD-Vantage* vials (only 500 mg, 1 g, 2 g). *Rx.*
Use: Anti-infective, penicillin.

Omniscan. (Nycomed Amersham) Gadodiamide 287 mg/mL, preservative free. Inj. Vial 10 mL, 20 mL, 50 mL, 5 mL fill in 10 mL vials, 15 mL fill in 20 mL vials, 10 mL fill in 20 mL prefilled syringe, 15 mL fill in 20 mL prefilled syringe. Prefilled Syringe 20 mL. *Rx.*
Use: Radiopaque agent, parenteral.

Omnitabs. (Halsey Drug) Vitamins A 5000 units, D 400 units, C 50 mg, B_1 3 mg, B_2 2.5 mg, niacin 20 mg, B_6 1 mg, B_{12} 1 mcg, pantothenic acid 0.9 mg Tab. Bot. 100s. *OTC.*
Use: Vitamin supplement.

Omnitabs with Iron. (Halsey Drug) Vitamins A 5000 units, D 400 units, B_1 3 mg, B_2 2.5 mg, B_6 1 mg, B_{12} 1 mcg, C 50 mg, niacinamide 20 mg, calcium pantothenate 1 mg, Fe 15 mg. Tab. Bot. 100s. *OTC.*
Use: Mineral, vitamin supplement.

• **omoconazole nitrate.** (oh-moe-KAHN-ah-zole) USAN.
Use: Antifungal.

Oncaspar. (Enzon) Pegaspargase 750 units/mL in a phosphate buffered saline solution. Inj. Single-use vials. *Rx.*
Use: Antineoplastic agent.

Oncet. (Wakefield) Hydrocodone bitartrate 5 mg, acetaminophen 500 mg. Cap. Bot. 100s. *c-III.*
Use: Analgesic; antitussive.
OncoRad ov103.
Use: Antineoplastic. [Orphan Drug]
OncoScint CR/OV. (Cytogen) Satumomab pendetide labeled with indium-111, obtained separately. Kit with 1 mg/2 mL satumomab vial, vial of sodium acetate buffer, and filter.
Oncovin. (Eli Lilly) Vincristine sulfate for inj. 1 mg/mL, 2 mg/2 mL, or 5 mg/5 mL. Soln. Ctn. 10s. Hyporets 1 mg/Pkg 3s; 2 mg/Pkg 3s. *Rx.*
Use: Antineoplastic.
Oncovite. (Mission Pharmacal) Vitamin A 10,000 units, C 500 mg, D_3 400 units, E 200 units, B_1 0.37 mg, B_2 0.5 mg, B_6 25 mg, B_{12} 1.5 mcg, folate 0.4 mg, Zn 7.5 mg, sugar. Tab. Bot. 120s. *OTC.*
Use: Vitamin supplement.
• **ondansetron hydrochloride.** (ahn-DAN-SEH-trahn) USAN.
Use: Anxiolytic; antiemetic; antischizophrenic.
See: Zofran.
Zofran ODT.
Ondrox. (LSI) Ca 50 mg, vitamins A 6000 units, D 300 units, E 50 units, B_1 0.75 mg, B_2 0.75 mg, B_3 10 mg, B_5 5 mg, B_6 1 mg, B_{12} 3 mcg, C 125 mg, folic acid 200 mcg, biotin 15 mcg, I, Mg, Cu, P, vitamin K, Cr, Mn, Mo, Se, V, B, Si, Zn 7.5 mg, inositol, citrus bioflavonoids, N-acetylcysteine, l-methionine, l-glutamine, taurine. Tab. Bot. 60s, 180s. *OTC.*
Use: Mineral, vitamins supplements.
One-A-Day Essential. (Bayer) Vitamins A 5000 units, E 30 units, C 60 mg, folic acid 0.4 mg, B_1 1.5 mg, B_2 1.7 mg, B_3 20 mg, B_6 2 mg, B_{12} 6 mcg, B_5 10 mg, D 400 units. Tab. Sodium free. Bot. 75s, 130s. *OTC.*
Use: Vitamin supplement.
One-A-Day Extras Antioxidant. (Bayer) Vitamin E 200 units, C 250 mg, A 5000 units, Zn 7.5 mg, Cu, Se, Mn, tartrazine. Softgel Cap. Bot. 50s. *OTC.*
Use: Vitamin supplement.
One-A-Day Extras Vitamin E. (Bayer) Vitamin E 400 units. Softgel Cap. Bot. 60s. *OTC.*
Use: Vitamin supplement.
One-A-Day 55 Plus. (Bayer) Vitamin A 6000 units, C 120 mg, B_1 4.5 mg, B_2 3.4 mg, B_3 20 mg, D 400 units, E 60 units, B_6 6 mg, folic acid 0.4 mg, biotin 30 mcg, B_5 20 mg, K 25 mcg, Ca 220 mg, I, Mg, Cu, Zn 15 mg, Cr, Se, Mo, Mn, K, Cl. Tab. Bot. 50s, 80s. *OTC.*
Use: Mineral, vitamin supplement.
One-A-Day Kids. (Bayer) Vitamin A 5000 units, C 60 mg, D 400 units, E 30 units, B_1 1.5 mg, B_2 1.7 mg, B_3 20 mg, B_5 10 mg, B_6 2 mg, B_{12} 6 mcg, folic acid 400 mcg, biotin 40 mcg, calcium 100 mg, iron 18 mg, phosphorus 100 mg, iodine 150 mcg, magnesium 20 mg, zinc 15 mg, copper 2 mg, sorbitol, aspartame, phenylalanine. Chew. Tab. 50s. *OTC.*
Use: Vitamin, mineral supplement.
One-A-Day Kids Scooby-Doo! Fizzy Vites. (Bayer) Ca 50 mg, Fe (as ferrous fumarate) 9 mg, vitamin A 1500 units, D 200 units, E 15 units, B_1 0.75 mg, B_2 0.85 mg, B_3 7.5 mg, B_5 5 mg, B_6 1 mg, B_{12} 3 mcg, C 170 mg, FA 200 mcg, biotin 20 mcg, P, I, Mg, Zn, Cu, Na. Aspartame, phenylalanine, sucrose, vegetable oil. Chew. Tab. 60s. *OTC.*
Use: Multivitamin.
One-A-Day Maximum Formula. (Bayer) Fe 18 mg, vitamins A 5000 units, D 400 units, E 30 units, B_1 1.5 mg, B_2 1.7 mg, B_3 20 mg, B_5 10 mg, B_6 2 mg, B_{12} 6 mcg, C 60 mg, folic acid 0.4 mg, Ca, Cl, Cr, Cu, I, K, Mg, Mn, Mo, P, Se, Zn 15 mg, biotin 30 mcg. Tab. Bot. 60s, 100s. *OTC.*
Use: Mineral, vitamin supplement.
One-A-Day Men's Vitamins. (Bayer) Vitamin A 5000 units, C 200 mg, B_1 2.25 mg, B_2 2.55 mg, B_3 20 mg, D 400 units, E 45 units, B_6 3 mg, folic acid 0.4 mg, B_{12} 9 mcg, B_5 10 mg. Tab. Bot. 60s, 100s. *OTC.*
Use: Mineral, vitamin supplement.
One-A-Day Weight Smart. (Bayer) Ca 300 mg, Fe (as ferrous fumarate) 18 mg, vitamin A 2500 units, D 400 units, E 30 units, B_1 1.9 mg, B_2 2.125 mg, B_3 25 mg, B_5 12.5 mg, B_6 2.5 mg, B_{12} 7.5 mcg, FA 400 mcg, vitamin K, Mg, Zn, Se, Cu, Mn, Cr, EGCG, dextrose, glucose. Tab. 50s, 100s. *OTC.*
Use: Multivitamin.
One-A-Day Women's Formula. (Bayer) Ca 450 mg, Fe 27 mg, vitamins A 5000 units, D 400 units, E 30 mg, B_1 1.5 mg, B_2 1.7 mg, B_3 20 mg, B_5 10 mg, B_6 2 mg, B_{12} 6 mcg, C 60 mg, folic acid 0.4 mg, Zn 15 mg, tartrazine. Tab. Bot. 60s, 100s. *Rx.*
Use: Mineral, vitamin supplement.
1+1-F Creme. (Oxypure) Hydrocortisone 1%, pramoxine hydrochloride 1%, iodochlorhydroxyquin 3%. Tube 30 g. *Rx.*

Use: Corticosteroid; anesthetic, local; antifungal, topical.

●**onercept.** (O-ner-sept) USAN.
Use: Anti-tumor-necrosis factor activity.

One-Tablet-Daily. Various Mfr. Vitamins A 5000 units, D 400 units, E 30 mg, B_1 1.5 mg, B_2 1.7 mg, B_3 20 mg, B_5 10 mg, B_6 2 mg, B_{12} 6 mcg, C 60 mg, folic acid 0.4 mg. Tab. Bot. 30s, 100s, 250s, 365s, 1000s. *OTC.*
Use: Vitamin supplement.

One-Tablet-Daily Plus Iron. Various Mfr. Iron 18 mg, vitamins A 5000 units, D 400 units, E 15 mg, B_1 1.5 mg, B_2 1.7 mg, B_3 20 mg, B_6 2 mg, B_{12} 6 mcg, C 60 mg, folic acid 0.4 mg. Tab. Bot. 100s, 250s, 365s. *OTC.*
Use: Mineral, vitamin supplement.

One-Tablet-Daily with Iron. (Ivax) Fe 18 mg, A 5000 units, D 400 units, E 30 mg, B_1 1.5 mg, B_2 1.7 mg, B_3 20 mg, B_5 10 mg, B_6 2 mg, B_{12} 6 mcg, C 60 mg, folic acid 0.4 mg. Tab. Bot. 100s. *OTC.*
Use: Mineral, vitamin supplement.

One-Tablet-Daily with Minerals. (Ivax) Fe 18 mg, vitamins A 5000 units, D 400 units, E 30 units, B_1 1.5 mg, B_2 1.7 mg, B_3 20 mg, B_5 10 mg, B_6 2 mg, B_{12} 6 mcg, C 60 mg, folic acid 0.4 mg, Ca, Cl, Cr, Cu, I, K, Mg, Mn, Mo, P, Se, Zn 15 mg, biotin 30 mcg. Tab. Bot. 100s, 1000s. *OTC.*
Use: Mineral, vitamin supplement.

1000-BC, IM, or IV. (Solvay) Vitamins B_1 25 mg, B_2 2.5 mg, B_6 5 mg, panthenol 5 mg, B_{12} 500 mcg, niacinamide 75 mg, C 100 mg/mL. Vial 10 mL. *Rx.*
Use: Vitamin supplement.

1-2-3 Ointment No. 20. (Durel) Burow's solution, lanolin, zinc oxide (Lassar's paste). Jar oz, 1 lb, 6 lb. *OTC.*
Use: Anti-inflammatory, topical.

1-2-3 Ointment No. 21. (Durel) Burow's solution 1 part, lanolin 2, zinc oxide (Lassar's paste) 1.5 oz, cold cream 1.5 oz. Jar oz, 1 lb, 6 lb. *OTC.*
Use: Anti-inflammatory, topical.

Onoton Tablets. (Sanofi-Synthelabo) Pancreatin, hemicellulose, ox bile extracts. *OTC.*
Use: Digestive aid.

●**onsifocon A.** (on-si-FOE-kon) USAN.
Use: Hydrophobic.

Ontak. (Ligand) Denileukin diftitox 150 mcg/mL. Soln. for Inj, frozen, EDTA. Single-use vial. *Rx.*
Use: Antineoplastic; biological resonse modifier.

●**ontazolast.** (ahn-TAH-zoe-last) USAN.
Use: Antiasthmatic, leukotriene antagonist.

ontosein.
See: Orgotein.

Onxol. (Ivax) Paclitaxel 6 mg/mL, polyoxyl 35 castor oil 527 mg/mL, dehydrated alcohol 49.7%. Inj. Multi-dose vial 5 mL, 25 mL, 50 mL. *Rx.*
Use: Antimitotic agent; taxoid.

Opcon. (Bausch & Lomb) Naphazoline hydrochloride 0.1%. Soln. Bot. 15 mL. *OTC.*
Use: Mydriatic; vasoconstrictor.

Opcon-A. (Bausch & Lomb) 0.027% nephazoline hydrochloride, 0.315% pheniramine maleate, 0.5% hydroxypropyl methylcellulose, 0.01% benzalkonium chloride, 0.1% EDTA, NaCl, boric acid, sodium buffers. Soln. Bot. 15 mL. *OTC.*
Use: Mydriatic; vasoconstrictor; antihistamine.

o,p'-DDD.
Use: Miscellaneous antineoplastic.
See: Lysodren

●**opebacan.** (oh-PE-bay-kan) USAN.
Use: Antimicrobial

Operand. (Aplicare) **Aerosal:** Iodine 0.5%. 90 mL. **Skin cleanser:** Iodine 1%. 90 mL. **Oint.:** Iodine 1%. 30 g, lb, packette 1.2 g, 2.7 g. **Perineal wash conc.:** Iodine 1%. 240 mL. **Prep soln.:** Iodine 1%. 60 mL, 120 mL, 240 mL, pt, qt. **Soln:** Prep pad 100s, swab stick 25s. **Surgical scrub:** Povidone-iodine 7.5%. 60 mL, 120 mL, 240 mL, pt, qt, gal, packette 22.5 mL. **Whirlpool conc.:** Iodine 1%. Gal. *OTC.*
Use: Antiseptic; antimicrobial.

Operand Douche. (Aplicare) Povidone-iodine. Soln. Bot. 60 mL, 240 mL, UD 15 mL. *OTC.*
Use: Vaginal agent.

o-phenylphenol.
W/Amyl complex, phenylmercuric nitrate.
See: Lubraseptic Jelly.

Ophthacet. (Vortech Pharmaceuticals) Sodium sulfacetamide 10%. Soln. 15 mL. *Rx.*
Use: Anti-infective, ophthalmic.

ophthalmic agents.
See: Alamast.
   Alocril.
   Nedocromil Sodium.
   Pemirolast Potassium.

ophthalmic antihistaminic agents.
See: Azelastine hydrochloride.
   Epinastine hydrochloride.

ophthalmic decongestant agents.
See: Azelastine hydrochloride.
   Optivar.

ophthalmic diagnostic products.
See: Fluorexon.
Indocyanine Green.
Rose Bengal.
Tear Test Strips.
ophthalmic phototherapy.
See: Verteporfin.
ophthalmic surgical adjuncts.
See: Botox.
Botulinum Toxin Type A.
Trypan Blue.
Ophtha P/S. (Edwards) Prednisolone acetate 0.5%, sodium sulfacetamide 10%, hydroxyethyl cellulose, EDTA, polysorbate 80, sodium thiosulfate, benzalkonium chloride 0.025%. Susp. Bot. 5 mL. *Rx.*
Use: Corticosteroid; anti-infective, ophthalmic.
Ophtha P/S Ophthalmic Suspension. (Edwards) Sodium sulfacetamide 10%, prednisolone acetate 0.5%. Bot. 5 mL w/dropper. *Rx.*
Use: Corticosteroid; anti-infective, ophthalmic.
Ophthetic. (Allergan) Proparacaine hydrochloride 0.5%. Bot. 15 mL. *Rx.*
Use: Anesthetic, ophthalmic.
opioid analgesics.
See: Alfentanil Hydrochloride.
Codeine.
Fentanyl Citrate.
Fentanyl Transdermal System.
Hydromorphone Hydrochloride.
Levomethadyl Acetate Hydrochloride.
Levorphanol Tartrate.
Meperidine Hydrochloride.
Methadone Hydrochloride.
Morphine Sulfate.
Opium.
Oxycodone Hydrochloride.
Oxymorphone Hydrochloride.
Propoxyphene.
Remifentanil Hydrochloride.
Sufentanil Citrate.
Tramadol Hydrochloride.
• **opipramol hydrochloride.** (oh-PIH-prah-mole) USAN.
Use: Antipsychotic; antidepressant; tranquilizer.
• **opium.** (OH-pee-uhm) *USP 28.*
Use: Opioid analgesic; pharmaceutic necessity for powdered opium.
See: Opium Tincture, Deodorized.
Paregoric.
opium and belladonna. (Wyeth) Powdered opium 60 mg, extract of belladonna 15 mg. Supp. Box 20s. *c-II.*
Use: Analgesic, narcotic; anticholinergic; antispasmodic.

• **opium powdered.** *USP 28.*
Use: Pharmaceutical necessity for Paregoric.
W/Albumin tannate, colloidal kaolin, pectin.
See: Ekrised.
W/Belladonna extract.
See: B & O.
W/Bismuth subgallate, kaolin, pectin, zinc phenolsulfonate.
See: Diastay.
opium tincture.
W/Homatropine MBr, Pectin.
See: Dia-Quel.
opium tincture, camphorated.
Use: Antidiarrheal.
See: Paregoric.
opium tincture, deodorized. (Ranbaxy) Anhydrous morphine equivalent to 10 mg/mL, alcohol 19%. Liq. Bot. 120 mL, 473 mL. *c-II.*
Use: Opioid analgesic.
• **oprelvekin.** (oh-PRELL-veh-kin) USAN.
Use: Hematopoietic, interleukin.
See: Neumega.
Opti-Bon Eye Drops. (Barrows) Phenylephrine hydrochloride, berberine sulfate, boric acid, sodium Cl, sodium bisulfite, glycerin, camphor, water, peppermint water, thimerosal 0.004%. Bot. 1 oz. *OTC.*
Use: Ophthalmic.
Opticaps. (Health for Life Brands) Vitamins A 32,500 units, D 3250 units, B_1 15 mg, B_2 5 mg, B_6 0.5 mg, C 150 mg, E 5 units, calcium pantothenate 3 mg, niacinamide 150 mg, B_{12} 20 mcg, Fe 11.26 mg, choline bitartrate 30 mg, inositol 30 mg, pepsin 32.5 mg, diastase 22.5 mg, Ca 30 mg, P 25 mg, Mn 0.7 mg, Fr. dicalcium phosphate 110 mg, Mn 1.3 mg, K 0.68 mg, Zn 0.45 mg, hesperidin compound 25 mg, biotin 20 mcg, brewer's yeast 50 mg, wheat germ oil 20 mg, hydrolyzed yeast 81.25 mg, protein digest 47.04 mg, amino acids 34.21 mg. Cap. Bot. 30s, 60s, 90s, 1000s. *OTC.*
Use: Mineral, vitamin supplement.
Opticare PMS. (Standard Drug Co.) Fe 2.5 mg, vitamins 2083 units, D 17 units, E 14 units, B_1 4.2 mg, B_2 4.2 mg, B_3 4.2 mg, B_5 4.2 mg, B_6 50 mg, B_{12} 10.4 mcg, C 250 mg, folic acid 0.03 mg, Cr, Cu, I, K, Mg, Mn, Se, Zn 4.2 mg, biotin 10.4 mcg, choline bitartrate, bioflavonoids, inositol, PABA, rutin, Ca, amylase activity, protease activity, lipase activity, betaine, tartrazine. Bot. 150s. *OTC.*
Use: Mineral, vitamin supplement.

Opti-Clean. (Alcon) Tween 21, polymeric cleaners, hydroxyethyl cellulose, thimerosal 0.004%, EDTA 0.1%. Bot 12 mL, 20 mL. *OTC.*
Use: Contact lens care.

Opti-Clean II. (Alcon) Polymeric cleaning agent, Tween 21, EDTA 0.1%, polyquaternium 1 0.001%, thimerosal free. Bot. 12 mL, 20 mL. *OTC.*
Use: Contact lens care.

Opti-Clean II Especially For Sensitive Eyes. (Alcon) EDTA 0.1%, polyquaternium 1 0.001%, polymeric cleaners, Tween 21. Thimerosal free. Bot. 12 mL, 20 mL. *OTC.*
Use: Contact lens care.

Opticyl. (Optopics) Tropicamide 0.5%, 1%. Soln. Bot. 2 mL, 15 mL. *Rx.*
Use: Cycloplegic; mydriatic.

Opti-Free Enzymatic Cleaner. (Alcon) Highly purified pork pancreatin. Tab. Pkg. 6s, 12s, 18s. *OTC.*
Use: Contact lens care.

Opti-Free Express Multi-Purpose. (Alcon) Isotonic myristamidopropyl dimethylamine 0.0005%, polyquaternium-1 0.001%, citrate, sodium chloride, boric acid, sorbitol, EDTA. Soln. 118 mL. *OTC.*
Use: Soft contact lens rewetting solution.

Opti-Free Non-Hydrogen Peroxide-Containing System. (Alcon) Citrate buffer, NaCl, EDTA 0.05%, polyquaternium 1 0.001%. Soln. 118 mL, 237 mL, 355 mL. *OTC.*
Use: Ophthalmic.

Opti-Free Rewetting Solution. (Alcon) Citrate buffer, sodium Cl, EDTA 0.05%, polyquaternium 1 0.001%. Soln. Bot. 10 mL, 20 mL. *OTC.*
Use: Contact lens care.

Opti-Free Surfactant Cleaning Solution. (Alcon) EDTA 0.01%, polyquaternium 1 0.001%, microclens polymeric cleaners, Tween 21. Thimerosal free. Soln. Bot. 12 mL, 20 mL. *OTC.*
Use: Contact lens care.

Optigene. (Pfeiffer) Sodium Cl, mono- and dibasic sodium phosphate, benzalkonium Cl, EDTA. Soln. Bot. 118 mL. *OTC.*
Use: Irrigant, ophthalmic.

Optigene 3. (Pfeiffer) Tetrahydrozoline hydrochloride 0.05%. Soln. Bot. 15 mL. *OTC.*
Use: Mydriatic, vasoconstrictor.

Optilets-500. (Abbott) Vitamins B_1 15 mg, B_2 10 mg, B_3 100 mg, B_5 20 mg, B_6 5 mg, C 500 mg, A 10,000 units, D 400 units, E 30 units, B_{12} 12 mcg.

Filmtab. Bot. 120s. *OTC.*
Use: Mineral, vitamin supplement.

Optilets-M-500. (Abbott) Vitamins C 500 mg, B_3 100 mg, B_5 20 mg, $B_1$15 mg, A 5000 units, B_2 10 mg, B_6 5 mg, D 400 units, B_{12} 12 mcg, E 30 units, Fe 20 mg, Mg, Zn 1.5 mg, Cu, Mn, I. Filmtab. Bot. 120s. *OTC.*
Use: Mineral, vitamin supplement.

OptiMARK. (Mallinckrodt) Gadoversetamide 330.9 mg, preservative free. Inj. Bot. 50 mL. *Rx.*
Use: Radiopaque agent, parenteral.

Optimental. (Ross) Protein 12.2 g, fat 6.7 g, carbohydrate 32.9 g, vitamin A 1950 units, D 67 units, E 50 units, K 20 mcg, C 50 mg, folic acid 135 mcg, B_1 0.5 mg, B_2 0.57 mg, B_6 0.67 mg, B_{12} 2 mcg, B_3 6.7 mg, choline 100 mg, biotin 100 mcg, B_5 3.4 mg, Na 250 mg, K 420 mg, chloride 320 mg, Ca 250 mg, P 250 mg, Mg 100 mg, I 38 mcg, Mn 0.84 mg, Cu 0.34 mg, Zn 3.8 mg, Fe 3 mg, Se 12 mcg, Cr 20 mcg, Mo 25 mcg, sucrose, canola oil, soy oil. Liq. Bot. 237 mL. *OTC.*
Use: Nutritional therapy, enteral.

Optimine. (Key) Azatadine maleate 1 mg, lactose. Tab. Bot. 100s. *Rx.*
Use: Antihistamine, non-selective piperidine.

Optimox Prenatal. (Optimox) Ca 100 mg, iron 5 mg, vitamins A 833 units, D 67 units, E 2 mg, B_1 0.5 mg, B_2 0.6 mg, B_3 6.7 mg, B_5 3.3 mg, B_6 0.73 mg, B_{12} 0.87 mcg, C 30 mg, folic acid 0.13 mg, Cr, Cu, I, K, Mg, Mn, Se, Zn 3.17 mg. Tab. Bot. 360s. *OTC.*
Use: Mineral, vitamin supplement.

Optimyd. (Schering-Plough) Prednisolone phosphate 0.5%, sodium sulfacetamide 10%, sodium thiosulfate. Sterile Soln. Drop Bot. 5 mL. *Rx.*
Use: Anti-infective; corticosteroid; ophthalmic.

Opti-One. (Alcon) EDTA 0.05%, polyquaternium 1 0.001%, NaCl, sodium citrate. Buffered, isotonic. Soln. 120 mL. *OTC.*
Use: Contact lens care.

Opti-One Multi-Purpose. (Alcon) EDTA 0.05%, polyquaternium 0.001%, NaCl, mannitol. Buffered, isotonic. Soln. Bot. 118 mL, 237 mL, 355 mL, 473 mL. *OTC.*
Use: Contact lens care.

Opti-One Rewetting. (Alcon) EDTA 0.05%, polyquaternium 1 0.001%, sodium chloride, citrate buffer, isotonic. Drops. Bot. 10 mL. *OTC.*
Use: Contact lens care.

OptiPranolol. (Bausch & Lomb) Metipranolol hydrochloride 0.3%, benzalkonium chloride 0.004%, glycerin, EDTA, povidone, hydrochloric acid, sodium chloride, sodium hydroxide and/or hydrochloric acid. Soln. Bot. 5 mL, 10 mL w/dropper. *Rx.*
Use: Antiglaucoma agent; beta-adrenergic blocker.

Optiray 160. (Mallinckrodt) Ioversol 339 mg, iodine 160 mg/mL, EDTA. Inj. Bot. 50 mL, 100 mL. *Rx.*
Use: Radiopaque agent, parenteral.

Optiray 300. (Mallinckrodt) Ioversol 636 mg, iodine 300 mg/mL, EDTA. Inj. Bot. 50 mL, 100 mL, 150 mL. 200 mL fill in 250 mL Bot. Hand–held syr. 50 mL. 100 mL fill in 125 mL Power Injector Syringe. *Rx.*
Use: Radiopaque agent, parenteral.

Optiray 350. (Mallinckrodt) Ioversol 741 mg, iodine 350 mg/mL, EDTA. Inj. Bot. 50 mL, 100 mL, 150 mL. 75 mL fill in 150 mL Bot., 200 mL fill in 250 mL Bot. Hand-held Syringe 30 mL, 50 mL. 50 mL fill in 125 mL, 75 mL fill in 125 mL, 100 mL fill in 125 mL Power Injector Syringe. Power Injector Syringe 125 mL. *Rx.*
Use: Radiopaque agent, parenteral.

Optiray 320. (Mallinckrodt) Ioversol 678 mg, iodine 320 mg/mL, EDTA. Inj. Vial 20 mL, 30 mL. Bot. 50 mL, 100 mL, 150 mL. 75 mL fill in 150 mL Bot. 200 mL fill in 250 mL Bot. Hand-held Syringe 30 mL, 50 mL. 50 mL fill in 125 mL, 75 mL fill in 125 mL, 100 mL fill in 125 mL Power Injector Syringe. Power Injector Syringe 125 mL. *Rx.*
Use: Radiopaque agent, parenteral.

Optiray 240. (Mallinckrodt) Ioversol 509 mg, iodine 240 mg/mL, EDTA. Inj. Bot. 50 mL, 100 mL, 150 mL, 200 mL fill in 250 mL Bot. Hand-held Syringe 50 mL. Power Injector Syringe 125 mL. *Rx.*
Use: Radiopaque agent, parenteral.

Opti-Soft. (Alcon) Isotonic soln of sodium Cl, borate buffer, EDTA 0.1%, polyquaternium 1 0.001%. Thimerosal free. Soln. Bot. 237 mL, 355 mL. *OTC.*
Use: Contact lens care.

Opti-Soft Especially for Sensitive Eyes. (Alcon) Buffered, isotonic. EDTA 0.1%, polyquaternium 1 0.001%, NaCl, borate buffer. For lenses w/≤ 45% water content. Soln. Bot. 118 mL, 237 mL, 355 mL. *OTC.*
Use: Contact lens care.

Opti-Tears. (Alcon) Isotonic solution with dextran, sodium Cl, potassium Cl,

hydroxypropyl methylcellulose, EDTA 0.1%, polyquaternium 1 0.001%. Thimerosal and sorbic acid free. Soln. Bot. 15 mL. *OTC.*
Use: Contact lens care.

Optivar. (MedPointe Healthcare) Azelastine hydrochloride 0.5 mg/mL, benzalkonium chloride 0.125 mg, EDTA, dihydrate, hydroxypropylmethylcellulose, sodium hydroxide. Soln. Cont. 10 mL w/6 mL soln. w/dropper. *Rx.*
Use: Ophthalmic decongestant, antihistamine.

Optivite for Women. (Optimox) Vitamins A 2083 units, D 16.7 units, E 14 mg, B_1 4.2 mg, B_2 4.2 mg, B_3 4.2 mg, B_5 4.2 mg, B_6 50 mg, B_{12} 10.4 mcg, C 250 mg, Fe 2.5 mg, folic acid 0.03 mg, Zn 4.2 mg, choline 52 mg, inositol 10 mg, Cr, Cu, I, K, Mg, Mn, Se, citrus bioflavonoids, PABA, rutin, pancreatin, biotin. Tab. Bot. 180s. *OTC.*
Use: Mineral, vitamin supplement.

Optivite P.M.T. (Optimox) Vitamins A 2083 units, D, E 16.7 mg, B_1 4.2 mg, B_2 4.2 mg, B_3 4.2 mg, B_5 4.2 mg, B_6 50 mg, B_{12} 10.4 mcg, C 250 mg, Fe 2.5 mg, FA 0.03 mg, Zn 4.2 mg, choline, Ca, Cr, Cu, I, K, Mg, Mn, Se, bioflavonoids, betaine, PABA, rutin, pancreatin, biotin, inositol. Tab. Bot. 180s. *OTC.*
Use: Mineral, vitamin supplement.

OptiZen. (InnoZen) Polysorbate 80 0.5%, EDTA, NaCl, sodium phosphate, sorbic acid. Drops. 10 mL. *OTC.*
Use: Artificial tears.

Opti-Zyme Enzymatic Cleaner Especially For Sensitive Eyes. (Alcon) Pork pancreatin tablets. Pak 8s, 24s, 36s, 56s. *OTC.*
Use: Contact lens care.

Orabase. (Colgate Oral) Gelatin, pectin, sodium carboxymethylcellulose in hydrocarbon gel w/polyethylene and mineral oil. 0.75 g Pkt. Box 100s. Tube 5 g, 15 g. *OTC.*
Use: Mouth preparation.

Orabase-B. (Colgate Oral) Benzocaine 20%, mineral oil. Paste. 5 g, 15 g. *OTC.*
Use: Mouth and throat preparation.

Orabase Baby. (Colgate Oral) Benzocaine 7.5%, alcohol free, fruit flavor. Gel. Tube 7.2 mL. *OTC.*
Use: Anesthetic, local.

Orabase Gel. (Colgate Oral) Benzocaine 15%, ethyl alcohol, tannic acid, salicylic acid, saccharin. Gel. Tube 7 mL. *OTC.*
Use: Anesthetic, local.

Orabase HCA. (Colgate Oral) Hydrocortisone acetate 0.5%, polyethylene 5%, mineral oil. Gel. Tube 5 mL. *Rx.*
Use: Corticosteroid, dental.

Orabase Lip. (Colgate Oral) Benzocaine 5%, allantoin 1.5%, menthol 0.5%, petrolatum, lanolin, parabens, camphor, phenol/g. Cream. Tube 10 g. *OTC.*
Use: Anesthetic, local.

Orabase Plain. (Colgate Oral) Gelatin, pectin & sodium carboxymethyl cellulose in polyethylene and mineral gel. Paste. Tube 5 g, 15 g. *OTC.*
Use: Mouth and throat preparation.

Orabase with Benzocaine. (Colgate Oral) Benzocaine 20% in gelbase. Gel. Pkt. 0.75 g, Box 100s. Tube 5 mL, 15 mL. *OTC.*
Use: Anesthetic, local.

Oracit. (Carolina Medical Products) Sodium citrate 490 mg, citric acid 640 mg/5 mL, (sodium 1 mEq/mL equivalent to 1 mEq bicarbonate), alcohol 0.25%. Soln. Bot. Pt, UD 15 mL, 30 mL. *Rx.*
Use: Alkalinizer, systemic.

Oraderm Lip Balm. (Schattner) Sodium phenolate, sodium tetraborate, phenol, base containing an anionic emulsifier. ⅛ oz. *OTC.*
Use: Anesthetic; antiseptic, local.

ORA5. (McHenry Laboratories, Inc.) Copper sulfate, iodine, potassium iodide, alcohol 1.5%. Liq. Bot. 3.75 mL, 30 mL. *OTC.*
Use: Mouth preparation.

Orafix Medicated. (GlaxoSmithKline) Allantoin 0.2%, benzocaine 2%. Tube 0.75 oz. *OTC.*
Use: Anesthetic, local; denture adhesive.

Orafix Original. (GlaxoSmithKline) Tube 1.5 oz, 2.5 oz, 4 oz. *OTC.*
Use: Denture adhesive.

Orafix Special. (GlaxoSmithKline) Tube 1.4 oz, 2.4 oz. *OTC.*
Use: Denture adhesive.

Oragrafin Calcium Granules. (Bristol-Myers Squibb) Ipodate calcium (61.7% iodine) 3 g/8 g Pkg. 25 × 1 dose pkg.
Use: Radiopaque agent.

Orahesive. (Colgate Oral) Gelatin, pectin, sodium carboxymethylcellulose. Pow. Bot. 25 g. *OTC.*
Use: Denture adhesive.

Orajel. (Del) Benzocaine 10% in a special base. Gel. Tube 0.2 oz, 0.5 oz. *OTC.*
Use: Anesthetic, local.

Orajel D. (Del) Benzocaine 10%, saccharin. Gel. Tube 9.45 mL. *OTC.*
Use: Anesthetic, local.

Orajel Mouth-Aid. (Del) Benzocaine 20%. **Liq.:** Cetylpyridinium 0.1%, ethyl alcohol 70%, tartrazine, saccharin, 13.5 mL. **Gel:** Benzalkonium Cl 0.02%, zinc Cl 0.1%, EDTA, saccharin. 5.6 g, 10 g. *OTC.*
Use: Anesthetic, local.

Orajel Perioseptic. (Del) Carbamide peroxide 15%, saccharin, methylparaben, EDTA, sorbitol, ethyl alcohol. Liq. Bot. 240 mL. *OTC.*
Use: Mouth and throat product.

Orajel P.M. Nighttime Formula Toothache Pain Relief. (Del) Benzocaine 20%, menthol, methyl salicylate, saccharin. Cream. 5.4 g. *OTC.*
Use: Mouth and throat product.

Oral-B Muppets Fluoride Toothpaste. (Oral-B) Fluoride 0.22%. Pump 4.3 oz. *OTC.*
Use: Dental caries agent.

oralcid.
See: Acetarsone.

oral contraceptives.
See: Alesse.
    Apri.
    Aviane.
    Brevicon.
    Demulen 1/35.
    Demulen 1/50.
    Desogen.
    Enovid-E.
    Estrostep 21.
    Estrostep Fe.
    GenCept.
    Jenest-28.
    Levlen.
    Levlite.
    Levora.
    Loestrin 21 1/20.
    Loestrin 21 1.5/30.
    Loestrin Fe 1/20.
    Loestrin Fe 1.5/30.
    Lo/Ovral.
    Low-Ogestrel.
    Microgestin Fe 1/20.
    Microgestin Fe 1.5/30.
    Micronor.
    Mircette.
    Modicon.
    MonoNessa.
    Nelulen.
    Necon 0.5/35.
    Necon 1/35.
    Necon 1/50.
    Necon 10/11.
    Nelova 0.5/35E.
    Nelova 1/35E.
    Nelova 1/50M.
    Nelova 10/11.
    Nor-Q.D.

Norethin 1/35 E.
Norethin 1/50 M.
Nordette.
Norinyl 1+35.
Norinyl 1+50.
Norlestrin.
Nortrel 0.5/35.
Nortrel 1/35.
Ogestrel.
Ortho Cept.
Ortho-Cyclen.
Ortho Tri-Cyclen.
Ortho-Novum 1/35.
Ortho-Novum 1/50.
Ortho-Novum 7/7/7.
Ortho-Novum 10/11.
Ovcon-35.
Ovcon-50.
Ovral-28.
Ovrette.
Ovulen
Plan B.
Preven.
Tri-Levlen.
Tri-Norinyl.
Triphasil.
Trivora-28.
Yasmin.
Zovia 1/35E.
Zovia 1/50E.
Oral Drops/Canker Sore Relief. (Weeks & Leo) Carbamide peroxide 10% in anhydrous glycerin base. Bot. 30 mL. *OTC.*
Use: Mouth preparation.
Oralone Dental. (Thames Pharmacal) Triamcinolone acetonide 0.1%. Paste 5 g. *Rx.*
Use: Corticosteroid, dental.

oral rehydration salts.
Use: Electrolyte combination.
Oral Wound Rinse. (Carrington) Acemannan hydrogel. Fructose. Mouthwash. 7.4 g. *OTC.*
Use: Mouth and throat product.
Oramide. (Major) Tolbutamide 0.5 g. Tab. Bot. 100s, 1000s. *Rx.*
Use: Antidiabetic.
Oraminic II. (Vortech Pharmaceuticals) Brompheniramine maleate 10 mg/mL. Inj. Vial. 10 mL multidose. *Rx.*
Use: Antihistamine.
Oramorph SR. (aaiPharma) Morphine sulfate 15 mg, 30 mg, 60 mg, 100 mg, lactose. CR Tab. Bot. 50s (30 mg only), 100s, 250s (30 mg only), 500s (15 mg only), UD 25s (60 mg and 100 mg only), 100s (15 mg and 30 mg only). *c-II.*
Use: Opioid analgesic.

orange flower oil. *NF 23.*
Use: Flavor; perfume; vehicle.
orange flower water. *NF 23.*
Use: Flavor; perfume.
• **orange oil.** *NF 23.*
Use: Flavor.
• **orange peel tincture, sweet.** *NF 23.*
Use: Flavor.
orange spirit, compound. *NF 23.*
Use: Flavor.
• **orange syrup.** *NF 23.*
Use: Flavored vehicle.
Orap. (Teva) Pimozide 1 mg, 2 mg, lactose. Tab. Bot. 100s. *Rx.*
Use: Antipsychotic.
Oraphen-PD. (Great Southern) Acetaminophen 120 mg/5 mL, alcohol 5%, cherry flavor. Elix. 120 mL. *OTC.*
Use: Analgesic.
Orapred. (BioMarin) Prednisolone base 15 mg (prednisolone sodium phosphate 20.2 mg)/5 mL, dye free, alcohol 2%, fructose, sorbitol, grape flavor. Oral Soln. Bot. 237 mL. *Rx.*
Use: Corticosteroid.
orarsan.
See: Acetarsone.
Orasept. (Pharmakon) Tannic acid 12.16%, methyl benzethonium hydrochloride 1.53%, ethyl alcohol 53.31%, camphor, menthol, benzyl alcohol, spearmint oil, cassia oil. Liq. Bot. 15 mL. *OTC.*
Use: Mouth and throat preparation.
Orasept, Throat. (Pharmakon) Benzocaine 0.996%, methyl benzethonium Cl 1.037%, sorbitol 70%, menthol, peppermint, saccharin. Throat spray. 45 mL. *OTC.*
Use: Mouth and throat preparation.
Orasol. (Ivax) Benzocaine 6.3%, phenol 0.5%, alcohol 70%, povidone-iodine. Liq. Bot. 14.79 mL. *OTC.*
Use: Anesthetic, local.
Orasone. (Solvay) Prednisone. Tab. **1 mg, 5 mg, 10 mg, 20 mg:** Bot. 100s, 1000s, UD 100s. **50 mg:** Bot. 100s, UD 100s. *Rx.*
Use: Corticosteroid.
OraSure HIV-1. (Epitope) Collection kit: Cotton fiber on a stick with collection vial. Device for oral specimen collection. For professional use only.
Use: Diagnostic aid.
Orazinc. (Mericon Industries) Zinc sulfate 220 mg. Cap. Bot. 100s, 1000s. *OTC.*
Use: Mineral supplement.
orbenin. Sodium cloxacillin.
Use: Anti-infective.
See: Cloxapen.

Orbiferrous. (Orbit) Ferrous fumarate 300 mg, vitamins B_{12} 12 mcg, C 50 mg, B_1 3 mg, defatted desiccated liver 50 mg. Tab. Bot. 60s, 500s. *OTC.*
Use: Mineral, vitamin supplement.

Orbit. (Spanner) Vitamins A 6250 units, D 400 units, B_1 3 mg, B_2 3 mg, B_6 2 mg, B_{12} 5 mcg, C 75 mg, niacinamide 20 mg, calcium pantothenate 10 mg, E 15 units, biotin 15 mcg, Fe 20 mg. Tab. Bot. 100s. *OTC.*
Use: Mineral, vitamin supplement.

● **orbofiban acetate.** (ore-boe-FIE-ban) USAN.
Use: Fibrinogen receptor antagonist; platelet aggregation inhibitor, antithrombotic.

● **orconazole nitrate.** (ahr-KOE-nah-zole NYE-trate) USAN.
Use: Antifungal.

● **oregovomab.** (oh-re-GOE-voe-mab) USAN.
Use: Monoclonal antibody (ovarian cancer).

Oretic. (Abbott) Hydrochlorothiazide 25 mg, 50 mg. Tab. Bot. 100s, 1000s, UD 100s. *Rx.*
Use: Diuretic.

Orexin. (Roberts) Vitamins B_1 8.1 mg, B_6 4.1 mg, B_{12} 25 mcg. Chew. Tab. Bot. 100s. *OTC.*
Use: Vitamin supplement.

Organidin. (Wallace) **Tab.:** 30 mg. Bot. 100s. **Elix.:** 60 mg/5 mL. 21.75% alcohol, glucose, saccharin. Bot. Pt., gal. **Soln.:** 50 mg/mL. Bot. 30 mL w/dropper.
Use: Expectorant.

Organidin NR. (Medpointe) Guaifenesin 100 mg/5 mL, saccharin, sorbitol, raspberry flavor. Liq. Bot. 473 mL. *Rx.*
Use: Expectorant.

Orglagen. (Ivax) Orphenadrine citrate 100 mg. Tab. Bot. 100s, 1000s. *Rx.*
Use: Muscle relaxant.

● **orgotein.** (ORE-go-teen) USAN. A group of soluble metalloproteins isolated from liver, red blood cells, and other mammalian tissues.
Use: Anti-inflammatory; antirheumatic.

orgotein. (Diagnostic Data) Pure water-soluble protein with a compact conformation maintained by 4 g atoms of chelated divalent metals, produced from bovine liver as a Cu-Zn mixed chelate having superoxide dismutase activity. Ontosein, Palosein.

oriental ginseng.
See: Asian Ginseng, *NF 20.*

Original Alka-Seltzer Effervescent. (Bayer Corp. (Consumer Div.)) 1700 mg sodium bicarbonate, 325 mg aspirin, 1000 mg citric acid, 9 mg phenylalanine, 506 mg Na, aspartame. Tab. Pkg. 24s. *OTC.*
Use: Antacid.

Original Eclipse Sunscreen. (Tri Tec) Padimate O, glyceryl PABA, SPF 10. Lot. Bot. 100s. *OTC.*
Use: Sunscreen.

Original Sensodyne. (Block Drug) Strontium chloride hexahydrate 10%, saccharin, sorbitol. Toothpaste. Tube 59.5 g. *OTC.*
Use: Mouth and throat preparation.

Orinase. (Pharmacia) Tolbutamide 500 mg. Tab. Bot. 200s, unit-of-use 100s. *Rx.*
Use: Antidiabetic.

Orinase Diagnostic. (Pharmacia) Tolbutamide sodium 1 g/vial. Pow. for Inj. Vial. *Rx.*
Use: In vivo diagnostic aid.

Orisul. (Novartis) Sulfaphenazole. A sulfonamide under study.

● **oritavancin diphosphate.** USAN.
Use: Antibacterial.

● **orlistat.** (ORE-lih-stat) USAN.
Use: Inhibitor, pancreatic lipase.
See: Xenical.

● **ormaplatin.** (ORE-mah-PLAT-in) USAN.
Use: Antineoplastic.

● **ormetoprim.** (ore-MEH-toe-PRIM) USAN.
Use: Anti-infective.

Ornex No Drowsiness. (B.F. Ascher) Pseudoephedrine hydrochloride 30 mg, acetaminophen 325 mg. Tab. Bot. 24s, 48s. *OTC.*
Use: Upper respiratory combination, analgesic, decongestant.

Ornex No Drowsiness Maximum Strength. (B.F. Ascher) Pseudoephedrine hydrochloride 30 mg, acetaminophen 500 mg. Tab. Bot. 24s, 48s. *OTC.*
Use: Upper respiratory combination, analgesic, decongestant.

● **ornidazole.** (ahr-NIH-DAH-zole) USAN.
Use: Anti-infective.

Ornidyl. (Hoechst) Eflornithine hydrochloride 200 mg/mL. Inj. Vial. 100 mL. *Rx.*
Use: Antiprotozoal.

● **orpanoxin.** (AHR-pan-OX-in) USAN.
Use: Anti-inflammatory.

Orpeneed VK. (Hanlon) Penicillin, buffered, 400,000 units. Tab. Bot. 100s. *Rx.*
Use: Anti-infective, penicillin.

•**orphenadrine citrate.** (ore-FEN-uh-dreen) *USP 28.*
Use: Antihistamine, muscle relaxant.
See: Banflex.
  Flexoject.
  Flexon.
  Myolin.
  Norflex.
  Orphanate.
W/Aspirin, caffeine.
  See: Orphengesic.
  Orphengesic Forte.
W/Aspirin, phenacetin, caffeine.
  See: Norgesic.
  Norgesic Forte.
orphenadrine citrate. (Various Mfr.)
Orphenadrine citrate. **Inj:** 30 mg/mL.
Amps 2 mL, vial 10 mL. **Tab.:** 100 mg.
Bot. 30s, 100s, 500s, 1000s. *Rx.*
Use: Antihistamine; muscle relaxant
Orphengesic. (Various Mfr.) Orphena-drine citrate 25 mg, aspirin 385 mg,
caffeine 30 mg, lactose. Tab. Bot. 100s,
500s, UD 100s. *Rx.*
Use: Analgesic, muscle relaxant.
Orphengesic Forte. (Various Mfr.)
Orphenadrine citrate 50 mg, aspirin
770 mg, caffeine 60 mg, lactose. Tab.
Bot. 100s, 500s. *Rx.*
Use: Analgesic, muscle relaxant.
Ortac-DM. (ION Laboratories, Inc.) Dex-tromethorphan 10 mg, phenylephrine
hydrochloride 5 mg, guaifenesin
100 mg/5 ml. Liq. Bot. 4 oz. *OTC.*
Use: Antitussive, decongestant,
expectorant.
ortal sodium. Sodium 5-ethyl-5-hexyl-barbiturate. Hexethal sodium.
ortedrine.
See: Amphetamine.
orthesin.
See: Benzocaine.
Ortho All-Flex Diaphragm. (Ortho-McNeil) Diaphragm kit (all flex arcing
spring) in plastic compact, sizes 55, 60,
65, 70, 75, 80, 85, 90, 95 mm. *Rx.*
Use: Contraceptive.
orthocaine.
See: Orthoform.
Ortho-Cept. (Ortho-McNeil) Desogestrel
0.15 mg, ethinyl estradiol 30 mcg, lac-tose. Tab. *Dialpak* and *Veridate* 28s.
Rx.
Use: Sex hormone, contraceptive
hormone.
Orthoclone OKT3. (Ortho Biotech) Muro-monab-CD3 5 mg/5 mL. Polysorbate
80 1 mg. Inj. Amps 5 mL. *Rx.*
Use: Immunosuppressant.
Ortho-Cyclen. (Ortho-McNeil) Norgesti-mate 0.25 mg, ethinyl estradiol 35 mcg,

lactose. Tab. *Dialpak* and *Veridate* 28s.
Rx.
Use: Sex hormone, contraceptive
hormone.
Ortho Diaphragm. (Ortho-McNeil) Dia-phragm kit, coil spring sizes 50, 55,
60, 65, 70, 75, 80, 85, 90, 95, 100,
105 mm. *Rx.*
Use: Contraceptive.
Ortho Diaphragm-White. (Ortho-McNeil)
Diaphragm kit, flat spring sizes 55, 60,
65, 70, 75, 80, 85, 90, 95 mm. *Rx.*
Use: Contraceptive.
Ortho Dienestrol Vaginal Cream.
(Ortho-McNeil) Dienestrol 0.01%.
Cream. Tube 78 g with or without
applicator. *Rx.*
Use: Estrogen.
Ortho-Est. (Women First Healthcare)
Estropipate 0.75 mg, 1.5 mg, lactose.
Tab. Bot. 100s. *Rx.*
Use: Estrogen.
Ortho Evra. (Ortho-McNeil) Norelgestro-min 6 mg, ethinyl estradiol 0.75 mg/
patch. Transdermal system. Box cycles
(3 patches), single patches. *Rx.*
Use: Sex hormone, contraceptive
hormone.
Orthoflavin. (Enzyme Process) Vitamins
C 150 mg, E 25 mg. Tab. Bot. 100s,
250s. *OTC.*
Use: Vitamin supplement.
Orthoform. (Columbus) Tyrothricin
0.5 mg, tetracaine hydrochloride 0.5%,
epinephrine 1/1000 Soln. 2%/g. Oint.
Tube oz. *Rx.*
Use: Anti-infective, ophthalmic.
Ortho-Gynol Contraceptive. (Johnson
& Johnson) Oxtoxynol 9. Gel. Tube.
75 g w/applicator and 75 g, 114 g re-fills. *OTC.*
Use: Contraceptive.
ortho-hydroxybenzoic acid. Salicylic
Acid.
orthohydroxyphenylmercuric chloride.
Use: Antiseptic.
W/Benzocaine, ephedrine hydrochloride.
  See: Myrimgacaine.
W/Benzocaine, parachlorometaxylenol,
benzalkonium Cl, phenol.
  See: Unguentine.
W/Benzoic acid, salicylic acid.
  See: NP-27.
Ortho Micronor. (Ortho-McNeil) Nor-ethindrone 0.35 mg, lactose. Tab.
Dialpak 28s. *Rx.*
Use: Sex hormone, contraceptive
hormone.
Ortho-Novum 1/50. (Ortho-McNeil) Nor-ethindrone 1 mg, mestranol 50 mcg,
lactose. Tab. *Dialpak* 28s. *Rx.*
Use: Sex hormone, contraceptive
hormone.

Ortho-Novum 1/35. (Ortho-McNeil) Norethindrone 1 mg, ethinyl estradiol 35 mcg. lactose. Tab. *Dialpak* and *Veridate* 28s. *Rx.*
Use: Sex hormone, contraceptive hormone.

Ortho-Novum 7/7/7. (Ortho-McNeil) **Phase 1:** Norethindrone 0.5 mg, ethinyl estradiol 35 mcg. **Phase 2:** Norethindrone 0.75 mg, ethinyl estradiol 35 mcg. **Phase 3:** Norethindrone 1 mg, ethinyl estradiol 35 mcg. Lactose. Tab. *Dialpak* and *Veridate* 28s. *Rx.*
Use: Sex hormone, contraceptive hormone.

Ortho-Novum 10/11. (Ortho-McNeil) **Phase 1:** Norethindrone 0.5 mg, ethinyl estradiol 35 mcg. **Phase 2:** Norethindrone 1 mg, ethinyl estradiol 35 mcg, lactose. Tab. *Dialpak* and *Veridate* 28s. *Rx.*
Use: Sex hormone, contraceptive hormone.

Ortho Personal Lubricant. (Johnson & Johnson) Greaseless, water-soluble, and non-staining aqueous hydrocolloid gel. Acid buffered to vaginal pH. Tube 2 oz, 4 oz. *OTC.*
Use: Lubricant.

Ortho Tri-Cyclen. (Ortho-McNeil) **Phase 1:** Norgestimate 0.18 mg, ethinyl estradiol 35 mcg. **Phase 2:** Norgestimate 0.215 mg, ethinyl estradiol 35 mcg. **Phase 3:** Norgestimate 0.25 mg, ethinyl estradiol 35 mcg.Lactose. Tab. *Dialpak* and *Veridate* 28s. *Rx.*
Use: Sex hormone, contraceptive hormone.

Ortho Tri-Cyclen Lo. (Ortho-McNeil) **Phase 1:** Norgestimate 0.18 mg, ethinyl estradiol 25 mcg. **Phase 2:** Norgestimate 0.215 mg, ethinyl estradiol 25 mcg. **Phase 3:** Norgestimate 0.25 mg, ethinyl estradiol 25 mcg.Talc, lactose. Tab. *Dialpak* and *Veridate* 28s. *Rx.*
Use: Sex hormone, contraceptive hormone.

Orthovisc. (Ortho Biotech) Hyaluronan 30 mg (molecular weight is 1,000,000 to 2,900,000 daltons); sodium chloride 18 mg. Inj. Single-use vials. 2 mL. *Rx.*
Use: Treatment of pain in osteoarthritis.

OrthoWash. (Omnil Oral) Sodium fluoride (as acidulated phosphate solution) 0.044%. Grape flavor. Rinse. 480 mL. *Rx.*
Use: Prevention of dental caries.

orthoxine. Methoxyphenamine.

orticalm.
Use: Hypotensive; tranquilizer.

See: Serpasil.

Orudis KT. (Whitehall-Robins) Ketoprofen 12.5 mg, tartrazine, sugar. Tab. Bot. 24s, 50s, 100s. *OTC.*
Use: Analgesic, NSAID.

Oruvail. (Wyeth) Ketoprofen 100 mg, 150 mg, 200 mg, sucrose. ER Cap. Bot. 100s. *Rx.*
Use: Analgesic, NSAID.

orvus.
See: Gardinol Type Detergents.

osarsal.
See: Acetarsone.

Os-Cal 500. (GlaxoSmithKline Consumer) Calcium carbonate 1250 mg (elemental calcium 500 mg). **Tab.:** Oyster shell powder, corn syrup, parabens. Bot. 75s. **Chew. Tab.:** Dextrose. Bot. 60s. *OTC.*
Use: Mineral supplement.

Os-Cal 500 + D. (GlaxoSmithKline Consumer) Calcium 500 mg, vitamin D 200 units, corn syrup, parabens, polydextrose. Tab. Bot. 75s, 160s. *OTC.*
Use: Mineral, vitamin supplement.

Os-Cal Fortified. (GlaxoSmithKline Consumer) Ca 250 mg, Fe (as ferrous fumarate) 5 mg, Mg, Mn, zinc 0.5 mg, D 125 units, B_1 1.7 mg, B_2 1.7 mg, B_3 15 mg, B_6 2 mg, C 50 mg, E 0.8 units, parabens, corn syrup solids, EDTA. Tab. Bot. 100s. *OTC.*
Use: Mineral, vitamin supplement.

Os-Cal Fortified Multivitamin & Minerals. (GlaxoSmithKline) Vitamins A 1668 units, D 125 units, E 0.8 units, B_1 1.7 mg, B_2 1.7 mg, B_3 15 mg, B_6 2 mg, C 50 mg, Fe 5 mg, Ca 250 mg, Zn 0.5 mg, Mn, Mg, EDTA, parabens. Tab. Bot. 100s. *OTC.*
Use: Mineral, vitamin supplement.

Os-Cal Plus. (GlaxoSmithKline) Ca 250 mg, vitamins D 125 units, A 1666 units, C 33 mg, B_2 0.66 mg, B_1 0.5 mg, B_6 0.5 mg, niacinamide 3.33 mg, Zn 0.75 mg, Mn 0.75 mg, Fe 16.6 mg. Tab. Bot. 100s. *OTC.*
Use: Mineral, vitamin supplement.

Os-Cal 250. (Hoechst) Oyster shell powder as calcium 250 mg, vitamin D 125 units, and trace minerals (Cu, Fe, Mg, Mn, Zn, silica). Tab. Bot. 100s, 240s, 500s, 1000s. *OTC.*
Use: Mineral, vitamin supplement.

Os-Cal 250 + D. (GlaxoSmithKline Consumer) Calcium carbonate 625 mg, vitamin D 125 units. Tab. Bot. 100s. *OTC.*
Use: Mineral, vitamin supplement.

Os-Cal Ultra. (GlaxoSmithKline Consumer) Ca 600 mg, vitamin D 200 units, C 60 mg, E 15 units, Mg 20 mg, Zn

7.5 mg, Cu, Mn, boron 250 mcg. Lactose, sucrose. Tab. 120s. *OTC.*
Use: Nutritional supplement.

•oseltamivir phosphate. (oh-sel-TAM-i-vir) USAN.
Use: Antiviral.
See: Tamiflu.

Osmitrol. (Baxter PPI) Mannitol in water. **5%:** 1000 mL. **10%:** 500 mL, 1000 mL. **15%:** 150 mL, 500 mL. **20%:** 250 mL, 500 mL. Mannitol in 0.3% Na. **5%:** 1000 mL. Mannitol in 0.45% Na. **20%:** 500 mL. *Rx.*
Use: Diuretic.
See: Mannitol.

Osmoglyn. (Alcon) Glycerin 50% in flavored aqueous vehicle. Plastic Bot. 6 oz. *Rx.*
Use: Diuretic.

Osmolite. (Ross) Isotonic liquid food containing 1.06 calories/mL. Two quarts (2000 calories) provides 100% US RDA vitamins and minerals for adults and children. Osmolality: 300 mOsm/kg water. Ready-to-Use: Bot. Can 8 fl oz, 32 fl oz. *OTC.*
Use: Nutritional supplement.

Osmolite HN. (Ross) High nitrogen isotonic liquid food containing 1.06 calories/mL; 1400 calories provides 100% USRDA vitamins and minerals for adults and children. Osmolality: 300 mOsm/kg water. Ready-to-Use: Bot. 8 fl oz. Can 8 fl oz, 32 fl oz. *OTC.*
Use: Nutritional supplement.

Osmotic Diuretics.
See: Ismotic.
Mannitol.
Osmitrol.
Osmoglyn.
Ureaphil.

ospolot.
Use: Anticonvulsant drug; pending release.

Ossonate. (Marcen) Cartilage mucopolysaccharide extract, chondroitin sulfate 50 mg. Cap. Bot. 100s, 500s, 1000s.

Ossonate-Plus. (Marcen) Ossonate-mucopolysaccharide extract 50 mg, acetaminophen 300 mg, salicylamide 200 mg. Cap. Bot. 100s, 500s, 1000s. *OTC.*
Use: Antiarthritic.

Ossonate-Plus, Inj. (Marcen) Ossonate cartilage mucopolysaccharide extract 12.5 mg, case in hydrolysates 80 mg, sulfur 20 mg, sodium citrate 5 mg, benzyl alcohol 0.5%, phenol 0.5%/mL. Multidose 10 mL vial. *Rx.*
Use: Muscle relaxant, pain reliever.

Ossonate-75. (Marcen) Chondroitin sulfate 37.5 mg, benzyl alcohol 0.5%, phenol 0.5%, sodium citrate 5 mg/mL. Vial 10 mL. *Rx.*
Use: Infantile and atopic eczemas; drug allergies; dermatoses associated with intestinal toxemias.

Osteocalcin. (Arcola) Calcitonin-salmon 200 units, phenol 5 mg/mL. Inj. Vial 2 mL. *Rx.*
Use: Hormone.

Osteo-D. (Teva)
See: Secalciferol.

Osteolate. (Fellows) Sodium thiosalicylate 50 mg, benzyl alcohol 2%/mL. Inj. Vial 30 mL. *Rx.*
Use: Analgesic.

Osteo-Mins. (Tyson) **Pow.:** Vitamin C 500 mg, Ca 250 mg, Mg 250 mg, K 16 mg, 100 units D/4.5 g, sugar free, 200 g. *OTC.*
Use: Vitamin supplement.

Osteon/D. (Taylor Pharmaceuticals) Ca 600 mg, P 400 mg, Mg 240 mg, vitamin D 400 units. Tab. Bot. 180s. *Rx.*
Use: Mineral, vitamin supplement.

Ostiderm Roll-On. (Pedinol Pharmacal) Aluminum chlorohydrate, camphor, alcohol, EDTA, diazolidinyl urea. Bot. 88.7 mL. *OTC.*
Use: Antipruritic; astringent, topical.

Osto-K. (Parthenon) Potassium 1 mEq (39 mg from gluconate, Cl, and citrate), vitamin C 25 mg, sodium 0.52 mg. Tab. Bot. 60s. *OTC.*
Use: Mineral, vitamin supplement.

osvarsan.
See: Acetarsone.

Otic-Care. (Parmed Pharmaceuticals, Inc.) Hydrocortisone 1%, neomycin sulfate 5 mg, polymyxin B sulfate 10,000 units/mL, glycerin, hydrochloric acid, propylene glycol, potassium metabisulfite. Soln. Bot. *Rx.*
Use: Otic.

Otic Domeboro. (Bayer) Acetic acid 2%, aluminum acetate solution. Plastic Dropper Bot. 2 oz. *Rx.*
Use: Otic.

Otic-HC. (Roberts) Chloroxylenol 1 mg, pramoxine hydrochloride 10 mg, hydrocortisone alcohol 10 mg, benzalkonium Cl 0.2 mg/mL. Bot. 12 mL. *Rx.*
Use: Otic.

Otic-Neo-Cort Dome.
See: Neo-Cort Dome.

Otic-Plain. (Roberts) Chloroxylenol 1 mg, pramoxine hydrochloride 10 mg, benzalkonium Cl 0.2 mg/mL. Bot. 12 mL. *Rx.*
Use: Otic.

Otic Solution No. 1. (Foy Laboratories) Hydrocortisone alcohol 10 mg, pramoxine hydrochloride 10 mg, benzalkonium Cl 0.2 mg, acetic acid glacial 20 mg/mL w/propylene glycol q.s. Bot. *Rx.*
Use: Otic.

Oti-Med. (Hyrex) Chloroxylenol 1 mg, pramoxine hydrochloride 10 mg, hydrocortisone 10 mg/mL, propylene glycol, benzalkonium chloride. Drops. Vial 10 mL. *Rx.*
Use: Otic.

Otobiotic Otic Solution. (Schering-Plough) Polymyxin B, hydrocortisone in propylene glycol and glycerin vehicle w/edetate disodium, sodium bisulfite, anhydrous sodium sulfite, purified water. Bot. w/dropper 15 mL. *Rx.*
Use: Otic.

Otocain. (Holloway) Benzocaine 20%, benzethonium Cl 0.1%, glycerin 1%, polyethylene glycol. Soln. Bot. 15 mL. *Rx.*
Use: Otic.

Otocalm-H Ear Drops. (Parmed Pharmaceuticals, Inc.) Pramoxine hydrochloride 10 mg, hydrocortisone alcohol 10%, p-chloro-m-xylenol 1 mg, benzalkonium Cl 0.2 mg, acetic acid glacial 20 mg, propylene glycol/mL. Bot. 10 mL. *Rx.*
Use: Otic.

Otocort Sterile Solution. (Teva) Neomycin sulfate equivalent to 3.5 mg neomycin base, polymyxin B sulfate 10,000 units, hydrocortisone 10 mg/mL, propylene glycol, glycerin, potassium metabisulfite, hydrochloride, purified water. Bot. 10 mL. *Rx.*
Use: Otic.

Otocort Sterile Suspension. (Teva) Neomycin sulfate equivalent to 3.5 mg neomycin base, polymyxin B sulfate 10,000 units, hydrocortisone 10 mg/mL, cetyl alcohol, propylene glycol, polysorbate 80, thimerosal, water for injection. Bot. 10 mL. *Rx.*
Use: Otic.

Otogesic HC Solution. (Lexis Laboratories) Polymyxin B sulfate 10,000 units, neomycin sulfate 3.5 mg, hydrocortisone 10 mg/mL, potassium metabisulfite 0.1%. Bot. 10 mL. *Rx.*
Use: Otic.

Otogesic HC Suspension. (Lexis Laboratories) Polymyxin B sulfate 10,000 units, neomycin sulfate 3.5 mg, hydrocortisone 10 mg/mL, benzalkonium Cl 0.01%. Bot. 10 mL. *Rx.*
Use: Otic.

Otomar-HC. (Marnel) Chloroxylenol 1 mg, hydrocortisone 10 mg, pramoxine hydrochloride 10 mg/mL. Otic Soln. Plastic dropper vials 10 mL. *Rx.*
Use: Otic preparation.

Otomycin-HPN. (Edwards) Polymyxin B sulfate 10,000 units, neomycin sulfate 3.5 mg, hydrocortisone 10 mg/mL. Bot. w/dropper 10 mL. *Rx.*
Use: Otic.

Otrivin. (Novartis) Xylometazoline hydrochloride 0.1%, benzalkonium chloride, sodium chloride, EDTA. Soln. Dropper Bot. 25 mL. Spray Bot. 20 mL. *OTC.*
Use: Nasal decongestant, imidazoline.

Otrivin Pediatric Nasal. (Novartis) Xylometazoline hydrochloride 0.05%, benzalkonium chloride, EDTA. Soln. Dropper Bot. 25 mL. *OTC.*
Use: Nasal decongestant, imidazoline.

ouabain octahydrate. Ouabain.

ovarian extract. Aqueous extract of whole ovaries of cattle. *Rx.*
Use: Estrogen.

ovarian substance. (Various Mfr.) Whole ovarian substance from cattle, sheep, or swine. *Rx.*
Use: Estrogen.

Ovastat. (Medac GmbH c/o Princeton Regulatory Assoc.)
See: Treosulfan.

Ovcon-50. (Warner Chilcott) Norethindrone 1 mg, ethinyl estradiol 50 mcg, lactose. Tab. Pack 28s. *Rx.*
Use: Sex hormone, contraceptive hormone.

Ovcon-35. (Warner Chilcott) Norethindrone 0.4 mg, ethinyl estradiol 35 mcg, lactose. Tab. Pack 28s. *Rx.*
Use: Sex hormone, contraceptive hormone.

Overtime. (BDI) Caffeine 200 mg. Tab. Bot. 100s, 500s. *OTC.*
Use: CNS stimulant, analeptic.

Ovide. (Medicis) Malathion 0.5%. In a vehicle of isopropyl alcohol 78%, terpineol, dipentene, and pine needle oil. Lot. Bot. 59 mL. *Rx.*
Use: Pediculicide, scabicide.

Ovidrel. (Serono) Choriogonadotropin alfa 250 mcg/0.5 mL, mannitol 28.1 mg, 85% O-phosphoric acid 505 mcg. Inj. Single-dose prefilled syringes. *Rx.*
Use: Sex hormone, ovulation stimulant.

ovifollin.
See: Estrone.

Ovlin. (Sigma-Tau) **Tab.:** Ethinyl estradiol 0.02 mg, conjugated estrogens 0.2 mg. Bot. 100s, 1000s. **Inj.:** Estrone 2 mg, ethinyl estradiol 0.05 mg, vitamin B_{12} 1000 mcg/mL. Vial 30 mL. *Rx.*

Use: Estrogen.

Ovocylin Dipropionate. (Novartis) Estradiol dipropionate. *Rx.*
Use: Estrogen.

Ovral. (Wyeth-Ayerst) Norgestrel 0.5 mg, ethinyl estradiol 50 mcg, lactose. Tab. *Pilpak* 21s, 28s. *Rx.*
Use: Sex hormone, contraceptive hormone.

Ovrette. (Wyeth-Ayerst) Norgestrel 0.075 mg, lactose, tartrazine. Tab. *Pilpak* 28s. *Rx.*
Use: Sex hormone, contraceptive hormone.

ovulation stimulants.
See: Choriogonadotropin Alfa.
Chorionic Gonadotropin.
Clomiphene Citrate.
Gonadotropins.
Lutropin Alfa.
Menotropins.

ovulation tests.
See: Answer Ovulation.
Clearblue Easy Ovulation Test.
First Response Ovulation Predictor Test Kit.
Fortel Home Ovulation Test.

Ovulen-28. (Pharmacia) Ethynodiol diacetate 1 mg, mestranol 0.1 mg. Tab. w/7 inert Tab. Compack 28s: 21 active tab., 7 placebo tab. Compack dispenser 28s. Box 6 × 28. Refill 28s, Box 12 × 28. *Rx.*
Use: Contraceptive.

Ovulen-21. (Pharmacia) Ethynodiol diacetate 1 mg, mestranol 0.1 mg. Tab. Compack Disp. 21s, 6 × 21, 24 × 21. Refill 21s, 12 × 21. *Rx.*
Use: Contraceptive.

Ovustick Self-Test. (Monoclonal Antibodies) Home test for ovulation. Test kit 10s.
Use: Diagnostic aid.

Oxabid. (Jamieson-McKames) Magnesium oxide 140 mg or magnesium oxide heavy 400 mg. Cap. Bot. 100s. *OTC.*
Use: Antacid.

● **oxacillin sodium.** (ox-uh-SILL-in) *USP 28.*
Use: Anti-infective.

oxacillin sodium. (Various Mfr.) **Pow. for Inj.:** 500 mg, 1 g, 2 g, 10 g. Vial (except 10 g), piggyback vial (1 g, 2 g only), *ADD-Vantage* vials (1 g, 2 g only), Bulk Vial (10 g only). **Pow. for Oral Soln.:** Oxacillin sodium 250 mg/5 mL when reconstituted. Bot. 100 mL. *Rx.*
Use: Anti-infective, penicillin.

oxadimedine hydrochloride.
Use: Antiarrhythmic.

oxafuradene. (OX-ah-FYOOR-ah-deen)
Name used for Nifuradene.
Use: Platelet aggregation agent.

● **oxagrelate.** (OX-ah-greh-LATE) USAN.
Use: Platelet aggregation inhibitor.

oxaliplatin. (ocks-AL-ih-pla-tin)
Use: Antineoplastic. [Orphan Drug]
See: Eloxatin.

oxalodinones.
Use: Anti-infective.
See: Linezolid.

● **oxamarin hydrochloride.** (OX-ah-mah-rin) USAN.
Use: Hemostatic.

● **oxamisole hydrochloride.** (ox-AM-ih-sole) USAN.
Use: Immunoregulator.

● **oxamniquine.** (ox-AM-nih-kwin) *USP 28.*
Use: Antischistosomal. Treatment of schistosomiasis.

oxanamide.
Use: Anxiolytic.

Oxandrin. (Savient) Oxandrolone 2.5 mg, 10 mg, lactose. Tab. Bot. 100s (2.5 mg only), 60s (10 mg only). *c-III.*
Use: Anabolic steroid.

● **oxandrolone.** (ox-AN-droe-lone) *USP 28.*
Use: Androgen, anabolic. [Orphan Drug]
See: Oxandrin.

● **oxantel pamoate.** (OX-an-tell PAM-oh-ate) USAN.
Use: Anthelmintic.

● **oxaprotiline hydrochloride.** (OX-ah-PRO-tih-leen) USAN.
Use: Antidepressant.

● **oxaprozin.** (OX-ah-pro-zin) *USP 28.*
Use: Anti-inflammatory, NSAID.
See: Daypro.
Daypro ALTA.

oxaprozin. (EON) Oxaprozin 600 mg. Tab. Bot. 100s, 500s, 1000s, blister 100s. *Rx.*
Use: Anti-inflammatory, NSAID.

● **oxarbazole.** (ox-AHR-bah-zole) USAN.
Use: Antiasthmatic.

● **oxatomide.** (ox-AT-ah-mid) USAN.
Use: Antiallergic, antiasthmatic.

● **oxazepam.** (ox-AZE-uh-pam) *USP 28.*
Use: Anxiolytic, sedative.

oxazepam. (Various Mfr.) Oxazepam 10 mg, 15 mg, 30 mg. Cap. 100s, 500s, UD 100s. *c-IV.*
Use: Anxiolytic.

ox bile extract. Purified ox gall.
See: Bile Extract.

● **oxcarbazepine.** (ox-kar-BAY-ze-peen) USAN.

Use: Anticonvulsant; antiepileptic.
See: Trileptal.

●**oxendolone.** (OX-en-doe-LONE) USAN.
Use: Antiandrogen (benign prostatic hypertrophy).

●**oxethazaine.** (OX-ETH-ah-zane) USAN.
Use: Anesthetic, local.

●**oxetorone fumarate.** (ox-EH-toe-rone) USAN.
Use: Antimigraine.

●**oxfendazole.** (ox-FEN-DAH-zole) USAN.
Use: Anthelmintic.

oxfenicine. (OX-FEN-ih-seen) USAN.
Use: Vasodilator.

ox gall.
See: Bile Extract.

●**oxibendazole.** (ox-ee-BEND-ah-zole) USAN.
Use: Anthelmintic.

●**oxiconazole nitrate.** (ox-ee-KAHN-ah-zole) USAN.
Use: Antifungal.
See: Oxistat.

oxidized bile acids.
See: Bile Acids, Oxidized.

oxidized cellulose. Absorbable cellulose. Cellulosic acid.
Use: Hemostatic.
See: Oxycel.
Surgicel.

●**oxidopamine.** (OX-ih-DOE-pah-meen) USAN.
Use: Adrenergic (ophthalmic).

●**oxidronic acid.** (OX-ih-DRAHN-ik) USAN.
Use: Regulator (calcium).

Oxi-Freeda. (Freeda) Vitamin A 5000 units, E 150 mg, B_3 40 mg, C 100 mg, B_1 20 mg, B_2 20 mg, B_5 20 mg, B_6 20 mg, B_{12} 10 mcg, Zn 15 mg, Se, glutathione, L-cysteine. Tab. Bot. 100s, 250s. *OTC.*
Use: Mineral, vitamin supplement.

●**oxifungin hydrochloride.** (OX-ih-FUN-jin) USAN.
Use: Antifungal.

●**oxilorphan.** (ox-ih-LORE-fan) USAN.
Use: Narcotic antagonist.

●**oximonam.** (OX-ih-MOE-nam) USAN.
Use: Anti-infective.

●**oximonam sodium.** (OX-ih-MOE-nam) USAN.
Use: Anti-infective.

oxine.
See: Oxyquinoline Sulfate.

●**oxiperomide.** (ox-ih-PURR-oh-mide) USAN.
Use: Antipsychotic.

Oxipor VHC. (Medtech) Coal tar soln. 25% (equiv. to 5% coal tar), alcohol 79%. Lot. Bot. 56 mL. *OTC.*
Use: Antipsoriatic.

●**oxiramide.** (ox-EER-am-ide) USAN.
Use: Cardiovascular agent.

Oxistat. (GlaxoSmithKline) Oxiconazole nitrate 1%. Cream. Tube 15 g, 30 g, 60 g; Lot. Bot. 30 mL. *Rx.*
Use: Antifungal, topical.

●**oxisuran.** (OX-ih-SUH-ran) USAN.
Use: Antineoplastic.

●**oxmetidine hydrochloride.** (ox-MEH-tih-DEEN) USAN.
Use: Antiulcerative.

●**oxmetidine mesylate.** (ox-MEH-tih-DEEN) USAN.
Use: Antiulcerative.

●**oxogestone phenpropionate.** (ox-oh-JESS-tone fen-PRO-pih-oh-nate) USAN.
Use: Hormone, progestin.

Oxolamine. (Arcum) Crystalline hydroxy-cobalamin 1000 mcg/mL. Vial 10 mL. *Rx.*
Use: Vitamin supplement.

●**oxolinic acid.** (ox-oh-LIH-nik acid) USAN.
Use: Anti-infective.

Oxothiazolidine Carboxylate. (Clintec Nutrition) Phase I restoration of glutathione depletion in HIV, ARC, AIDS; prevention of inflammation-induced HIV replication. *Rx.*
Use: Immunomodulator.

l-2-oxothiazolidine$_4$-carboxylicacid.
Use: Treatment of adult respiratory distress syndrome. [Orphan Drug]
See: Procysteine.

●**oxprenolol hydrochloride.** (ox-PREH-no-lole) *USP 28.* Under study.
Use: Beta-adrenergic receptor blocker, vasodilator (coronary).

Oxsoralen. (ICN Pharmaceuticals) Methoxsalen 1% (10 mg/mL), acetone, alcohol 71%. Lot. Bot. 30 mL. *Rx.*
Use: Dermatologic.

Oxsoralen-Ultra. (ICN Pharmaceuticals) Methoxsalen 10 mg. Soft Gelatin Cap. Bot. 50s. *Rx.*
Use: Dermatologic.

●**oxtriphylline.** (ox-TRY-fih-lin) *USP 28.*
Use: Bronchodilator.
W/Guaifenesin.
See: Brondecon.

oxtriphylline and guaifenesin elixir. (Alra) Oxtriphylline 300 mg, guaifenesin 150 mg, alcohol 20%/15 mL. Elix. Bot. Pt, gal. *Rx.*
Use: Bronchodilator, expectorant.

● **oxybenzone.** (ox-ee-BEN-zone) *USP 28.*
Use: Ultraviolet screen.
W/Dioxybenzone, benzophenone.
See: Solbar.
oxybenzone with combinations.
See: Coppertone.
Noskote.
Shade.
Super Shade.
● **oxybutynin chloride.** (OX-ee-BYOO-tih-nin) *USP 28.*
Use: Anticholinergic.
See: Ditropan.
Ditropan XL.
Oxytrol.
oxybutynin chloride. (Various Mfr.) Oxybutynin chloride. **Tab.:** 5 mg. Bot. 100s, 500s, 1000s, blister pack 25s, UD 100s, 9vr.; 5 mg/5 ml. Bot. 473 mL. *Rx.*
Use: Antispasmodic; anticholinergic.
Oxycel. (Becton Dickinson & Co.) Cellulosic acid in absorbable hemostatic agent prepared from cellulose. Resembles ordinary surgical gauze or cotton. Pledget 2 × 1 × 1 inch. 10s. Pad 3 × 3 inch. 8 ply. 10s. Strip 5 × 0.5 inch. 4 ply. 18 × 2 inch. 4 ply. 10s. 36 × 0.5 inch. 4 ply. *Rx.*
Use: Hemostatic, topical.
Oxycet. (Halsey Drug) Oxycodone hydrochloride 5 mg, acetaminophen 325 mg. Tab. Bot. 100s, 500s, Hospital pack 250s. *c-II.*
Use: Narcotic analgesic combination.
Oxy-Chinol. (Ferndale) Potassium oxyquinoline sulfate 1 g. Tab. Bot. 100s, 1000s. *OTC.*
Use: Antimicrobial, deodorant.
● **oxychlorosene.** (OCK-sih-KLOR-ah-seen) USAN. Monoxychlorosene. Hydrocarbon derivative containing 14 carbons and hypochlorous acid. The hydrocarbon chain also has a phenyl substituent which in turn holds a sulfonic acid group.
Use: Anti-infective, topical.
See: Clorpactin.
● **oxychlorosene sodium.** (OCK-sih-KLOR-ah-seen) USAN. Sodium salt of the complex derived from hypochlorous acid and tetradecylbenzene sulfonic acid. Action of active chlorine.
Use: Anti-infective, topical.
Oxy Clean Lathering Facial. (GlaxoSmithKline) Sodium tetraborate decahydrate dissolving particles in a base of surfactant cleaning agents. Soap free. Scrub 79.5 g. *OTC.*
Use: Dermatologic, acne.

Oxy Clean Medicated Cleanser and Pads. (GlaxoSmithKline) **Cleanser and reg. strength pads:** Salicylic acid 0.5%, SD alcohol 40B 40%, citric acid, menthol, sodium lauryl sulfate. **Max. strength pads:** Salicylic acid 2%, SD alcohol 40B 50%, citric acid, menthol, sodium lauryl sulfate. Cleanser 120 mL. Pad. 50s. *OTC.*
Use: Dermatologic, acne.
Oxy Clean Medicated Pads for Sensitive Skin. (GlaxoSmithKline) Salicylic acid 0.5%, SD alcohol 40B 16%. Jar 50s. *OTC.*
Use: Dermatologic, acne.
Oxy Clean Scrub. (GlaxoSmithKline) Sodium tetraborate decahydrate dissolving particles in a base of surfactant cleaning agents. Soap Free. Lot. Bot. 79.5 g. *OTC.*
Use: Dermatologic, acne.
Oxy Clean Soap. (GlaxoSmithKline) Salicylic acid 3.5%, sodium borate. Bar 97.5 g. *OTC.*
Use: Dermatologic, acne.
● **oxycodone.** (OX-ee-KOE-dohn) USAN.
Use: Analgesic, narcotic w/combinations.
See: Endocet.
oxycodone and acetaminophen. (Mallinckrodt) Oxycodone hydrochloride/acetaminophen 7.5 mg/325 mg, 7.5 mg/500 mg, 10 mg/325 mg, 10 mg, 650 mg. Tab. 20s, 100s, 500s, 1,000s, UD 100s. *c-II.*
Use: Narcotic analgesic.
oxycodone and acetaminophen. (OX-ee-KOE-dohn and ass-cet-ah-MEE-noe-fen) (Various Mfr.) **Cap.:** Oxycodone hydrochloride 5 mg, acetaminophen 500 mg. Bot. 100s, 500s, 1000s, UD 25s. **Tab.:** Oxycodone hydrochloride 5 mg, acetaminophen 325 mg. Bot. 100s, 500s, 1000s, UD 25s. *c-II.*
Use: Analgesic combination, narcotic.
oxycodone and aspirin. (Various Mfr.) Oxycodone hydrochloride 4.5 mg, oxycodone terephthalate 0.38 mg, aspirin 325 mg. Tab. Bot. 100s, 500s, 1000s, UD 25s. *c-II.*
Use: Analgesic combination, narcotic.
● **oxycodone hydrochloride.** (OX-ee-KOE-dohn) *USP 28.*
Use: Opioid analgesic.
See: Dihydrohydroxycodeinone hydrochloride.
M-Oxy.
OxyContin.
Oxydose.
OxyFAST.

OxyIR.
Roxicodone.
Roxicodone Intensol.
W/Combinations.
See: Combunox.
Endocet.
Percocet.
Tylox.
oxycodone hydrochloride. (Amide) Oxycodone hydrochloride 15 mg, 30 mg. Lactose. IR Tab. 100s, UD 100s. *c-II.*
Use: Opioid analgesic.
oxycodone hydrochloride. (Endo) Oxycodone hydrochloride 10 mg, 20 mg, 40 mg. CR Tab. 30s, 500s. *c-II.*
Use: Opioid analgesic.
oxycodone hydrochloride. (Ethex) Oxycodone hydrochloride 5 mg. Lactose. IR Cap. 100s, UD 100s. *c-II.*
Use: Opioid analgesic.
oxycodone hydrochloride. (Teva) Oxycodone hydrochloride 80 mg. Lactose. Film-coated. ER Tab. 100s. *c-II.*
Use: Opioid analgesic.
oxycodone hydrochloride. (Various Mfr.) Oxycodone hydrochloride. **CR Tab.:** 80 mg. Lactose. 100s, 500s, 1,000s. **Oral Soln.:** 5 mg/5 mL. 500 mL. **Soln. Concentrate:** 20 mg/mL. 30 mL. **Tab.:** 5 mg. Bot. 100s, 500s, UD 100s. *c-II.*
Use: Analgesic, narcotic agonist.
•**oxycodone terephthalate.** (OX-ee-KOE-dohn teh-REFF-thah-late) *USP 28.*
Use: Analgesic, narcotic.
OxyContin. (Purdue Pharma LP) Oxycodone hydrochloride 10 mg, 20 mg, 40 mg, 80 mg. Lactose. CR Tab. Bot. 100s, UD 25s. *c-II.*
Use: Opioid analgesic.
Oxy Cover. (GlaxoSmithKline) Benzoyl peroxide 10%. Cream. 30 g. *OTC.*
Use: Dermatologic, acne.
Oxydose. (Ethex) Oxycodone hydrochloride 20 mg/mL, saccharin, sorbitol, berry flavor. Conc. Soln. Bot. 30 mL w/dropper. *c-II.*
Use: Opioid analgesic.
oxyethylene oxypropylene polymer.
See: Poloxalkol.
W/Danthron, vitamin B₁, carboxymethyl cellulose.
See: Evactol.
OxyFAST. (Purdue Pharma LP) Oxycodone hydrochloride 20 mg/mL, saccharin. Conc. Soln. Dropper Bot. 30 mL. *c-II.*
Use: Opioid analgesic.
•**oxyfilcon a.** (OX-ee-FILL-kahn A) USAN.
Use: Contact lens material (hydrophilic).

Oxy 5 Acne-Pimple Medication. (GlaxoSmithKline) Benzoyl peroxide 5% in lotion base. Lot. Bot. oz. *OTC.*
Use: Dermatologic, acne.
•**oxygen.** *USP 28.*
Use: Gas, medicinal.
•**oxygen 93 percent.** *USP 28.*
Use: Gas, medicinal.
OxyIR. (Purdue Pharma) Oxycodone hydrochloride 5 mg, sucrose. IR Cap. Bot. 100s. *c-II.*
Use: Opioid analgesic.
Oxy Medicated Cleanser and Maximum Strength Pads. (GlaxoSmithKline) Salicylic acid 2%, SD alcohol 44%, citric acid, menthol, propylene glycol. Cleanser. Bot. 120 mL. Pads 50s, 90s. *OTC.*
Use: Dermatologic, acne.
Oxy Medicated Cleanser and Regular Strength Pads. (GlaxoSmithKline) Salicylic acid 0.5%, SD alcohol 28%, citric acid, menthol, propylene glycol. Cleanser. Bot. 120 mL. Pads 50s, 90s. *OTC.*
Use: Dermatologic, acne.
Oxy Medicated Cleanser and Sensitive Skin Pads. (GlaxoSmithKline) Salicylic acid 0.5%, alcohol 22%, disodium lauryl sulfosuccinate, menthol, trisodium EDTA. Cleanser. Bot. 120 mL. Pads 50s, 90s. *OTC.*
Use: Dermatologic, acne.
Oxy Medicated Soap. (GlaxoSmithKline) Triclosan 1%, bentonite, cocoamphodipropionate, iron oxides, glycerin, magnesium silicate, sodium borohydride, sodium cocoate, sodium tallowate, talc, EDTA, titanium dioxide. Bar. 97.5 g. *OTC.*
Use: Dermatologic, acne.
•**oxymetazoline hydrochloride.** (OX-ee-MET-azz-oh-leen) *USP 28.*
Use: Nasal decongestant, imidazoline; adrenergic (vasoconstrictor); mydriatic.
See: Afrin No-Drip Sinus with Vapornase.
Afrin No-Drip 12–Hour.
Afrin No-Drip 12–Hour Extra Moisturizing.
Afrin No-Drip 12–Hour Severe Congestion with Menthol.
Afrin Severe Congestion with Menthol.
Afrin Sinus with Vapornase.
Afrin 12–Hour Original.
Afrin 12–Hour Original Pump Mist.
Dristan 12–Hr Nasal.
Duramist Plus 12–Hr Decongestant.

Duration.
Duration Nose Drops.
Duration Nose Drops for Children.
Genasal.
Nasal Decongestant, Maximum
Strength.
Nasal Relief.
Neo-Synephrine 12–Hour.
Neo-Synephrine 12–Hour Extra Mois-
turizing.
Nōstrilla 12–Hour.
Ocuclear.
St Joseph Nasal Spray for Children.
St Joseph Nose Drops for Children.
12 Hour Nasal.
Twice-A-Day 12–Hour Nasal.
Vicks Sinex 12–Hour Long-Acting.
Vicks Sinex 12–Hour Ultra Fine Mist
for Sinus Relief
Visine.
oxymetazoline hydrochloride. (Various
Mfr.) Oxymetazoline hydrochloride
0.05%. Soln. Spray Bot. 15 mL, 30 mL.
OTC.
Use: Nasal decongestant, imidazoline.
●**oxymetholone.** (OCK-sih-METH-oh-
lone) *USP 28.*
Use: Anabolic steroid.
See: Anadrol-50.
●**oxymorphone hydrochloride.** (ox-ee-
MORE-fone) *USP 28.*
Use: Opioid analgesic.
See: Numorphan.
Oxy Night Watch. (GlaxoSmithKline)
Salicylic acid 1%, cetyl alcohol, silica,
propylene glycol, stearyl alcohol, so-
dium laureth sulfate, parabens, EDTA.
Lot. Bot. 60 mL. *OTC.*
Use: Dermatologic, acne.
Oxy Night Watch Maximum Strength.
(GlaxoSmithKline) Salicylic acid 2%,
cetyl alcohol, EDTA, parabens, stearyl
alcohol. Lot. Bot. 60 mL. *OTC.*
Use: Dermatologic, acne.
Oxy Night Watch Sensitive Skin.
(GlaxoSmithKline) Salicylic acid 1%,
cetyl alcohol, EDTA, stearyl alcohol,
parabens. Lot. Bot. 60 mL. *OTC.*
Use: Dermatologic, acne.
**Oxy Oil-Free Maximum Strength Acne
Wash.** (GlaxoSmithKline) Benzoyl per-
oxide 10%, parabens, diazolidinyl urea.
Liq. 237 mL. *OTC.*
Use: Dermatologic, acne.
●**oxypertine.** (OX-ee-PURR-teen) USAN.
Integrin hydrochloride.
Use: Psychotherapeutic agent, antide-
pressant.
●**oxyphenbutazone.** (ox-ee-fen-BYOO-
tah-zone) *USP 28.*

Use: Analgesic, antiarthritic, anti-inflam-
matory, antipyretic, antirheumatic.
●**oxyphenisatin acetate.** (OX-ee-fen-
EYE-sah-tin) USAN.
Use: Laxative.
See: Endophenolphthalein.
Isacen.
Prulet.
●**oxypurinol sodium.** (OX-ee-PYOO-ree-
nahl) USAN.
Use: Investigational xanthine oxidase
inhibitor.
●**oxyquinoline.** (OX-ih-KWIN-oh-lin)
USAN.
Use: Disinfectant.
oxyquinoline benzoate. (Merck & Co.)
Pkg. lb.
W/Alkyl aryl sulfonate, disodium edetate,
aminacrine hydrochloride, copper sul-
fate, sodium sulfate.
See: NP-27.
●**oxyquinoline sulfate.** (OX-ih-KWIN-oh-
lin) *NF 23.*
Use: Disinfectant, pharmaceutic aid
(complexing agent).
See: Chinositol.
oxyquinoline sulfate w/combinations.
See: Acid Jelly.
Aci-jel
Fem ph.
Oxyzal Wet Dressing.
Rectal Medicone.
Rectal Medicone Unguent.
Rectal Medicone HC.
Oxy-Scrub. (GlaxoSmithKline) Abradant
cleanser containing dissolving abrad-
ant particles of sodium tetraborate
decahydrate. Tube 2.65 oz. *OTC.*
Use: Dermatologic, acne.
Oxysept. (Allergan) **Disinfecting Soln.:**
Hydrogen peroxide 3%, sodium stan-
nate, sodium nitrate, phosphate buffer.
Bot. 240 mL, 360 mL. **Neutralizer Tab.:**
Catalase, buffering agents. In 12s
(w/*Oxy-Tab* cup), 36s. *OTC.*
Use: Contact lens care.
Oxysept 1. (Allergan) Microfiltered hydrogen peroxide 3% w/sodium tannate and
sodium nitrate, preservative free, buffered. Soln. Bot. 355 mL. *OTC.*
Use: Contact lens care.
Oxysept 2. (Allergan) Catalytic neutralizing agent, EDTA, sodium Cl, mono- and
dibasic sodium phosphates. Buffered,
preservative free. Soln. In 15 mL single-
use containers(25s). *OTC.*
Use: Contact lens care.
●**oxytetracycline.** (ox-ee-teh-trah-SIGH-
kleen) *USP 28.*
Use: Anti-infective.

See: Terramycin.
oxytetracycline and hydrocortisone acetate ophthalmic suspension.
Use: Anti-infective, anti-inflammatory.
oxytetracycline and nystatin capsules.
Use: Anti-infective, antifungal.
oxytetracycline and nystatin for oral suspension.
Use: Anti-infective, antifungal.
oxytetracycline and phenazopyridine hydrochlorides and sulfamethizole capsules.
Use: Analgesic; anti-infective; antispasmodic, urinary.
•**oxytetracycline calcium.** *USP 28.*
Use: Anti-infective.
•**oxytetracycline hydrochloride.** *USP 28.*
An antibiotic from *Streptomyces rimosus.*
Use: Anti-infective; antirickettsial.
See: Terramycin hydrochloride.
Urobiotic.
oxytetracycline hydrochloride and hydrocortisone ointment.
Use: Anti-infective; anti-inflammatory.
oxytetracycline hydrochloride and polymyxin B sulfate.
Use: Anti-infective.
oxytetracycline hydrochloride and polymyxin B sulfate ophthalmic ointment.
Use: Anti-infective.
oxytetracycline hydrochloride and polymyxin B sulfate topical powder.
Use: Anti-infective.
•**oxytetracycline hydrochloride and polymyxin B sulfate vaginal inserts.** *USP 28.*
Use: Anti-infective.
oxytetracycline-polymyxin B. Mix of oxytetracycline hydrochloride and polymyxin B sulfate.
Use: Anti-infective.
See: Terramycin hydrochloride w/Polymyxin B.
oxytocics.
See: Oxytocin, Parenteral.
•**oxytocin.** (ox-ih-TOE-sin) *USP 28.*
Use: Oxytocic.
See: Pitocin.
oxytocin. (Various Mfr.) Oxytocin 10 units/mL. Inj. Vials. 3 mL, 10 mL. *Rx.*
Use: Uterine active agent.

oxytocin nasal solution. (ox-ih-TOE-sin)
Use: Oxytocic.
oxytocin, synthetic. (ox-ih-TOE-sin)
See: Pitocin.
Oxytrol. (Watson) Oxybutynin 36 mg (delivers 3.9 mg/day over 3 to 4 days). Transdermal Patch. 8s. *Rx.*
Use: Anticholinergic.
Oxy Wash. (GlaxoSmithKline) Benzoyl peroxide 10%. Liq. Bot. 120 mL. *OTC.*
Use: Dermatologic, acne.
Oxyzal Wet Dressing. (Gordon Laboratories) Benzalkonium Cl 1:2000, oxyquinoline sulfate, distilled water. Dropper bot. 1 oz, 4 oz. *OTC.*
Use: Dermatologic, counterirritant.
Oysco D. (Rugby) Ca 250 mg, D 125 units. Tab. Bot. 100s, 250s, 1000s. *OTC.*
Use: Mineral, vitamin supplement.
Oysco 500. (Rugby) Calcium carbonate 1250 mg (elemental calcium 500 mg), as oyster shell calcium. Tab. Bot. 60s, 250s. *OTC.*
Use: Mineral supplement.
Oyst-Cal-D. (Ivax) Calcium 250 mg, vitamin D 125 units. Tab. Bot. 100s, 1000s. *OTC.*
Use: Mineral, vitamin supplement.
Oyst-Cal 500. (Goldline) Calcium carbonate 1250 mg (elemental calcium 500 mg), as oyster shell calcium, preservative free, tartrazine. Tab. Bot. 60s, 120s. *OTC.*
Use: Mineral supplement.
Oyster Calcium. (NBTY) Ca 275 mg, D 200 units, A 800 units. Tab. Bot. 100s. *OTC.*
Use: Mineral, vitamin supplement.
Oystercal-D. (NBTY) Calcium 250 mg, vitamin D 125 units. Tab. Bot. 100s, 250s. *OTC.*
Use: Mineral, vitamin supplement.
Oyster Shell Calcium. (Various Mfr.) Calcium carbonate 1250 mg (elemental calcium 500 mg). Tab. Bot. 60s, 150s, 300s, 1000s, UD 100s. *OTC.*
Use: Mineral supplement.
oyster shells.
See: Os-Cal.
•**ozolinone.** (oh-ZOE-lih-NOHN) *USAN.*
Use: Diuretic.

P

Pabalate-SF. (Wyeth) Potassium salicylate 300 mg, potassium aminobenzoate 300 mg. Tab. Bot. 100s, 500s. *OTC.*
Use: Antirheumatic.
PABA-Salicylate. (Various Mfr.) Sodium salicylate, p-aminobenzoate, vitamin C. Tab. Bot. 100s, 500s. *OTC.*
Use: Analgesic; vitamin combination.
PABA sodium. (Various Mfr.) Sodium p-aminobenzoate. *OTC.*
Use: Vitamin supplement.
Pabasone. (Pinex) Sodium salicylate 5 g, para-aminobenzoic acid 5 g, ascorbic acid 20 mg. Tab. Bot. 100s. *OTC.*
Use: Analgesic; vitamin supplement.
P-A-C. Preparations of phenacetin, aspirin, caffeine.
Use: A.P.C. Preparations, Empirin Preparations.
P-A-C Analgesic. (Lee) Aspirin 400 mg, caffeine 32 mg. Tab. Bot. 100s, 1000s. *OTC.*
Use: Analgesic combination.
Pacemaker Prophylaxis Pastes with Fluoride. (Pacemaker) Silicone dioxide and diatomaceous earth, sodium fluoride 4.4%. Light abrasive, cinnamon/cherry. Medium abrasive, orange. Heavy abrasive, mint. Paste. Bot. 8 oz.
Use: Dental caries agent.
Pacerone. (Upsher-Smith) Amiodarone hydrochloride 100 mg, 200 mg, 400 mg, lactose. Tab. Bot. 30s (100 mg, 400 mg only), 60s (200 mg only), 90s (200 mg only), 100s (400 mg only), 500s (except 100 mg), UD 100s. *Rx.*
Use: Antiarrhythmic.
p-acetylaminobenzaldehyde thiosemicarbazone.
Use: Antituberculous.
See: Amithiozone, Antib, Berculon A, Benzothiozon, Conteben, Myuizone, Neustab, Tebethion, Thiomicid, Thioparamizone, Thiacetazone.
Packer's Pine Tar. (GenDerm) Pine tar, pine oil. Soap base. 99 g. *OTC.*
Use: Dermatologic.
Paclin VK. (Armenpharm Ltd.) Penicillin phenoxymethyl 125 mg, 250 mg. Tab. Bot. 100s, 1000s. *Rx.*
Use: Anti-infective, penicillin.
• **paclitaxel.** (pak-lih-TAX-uhl) *USP 28.*
Use: Antineoplastic.
See: Abraxane.
Onxol.
Taxol.
paclitaxel. (SuperGen) Paclitaxel 6 mg/mL. Polyoxyethylated castor oil 527 mg/mL, dehydrated alcohol 49.7%.

Inj. Multidose vials. 5 mL, 16.7 mL. *Rx.*
Use: Antimitotic agent.
• **paclitaxel poliglumex.** (pak-lih-TAX-uhl pol-ee-GLOO-mex) USAN.
Use: Antineoplastic.
P-A-C Revised Formula Analgesic. (Pharmacia) Aspirin 400 mg, caffeine 32 mg. Tab. Bot. 100s, 1000s. *OTC.*
Use: Analgesic.
• **padimate a.** (PAD-ih-mate) USAN.
Use: Ultraviolet screen.
• **padimate O.** *USP 28.*
Use: Ultraviolet screen.
See: Coppertone.
Eclipse.
Noskote.
Shade.
Super Shade.
Tropical Blond Sunscreen.
W/Combinations.
See: Glyquin.
• **paflufocon A.** (pah-flew-FOE-kahn) USAN.
Use: Contact lens material, hydrophobic.
• **paflufocon B.** USAN.
Use: Contact lens material, hydrophobic.
• **paflufocon C.** USAN.
Use: Contact lens material, hydrophobic.
• **paflufocon D.** USAN.
Use: Contact lens material, hydrophobic.
• **paflufocon E.** USAN.
Use: Contact lens material, hydrophobic.
• **pagoclone.** (PAG-oh-klone) USAN.
Use: Anxiolytic.
PAH.
See: Sodium aminohippurate.
Painaid. (Zee Medical) Aspirin 162 mg, salicylamide 152 mg, acetaminophen 110 mg, caffeine 32.4 mg. Tab. 24s.
OTC.
Use: Nonnarcotic analgesic.
Painaid BRF Back Relief Formula. (Zee Medical) Magnesium salicylate tetrahydrate 250 mg, acetaminophen 250 mg. Tab. 24s. *OTC.*
Use: Nonnarcotic analgesic.
Painaid ESF Extra-Strength Formula. (Zee Medical) Acetaminophen 250 mg, aspirin 250 mg, caffeine 65 mg. Tab. 24s. *OTC.*
Use: Nonnarcotic analgesic.
Painaid PMF Premenstrual Formula. (Zee Medical) Acetaminophen 500 mg, pamabrom 25 mg. Tab. 24s. *OTC.*
Use: Nonnarcotic analgesic.

Pain and Fever. (Wyeth) Acetaminophen. **Cap.:** 500 mg. Bot. 50s, 100s. **Liq.:** 160 mg/5 mL (children's strength). Unit-of-use 4 oz, Bot. 16 oz. **Tab.: 325 mg:** Bot. 100s, 1000s. **Tab.: 500 mg:** Bot. 50s, 100s. *OTC.*
Use: Analgesic.

Pain Bust-R II. (Continental Consumer Products) Methyl salicylate 17%, menthol 12%. Cream. Jar 90 g. *OTC.*
Use: Liniment.

Pain Doctor. (E. Fougera) Capsaicin 0.025%, methyl salicylate 25%, menthol 10%, parabens, propylene glycol. Cream. Tube 60 g. *OTC.*
Use: Anesthetic, local.

Pain Gel Plus. (Mentholatum Co.) Menthol 4%, aloe, vitamin E. Gel. Tube 57 g. *OTC.*
Use: Liniment.

Pain Relief. (Walgreen) Methyl salicylate 15%, menthol 10%. Oint. Tube 1.5 oz, 3 oz. *OTC.*
Use: Analgesic, topical.

Pain Relief, Aspirin Free. (Hudson Corp.) Acetaminophen 325 mg. Tab. Bot. 100s, 200s. *OTC.*
Use: Analgesic, local.

Pain Relievers-Tension Headache Relievers. (Weeks & Leo) Acetaminophen 325 mg, phenyltoloxamine citrate 30 mg. Tab. Bot. 40s, 100s. *OTC.*
Use: Analgesic combination.

Pain-X. (B.F. Ascher) Capsaicin 0.05%, menthol 5%, camphor 4%, alcohols, parabens. Gel. Tube 42.5 g. *OTC.*
Use: Pain reliever, topical.

Palbar No. 2. (Roberts) Atropine sulfate 0.012 mg, scopolamine HBr 0.005 mg, hyoscyamine HBr 0.018 mg, phenobarbital 32.4 mg. Tab. Bot. 100s. *Rx.*
Use: Anticholinergic; antispasmodic; sedative; hypnotic.

Palcaps 10. (Breckenridge) Lipase 10,000 units, protease 37,500 units, amylase (porcine-derived enzymes) 33,200 units. Sucrose. Enteric-coated microspheres. DR Cap. 100s, 250s. *Rx.*
Use: Digestive enzyme.

Palcaps 20. (Breckenridge) Lipase 4,500 units, protease 75,000 units, amylase (porcine-derived enzymes) 66,400 units. Sucrose. Enteric-coated microspheres. DR Cap. 100s, 250s. *Rx.*
Use: Digestive enzyme.

• **paldimycin.** (pal-dih-MY-sin) USAN.
Use: Anti-infective.

palestrol.
See: Diethylstilbestrol.

Palgic. (Pamlab) Carbinoxamine maleate 4 mg/5 mL. Parabens. Sugar free. Bubble gum flavor. Liq. 118 mL, 473 mL. *Rx.*
Use: Antihistamine.

Palgic-D. (Pan American) Pseudoephedrine hydrochloride 80 mg, carbinoxamine maleate 8 mg. ER Tab. Bot. 100s. *Rx.*
Use: Upper respiratory combination, antihistamine, decongestant.

Palgic DS. (Pan American) Carbinoxamine maleate 2 mg, pseudoephedrine hydrochloride 15 mg/5 mL, strawberry/pineapple flavor. Syr. Bot. 15 mL, 473 mL. *Rx.*
Use: Upper respiratory combination, antihistamine, decongestant.

• **palifermin.** (pal-ee-FER-min) USAN.
Use: Keratinocyte growth factor.
See: Kepivance.

• **palinavir.** (pal-LIH-nah-veer) USAN.
Use: Antiviral.

palinum.
Use: Hypnotic; sedative.
See: Cyclobarbital calcium.

• **paliperidone palmitate.** (pal-ee-PER-i-done) USAN.
Use: Antipsychotic, schizophrenia.

palivizumab.
Use: Antibody.
See: Synagis.

Palladone. (Purdue Pharma) Hydromorphone hydrochloride 12 mg, 16 mg, 24 mg, 32 mg. Pellet filled. ER Cap. 60s, UD 20s. *c-II.*
Use: Opioid analgesic.

Palmitate-A 5000. (Akorn) Vitamin A 5000 units. Tab. Bot. 100s. *OTC.*
Use: Vitamin supplement.

• **palmoxirate sodium.** (pal-MOX-ihr-ate) USAN.
Use: Antidiabetic.

• **palonosetron hydrochloride.** (pal-oh-NO-seh-trahn) USAN.
Use: 5-HT$_3$ receptor antagonist; antiemetic; antinauseant.
See: Aloxi.

PALS. (Palisades Pharmaceuticals) Chlorophyllin copper complex 100 mg. Tab. Bot. 30s, 100s, 1000s, UD 30s. *OTC.*
Use: Deodorant, systemic.

PAM.
See: Melphalan.

• **pamabrom.** USAN.
See: Maximum Strength Aqua-Ban. W/Acetaminophen.
See: Fem-1.
Midol Teen Maximum Strength.
Painaid PMF Premenstrual Formula.
Women's Tylenol Multi-Symptom Menstrual Relief.

W/Acetaminophen, magnesium salicylate.
See: Pamprin Maximum Pain Relief.
W/Acetaminophen, pyrilamine maleate.
See: Cardui.
Fem-1.
Midol Maximum Strength PMS.
Pamprin Multi-Symptom Maximum Strength.
Prēmsyn PMS.
Sunril.
Vitelle Lurline PMS.
W/Pyrilamine maleate, homatropine methylbromide, hyoscyamine sulfate, scopolamine HBr, methamphetamine hydrochloride.
See: Aridol.
• **pamaqueside.** (pam-ah-KWEH-side) USAN
Use: Antiatherosclerotic; hypocholesterolemic.
• **pamatolol sulfate.** (PAM-ah-TOE-lole) USAN.
Use: Anti-adrenergic, β-receptor.
Pamelor. (Novartis) Nortriptyline hydrochloride. **Cap.:** 10 mg, 25 mg, 50 mg, 75 mg, benzyl alcohol, EDTA, parabens. Bot. 100s, 500s (25 mg only), UD 100s (except 75 mg). **Soln.:** 10 mg base/5 mL, alcohol 3.4%. Bot. 480 mL. Rx.
Use: Antidepressant.
• **pamidronate disodium.** (pam-IH-DROE-nate) USAN.
Use: Bisphosphonate.
See: Aredia.
pamidronate disodium. (Mayne Pharma) Pamidronate disodium 6 mg/ mL, mannitol 100 mg. Inj. Vials 10 ml Rx.
Use: Bisphosphonate.
pamidronate disodium. (Various Mfr.) Pamidronate disodium 3 mg/mL, 9 mg/ mL, may contain parabens. Inj. Vials 10 mL. Rx.
Use: Bisphosphonate.
Pamine. (Kenwood/Bradley) Methscopolamine bromide 2.5 mg. Tab. Bot. 100s, 500s. Rx.
Use: Anticholinergic/antispasmodic.
Pamine Forte. (Kenwood Therapeutics) Methscopolamine bromide 5 mg. Tab. 60s. Rx.
Use: Anticholinergic/antispasmodic.
p-aminosalicylic acid salts.
See: Aminosalicylic acid salts.
Pamprin Extra Strength Multi-Symptom Relief Formula. (Chattem) Acetaminophen 400 mg, pamabrom 25 mg, pyrilamine maleate 15 mg. Tab. Bot.

12s, 24s, 48s. OTC.
Use: Analgesic combination.
Pamprin Maximum Cramp Relief Formula Caplets. (Chattem) Acetaminophen 500 mg, pamabrom 25 mg, pyrilamine maleate 15 mg. Tab. Bot. 8s, 16s, 32s. OTC.
Use: Analgesic combination.
Pamprin Maximum Pain Relief Caplets. (Chattem) Acetaminophen 250 mg, magnesium salicylate 250 mg, pamabrom 25 mg. Tab. Bot. 16s, 32s. OTC.
Use: Analgesic combination.
Pamprin Multi-Symptom Maximum Strength. (Chattem) Acetaminophen 500 mg, pamabrom 25 mg, pyrilamine maleate 15 mg. **Cap.:** Bot. 24s, 48s. **Tab.:** Bot. 12s, 24s, 48s. OTC.
Use: Analgesic combination.
Panacet 5/500. (ECH) Hydrocodone bitartrate 5 mg, acetaminophen 500 mg. Tab. Bot. 100s. c-III.
Use: Analgesic combination; narcotic.
• **panadiplon.** (pan-ad-IH-plone) USAN.
Use: Anxiolytic.
Panadol. (Bayer Corp. (Consumer Div.)) Acetaminophen 500 mg. **Tab.:** Bot. 2s, 30s, 60s, 100s. **Cap.:** Bot. 10s, 24s, 48s. OTC.
Use: Analgesic.
Panadol, Children's. (Bayer Corp. (Consumer Div.)) Acetaminophen. **Tab.:** 80 mg. Bot. 30s. **Liq.:** 80 mg/0.8 mL. Bot. 2 oz, 4 oz. **Drops.** 80 mg/0.5 oz. Bot. 0.5 oz. OTC.
Use: Analgesic.
Panadol, Infants'. (Bayer Corp. (Consumer Div.)) Acetaminophen 100 mg/ ml. Drops. Bot. 15 ml. with 0.8 mL dropper. OTC.
Use: Analgesic.
Panadol, Jr. (Bayer Corp. (Consumer Div.)) Acetaminophen 160 mg. Cap. Box. 30s. OTC.
Use: Analgesic.
Panafil. (Healthpoint) **Oint.:** Papain ≥ 521,700 units, urea 10%, chlorophyllin copper complex sodium 0.5%/g in a hydrophilic base, propylene glycol, white petrolatum, stearyl alcohol, boric acid, chlorobutanol (anhydrous). Oint. Tube 30 g. **Spray:** Papain ≥ 521,700 units, urea 10%, chlorophyllin copper complex sodium 0.5%/g. Glycerin, cetearyl alcohol, lactose (anhydrous), mineral oil, parabens. 33 mL. Rx.
Use: Enzyme preparation, topical.
Panafil White. (Rystan) Papain 10,000 units enzyme activity, hydrophilic base/g, urea 10%. Oint. Tube oz.

Rx.
Use: Enzyme, topical.
Panalgesic. (ECR) **Cream:** Methyl salicylate 35%, menthol 4%. Jar 4 oz. **Liq.:** Methyl salicylate 55.01%, menthol 1.25%, camphor 3.1%, in alcohol 22%, emollients, color. Bot. 4 oz, pt, 0.5 gal. *OTC.*
Use: Analgesic, topical.
Panasal 5/500. (Whitehall-Robins) Hydrocodone bitartrate 5 mg, aspirin 500 mg. Tab. Bot. 100s. *c-III.*
Use: Analgesic combination; narcotic.
Panasol. (Seatrace) Prednisone 5 mg. Tab. Bot. 100s. *Rx.*
Use: Corticosteroid.
Panasol-S. (Seatrace) Prednisone 1 mg. Tab. Bot. 100s, 1000s. *Rx.*
Use: Corticosteroid.
Pan C Ascorbate. (Freeda) Vitamin C 200 mg, hesperiden 100 mg, citrus bioflavonoids 100 mg. Tab. Bot. 100s. *OTC.*
Use: Vitamin supplement.
Pan C-500. (Freeda) Hesperidin 100 mg, citrus bioflavonoids 100 mg, vitamin C 500 mg, sodium free. Tab. Bot. 100s, 250s, 500s. *OTC.*
Use: Vitamin supplement.
Pancof. (Pan American) Dihydrocodeine bitartrate 7.5 mg, chlorpheniramine maleate 2 mg, pseudoephedrine hydrochloride 15 mg/5 mL, saccharin, sorbitol, alcohol free, dye free. Syr. 473 mL. *c-III.*
Use: Antitussive combination.
Pancof-EXP. (Pan American) Dihydrocodeine bitartrate 7.5 mg, guaifenesin 100 mg, pseudoephedrine 15 mg/5 mL, saccharin, sorbitol, menthol. Alcohol, sugar, and dye free. Syr. Bot. 25 mL, 473 mL. *Rx.*
Use: Upper respiratory combination, antitussive, expectorant, decongestant.
Pancof-HC. (Pan American) Hydrocodone bitartrate 3 mg, chlorpheniramine maleate 2 mg, pseudoephedrine hydrochloride 15 mg/5 mL, dye and alcohol free. Liq. Bot. 480 mL, pt. *c-III.*
Use: Upper respiratory combination, antihistamine, antitussive, decongestant.
Pancof PD. (Pan American) Dihydrocodeine bitartrate 3 mg, chlorpheniramine maleate 2 mg, phenylephrine hydrochloride 7.5 mg/5 mL. Syr. 120 mL. *c-v.*
Use: Antitussive combination.
Pancof XP. (Pan American) Hydrocodone bitartrate 3 mg, guaifenesin 100 mg, pseudoephedrine hydrochloride 15 mg/5 mL, alcohol and dye free. Liq. Bot.

473 mL. *c-III.*
Use: Upper respiratory combination, antitussive, expectorant, decongestant.
•**pancopride.** (PAN-koe-pride) USAN.
Use: Antiemetic, anxiolytic, peristaltic stimulant.
Pancrease. (McNeil) Enteric-coated capsules. **Regular:** Lipase 4500 units, amylase 20,000 units, protease 25,000 units. Sucrose. Dye free. Bot. 100s, 250s. **MT 4 Capsules:** Lipase 4000 units, amylase 12,000 units, protease 12,000 units. Bot. 100s. **MT 10 Capsules:** Lipase 10,000 units, amylase 30,000 units, protease 30,000 units. Bot. 100s. **MT 16 Capsules:** Lipase 16,000 units, amylase 48,000 units, protease 48,000 units. Bot. 100s. **MT 20 Capsules:** Lipase 20,000 units, amylase 56,000 units, protease 44,000 units. Bot. 100s. *Rx.*
Use: Digestive enzyme.
pancreatic enzyme.
See: Pepsin, ox bile.
pancreatic substance. Substance from fresh pancreas of hog or ox, containing the enzymes amylopsin, trypsin, steapsin.
W/Bile extract, dl-methionine, choline bitartrate.
See: Pancobile.
W/Lipase.
See: Cotazym.
•**pancreatin.** (PAN-kree-ah-tin) *USP 28.* Pancreatic enzymes obtained from hog or cattle pancreatic tissue.
Use: Enzyme (digestant adjunct).
Pancrecarb MS-8 Delayed-Release Capsules. (Digestive Care) Lipase 8000 units, protease 45,000 units, amylase 40,000 units. Cap. Bot. 100s, 250s. *Rx.*
Use: Digestive enzyme.
Pancrecarb MS-4 Delayed-Release Capsules. (Digestive Care) Lipase 4000 units, protease 25,000 units, amylase 25,000 units. Cap. Bot. 100s. *Rx.*
Use: Digestive enzyme.
Pancrecarb MS-16. (Digestive Care) Lipase 16,000 units, protease 52,000 units, amylase 52,000 units. Enteric-coated microspheres. DR Cap. 100s, 250s. *Rx.*
Use: Digestive enzymes.
•**pancrelipase.** (pan-KREE-lih-pace) *USP 28.* Preparation of hog pancreas with high content of steapsin and adequate amounts of pancreatic enzymes.
Use: Enzyme (digestant adjunct).

See: Cotazym.
Ultrase.
Ultrase MT18.
Ultrase MT12.
Ultrase MT20.
Viokase.
pancrelipase. (Various Mfr.) **Cap.:** Lipase 4500 units, protease 25,000 units, amylase 20,000 units; lipase 16,000 units, protease 48,000 units, amylase 48,000 units. Bot. 100s, 250s. **Tab.:** Lipase 8000 units, protease 30,000 units, amylase 30,000 units; lipase 16,000 units, protease 60,000 units, amylase 60,000 units. May contain lactose. Bot. 100s, 500s. *Rx.*
Use: Digestive enzyme.
Pancretide. (Baxter PPI) Pancreatic polypeptide in normal saline.
Use: Fibrinolytic conditions.
pancuronium.
See: Pancuronium bromide.
•**pancuronium bromide.** (PAN-cue-ROW-nee-uhm) USAN.
Use: Neuromuscular blocker, muscle relaxant.
pancuronium bromide. (Various Mfr.) Pancuronium bromide. **1 mg/mL:** Vials 10 mL with benzyl alcohol. **2 mg/mL:** Benzyl alcohol. Vials 2 mL, 5 mL. Amps with benzyl alcohol. *Rx.*
Use: Neuromuscular blocker, muscle relaxant.
Pandel. (Collagenex) Hydrocortisone probutate 0.1%, white petrolatum, light mineral oil, stearyl alcohol, parabens. Cream. Tube 15 g, 45 g, 80 g. *Rx.*
Use: Corticosteroid, topical.
P and S. (Ivax) Liq. Bot. 4 oz, 8 oz. *OTC.*
Use: Antiseborrheic.
P and S Shampoo. (Ivax) Salicylic acid 2%, lactic acid 0.5%. Liq. Bot. 4 oz. *OTC.*
Use: Antiseborrheic.
Panfil G. (Pan American) **Cap.:** Dyphylline 200 mg, guaifenesin 100 mg, lactose. Bot. 100s. **Syr.:** Dyphylline 100 mg, guaifenesin 50 mg/5 mL, parabens, sorbitol, sucrose, vanilla flavor. Bot. 473 mL. *Rx.*
Use: Antiasthmatic; expectorant.
Panglobulin. (American Red Cross) Immune globulin intravenous (IGIV) 6 g, 12 g, sucrose ≈ 1.67 g, sodium chloride < 20 mg/g, preservative free, filtrated. Pow. for Inj., lyophilized. Vial. *Rx.*
Use: Immune globulin.
Panglobulin NF. (American Red Cross) Immune globulin IV 1 g, 3 g, 6 g, 12 g. Preservative-free. With 1.67 g sucrose/

g protein. Pow. for Inj., lyophilized. Vials 1 g, 3 g, 6 g, 12 g. *Rx.*
Use: Immune globulin.
Panhematin. (Ovation) Hematin 301 mg/vial (equivalent to hematin 7 mg/mL) after reconstitution w/Sterile Water for Injection 43 mL, sorbitol 300 mg, preservative free. Pow. for Inj. Single-dose dispensing vial 100 mL. *Rx.*
Use: Hematinic.
Panitol. (Wesley) Allylisobutyl barbituric acid 15 mg, acetaminophen 300 mg. Tab. Bot. 100s, 1000s. *Rx.*
Use: Analgesic; hypnotic; sedative.
•**panitumumab.** (pan-i-TUE-moo-mab) USAN.
Use: Antineoplastic.
Panlor DC. (Pan American) Acetaminophen 356.4 mg, caffeine 30 mg, dihydrocodeine bitartrate 16 mg. Cap. Bot. 100s. *c-III.*
Use: Analgesic.
Panlor SS. (Pan American) Dihydrocodeine bitartrate 32 mg, acetaminophen 712.8 mg, caffeine 60 mg. Tab. 100s. *c-III.*
Use: Narcotic analgesic.
PanMist-DM. (Pan American) **Syr.:** Dextromethorphan HBr 15 mg, guaifenesin 100 mg, pseudoephedrine hydrochloride 40 mg/5 mL, strawberry flavor, alcohol and dye free. Bot. 15 mL, 473 mL. **ER Tab.:** Dextromethorphan HBr 32 mg, guaifenesin 595 mg, pseudoephedrine hydrochloride 48 mg. Bot. 100s. *Rx.*
Use: Upper respiratory combination, antitussive, expectorant, decongestant.
PanMist JR. (Pan American) Pseudoephedrine hydrochloride 48 mg, guaifenesin 595 mg, dye free. ER Tab. Bot. 100s. *Rx.*
Use: Upper respiratory combination, decongestant, expectorant.
PanMist LA. (Pan American) Pseudoephedrine hydrochloride 85 mg, guaifenesin 795 mg. ER Tab. Bot. 100s. *Rx.*
Use: Upper respiratory combination, decongestant, expectorant.
PanMist-S. (Pan American) Pseudoephedrine hydrochloride 40 mg, guaifenesin 200 mg/5 mL, alcohol free, grape flavor. Syr. Bot. 15 mL, 473 mL. *Rx.*
Use: Upper respiratory combination, decongestant, expectorant.
Panmycin. (Pharmacia) Tetracycline hydrochloride 250 mg. Cap. Bot. 100s, 1000s. *Rx.*
Use: Anti-infective, tetracycline.

Pannaz. (Pan American) Pseudoephedrine hydrochloride 90 mg, carbinoxamine maleate 8 mg, methscopolamine nitrate 2.5 mg. ER Tab. Bot. 100s. *Rx.*
Use: Upper respiratory combination, anticholinergic, antihistamine, decongestant.

Pannaz S. (Pan American) Pseudoephedrine hydrochloride 15 mg, carbinoxamine maleate 2 mg, methscopolamine nitrate 1.25 mg/5 mL, blueberry flavor. Syr. Bot. 15 mL, 473 mL. *Rx.*
Use: Upper respiratory combination, decongestant, antihistamine, anticholinergic.

Panocaps. (Breckenridge) Lipase 4,500 units, protease 25,000 units, amylase (porcine-derived enzymes) 20,000 units. Sucrose. Enteric-coated microspheres. DR Cap. 100s, 250s. *Rx.*
Use: Digestive enzyme.

Panocaps MT 16. (Breckenridge) Lipase 16,000 units, protease 48,000 units, amylase (porcine-derived enzymes) 48,000 units. Sucrose. Enteric-coated microspheres. DR Cap. 100s. *Rx.*
Use: Digestive enzymes.

Panocaps MT 20. (Breckenridge) Lipase 20,000 units, protease 44,000 units, amylase (porcine-derived enzymes) 56,000 units. Sucrose. Enteric-coated microspheres. DR Cap. 100s. *Rx.*
Use: Digestive enzyme.

Panokase Tablets. (Breckenridge) Lipase 8000 units, protease 30,000 units, amylase 30,000 units, lactose. Tab. Bot. 100s, 500s. *Rx.*
Use: Digestive enzyme.

PanOxyl AQ 2½, 5, 10. (Stiefel) Benzoyl peroxide 2.5%, 5%, 10%, methylparaben, EDTA, glycerin. Gel. Tube 57 g, 113 g. *Rx.*
Use: Dermatologic, acne.

PanOxyl Bar. (Stiefel) Benzoyl peroxide 5%, 10%, cetostearyl alcohol, glycerin, castor oil, mineral oil in a rich lathering, mild surfactant cleansing base. Soap-free. Bar 113 g. *OTC.*
Use: Dermatologic, acne.

PanOxyl 5, 10. (Stiefel) Benzoyl peroxide 5% (alcohol 12%), 10% (alcohol 20%). Gel. Tube 56.7 g, 113.4 g. *Rx.*
Use: Dermatologic, acne.

panparnit hydrochloride. Caramiphen hydrochloride.
Use: Antiparkinsonian.

Panretin. (Ligand) Alitretinoin 0.1%. Gel. Tube 60 g. *Rx.*
Use: Antineoplastic, retinoid.

Panscol. (Ivax) Salicylic acid 3%, lactic acid 2%, phenol (< 1%). **Oint.:** Jar 3 oz. **Lot.:** Bot. 4 oz. *OTC.*
Use: Emollient.

•**panthenol.** (PAN-theh-nahl) *USP 28.* Alcohol corresponding to pantothenic acid. Pantothenol. Pantothenylol.
Use: Treatment of paralytic ileus and postoperative distention; vitamin.
See: Ilopan.
Panthoderm.

panthenol w/combinations.
See: Lifer-B.

Panthoderm. (Aventis) Dexpanthenol 2% in water-miscible cream. Cream. Tube 1 oz. Jar 2 oz, lb. *OTC.*
Use: Emollient.

pantocaine.
See: Tetracaine hydrochloride.

Pantocrin-F. (Spanner) Plurigland, ovarian, anterior and posterior pituitary, adrenal, thyroid extracts. Vial 30 mL. *Rx.*
Use: Hormone.

Pantopaque. (Alcon) Iophendylate, ethyl iodophenylundecanoate. Amp. 3 mL 3s; 6 mL 6s; 1 mL 2s.
Use: Radiopaque agent.

•**pantoprazole.** (pahn-TOE-prazz-ole) USAN.
Use: Antiulcerative.

•**pantoprazole sodium.** USAN.
Use: Proton pump inhibitor.
See: Protonix.
Protonix I.V.

pantothenic acid.
Use: Vitamin B$_5$ supplement.
See: Calcium Pantothenate.

pantothenic acid salts.
See: Calcium pantothenate.
Sodium pantothenate.

pantothenol.
See: Panthenol.

pantothenyl alcohol.
See: Panthenol.

pantothenylol.
See: Panthenol.

PAN-2400. (Bio-Tech) Lipase 9,816 units, protease 60,214 units, amylase 75,900. Cap. 100s. *OTC.*
Use: Digestive enzyme.

Panvitex Geriatric. (Forest) Safflower oil 340 mg, vitamins A 10,000 units, D 400 units, B$_1$ 5 mg, B$_6$ 1 mg, B$_2$ 2.5 mg, B$_{12}$ activity 2 mcg, C 75 mg, niacinamide 40 mg, calcium pantothenate 4 mg, E 2 units, inositol 15 mg, choline bitartrate 31.4 mg, Ca 75 mg, P 58 mg, Fe 30 mg, Mn 0.5 mg, K 2 mg, Zn 0.5 mg, Mg 3 mg. Cap. Bot. 100s, 1000s. *OTC.*
Use: Mineral, vitamin supplement.

Panvitex Plus Minerals. (Forest) Vitamins A 5000 units, D 400 units, B_1 3 mg, B_2 2.5 mg, niacinamide 20 mg, B_6 1.5 mg, calcium pantothenate 5 mg, B_{12} 2.5 mcg, C 50 mg, E 3 units, Ca 215 mg, P 166 mg, Fe 13.4 mg, Mg 7.5 mg, Mn 1.5 mg, K 5 mg, Zn 1.4 mg. Cap. Bot. 100s, 1000s. *OTC.*
Use: Mineral, vitamin supplement.

Panvitex Prenatal. (Forest) Ferrous fumarate 150 mg, cobalamin concentration 2 mcg, vitamins A 6000 units, D 400 units, B_1 1.5 mg, B_2 2.5 mg, niacinamide 15 mg, B_6 3 mg, C 100 mg, Ca 250 mg, calcium pantothenate 5 mg, folic acid 0.2 mg. Cap. Bot. 100s, 1000s. *OTC.*
Use: Mineral, vitamin supplement.

Panvitex T-M. (Forest) Vitamins A 10,000 units, D 400 units, D_1 10 mg, B_6 1 mg, B_2 5 mg, B_{12} 5 mcg, C 150 mg, niacinamide 100 mg, Ca 103 mg, P 80 mg, Fe 10 mg, Mn 1 mg, K 5 mg, Zn 1.4 mg, Mg 5.56 mg. Cap. Bot. 100s, 1000s. *OTC.*
Use: Mineral, vitamin supplement.

PAP. (Abbott Diagnostics) Enzyme immunoassay for measurement of prostatic acid phosphatase. Test kit 100s.
Use: Diagnostic aid.

Papadeine #3. (Vangard Labs, Inc.) Codeine phosphate 30 mg, acetaminophen 300 mg. Tab. Bot. 100s, 1000s.
Use: Analgesic combination; narcotic.

•**papain.** (pap-ANE) *USP 28.* A proteolytic substance derived from *Carlica papaya.*
Use: Proteolytic enzyme.

papain-urea-chlorophyllin. (Cypress) Papain ≥ 521,700 units, urea 10%, chlorophyllin copper complex sodium 0.5%/g. Glycerin, parabens. Oint. Tube 30 g. *Rx.*
Use: Enzyme preparation, topical.

papain w/combinations.
See: Accuzyme.
Ethezyme 830.
Gladase.
Gladase-C.
Panafil.

Pap-a-Lix. (Freeport) n-acetyl-aminophenol 120 mg, alcohol 10%/5 mL. Bot. 4 oz, gal. *OTC.*
Use: Analgesic.

•**papaverine hydrochloride.** (pap-PAV-uhr-een) *USP 28.*
Use: Muscle relaxant.
See: BP-Papaverine.
Cerespan.
Cirbed.
Delapav.

Myobid.
Pavabid.
Pavacap.
Pavacaps.
Pavacen Cenules.
Pavaclor.
Pavadel.
Pavadyl.
Pavakey S.A.
Pavakey 300.
Pava-lyn.
Pava Par.
Pavasule.
Pavatest T.D.
Pavatym.
Pavatran T.D.
P-200.
Vasocap.
W/Codeine sulfate.
See: Vatnsan.
W/Codeine sulfate, aloin, sodium salicylate.
See: Copavin.
W/Codeine sulfate, emetine hydrochloride, ephedrine hydrochloride.
See: Copavin Compound.
W/Phenobarbital.
See: Golacol.
Pavadel PB.

papaverine hydrochloride. (Apotex) Papaverine hydrochloride 30 mg/mL, EDTA. Inj. Vial 2 mL, multiple-dose vial 10 mL (chlorobutanol 0.5%). *Rx.*
Use: Muscle relaxant.

Paplex Ultra. (Medicis) Salicylic acid 26% in flexible collodion. Bot. 15 mL. *OTC.*
Use: Keratolytic.

para-aminobenzoic acid (PABA).
Use: Sunscreen; agent for scleroderma.
See: Potaba.

para-aminobenzoic acid. (Various Mfr.) para-aminobenzoic acid. **Tab.:** 100 mg. Bot. 100s, 250s. **SR Tab.:** 100 mg. Bot. 100s. *OTC.*
Use: Sunscreen; agent for scleroderma.

•**para-aminosalicylic acid.** *USP 28.* Aminosalicylic acid. *Rx.*
Use: Antituberculosis.

Parabaxin. (Parmed Pharmaceuticals, Inc.) Methocarbamol 500 mg, 750 mg. Tab. Bot. 100s. *Rx.*
Use: Muscle relaxant.

parabrom.
See: Pyrabrom.

parabromidylamine.
See: Brompheniramine, Dimetane.

paracarbinoxamine maleate. Carbinoxamine.

paracetaldehyde. *USP 28.*
See: Paraldehyde.

Paracet Forte. (Major) Chlorzoxazone, acetaminophen. Tab. Bot. 100s, 1000s. *Rx.*
Use: Muscle relaxant.

parachloramine hydrochloride. Meclizine hydrochloride.
See: Bonine.

parachlorometaxylenol.
Use: Phenolic antiseptic.
See: D-Seb.
Nu-Flow.
W/9-aminoacridine hydrochloride, methyldodecylbenzyl-trimethyl ammonium Cl, pramoxine hydrochloride, hydrocortisone, acetic acid.
See: Drotic No. 2.
W/Benzocaine.
See: TPO 20.
W/Coconut oil, pine oil, castor oil, lanolin, cholesterols, lecithin.
See: Sebacide.
W/Hydrocortisone, pramoxine hydrochloride, benzalkonium Cl, acetic acid.
See: Oto Drops.
W/Lidocaine, phenol, zinc oxide.
See: Unguentine Plus.
W/Pramoxine hydrochloride, hydrocortisone, benzalkonium Cl, acetic acid.
See: My Cort Otic #2.
Rezamid.

•**parachlorophenol.** (par-ah-KLOR-oh-feh-nole) *USP 28.*
Use: Anti-infective, topical.

•**parachlorophenol, camphorated.** *USP 28.*
Use: Anti-infective, topical.

paracodin.
See: Dihydrocodeine.

Paraeusal Liquid. (Paraeusal) Liq. Bot. 2 oz, 6 oz, 12 oz.
Use: Minor skin irritations.

Paraeusal Solid. (Paraeusal) Oint. Jar 1 oz, 2 oz, 16 oz.
Use: Dermatologic, counterirritant.

•**paraffin.** (PAR-ah-fin) *NF 23.*
Use: Pharmaceutic aid (stiffening agent).

•**paraffin, synthetic.** *NF 23.*
Use: Pharmaceutic aid (stiffening agent).

Paraflex. (Ortho-McNeil) Chlorzoxazone 250 mg. Tab. Bot. 100s. *Rx.*
Use: Muscle relaxant.

Parafon Forte DSC. (Ortho-McNeil) Chlorzoxazone 500 mg. Cap. Bot. 100s, 500s, UD 100s. *Rx.*
Use: Muscle relaxant.

paraform. Paraformaldehyde (No Manufacturer Available).

paraformaldehyde.
Use: Essentially the same as formaldehyde.
See: Formaldehyde.
Trioxymethylene (an incorrect term for paraformaldehyde).

paraglycylarsanilic acid. N-carbamyl-methyl-p-aminobenzenearsonic acid, the free acid of tryparsamide.

Parahist HD. (Pharmics) Phenylephrine hydrochloride 5 mg, chlorpheniramine maleate 2 mg, hydrocodone bitartrate 1.67 mg, alcohol free. Liq. Bot. 473 mL. *c-III.*
Use: Antihistamine; antitussive; decongestant.

Para-Jel. (Health for Life Brands) Benzocaine 5%, cetyl dimethyl benzyl ammonium Cl. Tube 0.25 oz. *OTC.*
Use: Anesthetic, local.

•**paraldehyde.** (par-AL-deh-hide) *USP 28.*
Use: Hypnotic; sedative.
See: Paral.

Paral Oral. (Forest) Paraldehyde 30 mL. Bot. 12s, 25s. *c-IV.*
Use: Hypnotic; sedative.

paramephrin.
See: Epinephrine.

•**paramethasone acetate.** (PAR-ah-meth-ah-zone) *USP 28.*
Use: Corticosteriod, topical.
See: Haldrone.

para-monochlorophenol.
See: Camphorated para-chlorophenol.

•**paranyline hydrochloride.** (PAR-ah-NYE-leen) USAN.
Use: Anti-inflammatory.

•**parapenzolate bromide.** (pa-rah-PEN-zoe-late) USAN.
Use: Anticholinergic.

Paraplatin. (Bristol-Myers Squibb Oncology) Carboplatin. **Inj.:** 10 mg/mL. Single-dose vials. 5 mL, 15 mL, 45 mL. **Pow. for Inj., lyophilized:** 50 mg, 150 mg, 450 mg. Mannitol. Single-dose vial. *Rx.*
Use: Antineoplastic.

pararosaniline embonate. Pararosaniline pamoate.

•**pararosaniline pamoate.** (par-ah-row-ZAN-ih-lin PAM-oh-ate) USAN.
Use: Antischistosomal.

parasympatholytic agents. Cholinergic blocking agents.
See: Anticholinergic agents.
Antispasmodics.
Mydriatics.
Parkinsonism agents.

parasympathomimetic agents.
See: Cholinergic agents.

• **parathyroid hormone.** (par-a-THYE-roid) USAN.
Use: Anti-osteoporotic.

Paratrol. (Walgreen) Pyrethrins 0.2%, piperonyl butoxide technical 2%, deodorized kerosene 0.8%. Liq. Bot. 2 oz. *OTC.*
Use: Pediculicide.

Parazone. (Henry Schein) Chlorzoxazone 250 mg, acetaminophen 300 mg. Tab. Bot. 100s, 1000s. *Rx.*
Use: Muscle relaxant; analgesic.

• **parbendazole.** (par-BEN-dah-ZOLE) USAN. Under study.
Use: Anthelmintic.

Parcillin. (Parmed Pharmaceuticals, Inc.) Crystalline potassium penicillin G 240 mg, 400,000 units. Tab. Bot. 100s, 1000s. Pow. for Syr. 400,000 units/ 5 mL. 80 mL. *Rx.*
Use: Anti-infective, penicillin.

• **parconazole hydrochloride.** (par-KOE-nah-zole) USAN.
Use: Antifungal.

Parcopa. (Schwarz Pharma) Carbidopa/levodopa 10 mg/100 mg (phenylalanine 3.4 mg), 25 mg/100 mg (phenylalanine 3.4 mg), 25 mg/250 mg (phenylalanine 8.4 mg). Aspartame, mannitol. Mint flavor. Orally Disintegrating Tab. 100s. *Rx.*
Use: Antiparkinson agent.

• **parecoxib.** (pa-re-KOX-ib) USAN.
Use: Anti-inflammatory; analgesic.

Paredrine. (Pharmics) Hydroxyamphetamine HBr 1%. Bot. 15 mL. *Rx.*
Use: Mydriatic.

• **paregoric.** (par-eh-GORE-ik) *USP 28.*
Opioid antitussive.
paregoric. (Various Mfr.) Morphine anhydrous equivalent 2 mg/5 mL, alcohol 45%, may contain benzoic acid. Liq. Bot. 473 mL. *c-iii.*
Use: Antiperistaltic; opioid analgesic.

Paremyd. (Allergan) Hydroxyamphetamine HBr 1%, tropicamide 0.25%. Soln. Bot. 5 mL, 15 mL. *Rx.*
Use: Cycloplegic, mydriatic.

parenabol. Boldenone undecylenate.

• **pareptide sulfate.** (PAR-epp-tide) USAN.
Use: Antiparkinsonian.

Par Estro. (Parmed Pharmaceuticals, Inc.) Conjugated estrogens 1.25 mg. Tab. Bot. 100s. *Rx.*
Use: Estrogen.

parethoxycaine hydrochloride.
W/Zirconium oxide, calamine.
See: Zotox.

Par-F. (Pharmics) Fe 60 mg, Ca 250 mg, vitamins C 120 mg, A 5000 units, D

400 units, B_1 3 mg, B_2 3.4 mg, B_{12} 12 mcg, B_6 12 mg, B_3 20 mg, Cu, I, Mg, Zn 15 mg, E 30 units, folic acid 1 mg. Tab. Bot. 100s. *Rx.*
Use: Mineral, vitamin supplement.

Par Glycerol. (Par Pharmaceuticals) Iodinated glycerol 60 mg/5 mL. Alcohol 21.75%, peppermint oil, corn syrup, saccharin. Caramel-mint flavor. Elix. Bot. Pt. *Rx.*
Use: Expectorant.

• **pargyline hydrochloride.** (PAR-jih-leen) *USP 28.*
Use: Antihypertensive.

• **paricalcitol.** (pah-ri-KAL-si-tole) *USP 28.*
Use: Hyperparathyroidism.
See: Zemplar.

Parkelp. (Phillip R. Park) Pacific sea kelp.
Tab.: Bot. 100s, 200s, 500s, 800s.
Gran.: Bot. 2 oz, 7 oz, 1 lb, 3 lb. *OTC.*
Use: Nutritional supplement.

parkinsonism, agents for. Parasympatholytic agents.
See: Akineton.
Artane.
Benztropine mesylate.
Caramiphen hydrochloride.
Cogentin.
Dopar.
Eldepryl.
Kemadrin.
Larodopa.
Lodosyn.
Parlodel.
Permax.
Sinemet.
Symmetrel.
Trihexyphenidyl hydrochloride.
Trihexy-2

Parlodel. (Novartis) Bromocriptine mesylate. Lactose. **Tab.:** 2.5 mg. Bot. 30s, 100s. **Cap.:** 5 mg. Bot. 30s, 100s. *Rx.*
Use: Antiparkinsonian.

Parmeth. (Parmed Pharmaceuticals, Inc.) Promethazine hydrochloride 50 mg. Cap. Bot. 100s, 1000s. *Rx.*
Use: Antiemetic; antihistamine; antivertigo.

parminyl. Salicylamide, phenacetin, caffeine, acetaminophen.

Par-Natal-FA. (Parmed Pharmaceuticals, Inc.) Vitamins A 4000 units, D 400 units, thiamine hydrochloride 2 mg, riboflavin 2 mg, pyridoxine hydrochloride 0.8 mg, ascorbic acid 50 mg, niacinamide 10 mg, I 0.15 mg, folic acid 0.1 mg, cobalamin concentrate 2 mcg, Fe 50 mg, Ca 240 mg. Cap. Bot. 100s, 1000s. *OTC.*
Use: Mineral, vitamin supplement.

Par-Natal Plus 1 Improved. (Parmed Pharmaceuticals, Inc.) Elemental calcium 200 mg, elemental iron 65 mg, vitamins A 4000 units, D 400 units, E 11 mg, B_1 1.5 mg, B_2 3 mg, B_3 20 mg, B_6 10 mg, B_{12} 12 mcg, C 120 mg, folic acid 1 mg, Zn 25 mg, Cu. Tab. Bot. 500s. *Rx.*
Use: Mineral, vitamin supplement.

Parnate. (GlaxoSmithKline) Tranylcypromine sulfate 10 mg. Tab. Bot. 100s. *Rx.*
Use: Antidepressant.

parodyne.
See: Antipyrine.

paroleine.
See: Petrolatum Liquid.

• **paromomycin sulfate.** (par-oh-moe-MY-sin) *USP 28.* An antibiotic substance obtained from cultures of certain *Streptomyces* species, one of which is *Streptomyces rimosus.*
Use: Antiamebic.
See: Humatin.

parothyl. (Henry Schein) Meprobamate 400 mg, tridihexethyl Cl 25 mg. Tab. Bot. 100s. *c-iv.*
Use: Anticholinergic; anxiolytic; antispasmodic.

paroxetine. (Various Mfr.) Paroxetine hydrochloride 10 mg, 20 mg, 30 mg, 40 mg. Tab. 30s, 100s, 1000s, UD 100s. *Rx.*
Use: Antidepressant, selective serotonin reuptake inhibitor.

• **paroxetine hydrochloride.** (puh-ROX-eh-teen) *USP 28.*
Use: Antidepressant, selective serotonin reuptake inhibitor.
See: Paxil.
   Paxil CR.
   Pexeva.

• **paroxetine mesylate.** (puh-ROX-eh-teen) USAN.
Use: Antidepressant.

paroxyl.
See: Acetarsone.

parpanit.
See: Caramiphen hydrochloride.

parsley concentrate. Garlic concentrate. *Rx.*

Par-Supp. (Parmed Pharmaceuticals, Inc.) Estrone 0.2 mg, lactose 50 mg. Vaginal Supp. Pkg. 12s.
Use: Estrogen.

• **partricin.** (PAR-trih-sin) USAN. Antibiotic produced by *Streptomyces aureofaciens.*
Use: Antifungal; antiprotozoal.

Partuss A.C. (Parmed Pharmaceuticals, Inc.) Guaifenesin 100 mg, pheniramine maleate 7.5 mg, codeine phosphate 10 mg, alcohol 3.5%/5 mL. Bot. 4 oz. *c-v.*
Use: Antihistamine; antitussive; expectorant.

Parvlex. (Freeda) Iron 100 mg, vitamins B_1 20 mg, B_2 20 mg, B_3 20 mg, B_5 1 mg, B_6 10 mg, B_{12} 50 mcg, folic acid 0.1 mg, Cu, Mn. Tab. Bot. 100s, 250s. *OTC.*
Use: Mineral, vitamin supplement.

Pas-C. (Hellwig) Pascorbic. p-aminosalicylic acid 0.5 g with vitamin C. Tab. Bot. 1000s. *Rx.*
Use: Antituberculosal.

• **pascolizumab.** (pas-co-LIZ-oo-mab) USAN.
Use: Asthma.

Paser. (Jacobus) Aminosalicylic acid 4 g. DR Gran. Pkt. *Rx.*
Use: Adjunctive tuberculosis agent.

passiflora. Dried flowering and fruiting tops of *Passiflora incarnata.* Phenobarbital, valerian, hyoscyamus.

Patanol. (Alcon) Olopatadine hydrochloride 0.1%. Soln. *Drop-Tainer* 5 mL. *Rx.*
Use: Antihistamine, ophthalmic.

Path. (Parker) Buffered neutral formalin soln. 10%. Bot. 1 gal, 5 gal. Jar 4 oz.
Use: Tissue specimen fixative.

Pathocil. (Wyeth) Dicloxacillin sodium.
Cap.: 250 mg, 500 mg. Bot. 50s (500 mg only), 100s (250 mg only).
Pow. for Oral Susp.: 62.5 mg/5 mL. Bot. to make 100 mL. *Rx.*
Use: Anti-infective, penicillin.

• **paulomycin.** (PAW-low-MY-sin) USAN.
Use: Anti-infective.

Pavabid Plateau. (Hoechst) Papaverine hydrochloride 150 mg. TR Cap. Bot. 100s, 250s, 1000s, UD 100s. *Rx.*
Use: Vasodilator.

Pavacaps. (Freeport) Papaverine hydrochloride 150 mg. TR Cap. Bot. 1000s. *Rx.*
Use: Vasodilator.

Pavacen Cenules. (Schwarz Pharma) Papaverine hydrochloride 150 mg. TR Cap. Bot. 100s. *Rx.*
Use: Vasodilator.

Pavadel. (Canright) Papaverine hydrochloride 150 mg. Cap. Bot. 100s, 1000s. *Rx.*
Use: Vasodilator.

Pavadel PB. (Canright) Papaverine hydrochloride 150 mg, phenobarbital 45 mg. Cap. Bot. 100s. *Rx.*
Use: Vasodilator.

Pavadyl. (Sanofi-Synthelabo) Papaverine hydrochloride 150 mg. Cap. Bot. 100s. *Rx.*

Use: Vasodilator.
Pavagen. (Rugby) Papaverine 150 mg.
TR Cap. Bot. 500s, 1000s, UD 100s.
Rx.
Use: Vasodilator.
Pava-Lyn. (Lynwood) Papaverine hydrochloride 150 mg. Cap. Bot. 100s. *Rx.*
Use: Vasodilator.
Pavatine. (Major) Papaverine 300 mg.
Tab. Bot. 100s. *Rx.*
Use: Vasodilator.
Pavatine T.D. (Major) Papaverine
150 mg. TD Cap. Bot. 100s, 1000s. *Rx.*
Use: Vasodilator.
Paxarel. (Circle) Acetylcarbromal
250 mg. Tab. Bot. 100s. *Rx.*
Use: Hypnotic; sedative.
Paxil. (GlaxoSmithKline) Paroxetine hydrochloride. **Tab.:** 10 mg, 20 mg,
30 mg, 40 mg. Film-coated. Bot. 30s;
100s (20 mg only), SUP 100s (20 mg
only). **Oral Susp.:** 10 mg/5 mL, parabens, saccharin, sorbitol, orange flavor.
Bot. 250 mL. *Rx.*
Use: Antidepressant, selective serotonin reuptake inhibitor.
Paxil CR. (GlaxoSmithKline) Paroxetine
hydrochloride 12.5 mg, 25 mg,
37.5 mg, lactose. CR Tab. Bot. 30s,
100s (except 37.5 mg), SUP 100s
(25 mg only). *Rx.*
Use: Antidepressant, selective serotonin reuptake inhibitor.
• **pazinaclone.** (pah-ZIN-ah-klone) USAN.
Use: Anxiolytic.
Pazo Hemorrhoid. (Bristol-Myers
Squibb) Zinc oxide 5%, ephedrine sulfate 0.2%, camphor 2% in lanolin-petrolatum base. Oint. Tube 28 g. *OTC.*
Use: Anorectal preparation.
• **pazoxide.** (pay-ZOX-ide) USAN.
Use: Antihypertensive.
PB 100. (Schlicksup) Phenobarbital
1.5 g. Tab. Bot. 1000s. *c-iv.*
Use: Hypnotic; sedative.
PBZ. (Novartis) Tripelennamine hydrochloride 25 mg, 50 mg. Tab. Bot. 100s.
Rx.
Use: Antihistamine.
PBZ-SR. (Novartis) Tripelennamine hydrochloride 100 mg. SR Tab. Bot.
100s. *Rx.*
Use: Antihistamine.
PCE Dispertab. (Abbott) Erythromycin
333 mg (lactose), 500 mg. Polymer-coated particles. Tab. Bot. 60s (333 mg
only), 100s (500 mg only). *Rx.*
Use: Anti-infective, erythromycin.
p-chlorometaxylenol. Benzocaine,
benzyl alcohol, propylene glycol.
W/Hydrocortisone, pramoxine
hydrochloride.

See: 20-Caine Burn Relief.
p-chlorophenol.
See: Parachlorophenol.
PCMX.
See: Parachlorometaxylenol.
PC-Tar. (Geritrex) Coal tar 1%. EDTA.
Shampoo. 180 mL. *OTC.*
Use: Photochemotherapy.
PDP Liquid Protein. (Wesley) Protein
15 g (from protein hydrolysates), cal
60/30 mL. Bot. Pt, qt, gal. *OTC.*
Use: Protein supplement.
Peacock's Bromides. (Natcon) **Liq.:** Potassium bromide 6 g, sodium bromide
6 g, ammonium bromide 3 g/5 mL. Bot.
8 oz. **Tab.:** Potassium bromide 3 g, sodium bromide 3 g, ammonium bromide
1.5 g. Bot. 100s. *Rx.*
Use: Hypnotic; sedative.
• **peanut oil.** *NF 23.*
Use: Pharmaceutic aid (solvent).
Pectamol. (British Drug House) Diethyl-aminoethoxyethyl-a,a-diethylphenylacetate citrate. Bot. 4 fl oz, 16 fl oz, 80 fl
oz, 160 fl oz.
Use: Antitussive.
• **pectin.** (PECK-tin) *USP 28.*
Use: Protectant; pharmaceutic aid, suspending agent.
pectin w/combinations.
See: Donnagel.
Furoxone.
Kaopectate.
Pedameth. (Forest) Racemethionine.
Cap.: 200 mg. Bot. 30s, 500s. **Liq.:**
75 mg/5 mL. Bot. Pt. *Rx.*
Use: Diaper rash preparation.
Pedenex. (Health for Life Brands) Caprylic acid, zinc undecylenate, sodium
propionate. Tube 1.5 oz. Foot pow.
spray 5 oz. *OTC.*
Use: Antifungal, topical.
PediaCare Children's Cold & Allergy.
(Pharmacia) Pseudoephedrine hydrochloride 15 mg, chlorpheniramine
maleate 1 mg/5 mL, corn syrup, sorbitol, bubble-gum flavor, alcohol free.
Liq. Bot. 120 mL. *OTC.*
Use: Upper respiratory combination;
decongestant, antihistamine.
**PediaCare Children's Long-Lasting
Cough Plus Cold.** (Pharmacia)
Pseudoephedrine hydrochloride 15 mg,
dextromethorphan HBr 7.5 mg/5 mL,
corn syrup, sorbitol, grape flavor, alcohol free. Liq. Bot. 120 mL. *OTC.*
Use: Upper respiratory combination,
decongestant, antitussive.
**PediaCare Children's Multi-Symptom
Cold.** (Pharmacia) Pseudoephedrine
hydrochloride 15 mg, chlorpheniramine

maleate 1 mg, dextromethorphan HBr 5 mg, aspartame, phenylalanine, sucrose, cherry flavor. Chew. Tab. 18s. *OTC.*
Use: Antitussive combination.

PediaCare Cold Allergy. (McNeil Consumer) Pseudoephedrine hydrochloride 15 mg, chlorpheniramine maleate 1 mg, aspartame, phenylalanine 8 mg. Chew. Tab. Pkg. 18s. *OTC.*
Use: Antihistamine; decongestant.

PediaCare Cough-Cold. (Pharmacia) **Chew. Tab.:** Pseudoephedrine hydrochloride 15 mg, chlorpheniramine maleate 1 mg, dextromethorphan HBr 5 mg, aspartame (phenylalanine 6 mg), dextrose, sucrose. Fruit flavor. Pkg. 16s. **Liq.:** Pseudoephedrine hydrochloride 15 mg, chlorpheniramine maleate 1 mg, dextromethorphan HBr 5 mg/ 5 mL, corn syrup, sorbitol. Alcohol free. Cherry flavor. Bot. 118 mL. *OTC.*
Use: Upper respiratory combination, antihistamine, antitussive, decongestant.

PediaCare Decongestant Infants'. (Pharmacia) Pseudoephedrine hydrochloride 7.5 mg/0.8 mL, alcohol free, fruit flavor, sorbitol, sucrose. Drops. Bot. 15 mL w/dropper. *OTC.*
Use: Nasal decongestant, arylalkylamine.

PediaCare Fever. (Pharmacia) Ibuprofen. **Susp.:** 100 mg/5 mL, sucrose, berry flavor. Bot. 120 mL. **Oral Drops:** 40 mg/mL, sorbitol, sucrose, berry flavor. Bot. 15 mL. *OTC.*
Use: Anti-inflammatory; NSAID.

PediaCare Infants' Decongestant & Cough. (Pharmacia) Pseudoephedrine hydrochloride 9.375 mg dextromethorphan HBr 3.125 mg/mL, sorbitol, cherry flavor, alcohol free. Drops. Bot. 15 mL w/dropper. *OTC.*
Use: Upper respiratory combination, decongestant, antitussive.

PediaCare Infants' Long-Acting Cough. (Pfizer Consumer Health) Dextromethorphan hydrobromide 7.5 mg per 0.8 mL. Alcohol free. Glycerin, sorbitol. Grape flavor. Drops. 15 mL. *OTC.*
Use: Nonnarcotic antitussive.

PediaCare Multi-Symptom Cold. (Pharmacia) Pseudoephedrine hydrochloride 15 mg, chlorpheniramine maleate 1 mg, dextromethorphan HBr 5 mg/ 5 mL, corn syrup, sorbitol, cherry flavor, alcohol free. Liq. Bot. 120 mL. *OTC.*
Use: Upper respiratory combination, decongestant, antihistamine, antitussive.

PediaCare NightRest. (Pharmacia) Pseudoephedrine hydrochloride 15 mg, chlorpheniramine maleate 1 mg, dextromethorphan HBr 7.5 mg/5 mL, sorbitol, corn syrup. Alcohol free. Cherry flavor. Liq. Bot. 120 mL. *OTC.*
Use: Upper respiratory combination, antihistamine, antitussive, decongestant.

Pediacof. (Sanofi-Synthelabo) Codeine phosphate 5 mg, phenylephrine hydrochloride 2.5 mg, chlorpheniramine maleate 0.75 mg, potassium iodide 75 mg/5 mL, sodium benzoate 0.2%, alcohol 5%. Syr. Bot. 16 fl oz. *c-v.*
Use: Antihistamine; antitussive; decongestant; expectorant.

Pediaflor Fluoride Drops. (Ross) Fluoride 0.5 mg/mL as sodium fluoride 1.1 mg/mL. Bot. 50 mL. *Rx.*
Use: Dental caries agent.

Pediahist DM. (Boca) **Drops:** Pseudoephedrine hydrochloride 15 mg, brompheniramine maleate 1 mg, dextromethorphan hydrobromide 4 mg/mL. Sorbitol. Grape flavor. 30 mL with dropper. **Syrup.:** Pseudoephedrine hydrochloride 30 mg, brompheniramine maleate 2 mg, dextromethorphan hydrobromide 5 mg, guaifenesin 50 mg per 5 mL. Alcohol free. Corn syrup. Grape flavor. 473 mL. *Rx.*
Use: Antitussive combination; antitussive and expectorant.

Pedialyte. (Ross) Na 45 mEq, K 20 mEq, chloride 35 mEq, citrate 30 mEq, dextrose 25 g/L. 100 calories/L. **Plastic Bot.:** 8 fl oz. (unflavored), 32 fl oz. (unflavored, fruit). **Nursing Bot.:** Hospital use. Bot. 8 fl oz. *OTC.*
Use: Electrolytes, mineral supplement.

Pedialyte Electrolyte. (Ivax) Dextrose 25 g, K 20 mEq, Cl 35 mEq, Na 45 mEq, citrate 30 mEq, 100 cal/L. Oral Soln. Bot. 1 L. *OTC.*
Use: Electrolytes, mineral supplement.

Pedialyte Freezer Pops. (Ross) Na 45 mEq, K 20 mEq, Cl 35 mEq, citrate 30 mEq, dextrose 25 g/L, phenylalanine, aspartame. Liq. Ready-to-freeze pops. 2.1 fl oz. Box. 16s. *OTC.*
Use: Electrolytes, mineral supplement.

Pediamycin. (Ross) Erythromycin ethylsuccinate for oral suspension 100 mg/ 2.5 mL. Drops. Bot. 50 mL (Dropper enclosed). *Rx.*
Use: Anti-infective, erythromycin.

Pediapred. (Medeva) Prednisolone sodium phosphate 6.7 mg/5 mL. Liq. Bot. 4 oz. *Rx.*
Use: Corticosteroid.

Pedia Relief Decongestant Plus Cough. (Major) Pseudoephedrine hydrochloride 9.375 mg, dextromethorphan HBr 3.125 mg/mL, sorbitol, cherry flavor, alcohol free. Drops. Bot. 15 mL w/dropper. *OTC.*
Use: Upper respiratory combination, decongestant, antitussive.

Pediarix. (SmithKline Beecham) Diphtheria toxoid 25 Lf, tetanus toxoid 10 Lf, inactivated pertussis toxin 25 mcg, filamentous hemagglutinin 25 mcg, pertactin 8 mg, hepatitis B surface antigen 10 mcg, D-antigen units type 1 poliovirus 40, DU type 2 poliovirus 8, DU type 3 poliovirus 32, 2-phenoxyethanol 2.5 mg, sodium chloride 4.5 mg, aluminum adjuvant per 0.5 mL. Vials. Single-dose, prefilled syringes. *Rx.*
Use: Vaccine.

PediaSure. (Ross) Protein 30 g (Na caseinate, whey protein concentrate), carbohydrate 109.8 g (hydrolyzed cornstarch, sucrose), fat 49.8 g (hi-oleic safflower oil, soy oil, MCT [fractionated coconut oil], mono- and diglycerides, soy lecithin), Na 380 mg, K 1308 mg/L, vitamins A, B_1, B_2, B_3, B_5, B_6, B_{12}, C, D, E, K, inositol, Cl, Ca, P, Mg, I, Mn, Cu, Zn, Fe, biotin, choline, folic acid. < 310 mOsm/kg H_2O, 1 cal/mL. Gluten free. Vanilla flavor. Ready-to-use can 240 ml. *OTC.*
Use: Nutritional supplement.

PediaSure with Fiber. (Ross) Protein 30 g (sodium caseinate, low-lactose whey, carnitine, taurine), carbohydrate 113.5 g (maltodextrin, sucrose, soy fiber [total dietary fiber 5 g]), fat 49.7 g (high-oleic safflower oil, soy oil, medium chain triglyceride oil, lecithin)/L, vitamins A, B_1, B_2, B_3, B_6, B_{12}, C, D, E, K, folic acid, Ca, Fe, I, Mg, P, Se, Zn, Na 380 mg (16.5 mEq), K 1310 mg (33.5 mEq), cal 1/L, vanilla flavor, lactose and gluten free. Liq. Bot. 8 oz. *OTC.*
Use: Enteral nutritional therapy, defined formula diet.

Pediatex. (Zyber Pharmaceuticals) Carbinoxamine maleate 1.75 mg/5 mL. Parabens, cotton candy flavor. Liq. *Rx.*
Use: Antihistamine, nonselective ethanolamine.

Pediatex-D. (Zyber Pharmaceuticals) Pseudoephedrine hydrochloride 20 mg, carbinoxamine maleate 2 mg/5 mL, alcohol and dye free, cotton candy flavor. Liq. Bot. 20 mL, 473 mL. *Rx.*
Use: Upper respiratory combination, decongestant, antihistamine.

Pediatex-DM. (Zyber Pharmaceuticals) Pseudoephedrine hydrochloride 15 mg, carbinoxamine maleate 2 mg, dextromethorphan HBr 15 mg/5 mL, saccharin, sorbitol, cotton candy flavor. Liq. Bot. 20 mL, 473 mL. *Rx.*
Use: Upper respiratory combination, decongestant, antihistamine, antitussive.

Pediatex 12. (Zyber) Carbinoxamine tannate 3.6 mg/5 mL. Methylparaben, saccharin, sucrose. Candy apple flavor. Oral Susp. 473 mL. *Rx.*
Use: Antihistamine.

Pediatric Advil Drops. (Whitehall-Robins) Ibuprofen 100 mg/2.5 mL, EDTA, glycerin, sorbitol, sucrose, grape flavor. Oral Susp. Bot. 7.5 mL. *OTC.*
Use: Antiinflammatory.

Pediatric Cough Syrup. (Weeks & Leo) Ammonium Cl 300 mg, sodium citrate 600 mg/oz. Syr. Bot. 4 oz. *OTC.*
Use: Expectorant.

Pediatric Electrolyte. (Ivax) Dextrose 25 g, K 20 mEq, Cl 35 mEq, Na 45 mEq, citrate 48 mEq, calories 100/L. Soln. Bot. 1 L. *OTC.*
Use: Nutritional supplement, enteral.

Pediatric Maintenance Solution. (Abbott) IV solution w/dose calculated according to age, weight, clinical condition. Bot. 250 mL. *Rx.*
Use: Electrolytes, nutrient replacement.

Pediatric Multiple Trace Element. (American Regent) Zn (as sulfate) 0.5 mg, Cu (as sulfate) 0.1 mg, Mn (as sulfate) 0.03 mg, Cr (as chloride) 1 mcg/mL. Soln. Vial 10 mL. *Rx.*
Use: Nutritional supplement, parenteral.

Pediatric Triban. (Great Southern) Trimethobenzamide hydrochloride 100 mg, benzocaine 2%. Ped. Supp. Pkg. 10s. *Rx.*
Use: Antiemetic/antivertigo agent.

Pediatric Vicks 44D Dry Hacking Cough and Head Congestion. (Procter & Gamble) Dextromethorphan HBr 15 mg/15 mL (1 mg/mL), sorbitol, sucrose, cherry flavor, alcohol free. Syr. Bot. 120 mL. *OTC.*
Use: Antitussive.

Pediazole. (Ross) Erythromycin ethylsuccinate 200 mg, sulfisoxazole acetyl 600 mg/5 mL. Bot. Gran. reconstituted to 100 mL, 150 mL, 200 mL suspension. *Rx.*
Use: Anti-infective, erythromycin.

Pedi-Boot Mist Kit. (Pedinol Pharmacal) Cetylpyridinium Cl, triacetin, chloroxylenol. Bot. 2 oz. *OTC.*

Use: Antifungal; antiseptic; deodorant.
Pedi-Boro Soak Paks. (Pedinol Pharmacal) Astringent wet dressing w/aluminum sulfate, calcium acetate, coloring agent. Box 12s, 100s. *OTC.*
Use: Dermatologic, counterirritant.
Pedicran with Iron. (Scherer) Vitamin B$_{12}$ (crystallized) 25 mcg, ferric pyrophosphate, soluble (elemental iron 30 mg) 250 mg, thiamine mononitrate 10 mg, nicotinamide 10 mg, alcohol 1%/5 mL. Bot. 4 oz, pt. *OTC.*
Use: Mineral, vitamin supplement.
pediculicides/scabicides.
See: Elimite.
    Eurax.
    Lindane.
    Nix.
    Ovide.
    Pronto Concentrate, Shampoo.
    RID.
    Tisit.
Pedi-Dri. (Pedinol Pharmacal) Nystatin 100,000 units/g, talc. Pow. Plastic Bot. w/shaker cap. 56.7 g. *Rx.*
Use: Antifungal; antiperspirant; deodorant; foot powder.
Pediotic. (GlaxoSmithKline) Hydrocortisone 1%, neomycin 3.5 mg (as sulfate), polymyxin B sulfate 10,000 units/mL. Susp. Bot 7.5 mL with dropper. *Rx.*
Use: Otic.
Pediox. (Atley) Pseudoephedrine hydrochloride 15 mg, chlorpheniramine maleate 2 mg, aspartame, phenylalanine, mannitol, sorbitol, xylitol, grape flavor. Chew. Tab. 100s. *Rx.*
Use: Decongestant and antihistamine.
Pedi-Pro. (Pedinol) Benzalkonium chloride, menthol. Pow. 56.7 g. *OTC.*
Use: Antifungal; antiperspirant; deodorant.
Pedituss Cough. (Major) Phenylephrine hydrochloride 2.5 mg, chlorpheniramine maleate 0.75 mg, codeine phosphate 5 mg, potassium iodide 75 mg/5 mL, alcohol 5%, saccharin, sorbitol, sucrose. Syr. Bot. Pt., gal. *c-v.*
Use: Antihistamine; antitussive; decongestant; expectorant.
Pedolatum. (King) Salicylic acid, sodium salicylate. Oint. Pkg. 0.5 oz. *OTC.*
Use: Analgesic, topical.
Pedric Senior. (Pal-Pak, Inc.) Acetaminophen 320 mg. *OTC.*
Use: Analgesic.
PedTE-PAK-4. (SoloPak Pharmaceuticals, Inc.) Zn 1 mg, Cu 0.1 mg, Mn 0.025 mg, Cr 1 mcg. Vial 3 mL. *Rx.*
Use: Nutritional supplement, parenteral.

Pedtrace-4. (Fujisawa Healthcare) Zinc 0.5 mg, copper 0.1 mg, chromium 0.85 mcg, manganese 0.025 mg/mL. Vial 3 mL, 10 mL. *Rx.*
Use: Nutritional supplement, parenteral.
PedvaxHIB. (Merck & Co.) Purified capsular polysaccharide of *Haemophilus influenzae* type b, *Neisseria meningitidis* OMPC 250 mcg/dose when reconstituted, sodium chloride 0.9%, lactose 2 mg, thimerosal 1:20,000. Pow. for Inj. or Soln. Single-dose vial with vial of aluminum hydroxide diluent or single-dose vial. *Rx.*
Use: Immunization.
●**pefloxacin.** (PEH-FLOX-ah-sin) USAN.
Use: Anti-infective.
●**pefloxacin mesylate.** USAN.
Use: Anti-infective.
PEG. (Medco Lab) Polyethylene glycol. Oint. Jar 16 oz. *OTC.*
Use: Pharmaceutical aid, ointment base.
●**pegademase bovine.** (peg-AD-ah-MASE BOE-vine) USAN.
Use: Replacement therapy (adenosine deaminase deficiency); modified enzyme for use in ADA deficiency. [Orphan Drug]
See: Adagen.
●**pegamotecan.** (peg-am-oh-TEE-kan) USAN.
Use: Gastrointestinal.
Peganone. (Ovation) Ethotoin 250 mg, 500 mg. Tab. Bot. 100s. *Rx.*
Use: Anticonvulsant.
●**pegaptanib octasodium.** (pag-AP-ta-nib) USAN.
Use: Age-related macular degeneration disease.
●**pegaptanib sodium.** (pag-AP-ta-nib) USAN.
Use: Age-related macular degeneration disease.
See: Macugen.
●**pegaspargase.** (peh-ASS-par-jase) USAN.
Use: Antineoplastic. [Orphan Drug]
See: Oncaspar.
Pegasys. (Roche) Peginterferon alfa-2a 180 mcg/mL. Inj. Single-dose vials (sodium chloride 8 mg, polysorbate 80 0.05 mg, benzyl alcohol 10 mg) and monthly convenience packs (4 single-use vials, 4 1-mL syringes with needles, and 8 alcohol swabs). *Rx.*
Use: Immunologic agent, immunomodulator.
pegfilgrastim.
Use: Hematopoietic, colony stimulating factor.

See: Neulasta.
PEG-glucocerebrosidase. (Enzon)
Use: Treatment of Gaucher disease.
[Orphan Drug]
●**peginterferon alfa-2a.** (peg-IN-ter-
FEER-ahn AL-fuh-2a) USAN.
Use: Immunologic agent, immunomodu-
lator.
See: Pegasys.
●**peginterferon alfa-2b.** USAN.
Use: Immunologic agent, immunomodulator.
See: PEG-Intron.
PEG-interleukin-2. (Cetus)
Use: Immunomodulator. [Orphan Drug]
PEG-Intron. (Schering) Peginterferon
alfa-2b 50 mcg/0.5 mL, 80 mcg/0.5 mL,
120 mcg/0.5 mL, 150 mcg/0.5 mL,
polysorbate 80, dibasic and monobasic
sodium phosphate dihydrate. Pow. for
Inj., lyophilized. Vial 2 mL (contains dibasic and monobasic sodium phosphate 1.11 mg, polysorbate 80
0.074 mg, and sucrose 59.2 mg) with
1 mL diluent vial, 2 syringes, and 2 alcohol swabs and *Redipen* (contains dibasic and monobasic sodium phosphate 1.013 mg, polysorbate 80
0.0675 mg, and sucrose 54 mg) with
1 B-D needle and 2 alcohol swabs. *Rx.*
Use: Immunologic agent, immunomodulator.
PEG-L-asparaginase. (Enzon) *Rx.*
Use: Antineoplastic.
●**peglicol 5 oleate.** (PEG-lih-kahl 5 OH-
lee-ate) USAN.
Use: Pharmaceutic aid, emulsifying
agent.
●**pegorgotein.** (peg-AHR-gah-teen)
USAN.
Use: Free oxygen radical scavenger.
●**pegoterate.** (PEG-oh-TEER-ate) USAN.
Use: Pharmaceutic aid, suspending
agent.
●**pegoxol 7 stearate.** (peg-OX-ole 7
STEE-ah-rate) USAN.
Use: Pharmaceutic aid, emulsifying
agent.
●**pegsunercept.** (peg-SOO-ner-sept)
USAN.
Use: TNF-inhibitor; anti-inflammatory
(Crohn disease, RA).
●**PEG 3350.**
Use: Laxative.
See: GlycoLax.
●**pegvisomant.** (peg-VI-soe-mant) USAN.
Use: Acromegaly; proliferative diabetic
retinopathy.
●**pelanserin hydrochloride.** (peh-LAN-
ser-in) USAN.

Use: Antihypertensive; vasodilator (serotonin S_2 and α_1 adrenergic receptor blocker).
●**peldesine.** (PELL-deh-seen) USAN.
Use: Antineoplastic; antipsoriatic.
pelentan. Ethyl Biscoumacetate. (No
Manufacturer Available).
●**peliomycin.** (PEE-lee-oh-MY-sin) USAN.
An antibiotic derived from *Streptomycin
luteogriseus.*
Use: Antineoplastic.
●**pelitinib.** (pel-i-TYE-nib) USAN.
Use: Antineoplastic.
●**pelitrexol.** (PEL-i-trex-ol) USAN.
Use: Antineoplastic.
●**pelretin.** (PELL-REH-tin) USAN.
Use: Antikeratinizer.
●**pelrinone hydrochloride.** (PELL-rih-
nohn) USAN.
Use: Cardiovascular agent.
PemADD. (Mallinckrodt) Pemoline
18.75 mg, 37.5 mg, 75 mg, lactose.
Tab. Bot. 100s. *c-iv.*
Use: CNS stimulant.
PemADD CT. (Mallinckrodt) Pemoline
37.5 mg. Chew. Tab. Bot. 100s. *c-iv.*
Use: CNS stimulant.
●**pemedolac.** (peh-MEH-doe-LACK)
USAN.
Use: Analgesic.
●**pemerid nitrate.** (PEM-eh-rid) USAN.
Use: Antitussive.
pemetrexed.
Use: Antimetabolite.
See: Alimta.
●**pemetrexed disodium.** (pem-eh-TREX-
ehd) USAN.
Use: Antineoplastic.
●**pemirolast potassium.** (peh-mihr-OH-
last) USAN.
Use: Antiallergic; inhibitor (mediator
release).
●**pemoline.** (PEM-oh-leen) USAN.
Use: CNS stimulant (central); childhood
attention-deficit syndrome, hyperki-
netic syndrome.
See: Cylert.
PemADD.
PemADD CT.
pemoline. (Apothecon, Mallinckrodt)
Pemoline 18.75 mg, 37.5 mg, 75 mg,
lactose. Tab. Bot. 100s. *c-iv.*
Use: CNS stimulant.
Penagen-VK. (Grafton) Penicillin V. **Tab.:**
250 mg. Bot. 100s. **Pow.:** 250 mg/
100 mL. *Rx.*
Use: Anti-infective, penicillin.
●**penamecillin.** (PEN-ah-meh-SILL-in)
USAN.

Use: Anti-infective.
●**penbutolol sulfate.** (pen-BYOO-toe-lole) USP 28.
Use: Antiadrenergic/sympatholytic, beta-adrenergic blocking agent.
See: Levatol.
●**penciclovir.** (pen-SIGH-kloe-VEER) USAN.
Use: Antiviral.
See: Denavir.
Penecare. (Schwarz Pharma) **Cream:** Lactic acid, mineral oil, imidurea. Tube 120 g. **Lot.:** Lactic acid, imidurea. Bot. 240 mL. OTC.
Use: Emollient.
Penecort. (Allergan) Hydrocortisone 1%, 2.5%, benzyl alcohol, petrolatum, stearyl alcohol, propylene glycol, isopropyl myristate, polyoxyl 40 stearate, carbomer 934, sodium lauryl sulfate, edetate disodium w/sodium hydroxide to adjust pH, purified water. Cream. **1%:** Tube 30 g, 60 g. **2.5%:** Tube 30 g. Rx.
Use: Corticosteroid, topical.
●**penfluridol.** (pen-FLEW-rih-dahl) USAN.
Use: Antipsychotic.
●**penicillamine.** (PEN-ih-SILL-ah-meen) USP 28.
Use: Chelating agent; metal complexing agent, cystinuria, rheumatoid arthritis.
See: Cuprimine.
Depen.
penicillin. (pen-ih-SILL-in) Unless clarified, it means an antibiotic substance or substances produced by growth of the molds Penicillium notatum or P. chrysogenum. Rx.
Use: Anti-infective.
penicillin aluminum. Rx.
Use: Anti-infective, penicillin.
penicillinase-resistant penicillins.
Use: Anti-infective.
See: Dicloxacillin Sodium.
Nafcillin Sodium.
Oxacillin Sodium.
●**penicillin calcium.** USP 28. Rx.
Use: Anti-infective, penicillin.
penicillin, dimethoxy-phenyl. Methicillin sodium.
Use: Anti-infective, penicillin.
penicillin g, aqueous.
Use: Anti-infective.
See: Penicillin G potassium.
Pfizerpen.
●**penicillin G benzathine.** (pen-ih-SILL-in G BENZ-ah-theen) USP 28.
Use: Anti-infective.
See: Bicillin L-A.
Permapen.

penicillin G benzathine and procaine combined.
Use: Anti-infective.
See: Bicillin C-R.
Bicillin C-R 900/300.
●**penicillin G potassium.** USP 28.
Use: Anti-infective.
See: Pfizerpen.
penicillin G potassium. (Baxter PPI) Penicillin G potassium 1,000,000 units, 2,000,000 units, 3,000,000 units. Premixed frozen Inj. Galaxy cont. 50 mL. Rx.
Use: Anti-infective, penicillin.
penicillin G potassium. (Marsam) Penicillin G potassium 1,000,000 units, 5,000,000 units, 10,000,000 units, 20,000,000 units/vial. Pow. for Inj. Vial. Rx.
Use: Anti-infective, penicillin.
●**penicillin G procaine.** (pen-ih-SILL-in G PRO-cane) USP 28.
Use: Anti-infective.
penicillin G procaine. (Monarch) Penicillin G procaine 600,000 units/vial. Inj. 1 mL Tubex; 1,200,000 units/vial. Inj. 2 mL Tubex. Parabens, povidone. Rx.
Use: Anti-infective, penicillin.
penicillin G procaine and dihydrostreptomycin sulfate intramammary infusion.
Use: Anti-infective.
penicillin G procaine and dihydrostreptomycin sulfate suspension, sterile.
Use: Anti-infective.
penicillin G procaine and novobiocin sodium intramammary infusion.
Use: Anti-infective.
penicillin G procaine combinations.
See: Bicillin C-R.
penicillin G procaine, dihydrostreptomycin sulfate, and prednisolone suspension, sterile.
Use: Anti-infective; anti-inflammatory.
penicillin G procaine, dihydrostreptomycin sulfate, chlorpheniramine maleate, and dexamethasone suspension, sterile.
Use: Anti-infective; antihistamine; anti-inflammatory.
penicillin G procaine, neomycin and polymyxin B sulfates, and hydrocortisone acetate topical suspension.
Use: Anti-infective; anti-inflammatory.
penicillin G procaine, sterile. Sterile Susp., Intramammary infusion, Procaine Penicillin.
Use: Anti-infective.
W/Parenteral, Aqueous Susp., (Procaine

Penicillin, for Aqueous Inj.,) Procaine Penicillin and Buffered Penicillin for Aqueous, Inj.
See: Wycillin.
W/Parenteral, in oil w/aluminum monostearate.
See: Penicillin Procaine in Oil Inj.
penicillin G procaine w/aluminum stearate suspension, sterile.
Use: Anti-infective.
penicillin G sodium. (Marsam) Penicillin G sodium 5,000,000 units/Vial. Pow. for Inj. Vial. *Rx.*
Use: Anti-infective, penicillin.
•**penicillin G sodium for injection.**
USP 28.
Use: Anti-infective.
penicillin hydrabamine phenoxymethyl.
Use: Anti-infective.
penicillin O chloroprocaine.
Use: Anti-infective, penicillin.
penicillin O, sodium. Allylmercaptomethyl penicillin.
Use: Anti-infective.
penicillin, phenoxyethyl.
Use: Anti-infective, penicillin.
penicillin phenoxymethyl benzathine.
Use: Anti-infective, penicillin.
See: Penicillin V benzathine.
penicillin phenoxymethyl hydrabamine.
Use: Anti-infective, penicillin.
See: Penicillin V hydrabamine.
penicillins.
Use: Anti-infective.
See: Aminopenicillins.
Amoxicillin.
Amoxicillin and Potassium Clavulanate.
Ampicillin.
Ampicillin Sodium and Sulbactam Sodium.
Carbenicillin Indanyl Sodium.
Dicloxacillin Sodium.
Extended-Spectrum Pencillins.
Nafcillin Sodium.
Natural Penicillins.
Oxacillin Sodium.
Penicillinase-Resistant Penicillins.
Penicillin G (Aqueous).
Pencillin G Benzathine and Procaine Combined, Intramuscular.
Penicillin G Benzathine, Intramuscular.
Penicillin G Procaine, Injectable.
Pencillin V (Phenoxymethyl Penicillin).
Piperacillin Sodium.
Piperacillin Sodium and Tazobactam Sodium.
Ticarcillin and Clavulanate Potassium.

Ticarcillin Disodium.
penicillin S benzathine and penicillin G procaine suspension, sterile.
Use: Anti-infective.
penicillins, extended spectrum.
Use: Anti-infective.
See: Carbenicillin Indanyl Sodium.
Piperacillin Sodium.
Piperacillin Sodium and Tazobactam Sodium.
Ticarcillin and Clavulanate Potassium.
Ticarcillin Disodium.
penicillins, natural.
Use: Anti-infective.
See: Penicillin G (Aqueous).
Penicillin G Benzathine and Procaine Combined, Intramuscular.
Penicillin G Benzathine, Intramuscular.
Penicillin G Procaine, Injectable.
Penicillin V (Phenoxymethyl Penicillin).
•**penicillin V.** *USP 28. Formerly Penicillin Phenoxymethyl. A biosynthetic penicillin formed by fermentation, with suitable precursors of Penicillin notatum.*
Use: Anti-infective.
See: Penicillin VK.
Veetids.
•**penicillin V benzathine.** (pen-ih-SILL-in V BEN-zah-theen) *USP 28. Formerly Penicillin Benzathine Phenoxymethyl.*
Use: Anti-infective.
See: Pen Vee.
•**penicillin V hydrabamine.** (pen-ih-SILL-in V HIGH-drah-BAM-een) *USP 28. Formerly Penicillin Hydrabamine Phenoxymethyl.*
Use: Anti-infective.
Penicillin VK. (Various Mfr.) Penicillin v.
Tab.: 250 mg, 500 mg. Bot. 100s, 500s (500 mg only), 1000s (250 mg only).
Pow. for Oral Soln.: 125 mg/5 mL, 250 mg/5 mL when reconstituted. Bot. 100 mL, 200 mL. *Rx.*
Use: Anti-infective, penicillin.
•**penicillin V potassium.** *USP 28. Formerly Penicillin Potassium Phenoxymethyl.*
Use: Anti-infective.
See: Beepen VK.
Betapen VK.
Bopen, V-K.
Pen-Vee K.
Pfizerpen VK.
Suspen.
V-Cillin K.
Veetids.
penidural.
Use: Anti-infective.

Pen-Kera Creme with Keratin Binding Factor. (B.F. Ascher) Bot. 8 oz. *OTC.*
Use: Emollient.

Penlac Nail Lacquer. (Dermik Labs) Ciclopirox 8%, isopropyl alcohol. Top. Soln. Bot. 3.3 mL, 6.6 mL w/brushes. *Rx.*
Use: Anti-infective, topical; antifungal.

Penntuss. (Medeva) Codeine (as polistirex) 10 mg, chlorpheniramine maleate 4 mg/5 mL. Bot. Pt. *c-v.*
Use: Antitussive; antihistamine.

• **pentabamate.** (PEN-tah-BAM-ate) USAN.
Use: Anxiolytic.

Pentacarinat. (Aventis) Pentamidine isethionate 300 mg. Inj. Single-dose vial. *Rx.*
Use: Anti-infective.

pentacosactride.
Use: Corticotrophic peptide.

• **pentaerythritol tetranitrate diluted.** (pen-tuh-eh-Rith-rih-tole teh-truh-NYE-trate) *USP 28.*
Use: Vasodilator.
See: Arcotrate Nos. 1 and 2.
   Duotrate 45.
   Pentetra.
   Peritrate.
   Petro-20 mg.
   Tetratab.
   Tetratab No. 1.
   Vasolate.
   Vasolate-80.

pentaerythritol tetranitrate w/combinations.
See: Arcotrate No. 3.
   Bitrate.
   Dimycor.
   Pentetra w/Phenobarbital.
   Peritrate w/Nitroglycerin.

• **pentafilcon a.** (PEN-tah-FILL-kahn A) USAN.
Use: Contact lens material, hydrophilic.

• **pentalyte.** (PEN-tah-lite) USAN.
Use: Electrolyte combination.

pentamidine isethionate. (pen-TAM-ih-deen ice-uh-THIGH-uh-nate) (Abbott) Pentamidine isethionate 300 mg. Pow. for Inj., lyophilized. Single-dose fliptop vials. *Rx.*
Use: Anti-infective. [Orphan Drug]
See: Pentam 300.
   Pentacarinat.

pentamidine isethionate (inhalation).
Use: Anti-infective. [Orphan Drug]

• **pentamorphone.** (PEN-tah-MORE-fone) USAN.
Use: Analgesic; narcotic.

pentamoxane hydrochloride.
Use: Anxiolytic.

Pentam 300. (American Pharmaceutical Partners) Pentamidine isethionate 300 mg/Vial. *Rx.*
Use: Anti-infective.

• **pentamustine.** (PEN-tah-MUSS-teen) USAN.
Use: Antineoplastic.

pentaphonate. Dodecyltriphenylphosphonium pentachlorophenolate.
Use: Anti-infective.

• **pentapiperium methylsulfate.** (PEN-tah-PIP-ehr-ee-uhm METH-ill-SULL-fate) USAN.
Use: Anticholinergic.

pentapyrrolidinium bitartrate.
See: Pentolinium tartrate.

Pentasa. (Shire US) Mesalamine 250 mg, 500 mg. Sugar and talc (500 mg only). CR Cap. Bot. 120s (500 mg only), 240s (250 mg only), UD 80s. *Rx.*
Use: Anti-inflammatory.

pentasodium colistinmethanesulfonate. *USP 28.* Sterile Colistimethate Sodium.

• **pentastarch.** (PEN-tah-starch) USAN.
Use: Leukopheresis adjunct, red cell sedimenting agent. [Orphan Drug]

Penta-Stress. (Penta) Vitamins A 10,000 units, D 500 units, B_1 10 mg, B_2 10 mg, B_6 1 mg, calcium pantothenate 5 mg, niacinamide 50 mg, C 100 mg, E 2 units, B_{12} 3.3 mcg. Cap. Bot. 90s, 1000s, Jar 250s. *OTC.*
Use: Mineral, vitamin supplement.

Penta-Viron. (Penta) Calcium carbonate 500 mg, ferrous fumarate 100 mg, vitamins C 50 mg, D 167 units, A 3.333 units, B_1 3.3 mg, B_2 3.3 mg, B_6 2 mg, calcium pantothenate 1.6 mg, niacinamide 16.7 mg, E 2 units. Cap. Bot. 100s, 1000s, Jar 250s. *OTC.*
Use: Mineral, vitamin supplement.

Pentazine. (Century) Promethazine 50 mg/mL. Inj. Vial 10 mL. *Rx.*
Use: Antihistamine.

Pentazine VC w/Codeine. (Century) Promethazine hydrochloride 6.25 mg, codeine phosphate 10 mg. Liq. Bot. 118 mL, pt, gal. *c-v.*
Use: Antihistamine; antitussive.

Pentazine w/Codeine. (Century) Promethazine expectorant. Bot. 4 oz, 16 oz, gal.
Use: Antihistamine.

• **pentazocine.** (pen-TAZ-oh-seen) *USP 28.*
Use: Narcotic agonist-antagonist analgesic.

See: Talwin.
- **pentazocine and aspirin.** *USP 28.* Formerly pentazocine hydrochloride and aspirin.
  Use: Analgesic.
  See: Talwin Compound.
- **pentazocine and naloxone.** *USP 28.* Formerly pentazocine and naloxone hydrochloride.
  Use: Analgesic.

pentazocine and naloxone. (Royce) Pentazocine 50 mg, naloxone hydrochloride 0.5 mg. Tab. Box. 100s, 500s, 1000s. *Rx.*
  Use: Analgesic.
  See: Talwin NX.
- **pentazocine hydrochloride.** *USP 28.*
  Use: Analgesic.
  W/Acetaminophen
  See: Talacen.

pentazocine hydrochloride and acetaminophen. (Watson) Pentazocine hydrochloride 25 mg, acetaminophen 650 mg. Tab. Bot. 100s, 500s, 1000s. *c-IV.*
  Use: Analgesic combination.
- **pentazocine injection.** *USP 28.* Formerly pentazocine lactate injection.
  Use: Analgesic.
  See: Talwin Injection.
- **pentetate calcium trisodium.** (PEN-teh-tate KAL-see-uhm try-SO-dee-uhm) USAN.
  Use: Chelating agent, plutonium.

pentetate calcium trisodium. (Hameln Pharmaceuticals) Pentetate calcium trisodium 200 mg/mL. Inj. 5 mL single-use ampules. *Rx.*
  Use: Chelating agent, plutonium, americium, or curium.
- **pentetate calcium trisodium Yb 169.** USAN.
  Use: Radiopharmaceutical.
- **pentetate indium disodium In 111.** (PEN-teh-tate IN-dee-uhm) USAN.
  Use: Diagnostic aid, radiopharmaceutical.

pentetate zinc trisodium.
  Use: Detoxification agent, chelating agent.

pentetate zinc trisodium. (Hameln Pharmaceuticals) Pentetate zinc trisodium 200 mg/mL. Inj. 5 mL single-use ampules. *Rx.*
  Use: Detoxification agent, chelating agent.
- **pentetic acid.** (PEN-teh-tick) *USP 28.*
  Use: Diagnostic aid.

Pentetra-Paracote. (Paddock) Pentaerythritol tetranitrate 30 mg, 80 mg.

Cap. Bot. 100s, 500s, 1000s. *Rx.*
  Use: Antianginal.

pentetreotide.
  Use: Radiopaque agent, parenteral.
  See: OctreoScan.

Penthrane. (Abbott Hospital Products) Methoxyflurane. Bot. 15 mL, 125 mL. *Rx.*
  Use: Anesthetic, general.
- **pentiapine maleate.** (pen-TIE-ah-PEEN) USAN.
  Use: Antipsychotic.
- **pentigetide.** (pent-EYE-jeh-TIDE) USAN.
  Use: Antiallergic.

Pentina. (Freeport) Rauwolfia serpentina, 100 mg. Tab. Bot. 1000s. *Rx.*
  Use: Antihypertensive.
- **pentisomicin.** (pent-IH-so-MY-sin) USAN.
  Use: Anti-infective.
- **pentizidone sodium.** (pen-TIH-ZIH-dohn) USAN.
  Use: Anti-infective.
- **pentobarbital.** (pen-toe-BAR-bih-tahl) *USP 28.*
  Use: Hypnotic; sedative.
  See: Nembutal.
  Penta.

pentobarbital combinations.
  Use: Sedative; hypnotic.
  See: Cafergot P-B.
  Nembutal.
- **pentobarbital sodium.** *USP 28.*
  Use: Hypnotic; sedative.
  See: Maso-Pent.
  Nembutal Sodium.
  Night-Caps.
  W/Adiphenine hydrochloride, pharmasorb, aluminum hydroxide.
  See: Ephedrine and Nembutal-25.
  W/Ergotamine tartrate, caffeine alkaloid, bellafoline.
  See: Cafergot-P.B.
  W/Homatropine methylbromide, dehydrocholic acid, ox bile extract.
  See: Homachol.
  W/Pyrilamine maleate.
  See: A-N-R, Rectorette.

pentobarbital sodium. (Various Mfr.) Pentobarbital sodium 100 mg. Cap. Bot. 100s. *c-II.*
  Use: Hypnotic; sedative.

pentobarbital sodium. (Wyeth) Pentobarbital sodium 50 mg/mL. Inj. *Tubex* 2 mL. *c-II.*
  Use: Hypnotic; sedative.

pentobarbital, soluble.
  See: Pentobarbital Sodium, USP.

Pentolair. (Bausch & Lomb) Cyclopentolate hydrochloride 1%. Soln.

Squeeze Bot. 2 mL, 15 mL. *Rx.*
Use: Cycloplegic, mydriatic.

pentolinium tartrate. Pentamethylene-1:5-bis (1'-methylpyrrolidinium bitartrate).
Use: Antihypertensive.

Pentol Tabs. (Major) Pentaerythritol tetranitrate. **Tab.: 10 mg:** Bot. 1000s. **Tab.: 20 mg:** Bot. 100s, 1000s. **SA Tab.: 80 mg:** Bot. 250s, 1000s. *Rx.*
Use: Antianginal.

• **pentomone.** (PEN-toe-MONE) USAN.
Use: Prostate growth inhibitor.

• **pentopril.** (PEN-toe-prill) USAN.
Use: Enzyme inhibitor, angiotensin-converting.

• **pentosan polysulfate sodium.** (PEN-toe-san PAHL-in-SULL-fate) USAN.
Use: Anti-inflammatory, interstitial cystitis.

pentosan sodium polysulfate.
Use: Treatment of interstitial cystitis. [Orphan Drug]
See: Elmiron.

• **pentostatin.** (PEN-toe-STAT-in) USAN.
Use: Potentiator; leukemia; antineoplastic. [Orphan Drug]
See: Nipent.

Pentothal. (Abbott) **Pow. for Inj.:** Thiopental sodium 20 mg/mL. In 1, 2.5, 5 g kits, 400 mg syringes; 25 mg/mL. In 1, 2.5, 5 g, 500 mg kits, 250, 400, 500 mg syringes. **Rectal Susp.:** Thiopental sodium 400 mg/g. In 2 g syringe. *Rx.*
Use: Anesthetic.

• **pentoxifylline.** (pen-TOX-IH-fill-in) *USP 28.*
Use: Hemorrheologic, vasodilator.
See: Trental.

pentoxifylline. (Copley) Pentoxifylline 400 mg. CR Tab. Bot. 100s, 500s, bulk pack 5000s. *Rx.*
Use: Hemorrheologic, vasodilator.

pentoxifylline extended-release. (Various Mfr.) Pentoxifylline 400 mg. ER Tab. Bot. 100s, 500s, 1000s, bulk pack 5000s. *Rx.*
Use: Hemorrheologic, vasodilator.

Pentrax. (Medicis) Coal tar extract 5%. Shampoo. Bot. 236 mL. *OTC.*
Use: Antiseborrheic.

• **pentrinitrol.** (pen-TRY-nye-TROLE) USAN.
Use: Vasodilator, coronary.

Pent-T-80. (Mericon Industries) Pentaerythritol tetranitrate 80 mg. TD Cap. Bot. 100s, 1000s. *Rx.*
Use: Antianginal.

Pen-V. (Ivax) Penicillin 250 mg, 500 mg. Tab. Bot. 100s, 1000s. *Rx.*
Use: Anti-infective, penicillin.

Pen-Vee K. (Wyeth) Penicillin V 250 mg, 500 mg Tab. Bot. 100s, 500s, UD 100s. *Rx.*
Use: Anti-infective, penicillin.

Pen-Vee K for Oral Solution. (Wyeth) Penicillin V 125 mg/5 mL, 250 mg/5 mL. Bot. 100 mL, 150 mL (250 mg/5 mL only), 200 mL. *Rx.*
Use: Anti-infective, penicillin.

Pepcid. (Merck) Famotidine. **Tab.:** 20 mg, 40 mg. Film coated. Bot. 1000s, 10,000. Unit-of-use 30s, 90s, 100s. UD 100s. *Uniblister* 31s. **Pow. for Oral Susp.:** 40 mg/5 mL when reconstituted. Parabens, sucrose, cherry-banana-mint flavor. Bot. 400 mg. **Inj. premixed:** 20 mg/50 mL, preservative free. Single-dose *Galaxy* containers. 50 mL. **Inj.:** 10 mg/mL, mannitol. Single-dose vial 2 mL (preservative free). Multidose vial 4 mL, 20 mL (benzyl alcohol 0.9%). *Rx.*
Use: Histamine H_2 antagonist.

Pepcid AC. (J & J Merck) Famotidine. **Chew. Tab.:** 10 mg, phenylalanine 1.4 mg, lactose, aspartame, mannitol. Pkg. 6s, 18s, 30s, 50s, 60s, 68s. **Gelcap:** 10 mg. Bot. 30s, 50s, 60s, 90s. **Tab.:** 10 mg. Pkg. 2s, 6s, 18s, 30s, 60s, 90s. *OTC.*
Use: Histamine H_2 antagonist.

Pepcid AC Maximum Strength. (J&J Merck) Famotidine 20 mg. Tab. 25s. *OTC.*
Use: Histamine H_2 antagonist.

Pepcid RPD. (Merck) Famotidine 20 mg, 40 mg. Aspartame, mint flavor, mannitol, phenylalanine 1.05 mg (20 mg only), 2.1 mg (40 mg only). Orally disintegrating Tab. UD 30s, 100s. *Rx.*
Use: Histamine H_2 antagonist.

• **peplomycin sulfate.** (PEP-low-MY-sin) USAN.
Use: Antineoplastic.

• **peppermint.** *NF 23.*
Use: Pharmaceutic aid, flavor, perfume; antitussive; expectorant; nasal decongestant.
See: Vicks Prods.

• **peppermint oil.** *NF 23.*
Use: Pharmaceutic aid, flavor.

• **peppermint spirit.** *USP 28.*
Use: Pharmaceutic aid, flavor, perfume.

• **peppermint water.** *NF 23.*
Use: Pharmaceutic aid, vehicle, flavored.

Pepsamar. (Sanofi-Synthelabo) **Liq.:** Aluminum hydroxide. **Susp.:** Aluminum hydroxide, magnesium hydroxide, sorbi-

tol. **Tab.:** Aluminum hydroxide. *OTC.*
Use: Antacid.

Pepsamar Comp. Tablets. (Sanofi-Synthelabo) Aluminum hydroxide, magnesium hydroxide. *OTC.*
Use: Antacid.

Pepsamar Esp. (Sanofi-Synthelabo) **Liq.:** Aluminum hydroxide, glycerin. **Tab.:** Aluminum hydroxide, magnesium hydroxide, mannitol powder. *OTC.*
Use: Antacid.

Pepsamar HM. (Sanofi-Synthelabo) Aluminum hydroxide, starch. Tab. *OTC.*
Use: Antacid.

Pepsicone. (Sanofi-Synthelabo) **Gel:** Aluminum hydroxide, magnesium hydroxide, simethicone. **Tab.:** Aluminum hydroxide, magnesium hydroxide, simethicone. *OTC.*
Use: Antacid; antiflatulent.

pepsin.
Use: Digestive aid.

pepsin w/combinations.
See: Biloric.
Donnazyme.
Enzobile.
Leber Taurine.

•**pepstatin.** (pep-STAT-in) USAN.
Use: Enzyme inhibitor, pepsin.

Peptamen. (Clintec Nutrition) Enzymatically hydrolyzed whey proteins, maltodextrin, starch, MCT, sunflower oil, lecithin, vitamins A, B_1, B_2, B_3, B_5, B_6, B_{12}, C, D, E, K, folic acid, biotin, choline, Ca, Cl, Cu, Fe, I, Mg, Mn, P, Zn. Liq. Can 500 mL. *OTC.*
Use: Nutritional supplement.

Peptenzyme. (Schwarz Pharma) Alcohol 16%. Pleasantly aromatic. Bot. Pt.
Use: Pharmaceutic aid.

Peptic Relief. (Rugby) Bismuth subsalicylate. **Chew. Tab.:** 262 mg, dextrose, sorbitol. Bot. 30s. **Liq.:** 87.3 mg/5 mL, saccharin, sorbitol. Bot. 237 mL. *OTC.*
Use: Antidiarrheal.

Peptinex. (Novartis Nutrition) Protein (whey protein hydrolysate, taurine, L-carnitine) 50 g, carbohydrate (hydrolyzed cornstarch) 160 g, fat (soybean oil, medium chain triglycerides, soy lecithin) 17 g/L, vitamins A, B_1, B_2, B_3, B_5, B_6, B_{12}, C, D, E, K, biotin, choline, folic acid, Ca, Cl, Cr, Cu, Fe, I, Mg, Mn, Mo, P, Se, Zn, Na 1010 mg (44 mEq), K 1490 mg (38 mEq)/L, H_2O 320 mOsm/kg, 1 cal/mL, vanilla flavor. Liq. *Tetra Brik* Paks 8 oz. *OTC.*
Use: Enteral nutritional therapy.

Peptinex DT. (Novartis Nutrition) Protein (casein hydrolysate, amino acids) 50 g,

carbohydrate (maltodextrin, modified cornstarch) 164 g, fat (medium chain triglycerides, soybean oil) 17.4 g/L, vitamins A, B_1, B_2, B_3, B_5, B_6, B_{12}, C, D, E, K, biotin, choline, folic acid, Ca, Cl, Cr, Cu, Fe, I, Mg, Mn, Mo, P, Se, Zn, Na 1700 mg (74 mEq), K 800 mg (21 mEq)/L, H_2O 460 mOsm/kg, 1 cal/mL, lactose and gluten free. Liq. Can 250 mL; closed system containers 1 L, 1.5 L. *OTC.*
Use: Enteral nutritional therapy.

Pepto-Bismol. (Procter & Gamble) **Chew. Tab.:** Bismuth subsalicylate 262.5 mg. Pkg. 24s, 42s. **Liq.:** Bismuth subsalicylate 262 mg/15 mL. Bot. 4 oz, 8 oz, 12 oz, 16 oz. **Tab.:** Bismuth subsalicylate 262 mg, < 2 mg sodium. Capl. Sugar free. Bot. 24s, 40s. *OTC.*
Use: Antidiarrheal.

Pepto-Bismol Maximum Strength. (Procter & Gamble) 524 mg/15 mL. Liq. Bot. 120 mL, 240 mL, 360 mL. *OTC.*
Use: Antidiarrheal.

•**peramivir.** (per-AM-i-vir) USAN.
Use: Neuromindase inhibitor.

Perandren Phenylacetate. (Novartis) Testosterone phenylacetate. *c-III.*
Use: Androgen.

percaine.
Use: Local anesthetic.
See: Dibucaine hydrochloride.

•**perchloroethylene.** USP 28.
See: Tetrachlorethylene.

perchlorperazine.
See: Compazine.

Percocet. (Endo) Oxycodone hydrochloride 2.5 mg, acetaminophen 325 mg; oxycodone hydrochloride 5 mg, acetaminophen 325 mg; oxycodone hydrochloride 7.5 mg, acetaminophen 500 mg; oxycodone hydrochloride 10 mg, acetaminophen 325 mg; oxycodone hydrochloride 10 mg, acetaminophen 650 mg. Tab. Bot. 100s, 500s, UD 100s. *c-II.*
Use: Analgesic combination; narcotic.

Percodan. (DuPont) Oxycodone hydrochloride 4.5 mg, oxycodone terephthalate 0.38 mg, aspirin 325 mg. Tab. Bot. 100s, 500s, 1000s, UD 250s. *c-II.*
Use: Analgesic combination; narcotic.

Percodan-Demi. (DuPont) Oxycodone hydrochloride 2.25 mg, oxycodone terephthalate 0.19 mg, aspirin 325 mg. Tab. Bot. 100s. *c-II.*
Use: Analgesic combination; narcotic.

Percogesic. (Medtech) Acetaminophen 325 mg, phenyltoloxamine citrate 30 mg, sucrose. Tab. Bot. 24s, 50s, 90s. *OTC.*

Use: Upper respiratory combination, analgesic, antihistamine.

Percogesic Extra Strength. (Medtech) Diphenhydramine hydrochloride 12.5 mg, acetaminophen 500 mg, dextrose. Tab. Bot. 40s. *OTC.*
Use: Upper respiratory combination, antihistamine, analgesic.

Percomorph Liver Oil. May be blended with 50% other fish liver oils; each g contains vitamins A 60,000 units, D 8500 units.

Percy Medicine. (Merrick Medicine) Bismuth subnitrate 959 mg, calcium hydroxide 21.9 mg/10 mL, alcohol 5%. *OTC.*
Use: Antidiarrheal.

Perdiem. (Aventis) Blend of psyllium 82%, senna 18% as active ingredients in granular form. Sodium content (0.08 mEq) 1.8 mg/rounded tsp. (6 g). Can. 100 g, 250 g, UD 6 g. *OTC.*
Use: Laxative.

Perdiem Fiber Therapy. (Novartis) Psyllium 4.03 g, sodium 1.8 mg, potassium 36.1 mg, 4 cal/6 g, sucrose, dye free, mint flavor. Gran. Can. 100 g, 250 g. *OTC.*
Use: Laxative.

Perdiem Overnight Relief. (Novartis) Psyllium 3.25 g, senna 0.74 g, sodium 1.8 mg, potassium 35.5 mg, 4 cal/rounded tsp., dye free, sucrose, mint flavor. Gran. Bot. 100 g, 250 g, 400 g. *OTC.*
Use: Laxative.

Pere-Diosate. (Towne) Docusate sodium 100 mg, casanthranol 30 mg. Cap. Bot. 100s. *OTC.*
Use: Laxative.

Perestan. (Henry Schein) Docusate sodium 100 mg, casanthranol 30 mg. Cap. Bot. 100s, 1000s. *OTC.*
Use: Laxative.

•**perfilcon a.** (per-FILL-kahn A) USAN.
Use: Contact lens material, hydrophilic.

•**perflenapent.** (per-FLEN-ah-pent) USAN.
Use: Diagnostic aid, ultrasound contrast agent.

•**perflexane.** (per-FLEKS-ane) USAN.
Use: Diagnostic aid, ultrasound contrast agent.

•**perflisopent.** (per-FLYE-soh-pent) USAN.
Use: Diagnostic aid, ultrasound contrast agent.

•**perflubrodec.** (per-FLOO-broe-deck) USAN.
Use: Anemia.

•**perflubron.** (per-FLEW-brahn) *USP 28.*
Use: Contrast agent; blood substitute.

•**perflutren.** (per-FLOO-tren) *USP 28.*
Use: Radiopaque agent, parenteral.
See: Definity.

•**perflutren protein-type A microspheres injectable suspension.** *USP 28.* Formerly perflutren protein-type A microspheres for injection.
Use: Diagnostic aid.

•**perfosfamide.** (per-FOSS-fam-ide) USAN.
Use: Antineoplastic. [Orphan Drug]

pergalen.
See: Sodium Apolate.

•**pergolide mesylate.** (PURR-go-lide) *USP 28.*
Use: Antiparkinson agent.
See: Permax.

pergolide mesylate. (Teva) Pergolide mesylate 0.05 mg, 0.25 mg, 1 mg, lactose. Tab. Bot. 100s. *Rx.*
Use: Antiparkinson agent.

Pergonal. (Serono) Follicle-stimulating hormone (FSH) and luteinizing hormone (LH) 75 units, 150 units. Pow. or pellet for inj., lyophilized. Amps with diluent. *Rx.*
Use: Sex hormone, ovulation stimulant.

Pergrava. (Arcum) Vitamins A 2000 units, D 300 units, B$_1$ 2 mg, B$_2$ 2 mg, nicotinamide 10 mg, B$_6$ 2 mg, B$_{12}$ 5 mcg, C 60 mg, Ca 40 mg. Cap. Bot. 100s, 1000s. *OTC.*
Use: Mineral, vitamin supplement.

Pergrava No. 2. (Arcum) Vitamins A 2000 units, D 300 units, B$_1$ 2 mg, B$_2$ 2 mg, nicotinamide 10 mg, B$_6$ 2 mg, C 60 mg, calcium lactate monohydrate 200 mg, ferrous gluconate 31 mg, folic acid 0.1 mg. Cap. Bot. 100s, 1000s. *OTC.*
Use: Mineral, vitamin supplement.

perhexiline. (per-HEX-ih-leen)
Use: Antianginal.

•**perhexiline maleate.** (per-HEX-ih-leen) USAN.
Use: Vasodilator, coronary.

perhydrol.
See: Hydrogen Peroxide 30%.

Periactin. (Merck & Co.) Cyproheptadine hydrochloride. **Tab.:** 4 mg, lactose. Bot. 100s. **Syr.:** 2 mg/5 mL, alcohol 5%, sucrose, saccharin. Bot. 473 mL. *Rx.*
Use: Antihistamine, nonselective piperidine.

Peri-Care. (Sween) Vitamins A and D in petroleum ointment base. Tube 0.5 oz, 1.75 oz. Jar 2 oz, 5 oz, 8 oz. *OTC.*
Use: Emollient.

Peri-Colace. (Purdue) Docusate sodium 50 mg, sennosides 8.6 mg. Tab. 10s, 30s, 60s. *OTC.*
Use: Laxative.

Peridex. (Procter & Gamble) Chlorhexidine gluconate 0.12%, alcohol 11.6%, glycerin, PEG-40 sorbitan diisostearate, flavor, sodium saccharin, FD&C blue No. 1, water. Bot. 480 mL. *Rx.*
Use: Mouth preparation.

Peridin-C. (Beutlich) Hesperidin methyl cholcone 50 mg, hesperidin complex 150 mg, ascorbic acid 200 mg. Tab. Bot. 100s, 500s. *OTC.*
Use: Vitamin supplement.

Peries. (Xttrium) Medicated pads w/witch hazel, glycerin. Jar pad 40s. *OTC.*
Use: Hygienic wipe and local compress.

• **perindopril.** (per-IN-doe-prill) USAN.
Use: ACE inhibitor.

• **perindopril erbumine.** (per-IN-doe-prill ehr-BYOO-meen) USAN.
Use: Antihypertensive.
See: Aceon.

PerioChip. (AstraZeneca) Chlorhexidine gluconate 2.5 mg. Chip Blister pack 10s. *Rx.*
Use: Anesthetic.

Perio-Eze 20. (Moyco Union Broach Division) Oral paste.
Use: Analgesic, topical.

PerioGard. (Colgate Oral) Chlorhexidine gluconate 0.12%, alcohol 11.6%, glycerin, PEG 40, sorbitol diisostearate, saccharin. Rinse. Bot. 473 mL w/15 mL dose cup. *Rx.*
Use: Anesthetic.

PerioMed. (Omnii Oral) Stannous fluoride concentrate 0.64%. Alcohol-free. Tropical fruit, mint, and cinnamon flavor. Rinse. 283.5 g. *Rx.*
Use: Prevention of dental caries.

Periostat. (CollaGenex) Doxycycline hyclate 20 mg, lactose. Tab. Bot. 60s, 100s, 1000s. *Rx.*
Use: Anti-infective; mouth and throat product.

Peri Sofcap. (Alton) Docusate sodium with peristim. Bot. 100s, 1000s. *OTC.*
Use: Laxative.

Peritinic. (Wyeth) Elemental iron 100 mg, docusate sodium 100 mg, vitamins B_1 7.5 mg, B_2 7.5 mg, B_6 7.5 mg, B_{12} 50 mcg, C 200 mg, niacinamide 30 mg, folic acid 0.05 mg, pantothenic acid 15 mg. Tab. Bot. 60s. *OTC.*
Use: Mineral, vitamin supplement; laxative.

Peritrate. (Parke-Davis) Pentaerythritol tetranitrate. **Tab.: 10 mg:** Bot. 100s, 1000s. **Tab.: 20 mg:** Bot. 100s, 1000s,

UD 100s. **Tab.: 40 mg:** Bot. 100s. *Rx.*
Use: Antianginal.

Peritrate S.A. (Parke-Davis) Pentaerythritol tetranitrate 80 mg (20 mg in immediate-release layer, 60 mg in sustained-release base). Tab. Bot. 100s, 1000s, UD 100s. *Rx.*
Use: Antianginal.

Peri-Wash. (Sween) Bot. 4 oz, 8 oz, 1 gal., 5 gal., 30 gal., 55 gal.
Use: Anorectal preparation.

Peri-Wash II. (Sween) Bot. 4 oz, 8 oz, 1 gal., 5 gal., 30 gal., 55 gal.
Use: Anorectal preparation.

• **perlapine.** (PURR-lah-peen) USAN.
Use: Hypnotic; sedative.

perlatan.
See: Estrone.

‡ **permanganic acid, potassium salt.**
USP 28. Potassium permanganate.

Permapen. (Roerig) Penicillin G benzathine 1,200,000 units/dose with polyvinylpyrrolidone, parabens. Inj. *Isoject* 2 mL. *Rx.*
Use: Anti-infective, penicillin.

Permax. (Amarin) Pergolide mesylate. 0.05 mg, 0.25 mg, 1 mg, lactose. Tab. Bot. 30s (0.05 mg only), 100s (except 0.05 mg). *Rx.*
Use: Antiparkinson agent.

• **permethrin.** (per-METH-rin) USAN. Synthetic pyrethrin.
Use: Pediculicide for treatment of head lice, ectoparasiticide.
See: Acticin.
Elimite.
Nix.

permethrin. (Various Mfr.) Permethrin. **Cream:** 5%. 60 g. **Lot.:** 1%. 60 mL with comb. *OTC.*
Use: Scabicide, pediculicide.

Permitil. (Schering) Fluphenazine hydrochloride. **Concentrate:** 5 mg/mL, alcohol 1%, parabens. Dropper Bot. 118 mL. **Tab.:** 2.5 mg, 5 mg, 10 mg, lactose. Bot. 100s (except 10 mg), 1000s (10 mg only). *Rx.*
Use: Antipsychotic.

Pernox. (Bristol-Myers Squibb) Microfine granules of polyethylene 20%, sulfur 2%, salicylic acid 2% in a combination of soapless cleansers and wetting agents. Lot. Bot. 6 oz. *OTC.*
Use: Dermatologic, acne.

Pernox Lathering Abradant Scrub. (Bristol-Myers Squibb) Sulfur, salicylic acid. Lot. Bot. 141 g. *OTC.*
Use: Dermatologic, acne.

Pernox Medicated Lathering Scrub Cleanser. (Bristol-Myers Squibb) Poly-

ethylene granules 26%, sulfur 2%, salicylic acid 1.5% w/soapless surface-active cleansers and wetting agents. Regular or lemon. Tube 2 oz, 4 oz. *OTC.*
Use: Dermatologic, acne.
Pernox Scrub for Oily Skin. (Bristol-Myers Squibb) Sulfur, salicylic acid, EDTA. Cleanser. 56 g, 113 g. *OTC.*
Use: Dermatologic, acne.
Pernox Shampoo. (Bristol-Myers Squibb) Sodium laureth sulfate, water, lauramide DEA, quaternium 22, PEG-75 lanolin/hydrolyzed animal protein, fragrance, sodium Cl, lactic acid, sorbic acid, disodium EDTA, FD&C yellow No. 6 and blue No. 1. Bot. 8 oz. *OTC.*
Use: Cleanser; conditioner.
peroxidase.
W/Glucose oxidase, potassium, iodide.
See: Diastix Reagent Strips.
peroxide, dibenzoyl. Benzoyl Peroxide, Hydrous.
peroxides.
See: Hydrogen Peroxide.
Urea Peroxide.
Zinc Peroxide.
Peroxyl. (Colgate Oral) Hydrogen peroxide 1.5% in a mint-flavored base. Gel. Tube 15 mL. *OTC.*
Use: Mouth preparation.
Peroxyl Dental Rinse. (Colgate Oral) Hydrogen peroxide 1.5% in mint-flavored base, alcohol 6%. Bot. 240 mL, pt. *OTC.*
Use: Mouth preparation.
•**perphenazine.** (per-FEN-uh-ZEEN) *USP 28.*
Use: Antiemetic; antipsychotic; anxiolytic.
See: Trilafon.
perphenazine. (Pharmaceutical Associates) Perphenazine 16 mg/5 mL, sucrose, berry flavor. Oral Concentrate. Bot. 118 mL w/graduated calibrated dropper. *Rx.*
Use: Antispychotic.
perphenazine. (Various Mfr.) Perphenazine 2 mg, 4 mg, 8 mg, 16 mg, sorbitol. Tab. Bot. 100s, 500s (4 mg, 8 mg only), 1000s, UD 100s. *Rx.*
Use: Antipsychotic.
perphenazine/amitriptyline.
See: Etrafon.
Etrafon-A.
Etrafon-Forte.
Etrafon 2-10.
perphenazine/amitriptyline. (Various Mfr.) Perphenazine/amitriptyline 2 mg/10 mg, 2 mg/25 mg, 4 mg/10 mg, 4 mg/25 mg, 4 mg/50 mg. Tab. Bot. 21s

(2 mg/10 mg only), 100s, 250s (4 mg/10 mg and 4 mg/50 mg only), 500s (except 4 mg/50 mg), 800s (4 mg/25 mg only), 1,000s (except 4 mg/50 mg).
Use: Miscellaneous psychotherapeutic.
Persangue. (Arcum) Ferrous gluconate 192 mg, vitamins C 150 mg, B_1 3 mg, B_2 3 mg, B_{12} 50 mcg. Cap. Bot. 100s, 500s. *OTC.*
Use: Mineral, vitamin supplement.
Persantine. (Boehringer Ingelheim) Dipyridamole 25 mg, 50 mg, 75 mg. Tab. **25 mg , 50 mg:** Bot. 100s, 1000s, UD 100s. **75 mg:** Bot. 100s, 500s, UD 100s. *Rx.*
Use: Antiplatelet.
Persantine IV. (DuPont) Dipyridamole. Inj. For evaluation of coronary artery disease.
Use: Diagnostic aid.
•**persic oil.** (PER-sik) *NF 23.*
Use: Vehicle.
pertechnetic acid, sodium salt. Sodium Pertechnetate Tc-99m Solution.
Pertscan-99m. (Abbott Diagnostics) Radiodiagnostic. Inj. Tc-99m.
Use: Diagnostic aid.
Pertussin. (Pertussin) Dextromethorphan HBr 15 mg/5 mL, alcohol 9.5%. Syr. Bot. 3 oz, 6 oz. *OTC.*
Use: Antitussive.
Pertussin All-Night PM. (Pertussin) Acetaminophen 167 mg, doxylamine succinate 1.25 mg, pseudoephedrine hydrochloride 10 mg, dextromethorphan HBr 5 mg/5 mL, alcohol 25%. Liq. Bot. 240 mL. *OTC.*
Use: Analgesic; antihistamine; antitussive; decongestant.
Pertussin CS. (Pertussin) Dextromethorphan HBr 3.5 mg, guaifenesin 25 mg/5 mL, 8.5% alcohol. Bot. 90 mL. *OTC.*
Use: Antitussive; expectorant.
Pertussin ES. (Pertussin) Dextromethorphan HBr 15 mg/5 mL, alcohol 9.5%, sugar, sorbitol. Liq. Bot. 120 mL. *OTC.*
Use: Antitussive.
•**pertussis immune globulin.** (per-TUSS-iss) *USP 28. Formerly Pertussis Immune Human Globulin.*
Use: Immunization.
•**pertussis vaccine.** *USP 28.*
Use: Immunization.
W/diphtheria and tetanus toxoids.
See: Daptacel.
Infanrix.
Tripedia.
W/Diphtheria, tetanus toxoids, Haemophilus influenzae type b.
See: TriHIBit.

pertussis vaccine. (Michigan Department of Health) Vial 5 mL.
Use: Immunization.
- **pertussis vaccine adsorbed.** *USP 28.*
Use: Immunization.
pertussis vaccine and diphtheria and tetanus toxoids, combined.
Use: Immunization.
See: Daptacel.
Infanrix.
Tripedia.
- **pertuzumab.** (per-TUE-zue-mab) USAN.
Use: Antineoplastic.
peruvian balsam.
Use: Local protectant, rubefacient.
W/Benzocaine, zinc oxide, bismuth subgallate, boric acid.
See: Hemorrhoidal Oint.
W/Ephedrine sulfate, belladonna extract, zinc oxide, boric acid, bismuth oxyiodide, subcarbonate.
See: Wyanoids.
W/Lidocaine, bismuth subgallate, zinc oxide, aluminum subacetate.
See: Xylocaine.
- **perzinfotel.** (per-zin-FOE-tel) USAN.
Use: NMDA receptor antagonist.
peson. Sodium Lyapolate. Polyethylene sulfonate sodium.
Use: Anticoagulant.
Peterson's Ointment. (Peterson) Carbolic acid, camphor, tannic acid, zinc oxide. Tube w/pipe 1 oz. Jar 16 oz. Can 1.4 oz, 3 oz. *OTC.*
Use: Anorectal preparation.
Pethadol. (Halsey Drug) Meperidine hydrochloride 50 mg, 100 mg. Tab. Bot. 100s, 1000s. *c-II.*
Use: Analgesic; narcotic.
- **pethidine hydrochloride.** *USP 28.*
See: Meperidine hydrochloride.
PETN.
See: Pentaerythritol tetranitrate.
petrichloral. Pentaerythritol chloral.
Use: Sedative.
- **petrolatum.** (pe-troe-LAY-tum) *USP 28.*
Use: Pharmaceutic aid (ointment base).
See: Lipkote.
petrolatum gauze.
Use: Surgical aid.
- **petrolatum, hydrophilic.** *USP 28.*
Use: Pharmaceutic aid, absorbent, ointment base; topical protectant.
See: Lipkote.
- **petrolatum, liquid.** *USP 28.* Mineral Oil, Light Mineral Oil, Adepsine Oil, Glymol, Liquid Paraffin, Parolein, White Mineral Oil, Heavy Liquid Petrolatum.
Use: Laxative.

See: Fleet Mineral Oil Enema.
Mineral Oil.
Saxol.
petrolatum, liquid, emulsion.
Use: Lubricant, laxative.
See: Milkinol.
W/Agar-Gel.
See: Agoral Plain.
Milkinol.
W/Irish moss, casanthranol.
See: Haley's M. O.
W/Phenolphthalein.
See: Agoral.
Phenolphthalein in liquid Petrolatum Emulsion.
petrolatum, red veterinarian. (AstraZeneca) Also known as RVP.
W/Micasorb.
See: RV Plus.
W/N-diethyl metatoluamide.
See: RV Pellent.
W/Zinc oxide, 2-ethoxyethyl p-methoxycinnamate.
See: RV Paque.
- **petrolatum, white.** *USP 28.*
Use: Pharmaceutic aid, oleaginous ointment base; topical protectant.
See: Moroline.
Petro-Phyllc Soap. (Doak Dermatologics) Hydrophilic Petrolatum. Cake 4 oz.
Use: Emollient; anti-infective, topical.
Petro-20. (Foy Laboratories) Pentaerythritol tetranitrate 20 mg. Tab. Bot. 100s, 1000s. *Rx.*
Use: Antlanginal.
- **pexelizumab.** (peks-e-li-ZOO-mab) USAN.
Use: Monoclonal antibody.
Pexeva. (Synthon) Paroxetine mesylate 10 mg, 20 mg, 30 mg, 40 mg. Tab. 30s, 100s (20 mg only), 500s (20 mg only). *Rx.*
Use: Antidepressant, selective serotonin reuptake inhibitor.
Pfeiffer's Cold Sore. (Pfeiffer) Gum benzoin 7%, camphor, menthol, thymol, eucalyptol, alcohol 85%. Lot. Bot. 15 mL. *OTC.*
Use: Cold sores; fever blisters; moisturizer.
PF4RIA. (Abbott Diagnostics) Platelet factor 4 radioimmunoassay for the quantitative measurement of total PF4 levels in plasma.
Use: Diagnostic aid.
Pfizerpen. (Pfizer) Penicillin G potassium 5,000,000 units, 20,000,000 units/vial, sodium $\approx$ 6.8 mg (0.3 mEq), potassium 65.6 mg (1.68 mEq)/million units. Pow. for Inj. Vial. *Rx.*
Use: Anti-infective, penicillin.

Pfizerpen VK. (Pfizer) Penicillin V potassium. Tab. **250 mg:** Bot. 1000s.
500 mg: Bot. 100s. *Rx.*
Use: Anti-infective, penicillin.
•**PGA.** *USP 28.*
See: Folic acid.
PGE.
Use: Prostaglandin.
See: Alprostadil.
pH acid. (Ivax) Bot. 8 oz.
Use: Dermatologic.
Phadiatop RIA Test. (Pharmacia) Determination of IgE antibodies specific to inhalant allergens in human serum. Kit 60s.
Use: Diagnostic aid.
Phanatuss Cough. (Pharmakon) Dextromethorphan HBr 10 mg, guaifenesin 85 mg, potassium citrate 75 mg, citric acid 35 mg/5 mL, sorbitol, menthol. Syr. Bot. 118 mL. *OTC.*
Use: Antitussive; expectorant.
Phanatuss DM Cough. (Pharmakon) Dextromethorphan HBr 10 mg, guaifenesin 100 mg/5 mL, parabens, saccharin, menthol, alcohol free. Syr. Bot. 118 mL. *OTC.*
Use: Upper respiratory combination, antitussive, expectorant.
pH Antiseptic Skin Cleanser. (Walgreen) Alcohol 63%. Bot. 16 oz. *OTC.*
Use: Astringent; cleanser.
Pharazine. (Halsey Drug) Bot. 4 oz, pt, gal.
Use: A series of cough and cold products.
Pharmadine. (Sherwood Davis & Geck) Povidone-iodine. **Oint.:** Pkt. 1 g, 1.5 g, 2 g, 30 g, 1 lb. **Perineal wash:** 240 mL. **Skin cleanser:** 240 mL. **Soln.:** 15 mL, 120 mL, 240 mL, pt, qt. **Soln., swabs:** 100s. **Soln., swabsticks:** 1 or 3/packet in 250s. **Spray:** 120 g. **Surgical scrub:** 30 mL, pt, qt, gal, foil-pack 15 mL. **Surgical scrub sponge/brush:** 25s. **Swabsticks, lemon glycerin:** 100s. **Whirlpool soln.:** Gal. *OTC.*
Use: Antiseptic.
Pharmaflur. (Pharmics) Sodium fluoride 2.21 mg. Tab. Bot. 1000s. *Rx.*
Use: Dental caries agent.
Pharmalgen Hymenoptera Venoms. (ALK) Freeze-dried venom or venom protein. Vials of 120 mcg, 1100 mcg for each of honey bee, white-faced hornet, yellow hornet, yellow jacket, or wasp. Vials of 360 mcg, 3300 mcg for mixed vespids (white-faced hornet, yellow hornet, yellow jacket). Diagnostic kit: 5 × 1 mL vial. Treatment kit: 6 × 1 mL vial or 1 × 1.1 mg multiple-dose

vial. Starter Kit: 6 × 1 mL, prediluted 0.01 mcg to 100 mcg/mL.
Use: Antivenom.
Pharmalgen Standardized Allergenic Extracts. (ALK) 100,000 allergenic units. Vial. Box 5 × 1 mL.
Use: Diagnostic aid.
Phazyme. (Schwarz Pharma) Simethicone. **Drops:** 40 mg/0.6 mL, saccharin. Bot. 30 mL w/dropper. **Tab.:** 60 mg. Bot. 50s, 100s, 1000s. *OTC.*
Use: Antiflatulent.
Phazyme 95. (Schwarz Pharma) Simethicone 95 mg. Tab. Bot. 100s. *OTC.*
Use: Antiflatulent.
Phazyme 125. (Schwarz Pharma) Simethicone 125 mL. Cap. Bot. 50s. *OTC.*
Use: Antiflatulent.
•**phemfilcon a.** (FEM-fill-kahn A) USAN.
Use: Contact lens material, hydrophilic.
•**phenacaine hydrochloride.** *USP 28.*
Use: Anesthetic, local.
Phenacal. (NeuroGenesis/Matrix Tech.) D,l-phenylalanine 500 mg, l-glutamine 15 mg, l-tyrosine 25 mg, l-carnitine 10 mg, l-arginine pyroglutamate 10 mg, l-ornithine/l-aspartate 10 mg, Cr 0.033 mg, Se 0.012 mg, vitamin B_1 0.33 mg, B_2 5 mg, B_3 3.3 mg, B_5 0.33 mg, B_6 0.33 mg, B_{12} 1 mcg, E 5 units, biotin 0.05 mg, folic acid 0.066 mg, Fe 1 mg, Zn 2.5 mg, Ca 35 mg, I 0.25 mg, Cu 0.33 mg, Mg 25 mg. Cap. Bot. 42s, 180s. *OTC.*
Use: Nutritional supplement.
phenacetin. Acetophenetidin. Ethoxyacetanilide.
Note: This drug has been withdrawn from the market because of liver and kidney toxicity. This drug is no longer official in the USP.
Use: Antipyretic; analgesic.
Phenadex Senior. (Alra) Dextromethorphan HBr 10 mg, guaifenesin 200 mg/5 mL. Liq. Bot. 118 mL. *OTC.*
Use: Antitussive; expectorant.
Phenadoz. (Paddock) Promethazine 12.5 mg, 25 mg. Cocoa butter. Supp. 12s. *Rx.*
Use: Antihistamine.
phenamazoline hydrochloride.
Use: Vasoconstrictor.
Phenameth. (Major) Promethazine 25 mg. Tab. Bot. 1000s. *Rx.*
Use: Antiemetic; antihistamine.
Phenameth DM. (Major) Promethazine hydrochloride 6.25 mg, dextromethorphan HBr 15 mg/5 mL, alcohol. Syr. Bot. 120 mL. *Rx.*
Use: Antihistamine; antitussive.

Phenameth VC w/Codeine. (Major) Phenylephrine hydrochloride 5 mg, promethazine hydrochloride 6.25 mg, codeine phosphate 10 mg/5 mL, alcohol 7%. Syr. Bot. Pt, gal. *c-v.*
Use: Antihistamine; antitussive; decongestant.

Phenameth w/Codeine. (Major) Promethazine hydrochloride 6.25 mg, codeine phosphate 10 mg/5 mL, alcohol 7%. Syr. Bot. 4 oz, pt, gal. *c-v.*
Use: Antihistamine; antitussive.

phenantoin. Mephenytoin.
See: Mesantoin.

Phenapap. (Rugby) Pseudoephedrine hydrochloride 30 mg, acetaminophen 325 mg. Tab. Bot. 100s. *OTC.*
Use: Upper respiratory combination, decongestant, analgesic.

Phenapap Sinus Headache & Congestion. (Rugby) Pseudoephedrine hydrochloride 30 mg, chlorpheniramine 2 mg, acetaminophen 325 mg. Tab. Bot. 30s, 100s, 1000s. *OTC.*
Use: Analgesic; antihistamine; decongestant.

phenaphthazine. Sodium dinitro phenylazonaphthol disulfonate.
See: Nitrazine Paper.

phenarsone sulfoxylate. Methanesulfinic acid disodium salt.
Use: Antiamebic.

Phenaseptic. (Rugby) Phenol 1.4%, saccharin, cherry flavor. Throat spray. Bot. 177 mL. *OTC.*
Use: Mouth and throat product.

Phenaspirin Compound. (Davis & Sly) Phenobarbital 0.25 g, aspirin 3.5 g. Cap. Bot. 1000s. *Rx.*
Use: Analgesic; hypnotic; sedative.

PhenaVent D. (Ethex) Phenylephrine hydrochloride 40 mg, guaifenesin 1200 mg. Tab. 100s. *Rx.*
Use: Decongestant, expectorant.

PhenaVent LA. (Ethex) Phenylephrine hydrochloride 30 mg, guaifenesin 400 mg. Sucrose. ER Cap. 30s. *Rx.*
Use: Decongestant, expectorant.

phenazocine hydrobromide.
Use: Analgesic.

phenazone.
See: Antipyrine.

•**phenazopyridine hydrochloride.** (fen-AZZ-oh-PIH-rih-deen) *USP 28.*
Use: Analgesic, urinary.
See: Azo-Standard.
Pyridium.
W/Combinations.
See: Azo Gantanol.
Azo Gantrisin.
Azo-sulfisoxazole.

Phenazopyridine Plus.
Pyridium Plus.
Triurisul.
Uridium.
Urisan-P.
Urobiotic.
Urogesic.

Phenazopyridine Plus. (Breckenridge) Phenazopyridine hydrochloride 150 mg, hyoscyamine hydrobromide 0.3 mg, butabarbital 15 mg. Tab. 30s. *Rx.*
Use: Interstitial cystitis agent.

•**phenbutazone sodium glycerate.** (fen-BYOO-tah-zone so-dee-uhm GLIH-seh-rate) *USAN.*
Use: Anti-inflammatory.

•**phencarbamide.** (FEN-car-BAM-id) *USAN.*
Use: Anticholinergic, spasmolytic.

Phenchlor-Eight. (Freeport) Chlorpheniramine maleate 8 mg. TR Cap. Bot. 1000s. *Rx.*
Use: Antihistamine.

Phenchlor-Twelve. (Freeport) Chlorpheniramine maleate 12 mg. TR Cap. Bot. 1000s. *Rx.*
Use: Antihistamine.

•**phencyclidine hydrochloride.** (fen-SIGH-klih-deen) *USAN.*
Use: Anesthetic.

phendimetrazine. (Various Mfr.) Phendimetrazine tartrate 35 mg. Tab. Bot. 100s, 1000s, 5000s. *c iii*
Use: CNS stimulant, anorexiant.

•**phendimetrazine tartrate.** (fen-die-MEH-trah-zeen) *USP 28.*
Use: CNS stimulant, anorexiant.
See: Anorex.
Bontril PDM.
Bontril Slow Release.
Delcozine.
Di-Ap-Trol.
Elphemet.
Melfiat-105 Unicelles.
Obepar.
Obe-Tite.
Phendimetrazine.
Phen-70.
Prelu-2.
Reducto.
Rexigen Forte.
Slim-Tabs.

Phendry. (LuChem Pharmaceuticals, Inc.) Diphenhydramine hydrochloride 12.5 mg/5 mL, alcohol 14%. Elix. Bot. Pt, gal. *OTC.*
Use: Antihistamine.

Phendry Children's Allergy Medicine. (LuChem Pharmaceuticals, Inc.)

Diphenhydramine hydrochloride 12.5 mg/5 mL, alcohol 14%. Elix. Bot. 120 mL. *OTC.*
Use: Antihistamine.

phenelzine dihydrogen sulfate.
See: Nardil.

●**phenelzine sulfate.** (FEN-uhl-zeen) *USP 28.*
Use: Antidepressant.
See: Nardil.

Phenerbel-S. (Rugby) Phenobarbital 40 mg, ergotamine tartrate 0.6 mg, l-alkaloids of belladonna 0.2 mg. Tab. Bot. 100s. *Rx.*
Use: Anticholinergic; hypnotic; sedative.

Phenergan. (Wyeth) Promethazine hydrochloride. **Inj.:** 25 mg, 50 mg/mL, EDTA, sodium metabisulfite 0.25 mg/mL. Inj. Amp. 1 mL. **Supp.:** 12.5 mg, 25 mg, 50 mg, cocoa butter. Box. 12s. **Tab.:** 25 mg, 50 mg, lactose, saccharin (except 50 mg). Tab. Bot. 100s. Blister pack 100s (25 mg only). *Rx.*
Use: Antihistamine, nonselective phenothiazine.

Phenergan Injection. (Wyeth) *Rx.*
Use: Antihistamine.

Phenergan with Codeine. (Wyeth) Promethazine hydrochloride 6.25 mg, codeine phosphate 10 mg/5 mL. Bot. 4 oz, 6 oz, 8 oz, pt, gal. *c-v.*
Use: Antihistamine; antitussive.

Phenergan with Dextromethorphan. (Wyeth) Promethazine hydrochloride 6.25 mg, dextromethorphan HBr 15 mg/5 mL, alcohol 7%. Bot. 4 oz, 6 oz, pt, gal. *Rx.*
Use: Antihistamine; antitussive.

pheneridine.
Use: Analgesic.

i-phenethylbiguanide monohydrochloride. Phenformin hydrochloride.

Phenex-1. (Ross) Protein 15 g, fat 23.9 g, carbohydrates 46.3 g, linoleic acid 1800 mg, Fe 9 mg, Na 190 mg, K 675 mg, Cal 480/100 g. With appropriate vitamins and minerals. Phenylalanine free. Pow. Can 350 g. *OTC.*
Use: Nutritional supplement.

Phenex-2. (Ross) Protein 30 g, fat 15.5 g, carbohydrates 30 g, Na 880 mg, K 1370 mg, Cal 410/mL. With appropriate vitamins and minerals. Phenylalanine free. Pow. Can 325 g. *OTC.*
Use: Nutritional supplement.

phenformin hydrochloride. *Rx.*
Note: Withdrawn from market in 1977. Available under IND exemption.
Use: Hypoglycemic.

Phenhist DH w/Codeine. (Rugby) Pseudoephedrine hydrochloride 30 mg, chlorpheniramine maleate 2 mg, codeine phosphate 10 mg/5 mL, alcohol 5%. Liq. Bot. 120 mL, 480 mL. *c-v.*
Use: Antihistamine; antitussive; decongestant.

Phenhist Expectorant. (Rugby) Pseudoephedrine hydrochloride 30 mg, codeine phosphate 10 mg, guaifenesin 100 mg/5 mL, alcohol 7.5%. Liq. Bot. 118 mL, pt, gal. *c-v.*
Use: Antihistamine; antitussive; decongestant.

pheniform.
See: Phenformin hydrochloride.

●**phenindamine tartrate.** USAN.
Use: Antihistamine, nonselective piperazine.
See: Nolahist.
W/Phenylephrine hydrochloride, aspirin, caffeine, aluminum hydroxide, magnesium carbonate.
See: Dristan.
W/Phenylephrine hydrochloride, caramiphen ethanedisulfonate.
See: Dondril.
W/Phenylephrine hydrochloride, chlorpheniramine maleate, drytane.
See: Comhist.
W/Phenylephrine hydrochloride, chlorpheniramine maleate, belladonna alkaloids.
See: Comhist L.A.
W/Phenylephrine hydrochloride, pyrilamine maleate, chlorpheniramine maleate, dextromethorphan HBr.
See: Histalet, Histalet-DM, Histalet-Forte.

pheniodol.
See: Iodoalphionic acid.

peniprazine hydrochloride.
Use: Antihypertensive.

●**pheniramine maleate.** *USP 28.*
Use: Antihistamine.
See: Citra Forte.
Partuss AC.
Thor.
Tritussin.
W/Combinations.
See: Dristan Fast Acting Formula.
Iohist D.
Poly-Histine.
Quadra-Hist D.
Quadra-Hist D PED.
Scot-Tussin Original Clear 5-Action Cold and Allergy Formula.
Scot-Tussin Original 5-Action Cold and Allergy Formula.
Statuss Green.
Tri-P Oral Infant Drops.
Tussirex.

Tussirex Sugar Free.
Vetuss HC.
● **phenmetrazine hydrochloride.** (fen-MEH-trah-zeen) *USP 28.*
Use: Anorexic.
● **phenobarbital.** (fee-no-BAR-bih-tahl) *USP 28.*
Use: Anticonvulsant; hypnotic; sedative.
See: Solfoton.
W/Combinations.
See: Donnatal.
Donnatal Extentabs.
phenobarbital. (Various Mfr.) Phenobarbital. **Tab.: 15 mg, 30 mg:** Bot. 100s, 1000s, 5000s, UD 100s. **Tab.: 60 mg:** Bot. 100s, 1000s, UD 100s. **Tab.: 100 mg:** 100s, 1000s. **Elix.:** 20 mg/5 mL. Bot. Pt, gal, UD 5 mL, UD 7.5 mL.
Use: Anticonvulsant; hypnotic; sedative.
phenobarbital. (Pharmaceutical Associates) Phenobarbital 15 mg/5 mL. Elix. Bot. Pt, UD 5 mL, 10 mL, 20 mL. *c-iv.*
Use: Anticonvulsant; hypnotic; sedative.
phenobarbital and theobromine combinations.
See: Theobromine w/phenobarbital combinations.
phenobarbital combinations.
See: Aminophylline w/phenobarbital, combinations.
Aspirin-barbiturate, combinations.
Atropine-hyoscine-hyoscyamine combinations.
Atropine sulfate w/phenobarbital.
Belladonna extract combinations.
Belladonna products and phenobarbital combinations.
Bellamine.
Bellatal.
Folergot-DF.
Homatropine methylbromide and phenobarbital combinations.
Hyoscyamus products and phenobarbital combinations.
Mannitol hexanitrate w/phenobarbital combinations.
Mephenesin and barbiturates combinations.
Phenobarbital w/central nervous system stimulants.
Secobarbital combinations.
Sodium nitrite combinations.
Theobromine w/phenobarbital combinations.
Theophylline w/phenobarbital combinations.
Veratrum viride w/phenobarbital combinations.

● **phenobarbital sodium.** *USP 28.*
Use: Anticonvulsant; hypnotic; sedative.
See: Luminal Sodium, Inj.
phenobarbital sodium. (Wyeth) Phenobarbital sodium Inj. **30 mg/mL, 60 mg/mL:** *Tubex* 1 mL. **65 mg/mL:** Vial 1 mL. *c-iv.*
Use: Anticonvulsant; hypnotic; sedative.
phenobarbital sodium in propylene glycol. Vitarine. Amp. 0.13 g: 1 mL, Box 25s, 100s. *c-iv.*
Use: Anticonvulsant; hypnotic; sedative.
phenobarbital w/aminophylline.
See: Aminophylline.
phenobarbital w/atropine sulfate.
See: Atropine sulfate.
phenobarbital w/belladonna.
See: Belladonna products and phenobarbital combinations.
phenobarbital w/central nervous system stimulants.
See: Arcotrate No. 3.
Sedamine.
Spabelin.
phenobarbital w/homatropine methylbromide.
See: Homatropine methylbromide and phenobarbital combinations.
phenobarbital w/hyoscyamus.
See: Hyoscyamus products and phenobarbital combinations.
phenobarbital w/mannitol hexanitrate.
Use: Anticonvulsant; sedative; hypnotic.
See: Mannitol hexanitrate w/phenobarbital combinations.
phenobarbital w/theophylline.
See: Theophylline w/phenobarbital combinations.
phenobarbital w/veratrum viride.
See: Veratrum viride w/phenobarbital combinations.
Pheno-Bella. (Ferndale) Belladonna extract 10.8 mg, phenobarbital 16.2 mg. Tab. Bot. 100s, 1000s. *Rx.*
Use: Anticholinergic; antispasmodic; hypnotic; sedative.
● **phenol.** (FEE-nole) *USP 28.*
Use: Pharmaceutic aid, preservative; topical antipruritic; mouth and throat product.
See: Green Throat Spray.
Phenaseptic.
Red Throat Spray.
Triaminic Sore Throat Spray.
W/Aluminum hydroxide, zinc oxide, camphor, eucalyptol, ichthammol, thyme oil.
See: Solarcaine Pump Spray.

W/Dextromethorphan.
See: Chloraseptic DM.
W/Resorcinol.
See: Black & White.
W/Resorcinol, boric acid, basic fuchsin, acetone.
See: Castellani's Paint.
●**phenolate sodium.** (FEEN-oh-late) USAN.
Use: Disinfectant.
Phenolax. (Pharmacia) Phenolphthalein 64.8 mg. Wafer. Bot. 100s. *OTC.*
Use: Laxative.
●**phenol, camphorated topical gel.** (FEEnole) *USP 28.*
Use: Topical antipruritic.
●**phenol, liquefied.** *USP 28.*
Use: Topical antipruritic.
●**phenolphthalein.** (fee-nahl-THAY-leen) *USP 28.*
Use: Laxative.
●**phenolphthalein yellow.** *USP 28.*
Use: Laxative.
phenolsulfonates.
See: Sulfocarbolates.
phenolsulfonic acid. Sulfocarbolic acid. Used in Sulphodine. (Strasenburgh).
phenoltetrabromophthalein. Disulfonate Disodium.
See: Sulfobromophthalein Sodium, USP.
Pheno Nux. (Pal-Pak, Inc.) Phenobarbital 16.2 mg, nux vomica extract 8.1 mg, calcium carbonate 194.4 mg. Tab. Bot. 1000s. *c-iv.*
Use: Sedative; hypnotic; antacid.
Phenoptic. (Optopics) Phenylephrine hydrochloride 2.5%. Soln. Bot. 2 mL, 5 mL, 15 mL. *Rx.*
Use: Mydriatic, vasoconstrictor.
phenothiazine. Thiodiphenylamine.
phenothiazine derivatives.
See: Chlorpromazine Hydrochloride.
Fluphenazine.
Mesoridazine.
Perphenazine.
Prochlorperazine.
Thioridazine Hydrochloride.
Trifluoperazine Hydrochloride.
phenothiazines, nonselective.
See: Promethazine Hydrochloride.
Phenoturic. (Truett) Phenobarbital 40 mg/5 mL. Elix. Bot. Pt, gal. *c-iv.*
Use: Hypnotic; sedative.
●**phenoxybenzamine hydrochloride.** (fen-ox-ee-BEN-zuh-meen) *USP 28.*
Use: Antihypertensive.
See: Dibenzyline.
phenoxymethyl penicillin.
See: Penicillin V.

phenoxymethyl penicillin potassium.
See: Penicillin V potassium.
phenoxynate. Mixture of phenylphenols 17% to 18%, octyl and related alkylphenols 2% to 3%.
●**phenprocoumon.** (fen-PRO-koo-mahn) USAN.
Use: Anticoagulant.
Phen-70. (Parmed Pharmaceuticals, Inc.) Phendimetrazine tartrate 70 mg. Tab. Bot. 100s, 1000s. *c-iii.*
Use: Anorexiant.
Phental. (Armenpharm Ltd.) Belladonna alkaloids, phenobarbital 0.25 g. Tab. Bot. 1000s. *c-iv.*
Use: Anticholinergic; antispasmodic; hypnotic; sedative.
Phentamine. (Major) Phentermine hydrochloride 30 mg. Cap. (equivalent to 24 mg base). Bot. 100s. *c-iv.*
Use: Anorexiant.
●**phentermine.** (FEN-ter-meen) USAN.
Use: Anorexic.
See: Adipex.
Adipex-P.
Tora.
Wilpowr.
phentermine as resin complex.
See: Ionamin.
●**phentermine hydrochloride.** *USP 28.*
Use: CNS stimulant, anorexiant.
See: Adipex-P.
Pro-Fast HS.
Pro-Fast SA.
Pro-Fast SR.
phentermine hydrochloride. (Various Mfr.) **Tab.:** Phentermine hydrochloride 8 mg, 37.5 mg (equivalent to 30 mg phentermine base). Bot. 100s (37.5 mg only), 1000s. **Cap.:** Phentermine resin 15 mg. Bot. 100s, 1000s. Phentermine hydrochloride 18.75 mg (equivalent to 15 mg phentermine base), 30 mg (equivalent to 24 mg phentermine base), 37.5 mg (equivalent to 30 mg phentermine base). Bot. 100s (except 18.75 mg), 1000s. *c-iv.*
Use: CNS stimulant, anorexiant.
phentetiothalein sodium. Iso-Iodeikon.
Use: Radiopaque agent.
phentolamine hydrochloride.
Use: Antihypertensive.
See: Regitine hydrochloride.
●**phentolamine mesylate.** (fen-TOLE-uh-meen) *USP 28. Formerly Phentolamine Methanesulfonate.*
Use: Antiadrenergic.
phentolamine mesylate for injection. (Bedford) Phentolamine mesylate 5 mg, mannitol. Pow. for Inj. Vial 2 mL.

Rx.
Use: Antiadrenergic.
phentolamine methanesulfonate.
USP 28. Phentolamine mesylate.
Phentolox w/APAP. (Global Source)
Phenyltoloxamine citrate 30 mg, aceta-
minophen 325 mg. Tab. Bot. 1000s.
Rx.
Use: Antihistamine; analgesic.
phentydrone.
Use: Systemic fungicide.
n-phenylacetamide.
See: Acetanilid.
•**phenylalanine.** (fen-ill-AL-ah-NEEN)
USP 28.
Use: Amino acid.
W/Combinations.
See: Alka-Seltzer Plus Children's Cold
Alka-Seltzer Plus Cold & Sinus.
Amoxillin.
Amoxil.
Benadryl Children's Allergy Fastmelt.
Pepcid AC.
phenylalanine ammonia-lyase.
Use: Hyperphenylalaninemia. [Orphan
Drug]
phenylalanine mustard.
See: Melphalan, USP, analgesic.
•**phenyl aminosalicylate.** (FEN-ill ah-
MEE-no-sah-LIH-sih-late) USAN.
Use: Anti-infective.
phenylazo. (A.P.C.) Phenylazodiamino-
pyridine hydrochloride 1.5 g. Tab. Bot.
1000s. *Rx.*
Use: Analgesic, urinary.
phenylazodiaminopyridine.
See: Phenazopyridine.
**phenylazodiaminopyridine hydrochlo-
ride or HBr.**
See: Phenazopyridine hydrochloride or
HBr.
phenylazo sulfisoxazole. (A.P.C.) Sulfisoxazole 0.5 g, phenylazopyridine
50 mg. Tab. Bot. 1000s. *Rx.*
Use: Anti-infective, sulfonamide.
phenylbenzimidazole sulfonic acid.
See: Ensulizole.
•**phenylbutazone.** (fen-ill-BYOO-tah-
zone) *USP 28.*
Use: Antirheumatic.
phenylbutylpiperadine derivatives.
Use: Antipsychotic.
See: Haloperidol.
Pimozide.
phenylbutyrate sodium.
Use: Treatment of blood disorders.
[Orphan Drug]
phenylcarbinol.
See: Benzyl Alcohol, NF.
phenylcinchoninic acid. Name used for
cinchophen.

phenylephedrine w/combinations.
See: Diabetic Tussin.
•**phenylephrine hydrochloride.** (fen-ill-
EFF-rin) *USP 28.*
Use: Adrenergic; mydriatic; sympatho-
mimetic; vasoconstrictor; nasal de-
congestant, arylalkylamine.
See: Afrin Children's Pump Mist.
AH-Chew.
AH-Chew D.
AK-Dilate.
Alcon-Efrin.
Allerest Nasal Spray.
Coricidin Decongestant Nasal Mist.
Formulation R.
4-Way Fast Acting.
Isopto Frin.
Little Colds for Infants and Children.
Little Noses Gentle Formula, Infants &
Children.
Lusonal.
Mydfrin 2.5%.
Neo-Synephrine 4-Hour Extra
Strength.
Neo-Synephrine 4-Hour Mild Formula.
Neo-Synephrine 4-Hour Regular
Strength.
Neo-Synephrine hydrochloride.
Phenoptic.
Prefrin Liquifilm Ophth.
Relief.
Rhinall.
Sinarest.
Sudafed PE.
Super-Anahist Nasal Spray.
Vicks Sinex Ultra Fine Mist.
W/Combinations.
See: 4-Way.
AccuHist LA.
AccuHist PDX.
Acotus.
AeroHist Plus.
AeroKid.
AH-chew.
Alacol DM.
Alka-Seltzer Plus Cold & Cough
Medicine.
Alka-Seltzer Plus Cold Medicine.
Alka-Seltzer Plus Cold & Sinus.
Alka-Seltzer Plus Night-Time Cold
Medicine.
Alka-Seltzer Plus Nose & Throat.
Amerituss AD.
Atuss DM.
Atuss G.
Atuss HC.
Atuss HD.
Atuss MS.
Bellahist-D LA.
Bromfed.
Bromhist-PDX Syrup.

Bur-Tuss Expectorant.
Chlor-Trimeton Expectorant.
Chlor-Trimeton Expectorant
  w/Codeine.
Codal-DH.
Codal-DM.
Codimal DH.
Codimal DM.
Codimal PH.
Coldloc.
Comtussin HC.
Coricidin Demilets.
Crantex ER.
Cytuss HC.
D.A.
D.A. II.
Dallergy.
Dallergy-JR.
Decodult.
Decolate.
Deconhist L.A.
Deconsal II.
Dehistine.
Demazin.
Diabetic Tussin.
Dicomal-DH.
Dicomal-DM.
Dimetane Decongestant.
Dimetane Expectorant.
Dimetane Expectorant-DC.
Dimetapp.
DMax.
Doktors.
Donatussin.
Donatussin DC.
DriHist-SR.
Dristan Cold Multi-Symptom Formula.
Dristan Fast Acting Formula.
Dryphen, Multi-Symptom Formula.
Duradryl.
Dura-Gest.
Duraphen II.
Duratuss.
Duratuss GP.
Duratuss HD.
Ed A-Hist.
ED-TLC.
ED Tuss HC.
Endagen-HD.
Endal.
Endal Expectorant.
Entex.
Entex HC.
Entex LA.
ExeFen-PD.
Ex-Histine.
Extendryl.
Extendryl JR.
Extendryl SR.
Father John's Medicine Plus.
Furacin Nasal Soln.

GFN 600/Phenylephrine 20.
Guaifenex.
Guiatex.
Histatab Plus.
Hista-Vent DA.
Histex SR.
Histinex HC.
Histussin HC.
Hydrocodone CP.
Hydrocodone HD.
Hydrocodone PA.
Hydron CP.
Hydro-DP.
Hydro-PC.
Hydro-PC II.
Levall 5.0.
Liquibid-D.
Liquibid-D 1200.
Liquibid-PD.
Levall.
Lortuss DM.
Lortuss HC.
Maxi-Tuss HC.
Maxi-Tuss HCX.
MAXIPHEN DM.
Mydfrin Ophthalmic.
Nalex-A.
Nalex DH.
Nasahist.
Nasop.
Norel.
Norel DM.
Norel LA.
Notuss PD.
OMNIhist L.A.
Pancof PD.
Pediacof.
PhenaVent D.
PhenaVent LA.
Phenoptic.
Phenylzin Drops.
Phenergan VC.
Poly-Tussin.
Pre-Hist-D.
Preparation H Cooling.
Prometh VC w/Codeine Cough.
Prometh VC Plain.
Promethazine hydrochloride and
  phenylephrine hydrochloride.
Promethazine VC w/Codeine Cough.
Rescon-GG.
Rescon-Jr.
Rhinall.
Rymed.
Scot-Tussin Original Clear 5-Action
  Cold and Allergy Formula.
Scot-Tussin Original 5-Action Cold
  and Allergy Formula.
Sil-Tex.
Sinex.
Singlet.

SINUtuss DM.
SINUvent PE.
Spec-T Sore Throat-Decongestant
Loz.
Stahist.
Statuss Green.
Sucrets Cold Decongestant Loz.
Triaminic Chest & Nasal Congestion.
Triaminic Flu, Cough, & Fever.
Triaminic Night Time Cough & Cold.
Trind.
Turbispan Leisurecaps.
Tussafed EX.
Tussafed HC.
TUSSI-PRES.
Tussirex.
Tussirex Sugar Free.
Tympagesic.
Vanex HD.
Vaoooidin.
Vasosulf.
Vetuss HC.
Z-Cof HC.

phenylephrine hydrochloride. (Various
Mfr.) Phenylephrine hydrochloride 1%.
Soln. Bot. 480 mL. *OTC.*
Use: Nasal decongestant, arylalkyl-
amine.
W/Combinations.
See: DMax Pediatric.

phenylephrine hydrochloride. (Various
Mfr.) Phenylephrine hydrochloride.
Ophth. Soln. 2.5%: Bot. 15 mL. **10%:**
Bot. 2 mL, 5 ml **Inj. 1%:** Vial 5 mL.
Rx.
Use: Adrenergic, mydriatic, sympatho-
mimetic, vasoconstrictor.

**phenylephrine tannate, chlorphenir-
amine tannate and pyrilamine tannate.** (Ivax) Phenylephrine tannate
25 mg, chlorpheniramine tannate 8 mg,
pyrilamine tannate 25 mg. Tab. Bot.
100s, 500s. *Rx.*
Use: Antihistamine; decongestant.

**phenylephrine tannate/chlorphenir-
amine tannate/pyrilamine tannate
pediatric.** (Duramed) Phenylephrine
tannate 5 mg, pyrilamine tannate
12.5 mg, chlorpheniramine tannate
2 mg/5 mL, methylparaben, saccharin,
sucrose, strawberry-blackberry-currant
flavor. Susp. Unit of use 118 mL, Bot.
473 mL. *Rx.*
Use: Upper respiratory combination,
decongestant, antihistamine.

**phenylephrine tannate w/combina-
tions.**
See: AlleRx.
C-Tanna 12 D.
Dallergy-Jr.
Duonate-12.

Dytan-CS.
Dytan-D.
Exratuss.
Gelhist Pediatric.
Nalex-A.
Nuhist.
Phenylephrine tannate/chlorphenir-
amine tannate/pyrilamine tannate
pediatric.
Quad Tann.
Rhinatate-NF Pediatric.
Rhinatate Pediatric.
R-Tanna.
R-Tanna S Pediatric.
Ryna-12.
Ryna-12 S.
Rynatan.
Rynatuss Pediatric.
Tannate Pediatric.
Tannic-12.
Triotann Pediatric.
Triotann-S Pediatric.
Tussi-12.
Tuss-Tan Pediatric.
Tuss-12 D.
Tuss-12D S.
Viravan-DM.
Viravan-S.
Viravan-T.

●**phenylethyl alcohol.** (fen-ill-ETH-ill)
USP 28.
Use: Pharmaceutic aid, antimicrobial.

phenyl-ethyl-hydrazine, beta. Phenelzine dihydrogen sulfate.
See: Nardil.

phenylethylmalonylurea.
See: Phenobarbital.

Phenyl-Free 1. (Mead Johnson Nutritionals) Corn syrup solids 49.2%, casein hydrolysate 18.7% (enzymic digest of casein containing amino acids and small
peptides), corn oil 18%, modified tapioca starch 9.57%, protein equivalent
15%, fat 18%, carbohydrate 60%, minerals (ash) 3.6%, phenylalanine 75 mg/
100 g pow., vitamins A 1600 units, D
400 units, E 10 units, C 52 mg, folic acid
100 mcg, B_1 0.5 mg, B_2 0.6 mg, niacin 8 mg, B_6 0.4 mg, B_{12} 2 mcg, biotin
0.05 mg, pantothenic acid 3 mg, vitamin K-1 100 mcg, choline 85 mg, inositol 30 mg, Ca 600 mg, P 450 mg, I
45 mcg, Fe 12 mg, Mg 70 mg, Cu
0.6 mg, Zn 4 mg, Mn 1 mg, C 450 mg,
K 650 mg, Na 300 mg/qt. at normal
dilution of 20 k cal/fl oz, Can 2 1/2 lb.
OTC.
Use: Nutritional supplement.

Phenylgesic. (Ivax) Phenyltoloxamine
citrate 30 mg, acetaminophen 325 mg.
Tab. Bot. 100s, 1000s. *OTC.*

Use: Upper respiratory combination, analgesic, antihistamine.

phenylic acid.
See: Phenol, USP.

●**phenylmercuric acetate.** (fen-ill-mer-CURE-ik ASS-eh-tate) *NF 23.*
Use: Pharmaceutic aid, antimicrobial; preservative, bacteriostatic.
W/9-Aminoacridine hydrochloride, tyrothricin, urea, lactose.
See: Trinalis.
W/Benzocaine, chlorothymol, resorcin.
See: Lanacane.
W/Boric acid, polyoxyethylenenonylphenol or oxyquinoline benzoate.
See: Koromex.

phenylmercuric acetate. (Various Mfr.)
Phenylmercuric acetate. Bot. 1 lb, 5 lb, 10 lb.
Use: Pharmaceutic aid, antimicrobial; preservative, bacteriostatic.

phenylmercuric borate. (F. W. Berk)
Pkg. Custom packed.
W/Benzyl alcohol, benzocaine, butyl p-aminobenzoate.
See: Dermathyn.

phenylmercuric chloride. Chlorophenylmercury.

●**phenylmercuric nitrate.** *NF 23.*
Use: Pharmaceutic aid, antimicrobial; preservative, bacteriostatic.
See: Preparation H.
W/Amyl, phenylphenol complex.
See: Lubraseptic Jelly.

phenylmercuric nitrate. (A.P.L.) Phenylmercuric nitrate. **Oint. 1:1500:** 1 oz, 4 oz, lb. (Chicago Pharm) Loz. w/benzocaine. Bot. 100s, 1000s.
Ophth. Oint., 1:3000: Tube ⅛ oz. **Soln. 1:20,000:** Bot. pt, gal. **Vaginal supp., 1:5000:** Box 12s.
Use: Pharmaceutic aid, antimicrobial; preservative, bacteriostatic.

phenylmercuric picrate.
Use: Antimicrobial.

phenylphenol-o.
W/Amyl complex, phenylmercuric nitrate.
See: Lubraseptic.

phenylpropylmethylamine hydrochloride. Vonedrine hydrochloride.

phenyl salicylate. Salol.
W/Combinations.
See: Rayderm.
Urised.

phenyl-tert-butylamine.
See: Phentermine.

phenylthilone.
Use: Anticonvulsant.

●**phenyltoloxamine citrate.** *USP 28.*
Use: Antihistamine.

W/Combinations.
See: Aceta-Gesic.
Duraxin.
Ed-Flex.
FemBack.
Flextra-DS.
Hyflex 650.
Iohist D.
Levacet.
Major-gesic.
Meditussin-X.
Mobigesic.
Naldecon.
Nalex-A.
Novasal.
Percogesic.
Phenylgesic.
Poly-Histine.
Quadra-Hist D.
Quadra-Hist D PED.
Relagesic.

phenyltoloxamine resin w/combinations.
See: Tussionex.

Phenylzin. (Ciba Vision) Zinc sulfate 0.25%, phenylephrine hydrochloride 0.12%. Bot. 15 mL. *Rx.*
Use: Decongestant, ophthalmic.

●**phenyramidol hydrochloride.** (FEN-ih-RAM-ih-dole) USAN.
Use: Analgesic; muscle relaxant.

Phenytek. (Bertek) Phenytoin extended 200 mg, 300 mg. Cap. Bot. 30s, 100s. *Rx.*
Use: Anticonvulsant, hydantoin.

●**phenytoin.** (FEN-ih-toe-in) *USP 28.* Formerly Diphenylhydantoin.
Use: Anticonvulsant.
See: Dilantin.
Phenytek.

phenytoin. (Alra) Phenytoin 125 mg/5 mL. Oral Susp. Bot. 240 mL. *Rx.*
Use: Anticonvulsant.

●**phenytoin sodium.** *USP 28.* Formerly Diphenylhydantoin Sodium.
Use: Anticonvulsant; cardiac depressant, antiarrhythmic.
See: Dilantin Sodium.

phenytoin sodium w/phenobarbital.
Use: Anticonvulsant.
See: Dilantin with Phenobarbital Kapseals.

pheochromocytoma, agents for.
See: Demser.
Dibenzyline.
Regitine.

Pherazine DM. (Halsey Drug) Promethazine 6.25 mg, dextromethorphan HBr 15 mg, alcohol 7%/5 mL. Bot. 4 oz, 6 oz, pt, gal. *Rx.*

Use: Antihistamine; antitussive.

Pherazine VC. (Halsey Drug) Phenylephrine hydrochloride 5 mg, promethazine hydrochloride 6.25 mg, alcohol 7%/5 mL. Syr. Bot. Pt, gal. *Rx.*
Use: Antihistamine; decongestant.

Pherazine VC with Codeine. (Halsey Drug) Phenylephrine hydrochloride 5 mg, promethazine hydrochloride 6.25 mg, codeine phosphate 10 mg, alcohol 7%/5 mL. Syr. Bot. Pt, gal. *c-v.*
Use: Antihistamine; antitussive; decongestant.

Pherazine w/Codeine. (Halsey Drug) Promethazine hydrochloride 6.25 mg, codeine phosphate 10 mg/5 mL, alcohol 7%, sorbitol, sucrose. Syr. Bot. 120 mL, pt, gal. *c-v.*
Use: Antihistamine; antitussive.

phethenylate. Also sodium salt.

Phicon. (T.E. Williams Pharmaceuticals) Pramoxine hydrochloride 0.5%, vitamin A 7500 units, E 2000 units/30 g. Cream. Tube 60 g. *OTC.*
Use: Emollient.

Phicon F. (T.E. Williams Pharmaceuticals) Undecylenic acid 8%, pramoxine hydrochloride 0.05%. Cream. 60 g. *OTC.*
Use: Anesthetic, local; antifungal.

Phillips' Chewable. (Bayer Corp. (Consumer Div.)) Magnesium hydroxide 311 mg. Tab. 100s, 200s.
Use: Laxative, antacid.

Phillips' LaxCaps. (Bayer Corp. (Consumer Div.)) Docusate sodium 83 mg, phenolphthalein 90 mg. Cap. Bot. 8s, 24s, 48s. *OTC.*
Use: Laxative.

Phillips' Liqui-Gels. (Bayer Corp. (Consumer Div.)) Docusate sodium 100 mg, parabens, sorbitol. Softgel Cap. Bot. 10s, 30s, 50s. *OTC.*
Use: Laxative.

Phillips' Milk of Magnesia. (Bayer Corp. (Consumer Div.)) Magnesium hydroxide 400 mg/5 mL, saccharin (mint), sorbitol, sugar (cherry), mint, cherry, regular flavors. Susp. Bot. 120 mL, 360 mL, 780 mL. *OTC.*
Use: Laxative; antacid.

Phillips' Milk of Magnesia Concentrated. (Bayer Corp. (Consumer Div.)) Magnesium hydroxide 800 mg/5 mL, sorbitol, sugar, strawberry creme flavor. Susp. Bot. 240 mL. *OTC.*
Use: Laxative; antacid.

Phish Omega. (Pharmics) Natural salmon oil concentrate containing EPA 120 mg, DHA 100 mg. Cap. Bot. 60s. *OTC.*

Use: Vitamin supplement.

Phish Omega Plus. (Pharmics) Natural fish oil concentrate containing EPA 300 mg, DHA 200 mg. Cap. Bot. 60s. *OTC.*
Use: Vitamin supplement.

pHisoDerm. (Chattem) Sodium octoxynol-2 ethane sulfonate, white petrolatum, water, mineral oil (with lanolin alcohol and oleyl alcohol), sodium benzoate, octoxynol-3, tetrasodium EDTA, methylcellulose, cocamide MEA, imidazolidinyl urea. **Regular:** 150 mL, 270 mL, 480 mL, gal. **Oily skin:** 150 mL, 480. *OTC.*
Use: Dermatologic, cleanser.

pHisoDerm for Baby. (Chattem) Sodium octoxynol-2 ethane sulfonate, petrolatum, octoxynol-3, mineral oil (with lanolin alcohol and oleyl alcohol), cocamide MEA, imidazolidinyl urea, sodium benzoate, tetrasodium EDTA, methylcellulose, hydrochloric acid. Liq. Bot. 150 mL, 270 mL. *OTC.*
Use: Dermatologic, cleanser.

pHisoHex. (Sanofi-Synthelabo) Entsufon sodium, hexachlorophene 3%, petrolatum, lanolin cholesterols, methylcellulose, polyethylene glycol, polyethylene glycol monostearate, lauryl myristyl diethanolamide, sodium benzoate, water, pH adjusted with hydrochloric acid. Emulsion, Bot. 5 oz, pt, gal. Wall dispensers pt. Unit packets 0.25 oz. Box 50s, Pedal operated dispenser 30 oz. *OTC.*
Use: Antimicrobial, antiseptic.

pHisoMed. (Sanofi-Synthelabo) Hexachlorophene. *OTC.*
Use: Antimicrobial; antiseptic.

pHisoPuff. (Sanofi-Synthelabo) Nonmedicated cleansing sponge. Box sponge 1s. *OTC.*
Use: Dermatologic, cleanser.

PhosChol. (American Lecithin) Phosphatidylcholine (highly purified lecithin). **Softgel:** 565 mg, 900 mg. Bot. 100s, 300s. **Liq. Conc.:** 3000 mg/5 mL. Bot. 240 mL, 480 mL. *OTC.*
Use: Nutritional supplement.

phoscolic acid.
Use: Adjuvant.

Phos-Flur Oral Rinse Supplement. (Colgate Oral) Acidulated phosphate sodium fluoride 0.05%, fluoride 1 mL/5 mL. Bot. 250 mL, 500 mL, gal. *Rx.*
Use: Dental caries preventative.

PhosLo. (Nabi) Calcium acetate. **Tab.:** 667 mg (elemental calcium 169 mg), polyethylene glycol 8000. Bot. 200s. **Cap.:** 333.5 mg (half-size) (elemental

calcium 84.5 mg), 667 mg (elemental calcium 169 mg), polyethylene glycol 8000. Bot. 200s (667 mg only), 400s (333.5 mg only). **Gelcap:** 667 mg (elemental calcium 169 mg), polyethylene glycol 8000. Bot. 200s. *Rx.*
Use: Electrolytes, mineral supplement.

PHOS-NaK. (Cypress) Potassium 280 mg, phosphorus 250 mg, sodium 160 mg/packet, fruit flavor. Pow. Packets. 1.5 g (100s). *OTC.*
Use: Phosphorus replacement.

phosphate.
See: Potassium phosphate.
Sodium phosphate.

phosphate binders.
Use: Phosphate reduction.
See: Lanthanum Carbonate.

phosphentaside. Adenosine-5-monophosphate. Adenylic acid.
W/Vitamin B$_{12}$, niacin.
See: Denylex Gel.
W/Vitamin B$_{12}$, niacin, B$_1$.
See: Adenolin.

phosphocol P 32. (Mallinckrodt) Chromic phosphate P 32: 15 mCi with a concentration of up to 5 mCi/mL and specific activity of up to 5 mCi/mg at time of standardization. Susp. Vial 10 mL.
Use: Radiopharmaceutical.

phosphocysteamine.
Use: Cystinosis. [Orphan Drug]

Phospholine Iodide. (Wyeth-Ayerst) Echothiophate iodide 6.25 mg to make 0.125%. Pow. for Reconstitution with 5 mL diluent (potassium acetate, chlorobutanol 0.55%, mannitol 1.2%). *Rx.*
Use: Glaucoma agent.

phosphonoformic acid.
See: Foscarnet sodium.

phosphorated carbohydrate solution.
See: Emetrol.
Nausea Relief.
Nausetrol.

• **phosphoric acid.** (fos-FORE-ik) *NF 23.*
Use: Pharmaceutic aid, solvent.

phosphoric acid, diluted.
Use: Pharmaceutic aid, solvent.

phosphorus.
Use: Phosphorus replacement.
See: K-Phos Neutral.
Neutra-Phos.
Neutra-Phos K.
PHOS-NaK.
Uro-KP-Neutral.

Phospho-Soda. (C.B. Fleet) Sodium biphosphate 48 g, sodium phosphate 18 g/100 mL. Bot. 1.5 oz, 3 oz, 8 oz. Flavored, unflavored. *OTC.*
Use: Laxative.

Phosphotec. (Bristol-Myers Squibb) Technetium Tc-99m pyrophosphate kit. 10 vials/kit.
Use: Radiodiagnostic.

photochemotherapy.
See: Aminolevulinic acid hydrochloride.
Methoxasalen.
Psoralens.
Tar-containing preparations.

photochemotherapy, ophthalmic.
See: Verteporfin.
Visudyne.

Photofrin. (Axican Scandipharm) Porfimer sodium 75 mg. Preservative-free. Freeze-dried cake or Pow. for Inj. Vial. *Rx.*
Use: Antineoplastic.

Photoplex Sunscreen. (Allergan) Butyl methoxydibenzoylmethane 3%, padimate O 7%. Lot. 120 mL. *OTC.*
Use: Sunscreen.

Phrenilin. (Carnrick) Butalbital 50 mg, acetaminophen 325 mg. Tab. Bot. 100s, 500s. *Rx.*
Use: Analgesic; hypnotic; sedative.

Phrenilin Forte. (Carnrick) Acetaminophen 650 mg, butalbital 50 mg, benzyl alcohol, parabens, EDTA. Cap. Bot. 100s, 500s. *Rx.*
Use: Analgesic; hypnotic; sedative.

Phresh 3.5 Finnish Cleansing Liquid. (3M) Water, cocamidopropyl betaine, lactic acid, polyoxyethylene distearate, polyoxyethylene monostearate, hydroxyethyl cellulose, sodium phosphate, methylparaben. Bot. 6 oz. *OTC.*
Use: Soapless cleansing agent.

pH-Stabil. (Healthpoint Medical) Skin protection cream. Bot. 8 oz. Cream. Tube 2 oz. *OTC.*
Use: Dermatologic.

Phthalamaquin. (Penick) Quinetolate.
Use: Antiasthmatic.

• **phthalazine, i-hydrazino-, monohydrochloride.** *USP 28.* Hydralazine hydrochloride.

phthalazinones, peripherally selective.
Use: Antihistamine.
See: Azelastine Hydrochloride.

phylcardin.
See: Aminophylline.

phyllindon.
See: Aminophylline.

Phylorinol. (Schaffer) Phenol 0.6%, boric acid, strong iodine solution, sorbitol 70% solution, sodium copper chlorophyll. Liq. Bot. 240 mL. *OTC.*
Use: Mouth and throat preparation.

Phylorinol Mouthwash. (Schaffer) Phenol 0.6%, methyl salicylate, sorbitol. Bot. 240 mL. *OTC.*

Use: Mouth and throat preparation.
physical adjuncts.
See: Hyaluronic Acid.
Hyaluronic Acid Derivatives.
Hyaluronidase.
Poly-l-lactic Acid.
physiological irrigating solution.
See: Physiolyte.
Physiosol.
TIS-U-SOL.
Physiolyte. (McGaw) Sodium Cl 530 mg, sodium acetate 370 mg, sodium gluconate 500 mg, potassium Cl 37 mg, magnesium Cl 30 mg/100 mL. Soln. Bot. 500 mL, 2 L, 4 L. *Rx.*
Use: Irrigant, ophthalmic.
Physiosol Irrigation. (Abbott Hospital Products) Bot. 250 mL, 500 mL, 1000 mL glass or Aqualite (semirigid) containers. *Rx.*
Use: Irrigant, ophthalmic.
• **physostigmine salicylate.** (fie-zoe-STIG-meen) *USP 28.*
Use: Cholinergic, ophthalmic; parasympathomimetic agent, Friedreich and other inherited ataxias. [Orphan Drug]
See: Antilirium.
Isopto-Eserine.
W/I-Hyoscyamine HBr.
See: Phyatromine-H.
W/Pilocarpine, methylcellulose.
See: Isopto P-ES.
physostigmine salicylate. (Taylor) Physostigmine salicylate 1 mg/mL. Benzyl alcohol 2%, sodium metabisulfite 0.1%. Inj. Amp. 2 mL. *Rx.*
Use: Cholinergic, antidote.
• **physostigmine sulfate.** *USP 28.*
Use: Cholinergic, ophthalmic.
• **phytate persodium.** (FIE-tate per-SO-dee-uhm) *USAN.*
Use: Pharmaceutic aid.
• **phytate sodium.** *USAN.* Sodium salt of inositol hexaphosphoric acid.
Use: Chelating agent, calcium.
phytic acid. Inositol hexophosphoric acid.
• **phytonadione.** (fye-toe-nuh-DIE-ohn) *USP 28.*
Use: Vitamin, prothrombogenic.
See: Aquamephyton.
Mephyton.
phytonadione. (I.M.S., Ltd.) Phytonadione 2 mg/mL. Inj. 0.5 mL, *Min-I-ject* prefilled syringes. *Rx.*
Use: Vitamin, prothrombogenic.
• **piboserod hydrochloride.** (pi-BOE-ser-od) *USAN.*
Use: Irritable bowel syndrome.

• **picenadol hydrochloride.** (pih-SEN-AID-ole) *USAN.*
Use: Analgesic.
• **piclamilast.** (pih-KLAM-ill-ast) *USAN.*
Use: Antiasthmatic, type IV phosphodiesterase inhibitor.
• **picotrin diolamine.** (PIH-koe-trin die-OH-lah-meen) *USAN.*
Use: Keratolytic.
picric acid, trinitrophenol.
See: Silver Salts.
picrotoxin. Cocculin.
Use: Respiratory.
• **picumeterol fumarate.** (PIKE-you-MEH-teh-role) *USAN.*
Use: Bronchodilator.
• **pifarnine.** (pih-FAR-neen) *USAN.*
Use: Antiulcerative, gastric.
pigment agent combinations.
See: Eldoquin.
Tri-Luma.
pigment agents.
See: Dihydroxyacetone.
Hydroquinone.
Monobenzone.
Pilocar. (Novartis Ophthalmic) Pilocarpine hydrochloride 0.5%, 1%, 2%, 3%, 4%, 6%. Bot. 15 mL; Twinpack 2 × 15 mL 0.5%, 1%, 2%, 3%, 4%, 6%; 1 mL Dropperettes 1%, 2%, 4%. *Rx.*
Use: Antiglaucoma.
• **pilocarpine.** (pie-low-CAR-peen) *USP 28.*
Use: Antiglaucoma; ophthalmic cholinergic; miotic.
See: Ocusert Pilo-20, Pilo-40.
• **pilocarpine hydrochloride.** *USP 28.*
Use: Cholinergic, ophthalmic; topically as a miotic, xerostomia and keratoconjunctivitis sicca; mouth and throat product. [Orphan Drug]
See: Almocarpine.
Isopto Carpine.
Mi-Pilo.
Pilocar.
Pilomiotin.
Piloptic.
Salagen.
W/Physostigmine salicylate, methylcellulose.
See: Isopto P-ES.
pilocarpine hydrochloride. (Sandoz) Pilocarpine hydrochloride 5 mg. Tab. 100s. *Rx.*
Use: Treatment of dry mouth.
pilocarpine hydrochloride. (Various Mfr.) Pilocarpine hydrochloride. **0.5%:** 15 mL, 30 mL. **1%:** 2 mL, 15 mL, 30 mL, UD 1 mL. **2%, 4%:** 2 mL, 15 mL, 30 mL. **6%:** 15 mL. **8%:** 2 mL.
Use: Cholinergic, ophthalmic; topically

as a miotic, xerostomia and kerato-conjunctivitis sicca. [Orphan Drug]

Pilopine. (International Pharm) Pilocarpine hydrochloride 1%, 2%, 4%. Soln. Bot. 15 mL. *Rx.*
Use: Antiglaucoma.

Pilopine HS. (Alcon) Pilocarpine hydrochloride 4%. Gel. Tube 3.5 g. *Rx.*
Use: Antiglaucoma.

Piloptic. (Optopics) Pilocarpine hydrochloride 0.5%, 1%, 2%, 3%, 4%, 6%. Soln. Bot. 15 mL. *Rx.*
Use: Antiglaucoma.

Pilostat. (Bausch & Lomb) Pilocarpine hydrochloride 0.5%, 1%, 2%, 3%, 4%, 6%. Soln. Bot. 15 mL, twinpack 2 × 15 mL. *Rx.*
Use: Antiglaucoma.

Pima. (Fleming & Co.) Potassium iodide 325 mg/5 mL, sugar. Syr. Bot. Pt, gal. *Rx.*
Use: Expectorant.

•**pimagedine hydrochloride.** (pih-MAH-jeh-deen) USAN.
Use: Inhibitor (advanced glycosylation end-product formation inhibitors).

pimecrolimus.
Use: Immunomodulator, topical.
See: Elidel.

•**pimetine hydrochloride.** (PIM-eh-teen) USAN.
Use: Antihyperlipoproteinemic.

piminodine esylate.
Use: Analgesic.

piminodine ethanesulfonate.
Use: Analgesic; narcotic.

•**pimobendan.** (pie-MOE-ben-dan) USAN.
Use: Cardiovascular agent.

•**pimozide.** (pih-moe-ZIDE) *USP 28.*
Use: Antipsychotic.
See: Orap.

•**pinacidil.** (pie-NASS-ih-DILL) USAN.
Use: Antihypertensive.

•**pinadoline.** (pih-nah-DOE-leen) USAN.
Use: Analgesic.

•**pindolol.** (PIN-doe-lahl) *USP 28.*
Use: Antiadrenergic/sympatholytic, beta-adrenergic blocking agent, vasodilator.
See: Visken.

pindolol. (Various Mfr.) Pindolol 5 mg, 10 mg. Tab. Bot. 100s, 500s, 1000s. *Rx.*
Use: Antiadrenergic/sympatholytic, beta-adrenergic blocker.

pine needle oil. *NF 23.*
Use: Perfume; flavor.

pine tar. *USP 28.*
Use: Local antieczematic; rubefacient.

Pinex Concentrate Cough. (Last) Dextromethorphan HBr 7.5 mg/5 mL (after diluting 3 oz. concentrate to make 16 oz. solution). Syr. Bot. 3 oz. *OTC.*
Use: Antitussive.

Pinex Cough. (Last) Dextromethorphan HBr 7.5 mg/5 mL. Syr. Bot. 3 oz, 6 oz. *OTC.*
Use: Antitussive.

Pinex Regular. (Last) Potassium guaiacolsulfonate, oil of pine and eucalyptus, extract of grindelia, alcohol 3%/30 mL. Syr. Bot. 3 oz, 8 oz. Also cherry flavored 3 oz. Super and concentrated 3 oz. *OTC.*
Use: Expectorant.

Pink Bismuth. (Ivax) Pink bismuth 130 mg/15 mL. Liq. Bot. 240 mL. *OTC.*
Use: Antidiarrheal.

•**pinoxepin hydrochloride.** (pih-NOX-eh-PIN) USAN.
Use: Antipsychotic.

Pin-Rid. (Apothecary Prods.) **Soft gel-cap:** Pyrantel pamoate 180 mg (equivalent to 62.5 mg pyrantel base). Pkg. 24s. **Liq.:** Pyrantel pamoate 144 mg/mL (equivalent to 50 mg/mL pyrantel base), saccharin, sucrose. Bot. 30 mL. *OTC.*
Use: Anthelmintic.

Pin-X. (Effcon) Pyrantel base (as pamoate) 50 mg/mL, sorbitol. Liq. Bot. 30 mL. *OTC.*
Use: Anthelmintic.

•**pioglitazone hydrochloride.** (PIE-oh-GLIH-tah-zone) USAN.
Use: Antidiabetic.
See: Actos.

•**pipamperone.** (pih-PAM-peer-OHN) USAN. *Formerly Floropipamide.*
Use: Antipsychotic.

•**pipazethate.** (pip-AZZ-eh-thate) USAN.
Use: Cough suppressant; antitussive.

pipazethate hydrochloride.
Use: Antitussive.

•**piperacetazine.** (pih-PURR-ah-SET-ah-zeen) USAN.
Use: Antipsychotic.

•**piperacillin.** (PIH-per-uh-SILL-in) *USP 28.*
Use: Anti-infective.

•**piperacillin sodium.** *USP 28.*
Use: Anti-infective.
W/Tazobactam.
See: Zosyn.

piperacillin sodium. (American Pharmaceutical Partners) Piperacillin sodium (as base) 2 g, 3 g, 4 g, 40 g. Contains 1.85 mEq (42.5 mg) sodium/g. Pow. for Inj. Vials (except 40 g). Pharmacy bulk vials (40 g only). *Rx.*

Use: Anti-infective.
piperacillin sodium and tazobactam sodium.
Use: Anti-infective.
See: Zosyn.
●**piperamide maleate.** (PIH-per-ah-mid) USAN.
Use: Anthelmintic.
●**piperazine.** (pie-PEAR-ah-zeen) *USP 28.*
Use: Anthelmintic.
●**piperazine citrate.** *USP 28.* Piperazine Citrate Telra Hydrous Tripiperazine Dicitrate.
Use: Anthelmintic.
See: Bryrel.
Ta-Verm.
●**piperazine edetate calcium.** USAN.
Use: Anthelmintic.
piperazine estrone sulfate.
See: Estropipate.
piperazine hexahydrate. Tivazine.
piperazine, peripherally selective.
Use: Antihistamine.
See: Cetirizine Hydrochloride.
piperazine phosphate.
Use: Anthelmintic.
piperazines, nonselective.
Use: Antihistamine.
See: Hydroxyzine.
Phenindamine Tartrate.
piperidine phosphate.
Use: Psychiatric drug.
piperidines, nonselective.
Use: Antihistamine.
See: Azatadine Maleate.
Cyproheptadine Hydrochloride.
Phenindamine Tartrate.
piperidines, peripherally selective.
Use: Antihistamine.
See: Desloratidine,
Fexofenadine Hydrochloride.
Loratadine.
piperidolate hydrochloride.
Use: Anticholinergic.
piperoxan hydrochloride. Fourneau 933. Benzodioxane. Diagnosis of hypertension.
Use: Diagnostic aid.
pipethanate hydrochloride.
Use: Anxiolytic.
●**piposulfan.** (PIP-oh-SULL-fan) USAN.
Use: Antineoplastic.
●**pipotiazine palmitate.** (PIP-oh-TIE-ah-zeen PAL-mih-tate) USAN.
Use: Antipsychotic.
●**pipoxolan hydrochloride.** (pih-POX-oh-lan) USAN.
Use: Muscle relaxant.

●**piprozolin.** (PIP-row-ZOE-lin) USAN.
Use: Choleretic.
●**piquindone hydrochloride.** (PIH-kwin-dohn) USAN.
Use: Antipsychotic.
●**piquizil hydrochloride.** (PIH-kwih-zill) USAN.
Use: Bronchodilator.
●**piracetam.** (PIHR-ASS-eh-tam) USAN.
Use: Cognition adjuvant; cerebral stimulant, myoclonus. [Orphan Drug]
●**pirandamine hydrochloride.** (pih-RAN-dah-meen) USAN.
Use: Antidepressant.
●**pirazmonam sodium.** (pihr-AZZ-moe-nam) USAN.
Use: Antimicrobial.
●**pirazolac.** (PIHR-AZE-oh-lack) USAN.
Use: Antirheumatio.
●**pirbenicillin sodium.** (pihr-ben-IH-SILL-in) USAN.
Use: Anti-infective.
●**pirbuterol acetate.** (pihr-BYOO-tuh-role) USAN.
Use: Bronchodilator, sympathomimetic.
See: Maxair Inhaler.
●**pirbuterol hydrochloride.** USAN.
Use: Bronchodilator.
●**pirenperone.** (PIHR-en-PURR-ohn) USAN.
Use: Anxiolytic.
●**pirenzepine hydrochloride.** (PIHR-en-zeh-PEEN) USAN.
Use: Antiulcerative.
●**piretanide.** (pihr-ETT-ah-nide) USAN.
Use: Diuretic.
●**pirfenidone.** (PEER-FEN-ih-dohn) USAN.
Use: Analgesic; anti-inflammatory; anti-pyretic.
piridazol.
See: Sulfapyridine.
●**piridicillin sodium.** (pihr-RIH-dih-SILL-in) USAN.
Use: Anti-infective.
●**piridronate sodium.** (pihr-IH-DROE-nate) USAN.
Use: Regulator, calcium.
●**piriprost.** (PIHR-ih-prahst) USAN.
Use: Antiasthmatic.
●**piriprost potassium.** USAN.
Use: Antiasthmatic.
piriton.
See: Chlorpheniramine.
●**piritrexim isethionate.** (pih-rih-TREX-im eye-seh-THIGH-oh-nate) USAN.
Use: Antiproliferative. [Orphan Drug]

•**pirlimycin hydrochloride.** (PIHR-lih-MY-sin) USAN.
Use: Anti-infective.

•**pirmagrel.** (PIHR-mah-GRELL) USAN.
Use: Inhibitor, thromboxane synthetase.

•**pirmenol hydrochloride.** (PIHR-MEH-nahl) USAN.
Use: Cardiovascular agent, antiarrhythmic.

•**pirnabine.** (PIHR-NAH-bean) USAN.
Use: Antiglaucoma agent.

•**piroctone.** (pihr-OCK-TONE) USAN.
Use: Antiseborrheic.

•**piroctone olamine.** USAN.
Use: Antiseborrheic.

•**pirodavir.** (pih-ROW-dav-ihr) USAN.
Use: Antiviral.

•**pirogliride tartrate.** (PIHR-oh-GLIE-ride) USAN.
Use: Antidiabetic.

•**pirolate.** (PIHR-oh-late) USAN.
Use: Antiasthmatic.

•**pirolazamide.** (PIHR-ole-aze-ah-mide) USAN.
Use: Cardiovascular agent, antiarrhythmic.

•**piroxantrone hydrochloride.** (PIH-row-ZAN-trone) USAN.
Use: Antineoplastic.

•**piroxicam.** (pihr-OX-ih-kam) *USP 28.*
Use: Anti-inflammatory.
See: Feldene.

piroxicam. (Various Mfr.) Piroxicam 10 mg, 20 mg. Cap. Bot. 100s, 500s, 1000s, UD 100s. *Rx.*
Use: Anti-inflammatory; NSAID.

•**piroxicam betadex.** USAN.
Use: Analgesic; anti-inflammatory; antirheumatic.

•**piroxicam cinnamate.** USAN.
Use: Anti-inflammatory.

•**piroxicam olamine.** USAN.
Use: Anti-inflammatory; analgesic.

•**piroximone.** (PIHR-ox-ih-MONE) USAN.
Use: Cardiovascular agent.

•**pirprofen.** (pihr-PRO-fen) USAN.
Use: Anti-inflammatory.

•**pirquinozol.** (PIHR-KWIN-oh-zole) USAN.
Use: Antiallergic.

•**pirsidomine.** (pihr-SIH-doe-meen) USAN.
Use: Vasodilator.

pitayine.
See: Quinidine.

Pitocin. (Monarch) Oxytocin. Inj. 1 mL amps (chlorobutanol 0.5%), 1 mL *Steri-Dose* disposable syringes, 1 mL *Steri-*

Vials. 10 units/mL. *Rx.*
Use: Oxytocic.

Pitressin. (Monarch) Vasopressin 20 pressor units/mL, chlorobutanol 0.5%. Inj. Amp, vial 1 mL. *Rx.*
Use: Hormone, posterior pituitary.

Pitts Carminative. (Del) Bot. 2 oz.
Use: Antiflatulent.

pituitary, anterior. The anterior lobe of the pituitary gland supplies protein hormones classified under following headings.
See: Corticotropin.
 Gonadotropin.
 Growth hormone.
 Thyrotropic Principle.

Pituitary Function Test.
See: Metopirone.

pituitary, posterior, hormones.
W/Vasopressin. Pressor principle, β-hypophamine, postlobin-V.
See: Pitressin.
W/Oxytocin. Oxytocic principle. α-hypophamine, postiobin-O.
See: Oxytocin.
 Pitocin.

•**pituitary, posterior, injection.** *USP 28.*
Use: Hormone, antidiuretic.

•**pivampicillin hydrochloride.** (pihv-AM-pih-SILL-in) USAN.
Use: Anti-infective.

•**pivampicillin pamoate.** USAN.
Use: Anti-infective.

•**pivampicillin probenate.** USAN.
Use: Anti-infective.

•**pivopril.** (PIH-voe-PRILL) USAN.
Use: Antihypertensive.

•**pixantrone.** (PIX-an-trone) USAN.
Use: Antineoplastic.

pix carbonis.
See: Coal tar.

pix juniperi.
Use: Sunscreen; moisturizer.
See: Juniper tar.

•**pizotyline.** (pih-ZOE-tih-leen) USAN.
Use: Anabolic; antidepressant; serotonin inhibitor, migraine.

placebo capsules. (Cowley) No. 3 orange red; No. 4 yellow. Bot. 1000s.
Use: Placebo.

placebo tablets. (Cowley) 1 g white; 2 g white; 3 g white, red or yellow, pink, orange; 4 g white; 5 g white. Bot. 1000s.
Use: Placebo.

Plan B. (Duramed) Levonorgestrel 0.75 mg, lactose. Tab. Blister pack 2s. *Rx.*
Use: Sex hormone, contraceptive hormone.

planocaine.
See: Procaine hydrochloride.
planochrome.
See: Merbromin.
plantago, ovata coating.
See: Konsyl.
L.A. Formula.
Metamucil.
•**plantago seed.** (PLAN-tah-go seed)
USP 28.
Use: Laxative.
Plaquenil. (Sanofi Synthelabo) Hydroxy-
chloroquine sulfate 200 mg (equiv. to
155 mg base). Film-coated. Tab. Bot.
100s. Rx.
Use: Antimalarial; antirheumatic; lupus
erythematosus suppressant.
Plaretase 8000. (Ethex) Lipase
8000 units, protease 30,000 units,
amylase 30,000 units. Tab. Bot. 100s,
500s. Rx.
Use: Digestive enzyme.
Plasbumin-5. (Bayer Corp. (Consumer
Div.)) Normal serum albumin (human)
5% USP fractionated from normal serum plasma, heat treated against
hepatitis virus. Albumin 12.5 g/250 mL.
Inj. Vial 50 mL. Bot. with IV set
250 mL, 500 mL. Rx.
Use: Plasma protein fraction.
Plasbumin-25. (Bayer Corp. (Consumer
Div.)) Normal serum albumin (human)
25% USP fractionated from normal serum plasma, heat treated against
hepatitis virus. Albumin 12.5 g/50 mL.
Inj. Vial 20 mL. Bot. with IV set 50 mL,
100 mL. Rx.
Use: Plasma protein fraction.
plasma.
See: Normal human plasma.
plasma expanders or substitutes.
See: Dextran 6% and LMD 10%.
Macrodex.
Plasma-Lyte A ph 7.4. (Baxter PPI) Na
140 mEq, K 5 mEq, Mg 3 mEq, Cl
98 mEq, acetate 27 mEq, gluconate
23 mEq, osmolarity 294 mOsm/L, pH
7.4. Soln. Plastic Bot. 500 mL,
1000 mL. Rx.
Use: Intravenous nutritional therapy,
intravenous replenishment solution.
Plasma-Lyte 56 and 5% Dextrose. (Baxter PPI) Na 40 mEq, K 13 mEq, Mg
3 mEq, Cl 40 mEq, acetate 16 mEq,
dextrose 50 g, calories 170, osmolarity
363 mOsm/L. Soln. Plastic Bot.
500 mL, 1000 mL. Rx.
Use: Intravenous nutritional therapy,
intravenous replenishment solution.
Plasma-Lyte 56 in Water. (Baxter PPI)
Na 40 mEq, K 13 mEq, Mg 3 mEq, Cl

40 mEq, acetate 16 mEq/L. Plastic Bot.
500 mL, 1000 mL. Rx.
Use: Nutritional supplement, parenteral.
Plasma-Lyte M and 5% Dextrose. (Baxter PPI) Na 40 mEq, K 16 mEq, Ca
5 mEq, Mg 3 mEq, Cl 40 mEq, acetate
12 mEq, lactate 12 mEq, dextrose
50 g, calories 180, osmolarity
377 mOsm/L. Soln. Plastic Bot. 500 mL,
1000 mL. Rx.
Use: Intravenous nutritional therapy,
intravenous replenishment solution.
Plasma-Lyte 148. (Baxter PPI) Na
140 mEq, K 5 mEq, Mg 3 mEq, Cl
98 mEq, acetate 27 mEq, gluconate
23 mEq, osmolarity 294 mOsm/L, ph
≈ 5.5. Soln. Bot. 500 mL, 1000 mL. Rx.
Use: Intravenous nutritional therapy,
intravenous replenishment solution.
Plasma-Lyte 148 and 5% Dextrose.
(Baxter PPI) Dextrose 50 g, calories
190, Na 140 mEq, K 5 mEq, Mg 3 mEq,
Cl 98 mEq, acetate 27 mEq, osmolarity 547 mOsm, gluconate 23 mEq/L.
Soln. Bot. 500 mL, 1000 mL. Rx.
Use: Intravenous nutritional therapy,
intravenous replenishment solution.
Plasma-Lyte R. (Baxter PPI) Na
140 mEq, K 10 mEq, Ca 5 mEq, Mg
3 mEq, Cl 103 mEq, acetate 47 mEq,
lactate 8 mEq, osmolarity 312 mOsm/L,
ph ≈ 5.5. Soln. Bot. 1000 mL. Rx.
Use: Intravenous nutritional therapy,
intravenous replenishment solution.
Plasma-Lyte R and 5% Dextrose. (Baxter Healthcare) Dextrose 50 g, calories
180, Na⁺ 140 mEq, K⁺ 10 mEq, Ca⁺⁺
5 mEq, Mg⁺⁺ 3 mEq, Cl⁻ 103 mEq, lactate 8 mEq, acetate 47 mEq, osmolarity 564 mOsm/L, sodium bisulfite. Soln.
Bot. 1000 mL. Rx.
Use: Intravenous nutritional therapy,
intravenous replenishment solution.
Plasma-Lyte R Injection. (Baxter PPI)
Na 140 mEq, K 10 mEq, Ca 5 mEq,
Mg 3 mEq, Cl 103 mEq, acetate
47 mEq, lactate 8 mEq/L. Bot. 1000 mL.
Rx.
Use: Nutritional supplement, parenteral.
Plasmanate. (Bayer Corp. (Consumer
Div.)) Plasma protein fraction (human)
5%. USP Vial 50 mL. Bot. 250 mL,
500 mL with set. Rx.
Use: Plasma protein fraction.
Plasma-Plex. (Centeon) Plasma protein
fraction 5%. Inj. Vial 250 mL, 500 mL.
Rx.
Use: Plasma protein fraction.
•**plasma protein fraction.** USP 28. For-
merly Plasma Protein Fraction, Human.
Use: Blood-volume supporter.

See: Plasmanate.
 Plasma-Plex.
 Plasmatein.
 Protenate.
plasma protein fraction. (Baxter PPI) For the plasma protein preparation obtained from human plasma using the Cohn fractionation technique. Bot. 250 mL.
 Use: Blood volume supporter.
Plasmatein. (Alpha Therapeutic) Plasma protein fraction 5%. Inj. Vial w/injection set 250 mL, 500 mL. *Rx.*
 Use: Plasma protein fraction.
plasmochin naphthoate. Pamaquine naphthoate.
 Use: Antimalarial.
•**platelet concentrate.** *USP 28.*
 Use: Platelet replenisher.
Platelet Factor 4. (Abbott Diagnostics) Radioimmunoassay for quantitative measurement of total PF4 levels in plasma. Test kit 100s.
 Use: Diagnostic aid.
Platinol-AQ. (Bristol-Myers Squibb Oncology) Cisplatin 1 mg/mL, sodium chloride 9 mg, preservative free. Inj. Multidose vial. 50 mL, 100 mL. *Rx.*
 Use: Antineoplastic.
platinum coordination complex.
 Use: Antineoplastic.
 See: Carboplatin.
 Cisplatin.
 Oxaliplatin.
Plavix. (Bristol-Myers Squibb) Clopidogrel 75 mg (as base), lactose, castor oil, mannitol. Tab. Bot. 30s, 90s, 500s, UD 100s. *Rx.*
 Use: Antiplatelet.
•**pleconaril.** (pleh-KOE-nah-rill) USAN.
 Use: Antiviral.
Plegisol. (Abbott Hospital Products) Calcium Cl dihydrate 17.6 mg, magnesium Cl hexahydrate 325.3 mg, potassium Cl 119.3 mg, sodium Cl 643 mg/ 100 mL. Approximately 260 mOsm/L. Single-dose container 1000 mL without sodium bicarbonate. *Rx.*
 Use: Cardiovascular agent.
Plenaxis. (Praecis) Abarelix 113 mg. Preservative-free. Pow. for Inj. Kits with a single-use 10 mL diluent vial of 0.9% sodium chloride injection, one 3 mL syringe with an 18-gauge 1½ inch needle, and one 22-gauge 1½ *Safety Glide* injection needle. *Rx.*
 Use: Gonadotropin-releasing hormone antagonists.
Plendil. (AstraZeneca) Felodipine 2.5 mg, 5 mg, 10 mg, lactose. ER Tab. Bot. 30s, 100s, UD 100s. *Rx.*

 Use: Calcium channel blocker.
Pletal. (Otsuka America Pharmaceutical) Cilostazol 50 mg, 100 mg. Tab. Bot. 60s, UD 100s. *Rx.*
 Use: Antiplatelet.
Plewin. (Sanofi-Synthelabo) Glycobiarsol, chloroquine phosphate. Tab. *Rx.*
 Use: Amebicide.
Plexion. (Medicis) Sulfur 5%, sodium sulfacetamide 10%, cetyl alcohol, stearyl alcohol, EDTA, parabens. Cleanser. Bot. 170 g, 340 g. *Rx.*
 Use: Keratolytic.
Plexion Cleansing Cloths. (Medicis) Sulfur 5%, sodium sulfacetamide 10%. Glycerine, glyceryl stearate, propylene glycol, propylene glycol oleate, alcohols, EDTA, parabens. Cloths. 30s. *Rx.*
 Use: Keratolytic agent.
Plexion SCT. (Medicis) Sulfur 5%, sodium sulfacetamide 10%, witch hazel, benzyl alcohol. Cream. Tube 120 g. *Rx.*
 Use: Keratolytic.
Plexion TS. (Medicis) Sulfur 5%, sodium sulfacetamide 10%. Mineral oil, glyceryl stearate, propylene glycol, propylene glycol oleate, alcohols, EDTA, sodium thiosulfate, coco-glycerides. Susp. Topical. 30 g. *Rx.*
 Use: Keratolytic agent.
Plexolan. (Last) Zinc oxide, lanolin. Cream. Tube 1.25 oz, 3 oz. Jar 16 oz. *OTC.*
 Use: Dermatologic.
Plexon. (Sigma-Tau) Testosterone 10 mg, estrone 1 mg, liver 2 mcg, pyridoxine hydrochloride 10 mg, panthenol 10 mg, inositol 20 mg, choline Cl 20 mg, vitamin B_2 2 mg, B_{12} 100 mcg, procaine hydrochloride 1%, niacinamide 100 mg/mL. Vial 10 mL.
 Use: Hormone; mineral, vitamin supplement.
Pliagel. (Alcon) NaCl, KCl, poloxamer 407, sorbic acid 0.25%, EDTA 0.5%. Soln. Bot. 25 mL. *OTC.*
 Use: Contact lens care.
•**plomestane.** (PLOE-mess-TANE) USAN.
 Use: Antineoplastic, aromatase inhibitor.
Plova. (Washington Ethical) Psyllium mucilloid. Pow. (flavored) 12 oz., (plain) 10 0.5 oz. *OTC.*
 Use: Laxative.
Pluravit. (Sanofi-Synthelabo) Multivitamin. Drops.
 Use: Vitamin supplement.
PMB 400. (Wyeth) Conjugated estrogens 0.45 mg, meprobamate 400 mg, lactose, sucrose. Tab. Bot. 100s. *Rx.*
 Use: Anxiolytic, estrogen.

PMB 200. (Wyeth) Conjugated estrogens 0.45 mg, meprobamate 200 mg, lactose, sucrose. Tab. Bot. 60s. *Rx.*
Use: Anxiolytic, estrogen.

P.M.P. Compound. (Mericon Industries) Chlorpheniramine maleate 4 mg, phenylephrine hydrochloride 15 mg, salicylamide 300 mg, scopolamine methylnitrate 0.8 mg. Tab. Bot. 100s, 1000s. *Rx.*
Use: Analgesic; antihistamine; decongestant.

PMP Expectorant. (Mericon Industries) Codeine phosphate 10 mg, phenylephrine hydrochloride 10 mg, guaifenesin 40 mg, chlorpheniramine maleate 2 mg/5 mL. Bot. Gal. *c-v.*
Use: Antihistamine; antitussive; decongestant; expectorant.

pneumococcal 7 valent conjugate vaccine.
Use: Immunization.
See: Prevnar.

pneumococcal vaccine, polyvalent. (new-moe-KAH-kuhl)
Use: Immunization.
See: Pneumovax 23.

Pneumomist. (ECR) Guaifenesin 600 mg. SR Tab. Bot. 100s. *Rx.*
Use: Expectorant.

Pneumotussin. (ECR) Hydrocodone bitartrate 2.5 mg, guaifenesin 300 mg, dye free. Tab. Bot. 100s. *c-III.*
Use: Upper respiratory combination, antitussive, expectorant.

Pneumotussin 2.5 Cough. (ECR) Hydrocodone bitartrate 2.5 mg, guaifenesin 200 mg/5 mL, cherry punch flavor, alcohol and dye free. Syr. Bot. 473 mL. *c-III.*
Use: Upper respiratory combination, antitussive, expectorant.

Pneumotussin HC. (ECR) Hydrocodone bitartrate 5 mg, guaifenesin 100 mg/5 mL. Syr. Bot. 120 mL, 480 mL. *c-III.*
Use: Antitussive; expectorant.

Pneumovax 23. (Merck) 23 polysaccharide isolates 25 mcg each/0.5 mL, phenol 0.25%. Inj. Vial 1-dose, 5-dose. *Rx.*
Use: Vaccine.

PNS Unna Boot. (Pedinol Pharmacal) Nonsterile gauze bandage 10 yds × 3". Box 12s.
Use: Ambulatory procedure in treatment of leg ulcers and varicosities.

•**pobilukast edamine.** (poe-BIH-loo-kast EH-dah-meen) USAN.
Use: Antiasthmatic, leukotriene antagonist.

pochlorin. Prophyrinic and chlorophyllic compound.

Use: Antihypercholesteremic agent.

Pod-Ben-25. (C & M Pharmacal) Podophyllin 25% in benzoin tincture. Bot. 1 oz. *Rx.*
Use: Keratolytic.

Podoben. (American Pharmaceutical) Podophyllum resin extract 25%. Bot. 5 mL. *Rx.*
Use: Keratolytic.

Podocon-25. (Paddock) Podophyllum resin 25% in benzoin tincture. Soln. 15 mL. *Rx.*
Use: Keratolytic.

•**podofilox.** (pah-dah-FILL-ox) USAN.
Use: Antimitotic.
See: Condylox.

podofilox. (Various Mfr.) Podofilox 0.5%. Alcohol 95%. Top. Soln. 3.5 mL. *Rx.*
Use: Antimitotic.

podophyllin.
See: Podophyllum resin.

•**podophyllum.** (poe-doe-FILL-uhm) *USP 28.*
Use: Pharmaceutic necessity.

•**podophyllum resin.** *USP 28.*
Use: Caustic.
See: Podoben.

podophyllum resin. (Various Mfr.) Podophyllin. Pkg. 1 oz, 0.25 lb, 1 lb.
Use: Caustic.

Point-Two Mouthrinse. (Colgate Oral) Sodium fluoride 0.2% in a flavored neutral liquid. Bot. 120 mL. *Rx.*
Use: Dental caries agent.

•**poison ivy extract, alum precipitated.** (poy-zuhn EYE-vee EX-tract, AL-uhm pree-SIP-ih-tay-tehd) USAN.
Use: Ivy poisoning counteractant.

•**polacrilin.** (pahl-ah-KRILL-in) USAN. Methacrylic acid with divinylbenzene. A synthetic ion-exchange resin, supplied in the hydrogen or free acid form. Amberlite IRP-64.
Use: Pharmaceutic aid.

•**polacrilin potassium.** *NF 23.* A synthetic ion-exchange resin, prepared through the polymerization of methacrylic acid and divinylbenzene, further neutralized with potassium hydroxide to form the potassium salt of methacrylic acid and divinylbenzene. Supplied as a pharmaceutical-grade ion-exchange resin in a particle size of 100- to 500-mesh.
Use: Pharmaceutic aid, tablet disintegrant.
See: Amberlite IRP-88.

Poladex Tabs. (Major) Dexchlorpheniramine maleate. Tab. **4 mg:** Bot. 100s, 250s, 1000s. **6 mg:** Bot. 100s, 1000s. *Rx.*

Use: Antihistamine.

polamethene resin caprylate. The physiochemical complex of the acid-binding ion exchange resin, polyamine-methylene resin and caprylic acid.

Polaramine. (Schering-Plough) Dexchlorpheniramine maleate, lactose. **Tab.:** 2 mg, lactose. Bot. 100s. **Syr.:** 2 mg/5 mL alcohol 6%, sorbitol, menthol, parabens, sugar, orange-like flavor. Bot. 473 mL. *Rx.*
Use: Antihistamine, nonselective alkylamine.

Polaramine Expectorant. (Schering-Plough) Dexchlorpheniramine maleate 2 mg, pseudoephedrine sulfate 20 mg, guaifenesin 100 mg/5 mL, alcohol 7.2%, menthol, sorbitol, sugar. Liq. Bot. 473 mL. *Rx.*
Use: Upper respiratory combination, antihistamine, decongestant, expectorant.

Polaramine Repetabs. (Schering-Plough) Dexchlorpheniramine maleate 4 mg, 6 mg, parabens, lactose, sugar. TR Tab. Bot. 100s. *Rx.*
Use: Antihistamine, nonselective alkylamine.

Poldeman. (Sanofi-Synthelabo) Kaolin. Susp. *OTC.*
Use: Antidiarrheal.

Poldeman AD. (Sanofi-Synthelabo) Kaolin. Susp. *OTC.*
Use: Antidiarrheal.

Poldemicina. (Sanofi-Synthelabo) Kaolin. Susp. *OTC.*
Use: Antidiarrheal.

•**poldine methylsulfate.** (POLE-deen METH-ill-SULL-fate) *USP 28.*
Use: Anticholinergic.

•**policapram.** (PAH-lee-CAP-ram) USAN.
Use: Pharmaceutic aid, tablet binder.

Polident Dentu-Grip. (Block Drug) Carboxymethylcellulose gum, ethylene oxide polymer. Pkg. 0.675 oz, 1.75 oz, 3.55 oz. *OTC.*
Use: Denture adhesive.

•**polifeprosan 20.** (pahl-ee-FEH-pro-SAHN 20) USAN.
Use: Pharmaceutic aid, biodegradable polymer for controlled drug delivery.

•**poligeenan.** (PAHL-ih-JEE-nan) USAN. Polysaccharide produced by extensive hydrolysis of carragheen from red algae.
Use: Pharmaceutic aid, dispersing agent.

•**poliglecaprone 90.** USAN.
Use: Surgical aid, surgical suture coating (absorbable).

•**poliglecaprone 25.** (poe-lih-GLEH-kah-prone) USAN.
Use: Surgical aid, surgical suture material (absorbable).

•**poliglusam.** (pahl-ee-GLUE-sam) USAN.
Use: Antihemorrhagic, hemostatic; dermatologic, wound therapy.

•**polignate sodium.** (poe-LIG-nate) USAN.
Use: Enzyme inhibitor, pepsin.

Poli-Grip. (Block Drug) Karaya gum, magnesium oxide in petrolatum mineral oil base, peppermint and spearmint flavor. Tube 0.75 oz, 1.5 oz, 2.5 oz. *OTC.*
Use: Denture adhesive.

poliomyelitis vaccine, inactivated. (Aventis Pasteur) (Purified, Salk Type IPV) Poliovirus vaccine, inactivated. Amp. 5 × 1 mL. Vial 10 dose. *Rx.*
Use: Immunization.
See: IPOL.
Poliovirus vaccine, inactivated

•**poliovirus vaccine, inactivated.** (POE-lee-oh-VYE-russ) *USP 28. Formerly Poliomyelitis Vaccine.*
Use: Immunization.
See: IPOL.

poliovirus vaccine, inactivated. (Aventis Pasteur) Amp. 1 mL. Box 5s. Vial 10 dose. Subcutaneous administration.
Use: Agent for immunization, active.

poliovirus vaccine, inactivated, combined, diphtheria and tetanus toxoids and acellular pertussis adsorbed, hepatitis B (recombinant).
Use: Active immunization, toxoid.
See: Diphtheria and tetanus toxoids and acellular pertussis adsorbed, hepatitis B (recombinant), inactivated poliovirus vaccine combined.

•**polipropene 25.** (pahl-ee-PRO-peen 25) USAN.
Use: Pharmaceutic aid, tablet excipient.

•**polixetonium chloride.** (pahl-ix-eh-TOE-nee-uhm) USAN.
Use: Pharmaceutic aid, preservative.

Polocaine. (AstraZeneca) Mepivacaine hydrochloride. **1%, 2%:** Mannitol. Inj. Multidose vial 50 mL. **3%:** Sodium bisulfite. Inj. Dental cartridge 1.8 mL. *Rx.*
Use: Anesthetic, local amide.

Polocaine MPF. (AstraZeneca) Mepivacaine hydrochloride. **1%, 1.5%:** Inj. Methylparaben. Single-dose vial 30 mL. **2%:** Inj. Single-dose vial 20 mL. *Rx.*
Use: Anesthetic, local amide.

Polocaine with Levonordefrin. (AstraZeneca) Mepivacaine hydrochloride

2%, levonordefrin 1:20,000, sodium metabisulfite. Inj. Dental cart. 1.8 mL. *Rx.*
Use: Anesthetic, local amide.

Poloris Poultices. (Block Drug) Benzocaine 7.5 mg, capsicum 4.6 mg in poultice base. Pkg. 5 unit, 12 unit. *Rx.*
Use: Anesthetic, local.

•**poloxalene.** (PAHL-OX-ah-leen) *USP 28.* Liquid nonionic surfactant polymer of polyoxypropylene polyoxyethylene type.
Use: Pharmaceutic aid, surfactant.

poloxalkol. Polyoxyethylene polyoxypropylene polymer.
See: Magcyl.
W/Casanthrol.
See: Casakol.

•**poloxamer.** (pahl-OX-ah-mer) *NF 23.*
Use: Pharmaceutic aid (ointment and suppository base, surfactant, tablet binder and coating agent, emulsifying agent).

poloxamer-iodine.
See: Prepodyne.

poloxamer 188.
Use: Cathartic; sickle cell crisis; severe burns. [Orphan Drug]

poloxamer 188 lf.
Use: Pharmaceutic aid, surfactant.

poloxamer 182 d.
Use: Pharmaceutic aid, surfactant.

poloxamer 182 lf.
Use: Food additive; pharmaceutic aid.

poloxamer 331.
Use: Food additive, surfactant; AIDS-related toxoplasmosis. [Orphan Drug]

polyamine resin.
See: Polyamine-Methylene Resin.

polyanhydroglucose. Polyanhydroglucuronic acid.
See: Dextran.

Polybase. (Paddock) Preblended polyethylene glycol suppository base for incorporation of medications where a water-soluble base is indicated. Jar 1 lb, 5 lb.
Use: Pharmaceutical aid, suppository base.

polybenzarsol. Benzocal.

Poly-Bon Drops. (Barrows) Vitamins A 3000 units, D 400 units, C 60 mg, B₁ 1 mg, B₂ 1.2 mg, niacinamide 8 mg/ 0.6 mL. Bot. 50 mL. *OTC.*
Use: Vitamin supplement.

•**polybutester.** (PAHL-ee-byoot-ESS-ter) USAN.
Use: Surgical aid, surgical suture material.

•**polybutilate.** (PAHL-ee-BYOO-tih-late) USAN.

Use: Surgical aid, surgical suture coating.

•**polycarbophil.** *USP 28.*
Use: Laxative.
See: Bulk Forming Fiber Laxative.
Equalactin.
FiberCon.
Fiber-Lax.
FiberNorm.
Konsyl Fiber.
Mitrolan.

Polycillin. (Bristol-Myers Squibb) Ampicillin trihydrate. **Cap.: 250 mg:** Bot. 100s, 500s, 1000s, UD 100s. **Cap.: 500 mg:** Bot. 100s, 500s, UD 100s. **Pediatric Drops:** 100 mg/mL. Dropper bot. 20 mL. **Susp.: 125 mg/5 mL:** Bot. 80 mL, 100 mL, 150 mL, 200 mL, UD 5 mL. **Susp.: 250 mg/5 mL:** Bot. 80 mL, 100 mL, 150 mL, 200 mL, UD 5 mL. **Susp.: 500 mg/5 mL:** Bot. 100 mL, UD 5 mL. *Rx.*
Use: Anti-infective, penicillin.

Polycitra. (Baker Norton) Potassium citrate monohydrate 550 mg, sodium citrate dihydrate 500 mg, citric acid monohydrate 334 mg, potassium ion 5 mEq, sodium ion 5 mEq/5 mL. Syr. Bot. 4 oz, pt. *Rx.*
Use: Alkalinizer, systemic.

Polycitra K. (Baker Norton) Potassium citrate monohydrate 1100 mg, citric acid monohydrate 334 mg, potassium ion 10 mEq/5 mL. Bot. 4 oz, pt. *Rx.*
Use: Alkalinizer, systemic.

Polycitra K Crystals. (Baker Norton) Potassium citrate monohydrate 3300 mg, citric acid 1002 mg, potassium ion 30 mEq, equivalent to 30 mEq bicarbonate. UD pkg. Sugar free. Box 100s. *Rx.*
Use: Alkalinizer, systemic.

Polycitra LC. (Baker Norton) Potassium citrate monohydrate 550 mg, sodium citrate dihydrate 500 mg, citric acid monohydrate 334 mg, potassium ion 5 mEq, sodium ion 5 mEq/5 mL. Bot. 4 oz, pt. *Rx.*
Use: Alkalinizer, systemic.

Polycose. (Ross) **Pow.:** Glucose polymers derived from controlled hydrolysis of corn starch. Calories 380, carbohydrate 94 g, water 6 g, Na 110 mg, K 10 mg, Cl 223 mg, Ca 30 mg, P 5 mg/ 100 g. Can 12.3 oz. Case 6s. **Liq.:** Calories 200, carbohydrate 50 g, water 70 g, Na 70 mg, K 6 mg, Cl 140 mg, Ca 20 mg, P 3 mg/100 mL. Bot. 4 oz. Case 48s. *OTC.*
Use: Nutritional supplement.

• **polydextrose.** (PAH-lee-DEX-trose) USAN.
Use: Food additive.

polydimethylsiloxane (silicone oil).
Use: Ophthalmic.
See: AdatoSil 5000.

Polydine. (Century) Povidone-iodine in ointment base. Oint. Jar 1 oz, 4 oz, lb. *OTC.*
Use: Anti-infective, topical.

Polydine. (Century) Povidone-iodine solution. Soln. Bot. 1 oz, 4 oz, 8 oz, pt, gal. *OTC.*
Use: Antiseptic.

Polydine Scrub. (Century) Povidone-iodine in scrub solution. Bot. 1 oz, 4 oz, 8 oz, pt, gal. *OTC.*
Use: Antiseptic.

• **polydioxanone.** (PAHL-ee-die-OX-ah-nohn) USAN.
Use: Surgical aid, surgical suture material (absorbable).

Poly ENA Test System for RNP and SM. (Wampole) Qualitative identification of auto antibodies to extractable nuclear antigens in human serum by gel precipitation technique. Aid in the diagnosis of SLE, MCTD, PSS, SS. Box test 48s.
Use: Diagnostic aid.

Poly ENA Test System for RNP, SM, SSA, and SSB. (Wampole) Qualitative identification of auto antibodies to extractable nuclear antigens in human serum by gel precipitation techniques. Aid in the diagnosis of SLE, MCTD, PSS, SS. Box test 96s.
Use: Diagnostic aid.

Poly ENA Test System for SSA and SSB. (Wampole) Qualitative identification of auto antibodies to extractable nuclear antigens in human serum by gel precipitation techniques. Aid in the diagnosis of SLE, MCTD, PSS, SS. Box test 48s.
Use: Diagnostic aid.

polyene antifungals.
See: Amphotericin B Desoxycholate.
Amphotericin B, Lipid-Based.
Nystatin.

• **polyethadene.** (PAHL-ee-ETH-ah-DEEN) USAN.
Use: Antacid.

• **polyethylene excipient.** (poli-eth-uh-leen) *NF 23.*
Use: Pharmaceutic aid, stiffening agent.

• **polyethylene glycol.** *NF 23.*
Use: Pharmaceutic aid (ointment and suppository base, tablet excipient, solvent, tablet and capsule lubricant).
See: MiralLax.

Zanfel.

polyethylene glycol. (Braintree) PEG 3350 255 g, 527 g. Pow. for Oral Soln. 16 oz (255 g only), 32 oz (527 g only). *Rx.*
Use: Laxative.

polyethylene glycol and electrolytes.
Use: Rehydration; bowel evacuant.
See: Colyte.
GoLYTELY.
MiraLax.
NuLYTELY.
OCL.

• **polyethylene glycol monomethyl ether.** *NF 23.*
Use: Pharmaceutic aid, excipient.

• **polyethylene granules.**
Use: Poison ivy treatment.
See: Zanfel.
Zanfel Wash.

• **polyethylene oxide.** *NF 23.*
Use: Pharmaceutic aid, suspending and viscosity agent, tablet binder.

• **polyferose.** (PAHL-ee-feh-rohs) USAN. An iron carbohydrate chelate containing approximately 45% of iron in which the metallic (Fe) ion is sequestered within a polymerized carbohydrate derived from sucrose.
Use: Hematinic.

Poly-F Fluoride. (Major) Fluoride 0.5 mg, vitamins A 1500 units, D 400 units, E 5 mg, B_1 0.5 mg, B_2 0.6 mg, B_3 8 mg, B_6 0.4 mg, B_{12} 2 mcg, C 35 mg/mL. Drops. Bot. 50 mL. *Rx.*
Use: Mineral, vitamin supplement.

Polygam S/D. (American Red Cross) Immune globulin intravenous (IGIV) 50 mg/mL, gammaglobulin 90%, glucose 20 mg, polyethylene glycol 2 mg, glycine 22.5 mg, tri-n-butylphosphate 1 mcg, octoxynol 9 1 mcg, polysorbate 80 100 mcg, albumin (human) 3 mg/mL, preservative free, solvent/detergent treated. Pow. for Inj. (freeze-dried). Single-use Bot. 2.5 g, 5 g, 10 g w/diluent, transfer device, administration set. *Rx.*
Use: Immunization.

• **polyglactin 910.** (PAHL-ee-GLAHK-tin) USAN.
Use: Surgical aid, surgical suture coating (absorbable).

• **polyglactin 370.** USAN. Lactic acid polyester with glycolic acid.
Use: Surgical aid, surgical suture coating (absorbable).

• **polyglycolic acid.** (PAHL-ee-glie-KAHL-ik) USAN.
Use: Surgical aid, surgical suture material.

See: Dexone Sterile Suture.
- **polyglyconate.** (PAHL-ee-GLIE-koe-nate) USAN.
  Use: Surgical aid, surgical suture material (absorbable).

Poly-Histine. (Sanofi-Synthelabo) Pheniramine maleate 4 mg, pyrilamine maleate 4 mg, phenyltoloxamine citrate 4 mg/5 mL, alcohol 4%, lemon-lime flavor. Elix. Bot. 473 mL. *Rx.*
  Use: Antihistamine.

poly I; poly C12U.
  Use: AIDS; antineoplastic. [Orphan Drug]

poly-l-lactic acid.
  Use: Restoration/correction of facial fat loss in individuals with HIV.
  See: Sculptra.

- **polymacon** (PAHL ın MAY-kahn) USAN.
  Use: Contact lens material, hydrophilic.

polymeric oxygen.
  Use: Sickle cell disease. [Orphan Drug]

polymeric phosphate binders.
  Use: Treatment of hyperphosphatemia.
  See: Sevelamer hydrochloride.

- **polymetaphosphate p 32.** (pahl-ee-met-ah-FOSS-fate) USAN.
  Use: Radiopharmaceutical.

Polymox. (Bristol-Myers Squibb) Amoxicillin trihydrate. **Cap.:** 250 mg. Bot. 100s, 500s, UD 100s; 500 mg. Bot. 50s, 100s, 500s, UD 100s. **Oral Susp.:** 125 mg, 250 mg/5 mL. Bot. 80 mL, 100 mL, 150 mL. **Ped. Drops:** 50 mg/mL. Bot. 15 mL. *Rx.*
  Use: Anti-infective, penicillin.

polymyxin B. (Various Mfr.) Antimicrobial substances produced by *Bacillus polymyxa.*

- **polymyxin B sulfate.** (pahl-ee-mix-in) USP 28.
  Use: Anti-infective.
  See: Aerosporin.

polymyxin B sulfate and bacitracin zinc.
  Use: Anti-infective, topical.
  See: Betadine First Aid Antibiotics Plus Moisturizer.
  Double Antibiotic.
  Polysporin.

polymyxin B sulfate and hydrocortisone.
  Use: Anti-infective; anti-inflammatory, otic.

- **polymyxin B sulfate and trimethoprim ophthalmic solution.** *USP 28.*
  Use: Anti-infective, ophthalmic.

polymyxin B sulfate sterile. (Roerig) Polymyxin B sulfate 500,000 units Ophth Soln. Vial 20 mL for reconstitution. *Rx.*
  Use: Anti-infective.

polymyxin B sulfate w/combinations.
  See: AK-Poly-Bac Oint.
  AK-Spore.
  AK-Trol.
  Aquaphor.
  Betadine First Aid Antibiotics Plus Moisturizer.
  Betadine Plus First Aid Antibiotics and Pain Reliever.
  Cortisporin.
  Dexacidin.
  Double Antibiotic.
  Lanabiotic.
  Maxitrol.
  Mycitracin.
  Neomycin and Polymyxin B Sulfates and Bacitracin Zinc Ophthalmic Ointment.
  Neosporin.
  Neosporin G.U. Irrigant.
  Neosporin Original.
  Neosporin Plus Pain Relief Maximum Strength.
  Neotal.
  Neo-Thrycex.
  Ocutricin.
  Otobiotic.
  Poly-Pred Liquifilm Ophthalmic Suspension.
  Polysporin.
  Polytrim Ophthalmic Solution.
  Pyocidin-Otic.
  Terak with Polymyxin B Sulfate Ophthalmic Ointment.
  Terramycin w/Polymyxin B Ophthalmic Ointment.
  Tigo.
  Tri-Biozene.
  Trimethoprim Sulfate and Polymyxin B Sulfate Ophthalmic.
  Trimixin.
  Triple Antibiotic.

polymyxin-neomycin-bacitracin. (Various Mfr.) Oint. *OTC.*
  Use: Anti-infective, topical.

polynoxylin. Anaflex.

polyoxyethylene 8 stearate. Myrj 45. (Zeneca Pharmaceuticals), Polyoxyl 8 Stearate.

polyoxyethylene 50 stearate.
  See: Polyoxyl 50 stearate.

polyoxyethylene 40 monostearate.
  See: Polyoxyl 40 stearate.
  Myrj 52 & Myrj 52S.

polyoxyethylene lauryl ether.
  W/Benzoyl peroxide, ethyl alcohol.
  See: Benzagel.
  Desquam-X.

W/Hydrocortisone, sulfur.
See: Fostril HC.
W/Sulfur.
See: Fostril.
polyoxyethylene nonyl phenol.
W/Sodium edetate, docusate sodium,
9-aminoacridine hydrochloride.
See: Vagisec Plus.
polyoxyethylene sorbitan monolaurate. Polysorbate 20.
W/Ferrous gluconate.
See: Simron.
W/Ferrous gluconate, vitamins.
See: Simron Plus.
polyoxyethylene 20 sorbitan monoleate.
See: Polysorbate 80, USP.
polyoxyethylene 20 sorbitan trioleate.
Tween 85. (Zeneca Pharmaceuticals),
Polysorbate 85.
polyoxyethylene 20 sorbitan tristearate. Tween 65. (Zeneca Pharmaceuticals), Polysorbate 65.
•**polyoxyl 8 stearate.** (PAHL-ee-OX-ill 8
STEE-ah-rate) USAN.
Use: Pharmaceutic aid, surfactant.
See: Myrj 45.
•**polyoxyl 50 stearate.** NF 23. Formerly
Polyxyethylene 50 stearate.
Use: Pharmaceutic aid, surfactant,
emulsifying agent.
•**polyoxyl 40 hydrogenated castor oil.**
NF 23.
Use: Pharmaceutic aid, surfactant,
emulsifying agent.
•**polyoxyl 40 stearate.** NF 23. Macrogic
Stearate 2000 (I.N.N.) Polyoxyethylene 40 monostearate.
Use: Pharmaceutic aid; hydrophilic
oint., surfactant; surface-active agent.
See: Myrj 52.
Myrj 52S.
•**polyoxyl 10 oleyl ether.** NF 23.
Use: Pharmaceutic aid, surfactant.
•**polyoxyl 35 castor oil.** NF 23.
Use: Pharmaceutic aid, surfactant,
emulsifying agent.
•**polyoxyl 20 cetostearyl ether.** NF 23.
Use: Pharmaceutic aid, surfactant.
•**polyoxypropylene 15 stearyl ether.**
USAN. Formerly PPG-15 Stearyl Ether.
Use: Pharmaceutic aid, solvent.
Poly-Pred Liquifilm. (Allergan) Prednisolone acetate 0.5%, neomycin sulfate
equivalent to 0.35% neomycin base,
polymyxin B sulfate 10,000 units/mL,
polyvinyl alcohol 1.4%, thimerosal
0.001%, polysorbate 80, propylene glycol, sodium acetate. Ophth. Susp. Bot.
5 mL, 10 mL. Rx.

Use: Anti-infective; corticosteroid,
ophthalmic.
polypropylene glycol. An addition polymer of propylene oxide and water.
Use: Pharmaceutic aid, suspending
agent.
polysaccharide-iron complex.
Use: Mineral supplement.
See: Ferrex 150.
Fe-Tinic 150.
Hytinic.
Niferex.
Nu-Iron 150.
polysaccharide iron complex. (Various
Mfr.) Iron (as polysaccharide iron complex) 150 mg. Cap. Bot. 100s. OTC.
Use: Mineral supplement.
polysonic lotion. (Parker) Multipurpose
ultrasound lotion with high coupling efficiency. Bot. 8.5 oz, gal.
Use: Diagnostic aid, therapeutic aid.
•**polysorbate 80.** (PAHL-ee-SORE-bate)
NF 23.
Use: Pharmaceutic aid, surfactant; artificial tears.
See: OptiZen.
•**polysorbate 85.** USAN.
Use: Pharmaceutic aid, surfactant.
•**polysorbate 40.** NF 23.
Use: Pharmaceutic aid, surfactant.
•**polysorbate 60.** NF 23.
Use: Pharmaceutic aid, surfactant.
•**polysorbate 65.** USAN.
Use: Pharmaceutic aid, surfactant.
•**polysorbate 20.** NF 23.
Use: Pharmaceutic aid, surfactant.
Polysorb Hydrate. (E. Fougera) Sorbitan sesquinoleate in a wax and petrolatum base. Cream. Tube 56.7 g, lb.
OTC.
Use: Emollients.
Polysporin. (Pfizer) Polymyxin B sulfate
10,000 units, bacitracin zinc 500 units/
g white petrolatum base. Oint. Tube
15 g, 30 g. OTC.
Use: Anti-infective, antibiotic, topical.
Polysporin Ophthalmic. (Monarch) Polymyxin B sulfate, 10,000 units, bacitracin
zinc 500 units/g, white petrolatum.
Ophth. Oint. Tube 3.5 g. Rx.
Use: Antibiotic, ophthalmic.
polysulfides. Polythionate.
Polytabs-F Chewable Vitamin. (Major)
Fluoride 1 mg, vitamins A 2500 units,
D 400 units, E 15 mg, B_1 1.05 mg, B_2
1.2 mg, B_3 13.5 mg, B_6 1.05 mg, B_{12}
4.5 mcg, C 60 mg, folic acid 0.3 mg.
Chew. Tab. Bot. 100s, 1000s. Rx.
Use: Mineral, vitamin supplement.

Polytar Shampoo. (Stiefel) Polytar 4.5% (coal tar soln., solubilized crude coal tar equiv. to 0.5% coal tar). Lanolin. 177 mL, 355 mL. *OTC.*
Use: Antiseborrheic.

Polytar Soap. (Stiefel) Coal tar soln. 2.5% (equiv. to coal tar 0.5%). Glycerin, ethyl alcohol, peanut oil. 113 g. *OTC.*
Use: Dermatologic.

• **polytef.** (PAHL-ee-teff) USAN.
Use: Prosthetic aid.

Polytinic. (Pharmics) Elemental iron 100 mg, vitamin C 300 mg, folic acid 1 mg. tab. Bot. 100s. *Rx.*
Use: Mineral, vitamin supplement.

Polytrim. (Allergan) Polymyxin B sulfate 10,000 units, trimethoprim 1 mg/mL, benzalkonium chloride 0.04 mg/mL, sodium chloride, sodium hydroxide. Bot. 5 mL, 10 mL. *Rx.*
Use: Anti-infective, ophthalmic.

Polytuss-DM. (Rhode) Dextromethorphan HBr 15 mg, chlorpheniramine maleate 1 mg, guaifenesin 25 mg/5 mL. Bot. 4 oz, 8 oz. *OTC.*
Use: Antihistamine; antitussive; expectorant.

Poly-Tussin. (Pharmakon) Hydrocodone bitartrate 5 mg, chlorpheniramine maleate 2 mg, phenylephrine hydrochloride 4 mg/5 mL, ethyl alcohol 5%, saccharin, sorbitol, dye free, wintergreen spice flavor. Syr. 473 mL. *c-III.*
Use: Antitussive combination.

• **polyurethane foam.** (PAHL-ih-you-ree-thane foam) USAN.
Use: Prosthetic aid, internal bone splint.

polyvidone.
See: Polyvinylpyrrolidone.

Poly-Vi-Flor 1 mg. (Bristol-Myers Squibb) Vitamins A 2500 units, D 400 units, E 15 units, C 60 mg, B_1 1.05 mg, B_2 1.2 mg, B_3 13.5 mg, B_6 1.05 mg, B_{12} 4.5 mcg, fluoride 1 mg, folic acid 0.3 mg, sucrose. Chew. Tab. Bot. 100s, 1,000s. **With Iron:** Above formula plus Fe 12 mg, Cu 1 mg, Zn 10 mg. Tab. *Rx.*
Use: Mineral, vitamin supplement; dental caries agent.

Poly-Vi-Flor 0.5 mg. (Bristol-Myers Squibb) **Chew. Tab.:** Vitamins A 2500 units, D 400 units, E 15 units, C 60 mg, B_1 1.05 mg, B_2 1.2 mg, B_3 13.5 mg, B_6 1.05 mg, B_{12} 4.5 mcg, fluoride 0.5 mg, folic acid 0.3 mg. Bot. 100s. **Chew. Tab. With Iron:** Above formula plus Fe 12 mg, Cu, Zn 10 mg. Tab. Bot. 100s. **Drops:** Vitamins A 1500 units, D 400 units, E 5 units, C 35 mg, B_1 0.5 mg, B_2 0.6 mg, B_6

0.4 mg, niacin 8 mg, B_{12} 2 mcg, fluoride 0.5 mg/mL. Dropper Bot. 30 mL, 50 mL. **Tab.:** Fluoride 0.5 mg, vitamins A 2500 units, D 400 units, E 15 mg, B_1 1.05 mg, B_2 1.2 mg, B_3 13.5 mg, B_6 1.05 mg, B_{12} 4.5 mcg, C 60 mg, folic acid 0.3 mg, Cu, Fe 12 mg, Zn 10 mg, sucrose. Bot. 100s. *Rx.*
Use: Mineral, vitamin supplement; dental caries agent.

Poly-Vi-Flor 0.5 mg w/Iron. (Bristol-Myers Squibb) **Drops:** Vitamins A 1500 units, D 400 units, E 5 units, C 35 mg, B_1 0.5 mg, B_2 0.6 mg, B_3 8 mg, B_6 0.4 mg, fluoride 0.5 mg, Fe 10 mg/mL. Dropper Bot. 50 mL. **Chew. Tab.:** Vitamins A 2500 units, D 400 units, E 15 units, B_1 1.05 mg, B_2 1.2 mg, B_3 13.5 mg, B_6 1.05 mg, B_{12} 4.5 mcg, C 60 mg, folic acid 0.3 mg, fluoride 0.5 mg, Fe 12 mg, Cu, Zn 10 mg, lactose, sucrose. Bot. 100s. *Rx.*
Use: Mineral, vitamin supplement; dental caries agent.

Poly-Vi-Flor 0.25 mg. (Bristol-Myers Squibb) **Drops:** Vitamins A 1500 units, D 400 units, E 5 units, C 35 mg, B_1 0.5 mg, B_2 0.6 mg, B_6 0.4 mg, B_3 8 mg, B_{12} 2 mcg, fluoride 0.25 mg/mL. Dropper Bot. 50 mL. **Chew. Tab.:** Vitamins A 2500 units, D 400 units, E 15 units, B_1 1.05 mg, B_2 1.2 mg, B_3 13.5 mg, B_6 1.05 mg, B_{12} 4.5 mcg, C 60 mg, folic acid, 0.3 mg, fluoride 0.25 mg, lactose, sucrose. Bot. 100s. *Rx.*
Use: Mineral, vitamin supplement; dental caries agent.

Poly-Vi-Flor 0.25 mg w/Iron. (Bristol-Myers Squibb) **Drops:** Vitamins A 1500 units, D 400 units, E 5 units, C 35 mg, B_1 0.5 mg, B_2 0.6 mg, B_6 0.4 mg, niacin 8 mg, fluoride 0.25 mg, Fe 10 mg/mL. Bot. 50 mL. **Chew. Tab.:** Vitamins A 2500 units, D 400 units, E 15 units, B_1 1.05 units, B_2 1.2 mg, B_3 13.5 mg, B_6 1.05 mg, B_{12} 4.5 mcg, C 60 mg, folic acid 0.3 mg, fluoride 0.25 mg, Cu, Fe 12 mg, Zn 10 mg, lactose, sucrose. Bot. 100s. *Rx.*
Use: Mineral, vitamin supplement; dental caries agent.

• **polyvinyl acetate phthalate.** (pahl-ee-VYE-nil) *NF 23.*
Use: Pharmaceutic aid, coating agent.

• **polyvinyl alcohol.** *USP 28.* Ethanol, homopolymer.
Use: Pharmaceutic aid, viscosity-increasing agent.
See: Liquifilm Forte.
  Liquifilm Tears.
  Puralube Tears.

W/Hydroxypropyl methylcellulose. *See:* Liquifilm Wetting.

polyvinylpyrrolidone vinylacetate copolymers.

Poly-Vi-Sol. (Bristol-Myers Squibb) **Drops:** Vitamins A 1500 units, D 400 units, C 35 mg, B_1 0.5 mg, B_2 0.6 mg, E 5 units, B_6 0.4 mg, B_3 8 mg, B_{12} 2 mcg/mL. Bot. 50 mL. **Chew. Tab.:** Vitamins A 2500 units, E 15 units, D 400 units, C 60 mg, B_1 1.05 mg, B_2 1.2 mg, B_3 13.5 mg, B_6 1.05 mg, B_{12} 4.5 mcg, folic acid 0.3 mg. Bot. 100s. **Chew. Tab. With Iron:** Above formula plus Fe 12 mg, Zn 8 mg. Tab. Bot. 100s. Circus shape Tab. Bot. 100s. *OTC.*
Use: Vitamin supplement.

Poly-Vi-Sol w/Iron. (Bristol-Myers Squibb) **Chew. Tab.:** Fe 12 mg, vitamins A 2500 units, D 400 units, E 15 mg, B_1 1.05 mg, B_2 1.2 mg, B_3 13.5 mg, B_6 1.05 mg, B_{12} 4.5 mcg, C 60 mg, folic acid 0.3 mg, Cu, Zn 8 mg, sugar. Bot. 100s. **Drops:** Vitamins A 1500 units, D 400 units, E 5 units, C 35 mg, B_1 0.5 mg, B_2 0.6 mg, B_3 8 mg, B_6 0.4 mg, Fe 10 mg/mL. Bot. 50 mL. *OTC.*
Use: Mineral, vitamin supplement.

Poly-Vi-Sol w/Minerals. (Bristol-Myers Squibb) Fe 12 mg, vitamins A 2500 units, D 400 units, E 15 mg, B_1 1.05 mg, B_2 1.2 mg, B_3 13.5 mg, B_6 1.06 mg, B_{12} 4.5 mcg, C 60 mg, folic acid 0.3 mg, Cu, Zn 8 mg. Chew. Tab. Bot. 60s, 100s. *OTC.*
Use: Mineral, vitamin supplement.

Poly-Vitamin Drops. (Schein) Vitamins A 1500 units, D 400 units, E 5 units, B_1 0.5 mg, B_2 0.6 mg, B_3 8 mg, B_6 0.4 mg, B_{12} 1.5 mcg, C 35 mg/mL. Dropper. Bot. 50 mL. *OTC.*
Use: Vitamin supplement.

Polyvitamin Drops with Iron. (Various Mfr.) Fe 10 mg, vitamins A 1500 units, D 400 units, E 5 mg, B_1 0.5 mg, B_2 0.6 mg, B_3 8 mg, B_6 0.4 mg, C 35 mg/mL. Bot. 50 mL. *OTC.*
Use: Mineral, vitamin supplement.

Polyvitamin Drops w/Iron and Fluoride. (Various Mfr.) Fluoride 0.25 mg, Vitamins A 1500 units, D 400 units, E 5 units, B_1 0.5 mg, B_2 0.6 mg, B_3 8 mg, B_6 0.4 mg, C 35 mg, Fe 10 mg. Bot. 50 mL. *Rx.*
Use: Mineral, vitamin supplement; dental caries agent.

Polyvitamin Fluoride. (Various Mfr.) Fluoride 0.25 mg, vitamins A 1500 units, D 400 units, E 5 units, B_1 0.5 mg, B_2

0.6 mg, B_3 8 mg, B_6 0.4 mg, B_{12} 2 mcg, C 35 mg/mL. Dropper. Bot. 50 mL. *Rx.*
Use: Mineral, vitamin supplement; dental caries agent.

Polyvitamin Fluoride w/Iron. (Various Mfr.) Fluoride 1 mg, vitamins A 2500 units, D 400 units, E 15 mg, B_1 1.05 mg, B_2 1.2 mg, B_3 13.5 mg, B_6 1.05 mg, B_{12} 4.5 mcg, C 60 mg, folic acid 0.3 mg, Fe 12 mg, Cu, Zn 10 mg. Tab. Bot. 100s, 1000s. *Rx.*
Use: Mineral, vitamin supplement; dental caries agent.

Poly-Vitamins w/Fluoride. (Various Mfr.) Fluoride 1 mg, vitamins A 2500 units, D 400 units, E 15 mg, B_1 1.05 mg, B_2 1.2 mg, B_3 13.5 mg, B_6 1.05 mg, B_{12} 4.5 mcg, C 60 mg, folic acid 0.3 mg. Chew. Tab. Bot. 100s, 1000s. *Rx.*
Use: Mineral, vitamin supplement; dental caries agent.

Poly-Vitamins w/Fluoride 0.5 mg. (Various Mfr.) **Drops:** Fluoride 0.5 mg, vitamins A 1500 units, D 400 units, E 5 units, B_1 0.5 mg, B_2 0.6 mg, B_3 8 mg, B_6 0.4 mg, B_{12} 2 mcg, C 35 mg/mL. Bot. 50 mL. **Tab.:** Fluoride 0.5 mg, vitamins A 2500 units, D 400 units, E 15 mg, B_1 1 mg, B_2 1.2 mg, B_3 13.5 mg, B_6 1 mg, B_{12} 4.5 mcg, C 60 mg, folic acid 0.3 mg. Bot. 100s, 1000s. *Rx.*
Use: Mineral, vitamin supplement; dental caries agent.

Polyvitamins w/Fluoride 0.5 mg and Iron. (Rugby) Fluoride 0.5 mg, vitamins A 2500 units, D 400 units, E 15 units, B_1 1.05 mg, B_2 1.2 mg, B_3 13.5 mg, B_6 1.05 mg, B_{12} 4.5 mcg, C 60 mg, folic acid 0.3 mg, Cu, Fe 12 mg, Zn 10 mg, sucrose. Tab. Bot. 100s. *Rx.*
Use: Mineral, vitamin supplement; dental caries agent.

Polyvitamin w/Fluoride. (Rugby) Fluoride 0.5 mg, vitamins A 1500 units, D 400 units, E 5 mg, B_1 0.5 mg, B_2 0.6 mg, B_3 8 mg, B_6 0.4 mg, B_{12} 2 mcg, C 35 mg/mL. Dropper Bot. 50 mL. *Rx.*
Use: Mineral, vitamin supplement; dental caries agent.

Polyvite with Fluoride. (Geneva) Fluoride 0.25 mg, vitamins A 1500 units, D 400 units, E 5 mg, B_1 0.5 mg, B_2 0.6 mg, B_3 8 mg, B_6 0.4 mg, B_{12} 2 mcg, C 35 mg/mL. Dropper. Bot. 50 mL. *Rx.*
Use: Mineral, vitamin supplement; dental caries agent.

•**ponalrestat.** (poe-NAHL-ress-TAT) USAN.
Use: Antidiabetic.

Ponaris. (Jamol Lab Inc.) Nasal emollient of mucosal lubricating and mois-

turizing botanical oils. Cajeput, eucalyptus, peppermint in iodized cottonseed oil. Bot. 1 oz w/dropper. *OTC.*
Use: Moisturizer, nasal.

Ponstel. (Parke-Davis) Mefenamic acid 250 mg, lactose. Cap. Bot. 100s. *Rx.*
Use: Analgesic; NSAID.

Pontocaine. (Sanofi-Synthelabo) **Cream:** Tetracaine hydrochloride 1%, glycerin, light mineral oil, methylparaben, sodium metabisulfite. Tube 28.35 g. **Oint.:** Tetracaine 0.5%, menthol, white petrolatum. Tube 28.35 g. *OTC.*
Use: Anesthetic, topical.

Pontocaine Hydrochloride. (Hospira) Tetracaine hydrochloride. **Inj. 0.2%:** Dextrose 6%. Amp 2 mL. **0.3%:** Dextrose 6%. Amp 5 mL. **1%:** Acetone sodium bisulfite. Amp 2 mL. **Pow. for reconstitution:** Niphanoid (Instantly soluble). Amp. *Rx.*
Use: Anesthetic, injectable local.

Pontocaine Hydrochloride in Dextrose (Hyperbaric). (Sanofi-Synthelabo) **0.2%:** Tetracaine hydrochloride 2 mg/mL in a sterile solution containing dextrose 6%. Amp. 2 mL, 10s. **0.3%:** Tetracaine hydrochloride 3 mg/mL in a sterile solution containing dextrose 6%. Amp. 5 mL, 10s. *Rx.*
Use: Anesthetic, local.

Pontocaine Hydrochloride 0.5% Solution for Ophthalmology. (Sanofi-Synthelabo) Tetracaine hydrochloride 0.5%. Bot. 15 mL, 59 mL. *Rx.*
Use: Anesthetic, local.

Pontocaine 2% Aqueous Solution. (Sanofi-Synthelabo) Tetracaine hydrochloride 20 mg, chlorobutanol 4 mg/mL of 2% soln. Bot. 30 mL. Box 12s. Bot 118 mL, Box 6s. *Rx.*
Use: Anesthetic, local.

Po-Pon-S. (Shire US) Vitamins A 2000 units, D 100 units, E 5 mg, B_1 5 mg, B_2 3 mg, B_3 35 mg, B_5 15 mg, B_6 4 mg, B_{12} 6 mcg, C 100 mg, Ca, P. Tab. Bot. 60s, 240s. *OTC.*
Use: Vitamin, mineral supplement.

poppy-seed oil. The ethyl ester of the fatty acids of the poppy w/iodine.

poractant alfa.
Use: Lung surfactant.
See: Curosurf.

porcine islet preparation, encapsulated.
Use: For type I diabetes patients already on immunosuppression. [Orphan Drug]

• **porfimer sodium.** (PORE-fih-muhr) USAN.
Use: Antineoplastic.

See: Photofrin.

porfimer sodium. (PORE-fih-muhr) USAN.
Use: Antineoplastic. [Orphan Drug]
See: Photofrin.

• **porfiromycin.** (par-FIH-row-MY-sin) USAN.
Use: Anti-infective; antineoplastic.

Pork NPH Iletin II. (Eli Lilly) Purified pork insulin 100 units/mL in isophane insulin suspension (insulin w/protamine and zinc). Inj. Bot. 10 mL.
Use: Antidiabetic.

Pork Regular Iletin II. (Eli Lilly) Insulin 100 units/mL. Purified pork. Inj. Vial 10 mL.
Use: Antidiabetic.

• **porofocon a.** (PAR-oh-FOE-kahn) USAN.
Use: Contact lens material, hydrophobic.

• **porofocon b.** USAN.
Use: Contact lens material, hydrophobic.

Portabiday. (Washington Ethical) Concentrated soln. of alkylamine lauryl sulfate, a mild detergent with pH approx. 6 for use with *Portabiday* Vaginal Cleansing Kit. Bot. 3 oz. *OTC.*
Use: Vaginal agent.

Portagen. (Bristol-Myers Squibb) A nutritionally complete dietary powder containing as a % of the calories protein 14% as caseinate, fat 41% (medium chain triglycerides 86%, corn oil 14%), carbohydrate 45% as corn syrup solids and sucrose, vitamins A 5000 units, D 500 units, E 20 units, C 52 mg, B_1 1 mg, B 1.2 mg, B 1.4 mg, B 4 mcg, niacin 13 mg, folic acid 0.1 mg, choline 83 mg, biotin 0.05 mg, Ca 600 mg, P 450 mg, Mg 133 mg, Fe 12 mg, I 47 mcg, Cu 1 mg, Zn 6 mg, Mn 0.8 mg, Cl 550 mg, Na 300 mg, K 800 mg, pantothenic acid 6.7 mg, K-1 0.1 mg/qt. 20 Kcal/fl oz. Can 1 lb. *OTC.*
Use: Nutritional supplement, enteral.

Portia. (Barr) Levonorgestrel 0.1 mg, ethinyl estradiol 30 mcg, lactose. Tab. Packs. 21s, 28s. *Rx.*
Use: Sex hormone, contraceptive hormone.

porton asparaginase.
See: Erwinia L-asparaginase.

• **posaconazole.** (poe-sa-KONE-a-zole) USAN.
Use: Antifungal.

positive and negative hCG urine controls. (Wampole) Positive and negative human urine controls for (Wam-

pole) urine pregnancy tests. 1 set, 1 vial each.
Use: Diagnostic aid.
Poslam Psoriasis Ointment. (Last) Sulfur 5%, salicylic acid 2%. Jar 1 oz.
Use: Antipsoriatic.
posterior pituitary hormones.
See: Concentraid.
DDAVP.
Desmopressin Acetate.
Diapid.
Pitressin.
Pitressin Tannate in Oil.
Stimate.
Vasopressin.
posterior pituitary injection.
Use: Hormone, antidiuretic.
postlobin-o.
See: Pituitary, Posterior, Hormone (b).
postlobin-v.
See: Pituitary, Posterior, Hormone (a).
Posture. (Iverness Medical) Elemental calcium 600 mg, preservative free. Tab. Bot. 90s. *OTC.*
Use: Mineral supplement, calcium.
Posture D 600. (Wyeth) Calcium phosphate 600 mg, vitamin D 125 units. Tab. Bot. 60s. *OTC.*
Use: Mineral supplement.
Potaba. (Glenwood) Potassium aminobenzoate. **Cap.:** 500 mg. Bot. 250s, 1000s. **Tab.:** 500 mg. Bot. 100s, 1000s. **Envule (Pow.):** 2 g. Box 50s. *Rx.*
Use: Nutritional supplement.
Potachlor 10%. (Rosemont) Potassium and chloride 20 mEq/15 mL. Alcohol 5%. Bot. Pt, gal. Alcohol 3.8%. Bot. Pt, gal, UD 15 mL, 30 mL. *Rx.*
Use: Electrolyte supplement.
Potachlor 20%. (Rosemont) Potassium and chloride 40 mEq/15 mL. Alcohol free. Liq. Bot. pt, gal. *Rx.*
Use: Electrolyte supplement.
•**potash, sulfurated.** *USP 28.*
Use: Source of sulfide.
potassic saline lactated injection.
Use: Electrolyte replacement.
•**potassium acetate.** (poe-TASS-ee-um) *USP 28.* Acetic acid, potassium salt.
Use: Electrolyte replacement; to avoid Cl when high concentration of potassium is needed.
potassium acetate. (Various Mfr.) Potassium acetate. **Inj.:** 40 mEq, 20 mL in 50 mL Vial.
Use: Electrolyte replacement; to avoid Cl when high concentration of potassium is needed.
potassium acid phosphate.
See: K-Phos.
Uro-K.

potassium acid phosphate/sodium acid phosphate.
Use: Genitourinary.
See: K-Phos M.F.
K-Phos No. 2.
•**potassium aspartate and magnesium aspartate.** USAN.
Use: Nutrient.
•**potassium benzoate.** *NF 23.*
Use: Pharmaceutic aid, preservative.
•**potassium bicarbonate.** *USP 28.*
Use: Pharmaceutic necessity; electrolyte replacement.
potassium bicarbonate and potassium chloride effervescent tablets for oral solution.
Use: Electrolyte supplement.
potassium bicarbonate and potassium chloride for effervescent oral solution.
Use: Electrolyte supplement.
potassium bicarbonate and sodium bicarbonate and citric acid effervescent tablets for oral solution.
Use: Electrolyte supplement.
potassium bicarbonate effervescent tablets for oral solution.
Use: Electrolyte supplement.
•**potassium bitartrate.** *USP 28.*
Use: Cathartic.
•**potassium carbonate.** *USP 28.*
Use: Potassium therapy; pharmaceutic aid, alkalizing agent.
•**potassium chloride.** *USP 28.*
Use: Electrolyte replacement; potassium deficiency, hypopotassemia.
See: Cena-K.
Choice 10 and 20.
Effervescent Potassium/Chloride.
Kaochlor.
Kaochlor-Eff.
Kaon.
Kaon-Cl 20%.
Kaon Controlled Release.
Kato.
Kay Ciel.
Kay Ciel.
K+8.
K-Lor.
Klor-Con.
Klorvess.
Klotrix.
Klowess.
K-Lyte/Cl.
K-Lyte/Cl 50.
K-Tab.
Micro-K Extencaps.
Pan-Kloride.
Potage.
Potassine.

Ten-K.
potassium chloride. (Abbott) Potassium chloride. **Ampules:** 20 mEq, 10 mL; 40 mEq, 20 mL. **Pintop Vials:** 10 mEq, 5 mL in 10 mL; 20 mEq, 10 mL in 20 mL; 30 mEq, 12.5 mL in 30 mL; 40 mEq, 12.5 mL in 30 mL. **Fliptop Vials:** 20 mEq, 10 mL in 20 mL; 40 mEq, 20 mL in 50 mL. **Univ. Add. Syr.:** 5 mEq/5 mL, 20 mEq/10 mL, 30 mEq/20 mL, 40 mEq/20 mL (Eli Lilly and Co.) Amp. (40 mEq) 20 mL, 6s, 25s. *Rx.*
Use: Nutritional therapy.

potassium chloride. (Roxane) Postassium chloride. **Oral soln.:** Sugar free. 40 mEq/30 mL. Bot. 6 oz, 500 mL, 1 L, 5 L 20%. 80 mEq/30 mL. Bot. 500 mL, 1 L, 5 L. **Pow.:** 20 mEq/4 g. Pkt. 30s, 100s. *Rx.*
Use: Electrolyte supplement.

potassium chloride. (Wyeth) Potassium Cl 10%, 20%. Sugar free. Soln. Bot. 16 oz, gal. *Rx.*
Use: Electrolyte supplement.

potassium chloride in dextrose and sodium chloride injection.
Use: Electrolyte supplement.

potassium chloride in 5% dextrose. (Various Mfr.) Dextrose 50 g; calories 170; K$^+$ 10, 20, 30, or 40 mEq; Cl$^-$ 10, 20, 30, or 40 mEq, osmolarity ≈ 272, 292 to 295, 310 to 312, or 330 to 333 mOsm/L. Soln. Bot. 500 mL (330 to 333 mOsm only); 1000 mL. *Rx.*
Use: Intravenous nutritional therapy, intravenous replenishment solution.

potassium chloride in 5% dextrose and lactated Ringer's. (Baxter Healthcare) Dextrose 50 g, calories 170, Na$^+$ 130 mEq, K$^+$ 24 or 44 mEq, Ca 3 mEq, Cl$^-$ 129 or 149 mEq, lactate 28 mEq, osmolarity 565 or 605 mOsm/L. Soln. Bot. 1000 mL. *Rx.*
Use: Intravenous nutritional therapy, intravenous replenishment solution.

potassium chloride in 5% dextrose and lactated ringers. (Hospira) Dextrose 50 g, kcal 179, Na+ 130 mEq, K+ 24 mEq, Ca++ 2.7 mEq, Cl– 129 mEq, lactate 28 mEq, 563 mOsm per liter. Inj. 1,000 mL. *Rx.*
Use: Intravenous nutritional therapy.

potassium chloride in 5% dextrose and 0.45% sodium chloride. (Various Mfr.) Dextrose 50 g; calories 170; Na$^+$ 77 mEq; K$^+$ 10, 20, 30, or 40 mEq; Cl$^-$ 87, 97, 107, or 117 mEq; osmolarity ≈ 425, 445 to 447, ≈ 465, or 487 to 490 mOsm/L. Soln. Bot. 500 mL (445 to 447 mOsm only); 1000 mL. *Rx.*

Use: Intravenous nutritional therapy, intravenous replenishment solution.

potassium chloride in 5% dextrose and 0.9% sodium chloride. (Various Mfr.) Dextrose 50 g; calories 170; Na$^+$ 154 mEq; K$^+$ 20 or 40 mEq, Cl$^-$ 174 or 194 mEq; osmolarity ≈ 600 or 640 mOsm/L. Soln. Bot. 1000 mL. *Rx.*
Use: Intravenous nutritional therapy, intravenous replenishment solution.

potassium chloride in 5% dextrose and 0.33% sodium chloride. (Various Mfr.) Dextrose 50 g; calories 170; Na$^+$ 56 mEq; K$^+$ 20, 30, or 40 mEq, Cl$^-$ 76, 86, or 96 mEq; osmolarity 405, 425, or 446 mOsm/L. Soln. Bot. 500 mL (405 mOsm only); 1000 mL. *Rx.*
Use: Intravenous nutritional therapy, intravenous replenishment solution.

potassium chloride in 5% dextrose and 0.2% sodium chloride. (Various Mfr.) Dextrose 50 g; calories 170; Na$^+$ 34 mEq; K$^+$ 10, 20, 30, or 40 mEq, Cl$^-$ 44, 54, 64, or 74 mEq; osmolarity ≈ 340, 360, 380, or 400 mOsm/L. Soln. Bot. 250 mL, 500 mL (≈ 360 mOsm only); 1000 mL. *Rx.*
Use: Intravenous nutritional therapy, intravenous replenishment solution.

potassium chloride in lactated Ringer's and dextrose injection.
Use: Electrolyte supplement.

potassium chloride in sodium chloride injection.
Use: Electrolyte supplement.

potassium chloride in 10% dextrose and 0.2% sodium chloride. (B. Braun) Dextrose 100 g, calories 340, Na$^+$ 34 mEq; K$^+$ 20 mEq, Cl$^-$ 54 mEq; osmolarity 615 mOsm/L. Soln. Bot. 250 mL. *Rx.*
Use: Intravenous nutritional therapy, intravenous replenishment solution.

potassium chloride in 3.3% dextrose and 0.3% sodium chloride. (B. Braun) Dextrose 33 g, calories 110, Na$^+$ 51 mEq, K$^+$ 20 mEq, Cl$^-$ 71 mEq, osmolarity 310 mOsm/L. Soln. Bot. 1000 mL. *Rx.*
Use: Intravenous nutritional therapy, intravenous replenishment solution.

potassium chloride in 0.9% sodium chloride. (Various Mfr.) Na$^+$ 154 mEq, K$^+$ 20 or 40 mEq, Cl$^-$ 174 or 194 mEq, osmolarity ≈ 350 or 390 mOsm/L. Soln. Bot. 1000 mL. *Rx.*
Use: Intravenous nutritional therapy, intravenous replenishment solution.

• **potassium chloride K 42.** USAN.
Use: Radiopharmaceutical.

potassium chloride, sodium chloride, and calcium carbonate.
Use: Salt replacement.
See: Sustain.

potassium chloride with potassium gluconate.
See: Kolyum.

•**potassium citrate.** *USP 28.* Tripotassium citrate.
Use: Alkalizer. [Orphan Drug]
See: Urocit-K.
W/Sodium citrate.
See: Bicitra.
W/Sodium citrate, citric acid.
See: Cytra.
Polycitra K.
Polycitra LC.

potassium clavulanate/amoxicillin.
Use: Anti-infective, penicillin.
See: Amoclan.
Amoxicillin and potassium clavulanate.
Augmentin.

potassium clavulanate/ticarcillin.
Use: Anti-infective, penicillin.
See: Ticarcillin and clavulanate potassium.

•**potassium glucaldrate.** USAN.
Use: Antacid.

•**potassium gluconate.** *USP 28.*
Use: Electrolyte replacement.
See: Kaon.

potassium gluconate and potassium chloride. Oral Soln.
Use: Replacement therapy.

potassium gluconate and potassium chloride for oral solution.
Use: Replacement therapy.

potassium gluconate. (Various Mfr.) Potassium 40 mEq provided by potassium gluconate 9.36 g/30 mL, alcohol 5%. Elix. Bot. Pt, Patient-Cup 15 mL. *Rx.*
Use: Electrolyte supplement.

potassium gluconate and potassium citrate oral solution.
Use: Electrolyte supplement.

potassium gluconate, potassium citrate, and ammonium chloride oral solution.
Use: Electrolyte supplement.

potassium glutamate. The monopotassium salt of l-glutamic acid.

potassium G penicillin.
See: Penicillin G potassium, USP.

•**potassium guaiacolsulfonate.** *USP 28.*
Sulfoguaiacol. Potassium Hydroxymethoxybenzene sulfonate. Used in many cough preps.
Use: Expectorant.
See: Conex.

Pinex Regular.
W/Combinations.
See: Humibid DM.
Humibid L.A.
Hydron KGS.
Lemotussin DM.
Marcof Expectorant.
Prolex DH.
Tusquelin.

•**potassium hydroxide.** *NF 23.*
Use: Pharmaceutic aid, alkalinizing agent.

potassium in sodium chloride. (Various Mfr.) Potassium Cl 0.15%, 0.22%, 0.3% in sodium Cl 0.9%. Soln. for Inj. 1000 mL. *Rx.*
Use: Intravenous replenishment solution, nutritional supplement.

•**potassium iodide.** *USP 28.*
Use: Expectorant; antifungal; supplement, iodine.
See: Pima Expectorant.

potassium iodide w/combinations.
See: Diastix, Reagent Strips.
Elixophyllin-KI.
KIE.
Mudrane.
Mudrane-2.

•**potassium metabisulfite.** *NF 23.*
Use: Pharmaceutic aid, antioxidant.

•**potassium metaphosphate.** *NF 23.*
Use: Pharmaceutic aid, buffering agent.

•**potassium nitrate.** *USP 28.*
W/Combinations.
See: Arszol Silver Nitrate Applicators.

potassium p-aminobenzoate.
See: Potaba.
W/Potassium salicylate.
See: Pabalate-SF.
W/Pyridoxine.
See: Potaba Plus 6.

potassium penicillin G.
Use: Anti-infective, penicillin.
See: Penicillin G, Potassium, USP.

potassium penicillin V.
Use: Anti-infective, pencillin.
See: Phenoxymethyl penicillin potassium, USP.

•**potassium permanganate.** *USP 28.*
Permanganic acid, potassium salt.
Use: Anti-infective, topical.

•**potassium phenethicillin.** *USP 28.*
Phenethicillin potassium.
Use: Anti-infective.

potassium phenoxymethyl penicillin.
Use: Anti-infective.
See: Penicillin V potassium, USP.

•**potassium phosphate, dibasic.**
USP 28.
Use: Calcium regulator.

• **potassium phosphate, monobasic.**
NF 23. Dipotassium hydrogen phosphate.
Use: Pharmaceutic aid, buffering agent; source of potassium.

potassium phosphate, monobasic.
(Abbott) Potassium phosphate monobasic 15 mM, 5 mL in 10 mL Vial; 45 mM, 15 mL in 20 mL/Inj. Vial.
Use: Pharmaceutic aid, buffering agent; source of potassium.

potassium reagent strips. (Bayer Corp. (Consumer Div.)) Quantitative dry reagent strip test for potassium in serum or plasma. Bot. 50s.
Use: Diagnostic aid.

potassium-removing resins.
See: Kayexalate.
Sodium Polystyrene Sulfonate.
SPS.

potassium rhodanate.
See: Potassium Thiocyanate.

potassium salicylate.
See: Neocylate.
W/Potassium bromide, methapyrilene hydrochloride, vitamins.
See: Alva-Tranquil.
W/Potassium p-aminobenzoate.
See: Pabalate-SF.

potassium salt.
See: Potassium sorbate.

• **potassium sodium tartrate.** *USP 28.*
Use: Laxative.

• **potassium sorbate.** *NF 23.*
Use: Pharmaceutic aid, antimicrobial.

potassium sulfocyanate. Potassium Rhodanate.
See: Potassium thiocyanate.

potassium thiocyanate. Potassium sulfocyanate, potassium rhodanate.

potassium thiphencillin
Use: Anti-infective.

potassium troclosene. (Monsanto) Potassium dichloroisocyanurate.
Use: Anti-infective.

• **povidone.** (POE-vih-dohn) *USP 28.* Formerly Polyvidone, Polyvinylpyrrolidone.
Use: Pharmaceutic aid, dispersing and suspending agent.

• **povidone-iodine.** *USP 28.*
Use: Anti-infective, topical.
See: Betadine.
Betadine PrepStick.
Betadine PrepStick Plus.
Massengill Medicated.

povidone-iodine complex.
See: Betadine.

• **povidone I 131.** USAN.
Use: Radiopharmaceutical.

• **povidone I 125.** USAN.
Use: Radiopharmaceutical.

PowerMate. (Green Turtle Bay Vitamin Co.) Vitamins A 5000 units, E 100 units, B_3 12.5 mg, C 250 mg, Zn 2.5 mg, Se 7.5 mcg, n-acetyl-L-cysteine 25 mg, glutathione 5 mg, gingko biloba 5 mg, green tea extract 100 mg, pine bark extract 5 mg, echinacea 50 mg, golden seal root 20 mg, coenzyme Q10 2 mg, yeast free. Tab. Bot. 50s. *OTC.*
Use: Amino acid

PowerSleep. (Green Turtle Bay Vitamin Co.) L-glutamine 250 mg, 5-HTP 25 mg, melatonin 0.25 mg, vitamin B_3 25 mg, B_6 5 mg, inositol 100 mg, Ca 25 mg, passion flower extract 100 mg, valerian powder 75 mg. Tab. Bot. 60s. *OTC.*
Use: Amino acid.

PowerVites. (Green Turtle Bay Vitamin Co.) Vitamin A 2500 units, D 150 units, E 12.5 units, C 125 mg, B_1 6.3 mg, B_2 6.3 mg, B_3 25 mg, B_5 25 mg, B_6 12.5 mg, B_{12} 6.3 mcg, biotin, folic acid 0.15 mg, Ca, Mg, Cu, Zn 2.5 mg, Cr, Mn, K, Se, betaine, hesperidin. Tab. Bot. 40s, 100s, 200s. *OTC.*
Use: Mineral, vitamin supplement.

Poyaliver Stronger. (Forest) Liver inj. (equivalent to 10 mcg B_{12}), vitamin B_{12} 100 mcg, folic acid 10 mcg, niacinamide 1%/mL. Vial 10 mL. *Rx.*
Use: Nutritional supplement, parenteral.

Poyamin Jel Injection. (Forest) Cyanocobalamin 1000 mcg/mL. Vial 10 mL.
Use: Nutritional supplement, parenteral.

Poyaplex. (Forest) Vitamins B_1 100 mg, niacinamide 100 mg, B_6 10 mg, B_2 1 mg, panthenol 10 mg, B_{12} 5 mcg/mL. Vial 10 mL, 30 mL. *Rx.*
Use: Nutritional supplement, parenteral.

P.P.D. tuberculin.
See: Tuberculin, Purified Protein Derivative, USP.

P.P. factor (pellagra preventive factor).
See: Nicotinic acid.

ppg-15 stearyl ether.
Use: Pharmaceutic aid, surfactant.

PPI-002.
Use: Malignant mesothelioma. [Orphan Drug]

• **practolol.** (PRAK-toe-lole) USAN.
Use: Antiadrenergic, β-receptor.

• **pralatrexate.** (PRAL-a-TREX-ate) USAN.
Use: Cytotoxic agent.

• **pralidoxime chloride.** (pra-lih-DOCK-seem) *USP 28.*
Use: Cholinesterase reactivator; antidote.
See: Protopam chloride.

pralidoxime chloride. (Survival Technical) Pralidoxime chloride 600 mg, benzyl alcohol, aminocaproic acid. Inj. Vial 2 mL. *Rx.*
Use: Antidote.
●**pralidoxime iodide.** USAN.
Use: Cholinesterase reactivator.
See: Protopam iodide.
●**pralidoxime mesylate.** USAN.
Use: Cholinesterase reactivator.
pralidoxime methiodide.
See: Pralidoxime Iodide.
●**pralmorelin dihydrochloride.** (pralmore-ELL-in die-HIGH-droe-KLOR-ide) USAN.
Use: Growth hormone-releasing factor.
●**pralnacasan.** (PRAL-na-ka-san) USAN.
Use: Rheumatoid arthritis.
PrameGel. (Bioglan) Pramoxine hydrochloride 1%, menthol 0.5% in base w/benzyl alcohol. Gel. Bot. 118 mL. *OTC.*
Use: Anesthetic, local.
Pramilet FA. (Ross) Vitamins A 4000 units, B_1 3 mg, B_2 2 mg, B_6 3 mg, B_{12} 3 mcg, C 60 mg, D 400 units, B_5 1 mg, B_3 10 mg, Ca 250 mg, Cu, I, Fe 40 mg, Mg, Zn, folic acid 1 mg. Filmtab. Bot. 100s. *Rx.*
Use: Mineral, vitamin supplement.
●**pramipexole.** (pram-ih-PEX-ole) USAN. (Pharmacia)
Use: Antidepressant, dopamine agonist; antiparkinsonian; antischizophrenic.
See: Mirapex.
●**pramipexole dihydrochloride.** USAN.
Use: Antiparkisonian; antischizophrenic; antidepressant.
See: Mirapex.
●**pramiracetam hydrochloride.** (PRAM-ih-RASS-eh-tam) USAN. *Formerly Amacetam Hydrochloride.*
Use: Cognition adjuvant.
●**pramiracetam sulfate.** USAN. *Formerly Amacetam Sulfate.*
Use: Cognition adjuvant.
●**pramlintide acetate.** (PRAM-lin-tide) USAN.
Use: Antidiabetic.
See: Symlin.
Pramosone Cream 1%. (Ferndale) Hydrocortisone acetate 1%, pramoxine hydrochloride 1% in cream base. Tube 1 oz, 4 oz. Jar 4 oz, lb. *Rx.*
Use: Corticosteroid; anesthetic, local.
Pramosone Cream 2.5%. (Ferndale) Hydrocortisone acetate 2.5%, pramoxine hydrochloride 1% in cream base. Tube 1 oz, 4 oz. Jar lb. *Rx.*

Use: Corticosteroid; anesthetic, local.
Pramosone Cream 0.5%. (Ferndale) Hydrocortisone acetate 0.5%, pramoxine hydrochloride 1% in cream base. Tube 1 oz, 4 oz. Jar 4 oz, lb.
Use: Corticosteroid; anesthetic, local.
Pramosone Lotion 1%. (Ferndale) Hydrocortisone acetate 1%, pramoxine hydrochloride 1% in lotion base. Bot. 2 oz, 4 oz, 8 oz. *Rx.*
Use: Corticosteroid; anesthetic, local.
Pramosone Lotion 2.5%. (Ferndale) Hydrocortisone acetate 2.5%, pramoxine hydrochloride 1% in lotion base. Bot 2 oz, gal. *Rx.*
Use: Corticosteroid; anesthetic, local.
Pramosone Lotion 0.5%. (Ferndale) Hydrocortisone acetate 0.5%, pramoxine hydrochloride 1% in lotion base. Bot. 1 oz, 4 oz, 8 oz. *Rx.*
Use: Corticosteroid; anesthetic, local.
Pramosone Ointment 1%. (Ferndale) Hydrocortisone acetate 1%, pramoxine hydrochloride 1% in ointment base. Tube 1 oz, 4 oz. Jar 4 oz, lb. *Rx.*
Use: Corticosteroid; anesthetic, local.
Pramoxine HC. (Rugby) Pramoxine hydrochloride 1%, hydrocortisone acetate 1%. Aerosol foam. 10 g w/applicator. *Rx.*
Use: Anorectal preparation.
●**pramoxine hydrochloride.** (pram-OX-een) *USP 28.*
Use: Anesthetic, topical.
See: AmLactin AP.
    Campho-Phenique Cold Sore Treatment and Scab Relief.
    Itch-X.
    Prax.
    ProctoFoam.
    Tronothane hydrochloride.
W/Combinations.
See: Anti-Itch.
    Bactine Pain Relieving Cleansing.
    Band-Aid Plus.
    Betadine Plus First Aid Antibiotics and Pain Reliever.
    Caladryl.
    Cortic.
    Gentz.
    HC Pramoxine.
    Lanabiotic.
    Mediotic-HC.
    Neosporin Plus Pain Relief Maximum Strength.
    1 + 1 Creme.
    1 +1-F Creme.
    Oti-Med.
    Otocalm-H Ear Drops.
    Proctofoam-HC.
    Tri-Biozene.

Tri-Otic.
Triple Antibitoc Plus.
Zoto-HC.
Prandin. (Novo Nordisk) Repaglinide 0.5 mg, 1 mg, 2 mg. Tab. Bot. 100s, 500s, 1000s. *Rx.*
Use: Antidiabetic, meglitinide.
●**pranolium chloride.** (pray-NO-lee-uhm) USAN.
Use: Cardiovascular agent, antiarrhythmic.
●**prasugrel hydrochloride.** (pra-SOO-grel) USAN.
Use: Platelet antagonist.
Pravachol. (Bristol-Myers Squibb) Pravastatin sodium 10 mg, 20 mg, 40 mg, 80 mg, lactose. Tab. Bot. 90s; 500s (80 mg only); 1000s, UD 100s (20 mg, 40 mg only). *Rx.*
Use: Antihyperlipidemic, HMG-CoA reductase inhibitor.
●**pravadoline maleate.** (pray-AH-doe-leen) USAN.
Use: Analgesic.
pravastatin/aspirin.
Use: Antihyperlipidemic combination.
See: Pravigard PAC.
●**pravastatin sodium.** (PRUH l-vuh-stuh-tin) USAN.
Use: Antihyperlipidemic, HMG-CoA reductase inhibitor.
See: Pravachol.
Pravigard PAC. (Bristol-Myers Squibb) Aspirin (buffered) 81 mg with pravastatin 20 mg, 40 mg, or 80 mg. Aspirin (buffered) 325 mg with pravastatin 20 mg, 40 mg, or 80 mg. Mineral oil, lactose. Tab. Blister pack. 5s. *Rx.*
Use: Antihyperlipidemic, HMG-CoA reductase inhibitor.
Prax. (Ferndale) Pramoxine hydrochloride 1%. **Cream:** Glycerin, cetyl alcohol, white petrolatum. Jar 13.4 g. **Lot.:** Potassium sorbate, sorbic acid, mineral oil, cetyl alcohol, glycerin, lanolin. Bot. 15 mL, 120 mL, 240 mL. *OTC.*
Use: Anesthetic, local.
praziquantel.
Use: Anthelmintic.
See: Biltricide.
●**prazosin hydrochloride.** (PRAY-zoe-sin) USP 28.
Use: Antihypertensive, antiadrenergic.
See: Minipress.
prazosin hydrochloride. (Various Mfr.) Prazosin hydrochloride 1 mg, 2 mg, 5 mg. Cap. Bot. 100s, 250s, 500s, 1000s (except 5 mg).
Use: Antihypertensive, antiadrenergic.
Pre-Attain. (Sherwood Davis & Geck)

Sodium caseinate, maltodextrin, corn oil, soy lecithin, vitamins A, B_1, B_2, B_3, B_5, B_6, B_{12}, C, D, E, K, folic acid, Ca, Cl, Cu, Fe, I, Mg, Mn, P, Zn. Liq. Can 250 mL, closed system 1000 mL. *OTC.*
Use: Nutritional supplement.
PreCare. (Ther-Rx) Vitamin C 50 mg, Ca 250 mg, Fe 40 mg, D_3 6 mcg, E 3.5 mg, B_6 2 mg, folic acid 1 mg, Mg, Zn 15 mg, Cu, mannitol, sucrose, vanilla flavor. Chew. Tab. UD 100s. *Rx.*
Use: Vitamin, mineral supplement.
PreCare Conceive. (Ther-Rx) Vitamin C 60 mg, Ca 200 mg, Fe 30 mg, E 30 units, thiamin 3 mg, riboflvin 3.4 mg, niacin 20 mg, pyridoxine 50 mg, folic acid 1 mg, Mg, cyanocobalamin 12 mcg, Zn 15 mg, Cu, lactose. Tab. UD 100s. *Rx.*
Use: Vitamin, mineral supplement.
PreCare Prenatal. (Ther-Rx) Ca 250 mg, Fe (as ferrous fumarate) 40 mg, E (dl-alpha tocopheryl acetate) 3.5 mg, D_3 6 mcg, B_1 3 mg, B_2 3.4 mg, B_3 20 mg, B_6 12 mcg, C 50 mg, folic acid 1 mg, Mg, Zn 15 mg, Cu. Dye free. Tab. UD 100s. *Rx.*
Use: Vitamin, mineral supplement.
Precedex. (Abbott) Dexmedetomidine hydrochloride 100 mcg/mL, sodium chloride 9 mg, preservative free. Inj. Vial 2 mL. *Rx.*
Use: Sedative; hypnotic (nonbarbiturate).
Precef for Injection. (Bristol Myers Squibb) Ceforanide 500 mg, 1 g/Vial or piggyback. *Rx.*
Use: Anti-infective, cephalosporin.
Precision High Nitrogen Diet. (Novartis) Vanilla flavor: Maltodextrin, pasteurized egg white solids, sucrose, natural and artificial flavors, medium chain triglycerides, partially hydrogenated soybean oil, polysorbate 80, mono- and diglycerides, vitamins, minerals. Pow. Packet 2.93 oz. *OTC.*
Use: Nutritional supplement.
Precision LR Diet. (Novartis) Orange flavor: Maltodextrin, pasteurized egg white solids, sucrose, medium chain triglycerides, partially hydrogenated soybean oil with BHA, citric acid, natural and artificial flavors, mono- and diglycerides, polysorbate 80, FD&C Yellow No. 5 and No. 6, vitamins, minerals. Pow. Packet 3 oz. *OTC.*
Use: Nutritional supplement.
Precose. (Bayer) Acarbose 25 mg, 50 mg, 100 mg. Tab. Bot. 100s, UD 100s (except 25 mg). *Rx.*
Use: Antidiabetic.

Predamide Ophthalmic. (Maurry) Sodium sulfacetamide 10%, prednisolone acetate 0.5%, hydroxyethyl cellulose, polysorbate 80, sodium thiosulfate, benzalkonium Cl 0.025%. Bot. 5 mL, 15 mL. *Rx.*
Use: Anti-infective; corticosteroid, ophthalmic.

Predcor-50. (Roberts) Prednisolone acetate 50 mg/mL. Inj. Vial 10 mL. *Rx.*
Use: Corticosteroid.

Pred Forte. (Allergan) Prednisolone acetate 1%. Susp. Bot. 1 mL, 5 mL, 10 mL, 15 mL. *Rx.*
Use: Corticosteroid, ophthalmic.

Pred-G. (Allergan) Prednisolone acetate 1%, gentamicin sulfate 0.3%, benzalkonium chloride 0.005%, polyvinyl alcohol 1.4%, EDTA, hydrochloric acid, hydroxypropyl methylcellulose, sodium chloride, polysorbate 80, sodium citrate dihydrate, sodium hydroxide. Ophth. Susp. Bot. 2 mL, 5 mL, 10 mL. *Rx.*
Use: Corticosteroid; anti-infective, ophthalmic.

Pred-G S.O.P. (Allergan) Prednisolone acetate 0.6%, gentamicin sulfate 0.3%, chlorobutanol 0.5%. Oint. Tube 3.5 g. *Rx.*
Use: Anti-infective; corticosteroid, ophthalmic.

Predicort-AP. (Oxypure) Prednisolone sodium phosphate 20 mg, prednisolone acetate 80 mg/mL. Vial 10 mL. *Rx.*
Use: Corticosteroid.

Predicort-RP. (Oxypure) Prednisolone sodium phosphate equivalent to prednisolone phosphate 20 mg, niacinamide 25 mg/mL. Vial 10 mL. *Rx.*
Use: Corticosteroid.

Pred Mild. (Allergan) Prednisolone acetate 0.12%. Susp. Bot. 5 mL, 10 mL. *Rx.*
Use: Corticosteroid, ophthalmic.

•**prednazate.** (PRED-nah-zate) USAN.
Use: Anti-inflammatory.

•**prednicarbate.** (PRED-nih-CAR-bate) USAN.
Use: Corticosteroid, topical.
See: Dermatop.

Prednicen-M. (Schwarz Pharma) Prednisone 5 mg. Tab. Bot. 100s, 1000s. *Rx.*
Use: Corticosteroid.

•**prednimustine.** (PRED-nih-MUSS-teen) USAN.
Use: Antineoplastic. [Orphan Drug]

•**prednisolone.** (pred-NISS-oh-lone) *USP 28.* Metacortandralone.
Tall Man: PrednisoLONE

Use: Corticosteroid.
See: Cordrol.
   Delta-Cortef.
   Fernisolone.
   Orapred.
   Orasone.
   Orasone 50.
   Prednis.
   Prelone.
W/Aluminum hydroxide gel, dried.
   See: Predoxide.
W/Chloramphenicol.
   See: Chloroptic-P.
   Neo-Deltef.

prednisolone. (Halsey Drug) Prednisolone 15 mg/5 mL, alcohol 5%. Syr. Bot. 236 mL, 473 mL. *Rx.*
Use: Corticosteroid.

•**prednisolone acetate.** *USP 28.*
Tall Man: PrednisoLONE
Use: Corticosteroid, topical.
See: Econopred.
   Key-Pred.
   Pred.
   Pred Forte.
   Pred Mild.
   Predicort.
   Sigpred.
   Steraject.

prednisolone acetate and prednisolone sodium phosphate. (Various Mfr.) Prednisolone acetate 80 mg, prednisolone sodium phosphate 20 mg/mL. Inj. Vial 10 mL. *Rx.*
Use: Corticosteroid.

prednisolone acetate ophthalmic. (Falcon Ophthalmics) Prednisolone acetate 1% Ophth. Susp. Bot. 5 mL, 10 mL. *Rx.*
Use: Corticosteroid, topical.

prednisolone acetate w/combinations.
See: Blephamide Liquifilm.
   Blephamide S.O.P.
   Cetapred.
   Isopto Cetapred.
   Metimyd.
   Poly-Pred Liquifilm Ophthalmic Suspension.
   Pred-G Ophthalmic Suspension.
   Vasocidin.

prednisolone acetate ophthalmic suspension. (Falcon Ophthalmics) Prednisolone 1%, benzalkonium Cl 0.01%, EDTA. Susp. Bot. 5 mL, 10 mL. *Rx.*
Use: Corticosteroid.

prednisolone butylacetate.
Use: Corticosteroid.

prednisolone cyclopentylpropionate.
Use: Corticosteroid.

•**prednisolone hemisuccinate.** *USP 28.*
Tall Man: PrednisoLONE

Use: Corticosteroid, topical.
●**prednisolone sodium phosphate.**
USP 28.
Tall Man: PrednisoLONE
Use: Corticosteroid, topical.
See: AK-Pred.
Alto-Pred Soluble.
Inflamase Forte.
Inflamase.
Key-Pred SP.
Liquid Pred.
Metreton.
Orapred.
Pediapred.
P.S.P. IV (Four).
Savacort-S.
W/Neomycin sulfate.
See: P.SP IV.
W/Prednisolone acetate.
See: Optimyd.
Vasocidin.
prednisolone sodium phosphate. (Up-
state Pharma) Prednisolone sodium
phosphate 6.75 mg (prednisolone 5 mg)
per 5 mL. EDTA, methylparaben, sorbi-
tol. Dye free. Raspberry flavor. Oral
Soln. 120 mL. *Rx.*
Use: Adrenocortical steroid.
prednisolone sodium phosphate.
(Various Mfr.) Prednisolone sodium
phosphate 0.125%, 1%. Soln. Bot.
5 mL, 10 mL, 15 mL. *Rx.*
Use: Corticosteroid, topical.
**prednisolone sodium succinate for
injection.** *USP 28.*
Tall Man: PrednisoLONE
Use: Corticosteroid, topical.
●**prednisolone tebutate.** *USP 28.*
Tall Man: PrednisoLONE
Use: Corticosteroid, topical.
See: Metalone.
prednisolone tertiary-butylacetate.
See: Prednisolone Tebutate, USP.
Prednisol TBA. (Taylor Pharmaceuticals)
Prednisolone tebutate 20 mg/mL. Vial
10 mL. *Rx.*
Use: Corticosteroid.
●**prednisone.** (PRED-nih-sone) *USP 28.*
Tall Man: PredniSONE
Use: Corticosteroid.
See: Delta-Dome.
Deltasone.
Keysone.
Maso-Pred.
Meticorten.
Orasone.
Sterapred.
Sterapred DS.
W/Chlorpheniramine maleate.
See: Histone.

●**prednisone.** (Roxane) Prednisone
2.5 mg. Lactose. Tab. 100s, UD 100s.
Rx.
Use: Glucocorticoid.
prednisone. (Various Mfr.) Prednisone
1 mg, 5 mg, 20 mg. Tab. Bot. 100s,
1000s, UD 100s. *Rx.*
Use: Corticosteroid, topical.
Prednisone Intensol. (Roxane) Prednisone concentrated oral solution 5 mg/
mL. Bot. 30 mL w/calibrated dropper.
Rx.
Use: Corticosteroid.
●**prednival.** (PRED-nih-val) *USAN.*
Use: Corticosteroid.
Predsulfair. (Bausch & Lomb) **Drops:**
Prednisolone acetate 0.5%, sodium
sulfacetamide 10%, hydroxypropyl
methylcellulose, polysorbate 80 0.5%,
sodium thiosulfate, benzalkonium Cl
0.01%. Bot. 5 mL, 15 mL. **Oint.:** Prednisolone acetate 0.5%, sodium sulfacetamide 10%, mineral oil, white petrolatum, lanolin, parabens. 3.5 g. *Rx.*
Use: Anti-infective; corticosteroid, ophthalmic.
Prefest. (Barr/Duramed) Estradiol 1 mg;
estradiol 1 mg/norgestimate 0.09 mg,
lactose. Tab. Blister card 30s (15 each
tablet). *Rx.*
Use: Sex hormone, estrogen and progestin combination.
**Preflex Daily Cleaning Especially for
Sensitive Eyes.** (Alcon) Isotonic,
aqueous solution of sorbic acid, sodium
phosphates, sodium Cl, tyloxapol,
hydroxyethyl cellulose, polyvinyl alcohol, EDTA. Bot. 30 mL. *OTC.*
Use: Contact lens care.
Prefrin Liquifilm. (Allergan) Phenylephrine hydrochloride 0.12%. Bot.
20 mL. *OTC.*
Use: Mydriatic, vasoconstrictor.
●**pregabalin.** (preh-GAB-ah-lin) *USAN.*
Use: Anticonvulsant.
Pregestimil. (Bristol-Myers Squibb) Protein hydrolysate formula supplies
640 calories/qt. protein 18 g, fat 26 g,
carbohydrate 86 g, vitamins A
2000 units, D 400 units, E 15 units, C
52 mg, folic acid 100 mcg, thiamine hydrochloride 0.5 mg, riboflavin 0.6 mg,
niacin 8 mg, B_6 0.4 mg, B_{12} 2 mg, biotin 0.05 mg, pantothenic acid 3 mg, K-
1 100 mcg, choline 85 mg, inositol
30 mg, Ca 600 mg, P 400 mg, I 45 mcg,
Fe 12 mg, Mg 70 mg, Cu 0.6 mg, Zn
4 mg, Mn 0.2 mg, Cl 550 mg, K 700 mg,
Na 300 mg/qt. (20 Kcal/fl oz.). Pow.
Can lb. *OTC.*
Use: Nutritional supplement, enteral.

Pregnaslide Latex hCG Test with Fast Trak Slides. (Wampole) Latex agglutination slide test for the qualitative detection of hCG in urine. Test 24s. Test kit 96s.
Use: Diagnostic aid.

pregneninolone.
See: Ethisterone.

pregnenolone.
Use: Treatment of rheumatoid arthritis.

• **pregnenolone succinate.** (preg-NEN-oh-lone) USAN.
Use: Nonhormonal sterol derivative.

Pregnosis Slide Test. (Roche) Latex agglutination inhibition slide test. 50s, 200s.
Use: Diagnostic aid.

Pregnyl. (Organon) Chorionic gonadotropin 10,000 units/vial with diluent 10 mL (1,000 units per mL), benzyl alcohol 0.9%. Vial 10 mL. *Rx.*
Use: Ovulation stimulant.

Pre-Hist-D. (Marnel) Phenylephrine hydrochloride 20 mg, chlorpheniramine maleate 8 mg, methscopolamine nitrate 2.5 mg. SR Tab. Bot. 100s. *Rx.*
Use: Upper respiratory combination, anticholinergic, antihistamine, decongestant.

Preject Preinjection Topical Anesthetic. (Colgate Oral) Benzocaine 20% in polyethylene glycol base. Jar 2 oz. *OTC.*
Use: Anesthetic, local.

Prelestrin. (Taylor Pharmaceuticals) Conjugated estrogens 0.625 mg, 1.25 mg. Tab. Bot. 100s, 1000s. *Rx.*
Use: Estrogen.

Prelone. (Aero) Prednisolone 15 mg/5 mL. Alcohol 5%. Syrup. Plast. Bot. 240 mL. *Rx.*
Use: Corticosteroid.

Prelu-2. (Roxane) Phendimetrazine tartrate 105 mg, sucrose. Cap. Bot. 100s. *c-III.*
Use: CNS stimulant, anorexiant.

Premarin. (Wyeth-Ayerst) Conjugated estrogens. 0.3 mg, 0.45 mg, 0.625 mg, 0.9 mg, 1.25 mg, lactose, sucrose. Tab. Bot. 100s, 1000s (except 0.45 mg, 0.9 mg), UD 100s (0.45 mg, 0.625 mg only). *Rx.*
Use: Estrogen.

Premarin Intravenous. (Wyeth-Ayerst) Conjugated estrogens 25 mg. Inj. *Secules* each with 5 mL sterile diluent. Lactose 200 mg, simethicone 0.2 mg, sodium citrate 12.2 mg, benzyl alcohol 2%. *Rx.*
Use: Estrogen.

Premarin Vaginal. (Wyeth-Ayerst) Conjugated estrogens 0.625 mg/g w/benzyl alcohol, cetyl alcohol, mineral oil. Cream. Tube w/applicator 42.5 g. *Rx.*
Use: Estrogen.

Premarin w/Meprobamate.
See: PMB 200 and 400.

PremesisRx. (Ther-Rx) Vitamin B_6 75 mg, B_{12} 12 mcg, folic acid 1 mg, Ca 200 mg. Tab. Bot. 100s. *Rx.*
Use: Vitamin supplement.

Premphase. (Wyeth-Ayerst) Conjugated estrogens 0.625 mg. Medroxyprogesterone acetate 5 mg, conjugated estrogens 0.625 mg. Lactose, sucrose. Tab. Dial pack 28s (14 of each tablet). *Rx.*
Use: Sex hormone, estrogen, progestin combination.

Prempro. (Wyeth-Ayerst) Conjugated estrogen 0.3 mg/medroxyprogesterone acetate 1.5 mg, conjugated estrogen 0.45 mg/medroxyprogesterone acetate 1.5 mg, conjugated estrogen 0.625 mg/medroxyprogesterone acetate 2.5 mg (lactose, sucrose), conjugated estrogen 0.625 mg/medroxyprogesterone acetate 5 mg (lactose, sucrose). Tab. Dial pack 28s (except 0.45 mg/1.5 mg), *EZ Dial* 28s (0.45 mg/1.5 mg only). *Rx.*
Use: Sex hormone, estrogen, progestin combination.

Prēmsyn PMS. (Chattem) Acetaminophen 500 mg, pamabrom 25 mg, pyrilamine maleate 15 mg. Cap. Bot. 20s, 40s. *OTC.*
Use: Analgesic; antihistamine; diuretic.

• **prenalterol hydrochloride.** (PREE-NAL-teh-role) USAN.
Use: Adrenergic.

Prenatabs RX. (Cypress) Ca 200 mg, Fe (as carbonyl iron) 29 mg, vitamin A 4000 units, D 400 units, E (dl-alpha tocopheryl acetate) 30 units, B_1 3 mg, B_2 3 mg, B_3 20 mg, B_5 7 mg, B_6 3 mg, B_{12} 8 mcg, C 120 mg, folic acid 1 mg, biotin 30 mcg, Zn 15 mg, Cu, I, Mg. Tab. Bot. 90s. *Rx.*
Use: Mineral, vitamin supplement.

Prenatal AD. (Cypress) Ca 200 mg, Fe (carbonyl iron) 90 mg, vitamin A 2700 units, D_3 400 units, E (dl-alpha tocopheryl acetate) 30 units, B_1 3 mg, B_2 3.4 mg, B_3 20 mg, B_6 20 mg, B_{12} 12 mcg, C 120 mg, folic acid 1 mg, Zn 25 mg, Cu, Mg, docusate sodium 50 mg. Tab. Bot. 90s. *Rx.*
Use: Mineral, vitamin supplement.

Prenatal Folic Acid + Iron. (Everett) Vitamins, minerals, folic acid 1 mg. Tab. Bot. 100s. *Rx.*
Use: Mineral, vitamin supplement.

Prenatal-H. (Cypress) Fe (as ferrous fumarate) 106.5 mg, vitamin B_1 10 mg, B_2 6 mg, B_3 30 mg, B_5 10 mg, B_6 5 mg, B_{12} 15 mcg, C 200 mg, folic acid 1 mg, Cu, Mg, Mn, Zn 18.2 mg. Cap. Bot. 100s. *Rx.*
Use: Mineral, vitamin supplement.

Prenatal H.P. (Mission Pharmacal) Vitamins A 4000 units, C 100 mg, D_3 400 units, B_1 4 mg, B_2 2 mg, B_3 10 mg, B_5 1 mg, B_6 20 mg, B_{12} 2 mcg, folate 0.8 mg, Ca 50 mg, Fe 30 mg, sugar. Tab. Bot. 100s. *OTC.*
Use: Mineral, vitamin supplement.

Prenatal Maternal. (Ethex) Ca 250 mg, Fe 4 mg, B_2 60 mg, vitamins A 5000 units, D 400 units, E 30 mg, B_1 2.9 mg, B_2 3.4 mg, B_3 20 mg, B_5 10 mg, B_6 12.2 mg, B_{12} 12 mcg, C 100 mg, folic acid 1 mg, Cr, Cu, I, Mg, Mn, Mo, Zn 25 mg, biotin 30 mcg. Tab. Bot. 100s. *Rx.*
Use: Mineral, vitamin supplement.

Prenatal MR 90. (Ethex) Ca 250 mg, Fe 90 mg, vitamins A 4000 units, D 400 units, E 30 mg, B_1 3 mg, B_2 3.4 mg, B_3 20 mg, B_6 20 mg, B_{12} 12 mcg, C 120 mg, folic acid 1 mg, Zn 25 mg, I, Cu, DSS. Tab. Bot. 100s. *Rx.*
Use: Mineral, vitamin supplement.

Prenatal 19. (Cypress) Ca 200 mg, Fe 29 mg, vitamin A 1000 units, D 400 units, E (dl-alpha tocopheryl acetate) 30 units, B_1 3 mg, B_2 3 mg, B_3 15 mg, B_5 7 mg, B_6 20 mg, B_{12} 12 mcg, C 100 mg, folic acid 1 mg, Zn 20 mg, docusate sodium 25 mg. Tab. Bot. 100s. *Rx.*
Use: Mineral, vitamin supplement.

Prenatal 19 Chewable. (Cypress) Ca 200 mg, Fe 29 mg, vitamin A 1000 units, D 400 units, E (dl-alpha tocopheryl acetate) 30 units, B_1 3 mg, B_2 3 mg, B_3 15 mg, B_5 7 mg, B_6 20 mg, B_{12} 12 mcg, C 100 mg, folic acid 1 mg, Zn 20 mg, docusate sodium 25 mg, orange flavor. Tab. Bot. 100s. *Rx.*
Use: Mineral, vitamin supplement.

Prenatal-1 + Iron. (Various Mfr.) Ca 200 mg, Fe 65 mg, vitamins A 4000 units, D 400 units, E 11 mg, B_1 1.5 mg, B_2 3 mg, B_3 20 mg, B_6 10 mg, B_{12} 12 mcg, C 120 mg, folic acid 1 mg, Cu, Zn 25 mg. Tab. Bot. 100s, 500s. *Rx.*
Use: Mineral, vitamin supplement.

Prenatal PC 40. (Integrity) Ca 250 mg, Fe (as ferrous fumarate and carbonyl iron) 40 mg, vitamin D_3 6 mcg, E (dl-alpha tocopheryl acetate) 3.5 mg, B_1 3 mg, B_2 3.4 mg, B_3 20 mg, B_6

20 mg, B_{12} 12 mcg, C 50 mg, folic acid 1 mg, Zn 15 mc, CU, Mg, polydextrose. Tab. UD 100s. *Rx.*
Use: Multivitamin.

Prenatal Plus. (Ivax) Vitamins A (as acetate and carotene) 4000 units, D 400 units, E 22 mg, C 120 mg, folic acid 1 mg, B_1 1.84 mg, B_2 3 mg, B_3 20 mg, B_6 10 mg, B_{12} 12 mcg, Ca 200 mg, Fe 65 mg, Cu 2 mg, Zn 25 mg. Tab. Bot. 100s. *Rx.*
Use: Mineral, vitamin supplement.

Prenatal Plus-Improved. (Rugby) Ca 200 mg, Fe 65 mg, vitamins A 4000 units, D 400 units, E 11 mg, B_1 1.5 mg, B_2 3 mg, B_3 20 mg, B_6 10 mg, B_{12} 12 mcg, C 120 mg, folic acid 1 mg, Cu, Zn 25 mg. Tab. Bot. 100s. *Rx.*
Use: Mineral, vitamin supplement.

Prenatal Plus Iron. (Major) Vitamins A 4000 units, D 400 units, E 22 mg, C 120 mg, folic acid 1 mg, B_1 1.84 mg, B_2 3 mg, niacinamide 20 mg, B_6 10 mg, B_{12} 12 mcg, Ca 200 mg, Cu 2 mg, Fe 27 mg, Zn 25 mg. Tab. Bot. 100s. *Rx.*
Use: Vitamin, mineral supplement.

Prenatal Rx. (Mission Pharmacal) Vitamins A 3000 units (as acetate), D_3 400 units, C 240 mg (as ascorbic and calcium ascorbate), B_1 4 mg, B_2 2 mg, B_3 20 mg, B_5 10 mg, B_6 20 mg, B_{12} 8 mcg, folic acid 1 mg, Fe 29.5 mg (as ferrous fumarate), Ca 175 mg (as carbonate and ascorbate), I 0.3 mg (as potassium iodide), Zn 15 mg (as zinc sulfate), Cu 2 mg (as cupric oxide). Tab. Bot. 100s. *Rx.*
Use: Mineral, vitamin supplement.

Prenatal Rx with Beta Carotene. (Various Mfr.) Ca 200 mg, Fe 60 mg, vitamins A 4000 units, D 400 units, E 15 mg, B_1 1.5 mg, B_2 1.6 mg, B_3 17 mg, B_5 7 mg, B_6 4 mg, B_{12} 2.5 mcg, C 80 mg, folic acid 1 mg, biotin 30 mcg, Cu, Mg, Zn 25 mg. Tab. Bot. 100s, 500s. *Rx.*
Use: Mineral, vitamin supplement.

Prenatal-S. (Ivax) Ca 200 mg, Fe 60 mg, vitamins A 4000 units, D 400 units, E 11 mg, B_1 1.5 mg, B_2 1.7 mg, B_3 18 mg, B_6 2.6 mg, B_{12} 4 mcg, C 100 mg, folic acid 0.8 mg, Zn 25 mg. Tab. Bot. UD 100s. *OTC.*
Use: Mineral, vitamin supplement.

Prenatal with Folic Acid. (Geneva) Ca 200 mg, Fe 60 mg, vitamins A 4000 units, D 400 units, E 11 mg, B_1 1.5 mg, B_2 1.7 mg, B_3 18 mg, B_6 2.6 mg, B_{12} 4 mcg, C 100 mg, folic acid 0.8 mg, Zn 25 mg. Tab. Bot. 100s. *OTC.*
Use: Mineral, vitamin supplement.

Prenatal with Folic Acid. (Eon Labs)
Vitamins A 6000 units, D 400 units, E
30 units, folic acid 1 mg, C 60 mg, B_1
1.1 mg, B_2 1.8 mg, B_6 2.5 mg, B_{12}
5 mcg, niacin 15 mg, Ca 125 mg, Fe
65 mg. Tab. Bot. 100s, 1000s. *Rx.*
Use: Mineral, vitamin supplement.

Prenatal Z. (Ethex) Ca 300 mg, Fe
65 mg, vitamins A 5000 units, D
400 units, E 30 mg, B_1 3 mg, B_2 3 mg,
B_3 20 mg, B_6 12.2 mg, B_{12} 12 mcg, C
80 mg, folic acid 1 mg, Zn 20 mg, I, Mg.
Tab. Bot. 100s. *Rx.*
Use: Mineral, vitamin supplement.

Prenatal Z Advanced Formula. (Ethex)
Vitamin A 3000 units, ascorbic acid
70 mg, calcium carbonate 200 mg, ferrous fumarate 65 mg, cholecalciferol
400 units, dl-alpha tocopheryl acetate
10 units, B_1 1.5 mg, B_2 1.6 mg, B_3
17 mg, B_6 2.2 mg, folic acid 1 mg, B_{12}
2.2 mcg, potassium iodide 175 mcg,
magnesium oxide 100 mg, zinc oxide
15 mg. Tab. Bot. 100s. *Rx.*
Use: Mineral, vitamin supplement.

Prenate 90. (Sanofi-Synthelabo) Vitamins A 4000 units, D 400 units, E
30 mg, C 120 mg, folic acid 1 mg, B_1
3 mg, B_2 3.4 mg, B_6 20 mg, B_{12} 12 mcg,
B_3 20 mg, DSS, Ca 250 mg, I, Fe
90 mg, Cu, Zn 20 mg. FC Tab. Bot.
100s, 1000s. *Rx.*
Use: Mineral, vitamin supplement.

Prenavite. (Rugby) Ca 200 mg, Fe
60 mg, vitamins A 4000 units, D
400 units, E 11 mg, B_1 1.5 mg, B_2
1.7 mg, B_3 18 mg, B_6 2.6 mg, B_{12}
4 mcg, C 100 mg, folic acid 0.8 mg, Zn
25 mg. Tab. Bot. 100s, 500s. *OTC.*
Use: Mineral, vitamin supplement.

•**prenylamine.** (PREH-nill-ah-meen)
USAN. Segontin; synadrin lactate.
Use: Coronary vasodilator.

Preparation H. (Whitehall-Robins)
Cream: Petrolatum 18%, glycerin 12%,
shark liver oil 3%, phenylephrine hydrochloride 0.25%, cetyl and stearyl alcohol, EDTA, parabens, lanolin. Tube
27 g, 54 g. **Oint.:** Petrolatum 71.9%,
mineral oil 14%, shark liver oil 3%,
phenylephrine hydrochloride 0.25%,
corn oil, glycerin, lanolin, lanolin alcohol, parabens, tocopherol. 30 g, 60 g.
Supp.: Shark liver oil 3%, cocoa butter 79%, corn oil, EDTA, parabens, tocopherol. 12s, 24s, 36s, 48s. *OTC.*
Use: Anorectal preparation.

Preparation H Cooling. (Whitehall-
Robins) Witch hazel 50%, phenyl-
ephrine hydrochloride 0.25%, alcohol
7.5%, EDTA, parabens. Gel. Tube 51 g.
OTC.
Use: Anorectal preparation.

Prepcat. (Mallinckrodt) Barium sulfate
1.5%, simethicone, sorbitol, strawberry
flavor. Susp. Bot. 450 mL. *Rx.*
Use: Radiopaque agent, GI contrast
agent.

Prepcat 2000. (Lafayette) Barium sulfate
1.2% w/w suspension. Bot. 2000 mL,
Case Bot. 4s.
Use: Radiopaque agent.

Prepcort. (Whitehall-Robins) Hydrocortisone 0.5%. Cream. Tube 0.5 oz, 1 oz.
Use: Corticosteroid.

Pre-Pen. (Schwarz Pharma) Benzylpeni-
cilloyl-polylysine 0.25 mL/Amp. *Rx.*
Use: Diagnostic aid.

Pre-Pen/MDM. (Schwarz Pharma)
See: Benzylpenicillin, Benzylpenicilloic,
Benzylpenilloic Acid.

Prepidil. (Pharmacia) Dinoprostone
0.5 mg. Gel. Syringes (with 2 shielded
catheters 10 and 20 mm tip) 3 g. *Rx.*
Use: Cervical ripening.

Prepodyne. (West) Titratable iodine.
Soln.: 1%. Bot. Pt, gal. **Scrub:** 0.75%.
Bot. 6 oz, gal. **Swab:** Saturated with
soln. Pkt. 1s, Box 100s. **Swabsticks:**
Saturated with soln. Pkt. 1s, Box 50s.
Pkt. 3s, Box 75s.
Use: Antiseptic, topical.

Presalin. (Roberts) Aspirin 260 mg, salicylamide 120 mg, acetaminophen
120 mg, aluminum hydroxide 100 mg.
Tab. Bot. 50s. *OTC.*
Use: Analgesic combination; antacid.

Prescription Strength Desenex. (Novartis) **Spray Liq.:** Miconazole nitrate 2%.
105 mL. **Spray Pow.:** Miconazole nitrate 2%. 90 mL. **Cream:** Clotrimazole
1%. Tube 15 g. *OTC.*
Use: Antifungal, topical.

Preservative Free Moisture Eyes.
(Bausch & Lomb) Propylene glycol
0.95%, boric acid, NaCl, KCl, sodium
borate, EDTA. Soln. UD 32s. *OTC.*
Use: Artificial tear solution.

pressor agents.
See: Sympathomimetic agents.

Pressorol. (Baxter PPI) Metaraminol bitartrate 10 mg/mL. Inj. Vial 10 mL. *Rx.*
Use: Vasoconstrictor.

PreSun Active. (Bristol-Myers Squibb)
Octyl methoxycinnamate, oxybenzone,
octyl salicylate, 69% SD alcohol 40.
PABA free. Waterproof. SPF 15, 30.
Gel. 120 g. *OTC.*
Use: Sunscreen.

PreSun 8 Creamy. (Bristol-Myers
Squibb) Padimate O 5%, oxybenzone
2%. Waterproof. SPF 8. Bot. 4 oz. *OTC.*
Use: Sunscreen.

OTC.
Use: Anorectal preparation.

PreSun 8 Lotion. (Bristol-Myers Squibb) Padimate O 7.3%, oxybenzone 2.3%, SD alcohol 40 60%. SPF 8. Bot. 4 oz. *OTC.*
Use: Sunscreen.

PreSun 15 Creamy. (Bristol-Myers Squibb) Padimate O 8%, oxybenzone 3%, benzyl alcohol. Waterproof. SPF 15. Bot. 4 oz. *OTC.*
Use: Sunscreen.

PreSun 15 Facial Sunscreen. (Bristol-Myers Squibb) Padimate O (octyl dimethyl PABA) 8%, oxybenzone 3%. SPF 15. Bot. 2 oz. *OTC.*
Use: Sunscreen.

PreSun 15 Facial Sunscreen Stick. (Bristol-Myers Squibb) Octyl dimethyl PABA 8%, oxybenzone 3%. SPF 15. Stick 0.42 oz. *OTC.*
Use: Sunscreen.

PreSun 15 Lip Protector. (Bristol-Myers Squibb) Padimate O 8%, oxybenzone 3%. SPF 15. Stick 4.5 g. *OTC.*
Use: Sunscreen.

PreSun 15 Lotion. (Bristol-Myers Squibb) Padimate O 5%, PABA 5%, oxybenzone 3%, SD alcohol 40 58%. SPF 15. Bot. 4 oz. *OTC.*
Use: Sunscreen.

PreSun 15 Sensitive Skin Sunscreen. (Bristol-Myers Squibb) Octyl methoxycinnamate, oxybenzone, octyl salicylate, cetyl alcohol, PABA free, waterproof, SPF 15. Cream. Bot. 120 mL. *OTC.*
Use: Sunscreen.

PreSun for Kids. (Bristol-Myers Squibb) **Cream:** Octyl methoxycinnamate, oxybenzone, octyl salicylate, cetyl alcohol, PABA free. Waterproof. SPF 29. Bot. 120 mL. **Liq.:** Padimate O, octyl methoxycinnamate, oxybenzone, octyl salicylate, SD alcohol 40 19%. Waterproof. SPF 23. Spray Bot. 105 mL. *OTC.*
Use: Sunscreen.

PreSun 4 Creamy. (Bristol-Myers Squibb) Padimate O 1.4%, alcohol, titanium dioxide. Waterproof. Lot. SPF 4. Bot. 4 oz. *OTC.*
Use: Sunscreen.

PreSun Moisturizing. (Bristol-Myers Squibb) Octyl dimethyl PABA, oxybenzone, cetyl alcohol, diazolidinyl urea. SPF 46. Lot. Bot. 120 mL. *OTC.*
Use: Sunscreen.

PreSun Moisturizing Sunscreen with Keri, SPF 15. (Bristol-Myers Squibb) Octyl dimethyl PABA, oxybenzone, cetyl alcohol, diazolidinyl urea. Waterproof. Lot. Bot. 120 mL. *OTC.*

Use: Sunscreen.

PreSun Moisturizing Sunscreen with Keri, SPF 25. (Bristol-Myers Squibb) Octyl methoxycinnamate, oxybenzone, octyl salicylate, petrolatum, cetyl alcohol, diazolidinyl urea. Waterproof. Lot. Bot. 120 mL. *OTC.*
Use: Sunscreen.

PreSun Spray Mist. (Bristol-Myers Squibb) Octyl dimethyl PABA, octyl methoxycinnamate, oxybenzone, octyl salicylate, 19% SD alcohol 40, C12-15 alcohols benzoate. Waterproof. SPF 23. Liq. Bot. 120 mL. *OTC.*
Use: Sunscreen.

PreSun 39 Creamy Sunscreen. (Bristol-Myers Squibb) Padimate O, oxybenzone, cetyl alcohol. Waterproof. SPF 39. Cream. Bot. 120 mL. *OTC.*
Use: Sunscreen.

PreSun 29 Sensitive Skin Sunscreen. (Bristol-Myers Squibb) Octyl methoxycinnamate, oxybenzone, octyl salicylate. Waterproof. SPF 29. Bot. 4 oz. *OTC.*
Use: Sunscreen.

PreSun 23. (Bristol-Myers Squibb) Padimate O, octyl methoxycinnamate, oxybenzone, octyl salicylate, SD alcohol 40 19%. Waterproof. SPF 23. Spray mist. Bot. 105 mL. *OTC.*
Use: Sunscreen.

PreSun Ultra. (Westwood Squibb) Avobenzone 3%, octyl methoxycinnamate 7.5%, octyl salicylate 5%, oxybenzone 6%. SPF 30. SD alcohol 65.5%. Gel. 120 mL. *OTC.*
Use: Sunscreen.

Pretend-U-Ate. (Vitalax) Enriched candy-appetite pacifier. Pkg. 20s. *OTC.*
Use: Dietary aid.

prethcamide. Mixture of crotethamide and cropropamide.
See: Micoren.

Pretts Diet Aid. (Milance Laboratories, Inc.) Alginic acid 200 mg, sodium carboxymethylcellulose 100 mg, sodium bicarbonate 70 mg. Chew. Tab. Bot. 60s. *OTC.*
Use: Dietary aid.

Pretty Feet & Hands. (B.F. Ascher) Paraffin, triethanolamine, parabens. Cream 90 g. *OTC.*
Use: Emollient.

Pretz-D. (Parnell) Ephedrine sulfate 0.25%, yerba santa. Soln. Spray Bot. 50 mL. *OTC.*
Use: Nasal decongestant, arylalkylamine.

Pretz Irrigation. (Parnell) Sodium chloride, yerba santa. Soln. Spray bot.

273 mL. *OTC.*
Use: Nasal decongestant.
Pretz Moisturizing. (Parnell) Sodium chloride, glycerin, yerba santa. Soln. Spray bot. 50 mL. *OTC.*
Use: Nasal decongestant.
Prevacid. (TAP Pharma) Lansoprazole. **DR Cap.:** 15 mg, 30 mg, enteric-coated granules, sugar spheres, sucrose. Bot. 100s (30 mg only), 1000s, unit-of-use 30s, (15 mg only) UD 100s. **Gran. for DR Oral Susp.:** 15 mg, 30 mg, enteric-coated granules, sugar, mannitol, docusate sodium, strawberry flavor. UD 30s. **Orally Disintegrating DR Tab.:** 15 mg (phenylalanine 2.5 mg), 30 mg (5.1 mg). Mannitol, lactose, aspartame, strawberry flavor. Enteric-coated granules. UD 30s. *Rx.*
Use: Proton pump inhibitor.
Prevacid IV. (TAP Pharm) Lansoprazole 30 mg/vial, mannitol 60 mg, meglumine 10 mg. Pow. for Inj., lyophilized. Single-dose vials with in-line filters. *Rx.*
Use: Proton pump inhibitor.
Prevacid NapraPAC. (TAP) Naproxen (Tab.)/lansoprazole (DR Cap.) 375 mg/ 15 mg, 500 mg/15 mg. Sucrose. Kit. Blister cards. *Rx.*
Use: Nonnarcotic analgesic.
Prevacid SoluTab. (TAP Pharma) Lansoprazole 15 mg (phenylalanine 2.5 mg), 30 mg (phenylalanine 5.1 mg). Mannitol, lactase, aspartame, strawberry flavor. DR Orally Disintegrating Tab. UD 30s. *Rx.*
Use: Proton pump inhibitor.
Prevalite. (Upsher Smith) Cholestyramine 4 g (as anhydrous cholestyramine resin)/5.5 g powder, aspartame, phenylalanine 14.1 mg/5.5 g, orange flavor. Pow. for Susp. Box. 5.5 g single-dose packet (42s, 60s). Can. 231 g (42 doses). *Rx.*
Use: Antihyperlipidemic; bile acid sequestrant.
Preven. (Gynetics) Levonorgestrel 0.25 mg, ethinyl estradiol 0.05 mg, lactose. Tab. Blister pkg. 4s. *Rx.*
Use: Sex hormone, contraceptive hormone.
Prevident Disclosing. (Colgate Oral) Erythrosine sodium 1%. **Drops:** Bot. 1 oz. **Tab.:** UD strip 1000s.
Use: Diagnostic aid, dental plaque.
Prevident 5000 Plus. (Colgate Oral) Sodium fluoride 1.1%, sorbitol, saccharin, spearmint and fruit flavors. Dental Cream. Tube 51 g (1s, 2s). *Rx.*
Use: Caries prevention.

Prevident Prophylaxis Paste. (Colgate Oral) Sodium fluoride containing 1.2% fluoride ion w/pumice and alumina abrasives. Cup 2 g, Box 200s. Jar 9 oz. *Rx.*
Use: Dental caries agent.
Prevident Rinse. (Colgate Oral) Neutral sodium fluoride 0.2%, alcohol 6%. Sol. Bot. 250 mL, gal (w/pump dispenser). *Rx.*
Use: Dental caries agent.
Preview. (Lafayette) Barium sulfate 60% w/v suspension. Bot. 355 mL, Case 24 bot.
Use: Radiopaque agent.
Preview 2000. Barium sulfate 60% w/v suspension. Bot. 2000 mL, Case 4 Bot.
Use: Radiopaque agent.
Prevision. Mestranol, USP.
Prevnar. (Wyeth Lederle Vaccines) 6 polysaccharide isolates 2 mcg each, 1 polysaccharide isolate 4 mcg per 0.5 mL, aluminum 0.125 mg/dose. Inj. Vial 0.5 mL. *Rx.*
Use: Immunization.
Prevpac. (TAP Pharmaceuticals) Two *Prevacid* (lansoprazole) 30 mg Cap. Four *Trimox* (amoxicillin) 500 mg Cap. Two *Biaxin* (clarithromycin) 500 mg. Tab. Daily administration pack.
Use: H. pylori eradication.
Prexonate. (Tennessee Pharmaceutic) Vitamins A acetate 5000 units, D 500 units, B_6 2 mg, B_1 5 mg, B_2 2 mg, C 100 mg, B_{12} 2.5 mcg, calcium pantothenate 1 mg, niacinamide 15 mg, folic acid 1 mg, Fe 45 mg, Ca 500 mg, intrinsic factor 3 mg. Tab. Bot. 100s, 1000s. *Rx.*
Use: Mineral, vitamin supplement.
•**prezatide copper acetate.** (PREH-zat-IDE KAH-per) USAN.
Use: Immunomodulator.
Prialt. (Elan) Ziconotide 25 mcg/mL (used onlly for ziconotide-naive pump priming), 100 mcg/mL. Preservative free. L-methionine. Inj. Single-use vials. 1 mL, 2 mL, 5 mL (100 mcg/mL only); 20 mL (25 mcg/mL only). *Rx.*
Use: Management of severe chronic pain.
•**pridefine hydrochloride.** (PRIH-deh-FEEN) USAN.
Use: Antidepressant.
Prid Salve. (Walker) Ichthammol, Phenol, Lead Oleate, Rosin, Beeswax, Lard. Tin 20 g. *OTC.*
Use: Drawing salve.
•**prifelone.** (PRIH-feh-LONE) USAN.
Use: Anti-inflammatory, dermatologic.

Priftin. (Aventis) Rifapentine 150 mg. EDTA, polyethylene glycol. Tab. Bot. 32s. *Rx.*
Use: Antituberculosal.

•**priliximab.** (prih-LICK-sih-mab) USAN.
Use: Monoclonal antibody (autoimmune lymphoproliferative diseases, organ transplantation).

•**prilocaine.** (PRILL-oh-cane) USAN.
Use: Anesthetic, local.
W/Lidocaine.
See: EMLA Anesthetic.

prilocaine and epinephrine injection.
Use: Anesthetic, local.

•**prilocaine hydrochloride.** *USP 28.*
Use: Anesthetic, local amide.
See: Citanest Forte.
Citanest Plain.

Prilosec. (AstraZeneca) Omeprazole 10 mg, 20 mg, 40 mg, lactose, mannitol. Enteric-coated granules. DR Cap. Bot. 100s (40 mg only), 1000s, unit-of-use 30s. *Rx.*
Use: Antiulcerative; proton pump inhibitor.

Prilosec OTC. (Proctor and Gamble) Omeprazole magnesium 20 mg. Sucrose, talc. DR Tab. 14s, 28s, 42s. *OTC.*
Use: Proton pump inhibitor.

primacaine.
Use: Anesthetic, local.

Primacor. (Sanofi-Synthelabo) Milrinone lactate. **Inj..** 1 mg/mL, anhydrous dextrose 47 mg. Single-dose vial 10 mL, 20 mL. **Inj., Premixed:** 200 mcg/mL in dextrose 5%, lactic acid 0.282 mg/mL. Vial 100 mL. *Rx.*
Use: Cardiovascular agent; inotropic agent.
See: Milrinone.

•**primaquine phosphate.** (PRIM-uh-kween) *USP 28.*
Use: Antimalarial.

primaquine phosphate. (Sanofi-Synthelabo) Primaquine phosphate 26.3 mg. Tab. Bot. 100s.
Use: Antimalarial.

primaquine phosphate. (Sanofi-Synthelabo)
Use: Treatment of AIDS-associated PCP. [Orphan Drug]

Primatene. (Whitehall-Robins) Ephedrine hydrochloride 12.5 mg, guaifenesin 200 mg. Tab. Bot. 24s, 60s. *OTC.*
Use: Upper respiratory combination, decongestant, expectorant.

Primatene M. (Whitehall-Robins) Theophylline 118 mg, ephedrine hydrochloride 24 mg, pyrilamine maleate 16.6 mg. Tab. Bot. 24s, 60s. *OTC.*
Use: Antihistamine, bronchodilator.

Primatene Mist. (Whitehall-Robins) Epinephrine 0.22 mg/spray, alcohol 34%. Aer. Bot. 15 mL w/mouthpiece or 15 mL, 22.5 mL refills. *OTC.*
Use: Bronchodilator, sympathomimetic.

Primatene Mist Suspension. (Whitehall-Robins) Epinephrine bitartrate 0.3 mg. Bot. 10 mL w/mouthpiece. Spray. *OTC.*
Use: Bronchodilator.

Primatene P. (Whitehall-Robins) Theophylline 118 mg, ephedrine hydrochloride 24 mg, phenobarbital 8 mg. Tab. Bot. 24s, 60s. *OTC.*
Use: Bronchodilator; hypnotic; sedative.

Primatuss Cough Mixture 4. (Rugby) Doxylamine succinate 3.75 mg, dextromethorphan HBr 7.5 mg/5 mL, alcohol 10%. Liq. Bot. 180 mL. *OTC.*
Use: Antihistamine; antitussive.

Primatuss Cough Mixture 4D. (Rugby) Pseudoephedrine hydrochloride 20 mg, dextromethorphan HBr 10 mg, guaifenesin 67 mg/5 mL, alcohol 10%. Liq. Bot. 120 mL. *OTC.*
Use: Antitussive; decongestant; expectorant.

Primaxin. (Merck & Co.) Imipenem (anhydrous equivalent), cilastatin w/sodium bicarbonate buffer. **250-250:** *ADD-Vantage* Vial, Tray 10s, 25s. Tray 10 infusion bottles. **500-500:** *ADD-Vantage* Vial, Tray 10s, 25s. Tray 10 infusion bottles. *Rx.*
Use: Anti-infective.

Primaxin I.M. (Merck & Co.) Imipenem 500 mg, cilastatin 500 mg, Na 1.4 mEq. Imipenem 750 mg, cilastatin 750 mg, Na 2.1 mEq. Pow. for Inj. Vial. *Rx.*
Use: Anti-infective.

Primaxin I.V. (Merck & Co.) Imipenem 250 mg, cilastatin 250 mg, Na 0.8 mEq. Imipenem 500 mg, cilastatin 500 mg, Na 1.6 mEq. Pow. for Inj. Infusion bot., *ADD-Vantage* vial. *Rx.*
Use: Anti-infective.

•**primidolol.** (prih-MID-oh-lahl) USAN.
Use: Antianginal; antihypertensive; cardiovascular agent, antiarrhythmic.

•**primidone.** (PRIM-ih-dohn) *USP 28.*
Use: Anticonvulsant.
See: Mysoline.

primidone. (Lannett) Primidone 50 mg. Tab. 100s, 500s, 1000s. *Rx.*
Use: Anticonvulsant.

primidone. (Various Mfr.) Primidone 250 mg. Tab. Bot. 100s, 500s, 1000s. *Rx.*

Use: Anticonvulsant.

primostrum. A prep. of primiparous colostrum.

Primsol. (Ascent Pediatrics) Trimethoprim 50 mg/5 mL, parabens, sorbitol, alcohol free, bubble gum flavor. Oral Soln. Bot. 473 mL. *Rx.*
Use: Anti-infective.

Principen. (Geneva) Ampicillin trihydrate. **Cap.:** 250 mg, 500 mg, lactose. Bot. 100s, 500s, UD 100s. **Pow. for Oral Susp.:** 125 mg/5 mL, 250 mg/5 mL, sucrose, fruit flavor. Bot. 100 mL, 150 mL (125 mg/5 mL only), 200 mL. *Rx.*
Use: Anti-infective, penicillin.

Principen with Probenecid. (Bristol-Myers Squibb) Ampicillin (as trihydrate) 3.5 g, probenecid 1 g/regimen. Single-dose Bot. 9s. *Rx.*
Use: Anti-infective, penicillin.

Prinivil. (Merck) Lisinopril 2.5 mg, 5 mg, 10 mg, 20 mg, 40 mg, mannitol. Tab. Bot. 1000s (5 mg, 10 mg, 20 mg), 10,000s (5 mg, 10 mg, 20 mg), unit-of-use 30s (2.5 mg, 10 mg, 20 mg only), 90s (5 mg, 10 mg, 20 mg only), 100s, UD 100s (except 40 mg), blister pack 31s (except 2.5 mg, 40 mg). *Rx.*
Use: Antihypertensive.

• **prinomastat.** (pri-NOE-ma-stat) USAN.
Use: Antineoplastic; antiangiogenic; retinal and subfoveal choroidal neovascularization.

• **prinomide tromethamine.** (PRIH-no-MIDE troe-METH-ah-meen) USAN.
Use: Antirheumatic.

• **prinoxodan.** (prin-OX-oh-dan) USAN.
Use: Cardiovascular agent.

Prinzide. (Merck & Co.) Lisinopril 10 mg, 20 mg, hydrochlorothiazide 12.5 mg. Tab. Lisinopril 20 mg, hydrochlorothiazide 25 mg. Tab. Bot. 30s, 100s. *Rx.*
Use: Antihypertensive.

Privine. (Heritage) Naphazoline hydrochloride, benzalkonium chloride, EDTA. Soln. Dropper bot. 25 mL. Spray bot. 20 mL. *OTC.*
Use: Nasal decongestant, imidazoline.

• **prizidilol hydrochloride.** (PRIH-zie-DILL-ole) USAN.
Use: Antihypertensive.

Pro-Acet Douche Concentrate. (Pro-Acet) Lactic, citric, and acetic acids, sodium lauryl sulfate, lactose, dextrose, sodium acetate. Pkg. polyethylene envelope 10 mL. Contents of 1 envelope to be diluted with 2 quarts of water. Douche 6 oz, 12 oz. Travel Packet 10 mL. *OTC.*
Use: Vaginal agent.

• **proadifen hydrochloride.** (pro-AD-ih-fen) USAN.
Use: Synergist, nonspecific.

ProAmatine. (Shire) Midodrine hydrochloride 2.5 mg, 5 mg, 10 mg. Tab. Bot. 100s. *Rx.*
Use: Orthostatic hypotension.

Pro-Banthine. (Schiapparelli Searle) Propantheline bromide. Tab. **7.5 mg:** Bot. 100s. **15 mg:** Bot. 100s, 500s, UD 100s. *Rx.*
Use: Anticholinergic.

Probarbital Sodium. 5-Ethyl-5-isopropyl-barbiturate sodium.

Probax. (Fischer) Propolis 2%, petrolatum, mineral oil, lanolin. Gel. Tube 3.5 g. *OTC.*
Use: Mouth and throat preparation.

Probec-T. (Roberts) Vitamins B_1 12.2 mg, B_2 10 mg, B_3 100 mg, B_5 18.4, B_6 4.1 mg, B_{12} 5 mcg, C 600 mg. Tab. Bot. 60s. *OTC.*
Use: Mineral, vitamin supplement.

Proben-C. (Rugby) Probenecid 500 mg, colchicine 0.5 mg. Tab. Bot. 100s, 1000s. *Rx.*
Use: Antigout agent.

• **probenecid.** (pro-BEN-uh-sid) *USP 28.*
Use: Uricosuric.
W/Ampicillin.
 See: Amcill-GC.
  Principen w/Probenecid.

probenecid and colchicine.
Use: Agent for gout.

probenecid and colchicine. (Various Mfr.) Probenecid 500 mg, colchicine 0.5 mg. Tab. Bot. 100s, 1000s. *Rx.*
Use: Agent for gout.

• **probicromil calcium.** (pro-BYE-KROE-mill) USAN.
Use: Antiallergic, prophylactic.

Pro-Bionate. (NaTREN) *Lactobacillus acidophilus* strain NAS 2 billion units/g. **Pow.:** 52.5 g, 90 g. **Cap.:** Bot. 30s, 60s. *OTC.*
Use: Antidiarrheal; nutritional supplement.

• **probucol.** (PRO-byoo-kahl) *USP 28.*
Use: Antihyperlipidemic.
 See: Lorelco.

• **probutate.** (pro-BYOO-tate) USAN. Formerly buteprate.
Use: Radical.

procainamide hydrochloride. (Various Mfr.) Procainamide hydrochloride. **Cap.:** 250 mg, 375 mg, 500 mg. Bot. 100s, 250s, 1000s. **ER Tab.:** 250 mg, 500 mg, 750 mg, 1000 mg. Bot. 100s, 500s (except 1000 mg). **Inj.:** 500 mg/mL. Vial 2 mL. *Rx.*

Use: Antiarrhythmic.

• **procainamide hydrochloride.** (pro-CANE-uh-mide) *USP 28.*
Use: Cardiovascular agent, antiarrhythmic.
See: Procanbid.

procaine and phenylephrine hydrochlorides injection.
Use: Anesthetic, local.

procaine and tetracaine hydrochlorides and levonordefrin injection.
Use: Anesthetic, local.

procaine base.
Use: Anesthetic, local.
See: Anucaine.

• **procaine hydrochloride.** (pro-CANE) *USP 28.* Bernocaine, Chlorocaine, Ethocaine, Irocaine, Kerocaine, Syncaine
Use: Anesthetic, injectable local.
See: Novocain.

procaine hydrochloride. (Various Mfr.) Procaine hydrochloride 1%, 2%, may contain sodium metabisulfite. Inj. Multiple-dose vials. 30 mL.
Use: Anesthetic, injectable local.

procaine hydrochloride and epinephrine injection.
Use: Anesthetic, local.

procaine hydrochloride and levonordefrin injection.
Use: Anesthetic, local.

procaine, penicillin G suspension, sterile.
Use: Anti-infective, penicillin.
See: Penicillin G, Procaine.
Pfizerpen.

procaine, penicillin G w/aluminum stearate suspension, sterile.
Use: Anti-infective, penicillin.
See: Penicillin G Procaine with Aluminum Stearate, Sterile, USP.

procaine, tetracaine and nordefrin hydrochlorides injection.
Use: Anesthetic, local.

procaine, tetracaine and phenylephrine hydrochlorides injection.
Use: Anesthetic.

ProcalAmine Injection. (McGaw) Injection of amino acid 3%, glycerin 3%, electrolytes. Bot. 1000 mL. *Rx.*
Use: Nutritional supplement, parenteral.

Procanbid. (Monarch) Procainamide 500 mg, 1000 mg. SR Tab. Bot. 60s, UD 100s. *Rx.*
Use: Antiarrhythmic.

• **procarbazine hydrochloride.** (pro-CAR-buh-ZEEN) *USP 28.* (Roche) Natulan.
Use: Cytostatic; antineoplastic.
See: Matulane.

Procardia. (Pfizer) Nifedipine 10 mg. Saccharin. Cap. Bot. 100s, 300s. *Rx.*
Use: Calcium channel blocker.

Procardia XL. (Pfizer) Nifedipine. ER Tab. **30 mg, 60 mg:** Bot. 100s, 300s, 5000s, UD 100s. **90 mg:** Bot 100s, UD 100s. *Rx.*
Use: Calcium channel blocker.

• **procaterol hydrochloride.** (PRO-CAT-ehr-ole) USAN.
Use: Bronchodilator.

Proception Sperm Nutrient Douche. (Milex) Ringer type glucose douche. Bot. sufficient for 10 douches. *OTC.*
Use: Vaginal agent.

Prochieve. (Columbia) Progesterone 4% (45 mg), 8% (90 mg), glycerin, mineral oil. Vaginal Gel. Single-use prefilled disposable applicators delivering 1.125 g gel. 6s, 18s (8% only). *Rx.*
Use: Progestin, sex hormone.

• **prochlorperazine.** (pro-klor-PURR-uh-zeen) *USP 28.*
Use: Antiemetic, antipsychotic.
See: Compazine.
Compro.

prochlorperazine. (Various Mfr.) Prochlorperazine 25 mg. Supp. 12s. *Rx.*
Use: Antiemetic, antipsychotic.

• **prochlorperazine edisylate.** *USP 28.*
Use: Antipsychotic; antiemetic.
See: Compazine.

prochlorperazine edisylate. (Various Mfr.) Prochlorperazine edisylate 5 mg/mL. Inj. 2 mL vials. *Rx.*
Use: Antipsychotic.

prochlorperazine ethanedisulfonate. Prochlorperazine Edisylate, USP.
Use: Anxiolytic.

prochlorperazine/isopropamide. (Various Mfr.) Isopropamide iodide 5 mg, prochlorperazine maleate 10 mg. Cap. Bot. 100s, 500s, 1000s, UD 100s. *Rx.*
Use: Anticholinergic; antispasmodic; antiemetic; antivertigo.

• **prochlorperazine maleate.** *USP 28.*
Use: Antiemetic; antipsychotic.
See: Compazine.

prochlorperazine maleate. (Various Mfr.) Prochlorperazine maleate 5 mg, 10 mg. Tab. Bot. 100s, 500s, 1000s, UD 100s. Blister packs. 25s. *Rx.*
Use: Antipsychotic.

• **procinonide.** (pro-SIN-oh-nide) USAN.
Use: Adrenocortical steroid.

• **proclonol.** (PRO-klah-nole) USAN. Under study.
Use: Anthelmintic; antifungal.

Pro Comfort Athlete's Foot Spray. (Scholl) Tolnaftate 1%. Aer. Can 4 oz. *OTC.*
Use: Antifungal, topical.

Pro Comfort Jock Itch Spray Powder. (Scholl) Tolnaftate 1%. Aer. Can 3.5 oz. *OTC.*
Use: Antifungal, topical.

Procort. (Roberts) Hydrocortisone 1%. **Cream:** Tube 30 g. **Spray:** Can. 45 mL. *OTC.*
Use: Corticosteroid, topical.

Procrit. (Ortho Biotech) Epoetin alfa, recombinant 2,000 units/mL, 3,000 units/mL , 4,000 units/mL, 10,000 units/mL, 20,000 units/mL, 40,000 units/mL. Inj. Single-dose vials. 1 mL, preservative free with albumin (human) 2.5 mg/mL (except 20,000 units/mL). Multidose vials. 1 mL (20,000 units/mL only) and 2 mL (10,000 units only), preserved with benzyl alcohol 1% and with albumin (human) 2.5 mg/mL. *Rx.*
Use: Hematopoietic.

Proctocort. (Salix) Hydrocortisone. Cream 30 g w/rectal applicator. Hydrocortisone acetate 30 mg. Supp. Box. 12s. *Rx.*
Use: Corticosteroid.

ProctoCream-HC 2.5%. (Schwarz Pharma) Hydrocortisone 2.5%, glyceryl monostearate, glycerin, stearyl alcohol, benzyl alcohol. Cream. Tube 30 g. *Rx.*
Use: Corticosteroid.

ProctoFoam. (Schwarz Pharma) Pramoxine hydrochloride 1% in an anesthetic muco adhesive foam base. Foam. Can. 15 g. *OTC.*
Use: Anorectal preparation.

ProctoFoam-HC. (Schwarz Pharma) Hydrocortisone acetate 1%, pramoxine hydrochloride 1% in hydrophilic foam base. Bot. aerosol container, Aerosol foam 10 g w/applicator. *Rx.*
Use: Corticosteroid; anesthetic, local.

ProctoFoam NS. (Schwarz Pharma) Pramoxine hydrochloride 1%. Aer. Bot. 15 g w/applicator. *OTC.*
Use: Anesthetic, local.

Pro-Cute. (Ferndale) Silicone, hexachlorophene, lanolin. Cream. 2 oz, lb. *OTC.*
Use: Emollient.

ProCycle Gold. (Cyclin) Vitamins A 833.3 units, D 66.7 units, E 66.7 units, C 30 mg, B_1 1.7 mg, B_2 1.7 mg, B_3 3.3 mg, B_5 1.7 mg, B_6 3.3 mg, B_{12} 21 mcg, folic acid 66.7 mg, Ca 166.7 mg, Fe 3 mg, Zn 2.5 mg, B, Cu,

Cr, I, Mg, Mn, Se, PABA, inositol, rutin, biotin, hesperidin, pancreatin, betaine. Tab. Sugar free. Bot. 100s. *OTC.*
Use: Mineral, vitamin supplement.

•**procyclidine hydrochloride.** (pro-SI-klih-deen) *USP 28.*
Use: Muscle relaxant; antiparkinsonian.
See: Kemadrin.

Procysteine. (Free Radical Sciences)
See: L_2-Oxothiazolidine$_4$-carboxylic acid.

Proderm Topical Dressing. (Dow Hickam) Castor oil 650 mg, peruvian balsam 72.5 mg/0.82 mL. Aer. 4 oz. *OTC.*
Use: Dermatologic, wound therapy.

•**prodilidine hydrochloride.** (pro-DIH-lih-deen) USAN.
Use: Analgesic.

Prodium. (Breckenridge) Phenazopyramide hydrochloride 90 mg. Tab. Pkg. 12s, Bot. 30s. *OTC.*
Use: Analgesic.

•**prodolic acid.** (PRO-dole-ik acid) USAN.
Use: Anti-inflammatory.

Pro-Est. (Burgin-Arden) Progesterone 25 mg, estrogenic substance 25,000 units, sodium carboxymethylcellulose 1 mg, sodium Cl 0.9%, benzalkonium Cl 1:10,000, sodium phosphate dibasic 0.1% in water. *Rx.*
Use: Estrogen, progestin combination.

•**profadol hydrochloride.** (PRO-fah-dahl) USAN.
Use: Analgesic.

profamina.
See: Amphetamine.

Profasi. (Serono) Chorionic gonadotropin 5000 units/per vial with 10 mL diluent (500 units per mL), 10,000 units/per vial with 10 mL diluent (1,000 units per mL). Mannitol, benzyl alcohol 0.9%. Pow. for Inj. Vials. 10 mL. *Rx.*
Use: Ovulation stimulant.

Pro-Fast HS. (American Pharmaceutical) Phentermine hydrochloride 18.75 mg (equivalent to 15 mg phentermine base), EDTA, benzyl alcohol, parabens. Cap. Bot. 100s. *c-IV.*
Use: CNS stimulant, anorexiant.

Pro-Fast SA. (American Pharmaceutical) Phentermine hydrochloride 8 mg, lactose, tartrazine. Tab. Bot. 100s. *c-IV.*
Use: CNS stimulant, anorexiant.

Pro-Fast SR. (American Pharmaceutical) Phentermine hydrochloride 37.5 mg (equivalent to 30 mg phentermine base), sugar, tartrazine, EDTA, benzyl alcohol, parabens. Cap. Bot. 100s. *c-IV.*

Use: CNS stimulant, anorexiant.
Profenal. (Alcon) Suprofen 1%. Soln.
Drop-Tainer 2.5 mL. *Rx.*
Use: NSAID, ophthalmic.
Profen II. (IVAX) Pseudoephedrine hydrochloride 45 mg, guaifenesin 800 mg. ER Tab. Bot. 100s. *Rx.*
Use: Upper respiratory combination, decongestant, expectorant.
Profen II DM. (IVAX) Pseudoephedrine hydrochloride 45 mg, guaifenesin 800 mg, dextromethorphan HBr 30 mg. ER Tab. Bot. 100s. *Rx.*
Use: Upper respiratory combination, antitussive, decongestant, expectorant.
Profen Forte. (IVAX) Pseudoephedrine hydrochloride 90 mg, guaifenesin 800 mg. ER Tab. Bot. 100s *Rx.*
Use: Upper respiratory combination; decongestant, expectorant.
Profen Forte DM. (IVAX) Pseudoephedrine hydrochloride 90 mg, dextromethorphan HBr 60 mg, guaifenesin 800 mg. SR Tab. Bot. 100s. *Rx.*
Use: Upper respiratory combination, antitussive, antihistamine, decongestant, expectorant.
Professional Care Lotion, Extra Strength. (Walgreen) Zinc oxide 0.25% in a lotion base. Lot. Bot. 16 oz. *OTC.*
Use: Astringent; antiseptic, dermatologic.
Profiber. (Sherwood Davis & Geck) Sodium caseinate, dietary fiber from soy, calcium caseinate, hydrolyzed cornstarch, corn oil, soy lecithin, vitamins A, B$_1$, B$_2$, B$_3$, B$_5$, B$_6$, B$_{12}$, C, D, E, K, folic acid, biotin, choline, Ca, Cl, Cr, Cu, Fe, I, Mg, Mn, Mo, P, Se, Zn. Liq. Can 250 mL, closed system 1000 mL. *OTC.*
Use: Nutritional supplement.
Profilnine SD. (Grifols) Sterile, lyophilized concentrate of Factor IX, plasma-derived. Preservative and heparin free. Solvent/detergent treated. Pow. for Inj. Single-dose vials 250 U, 500 U, 1000 U with diluent. *Rx.*
Use: Antihemophilic.
proflavine dihydrochloride. 3,6-Diaminoacridine dihydrochloride.
proflavine sulfate. 3,6-Diaminoacridine sulfate.
ProFree/GP Weekly Enzymatic Cleaner. (Allergan) Papain, sodium Cl, sodium borate, sodium carbonate, edetate disodium. Kit 16s or 24s with vials. *OTC.*
Use: Contact lens care.
•**progabide.** (pro-GAB-ide) USAN.
Use: Anticonvulsant, muscle relaxant.

Progens. (Major) Conjugated estrogens. Tab. **0.625 mg:** Bot. 100s, 1000s. **1.25 mg:** Bot. 1000s. **2.5 mg:** Bot. 100s, 1000s. *Rx.*
Use: Estrogen.
Pro-Gesic. (Nastech) Trolamine salicylate 10%, propylene glycol, methylparahydroxybenzoic acid, propyl parahydroxybenzoic acid, EDTA. Liq. Bot. 75 mL. *OTC.*
Use: Liniment.
Progestasert. (Alza) T-shaped intrauterine device (IUD) unit containing a reservoir of progesterone 38 mg with barium sulfate dispersed in medical grade silicone fluid. Intrauterine system. In 6s w/inserter. *Rx.*
Use: Contraceptive.
•**progesterone.** (pro-JESS-ter-ohn) /HSP'sn Flavolutan, Luteogan, Lutean-san, Lutren.
Use: Hormone, progestin.
See: Crinone.
W/Aqueous. Susp.
See: Prorone.
W/Estradiol, testosterone, procaine hydrochloride, procaine base.
See: Hormo-Triad.
W/Oil.
See: Crinone.
Femotrone.
Lipo-Lutin.
Prochieve.
Progestin.
Prometrium.
Prorone.
progesterone. (Various Mfr.) Progesterone Pow. 1 g, 10 g, 25 g, 100 g, 1000 g.
Use: Hormone, progestin.
progesterone in oil. (Various Mfr.) Progesterone 50 mg/mL. In sesame or peanut oil with benzyl alcohol. Inj. Vials 10 mL. Multidose vials 10 mL. *Rx.*
Use: Hormone, progestin.
progesterone intrauterine contraceptive system.
Use: Contraceptive.
progestins. Progesterone.
Use: Sex hormone.
See: Estrogens and progestins.
Medroxyprogesterone.
Medroxyprogesterone acetate.
Megestrol.
Megestrol acetate.
Micronor.
Norethindrone.
Norethindrone acetate.
Nor-QD.
Ovrette.
Progesterone.

•**proglumide.** (pro-GLUE-mid) USAN. (Wallace)
Use: Anticholinergic.
Proglycem. (Baker Norton) **Cap.:** Diazoxide 50 mg. Bot. 100s. **Oral Susp.:** Diazoxide 50 mg/mL. Bot. 30 mL w/calibrated dropper. *Rx.*
Use: Hyperglycemic.
Prograf. (Fujisawa) Tacrolimus. **Cap.:** 0.5 mg, 1 mg, 5 mg, lactose. Bot. 60s (0.5 mg only), 100s, blister cards of 100 (except 0.5 mg). **Inj.:** 5 mg/mL, polyoxyl 60 hydrogenated castor oil (HCO-60) 200 mg/mL, dehydrated alcohol 80%. Amp. 1 mL. *Rx.*
Use: Immunosuppressant.
proguanil hydrochloride.
See: Chloroguanide hydrochloride.
W/Atovaquone.
See: Malarone.
Malarone Pediatric.
ProHance. (Bracco Diagnostics) Gadoteridol 279.3 mg/mL, preservative free. Inj. Vial 5 mL fill in 15 mL; 10 mL, 15 mL, 20 mL fill in 30 mL. Prefilled syr. 10 mL, 17 ml fill in 20 mL. *Rx.*
Use: Radiopaque agent, parenteral.
ProHIBiT. (Aventis Pasteur) Purified capsular polysaccharide of *Haemophilus influenzae* type b 25 mcg, conjugated diphtheria toxoid protein 18 mcg/0.5 mL dose. Also called PRP-D. Inj. Vial 0.5 mL, 2.5 mL, 5 mL. Syr. 0.5 mL. *Rx.*
Use: Immunization.
•**proinsulin human.** (PRO-in-suh-LIN HYOO-muhn) USAN.
Use: Antidiabetic.
Prolactin RIA. (Abbott Diagnostics) Quantitative measurement of total circulating human prolactin. Test unit 50s, 100s.
Use: Diagnostic aid.
Prolactin RIAbead. (Abbott Diagnostics) Radioimmunoassay for the quantitative measurement of prolactin in human serum and plasma.
Use: Diagnostic aid.
proladyl. Pyrrobutamine.
Use: Antihistamine.
prolase. Proteolytic enzyme from *Carica papaya.*
See: Papain.
Prolastin. (Bayer) Alpha$_1$-proteinase inhibitor 500 mg, 1000 mg ($\geq$ 20 mg alpha$_1$-PI/mL when reconstituted). Preservative free w/polyethylene glycol, sucrose and small amounts of other plasma proteins. Pow. for Inj., lyophilized. Single-dose vial w/20 mL diluent (500 mg only), w/40 mL diluent (1000 mg only). *Rx.*

Use: Alpha$_1$-proteinase inhibitor.
Proleukin. (Chiron) Aldesleukin (interleukin-2). Pow. for Inj., lyophilized. 22 $\times$ 10^6 units/vial (18 million units [1.1 mg/ mL] when reconstituted). Mannitol 50 mg, sodium dodecyl sulfate 0.18 mg, monobasic 0.17 mg and dibasic 0.89 mg sodium phosphate. Preservative-free. Single-use vial. *Rx.*
Use: Antineoplastic.
Prolex DH. (Blansett Pharmacal) Hydrocodone bitartrate 4.5 mg, potassium guaiacolsulfonate 300 mg/5 mL, saccharin, sorbitol, menthol, tropical fruit punch flavor, alcohol free. Liq. Bot. 25 mL, 118 mL, 473 mL. *c-III.*
Use: Upper respiratory combination, antitussive, expectorant.
•**proline.** (PRO-leen) *USP 28.*
Use: Amino acid.
•**prolintane hydrochloride.** (pro-LIN-tane) USAN.
Use: Antidepressant.
Prolixin. (Apothecon) Fluphenazine hydrochloride. **Tab.:** 1 mg, 2.5 mg, 5 mg, 10 mg. Bot. 50s, 100s, 500s, UD 100s. **Elixir:** 2.5 mg/5 mL, alcohol 14%, sucrose. Dropper Bot. 60 mL. Bot. 473 mL. **Conc.:** 5 mg/mL, alcohol 14%, Dropper Bot. 120 mL. **Inj.:** 2.5 mg/mL. Vial 10 mL w/methyl- and propylparabens. *Rx.*
Use: Antipsychotic.
Prolixin Decanoate. (Apothecon) Fluphenazine decanoate 25 mg/mL (in sesame oil with benzyl alcohol). Multidose vial 5 mL. *Rx.*
Use: Antipsychotic.
Proloprim. (GlaxoSmithKline) Trimethoprim 100 mg. Tab. Bot. 100s, UD 100s (in sesame oil with benzyl alcohol). *Rx.*
Use: Anti-infective, urinary.
Promacet. (MCR American) Acetaminophen 650 mg, butalbital 50 mg. Tab. 100s. *Rx.*
Use: Nonnarcotic analgesic.
Promachlor. (Geneva) Chlorpromazine hydrochloride 10 mg, 25 mg, 50 mg, 100 mg, 200 mg. Tab. Bot. 100s, 1000s. *Rx.*
Use: Antiemetic; antivertigo; antipsychotic.
Promega. (Parke-Davis) Omega-3 (N-3) polyunsaturated fatty acids 1000 mg, containing EPA 350 mg, DHA 150 mg, vitamins E (3% RDA), A, B$_1$, B$_2$, B$_3$, Ca, Fe (< 2% RDA). Cap., cholesterol and sodium free. Bot. 30s. *OTC.*
Use: Mineral, vitamin supplement.
Promega Pearls. (Parke-Davis) EPA 168 mg, DHA 72 mg, < cholesterol

2 mg, E 1 units, < 2% RDA of A, B₁, B₂, B₃, Fe, Ca. Cap. Bot. 60s, 90s. *OTC.*
Use: Vitamin supplement.
Prometa. (Muro) Metaproterenol sulfate 10 mg/5 mL, with saccharin and sorbitol, strawberry flavor. Syr. Bot. 480 mL. *Rx.*
Use: Bronchodilator.
•**promethazine.** (pro-METH-uh-zeen) *USP 28.*
Use: Antiemetic; antihistamine, nonselective phenothiazine.
See: Pentazine.
Phenadoz.
Phenergan.
Sigazine.
promethazine. (Alpharma) Promethazine 25 mg, hard fat. Supp. 12s. *Rx.*
Use: Antihistamine, nonselective phenothiazine.
promethazine. (Various Mfr.) Promethazine. **Tab.:** 25 mg, 50 mg. Bot. 100s, 1000s (25 mg only). **Syr.:** 6.25 mg/5 mL, alcohol. Bot. 473 mL. **Supp.:** 50 mg. Pkg. 12s. **Inj.:** 25 mg/mL, 50 mg/mL, may contain EDTA. Amp. 1 mL. *Rx.*
Use: Antiemetic; antihistamine, nonselective phenothiazine; sedative.
promethazine hydrochloride. (Able) Promethazine hydrochloride 12.5 mg. May contain lactose. Tab. 30s, 100s, 500s, 1,000s. *Rx.*
Use: Antihistamine.
promethazine hydrochloride. (Ivax) Promethazine hydrochloride 12.5 mg. May contain hard fat. Supp. 12s. *Rx.*
Use: Antihistamine.
promethazine hydrochloride and phenylephrine hydrochloride.
(Various Mfr.) Phenylephrine hydrochloride 5 mg, promethazine hydrochloride 6.25 mg/5 mL, alcohol 7%, may contain sorbitol, sugar, parabens. Syr. Bot. 118 mL, 473 mL, 3.8 L. *Rx.*
Use: Upper respiratory combination, decongestant, antihistamine.
promethazine hydrochloride w/codeine. (Various Mfr.) Codeine phosphate 10 mg, promethazine hydrochloride 6.25 mg/5 mL. Syr. Bot. 118 mL, 473 mL. *c-v.*
Use: Upper respiratory combination, antitussive, antihistamine.
promethazine hydrochloride w/combinations.
Use: Antiemetic; antihistamine; antivertigo.
See: Prometh VC w/Codeine Cough.
Prometh w/Codeine Cough.

Prometh w/Dextromethorphan.
Prometh w/Dextromethorphan Cough.
Promethazine Hydrochloride w/Codeine.
Promethazine Hydrochloride and Phenylephrine Hydrochloride.
Promethazine VC w/Codeine Cough.
Promethazine w/Dextromethorphan Cough.
Promethazine VC Plain. (Various Mfr.) Phenylephrine hydrochloride 5 mg, promethazine hydrochloride 6.25 mg/5 mL. Syr. Bot. 473 mL. *Rx.*
Use: Antihistamine; decongestant.
Promethazine VC w/Codeine Cough. (URL) Promethazine hydrochloride 6.25 mg, phenylephrine hydrochloride 5 mg, codeine phosphate 10 mg/5 mL, alcohol 7.1%, EDTA, sugar, methylparaben, cherry/raspberry flavor. Syr. Bot. 473 mL. *c-v.*
Use: Upper respiratory combination, antihistamine, antitussive, decongestant.
promethazine w/dextromethorphan cough. (Morton Grove) Dextromethorphan HBr 15 mg, promethazine hydrochloride 6.25 mg/5 mL, alcohol 7.1%, saccharin, pineapple flavor. Syr. Bot. 118 mL, 473 mL. *Rx.*
Use: Upper respiratory combination, antitussive, antihistamine.
promethestrol dipropionate.
Use: Estrogen.
Prometh VC Plain. (Alpharma) Phenylephrine hydrochloride 5 mg, promethazine hydrochloride 6.25 mg/5 mL, alcohol 7%. Syr. Bot. 3.8 L. *Rx.*
Use: Upper respiratory combination, antihistamine, decongestant.
Prometh VC w/Codeine Cough. (Alpharma) Codeine phosphate 10 mg, promethazine hydrochloride 6.25 mg, phenylephrine hydrochloride 5 mg/5 mL, alcohol 7%, parabens, sugar, saccharin. Syr. Bot. 118 mL, 237 mL, 473 mL, 3.8 L. *c-v.*
Use: Upper respiratory combination, antitussive, antihistamine, decongestant.
Prometh w/Codeine Cough. (Alpharma) Codeine phosphate 10 mg, promethazine hydrochloride 6.25 mg/5 mL, alcohol 7%, corn syrup, parabens, saccharin. Syr. Bot. 118 mL. *c-v.*
Use: Upper respiratory combination, antitussive, antihistamine.
Prometh w/Dextromethorphan. (Alpharma) Dextromethorphan HBr 15 mg, promethazine hydrochloride 6.25 mg/5 mL, alcohol 7%, parabens, saccharin,

lemon/mint flavor. Syr. Bot. 118 mL, 237 mL, 473 mL, 3.8 L. *Rx.*
Use: Upper respiratory combination, antitussive, antihistamine.

Prometol. (Viobin) Concentrated wheat germ oil. **3 min/Cap.:** Bot. 100s, 250s. **10 min/Cap.:** Bot. 100s. *OTC.*
Use: Supplement.

Prometrium. (Solvay) Progesterone (micronized) 100 mg, 200 mg, peanut oil, glycerin. Cap. Bot. 100s. *Rx.*
Use: Progestin.

prominal.
See: Mephobarbital.

Promine. (Major) Procainamide 250 mg, 375 mg, 500 mg. Cap. Bot. 100s, 250s, 1000s, UD.100s (375 mg/Cap. w/500s instead of 250s). *Rx.*
Use: Antiarrhythmic.

Promine S.R. (Major) Procainamide. **SR Tab.:** 250 mg. Bot. 100s, 250s; 500 mg. Bot. 100s, 250s, 1000s; 750 mg. **SR Cap.:** 250 mg, 375 mg, 500 mg. Bot. 100s, 250s. *Rx.*
Use: Antiarrhythmic.

Promist HD. (UCB) Hydrocodone bitartrate 2.5 mg, pseudoephedrine hydrochloride 30 mg, chlorpheniramine maleate 2 mg/5 mL, alcohol 5%, menthol, saccharin, sorbitol. Bot. Pt. *c-III.*
Use: Antihistamine; antitussive; decongestant.

Promist LA. (UCB) Pseudoephedrine hydrochloride 120 mg, guaifenesin 500 mg. Tab. Bot. 100s. *Rx.*
Use: Decongestant; expectorant.

Promit. (Pharmacia) Dextran 1 150 mg/mL Inj. Vial 20 mL. *Rx.*
Use: Antiallergic.

Pro-Mix R.D.P. (Navaco) Protein 15 g (from whey protein), fat 0.8 g, carbohydrate 1 g, Na 46 mg, K 165 mg, Cl 46 mg, Ca 73.6 mg, P 64.4 mg, Fe 0.3 mg, Cr, Cu, Mg, Mn, Mo, Se, Zn, 72 Cal./5 Tbsp. (20 g). Pow. Packet 20 g, can 300 g. *OTC.*
Use: Nutritional supplement.

ProMod. (Ross) Protein supplement. Nine scoops provides protein 45 g, 100% US RDA. Pow. Can 9.7 oz. *OTC.*
Use: Nutritional supplement.

Promylin Enteric Coated Microzymes. (Shear/Kershman) Enteric-coated pancrelipase. Lipase 4000 units, amylase 20,000 units, protease 25,000 units. *Rx.*
Use: Digestive enzymes.

Pro-Nasyl. (Progonasyl) o-Iodobenzoic acid 0.5%, triethanolamine 5.5% in a special neutral hydrophilic base compounded from oleic acid, mineral oil, vegetable oil. Bot. 15 mL, 60 mL.

Use: Treatment of sinusitis.

Pronemia Hematinic. (Wyeth) Iron 115 mg, B_{12} 15 mcg, IFC 75 mg, C 150 mg, folic acid 1 mcg. Cap. Bot. 30s. *Rx.*
Use: Iron w/B_{12} and intrinsic factor.

Pronestyl. (Bristol-Myers Squibb) Procainamide. **Cap.:** 250 mg. Bot. 100s, 1000s; 375 mg. Bot. 100s; 500 mg. Bot. 100s, 1000s. **Inj.:** 100 mg/mL w/benzyl alcohol 0.9%, sodium bisulfite 0.09%. Vial 10 mL; 500 mg/mL w/methylparaben 0.1%, sodium bisulfite 0.2%. Vial 2 mL. **Tab.:** 250 mg. Bot. 100s, 1000s, Unimatic 100s; 375 mg. Bot. 100s; 500 mg. Bot. 100s, 1000s, Unimatic 100s. *Rx.*
Use: Antiarrhythmic.

Pronestyl-SR. (Bristol-Myers Squibb) Procainamide 500 mg. Tab. Bot. UD 100s. *Rx.*
Use: Antiarrhythmic.

Pronto. (Del) Pyrethrins 0.33%, piperonyl butoxide 4%, benzyl alcohol, decyl alcohol, isopropyl alcohol. Shampoo. 60 mL, 120 mL with comb. *OTC.*
Use: Pediculicide.

Propac. (Biosearch Medical Products) Protein 3 g (from whey protein), carbohydrate 0.2 g, fat 0.3 g, Cl 3 mg, K 20 mg, Na 9 mg, Ca 24 mg, P 12 mg, 16 Cal/Tbsp. (4 g). Pow. Packet 19.5 g, Can 350 g. *OTC.*
Use: Nutritional supplement.

Propacet 100. (Teva) Propoxyphene napsylate 100 mg, acetaminophen 650 mg. Tab. Bot. 100s, 500s. *c-IV.*
Use: Analgesic combination; narcotic.

propaesin. (Various Mfr.) Propyl p-Aminobenzoate.

• **propafenone hydrochloride.** (pro-pah-FEN-ohn) *USP 28.*
Use: Antiarrhythmic agent.
See: Rythmol.
Rythmol SR.

propafenone hydrochloride. (Various Mfr.) Propafenone 150 mg, 225 mg, 300 mg. Tab. Bot. 100s, 500s (except 300 mg). *Rx.*
Use: Antiarrhythmic agent.

Propagon-S. (Spanner) Estrone 2 mg, 5 mg/mL. Vial 10 mL. *Rx.*
Use: Estrogen.

Propain HC. (Springbok) Acetaminophen 500 mg, hydrocodone bitartrate 5 mg. Cap. Bot. 100s, 500s. *c-III.*
Use: Analgesic combination; narcotic.

• **propane.** (PROE-pane) *NF 23.*
Use: Aerosol propellant.

propanediol diacetate, 1,2.
See: VoSoL.

1,2,3-propanetriol, trinitrate. Nitroglycerin Tab., USP.
•**propanidid.** (pro-PAN-ih-did) USAN.
Use: Anesthetic, intravenous.
propanolol. Propranolol.
•**propantheline bromide.** (pro-PAN-thuh-leen) *USP 28.*
Use: Anticholinergic.
See: Pro-Banthine.
W/Phenobarbital.
See: Probital.
W/Thiopropazate dihydrochloride.
See: Pro-Banthine W/Dartal.
propantheline bromide. (Various Mfr.)
Propantheline bromide 15 mg. Tab.
100s, 500s, 1,000, UD 100s. *Rx.*
Use: Anticholinergic.
PROPApH Astringent Cleanser Maximum Strength. (Del) Salicylic acid 2%, aloe vera gel, SD alcohol 40-2 55.1%. Liq. Bot. 355 mL. *OTC.*
Use: Dermatologic, acne.
PROPApH Cleansing for Oily Skin. (Del) Salicylic acid 0.6%, SD alcohol 40, EDTA, menthol. Lot. Bot. 180 mL. *OTC.*
Use: Dermatologic, acne.
PROPApH Cleansing for Sensitive Skin. (Del) Salicylic acid 0.5%, CD alcohol 40, aloe vera gel, EDTA, menthol. Pads. In 45s. *OTC.*
Use: Dermatologic, acne.
PROPApH Cleansing Lotion for Normal/Combination Skin. (Del) Salicylic acid 0.5%, SD alcohol 40, EDTA. Lot. Bot. 180 mL. Pads. 45s. *OTC.*
Use: Antiacne.
PROPApH Cleansing Maximum Strength. (Del) Salicylic acid 2%, SD alcohol 16, aloe vera gel, EDTA, propylene glycol, menthol. Pads. In 45s. *OTC.*
Use: Dermatologic, acne.
PROPApH Cleansing Pads. (Del) Salicylic acid 0.5%, SD alcohol 40, EDTA, menthol. Pads. 45s. *OTC.*
Use: Dermatologic, ance.
PROPApH Foaming Face Wash. (Del) Salicylic acid 2%, aloe vera gel, EDTA, menthol. Alcohol, oil and soap free. Liq. Bot. 180 mL. *OTC.*
Use: Dermatologic, acne.
PROPApH Maximum Strength Acne Cream. (Del) Salicylic acid 2%, acetylated lanolin alcohol, cetearyl alcohol, stearyl alcohol, EDTA, menthol. Tube 19.5 g. *OTC.*
Use: Dermatologic, acne.
PROPApH Medicated Acne Cream with Aloe. (Del) Salicylic acid 2%. Tube 1 oz. *OTC.*
Use: Dermatologic, acne.

PROPApH Medicated Acne Stick with Aloe. (Del) Salicylic acid 2%. Stick 0.05 oz. *OTC.*
Use: Dermatologic, acne.
PROPApH Medicated Cleansing Pads with Aloe. (Del) Salicylic acid 0.5%, SD alcohol 40 25%, aloe. Jar containing 45 pads. *OTC.*
Use: Dermatologic, acne.
PROPApH Peel-Off Acne Mask. (Del) Salicylic acid 2%, tartrazine, parabens, polyvinyl alcohol, vitamin E acetate, SD alcohol 40. Mask. 60 mL. *OTC.*
Use: Dermatologic, acne.
PROPApH Skin Cleanser with Aloe. (Del) Salicylic acid USP 0.5%, SD alcohol 40 25%. Liq. Bot. 6 oz, 10 oz. *OTC.*
Use: Dermatologic, acne.
•**proparacaine hydrochloride.** (pro-PAR-ah-cane) *USP 28.*
Use: Anesthetic local, ophthalmic.
See: Alcaine.
AK-Taine.
Fluoracain.
Ophthaine hydrochloride.
Ophthetic.
proparacaine hydrochloride. (Various Mfr.) Proparacaine hydrochloride 0.5% Mfr.) Soln. Bot. 2 mL, 15 mL, UD 1 mL.
Use: Anesthetic local, ophthalmic.
proparacaine hydrochloride and fluorescein sodium. (Taylor Pharmaceuticals) Proparacaine hydrochloride 0.5%, fluorescein sodium 0.25%, thimerosal 0.01%, EDTA. Soln. Bot. 5 mL. *Rx.*
Use: Anesthetic local, ophthalmic.
proparacaine hydrochloride/procaine hydrochloride
Use: Anesthetic.
See: Ravocaine and Novocain w/Levophed.
Ravocaine and Novocain w/Neocobefrin.
•**propatyl nitrate.** (PRO-pah-till) USAN. Investigational drug in US but available in England.
Use: Coronary vasodilator.
Propecia. (Merck) Finasteride 1 mg, lactose. Film coated. Tab. Unit-of-use 30s, *ProPak* carton of 3 unit-of-use bottles of 30. *Rx.*
Use: Androgen hormone inhibitor; hair growth.
•**propenzolate hydrochloride.** (pro-PEN-zoe-late) USAN.
Use: Anticholinergic.
propesin. Name used for *Risocaine.*
Prophene 65. (Halsey Drug) Propoxyphene hydrochloride 65 mg. Cap. Bot.

100s, 500s, 1000s. *c-iv.*
Use: Analgesic; narcotic.

prophenpyridamine.
See: Pheniramine.

prophenpyridamine maleate.
See: Pheniramine maleate.

prophenpyridamine maleate w/combinations.
See: Panadyl.
Trimahist.
Vasotus.

Pro-Phree. (Ross) Fat 31 g, carbohydrate 60 g, linoleic acid 2250 mg, Fe 11.9 mg, Na 250 mg, K 875 mg, with appropriate vitamins and minerals, 520 Cal/100 g. Protein free. Pow. Can 350 g. *OTC.*
Use: Nutritional supplement.

Prophyllin. (Rystan) Sodium propionate 5%, chlorophyll derivatives 0.0125%. Tube 1 oz. *Rx.*
Use: Anti-infective, topical.

•**propikacin.** (PRO-pih-KAY-sin) USAN.
Use: Anti-infective.

Propimex-1. (Ross) Protein 15 g, fat 23.9 g, carbohydrate 46.3 g, linoleic acid 1800 mg, Fe 9 mg, Na 190 mg, K 675 mg, with appropriate vitamins and minerals, 480 Cal/100 g. Methionine and valine free. Pow. Can 350 g. *OTC.*
Use: Nutritional supplement.

Propimex-2. (Ross) Protein 30 g, fat 15.5 g, carbohydrate 30 g, Na 880 mg, K 1370 mg, with appropriate vitamins and minerals, 410 Cal/mL. Methionine and valine free. Pow. Can 325 g. *OTC.*
Use: Nutritional supplement for propionic or methylmalonic acidemia.

Propine Sterile Ophthalmic. (Allergan) Dipivefrin hydrochloride 0.1%. Soln. Bot. 5 mL, 10 mL, 15 mL. *Rx.*
Use: Antiglaucoma.

propiodal.
See: Entodon.

•**propiolactone.** (PRO-pee-oh-LACK-tone) USAN.
Use: Disinfectant, sterilizing agent of vaccines and tissue grafts.

•**propionic acid.** (pro-pee-AHN-ik) *NF 23.*
Use: Antimicrobial; pharmaceutic aid, acidifying agent.

propionyl erythromycin lauryl sulfate.
See: Erythromycin Propionate Lauryl Sulfate.

•**propiram fumarate.** (PRO-pih-ram) USAN.
Use: Analgesic.

propisamine.
See: Amphetamine (Various Mfr.).

propitocaine. Prilocaine.
See: Citanest.

Proplex. (Baxter PPI) Plasma derived concentrate of clotting Factors II, VII, IX, X. Actual number of units shown on each bottle. Heat treated. Heparin. Pow. for Inj. Vial 30 mL w/diluent, needles. *Rx.*
Use: Antihemophilic.

Proplex T. (Baxter PPI) Factor IX complex, heat treated. W/Factors II, VII, IX and X. W/heparin. Dried concentrate. Vial w/diluent. *Rx.*
Use: Antihemophilic.

•**propofol.** (PRO-puh-FOLE) *USP 28.*
Use: Anesthetic, intravenous.
See: Diprivan.

propofol. (PRO-puh-FOLE) (Baxter Healthcare) Propofol 10 mg/mL, soybean oil 100 mg/mL, glycerol 22.5 mg/mL, egg yolk phospholipid 12 mg/mL, sodium metabisulfite 0.25 mg/mL, ph = 4.5 to 6.4. Inj. Emulsion. Single-use vial 20 mL; Single-use infusion vial 50 mL, 100 mL. *Rx.*
Use: Anesthetic.

Propoquin. Amopyroquin hydrochloride.
Use: Antimalarial.

propoxycaine and procaine hydrochlorides and levonordefrin injection.
Use: Anesthetic, local.

propoxycaine and procaine hydrochlorides and norepinephrine bitartrate injection.
Use: Anesthetic, local.

•**propoxycaine hydrochloride.** (pro-POX-ih-cane) *USP 28.*
Use: Anesthetic, local.

propoxychlorinol. Toloxychlorinol.

•**propoxyphene hydrochloride.** (pro-POX-ih-feen) *USP 28.*
Use: Analgesic.
See: Darvon Pulvules.
Dolene.
Pro-Gesic.

propoxyphene hydrochloride. (Various Mfr.) Propoxyphene hydrochloride 65 mg. Cap. Bot. 100s. *c-iv.*
Use: Opioid analgesic.

propoxyphene hydrochloride and acetaminophen tablets. (Various Mfr.) Propoxyphene hydrochloride 65 mg, acetaminophen 650 mg. Tab. Bot. 500s. *c-iv.*
Use: Analgesic.

propoxyphene hydrochloride and APC capsules.
Use: Analgesic.

propoxyphene hydrochloride, aspirin and caffeine capsules.
Use: Analgesic.

See: Darvon Compound 32.
propoxyphene hydrochloride w/combinations.
Use: Analgesic.
See: Darvon Compound.
Darvon Compound-65.
Darvon With A.S.A.
Dolene, AP-65.
Dolene Compound-65.
•**propoxyphene napsylate.** *USP 28.*
Use: Analgesic.
See: Darvocet-N.
Darvon-N.
W/Acetaminophen.
See: Darvocet A500.
Darvocet-N.
Trycet.
propoxyphene napsylate and acetaminophen. (Various Mfr.) Propoxyphene napsylate 50 mg, acetaminophen 325 mg. Tab. Bot. 100s, 500s, 550s, 1000s, UD 100s. Propoxyphene napsylate 100 mg, acetaminophen 650 mg. Tab. Bot. 30s, 50s, 100s, 500s, 1000s, UD 100s. *c-iv.*
Use: Analgesic.
propoxyphene napsylate and aspirin.
Use: Analgesic. Tab.
•**propranolol hydrochloride.** (pro-PRAN-oh-lahl) *USP 28.*
Use: Antiadrenergic/sympatholytic, beta-adrenergic blocker.
See: Inderal.
Inderal LA.
InnoPran XL.
Propranolol Intensol.
propranolol hydrochloride ER capsules. (Various Mfr.) Propranolol hydrochloride 60 mg, 80 mg, 120 mg, 160 mg. ER Cap. Bot. 100s; 1000s (exept 160 mg). *Rx.*
Use: Antiadrenergic/sympatholytic, beta-adrenergic blocker.
propranolol hydrochloride injection. (Various Mfr.) Propranolol hydrochloride 1 mg/mL. Inj. Vial 1 mL. *Rx.*
Use: Antiadrenergic/sympatholytic, beta-adrenergic blocker.
propranolol hydrochloride solution. (Roxane) Propranolol hydrochloride 4 mg/mL, 8 mg/mL, parabens, saccharin, sorbitol, dye free, strawberry-mint flavor. Oral Soln. Bot. 500 mL; UD 5 mL patient cups (40s) (4 mg only). *Rx.*
Use: Antiadrenergic/sympatholytic, beta-adrenergic blocker.
propranolol hydrochloride tablets. (Various Mfr.) Propranolol hydrochloride 10 mg, 20 mg, 40 mg, 60 mg, 80 mg, 90 mg. Tab. Bot. 100s, 500s; 1000s (except 60 mg, 90 mg), 5,000s (except

60 mg, 80 mg, 90 mg), UD 100s (except 90 mg). *Rx.*
Use: Antiadrenergic/sympatholytic, beta-adrenergic blocker.
propranolol hydrochloride and hydrochlorothiazide tablets. (Various Mfr.) Propranolol hydrochloride 40 mg, 80 mg, hydrochlorothiazide 25 mg. Bot. 100s, 1000s. *Rx.*
Use: Antihypertensive.
See: Inderide.
propranolol intensol. (Roxane) Propranolol hydrochloride 80 mg/mL, alcohol and dye free. Concentrated Oral Soln. Bot. 30 mL with dropper. *Rx.*
Use: Antiadrenergic/sympatholytic, beta-adrenergic blocker.
•**propylene carbonate.** (PRO-pih-leen CAR-boe-nate) *NF 23.*
Use: Pharmaceutic aid, gelling agent.
•**propylene glycol.** *USP 28.*
Use: Pharmaceutic aid, humectant, solvent, suspending agent.
•**propylene glycol alginate.** *NF 23.*
Use: Pharmaceutic aid, suspending, viscosity-increasing agent.
•**propylene glycol diacetate.** *NF 23.*
Use: Pharmaceutic aid, solvent.
•**propylene glycol monostearate.** *NF 23.*
Use: Pharmaceutic aid, emulsifying agent.
•**propyl gallate.** (PRO-pill GAL-ate) *NF 23.*
Use: Pharmaceutic aid; antioxidant.
•**propylhexedrine.** (pro-pill-HEX-ih-dreen) *USP 28.*
Use: Adrenergic, vasoconstrictor; appetite suppressant; antihistamine.
•**propyliodone.** (pro-pill-EYE-oh-dohn) *USP 28.*
Use: Diagnostic aid, radiopaque medium.
See: Dionosil Oily.
propylnoradrenaline-iso.
See: Isoproterenol.
propyl p-aminobenzoate. (Various Mfr.) Propaesin.
Use: Anesthetic, local.
•**propylparaben.** (pro-pill-PAR-ah-ben) *NF 23.* Propyl Chemosept (Chemo Puro).
Use: Pharmaceutic aid, antifungal agent.
•**propylparaben sodium.** *NF 23.*
Use: Pharmaceutic aid, antimicrobial preservative.
•**propylthiouracil.** (pro-puhl-thigh-oh-YOU-rah-sill) *USP 28.*
Use: Antithyroid agent.

propylthiouracil. (Abbott) Propylthiouracil 50 mg. Tab. Bot. 100s, 1000s. (Eli Lilly and Co.) 50 mg. Tab. Bot. 100s, 1000s. (ESI Lederle Generics) 50 mg. Tab. Bot. 100s, 1000s. 50 mg. Tab. Bot. 100s, 1000s, UD 100s.
Use: Antithyroid agent.

Pro-Q. (CollaGenex) Dimethicone, glycerin, parabens. Foam. 76 mL, 161 mL. *OTC.*
Use: Protectant.

•**proquazone.** (PRO-kwah-zone) USAN.
Use: Anti-inflammatory.

•**prorenoate potassium.** (pro-REN-ohate) USAN.
Use: Aldosterone antagonist.

Prorone. (Sigma-Tau) Progesterone 25 mg/mL. Aqueous or oil susp. Vial 10 mL. *Rx.*
Use: Hormone, progestin.

•**proroxan hydrochloride.** (pro-ROCKsan) USAN. *Formerly Pyrroxane, Pirrousan.*
Use: Antiadrenergic, α-receptor.

Proscar. (Merck) Finasteride 5 mg, lactose. Tab. 1,000s, Unit-of-use 30s, 100s, UD 100s. *Rx.*
Use: Androgen hormone inhibitor.

•**proscillaridin.** (pro-sih-LARE-ih-din) USAN. Talusin, Tradenal.
Use: Cardiovascular agent.

Prosed/DS. (Star) Methenamine 81.6 mg, phenyl salicylate 36.2 mg, methylene blue 10.8 mg, benzoic acid 9 mg, atropine sulfate 0.06 mg, hyoscyamine sulfate 0.06 mg. Tab. Bot. 100s, 1000s. *Rx.*
Use: Anti-infective, urinary.

ProSight Lutein. (Major) Ca 22 mg, vitamin E 30 units, C 60 mg, Zn 15 mg, Cu 2 mg. Cap. Bot. 36s. *OTC.*
Use: Nutritional combination product.

Pro Skin. (Marlyn Nutraceuticals) Vitamins A 6250 units, E 100 units, C 100 mg, B_5 10 mg, Zn 10 mg, Se. Cap., Bot. 60s. *OTC.*
Use: Mineral, vitamin supplement.

ProSobee. (Bristol-Myers Squibb) Milk free formula supplies 640 cal/qt, protein 19.2 g, fat 34 g, carbohydrate 64 g, vitamins A 2000 units, D 400 units, E 20 units, C 52 mg, folic acid 100 mcg, B_1 0.5 mg, B_2 0.6 mg, niacin 8 mg, B_6 0.4 mg, B_{12} 2 mcg, biotin 50 mg, pantothenic acid 3 mg, K-1 100 mcg, choline 50 mg, inositol 30 mg, Ca 600 mg, P 475 mg, I 65 mcg, Fe 12 mg, Mg 70 mg, Cu 0.6 mg, Zn 5 mg, Mn 1.6 mg, Cl 530 mg, K 780 mg, Na 230 mg/Qt. (20 Kcal/fl oz). Concentrated liq. can

13 fl oz; Ready-to-Use Liq. Can 8 fl oz, 32 fl oz. Pow., Can 14 oz. *OTC.*
Use: Nutritional supplement.

ProSobee Concentrate. (Bristol-Myers Squibb) P-soy protein isolate, I-methionine. CHO. corn syrup solids, soy and coconut oil, lecithin, mono- and diglycerides. Protein 20.3 g, CHO 65.4 g, fat 33.6 g, Fe 12 mg, 640 cal./serving. Concentrate 390 mL. *OTC.*
Use: Nutritional supplement.

Pro-Sof w/Casanthranol SG. (Vangard Labs, Inc.) Casanthranol 30 mg, docusate sodium 100 mg. Cap. Bot. 100s, 1000s.
Use: Laxative.

ProSom. (Abbott) Estazolam 1 mg, 2 mg. Lactose. Tab. Bot. 100s, UD 100s. *c-IV.*
Use: Sedative/hypnotic, nonbarbiturate.

prostacyclin analog.
Use: Vasodilator.
See: Iloprost.

prostaglandin agonist.
Use: Antiglaucoma agent.
See: Bimatoprost.
Latanoprost.
Lumigan.
Rescula.
Travatan.
Travoprost.

prostaglandin E_2.
See: Dinoprostone.

prostaglandins.
Use: Abortifacient; agent for impotence; agent for cervical ripening; patent ductus arteriosus; antiulcerative.
See: Carboprost Tromethamine.
Dinoprostone.
Misoprostol.

•**prostalene.** (PRAHST-ah-leen) USAN.
Use: Prostaglandin.

ProstaScint. (Cytogen) Pendetide 0.5 mg for conjugation w/indium-111. Kit. *Rx.*
Use: Radioimmunoscintigraphy agent.

Pro-Stat 101. (Medical Nutrition) Protein (collagen hydrolysate, amino acids [with histidine isoleucine, leucine, lysine, methionine, phenylalanine, threonine, tryptophan, valine, alanine, arginine, aspartic acid, cystine, glutamic acid, glycine, proline, serine, tyrosine, hydroxylysine, hydroxyproline]) 340 g. Fat 0 g, Na 2438 mg/mL, K 390 mg/mL. 3.4 cal/mL. Cl, Mg, P, Cu. Butterpecan and cherry flavors. Liq. 946 mL. *OTC.*
Use: Enteral nutrition therapy.

Pro-Stat 64. (Medical Nutrition) Protein (collagen hydrolysate, amino acids [with histidine isoleucine, leucine, ly-

sine, methionine, phenylalanine, threonine, tryptophan, valine, alanine, arginine, aspartic acid, cystine, glutamic acid, glycine, proline, serine, tyrosine, hydroxylysine, hydroxyproline]) 500 g. Carbohydrates (sorbitol, sucralose) 33 g, fat 0 g, Na 2438 mg/mL, K 390 mg/mL. 2.1 cal/mL. Cl, Mg, P, Cu. Butterpecan and cherry flavors. Liq. 946 mL. *OTC.*
Use: Enteral nutrition therapy.

ProStep. (Wyeth) Transdermal nicotine 11 mg, 22 mg/day. Patch 7s. *Rx.*
Use: Smoking deterrent.

Prostigmin. (ICN) Neostigmine methylsulfate 1:4000 (0.25 mg/mL), 1:2000 (0.5 mg/mL), 1:1000 (1 mg/mL). Inj. Amps. 1 mL with 0.2% methyl- and propylparabens (except 1:1000). Multidose vials. 10 mL with phenol 0.45%, sodium acetate 0.2 mg (except 1:4000). *Rx.*
Use: Muscle stimulant; urinary cholinergic.

Prostigmin Bromide. (AstraZeneca) Neostigmine bromide 15 mg. Tab. Bot. 100s, 1000s. *Rx.*
Use: Muscle stimulant.

Prostin E2. (Pharmacia) Dinoprost 20 mg. Supp. Containers of 1 each. *Rx.*
Use: Abortifacient.

Prostin VR Pediatric. (Pharmacia) Alprostadil 500 mcg/mL. Amp. 1 mL. *Rx.*
Use: Arterial patency agent.

Prostonic. (Seatrace) Thiamine hydrochloride 10 mg, alanine 130 mg, glutamic acid 130 mg, amino-acetic acid 130 mg. Cap. Bot. 100s. *Rx.*
Use: Palliative relief of benign prostatic hypertrophy.

Protabolin. (Taylor Pharmaceuticals) Methandriol dipropionate 50 mg/mL. Vial 10 mL. *Rx.*
Use: Hormone.

•**protamine sulfate.** (PRO-tuh-meen) *USP 28.*
Use: Antidote, heparin.
W/Insulin lispro.
See: Humalog Mix 50/50.
Humalog Mix 75/25.

protamine sulfate. (Various Mfr.) Protamine sulfate 10 mg/mL. Inj. Vials 5 mL, 25 mL.
Use: Antidote, heparin.

protargin mild.
See: Silver Protein, Mild.

Protargol. (Sterwin) Strong silver protein. Pow. Bot. 25 g. *Rx.*
Use: Antiseptic.

protease.
W/Amylase, lipase.

See: Kutrase.
Ku-Zyme.
Lipram.
Palcaps 10.
Palcaps 20.
Pancrelipase.
Panocaps.
Panocaps MT 16.
Panocaps MT 20.
PAN-2400.
Ultrase.
Ultrase MT 12.
Ultrase MT 18.
Ultrase MT 20.
Viokase.
W/Pancreatin, amylase.
See: Dizymes.
W/Vitamins B_1, B_{12}.
See: Arcoret.

protease inhibitors.
Use: Antiretroviral.
See: Amprenavir.
Atazanavir sulfate.
Fosamprenavir calcium.
Indinavir sulfate.
Ritonavir.
Saquinavir.
W/Combinations.
See: Lopinavir/Ritonavir.

proteasome inhibitors.
See: Bortezomib.

Protectol Medicated Powder. (Jones Pharma) Calcium undecylenate 15%. Bot. 2 oz. *OTC.*
Use: Diaper rash preparation.

Protegra Softgels. (Wyeth) Vitamins E 200 units, C 250 mg, beta-carotene 3 mg, Zn 7.5 mg, Cu, Se, Mn. Cap. Bot. 50s. *OTC.*
Use: Vitamin supplement.

proteinase inhibitor, alpha 1.
See: Prolastin.

protein C concentrate.
Use: Protein C deficiency. [Orphan Drug]

•**protein hydrolysate injection.** *USP 28.*
Use: Fluid, nutrient replacement.
See: Amigen.
Aminogen.
Lacotein.

protein hydrolysates oral.
Use: Enteral nutritional supplement.
See: Lofenalac.
Nutramigen.
Pregestimil.
Stuart Amino Acids.
W/Vitamin B_{12}.
See: Stuart Amino Acids and B_{12}.

protein-tyrosine kinase inhibitor.
See: Imatinib mesylate.

Protenate. (Baxter PPI) Plasma protein fraction (Human) 5%. Inj. Vial 250 mL, 500 mL w/administration set. *Rx.*
Use: Plasma protein fraction.
See: Arco-Lase.
   Kutrase.
   Ku-Zyme.
See: Arco-Lipase Plus.
Prothers. (ICN) Soap free. White petrolatum, disodium cocamido MIPA-sulfosuccinate, pentane, ammonium laureth sulfate, PEG-150 distearate, hydroxypropyl methylcellulose, imidazolidinyl urea, parabens, propylene glycol stearate, hydrogenated soy glyceride, sodium stearyl lactylate. Liq. Bot. 180 mL. *OTC.*
Use: Dermatologic, cleanser.
prothipendyl hydrochloride.
Use: Sedative.
Proticuleen. (Spanner) Vitamin B_{12} activity 10 mcg, folic acid 10 mg, B_{12} crystalline 50 mcg, niacinamide 75 mg/mL. Multiple-dose vial 10 mL. IM Inj. *Rx.*
Use: Nutritional supplement, parenteral.
•**protirelin.** (PRO-tie-reh-lin) USAN. *Formerly Lopremone.*
Protonix. (Wyeth-Ayerst) Pantoprazole sodium (as base) 20 mg, 40 mg, mannitol. DR Tab. Bot. 90s; 100s, 1000s, blister pack of 10 (10s) (40 mg only). *Rx.*
Use: Proton pump inhibitor.
Protonix I.V. (Wyeth-Ayerst) Pantoprazole sodium 40 mg (as base)/vial. EDTA. Pow. for Inj., freeze-dried. Vials. *Rx.*
Use: Proton pump inhibitor.
proton pump inhibitors.
See: Esomeprazole magnesium.
   Lansoprazole.
   Omeprazole.
   Pantoprazole sodium.
   Rabeprazole sodium.
Protopam Chloride. (Wyeth-Ayerst) Pralidoxime chloride 1 g. Pow. for Inj. Single-use vial. 20 mL. *Rx.*
Use: Antidote.
Protopic. (Fujisawa Healthcare) Tacrolimus 0.03%, 0.1%, mineral oil, white petrolatum. Oint. Tube 30 g, 60 g. *Rx.*
Use: Immunomodulator, topical.
Protosan. (Recsei) Protein 87.5%, lactose 0.5%, fat 1.3%, ash 3.5%, Na 0.02%. Jar 1 lb, 5 lb. *OTC.*
Use: Nutritional supplement.
Prot-O-Sea. (Barth's) Protein 90%, containing amino acids and minerals. Bot. 100s, 500s. *OTC.*
Use: Nutritional supplement.

Protostat. (Ortho-McNeil) Metronidazole. Tab. **250 mg:** Bot. 100s. **500 mg:** Bot. 50s. *Rx.*
Use: Anti-infective.
Protran Plus. (Vangard Labs, Inc.) Meprobamate 150 mg, ethoheptazine citrate 75 mg, aspirin 250 mg. Tab. Bot. 100s. *Rx.*
Use: Analgesic, anxiolytic combination.
•**protriptyline hydrochloride.** (pro-TRIP-tih-leen) *USP 28.*
Use: Antidepressant.
See: Vivactil.
protriptyline hydrochloride. (Various Mfr.) Protryptyline hydrochloride 5 mg, 10 mg, Tab. Bot. 100s, 1000s. *Rx.*
Use: Antidepressant.
Proventil. (Schering-Plough) Albuterol sulfate. **Soln.:** 0.083%, 0.5%. Soln. for Inh. UD vial 3 mL (0.083%). Bot. 20 mL w/dropper (0.5%). **Syr.:** 2 mg/5 mL, saccharin, strawberry flavor. Bot. 480 mL. **Tab.:** 2 mg, 4 mg, lactose. Bot. 100s, 500s. *Rx.*
Use: Bronchodilator, sympathomimetic.
Proventil Aerosol. (Schering-Plough) Albuterol 90 mcg/actuation. Aer. Canister 17 g (200 inhalations). *Rx.*
Use: Bronchodilator, sympathomimetic.
Proventil HFA. (Key) Albuterol sulfate 90 mcg/actuation. Aer. Can. 6.7 g/ (200 inhalations) contains no chlorofluorocarbons (CFCs). *Rx.*
Use: Bronchodilator, sympathomimetic.
Provera. (Pharmacia & Upjohn) Medroxyprogesterone acetate 2.5 mg, 5 mg, 10 mg. Lactose, sucrose. Tab. Bot. 30s, 100s; 500s, UD 10s (10 mg only). *Rx.*
Use: Hormone, progestin.
Provigil. (Cephalon) Modafinil 100 mg, 200 mg, lactose, talc. Tab. Bot. 100s. *c-IV.*
Use: CNS stimulant, analeptic.
Provocholine. (Methapharm) Methacholine Cl 100 mg/5 mL. Soln. for Inhalation. Vial 5 mL. *Rx.*
Use: Diagnostic aid.
Prox/APAP. (Forest) Propoxyphene hydrochloride 65 mg, acetaminophen 650 mg. Tab. Bot. 100s, 500s. *c-IV.*
Use: Analgesic combination; narcotic.
•**proxazole.** (PROX-ah-zole) USAN.
Use: Analgesic; anti-inflammatory; muscle relaxant.
•**proxazole citrate.** USAN.
Use: Relaxant, smooth muscle; analgesic; anti-inflammatory.
•**proxicromil.** (prox-ih-KROE-mill) USAN.
Use: Antiallergic.

Proxigel. (Schwarz Pharma) Carbamide peroxide 10% in a water-free gel base. Tube 34 g w/applicator. *OTC.*
Use: Antiseptic, cleanser.

•**proxorphan tartrate.** (PROX-ahr-fan TAR-trate) USAN.
Use: Analgesic; antitussive.

Proxy 65. (Parmed Pharmaceuticals, Inc.) Propoxyphene hydrochloride 65 mg, acetaminophen 650 mg. Tab. Bot. 100s, 500s. *c-iv.*
Use: Analgesic combination; narcotic.

Prozac. (Eli Lilly/Dista) Fluoxetine hydrochloride. **Pulvules:** 10 mg, 20 mg, 40 mg. Bot. 30s (except 10 mg); 100s, 2000s, blister card 31s (10 mg, 20 mg only); UD 100s (20 mg only). **Tab.:** 10 mg. Bot. 30s, 100s. **Oral Soln.:** 20 mg/5 mL, alcohol 0.23%, sucrose, mint flavor. Bot. 120 mL. *Rx.*
Use: Antidepressant, SSRI.

Prozac Weekly. (Eli Lilly/Dista) Fluoxetine hydrochloride 90 mg, sucrose, sugar spheres. DR Cap. Blister 4s. *Rx.*
Use: Antidepressant, SSRI.

•**prucalopride hydrochloride.** USAN.
Use: Constipation.

•**prucalopride succinate.** USAN.
Use: Constipation.

Prudents. (Bariatric) Acetylphenylisatin 5 mg. Chewable protein and amino acid. Tab. Bot. 30s, 100s. *OTC.*
Use: Laxative.

Prulet. (Mission Pharmacal) White phenolphthalein 60 mg. Tab. Strips 12s, 40s. *OTC.*
Use: Laxative.

prune powder concentrated dehydrated.
See: Diacetyldihydroxyphenylisatin.

Prurilo. (Whorton Pharmaceuticals, Inc.) Menthol 0.25%, phenol 0.25%, calamine lotion in special lubricating base. Bot. 4 oz, 8 oz. *OTC.*
Use: Dermatologic, counterirritant.

PSE CPM. (Boca) Pseudoephedrine hydrochloride 15 mg, chlorpheniramine maleate 2 mg. Aspartame, phenylalanine, sugar. Grape flavor. Chew. Tab. 100s. *Rx.*
Use: Decongestant, antihistamine.

PSE 120/MSC 2.5. (Cypress) Pseudoephedrine hydrochloride 120 mg, methscopolamine nitrate 2.5 mg. SR Tab. Bot. 60s. *Rx.*
Use: Upper respiratory combination, decongestant, anticholinergic.

Pseudo-Car DM. (Geneva) Pseudoephedrine hydrochloride 60 mg, carbinoxamine maleate 4 mg, dextromethorphan HBr 15 mg/5 mL, alcohol < 0.6%. Bot. Pt, gal. *Rx.*
Use: Antihistamine; antitussive; decongestant.

Pseudo-Chlor. (Various Mfr.) Pseudoephedrine hydrochloride 120 mg, chlorpheniramine maleate 8 mg. Cap. Bot. 100s, 250s. *Rx.*
Use: Antihistamine; decongestant.

•**pseudoephedrine hydrochloride.** (SUE-doe-eh-FED-rin) *USP 28.*
Use: Adrenergic, vasoconstrictor.
See: Allerest No Drowsiness.
Anatuss DM.
Aspirin-Free Bayer Select Head & Chest Cold.
Benylin Multi-Symptom.
Bromfenex.
Cenafed.
Claritin.
Coldrine.
Congestaid.
Cycofed Pediatric.
Decofed.
Dimetapp Decongestant Pediatric.
Dimetapp, Maximum Strength Non-Drowsy Liqui-Gels.
Dimetapp, Maximum Strength 12-Hour Non-Drowsy Extentabs.
Efidac 24 Hour Relief.
ElixSure Children's Congestion.
Genaphed.
Iofed.
Kid Kare.
Medi-First Sinus Decongestant.
Mini Thin Pseudo.
Nasal Decongestant, Children's Non-Drowsy.
Nasal Decongestant Oral.
Pediacare Decongestant, Infants'.
Pseudo.
Sildec-DM.
Silfedrine Children's.
Simply Stuffy.
Sinufed.
Sinus Relief.
Sinustop.
Sudafed.
Sudafed Children's Non-Drowsy.
Sudafed Non-Drowsy, Maximum Strength.
Sudafed Non-Drowsy 12 Hour Long-Acting.
Sudafed Non-Drowsy 24 Hour Long-Acting.
Sudafed SA.
Sudal.
Sudodrin.
Triaminic Allergy Congestion.
Triaminic Allergy Congestion Softchews.

Triaminic AM Decongestant Formula.
Triaminic Infant Oral Decongestant
 Drops.
Unifed.
Ursinus.
W/Combinations.
 See: AccuHist.
 AccuHist DM Pediatric.
 AccuHist PDX.
 Actifed Cold & Allergy.
 Actifed Cold & Sinus Maximum
  Strength.
 Advil Allergy Sinus.
 Advil Cold & Flu.
 Advil Cold & Sinus.
 Advil Cold & Sinus Liqui-gels.
 Advil Flu & Body Ache.
 Aleve Cold & Sinus.
 Aleve Sinus & Headache.
 Alka-Seltzer Plus Cold & Flu.
 Alka-Seltzer Plus Cold & Cough.
 Alka-Seltzer Plus Cold & Sinus.
 Alka-Seltzer Plus Cold Medicine.
 Alka-Seltzer Plus Liqui-Gels Flu
  Medicine.
 Alka-Seltzer Plus Night Time Cold.
 Alka-Seltzer Plus & Sinus.
 Allegra-D 12 Hour Tablets.
 Allegra-D 24 Hour.
 Allerest Allergy & Sinus Relief Maxi-
  mum Strength.
 Allerest Maxiumum Strength.
 Allerest No Drowsiness.
 Allerfrim.
 AlleRx.
 AlleRx-D.
 All Nite.
 AMBI 60/580.
 AMBI 60/580/30.
 Amerifed.
 Anaplex-DM.
 Anaplex HD.
 Andehist DM NR.
 Andehist-DM.
 Aprodine.
 AquaTab C.
 AquaTab D.
 Aspirin-Free Bayer Select Head &
  Chest Cold.
 Atridine.
 Balamine DM.
 Banophen Decongestant.
 Benadryl Allergy & Cold.
 Benadryl Allergy & Sinus.
 Benadryl Allergy & Sinus Headache.
 Benadryl Children's Allergy & Cold.
 Benadryl Children's Allergy & Sinus.
 Benadryl Maximum Strength Severe
  Allergy & Sinus Headache.
 Biohist LA.
 Brexin EX.

Bromanate.
Bromanate DM Cold & Cough.
Bromatane DX.
Bromfed.
Bromfed DM Cough.
Bromfed-PD.
Bromfenex.
Bromfenex PD.
Bromhist-DM.
Bromhist-NR.
Bromhist PDX Drops.
Brompheniramine maleate/pseudo-
 ephedrine hydrochloride.
Carbinoxamine.
Carbodex DM.
Carbofed DM.
Carbofed DM.
Cardec DM.
Cardec-S.
Cenafed Plus.
Cēpacol Sore Throat.
Children's Elixir DM Cough & Cold.
Children's Ibuprofen Cold.
Children's Motrin Cold.
Claritin-D.
Chlorpheniramine maleate/pseudo-
 ephedrine hydrochloride.
Chlor-Trimeton Allergy-D 4 Hour.
Chlor-Trimeton Allergy-D 12 Hour.
Claritin-D 12 Hour.
Claritin-D 24 Hour.
Clorfed.
Cold & Cough Tussin.
Cold Symptoms Relief Maximum
 Strength.
Coldec D.
Coldec DM.
Coldmist JR.
Coldmist LA.
Coldrine.
Colfed-A.
Comtrex Acute Head Cold & Sinus
 Pressure Relief, Multi-Symptom
 Maximum Strength.
Comtrex Allergy-Sinus Treatment,
 Maximum Strength.
Comtrex Cough and Cold Relief,
 Multi-Symptom Maximum Strength.
Comtrex Day & Night Cold & Cough
 Relief, Multi-Symptom Maximum
 Strength.
Comtrex Day/Night Flu Therapy Maxi-
 mum Strength Caplets.
Comtrex Maximum Strength Night-
 time Cold & Cough.
Comtrex Multi-Symptom Deep Chest
 Cold & Congestion Relief.
Comtrex Multi-Symptom Maximum
 Strength Non-Drowsy Cold &
 Cough Relief.
Congestac.

Contac Day & Night Allergy/Sinus Relief.
Contac Day & Night Cold & Flu.
Contac Severe Cold & Flu Maximum Strength.
Coricidin D Cold, Flu, & Sinus.
C.P.-DM.
CPM 8/PSE 90/MSC 2.5.
Cydec.
Cydec-DM.
Cycofed.
Cycofed Pediatric.
DALLERGY-JR.
Decohstine DH.
Deconamine.
Deconamine SR.
Deconomed SR.
Deconsal Pediatric.
Decohistine.
DEKA.
DEKA Pediatric.
Detussin.
Dihistine.
Dihistine DH.
Dilotab.
Dimaphen.
Dimaphen DM Cold & Cough.
Dimetapp DM Children's Cold & Cough.
Dimetapp Children's Nighttime Flu.
Dimetapp Children's Non-Drowsy Flu.
Dimetapp Cold & Allergy.
Dimetapp Decongestant Plus Cough Infant.
Dimetapp Long Acting Cough Plus Cold.
Dorcol.
Dristan Cold Non-Drowsy Maximum Strength.
Dristan Sinus.
Drixomed.
Drixoral Allergy Sinus.
Drixoral Cold & Allergy.
Duraflu.
Durahist.
Duratuss.
Durasal II.
Dynex.
Entex PSE.
Entex PSE 120.
Fedahist Expectorant.
Genac.
Genacol Maximum Strength Cold & Flu Relief.
GFN 550/PSE 60/DM 30.
GFN/PSE.
GFN 1200/DM 60/PSE.
Good Sense Maximum Strength Dose Sinus.
Good Sense Maximum Strength Pain Relief Allergy Sinus.

GP-500.
G/P 1200/60.
GRN/PSE.
Guaifed.
Guaifed-PD.
Guaifenesin/Pseudoephedrine Hydrochloride.
Guaifenex GP.
Guaifenex PSE 60.
Guaifenesin DAC.
Guaifenex.
Guaifenex PSE 120.
Guaimax-D.
Guaipax PSE.
Guaitex PSE.
Guaivent.
Guaivent PD.
Guai-Vent/PSE.
Guiatuss DAC.
II 9000 SR.
Halotussin DAC.
Histacol DM.
Histade.
Histex HC.
Histex SR.
Histinex-D.
Histinex PV.
Histenol-Forte.
Histussin D.
H-Tuss-D.
Hydrocodone bitartrate 5 mg/pseudo-ephedrine hydrochloride 30 mg/car-binoxamine maleate 2 mg.
Hydron PSC.
Hydro-Tussin HC.
Hydro-Tussin HD.
Hyphed.
Iofed.
Iosal II.
Kid Kare Children's Cough/Cold.
Kolephrin/DM.
Kronofed-A.
Kronofed-A Jr.
Lemotussin-DM.
Lodrane.
Lodrane LD.
Mapap Cold Formula.
Mapap Sinus Maximum Strength.
Maxifed.
Maxifed DM.
Maxifed DMX.
Maxifed-G.
Maximum Strength Dynafed Plus.
MED-Rx.
Miraphen PSE.
Motrin Children's Cold.
Motrin Sinus Headache.
Mytussin DAC.
Nalex Expectorant.
Nasabid.
Nasabid Sr.

Nasatab LA.
Nasal Decongestatnt Sinus Non-
Drowsy.
Nite Time Children's.
Nite Time Cold Formula for Adults.
Novagest Expectorant with Codeine.
Novahistine Sinus.
Nucofed.
Nucofed Expectorant.
Nucofed Pediatric Expectorant.
Nucotuss Expectorant.
Nucotuss Pediatric Expectorant.
Ornex No Drowsiness.
Ornex No Drowsiness Maximum
Strength.
Palgic-D.
Palgic-DS.
Pancof.
Pancof-EXP.
Pancof-HC.
Pancof-XP.
PanMist-DM.
PanMist LA.
Panmist JR.
PanMist-S.
Pannaz.
Pannaz S.
Pedia Care Children's Cold & Allergy.
Pedia Care Children's Long-Lasting
Cough Plus Cold.
PediaCare Children's Multi-Symptom
Cold.
Pedia Care Cough-Cold.
Pedia Care Infants' Decongestant &
Cough.
Pedia Care Multi-Symptom Cold.
Pedia Care NightRest Cough & Cold.
Pediahist DM.
Pedia Relief Decongestant Plus
Cough.
Pediatex-D.
Pediatex-DM.
Pediox.
Phenapap.
Phenergan-D.
Profen II.
Profen II DM.
Profen Forte.
Profen Forte DM.
PSE CPM.
PSE 120/MSC 2.5.
Pseudovent.
Pseudovent-PED.
P-V-Tussin.
Quadra-Hist D.
Quadra-Hist D PED.
QDALL.
Refensen Plus Severe Strength
Cough & Cold Medicine.
Rescon-DM.
Respaire-60 SR.

Respaire-120 SR.
Robafen CF.
Robafen PE.
Robitussin Allergy & Cough.
Robitussin CF.
Robitussin Cold & Cough.
Robitussin Cold, Cold & Congestion.
Robitussin Cold, Cold & Cough.
Robitussin Cold, Multi-Symptom Cold
& Flu.
Robitussin Cold Sinus & Congestion.
Robitussin Cough & Cold Infant.
Robitussin-DAC.
Robitussin Flu.
Robitussin Honey Cough & Cold.
Robitussin Honey Flu Multi-
Symptom.
Robitussin Honey Flu Night Time.
Robitussin Honey Flu Non-Drowsy.
Robitussin Maximum Strength Cough
& Cold.
Robitussin Night Relief.
Robitussin PE.
Robitussin Pediatric Cough & Cold
Formula.
Robitussin Pediatric Night Relief
Cough & Cold.
Robitussin PM Cough & Cold.
Robitussin Severe Congestion.
Rondamine DM.
Rondec.
Rondec D.
Rondec DM
Rondec-TR.
Scot-Tussin Hayfebrol.
Semprex-D.
Severe Congestion Tussin.
Silafed.
Sildec-DM.
Simplet.
Sine-Aid IB.
Sine-Off Night Time Formula Sinus,
Cold & Flu Medicine.
Sine-Off No Drowsiness Formula.
Sine-Off Sinus Medicine.
Singlet for Adults.
Sinus Relief Maximum Strength.
Sinutab Sinus Allergy, Maximum
Strength.
Sinutab Sinus Without Drowsiness
Maximum Strength.
Sinutab Sinus Without Drowsiness
Regular Strength.
Sinus Relief.
Sinutab Non-Drying.
666 Cold Preparation, Maximum
Strength.
Stahist.
Stamoist E.
Statuss Green.
Sudafed Children's Non-Drowsy Cold
& Cough.

Sudafed Cold & Allergy Maximum Strength.
Sudafed Cold & Sinus Non-Drowsy.
Sudafed Maximum Strength Sinus Nighttime Plus Pain Relief.
Sudafed Multi-Symptom Cold & Cough.
Sudafed Non-Drowsy Non-Drying Sinus.
Sudafed Non-Drowsy Severe Cold Formula Maximum Strength.
Sudafed Sinus Headache Non-Drowsy.
Sudafed Sinus Nighttime Maximum Strength.
Sudal 60/500.
SudoGest Sinus Maximum Strength.
Sudal.
Su-Tuss IID.
Syn-Rx.
Tanafed DP.
Tavist Allergy/Sinus/Headache.
Tavist Sinus Maximum Strength.
TheraFlu Cold & Cough Night Time.
TheraFlu Flu and Chest Congestion Non-Drowsy.
TheraFlu Flu & Cold Medicine for Sore Throat, Maximum Strength.
TheraFlu Flu and Cold Medicine Original Formula.
TheraFlu Flu & Cough Night Time, Maximum Strength.
TheraFlu Flu & Sore Throat, Maximum Strength.
TheraFlu Flu & Sore Throat Night Time, Maximum Strength.
TheraFlu Flu, Cold & Cough Night Time, Maximum Strength.
TheraFlu Flu, Cold & Cough and Sore Throat, Maximum Strength.
TheraFlu Maximum Strength Flu, Cold, & Cough.
TheraFlu Maximum Strength Night Time Formula Flu, Cold, & Cough Medicine.
TheraFlu Non-Drowsy Flu, Cold, & Cough Maximum Strength.
TheraFlu Non-Drowsy Formula Maximum Strength.
TheraFlu Severe Cold & Congestion Night Time, Maximum Strength.
TheraFlu Severe Cold & Congestion Non-Drowsy, Maximum Strength.
Thera-Hist Cold & Allergy.
Thera-Hist Cold & Cough.
Thera-Hist Expectorant Chest Congestion.
Time-Hist.
Top Care Liquicaps Nite Time Multi-Symptom Cold/Flu Relief.

Top Care Maximum Strength Flu, Cold & Cough Medicine Night Time.
Top Care Maximum Strength Soothing Cough & Head Congestion Relief D.
Top Care Multi-Symptom Pain Relief Cold.
Touro Allergy.
Touro CC.
Touro LA.
Triacin-C Cough.
Tri-Acting Cold & Allergy.
Tri-Acting Cold & Cough.
Triacting.
Triacting Cold & Allergy.
Triaminic AM Cough & Decongestant Formula.
Triaminic AM Non-Drowsy Cough & Decongestant.
Triaminic Cold, Allergy, Sinus Medicine.
Triaminic Cold & Allergy.
Triaminic Cold & Cough.
Triaminic Cough.
Triaminic Cough & Sore Throat.
Triaminic Softchews Allergy Sinus & Headache.
Triaminic Softchews Cold & Sore Throat.
Triaminic Throat Pain & Cough.
Trinalin Repetabs.
Triprolidine hydrochloride with pseudoephedrine hydrochloride.
Tussafed.
Tussafed Expectorant.
Tussafed-LA.
Tussend.
Tylenol Allergy Sinus, Maximum Strength.
Tylenol Flu Night Time , Maximum Strength.
Tylenol Children's Cold.
Tylenol Children's Cold Plus Cough.
Tylenol Children's Flu.
Tylenol Children's Sinus.
Tylenol Cold Complete Formula.
Tylenol Cold Non-Drowsy Formula.
Tylenol Flu, Maximum Strength.
Tylenol Flu Maximum Strength Non-Drowsy.
Tylenol Flu NightTime, Maximum Strength.
Tylenol Infant's Cold.
Tylenol Infants' Cold Decongestant & Fever Reducer Plus Cough Concentrated.
Tylenol Multi-Symptom Cold Severe Congestion.
Tylenol Sinus Nighttime, Maximum Strength.
Tylenol Sinus Non-Drowsy Maximum Strength.

Tylenol Sinus Severe Congestion.
Tyrodone.
ULTRAbrom.
ULTRAbrom PD.
V-Dec-M.
Versacaps.
Vicks Children's NyQuil Cold/Cough Relief.
Vicks DayQuil LiquiCaps Multi-Symptom Cold/Flu Relief.
Vicks DayQuil Liqui-Gels Flu Medicine.
Vicks DayQuil Multi-Symptom.
Vicks DayQuil Multi-Symptom Cold/Flu Relief.
Vicks 44D Cough & Head Congestion.
Vicks 44M Cough, Cold, & Flu Relief Liquicaps.
Vicks NyQuil Multi-Symptom Cold/Flu Relief.
Vicks Pediatric 44M Cough & Cold Relief.
Z-Cof DM.
Zephrex.
Zephrex LA.
ZTuss Expectorant.
Zyrtec-D 12 Hour.

pseudoephedrine hydrochloride.
(Various Mfr.) Pseudoephedrine hydrochloride. **Tab.:** 30 mg, 60 mg. Bot. 24s (30 mg only), 100s, 1000s, blister pack 100s. **Liq.:** 30 mg/5 mL. Bot. 120 mL, 473 mL. *OTC.*
Use: Nasal decongestant, arylalylamine.

pseudoephedrine hydrochloride and triprolidine hydrochloride. (Various Mfr.) Pseudoephedrine hydrochloride 60 mg, triprolidine hydrochloride 2.5 mg. Tab. Bot. 100s, 1000s, UD 100s. *Rx.*
Use: Antihistamine; decongestant.

pseudoephedrine hydrochloride and triprolidine hydrochloride. (Various Mfr.) Pseudoephedrine hydrochloride 60 mg, triprolidine hydrochloride 2.5 mg. Tab. Bot. 100s, 1000s, UD 100s. *Rx.*
Use: Antihistamine; decongestant.

•**pseudoephedrine hydrochloride, carbinoxamine maleate, and dextromethorphan hydrobromide oral solution.** *USP 28.*
Use: Decongestant, antihistamine, antitussive.

pseudoephedrine hydrochloride/guaifenesin LA. (URL) Pseudoephedrine 85 mg, guaifenesin 795 mg. TR Tab. 100s. *Rx.*
Use: Decongestant, expectorant.

pseudoephedrine hydrochloride/guaifenesin SR. (URL) Pseudoephedrine hydrochloride 48 mg, guaifenesin 595 mg. ER Tab. 100s. *Rx.*
Use: Decongestant, expectorant.

•**pseudoephedrine polistirex.** USAN.
Use: Decongestant, nasal.
W/Combinations.
See: Atuss-12 DM.

•**pseudoephedrine sulfate.** *USP 28.*
Use: Bronchodilator.
See: Afrinol Repetabs.
Drixoral 12 Hour Non-Drowsy Formula.
W/Combinations.
See: Alavert Allergy & Sinus D-12 Hour.
Chlor-trimeton Decongestant.
Clarinex-D 24 Hour.
Disophrol Chronotabs.
Drixoral S.A.
Polaramine Expectorant.
Rynatan.

pseudoephedrine tannate w/combinations.
See: Chlorpheniramine tannate/pseudoephedrine tannate.
C-PHED Tannate.
CP-TANNIC.
Lodrane D.
Tanafed DMX.

Pseudo-Gest. (Major) Pseudoephedrine hydrochloride 30 mg, 60 mg. Tab. Bot. 24s, 100s. *OTC.*
Use: Decongestant.

Pseudo-Gest Plus. (Major) Pseudoephedrine hydrochloride 60 mg, chlorpheniramine maleate 4 mg. Tab. Bot. 24s, 100s, 200s. *OTC.*
Use: Antihistamine; decongestant.

Pseudo-Hist. (Holloway) Pseudoephedrine hydrochloride 30 mg, chlorpheniramine maleate 10 mg. Cap. Bot. 100s. *OTC.*
Use: Antihistamine; decongestant.

Pseudo-Hist Expectorant. (Holloway) Pseudoephedrine 15 mg, hydrocodone bitartrate 2.5 mg, guaifenesin 100 mg, alcohol 5%. Bot. 480 mL. *c-III.*
Use: Antitussive; decongestant; expectorant.

pseudomonas hyperimmune globulin (mucoid exopolysaccharide).
Use: Pulmonary infection in cystic fibrosis. [Orphan Drug]

pseudomonas test.
Use: Urine test.
See: Isocult for *Pseudomonas aeruginosa.*

pseudomonic acid A.
Use: Anti-infective, topical.
See: Bactroban.

Pseudo Plus. (Weeks & Leo) Pseudoephedrine hydrochloride 60 mg, chlorpheniramine maleate 4 mg. Tab. Bot. 40s. *OTC.*
Use: Antihistamine; decongestant.

Pseudo Syrup. (Major) Pseudoephedrine 30 mg/5 mL. Liq. Bot. 120 mL, pt, gal. *OTC.*
Use: Decongestant.

Pseudovent. (Ethex) Pseudoephedrine hydrochloride 120 mg, guaifenesin 250 mg, EDTA, sucrose, methylparaben. SR Cap. Bot. 100s. *Rx.*
Use: Upper respiratory combination, decongestant, expectorant.

Pseudovent-PED. (Ethex) Pseudoephedrine hydrochloride 60 mg, guaifenesin 300 mg, EDTA, parabens, sucrose. SR Cap. Bot. 100s. *Rx.*
Use: Upper respiratory combination; decongestant, expectorant.

psoralens.
See: Methoxsalen.

Psor-a-set. (Hogil) Salicylic acid 2%. Soap. Bar 97.5 g. *OTC.*
Use: Keratolytic.

Psorcon E. (Dermik) Diflorasone diacetate 0.05%. Oint.. Emollient, occlusive base, lanolin alcohol, white petrolatum. Tube 15 g, 30 g, 60 g. **Cream:** Hydrophilic base, stearyl alcohol, cetyl alcohol, mineral oil. Tube 15 g, 30 g, 60 g. *Rx.*
Use: Corticosteroid, topical.

Psoriatec Cream. (Sirius) Anthralin 1%. Cream. Tube. 50 g. *Rx.*
Use: Dermatologic.

PsoriGel. (Healthpoint) Coal tar soln. 7.5%, alcohol 28.3%. Gel. 113 g. *OTC.*
Use: Dermatologic.

Psorinail. (Summers) Coal tar solution w/isopropyl alcohol 2.5%, 3-butylene glycol l, acetyl mandelic acid. Liq. Bot. 30 mL. *OTC.*
Use: Antipsoriatic, topical.

Psorion. (ICN) Betamethasone dipropionate 0.05%, mineral oil, white petrolatum, propylene glycol. Cream. Tube 15 g, 45 g. *Rx.*
Use: Corticosteroid, topical.

psychotherapeutic agents.
See: Olanzapine and fluoxetine hydrochloride.
Sodium Oxybate.
Tranquilizers.

psyllium.
Use: Laxative.
See: Fiberall Orange Flaor.
Fiberall Tropical Fruit Flavor.
Genfiber.
Genfiber, Orange Flavor.
Hydrocil Instant.
Konsyl.
Konsyl-D.
Konsyl Easy Mix Formula.
Konsyl-Orange.
Metamucil.
Metamucil Orange Flavor, Original Texture.
Metamucil Orange Flavor, Smooth Texture.
Metamucil Original Texture.
Metamucil, Sugar Free, Orange Flavor, Smooth Texture.
Metamucil, Sugar Free, Smooth Texture.
Modane Bulk.
Natural Fiber Laxative.
Perdiem Fiber Therapy.
Perdiem Overnight Relief.
Reguloid.
Reguloid, Orange.
Reguloid, Sugar Free Orange.
Reguloid, Sugar Free Regular.
Serutan.
Syllact.

• **psyllium hemicellulose.** (SILL-i-yum) USAN
Use: Laxative.

• **psyllium husk.** *USP 28.*
Use: Laxative, cathartic.

psyllium hydrocolloid.
Use: Laxative.

psyllium seed gel.
Use: Laxative.

PTE-5. (Fujisawa Healthcare) Zn 1 mg, Cu 0.1 mg, Cr 1 mcg, Mn 25 mcg, Se 15 mcg/mL. Vial 3 mL, 10 mL. *Rx.*
Use: Mineral supplement.

PTE-4. (Fujisawa Healthcare) Zn 1 mg, Cu 0.1 mg, Cr 1 mcg, Mn 25 mcg/mL. Vial 3 mL. *Rx.*
Use: Mineral supplement.

pteroic acid. The compound formed by the linkage of carbon 6 of 2-amine-4-hydroxypteridine by means of a methylene group with the nitrogen of p-aminobenzoic acid.

pteroylglutamic acid.
See: Folic acid.

pteroylmonoglutamic acid. Pteroylglutamic acid.
See: Folic acid.

PTFE. (Ethicon) Polytef.

PTU.
See: Propylthiouracil.

Pulmicort Respules. (AstraZeneca) Budesonide 0.25 mg/2 mL, 0.5 mg/2 mL, EDTA. Inh. Susp. Pkg. 30s. *Rx.*
Use: Respiratory inhalant, corticosteroid.

Pulmicort Turbuhaler. (AstraZeneca) Budesonide 200 mcg (≈ 160 mcg per actuation). Pow. *Turbuhaler* 200 doses. *Rx.*
Use: Respiratory inhalant, corticosteroid.

Pulmocare. (Ross) High-fat, low-carbohydrate liquid diet for pulmonary patients containing 1500 calories/L; 1420 calories provides 100% US RDA vitamins and minerals. Cal/Nitrogen ratio is 150:1. Osmolarity: 490 mOsm/kg water. Can 8 fl oz. *OTC.*
Use: Nutritional supplement.

pulmonary surfactant replacement. (Scios Nova)
Use: Diagnostic aid, thyroid. [Orphan Drug]

pulmonary surfactant replacement, porcine.
Use: Diagnostic aid, thyroid. [Orphan Drug]
See: Curosurf.

Pulmosin. (Spanner) Guaiacol 0.1 g, eucalyptol 0.08 g, camphor 0.05 g, iodoform 0.02 g/2 mL. Multiple-dose vial 30 mL. IM. Inj. *Rx.*

Pulmozyme. (Genentech) Dornase alfa 1 mg, calcium chloride dihydrate 0.15 mg, NaCl 8.77 mg/mL. Soln. for Inh. Amps. Single-use 2.5 mL. *Rx.*
Use: Anti-infective.

•**pumice.** (PUM-iss) *USP 28.*
Use: Abrasive, dental.

punctum plug. (Eagle Vision) Silicone plug. 0.5 mm, 0.6 mm, 0.7 mm, 0.8 mm. Pkg. 2 plugs, 1 inserter tool. *Rx.*
Use: Punctal plug.

Puralube. (E. Fougera) White petrolatum, light mineral oil. Oint. Tube 3.5 g. *OTC.*
Use: Lubricant, ophthalmic.

Puralube Tears. (E. Fougera) Polyvinyl alcohol 1%, polyethylene glycol 400 1%, EDTA, benzalkonium Cl. Soln. Bot. 15 mL. *OTC.*
Use: Lubricant, ophthalmic.

Puresept Murine Saline. (Ross) **Disinfecting soln.:** Sterile hydrogen peroxide solution 3%, sodium stannate, sodium nitrate, phosphate buffers, thimerosal free. 237 mL. **Murine Saline Soln.:** Buffered isotonic solution w/borate buffers, NaCl, sorbic acid 0.1%, EDTA 0.1%. 60, 237, 355 mL. Includes cups and lens holder. *OTC.*
Use: Contact lens care.

Puri-Clens. (Sween) UD 2 oz. Bot. 8 oz.
Use: Dermatologic, wound therapy.

purified oxgall.
See: Bile Extract, Ox.

purified protein derivative of tuberculin.
Use: Mantoux TB test.
See: Aplisol.
Aplitest.
Tubersol.

purified type II collagen.
Use: Juvenile rheumatoid arthritis. [Orphan Drug]

purine analogs and related agents.
Use: Antimetabolite.
See: Allopurinol.
Cladribine.
Clofarabine.
Fludarabine Phosphate.
Mercaptopurine.
Pentostatin.
Rasburicase.
Thioguanine.

Purinethol. (GlaxoSmithKline) Mercaptopurine 50 mg. Tab. Bot. 25s, 250s. *Rx.*
Use: Antineoplastic.

•**puromycin.** (PURE-oh-MY-sin) USAN.
Use: Antineoplastic; antiprotozoal, trypanosoma.

•**puromycin hydrochloride.** USAN.
Use: Antineoplastic; antiprotozoal, trypanosoma.

purple foxglove.
See: Digitalis.

Purpose Shampoo. (Johnson & Johnson) Water, amphoteric-19, PEG-44 sorbitan laurate, PEG-150 distearate, sorbitan laurate, boric acid, fragrance, benzyl alcohol. Bot. 8 oz. *OTC.*
Use: Dermatologic.

Purpose Soap. (Johnson & Johnson) Sodium tallowate, sodium cocoate, glycerin, NaCl, BHT, EDTA. Bar 108 g, 180 g. *OTC.*
Use: Dermatologic, cleanser.

Pursettes Premenstrual. (DEP Corp.) Acetaminophen 500 mg, pamabrom 25 mg, pyrilamine maleate 15 mg. Tab. Bot. 24s. *OTC.*
Use: Analgesic; antihistamine; diuretic.

PVP-I. (Day-Baldwin) Povidone-iodine. Oint. Tube 1 oz, Jar lb, Foilpac 1.5 g. *OTC.*
Use: Antiseborrheic; antiseptic.

P-V-Tussin. (Numark) **Syr.:** Hydrocodone bitartrate 2.5 mg, pseudoephedrine hydrochloride 30 mg, chlorpheniramine maleate 2 mg/5 mL, alcohol 5%, glucose, parabens, saccharin, sorbitol, sucrose, banana flavor. Bot. 473 mL, 3.8 L. **Tab.:** Hydrocodone bitartrate 5 mg, pseudoephedrine hydrochloride 60 mg, lactose. Tab. Bot. 100s. *c-III.*

Use: Upper respiratory combination, antihistamine, antitussive, decongestant.

Py-Co-Pay Tooth Powder. (Block Drug) Sodium Cl, sodium bicarbonate, calcium carbonate, magnesium carbonate, tricalcium phosphate, eugenol, methyl salicylate. Can 7 oz. *OTC.*
Use: Dentifrice.

Pyocidin-Otic. (Forest) Hydrocortisone 5 mg, polymyxin B sulfate 10,000 USP units/mL in a vehicle containing water and propylene glycol. Otic Soln. Bot. 10 mL w/sterile dropper. *Rx.*
Use: Anti-infective; corticosteroid; otic.

•**pyrabrom.** (PEER-ah-brahm) USAN.
Use: Antihistamine.

Pyracol. (Davis & Sly) Pyrathyn hydrochloride 0.00 g, ammonium Cl 0.778 g, citric acid 0.52 g, menthol 0.006 g/fl oz. Bot. pt.

pyraminyl.
See: Pyrilamine maleate.

pyranilamine maleate.
See: Pyrilamine maleate.

pyranisamine bromotheophyllinate.
See: Pyrabrom.

pyranisamine maleate.
See: Pyrilamine maleate.

•**pyrantel pamoate.** (pie-RAN-tell) *USP 28.*
Use: Anthelmintic.
See: Pin-Rid.
Pin-X.

•**pyrantel tartrate.** USAN.
Use: Anthelmintic.

•**pyrazinamide.** (peer-uh-ZIN-uh-mide) *USP 28.* Aldinamide, Zinamide.
Use: Anti-infective; tuberculostatic.

pyrazinamide. (ESI Lederle Generics, UDl) Pyrazinamide 500 mg. Tab. UD 100s.
Use: Anti-infective; tuberculostatic.

•**pyrazinecarboxamide.** *USP 28.* Pyrazinamide.

•**pyrazofurin.** (pihr-AZZ-oh-FYOO-rin) USAN.
Use: Antineoplastic.

pyrazoline.
See: Antipyrine.

pyrbenzindole.
See: Benzindopyrine hydrochloride.

•**pyrethrum extract.** USAN.
Use: Pediculicide.

pyribenzamine.
See: PBZ, Prods.

Pyridamole. (Major) Dipyridamole. Tab. **25 mg:** Bot. 1000s, 2500s. **50 mg, 75 mg:** 100s, 1000s. *Rx.*
Use: Antianginal; antiplatelet.

Pyridate. (Major) Phenazopyridine 100 mg, 200 mg. Tab. Bot. 1000s. *Rx.*
Use: Analgesic; anti-infective, urinary.

Pyridene. (Health for Life Brands) Phenylazo Diamino Pyridine hydrochloride 100 mg. Tab. Bot. 24s, 100s, 1000s. *Rx.*
Use: Analgesic, urinary.

Pyridium. (Warner Chilcott) Phenazopyridine hydrochloride 100 mg, 200 mg. Tab. Bot. 100s, 1000s, UD 100s. *Rx.*
Use: Analgesic; anti-infective, urinary.
W/Hyoscyamine HBr, butabarbital.
See: Pyridium Plus.

Pyridium Plus. (Warner Chilcott) Phenazopyridine hydrochloride 150 mg, hyoscyamine HBr 0.3 mg, butabarbital 15 mg, lactose. Tab. Bot. 30s, 100s. *Rx.*
Use: Analgesic; anti-infective.

•**pyridostigmine bromide.** (pihr-id-oh-STIG-meen) *USP 28.*
Use: Cholinergic.
See: Mestinon.

pyridostigmine bromide. (Various Mfr.) Pyridostigmine bromide 60 mg. Tab. 100s, 500s. *Rx.*
Use: Cholinergic.

Pyridox. (Oxford Pharmaceutical Services) **No. 1:** Pyridoxine hydrochloride 100 mg. Tab. **No. 2:** Pyridoxine hydrochloride 200 mg. Tab. Bot. 100s. *OTC.*
Use: Vitamin supplement.

pyridoxal. Vitamin B$_6$. *OTC.*
Use: Vitamin supplement.

pyridoxamine. Vitamin B$_6$. *OTC.*
Use: Vitamin supplement.
See: Pyridoxine.

•**pyridoxine hydrochloride.** (peer-ih-DOX-een) *USP 28.*
Use: Enzyme co-factor vitamin.
See: Aminoxin.
Vitamin B$_6$.
Vitelle Nestrex.
W/Combinations.
See: Vitelle Lurline PMS.

pyridoxine hydrochloride. (Various Mfr.) Pyridoxine hydrochloride 100 mg/mL, chorobutanol anhydrous 5 mg. Inj. Vials. 1 mL. *Rx.*
Use: Enzyme co-factor vitamin.

pyridoxol.
See: Pyridoxine, Vitamin B$_6$.

pyrilamine bromotheophyllinate.
See: Bromaleate.
Pyrabrom.

pyrilamine maleate w/combinations.
See: Codal-DH.
Codal-DM.
Codimal DH.
Codimal DM.
Codimal PH.

Dicomal-DH.
Dicomal-DM.
Iohist D.
Midol Maximum Strength Menstrual.
Midol Maximum Strength PMS.
Pamprin Multi-Symptom Maximum
 Strength.
Poly-Histine.
Prēmsyn PMS.
Robitussin Night Relief.
Quadra-Hist D.
Quadra-Hist D PED.
Statuss Green.
Tricodene Cough & Cold.
Tri-P Oral Infant Drops.
Vetuss HC.
Z-Xtra.
pyrilamine tannate w/combinations.
 See: AlleRx.
 C-Tanna 12D.
 Duonate-12.
 Gelhist Pediatric.
 Nalex-A.
 Phenylephrine tannate/chlorpheniramine tannate/pyrilamine tannate
  pediatric.
 Rhinatate Pediatric.
 R-Tanna 12.
 Ryna-12.
 Ryna-12 S.
 Tannate Pediatric.
 Triotann Pediatric.
 Triotann-S Pediatric.
 Tussi-12 D.
 Tussi-12D S.
 Viravan-DM.
 Viravan-S.
 Viravan-T.
● **pyrimethamine.** (pihr-ih-METH-ah-meen) *USP 28.*
 Use: Antimalarial.
 See: Daraprim.
 W/Sulfadoxine.
 See: Fansidar.
pyrimidine analogs.
 Use: Antimetabolite.
 See: Capecitabine.
 Cytarabine.
 Floxuridine.
 Fluorouracil.
 Gemcitabine Hydrochloride.
● **pyrimidine antagonist, topical.**
 Use: Antineoplastic.
 See: Fluorouracil.
● **pyrinoline.** (PIHR-ih-NO-leen) USAN.
 Use: Cardiovascular agent, antiarrhythmic.
Pyrinyl Plus. (Rugby) Pyrethrins 0.33%,
 piperonyl butoxide 4%, benzyl alcohol.
 Shampoo. 59 mL. *OTC.*
 Use: Pediculicide.
pyrithen.
 See: Chlorothen Citrate.

● **pyrithione sodium.** (PEER-ih-THIGH-ohn) USAN.
 Use: Antimicrobial, topical.
● **pyrithione zinc.** (PEER-ih-THIGH-ohn
 zingk) USAN. Zinc Omadine.
 Use: Antifungal; anti-infective; antiseborrheic.
 See: Denorex Everyday Dandruff.
 Dermazine.
 DHS Zinc.
 Head & Shoulders.
 Zincon.
 ZNP Bar.
Pyrogallic Acid. (Gordon Laboratories)
 Pyrogallic acid 25%, chlorobutanol.
 Oint. Jar 1 oz, 1 lb.
 Use: Dermatologic, wart therapy.
pyrogallol. Pyrogallic acid.
Pyrohep. (Major) Cyproheptadine hydrochloride 4 mg. Tab. Bot. 250s, 500s.
 Rx.
 Use: Antihistamine.
pyrophenindane. (Bristol-Myers Squibb)
● **pyrovalerone hydrochloride.** (PIE-row-val-EH-rone) USAN.
 Use: Central stimulant.
● **pyroxamine maleate.** (pihr-OX-ah-meen) USAN.
 Use: Antihistamine.
● **pyroxylin.** (pihr-OX-ih-lin) *USP 28.*
 Soluble gun cotton. Cellulose nitrate.
 Use: Pharmaceutic necessity for collodion.
● **pyrrobutamine phosphate.** *USP 28.*
 Use: Antihistamine.
 W/Clopane hydrochloride, histadyl.
 See: Co-Pyronil.
● **pyrrocaine.** (PIHR-oh-cane) USAN.
 Use: Anesthetic, local.
pyrrocaine hydrochloride.
 Use: Anesthetic, local.
pyrrocaine hydrochloride and epinephrine injection.
 Use: Anesthetic, local.
● **pyrroliphene hydrochloride.** (pihr-OLE-ih-feen) USAN.
 Use: Analgesic.
● **pyrrolnitrin.** (pihr-OLE-nye-trin) USAN.
 Under study.
 Use: Antifungal.
● **pyrvinium pamoate.** (pihr-VIN-ee-uhm
 PAM-oh-ate) *USP 28.*
 Use: Anthelmintic.
PYtest. (Tri-Med) 1 mCi[14]-C-urea. Cap.
 UD 1s, 10s, 100s. *Rx.*
 Use: Diagnostic aid.
PYtest Kit. (Tri-Med) Breath test for detecting *H. pylori.* Kit. 1 PYtest Cap. and
 breath collection equipment. *Rx.*
 Use: Diagnostic aid.

Q

QB. (Major) Theophylline 150 mg, guaifenesin 90 mg. Liq. Bot. Pt, gal. *Rx.*
Use: Bronchodilator, expectorant.

QDALL. (Atley) Pseudoephedrine hydrochloride 100 mg, chlorpheniramine maleate 12 mg, sucrose. ER Cap. 100s. *Rx.*
Use: Decongestant and antihistamine.

Q.T. Quick Tanning Suntan by Coppertone. (Schering-Plough) Ethylhexyl p-methoxycinnamate, dihydroxyacetone. SPF 2. Lot. Bot. 120 mL. *OTC.*
Use: Sunscreen.

Qua-Bid. (Quaker City Pharmacal) Papaverine hydrochloride 150 mg. TR Cap. Bot. 100s, 1000s. *OTC.*
Use: Vasodilator.

•**quadazocine mesylate.** (kwad-AZE-oh-SEEN MEH-sih-LATE) USAN.
Use: Opioid antagonist.

Quadra-Hist D. (Ethex) Pseudoephedrine hydrochloride 80 mg, phenyltoloxamine citrate 16 mg, pyrilamine maleate 16 mg, pheniramine maleate 16 mg, sucrose. ER Cap. Bot. 100s *Rx*
Use: Upper respiratory combination, decongestant, antihistamine.

Quadra-Hist D PED. (Ethex) Pseudoephedrine hydrochloride 40 mg, phenyltoloxamine citrate 8 mg, pyrilamine maleate 8 mg, pheniramine maleate 8 mg, sucrose. ER Cap. Bot. 100s. *Rx.*
Use: Upper respiratory combination, decongestant, antihistamine.

Quadramet. (DuPont) Samarium SM 153 lexidronam 1850 MBq/mL (50 mCi/mL) at calibration. Inj. Frozen, single-dose vial. 10 mL. In 2 mL fill (3700 MBq), 3 mL fill (5550 MBq). *Rx.*
Use: Treatment for bone lesions.

quadruple sulfonamides.
See: Sulfonamide.

Quad Tann. (Breckenridge Pharm.) Carbetapentane tannate 60 mg, chlorpheniramine tannate 5 mg, phenylephrine tannate 10 mg, ephedrine tannate 10 mg. Tab. Bot. 100s. *Rx.*
Use: Upper respiratory combination, antitussive, antihistamine, decongestant.

•**quazepam.** (KWAY-zuh-pam) *USP 28.*
Use: Sedative/hypnotic, nonbarbiturate.
See: Doral.

•**quazinone.** (KWAY-zih-NOHN) USAN.
Use: Cardiovascular agent.

•**quazodine.** (KWAY-zoe-deen) USAN.
Use: Cardiovascular agent.

•**quazolast.** (KWAY-ZOLE-ast) USAN.
Use: Antiasthmatic mediator release inhibitor.

Quelicin. (Abbott Hospital Products) Succinylcholine Cl. **20 mg/mL:** Fliptop vial 10 mL, *Abboject* Syringe 5 mL. **50 mg/mL:** Amp. 10 mL. **100 mg/mL:** Amp. 10 mL. **Quelicin-500:** 5 mL in Pintop vial 10 mL. **Quelicin-1000:** 10 mL in Pintop vial 20 mL. *Rx.*
Use: Muscle relaxant.

Quelidrine Cough. (Abbott) Dextromethorphan HBr 10 mg, chlorpheniramine maleate 2 mg, ephedrine hydrochloride 5 mg, phenylephrine hydrochloride 5 mg, ammonium Cl 40 mg, ipecac fluid extract 0.005 mL, ethyl alcohol 2%/ 5 mL. Syr. Bot. 4 oz. *Rx.*
Use: Antihistamine; antitussive; bronchodilator; decongestant; expectorant.

Quercetin. (Freeda) Quercetin (from eucalyptus) 50 mg, 250 mg, sodium free. Tab. Bot. 100s, 250s. *OTC.*
Use: Vitamin supplement.

Quertine.
Use: Bioflavonoid supplement.

Questran. (Par) Cholestyramine resin 4 g/9 g powder, sucrose. Pow. for Susp. Single-dose Pkt. 9 g (60s). Can 378 g. *Rx.*
Use: Antihyperlipidemic; bile acid sequestrant; antipruritic.

Questran Light. (Par) Anhydrous cholestyramine resin 4 g/6.4 g powder, maltodextrin, aspartame, phenylalanine 28 mg/6.4 g, orange vanilla flavor. Pow. Pkt 6.4 g (60s). *Rx.*
Use: Antihyperlipidemic; bile acid sequestrant.

•**quetiapine fumarate.** (cue-TIE-ah-peen FEW-mah-rate) USAN.
Use: Antipsychotic, dibenzapine derivative.
See: Seroquel.

Quiagel. (Rugby) Kaolin 6 g, pectin 142.8 mg, hyoscyamine sulfate 0.1037 mg, atropine sulfate 0.0194 mg, scopolamine HBr 0.0065 mg/30 mL. Susp. Bot. Pt, gal. *Rx.*
Use: Antidiarrheal.

Quibron. (Roberts) Theophylline (anhydrous) 150 mg, guaifenesin 90 mg. Cap. Bot. 100s, 1000s, UD 100s. *Rx.*
Use: Bronchodilator; expectorant.

Quibron Plus. (Bristol-Myers Squibb) Ephedrine hydrochloride 25 mg, theophylline (anhydrous) 150 mg, butabarbital 20 mg, guaifenesin 100 mg. Cap. Bot. 100s. *Rx.*
Use: Antiasthmatic combination.

Quibron Plus Elixir. (Bristol-Myers Squibb) Theophylline 150 mg, ephedrine hydrochloride 25 mg, guaifenesin 100 mg, butabarbital 20 mg, alcohol 15%. Elix. Bot. Pt. *Rx.*
Use: Antiasthmatic combination.

Quibron-T Dividose Tablets. (Roberts) Theophylline anhydrous 300 mg. Tab. Dividose design breakable into 100, 150, or 200 mg portions. Immediate-release. Bot. 100s. *Rx.*
Use: Bronchodilator.

Quibron-300. (Roberts) Theophylline (anhydrous) 300 mg, guaifenesin 180 mg. Cap. Bot. 100s. *Rx.*
Use: Bronchodilator; expectorant.

Quibron-T/SR Dividose Tablets. (Roberts) Theophylline anhydrous 300 mg. Tab. Dividose design breakable into 100 mg, 150 mg, or 200 mg portions. Sustained-release. Bot. 100s. *Rx.*
Use: Bronchodilator.

Quick CARE. (Novartis) **Disinfecting solution:** Isopropanol, sodium Cl, polyoxypropylenepolyoxyethylene block copolymer, disodium lauroamphodiacetate. Bot. 15 mL. **Rinse and neutralizer:** Sodium borate, boric acid, sodium perborate (generating up to 0.006% hydrogen peroxide), phosphoric acid. Bot. 360 mL. *OTC.*
Use: Contact lens care.

Quick-K. (Western Research) Potassium bicarbonate 650 mg (potassium 6.5 mEq). Tab. Bot. 30s, 100s. *Rx.*
Use: Electrolyte supplement.

Quiebar. (Nevin) Butabarbital sodium. **Spantab:** 1.5 gr. TR Spantab. Bot. 50s, 500s. **Elix.:** 30 mg/5 mL. Bot. pt, gal. **Tab.:** 15 mg. Bot. 100s, 1000s; 30 mg. Bot. 1000s. **A.C. Cap.:** Bot. 100s, 500s. *c-III.*
Use: Hypnotic; sedative.

Quiebel. (Nevin) Butabarbital sodium 15 mg, belladonna extract 15 mg. Cap. Bot. 100s, 1000s. Elix. Pt, gal. *c-III.*
Use: Anticholinergic; antispasmodic; hypnotic; sedative.

Quiecof. (Nevin) Dextromethorphan HBr 7.5 mg, chlorpheniramine maleate 0.75 mg, guaiacol glyceryl ether 25 mg/5 mL. Bot. 4 oz, pt, gal. *OTC.*
Use: Antitussive; antihistamine; expectorant.

Quiet Night. (Rosemont) Pseudoephedrine hydrochloride 10 mg, doxylamine succinate 1.25 mg, dextromethorphan HBr 5 mg, acetaminophen 167 mg/5 mL. Liq. Bot. 180 mL, 300 mL. *OTC.*
Use: Analgesic; antihistamine; antitussive; decongestant.

Quiet Time. (Whiteworth Towne) Acetaminophen 600 mg, ephedrine sulfate 8 mg, dextromethorphan HBr 15 mg, doxylamine succinate 7.5 mg, alcohol 25 mg/30 mL. Bot. 180 mL. *OTC.*
Use: Analgesic; antihistamine; antitussive; decongestant.

•**quiflapon sodium.** (KWIH-flap-ahn SO-dee-uhm) USAN.
Use: Antiasthmatic; inflammatory bowel disease suppressant.

Quik-Cept. (Laboratory Diagnostics) Slide test for pregnancy, rapid latex inhibition test. Kit 25s, 50s, 100s.
Use: Diagnostic aid.

Quik-Cult. (Laboratory Diagnostics) Slide test for fecal occult blood. Kit 150s, 200s, 300s, and tape test.
Use: Diagnostic aid.

•**quilostigmine.** (Kwill-oh-STIG-meen) USAN.
Use: Cholinergic, cholinesterase inhibitor; treatment of Alzheimer disease.

Quinaglute Dura-Tabs. (Berlex) Quinidine gluconate 324 mg. Tab. Bot. 100s, 250s, 500s, UD 100s. Unit-of-use 90s, 120s. *Rx.*
Use: Antiarrhythmic.

•**quinaldine blue.** (kwin-AL-deen) USAN.
Use: Diagnostic agent, obstetrics.

•**quinaprilat.** (KWIN-ah-PRILL-at) *USP 28.*
Use: Antihypertensive; enzyme inhibitor, angiotensin-converting.

•**quinapril hydrochloride.** (KWIN-uh-PRILL) USAN.
Use: Antihypertensive; enzyme inhibitor, angiotensin-converting.
See: Accupril.
W/Hydrochlorothiazide.
See: Accuretic.

quinapril hydrochloride. (Various Mfr.) Quinapril hydrochloride 5 mg, 10 mg, 20 mg, 40 mg. May contain lactose. Tab. 90s. *Rx.*
Use: Angiotensin-converting enzyme inhibitor.

Quinaretic. (Amide) Hydrochlorothiazide/quinapril hydrochloride 12.5 mg/10 mg, 12.5 mg/20 mg, 25 mg/20 mg. Film coated. Tab. 30s, 100s, 500s. *Rx.*
Use: Antihypertensive combination.

•**quinazosin hydrochloride.** (kwin-AZZ-oh-sin) USAN.
Use: Antihypertensive.

•**quinbolone.** (KWIN-bole-ohn) USAN.
Use: Anabolic.

•**quindecamine acetate.** (kwin-DECK-ah-meen) USAN.
Use: Anti-infective.

•**quindonium bromide.** (kwin-DOE-nee-uhn) USAN.
Use: Cardiovascular agent, antiarrhythmic.

•**quinelorane hydrochloride.** (kwih-NELL-oh-RANE) USAN.
Use: Antihypertensive; antiparkinsonian.

•**quinetolate.** (Kwin-EH-toe-late) USAN.
Use: Muscle relaxant.

•**quinfamide.** (KWIN-fah-mide) USAN.
Use: Antiamebic.

•**quingestanol acetate.** (kwin-JESS-tan-ahl) USAN.
Use: Hormone, progestin.

•**quingestrone.** (kwin-JESS-trone) USAN.
Use: Hormone, progestin.

Quinidex L-A.
See: Quinidex Extentabu.

quinidine.
Use: Antiarrhythmic.
See: Quinidine Gluconate.
Quinidine Sulfate.

•**quinidine gluconate.** (KWIN-ih-deen) *USP 28.*
Use: Cardiovascular agent, antiarrhythmic.

quinidine gluconate. (Lilly) Quinidine gluconate 80 mg/mL (50 mg/mL quinidine), EDTA 0.005%, phenol 25%. Inj. Vials. 10 mL multidose. *Rx.*
Use: Antiarrhythmic.

quinidine gluconate. (Various Mfr.) Quinidine gluconate 324 mg. SR Tab. Bot. 100s, 250s, 500s. *Rx.*
Use: Antiarrhythmic.

•**quinidine sulfate.** (KWIN-ih-deen SULL-fate) *USP 28.*
Use: Cardiovascular agent, antiarrhythmic.

quinidine sulfate. (Various Mfr.) Quinidine sulfate. **Tab.:** 200 mg, 300 mg. Bot. 100s, 1000s. **SR Tab.:** 300 mg. 100s, 250s. *Rx.*
Use: Cardiovascular agent, antiarrhythmic.

quinine and urea hydrochloride. (KWIE-nine and you-REE-ah HIGH-droe-KLOR-ide)
Use: Sclerosing agent.

•**quinine ascorbate.** (KWIE-nine ass-CORE-bate) USAN. *Formerly quinine biascorbate.*
Use: Smoking deterrent.

quinine bisulfate. (KWIE-nine)
Use: Analgesic; antimalarial; antipyretic.

quinine dihydrochloride. (KWIE-nine)
Use: Antimalarial.

quinine ethylcarbonate. (KWIE-nine)
See: Euquinine.

quinine glycerophosphate. (KWIE-nine) Quinine compound with glycerol phosphate.

•**quinine sulfate.** (KWIE-nine) *USP 28.*
Use: Antimalarial.
W/Aminophylline.
See: Strema.
W/Atropine sulfate, emetine hydrochloride, aconitine, camphor monobromate.
See: Coryza.

quinine sulfate. (Various Mfr.) Quinine sulfate. **Cap.:** 200 mg, 260 mg, 325 mg. Bot. 100s, 500s, 1000s. **Tab.:** 260 mg. Bot. 100s, 500s, 1000s. *Rx.*
Use: Antimalarial; cinchona alkaloid.

quinisocaine.
See: Dimethisoquin hydrochloride.

quinolinone derivatives.
Use: Antipsychotic.
See: Aripiprazole.

quinophan.
See: Cinchophen.

Quinora. (Key) Quinidine sulfate 300 mg. Tab. Bot. 100s, 1000s, UD 100s. *Rx.*
Use: Antiarrhythmic.

quinoxyl.
See: Chiniofon.

•**quinpirole hydrochloride.** (KWIN-pihr-ole) USAN.
Use: Antihypertensive.

quinprenaline. Quinterenol Sulfate.

Quin-Release. (Major) Quinidine gluconate 324 mg. SR Tab. Bot. 100s, 250s, 500s, UD 100s. *Rx.*
Use: Antiarrhythmic.

Quinsana Plus. (Stephan) Tolnafate 1%, cornstarch, talc. Pow. In 90 g. *OTC.*
Use: Antifungal, topical.

Quintabs. (Freeda) Vitamins A 10,000 units, D 400 units, E 29 mg, B_1 25 mg, B_2 25 mg, B_3 100 mg, B_5 25 mg, B_6 25 mg, B_{12} 25 mcg, C 300 mg, folic acid 0.1 mg, inositol, PABA. Tab. Bot. 100s, 250s. *OTC.*
Use: Vitamin supplement.

Quintabs-M. (Freeda) Iron 15 mg, Vitamins A 10,000 units, D 400 units, E 50 mg, B_1 30 mg, B_2 30 mg, B_3 150 mg, B_5 30 mg, B_6 30 mg, B_{12} 30 mcg, C 300 mg, folic acid 0.4 mg, Ca, Cu, K, Mg, Mn, Se, Zn 30 mg, PABA. Tab. Bot. 100s, 250s, 500s. *OTC.*
Use: Mineral, vitamin supplement.

•**quinterenol sulfate.** (kwin-TER-en-ahl) USAN.
Use: Bronchodilator.

•**quinuclium bromide.** (kwih-NEW-klee-uhm) USAN.
Use: Antihypertensive.

•**quinupristin.** (kwih-NEW-priss-tin) USAN.
Use: Anti-infective.
quinupristin/dalfopristin. (kwih-NEW-priss-tin dal-FOE-priss-tin)
Use: Anti-infective
See: Synercid.
•**quipazine maleate.** (KWIP-ah-zeen) USAN.
Use: Antidepressant; oxytocic.
quipenyl naphthoate.
See: Plasmochin naphthoate.

Quixin. (Santen) Levofloxacin 0.5% (5 mg/mL), benzalkonium chloride 0.005%. Soln. Bot. 2.5 mL, 5 mL. *Rx.*
Use: Antibiotic.
QVAR. (IVAX) Beclomethasone dipropionate 40 mcg, 80 mcg per actuation. Aer. Can. 7.3 g (100 actuations w/actuator). *Rx.*
Use: Respiratory inhalant, corticosteroid.

R

RabAvert. (Chiron Therapeutics) Rabies antigen 2.5 units, < 1 mcg neomycin, < 20 ng chlortetracycline, < 2 ng amphotericin B, < 3 ng ovalbumin. Inj. *Rx.*
Use: Immunization.

●**rabeprazole sodium.** (rab-EH-pray-zahl) USAN.
Use: Proton pump inhibitor.
See: Aciphex.

rabies antigen.
Use: Immunization.

●**rabies immune globulin.** (RAY-beez-ih-MYOON GLAB-byoo-lin) *USP 28.*
Use: Immunization.
See: BayRab.
Imogam Rabies-HT.

rabies immune globulin (RIG), human.
See: Rabies immune globulin.

●**rabies vaccine.** (RAY-beez vaccine) *USP 28.*
Use: Immunization.
See: Imovax Rabies.
RabAvert.
Rabies Vaccine Adsorbed.

rabies vaccine (adsorbed). (Michigan Department of Health) Challenge virus standard (CVS) Kissling/MDPH Strain. Inj. Vial 1 mL. *Rx.*
Use: Immunization.

●**racemethionine.** (RAY-see-meh-THIGH-oh-neen) *USP 28.* Formerly Methionine.
Use: Acidifier, urinary.
See: Pedameth.

racemic calcium pantothenate.
See: Calcium Pantothenate, Racemic.

racemic desoxynorephedrine.
See: Amphetamine.

racemic ephedrine hydrochloride. Racephedrine hydrochloride.

racemic pantothenic acid.
See: Vitamin, Preps.

●**racephedrine hydrochloride.** USAN.
Use: Vasoconstrictor; decongestant, nasal.
See: Ephedrine Combinations.
W/Aminophylline, Phenobarbital.
See: Amodrine.

racephedrine hydrochloride. (Pharmacia) Racephedrine hydrochloride **Cap.:** ⅜ gr. Bot. 40s, 250s, 1000s. **Soln.:** 1%. Bot. 1 fl oz, pt, gal.
Use: Vasoconstrictor; decongestant, nasal.

●**racephenicol.** (ray-see-FEN-ih-KAHL) *USP 28.*
Use: Anti-infective.

●**racepinephrine hydrochloride.** (race-epp-ih-NEFF-rin) *USP 28.*
Use: Bronchodilator.

●**raclopride C11.** (RACK-low-pride) *USP 28.*
Use: Radiopharmaceutical.

●**radaxafine hydrochloride.** (rad-a-FAX-een) USAN.
Use: Antidepressant, antianxiety.

radioactive isotopes.
See: Albumin, Aggregated Iodinated, Human I-131.
Chlormerodrin Hg-197.
Chlormerodrin Hg-203.
Cyanocobalamin Co-57.
Cyanocobalamin Co-60.
Gold Au-198.
Medotope.
Radio-Iodinated Serum Albumin.
Selenomethionine Se-75.
Sodium Chromate Cr 51.
Sodium Iodide I-131.
Sodium Iodide I-125.
Sodium Phosphate P-32.
Sodium Radio-Chromate.
Sodium Radio-Iodide.
Sodium Radio Phosphate.
Sodium Rose Bengal I-131.
Strontium Nitrate Sr-85.
Technetium Tc-99m.
Triolein I-131.
Xenon Xe-133.

radiogold (^{198}Au), solution. *USP 28.*
Gold Au-198 Injection.
Use: Irradiation therapy.

radio-iodide (^{131}I), sodium.
Use: Radiopharmaceutical.
See: Iodotope.

radio-iodinated (^{131}I) serum albumin. (Human) Iodinated I-131 Albumin Injection.

radio-iodinated serum albumin (human), (^{125}I).
See: Albumotope (^{125}I).

radiopaque agents.
See: Anatrast.
Baricon.
Barobag.
Barium Sulfate.
Barium Sulfate, USP.
Baro-cat.
Baros.
Barosperse.
Bear•E•Yum CT.
Bear•E•Yum GI.
Cheetah.
Cholografin Meglumine.
Cystografin.
Cystografin Dilute.
Definity.
Diatrizoate Meglumine and Diatrizoate Sodium.

Diatrizoate Meglumine 18%.
Diatrizoate Meglumine 52% and Diatrizoate Sodium 8%.
Diatrizoate Meglumine 52.7% and Iodipamide Meglumine 26.8%.
Diatrizoate Meglumine 60%.
Diatrizoate Meglumine 66% and Diatrizoate Sodium 10%.
Diatrizoate Meglumine 30%.
Diatrizoate Sodium.
Diatrizoate Sodium 50%.
Enecat CT.
Enhancer.
Entrobar.
Entroease.
EntroEase Dry.
Epi-C.
Ethiodized Oil.
Ethiodol.
Feridex IV.
Ferumoxides.
Flo-coat.
Gadodiamide.
Gadopentetate Dimeglumine.
Gadoteridol.
Gadoversetamide.
Gastrografin.
GI Contrast Agents.
HD 85.
HD 200 Plus.
Hexabrix.
Hypaque-Cysto.
Hypaque-76.
Hypaque Sodium
Hypaque Sodium 50%.
Imager ac.
Intropaste.
Iodipamide Meglumine 52%.
Iodixanol.
Iohexol.
Iopamidol 51%.
Iopamidol 41%.
Iopamidol 76%.
Iopamidol 61%.
Iopromide.
Ioversol 51%.
Ioversol 74%.
Ioversol 68%.
Ioversol 64%.
Ioversol 34%.
Ioxaglate Meglumine 39.3% and Ioxaglate Sodium 19.6%.
Isosulfan Blue.
Isovue-300.
Isovue-370.
Isovue-200.
Isovue-250.
Isovue-M 300.
Isovue-M 200.
Liqui-coat HD.
Liquid Barosperse.

Lymphazurin 1%.
Magnevist.
Mangafodipir Trisodium.
MD-Gastroview.
MD-76 R.
Medebar Plus.
Medescan.
Octreoscan.
Omnipaque 180.
Omnipaque 140.
Omnipaque 300.
Omnipaque 350.
Omnipaque 240.
Omniscan.
OptiMARK.
Optiray 160.
Optiray 300.
Optiray 350.
Optiray 320.
Optiray 240.
Oral Cholecystographic Agents.
Pediatric Bear•E•Bag.
Pentereotide.
Perflutren.
Prepcat.
ProHance.
Radiopaque Polyvinyl Chloride.
Reno-60.
Reno-30.
RenoCal-76.
Reno-Dip.
Renografin-60.
Sinografin.
Sitzmarks.
Sodium Bicarbonate and Tartaric Acid.
Telepaque.
Teslascan.
Tomocat.
Tonopaque.
Ultravist 150.
Ultravist 300.
Ultravist 370.
Ultravist 240.
Visipaque 320.
Visipaque 270.
radiopaque polyvinyl chloride.
   Use: Radiopaque agent, GI contrast
   agent.
   See: Sitzmarks.
radio-phosphate (^{32}P), sodium.
   Use: Radiopharmaceutical.
radioselenomethionine 75 Se. Seleno-
   methionine Se 75.
radiotolpovidone I-131. Tolpovidone
   I-131.
• **rafoxanide.** (ray-FOX-ah-nide) USAN.
   Use: Anthelmintic.
Ragus. (Miller Pharmacal Group) Mg
   27 mg, vitamins C 100 mg, Ca 580 mg,
   P 450 mg, l-lysine 25 mg, dl-methionine 50 mg, A 5000 units, D 400 units,

E 10 mg, B₁ 20 mg, B₂ 3 mg, B₆ 5 mg, B₁₂ 9 mcg, niacinamide 80 mg, pantothenic acid 5 mg, Fe 20 mg, Cu 1 mg, Mn 2 mg, K 10 mg, Zn 2 mg, I 0.1 mg/ 3 Tab. Bot. 100s. *OTC.*
Use: Mineral, vitamin supplement.

• **ralitoline.** (rah-LIT-oh-leen) USAN.
Use: Anticonvulsant.

R A Lotion. (Medco Lab) Resorcinol 3%, alcohol 43%. Lot. Plastic Bot. 120 mL, 240 mL, 480 mL. *OTC.*
Use: Dermatologic, acne.

• **raloxifene hydrochloride.** (ral-OX-ih-FEEN) USAN. Formerly Keoxifene hydrochloride.
Use: Antiestrogen.
See: Evista.

• **raltitrexed.** (ral-tih-TREX-ehd) USAN.
Use: Advanced colorectal cancer treatment (thymidylate synthase inhibitor), antineoplastic.

• **raluridine.** (ral-YOUR-ih-deen) USAN.
Use: Antiviral.

• **ramelteon.** (ram-EL-tee-on) USAN.
Use: Sleep disorders.
See: Rozerem.

• **ramipril.** (ruh-MIH-prill) USAN.
Use: Antihypertensive, enzyme inhibitor (angiotensin-converting), congestive heart failure.
See: Altace.

• **ramoplanin.** (ram-oh-PLAN-in) USAN.
Use: Investigational anti-infective.

Randolectil. (Farbenfabriken Bayer Corp.) Butaperazine. *Rx.*
Use: Psychotherapeutic agent.

ranestol. Triclofenol piperazine.
Use: Anthelmintic.

• **ranibizumab.** (ra-NIB-i-ZUE-mab) USAN.
Use: Age-related macular degeneration.

Raniclor. (Ranbaxy) Cefaclor 125 mg (phenylalanine 2.8 mg), 187 mg (phenylalanine 4.2 mg), 250 mg (phenylalanine 5.6 mg), 375 mg (phenylalanine 8.4 mg). Aspartame, mannitol, tartrazine. Fruity flavor. Chew. Tab. 20s, 30s (125 mg and 250 mg only), 250s, UD 100s. *Rx.*
Use: Antibiotic.

• **ranimycin.** (ran-ih-MY-sin) USAN.
Use: Anti-infective.

ranitidine. (Various Mfr.) Ranitidine (as base) 75 mg, 150 mg, 300 mg. Tab. Bot. 30s (except 150 mg), 60s (150 mg only), 100s (except 75 mg), 250s (300 mg only), 500s (except 75 mg), 1,000s (except 75 mg), 2,500s (300 mg only), 5,000s (150 mg only), UD 100s (except 75 mg). *OTC.*

Use: Histamine H₂ antagonist.

• **ranitidine hydrochloride.** (ran-EYE-tih-DEEN) *USP 28.*
Use: Histamine H₂ antagonist.
See: Zantac.
Zantac Efferdose.
Zantac 150.
Zantac 75.

ranitidine hydrochloride. (Various Mfr.) Randitidine hydrochloride (as base) 15 mg/mL. May contain alcohol. Syrup. Bot. UD 10 mL. *Rx.*
Use: Histamine H₂ antagonist.

ranitidine hydrochloride in sodium chloride injection.
Use: Antiulcerative.
See: Zantac.

• **ranolazine hydrochloride.** (RAY-no-lah-ZEEN) USAN.
Use: Antianginal.

Rapamune. (Wyeth Laboratories) Sirolimus. **Oral Soln.:** 1 mg/mL, ethanol. 60 mL and 150 mL bot. with oral syringe adaptor. Pouches 1 mL, 2 mL, and 5 mL in 30s. **Tab.:** 1 mg, 2 mg, sucrose, lactose. Bot. 100s, *Redipak* UD 100s. *Rx.*
Use: Immunologic, immunosuppressive.

Rapid Test Strep. (SmithKline Diagnostics) Latex slide agglutination test for identification of group A streptococci. Box. 25s, 100s.
Use: Diagnostic aid.

Raptiva. (Genentech) Efalizumab 150 mg (125 mg/1.25 mL). Preservative-free. Pow. for Inj., lyophilized. Single-use vials (sucrose 123.2 mg, L-histidine hydrochloride monohydrate 6.8 mg, L-histidine 4.3 mg) with 1 single-use prefilled diluent syr. containing 1.3 mL sterile water for injection, 2 25-gauge × ⅝ inch needles, and 2 alcohol prep pads. *Rx.*
Use: Immunosuppressive.

• **rasagiline mesylate.** (rass-AH-jih-leen MEH-sih-late) USAN.
Use: Investigational antiparkinson agent.

• **rasburicase.** (raz-BYORR-ih-kays) USAN.
Use: Antimetabolite.
See: Elitek.

rastinon. Tolbutamide.
Use: Antidiabetic.

rattlesnake bite therapy.
See: Antivenin (crotalidae).

Rauneed. (Hanlon) Rauwolfia 50 mg, 100 mg. Tab. Bot. 100s. *Rx.*
Use: Antihypertensive.

Raunescine. (Penick) An alkaloid of rauwolfia serpentina. Under study.
Use: Antihypertensive.

Raunormine. (Penick) 11-Desmethoxy reserpine. *Rx.*

Raurine. (Westerfield) Reserpine. **Tab.:** 0.1 mg. Bot. 100s. **Delayed-Action Cap.:** 0.5 mg. Bot. 100s. *Rx.*
Use: Antihypertensive.

Rauserfia. (New Eng. Phr. Co.) Rauwolfia serpentina 50 mg, 100 mg. Tab. Bot. 100s. *Rx.*
Use: Antihypertensive.

Rautina. (Fellows) Rauwolfia serpentina whole root 50 mg, 100 mg. Tab. Bot. 1000s. *Rx.*
Use: Antihypertensive.

Rauval. (Pal-Pak, Inc.) Rauwolfia whole root 50 mg, 100 mg. Tab. Bot. 100s, 500s, 1000s. *Rx.*
Use: Antihypertensive.

rauwolfia/bendroflumethiazide. (Various Mfr.) Bendroflumethiazide 4 mg, powdered rauwolfia serpentina 50 mg. Tab. Bot. 100s. *Rx.*
Use: Antihypertensive.
See: Rauzide.

• **rauwolfia serpentina.** (rah-WOOL-fee-ah ser-pen-TEE-nah) *USP 28.*
Use: Antihypertensive.
See: Raudixin.
  Rauneed.
  Rauval.
  Rawfola.
  T-Rau.
  Wolfina.
  W/Bendroflumethiazide.
  See: Rauzide.

rauwolfia serpentina active principles (alkaloids). Deserpidine, Rescinnamone.
See: Reserpine.

rauwolscine. An alkaloid of *Rauwolfia canescens.* Under study.
Use: Antihypertensive.

Rauzide. (Bristol-Myers Squibb) Rauwolfia serpentina pow. 50 mg, bendroflumethiazide 4 mg, tartrazine. Tab. Bot. 100s. *Rx.*
Use: Antihypertensive.

Ravocaine. (Cook-Waite Laboratories, Inc.) Propoxycaine hydrochloride 4 mg, procaine 20 mg, norepinephrine bitartrate equivalent to 0.033 mg levophed base, sodium Cl 3 mg, acetone sodium bisulfite not more than 2 mg. Cartridge 1.8 mL. *Rx.*
Use: Anesthetic, local.

ravuconazole.
Use: Antifungal.

Rawfola. (Foy Laboratories) Rauwolfia serpentina 50 mg. Tab. Bot. 1000s. *Rx.*
Use: Antihypertensive.

Rawl Vite. (Rawl) Vitamins A 10,000 units, D 500 units, B_1 10 mg, B_2 5 mg, B_6 1 mg, calcium pantothenate 5 mg, nicotinamide 50 mg, C 125 mg, E 2.5 units. Tab. Bot. 100s. *OTC.*
Use: Mineral, vitamin supplement.

Rawl Whole Liver Vitamin B Complex. (Rawl) Whole liver 500 mg, amino acids found in the whole liver, vitamins B_1 1 mg, B_2 2 mg, niacinamide 5 mg, choline Cl 12 mg, B_6 0.2 mg, calcium pantothenate 0.2 mg, inositol 5 mg, biotin 0.6 mcg, B_{12} 0.3 mcg. Cap. Bot. 100s, 500s. *OTC.*
Use: Mineral, vitamin supplement.

• **raxibacumab.** (RAX-ee-BAK-ue-mab) USAN.
Use: Anthrax infection.

Ray Block. (Del-Ray) Octyl dimethyl PABA 5%, benzophenone-3 3%, SD alcohol. Lot. Bot. 118.3 mL. *OTC.*
Use: Sunscreen.

Ray-D. (Nion Corp.) Vitamin D 400 units, thiamine mononitrate 1 mg, riboflavin 2 mg, niacin 10 mg, I 0.1 mg, Ca 375 mg, P 300 mg/6 Tab. In base of brewer's yeast. Bot. 100s, 500s. *OTC.*
Use: Mineral, vitamin supplement.

Rayderm. (Velvet Pharmacal) Euphorbia extract, phenyl salicylate, neatsfoot oil, olive oil, lanolin in emulsion base preserved with methyl- and propylparabens. Oint. Tube 1.5 oz, Jar lb. *OTC.*
Use: Burn therapy.

• **rayon, purified.** (RAY-ahn) *USP 28.*
Use: Surgical aid.

raythesin. (Raymer)
See: Propyl p-Aminobenzoate.

Razadyne. (Janssen) Galantamine hydrobromide. **Tab.:** 4 mg, 8 mg, 12 mg, lactose. Bot. 60s. **Oral Soln.:** 4 mg/mL, saccharin. Bot. 100 mL with calibrated pipette. *Rx.*
Use: Cholinesterase inhibitor.

Razadyne ER. (Janssen) Galantamine hydrobromide 8 mg, 16 mg, 24 mg. Sucrose. ER Cap. 30s. *Rx.*
Use: Cholinesterase inhibitor.

• **razaxaban hydrochloride.** (ra-ZAX-aban) USAN.
Use: Anticoagulant.

Razepam. (Major) Temazepam 15 mg, 30 mg. Cap. Bot. 100s. *c-iv.*
Use: Hypnotic; sedative.

RCF. (Ross) Carbohydrate free low iron soy protein formula base. Carbohydrate and water must be added. For infants unable to tolerate the amount or

type of carbohydrate in conventional formulas. Can 14 fl oz. (Concentrated liq.). *OTC.*
Use: Nutritional supplement.

Reabilan. (Elan) Protein 31.5 g, fat 39 g, carbohydrates 131.5 g, Na 702 mg, K 1.252 g/L, lactose free. With appropriate vitamins and minerals. Liq. Bot. 375 mL. *OTC.*
Use: Nutritional supplement.

Reabilan HN. (Elan) Protein 58.2 g, fat 52 g, carbohydrates 158 g, Na 1000 mg, K 1661 mg/L, lactose free. With appropriate vitamins and minerals. Liq. Bot. 375 mL. *OTC.*
Use: Nutritional supplement.

Rea-Lo. (Whorton Pharmaceuticals, Inc.) Urea in water-soluble moisturizing oil base. Lot 1th Bot 4 oz, pl. Cream. 30%. Jar 2 oz, 16 oz. *OTC.*
Use: Emollient.

Rebetol. (Schering) Ribavirin. **Cap.:** 200 mg, lactose. Bot 42s, 56s, 70s, 84s. **Oral Soln.:** 40 mg/mL. Sucrose, sorbitol. Bubble gum flavor. 100 mL. *Rx.*
Use: Antiviral.

Rebetron. (Schering) Interferon alfa-2b, recombinant 3 million units/0.5 mL, ribavirin 200 mg. Inj. Cap. *Intron A* in single-dose vials (6s), one 18 million units multidose vial or one 18 million units multidose pen. *Rebetol* Caps. 42s, 70s, 84s. *Rx.*
Use: Antineoplastic; immunologic, immunomodulator.

Rebif. (Serono) Interferon beta-1a 22 mcg/0.5 mL, 44 mcg/0.5 mL; human albumin 2 mg (22 mcg only), 4 mg (44 mcg only), mannitol 27.3 mg, sodium acetate 0.4 mg, preservative free. Pow. for Inj. Prefilled single-use syringe with diluent (Sterile Water for Injection) and needle. Box. 1s, 3s (44 mcg only); 12s. *Rx.*
Use: Immunologic, immunomodulator.

•**rebimastat.** (re-BIM-a-stat) USAN.
Use: Antineoplastic.

reboxetine mesylate.
Use: Antidepressant.

•**recainam hydrochloride.** (reh-CANE-am) USAN.
Use: Cardiovascular agent, antiarrhythmic.

•**recainam tosylate.** (reh-CANE-am TAH-sill-ate) USAN.
Use: Cardiovascular agent, antiarrhythmic.

•**reclazepam.** (reh-CLAY-zeh-pam) USAN.
Use: Hypnotic; sedative.

Reclomide. (Major) Metoclopramide hydrochloride 10 mg. Tab. Bot. 100s, 500s, 1000s, UD 100s. *Rx.*
Use: Antiemetic, gastrointestinal stimulant.

recombinant human activated protein C.
Use: Thrombolytic agent.
See: Drotrecogic Alfa (activated).

recombinant human erythropoietin.
Use: Hemotopoietic.
See: Darbepoetin Alfa.
  Epoetin Alfa, Recombinant.

recombinant human insulin-like growth factor I.
Use: Antibody-mediated growth hormone resistance. [Orphan Drug]

recombinant tissue plasminogen activator. *Rx.*
See: Activase.

recombinant vaccinia (human papillomavirus).
Use: Cervical cancer. [Orphan Drug]

Recombinate. (Baxter) Concentrated recombinant antihemophilic factor. When reconstituted, contains albumin (human)12.5 mg/mL, polyethylene glycol 1.5 mg, sodium 180 mEq/L, histidine 55 mM, calcium 0.2 mg/mL. Monoclonal purified. Pow. for Inj., lyophilized. Single-dose bot. 250 IU, 500 IU, 1,000 IU with diluent, double-ended needle, and filter needle. Actual number of antihemophilic factor units indicated on vial. *Rx.*
Use: Antihemophilic.

Recombivax HB. (Merck & Co.) Hepatitis B vaccine recombinant. Hepatitis B surface antigen. **Pediatric/Adolescent:** 5 mcg/0.5 mL, preservative free. Inj. Single-dose vial 0.5 mL. **Adult:** 10 mcg/mL, thimerosal 50 mcg. Single-dose vial 1 mL, multi-dose vial 3 mL, prefilled, single-dose syringe 1 mL. **Dialysis:** 40 mcg/mL, thimerosal 50 mcg. Single-dose vial 1 mL. *Rx.*
Use: Immunization, viral vaccine.

Recortex 10X in Oil. (Forest) 1000 mcg/mL. Vial 10 mL. *Rx.*

Recover. (Dermik) Bot. 2.25 oz. *OTC.*
Use: Dermatologic.

Rectagene. (Pfeiffer) Live yeast cell derivative supplying 2000 units Skin Respiratory Factor/oz, shark liver oil in a cocoa butter base. Supp. 12s. *OTC.*
Use: Anorectal preparation.

Rectagene Medicated Rectal Balm. (Pfeiffer) Live yeast cell derivative that supplies 2000 units Skin Respiratory Factor/30 g, refined shark liver oil 3%, white petrolatum, lanolin, thyme oil, 1:10,000 phenylmercuric nitrate. Oint.

Tube. 56.7 g. *OTC.*
Use: Anorectal preparation.

Rectal Medicone. (Medicore) Benzocaine 2 g, balsam peru 1 g, hydroxyquinoline sulfate 0.25 g, menthol $\frac{1}{7}$ g, zinc oxide 3 g. Supp. Box 12s, 24s. *OTC.*
Use: Anesthetic; antiseptic, topical.

Rectal Medicone Unguent. (Medicore) Benzocaine 20 mg, oxyquinoline sulfate 5 mg, menthol 4 mg, zinc oxide 100 mg, balsam peru 12.5 mg, petrolatum 625 mg, lanolin 210 mg/g. Tube 1.5 oz. *OTC.*
Use: Anorectal preparation.

red blood cells. Human red blood cells given by IV infusion.
Use: Blood replenisher.

red cell tagging solution.
See: A-C-D.

Red Cross Toothache Kit. (Mentholatum Co.) Eugenol 85%, sesame oil. Drops. Bot. 3.7 mL w/cotton pellets and tweezers. *OTC.*
Use: Anesthetic, local.

red ferric oxide.
Use: Pharmaceutic aid (color).

Reditemp-C. (Wyeth) Ammonium nitrate, water, and special additives. Pkg. Large and small sizes. 4 × 10s. *OTC.*
Use: Cold compress.

Red Throat Spray. (Clay-Park Labs) Phenol 1.4%. Glycerin, saccharin. Alcohol-free. Throat spray. 177 mL. *OTC.*
Use: Mouth and throat product.

Reducto, Improved. (Arcum) Phendimetrazine bitartrate 35 mg. Tab. Bot. 100s, 1000s. *c-III.*
Use: Anorexiant.

Redutemp. (International Ethical Labs) Acetaminophen 500 mg. Tab. Bot. 60s. *OTC.*
Use: Analgesic.

Reese's Pinworm. (Reese) Pyrantel pamoate 144 mg. Liq. 30 mL. *OTC.*
Use: Anthelmintic.

ReFacto. (Genetics Institute) Recombinant antihemophilic factor. When reconstituted, contains L-histidine, CaCl, polysorbate 80, sodium chloride, sucrose, preservative free. Pow. for Inj., lyophilized. Single-use vial with 250 IU, 500 IU, 1,000 IU/vial, with diluent, double-ended needle, fliter needle for withdrawal, infusion set, alcohol swabs. *Rx.*
Use: Antihemophilic agent.

Refenesen Plus Severe Strength Cough & Cold Medicine. (Reese) Pseudoephedrine hydrochloride 60 mg, guaifenesin 400 mg. Tab. Pkg. 16s.

OTC.
Use: Upper respiratory combination, decongestant, expectorant.

Refludan. (Hoechst-Marion Roussel) Lepirudin 50 mg, mannitol. Pow. for Inj. Boxes of 10s. *Rx.*
Use: Thrombin inhibitor.

Refresh. (Allergan) Polyvinyl alcohol 1.4%, povidone 0.6%, sodium Cl. UD 30s, 50s (0.3 mL single-dose container). *OTC.*
Use: Artificial tears.

Refresh Plus. (Allergan) Carboxymethylcellulose sodium 0.5%, NaCl. Preservative-free. Soln. 0.3 mL/single-use container 4s, 30s. *OTC.*
Use: Artificial tears.

Refresh PM. (Allergan) White petrolatum 56.8%, mineral oil 41.5%, lanolin alcohol, sodium Cl. Tube 3.5 g. *OTC.*
Use: Lubricant, ophthalmic.

Refresh Tears. (Allergan) Carboxymethylcellulose 0.5%. Drops. Bot. 15 mL w/dropper. *OTC.*
Use: Artificial tears.

• **regadenoson.** (re-ga-DEN-oh-son) USAN.
Use: Cardiovascular agent.

Regain. (NCI Medical Foods) Protein 15 g, carbohydrates 52 g, fat 7 g, Na 45 mg, K 75 mg, Ca 200 mg, P 100 mg, Ca, Fe, vitamin B_{12}, Mg, folic acid, fructose. With dietary fiber. 300 calories. Lactose free. Vanilla, strawberry, and malt flavors. Bar 85 g. *OTC.*
Use: Nutritional supplement.

Reglan Injection. (Wyeth) Metoclopramide hydrochloride. **10 mg/2 mL:** Amp. 2 mL, 10 mL; **5 mg/mL:** Vial 2 mL, 10 mL, 30 mL. Inj. *Rx.*
Use: Antiemetic, gastrointestinal stimulant.

Reglan Tablets. (Schwarz Pharma) Metoclopramide hydrochloride 5 mg, 10 mg. Tab. Bot. 100s; 500s, *Dis-co Pak* 100s (10 mg only). *Rx.*
Use: Antiemetic, gastrointestinal stimulant.

• **regramostim.** (reh-GRAH-moe-STIM) USAN.
Use: Biological response modifier; antineoplastic adjunct; antineutropenic; hematopoietic stimulant.

Regranex. (Johnson & Johnson Wound Management) Becaplermin 100 mcg, parabens. Gel. Tube 2 mL, 7.5 mL, 15 mL. *Rx.*
Use: Diabetic neuropathic ulcers.

Regular Iletin II. (Lilly) Purified pork regular insulin 100 units/mL. Inj. Vials. 10 mL. *OTC.*

Use: Antidiabetic, insulin.

Regular Strength Bayer Enteric Coated Caplets. (Bayer Corp. (Consumer Div.)) Aspirin 325 mg. Bot. 50s, 100s. EC Tab. *OTC.*
Use: Analgesic.

Regular Strength Midol Multisymptom. (Bayer Corp. (Consumer Div.)) Acetaminophen 325 mg, pyrilamine maleate 12.5 mg. Tab. Bot. 30s. *OTC.*
Use: Analgesic combination.

Regulax SS. (Republic) Docusate sodium 100 mg. Cap. Bot. 60s, 100s, 1000s. *OTC.*
Use: Laxative.

Reguloid. (Rugby) Psyllium husk fiber 95% pure 3.4 g/5 mL, dextrose, 14 cal/tsp. Pow. Can. 369 g, 540 g. *OTC.*
Use: Laxative.

Reguloid, Orange. (Rugby) Psyllium mucilloid 3.4 g, sucrose, orange flavor/tbsp. Pow. Can. 369 g, 540 g. *OTC.*
Use: Laxative.

Reguloid, Sugar Free Orange. (Rugby) Psyllium hydrophilic mucilloid 3.4 g, aspartame, phenylalanine 30 mg/rounded tsp. Pow. Can. 284 g, 426 g. *OTC.*
Use: Laxative.

Reguloid, Sugar Free Regular. (Rugby) Psyllium hydrophilic mucilloid 3.4 g, aspartame, phenylalanine 6 mg/dose. Pow. Can. 284 g, 426 g. *OTC.*
Use: Laxative.

Rehydralyte. (Ross) Sodium 75 mEq, potassium 20 mEq, chloride 65 mEq, citrate 30 mEq, dextrose 25 g/L, 100 calories/L. Ready-to-use Bot. 8 oz. *Rx.*
Use: Fluid, electrolyte replacement.

Relafen. (GlaxoSmithKline) Nabumetone 500 mg, 750 mg. Tab. Bot. 180s, UD 100s. *Rx.*
Use: Analgesic, NSAID.

Relagesic. (International Ethical) Phenyltoloxamine citrate 50 mg, acetaminophen 650 mg. Tab. 100s. *Rx.*
Use: Antihistamine and analgesic.

relaxin. A purified ovarian hormone of pregnancy (obtained from sows) responsible for pubic relaxation or separation of the symphysis pubis in mammals.

Relenza. (GlaxoSmithKline) Zanamivir 5 mg, lactose 20 mg. Pow. for Inh. Blister. Box 4s w/5 *Rotadisks* and 1 *Diskhaler. Rx.*
Use: Antiviral.

Reliable Gentle Laxative. (Goldline Consumer) Bisacodyl. 5 mg, lactose, sugar. EC, DR Tab. Bot. 100s, 1000s. 10 mg. Supp. Bot. 100s, 1000s. *OTC.*
Use: Laxative.

Relief Eye Drops. (Allergan) Phenylephrine hydrochloride 0.12%, antipyrine 0.1%, polyvinyl alcohol 1.4%, edetate disodium. Bot. UD 0.3 mL. *OTC.*
Use: Decongestant, ophthalmic.

Relief Solution. (Allergan) Phenylephrine hydrochloride 0.12%, antipyrine 0.1%. Soln. Bot. 20 mL. *OTC.*
Use: Decongestant combination, ophthalmic.

• **relomycin.** (REE-low-MY-sin) USAN. A macrolide antibiotic produced by a variant strain of *Streptomyces hygroscopicus.*
Use: Anti-infective.

Relpax. (Pfizer) Eletriptan HBr 24.2 mg, 48.5 mg, lactose. Tab. Blistercard. 12s. *Rx.*
Use: Antimigraine agent, serotonin 5-HT$_1$ receptor agonist.

• **remacemide hydrochloride.** (rem-ASS-eh-MIDE) USAN.
Use: Anticonvulsant (neuroprotective).

Rem Cough Medicine. (Last) Dextromethorphan HBr 5 mg/5 mL. Bot. 3 oz, 6 oz. *OTC.*
Use: Antitussive.

Remegel Soft Chewable Antacid. (Warner Lambert) Aluminum hydroxide-magnesium carbonate 476.4 mg. Chew. Tab. Pkg. 8s, 24s. *OTC.*
Use: Antacid.

Remeron. (Organon Teknika) Mirtazapine 15 mg, 30 mg, 45 mg, lactose. Tab. Bot. 30s; 100s, UD 100s (15 mg and 30 mg only). *Rx.*
Use: Antidepressant, tetracyclic compound.

Remeron SolTab. (Organon) Mirtazapine 15 mg, 30 mg, 45 mg, aspartame, mannitol, phenylalanine 2.6 mg (15 mg), 5.2 mg (30 mg), 7.8 mg (45 mg). Orally disintegrating tab. UD 30s, 90s. *Rx.*
Use: Antidepressant, tetracyclic compound.

Remicade. (Centocor) Infliximab 100 mg, sucrose 500 mg. Preservative free. Pow. for Inj., lyophilized. Single-use vials. 20 mL. *Rx.*
Use: Crohn disease; rheumatoid arthritis; ankylosing spondylitis; immunologic agent; immunomodulator.

• **remifentanil hydrochloride.** (reh-mih-FEN-tah-nill) USAN.
Use: Opioid analgesic.
See: Ultiva.

• **remiprostol.** (reh-mih-PROSTE-ole) USAN.
Use: Antiulcerative.

Remivox. (Janssen) Lorcainide hydrochloride. *Rx.*
Use: Antiarrhythmic.

Remodulin. (United Therapeutics) Treprostinil sodium 1 mg/mL, 2.5 mg/mL, 5 mg/mL, sodium chloride 5.3 mg; 10 mg/mL, sodium chloride 4 mg. Multi-use vials. 20 mL. *Rx.*
Use: Antiplatelet agent.

•**remoxipride.** (reh-MOX-ih-PRIDE) USAN.
Use: Antipsychotic.

•**remoxipride hydrochloride.** (reh-MOX-ih-PRIDE) USAN.
Use: Antipsychotic.

Remular-S. (International Ethical Labs) Chlorzoxazone 250 mg. Tab. Bot. 100s. *Rx.*
Use: Muscle relaxant.

Renacidin. (Guardian Laboratories) The composition of this powder, as manufactured, is in terms of 156 to 171 g citric acid (anhydrous) and 21 to 30 g d-gluconic acid (as the lactone) w/purified magnesium hydroxycarbonate 75 to 87 g, magnesium acid citrate 9 to 15 g, calcium (as carbonate) 2 to 6 g, water 17 to 21 g per 300 g. Bot. 25 g 6s; 150 g, 300 g. *Rx.*
Use: Irrigant, genitourinary.

Renagel. (Genzyme) Sevelamer hydrochloride 400 mg, 800 mg. Film coated. Tab. Bot. 180s (800 mg only), 360s (400 mg only). *Rx.*
Use: Phosphate binder.

RenAmin. (Clintec Nutrition) Sterile hypertonic soln. of essential and nonessential amino acids. Soln. Bot. 250 mL, 500 mL. *Rx.*
Use: Nutritional supplement, parenteral.

renanolone. *Rx.*
Use: Steroid anesthetic.

Renax. (Everett) Vitamin E (as d-alpha tocopheryl succinate) 35 units, B_1 3 mg, B_2 2 mg, B_3 20 mg, B_5 10 mg, B_6 15 mg, B_{12} 12 mg, C 50 mg, folic acid 2.5 mg, Zn 20 mg, biotin 300 mcg, Cr, Se. Capl. Bot. 90s. *Rx.*
Use: Vitamin, mineral supplement.

Renbu. (Wren) Butabarbital sodium 32.4 mg. Tab. Bot. 100s, 1000s. *c-III.*
Use: Hypnotic; sedative.

Renese-R. (Pfizer) Polythiazide 2 mg, reserpine 0.25 mg. Tab. Bot. 100s, 1000s. *Rx.*
Use: Antihypertensive.

renin angiotensin system antagonists.
See: Accupril.
Angiotensin-Converting Enzyme Inhibitors.
Benazepril Hydrochloride.

Candesartan Cilexetil.
Captopril.
Enalapril Maleate.
Eplerenone.
Eprosartan Mesylate.
Fosinopril Sodium.
Irbesartan.
Lisinopril.
Losartan Potassium.
Moexipril hydrochloride.
Olmesartan Medoxomil.
Perindopril Erbumine.
Quinapril hydrochloride.
Ramipril.
Telmisartan.
Trandolapril.
Valsartan.

RenoCal-76. (Bracco Diagnostics) Diatrizoate meglumine 660 mg, diatrizoate sodium 100 mg, iodine 370 mg/mL, EDTA. Inj. Vial 50 mL. Bot. 100 mL, 150 mL, 200 mL. *Rx.*
Use: Radiopaque agent, GI contrast agent.

Reno-Dip. (Bracco Diagnostics) Diatrizoate meglumine 300 mg, iodine 141 mg/mL, EDTA. Inj. Bot. 300 mL with or without infusion set. *Rx.*
Use: Radiopaque agent, GI contrast agent.

renoform.
See: Epinephrine.

Renografin-60. (Bracco Diagnostics) Diatrizoate meglumine 520 mg, diatrizoate sodium 80 mg, iodine 292.5 mg/mL, EDTA. Inj. Vial 10 mL, 50 mL. Bot. 100 mL. *Rx.*
Use: Radiopaque agent, GI contrast agent.

Reno-M Dip. (Bracco Diagnostics) Diatrizoate meglumine 300 mg, iodine 141 mg/mL. Inj. Bot. 300 mL. *Formerly Renografin-Dip. Rx.*
Use: Radiopaque agent.

Renormax. (Novartis) Spirapril 3 mg, 6 mg, 12 mg, 24 mg. Tab. *Rx.*
Use: ACE inhibitor.

Reno-Sed. (Vita Elixir) Methenamine 2 g, salol 0.5 g, methylene blue $\frac{1}{10}$ g, benzoic acid $\frac{1}{8}$ g, atropine sulfate $\frac{1}{1000}$ g, hyoscyamine sulfate $\frac{1}{2000}$ g. Tab. *Rx.*
Use: Anti-infective, urinary.

Reno-60. (Bracco Diagnostics) Diatrizoate meglumine 600 mg, iodine 282 mg/mL, EDTA. Inj. Vial 10 mL, 50 mL. Bot. 100 mL, 150 mL (w/and w/o infusion sets). *Rx.*
Use: Radiopaque agent, GI contrast agent.

Reno-30. (Bracco Diagnostics) Diatrizoate meglumine 300 mg, iodine 141 mg/

mL, EDTA, parabens. Inj. Multi-dose
Vial 50 mL. *Rx.*
Use: Radiopaque agent.

Renova. (Ortho Dermatological) Tretinoin 0.02%, 0.05%, stearyl alcohol,
EDTA; parabensbenzyl alcohol, cetyl
alcohol (0.02% only); methylparabens
(0.05% only). Cream. Tube. 20 g
(0.05% only), 40 g, 60 g (0.05% only).
Rx.
Use: Retinoid.

Renovist. (Bracco Diagnostics) Diatrizoate methylglucamine 34.3%, diatrizoate sodium 35%, iodine 37%. Inj. Vial
50 mL, Box 25s.
Use: Radiopaque agent.

Renovist II. (Bracco Diagnostics) Diatrizoate sodium 29.1%, meglumine diatrizoate 29.5%, iodine 31%. Inj. Vial
30 mL, 60 mL, Box 25s.
Use: Radiopaque agent.

Renovue-Dip. (Bracco Diagnostics) Iodamide meglumide 24%, iodine 11.1%.
Infusion Bot. 300 mL.
Use: Radiopaque agent.

Renovue-65. (Bracco Diagnostics) Iodamide meglumide 65%, organically
bound iodine 30%, edetate disodium.
Vial 50 mL.
Use: Radiopaque agent.

Rentamine Pediatric. (Major) Phenylephrine tannate 5 mg, chlorpheniramine tannate 4 mg, carbetapentane
tannate/5 mL, saccharin, sucrose. Syr.
Bot. Pt. *Rx.*
Use: Antihistamine, antitussive, decongestant.

ReNu Effervescent Enzymatic Cleaner.
(Bausch & Lomb) Subtilisin, polyethylene glycol, sodium carbonate, sodium
Cl, tartaric acid. Tab. Bot. 10s, 20s, 30s.
OTC.
Use: Contact lens care.

ReNu Multi-Purpose. (Bausch & Lomb)
Isotonic soln. w/sodium Cl, sodium borate, boric acid, poloxamine, polyaminopropyl biguanide 0.00005%, EDTA.
Soln. Bot. 118 mL, 237 mL, 355 mL.
OTC.
Use: Contact lens care.

ReNu Saline. (Bausch & Lomb) Isotonic
buffered soln. of sodium Cl, boric acid,
polyaminopropyl biguanide 0.00003%,
EDTA. Soln. Bot. 355 mL. *OTC.*
Use: Contact lens care.

ReNu Thermal Enzymatic Cleaner.
(Bausch & Lomb) Subtilisin, sodium
carbonate, sodium Cl, boric acid. Tab.
16s. *OTC.*
Use: Contact lens care.

ReoPro. (Lilly) Abciximab 2 mg/mL in buffered solution of sodium phosphate
0.01 M, sodium chloride 0.15 M, polysorbate 80 0.001%. Inj. Vial 5 mL. *Rx.*
Use: Antiplatelet, glycoprotein IIb/IIIa
inhibitor.

•**repaglinide.** (re-pa-GLI-nide) *USP 28.*
Use: Antidiabetic, meglitinide.
See: Prandin.

Repan. (Everett) Butalbital 50 mg, caffeine 40 mg, acetaminophen 325 mg.
Tab. Bot. 100s. *Rx.*
Use: Analgesic; hypnotic; sedative.

Repan CF. (Everett) Acetaminophen
650 mg, butalbital 50 mg. Tab. Bot.
100s. *Rx.*
Use: Analgesic combination.

•**repifermin.** (re-pi-FER-min) USAN.
Use: Mucositis; wound healing.

•**repirinast.** (ruh-PIRE-ih-nast) USAN.
Use: Antiallergic; antiasthmatic.

Replete. (Clintec Nutrition) K caseinate,
Ca caseinate, maltodextrin, sucrose,
corn oil, lecithin, vitamins A, B_1, B_2, B_3,
B_5, B_6, B_{12}, C, D, E, K, folic acid, biotin, choline, Ca, Cl, Cu, Fe, I, Mg, Mn, P,
Zn. Liq. Bot. 250 mL. *OTC.*
Use: Nutritional supplement.

Reprieve. (Mayer Lab) Caffeine 32 mg,
salicylamide 225 mg, vitamin B_1
50 mg, homatropine methylbromide
0.5 mg. Tab. Bot. 8s, 16s. *Rx.*
Use: Analgesic combination.

•**repromicin.** (rep-ROW-MY-sin) USAN.
Use: Anti-infective.

Repronex. (Ferring) Follicle-stimulating
hormone and luteinzing hormone
75 units or 150 units. Pow. or pellet for
inj., lyophilized. Vial with diluent. *Rx.*
Use: Sex hormone, ovulation stimulant.

•**reproterol hydrochloride.** (rep-ROW-
TEE-role) USAN.
Use: Bronchodilator.

Reptilase-R. (Abbott Diagnostics) Diagnostic for the investigation of fibrin formation and disturbances in fibrin formation due to causes other than thrombin inhibition.
Use: Diagnostic aid.

Requa's Charcoal. (Requa, Inc.) Wood
charcoal 10 g. Tab. Pkg. 50s. Can
125s. *OTC.*
Use: Antiflatulent.

Requip. (GlaxoSmithKline) Ropinirole hydrochloride 0.25 mg, 0.5 mg, 1 mg,
2 mg, 5 mg, lactose. Tab. Bot. 30s,
100s. *Rx.*
Use: Antiparkinson agent.

Resa. (Vita Elixir) Reserpine 0.25 mg.
Tab. Bot. *Rx.*
Use: Antihypertensive.

Resaid. (Geneva) Phenylpropanolamine hydrochloride 75 mg, chlorpheniramine maleate 12 mg. Cap. Bot. 100s, 1000s. *Rx.*
Use: Antihistamine, decongestant.
Resaid S.R. (Geneva) Phenylpropanolamine hydrochloride 75 mg, chlorpheniramine maleate 12 mg. SR Cap. Bot. 100s, 1000s. *Rx.*
Use: Antihistamine, decongestant.
Rescaps-D S.R. (Geneva) Phenylpropanolamine hydrochloride 75 mg, caramiphen edisylate 40 mg. Cap. Bot. 100s. *Rx.*
Use: Antitussive, decongestant.
Rescon-DM. (Capellon) Dextromethorphan HBr 10 mg, pseudoephedrine hydrochloride 30 mg, chlorpheniramine maleate 2 mg/5 mL, alcohol and dye free. Liq. Bot. 118 mL, 473 mL. *OTC.*
Use: Upper respiratory combination, antihistamine, antitussive, decongestant.
Rescon-GG Capsules. (Capellon) Pseudoephedrine hydrochloride 120 mg, chlorpheniramine maleate 8 mg. Cap. Bot. 100s. *OTC.*
Use: Antihistamine, decongestant.
Rescon-GG Liquid. (Capellon) Phenylephrine hydrochloride 5 mg, guaifenesin 100 mg/5 mL, parabens, sorbitol, sugar, cherry flavor, alcohol and dye free. Liq. Bot 118 mL, 473 mL. *OTC.*
Use: Upper respiratory combination, decongestant, expectorant.
Rescon-JR. (Capellon) Phenylephrine hydrochloride 20 mg, chlorpheniramine maleate 4 mg. ER Tab. Bot. 100s. *Rx.*
Use: Upper respiratory combination, antihistamine, decongestant.
Rescon-MX. (Capellon) Phenylephrine hydrochloride 40 mg, chlorpheniramine maleate 8 mg, methscopolamine nitrate 2.5 mg. ER Tab. Bot. 100s. *Rx.*
Use: Upper respiratory combination, decongestant, antihistamine, anticholinergic.
Rescriptor. (Agouron) Delavirdine mesylate 100 mg, 200 mg, lactose. Tab. Bot. 180s (200 mg only), 360s (100 mg only). *Rx.*
Use: Antiretroviral, non-nucleoside reverse transcriptase inhibitor.
Resectisol. (McGaw) Mannitol soln. 5 g/1000 mL in distilled water (275 mOsm/L). In 2000 mL. *Rx.*
Use: Irrigant, genitourinary.
Reserpaneed. (Hanlon) Reserpine 0.25 mg. Tab. Bot. 100s, 1000s. *Rx.*
Use: Antihypertensive.

• **reserpine.** (reh-SER-peen) *USP 28.*
Use: Antihypertensive.
See: Arcum R-S.
Broserpine.
De Serpa.
Elserpine.
Raurine.
Reserpaneed.
Serpasil.
Sertabs.
Zepine.
W/Combinations.
See: Harbolin.
Hydropres-50.
Hydroserp.
Hydroserpine.
Hydrotensin-50.
Metatensin.
Renese-R.
Salutensin.
Salutensin-Demi.
Ser-Ap-Es.
Serpasil-Apresoline.
Serpasil-Esidrix.
reserpine and chlorothiazide tablets.
Use: Antihypertensive.
reserpine and hydrochlorothiazide tablets. (Various Mfr.) Hydrochlorothiazide 25 mg, 50 mg, reserpine 0.125 mg. Tab. Bot. 100s, 1000s. *Rx.*
Use: Antihypertensive.
reserpine, hydralazine hydrochloride, and hydrochlorothiazide.
Use: Antihypertensive.
resins, antacid.
See: Polyamine Methylene Resins.
resiquimod.
Use: Antiviral; antitumor.
• **reslizumab.** (res-li-ZOO-mab) USAN.
Use: Bronchial asthma.
• **resocortol butyrate.** (reh-so-CORE-tole BYOO-tih-rate) USAN.
Use: Corticosteroid; anti-inflammatory, topical.
Resol. (Wyeth) Na 50 mEq, K 20 mEq, Cl 50 mEq, citrate 34 mEq, Ca 4 mEq, Mg 4 mEq, phosphate 5 mEq, glucose 20 g/L. Contains 80 calories/L. Ctn. 32 fl oz. *Rx.*
Use: Fluid, electrolyte replacement.
Resolve/GP Daily Cleaner. (Allergan) Buffered solution with cocoamphocarboxyglycinate, sodium lauryl sulfate, hexylene glycol, alkyl ether sulfate, fatty acid amide surfactant cleaning agents, preservative free. Soln. Bot. 30 mL. *OTC.*
Use: Contact lens care.
Resonium-A. (Sanofi-Synthelabo) Sodium polystyrene sulfonate. *Rx.*
Use: Potassium removing resin.

resorcin.
See: Resorcinol.

• **resorcinol.** (reh-SORE-sih-nole)
USP 28.
Use: Keratolytic.
W/Combinations.
See: Adult Acnomel.
Bicozene.
Black and White.
Clearasil.
Lanacane.
RA.
Rezamid.
Unguentine Maximum Strength.

• **resorcinol and sulfur lotion.** USP 28.
Use: Antifungal; parasiticide; scabicide.

• **resorcinol and sulfur topical suspension.** USP 28.
Use: Antifungal; parasiticide; scabicide.

• **resorcinol monoacetate.** (re-SOR-sinole) USP 28.
Use: Antiseborrheic; keratolytic.
See: Euresol.

resorcinolphthalein sodium.
Use: Antiseborrheic, topical.
See: Fluorescein Sodium.

Resource. (Novartis Nutrition) Ca and Na caseinates, soy protein isolate 37 g, sugar, hydrolyzed cornstarch 140 g, corn oil, soy lecithin 37 g, Na 890 mg, K 1600 mg, A, B_1, B_2, B_3, B_5, B_6, B_{12}, C, D, E, K, Ca, P, I, Fe, Mg, Cu, Zn, Mn, Ol, gluten free, vanilla, chocolate, strawberry flavor. Liq. Bot. 237 mL. OTC.
Use: Nutritional supplement.

Resource Diabetic. (Novartis Nutrition) Protein (sodium and calcium caseinates, soy protein isolates, carnitine, taurine) 63 g, carbohydrate (hydrolyzed cornstarch, fructose) 99 g, fat (high oleic sunflower oil, soybean oil) 47 g/L, vitamins A, B_1, B_2, B_3, B_5, B_6, B_{12}, C, D, E, K, biotin, choline, folic acid, m-inositol, Ca, chloride, Cr, Cu, Fe, I, Mg, Mn, Mo, P, Se, Zn, Na 970 mg (42 mEq), K 1100 mg (29 mEq), H_2O 450 mOsm/Kg, 1.06 cal/mL, fiber 13 g/L, lactose-free, french vanilla, chocolate, strawberry, flavors. Liq. Tetra Brik Paks 237 mL (27s), closed system containers 1000 mL, 1500 mL (6s). OTC.
Use: Enteral nutritional therapy.

Resource Fruit Beverage. (Novartis Nutrition) Protein (whey protein concentrates) 38 g, carbohydrates (sugar, hydrolyzed cornstarch) 150 g/L, vitamins A, B_1, B_2, B_3, B_5, B_6, B_{12}, C, D, E, K, biotin, choline, folic acid, Ca, chloride,

Cu, Fe, I, Mg, Mn, P, Zn, Na < 295 mg (< 13 mEq), K < 93 mg (< 2.4 mEq), H_2O 700 mOsm/Kg, 0.76 cal/mL, lactose-free, orange, peach and wild berry flavors. Liq. Tetra Brik Paks 237 mL (27s). OTC.
Use: Enteral nutritional therapy.

Resource Instant Crystals. (Novartis Nutrition) Maltodextrin, sucrose, hydrogenated soy oil, sodium caseinate, calcium caseinate, soy protein isolate, potassium citrate, polyglycerol esters of fatty acids, vanilla and artificial flavors, vitamins and minerals. Instant Crystals. Pkt. 1.5 oz., 2 oz. OTC.
Use: Nutritional supplement.

Resource Just for Kids. (Novartis Nutrition) Protein (sodium and calcium caseinates, whey protein concentrate, carnitine, taurine) 30 g, carbohydrate (hydrolyzed cornstarch, sucrose) 110 g, fat (high oleic sunflower oil, soybean oil, medium chain triglycerides oil) 50 g, vitamins A, B_1, B_2, B_3, B_5, B_6, B_{12}, C, D, E, K, biotin, choline, folic acid, m-inositol, Ca, chloride, Cr, Cu, Fe, I, Mg, Mn, Mo, P, Se, Zn, Na 380 mg (17 mEq)/L, K 1300 mg (33 mEq)/L, H_2O 390 mOsm/Kg, 1 cal/mL, lactose-free, french vanilla, chocolate, strawberry flavors. Liq. Tetra Brik Paks 237 mL (27s). OTC.
Use: Enteral nutritional therapy.

Resource Plus. (Novartis Nutrition) Ca and Na caseinates, soy protein isolate 54.9 g, maltodextrin, sucrose 200 g, corn oil, lecithin 53.3 g, Na 899 mg, K 1740 mg, A, B_1, B_2, B_3, B_5, B_6, B_{12}, C, D, E, K, biotin, choline, Ca, P, I, Fe, Mg, Cu, Zn, Cl, Mn, gluten free, vanilla, chocolate, strawberry flavors. Liq. Bot. 8 oz. OTC.
Use: Nutritional supplement.

Respaire-120 SR. (Laser) Pseudoephedrine hydrochloride 120 mg, guaifenesin 250 mg. ER Cap. Bot. 100s. Rx.
Use: Upper respiratory combination, decongestant, expectorant.

Respaire-60 SR. (Laser) Pseudoephedrine hydrochloride 60 mg, guaifenesin 200 mg. ER Cap. Bot. 100s. Rx.
Use: Upper respiratory combination, decongestant, expectorant.

Respalor. (Bristol-Myers Squibb) Protein 75 g, carbohydrate 146 g, fat 70 g, Na 1248 mg, K 1456 mg, Fe 12.5 mg, cal/L 1498. Lactose free. Vanilla flavor. With appropriate vitamins and minerals. Liq. Bot. 237 mL. OTC.
Use: Nutritional supplement.

RespiGam. (MedImmune) RSV immuno-globulin (human) 50 ± 10 mg/mL, su-crose 5%, albumin (human) 1%, sodium 1 to 1.5 mEq/50 mL, preservative free, solvent/detergent treated. Inj. Single-use Vial 20 mL, 50 mL. *Rx.*
Use: Immunization.

Respihaler Decadron Phosphate. (Merck & Co.)
See: Decadron Phosphate.

Respiracult. (Orion) Culture test for group A beta-hemolytic streptococci. In 10s.
Use: Diagnostic aid.

Respiralex. (Orion) Latex agglutination test to detect group A streptococci in throat and nasopharynx. Kit 1s.
Use: Diagnostic aid.

respiratory enzymes.
See: Alpha₁-proteinase Inhibitor (Human).

respiratory gases.
See: INOmax.
Nitric oxide.

respiratory inhalant combination.
See: Fluticasone Propionate/Salme-terol.

respiratory inhalants.
See: Beclomethasone Dipropionate.
Budesonide.
Cromolyn Sodium.
Flunisolide.
Fluticasone Propionate.
Intranasal Steroids.
Mast Cell Stabilizers.
Mometasone Furoate Inhalation.
Mometasone Furoate Monohydrate.
Nedocromil Sodium.
Nitric Oxide.
Triamcinolone Acetonide.

respiratory syncytial virus immune globulin (human) (RSV-IG).
Use: Prophylaxis against respiratory tract infection.
See: RespiGam.

respiratory syncytial virus immune globulin intravenous (human) (RSV-IVIG).
Use: Respiratory syncytial virus im-mune serum.
See: RespiGam.

Restasis. (Allergan) Cyclosporine emul-sion 0.05%, glycerin, castor oil, poly-sorbate 80, preservative free. Single-use vials. 0.4 mL. *Rx.*
Use: Immunologic agent.

Rest Easy. (Walgreen) Acetaminophen 1000 mg, pseudoephedrine hydrochlo-ride 60 mg, dextromethorphan HBr 30 mg, doxylamine succinate 7.5 mg/ 30 mL. Bot. 6 oz, 16 oz. *OTC.*

Use: Analgesic; antihistamine; antitus-sive; decongestant.

Restoril. (Mallinckrodt) Temazepam 7.5 mg, 15 mg, 22.5 mg, 30 mg. Lac-tose. Cap. Bot. 30s (7.5 mg and 22.5 mg only), 100s, 500s (15 mg and 30 mg only). *c-ıv.*
Use: Sedative/hypnotic, nonbarbiturate.

Restylane. (Medicis Aesthetics) Hyal-uronic acid 20 mg/mL. Gel for Inj. Single-use prefilled syringes. *Rx.*
Use: Correction of facial wrinkles and folds.

•**retapamulin.** (re-TAP-a-MUE-lin) USAN.
Use: Antibiotic.

Retavase. (Centocor) Reteplase 10.4 units (18.1 mg). Pow. for Inj., ly-ophilized. Preservative-free. Kits with package insert, 2 single-use reteplase vials of 10.4 U (18.1 mg), 2 single-use diluent vials for reconstitution (10 mL sterile water for injection), 2 sterile 10 mL syringes, 2 sterile dispensing pins, 4 sterile needles, and 2 alcohol swabs. Half kits with package insert, 1 single-use reteplase vial 10.4 U (18.1 mg), 1 single-use diluent vial for reconstitution (10 mL sterile water for in-jection), and a sterile dispensing pin. *Rx.*
Use: Management of acute myocardial infarction.

•**reteplase, recombinant.** (RE-te-plase) USAN.
Use: Management of acute myocardial infarction; plasminogen activator.
See: Retavase.

Retin-A. (Ortho) **Cream:** Tretinoin 0.1%, 0.05%, 0.025%, stearyl alcohol (0.1% only). Cream. Tube 20 g, 45 g. **Gel:** Tretinoin 0.01%, 0.025%, alcohol 90%. Gel. Tube 15 g, 45 g. **Liq.:** Tretinoin 0.05%, alcohol 55%. Liq. Bot. 28 mL. *Rx.*
Use: Dermatologic; acne; retinoid.

Retin-A Micro. (Ortho) Tretinoin 0.04%, 0.1%, glycerin, propylene glycol, ben-zyl alcohol, EDTA. Gel. Tube 20 g, 45 g. *Rx.*
Use: Dermatologic; acne; retinoid.

retinoic acid. Tretinoin.
Use: Keratolytic.
See: Retin A.

retinoic acid, 9-cis.
Use: Acute promyelocytic leukemia. [Orphan Drug]

retinoids.
See: Acitretin.
Adapalene.
Alitretinoin.
Bexarotene.

Isotretinoin.
Tazarotene.
Tretinoin.
retinoin.
Use: Squamous metaplasia of the ocular surface epithelia with mucus deficiency and keratinization. [Orphan Drug]
Retinol. (NBTY) Vitamin A 100,000 units, glycol stearate, mineral oil, propylene glycol, lanolin oil, propylene glycol stearate SE, lanolin alcohol, retinol, parabens, EDTA. Cream. Tube 60 g. *OTC.*
Use: Emollient.
Retinol-A. (Young Again Products) Vitamin A palmitate 300,000 units/30 g. Cream. Tube 60 g. *OTC.*
Use: Emollient.
Retisert. (Bausch & Lomb) Fluocinolone acetonide 0.59 mg. Implant. Individual cartons. *Rx.*
Use: Corticosteroid, ophthalmic.
Retrovir. (GlaxoSmithKline) Zidovudine. **Tab.:** 300 mg. Bot. 60s. **Cap:** 100 mg. Bot. 100s. UD 100s. **Syrup:** 50 mg/5 mL, sodium benzoate 0.2%, sucrose, strawberry flavor. Bot. 240 mL. **Inj:** 10 mg/mL. Single-use Vial 20 mL. *Rx.*
Use: Antiretroviral, nucleoside reverse transcriptase inhibitor.
•**revaprazan hydrochloride.** (re-VA-prazan) USAN.
Use: Agent for GERD.
Reversol. (Organon Teknika) Edrophonium chloride 10 mg/mL. Inj. Vial. 10 mL. *Rx.*
Use: Muscle stimulant.
Revex. (Ohmeda) Nalmefene 100 mcg/mL, 1 mg/mL. Inj. **100 mcg/mL:** Amp 1 mL. **1 mg/mL:** Amp 2 mL. *Rx.*
Use: Narcotic antagonist; antidote.
Rēv-Eyes. (Bausch & Lomb) Dapiprazole hydrochloride 25 mg. Pow. Vial. 5 mL. *Rx.*
Use: Alpha-adrenergic blocker, ophthalmic.
ReVia. (Duramed) Naltrexone hydrochloride 50 mg. Tab. Bot. 30s, 100s. *Rx.*
Use: Antidote.
Revs Caffeine T.D. (Eon Labs) Caffeine 250 mg. Cap. Bot. 100s, 1000s. *OTC.*
Use: CNS stimulant.
Rexahistine. (Econo Med Pharmaceuticals) Phenylephrine hydrochloride 5 mg, chlorpheniramine maleate 1 mg, menthol 1 mg, sodium bisulfite 0.1%, alcohol 5%/5 mL. Bot. Gal. *OTC.*
Use: Antihistamine, decongestant.
Rexahistine DH. (Econo-Rx) Codeine phosphate 10 mg, phenylephrine hydrochloride 10 mg, chlorpheniramine

maleate 2 mg, menthol 1 mg, alcohol 5%/5 mL. Bot. Gal. *c-v.*
Use: Antihistamine, antitussive, decongestant.
Rexahistine Expectorant. (Econo-Rx) Codeine phosphate 10 mg, phenylephrine hydrochloride 10 mg, chlorpheniramine maleate 2 mg, guaifenesin 100 mg, menthol 1 mg, alcohol 5%/5 mL. Bot. Gal. *c-v.*
Use: Antihistamine, antitussive, decongestant, expectorant.
Rexigen Forte. (ION Laboratories, Inc.) Phendimetrazine tartrate 105 mg. SR Cap. Bot. 100s. *c-III.*
Use: Anorexiant.
rexinoids.
See: Bexarotene.
Targretin.
Reyataz. (Bristol-Myers Squibb) Atazanavir sulfate (as base) 100 mg, 150 mg, 200 mg. Lactose, alcohols, simethicone. Cap. 60s. *Rx.*
Use: Antiretroviral, protease inhibitor.
Rezamid. (Summers) Sulfur 5%, resorcinol 2%, SD alcohol 40 28%. Lot. Bot. 56.7 mL. *OTC.*
Use: Dermatologic; acne.
Rezine. (Marnel) Hydroxyzine hydrochloride 10 mg, 25 mg. Tab. Bot. 100s. *Rx.*
Use: Anxiolytic.
RF Latex Test. (Laboratory Diagnostics) Rapid latex agglutination test for the qualitative screening and semi-quantitative determination of rheumatoid factor. Kit 100s.
Use: Diagnostic aid.
R-Frone. (Serono)
See: Interferon Beta.
R-Gel. (Healthline Laboratories, Inc.) Capsaicin 0.025%, EDTA. Gel. Tube 15 mL, 30 mL. *OTC.*
Use: Analgesic, topical.
R-Gen. (Ivax) Iodinated glycerol 60 mg/5 mL, alcohol 21.75%. Elix. Bot. Pt. *Rx.*
Use: Expectorant.
R-Gene 10. (Pharmacia) Arginine hydrochloride 10% (950 mOsm/L) with Cl ion 47.5 mEq/100 mL. Inj. Vial 300 mL. *Rx.*
Use: Diagnostic aid; pituitary (growth hormone) function test.
R-HCTZ-H. (Wyeth) Reserpine 0.1 mg, hydrochlorothiazide 15 mg, hydralazine hydrochloride 25 mg. Tab. Bot. 100s, 500s. *Rx.*
Use: Antihypertensive.
Rheomacrodex. (Medisan) Dextran 40 10% in sodium Cl 0.9% or in dextrose 5%. Soln. Bot. 500 mL. *Rx.*
Use: Plasma expander.

Rheumatex. (Wampole) Latex agglutination test for the qualitative detection and quantitative determination of rheumatoid factor in serum. Kit 100s.
Use: Diagnostic aid.

Rheumaton. (Wampole) Two-minute hemagglutination slide test for the qualitative and quantitative determination of rheumatoid factor in serum or synovial fluid. Test kit 20s, 50s, 150s.
Use: Diagnostic aid.

Rheumatrex Dose Pack. (STADA Pharm) Methotrexate 2.5 mg. Tab. Pkg. 5 mg, 7.5 mg, 10 mg, 12.5 mg, 15 mg/week dose packs. *Rx.*
Use: Antipsoriatic; antirheumatic; antimetabolite.

Rhinall. (Scherer) Phenylephrine hydrochloride 0.25%, sodium bisulfite, chlorobutanol, benzalkonium chloride. Soln. Spray Bot. 40 mL. Dropper Bot. 30 mL. *OTC.*
Use: Nasal decongestant, arylalkylamine.

Rhinall 10. (Scherer) Phenylephrine hydrochloride 0.2%. Drop. Bot. oz. *OTC.*
Use: Decongestant.

Rhinaris Lubricating Mist. (Pharmascience) Polyethylene glycol 15%, propylene glycol 5% (spray only) 20% (gel only), benzalkonium chloride, sodium chloride. Soln. Spray Bot. 30 mL. Gel Tube. 28.35 g. *OTC.*
Use: Nasal decongestant.

Rhinatate. (Major) Phenylephrine tannate 25 mg, chlorpheniramine tannate 8 mg, pyrilamine tannate 25 mg. Tab. Bot. 100s, 250s. *Rx.*
Use: Antihistamine, decongestant.

Rhinatate-NF Pediatric. (Major) Phenylephrine tannate 5 mg, chlorpheniramine tannate 4.5 mg/5 mL, methylparaben, saccharin, sucrose. Susp. Bot. 473 mL. *Rx.*
Use: Upper respiratory combination, decongestant, antihistamine.

Rhinatate Pediatric. (Major) Phenylephrine tannate 5 mg, chlorpheniramine tannate 2 mg, pyrilamine tannate 12.5 mg/5 mL, methylparaben, saccharin, sucrose, strawberry-blackberry-currant flavor. Susp. Bot. 473 mL *Rx.*
Use: Upper respiratory combination, decongestant, antihistamine.

Rhinocort Aqua. (AstraZeneca) Budesonide 32 mcg/actuation, dextrose, polysorbate 80, EDTA. Spray. Bot. 8.6 g (120 metered sprays) with metered-dose pump. *Rx.*
Use: Respiratory inhalant, intranasal steroid.

Rhinolar-EX. (McGregor Pharmaceuticals, Inc.) Phenylpropanolamine hydrochloride 75 mg, chlorpheniramine maleate 8 mg. SR Cap. Dye free. Bot. 60s. *Rx.*
Use: Antihistamine, decongestant.

Rhinolar-EX 12. (McGregor Pharmaceuticals, Inc.) Phenylpropanolamine hydrochloride 75 mg, chlorpheniramine maleate 12 mg. SR Cap. Dye free. Bot. 60s. *Rx.*
Use: Antihistamine; decongestant.

Rhinosyn. (Great Southern) Pseudoephedrine hydrochloride 60 mg, chlorpheniramine maleate 4 mg/5 mL, alcohol 0.45%, sucrose. Liq. Bot. 120 mL, 473 mL. *OTC.*
Use: Antihistamine, decongestant.

Rhinosyn DM. (Great Southern) Pseudoephedrine hydrochloride 30 mg, chlorpheniramine maleate 2 mg, dextromethorphan HBr 15 mg/5 mL, alcohol 1.4%, sucrose. Liq. Bot. 120 mL. *OTC.*
Use: Antihistamine, antitussive, decongestant.

Rhinosyn DMX. (Great Southern) Dextromethorphan HBr 15 mg, guaifenesin 100 mg/5 mL, alcohol 1.4%. Syr. Bot. 120 mL. *OTC.*
Use: Antitussive, expectorant.

Rhinosyn-PD. (Great Southern) Pseudoephedrine hydrochloride 30 mg, chlorpheniramine maleate 2 mg/5 mL. Liq. Bot. 120 mL. *OTC.*
Use: Antihistamine, decongestant.

Rhinosyn-X. (Great Southern) Pseudoephedrine hydrochloride 30 mg, dextromethorphan HBr 10 mg, guaifenesin 100 mg/5 mL, alcohol 7.5%. Liq. Bot. 120 mL. *OTC.*
Use: Antitussive, decongestant, expectorant.

rhodanate.
See: Potassium Thiocyanate.

rhodanide. More commonly Rhodanate, same as thiocyanate.
See: Potassium Thiocyanate.

•RH$_o$(D) immune globulin. (RH$_o$D ih-MYOON GLAB-byoo-lin) *USP 28.*
Use: Immunization.
See: BayRh$_o$D Full Dose.
BayRh$_o$D Mini Dose.
Gamulin Rh.
MICRh$_o$GAM.
RhoGAM.
Rhophylac.
WinRho SD.
WinRho SDF.

RH$_o$(D) immune globulin. (RH$_o$D ih-MYOON GLAB-byoo-lin) *Formerly RH$_o$ Immune Human Globulin.*

Use: Immune thrombocytopenic purpura, immunizing agent (passive). [Orphan Drug]
See: WinRho SD.

RhoGAM. (Ortho Diagnostics) Rh₀(D) immune globulin ≈ 5% ± 1% gamma globulin, sodium chloride 2.9 mg, polysorbate 80 0.01%, glycine 15 mg/mL, filtrated, preservative free. Soln. for Inj. Pkg. Prefilled single-dose syringe, package insert, control form, patient ID card. 5s, 25s. Rx.
Use: Immunization.

Rhophylac. (ZLB Bioplasma) Rh₀(D) immune globulin IV (human) 1500 units. Preservative-free. Inj. Prefilled syringes 2 mL. Rx.
Use: Immunization.

Rhythmin. (Sidmak) Procainamide 250 mg, 500 mg. SR Tab. Bot. 100s, 500s, 1000s. Rx.
Use: Antiarrhythmic.

• **ribaminol.** (rye-BAM-ih-nahl) USAN.
Use: Memory adjuvant.

Ribaspheres. (Three Rivers) Ribavirin 200 mg. Lactose. Cap. 42s, 56s, 70s, 84s. Rx.
Use: Antiviral agents.

• **ribavirin.** (rye-buh-VIE-rin) USP 28.
Use: Antiviral.
See: Copegus.
Rebetol.
Ribaspheres.
Virazole.

ribavirin. (Various Mfr.) Ribavirin 200 mg. Cap. 42s, 56s, 70s, 84s, 100s. Rx.
Use: Antiviral agent.

ribavirin and interferon alfa-2b, recombinant.
Use: Antineoplastic.
See: Rebetron.

• **riboflavin.** (RYE-boh-FLAY-vin) USP 28.
Use: Vitamin (enzyme co-factor).

riboflavin. (Various Mfr.) Riboflavin 50 mg, 100 mg. Tab. Bot. 100s, 250s. OTC.
Use: Vitamin.

• **riboflavin 5'-phosphate sodium.** (RYE-boh-FLAY-vin 5'-FOSS-fate so-dee-oum) USP 28.
Use: Vitamin.

• **riboprine.** (RYE-boe-PREEN) USAN.
Use: Antineoplastic.

Ribozyme. (Fellows) Riboflavin-5-phosphate sodium 50 mg/mL Inj. Vial 10 mL. Rx.

ricin (blocked) conjugated murine mca. (ImmunoGen)
Use: Antineoplastic. [Orphan Drug]

ricin (blocked) conjugated murine moab.

Use: Antineoplastic. [Orphan Drug]

Ricolon Solution. (Sanofi-Synthelabo) Ricolon concentrate. Soln. Rx.
Use: Leucocytotic preparation.

RID. (Bayer) Pyrethrins 0.33%, piperonyl butoxide 4%. **Mousse:** Cetearyl alcohol, SD alcohol, isobutane. Bot. 165 mL w/comb. **Shampoo:** SD alcohol. 60 mL, 120 mL, 240 mL, and 120 mL kits containing gel, comb, and lice control spray. OTC.
Use: Pediculicide.

Rid•a•Pain•HP. (Pfeiffer) Capsaicin 0.075%, alcohols, parabens. Cream. Tube. 45 g. OTC.
Use: Analgesic.

Ridaura. (GlaxoSmithKline) Auranofin 3 mg. Cap. Bot. 60s. Rx.
Use: Antirheumatic.

Ridenol. (R.I.D., Inc.) Acetaminophen 80 mg/5 mL. Syr. Bot. 120 mL. OTC.
Use: Analgesic.

Rid Lice Control Spray. (Pfizer) Synthetic pyrethroids 0.5%, related compounds 0.065%, aromatic petroleum hydrocarbons 0.664%. Spray. Can 5 oz. OTC.
Use: Pediculicide.

Rid Lice Elimination System. (Pfizer) Rid lice killing shampoo, nit removal comb, Rid lice control spray and instruction booklet/unit. OTC.
Use: Pediculicide.

• **ridogrel.** (RYE-doe-grell) USAN.
Use: Thromboxane synthetase inhibitor.

• **rifabutin.** (RIFF-uh-BYOO-tin) USP 28.
Use: Anti-infective (antimycobacterial), MAC disease; antituberculosal.
See: Mycobutin.

Rifadin. (Aventis) Rifampin. **150 mg/Cap.:** Bot. 30s. **300 mg/Cap.:** Bot. 30s, 60s, 100s. **Pow. for Inj.:** 600 mg. Vials. Rx.
Use: Antituberculous.

• **rifalazil.** (RIFF-ah-lah-zill) USAN.
Use: Antibacterial.

Rifamate. (Aventis) Rifampin 300 mg, isoniazid 150 mg. Cap. Bot. 60s. Rx.
Use: Antituberculosal.

• **rifametane.** (RIFF-ah-met-ane) USAN.
Use: Anti-infective.

• **rifamexil.** (riff-ah-MEX-ill) USAN.
Use: Anti-infective.

• **rifamide.** (RIFF-am-ide) USAN.
Use: Anti-infective.

• **rifampin.** (RIFF-am-pin) USP 28. Rifampin, isoniazid, and pyrazinamide. Tablets.
Use: Anti-infective, antituberculostatic.

See: Rifadin.
Rifater.
Rimactane.
rifampin. (Various Mfr.) Rifampin 150 mg, 300 mg. Cap. Bot. 30s, 60s (300 mg only), 100s, 500s (300 mg only). *Rx.*
Use: Antituberculosal.
● **rifampin and isoniazid.** *USP 28.*
Use: Anti-infective (tuberculostatic).
See: Rifamate.
● **rifampin, isoniazid, and pyrazinamide.** *USP 28.*
Use: Anti-infective (tuberculostatic).
See: Rifater.
● **rifampin, isoniazid, pyrazinamide, and ethambutol hydrochloride.** *USP 28.*
Use: Anti-infective (tuberculostatic).
● **rifapentine.** (RIFF-ah-pen-teen) USAN.
Use: Anti-infective, antituberculosal.
See: Priftin.
rifapentine.
Use: Pulmonary tuberculosis; *mycobacterium avium* complex in AIDS patients. [Orphan Drug]
Rifater. (Aventis) Rifampin 120 mg, isoniazid 50 mg, pyrazinamide 300 mg. Tab. Bot. 60s. *Rx.*
Use: Antituberculosal.
● **rifaximin.** (riff-AX-ih-min) USAN.
Use: Anti-infective.
See: Xifaxan.
r-IFN-beta. (Biogen)
See: Interferon Beta (Recombinant).
RIG.
Use: Immunization, rabies.
See: Bayrab.
Imogam.
Rilutek. (Aventis) Riluzole 50 mg. Tab. *Rx.*
Use: Amyotrophic lateral sclerosis agent.
● **riluzole.** (RILL-you-zole) USAN.
Use: Amyotrophic lateral sclerosis agent. [Orphan Drug]
See: Rilutek.
Rimactane. (Novartis) Rifampin 300 mg. Cap. Bot. 30s, 60s, 100s. *Rx.*
Use: Antituberculous.
Rimadyl. (Roche) *Rx.*
Use: Analgesic, NSAID.
See: Carprofen.
● **rimantadine hydrochloride.** (rih-MAN-tuh-deen) *USP 28.*
Use: Antiviral.
See: Flumadine.
● **rimcazole hydrochloride.** (RIM-kazz-OLE) USAN.
Use: Antipsychotic.
● **rimexolone.** (rih-MEX-oh-lone) USAN.
Use: Anti-inflammatory.

See: Vexol.
● **rimiterol hydrobromide.** (RIH-mih-TER-ole) USAN.
Use: Bronchodilator.
Rimso-50. (Research Industries Corp.) Dimethyl sulfoxide in a 50% aqueous soln. Bot. 50 mL. *Rx.*
Use: Urinary tract agent.
Rinade. (Econo Med Pharmaceuticals) Chlorpheniramine maleate 8 mg, phenylephrine hydrochloride 20 mg, methscopolamine nitrate 2.5 mg. Cap. Bot. 120s. *Rx.*
Use: Anticholinergic; antihistamine, decongestant.
Ringer's in 5% dextrose. (Various Mfr.) Dextrose 50 g, calories 170, Na$^+$ $\approx$ 147 mEq, K$^+$ 4 mEq, Ca^{++} $\approx$ 4.5 mEq, Ca$^-$ $\approx$ 4.5 mEq, Cl$^-$ $\approx$ 156 mEq, osmolarity $\approx$ 560 mOsm/L. Soln. Bot. 500 mL. 1000 mL. *Rx.*
Use: Intravenous nutritional therapy, intravenous replenishment solution.
● **Ringer's injection.** *USP 28.*
Use: Fluid, electrolyte replacement; irrigant, ophthalmic.
Ringer's injection. (Various Mfr.) Na$^+$ $\approx$ 147 mEq, K$^+$ 4 mEq, Ca^{++} $\approx$ 4 mEq, Cl$^-$ $\approx$ 156 mEq, osmolarity $\approx$ 310 mOsm/L. Soln. Bot. 500 mL. 1000 mL. *Rx.*
Use: Intravenous nutritional therapy, intravenous replenishment solution.
Ringer's injection, lactated.
Use: Fluid, electrolyte replacement.
Ringer's irrigation. (Various Mfr.) Sodium chloride 0.86 g, potassium chloride 0.03 g, calcium chloride 0.033 g/ 100 mL. Bot. 1 liter. *Rx.*
Use: Irrigant, ophthalmic.
Riomet. (Ranbaxy) Metformin 500 mg/ 5 mL. Saccharin, cherry flavor. Oral Soln. Bot. 120 mL, 480 mL. *Rx.*
Use: Antidiabetic.
Riopan. (Whitehall-Robins) Magaldrate 540 mg, Na 0.1 mg/5 mL. Bot. 6 oz, 12 oz. Individual Cup 30 mL each. *OTC.*
Use: Antacid.
Riopan Plus Double Strength Suspension. (Whitehall-Robins) Magaldrate 1080 mg, simethicone 40 mg/5 mL. Bot. 360 mL. *OTC.*
Use: Antacid; antiflatulent.
Riopan Plus Double Strength Tablets. (Whitehall-Robins) Magaldrate 1080 mg, simethicone 20 mg. Chew. Tab. Bot. 60s. *OTC.*
Use: Antacid; antiflatulent.
Riopan Plus Tablets. (Whitehall-Robins) Magaldrate 480 mg, simethicone 20 mg. Chew. Tab. Bot. 50s, 100s.

OTC.
Use: Antacid; antiflatulent.

• **rioprostil.** (RYE-oh-PRAHS-till) USAN.
Use: Gastric antisecretory.

• **ripazepam.** (rip-AZE-eh-pam) USAN.
Use: Anxiolytic.

• **risedronate sodium.** (riss-ED-row-nate) USAN.
Use: Bisphosphonate.
See: Actonel.

• **rismorelin porcine.** (riss-more-ELL-in PORE-sine) USAN.
Use: Hormone, growth hormone-releasing.

• **risocaine.** (RIZZ-oh-cane) USAN.
Use: Anesthetic, local.

• **risotilide hydrochloride.** (rih-SO-tih-LIDE) USAN.
Use: Cardiovascular agent (antiarrhythmic).

Risperdal. (Janssen) Risperidone. **Tab.:** 0.25 mg, 0.5 mg, 1 mg, 2 mg, 3 mg, 4 mg, lactose. Bot. 60s, 500s (except 4 mg), blister pack 100s (except 0.25 mg, 0.5 mg). **Oral Soln.:** 1 mg/mL. Bot. 30 mL w/calibrated pipette. *Rx.*
Use: Antipsychotic, benzisoxazole derivative.

Risperdal Consta. (Janssen) Risperidone 25 mg, 37.5 mg, 50 mg. Pow. for Inj. Vials. Dose pack contains prefilled syringe and 2 mL of diluent. *Rx.*
Use: Antipsychotic, benzisoxazole derivatives.

Risperdal M-Tab. (Janssen) Risperidone 0.5 mg, phenylalanine 0.14 mg; 1 mg, phenylalanine 0.28 mg; 2 mg, phenylalanine 0.56 mg. Aspartame, mannitol, peppermint oil. Orally Disintegrating Tab. 7 blister packs of 4, bingo cards of 30 (except 2 mg). *Rx.*
Use: Antispychotic, benzisoxazole derivative.

• **risperidone.** (RISS-PURR-ih-dohn) USAN.
Use: Antipsychotic, neuroleptic, benzisoxazole deriative.
See: Risperdal.
Risperdal M-Tab.

• **ristianol phosphate.** (riss-TIE-ah-NOLE) USAN.
Use: Immunoregulator.

Ritalin. (Novartis) Methylphenidate hydrochloride 5 mg, 10 mg, 20 mg, lactose (except 20 mg), sucrose (20 mg only). Tab. Bot. 100s. *c-II.*
Use: CNS stimulant.

Ritalin LA. (Novartis) Methylphenidate hydrochloride 10 mg, 20 mg, 30 mg, 40 mg, sugar spheres. ER Cap. Bot.

100s. *c-II.*
Use: CNS stimulant.

Ritalin-SR. (Novartis) Methylphenidate hydrochloride 20 mg, lactose, alcohol, mineral oil, color-additive free. SR Tab. Bot. 100s. *c-II.*
Use: CNS stimulant.

• **ritanserin.** (rih-TAN-ser-in) USAN.
Use: Serotonin antagonist.

• **ritodrine.** (RIH-toe-DREEN) USAN.
Use: Muscle relaxant.

• **ritolukast.** (rih-tah-LOO-kast) USAN.
Use: Antiasthmatic (leukotriene antagonist).

• **ritonavir.** (rih-TON-a-veer) USAN.
Use: Antiretroviral, protease inhibitor.
See: Norvir.
W/Lopinavir.
See: Kaletra.

Rituxan. (IDEC/Genentech) Rituximab 10 mg/mL, polysorbate 80 0.7 mg, preservative free. Inj. Single-use Vial 10 mL, 50 mL. *Rx.*
Use: Antineoplastic; monoclonal antibody.

• **rituximab.** (rih-TUCK-sih-mab) USAN.
Use: Antineoplastic (microtubule inhibitor); monoclonal antibody.
See: Rituxan.

rivastigmine tartrate.
Use: Cholinesterase inhibitor.
See: Exelon.

• **rizatriptan benzoate.** (rye-zah-TRIP-tan BENZ-oh-ate) USAN.
Use: Antimigraine, serotonin 5-HT$_1$ receptor agonist.
See: Maxalt.
Maxalt-MLT.

• **rizatriptan sulfate.** (rye-zah-TRIP-tan) USAN.
Use: Antimigraine.

RMS. (Upsher-Smith) Morphine sulfate 5 mg, 10 mg, 20 mg, 30 mg. Rectal. Supp. Box 12s. *c-II.*
Use: Opioid analgesic.

Robafen. (Major) Guaifenesin 100 mg/ 5 mL, alcohol 3.5%. Syr. Bot. 118 mL, 240 mL, pt, gal. OTC.
Use: Expectorant.

Robafen AC Cough. (Major) Guaifenesin 100 mg, codeine phosphate 10 mg/ 5 mL, alcohol 3.5%, parabens. Syr. Bot. 473 mL. *c-v.*
Use: Antitussive; expectorant, narcotic.

Robafen CF. (Major) Psuedoephedrine hydrochloride 30 mg, dextromethorphan HBr 10 mg, guaifenesin 100 mg/ 5 mL, saccharin, sorbitol, alcohol free. Syr. Bot. 118 mL, 237 mL. OTC.

Use: Upper respiratory combination, antitussive, decongestant, expectorant.

Robafen DAC. (Major) Pseudoephedrine 30 mg, codeine phosphate 10 mg, guaifenesin 100 mg/5 mL, alcohol 1.4%. Liq. Bot. Pt. *c-v.*
Use: Antitussive, decongestant, expectorant.

Robafen DM. (Major) Dextromethorphan HBr 10 mg, guaifenesin 100 mg/5 mL, alcohol 1.4%. Syr. Bot. 473 mL. *OTC.*
Use: Antitussive; expectorant.

Robafen PE. (Major) Pseudoephedrine hydrochloride 30 mg, guaifenesin 100 mg/5 mL, glucose, corn syrup, saccharin, alcohol free. Liq. Bot. 118 mL. *OTC.*
Use: Upper respiratory combination, decongestant, expectorant.

robanul.
See: Robinul.

RoBathol Bath Oil. (Pharmaceutical Specialties) Cottonseed oil, alkyl aryl polyether alcohol. Lanolin free. Oil. Bot. 240 mL, 480 mL, gal. *OTC.*
Use: Dermatologic.

Robaxin Injection. (Wyeth) Methocarbamol 100 mg/mL of a 50% aqueous soln. of polyethylene glycol 300. Inj. Vial 10 mL. *Rx.*
Use: Muscle relaxant.

Robaxin-750. (Schwarz Pharma) Methocarbamol 750 mg. Tab. Bot. 100s, 500s, Dis-Co Pak 100s. *Rx.*
Use: Muscle relaxant.

Robaxin Tablets. (Schwarz Pharma) Methocarbamol 500 mg. Tab. Bot. 100s, 500s, UD 100s. *Rx.*
Use: Muscle relaxant.

Robimycin. (Wyeth) Erythromycin 250 mg. Tab. Bot. 100s, 500s. *Rx.*
Use: Anti-infective, erythromycin.

Robinul. (First Horizon) Glycopyrrolate 1 mg, lactose. Tab. Bot. 100s. *Rx.*
Use: Anticholinergic.

Robinul Forte. (First Horizon) Glycopyrrolate 2 mg, lactose. Tab. Bot. 100s. *Rx.*
Use: Anticholinergic.

Robinul Injectable. (Wyeth) Glycopyrrolate 0.2 mg/mL, benzyl alcohol 0.9%. Vial 1 mL, 2 mL, 5 mL, 20 mL. *Rx.*
Use: Anticholinergic.

Robitussin. (Wyeth) Guaifenesin 100 mg/5 mL, corn syrup, glucose, saccharin, menthol, alcohol free. Bot. 118 mL, 237 mL. *OTC.*
Use: Expectorant.

Robitussin A-C. (Whitehall-Robins) Guaifenesin 100 mg, codeine phosphate 10 mg/5 mL, alcohol 3.5%, saccharin, sorbitol. Bot. 2 oz, 4 oz, pt, gal. *c-v.*
Use: Antitussive, expectorant.

Robitussin Allergy & Cough. (Whitehall-Robins) Dextromethorphan HBr 10 mg, brompheniramine maleate 2 mg, pseudoephedrine hydrochloride 30 mg/5 mL, saccharin, sorbitol, alcohol and dye free. Liq. Bot 118 mL. *OTC.*
Use: Upper respiratory combination, antitussive, antihistamine, decongestant, analgesic.

Robitussin-CF. (Whitehall-Robins) Guaifenesin 100 mg, pseudoephedrine hydrochloride 30 mg, dextromethorphan HBr 10 mg/5 mL, alcohol free, saccharin, sorbitol. Syr. Bot. 355 mL. *OTC.*
Use: Upper respiratory combination, antitussive, decongestant, expectorant.

Robitussin Cold & Cough. (Whitehall-Robins) Guaifenesin 200 mg, pseudoephedrine hydrochloride 30 mg, dextromethorphan HBr 10 mg, sorbitol. Cap. Bot. 20s. *OTC.*
Use: Antitussive, expectorant, decongestant.

Robitussin Cold, Cold & Congestion. (Whitehall-Robins) Dextromethorphan HBr 10 mg, guaifenesin 200 mg, pseudoephedrine hydrochloride 30 mg. Softgel. Tab. Pkg. 20s. *OTC.*
Use: Upper respiratory combination, antitussive, expectorant, decongestant.

Robitussin Cold, Cold & Cough. (Whitehall-Robins) Dextromethorphan HBr 10 mg, guaifenesin 200 mg, pseudoephedrine hydrochloride 30 mg, sorbitol. Softgel. Pkg. 12s, 20s *OTC.*
Use: Upper respiratory combination, antitussive, expectorant, decongestant.

Robitussin Cold, Multi-Symptom Cold & Flu. (Whitehall-Robins) **Softgel:** Dextromethorphan HBr 10 mg, guaifenesin 100 mg, pseudoephedrine hydrochloride 30 mg, sorbitol. Pkg. 12s. **Tab.:** Dextromethorphan HBr 10 mg, guaifenesin 200 mg, pseudoephedrine hydrochloride 30 mg, acetaminophen 325 mg. Pkg. 20s. *OTC.*
Use: Upper respiratory combination, antitussive, expectorant, decongestant.

Robitussin Cold, Sinus & Congestion. (Whitehall-Robins) Pseudoephedrine hydrochloride 30 mg, guaifenesin 200 mg, acetaminophen 325 mg, lactose. Tab. Pkg. 20s. *OTC.*
Use: Upper respiratory combination, decongestant, expectorant, analgesic.

Robitussin Cough & Cold Infant. (Whitehall-Robins) Pseudoephedrine hydrochloride 6 mg, dextromethorphan

HBr 2 mg, guaifenesin 40 mg/mL, corn syrup, menthol, saccharin, sorbitol. Drops. Bot. 30 mL. *OTC.*
Use: Upper respiratory combination, decongestant, antitussive, expectorant.

Robitussin Cough & Congestion Formula. (Wyeth) Dextromethorphan HBr 10 mg, guaifenesin 200 mg, corn syrup, menthol, saccharin, sorbitol, alcohol free. Liq. Bot. 118 mL. *OTC.*
Use: Upper respiratory combination, antitussive, expectorant.

Robitussin Cough Calmers. (Whitehall-Robins) Dextromethorphan HBr 5 mg, corn syrup, sucrose, cherry flavor. Loz. Pkg. 16s. *OTC.*
Use: Antitussive.

Robitussin Cough Drops. (Whitehall-Robins) Menthol 7.4 mg, 10 mg, eucalyptus oil, ouoruuu, corn syrup 1 AT Pkg. 9s, 25s, menthol 10 mg, eucalyptus oil, sucrose, corn syrup, honey-lemon flavor. Loz. Pkg. 9s, 25s. *OTC.*
Use: Antitussive.

Robitussin CoughGels. (Wyeth) Dextromethorphan HBr 15 mg. Sorbitol. Gel Cap. 20s. *OTC.*
Use: Antitussive.

Robitussin-DAC. (Whitehall-Robins) Guaifenesin 100 mg, pseudoephedrine hydrochloride 30 mg, codeine phosphate 10 mg/5 mL, alcohol 1.9%, saccharin, sorbitol. Syr. Bot. 4 oz, pt. *c-v.*
Use: Antitussive, expectorant, decongestant.

Robitussin Dis-Co. (Whitehall-Robins) Guaifenesin 100 mg/5 mL, alcohol 3.5%. Syr. UD pack 5 mL, 10 mL, 15 mL. *OTC.*
Use: Expectorant.

Robitussin-DM. (Whitehall-Robins) Guaifenesin 100 mg, dextromethorphan HBr 10 mg/5 mL, glucose, corn syrup, saccharin. Syr. Bot. 118 mL, 237 mL, 360 mL, 473 mL. *OTC.*
Use: Upper respiratory combination, antitussive, expectorant.

Robitussin DM Infant. (Whitehall-Robins) Dextromethorphan HBr 2 mg, guaifenesin 40 mg/mL, corn syrup, saccharin, fruit punch flavor, alcohol free. Drops. Bot. 30 mL with oral syringe. *OTC.*
Use: Upper respiratory combination, antitussive, expectorant.

Robitussin Flu. (Whitehall-Robins) Dextromethorphan HBr 5 mg, chlorpheniramine maleate 1 mg, pseudoephedrine hydrochloride 15 mg, acetaminophen 160 mg/5 mL, alcohol free. Liq. Bot 118 mL. *OTC.*
Use: Upper respiratory combination, antitussive, antihistamine, decongestant, analgesic.

Robitussin Honey Cough & Cold. (Whitehall-Robins) Dextromethorphan HBr 10 mg, pseudoephedrine hydrochloride 20 mg/5 mL, saccharin. Liq. Bot. 118 mL. *OTC.*
Use: Upper respiratory combination, antitussive, decongestant.

Robitussin Honey Flu Multi-Symptom. (Whitehall-Robins) Dextromethorphan HBr 6.6 mg, pseudoephedrine hydrochloride 20 mg, acetaminophen 166.6 mg/5 mL, saccharin, corn syrup, menthol. Liq. Bot. 118 mL. *OTC.*
Use: Upper respiratory combination, antitussive, decongestant, analgesic.

Robitussin Honey Flu Nighttime. (Whitehall-Robins) Dextromethorphan HBr 20 mg, chlorpheniramine maleate 4 mg, pseudoephedrine hydrochloride 60 mg, acetaminophen 500 mg/5 mL, corn syrup, saccharin. Syr. Box. Pouch 6s. *OTC.*
Use: Upper respiratory combination, antitussive, antihistamine, decongestant, analgesic.

Robitussin Honey Flu Non-Drowsy. (Whitehall-Robins) Dextromethorphan HBr 20 mg, pseudoephedrine hydrochloride 60 mg, acetaminophen 500 mg/5 mL, corn syrup, saccharin. Syr. Pouch. Box 6s. *OTC.*
Use: Upper respiratory combination, antitussive, decongestant, analgesic.

Robitussin Liquid Center Cough Drops. (Whitehall-Robins) Menthol 10 mg, eucalyptus oil, corn syrup, honey, lemon oil, high fructose, parabens, sorbitol, sucrose. Loz. Pkg. 20s. *OTC.*
Use: Mouth and throat preparation.

Robitussin Maximum Strength Cough. (Whitehall-Robins) Dextromethorphan HBr 15 mg/5 mL, alcohol 1.4%, glucose, corn syrup, saccharin, cherry flavor. Liq. Bot. 118 mL, 273 mL. *OTC.*
Use: Antitussive.

Robitussin Maximum Strength Cough & Cold. (Whitehall-Robins) Dextromethorphan HBr 15 mg, pseudoephedrine hydrochloride 30 mg/5 mL, alcohol 1.4%, glucose, corn syrup, saccharin. Syr. Bot. 237 mL. *OTC.*
Use: Upper respiratory combination, antitussive, decongestant.

Robitussin Night Relief. (Whitehall-Robins) Acetaminophen 108.3 mg, pseudoephedrine hydrochloride 10 mg, pyrilamine maleate 8.3 mg, dextro-

methorphan HBr 5 mg/5 mL, alcohol free, saccharin, sorbitol, cherry flavor. Bot. 177 mL. *OTC.*
Use: Upper respiratory combination, analgesic, antihistamine, antitussive, decongestant.

Robitussin-PE. (Whitehall-Robins) Guaifenesin 100 mg, pseudoephedrine hydrochloride 30 mg/5 mL, saccharin, corn syrup, glucose. Liq. Bot. 118 mL, 237 mL. *OTC.*
Use: Upper respiratory combination, decongestant, expectorant.

Robitussin Pediatric Cough. (Whitehall-Robins) Dextromethorphan HBr 7.5 mg/5 mL, alcohol free, saccharin, sorbitol, cherry flavor. Liq. Bot. 118 mL. *OTC.*
Use: Antitussive.

Robitussin Pediatric Cough & Cold Formula. (Whitehall-Robins) Dextromethorphan HBr 7.5 mg, pseudoephedrine hydrochloride 15 mg/5 mL, corn syrup, saccharin, alcohol free, fruit punch flavor. Liq. Bot. 118 mL. *OTC.*
Use: Upper respiratory combination, antitussive, decongestant.

Robitussin Pediatric Night Relief Cough & Cold. (Whitehall-Robins) Pseudoephedrine hydrochloride 15 mg, chlorpheniramine maleate 1 mg, dextromethorphan HBr 7.5 mg/5 mL, corn syrup, saccharin, fruit punch flavor, alcohol free. Liq. Bot. 118 mL. *OTC.*
Use: Upper respiratory combination, decongestant, antihistamine, antitussive.

Robitussin PM Cough & Cold. (Wyeth Consumer) Dextromethorphan HBr 7.5 mg, chlorpheniramine maleate 1 mg, pseuodephrine hydrochloride 15 mg/5 mL, corn syrup, saccharin, alcohol free. Liq. 118 mL. *OTC.*
Use: Antitussive combination.

Robitussin Severe Congestion. (Whitehall-Robins) Guaifenesin 200 mg, pseudoephedrine hydrochloride 30 mg, mannitol, sorbitol. Liqui-gel. Pkg. 24s. *OTC.*
Use: Upper respiratory combination, decongestant, expectorant.

Robitussin Sugar Free Cough. (Whitehall-Robins) Dextromethorphan HBr 10 mg, guaifenesin 100 mg/5 mL, methylparaben, saccharin, alcohol and dye free. Liq. Bot. 118 mL *OTC.*
Use: Upper respiratory combination, antitussive, expectorant.

Robomol/ASA. (Major) Methocarbamol w/ASA. Tab. Bot. 100s, 500s. *Rx.*
Use: Muscle relaxant; analgesic.

Rocaltrol. (Roche) Calcitriol. **Cap.:** 0.25 mcg, 0.5 mcg, sorbitol, parabens. Bot. 30s (0.25 mcg only), 100s. **Oral Soln.:** 1 mcg/mL. Bot. 15 mL. *Rx.*
Use: Antihypocalcemic.

•**rocastine hydrochloride.** (row-KASS-teen) USAN.
Use: Antihistamine.

Rocephin. (Roche) Ceftriaxone sodium **Pow. for Inj.:** 250 mg, 500 mg, 1 g, 2 g, 10 g Vial. **250 mg, 500 mg:** Vial. **1 g, 2 g:** Vial, piggyback vial, *ADD-Vantage* vial. **10 g:** Bulk Containers. **Inj.: 1 g, 2 g, Frozen Premixed:** 50 mL plastic containers. *Rx.*
Use: Anti-infective; cephalosporin.

•**rocuronium bromide.** (row-kuhr-OH-nee-uhm) USAN.
Use: Neuromuscular blocker, muscle relaxant.
See: Zemuron.

•**rodocaine.** (ROW-doe-cane) USAN.
Use: Anesthetic, local.

roentgenography.
See: Iodine Products, Diagnostic.

Roferon-A. (Hoffman La-Roche) Interferon alfa-2a recombinant, sodium chloride, polysorbate 80, benzyl alcohol, ammonium acetate. **Inj. Soln. (Single Use):** 36 million units/vial. Vial. 1 mL single use. **Prefilled Syr.:** 3 million, 6 million, 9 million units/syringe. Single-use 0.5 mL syringes. 1s, 6s. *Rx.*
Use: Antineoplastic agent.

•**roflumilast.** (roe-FLUE-mi-last) USAN.
Use: Bronchial asthma; chronic obstructive pulmonary disease.

•**roflurane.** (row-FLEW-rane) USAN.
Use: Anesthetic, general.

Rogaine. (Pharmacia) Minoxidil 2% Topical Soln. Bot. 60 mL w/applicator. *OTC.*
Use: Antialopecia agent.

Rogaine Extra Strength for Men. (Pharmacia) Minoxidil 5%, alcohol. Soln. Bot. 60 mL w/dropper and sprayer applicators 2s. *OTC.*
Use: Antialopecia agent.

•**rogletimide.** (row-GLETT-ih-MIDE) USAN.
Use: Antineoplastic (aromatase inhibitor).

Rolaids. (Pfizer Consumer) Magnesium hydroxide 110 mg, calcium carbonate 550 mg. Dextrose, sucrose. Peppermint, spearmint, and cherry flavors. Chew. Tab. 12s, 36s, 150s, 250s, 300s. *OTC.*
Use: Antacid.

Rolaids Calcium Rich. (Warner Lambert) Calcium carbonate 412 mg, magnesium hydroxide 80 mg. Chew. Tab.

Bot. 12s, 36s, 75s, 150s. *OTC.*
Use: Antacid.

Rolaids Extra Strength. (Pfizer Consumer) Magnesium hydroxide 135 mg, calcium carbonate 675 mg. Dextrose, sucrose. Cool strawberry, freshmint, fruit, tropical punch flavors. Chew. Tab. 10s, 30s, 100s. *OTC.*
Use: Antacid.

Rolaids Extra Strength Softchews. (Pfizer Consumer) Calcium carbonate 1,177 mg. Corn syrup, sucrose. Vanilla creme and wild cherry flavors. Chew. Tab. 18s. *OTC.*
Use: Antacid.

Rolaids Multi-Symptom. (Pfizer Consumer) Magnesium hydroxide 135 mg, calcium carbonate 675 mg, simethicone 60 mg, dextrose, sucrose. Cool mint and berry flavors. Chew. Tab. 10s, 30s, 100s. *OTC.*
Use: Antacid.

Rolatuss Expectorant. (Huckaby Pharmacal) Phenylephrine hydrochloride 5 mg, chlorpheniramine maleate 2 mg, codeine phosphate 9.85 mg, ammonium Cl 33.3 mg/5 mL, alcohol 5%. Bot. 480 mL. *c-v.*
Use: Antihistamine, antitussive, decongestant, expectorant.

Rolatuss Plain. (Major) Phenylephrine hydrochloride 5 mg, chlorpheniramine maleate 2 mg/5 mL. Liq. Bot. 473 mL. *OTC.*
Use: Antihistamine, decongestant.

Rolatuss w/Hydrocodone. (Major) Phenylpropanolamine hydrochloride 3.3 mg, phenylephrine hydrochloride 5 mg, pyrilamine maleate 3.3 mg, pheniramine maleate 3.3 mg, hydrocodone bitartrate 1.67 mg/5 mL. Liq. Bot. 480 mL. *c-III.*
Use: Antihistamine, antitussive, decongestant.

• **roletamide.** (row-LET-am-ide) USAN.
Use: Hypnotic; sedative.

• **rolgamidine.** (role-GAM-ih-deen) USAN.
Use: Antidiarrheal.

Rolicap. (Arcum) Vitamins A acetate 5000 units, D_2 400 units, B_1 3 mg, B_2 2.5 mg, B_6 10 mg, C 50 mg, niacinamide 20 mg, B_{12} 1 mcg. Chew. Tab. Bot. 100s, 1000s. *OTC.*
Use: Vitamin supplement.

• **rolicyprine.** (ROW-lih-SIGH-preen) USAN.
Use: Antidepressant.

• **rolipram.** (ROLE-ih-pram) USAN.
Use: Anxiolytic.

• **rolitetracycline.** (ROW-lee-tet-rah-SIGH-kleen) USAN.
Use: Anti-infective.

• **rolitetracycline nitrate.** (ROW-lee-tet-rah-SIGH-kleen) USAN. Tetrim.
Use: Anti-infective.

• **rolodine.** (ROW-low-deen) USAN.
Use: Muscle relaxant.

Romach Antacid. (Last) Magnesium carbonate 400 mg, sodium bicarbonate 250 mg. Tab. Strip pack 60s, 500s. *OTC.*
Use: Antacid.

• **romazarit.** (row-MAZZ-ah-rit) USAN.
Use: Anti-inflammatory; antirheumatic.

Romazicon. (Hoffman-La Roche) Flumazenil 0.1 mg/mL, parabens, EDTA. Inj. Vials 5 mL, 10 mL. *Rx.*
Use: Antidotes.

Romex. (A.P.C.) **Troche:** Polymyxin B sulfate 1000 units, benzocaine 5 mg, cetalkonium Cl 2.5 mg, gramicidin 100 mcg, chlorphenira- mine maleate 0.5 mg, tyrothricin 2 mg. Pkg. 10s. **Liq.:** Guaifenesin 200 mg, dextromethorphan HBr 60 mg, chlorpheniramine maleate 12 mg, phenylephrine hydrochloride 30 mg/fl oz. Bot. 4 oz. *Rx.*
Use: Antihistamine, antitussive, decongestant, expectorant; anti-infective.

Romex Cough & Cold Capsules. (A.P.C.) Guaifenesin 65 mg, dextromethorphan HBr 10 mg, chlorpheniramine maleate 1.5 mg, pyrilamine maleate 12.5 mg, phenylephrine hydrochloride 5 mg, acetaminophen 160 mg. Cap. Bot. 21s. *OTC.*
Use: Antihistamine, antitussive, decongestant, expectorant.

Romex Cough & Cold Tablets. (A.P.C.) Dextromethorphan HBr 7.5 mg, phenylephrine hydrochloride 2.5 mg, ascorbic acid 30 mg. Tab. Box 15s. *OTC.*
Use: Antitussive, decongestant.

Romilar AC. (Scot-Tussin) Codeine phosphate 10 mg, guaifenesin 100 mg/5 mL, menthol, aspartame, parabens, phenylalanine, dye and alcohol free. Liq. Bot. 473 mL. *c-v.*
Use: Upper respiratory combination, antitussive, expectorant.

Rondamine-DM. (Major) **Drops:** Pseudoephedrine 25 mg, carbinoxamine maleate 2 mg, dextromethorphan HBr 4 mg/mL. Bot. 30 mL. **Syr.:** Dextromethorphan HBr 15 mg, brompheniramine maleate 4 mg, pseudoephedrine hydrochloride 60 mg/5 mL, alcohol < 0.2%, grape flavor. Bot. 120 mL. 473 mL, 3.8 L. *Rx.*

Use: Upper respiratory combination, antihistamine, antitussive, decongestant.

Rondec Chewable Tablets. (Dura) Brompheniramine maleate 4 mg, pseudoephedrine hydrochloride 60 mg, aspartame, phenylalanine 30.9 mg. Bot. 100s. *Rx.*
Use: Antihistamine, decongestant.

Rondec-DM. (Biovail) **Syrup:** Dextromethorphan HBr 15 mg, brompheniramine maleate 4 mg, pseduoephedrine hydrochloride 45 mg/5 mL, saccharin, sorbitol, grape, flavor. Bot. 118 mL, 473 mL. **Oral Drops:** Pseudoephedrine hydrochloride 15 mg, carbinoxamine maleate 1 mg, dextromethorphan 4 mg/mL, saccharin, sorbitol, grape flavor. Bot. 30 mL with dropper. *Rx.*
Use: Upper respiratory combination, antihistamine, antitussive, decongestant.

Rondec Oral Drops. (Biovail) Carbinoxamine maleate 1 mg, pseudoephedrine hydrochloride 15 mg/mL, saccharin, sorbitol, cherry flavor. Oral drops. Bot. 30 mL with dropper. *Rx.*
Use: Upper respiratory combination, antihistamine, decongestant.

Rondec Syrup. (Biovail) Brompheniramine maleate 4 mg, pseudoephedrine hydrochloride 45 mg/5 mL, saccharin, sorbitol, cherry flavor. Syr. Bot. 118 mL, 473 mL. *Rx.*
Use: Upper respiratory combination, antihistamine, decongestant.

Rondec Tablets. (Biovail) Pseudoephedrine hydrochloride 60 mg, carbinoxamine maleate 4 mg, lactose. Tab. Bot. 100s, 500s. *Rx.*
Use: Upper respiratory combination, antihistamine, decongestant.

Rondec-TR. (Biovail) Carbinoxamine maleate 8 mg, pseudoephedrine hydrochloride 120 mg, dextrose, lactose. Timed release. Tab. Bot. 100s. *Rx.*
Use: Upper respiratory combination, antihistamine, decongestant.

•**ronidazole.** (row-NYE-dazz-OLE) USAN.
Use: Antiprotozoal.

•**ronnel.** (RAHN-ell) USAN. Fenchlorphos.
Use: Insecticide (systemic).

Ronvet. (Armenpharm Ltd.) Erythromycin stearate 250 mg. Tab. Bot. 100s. *Rx.*
Use: Anti-infective, erythromycin.

•**ropinirole hydrochloride.** (row-PIN-ih-role) USAN.
Use: Antiparkinsonian (D$_2$ receptor agonist).
See: Requip.

•**ropitoin hydrochloride.** (ROW-pih-toe-in) USAN.
Use: Cardiovascular agent (antiarrhythmic).

ropivacaine hydrochloride.
Use: Anesthetic, local injectable.
See: Naropin.

•**ropizine.** (row-PIH-zeen) USAN.
Use: Anticonvulsant.

•**roquinimex.** (row-KWIH-nih-mex) USAN.
Use: Biological response modifier; immunomodulator; antineoplastic.

Rosac. (Stiefel) Sodium sulfacetamide 10%, sulfur 5%. Benzyl and cetostearyl alcohols, EDTA. Cream. 45 g. *Rx.*
Use: Keratolytic agent.

Rosanil. (Galderma) Sulfur 5%, sodium sulfacetamide 10%, EDTA, light mineral oil, parabens. Cleanser. 170 g. *Rx.*
Use: Keratolytic agent.

rosaniline dyes.
See: Fuchsin, Basic.
Methylrosaniline Cl.

•**rosaramicin.** (row-ZAR-ah-MY-sin) USAN. *Formerly Rosamicin.*
Use: Anti-infective.

•**rosaramicin butyrate.** (row-ZAR-ah-MY-sin BYOO-tih-rate) USAN. *Formerly Rosamicin Butyrate.*
Use: Anti-infective.

•**rosaramicin propionate.** (row-ZAR-ah-MY-sin PRO-pee-oh-nate) USAN. *Formerly Rosamicin Propionate.*
Use: Anti-infective.

•**rosaramicin sodium phosphate.** (row-ZAR-ah-MY-sin) USAN. *Formerly Rosamicin Sodium Phosphate.*
Use: Anti-infective.

•**rosaramicin stearate.** (row-ZAR-ah-MY-sin STEE-ah-rate) USAN. *Formerly Rosamicin Stearate.*
Use: Anti-infective.

rose bengal.
Use: Ophthalmic diagnostic product.
See: Rosets.

rose bengal. (Akorn) Rose bengal 1%. Bot. 5 mL.
Use: Diagnostic, tissue staining.

rose bengal. (Barnes-Hind) Rose bengal 1.3 mg. Strip. Box 100s. *OTC.*
Use: Diagnostic aid.

•**rose bengal sodium I-131 injection.** (rose BEN-gal) *USP 28.*
Use: Diagnostic aid (hepatic function), radiopharmaceutical.

•**rose bengal sodium I-125.** (rose BEN-gal) USAN.
Use: Radiopharmaceutical.

Rose-C. (Barth's) Vitamin C 300 mg, rose hip extract/5 mL. Liq. Dropper Bot. 2 oz,

8 oz. *OTC.*
Use: Vitamin supplement.

rose hips. (Burgin-Arden) Vitamin C 300 mg, in base of sorbitol. Bot. 4 oz, 8 oz. *OTC.*
Use: Vitamin supplement.

rose hips vitamin C. (Kirkman) Vitamin C 100 mg, 250 mg, 500 mg. Tab. Bot. 100s, 250s, 500s (except 100 mg). *OTC.*
Use: Vitamin supplement.

• **rose oil.** (rose) *NF 23.*
Use: Pharmaceutic aid; perfume.

Rosets. (Akorn) Rose bengal 1.3 mg. Strip. 100s. *OTC.*
Use: Diagnostic agent, ophthalmic.

rose water ointment.
Use: Emollient, ointment base.

• **rose water, stronger.** (rose) *NF 23.*
Use: Pharmaceutic aid; perfume.

• **rosiglitazone maleate.** (roe-sih-GLIH-tah-sone MAL-ee-ate) USAN.
Use: Antidiabetic.
See: Avandia.

• **rosiglitazone maleate and metformin hydrochloride.** (roe-sih-GLIH-tah-sone MAL-ee-ate/met-FORE-min)
Use: Antidiabetic.
See: Avandamet.

• **rosin.** (ROZZ-in) *USP 28.*
Use: Stiffening agent, pharmaceutical necessity.

• **rosoxacin.** (row-SOX-ah-sin) USAN.
Use: Anti-infective.
See: Rosoxacin.

Ross SLD. (Ross) Low-residue nutritional supplement for patients restricted to a clear liquid feeding or with fat malabsorption disorders. Packet 1.35 oz. Ctn. 6s. Case 4 ctn. Can 13.5 oz. Case 6s. *OTC.*
Use: Nutritional supplement.

• **rostaporfin.** (roe-sta-POR-fin) USAN.
Use: Cutaneous carcinomas; Kaposi sarcomas; choroidal neovascularization.

Rosula. (Doak Dermatologies) Sodium sulfacetamide 10%, sulfur 5% in a 10% urea vehicle. Gel. Tube. 45 mL. *Rx.*
Use: Keratolytic agent.

Rosula NS. (Doak) Sodium sulfacetamide 10% urea vehicle. EDTA, sodium thiosulfate. Pads. 30s. *Rx.*
Use: Keratolytic agent.

• **rosuvastatin calcium.** (roe-SOO-va-statin) USAN.
Use: Antihyperlipidemic.
See: Crestor.

Rotalex Test. (Orion) Latex slide agglutination test for detection of rotavirus in feces. Kit 1s.

Use: Diagnostic aid.

Rotazyme II. (Abbott Diagnostics) Enzyme immunoassay for detection of rotavirus antigen in feces. Test kit 50s.
Use: Diagnostic aid.

• **rotigotine.** (ROE-ti-goe-tine) USAN.
Use: Parkinson disease.

• **rotoxamine.** (row-TOX-ah-meen) USAN.
Use: Antihistamine.

• **rovelizumab.** (roe-ve-LYE-zue-mab) USAN.
Use: Immunomodulator. USAN.

Rowasa. (Solvay) **Enema:** Mesalamine 4 g/60 mL. EDTA, potassium acetate, potassium metabisulfite sodium benzoate, white petrolatum. 7s and 28s with lubricated applicator tip. **Rectal Susp.:** Mesalamine 4 g/60 mL. Units of 7 disposable Bot. **Supp.:** Mesalamine 500 mg. Box 12s, 24s. *Rx.*
Use: Anti-inflammatory.

• **roxadimate.** (rox-AD-ih-mate) USAN.
Use: Sunscreen.

Roxanol. (aaiPharma) Morphine sulfate 20 mg/mL. Oral Soln., concentrate. Bot. 30 mL, 120 mL w/calibrated dropper, *c-II.*
Use: Opioid analgesic.

Roxanol 100. (aaiPharma) Morphine sulfate 100 mg/5 mL. Oral Soln., concentrate. Bot. 240 mL with calibrated spoon. *c-II.*
Use: Opioid analgesic.

Roxanol T. (aaiPharma) Morphine sulfate 20 mg/mL, flavored. Oral Soln., concentrate. Bot. 30 mL, 120 mL with calibrated dropper. *c-II.*
Use: Opioid analgesic.

• **roxarsone.** (ROX-AHR-sone) USAN.
Use: Anti-infective.

• **roxatidine acetate.** (ROX-ah-tih-DEEN) USAN.
Use: Antiulcer.

Roxicet. (Roxane) **Oral Soln.:** Oxycodone hydrochloride 5 mg, acetaminophen 325 mg/5 mL. Bot. UD 5 mL, 500 mL. **Tab.:** Oxycodone hydrochloride 5 mg, acetaminophen 325 mg, 0.4% alcohol. Bot. 100s, 500s, UD 100s. *c-II.*
Use: Analgesic combination, narcotic.

Roxicet 5/500. (Roxane) Oxycodone hydrochloride 5 mg, acetaminophen 500 mg. Cap. Bot. 100s, UD 100s. *c-II.*
Use: Analgesic combination, narcotic.

Roxicodone. (aaiPharma) **Oral Soln.:** Oxycodone hydrochloride 5 mg/5 mL. Sorbitol. Bot. 500 mL, UD 5 mL. **Tab.:** Oxycodone hydrochloride 5 mg. Bot. 100s, UD 100s. **IR Tab.:** Oxycodone hy-

drochloride 15 mg, 30 mg. Lactose. Bot. 100s, UD 100s. *c-ii.*
Use: Opioid analgesic.

Roxicodone Intensol. (aaiPharma) Oxycodone hydrochloride 20 mg/mL. Conc. Soln. Bot. 30 mL with calibrated dropper. *c-ii.*
Use: Opioid analgesic.

• **roxifiban acetate.** (rox-ih-FIE-ban) USAN.
Use: Antithrombotic, fibrinogen receptor antagonist.

Roxilox. (Roxane) Oxycodone hydrochloride 5 mg, acetaminophen 500 mg. Cap. Bot. 100s. *c-ii.*
Use: Narcotic analgesic combination.

Roxiprin. (Roxane) Oxycodone hydrochloride 4.5 mg, oxycodone terephthalate 0.38 mg, aspirin 325 mg. Tab. Bot. 100s, 1000s, UD 100s. *c-ii.*
Use: Analgesic combination, narcotic.

• **roxithromycin.** (ROX-ith-row-MY-sin) USAN.
Use: Anti-infective.

Rozerem. (Takeda) Ramelteon 8 mg. Tab. Bot. 30s, 100s, 500s. *Rx.*
Use: Insomnia.

Rozex. (Galderma) Metronidazole 0.75%. Top. Emulsion. Tube. 60 g. *Rx.*
Use: Anti-inflammatory, dermatologic.

R/S. (Summers) Sulfur 5%, resorcinol 2%, alcohol 28%. Lot. Bot. 56.7 mL. *OTC.*
Use: Dermatologic; acne.

R-Tanna. (Prasco) Phenylephrine tannate 25 mg, chlorpheniramine tannate 9 mg. Tab. 100s. *Rx.*
Use: Decongestant and antihistamine.

R-Tannamine. (Qualitest) Phenylephrine tannate 25 mg, chlorpheniramine tannate 8 mg, pyrilamine tannate 25 mg. Tab. Bot. 100s. *Rx.*
Use: Antihistamine; decongestant.

R-Tannamine Pediatric. (Qualitest) Phenylephrine tannate 5 mg, chlorpheniramine tannate 2 mg, pyrilamine tannate 12.5 mg/5 mL, 120 mL, 473 mL. *Rx.*
Use: Antihistamine; decongestant.

R-Tanna S Pediatric. (Prasco) Phenylephrine tannate 5 mg, chlorpheniramine tannate 4.5 mg/mL, methylparaben, saccharin, sucrose, grape flavor. Susp. 118 mL. *Rx.*
Use: Decongestant and antihistamine.

R-Tannate. (Various Mfr.) Phenylephrine tannate 25 mg, chlorpheniramine tannate 8 mg, pyrilamine tannate 25 mg. Tab. Bot. 100s. *Rx.*
Use: Antihistamine; decongestant.

R-Tannate Pediatric. (Various Mfr.) Phenylephrine tannate 5 mg, chlorpheniramine tannate 2 mg, pyrilamine tannate 12.5 mg/5 mL, saccharin. Susp. Bot. 473 mL. *Rx.*
Use: Antihistamine; decongestant.

R-Tanna 12. (Duramed) Phenylephrine tannate 5 mg, pyrilamine tannate 30 mg/5 mL, saccharin, sucrose, methylparaben, strawberry-currant flavor. Susp. Unit of use 118 mL with oral syr. *Rx.*
Use: Upper respiratory combination, decongestant, antihistamine.

rt-PA.
Use: Tissue plasminogen.
See: Activase.

R-3 Screen Test. (Wampole) A three-minute latex-eosin slide test for the qualitative detection of rheumatoid factor activity in serum. Kit 100s.
Use: Diagnostic aid.

RII Retinamide.
Use: Myelodysplastic syndromes.
[Orphan Drug]

Rubacell. (Abbott Diagnostics) Passive hemagglutination (PHA) test for the detection of antibody to rubella virus in serum or recalcified plasma.
Use: Diagnostic aid.

Rubacell II. (Abbott) Passive hemagglutination (PHA) test to detect antibody to rubella in serum or recalcified plasma. In 100s, 1000s.
Use: Diagnostic aid.

Rubaquick Diagnostic Kit. (Abbott Diagnostics) Rapid passive hemagglutination (PHA) for the detection of antibodies to rubella virus in serum specimens.
Use: Diagnostic aid.

Ruba-Tect. (Abbott Diagnostics) Hemagglutination inhibition test for the detection and quantitation of rubella antibody in serum. In 100s.
Use: Diagnostic aid.

Rubatrope-57. (Bristol-Myers Squibb) Cyanocobalamin Co 57 Capsules; Soln U.S.P. 24. *OTC.*
Use: Vitamin supplement.

Rubazyme. (Abbott Diagnostics) Enzyme immunoassay for 1 gG antibody to rubella virus. Test kit 100s, 1000s.
Use: Diagnostic aid.

Rubazyme-M. (Abbott Diagnostics) Enzyme immunoassay for IgM antibody to rubella virus in serum. Test kit 50s.
Use: Diagnostic aid.

rubella & mumps virus vaccine, live.
Use: Immunization.
See: Biavax II.

- **rubella virus vaccine, live.** (roo-BELL-ah) *USP 28*.
Use: Immunization.
See: Meruvax II.
Rubex. (Bristol-Myers Squibb Oncology/Virology) Doxorubicin hydrochloride 100 mg, lactose 500 mg, preservative free. Pow. for Inj. lyophilized. Vial. *Rx.*
Use: Antibiotic.
- **rubidium chloride Rb 82 injection.** (roo-BIH-dee-uhm) *USP 28*.
Use: Diagnostic aid (radioactive, cardiac disease), radiopharmaceutical.
- **rubidium chloride Rb 86.** (roo-BIH-dee-uhm) USAN.
Use: Radiopharmaceutical.
- **rubitecan.** USAN.
Use: Antineoplastic.
RU 486.
Use: Antiprogesterone.
Ru-lets M 500. (Rugby) Vitamin C 500 mg, B_3 100 mg, B_5 20 mg, B_1 15 mg, B_2 10 mg, B_6 5 mg, A 10,000 units, B_{12} 12 mcg, D 400 units, E 30 mg, Mg, Fe 20 mg, Cu, Zn 1.5 mg, Mn, I. Tab. Bot. 100s. *OTC.*
Use: Mineral, vitamin supplement.
RuLox Plus. (Rugby) **Susp.:** Aluminum hydroxide 500 mg, magnesium hydroxide 450 mg, simethicone 40 mg/5 mL. Bot. 355 mL. **Tab.:** Aluminum hydroxide 200 mg, magnesium hydroxide 200 mg, simethicone 25 mg. Chew. Bot. 50s. *OTC.*
Use: Antacid; antiflatulent.
RuLox Suspension. (Rugby) Aluminum hydroxide 225 mg, magnesium hydroxide 200 mg/5 mL. Susp. Bot. 360 mL, 769 mL, gal. *OTC.*
Use: Antacid.
Rum-K. (Fleming & Co.) Potassium Cl 10 mEq/5 mL in butter rum flavored base. Bot. Pt, gal. *Rx.*
Use: Electrolyte supplement.
- **rupintrivir.** (roo-PIN-tri-veer) USAN.
Use: Antiviral.
- **ruplizumab.** (rue-PLYE-zue-mab) USAN.
Use: Immune thrombocytopenic purpura; systemic lupus erythematosus.
rust inhibitor.
See: Sodium Nitrite.
- **rutamycin.** (ROO-tah-MY-sin) USAN. From strain of *Streptomyces rutgersensis*. Under study.
Use: Antifungal.
rutgers 612.
See: Ethohexadiol.
rutin. (Various Mfr.) 3-Rhamnoglucoside of 5,7,3',4-tetrahydroxyflavonol. Eldrin, globulariacitrin, myrticalorin, oxyritin,

phytomelin, rutoside, sophorin. Tab. 20 mg, 50 mg, 60 mg, 100 mg. *Rx.*
Use: Vascular disorders.
rutoside.
See: Rutin.
Ru-Tuss II. (Knoll) Phenylpropanolamine hydrochloride 75 mg, chlorpheniramine maleate 12 mg. Cap. Bot. 100s. *Rx.*
Use: Antihistamine, decongestant.
RVPaque. (ICN) Red petrolatum, zinc oxide, cinoxate, in water-resistant base. Tube 15 g, 37.5 g. *OTC.*
Use: Sunscreen.
Rymed. (Edwards) **Cap.:** Pseudoephedrine hydrochloride 30 mg, guaifenesin 250 mg. Cap. Bot. 100s. **Liq.:** Pseudoephedrine hydrochloride 30 mg, guaifenesin 100 mg/5 mL, alcohol 1.4%. Bot. Pt. *OTC.*
Use: Decongestant, expectorant.
Rymed-TR. (Edwards) Phenylpropanolamine hydrochloride 75 mg, guaifenesin 400 mg. Tab. Bot. 100s. *OTC.*
Use: Decongestant, expectorant.
Ryna-CX. (Wallace) Guaifenesin 100 mg, pseudoephedrine hydrochloride 30 mg, codeine phosphate 10 mg, alcohol 7.5%, saccharin, sorbitol/5 mL. Bot. 4 oz, pt. *c-v.*
Use: Antitussive, decongestant, expectorant.
Rynatan. (Wallace) Phenylephrine tannate 5 mg, chlorpheniramine tannate 2 mg, pyrilamine tannate 12.5 mg/5 mL. Ped. Susp. Bot. 473 mL. *Rx.*
Use: Antihistamine, decongestant.
Rynatan Pediatric. (Wallace) Phenylephrine tannate 5 mg, carbetapentane tannate 30 mg, ephedrine tannate 5 mg, chlorpheniramine tannate 4 mg/5 mL, tartrazine, methylparaben, saccharin, sucrose, strawberry-currant flavor. Susp. Bot. 237 mL, 473 mL. *Rx.*
Use: Upper respiratory combination, decongestant, antihistamine, antitussive.
Rynatan-S Pediatric. (Wallace) Phenylephrine tannate 5 mg, chlorpheniramine tannate 2 mg, pyrilamine tannate 12.5 mg/5 mL. Susp. Bot. 120 mL w/syringe. *Rx.*
Use: Antihistamine, decongestant.
Rynatan Tablets. (Medpointe) Phenylephrine tannate 25 mg/chlorpheniramine tannate 9 mg. Tab. 100s. *Rx.*
Use: Decongestant, antihistamine upper respiratory combination.
Rynatuss. (Medpointe) Carbetapentane tannate 60 mg, chlorpheniramine tannate 5 mg, ephedrine tannate 10 mg, phenylephrine tannate 10 mg. Tab. Bot.

100s, 500s, 2000s. *Rx.*
Use: Upper respiratory combination, antihistamine, decongestant, anticholinergic.

Rynatuss Pediatric. (Wallace) Carbetapentane tannate 30 mg, chlorpheniramine tannate 4 mg, ephedrine tannate 5 mg, phenylephrine tannate 5 mg, saccharin, tartrazine/5 mL. Susp. Bot. 8 oz, pt. *Rx.*
Use: Antihistamine, antitussive, decongestant.

Ryna-12. (Wallace) Phenylephrine tannate 25 mg, pyrilamine tannate 60 mg, talc. Tab. 100s. *Rx.*
Use: Decongestant and antihistamine.

Ryna-12 S. (Wallace) Pyrilamine tannate 30 mg, phenylephrine tannate 5 mg/ 5 mL, methylparaben, saccharin, sucrose, strawberry-currant flavor. Susp. Unit-of-use 118 mL with oral syringe. *Rx.*
Use: Upper respiratory combination, antihistamine, decongestant.

Rythmol. (Reliant) Propafenone hydrochloride 150 mg, 225 mg, 300 mg. Film coated. Tab. Bot. 100s, UD 100s. *Rx.*
Use: Antiarrhythmic agent.

Rythmol SR. (Reliant) Propafenone hydrochloride 225 mg, 325 mg, 425 mg. ER Cap. 100s. *Rx.*
Use: Antiarrhythmic agent.

S

Saave+. (NeuroGenesis/Matrix Tech.) Vitamin D 40 mg, L-phenylalanine, L-glutamine 25 mg, vitamins A 333.3 units, B_1 2.417 mg, B_2 0.85 mg, B_3 33 mg, B_5 15 mg, B_6 3 mg, B_{12} 5 mcg, folic acid 0.067 mg, C 100 mg, E 5 units, biotin 0.05 mg, Ca 25 mg, Cr 0.01 mg, Fe 1.5 mg, Mg 25 mg, Zn 2.5 mg. Cap. Yeast and preservative free. Bot. 42s, 180s. OTC.
Use: Mineral, vitamin supplement.

• **sabcomeline hydrochloride.** (sab-KOE-meh-leen) USAN.
Use: Treatment of Alzheimer disease.

• **sabeluzole.** (sah-BELL-you-zole) USAN.
Use: Anticonvulsant; antihypoxic.

• **saccharin.** (SACK-ah-rin) NF 23.
Use: Pharmaceutic aid (flavor).

saccharin. (Merck & Co.) Saccharin. Pow. Pkg. 1 oz, 0.25 lb, 1 lb. (Bristol-Myers Squibb) Tab. 0.25 g, 0.5 g. Bot. 500s, 1000s; 1 g. Bot. 1000s.
Use: Pharmaceutic aid (flavor).

• **saccharin calcium.** USP 28.
Use: Non-nutritive sweetener.

• **saccharin sodium.** USP 28.
Use: Sweetener (non-nutritive).
See: Ril Sweet.
Sweeta.

saccharin sodium. (Various Mfr.) Saccharin sodium. Pow., Bot. 1 oz, 0.25 lb, 1 lb. Tab.
Use: Sweetener (non-nutritive).

saccharin soluble.
See: Saccharin Sodium.

Sac-500. (Western Research) Vitamin C 500 mg. TR Cap. Bot. 1000s. OTC.
Use: Vitamin supplement.

sacrosidase.
Use: Nutritional therapy.
See: Sucraid.

Saf-Clens. (Calgon Vestal Laboratories) Meroxapol 105, NaCl, potassium sorbate NF, DMDM hydantoin. Spray. Bot. 177 mL. OTC.
Use: Dermatologic, wound therapy.

Safeskin. (C & M Pharmacal) A dermatologically acceptable detergent for patients who are sensitive to ordinary detergents. No whiteners, brighteners, or other irritants. Bot. qt.
Use: Laundry detergent for sensitive skin.

Safe Suds. (Ar-Ex) Hypoallergenic, all-purpose detergent for patients whose hands or respiratory membranes are irritated by soaps or detergents. pH 6.8. No enzymes, phosphates, lanolin, fill-

ers, bleaches. Bot. 22 oz.
Use: Detergent.

Safe Tussin. (Kramer) Guaifenesin 100 mg, dextromethorphan HBr 15 mg/5 mL, sorbitol, menthol, mint flavor, alcohol and dye free. Liq. Bot. 120 mL. OTC.
Use: Upper respiratory combination, antitussive, expectorant.

Safety-Coated Arthritis Pain Formula. (Whitehall-Robins) Enteric coated aspirin 500 mg. Tab. Bot. 24s, 60s. OTC.
Use: Analgesic.

• **safflower oil.** USP 28.
Use: Pharmaceutic aid (vehicle, oleaginous).

safflower oil.
Use: Nutritional supplement.
See: Microlipid.

• **safingol.** (saff-IN-gole) USAN.
Use: Antineoplastic (adjunct); antipsoriatic.

• **safingol hydrochloride.** USAN.
Use: Antineoplastic (adjunct); antipsoriatic.

Saizen. (Serono) Somatropin 5 mg (≈ 15 units)/vial, sucrose. Pow. for Inj., lyophilized. Vial w/diluent (Bacteriostatic Water for Injection w/benzyl alcohol 0.9%). Rx.
Use: Hormone, growth.

SalAc Cleanser. (Medicis) Salicylic acid 2%, benzyl alcohol, glyceryl cocoate. Liq. Bot. 177 mL. OTC.
Use: Dermatologic, acne.

salacetin.
See: Acetylsalicylic Acid.

Sal-Acid. (Pedinol Pharmacal) Salicylic acid 40% in collodion-like vehicle. Plaster. Pkg. 14s. OTC.
Use: Keratolytic.

Salacid 60%. (Gordon Laboratories) Salicylic acid 60% in ointment base. Jar 2 oz. OTC.
Use: Keratolytic.

Salacid 25%. (Gordon Laboratories) Salicylic acid 25% in ointment base. Jar 2 oz, lb. OTC.
Use: Keratolytic.

Salactic Film. (Pedinol Pharmacal) Salicylic acid 16.7% in flexible collodion w/color. Liq. Applicator Bot. 15 mL. OTC.
Use: Keratolytic.

Salagen. (MGI Pharma) Pilocarpine hydrochloride 5 mg, 7.5 mg. Tab. Bot. 100s. Rx.
Use: Mouth and throat product.

Salazide. (Major) Hydroflumethiazide 50 mg, reserpine 0.125 mg. Tab. Bot.

100s, 500s, 1000s. *Rx.*
Use: Antihypertensive combination.
Salazide-Demi. (Major) Hydroflumethiazide 25 mg, reserpine 0.125 mg. Tab. Bot. 100s. *Rx.*
Use: Antihypertensive combination.
salbutamol.
See: Albuterol.
• **salcaprozate sodium.** (sal-KAP-roe-zate) USAN.
Use: Oral absorption promoter.
Salcegel. (Apco) Sodium salicylate 5 g, calcium ascorbate 25 mg, calcium carbonate 1 g, dried aluminum hydroxide gel 2 g. Tab. Bot. 100s. *OTC.*
Use: Analgesic.
Sal-Clens Acne Cleanser. (C & M Pharmacal) Salicylic acid 2%. Gel. Tube 240 g. *OTC.*
Use: Dermatologic, acne.
• **salcolex.** (SAL-koe-lex) USAN.
Use: Analgesic; anti-inflammatory; antipyretic.
• **salethamide maleate.** (sal-ETH-ah-MIDE) USAN. Under study.
Use: Analgesic.
saletin.
See: Acetylsalicylic Acid.
Saleto. (Mallard) Aspirin 210 mg, acetaminophen 115 mg, salicylamide 65 mg, caffeine 16 mg. Tab. Bot. 100s, 1000s, *Sani-Pak* 1000s. *OTC.*
Use: Analgesic.
Saleto-200. (Roberts) Ibuprofen 200 mg. Tab. Bot. 1000s, UD 50s. *OTC.*
Use: Analgesic; NSAID.
Salex. (Healthpoint) Salicylic acid.
Cream.: 6%. Alcohols, glycerin, parabens. Bot. 400 g. **Lot.:** 6%. Alcohols, EDTA, glycerin, mineral oil, parabens, PEG 100. 414 mL. *Rx.*
Use: Keratolytic agent.
Salflex. (Carnrick) Salsalate 500 mg, 750 mg. Tab. Bot. 100s. *Rx.*
Use: Analgesic.
• **salicyl alcohol.** (SAL-ih-sill AL-koe-hahl) USAN. *Formerly Saligenin, Saligenol, Salicain.*
Use: Anesthetic, local.
• **salicylamide.** *USP 28.*
Use: Analgesic.
W/Combinations.
See: Anodynos.
Dapco.
Decohist.
Ed-Flex.
Emersal.
Levacet.
Lobac.
Nokane.

Painaid.
Partuss T.D.
P.M.P. Compound.
Presalin.
Saleto.
Salipap.
Salocol.
Sinulin.
Sleep.
salicylanilide.
Use: Antifungal.
salicylated bile extract. Chologestin.
• **salicylate meglumine.** (suh-LIH-sih-late) USAN.
Use: Antirheumatic; analgesic.
salicylazosulfapyridine.
See: Sulfasalazine.
• **salicylic acid.** (sal-ih-SILL-ik) *USP 28.*
Use: Keratolytic.
See: Calicylic.
Clearasil Acne-Fighting Pads.
Compound W for Kids.
Compound W One Step Wart Remover for Kids.
Fung-O.
Maximum Strength Wart Remover.
MG217 Sal-Acid.
OFF-Ezy Corn & Callous Remover.
PROPApH Astringent Cleanser Maximum Strength.
Psor-a-set.
Sal-Acid.
Salactic Film.
Salex.
Salicylic Acid Acne Treatment.
Sal-Plant.
Scalpicin.
Sebulex.
Wart-Off.
salicylic acid & sulfur soap. (Stiefel) Salicylic acid 3%, sulfur 10%, EDTA. Cake 116 g. *OTC.*
Use: Antiseborrheic; keratolytic.
salicylic acid cleansing bar. (Stiefel) Salicylic acid 2%, EDTA. Cake 113 g. *OTC.*
Use: Antiseborrheic; keratolytic.
salicylic acid combinations.
See: Acnaveen.
Acno.
Akne Drying Lotion.
Bensal HP.
Clearasil.
Cuticura.
Duofilm.
Duo-WR.
Fostex.
Ionax.
Ionil.
Ionil T.
MG217 Medicated Tar Free.

MG217 Sal-Acid.
Neutrogena T/Sal.
Occlusal HP.
Oxy Clean Medicated Pads for Sensitive Skin.
Oxy Night Watch.
Pernox.
Propa pH.
Salicylic Acid Soap.
Sebulex Shampoo.
Therac.
Tinver.
•**salicylic acid topical foam.**
Use: Keratolytic.
•**salicylsalicylic acid.** USAN. Salsalate.
Use: Analgesic.
See: Arcylate.
Disalcid.
W/Aspirin.
See: Durageslo.
salicylsulphonic acid. Sulfosalicylic acid.
Saligenin. (City Chemical Corp.) Salicyl alcohol. Bot. 25 g, 100 g. *OTC.*
Saline. (Bausch & Lomb) Buffered isotonic. Thimerosal 0.001%, boric acid, NaCl, EDTA. Soln. Bot. 355 mL. *OTC.*
Use: Contact lens care.
saline laxatives.
See: Epsom Salt.
Fleet Phospho-soda.
Magnesium Citrate.
Milk of Magnesia.
Milk of Magnesia-Concentrated.
Phillips' Milk of Magnesia.
Phillips' Milk of Magnesia, Concentrated.
Saline Solution. (Akorn) Saline solution, isotonic, preserved. Bot. 12 oz. *OTC.*
Use: Contact lens care; rinsing
Saline Spray. (Akorn) Isotonic nonpreserved saline aerosol soln. Bot. 2 oz, 8 oz, 12 oz. *OTC.*
Use: Contact lens care.
SalineX. (Muro) Sodium chloride 0.4%, benzalkonium chloride, propylene glycol, polyethylene glycol, EDTA. Soln. Dropper bot. 15 mL. Mist bot. 50 mL. *OTC.*
Use: Nasal decongestant.
Salipap. (Freeport) Salicylamide 5 g, acetaminophen 5 g. Tab. Bot. 1000s. *OTC.*
Use: Analgesic.
Salithol. (Madland) Balm of methyl salicylate, menthol, camphor. Liq. Bot. pt, gal. Oint. Jar 1 lb, 5 lb. *OTC.*
Use: Analgesic, topical.
Salivart. (Gebauer) Sodium carboxymethylcellulose, sorbitol, NaCl, KCl, calcium Cl, magnesium Cl, dibasic po-

tassium phosphate, and nitrogen (as propellant), preservative free. Soln. Spray can 75 mL. *OTC.*
Use: Saliva substitute.
Saliva Substitute. (Roxane) Sorbitol, sodium carboxymethylcellulose, methylparaben. Soln. Spray Bot. 120 mL. *OTC.*
Use: Saliva substitute.
saliva substitutes.
Use: Mouth and throat product.
See: Entertainer's Secret.
Moi-Stir.
Moi-Stir Swabsticks.
MouthKote.
Salivart.
Saliva Substitute.
Salk vaccine.
See: IPOL.
Poliovirus Vaccine, Inactivated.
•**salmeterol xinafoate.** (sal-MEH-teh-role zin-AF-oh-ate) USAN.
Use: Bronchodilator, sympathomimetic.
See: Serevent Diskus.
W/Fluticasone propionate.
See: Advair Diskus.
•**salnacedin.** (sal-NAH-seh-din) USAN.
Use: Anti-inflammatory, topical.
Salocol. (Roberts) Acetaminophen 115 mg, aspirin 210 mg, salicylamide 65 mg, caffeine 16 mg. Tab. Bot. 1000s. *Rx.*
Use: Analgesic combination.
Salpaba w/Colchicine. (Madland) Sodium salicylate 0.25 g, para-aminobenzoic acid 0.25 g, vitamin C 20 mg, colchicine 0.25 mg. Tab. Bot. 100s, 1000s. *Rx.*
Use: Antigout.
Sal-Plant. (Pedinol Pharmacal) Salicylic acid 17% in flexible collodion vehicle. Gel. Tube 14 g. *OTC.*
Use: Keratolytic.
•**salsalate.** (SAL-sah-late) *USP 28.*
Use: Analgesic; anti-inflammatory.
See: Marthritic.
Salsitab. (Upsher-Smith) Salsalate 500 mg, 750 mg. Tab. Bot. 100s, 500s, UD 100s. *Rx.*
Use: Analgesic.
Salten. (Wren) Salicylamide 10 g. Tab. Bot. 100s, 1000s. *OTC.*
Use: Analgesic.
salt replacement products.
See: Slo-Salt.
Slo-Salt-K.
Sodium Chloride.
•**salts, rehydration, oral.** *USP 28.*
Use: Electrolyte combination.

salt substitutes.
Use: Sodium-free seasoning agent.
See: Adolph's Salt Substitute.
Adolph's Seasoned Salt Substitute.
Morton Salt Substitute.
Morton Seasoned Salt Substitute.
NoSalt.
Nu-Salt.
salt tablets. (Cross) Sodium Cl 650 mg.
Tab. Dispenser 500s. *OTC.*
Use: Salt replenisher.
Sal-Tropine. (Hope) Atropine sulfate
0.4 mg. Tab. Bot. 100s. *Rx.*
Use: Anticholinergic/antispasmodic.
Saluron. (Bristol-Myers Squibb) Hydroflu-methiazide 50 mg. Tab. Bot. 100s. *Rx.*
Use: Diuretic.
Salutensin. (Roberts) Hydroflumethia-zide 50 mg, reserpine 0.125 mg. Tab.
Bot. 100s, 1000s. *Rx.*
Use: Antihypertensive combination.
Salutensin-Demi. (Shire) Hydroflumeth-iazide 25 mg, reserpine 0.125 mg, lac-tose, sucrose. Tab. Bot. 100s. *Rx.*
Use: Antihypertensive combination.
Salvarsan.
Use: Antisyphilitic.
Salvite-B. (Faraday) Sodium chloride
7 g, dextrose 3 g, vitamin B$_1$ 1 mg. Tab.
Bot. 100s, 1000s. *OTC.*
• **samarium Sm 153 lexidronam injec-tion.** (sah-MARE-ee-uhm Sm 153 lex-IH-drah-nam) *USP 28.*
Use: Antineoplastic; radiopharmaceu-tical.
• **samarium Sm 153 lexidronam pentaso-dium.** USAN.
Use: Antineoplastic; radiopharmaceu-tical.
See: Quadramet.
Sanctura. (Various Mfr.) Trospium chlor-ide 20 mg. Lactose, sucrose. Tab. 60s,
500s. Blister 14s. *Rx.*
Use: Urinary incontinence.
Sancura. (Thompson Medical) Benzo-caine, chlorobutanol, chlorothymol,
benzoic acid, salicylic acid, benzyl al-cohol, cod liver oil, lanolin in a washable
petrolatum base. Oint. 30 g, 90 g.
Use: Anesthetic, local.
• **sancycline.** (SAN-SIGH-kleen) USAN.
Use: Anti-infective.
Sandimmune. (Novartis) Cyclosporine.
Oral soln.: 100 mg/mL. Alcohol 12.5%.
Bot. 50 mL with syringe. **Inj.:** 50 mg/
mL. Polyoxyethylated castor oil 650 mg/
mL, alcohol 32.9%. Amp. 5 mL. **Soft
Gelatin Cap.:** 25 mg, 100 mg. Sorbitol,
dehydrated alcohol ≤ 12.7%. UD 30s.
Rx.

Use: Immunosuppressant.
sandoptal. Isobutyl allylbarbituric acid.
See: Butalbital.
W/Caffeine, aspirin, phenacetin.
See: Fiorinal.
W/Caffeine, aspirin, phenacetin, codeine
phosphate.
See: Fiorinal w/Codeine.
Sandostatin. (Novartis) Octreotide ace-tate. **0.05 mg/mL, 0.1 mg/mL, 0.5 mg/
mL:** Inj. Amp 1 mL. **0.2 mg/mL, 1 mg/
mL:** 5 mL multidose vials. *Rx.*
Use: Antineoplastic, adjunctive.
Sanestro. (Sandia) Estrone 0.7 mg,
estradiol 0.35 mg, estriol 0.14 mg. Tab.
Bot. 100s, 1000s. *Rx.*
Use: Estrogen.
• **sanfetrinem cilexetil.** (san-FEH-trih-nem
sigh-LEX-eh-till) USAN.
Use: Anti-infective.
• **sanfetrinem sodium.** (san-FEH-trih-nem) USAN.
Use: Anti-infective.
SangCya. (SangStat) Cyclosporine
100 mg/mL, alcohol 10.5%. Oral Soln.
Bot. 50 mL. *Rx.*
Use: Immunosuppressive.
• **sanguinarium chloride.** (san-gwih-NARE-ee-uhm) USAN. *Formerly San-guinarine Chloride.*
Use: Antimicrobial; anti-inflammatory;
antifungal.
Sanguis. (Sigma-Tau) Liver 10 mcg, vita-min B$_{12}$ 100 mcg, folic acid 1 mcg/mL.
Vial 10 mL. *Rx.*
Use: Nutritional supplement.
Sani-Supp. (G & W) Glycerin. Supp.
Adults: Box 10s, 25s, 50s. **Pediatric:**
Box 10s, 25s. *OTC.*
Use: Laxative.
sanluol.
See: Arsphenamine.
Sanstress. (Sandia) Vitamins A
25,000 units, D 400 units, B$_1$ 10 mg, B$_2$
5 mg, niacinamide 100 mg, B$_6$ 1 mg,
B$_{12}$ 5 mcg, C 150 mg, Ca 103 mg, P
80 mg, Fe 10 mg, Cu 1 mg, I 0.1 mg,
Mg 5.5 mg, Mn 1 mg, K 5 mg, Zn
1.4 mg. Cap. Bot. 100s, 1000s. *OTC.*
Use: Mineral, vitamin supplement.
Santiseptic. (Santiseptic) Menthol, phe-nol, benzocaine, zinc oxide, calamine.
Lot. Bot. 4 oz. *OTC.*
Use: Dermatologic, counterirritant.
Santyl. (Knoll) Proteolytic enzyme de-rived from *Clostridium histolyticum*
250 units/g. Oint. Tube. 15 g, 30 g. *Rx.*
Use: Enzyme, topical.
• **saperconazole.** (SAP-ehr-KOE-nah-zole) USAN.

Use: Antifungal.

saponated cresol solution.
See: Cresol.

•**saprisartan potassium.** (sap-rih-SAHR-tan) USAN.
Use: Antihypertensive.

•**saquinavir mesylate.** (sack-KWIN-uh-vihr) *USP 28.*
Use: Antiviral.
See: Fortovase.
Invirase.

Sarafem. (Warner Chilcott) Fluoxetine hydrochloride 10 mg, 20 mg. Pulvule. Blister 28s. *Rx.*
Use: Antidepressant, SSRI.

•**sarafloxacin hydrochloride.** (sa-rah-FLOX-ah-SIN) USAN.
Use: Anti-infective (DNA gyrase inhibitor).

•**saralasin acetate.** (sare-AL-ah-sin) USAN.
Use: Antihypertensive.

Saratoga. (Blair) Boric acid, zinc oxide, eucalyptol, white petrolatum. Oint. Tube 1 oz, 2 oz. *OTC.*
Use: Dermatologic, counterirritant.

l-sarcolysin.
Use: Antineoplastic.
See: Alkeran.

Sardo Bath & Shower. (Schering-Plough) Mineral oil, tocopherol. Oil. Bot. 112.5 mL. *OTC.*
Use: Emollient.

Sardo Bath Oil Concentrate. (Schering-Plough) Mineral oil, isopropyl palmitate. Bot. 3.75 oz, 7.75 oz. *OTC.*
Use: Emollient.

Sardoettes. (Schering-Plough) Mineral oil, tocopherol, beta-carotene. Towelettes. Box 25s. *OTC.*
Use: Emollient.

Sardoettes Moisturizing Towelettes. (Schering-Plough) Mineral oil, isopropyl palmitate, impregnated towelling material. Individual packets. Box 25s. *OTC.*
Use: Emollient.

•**sargramostim.** (sar-GRUH-moe-STIM) USAN.
Use: Antineutropenic; hematopoietic stimulant; leukopoietic (granulocyte macrophage colony-stimulating factor).
See: Leukine.

Sarisol No. 2. (Halsey Drug) Butabarbital sodium 30 mg. Tab. Bot. 100s, 1000s. *c-III.*
Use: Hypnotic; sedative.

•**sarmoxicillin.** (sar-MOX-ih-SILL-in) USAN.

Use: Anti-infective.

Sarna. (Stiefel) Camphor 0.5%, menthol 0.5%, phenol 0.5% in a soothing emollient base. Bot. 7.4 oz. *OTC.*
Use: Emollient.

Sarna Anti-Itch. (Stiefel) Camphor 5%, menthol 5%, carbomer 940, cetyl alcohol, DMDM hydantoin. Foam. Bot. 105 mL. *OTC.*
Use: Emollient.

•**sarpicillin.** (sahr-PIH-SILL-in) USAN.
Use: Anti-infective.

SAStid soap. (Stiefel) Precipitated sulfur 10%. Bar 116 g. *OTC.*
Use: Dermatologic, acne.

satumomab pendetide.
Use: Detection of ovarian cancer. [Orphan Drug]
See: Oncoscint CR/OV.

saxol.
See: Petrolatum.

•**saw palmetto.** *NF 23.*
Use: Dietary supplement.

scabicides.
See: Benzyl Benzoate.
Eurax.

Scalpicin. (Combe) Salicylic acid 3%, menthol, SD alcohol 40. Shampoo. Bot. 45 mL, 75 mL, 120 mL. *OTC.*
Use: Corticosteroid, topical.

Scan. (Parker) Water-soluble gel. Bot. 8 oz, gal.
Use: Ultrasound aid.

Scar Cream Maximum Strength. (Clay-Park Labs) Octyl methoxycinnamate 7.5%, octyl salicylate 5%. Alcohols, mineral oil, parabens, urea. Cream. 28 g. *OTC.*
Use: Sunscreen.

Scarlet Red Ointment Dressings. (Sherwood Davis & Geck) 5% scarlet red, lanolin, olive oil, petrolatum. Gauze. 5" x 9" strips. *Rx.*
Use: Dermatologic, wound therapy.

Schamberg's. (C & M Pharmacal) Menthol 0.15%, phenol 1%, zinc oxide, peanut oil, lime water. Bot. Pt, gal. *OTC.*
Use: Antipruritic; counterirritant.

•**schick test control.** *USP 28.* Formerly *Diphtheria Toxin, Inactivated Diagnostic.*
Use: Diagnostic aid (dermal reactivity indicator).

Schirmer Tear Test. (Various Mfr.) Sterile tear flow test strips. 250s. *Rx.*
Use: Diagnostic aid, ophthalmic.

Schlesinger's Solution.
See: Morphine hydrochloride.

Sclerex. (Miller Pharmacal Group) Inositol 2 g, magnesium complex 34 mg,

vitamins C 100 mg, calcium succinate 25 mg, A 2500 units, D 200 units, E 100 units, B_1 5 mg, B_2 5 mg, B_6 5 mg, B_{12} 5 mcg, niacin 10 mg, niacinamide 30 mg, pantothenic acid 7.5 mg, folic acid 0.1 mg, Fe 10 mg, Cu 1 mg, Mn 2 mg, Zn 9 mg, I 0.10 mg/3 Tab. Bot. 60s. *OTC.*
Use: Mineral, vitamin supplement.

Scleromate. (Glenwood) Morrhuate sodium 50 mg/mL. Inj. Amps. 5 mL. Vials. 10 mL. 10 mL fill in 20 mL vials. *Rx.*
Use: Sclerosing agent.

sclerosing agents.
See: Ethanolamine Oleate.
Morrhuate Sodium.
Sodium Tetradecyl Sulfate.

Sclerosol. (Bryan) Talc 4 g. Aerosol. Single-use aluminum canister with 2 delivery tubes of 15 cm and 25 cm. *Rx.*
Use: Antineoplastic.

Scopace. (Hope Pharm) Scopolamine 0.4 mg. Tab. Bot. 100s. *Rx.*
Use: Antiparkinson; antiemetic/antivertigo agent; GI anticholinergic/antispasmodic.

• **scopafungin.** (SKOE-pah-FUN-jin) USAN.
Use: Antifungal; anti-infective.

Scope. (Procter & Gamble) Cetylpyridinium Cl, tartrazine, saccharin, SD alcohol 38F 67.9%. Liq. Bot. 90 mL, 180 mL, 360 mL, 720 mL, 1080 mL, 1440 mL. *OTC.*
Use: Mouthwash.

scopolamine. (skoe-PAHL-uh-meen) Hyoscine, I-Scopolamine, Epoxytropine tropate.
Use: Antiemetic/antivertigo agent.
See: Hyoscine.
Scopace.
Transderm-Scōp.

• **scopolamine hydrobromide.** (skoe-PAHL-uh-meen) *USP 28.* Formerly Hyoscine Hydrobromide.
Use: Anticholinergic (ophthalmic); cycloplegic; hypnotic; mydriatic; sedative; GI anticholinergic/antispasmodic.
See: Scopace.
Transderm-Scop
W/Combinations.
See: Aridol.
Atropine Sulfate.
Belladonna Alkaloids.
Bellahist-D LA.
Donnatal.
Donnatal Extentabs.
Isopto HBr.
Nilspasm.
Pedo-Sol.

Sedamine.
Sedapar.
Spasaid.
Stahist

scopolamine hydrobromide. (Invenex) Scopolamine HBr 0.3 mg/mL. Inj. Vial 1 mL. *Rx.*
Use: Amnestic; anxiolytic; sedative.

scopolamine hydrobromide. (GlaxoSmithKline) Scopolamine HBr 0.86 mg/mL. Inj. Vials. 1 mL. *Rx.*
Use: Amnestic; anxiolytic; sedative; GI anticholinergic/antispasmodic.

scopolamine hydrobromide. (Various Mfr.) Scopolamine HBr 0.3 mg/mL, 0.4 mg/mL, 1 mg/mL. Inj. Amps. 0.5 mL (0.4 mg/mL only). Vials. 1 mL. *Rx.*
Use: GI anticholinergic/antispasmodic.

scopolamine hydrobromide combinations.
See: Belladonna Products.
Hyoscine HBr.

scopolamine methobromide.
See: Methscopolamine Bromide.

scopolamine methyl nitrate.
See: Methscopolamine Nitrate.

scopolamine salts.
See: Belladonna Products.
Hyoscine Salts.

Scotavite. (Scot-Tussin) Vitamins A 25,000 units, D 400 units, B_1 10 mg, B_2 10 mg, B_6 5 mg, B_{12} 5 mcg, niacinamide 100 mg, calcium pantothenate 20 mg, C 200 mg, d-alpha tocopheryl 15 units, acid succinate iodine 0.15 mg. Tab. Bot. 100s, 500s. *OTC.*
Use: Mineral, vitamin supplement.

Scotcil. (Scot-Tussin) **Tab.:** Potassium penicillin 400,000 units w/calcium carbonate. Bot. 100s, 500s. **Pow.:** 80 mL, 150 mL. *Rx.*
Use: Anti-infective, penicillin.

Scotonic. (Scot-Tussin) Vitamins B_1 10 mg, B_2 5 mg, B_6 1 mg, niacinamide 50 mg, choline Cl 100 mg, inositol 100 mg, B_{12} 25 mcg, Ca 19 mg, Fe 50 mg, folic acid 0.15 mg, alcohol 15%, sodium benzoate 0.1%/45 mL. Bot. Pt, gal. *OTC.*
Use: Mineral, vitamin supplement.

Scott's Emulsion. (GlaxoSmithKline) Vitamins A 1,250 units, D 1,400 units/4 tsp. Bot. 6.25 oz, 12.5 oz. *OTC.*
Use: Vitamin supplement.

Scot-Tussin Allergy Relief Formula Clear. (Scot-Tussin) Diphenhydramine hydrochloride 12.5 mg/5 mL, parabens, menthol, alcohol and dye free, cherry-strawberry flavor. Liq. Bot. 118 mL. *OTC.*
Use: Antihistamine, nonselective ethanolamine.

Scot-Tussin DM. (Scot-Tussin) Dextromethorphan HBr 15 mg, chlorpheniramine maleate 2 mg/5 mL, parabens, alcohol and dye free. Liq. Bot. 118 mL, 237 mL, 473 mL, 3.8 L. *OTC.*
Use: Upper respiratory combination, antitussive, antihistamine.
Scot-Tussin DM Cough Chasers. (Scot-Tussin) Dextromethorphan HBr 5 mg, peppermint oil, sorbitol, dye free. Loz. Box 20s. *OTC.*
Use: Antitussive.
Scot-Tussin Expectorant. (Scot-Tussin) Guaifenesin 100 mg/5 mL, parabens, phenylalanine, menthol, aspartame, alcohol and dye free, grape flavor. Liq. Bot. 118 mL. *OTC.*
Use: Expectorant.
Scot-Tussin Hayfebrol. (Scot-Tussin) Pseudoephedrine hydrochloride 30 mg, chlorpheniramine maleate 2 mg/5 mL, parabens, menthol, alcohol and dye free. Liq. Bot. 120 mL. *OTC.*
Use: Upper respiratory combination, decongestant, antihistamine.
Scot-Tussin Original Clear 5-Action Cold and Allergy Formula. (Scot-Tussin) Phenylephrine hydrochloride 4.2 mg, pheniramine maleate 13.3 mg, sodium citrate 83.3 mg, sodium salicylate 83.3 mg, caffeine citrate 25 mg/5 mL, saccharin, parabens, cherry-strawberry flavor, alcohol and dye free. Syr. Liq. Bot. 118 mL, 473 mL, 3.8 L. *OTC.*
Use: Upper respiratory combination, decongestant, antihistamine, analgesic.
Scot-Tussin Original 5-Action Cold and Allergy Formula. (Scot-Tussin) Phenylephrine hydrochloride 4.2 mg, pheniramine maleate 13.3 mg, sodium citrate 83.3 mg, sodium salicylate 83.3 mg, caffeine citrate 25 mg/5 mL, sugar, parabens, sorbitol, grape flavor, alcohol free. Syr. Bot. 118 mL, 473 mL, 3.8 L. *OTC.*
Use: Upper respiratory combination, decongestant, antihistamine.
Scot-Tussin Pharmacal Allergy. (Scot-Tussin) Diphenhydramine hydrochloride 12.5 mg/5 mL, parabens, menthol. Liq. Dye free, sugar free. Bot. 120 mL. *OTC.*
Use: Antihistamine.
Scot-Tussin Pharmacal DM. (Scot-Tussin) Dextromethorphan HBr 15 mg, chlorpheniramine maleate 2 mg/5 mL, alcohol 10%, sugar free. Liq. Bot. 4 oz, 8 oz. *OTC.*
Use: Antihistamine.

Scot-Tussin Pharmacal DM Cough Chasers. (Scot-Tussin) Dextromethorphan HBr 2.5 mg, dye free, sorbitol. Loz. Pkg. 20s. *OTC.*
Use: Antitussive.
Scot-Tussin Pharmacal DM2. (Scot-Tussin) Dextromethorphan HBr 15 mg, guaifenesin 100 mg, alcohol 1.4%/5 mL. Syr. Bot. 120 mL, 240 mL. *OTC.*
Use: Antitussive; expectorant.
Scot-Tussin Pharmacal Expectorant. (Scot-Tussin) Guaifenesin 100 mg/5 mL, menthol, aspartame, phenylalanine, parabens, alcohol and dye free. Liq. Bot. 30 mL, 118.3 mL, 240 mL. *OTC.*
Use: Expectorant.
Scot-Tussin Pharmacal Senior Clear. (Scot-Tussin) Guaifenesin 200 mg, dextromethorphan HBr 15 mg/5 mL, parabens, phenylalanine, menthol, aspartame. Liq. Alcohol and sugar free. Bot 118.3 mL. *OTC.*
Use: Antitussive; expectorant.
Scot-Tussin Pharmacal Sugar-Free. (Scot-Tussin) Dextromethorphan HBr 15 mg, chlorpheniramine maleate 2 mg/5 mL. Bot. 4 oz, 8 oz, 16 oz, gal. *OTC.*
Use: Antitussive; antihistamine.
Scot-Tussin Pharmacal Sugar-Free Expectorant. (Scot-Tussin) Guaifenesin 100 mg/5 mL w/alcohol 3.5%. Dye, sodium free, and sugar free. *OTC.*
Use: Expectorant.
Scot-Tussin Pharmacal with Sugar. (Scot-Tussin) Phenylephrine hydrochloride 4.17 mg, pheniramine maleate 13.3 mg, sodium citrate 83.33 mg, sodium salicylate 83.33 mg, caffeine citrate 25 mg/5 mL. Bot. 4 oz, 8 oz, 16 oz, gal. *OTC.*
Use: Analgesic combination; antihistamine; decongestant.
Scot-Tussin Senior Clear. (Scot-Tussin) Guaifenesin 200 mg, dextromethorphan HBr 15 mg/5 mL, parabens, phenylalanine, aspartame, menthol, alcohol free. Liq. Bot. 118 mL. *OTC.*
Use: Upper respiratory combination, antitussive, expectorant.
Sculptra. (Dermik Laboratories) Poly-l-lactic acid (freeze dried). Pow. for Inj. Single-use vials. *Rx.*
Use: Restoration/correct of facial fat loss in individuals with HIV.
scurenaline.
See: Epinephrine.
scuroforme.
See: Butyl Aminobenzoate.
S.D.M. #50. (AstraZeneca) Isosorbide dinitrate 50% in lactose. *Rx.*

Use: Vasodilator.

S.D.M. #5. (AstraZeneca) Mannitol hexanitrate 7% in lactose. *Rx.*
Use: Vasodilator.

S.D.M. #40. (AstraZeneca) Isosorbide dinitrate 25% in lactose. *Rx.*
Use: Vasodilator.

S.D.M. #17. (AstraZeneca) Nitroglycerin 10% in lactose. *Rx.*
Use: Vasodilator.

S.D.M. #35. (AstraZeneca) Pentaerythritol tetranitrate 35% in mannitol. *Rx.*
Use: Vasodilator.

S.D.M. #37. (AstraZeneca) Nitroglycerin 10% in ethanol. *Rx.*
Use: Vasodilator.

S.D.M. #27. (AstraZeneca) Nitroglycerin 10% in propylene glycol. *Rx.*
Use: Vasodilator.

S.D.M. #23. (AstraZeneca) Pentaerythritol tetranitrate 20% in lactose. *Rx.*
Use: Vasodilator.

SDZ MSL-109. (Novartis)
Use: Antiparkinson. [Orphan Drug]

Sea & Ski Baby Lotion Formula. (Carter-Wallace) Octyl-dimethyl PABA. SPF 2. Lot. Bot. 120 mL. *OTC.*
Use: Sunscreen.

Sea & Ski Golden Tan. (Carter-Wallace) Padimate O. SPF 4. Lot. Bot. 120 mL. *OTC.*
Use: Sunscreen.

Sea Greens. (Modern Aids Inc.) Iodine 0.25 mg. Tab. Bot. 220s, 460s. *OTC.*

Sea Master. (Barth's) Vitamins A 10,000 units, D 400 units. Cap. Bot. 100s, 500s. *OTC.*
Use: Vitamin supplement.

Sea-Omega 50. (Rugby) Omega-3 polyunsaturated fatty acid 1000 mg. Cap. containing EPA 300 mg, DHA 200 mg, vitamin E 1 unit. Bot. 30s, 50s. *OTC.*
Use: Nutritional supplement.

Sea-Omega 30. (Rugby) N-3 fat content (mg) EPA 180, DHA 140. 100s. *OTC.*
Use: Nutritional supplement.

Seasonale. (Duramed) Levonorgestrel 0.15 mg, ethinyl estradiol 30 mcg. Lactose. Tab. 91s w/7 white inert tabs. *Rx.*
Use: Contraceptive hormone.

Seba-Lo. (Whorton Pharmaceuticals, Inc.) Acetone-alcohol cleanser. Bot. 4 oz. *OTC.*
Use: Skin cleanser.

Sebana. (Bristol-Myers Squibb) Salicylic acid 2%. Shampoo. Bot. 4 oz, 8 oz, pt, qt, 0.5 gal. *OTC.*
Use: Antiseborrheic.

Sebanatar. (Bristol-Myers Squibb) Salicylic acid 2%, liquor carbonis detergens 3%. Shampoo. Bot. 4 oz, 8 oz, pt,

qt, 0.5 gal, gal. *OTC.*
Use: Antiseborrheic.

Seba-Nil Cleansing Mask. (Galderma) Astringent face mask containing SD alcohol 40, sulfated castor oil, methylparaben. Tube 105 g. *OTC.*
Use: Dermatologic, acne.

Seba-Nil Liquid. (Galderma) Alcohol 49.7%, acetone, polysorbate 20. Liq. Bot. 240 mL, pt. *OTC.*
Use: Dermatologic, acne.

Seba-Nil Oily Skin Cleanser. (Galderma) SD alcohol, acetone. Liq. Bot. 240 mL, 473 mL. *OTC.*
Use: Dermatologic, acne.

Sebasorb. (Summers) Activated attapulgite 10%, salicylic acid 2%. Lot. Bot. 45 mL. *OTC.*
Use: Dermatologic, acne.

Sebulex with Conditioners. (Bristol-Myers Squibb) Sulfur 2%, salicylic acid 2%. Bot. 4 oz, 8 oz. *OTC.*
Use: Antiseborrheic.

• **secalciferol.** (seh-kal-SIFF-eh-ROLE) USAN.
Use: Regulator (calcium); treatment of familial hypophosphatemic rickets. [Orphan Drug]
See: Osteo-D.

• **seclazone.** (SEK-lah-zone) USAN.
Use: Anti-inflammatory; uricosuric.

• **secobarbital.** (see-koe-BAR-bih-tahl) *USP 28.*
Use: Hypnotic; sedative.

secobarbital combinations.
See: Efed.
Monosyl.

secobarbital elixir.
See: Seconal.

• **secobarbital sodium.** (see-koe-BAR-bih-tahl) *USP 28.*
Use: Hypnotic; sedative.

secobarbital sodium. (Wyeth) Secobarbital sodium 50 mg/mL. Inj. *Tubex* 2 mL. *c-II.*
Use: Hypnotic; sedative.

secobarbital sodium and amobarbital sodium capsules.
Use: Hypnotic; sedative.
See: Tuinal.

Seconal Sodium Pulvules. (Eli Lilly) Secobarbital sodium 100 mg. Cap. Bot. 100s, UD 100s. *c-II.*
Use: Hypnotic; sedative.

Secran. (Scherer) Vitamins B_1 10 mg, B_3 10 mg, B_{12} 25 mcg, alcohol 17%. Liq. Bot. 480 mL. *OTC.*
Use: Vitamin supplement.

SecreFlo. (RepliGen) Secretin 16 mcg. Mannitol 20 mg, L-cysteine 15 mg.

Pow. for Inj., lyophilized. Vials. *Rx.*
Use: Diagnostic aid, gastrointestinal
function test.
secretin.
Use: Diagnostic aid, gastrointestinal
function test.
See: SecreFlo.
Sectral. (ESP Pharma) Acebutolol hydrochloride 200 mg, 400 mg. Cap. Bot.
100s, *Redipak* 100s (200 mg only). *Rx.*
Use: Antiadrenergic/sympatholytic,
beta-adrenergic blocker.
sedaform.
See: Chlorobutanol.
Sedamine. (Health for Life Brands) Phos-
phorated carbohydrate soln. Bot. 4 oz.
OTC.
Use: Antinauseant.
Sedamine. (Oxypure) Hyoscyamine sul-
fate 0.1037 mg, atropine sulfate
0.0194 mg, hyoscine HBr 0.0065 mg,
phenobarbital 16.2 mg. Tab. Bot. 100s,
1000s. *Rx.*
Use: Antispasmodic; sedative.
Sedapap. (Merz) Acetaminophen
650 mg, butalbital 50 mg. Tab. Bot.
100s. *Rx.*
Use: Analgesic.
Sedapar. (Parmed Pharmaceuticals, Inc.)
Atropine sulfate 0.0195 mg, hyoscine
HBr 0.0065 mg, hyoscyamine sulfate
0.104 mg, phenobarbital 0.25 g. Tab.
Bot. 1000s. *Rx.*
Use: Antispasmodic; sedative.
sedative/hypnotic agents.
See: Barbiturates.
Bromides.
Butisol Sodium.
Carbamide (Urea) Compounds.
Chloral Hydrate.
Chlorobutanol.
Paraldehyde.
Phenergan hydrochloride.
Triazolam.
**sedative/hypnotic agents, nonbarbitu-
rate.**
See: Acetylcarbromal.
Benzodiazepines.
Chloral Hydrate.
Dexmedetomidine Hydrochloride.
Estazolam.
Eszopiclone.
Flurazepam Hydrochloride.
Glutethimide.
Imidazopyridines.
Paraldehyde.
Piperidine Derivatives.
Propiomazine Hydrochloride.
Pyrazolopyrimidine.
Quazepam.
Temazepam.
Tertiary Acetylenic Alcohols.
Triazolam.
Ureides.
Zaleplon.
Zolpidem Tartrate.
sedeval.
See: Barbital.
•**sedoxantrone trihydrochloride.** (sed-
OX-an-trone try-HIGH-droe-KLOR-ide)
USAN.
Use: Antineoplastic (DNA topoisomer-
ase II inhibitor).
Sedral. (Vita Elixir) Phenobarbital ⅛ g,
theophylline 2 g, ephedrine g. Tab. *Rx.*
Use: Bronchodilator; sedative.
•**seglitide acetate.** (SEH-glih-TIDE)
USAN.
Use: Antidiabetic.
selective cox-2 inhibitors.
Use: Anti-inflammatory; NSAID.
See: Celecoxib.
Rofecoxib.
Valdecoxib.
**selective estrogen receptor modu-
lator.**
Use: Sex hormone.
See: Raloxifene.
selective factor xa inhibitor.
Use: Anticoagulant.
See: Fondaparinux Sodium.
**selective serotonin reuptake inhibi-
tors.**
Use: Antidepressant.
See: Citalopram Hydrobromide.
Escitalopram Oxalate.
Fluoxetine Hydrochloride.
Fluvoxamine Maleate.
Paroxetine.
Sertraline Hydrochloride.
**selective vascular endothelial growth
factor antagonist.**
See: Pegaptanib Sodium.
•**selegiline hydrochloride.** (se-LE-ji-leen)
USAN.
Use: Antiparkinson agent.
See: Carbex.
Eldepryl.
selegiline hydrochloride. (Various Mfr.)
Selegiline hydrochloride 5 mg, lactose.
Tab. Bot. 60s, 500s. *Rx.*
Use: Antiparkinson agent.
Selenicel. (Taylor Pharmaceuticals) Sel-
enium yeast complex 200 mcg, vita-
mins C 100 mg, E 100 mg. Cap. Bot.
90s. *OTC.*
Use: Vitamin supplement.
•**selenious acid.** (seh-LEE-nee-us)
USP 28.
Use: Supplement (trace mineral).

selenium. (Nion Corp.) Selenium 50 mcg. Tab. Bot. 100s. *Rx.*
Use: Nutritional supplement, parenteral.

selenium disulfide.
See: Selenium Sulfide.

•**selenium sulfide.** (seh-LEE-nee-uhm SULL-fide) *USP 28.*
Use: Antidandruff; antifungal; antiseborrheic.
See: Head & Shoulders.
Selsun.

selenium sulfide. (Various Mfr.) Selenium sulfide. **Lot./Shampoo:** 1%. 210 mL. **Lot.:** 2.5%. 120 mL. *Rx-OTC.*
Use: Antidandruff; antiseborrheic.

•**selenomethionine Se 75.** (seh-LEE-no-meh-THIGH-oh-neen Se 75) USAN.
Use: Diagnostic aid (pancreas function determination), radiopharmaceutical.
See: Sethotope.

Sele-Pak. (SoloPak Pharmaceuticals, Inc.) Selenium 40 mcg/mL. Inj. Vial 10 mL, 30 mL. *Rx.*
Use: Nutritional supplement, parenteral.

Selepen. (American Pharmaceutical Partners) Selenium 40 mcg/mL. Vial 3 mL, 10 mL. *Rx.*
Use: Nutritional supplement, parenteral.

•**selfotel.** (SELL-fah-tell) USAN.
Use: NMDA antagonist.

•**selodenoson.** (sel-oh-DEN-oh-son) USAN.
Use: Cardiovascular agent.

Selora. (Sanofi-Synthelabo) Potassium Cl. Pow. *OTC.*
Use: Salt substitute.

Selsun. (Abbott) Selenium sulfide 2.5%. Lot. 120 mL. *Rx.*
Use: Antiseborrheic.

Selsun Blue Medicated Treatment. (Chattern) Selenium sulfide 1%. Menthol. Lot./Shampoo. 325 mL. *OTC.*
Use: Antiseborrheic.

•**sematilide hydrochloride.** (SEH-may-tih-LIDE) USAN.
Use: Cardiovascular agent (antiarrhythmic).

•**semaxanib.** (sem-AX-an-ib) USAN.
Use: Antineoplastic.

•**semduramicin.** (sem-DER-ah-MY-sin) USAN.
Use: Coccidiostat.

•**semduramicin sodium.** (sem-DER-ah-MY-sin) USAN.
Use: Coccidiostat.

Semicid. (Whitehall-Robins) Nonoxynol-9 100 mg. Vag. Supp. Box 9s, 18s. *OTC.*
Use: Contraceptive.

Semprex-D. (Celltech) Acrivastine 8 mg, pseudoephedrine hydrochloride 60 mg, lactose. Cap. Bot. 100s. *Rx.*
Use: Upper respiratory combination, decongestant, antihistimine.

•**semustine.** (SEH-muss-teen) USAN.
Use: Antineoplastic.

Senexon. (Rugby) Sennosides 8.6 mg, lactose. Tab. Bot. 100s, 1000s. *OTC.*
Use: Laxative.

Senilavite. (Defco) Vitamins A 5,000 units, C 100 mg, B$_1$ 2.5 mg, B$_2$ 2 mg, nicotinamide 10 mg, B$_6$ 1 mg, calcium pantothenate 5 mg, B$_{12}$ w/intrinsic factor concentrate 0.133 units, ferrous fumarate 150 mg, glutamic acid hydrochloride 150 mg, docusate sodium 50 mg. Cap. Bot. 100s. *OTC.*
Use: Nutritional supplement.

Senilezol. (Edwards) Vitamins B$_1$ 0.42 mg, B$_2$ 0.42 mg, B$_3$ 1.67 mg, B$_5$ 0.83 mg, B$_6$ 0.17 mg, B$_{12}$ 0.83 mcg, ferric pyrophosphate 3.3 mg/15 mL, alcohol 15%. Liq. Bot. 473 mL. *OTC.*
Use: Mineral, vitamin supplement.

•**senna.** (SEN-ah) *USP 28.*
Use: Laxative.

senna conc., standardized.
Use: Cathartic.
See: Senexon.
Senokot.
X-Prep.
W/Docusate sodium.
See: Gentlax S.
Senokap-DSS.
Senokot-S.
W/Guar gum.
See: Gentlax B.
W/Psyllium.
See: Perdiem.
Senokot W/Psyllium.

senna fruit extract, standarized.
Use: Cathartic.
See: Dosaflex.
Senokot.
X-Prep.

Senna-Gen. (Ivax) Sennosides 8.6 mg, lactose. Tab. Bot. 100s, 1000s. *OTC.*
Use: Laxative.

Senna Plus. (Contract Pharmacal) Docusate sodium 50 mg, senna concentrate (as sennosides) 8.6 mg. Tartrazine. Tab. 100s. *OTC.*
Use: Laxative.

•**sennosides.** (SEN-oh-sides) *USP 28.*
Use: Laxative.
See: Agoral.
Black Draught.
Evac-U-Gen.
ex-lax.
ex-lax chocolated.

Fletcher's Castoria.
Gentle Nature.
Lax-Pills.
Maximum Relief ex-lax.
Senexon.
Senna-Gen.
Senokot.
SenokotXTRA.
W/Docusate Sodium.
See: ex-lax Gentle Strength.
PeriColace.
Senna Plus.
Senokot. (Purdue) **Gran.:** Sennosides 15 mg/5 mL, sucrose. Can. 56 g, 170 g, 340 g. **Tab.:** Sennosides 8.6 mg, lactose. Bot. 10s, 20s, 50s, 100s, 1000s. UD 100s. **Syr.:** Sennosides 8.8 mg/5 mL, alcohol free, parabens, sucrose. Bot. 59 mL, 237 mL. *OTC.*
Use: Laxative.
Senokot-S. (Purdue) Docusate sodium 50 mg, senna concentrate 8.6 mg, lactose. Tab. Bot. 10s, 30s, 60s, 1000s, UD 100s. *OTC.*
Use: Laxative.
Senokot Suppositories. (Purdue) Standardized senna concentrate. Supp. Pkg. 6s. *OTC.*
Use: Laxative.
SenokotXTRA. (Purdue) Sennosides 17 mg, lactose. Tab. Bot. 12s, 36s. *OTC.*
Use: Laxative.
Sensipar. (Amgen) Cinacalcet hydrochloride (as base) 30 mg, 60 mg, 90 mg. Film-coated. Tab. 30s. *Rx.*
Use: Calcium receptor agonist.
Sensitive Eyes. (Bausch & Lomb) Sorbic acid 0.1%, EDTA 0.025%, NaCl, boric acid, sodium borate. Soln. Bot. 118 mL, 237 mL, 355 mL. *OTC.*
Use: Contact lens care.
Sensitive Eyes Daily Cleaner. (Bausch & Lomb) Sorbic acid 0.25%, EDTA 0.5%, NaCl, hydroxypropyl methylcellulose, poloxamine, sodium borate. Soln. Bot. 20 mL. *OTC.*
Use: Contact lens care.
Sensitive Eyes Drops. (Bausch & Lomb) Isotonic solution, sorbic acid 0.1%, EDTA 0.025%, NaCl, boric acid, sodium borate. Soln. Bot. 30 mL. *OTC.*
Use: Contact lens care.
Sensitive Eyes Plus. (Bausch & Lomb) Boric acid, sodium borate, KCl, NaCl, polyaminopropyl biguanide 0.00003%, EDTA 0.025%. Soln. Bot. 118 mL, 355 mL. *OTC.*
Use: Contact lens care.
Sensitive Eyes Saline. (Bausch & Lomb) NaCl, borate buffer, sorbic acid 0.1%,

EDTA. Soln. Bot. 118 mL, 237 mL, 355 mL. *OTC.*
Use: Contact lens care.
Sensitive Eyes Saline/Cleaning Solution. (Bausch & Lomb) Isotonic solution w/borate buffer, NaCl, poloxamine, sorbic acid 0.15%, sodium borate, boric acid, EDTA 0.1%. Soln. Bot. 237 mL. *OTC.*
Use: Contact lens care.
Sensodyne Fresh Mint Toothpaste. (Block Drug) Potassium nitrate 5%, sodium monofluorophosphate 0.76%, saccharin, sorbitol, mint flavor. Tube 2.4 oz, 4.6 oz. *OTC.*
Use: Dentrifice.
Sensodyne-SC Toothpaste. (Block Drug) Glycerin, sorbitol, sodium methylcocoyl taurate, PEG-40 stearate, strontium Cl hexahydrate 10%, methyl- and propylparabens. Tinted. Tube 2.1 oz, 4.0 oz. *OTC.*
Use: Dentrifice.
SensoGARD. (Block Drug) Benzocaine 20%, parabens. Gel. Tube 9.4 g. *OTC.*
Use: Anesthetic, local.
Sensorcaine. (AstraZeneca) Bupivacaine hydrochloride 0.25% or 0.5%. Bupivacaine hydrochloride 0.25% or 0.5%, epinephrine 1:200,000, methylparaben 1 mg/mL. Inj. Multidose vial 50 mL. *Rx.*
Use: Anesthetic, local amide.
Sensorcaine MPF. (AstraZeneca) Bupivacaine hydrochloride 0.25%, 0.5%, 0.75%. Inj. Single-dose amp. 30 mL (except 0.5%). Single-dose vials 10 mL, 30 mL. Bupivaccaine hydrochloride 0.25% or 0.5%, epinephrine 1:200,000. Inj. Single-dose amp. 5 mL (0.5% only). Single-dose vials 10 mL, 30 mL. *Rx.*
Use: Anesthetic, local amide.
Sensorcaine-MPF Spinal. (AstraZeneca) Bupivacaine hydrochloride 0.75%, dextrose 8.25%. Inj. Amp. 2 mL. *Rx.*
Use: Anesthetic, local amide.
• **sepazonium chloride.** (SEP-ah-ZOE-nee-uhm) USAN.
Use: Anti-infective, topical.
• **seperidol hydrochloride.** (seh-PURR-ih-dahl) USAN.
Use: Neuroleptic; antipsychotic.
• **seprilose.** (SEH-prih-LOHS) USAN.
Use: Antirheumatic.
• **seproxetine hydrochloride.** (sep-ROX-eh-teen) USAN.
Use: Antidepressant.
Septi-Chek. (Roche) Blood culture and simultaneous sub-culture system with

three media to support clinically significant pathogens. Quick and easy assembly forms a closed system to protect sub-cultures from contamination. *Use:* Diagnostic aid.

Septiphene. (SEP-tih-feen) (Monsanto) *Use:* Disinfectant.

Septi-Soft. (GlaxoSmithKline) Hexachlorophene 0.25%. Liq. Bot. 240 mL, pt, gal. *OTC.* *Use:* Antimicrobial; antiseptic.

Septisol. (GlaxoSmithKline) **Soln.:** Hexachlorophene 0.25%. Bot. 240 mL, qt, gal. **Foam:** Hexachlorophene 0.23%, alcohol 46%. In 180 mL, 600 mL. *OTC.* *Use:* Antimicrobial; antiseptic.

Septo. (Vita Elixir) Methylbenzethonium Cl, ethanol 2%, menthol. *OTC.* *Use:* Antimicrobial; antiseptic.

Septocaine. (Septodont) Articaine hydrochloride 4%, epinephrine 1:100,000, sodium metabisulfite 0.5 mg/mL, sodium chloride 1.6 mg/mL. Inj. Cartridge. 1.7 mL. Boxes and cans 50s. *Rx.* *Use:* Anesthetic, local amide.

Septra. (Monarch) Sulfamethoxazole 400 mg, trimethoprim 80 mg. Tab. Bot. 100s. *Rx.* *Use:* Anti-infective.

Septra DS. (Monarch) Trimethoprim 160 mg, sulfamethoxazole 800 mg. Tab. Bot. 100s, 250s, UD 100s. *Rx.* *Use:* Anti-infective.

Septra Grape Suspension. (GlaxoSmithKline) Trimethoprim 40 mg, sulfamethoxazole 200 mg/5 mL. Bot. 473 mL. *Rx.* *Use:* Anti-infective.

Septra I.V. (Monarch) Trimethoprim 80 mg, sulfamethoxazole 400 mg/5 mL. Amp. 5 mL, Vial 10 mL, 20 mL, multidose vials 20 mL. *Rx.* *Use:* Anti-infective.

Septra Suspension. (GlaxoSmithKline) Trimethoprim 40 mg, sulfamethoxazole 200 mg/5 mL. Bot. 20 mL, 100 mL, 150 mL, 200 mL, 473 mL. *Rx.* *Use:* Anti-infective.

• **seractide acetate.** (seer-ACK-tide) USAN. *Use:* Corticotrophic peptide, hormone (adrenocorticotrophic).

Ser-A-Gen. (Ivax) Hydrochlorothiazide 15 mg, reserpine 0.1 mg, hydralazine hydrochloride 25 mg. Tab. Bot. 100s, 1000s. *Rx.* *Use:* Antihypertensive combination.

Seralyzer. (Bayer Corp. (Consumer Div.)) A system for the measurement of enzymes, potassium levels, blood chemistries, and therapeutic drug assays consisting of a reflectance photometer and a series of solid-phase reagent strips. *Use:* Diagnostic aid.

Ser-Ap-Es. (Novartis) Reserpine 0.1 mg, hydralazine hydrochloride 25 mg, hydrochlorothiazide 15 mg. Tab. Bot. 100s, 1000s. *Rx.* *Use:* Antihypertensive combination.

• **seratrodast.** (seh-RAH-troe-dast) USAN. *Use:* Anti-inflammatory (non-antihistaminic); antiasthmatic (thromboxane receptor antagonist).

Serax. (Alpharma) Oxazepam. **Cap.:** 10 mg, 15 mg, 30 mg. Lactose. Bot. 100s. **Tab.:** 15 mg. Lactose. Bot. 100s. *c-IV.* *Use:* Anxiolytic.

• **serazapine hydrochloride.** (ser-AZE-ah-PEEN) USAN. *Use:* Anxiolytic.

Sereen. (Foy Laboratories) Chlordiazepoxide hydrochloride 10 mg. Cap. Bot. 500s, 1000s. *c-IV.* *Use:* Anxiolytic.

Sereine Cleaning Solution. (Optikem) Cocoamphodiacetate and glycols, EDTA 0.1%, benzalkonium Cl 0.01%. Soln. Bot. 60 mL. *OTC.* *Use:* Contact lens care.

Sereine Wetting/Soaking Solution. (Optikem) EDTA 0.1%, benzalkonium Cl 0.01%. Soln. Bot. 120 mL. *OTC.* *Use:* Contact lens care, soaking, wetting.

Sereine Wetting Solution. (Optikem) EDTA 0.1%, benzalkonium chloride 0.01%. Soln. Bot. 60 mL, 120 mL. *OTC.* *Use:* Contact lens care.

Serene. (Health for Life Brands) Salicylamide 2 g, scopolamine aminoxide HBr 0.2 mg. Cap. Bot. 24s, 60s. *Rx.* *Use:* Analgesic; sedative.

Serevent Diskus. (GlaxoSmithKline) Salmeterol xinafoate 50 mcg, lactose. Pow. for Inh. Blisters 28s, 60s. *Rx.* *Use:* Bronchodilator, sympathomimetic.

• **sergolexole maleate.** (SER-go-LEX-ole) USAN. *Use:* Antimigraine.

sericinase. A proteolytic enzyme.

• **serine.** (SER-een) *USP 28.* *Use:* Amino acid.

• **sermetacin.** (ser-MET-ah-sin) USAN. *Use:* Anti-inflammatory.

• **sermorelin acetate.** (SER-moe-REH-lin) USAN. *Use:* Growth hormone-releasing factor, diagnostic aid. [Orphan Drug]

Seromycin Pulvules. (Dura) Cycloserine 250 mg. Cap. Bot. 40s. *Rx.*

Use: Antituberculosal.

Serophene. (Serono) Clomiphene citrate 50 mg. Tab. Bot. 10s, 30s. *Rx.*
Use: Ovulation inducer; sex hormone.

Seroquel. (AstraZeneca) Quetiapine fumarate 25 mg, 100 mg, 200 mg, 300 mg, lactose. Tab. Bot. 60s (300 mg only), 100s (except 300 mg), UD 100s. *Rx.*
Use: Antipsychotic, dibenzapine derivative.

Serostim. (Serono) Somatropin 4 mg (≈ 12 units/vial), 5 mg (≈ 15 units/Vial), 6 mg (≈ 18 units/mL). Sucrose. Pow. for Injection, lyophilized. Single-use vial w/diluent. **8.8 mg:** ≈ 26.4 units/vial. Sucrose 60.2 mg and water for injection with metacresol 0.3%. In prefilled *one.click* auto-injector pen used with *ulluk.uuky* reconstitution device. *Rx.*
Use: Hormone, growth.

Serostim LQ. (Serono) Somatropin 6 mg (≈ 18 units) per 0.5 mL. Poloxamer 188 1.02 mg, sucrose 40.8 mg, citric acid 1.31 mg. Inj. Cartridges (1s or 7s). *Rx.*
Use: Growth hormone.

• **serotonin and norepinephrine reuptake inhibitors.**
Use: Antidepressant.
See: Cymbalta.

serotonin 5-ht₁ receptor agonists.
Use: Antimigraine.
See: Almotriptan Malate.
Eletriptan HBr.
Frovatriptan Succinate.
Naratriptan hydrochloride.
Rizatriptan Benzoate.
Sumatriptan Succinate.
Zolmitriptan.

serotonin reuptake inhibitors, selective.
Use: Antidepressant.
See: Paxil.
Prozac.
Zoloft.

Serpasil-Apresoline. (Novartis) **#1:** Reserpine 0.1 mg, hydralazine hydrochloride 25 mg. Tab. Bot. 100s. **#2:** Reserpine 0.2 mg, hydralazine hydrochloride 50 mg. Tab. Bot. 100s. *Rx.*
Use: Antihypertensive combination.

Serpasil-Esidrix. (Novartis) **#1:** Reserpine 0.1 mg, hydrochlorothiazide 25 mg. Tab. **#2:** Reserpine 0.1 mg, hydrochlorothiazide 50 mg. Tab. Bot. 100s, 1000s. *Rx.*
Use: Antihypertensive combination.

Serpazide. (Major) Reserpine 0.1 mg, hydralazine hydrochloride 25 mg, hydrochlorothiazide 15 mg. Tab. Bot. 100s, 1000s. *Rx.*

Use: Antihypertensive combination.

serratia marcescens extract (polyribosomes).
Use: Primary brain malignancies. [Orphan Drug]

Sertabs. (Table Rock) Reserpine 0.25 mg, 0.5 mg. Tab. Bot. 100s, 500s. *Rx.*
Use: Antihypertensive.

sertaconazole nitrate. (SIR-tah-KAHN-uh-zole)
Use: Antifungal.
See: Ertaczo.

Sertina. (Fellows) Reserpine 0.25 mg. Tab. Bot. 1000s, 5000s. *Rx.*
Use: Antihypertensive.

• **sertindole.** (ser-TIN-dole) USAN.
Use: Antipsychotic.

• **sertraline hydrochloride.** (SIR-truh-leen) USAN.
Use: Antidepressant, SSRI.
See: Zoloft.

serum, albumin, human, radioiodinated.
See: Albumin Injection.

serum, albumin, normal human.
See: Albumin Human.

serum, globulin (human), immune.
Use: Immunization.

Serutan. (GlaxoSmithKline) Psyllium 2.5 g, sodium < 0.03 g/heaping tsp, saccharin, sugar. Gran. Can. 170 g, 540 g. *OTC.*
Use: Laxative.

• **sesame oil.** *NF 23.*
Use: Pharmaceutic aid (solvent; vehicle, oleaginous).

Sesame Street Complete. (McNeil Consumer) Ca 80 mg, Fe 10 mg, vitamins A 2750 units, D 200 units, E 10 mg, B₁ 0.75 mg, B₂ 0.85 mg, B₃ 10 mg, B₅ 5 mg, B₆ 0.7 mg, B₁₂ 3 mcg, C 40 mg, folic acid 0.2 mg, biotin 15 mg, Cu, I, Mg, Zn 8 mg, lactose. Tab. Bot. 50s. *OTC.*
Use: Mineral, vitamin supplement.

Sesame Street Plus Iron. (McNeil Consumer) Fe 10 mg, vitamins A 2750 units, D 200 units, E 10 mg, B₁ 0.75 mg, B₂ 0.85 mg, B₃ 10 mg, B₅ 5 mg, B₆ 0.7 mg, B₁₂ 3 mcg, C 40 mg, folic acid 0.2 mg. Chew. Tab. Bot. 50s. *OTC.*
Use: Mineral, vitamin supplement.

Sesame Street Vitamins. (McNeil Consumer) **For ages 4 and older:** Vitamins A 5,000 units, B₁ 1.5 mg, B₁₂ 6 mcg, C 60 mg, D 400 units, E 30 units, folic acid 400 mcg, biotin 300 mcg. Chew. Tab. Bot. 60s. **For**

ages 2 to 3: Vitamins A 2,500 units, B_1 0.7 mg, B_2 0.8 mg, B_3 9 mg, B_5 5 mg, B_6 0.7 mg, B_{12} 3 mcg, C 40 mg, D 400 units, E 10 units, folic acid 200 mcg, biotin 150 mcg. Chew. Tab. Bot. 60s. *OTC.*
Use: Vitamin supplement.

Sesame Street Vitamins and Minerals. (McNeil Consumer) **For ages 4 and older:** Vitamins A 5,000 units, B_1 1.5 mg, B_2 1.7 mg, B_3 20 mg, B_5 10 mg, B_6 2 mg, B_{12} 6 mcg, C 60 mg, D 400 units, E 30 units, folic acid 400 mcg, biotin 300 mcg, Ca 100 mg, Fe 18 mg, I 150 mcg, Zn 15 mg, Cu 2 mg. Chew. Tab. Bot. 60s. **For ages 2 to 3:** Vitamins A 2,500 units, B_1 0.7 mg, B_{12} 3 mcg, C 40 mg, D 400 units, E 10 units, folic acid 200 mcg, biotin 150 mcg, Ca 80 mg, Fe 10 mg, I 70 mcg, Zn 8 mg, Cu 1 mg. Chew. Tab. Bot. 60s. *OTC.*
Use: Mineral, vitamin supplement.

Sethotope. (Bristol-Myers Squibb) Selenomethionine selenium 75; available as 0.25, 1 mCi.

•**setoperone.** (SEE-toe-per-OHN) USAN.
Use: Antipsychotic.

•**sevelamer hydrochloride.** (seh-VELL-ah-mer) USAN.
Use: Antihyperphosphatemic, control of hyperphosphatemia in end-stage renal disease (phosphate binder).
See: Renagel.

Severe Congestion Tussin. (AmerisourceBergen) Pseudoephedrine hydrochloride 30 mg, guaifenesin 200 mg, sorbitol. Softgel. Pkg. 12s. *OTC.*
Use: Upper respiratory combination, decongestant, expectorant.

•**sevirumab.** (seh-VIE-roo-mab) USAN.
Use: Monoclonal antibody (antiviral).

•**sevoflurane.** (SEE-voe-FLEW-rane) USAN.
Use: Anesthetic, general, volatile liquid.
See: Ultane.

sex hormones.
See: Abarelix.
Anabolic Steroids.
Androgen Hormone Inhibitor.
Androgens.
Biphasic Oral Contraceptives.
Cetrorelix Acetate.
Choriogonadotropin Alfa.
Chorionic Gonadotropin.
Clomiphene Citrate.
Contraceptive Hormones.
Danazol.
Dutasteride.
Emergency Contraceptives.

Esterified Estrogens.
Estradiol.
Estradiol Cypionate in Oil.
Estradiol Topical Emulsion.
Estradiol Transdermal System.
Estradiol Valerate in Oil.
Estrogen and Androgen Combinations.
Estrogens.
Estrogens and Progestins Combined.
Estrogens, Conjugated.
Estrogens, Miscellaneous Topical.
Estrogens, Miscellaneous Vaginal.
Estrogens, Synthetic Conjugated.
Estropipate.
Etonogestrel/Ethinyl Estradiol.
Finasteride.
Fluoxymesterone.
Follitropin Alfa.
Follitropin Beta.
Gonadorelin Acetate.
Gonadotropin-Releasing Hormone Antagonists.
Gonadotropin-Releasing Hormones.
Gonadotropins.
Intrauterine Progesterone Contraceptive System.
Levonorgestrel Implants.
Levonorgestrel-Releasing Intrauterine System.
Lutropin Alfa.
Medroxyprogesterone Acetate.
Medroxyprogesterone Acetate/Estradiol Cypionate.
Medroxyprogesterone Contraceptive Injection.
Megestrol Acetate.
Menotropins.
Methyltestosterone.
Monophasic Oral Contraceptives.
Nafarelin Acetate.
Nandrolone Decanoate.
Norelgestromine/Ethinyl Estradiol Transdermal System.
Norethindrone Acetate.
Oxandrolone.
Oxymetholone.
Ovulation Stimulants.
Progesterone.
Progestin-only Products.
Progestins.
Raloxifene.
Selective Estrogen Receptor Modulator.
Testosterone.
Testosterone Cypionate.
Testosterone Enanthate.
Triphasic Oral Contraceptives.
Urofollitropin.

•**sezolamide hydrochloride.** (seh-ZOLE-ah-MIDE) USAN.

Use: Carbonic anhydrase inhibitor.

SFC. USAN. (Stiefel) Soap free. Stearyl alcohol, PEG-75, sodium cocoyl isethionate, parabens. Lot. Bot. 237 mL, 480 mL. OTC.
Use: Dermatologic, cleanser.

Shade. (Schering-Plough) SPF 15. Contains one or more of the following ingredients: Padimate O, oxybenzone, ethylhexyl-p-methoxycinnamate. Bot. 118 mL, 120 mL, 240 mL. OTC.
Use: Sunscreen.

Shade Cream. (O'Leary) Jar 0.25 oz. OTC.
Use: Contouring cream.

Shade Sunblock Gel, 15 SPF. (Schering-Plough) Ethylhexyl p-methoxycinnamate, octyl salicylate, oxybenzone, SD alcohol 40. PABA free. SPF 15. Waterproof. Gel. Bot. 120 mL. OTC.
Use: Sunscreen.

Shade Sunblock Gel, 30 SPF. (Schering-Plough) Ethylhexyl p-methoxycinnamate, homosalate, oxybenzone, 73% SD alcohol 40. Bot. 120 mL. OTC.
Use: Sunscreen.

Shade Sunblock Gel, 25 SPF. (Schering-Plough) Ethylhexyl p-methoxycinnamate, octyl salicylate, homosalate, oxybenzone, SD alcohol 40. PABA free. Gel. Bot. 120 mL. OTC.
Use: Sunscreen.

Shade Sunblock Lotion, 15 SPF. (Schering Plough) Ethylhexyl p-methoxycinnamate, oxybenzone, benzyl alcohol, phenethyl alcohol. PABA free. Waterproof. Lot. Bot. 120 mL. OTC.
Use: Sunscreen.

Shade Sunblock Lotion, 45 SPF. (Schering-Plough) Ethylhexyl p-methoxycinnamate, oxybenzone, 2-ethylhexyl salicylate, benzyl alcohol, phenethyl alcohol. PABA free. Waterproof. Lot. Bot. 120 mL. OTC.
Use: Sunscreen.

Shade Sunblock Lotion, 30 SPF. (Schering-Plough) Ethylhexyl p-methoxycinnamate, 2-ethylhexyl salicylate, homosalate, oxybenzone, benzyl alcohol, phenethyl alcohol. PABA free. Waterproof. Lot. Bot. 120 mL. OTC.
Use: Sunscreen.

Shade Sunblock Stick, 30 SPF. (Schering-Plough) Ethylhexyl p-methoxycinnamate, oxybenzone, 2-ethylhexyl salicylate, homosalate. PABA free. Waterproof. Stick. 18 g. OTC.
Use: Sunscreen.

Shade UvaGuard. (Schering-Plough) Octyl methoxycinnamate 7.5%, avobenzone 3%, oxybenzone 3%. Waterproof. SPF 15. Lot. 120 mL. OTC.
Use: Sunscreen.

Sheik Elite. (Durex) Condom with nonoxynol-9 15%. 3s, 12s, 24s, 36s. OTC.
Use: Contraceptive.

•**shellac.** NF 23.
Use: Pharmaceutic aid (tablet coating agent).

Shellgel. (Cytosol Ophthalmics) Sodium hyaluronate 12 mg/mL, sodium chloride 9 mg/mL. Inj. Disposable syringes. 0.8 mL. Rx.
Use: Ophthalmic surgical adjunct.

Shepard's Cream Lotion. (Dermik) Creamy lotion with no lanolin or mineral oil, for entire body. Scented or unscented. Bot. 8 oz, 16 oz. OTC.
Use: Emollient.

Sherbul. (Sheryl) Phenylephrine hydrochloride, pyrilamine maleate. Tab. Bot. 100s. Liq. Bot. Pt.
Use: Decongestant; antihistamine.

Shernatal. (Sheryl) Phosphorus free calcium, non-irritating iron, trace minerals and essential vitamins. Tab. Bot. 100s. OTC.
Use: Mineral, vitamin supplement.

•**Shohl's Solution.** USP 28. Sodium Citrate and Citric Acid. Oral Soln.
Use: Alkalizer, systemic.

short chain fatty acid solution.
Use: Ulcerative colitis. [Orphan Drug]

Shur-Clens. (GlaxoSmithKline) Poloxamer 188 20%. Soln. Bot. UD 100 mL, 200 mL. OTC.
Use: Dermatologic.

Shur Seal Gel. (Milex) Nonoxynol-9 2. 24 UD gel paks. OTC.
Use: Contraceptive, spermicide.

Sibelium. (Janssen) Flunarizine hydrochloride. Rx.
Use: Vasodilator.

•**sibenadet hydrochloride.** (si-BEN-a-det) USAN.
Use: Chronic obstructive pulmonary disease.

•**sibopirdine.** (sih-BOE-pihr-deen) USAN.
Use: Nootropic; cognition enhancer (Alzheimer disease).

•**sibrafran.** (sib-rah-FIE-ban) USAN.
Use: Antithrombotic; fibrinogen receptor antagonist; platelet aggregation inhibitor.

•**sibutramine hydrochloride.** (sih-BYOO-trah-meen) USAN.
Use: Antidepressant, CNS stimulant, anorexic.
See: Meridia.

sickle cell test.
Use: Diagnostic aid.

See: Sickledex.

Sickledex. (Ortho-Clinical Diagnostics) Test kit 12s, 100s.
Use: Diagnostic aid to detect hemoglobin S.

Sigamine. (Sigma-Tau) Cyanocobalamin injection 1000 mcg/mL. Vial 10 mL, 30 mL. Also Sigamine L.A. Vial 10 mL. *Rx.*
Use: Vitamin supplement.

Sigazine. (Sigma-Tau) Promethazine hydrochloride 50 mg/mL. Vial 10 mL. *Rx.*
Use: Antihistamine.

Signa Creme. (Parker) Conductive cosmetic quality electrolyte cream. Bot. 5 oz, 2 L, 4 L. *OTC.*
Use: Diagnostic aid.

Signa Gel. (Parker) Conductive saline electrode gel. Tube 250 g.
Use: Diagnostic aid, gel.

Signa Pad. (Parker) Premoistened electrode pads.
Use: Diagnostic aid, pad.

Signatal C. (Sigma-Tau) Ca 230 mg, Fe 49.3 mg, vitamins A 4,000 units, D 400 units, B_1 2 mg, B_2 2 mg, B_6 1 mg, B_{12} 2 mcg, folic acid 0.1 mg, niacinamide 10 mg, C 50 mg, I 0.15 mg. SC Tab. Bot. 100s, 1000s. *OTC.*
Use: Mineral, vitamin supplement.

Signate. (Sigma-Tau) Dimenhydrinate 50 mg, propylene glycol 50%, benzyl alcohol 5%/mL. Vial 10 mL. *Rx.*
Use: Antiemetic; antivertigo.

Signef "Supps". (Fellows) Hydrocortisone 15 mg. Supp. 12s. w or w/o applicator. *Rx.*
Use: Corticosteroid, vaginal.

Sigpred. (Sigma-Tau) Prednisolone acetate. Vial 10 mL. *Rx.*
Use: Corticosteroid.

Sigtab. (Roberts) Vitamins A 5,000 units, D 400 units, B_1 10.3 mg, B_2 10 mg, C 333 mg, B_3 100 mg, B_6 6 mg, B_5 20 mg, folic acid 0.4 mg, B_{12} 18 mcg, E 15 mg. Tab. Bot. 90s, 500s. *OTC.*
Use: Vitamin supplement.

Sigtab-M. (Roberts) Vitamins A 6000 units, D_3 400 units, E 45 mg, C 100 mg, B_3 25 mg, B_1 5 mg, B_2 5 mg, B_6 3 mg, folic acid 400 mcg, B_5 0.015 mg, biotin 45 mcg, Ca 200 mg, P, Fe 18 mg, Mg, Cu, Zn 15 mg, Mn, K, Cl, Mo, Se, Cr, Ni, Sn, V, Si, B, vitamin K, I. Tab. Bot. 100s. *OTC.*
Use: Mineral, vitamin supplement.

Silace. (Silarx) Docusate sodium 60 mg/15 mL, alcohol ≤ 1%. Syr. Bot. 473 mL. *OTC.*
Use: Laxative.

Siladryl. (Silarx) Diphenhydramine hydrochloride 12.5 mg/5 mL, alcohol 5.6%, cherry flavor. Elix. Bot. 118 mL. *OTC.*
Use: Antihistamine, nonselective ethanolamine.

Silafed. (Silarx) Pseudoephedrine hydrochloride 30 mg, triprolidine hydrochloride 1.25 mg/5 mL, methylparaben, sucrose, saccharin. Syr. Bot. 118 mL, 237 mL. *OTC.*
Use: Upper respiratory combination, antihistamine, decongestant.

• **silafilcon a.** (SIH-lah-FILL-kahn A) USAN.
Use: Contact lens material (hydrophilic).

• **silafocon a.** (SIH-lah-FOH-kahn A) USAN.
Use: Contact lens material (hydrophobic).

• **silandrone.** (sil-AN-drone) USAN.
Use: Androgen.

Sildec-DM. (Silarx) **Drops, Pediatric:** Carbinoxamine maleate 2 mg, pseudoephedrine hydrochloride 15 mg, dextromethorphan HBr 4 mg/mL, saccharin, sorbitol, grape flavor, alcohol free. Bot. 30 mL w/dropper. **Syr.:** Pseudoephedrine hydrochloride 60 mg, dextromethorphan HBr 15 mg, brompheniramine maleate 4 mg/5 mL, saccharin, sorbitol, grape flavor, alcohol free. Bot. 473 mL. *Rx.*
Use: Upper respiratory combination, antihistamine, antitussive, decongestant.

• **sildenafil citrate.** (sill-DEN-ah-fil SIH-trate) USAN.
Use: Anti-impotence agent.
See: Viagra.

Silfedrine, Children's. (Silarx) Pseudoephedrine hydrochloride 30 mg/5 mL, methylparaben, saccharin, sucrose. Liq. Bot. 118 mL, 237 mL. *OTC.*
Use: Nasal decongestant, arylalkylamine.

• **silica, dental-type.** (SILL-ih-kah) *NF 23.*
Use: Pharmaceutic aid.

• **siliceous earth, purified.** (sih-LIH-shus) *NF 23.*
Use: Pharmaceutic aid (filtering medium).

• **silicon dioxide.** (SILL-ih-kahn die-OX-ide) *NF 23. Formerly Silica Gel.*
Use: Pharmaceutic aid (dispersing and suspending agent).

• **silicon dioxide, colloidal.** *NF 23.*
Use: Pharmaceutic aid (tablet/capsule diluent, suspending and thickening agent).

Silicone. (Dow Hickam) Dimethicone. Liq., Bot. oz. Bulk Pkg. Oint. W/Nitro-Cellulose, castor oil.
See: Allergex.
silicone oil.
See: Polydimethylsiloxane.
Silicone oil.
silicone ointment. Dimethicone Dimethyl Polysiloxane.
Silicone Ointment No. 2. (C & M Pharmacal) High viscosity silicone 10% in a blend of petrolatum and hydrophobic starch. Jar 2 oz, lb. *OTC.*
Use: Protective agent.
Silicone Powder. (Gordon Laboratories) Talc with silicone. Pkg. 4 oz, 1 lb, 5 lb. *OTC.*
Use: Dusting powder.
•**silodrate.** (SILL-oh-drate) USAN.
Uoo; Arilucid.
Silphen Cough. (Silarx) Diphenhydramine hydrochloride 12.5 mg/5 mL, alcohol 5%, menthol, sucrose, parabens, strawberry flavor. Syr. Bot. 118 mL. *OTC.*
Use: Antihistamine.
Silphen DM. (Silarx) Dextromethorphan HBr 10 mg/5 mL, alcohol 5%, menthol, methylparaben, sucrose. Syr. Bot. 118 mL. *OTC.*
Use: Antitussive.
Siltussin DAS. (Silarx) Guaifenesin 100 mg/5 mL. Strawberry flavor. Liq. 118 mL. *OTC.*
Use: Expectorant.
Siltussin DM. (Silarx) Dextromethorphan HBr 10 mg, guaifenesin 100 mg/5 mL, saccharin, sucrose, methylparaben, alcohol free. Syr. Bot. 118 mL. *OTC.*
Use: Upper respiratory combination, antitussive, expectorant.
Siltussin SA. (Silarx) Guaifenesin 100 mg/5 mL, strawberry flavor. Liq. 118 mL, 237 mL, 473 mL. *OTC.*
Use: Expectorant.
Silvadene. (Hoechst) Silver sulfadiazine (10 mg/g) 1%, base w/white petrolatum, stearyl alcohol, isopropyl myristate, sorbitan monooleate, polyoxyl 40 stearate, propylene glycol, methylparaben. Cream. Jar 50 g, 85 g, 400 g, 1000 g. Tube 20 g. *Rx.*
Use: Antimicrobial, topical.
silver compounds.
See: Silver Iodide, Colloidal.
Silver Nitrate.
Silver Protein, Mild.
Silver Protein, Strong.
•**silver nitrate.** (SILL-ver NYE-trate) *USP 28.*
Use: Anti-infective, topical.

W/Combinations
See: Arzol Silver Nitrate Applicators.
silver nitrate ointment. (Gordon Laboratories) Silver nitrate 1% in ointment base. Jar oz. *Rx.*
Use: Astringent; epithelial stimulant.
silver nitrate ophthalmic solution. Silver nitrate. Soln. 10%, 25%, 50%. Bot. oz. (Gordon Laboratories) Amp 1%, 100s (Eli Lilly and Co.) Cap 1%, 100s (Parke-Davis). *Rx.*
Use: Astringent; anti-infective.
silver nitrate topical sticks. (Graham Field) Silver nitrate, potassium nitrate 25%. Appl. 100s. *Rx.*
Use: Cauterizing agent.
•**silver nitrate, toughened.** (SILL-ver NYE-trate) *USP 28.*
Use: Caustic.
silver protein, mild. Argentum Vitellinum, Cargentos, Mucleinate Mild, Protargin Mild.
silver protein, strong.
See: Protargol.
silver sulfadiazine. (SILL-ver SULL-fah-DIE-ah-zeen)
Use: Anti-infective, topical.
See: Silvadene.
SSD.
SSD AF.
Thermazene.
•**simethicone.** (sih-METH-ih-cone) *USP 28.* Mixture of liquid dimethyl polysiloxanes with silica aerogel.
Use: Antiflatulent.
See: Degas.
Gas Relief.
Gas-X Extra Strength.
Maalox Anti-Gas.
Maalox Extra Strength Anti-Gas.
Mylanta.
Mylicon.
Mylicon-80.
Phazyme.
W/Combinations.
See: Di-Gel.
Gas-Ban.
Gas-X with Maalox.
Laxsil.
Maalox Anti-Gas Extra Strength.
Maalox Plus.
Mylanta, Mylanta II.
Phazyme.
Phazyme-95.
Rolaids Multi-Symptom.
Sidonna.
Trial AG.
simethicone-coated cellulose suspension.
Use: Diagnostic aid, gastrointestinal function test.

See: SonoRx.

Similac Human Milk Fortifier. (Ross) Protein (nonfat milk, whey protein concentrate) 1 g, carbohydrate (corn syrup solids) 1.8 g, fat (fractionated coconut oil [medium chain triglycerides], soy lecithin) 0.36 g per 4 packets (3.6 g), with vitamins A, B_1, B_2, B_3, B_5, B_6, B_{12}, C, D, E, K, folic acid (folacin), biotin, Ca, chloride, Cu, Fe, Mg, Mn, P, Zn, Na 15 mg, K 63 mg, 14 cal/3.6 g. Add to breast milk. Pow. Pkt. 0.9 g (50s). *OTC.*
Use: Enteral nutritional therapy.

Similac Low-Iron Liquid & Powder. (Ross) Protein 14.3 g, carbohydrates 72 g, fat 36 g, Fe 1.5 mg, with appropriate vitamins and minerals. **Liq.:** 390 mL concentrate, 240 mL and 1 qt. ready-to-use, 120 mL and 240 mL nursettes. **Pow.:** 1 lb. *OTC.*
Use: Nutritional supplement.

Similac Natural Care Human Milk Fortifier. (Ross) Liquid fortifier designed to be mixed with human milk or fed alternately with human milk to low-birthweight infants. Supplied as 24 Cal/fl oz. Bot. 4 fl oz. *OTC.*
Use: Nutritional supplement.

Similac PM 60/40. (Ross) Milk-based formula ready-to-feed or powder with 60:40 whey to casein ratio (20 Cal/fl oz). **Bot.:** Hospital use 4 fl oz. ready-to-feed. **Pow.:** Can lb. *OTC.*
Use: Nutritional supplement.

Similac Special Care 20. (Ross) Infant formula ready-to-feed (20 Cal/fl oz). Bot. 4 fl oz. *OTC.*
Use: Nutritional supplement.

Similac Special Care 24. (Ross) Infant formula ready-to-feed (24 Cal/fl oz). Bot. 4 fl oz. *OTC.*
Use: Nutritional supplement.

Similac 13/Similac 13 with Iron. (Ross) Milk-based infant formula ready-to-feed containing 13 calories/fl oz, 1.8 mg Fe/ 100 calories. Bot. 4 fl. oz. *OTC.*
Use: Nutritional supplement.

Similac 24 LBW. (Ross) Low-iron infant formula, ready-to-feed, 24 calories/fl oz. Bot. 4 fl oz. *OTC.*
Use: Nutritional supplement.

Similac 24/Similac 24 with Iron. (Ross) Milk-based infant formula ready-to-feed (24 cal/fl oz), Fe 1.8 mg/100 calories. Bot. 4 fl oz. *OTC.*
Use: Nutritional supplement.

Similac 27. (Ross) Milk-based ready-to-feed infant formula (27 cal/fl oz). Bot. 4 fl oz. *OTC.*
Use: Nutritional supplement.

Similac 20/Similac with Iron 20. (Ross) Milk-based infant formula. Standard dilution (20 cal/fl oz). Similac with iron: Fe 1.8 mg/100 cal. **Pow.:** Can lb. **Concentrated Liq.:** Can 13 fl oz. **Ready-to-feed:** Can 8 fl oz, 32 fl oz. Bot. 4 fl oz, 8 fl oz. *OTC.*
Use: Nutritional supplement.

Simplet. (Major) Pseudoephedrine hydrochloride 60 mg, chlorpheniramine maleate 4 mg, acetaminophen 650 mg. Tab. Bot. 100s. *OTC.*
Use: Upper respiratory combination, analgesic, antihistamine, decongestant.

Simply Cough. (McNeil PPC) Dextromethorphan HBr 5 mg/5 mL, corn syrup, sucralose, alcohol free, cherry berry flavor. Liq. 120 mL. *OTC.*
Use: Nonnarcotic antitussive.

Simply Saline. (Blairex) Sodium chloride. Soln. Spray bot. 44 mL. *OTC.*
Use: Nasal decongestant.

Simply Sleep. (McNeil) Diphenhydramine hydrochloride 25 mg. Tab. 24s, 48s. *OTC.*
Use: Nonprescription sleep aid.

Simply Stuffy. (McNeil PPC) Pseudoephedrine hydrochloride. **Liq.:** 15 mg/ 5 mL, corn syrup, sucralose, alcohol free, cherry berry flavor. 120 mL. **Tab.:** 30 mg, lactose. Pkg. 24s. *OTC.*
Use: Nasal decongestant, arylalkylamine.

Simron Plus. (GlaxoSmithKline) Fe 10 mg, vitamins B_{12} 3.33 mcg, C 50 mg, B_6 1 mg, folic acid 0.1 mg. Cap. Parabens. Bot. 100s. *OTC.*
Use: Mineral supplement.

•**simtrazene.** (SIM-trah-seen) USAN.
Use: Antineoplastic.

Simulect. (Novartis) Basiliximab 200 mg, sucrose, mannitol, potassium phosphate, sodium chloride, preservative free. Pow. for Inj., lyophilized. Single-use vial. *Rx.*
Use: Immunologic, immunosuppressive.

•**simvastatin.** (SIM-vuh-STAT-in) *USP 28.* Formerly Synvinolin.
Use: Antihyperlipidemic, HMG-CoA reductase inhibitor.
See: Zocor.
W/Ezetimibe.
See: Vytorin.

•**sinapultide.** (si-na-PUL-tide) USAN.
Use: Treatment of respiratory distress syndrome (pulmonary surfactant).

Sinarest Decongestant. (Novartis) Oxymetazoline hydrochloride 0.05%. Spray. Bot. 0.5 oz. *OTC.*
Use: Decongestant.

Sinarest Extra-Strength. (Novartis) Acetaminophen 500 mg, chlorpheniramine maleate 2 mg, pseudoephedrine hydrochloride 30 mg. Tab. 24s. *OTC.*
Use: Analgesic; antihistamine; decongestant.

Sinarest No Drowsiness. (Novartis) Pseudoephedrine hydrochloride 30 mg, acetaminophen 500 mg. Tab. Pkg. 20s. *OTC.*
Use: Analgesic; decongestant.

Sinarest Sinus. (Novartis) Acetaminophen 325 mg, chlorpheniramine maleate 2 mg, pseudoephedrine hydrochloride 30 mg. Tab. Pkg. 20s, 40s, 80s. *OTC.*
Use: Analgesic; antihistamine; decongestant.

Sinarest 12 Hour. (Novartis) Oxymetazoline hydrochloride 0.05%. Nasal Spray Bot. 15 mL. *OTC.*
Use: Decongestant.

• **sincalide.** (SIN-kah-lide) USAN.
Use: Choleretic, diagnostic aid, gastrointestinal function test.
See: Kinevac.

Sine-Aid IB. (McNeil Consumer) Pseudoephedrine 30 mg, ibuprofen 200 mg. Capl. Pkg. 20s. *OTC.*
Use: Analgesic; decongestant.

Sine-Aid Sinus Headache. (McNeil Consumer) Acetaminophen 325 mg, pseudoephedrine hydrochloride 30 mg. Tab. Bot. 24s, 50s, 100s. *OTC.*
Use: Analgesic; decongestant.

Sine-Aid Sinus Headache, Extra Strength. (McNeil Consumer) Acetaminophen 500 mg, pseudoephedrine hydrochloride 30 mg. Capl. Bot. 24s, 50s. *OTC.*
Use: Analgesic; decongestant.

• **sinefungin.** (sih-neh-FUN-jin) USAN.
Use: Antifungal.

Sinemet CR. (Bristol-Myers Squibb) Carbidopa 25 mg, 50 mg, levodopa 100 mg, 200 mg. ER Tab. Bot. 100s, 500s, UD 100s. *Rx.*
Use: Antiparkinson agent.

Sinemet 10/100. (Bristol-Myers Squibb) Carbidopa 10 mg, levodopa 100 mg. Tab. Bot. 100s, UD 100s. *Rx.*
Use: Antiparkinson agent.

Sinemet 25/100. (Bristol-Myers Squibb) Carbidopa 25 mg, levodopa 100 mg. Tab. Bot. 100s, UD 100s. *Rx.*
Use: Antiparkinson agent.

Sinemet 25/250. (Bristol-Myers Squibb) Carbidopa 25 mg, levodopa 250 mg. Tab. Bot. 100s, UD 100s. *Rx.*
Use: Antiparkinson agent.

Sine-Off Night Time Formula Sinus, Cold & Flu Medicine. (Hogil Pharm.) Pseudoephedrine hydrochloride 30 mg, diphenhydramine hydrochloride 25 mg, acetaminophen 500 mg. Geltab. Pkg. 10s. *OTC.*
Use: Upper respiratory combination, decongestant, antihistimine.

Sine-Off No Drowsiness Formula. (Hogil) Pseudoephedrine hydrochloride 30 mg, acetaminophen 500 mg. Tab. Pkg. 24s, 96s. *OTC.*
Use: Upper respiratory combination, decongestant, analgesic.

Sine-Off Sinus Medicine. (Hogil) Chlorpheniramine maleate 2 mg, pseudoephedrine hydrochloride 30 mg, acetaminophen 500 mg. Tab. Pkg. 24s, 96s. *OTC.*
Use: Upper respiratory combination, analgesic, antihistamine, decongestant.

Sinequan. (Roerig) Doxepin hydrochloride. **Cap.:** 10 mg, 25 mg, 50 mg, 75 mg, 100 mg, 150 mg. Bot. 50s (150 mg only), 100s (except 150 mg), 500s (150 mg only), 1000s (except 150 mg), 5000s (25 mg, 50 mg only). *Rx.*
Use: Antidepressant.

Sinex. (Procter & Gamble) Phenylephrine hydrochloride 0.5%, cetylpyridinium Cl 0.04% w/thimerosal 0.001% preservative. Nasal Spray. Bot. 0.5 oz, 1 oz. *OTC.*
Use: Decongestant.

Singlet for Adults. (GlaxoSmithKline) Pseudoephedrine hydrochloride 60 mg, chlorpheniramine maleate 4 mg, acetaminophen 650 mg, sucrose. Tab. Bot. 100s. *OTC.*
Use: Upper respiratory combination, analgesic, antihistamine, decongestant.

Singulair. (Merck) Montelukast sodium. **Tab.:** 10 mg, lactose. Unit-of-use 30s, 90s, UD 100s. **Chew. Tab.:** 4 mg, 5 mg, aspartame, mannitol, phenylalanine 0.674 mg (4 mg only), 0.842 mg (5 mg only), cherry flavor. Bot. 100s. Unit-of-use 30s, 90s, 100s, UD 100s. **Gran.:** 4 mg/packet, mannitol. 30 packets. *Rx.*
Use: Leukotriene receptor antagonist.

Sino-Eze MLT. (Global Source) Salicylamide 3.5 g, acetaminophen 100 mg, phenylephrine hydrochloride 5 mg, chlorpheniramine maleate 2 mg. Tab. Bot. 1000s. *Rx.*
Use: Upper respiratory combination, analgesic, antihistamine, decongestant.

Sinografin. (Bracco Diagnostics) Diatrizoate meglumine 527 mg, iodipamide meglumine 268 mg, iodine 380 mg/mL, EDTA. Inj. Vial 10 mL. *Rx.*

Use: Radiopaque agent.

Sinufed Timecelle. (Roberts) Pseudoephedrine hydrochloride 60 mg, guaifenesin 300 mg. Cap. Bot. 100s. *Rx.*
Use: Upper respiratory combination, decongestant, expectorant.

Sinumist-SR. (Roberts) Guaifenesin
600 mg. Tab. Bot. 100s. *Rx.*
Use: Upper respiratory combination, expectorant.

Sinupan. (ION Laboratories, Inc.)
Phenylephrine hydrochloride 40 mg,
guaifenesin 200 mg. SR Cap. Bot.
100s. *Rx.*
Use: Upper respiratory combination, decongestant, expectorant.

Sinus Excedrin Extra Strength. (Bristol-
Myers Squibb) Pseudoephedrine hydrochloride 30 mg, acetaminophen
500 mg. Tab or Cap. Bot. 50s. *OTC.*
Use: Upper respiratory combination, decongestant, analgesic.

Sinus Headache & Congestion.
(Rugby) Pseudoephedrine hydrochloride 30 mg, chlorpheniramine maleate
2 mg, acetaminophen 500 mg. Tab. Bot.
100s, 1000s. *OTC.*
Use: Upper respiratory combination, decongestant, antihistamine, analgesic.

Sinus Pain Formula Allerest. (Medeva)
Pseudoephedrine hydrochloride 30 mg,
chlorpheniramine maleate 2 mg, acetaminophen 500 mg. **Cap.:** Bot. 24s,
50s. **Gelcap:** Bot. 20s, 40s. *OTC.*
Use: Upper respiratory combination, analgesic, antihistamine, decongestant.

Sinus Relief. (Major) Pseudoephedrine
hydrochloride 30 mg, acetaminophen
325 mg. Tab. Bot. 24s, 100s, 1000s.
OTC.
Use: Upper respiratory combination, decongestant, analgesic.

Sinus-Relief Maximum Strength. (Major) Pseudoephedrine hydrochloride
30 mg, acetaminophen 500 mg, dextrose. Tab. Pkg. 24s. *OTC.*
Use: Upper respiratory combination, decongestant, analgesic.

Sinus Tablets. (Walgreen) Acetaminophen 325 mg, chlorpheniramine
maleate 2 mg, pseudoephedrine hydrochloride mg. Tab. Bot. 30s. *OTC.*
Use: Upper respiratory combination, analgesic, antihistamine, decongestant.

Sinustop. (Nature's Way) Pseudoephedrine hydrochloride 60 mg, echinacea
purpura, ginger, goldenseal root. Cap.
Pkg. 20s. *OTC.*
Use: Nasal decongestant, arylalkylamine.

**Sinutab Maximum Strength Sinus Al-
lergy.** (Warner Lambert) Acetaminophen 500 mg, pseudoephedrine hydrochloride 30 mg, chlorpheniramine
maleate 2 mg. Tab. or Capl. Blister pack
24s. *OTC.*
Use: Upper respiratory combination, analgesic, antihistamine, decongestant.

Sinutab Non-Drying. (Warner Lambert)
Pseudoephedrine hydrochloride 30 mg,
guaifenesin 200 mg, sorbitol, liquid
filled. Cap. (Liquid) Pkg. 24s. *OTC.*
Use: Upper respiratory combination, decongestant, expectorant.

**Sinutab Sinus Allergy, Maximum
Strength.** (Warner Lambert) Pseudoephedrine hydrochloride 30 mg, chlorpheniramine maleate 2 mg, acetaminophen 500 mg. Tab. Pkg. 24s. *OTC.*
Use: Upper respiratory combination, decongestant, antihistimine, analgesic.

**Sinutab Sinus Maximum Strength
Without Drowsiness Formula.**
(Warner Lambert) Acetaminophen
500 mg, pseudoephedrine hydrochloride 30 mg. Tab or Cap. Pack 24s. *OTC.*
Use: Upper respiratory combination,
analgesic, decongestant.

**Sinutab Sinus Regular Strength With-
out Drowsiness.** (Warner Lambert)
Pseudoephedrine hydrochloride 30 mg,
acetaminophen 325 mg. Tab. Bot. 24s.
OTC.
Use: Upper respiratory combination, analgesic, decongestant.

**Sinutab Sinus Without Drowsiness
Maximum Strength.** (Warner Lambert)
Pseudoephedrine hydrochloride 30 mg,
acetaminophen 500 mg. Tab. Pkg. 24s,
48s. *OTC.*
Use: Upper respiratory combination, decongestant, analgesic.

**Sinutab Sinus Without Drowsiness
Regular Strength.** (Warner Lambert)
Pseudoephedrine hydrochloride 30 mg,
acetaminophen 325 mg. Tab. Pkg. 24s.
OTC.
Use: Upper respiratory combination, de-
congestant, analgesic.

SINUtuss DM. (WE Pharmaceuticals)
Dextromethorphan HBr 30 mg, guai-
fenesin 600 mg, phenylephrine hydro-
chloride 15 mg. Dye-free. Tab. 100s.
Rx.
Use: Upper respiratory combination.

SINUvent PE. (WE Pharm) Phenylephrine hydrochloride 15 mg, guaifenesin 600 mg. ER Tab. 100s. *Rx.*
Use: Decongestant and expectorant.

•**siplizumab.** (sip-LIZ-oo-mab) USAN.
Use: Monoclonal antibody.

Siroil. (Siroil) Mercuric oleate, cresol, vegetable and mineral oil. Emulsion Bot. 8 oz. *OTC.*
Use: Antiseptic.

sir-o-lene.
Use: Emollient.

•**sirolimus.** (SER-oh-lih-muss) USAN. *Formerly Rapamycin.*
Use: Immunologic, immunosuppressive.
See: Rapamune.

•**sisomicin.** (SIS-oh-MY-sin) USAN.
Use: Anti-infective.

•**sisomicin sulfate.** (SIS-oh-MY-sin) *USP 28.*
Use: Anti-infective.

Sitabs. (Canright) Lobeline sulfate 1.5 mg, benzocaine 2 mg, aluminum hydroxide magnesium carbonate codried gel 150 mg. Loz. Bot. 100s. *OTC.*
Use: Smoking deterrent.

•**sitafloxacin.** (si-ta-FLOKS-a-sin) USAN.
Use: Antibacterial.

•**sitaxsentan sodium.** USAN.
Use: Congestive heart failure; ischemic deficits; hypertension; prostate cancer.

•**sitogluside.** (SIGH-toe-GLUE-side) USAN.
Use: Antiprostatic hypertrophy.

Sitzmarks. (Konsyl) Radiopaque polyvinyl chloride radiopaque rings 24 (1 mm × 4.5 mm). Cap. Box. 10s. *Rx.*
Use: Radiopaque agent, GI contrast agent.

•**sivelestat.** (si-VEL-es-tat) USAN.
Use: Acute respiratory distress syndrome.

•**sivelestat sodium.** (si-VEL-es-tat) USAN.
Use: Acute respiratory distress syndrome.

Sixameen. (Spanner) Vitamins B₁ 100 mg, B₆ 100 mg/mL. Vial 10 mL. *OTC.*
Use: Vitamin supplement.

666 Cold Preparation, Maximum Strength. (Monticello Drug) Dextromethorphan HBr 3.3 mg, pseudoephedrine hydrochloride 10 mg, acetaminophen 108.3 mg/5 mL, saccharin, sucrose. Liq. Bot. 177 mL. *OTC.*
Use: Upper respiratory combination, antitussive, decongestant, analgesic.

Skeeter Stik. (Outdoor Recreation) Lidocaine 4%, phenol 2%, isopropyl alcohol 45.5% in a propylene glycol base. Stick 1s. *OTC.*
Use: Anesthetic, local.

Skelaxin. (King) Metaxalone 800 mg. Tab. Bot. 100s, 500s. *Rx.*
Use: Muscle relaxant.

skeletal muscle relaxants.
See: Baclofen.
 Carisoprodol.
 Chlorphenesin Carbamate.
 Chlorzoxazone.
 Cyclobenzapine hydrochloride.
 Dantrolene Sodium.
 Diazepam.
 Metaxalone.
 Methocarbamol.
 Orphenadrine Citrate.
 Tizanidine hydrochloride.

Skelid. (Sanofi-Synthelabo) Tiludronate disodium 240 mg (equivalent to tiludronic acid 200 mg), lactose. Tab. Foil Strips in Ctn of 56 tabs/ctn. *Rx.*
Use: Bisphosphonates.

Skin Degreaser. (Health & Medical Techniques) Freon 100%. Bot. 2 oz, 4 oz. *OTC.*
Use: Dermatologic, degreaser.

Skin Shield. (Del) Dyclonine hydrochloride 0.75%, benzethonium Cl 0.2%, acetone, amyl acetate, castor oil, SD alcohol 40 10%. Waterproof. Liq. Bot. 13.3 mL. *OTC.*
Use: Dermatologic, protectant.

skin test antigen, multiple.
See: Multitest CMI.

SK 110679. (GlaxoSmithKline)
Use: Hormone, growth. [Orphan Drug]

Sleep Cap. (Weeks & Leo) Diphenhydramine hydrochloride 50 mg. Cap. Bot. 25s, 50s. *OTC.*
Use: Sleep aid.

Sleep-Eze. (Whitehall-Robins) Diphenhydramine hydrochloride 25 mg. Tab. Pkg. 12s, 26s, 52s. *OTC.*
Use: Sleep aid.

Sleep Tablets. (Towne) Scopolamine aminoxide HBr 0.2 mg, salicylamide 250 mg. Tab. Bot. 36s, 90s. *Rx.*
Use: Sleep aid.

Sleep II. (Walgreen) Diphenhydramine hydrochloride 25 mg. Tab. Bot. 16s, 32s, 72s. *OTC.*
Use: Sleep aid.

Sleepwell 2-Nite. (Rugby) Diphenhydramine hydrochloride 25 mg. Tab. Bot. 72s. *OTC.*
Use: Sleep aid.

Slender. (Carnation) Skim milk, vegetable oils, caseinates, vitamins, minerals. Liq.: 220 Cal/10 oz. Can. **Pow.:** 173 or 200 Cal mixed w/6 oz skim or low fat milk. Pkg 1 oz. *OTC.*
Use: Dietary aid.

Slim-Fast. (Thompson Medical) Meal replacement powder mixed with milk to

replace 1, 2 or 3 meals a day. *OTC.*
Use: Dietary aid.

Slim-Line. (Thompson Medical) Benzocaine, dextrose. Chewing gum. Box 24s. *OTC.*
Use: Dietary aid.

Slim-Tabs. (Wesley) Phendimetrazine tartrate 35 mg. Tab. Bot. 1000s. *c-III.*
Use: Anorexiant.

Sloan's Liniment. (Warner Lambert) Capsicum oleoresin 0.62%, methyl salicylate 2.66%, oil of camphor 3.35%, turpentine oil 46.76%, oil of pine 6.74%. Bot. 2 oz, 7 oz. *OTC.*
Use: Analgesic, topical.

Slo-Niacin. (Upsher-Smith) Niacin. 250 mg, 500 mg, 750 mg. Sugar free. CR Tab. Bot. 100s. *OTC.*
Use: Vitamin supplement.

Slo-Phyllin. (Aventis) Theophylline anhydrous 100 mg, 200 mg. Tab. Bot. 100s, 1000s, UD 100s. *Rx.*
Use: Bronchodilator.

Slo-Phyllin 80. (Aventis) Theophylline anhydrous 80 mg/15 mL. Nonalcoholic. Syr. Bot. 4 oz, pt, gal, UD 15 mL. *Rx.*
Use: Bronchodilator.

Slo-Salt-K. (Mission Pharmacal) KCl 150 mg, NaCl 410 mg. Tab. Bot. 1000s. Strip 100s. *OTC.*
Use: Salt substitute.

Slow FE. (Ciba) Dried ferrous sulfate 160 mg (iron 50 mg). Lactose, cetostearyl alcohol. SR Tab. Bot. 30s. *OTC.*
Use: Mineral supplement.

Slow Fe Slow Release Iron With Folic Acid. (Novartis) Fe 50 mg, folic acid 0.4 mg. SR Tab. Bot. 20s. *OTC.*
Use: Mineral, vitamin supplement.

Slow-Mag. (Purdue) Magnesium 64 mg (as chloride hexahydrate), calcium carbonate. EC Tab. Bot. 60s. *OTC.*
Use: Mineral.

Slow Release Iron. (Cardinal Health) Ferrous sulfate exsiccated (dried) 160 mg (iron 50 mg). Maltodextrin, mineral oil. SR Tab. Bot. 30s. *OTC.*
Use: Mineral supplement.

SLT Tablets. (Western Research) Sodium levothyroxine 0.1 mg, 0.2 mg, 0.3 mg. Bot. 1000s.
Use: Hormone, thyroid.

Small Fry Chewable Tabs. (Health for Life Brands) Vitamins A 5000 units, D 1000 units, B_{12} 5 mcg, B_1 3 mg, B_2 2.5 mg, B_6 1 mg, C 50 mg, niacinamide 20 mg, calcium pantothenate 1 mg, E 1 unit, l-lysine 15 mg, biotin 10 mg. Chew. Tab. Bot. 100s, 250s, 365s. *OTC.*
Use: Mineral, vitamin supplement.

●**smallpox vaccine.** *USP 28.*
Use: Immunization.
See: Dryvax.

smoking deterrents.
See: Bupropion hydrochloride.
Nicotine.
Nicotine Gum.
Nicotine Inhalation System.
Nicotine Nasal Spray.
Nicotine Polacrilex.
Nicotine Transdermal System.

snakebite antivenins.
See: Antivenin (Crotalidae).
Antivenin (*Micurus fulvius*).

snake venom.
Use: SC, IM, orally; trypanosomiasis.

Snaplets-D. (Baker Norton) Pseudoephedrine hydrochloride 6.25 mg, chlorpheniramine maleate 1 mg. Pkt., taste free. Granules 30s. *OTC.*
Use: Antihistamine; decongestant.

Snaplets-FR. (Baker Norton) Acetaminophen 80 mg. Pkt. Granules. 32s packets. *OTC.*
Use: Analgesic.

Snootie by Sea & Ski. (Carter-Wallace) Padimate O. SPF 10. Lot. Bot. 30 mL. *OTC.*
Use: Sunscreen.

Snooze Fast. (BDI) Diphenhydramine hydrochloride 50 mg. Tab. Bot. 36s. *OTC.*
Use: Sleep aid.

SN-13, 272.
See: Primaquine Phosphate.

Soac-Lens. (Alcon) Thimerosal 0.004%, EDTA 0.1%, wetting agents. Soln. Bot. 118 mL. *OTC.*
Use: Contact lens care.

Soakare. (Allergan) Benzalkonium Cl 0.01%, edetate disodium, NaOH to adjust pH, purified water. Bot. 4 fl oz. *OTC.*
Use: Contact lens care.

●**soap, green.** *USP 28.*
Use: Detergent.

soaps, germicidal.
See: Dial.
Fostex.
pHisoHex.
Thylox.

soap substitutes.
See: Lowila.
pHisoDerm.

●**soda lime.** *NF 23.*
Use: Carbon dioxide absorbent.

Soda Mint. (Eli Lilly) Sodium bicarbonate 5 g, peppermint oil q.s. Tab. Bot. 100s. *OTC.*
Use: Antacid.

Sodasone. (Fellows) Prednisolone sodium phosphate 20 mg, niacinamide

25 mg/mL. Vial 10 mL. *Rx.*
Use: Corticosteroid.

•**sodium acetate.** (SO-dee-uhm ASS-eh-tate) *USP 28.*
Use: Pharmaceutic aid (in dialysis solutions).

•**sodium acetate c 11 injection.** (SO-dee-uhm ASS-eh-tate) *USP 28.*
Use: Radiopharmaceutical.

sodium acetosulfone. (SO-dee-uhm ah-SEE-toe-sull-FONE)
Use: Leprostatic agent.

sodium acid phosphate.
See: Sodium Biphosphate.

sodium actinoquinol. (SO-dee-uhm ack-TIH-no-kwin-OLE)
Use: Treatment of flash burns (ophthalmic).

•**sodium alginate.** (SO-dee-uhm AL-jih-nate) *NF 23.*
Use: Pharmaceutic aid (suspending agent).

sodium aminobenzoate.
Use: Dermatomyositis and scleroderma.

sodium aminopterin. Aminopterin sodium.

sodium aminosalicylate.
See: Aminosalicylate Sodium.

sodium amobarbital. Amobarbital sodium, *USP.*

•**sodium amylosulfate.** (SO-dee-uhm AM-ill-oh-sull-fate) USAN.
Use: Enzyme inhibitor.

sodium anazolene. (SO-dee-uhm an-AZE-oh-leen)
Use: Diagnostic aid.

sodium antimony gluconate. (Pentostam)
Use: Anti-infective.

•**sodium arsenate As 74.** (SO-dee-uhm AHR-seh-nate) USAN.
Use: Radiopharmaceutical.

•**sodium ascorbate.** (SO-dee-uhm ass-CORE-bate) *USP 28.*
Use: Vitamin (antiscorbutic).
See: Cenolate.
Vitac.

sodium aurothiomalate.
See: Gold Sodium Thiosulfate.

•**sodium benzoate.** (SO-dee-uhm BEN-zoe-ate) *NF 23.*
Use: Pharmaceutic aid (antifungal, preservative); antihyperammonemic.

sodium benzoate and sodium phenylacetate.
Use: Antihyperammonemic. [Orphan Drug]

sodium benzylpenicillin. Penicillin G Sodium, *USP.* Sodium Penicillin G.

Rx.
Use: Anti-infective; penicillin.

•**sodium bicarbonate.** (SO-dee-uhm by-CAR-boe-nate) *USP 28.*
Use: Alkalizer, systemic; antacid; electrolyte replacement.
W/Combinations.
See: Zee-Seltzer.
W/Sodium bitartrate.
See: Ceo-Two.
W/Sodium carboxymethylcellulose, alginic acid.
See: Pretts.

sodium bicarbonate. (Hospira) Sodium bicarbonate. Inj. 4.2% (5 mEq). Infant 10 mL Syringe. 7.5% (44.6 mEq). 50 mL Syringe or 50 mL Amp. 8.4% (10 mEq). Pediatric 10 mL Syringe or (50 mEq). 50 mL Syringe or 50 mL Vial.
Use: Alkalizer, systemic; antacid; electrolyte replacement.

sodium biphosphate.
Use: Cathartic.
See: Sodium Phosphate Monobasic.
W/Combinations.
See: UniSyn.

sodium biphosphate/ammonium phosphate sodium acid.
See: Ammonium biphosphate, sodium biphosphate and sodium acid pyrophosphate.

sodium bismuth tartrate.
See: Bismuth Sodium Tartrate.

sodium bisulfite. Sulfurous acid, monosodium salt. Monosodium sulfite.
Use: Antioxidant.

•**sodium borate.** *NF 23.*
Use: Pharmaceutic aid (alkalizing agent).

sodium butabarbital.
See: Butabarbital Sodium.
Sodium Butyrate.

•**sodium butyrate.** *USP 28.*

sodium calcium edetate.
See: Calcium Disodium Versenate.

•**sodium carbonate.** *NF 23.*
Use: Pharmaceutic aid (alkalizing agent).

sodium carboxymethylcellulose.
Carboxymethylcellulose Sodium, *USP.* CMC. Cellulose Gum.

sodium cellulose glycolate.
See: Carboxymethylcellulose, sodium.

sodium cephalothin. (SO-dee-uhm SEFF-ah-low-thin) Cephalothin Sodium, *USP.*
Use: Anti-infective.

•**sodium chloride.** (SO-dee-uhm KLOR-ide) *USP 28.*
Use: Pharmaceutic aid (tonicity agent);

bronchodilator, diluent; nasal decongestant.
See: Afrin Moisturizing Saline Mist.
Afrin Saline, Extra Moisturizing.
Ayr Saline.
Breathe Free.
HuMist Moisturizing Mist.
Mycinaire Saline Mist.
NaSal.
Nasal Moist.
Nasal Spray.
Normaline.
Ocean.
Ocean for Kids.
Pretz Irrigation.
Pretz Moisturizing.
Simply Saline.
sodium chloride. (Various Mfr.) Sodium chloride 0.9%, benzyl alcohol 9 mg. Inj. Vial 1 mL, 2 mL, 2.5 mL, 5 mL, 10 mL, 30 mL. *Rx.*
Use: Bronchodilator, diluent.
sodium chloride and dextrose combinations.
Use: Intravenous nutritional therapy, intravenous replenishment solution.
See: Dextrose 5% with 0.45% Sodium Chloride.
Dextrose 5% with 0.9% Sodium Chloride.
Dextrose 5% with 0.3% Sodium Chloride.
Dextrose 5% with 0.33% Sodium Chloride.
Dextrose 5% with 0.2% Sodium Chloride.
Dextrose 5% and 0.225% Sodium Chloride.
Dextrose 10% with 0.45% Sodium Chloride.
Dextrose 10% and 0.9% Sodium Chloride.
Dextrose 10% with 0.2% Sodium Chloride.
Dextrose 10% with 0.225% Sodium Chloride.
Dextrose 3.3% and 0.3% Sodium Chloride.
Dextrose 2.5% with 0.45% Sodium Chloride.
sodium chloride, calcium carbonate, and potassium chloride.
Use: Salt replacement.
See: Sustain.
sodium chloride, dextrose and potassium chloride combinations.
Use: Intravenous nutritional therapy, intravenous replenishment solution.
See: Potassium Chloride in 5% Dextrose and 0.45% Sodium Chloride.
Potassium Chloride in 5% Dextrose

and 0.9% Sodium Chloride.
Potassium Chloride in 5% Dextrose and 0.33% Sodium Chloride.
Potassium Chloride in 5% Dextrose and 0.2% Sodium Chloride.
Potassium Chloride in 10% Dextrose and 0.2% Sodium Chloride.
Potassium Chloride in 3.3% Dextrose and 0.3% Sodium Chloride.
•**sodium chloride injection.** *USP 28.*
Use: Fluid and irrigation; electrolyte replacement; isotonic vehicle.
sodium chloride injection. (Abbott) Normal saline 0.9% in 150 mL, 250 mL, 500 mL, 1000 mL cont. **Partial-fill:** 50 mL in 200 mL, 50 mL in 300 mL, 100 mL in 300 mL. **Fliptop vial:** 10 mL, 20 mL, 50 mL, 100 mL. **Bacteriostatic vial:** 10 mL, 20 mL, 30 mL; 50 mEq, 20 mL in 50 mL fliptop or pintop vial;100 mEq, 40 mL in 50 mL fliptop vial; 50 mEq, 20 mL univ. add. syr.; sodium Cl 0.45%, 500 mL, 1000 mL; sodium Cl 5%, 500 mL; sodium Cl irrigating solution, 250 mL, 500 mL, 1000 mL, 3000 mL; (Pharmacia & Upjohn) sodium Cl 9 mg/mL w/benzyl alcohol 9.45 mg. Vial 20 mL (Sanofi Winthrop Pharmaceuticals).
Carpuject: 2 mL fill cartridge, 22-gauge, 1 ¼-inch needle or 25-gauge, ⅝-inch needle.
Use: Fluid and irrigation; electrolyte replacement; isotonic vehicle.
•**sodium chloride Na 22.** (So-dee-uhm KLOR-ide) USAN.
Use: Radioactive agent.
sodium chloride substitutes.
See: Salt Substitute.
sodium chloride tablets. (Parke-Davis) Sodium Cl 15 ½ g. Tab. Bot. 1000s.
Use: Normal saline.
sodium chloride 0.45%. (Dey) Sodium chloride 0.45%, preservative free. Soln. Single-use vial 3 mL, 5 mL. *OTC.*
Use: Bronchodilator, diluent.
sodium chloride 0.9%. (Dey) Sodium chloride 0.9%, preservative free. Soln. Vial 3 mL, 5 mL, 15 mL. *OTC.*
Use: Bronchodilator, diluent.
sodium chlorothiazide for injection. (SO-dee-uhm KLOR-oh-thigh-AZZ-ide) Chlorothiazide Sodium for Injection.
Use: Diuretic.
•**sodium chromate Cr 51 injection.** (So-dee-uhm KROE-mate) *USP 28.*
Use: Diagnostic aid (blood volume determination); radiopharmaceutical.
See: Radio Chromate Cr 51 Sodium.

•**sodium citrate.** (SO-dee-uhm SIH-trate) *USP 28.*
Use: Alkalizer, systemic.
See: Anticoagulant Citrate Dextrose Solution.
Anticoagulant Citrate Phosphate Dextrose Solution.
W/Combinations.
See: Tussirex.
Tussirex Sugar Free.
Scot-Tussin Original Clear 5-Action Cold and Allergy Formula.
Scot-Tussin Original 5-Action Cold and Allergy Formula.

sodium citrate and citric acid. Shohl's Solution.
Use: Alkalinizer, systemic.

sodium cloxacillin. (SO-dee-uhm CLOX-ah-SILL-in)
See: Cloxacillin Sodium.

sodium colistimethate. Colistimethate Sodium, Sterile. Antibiotic produced by *Aerobacillus colistinus.*

sodium colistin methanesulfonate. Colistimethane Sodium, *USP.* The sodium methanesulfonate salt of an antibiotic substance elaborated by *Aerobacillus colistinus.*
Use: Anti-infective.

•**sodium dehydroacetate.** *NF 23.*
Use: Pharmaceutic aid (antimicrobial preservative).

sodium dextrothyroxine. (SO-dee-uhm DEX-troe-thigh-ROCK-seen)
Use: Anticholesteremic.

sodium diatrizoate. Diatrizoate Sodium, *USP 25.*
Use: Radiopaque medium.

sodium dichloroacetate.
Use: Treatment of lactic acidosis and familial hypercholesterolemia. [Orphan Drug]

sodium dicloxacillin. (SO-dee-uhm die-KLOX-ass-IH-lin) Dicloxacillin Sodium, *USP.*
Use: Anti-infective.

sodium dicloxacillin monohydrate.
Use: Anti-infective.
See: Pathocil.

sodium dihydrogen phosphate.
See: Sodium Biphosphate.

sodium dimethoxyphenyl penicillin.
See: Methicillin Sodium.

sodium dioctyl sulfosuccinate.
See: Docusate Sodium.

sodium diphenylhydantoin. Phenytoin Sodium, *USP.* Diphenylhydantoin Sodium.
Use: Anticonvulsant.

sodium edetate. (SO-dee-uhm eh-deh-TATE) Edetate Disodium, *USP.* Tet-
rasodium ethylenediaminetetraacetate.
Use: Chelating agent.
See: Vagisec.

sodium ethacrynate. (SO-dee-uhm ETH-ah-krih-nate) Ethacrynate Sodium for Injection, *USP.*
Use: Diuretic.

•**sodium ethasulfate.** (SO-dee-uhm ETH-ah-SULL-fate) USAN.
Use: Detergent.

sodium ethyl-mercuri-thio-salicylate.
See: Merthiolate.
Thimerosal.

•**sodium ferric gluconate complex.** (FER-ik GLOO-koe-nate) USAN.
Use: Iron product.
See: Ferrlecit.

•**sodium fluorescein.** *USP 28.* Fluorescein Sodium, *USP;* Resorcinolphthalein sodium.
Use: Diagnostic aid (corneal trauma indicator).

•**sodium fluoride.** (SO-dee-uhm) *USP 28.*
Use: Dental caries agent.
See: ControlRx.
DentaGel.
EtheDent.
Fluoride.
Flura.
Karidium.
Karigel.
Kari-Rinse.
Luride.
Mouthkote F/R.
NaFeen.
OrthoWash.
Pediaflor.
Prevident 5000 Plus.
T-Fluoride.
W/Vitamins.
See: Fluorac.
Mulvidren-F.
So-Flo.
W/Vitamins A, D, C.
See: Tri-Vi-Flor.

sodium fluoride. (Hi-Tech) Fluoride 0.5 mg per mL (from sodium fluoride 1.1 mg). Peach flavor. Drops. 50 mL. *Rx.*
Use: Prevention of dental caries.

sodium fluoride and phosphoric acid.
Use: Dental caries agent.

•**sodium fluoride f 18.** (SO-dee-uhm) *USP 28.*
Use: Radiopharmaceutical.

sodium folate. Monosodium folate.
Use: Water-soluble, hematopoietic vitamin.

•**sodium formaldehyde sulfoxylate.** (SO-dee-uhm) *NF 23.*

Use: Pharmaceutic aid (preservative).
sodium gamma-hydroxybutyric acid.
Under study.
Use: Anesthetic adjuvant, sleep disorders. [Orphan Drug]
sodium gentisate.
See: Gentisate Sodium.
•**sodium gluconate.** (SO-dee-uhm) *USP 28.*
Use: Electrolyte, replacement.
sodium glucosulfone inj.
Use: Leprostatic.
sodium glutamate.
See: Glutamate.
sodium glycerophosphate. Glycerol phosphate sodium salt.
Use: Pharmaceutic necessity.
sodium glycocholate, a bile salt.
See: Bile Salts.
W/Phenolphthalein, cascara sagrada extract, sodium taurocholate, aloin.
See: So-Nitri-Nacea.
•**sodium heparin.** *USP 28.* Heparin Sodium.
Use: Anticoagulant.
sodium hexobarbital.
Use: Intravenous general anesthetic.
sodium hyaluronate.
Use: Ophthalmic.
See: Amo Vitrax.
   Amvisc.
   Amvisc Plus.
   Healon.
   Hyalgan.
   Shellgel.
   Synvisc.
W/Chondroitin sulfate.
See: Viscoat.
sodium hyaluronate and fluorescein sodium.
Use: Surgical aid, ophthalmic.
See: Healon Yellow.
•**sodium hydroxide.** (SO-dee-uhm) *NF 23.*
Use: Pharmaceutic aid (alkalizing agent).
•**sodium hypochlorite solution.** (SO-dee-uhm high-poe-KLOR-ite) *USP 28.*
Use: Anti-infective, local; disinfectant.
See: Antiformin.
   Dakin's Soln.
   Hyclorite.
sodium hypophosphite. Sodium phosphinate.
Use: Pharmaceutic necessity.
sodium hyposulfite.
See: Sodium Thiosulfate.
W/Potassium guaiacolsufonate.
See: Guaiadol Aqueous.
W/Potassium guaiacolsulfonate, chlor-

pheniramine maleate, sodium bisulfite.
See: Gomahist.
•**sodium iodide.** (SO-dee-uhm) *USP 28.*
Use: Nutritional supplement.
•**sodium iodide I-131.** *USP 28.*
Use: Antineoplastic; diagnostic aid (thyroid function determination); radiopharmaceutical.
See: Iodotope.
sodium iodide I-131. (Mallinckrodt) 0.75 to 100 mCi. Cap. 3.5 to 150 mCi. Vial. *Rx.*
Use: Antithyroid agent.
•**sodium iodide I-125.** USAN.
Use: Diagnostic aid (thyroid function determination); radiopharmaceutical.
•**sodium iodide I-123.** *USP 28.*
Use: In vivo diagnostic aid, thyroid function test.
sodium iodide I-123. (Mallinckrodt Medical) Sodium iodide I^{123} 3.7 MBq, 7.4 MBq, sucrose. Cap. Pkg. 1s, 3s, 5s. *Rx.*
Use: In vivo diagnostic aid, thyroid function test.
sodium iodipamide.
Use: Radiopaque medium.
•**sodium iodomethane sulfonate.** *USP 28.* Methiodal Sodium.
•**sodium iothalamate.** *USP 28.* Iothalmate Sodium Inj.
Use: Radiopaque medium.
•**sodium ipodate.** (SO-dee-uhm EYE-poe-date) *USP 28.* Ipodate Sodium.
Use: Radiopaque.
See: Oragrafin Sodium.
sodium isoamylethylbarbiturate.
See: Amytal Sodium.
•**sodium lactate injection.** (SO-dee-uhm LACK-tate) *USP 28.*
Use: Fluid and electrolyte replacement.
sodium lactate injection. (Abbott) Sodium lactate 1/6 Molar, 250 mL, 500 mL, 1,000 mL; 50 mEq, 10 mL in 20 mL fliptop vial.
Use: Electrolyte replacement.
sodium lactate solution.
Use: Electrolyte replacement.
•**sodium lauryl sulfate.** (SO-dee-uhm LAH-rill SULL-fate) *NF 23.* Sulfuric acid monodecyl ester sodium salt. Sodium monododecyl sulfate.
Use: Pharmaceutic aid (surfactant).
See: Duponol.
W/Hydrocortisone.
See: Nutracort.
•**sodium levothyroxine.** *USP 28.* Levothyroxine Sodium.
Use: Hormone, thyroid.
See: Synthroid.
sodium liothyronine. Liothyronine Sodium, *USP.*

Use: Hormone, thyroid.

sodium Iyapolate. (LIE-app-OLE-ate) Polyethylene sulfonate sodium. Peson (Hoechst Marion Roussel).
Use: Anticoagulant.

sodium malonylurea.
See: Barbital Sodium.

sodium mercaptomerin. Mercaptomerin Sodium, *USP.*
Use: Diuretic.

• **sodium metabisulfite.** (SO-dee-uhm) *NF 23.*
Use: Pharmaceutic aid (antioxidant).

sodium methiodal. Methiodal Sodium, *USP.* Sodium monoiodomethanesulfonate. Sodium Iodomethanesulfonate, Inj.
Use: Radiopaque medium.

sodium methohexital for injection, Methohexital Sodium for Injection, *USP.*
Use: Anesthetic, general.
See: Brevital Sodium.

sodium methoxycellulose. Mixture of methylcellulose and sodium.

• **sodium monofluorophosphate.** (SO-dee-uhm mahn-oh-flure-oh-FOSS-fate) *USP 28.*
Use: Dental caries agent.

sodium morrhuate, injection Morrhuate Sodium Inj., *USP.*
Use: Sclerosing agent.

sodium nafcillin. (SO-dee-uhm naff-SILL-in) Nafcillin Sodium, *USP.*
Use: Anti-infective.

sodium nicotinate. (Various Mfr.).
Use: IV nicotinic acid therapy.

• **sodium nitrite.** (SO-dee-uhm NYE-trite) *USP 28.*
Use: Antidote to cyanide poisoning, antioxidant. Vasodilator and antidote-cyanide.
See: Cyanide Antidote Pkg.

sodium nitrite. (Hope) Sodium nitrite 30 mg/mL. Inj. Vials. 10 mL. *Rx.*
Use: Antidote, cyanide.

• **sodium nitroprusside.** (SO-dee-uhm NYE-troe-PRUSS-ide) *USP 28.*
Use: Antihypertensive.
See: Keto-Diastix.
Nitropress.

sodium nitroprusside. (Wyeth) Sodium nitroprusside. 50 mg. Pow. for Inj. 5 mL. *Rx.*
Use: Antihypertensive.

sodium novobiocin. Sodium salt of antibacterial substance produced by *Streptomyces niveus.* Novobiocin monosodium salt.
Use: Anti-infective.

See: Albamycin.

sodium ortho-iodohippurate. Iodohippurate Sodium, I-131 Injection, *USP.*
See: Hipputope.

• **sodium oxybate.** (SO-dee-uhm OX-eebate) USAN.
Use: Psychotherapeutic agent, miscellaneous.
See: Xyrem.

sodium pantothenate.
Use: Orally, dietary supplement.

sodium para-aminohippurate injection.
Use: IV, to determine kidney tubular excretion function.

sodium penicillin G. Penicillin G Sodium, Sterile, *USP.* Sodium benzylpenicillin.

sodium pentobarbital. Pentobarbital Sodium, *USP.*
Use: Hypnotic.

• **sodium perborate monohydrate.** (SO-dee-uhm) USAN.

sodium peroxyborate.
See: Sodium Perborate.

sodium peroxyhydrate.
See: Sodium Perborate.

• **sodium pertechnetate Tc 99m injection.** (SO-dee-uhm per-TEK-neh-tate) *USP 28.* Pertechnetic acid, sodium salt.
Use: Radiopharmaceutical.
See: Minitec.

sodium phenobarbital. Phenobarbital Sodium, *USP.*
Use: Anticonvulsant; hypnotic.

• **sodium phenylacetate.** (SO-dee-uhm FEN-ill-ASS-eh-tate) USAN.
Use: Antihyperammonemic.

• **sodium phenylbutyrate.** (SO-dee-uhm fen-ill-BYOOT-ih-rate) USAN.
Use: Antihyperammonemic.
See: Buphenyl.

sodium phenylethylbarbiturate. Phenobarbital Sodium, *USP.*

sodium phosphate. (Abbott) Disodium hydrogen phosphate. 3 mM P and 4 mEq sodium. 15 mL in 30 mL fliptop vial.
Use: Buffering agent; source of phosphate.
W/Gentamicin sulfate, monosodium phosphate, sodium Cl, benzalkonium Cl.
See: Garamycin Ophthalmic.
W/Sodium biphosphate.
See: Fleet Enema.
Phospho-Soda.

• **sodium phosphate, dibasic.** (SO-dee-uhm FOSS-fate) *USP 28.*
Use: Laxative.

See: Visicol.
- **sodium phosphate, dried.** *USP 28.*
  Use: Cathartic.
- **sodium phosphate, monobasic.** (SO-dee-uhm FOSS-fate) *USP 28.*
  Use: Cathartic.
  See: Visicol.
  W/Gentamicin sulfate, disodium phosphate, sodium Cl, benzalkonium Cl.
  See: Garamycin.
  W/Methenamine.
  See: Uro-Phosphate.
  W/Methenamine mandelate, levo-hyoscyamine sulfate.
  See: Levo-Uroquid.
  W/Methenamine, phenyl salicylate, methylene blue, hyoscyamine, alkaloid.
  See: Fleet Enema.
    Phospho-Soda.
  sodium phosphate P 32. (Mallinckrodt) Sodium phosphate P 32 0.67 mCi/mL. Vial. 5 mCi Inj. *Rx.*
  Use: Antineoplastic.
- **sodium phosphate P 32 solution.** (SO-dee-uhm FOSS-fate) *USP 28.*
  Use: Antineoplastic; antipolycythemic; diagnostic aid (neoplasm); radiopharmaceutical.
- **sodium phosphates rectal solution.** *USP 28.*
  sodium phytate. (SO-dee-uhm FYE-tate) Nonasodium phytate: Sodium cyclohexanehexyl (hexaphosphate).
  Use: Chelating agent.
- **sodium polyphosphate.** (SO-dee-uhm pahl-ee-FOSS-fate) USAN.
  Use: Pharmaceutic aid.
- **sodium polystyrene sulfonate.** (SO-dee-uhm pah-lee-STYE-reen SULL-fuh-nate) *USP 28.*
  Use: Ion exchange resin (potassium).
  See: Kayexalate.
    SPS.
  sodium polystyrene sulfonate. (Roxane) Sodium polystyrene sulfonate 15 g, sorbitol 14.1 g, alcohol 0.1%/60 mL. Susp. Bot. 60 mL, 120 mL, 200 mL, 500 mL. *Rx.*
  Use: Ion exchange resin (potassium).
  sodium polystyrene sulfonate. (Crookes-Barnes) Sodium polystyrene sulfonate 5% Soln. Eye drops. Lacrivial 15 mL.
  Use: Ion exchange resin (potassium).
- **sodium propionate.** (SO-dee-uhm PRO-pee-oh-nate) *NF 23.*
  Use: Pharmaceutic aid (preservative).
  W/Chlorophyll "a".
  See: Prophyllin.
  W/Neomycin sulfate.

See: Otobiotic.
  sodium psylliate.
  Use: Sclerosing agent.
- **sodium pyrophosphate.** (SO-dee-uhm pie-row-FOSS-fate) USAN.
  Use: Pharmaceutic aid.
  sodium radio chromate injection. Sodium Chromate Cr 51 Inj., *USP.*
  sodium radio iodide solution. Sodium Iodide I-131 Solution, *USP.*
  Use: Thyroid tumors; hyperthyroidism; cardiac dysfunction.
  sodium radio-phosphate, P-32. Radio-Phosphate P 32 Solution. Sodium phosphate P-32 Solution, *USP.*
  sodium removing resins.
  See: Resins.
  sodium rhodanate.
  See: Sodium Thiocyanate.
  sodium rhodanide.
  See: Sodium Thiocyanate.
  sodium saccharin. Saccharin Sodium, *USP.*
  Use: Noncaloric sweetener.
- **sodium salicylate.** (SO-dee-uhm) *USP 28.*
  Use: Analgesic; IV, gout.
  sodium salicylate combinations.
  See: Apcogesic.
    Bisalate.
    Bufosal.
    Corilin.
    Scot-Tussin Original Clear 5-Action Cold and Allergy Formula.
    Scot-Tussin Original 5-Action Cold and Allergy Formula.
    Tussirex.
    Tussirex Sugar Free.
  sodium salicylate, natural.
  Use: Analgesic.
  sodium secobarbital. Secobarbital Sodium, *USP.*
  Use: Hypnotic.
  sodium secobarbital and sodium amobarbital.
  Use: Sedative.
  See: Tuinal.
- **sodium starch glycolate.** (SO-dee-uhm) *NF 23.*
  Use: Pharmaceutic aid (tablet excipient).
- **sodium stearate.** (SO-dee-uhm) *NF 23.*
  Use: Pharmaceutic aid (emulsifying and stiffening agent).
- **sodium stearyl fumarate.** *NF 23.*
  Use: Pharmaceutic aid (tablet/capsule lubricant).
  sodium stibogluconate.
  Use: CDC anti-infective agent.

sodium succinate.
Use: Alkalinize urine & awaken patients following barbiturate anesthesia.
sodium sulamyd.
Use: Sulfonamide, ophthalmic.
See: Sodium Sulamyd.
Sodium Sulamyd Ophthalmic Oint.
10% Sterile. (Schering-Plough) Sulfacetamide sodium 10%. Ophth. Oint. Tube 3.5 g. *Rx.*
Use: Anti-infective, ophthalmic.
Sodium Sulamyd Ophthalmic Soln.
10% Sterile. (Schering-Plough) Sulfacetamide sodium 10%. Ophth. Soln. Bot. 5 mL, 15 mL. *Rx.*
Use: Anti-infective, ophthalmic.
Sodium Sulamyd Ophthalmic Soln.
30% Sterile. (Schering-Plough) Sulfacetamide sodium 30%. Ophth. Soln. Bot. 15 mL. Box 1s. *Rx.*
Use: Anti-infective, ophthalmic.
sodium sulfabromomethazine.
Use: Anti-infective.
sodium sulfacetamide.
See: Clenia.
Rosula NS.
Sulfacetamide Sodium.
W/Sulfur.
See: Plexion Cleansing Cloths.
Plexion TS.
Zetacet Wash.
sodium sulfadiazine.
See: Sulfadiazine Sodium.
sodium sulfamerazine.
See: Sulfamerazine Sodium.
sodium sulfapyridine.
See: Sulfapyridine Sodium.
•**sodium sulfate.** (SO-dee-uhm SULL-fate) *USP 28.*
Use: Calcium regulator.
•**sodium sulfate S 35.** (SO-dee-uhm SULL-fate) USAN.
Use: Radiopharmaceutical.
sodium sulfathiazole.
Use: Anti-infective.
See: Sulfathiazole Sodium.
•**sodium sulfide.** *USP 28.*
•**sodium sulfide gel.** *USP 28.*
sodium sulfoacetate.
See: Sebulex.
sodium sulfobromophthalein. Sulfobromophthalein Sodium, *USP.*
Use: Diagnostic aid (hepatic function determination).
sodium sulfocyanate.
See: Sodium Thiocyanate.
sodium sulfoxone. Sulfoxone Sodium, *USP.* Disodium sulfonyl-bis (p- phenyleneimino) dimethanesulfonate.

sodium suramin.
See: Suramin Sodium.
sodium taurocholate, a bile salt.
See: Bile Salts.
sodium tetradecyl sulfate.
Use: Sclerosing agent; bleeding esophageal varices. [Orphan Drug]
See: Sotradecol.
sodium tetraiodophenolphthalein.
See: Iodophthalein Sodium.
sodium thiamylal for injection. Thiamylal Sodium for Injection, *USP.*
Use: Anesthetic, general.
sodium thiocyanate. Sodium Sulfocyanate. Sodium Rhodanide.
sodium thiopental.
See: Thiopental Sodium.
•**sodium thiosulfate.** (SO-dee-uhm thigh-oh-SULL-fate) *USP 28.*
Use: For argyria, cyanide, and iodine poisoning; arsphenamine reactions; prevention of spread of ringworm of feet; antidote to cyanide poisoning.
W/Salicylic acid, hydrocortisone acetate, alcohol.
See: Tinver.
Versiclear.
W/Salicylic acid, resorcinol, alcohol.
See: Cyanide Antidote Pkg.
Mild Komed.
sodium thiosulfate. (American Regent) Sodium thiosulfate (as pentahydrate) 10% (100 mg/mL), 25% (250 mg/mL). Preservative-free. Inj. Single-dose vials. 10 ml (10% only), 50 mL (25% only). *Rx.*
Use: Antidote.
sodium l-thyroxine.
See: Synthroid.
sodium tolbutamide. Tolbutamide Sodium, *USP.*
Use: Diagnostic aid (diabetes).
sodium triclofos. (SO-dee-uhm TRY-kloe-foss) Sodium trichloroethylphosphate.
Use: Sedative; hypnotic.
•**sodium trimetaphosphate.** (SO-dee-uhm try-met-AH-FOSS-fate) USAN.
Use: Pharmaceutic aid.
sodium valproate.
See: Valproate Sodium.
sodium vinbarbital injection.
Use: Sedative.
sodium warfarin. Warfarin Sodium, *USP.*
Use: Anticoagulant.
Sod-Late 10. (Schlicksup) Sodium salicylate 10 g. Tab. Bot. 1000s. *OTC.*
Use: Analgesic.
Sodol Compound. (Major) Carisoprodol 200 mg, aspirin 325 mg. Tab. Bot. 100s, 500s. *Rx.*

Use: Muscle relaxant.

Sofcaps. (Alton) Docusate sodium 100 mg, 250 mg. Cap. Bot. 100s, 1000s. *OTC.*
Use: Laxative.

Sof-Lax. (Fleet) Docusate sodium 100 mg. Softgel Cap. 60s. *OTC.*
Use: Laxative.

Sof/Pro-Clean. (Sherman Pharmaceuticals, Inc.) Buffered, hypertonic solution with thimerosal 0.004%, EDTA 0.1%, ethylene and propylene oxide, octylphenoxypolyethoxyethanol, lauryl sulfate salt of imidazoline. Soln. Bot. 30 mL. *OTC.*
Use: Contact lens care.

Sof/Pro Clean SA. (Sherman Pharmaceuticals, Inc.) Hypertonic solution: salt buffers, copolymers of ethylene and propylene oxide, octylphenoxypolyethoxyethanol, lauryl sulfate salt of imidazoline, sodium bisulfite 0.1%, sorbic acid 0.1%, trisodium EDTA 0.25%, thimerosal free. Bot. 30 mL. *OTC.*
Use: Contact lens care.

Soft Mate Comfort Drops for Sensitive Eyes. (PBH Wesley Jessen) Borate buffered, potassium sorbate 0.13%, EDTA 0.1%, sodium Cl, hydroxyethylcellulose, octylphenoxyethanol. Drop. Bot. 15 mL. *OTC.*
Use: Contact lens care.

Soft Mate Consept 1. (PBH Wesley Jessen) Hydrogen peroxide 3% w/polyoxyl 40 stearate, sodium stannate, sodium nitrate, phosphate buffer. 240 mL. *OTC.*
Use: Contact lens care.

Soft Mate Consept 2. (PBH Wesley Jessen) **Soln:** Isotonic solution of sodium thiosulfate 0.5%, borate buffers, chlorhexidine gluconate 0.001%. Bot. 360 mL. **Spray:** Isotonic sodium thiosulfate 0.5%, borate buffers. Aer. 360 mL. *OTC.*
Use: Contact lens care.

Soft Mate Daily Cleaning for Sensitive Eyes. (PBH Wesley Jessen) Isotonic solution w/NaCl, octylphenoxy (oxyethylene) ethanol hydroxyethylcellulose w/potassium sorbate 0.13%, EDTA 0.2%. Soln. Bot. 1 mL, 30 mL. *OTC.*
Use: Contact lens care.

Soft Mate Daily Cleaning Solution. (PBH Wesley Jessen) Sterile aqueous isotonic solution w/sodium Cl, octylphenoxy (oxyethylene) ethanol, hydroxyethylcellulose, thimerosal 0.004%, edetate disodium 0.2%. Soln. Bot. 30 mL. *OTC.*
Use: Contact lens care.

Soft Mate Disinfecting Solution For Sensitive Eyes. (PBH Wesley Jessen) Sterile, aqueous, isotonic solution w/sodium Cl, povidone, octylphenoxy (oxyethylene) ethanol, chlorhexidine gluconate 0.005%, borate buffer, edetate disodium 0.1%. Thimerosal free. Soln. Bot. 240 mL. *OTC.*
Use: Contact lens care.

Soft Mate Disinfection and Storage Solution. (PBH Wesley Jessen) Sterile aqueous isotonic solution w/sodium Cl, povidone, octylphenoxl (oxyethylene) ethanol with a borate buffer, thimerosal 0.001%, edetate disodium 0.1%, chlorhexidine gluconate 0.005%. Soln. Bot. 8 oz. *OTC.*
Use: Contact lens care.

Soft Mate Enzyme Plus Cleaner. (PBH Wesley Jessen) Subtilisin, poloxamer 338, povidone, citric acid, potassium bicarbonate, sodium carbonate, sodium benzoate. Tab. Pkg. 8s. *OTC.*
Use: Contact lens care.

Soft Mate Lens Drops. (PBH Wesley Jessen) Sterile aqueous isotonic solution w/sodium Cl, potassium sorbate 0.13%, edetate disodium 0.025%. Thimerosal free. Drops. Bot. 2 oz. *OTC.*
Use: Contact lens care.

Soft Mate Preservative-Free Saline Solution. (PBH Wesley Jessen) Sterile aqueous isotonic solution w/sodium Cl, borate buffer. Contains no preservatives. Soln. Bot. 0.5 oz, 30 single use. *OTC.*
Use: Contact lens care.

Soft Mate PS Comfort Drops. (PBH Wesley Jessen) Sterile aqueous isotonic solution w/potassium sorbate 0.13%, edetate disodium 0.1%. Drops. Bot. 15 mL. *OTC.*
Use: Contact lens care.

Soft Mate PS Daily Cleaning Solution. (PBH Wesley Jessen) Sterile aqueous isotonic solution w/sodium Cl, octylphenoxy (oxyethylene)ethanol, hydroxyethyl cellulose, potassium sorbate 0.13%, edetate disodium 0.2%. Soln. Bot. 30 mL. *OTC.*
Use: Contact lens care.

Soft Mate PS Saline Solution. (PBH Wesley Jessen) Sterile aqueous isotonic solution w/sodium Cl, potassium sorbate 0.13%, edetate disodium 0.025%. Soln. Bot. 8 oz, 12 oz. *OTC.*
Use: Contact lens care.

Soft Mate Rinsing Solution. (PBH Wesley Jessen) Sterile aqueous isotonic solution w/sodium Cl, thimerosal 0.001%, edetate disodium 0.1%, chlorhexidine gluconate 0.005%. Soln. Bot. 8 oz.

OTC.
Use: Contact lens care.
Soft Mate Saline for Sensitive Eyes.
(PBH Wesley Jessen) Isotonic, sorbic acid 0.1%, EDTA 0.1%, NaCl, borate buffer. Soln. Bot. 360(2s), 480 mL. OTC.
Use: Contact lens care.
Soft Mate Saline Preservative-Free.
(PBH Wesley Jessen) Sodium Cl w/borate buffer. Soln. Bot. 15 mL. OTC.
Use: Contact lens care.
Soft Mate Saline Solution. (PBH Wesley Jessen) Sterile aqueous isotonic solution of sodium Cl. Preservative free. Soln. Bot. 8 oz, 12 oz. OTC.
Use: Contact lens care.
Soft Mate Soft Lens Cleaners. (PBH Wesley Jessen) Kit containing: Soft Mate daily cleaning solution II (4 oz); Soft Mate weekly cleaning solution (1.2 oz.); Hydra-Mat II cleaning and storage unit. OTC.
Use: Contact lens care.
Soft'n Soothe. (B.F. Ascher) Benzocaine, menthol, moisturizers. Tube 50 g. OTC.
Use: Anesthetic, local.
Soft Sense. (Bausch & Lomb) **Hand Lot.:** Petrolatum, vitamin E, aloe, parabens. Non-greasy. Bot. 444 mL. **Body Lot.:** Petrolatum, vitamin E, parabens. Non-greasy. Bot. 444 mL. OTC.
Use: Emollient.
SoftWear. (Ciba Vision) Isotonic, sodium Cl, boric acid, sodium borate, sodium perborate (generating up to 0.006% hydrogen peroxide stabilized with phosphoric acid). Soln. Bot. 120 mL, 240 mL, 360 mL. OTC.
Use: Contact lens care.
•**solabearon hydrochloride.** (soe-la-BEG-ron) USAN.
Use: Antidiabetic.
Solage. (Galderma) Mequinal 2%, tretinoin 0.01%, ethyl alcohol, EDTA. Top. Soln. 30 mL. Rx.
Use: Pigment agent.
Solaneed. (Hanlon) Vitamin A 25,000 units. Cap. Bot. 100s. Rx.
Use: Vitamin supplement.
Solaquin. (ICN) Hydroquinone 2% with sunscreens. Tube. 28.4 g. OTC.
Use: Dermatologic.
Solaquin Forte. (ICN) Hydroquinone 4%, dioxybenzone, padimate O, oxybenzone, EDTA, sodium metabisulfite, cetearyl alcohol, stearyl alcohol, lactic acid. **Cream:** Vanishing cream base. Tube. 28.4 g. **Gel:** Padimate O, dioxybenzone, EDTA, alcohol, sodium met-

bisulfite. Tube. 28.4g. Rx.
Use: Dermatologic.
Solar. (Doak Dermatologics) PABA, titanium dioxide, magnesium stearate in a flesh-colored, water-repellent base. Cream. Tube oz. OTC.
Use: Sunscreen.
Solaraze. (SkyePharma) Diclofenac sodium 3% (30 mg/g), benzyl alcohol. Gel. Tube. 25 g, 50 g. Rx.
Use: Keratolytic agent.
Solarcaine. (Schering-Plough) **Lot.:** Benzocaine, triclosan, mineral oil, alcohol, aloe extract, tocopheryl acetate, menthol, camphor, parabens, EDTA. 120 mL. **Spray (aerosol):** Benzocaine 20%, triclosan 0.13%, SD alcohol 40 35%, tocopheryl acetate. 90 mL, 120 mL. OTC.
Use: Anesthetic, local.
Solarcaine Aloe Extra Burn Relief. (Schering-Plough) **Cream:** Lidocaine 0.5%, aloe, EDTA, lanolin oil, lanolin, camphor, propylparaben, eucalyptus oil, menthol, tartrazine. 120 g. **Gel:** Lidocaine 0.5%, aloe vera gel, glycerin, EDTA, isopropyl alcohol, menthol, diazolidinyl urea, tartrazine. 120 g, 240 g. **Spray:** Lidocaine 0.5%, aloe vera gel, glycerin, EDTA, diazolidinyl urea, vitamin E, parabens. 135 mL. OTC.
Use: Anesthetic, local.
solargentum.
See: Mild Silver Protein.
Solar Shield 15 SPF. (Akorn) Ethylhexyl p-methoxy-cinnamate 7.5%, oxybenzone in a moisturizing base 5%, PABA free. Waterproof. Lot. Bot. 120 mL. OTC.
Use: Sunscreen.
Solar Shield 30 SPF. (Akorn) Ethylhexyl p-methoxycinnamate 7.5%, oxybenzone 6%, 2-ethylhexyl salicylate 5%, 3-diphenylacrylate 7.5%, 2-ethylhexyl-2-cyano-3 in a moisturizing base, PABA free. Waterproof. Lot. Bot. 120 mL. OTC.
Use: Sunscreen.
SolBar PF 15. (Person and Covey) Octyl methoxycinnamate 7.5%, oxybenzone 5%. SPF 15. Cream. Bot. 1 oz, 4 oz. OTC.
Use: Sunscreen.
SolBar PF 50. (Person and Covey) Oxybenzone, octyl methoxycinnamate, octocrylene, PABA free. Waterproof. SPF 50. Cream. Tube 120 g. OTC.
Use: Sunscreen.
SolBar PF Liquid. (Person and Covey) Octyl methoxycinnamate 7.5%, oxybenzone 6%, SD alcohol 40 76%, PABA

free. SPF 30. Liq. Bot. 120 mL. *OTC.*
Use: Sunscreen.
SolBar PF Paba Free 15. (Person and
Covey) Oxybenzone 5%, octyl me-
thoxycinnamate 7.5%. SPF 15. Cream.
Tube 2.5 oz. *OTC.*
Use: Sunscreen.
SolBar Plus 15. (Person and Covey)
Padimate 6%, oxybenzone 4%, dioxy-
benzone 2%. SPF 15. Cream. Tube
1 oz, 4 oz. *OTC.*
Use: Sunscreen.
Solex A15 Clear Lotion Sunscreen.
(Dermol Pharmaceuticals, Inc.) Octyl di-
methyl PABA 5%, benzophenone 33%,
SD alcohol. SPF 15. Lot. Bot. 120 mL.
OTC.
Use: Sunscreen.
Solfoton. (ECR) Phenobarbital 16 mg.
Tab. or Cap. Bot. 100s, 500s. *c-iv.*
Use: Hypnotic; sedative.
Solfoton S/C. (ECR) Phenobarbital
16 mg. SC Tab. Bot. 100s. *c-iv.*
Use: Hypnotic; sedative.
Solganal. (Schering-Plough) Aurothio-
glucose 50 mg/mL. Vial 10 mL. *Rx.*
Use: IM, gold therapy, antiarthritic.
Solia. (Prasco) Ethinyl estradiol 30 mcg,
desogestrel 0.15 mg. Lactose. Tab.
28s. *Rx.*
Use: Contraceptive hormone.
•**solifenacin succinate.** (sol-i-FEN-a-cin)
USAN.
Use: Overactive bladder.
See: Vesicare.
Soliwax. Docusate Sodium, *USP 25.*
Docusate Sodium, Solasulfone (I.N.N.).
Soltice Quick-Rub. (Chattem) Methyl sa-
licylate, camphor, menthol, eucalyptol.
Cream. Tube 1.33 oz, 3.75 oz. *OTC.*
Use: Analgesic, topical.
Solu-Barb 0.25. (Forest) Phenobarbital
0.25 g. Tab. Bot. 24s. *c-iv.*
Use: Hypnotic; sedative.
**soluble complement receptor
(recombinant human) type 1.**
Use: Prevention or reduction of adult
respiratory distress syndrome.
[Orphan Drug]
Solu-Cortef. (Pharmacia) **100 mg:**
Hydrocortisone sodium succinate,
w/benzyl alcohol. Plain vial, 5s, 25s.
100 mg/2 mL *Mix-O-Vial.* **250 mg:**
Hydrocortisone sodium succinate, benzyl alcohol. *Mix-O-Vial* 2 mL, 5s, 25s.
25-Pack, 25s, 50s. **500 mg:** Hydrocortisone sodium succinate, benzyl alcohol. *Mix-O-Vial,* 5s, 25s. **1000 mg:**
Hydrocortisone sodium succinate, benzyl alcohol. *Mix-O-Vial,* 5s, 25s. *Rx.*
Use: Corticosteroid.

Solu-Eze. (Forest) Hydroxyquinoline
0.12%, carbitol acetate 12.10%. Liq.
Bot. 3 oz. *Rx.*
Use: Dermatologic.
Solu-Medrol. (Pharmacia) **40 mg:**
Methylprednisolone sodium succinate,
benzyl alcohol. Univial 1 mL. **125 mg:**
Methylprednisolone sodium succinate,
benzyl alcohol. *Act-O-Vial* 2 mL, 5s,
25s. 25-Pack, 25s, 50s. **500 mg:**
Methylprednisolone sodium succinate,
benzyl alcohol. Vial 8 mL, vials w/di-
luent 8 mL. **1000 mg:** Methylprednisolone sodium succinate, benzyl alcohol. Vial 16 mL, vial w/diluent 16 mL.
2000 mg: Methylprednisolone sodium
succinate powder for injection, benzyl
alcohol. Vial 30.6 mL, vial w/diluent
30.6 mL. *Rx.*
Use: Corticosteroid.
Solumol. (C & M Pharmacal) Petrolatum, mineral oil, cetylstearyl alcohol, sodium lauryl sulfate, glycerin, propylene glycol, sorbic acid, purified water.
Jar lb. *OTC.*
Use: Pharmaceutical aid, ointment
base.
Solurex. (Hyrex) Dexamethasone sodium phosphate 4 mg/mL. Methyl- and
propylparabens, sodium bisulfite. Liq.
Vial 5 mL, 10 mL, 30 mL. *Rx.*
Use: Corticosteroid.
Solurex LA. (Hyrex) Dexamethasone
acetate 8 mg/mL w/polysorbate 80,
carboxymethylcellulose, sodium bisulfite, EDTA, benzyl alcohol. Susp. Vial
5 mL. *Rx.*
Use: Corticosteroid.
Soluvite C.T. (Pharmics) Vitamins A
2500 units, D 400 units, B_1 1.05 mg, B_2
1.2 mg, B_6 1.05 mg, B_{12} 4.5 mcg, C
60 mg, B_3 13.5 mg, E 15 units, fluoride
1 mg, folic acid 0.3 mg. Tab. Bot. 100s,
1000s. *Rx.*
Use: Mineral, vitamin supplement.
Soluvite-f. (Pharmics) Vitamins A
1500 units, D 400 units, C 35 mg, fluoride 0.25 mg/0.6 mL. Drops. Bot.
57 mL. *Rx.*
Use: Mineral, vitamin supplement.
Solvisyn-A. (Towne) Water-soluble vitamin A 10,000 units, 25,000 units,
50,000 units. Cap. Bot. 100s, 1000s.
Rx-OTC.
Use: Vitamin supplement.
•**solypertine tartrate.** (SAHL-ee-PURR-
teen) USAN.
Use: Antiadrenergic.
Soma. (Wallace) Carisoprodol 350 mg.
Tab. Bot. 100s, 500s, UD 500s. *Rx.*
Use: Muscle relaxant.

Soma Compound. (Wallace) Cariso-
prodol 200 mg, aspirin 325 mg. Tab.
Bot. 100s, 500s, UD 500s. *Rx.*
Use: Muscle relaxant.
Soma Compound w/Codeine. (Med-
pointe) Carisoprodol 200 mg, aspirin
325 mg, codeine phosphate 16 mg.
Tab. Sodium metabisulfite. Bot. 100s.
c-III.
Use: Muscle relaxant.
Somagard. (Roberts)
See: Deslorelin.
•**somantadine hydrochloride.** (sah-
MAN-tah-deen) USAN.
Use: Antiviral.
somatostatin.
Use: Digestive aid. [Orphan Drug]
See: Zecnil.
•**somatropin.** (OO muh TROE pin)
USAN. Growth hormone derived from
the anterior pituitary gland.
Use: Hormone, growth.
See: Genotropin.
  Genotropin MiniQuick.
  Humatrope.
  Norditropin.
  Nutropin.
  Nutropin AQ.
  Saizen.
  Serostim.
  Serostim LQ.
  Tev-Tropin.
  Zorbtive.
Somavert. (Pharmacia.) Pegvisomant
10 mg, 15 mg, 20 mg, mannitol 36 mg.
Pow. for Inj., lyophilized. Vials. Single-
dose. *Rx.*
Use: Acromegaly.
Sominex. (GlaxoSmithKline) Diphen-
hydramine hydrochloride. **Tab.:** 25 mg.
Blister pack 16s, 32s, 72s. **Capl.:**
50 mg. Blister pack 8s, 16s, 32s. *OTC.*
Use: Sleep aid.
Sominex Pain Relief Formula. (Glaxo-
SmithKline) Diphenhydramine hydro-
chloride 25 mg, acetaminophen
500 mg. Tab. Blister pack 16s. Bot. 32s.
OTC.
Use: Sleep aid; analgesic.
Somnote. (Breckenridge) Chloral hydrate
500 mg. Cap. 50s, UD 50s. *c-IV.*
Use: Sedative and hypnotic, nonbarbi-
turate.
Sonacide. (Wyeth) Potentiated acid
glutaraldehyde. Bot. 1 gal, 5 gal. *OTC.*
Use: Disinfectant; sterilizing agent.
Sonata. (King) Zaleplon 5 mg, 10 mg,
lactose, tartrazine. Cap. Bot. 100s. *c-IV.*
Use: Sedative; hypnotic.
Sonekap. (Eastwood) Cap. Bot. 100s.

soneryl.
See: Butethal.
SonoRx. (Bracco Diagnostics) Simethicone-coated cellulose 7.5 mg/mL, fructose, orange flavor. Susp. Glass bot.
400 mL. *Rx.*
Use: Diagnostic aid, gastrointestinal
function test.
Soothaderm. (Pharmakon) Pyrilamine
maleate 2.07 mg, benzocaine 2.08 mg,
zinc oxide 41.35 mg/mL, camphor,
menthol. Lot. Bot. 118 mL. *OTC.*
Use: Antihistamine; anesthetic, local.
Soothe. (Alcon) Tetrahydrozoline 0.05%,
benzalkonium Cl 0.004%, adsorbo-
base. Liq. Bot. 15 mL. *OTC.*
Use: Decongestant, ophthalmic.
Soothe. (Walgreen) Bismuth subsalicylate 100 mg. Tsp. Bot. 9 oz. *OTC.*
Use: Antidiarrheal.
•**soproxil.** USAN.
Use: Radical.
Soquette. (PBH Wesley Jessen) Polyvi-
nyl alcohol w/benzalkonium Cl 0.01%,
EDTA 0.2%. Bot. 4 fl oz. *OTC.*
Use: Contact lens care.
•**sorbic acid.** (SORE-bik) *NF 23.*
Use: Pharmaceutic aid (antimicrobial).
Sorbide T.D. (Merz) Isosorbide dinitrate
40 mg. TR Cap. Bot. 100s. *Rx.*
Use: Antianginal.
Sorbidon Hydrate. (Gordon Laborato-
ries) Water-in-oil ointment. Jar 2 oz,
0.5 oz, 1 lb, 5 lb. *OTC.*
Use: Emollient.
sorbimacrogol oleate 300.
See: Polysorbate 80.
•**sorbinil.** (SORE-bih-nill) USAN.
Use: Enzyme inhibitor (aldose reduc-
tase).
•**sorbitan monolaurate.** (SORE-bih-tan
MAHN-oh-LORE-ate) *NF 23.*
Use: Pharmaceutic aid (surfactant).
See: Span 20.
•**sorbitan monooleate.** (SORE-bih-tan
MAHN-oh-OH-lee-ate) *NF 23.*
Use: Pharmaceutic aid (surfactant).
See: Span 80.
**sorbitan monooleate polyoxyethylene
derivatives.**
See: Polysorbate 80.
•**sorbitan monopalmitate.** (SORE-bih-
tan MAHN-oh-PAL-mih-tate) *NF 23.*
Use: Pharmaceutic aid (surfactant).
See: Span 40.
•**sorbitan monostearate.** (SORE-bih-tan
MAHN-oh-STEE-ah-rate) *NF 23.*
Use: Pharmaceutic aid (surfactant).
See: Span 60.
sorbitans.
See: Polysorbate 80.

- **sorbitan sesquioleate.** (SORE-bih-tan SESS-kwih-OH-lee-ate) *NF 23.*
  Use: Pharmaceutic aid (surfactant).
  See: Arlacel C.
- **sorbitan trioleate.** (SORE-bih-tan TRY-OH-lee-ate) *NF 23.*
  Use: Pharmaceutic aid, surfactant.
  See: Span 85.
- **sorbitan tristearate.** (SORE-bih-tan TRY-STEE-ah-rate) USAN.
  Use: Pharmaceutic aid; surfactant.
  See: Span 65.
- **sorbitol.** *NF 23.*
  Use: Diuretic; dehydrating agent; humectant; pharmaceutic aid (sweetening agent, tablet excipient, flavor).
  See: Sorbo.
  W/Homatropine methylbromide.
  See: Probilagol.
  W/Mannitol.
  See: Sorbitol-mannitol Irrigation.
  Sorbitol-Mannitol. (Abbott) Mannitol 0.54 g, sorbitol 2.7 g. Liq. Bot. 100 mL, 1500 mL, 3000 mL. *Rx.*
  Use: Irrigant, genitourinary.
- **sorbitol solution.** *USP 28.*
  Use: Pharmaceutic aid (flavor, tablet excipient).
  Sorbo. (AstraZeneca) Sorbitol Solution, *USP 25.*
  Sorbsan. (Dow Hickam) Calcium alginate fiber 2 × 2, 3 × 3, 4 × 4, 4 × 8 inch. Box 1s. Wound packing fibers-calcium alginate fiber ¼ × 12 inch. Box 1s. *Rx.*
  Use: Dermatologic, wound therapy.
  sorethytan (20) monooleate.
  See: Polysorbate 80.
  Soriatane. (Connetics) Acitretin 10 mg, 25 mg. Capsule shells contain gelatin, iron oxide, titanium dioxide, may also contain benzyl alcohol. Cap. Bot. 30s. *Rx.*
  Use: Retinoid.
  Sosegon. (Sanofi-Synthelabo) Pentazocine. Soln., Susp., Tab. *c-iv.*
  Use: Analgesic.
  Soss-10. (Roberts) Sodium sulfacetamide 10%. Soln. Bot. 15 mL. *Rx.*
  Use: Anti-infective, ophthalmic.
- **sotalol hydrochloride.** (SOTT-uh-lahl) *USP 28.*
  Use: Antiadrenergic/sympatholytic, beta-adrenergic blocker.
  See: Betapace.
  Betapace AF.
  sotalol hydrochloride. (SOTT-uh-lahl) (Various Mfr.) Sotalol hydrochloride 80 mg, 120 mg, 160 mg, 240 mg, lactose. Tab. Bot. 100s, 500s, 1000s. *Rx.*

Use: Antiadrenergic/sympatholytic; beta-adrenergic blocker.
  sotalol hydrochloride AF. (Apotex) Sotalol hydrochloride 80 mg, 120 mg, 160 mg. Tab. 100s. *Rx.*
  Use: Beta-adrenergic blocking agent.
- **soterenol hydrochloride.** (so-TER-en-ole) USAN.
  Use: Bronchodilator.
  Sotradecol. (Bioniche Pharma) Sodium tetradecyl sulfate 10 mg/mL, 30 mg/mL. Benzyl alcohol 0.02 mL. Inj. Vials. 2 mL. *Rx.*
  Use: Sclerosing agent. [Orphan Drug]
  Sotret. (Ranbaxy) Isotretinion 10 mg, 20 mg, 30 mg, 40 mg. Parabens. Softgel Cap. 30s, 100s. *Rx.*
  Use: Retinoid.
  Soxa. (Vita Elixir) Sulfisoxazole 0.5 g. Tab. Bot. 100s, 1000s. *Rx.*
  Use: Anti-infective.
  Soxa-Forte. (Vita Elixir) Sulfisoxazole 0.5 g, phenazopyridine 50 mg. Tab. *Rx.*
  Use: Anti-infective.
  Soyalac. (Mt. Vernon Foods, Inc.) Infant formula based on an extract from whole soybeans containing all-essential nutrients. **Ready to Serve Liq.:** Can 32 fl oz. **Double Strength Conc.:** Can 13 fl oz. **Pow.:** Can 14 oz. *OTC.*
  Use: Nutritional supplement.
  Soyalac-I. (Mt. Vernon Foods, Inc.) Soy protein isolate infant formula containing no corn derivatives and a negligible amount of soy carbohydrates. Contains all essential nutrients in various forms. **Ready to Serve Liq.:** Can 32 fl oz. **Double Strength Conc.:** Can 13 fl oz. *OTC.*
  Use: Nutritional supplement.
  soya lecithin. Soybean extract. 100s.
  Use: Phosphorus therapy.
  See: Neo-Vadrin.
- **soybean oil.** *USP 28.*
  Use: Pharmaceutic aid.
  Spabelin. (Arcum) Hyoscyamine sulfate 81 mcg, atropine sulfate 15 mcg, scopolamine HBr 5 mcg, phenobarbital 16.2 mg/5 mL. Elix. Bot. 16 oz, gal. *Rx.*
  Use: Anticholinergic; antispasmodic; hypnotic; sedative.
  Spabelin No. 1. (Arcum) Phenobarbital 15 mg, belladonna powdered extract ⅛ g. Tab. Bot. 100s, 1000s. *Rx.*
  Use: Hypnotic; sedative.
  Spabelin No. 2. (Arcum) Phenobarbital 30 mg, belladonna powdered extract ⅛ g. Tab. Bot. 100s, 1000s. *Rx.*
  Use: Hypnotic; sedative.
  Span C. (Freeda) Citrus bioflavonoids 300 mg, vitamin C 200 mg. Tab. Bot.

100s, 250s, 500s. *OTC.*
Use: Vitamin supplement.
Span 80. (AstraZeneca) Sorbitan mono-oleate, *NF 20.*
Span 85. (AstraZeneca) Sorbitan triole-ate. Mixture of oleate esters of sorbi-tol and its anhydrides.
Use: Surface active agent.
Span 40. (AstraZeneca) Sorbitan Mono-palmitate, *NF 20.*
Span PD. (Lexis Laboratories) Phenter-mine hydrochloride 37.5 mg. Cap. Bot. 100s. *c-iv.*
Use: Anorexiant.
Span-RD. (Lexis Laboratories) d-meth-amphetamine hydrochloride 12 mg, dl-methamphetamine hydrochloride 6 mg, butabarbital 30 mg. Tab. Bot. 100s, 1000s. *c-iii.*
Use: Amphetamine; hypnotic; sedative.
Span 60. (AstraZeneca) Sorbitan Mono-stearate, *NF 20.*
Span 65. (AstraZeneca) Sorbitan tristea-rate. Mixture of stearate esters of sorbi-tol and its anhydrides.
Use: Surface active agent.
Span 20. (AstraZeneca) Sorbitan Mono-laurate, *NF 20.*
• **sparfloxacin.** (spar-FLOX-ah-sin) USAN.
Use: Anti-infective.
See: Zagam.
• **sparfosate sodium.** (spar-FOSS-ate) USAN.
Use: Antineoplastic.
Sparkles Effervescent Granules. (Lafayette) Sodium bicarbonate 2000 mg, citric acid 1500 mg, simethi-cone. Pkt. Bot. UD 50s. *OTC.*
Use: Antacid.
Sparkles Granules. (Lafayette) Efferves-cent granules 4 g/Packet or 6 g/Packet. Each 6 g produces 500 mL of carbon dioxide gas. Ctn. 25 packets. Pkg. 2.
Use: Diagnostic aid.
Sparkles Tablets. (Lafayette) Efferves-cent tablets. Each 4.3 g of tablets pro-duces 250 mL of carbon dioxide gas. Bot. 43 g (10 doses).
Use: Diagnostic aid.
• **sparsomycin.** (SPAR-so-MY-sin) USAN.
Use: Antineoplastic.
• **sparteine sulfate.** (SPAR-teh-een SULL-fate) USAN.
Use: Oxytocic.
W/Sodium Cl.
See: Tocosamine Sulfate.
Spasmatol. (Pharmed) Homatropine MBr 3 mg, pentobarbital 12 mg, mepho-barbital 8 mg. Tab. Bot. 100s, 1000s. *Rx.*

Use: Anticholinergic; antispasmodic; hypnotic; sedative.
Spasmolin. (Global Source) Phenobarbi-tal 16.2 mg, hyoscyamine sulfate 0.1037 mg, atropine sulfate 0.0194 mg, hyoscine HBr 0.0065 mg. Tab. Bot. 1000s. *Rx.*
Use: Anticholinergic; antispasmodic; hypnotic; sedative.
spasmolytic agents.
See: Antispasmodics.
Spasno-Lix. (Freeport) Phenobarbital 16.2 mg, hyoscyamine sulfate 0.1037 mg, atropine sulfate 0.0194 mg, hyoscine HBr 0.0065 mg, alcohol 21% to 23%/5 mL. Bot. 4 oz. *Rx.*
Use: Anticholinergic; antispasmodic; hypnotic; sedative.
S.P.B. (Sheryl) Therapeutic B complex formula with ascorbic acid 300 mg. Tab. Bot. 100s. *OTC.*
Use: Vitamin supplement.
SPD. (A.P.C.) Methyl salicylate, methyl nicotinate, dipropylene glycol salicy-late, oleoresin capsicum, camphor, menthol. Cream. Bot. 4 oz, Tube 1.5 oz. *OTC.*
Use: Analgesic, topical.
spearmint. *NF 23.*
Use: Flavor.
spearmint oil. *NF 23.*
Use: Flavor.
Special Shampoo. (Del-Ray) Non-medi-cated shampoo. *OTC.*
Use: Cleanser.
Spectazole. (Ortho Pharm Corp.) Econa-zole nitrate 1% in a water-miscible base, mineral oil. Cream. Tube 15 g, 30 g, 85 g. *Rx.*
Use: Antifungal, topical.
spectinomycin. (speck-TIN-oh-MY-sin) *Formerly Actinospectocin.* An antibi-otic isolated from broth cultures of *Streptomyces spectabilis. Rx.*
Use: Anti-infective.
See: Trobicin.
• **spectinomycin hydrochloride, sterile.** (speck-TIN-oh-MY-sin) *USP 28.*
Use: Anti-infective.
See: Trobicin.
Spectracef. (Purdue) Cefditoren pivoxil 200 mg, mannitol. Tab. Bot. 20s, 60s. *Rx.*
Use: Antibiotic, cephalosporin.
Spectra 360. (Parker) Salt-free electrode gel. Tube 8 oz.
Use: T.E.N.S. application, ECG pediat-ric, and long-term procedures.
Spectrobid. (Roerig) Bacampicill hydro-chloride 400 mg (equiv. to 280 mg ampicillin), lactose. Tab. 100s. *Rx.*

Use: Anti-infective, penicillin.

Spectro-Biotic. (A.P.C.) Bacitracin 400 units, neomycin sulfate 5 mg, polymyxin B sulfate 5000 units/g Oint. Tube 0.5 oz, 1 oz. *OTC.*
Use: Anti-infective, topical.

Spectro-Jel. (Recsei) Soap free. Iodomethylcellulose, carboxypolymethylene, cetyl alcohol, sorbitan monooleate, fumed silica, triethanolamine stearate, glycol polysiloxane, propylene glycol, glycerin, isopropyl alcohol 5%. Gel. Bot. 127.5 mL, pt, gal. *OTC.*
Use: Dermatologic, cleanser.

Spec-T Sore Throat Anesthetic. (Apothecon) Benzocaine 10 mg. Loz. Box 10s. *OTC.*
Use: Anesthetic, local.

spermaceti.
Use: Stiffening agent; pharmaceutic necessity for cold cream.

spermine. Diaminopropyltetramethylene.

Sperti. (Whitehall-Robins) Live yeast cell derivative supplying 2000 units skin respiratory factor/g w/shark liver oil 3%, phenylmercuric nitrate 1:10,000. Oint. Tube oz. *OTC.*
Use: Dermatologic, wound therapy.

Spherulin. (ALK) Coccidioidin: 1:100 equivalent, Vial 1 mL, 1:10 equivalent, Vial 0.5 mL. *Rx.*
Use: Diagnostic aid, skin test.

spider-bite antivenin.
See: Antivenin, Latrodectus Mactans.

Spider-Man Children's Chewable Vitamin. (NBTY) Vitamins A 2500 units, D 400 units, E 15 mg, B_1 1.05 mg, B_2 1.2 mg, B_3 13.5 mg, B_6 1.05 mg, B_{12} 4.5 mcg, C 60 mg, folic acid 0.3 mg, xylitol, sorbitol. Chew. Tab. Bot. 75s, 130s. *OTC.*
Use: Vitamin supplement.

• **spiperone.** (spih-per-OHN) USAN.
Use: Antipsychotic.

• **spiradoline mesylate.** (spy-RAH-doe-leen) USAN.
Use: Analgesic.

• **spiramycin.** (SPIH-rah-MY-sin) USAN. Antibiotic substance from cultures of *Streptomyces ambofaciens.*
Use: Anti-infective.

• **spiraprilat.** (SPY-rah-PRILL-at) USAN.
Use: ACE inhibitor.

• **spirapril hydrochloride.** (SPY-rah-prill) USAN.
Use: ACE inhibitor.
See: Renormax.

Spiriva. (Boehringer Ingelheim) Tiotropium bromide 18 mcg (as base). Pow. for Inh. Blister packs containing 6 capsules with inhaler. *Rx.*
Use: Bronchodilator, anticholinergic.

• **spirogermanium hydrochloride.** (SPY-row-JER-MAY-nee-uhm) USAN.
Use: Antineoplastic.

• **spiromustine.** (SPY-row-MUSS-teen) USAN. *Formerly spirohydantoin mustard.*
Use: Antineoplastic.

spironazide. (Schein) Spironolactone 25 mg, hydrochlorothiazide 25 mg. Tab. Bot. 100s, 1000s, UD 100s. *Rx.*
Use: Diuretic combination.

• **spironolactone.** (SPEER-oh-no-LAK-tone) *USP 28.*
Use: Diuretic, aldosterone antagonist.
See: Aldactone.
W/Hydrochlorothiazide.
See: Aldactazide.

spironolactone. (Various Mfr.) Spironolactone 50 mg, 100 mg. May contain lactose. Tab. 50s, 100s, 250s, 500s, 1,000s, UD 30s, UD 60s. *Rx.*
Use: Diuretic.

spironolactone w/hydrochlorothiazide. (Various Mfr.) Spironolactone 25 mg, hydrochlorothiazide 25 mg. Tab. Bot. 30s, 60s, 100s, 250s, 500s, 1000s, UD 32s, 100s. *Rx.*
Use: Diuretic combination.

spiropitan. (SPY-row-PLAT-in) (Janssen) Spiperone. *Rx.*
Use: Antipsychotic.

• **spiroplatin.** (SPY-row-PLAT-in) USAN.
Use: Antineoplastic.

spirotriazine hydrochloride.
Use: Anthelmintic.

• **spiroxasone.** (spy-ROX-ah-sone) USAN.
Use: Diuretic.

Spirozide. (Rugby) Spironolactone 25 mg, hydrochlorothiazide 25 mg. Tab. Bot. 100s, 500s, 1000s. *Rx.*
Use: Diuretic combination.

SPL-Serologic Types I and III. (Delmont) *Staphylococcus aureus* 120 to 180 million units, *staphylococcus bacteriophage* plaque-forming 100 to 1000 million units/mL. Soln. Amp. 1 mL, Vial 10 mL. *Rx.*
Use: Anti-infective.

Sporanox. (Janssen) Itraconazole 100 mg, sucrose, sugar. Bot. 30s, UD 30s, *PulsePak* 28s. *Rx.*
Use: Antifungal, triazole.

Sporanox. (Ortho Biotech) **Oral Soln.:** 10 mg/mL, saccharin, sorbitol, cherry/caramel flavor. Bot. 150 mL. **Inj.:** 10 mg/mL. Kit. Amp 25 mL, NaCl 0.9% bag 50 mL, filtered infusion set 1. *Rx.*
Use: Antifungal, triazole.

Sportscreme. (Thompson Medical) Triethanolamine salicylate 10% in a nongreasy base. Cream. 37.5 g, 90 g. *OTC.*
Use: Analgesic, topical.

Sports Spray Extra Strength. (Mentholatum Co.) Methyl salicylate 35%, menthol 10%, camphor 5%, alcohol 58%, isobutane. Spray. 90 mL. *OTC.*
Use: Analgesic, topical.

Spray Skin Protectant. (Morton International) Isopropyl alcohol, polyvinylpyrrolidone, vinyl alcohol, plasticizer & propellant. Aer. Can 6 oz. *OTC.*
Use: Dermatologic, protectant.

spreading factor.
See: Hyaluronidase.

Sprintec. (Barr) Norgestimate 0.25 mg, ethinyl estradiol 35 mcg, lactose. Tab. 20s. *Rx.*
Use: Sex hormone, contraceptive hormone.

• **sprodiamide.** (sprah-DIE-ah-mide) USAN.
Use: Diagnostic aid (paramagnetic).

SPRX-105. (Reid-Provident) Phendimetrazine tartrate 105 mg. SR Cap. Bot. 28s, 500s. *c-III.*
Use: Anorexiant.

SPS. (Carolina Medical Products) Sodium polystyrene sulfonate 15 g, sorbitol solution 21.5 mL, alcohol 0.3%/60 mL, propylene glycol, sodium saccharin, methylparaben, propylparaben, cherry flavor. Susp. Bot. 120 mL, 480 mL, UD 60 mL. *Rx.*
Use: Potassium-removing resin.

• **squalamine lactate.** (SKWAH-la-meen) USAN.
Use: Antineoplastic.

• **squalane.** (SKWAH-lane) *NF 23.*
Use: Pharmaceutic aid (vehicle, oleaginous).

SRC Expectorant. (Edwards) Hydrocodone bitartrate 5 mg, pseudoephedrine hydrochloride 60 mg, guaifenesin 200 mg w/alcohol 12.5%. Bot. Pt. *c-III.*
Use: Antitussive; decongestant; expectorant.

SSD. (Knoll) Silver sulfadiazine 1%. Cream. Jar 50 g, 85 g, 400 g, 1000 g. Tube 25 g. *Rx.*
Use: Burn therapy.

SSD AF. (Knoll) Silver sulfadiazine 1% in a cream base containing white petrolatum, stearyl alcohol, isopropyl myristate, sorbitan monooleate, polyoxyl 40 stearate, sodium hydroxide, propylene glycol, methylparaben 3%. Cream. Tube 50 g, 400 g, 1000 g. *Rx.*
Use: Burn therapy.

SSKI. (Upsher-Smith) Potassium iodide 300 mg/0.3 mL. Soln. Dropper Bot. 1 oz, 8 oz.
Use: Expectorant.

S-Spas. (Southern States) Pentobarbital 16.2 mg, atropine sulfate 0.0194 mg, hyoscyamine sulfate 0.1037 mg, hyoscine HBr 0.0065 mg. **Liq.:** 5 mL. Bot. Pt. **Tab.:** Bot. 100s, 1000s. *Rx.*
Use: Anticholinergic; antispasmodic; hypnotic; sedative.

S.S.S. High Potency Vitamin. (S.S.S. Company) Vitamins C 300 mg, B_1 7.5 mg, B_2 7.5 mg, B_3 50 mg, Ca 100 mg, Fe 27 mg, E 50 units, B_6 2.5 mg, folic acid 200 mcg, B_{12} 12.5 mg, Mg 50 mg, Zn 12 mg, Cu 1.5 mg, biotin 22.5 mcg, pantothenic acid 10 mg. Tab. Bot. 20s, 40s, 80s. *OTC.*
Use: Vitamin, mineral supplement.

S.S.S. Vitamin and Mineral Supplement. (S.S.S. Company) Vitamins A 833 units, C 20 mg, E 10 units, B_1 1.7 mg, B_2 0.57 mg, niacinamide 6.7 mg, B_6 0.67 mg, B_{12} 2 mcg, D_3 133 units, biotin 100 mcg, pantothenic acid 3 mg, I 50 mcg, Fe 3 mg, Zn 1 mg, Ma 0.8 mg, Cr 8 mcg, Mo 8 mcg/5 mL, alcohol 6.6%, sugar. Liq. Bot. 236 mL. *OTC.*
Use: Vitamin, mineral supplement.

Stadol. (Bristol-Myers Squibb) Butorphanol tartrate 1 mg/mL; Vial 1 mL. 2 mg/mL; Vial 1 mL, 2 mL, 10 mL (with benzethonium chloride 0.1 mg/mL). *c-IV.*
Use: Analgesic.

Staftabs. (Modern Aids Inc.) Fine bone flour containing calcium, phosphorus, iron, iodine, vitamin D, magnesium. Tab. Bot. 85s, 160s. *OTC.*
Use: Mineral, vitamin supplement.

Stagesic. (Huckaby Pharmacal) Hydrocodone bitartrate 5 mg, acetaminophen 500 mg. Cap. Bot. 100s. *c-III.*
Use: Analgesic combination, narcotic.

Stahist. (Huckaby Pharmacal) Phenylephrine hydrochloride 25 mg, chlorpheniramine maleate 8 mg, hyoscyamine sulfate 0.19 mg, atropine sulfate 0.04 mg, scopolamine HBr 0.01 mg, pseudoephedrine 40 mg, dye free. SR Tab. Bot. 100s. *Rx.*
Use: Upper respiratory combination, antihistamine, anticholinergic, decongestant.

stainless iodized ointment. (Day-Baldwin) Jar lb.

stainless iodized ointment with methyl salicylate 5%. (Day-Baldwin) Jar lb.

Stalevo 50. (Novartis) Carbidopa 12.5 mg, levodopa 50 mg, entacapone 200 mg, mannitol, sucrose. Tab. 100s, 250s. *Rx.*
Use: Antiparkinson agent.

Stalevo 100. (Novartis) Carbidopa 25 mg, levodopa 100 mg, entacapone 200 mg, mannitol, sucrose. Tab. 100s, 250s. *Rx.*
Use: Antiparkinson agent.

Stalevo 150. (Novartis) Carbidopa 37.5 mg, levodopa 150 mg, entacapone 200 mg, mannitol, sucrose. Tab. 100s, 250s. *Rx.*
Use: Antiparkinson agents.

•**stallimycin hydrochloride.** (stal-IH-MY-sin) USAN.
Use: Anti-infective.

Stamoist E. (Huckaby Pharmacal) Pseudoephedrine hydrochloride 120 mg, guaifenesin 500 mg. SR Tab. Bot. 100s. *Rx.*
Use: Upper respiratory combination, decongestant, expectorant.

Stamyl. (Sanofi-Synthelabo) Pancreatin. Tab.
Use: Digestive aid.

•**stannous chloride.** (STAN-uhs KLOR-ide) USAN.
Use: Pharmaceutic aid.

•**stannous fluoride.** (STAN-uhs FLOR-ide) *USP 28.*
Use: Dental caries agent.
See: PerioMed.

stannous fluoride. (Cypress) **Gel:** Stannous fluoride 0.4%, parabens, mint flavor. Tube 122 g. **Conc. Oral Rinse:** Stannous fluoride 0.63%, mint flavor. Bot. 283 g. *Rx-OTC.*
Use: Trace element.

•**stannous pyrophosphate.** (STAN-uhs PIE-row-FOSS-fate) USAN.
Use: Diagnostic aid (skeletal imaging).

•**stannous sulfur colloid.** (STAN-uhs SULL-fer KAHL-oyd) USAN.
Use: Diagnostic aid (bone, liver, and spleen imaging).

staphage lysate (SPL).
Use: Anti-infective.
See: SPL-Serologic Types I and III.

staphylococcus bacteriophage lysate.
See: Staphage Lysate.

staphylococcus test.
See: Isocult for *Staphylococcus Aureus.*

•**starch.** *NF 23.*
Use: Dusting powder; pharmaceutic aid.

starch glycerite.
Use: Emollient.

•**starch, pregelatinized.** *NF 23.*
Use: Pharmaceutic aid (tablet excipient).

•**starch, topical.** *USP 28.*
Use: Dusting powder.

Starlix. (Novartis) Nateglinide 60 mg, 120 mg. Lactose. Tab. Bot. 100s, 500s. *Rx.*
Use: Antidiabetic, meglitinide.

Star-Otic. (Star) Burrows soln. 10%, acetic acid 1%, boric acid 1%. Drop Bot. 15 mL. *OTC.*
Use: Otic.

•**statolon.** (STAY-toe-lone) USAN. Antiviral agent derived from *Penicillium stoloniferum.*
Use: Antiviral.

Statomin Maleate II. (Jones Pharma) Chlorpheniramine maleate 2 mg, acetaminophen 324 mg, caffeine 32 mg. Tab. Bot. 1000s. *Rx.*
Use: Antihistamine; analgesic.

Statuss Green. (Huckaby Pharmacal) Phenylephrine hydrochloride 5 mg, pyrilamine maleate 3.3 mg, hydrocodone bitartrate 2.5 mg, chlorpheniramine maleate 2 mg, pseudoephedrine hydrochloride 3.3 mg/5 mL, alcohol free. Liq. Bot. 473 mL. *c-III.*
Use: Upper respiratory combination, antihistamine, antitussive, decongestant.

•**stavudine.** (STAHV-you-deen) USAN.
Use: Antiretroviral.
See: Zerit.
Zerit XR.

Sta-Wake Dextabs. (Health for Life Brands) Caffeine 1.5 g, dextrose 3 g. Tab. Bot. 36s, 1000s. *OTC.*
Use: CNS stimulant.

Stay Alert. (Apothecary Prods.) Caffeine 200 mg. Tab. Bot. 24s, 48s. *OTC.*
Use: CNS stimulant

Stay Awake. (Major) Caffeine 200 mg, dextrose. Tab. Bot. 16s. *OTC.*
Use: CNS stimulant, analeptic.

Stay-Brite. (Sherman Pharmaceuticals, Inc.) EDTA 0.25%, benzalkonium Cl 0.01%. Spray. Bot. 30 mL. *OTC.*
Use: Contact lens care.

Stay Moist Lip Conditioner. Padimate O, oxybenzone, aloe vera, vitamin E, tropical fruit flavor. SPF 15. Lip Balm 48 g. *OTC.*
Use: Emollient.

Stay-Wet. (Sherman Pharmaceuticals, Inc.) Polyvinyl alcohol, hydroxyethylcellulose, povidone, sodium Cl, potassium Cl, sodium carbonate, benzalkonium Cl 0.01%, EDTA 0.025%. Soln. Bot. 30 mL. *OTC.*
Use: Contact lens care.

Stay-Wet 4. (Sherman Pharmaceuticals, Inc.) Benzyl alcohol 0.15%, EDTA

0.1%, NaCl, KCl, polyvinyl alcohol, hydroxyethyl cellulose. Thimerosal free. Soln. 30 mL. *OTC.*
Use: Contact lens care (RGP lenses).
Stay-Wet Rewetting. (Sherman Pharmaceuticals, Inc.) Polyvinyl alcohol, hydroxyethycellulose, povidone, NaCl, KCl, sodium carbonate, benzalkonium Cl 0.01%, EDTA 0.025%. Soln. Bot. *OTC.*
Use: Lubricant-ophthalmic.
Stay-Wet 3. (Sherman Pharmaceuticals, Inc.) Sodium and potassium Cl salts containing polyvinyl pyrrolidone, polyvinyl alcohol, hydroxyethylcellulose, sodium bisulfite 0.02%, benzyl alcohol 0.1%, sorbic acid 0.05%, EDTA 0.1%. Soln. 30 mL. *OTC.*
Use: Lubricant, ophthalmic.
Stay-Wet 3 Wetting. (Sherman Pharmaceuticals, Inc.) Polyvinyl alcohol, hydroxyethycellulose, povidone, sodium Cl, potassium Cl, sodium carbonate, benzalkonium Cl 0.01%, EDTA 0.025%. Soln. 30 mL. *OTC.*
Use: Lubricant, ophthalmic.
Staze. (Del) Karaya gum. Tube 1.75 oz, 3.5 oz. *OTC.*
Use: Denture adhesive.
S-T Cort Cream. (Scot-Tussin) Hydrocortisone 0.5%, water-washable base, parabens. 120 g. *Rx.*
Use: Corticosteroid, topical.
S-T Cort Lotion. (Scot-Tussin) Hydrocortisone 0.5%, water-washable, lanolin alcohol, mineral oil base. 60 mL, 120 mL. *Rx.*
Use: Corticosteroid, topical.
● **stearic acid.** (STEER-ik) *NF 23.* Octadecanoic acid.
Use: Pharmaceutic aid (emulsion adjunct, tablet/capsule lubricant).
● **stearyl alcohol.** (STEE-rill AL-koe-hahl) *NF 23.*
Use: Pharmaceutic aid (emulsion adjunct).
● **steffimycin.** (steh-fih-MY-sin) USAN.
Use: Anti-infective; antiviral.
● **stenbolone acetate.** (STEEN-bow-lone) USAN.
Use: Anabolic.
Steraject. (Merz) Prednisolone acetate 25 mg, 50 mg/mL. Inj. Vial 10 mL. *Rx.*
Use: Corticosteroid.
Sterapred. (Merz) Prednisone 5 mg. Tab. *Uni-Pak* 21s. Sterapred 12 day in *Uni-Pak* 48s. *Rx.*
Use: Corticosteroid
Sterapred DS. (Merz) Prednisone 10 mg. Tab. *Uni-pak* 21s. Sterapred DS 12 day

in *Uni-Pak* 48s. Sterapred DS 14 day in *Uni-Pak* 49s. *Rx.*
Use: Corticosteroid.
Sterapred-Unipak. (Merz) Prednisone 5 mg. Tab. Dosepak 21s. *Rx.*
Use: Corticosteroid.
sterculia gum.
See: Karaya Gum.
W/Vitamin B$_1$.
See: Imbicoll W/Vitamin B$_1$.
Stericol. (Alton) Isopropyl alcohol 91%. Soln. Bot. 16 oz, 32 oz, gal. *OTC.*
Use: Anti-infective, topical.
sterile aurothioglucose suspension. Aurothioglucose Injection. Gold thioglucose.
Use: Antirheumatic.
See: Solganal.
sterile erythromycin gluceptate. Erythromycin monoglucoheptonate (salt). Erythromycin glucoheptonate (1:1) (salt).
Use: Anti-infective.
Sterile Lens Lubricant. (Blairex) Isotonic w/borate buffer system, sodium Cl, hydroxypropyl methylcellulose, glycerin, sorbic acid 0.25%, EDTA 0.1%, thimerosal free. Soln. Bot. 15 mL. *OTC.*
Use: Lubricant, ophthalmic.
Sterile Saline. (Bausch & Lomb) Sodium Cl, borate buffer, EDTA, thimerosal free. Soln. Bot. 60 mL. *OTC.*
Use: Lubricant, ophthalmic.
Sterile Talc Powder. (Bryan) Talc 5 g. Pow. Glass Bot. 100 mL. *Rx.*
Use: Antineoplastic.
sterile thiopental sodium. Thiopental sodium, *USP 25.*
See: Pentothal Sodium.
sterile water for irrigation. (Various Mfr.) Sterile water for irrigation 0.45%, 0.9%. Soln. Bot. 150 mL, 250 mL, 500 mL, 1000 mL, 1500 mL, 2000 mL, 4000 mL. *Rx.*
Use: Irrigant, genitourinary.
Steri-Unna Boot. (Pedinol Pharmacal) Glycerin, gum acacia, zinc oxide, white petrolatum, amylum in an oil base. 10 yds. × 3.5 in. sterilized bandage.
Use: Treatment of leg ulcers, varicosities, sprains, strains & to reduce swelling after surgery.
steroid antibiotic combinations.
Use: Anti-inflammatory.
See: AK-Trol.
    Cortisporin.
    Dexacidin.
    Maxitrol.
    NeoDecadron.
    Neo-Dexameth.
    Neomycin and Polymyxin B Sulfates and Dexamethasone.

Poly-Pred Liquifilm.
Pred-G.
TobraDex.
S-T Forte 2. (Scot-Tussin) Hydrocodone
bitartrate 2.5 mg, chlorpheniramine
maleate 2 mg/5 mL, menthol, parabens,
alcohol and dye free. Liq. Bot. 473 mL,
3.8 L. *c-III.*
Use: Upper respiratory combination,
antitussive, antihistamine.
stilbamidine isethionate.
Use: Antiprotozoal.
•**stilbazium iodide.** (still-BAY-zee-uhm
EYE-oh-dide) USAN.
Use: Anthelmintic.
stilbestrol.
See: Diethylstilbestrol.
stilbestronate.
See: Diethylstilbestrol Dipropionate.
stilboestrol.
See: Diethylstilbestrol.
Stilboestrol DP.
See: Diethylstilbestrol Dipropionate.
•**stilonium iodide.** (STILL-oh-nee-uhm
EYE-oh-dide) USAN.
Use: Antispasmodic.
Stilronate.
See: Diethylstilbestrol Dipropionate.
Stimate. (Aventis Behring) Desmopressin
acetate 1.5 mg, chlorobutanol 5 mg, so-
dium Cl 9 mg/mL. Nasal Soln. Bot.
2.5 mL (25 doses of 150 mcg each).
Rx.
Use: Hormone.
stimulant laxatives.
See: Agoral.
Aromatic Cascara Fluidextract.
Bisac-Evac.
Bisacodyl.
Bisacodyl Uniserts.
Black Draught.
Caroid.
Cascara Aromatic.
Cascara Sagrada.
Correctol.
Dulcolax.
ex•lax.
ex•lax chocolated.
Feen-a-mint.
Fleet Laxative.
Fletcher's Castoria.
Maximum Relief ex•lax.
Modane.
Reliable Gentle Laxative.
Senexon.
Senna-Gen.
Sennosides.
Senokot.
SenokotXTRA.
Woman's Gentle Laxative.

Sting-Eze. (Wisconsin Pharmacal Co.)
Diphenhydramine hydrochloride, cam-
phor, phenol, benzocaine, eucalyptol.
Liq. Bot. 15 mL. *OTC.*
Use: Antihistamine, topical.
•**stinging nettle.** *USP 28.*
Use: Dietary supplement.
Sting-Kill. (Milance Laboratories, Inc.)
Benzocaine 18.9%, menthol 0.9%.
Swab 14 mL, 0.5 mL (5s). *OTC.*
Use: Anesthetic, local.
•**stiripentol.** (STY-rih-PEN-tole) USAN.
Use: Anticonvulsant.
•**St. John's wort, powdered extract.**
USP 28.
Use: Dietary supplement.
St. Joseph Adult Chewable Aspirin.
(Schering-Plough) Aspirin 81 mg, sac-
charin. Chew. Tab. Bot. 36s. *OTC.*
Use: Analgesic.
St. Joseph Aspirin for Adults. (Scher-
ing-Plough) Aspirin 5 g. Tab. Bot. 36s,
100s, 200s. *OTC.*
Use: Analgesic.
**St. Joseph Aspirin-Free Elixir for Chil-
dren.** (Schering-Plough) Acetamino-
phen 160 mg/5 mL. Alcohol free. Elix.
Bot. 2 oz, 4 oz. *OTC.*
Use: Analgesic.
**St. Joseph Aspirin-Free for Children
Chewable.** (Schering-Plough) Aceta-
minophen 80 mg, fruit flavor. Chew.
Tab. Bot. 30s. *OTC.*
Use: Analgesic.
St. Joseph Aspirin-Free Infant. (Scher-
ing-Plough) Acetaminophen 100 mg/
mL. Aspirin and sugar free. Drops. Bot.
w/dropper. 0.5 oz. *OTC.*
Use: Analgesic.
**St. Joseph Aspirin-Free Tablets for
Children.** (Schering-Plough) Aceta-
minophen 80 mg. Tab. Bot. 30s.
Use: Analgesic.
St. Joseph Cough Suppressant. (Sch-
ering-Plough) Dextromethorphan HBr
7.5 mg/5 mL, alcohol free, sucrose,
cherry flavor. Liq. Bot. 60 mL, 120 mL.
OTC.
Use: Antitussive.
St. Joseph Cough Syrup for Children.
(Schering-Plough) Dextromethorphan
HBr 7.5 mg/5 mL. Syr. Bot. 2 oz, 4 oz.
OTC.
Use: Antitussive.
Stomal. (Foy Laboratories) Phenobarbi-
tal 16.2 mg, hyoscyamine sulfate
0.1037 mg, atropine sulfate 0.0194 mg,
scopolamine HBr 0.0065 mg. Tab. Bot.
1000s. *Rx.*
Use: Anticholinergic; antispasmodic;
hypnotic; sedative.

Stool Softener. (Apothecary Prods.) Docusate calcium 240 mg. Cap. Bot. 50s. *OTC.*
Use: Laxative.
Stool Softener. (Rugby) Docusate sodium. **Cap.**: 100 mg, 250 mg lactose, tartrazine. Bot. 1000s. **Soft gel Cap.**: 250 mg, sorbitol, parabens. Bot. 100s, 1000s. *OTC.*
Use: Laxative.
Stool Softener DC. (Rugby) Docusate calcium 240 mg, sorbitol, parabens. Cap. Bot. 100s, 500s, 1000s. *OTC.*
Use: Laxative.
Stop. (Oral-B) Stannous fluoride 0.4%. Tube 2 oz. *Rx.*
Use: Dental caries agent.
Stopayne Capsules. (Springbok) Codeine phosphate 30 mg, acetaminophen 357 mg. Cap. Bot. 100s, 500s, UD 100s. *c-iii.*
Use: Analgesic; antitussive.
Stopayne Syrup. (Springbok) Acetaminophen 120 mg, codeine phosphate 12 mg/5 mL. Syr. Bot. 4 oz, 16 oz. *c-v.*
Use: Analgesic; antitussive.
Stop-Zit. (Purepac) Denatonium benzoate in a clear nail polish base. Bot. 0.75 oz. *OTC.*
Use: Nail-biting deterrent.
•**storax.** (STORE-ax) *USP 28.*
Use: Pharmaceutic necessity for benzoin tincture compound.
Stovarsol.
Use: Trichomonas vaginalis vaginitis; amebiasis; Vincent's angina.
See: Acetarsone.
Strattera. (Eli Lilly) Atomoxetine hydrochloride 10 mg, 18 mg, 25 mg, 40 mg, 60 mg. Cap. Bot. 30s. *Rx.*
Use: Psychotherapeutic agent.
Strema. (Foy Laboratories) Quinine sulfate 260 mg. Cap. Bot. 100s, 500s, 1000s.
Use: Antimalarial.
Stren-Tab. (Barth's) Vitamins C 300 mg, B_1 10 mg, B_2 10 mg, niacin 33 mg, B_6 2 mg, pantothenic acid 20 mg, B_{12} 4 mcg. Tab. Bot. 100s, 300s, 500s. *OTC.*
Use: Vitamin supplement.
Streptase. (Aventis Behring) Streptokinase 250,000 units, 750,000 units, 1,500,000 units, cross-linked gelatin polypeptides 25 mg, sodium l-glutamate 25 mg, human albumin 100 mg, preservative free. Pow. for Inj., lyophilized. Vial 6 mL, Infusion Bot. 50 mL (1,500,000 units only). *Rx.*
Use: Thrombolytic.
streptococcus immune globulin group B.

Use: Immunization. [Orphan Drug]
streptokinase.
Use: Thrombolytic.
See: Streptase.
Streptolysin O Test. (Laboratory Diagnostics) Reagent 6 x 10 mL, buffer 6 x 40 mL, Control Serum, 6 x 10 mL, or Kit.
Use: Diagnosis of "group A" streptococcal infections.
streptomycin calcium chloride. Streptomycin Calcium Chloride Complex.
•**streptomycin sulfate.**
Use: Antituberculosis agent.
streptomycin sulfate. (Pharma-Tek) Streptomycin sulfate 1 g. Cake, lyophilized. Vial. *Rx.*
Use: Antituberculosis agent.
Streptonase B. (Wampole) Tube test for determination of streptococcal infection by serum DNase-B antibodies. Kit 1.
Use: Diagnostic aid.
•**streptonicozid.** (STREP-toe-nih-KOE-zid) USAN.
Use: Anti-infective.
•**streptonigrin.** (strep-toe-NYE-grin) USAN. Antibiotic isolated from both filtrates of *Streptomyces flocculus.*
Use: Antineoplastic.
See: Nigrin.
streptovaricin. An antibiotic composed of several related components derived from cultures of *Streptomyces variabilis.*
•**streptozocin.** (STREP-toe-ZOE-sin) USAN.
Use: Antineoplastic.
See: Zanosar.
Streptozyme. (Wampole) Rapid hemagglutination slide test for the qualitative detection and quantitative determination of streptococcal extracellular antigens in serum, plasma, and peripheral blood. Kit 15s, 50s, 150s.
Use: Diagnostic aid, streptococcus.
Stress B-Complex. (H.L. Moore Drug Exchange) Vitamins E 30 units, B_1 15 mg, B_2 15 mg, B_3 100 mg, B_5 20 mg, B_6 20 mg, B_{12} 12 mcg, C 500 mg, folic acid 0.4 mg, Zn 23.9 mg, Cu, biotin 45 mcg. Tab. Bot. 60s. *OTC.*
Use: Mineral, vitamin supplement.
Stress B Complex with Vitamin C. (Mission Pharmacal) Vitamins B_1 13.8 mg, B_2 10 mg, B_3 50 mg, B_6 4.1 mg, C 300 mg, Zn 15 mg. Tab. Bot. 60s. *OTC.*
Use: Mineral, vitamin supplement.
Stress-Bee. (Rugby) Vitamins B_1 10 mg, B_2 10 mg, B_3 100 mg, B_5 20 mg, B_6 2 mg, B_{12} 6 mcg, C 300 mg. Cap. Bot. 100s. *OTC.*

Use: Vitamin supplement.

Stress Formula. (Various Mfr.) Vitamins E 30 mg, B_1 15 mg, $B_2$15 mg, B_3 100 mg, B_5 20 mg, B_6 5 mg, B_{12} 12 mcg, C 600 mg, folic acid 0.4 mg, biotin 45 mcg. Cap., Tab. **Cap.:** Bot. 60s, 100s, 1000s. **Tab.:** Bot. 30s, 60s, 100s, 250s, 300s, 400s, 1000s, UD 100s. *OTC.*
Use: Vitamin supplement.

Stress Formula 600. (Vangard Labs, Inc.) Vitamins E 30 units, B_1 15 mg, B_2 10 mg, B_3 100 mg, B_5 20 mg, B_6 5 mg, B_{12} 12 mcg, C 500 mg, folic acid 0.4 mg, biotin 45 mcg. Tab. Bot. UD 100s. *OTC.*
Use: Vitamin supplement.

Stress Formula "605". (NBTY) Vitamins E 30 mg, B_1 15 mg, B_2 15 mg, B_3 100 mg, B_5 20 mg, B_6 5 mg, B_{12} 12 mcg, C 605 mg, folic acid 0.4 mg, biotin 45 mg. Tab. Bot. 60s. *OTC.*
Use: Vitamin supplement.

Stress Formula "605" with Zinc. (NBTY) Vitamins E 30 mg, B_1 20 mg, B_2 10 mg, B_3 100 mg, B_5 25 mg, B_6 5 mg, B_{12} 12 mcg, C 605 mg, folic acid 0.4 mg, Zn 23.9 mg, Cu, biotin 45 mcg. Tab. Bot. 60s. *OTC.*
Use: Mineral, vitamin supplement.

Stress Formula 600 Plus Iron. (Schein) Iron 27 mg, vitamins E 30 units, B_1 15 mg, B_2 15 mg, B_3 100 mg, B_5 20 mg, B_6 5 mg, B_{12} 12 mcg, C 600 mg, folic acid 0.4 mg, biotin 45 mcg. Tab. Bot. 60s, 250s. *OTC.*
Use: Mineral, vitamin supplement.

Stress Formula 600 Plus Zinc. (Schein) Vitamins E 30 mg, B_1 20 mg, B_2 10 mg, B_3 100 mg, B_5 25 mg, B_6 5 mg, B_{12} 12 mcg, C 600 mg, folic acid 0.4 mg, zinc 23.9 mg, Cu, Mg, biotin 45 mcg. Tab. Bot. 60s, 250s. *OTC.*
Use: Mineral, vitamin supplement.

Stress Formula 600 w/Iron. (Halsey Drug)
Use: Vitamin supplement.

Stress Formula 600 w/Zinc. (Halsey Drug)
Use: Dietary supplement.

Stress Formula Vitamins. (Various Mfr.) Vitamins E 30 mg, B_1 10 mg, B_2 10 mg, B_3 100 mg, B_5 20 mg, B_6 5 mg, B_{12} 12 mcg, C 500 mg, folic acid 0.4 mg, biotin 45 mcg. Cap. Bot. 100s. Tab. Bot. 60s. *OTC.*
Use: Vitamin supplement.

Stress Formula with Iron. (NBTY) Vitamins C 500 mg, B_1 10 mg, B_2 10 mg, B_3 100 mg, B_5 20 mg, B_6 5 mg, B_{12} 12 mcg, E 30 units, Fe 27 mg, folic acid 0.4 mg, biotin 45 mcg. Tab. Bot. 60s. *OTC.*
Use: Mineral, vitamin supplement.

Stress Formula w/Zinc. (Various Mfr.) Vitamins E 30 units, B_1 10 mg, B_2 10 mg, B_3 100 mg, B_5 20 mg, B_6 5 mg, B_{12} 12 mcg, C 500 mg, folic acid 0.4 mg, biotin 45 mcg, Zn 23.9 mg, Cu. Tab. Bot. 60s. *OTC.*
Use: Mineral, vitamin supplement.

Stress Formula with Zinc. (Towne) Vitamins E 45 units, C 600 mg, folic acid 400 mcg, B_1 20 mg, B_2 10 mg, niacinamide 100 mg, B_6 10 mg, B_{12} 25 mcg, biotin 40 mcg, pantothenic acid 25 mg, Cu 3 mg, Zn 23.9 mg. Tab. Bot. 60s. *OTC.*
Use: Mineral, vitamin supplement.

Stress "1000". (NBTY) Vitamins E 22 mg, B_1 15 mg, B_2 15 mg, B_3 100 mg, B_5 20 mg, B_6 5 mg, B_{12} 12 mcg, C 1000 mg. Tab. Bot. 60s. *OTC.*
Use: Vitamin supplement.

Stress 600 w/Zinc. (Nion Corp.) Vitamins E 45 units, B_1 20 mg, B_2 10 mg, B_3 100 mg, B_5 25 mg, B_6 10 mg, B_{12} 25 mcg, C 600 mg, folic acid 0.4 mg, Zn 5.5 mg, Cu, biotin 45 mcg. Tab. Bot. 60s. *OTC.*
Use: Mineral, vitamin supplement.

Stresstabs. (Wyeth) Vitamins E 30 mg, B_1 10 mg, B_2 10 mg, B_3 100 mg, B_5 20 mg, B_6 5 mg, B_{12} 12 mcg, C 500 mg, folic acid 0.4 mg, biotin 45 mcg. Tab. Bot. 60s. *OTC.*
Use: Vitamin supplement.

Stresstabs + Iron. (Wyeth) Fe 18 mg, E 30 units, B_1 10 mg, B_2 10 mg, B_3 100 mg, B_5 20 mg, B_6 5 mg, B_{12} 12 mcg, C 500 mg, folic acid 0.4 mg, biotin 45 mcg. Tab. Bot. 60s. *OTC.*
Use: Mineral, vitamin supplement.

Stresstabs + Zinc. (Wyeth) Vitamins E 30 mg, B_1 10 mg, B_2 10 mg, B_3 100 mg, B_5 20 mg, B_6 5 mg, B_{12} 12 mcg, C 500 mg, folic acid 0.4 mg, Zn 23.9 mg, Cu, biotin 45 mcg. Tab. Bot. 60s. *OTC.*
Use: Mineral, vitamin supplement.

Stresstabs 600. (Wyeth) Vitamins B_1 15 mg, B_2 10 mg, B_6 5 mg, B_{12} 12 mcg, C 600 mg, niacinamide 100 mg, vitamin E 30 units, biotin 45 mcg, folic acid 400 mcg, calcium pantothenate 20 mg. Tab. Bot. 30s, 60s, UD 10 x 10s. *OTC.*
Use: Vitamin supplement.

Stresstabs 600 with Iron. (Wyeth) Ferrous fumarate 27 mg, vitamins E 30 units, B_1 15 mg, B_2 15 mg, B_3 100 mg, B_5 20 mg, B_6 5 mg, B_{12} 12 mcg, C 600 mg, folic acid 0.4 mg,

Stress Formula w/Zinc. (Various Mfr.)
Vitamins E 30 units, B_1 10 mg, B_2 10 mg, B_3 100 mg, B_5 20 mg, B_6 5 mg, B_{12} 12 mcg, C 500 mg, folic acid 0.4 mg, biotin 45 mcg. Tab. Bot. 60s. *OTC.*

biotin 45 mcg. Tab. Bot. 30s, 60s. *OTC.*
Use: Mineral, vitamin supplement.
Stresstabs 600 with Zinc. (Wyeth) Vitamins B_1 15 mg, B_2 10 mg, B_3 100 mg, B_5 20 mg, B_6 5 mg, B_{12} 12 mcg, C 600 mg, E 30 units, folic acid 0.4 mg, biotin 45 mcg, Cu, Zn 23.9 mg. Tab. Bot. 30s, 60s. *OTC.*
Use: Mineral, vitamin supplement.
Stresstein. (Novartis) Maltodextrin, medium chain triglycerides, l-leucine, soybean oil, l-isoleucine, l-valine, l-glutamic acid, l-arginine, l-lysine acetate, l-alanine, l-threonine, l-phenylalanine, l-aspartic acid, l-histidine, l-methionine, glycine, polyglycerol esters of fatty acids, l-serine, l-proline, sodium Cl, l-tryptophan, l-cysteine, sodium citrate, vitamins and minerals. Powder 3.4 oz. packets. *OTC.*
Use: High-protein, branched chain enriched tube feeding.
Striant. (Columbia) Testosterone 30 mg. Lactose. Buccal system. Blisterpacks of 10 systems. *Rx.*
Use: Androgen.
Stri-dex Antibacterial Cleansing. (Bayer Corp. (Consumer Div.)) Triclosan 1%, acetylated lanolin alcohol, EDTA. Bar. 105 g. *OTC.*
Use: Dermatologic, acne.
Stri-dex B.P. (Bayer Corp. (Consumer Div.)) Benzoyl peroxide 10%. in greaseless, vanishing cream base. *OTC.*
Use: Dermatologic, acne.
Stri-dex Clear. (Bayer Corp. (Consumer Div.)) Salicylic acid 2%, SD alcohol 9.3%, EDTA. Gel. Tube. 30 g. *OTC.*
Use: Dermatologic, acne.
Stri-dex Face Wash. (Bayer Corp. (Consumer Div.)) Triclosan 1%, glycerin, EDTA, alcohol free. Soln. Bot. 237 mL. *OTC.*
Use: Dermatologic, acne.
Stri-dex Lotion. (Bayer Corp. (Consumer Div.)) Salicylic acid 0.5%, alcohol 28%, sulfonated alkyl benzenes, citric acid, sodium carbonate, simethicone, water. Bot. 4 oz. *OTC.*
Use: Dermatologic, acne.
Stri-dex Maximum Strength. (Bayer Corp. (Consumer Div.)) Salicylic acid 2%, SD alcohol 44%, citric acid, menthol. Pad. Box 55s, 90s, dual-textured 32s. *OTC.*
Use: Antiacne.
Stri-dex Oil Fighting Formula. (Bayer Corp. (Consumer Div.)) Salicylic acid 2%, citric acid, menthol, SD alcohol 54%. Super Scrub Pads. Box 55s. *OTC.*

Use: Dermatologic, acne.
Stri-dex Regular Strength. (Bayer Corp. (Consumer Div.)) Salicylic acid 0.5%, SD alcohol 28%, citric acid, menthol. Pad. Box 55s. *OTC.*
Use: Dermatologic, acne.
Stri-dex Sensitive Skin. (Bayer Corp. (Consumer Div.)) Salicylic acid 0.5%, citric acid, aloe vera gel, menthol, SD alcohol 28%. Pad. Box 50s, 90s. *OTC.*
Use: Dermatologic, acne.
Stromectol. (Merck & Co.) Ivermectin 3 mg, 6 mg. Tab. UD 20s (3 mg only), 10s (6 mg only). *Rx.*
Use: Anthelmintic.
strong iodine tincture. (Various Mfr.) Iodine 7%, potassium iodide 5%, alcohol 83%. Soln. Bot. 500 mL, 4000 mL. *OTC.*
Use: Antimicrobial; antiseptic.
StrongStart. (Savage) Ca 200 mg, Fe 29 mg, vitamin A 1000 units, D 400 units, E 30 units, B_1 3 mg, B_2 3 mg, B_3 15 mg, B_5 7 mg, B_6 20 mg, B_{12} 12 mcg, C 100 mg, folic acid 1 mg, Zn 20 mg; docusate sodium 25 mg (Tab only). Tab., Chew. Tab. Bot. 30s, 100s. *Rx.*
Use: Vitamin, mineral supplement
strontium bromide. Strontium bromide Cryst. or Granule. Bot. 0.25 lb, 1 lb. Amp. 1 g/10 mL. *Rx.*
Use: Antiepileptic; sedative.
● **strontium chloride Sr 85.** (STRAHN-shee-uhm) USAN.
Use: Radiopharmaceutical.
● **strontium chloride Sr 89 injection.** (STRAHN-shee-uhm) *USP 28.*
Use: Antineoplastic; radiopharmaceutical.
See: Metastron.
● **strontium nitrate Sr 85.** (STRAHN-shee-uhm) USAN.
Use: Radiopharmaceutical.
strontium Sr 85 injection.
Use: Diagnostic aid (bone scanning).
Strovite. (Everett) Vitamins B_1 15 mg, B_2 15 mg, B_3 100 mg, B_5 18 mg, B_6 4 mg, B_{12} 5 mcg, C 500 mg, folic acid 0.5 mg. Tab. Bot. 100s. *OTC.*
Use: Mineral, vitamin supplement.
Strovite Advance. (Everett) Vitamin D_3 400 units, E 100 units, B_1 20 mg, B_2 5 mg, B_3 25 mg, B_5 15 mg, B_6 25 mg, B_{12} 50 mcg, C 300 mg, folic acid 1 mg, Zn 25 mg, carotenoids 3000 units, biotin 100 mcg, alpha lipoic acid 15 mg, lutein 5 mg, Cr, Cu, Mg, Mn, Se, mineral oil. Tab. Bot. 100s. *Rx.*
Use: Vitamin, mineral supplement.

Strovite Forte. (Everett) Fe 10 mg, vitamins A 3000 units (acetate), A 1000 units (beta-carotene), E 60 units, D_3 400 units, folic acid 1 mg, C 500 mg, B_1 20 mg, B_2 20 mg, B_6 25 mg, B_{12} 50 mcg, B_3 100 mg, biotin 0.15 mg, B_5 25 mg, Se 50 mcg, Mg 50 mg, Zn 15 mg, Mo 20 mcg, Cu 3 mg, Cr 0.05 mg. Tab. Bot. 100s. *Rx.*
Use: Vitamin, mineral supplement.

Strovite Plus. (Everett) Vitamins A 5000 units, E 30 mg, B_1 20 mg, B_2 20 mg, B_3 100 mg, B_5 25 mg, B_6 25 mg, B_{12} 50 mcg, C 500 mg, Fe 9 mg, folic acid 0.8 mg, Zn 22.5 mg, biotin 150 mcg, Cr, Cu, Mg, Mn. Bot. 100s. *OTC.*
Use: Mineral, vitamin supplement.

S.T. 37. (GlaxoSmithKline) Hexylresorcinol 0.1% in glycerin aqueous soln. Bot. 5.5 oz, 12 oz. *OTC.*
Use: Antiseptic, topical.

Stuart Formula. (J & J Merck Consumer Pharm.) Vitamins A 5000 units, B_1 1.5 mg, B_2 1.7 mg, B_3 20 mg, B_6 1 mg, B_{12} 3 mcg, C 50 mg, D 400 units, E 10 units, Fe 5 mg, Cu, folic acid 0.4 mg, Ca, I, P. Tab. Bot. 100s. *OTC.*
Use: Mineral, vitamin supplement.

StuartNatal Plus 3. (Integrity) Ca 200 mg, Fe (as ferrous fumarate) 28 mg, vitamin A 3000 units, D 400 units, E (as dl-alpha tocopheryl acetate) 22 mg, B_1 1.8 mg, B_2 4 mg, B_3 20 mg, B_6 25 mg, B_{12} 12 mcg, C 120 mg, folic acid 1 mg, Cu, Mg, Zn 25 mg. Tab. Bot. 100s. *Rx.*
Use: Vitamin, mineral supplement.

Stuart Prenatal. (Integrity) Vitamins A (100% as beta carotene) 4000 units, B_1 1.8 mg, B_2 1.7 mg, B_3 20 mg, B_6 2.6 mg, B_{12} 8 mcg, C 120 mg, D 400 units, E (dl-alpha tocopheryl acetate) 30 units, Fe (as ferrous fumarate) 28 mg, Ca 200 mg, Zn 25 mg, folic acid 800 mcg. Tab. Bot. 100s. *OTC.*
Use: Mineral, vitamin supplement.

Stulex. (Jones Pharma) Docusate sodium 250 mg. Tab. Bot. 100s, 1000s. *OTC.*
Use: Fecal softener.

S-2. (Nephron) Racepinephrine hydrochloride 2.25% (epinephrine base 1.125%), sodium bisulfite, potassium metabisulfite, chlorobutanol, benzoic acid, propylene glycol. Inh. Soln. Bot. 15 mL. *OTC.*
Use: Bronchodilator, sympathomimetic.

Stye. (Del) White petrolatum 55%, mineral oil 32%, boric acid, wheat germ oil, stearic acid. Oint. Bot. 3.5 g. *OTC.*

Use: Lubricant, ophthalmic.

Stypt-Aid. (Pharmakon) Benzocaine 28.71 mg, methylbenzethonium hydrochloride 9.95 mg, aluminum Cl hexahydrate 55.43 mg, ethyl alcohol 70.97%/mL in a glycerin, menthol base. Spray. 60 mL. *OTC.*
Use: Anesthetic, local.

styptirenal.
See: Epinephrine.

Stypto-Caine. (Pedinol Pharmacal) Hydroxyquinoline sulfate, tetracaine hydrochloride, aluminum Cl, aqueous glycol base. Soln. Bot. 2 oz. *Rx.*
Use: Hemostatic solution.

styrene polymer, sulfonated, sodium salt. Sodium Polystyrene Sulfonate, *USP 25.*

styronate resins. Ammonium and potassium salts of sulfonated styrene polymers.
Use: Conditions requiring sodium restriction.

Sublimaze. (Akorn) Fentanyl citrate (as base) 50 mcg/mL. Preservative free. Inj. Amp. 2 mL, 5 mL, 10 mL, 20 mL. *c-II.*
Use: Opioid analgesic.

Sublingual B Total. (Pharmaceutical Labs) Vitamins B_2 1.7 mg, B_3 20 mg, B_5 30 mg, B_6 2 mg, B_{12} 1000 mcg, C 60 mg. Liq. Bot. 30 mL. *OTC.*
Use: Vitamin supplement.

Suboxone. (Reckitt Benckiser) Buprenorphine base 2 mg/naloxone 0.5 mg, buprenorphine base 8 mg/naloxone 2 mg, lactose, acesulfame K, lemon/lime flavor. Tab, Sublingual. Bot. 30s. *c-III.*
Use: Analgesic.

substituted ureas.
Use: Antisickling agent.
See: Hydrea.
Hydroxyurea.

Subutex. (Reckitt Benckiser) Buprenorphine hydrochloride 2 mg, 8 mg, lactose. Tab, Sublingual. Bot. 30s. *c-III.*
Use: Analgesic.

Suby's Solution G. (Various Mfr.) Citric acid 3.24 g, sodium carbonate 0.43 g, magnesium oxide 0.38 g/100 mL. Soln. Bot. 1000 mL. *Rx.*
Use: Irrigant, genitourinary.

•**succimer.** (SUX-ih-mer) USAN.
Use: Diagnostic aid; cystine kidney stones, mercury and lead poisoning. [Orphan Drug]
See: Chemet.

succinimides.
Use: Anticonvulsant
See: Methsuximide.

• **succinylcholine chloride.** (suck-sin-ill-KOE-leen KLOR-ide) *USP 28.*
Use: Neuromuscular blocker.
See: Anectine Cl.
  Quelicins.
  Sucostrin.
succinylsulfathiazole.
Use: Anti-infective, intestinal.
Succus Cineraria Maritima. (Walker) Aqueous and glycerin solution of senecio compositae, hamamelis water and boric acid. Soln. Bot. 7 mL. *Rx.*
Use: Ophthalmic.
Sucostrin. (Apothecon) Succinylcholine Cl 20 mg/mL Inj. Vial 10 mL. *Rx.*
Use: Neuromuscular blocker.
Sucostrin Chloride. (Marsam) Succinylcholine Cl 20 mg/mL w/methylparaben 0.1%, propylparaben 0.01%. Vial 10 mL, High potency 100 mg/ml Vial 10 mL. *Rx.*
Use: Muscle relaxant.
Sucraid. (Orphan Medical) Sacrosidase 8500 units/mL. Soln. Bot. 118 mL. *Rx.*
Use: Nutritional therapy.
• **sucralfate.** (sue-KRAL-fate) *USP 28.*
Use: Antiulcerative; oral complications of chemotherapy. [Orphan Drug]
See: Carafate.
sucralfate. (Precision Dose) Sucralfate 1 g/10 mL. Methylparaben, sorbitol. Susp. Unit dose cups. 10 mL. *Rx.*
Use: Antiulcerative.
sucralfate. (Various Mfr.) Sucralfate 1 g. Tab. Bot. 100s, 500s. *Rx.*
Use: Antiulcerative.
Sucrets Children's Sore Throat. (GlaxoSmithKline) Dyclonine hydrochloride 1.2 mg. Corn syrup, sucrose, cherry flavor. Loz. Tin 24s. *OTC.*
Use: Sore throat treatment for children 3 years and older.
Sucrets Cough Control. (GlaxoSmithKline) Dextromethorphan HBr 5 mg. Loz. Tin 24s. *OTC.*
Use: Antitussive.
Sucrets 4-Hour Cough. (GlaxoSmithKline) Dextromethorphan 15 mg. Loz. Menthol, sucrose, corn syrup. Pkg. 20s. *OTC.*
Use: Antitussive.
Sucrets Maximum Strength. (GlaxoSmithKline) Dyclonine hydrochloride 3 mg. Loz. Corn syrup, menthol, sucrose. Loz. Tin 24s, 48s, 55s. *OTC.*
Use: Mouth and throat preparation.
Sucrets Sore Throat. (GlaxoSmithKline) Hexylresorcinol 2.4 mg. Loz. Tin 24s. *OTC.*
Use: Mouth and throat preparation.
Sucrets Sore Throat Spray. (Glaxo-

SmithKline) Dyclonine hydrochloride 0.1%, alcohol 10%, sorbitol. Spray. Bot. 90 mL, 120 mL. *OTC.*
Use: Mouth and throat preparation.
Sucrets Wintergreen. (GlaxoSmithKline) Dyclonine hydrochloride 0.1%, alcohol 10%, sorbitol. Spray Bot. 90 mL. *OTC.*
Use: Mouth and throat preparation.
• **sucrose.** (SUE-krose) *NF 23.*
Use: IV; diuretic & dehydrating agent; pharmaceutic aid (flavor, tablet excipient).
• **sucrose octaacetate.** *NF 23.*
Use: Pharmaceutic aid (alcohol denaturant).
• **sucrosofate potassium.** (sue-KROE-so-FATE) USAN.
Use: Antiulcerative.
Sudafed. (Warner Lambert) Pseudoephedrine hydrochloride. 30 mg, 60 mg. **30 mg:** Box 24s, 48s. Bot. 100s, 1000s. **60 mg:** Bot. 100s, 1000s. *OTC.*
Use: Decongestant.
Sudafed, Children's Non-Drowsy. (Warner Lambert) Pseudoephedrine hydrochloride. **Chew. Tab.:** 15 mg, aspartame, mannitol, phenylalanine 0.78 mg, orange-flavor. Pkg. 24s. **Liq.:** 15 mg/5 mL, EDTA, saccharin, sorbitol, grape flavor, alcohol free. Bot. 118 mL. *OTC.*
Use: Nasal decongestant, arylalkylamine.
Sudafed Children's Non-Drowsy Cold & Cough. (Warner Lambert) Pseudoephedrine hydrochloride 15 mg, dextromethorphan HBr 5 mg/5 mL, saccharin, sorbitol, cherry-berry flavor, alcohol free. Liq. Bot. 118 mL. *OTC.*
Use: Upper respiratory combination, decongestant, antitussive.
Sudafed Cold & Allergy Maximum Strength. (Warner Lambert) Pseudoephedrine hydrochloride 60 mg, chlorpheniramine maleate 4 mg, lactose. Tab. Pkg. 24s. *OTC.*
Use: Upper respiratory combination, decongestant, antihistamine.
Sudafed Cold & Sinus Non-Drowsy. (Warner Lambert) Pseudoephedrine hydrochloride 30 mg, acetaminophen 325 mg, sorbitol. Liqui-Caps. Pkg. 10s, 20s. *OTC.*
Use: Upper respiratory combination, decongestant, analgesic.
Sudafed Maximum Strength Sinus Nighttime Plus Pain Relief. (Warner Lambert) Pseudoephedrine hydrochloride 30 mg, diphenhydramine hydrochloride 25 mg, acetaminophen

500 mg. Tab. Pkg. 20s. *OTC.*
Use: Upper respiratory combination, decongestant, antihistamine, analgesic.

Sudafed Multi-Symptom Cold & Cough. (Warner Lambert) Dextromethorphan HBr 10 mg, guaifenesin 100 mg, pseudoephedrine hydrochloride 30 mg, acetaminophen 250 mg, sorbitol. Liquicaps. Pkg. 20s. *OTC.*
Use: Upper respiratory combination, antitussive, expectorant, decongestant, analgesic.

Sudafed Non-Drowsy, Maximum Strength. (Warner Lambert) Pseudoephedrine hydrochloride 30 mg, lactose, sucrose. Tab. Bot. 24s, 96s. *OTC.*
Use: Nasal decongestant, arylalkylamine.

Sudafed Non-Drowsy Non-Drying Sinus. (Warner Lambert) Pseudoephedrine hydrochloride 30 mg, guaifenesin 120 mg, sorbitol. Liqui-Caps. Pkg. 24s. *OTC.*
Use: Upper respiratory combination, decongestant, expectorant.

Sudafed Non-Drowsy Severe Cold Formula Maximum Strength. (Warner Lambert) Dextromethorphan HBr 15 mg, pseudoephedrine hydrochloride 30 mg, acetaminophen 500 mg. Tab. Pkg. 24s. *OTC.*
Use: Upper respiratory combination, decongestant, antihistamine, analgesic.

Sudafed Non-Drowsy 12 Hour Long-Acting. (Warner Lambert) Pseudoephedrine hydrochloride 120 mg. ER Tab. Pkg. 10s. *OTC.*
Use: Nasal decongestant, arylalkylamine.

Sudafed Non-Drowsy 24 Hour Long-Acting. (Warner Lambert) Pseudoephedrine hydrochloride 240 mg (immediate-release 60 mg, controlled-release 180 mg). CR Tab. Pkg. 10s. *OTC.*
Use: Nasal decongestant, arylalkylamine.

Sudafed PE. (Pfizer) Phenylephrine hydrochloride 10 mg. Acesulfame K. Tab. 18s. *OTC.*
Use: Nasal decongestant.

Sudafed Sinus Headache Non-Drowsy. (Warner Lambert) Pseudoephedrine hydrochloride 30 mg, acetaminophen 500 mg. Tab. 24s, 48s. *OTC.*
Use: Upper respiratory combination, analgesic, decongestant.

Sudafed Sinus Nighttime Maximum Strength. (Warner Lambert) Pseudoephedrine hydrochloride 60 mg, triprolidine hydrochloride 2.5 mg, lactose, sucrose. Tab. Pkg. 12s. *OTC.*

Use: Upper respiratory combination, decongestant, antihistamine.

Sudafed 12 Hour. (Warner Lambert) Pseudoephedrine hydrochloride 120 mg. SA Cap. Box 10s, 20s, 40s. *OTC.*
Use: Decongestant.

Sudal-DM. (Atley) Dextromethorphan HBr 30 mg, guaifenesin 500 mg, dye free. SR Tab. Bot. 100s. *Rx.*
Use: Upper respiratory combination, antitussive, expectorant.

Sudal 120/600. (Atley) Pseudoephedrine hydrochloride 120 mg, guaifenesin 600 mg. SR Tab. Bot. 100s. *Rx.*
Use: Upper respiratory combination, decongestant, expectorant.

Sudal 60/500. (Atley) Pseudoephedrine hydrochloride 60 mg, guaifenesin 500 mg. SR Tab. Bot. 100s. *Rx.*
Use: Upper respiratory combination, decongestant, expectorant.

Sudanyl. (Dover Pharmaceuticals) Pseudoephedrine hydrochloride. Tab. Sugar, lactose, and salt free. UD Box 500s.
Use: Decongestant.

Sudden Tan Lotion. (Schering-Plough) Padimate O, dihydroxyacetone, Bot. 4 oz. *OTC.*
Use: Artificial tanning; moisturizer; sunscreen.

Sudodrin. (Textilease Medique) Pseudoephedrine hydrochloride 30 mg. Tab. Bot. 250s, 1000s. *OTC.*
Use: Nasal decongestant, arylalkylamine.

SudoGest Sinus Maximum Strength. (Major) Pseudoephedrine hydrochloride 30 mg, acetaminophen 500 mg, dextrose. Tab. Pkg. 24s. *OTC.*
Use: Upper respiratory combination, decongestant, analgesic.

•**sudoxicam.** (sue-DOX-ih-kam) USAN.
Use: Anti-inflammatory.

Sudrin. (Jones Pharma) Pseudoephedrine hydrochloride 30 mg. Tab. Bot. 100s, 1000s. *OTC.*
Use: Decongestant.

Sufenta. (Taylor) Sufentanil citrate (as base) 50 mcg/mL. Preservative free. Inj. Amp. 1 mL, 2 mL, 5 mL. *c-ii.*
Use: Opioid analgesic.

•**sufentanil.** (sue-FEN-tuh-nill) USAN.
Use: Analgesic.

•**sufentanil citrate.** (sue-FEN-tuh-nill SIHtrate) *USP 28.*
Use: Opioid analgesic.
See: Sufenta.

sufentanil citrate. (Various Mfr.) Sufentanil citrate (as base) 50 mcg/mL. Inj. Amp. 1 mL, 2 mL, 5 mL. Vials. 1 mL, 2 mL, 5 mL. *c-II.*
Use: Opioid analgesic.

• **sufentanil citrate injection.** *USP 28.*
Use: Analgesic; narcotic.

• **sufotidine.** (sue-FOE-tih-DEEN) USAN.
Use: Antiulcerative.

Sufrex. (Janssen) Ketanserin tartrate. *Rx.*
Use: Serotonin antagonist.

• **sugammadex sodium.** (soo-GAM-madex) USAN.
Use: CNS agent.

• **sugar, compressible.** *NF 23.*
Use: Pharmaceutic aid (flavor; tablet excipient)

• **sugar, confectioner's.** *NF 23.*
Use: Pharmaceutic aid (flavor; tablet excipient).

• **sugar, invert, injection.** *USP 28.*
Use: Replenisher (fluid and nutrient).

• **sugar spheres.** *NF 23.*
Use: Pharmaceutic aid (vehicle, solid carrier).

• **sulamserod hydrochloride.** USAN.
Use: Urge incontinence; atrial fibrillations.

Sular. (First Horizon) Nisoldipine 10 mg, 20 mg, 30 mg, 40 mg, lactose. ER Tab. 100s, UD 100s (except 40 mg). *Rx.*
Use: Calcium channel blocker.

• **sulazepam.** (sull-AZE-eh-pam) USAN.
Use: Anxiolytic.

Sulazo. (Freeport) Sulfisoxazole 500 mg, phenylazodiaminopyridine hydrochloride 50 mg. Tab. Bot. 1000s. *Rx.*
Use: Analgesic; anti-infective.

• **sulbactam benzathine.** (sull-BACK-tam BENZ-ah-theen) USAN.
Use: Synergistic (penicillin/cephalosporin); inhibitor (β-lactamase).

• **sulbactam pivoxil.** (sull-BACK-tam pihv-OX-ill) USAN.
Use: Inhibitor (β-lactamase); synergist (penicillin/cephalosporin).

sulbactam sodium/ampicillin sodium.
Use: Anti-infective; penicillin.
See: Unasyn.

• **sulbactam sodium sterile.** (sull-BACK-tam) *USP 28.*
Use: Inhibitor (β-lactamase); synergist (penicillin/cephalosporin).

• **sulconazole nitrate.** (SULL-CONE-ah-zole) *USP 28.*
Use: Antifungal.

• **sulesomab.** (sue-LEH-so-mab) USAN.
Use: Monoclonal antibody (diagnostic aid for detection of infectious lesions).

• **sulfabenz.** (SULL-fah-benz) USAN.
Use: Anti-infective.

• **sulfabenzamide.** (SULL-fah-BENZ-ah-mid) *USP 28.*
Use: Anti-infective.

sulfabromethazine sodium.
Use: Anti-infective.

Sulfacet. (Dermik)
See: Sulfacetamide.

• **sulfacetamide.** (sull-fah-SEE-tah-mide) *USP 28.*
Use: Anti-infective.

sulfacetamide combinations.
See: Acet-Dia-Mer Sulfonamides.
Chero-Trisulfa (V).
Sulf-10.
Sulster.
Triurisul.

• **sulfacetamide sodium.** *USP 28.*
Use: Anti-infective.
See: AK-Sulf.
Bleph 10.
Cetamide.
Isopto Cetamide.
Ocusulf-10.
Sodium Sulamyd Ophthalmic 30%.
Sulf-15.
Sulf-10.
W/Fluorometholone.
See: FML-S.
W/Methylcellulose.
See: Sodium Sulamyd Ophth. 10%.
W/Phenylephrine hydrochloride, methylparaben, propylparaben.
See: Vasosulf.
W/Prednisolone.
See: Vasocidin.
W/Prednisolone acetate.
See: Blephamide S.O.P.
Metimyd.
W/Prednisolone acetate, phenylephrine.
See: Blephamide Liquifilm.
Optimyd, Sterile.
W/Prednisolone, methylcellulose.
See: Isopto Cetapred.
W/Prednisolone sodium phosphate, phenylephrine, sulfacetamide sodium.
See: Vasocidin.
W/Sulfur.
See: Novacet.
Plexion.
Plexion SCT.
Rosac.
Rosanil.
Rosula.
Sulfacet-R.
Vancocin.
Zetacet.

sulfacetamide sodium. (Various Mfr.)
Sulfacetamide sodium. **Soln.: 10%,**
30%: Bot. 15 mL. **Oint.:** 10% Tube
3.5 g.
Use: Anti-infective.
sulfacetamide sodium and predniso-
lone acetate.
Use: Anti-infective; anti-inflammatory,
ophthalmic.
See: Blephamide S.O.P.
Cetapred.
Metimyd.
Predsulfair.
Vasocidin.
sulfacetamide sodium and predniso-
lone sodium phosphate. (Schein)
Sulfacetamide sodium 10%, prednisolone sodium phosphate 0.25%. Soln.
5 mL, 10 mL. *Rx.*
Use: Anti-infective, ophthalmic.
sulfacetamide sodium 10% and sulfur
5%. (Glades) Sulfur 5%, sodium sulfacetamide 10%, cetyl alcohol, benzyl alcohol, EDTA. Bot. 25 mL. Tube 30 mL.
Rx.
Use: Dermatologic, acne.
sulfacetamide, sulfadiazine, & sulfa-
merazine.
See: Acet-dia-mer-sulfonamide.
Sulfacet-R. (Dermik) Sulfur 5%, sulfacetamide sodium 10%, parabens. Lot. Bot.
25 mL. *Rx.*
Use: Dermatologic, acne.
● **sulfacytine.** (SULL-fah-SIGH-teen)
USAN.
Use: Anti-infective.
sulfadiasulfone sodium. Acetosulfone
sodium.
● **sulfadiazine.** (SULL-fah-DIE-ah-zeen)
USP 28.
Tall Man: SulfADIAZINE
Use: Anti-infective. [Orphan Drug]
sulfadiazine. (Various Mfr.) Sulfadiazine
500 mg. Tab. Bot. 100s, 1000s, UD
100s. *Rx.*
Use: Anti-infective.
sulfadiazine and sulfamerazine. Citra-
sulfas.
sulfadiazine combinations. (SULL-fah-
DIE-ah-zeen)
See: Acet-dia-mer-sulfonamide.
Chemozine.
Chero-Trisulfa.
Meth-Dia-Mer Sulfonamides.
Silvadene.
Triple Sulfa.
● **sulfadiazine, silver.** (sull-fah-DIE-ah-
zeen) *USP 28.*
Tall Man: SulfADIAZINE
Use: Anti-infective, topical.

● **sulfadiazine sodium.** (SULL-fah-DIE-ah-
zeen) *USP 28.*
Tall Man: SulfADIAZINE
Use: Anti-infective.
See: Sodium Bicarbonate.
sulfadiazine, sulfamerazine, & sulf-
acetamide.
See: Acet-dia-mer-sulfonamide.
Coco Diazine.
● **sulfadimethoxine.** *USP 28.*
● **sulfadimethoxine sodium.** *USP 28.*
sulfadimidine.
See: Sulfamethazine.
sulfadine.
See: Sulfadimidine.
Sulfamethazine.
Sulfapyridine.
● **sulfadoxine.** (SULL-fah-DOX-een)
USP 28.
Use: Anti-infective.
W/Pyrimethamine.
See: Fansidar.
sulfadoxine and pyrimethamine.
Use: Anti-infective; antimalarial.
See: Fansidar.
sulfaguanidine.
Use: GI tract infections.
Sulfair 15. (Bausch & Lomb) Sodium
sulfacetamide 15%. Soln. Bot. 15 mL.
Rx.
Use: Anti-infective, ophthalmic.
● **sulfalene.** (SULL-fah-leen) USAN.
Use: Anti-infective.
● **sulfamerazine.** (sull-fah-MER-ah-zeen)
USP 28.
Use: Anti-infective.
sulfamerazine combinations.
Use: Anti-infective.
See: Chemozine.
Chero-Trisulfa-V.
sulfamerazine sodium.
Use: Anti-infective.
sulfamerazine, sulfadiazine, & sulfa-
methazine.
Use: Anti-infective.
See: Meth-Dia-Mer Sulfonamides.
sulfamerazine, sulfadiazine, & sulfa-
thiazole.
Use: Anti-infective.
● **sulfameter.** (SULL-fam-EE-ter) USAN.
Use: Anti-infective.
● **sulfamethazine.** (sull fa-METH-ah zeen)
USP 28.
Use: Anti-infective.
See: Sulfa-Plex.
W/Sulfadiazine, sulfamerazine.
See: Triple Sulfa.
sulfamethoprim. (Par Pharmaceuticals)
Sulfamethoxazole 400 mg, trimetho-
prim 80 mg. Tab. Bot. 100s, 500s. *Rx.*

Use: Anti-infective.
• **sulfamethoxazole.** (sull-fah-meth-OX-ah-zole) *USP 28.*
Use: Anti-infective.
W/Trimethoprim.
See: Bactrim.
Septra.
Septra DS.
sulfamethoxazole and phenazo-pyridine hydrochloride.
Use: Anti-infective, urinary.
sulfamethoxazole and trimethoprim for injection. (SULL-fah-meth-OX-ah-zole and try-METH-oh-prim)
Use: Anti-infective, urinary.
sulfamethoxazole and trimethoprim oral suspension. (Various Mfr.) Trimethoprim 40 mg, sulfamethoxazole 200 mg/5 ml. Bol. 150 mL, 200 mL, 480 mL. *Rx.*
Use: Anti-infective, urinary.
sulfamethoxazole and trimethoprim tablets. (Various Mfr.) Trimethoprim 80 mg, sulfamethoxazole 400 mg. Tab. Bot. 100s, 500s. *Rx.*
Use: Anti-infective, urinary.
sulfamethoxazole/trimethoprim DS. (Various Mfr.) Trimethoprim 160 mg, sulfamethoxazole 800 mg. Tab, double-strength. Bot. 100s, 500s. *Rx.*
Use: Anti-infective.
sulfamethoxydiazine. Sulfameter.
Use: Anti-infective.
sulfamethoxypyridazine acetyl.
Use: Anti-infective.
sulfamethylthiadiazole.
Use: Anti-infective.
See: Sulfamethizole.
sulfametin. *Formerly sulfamethoxydiazine.*
Use: Anti-infective.
sulfamezanthene.
Use: Anti-infective.
See: Sulfamethazine.
Sulfamide. (Rugby) Prednisolone acetate 0.5%, sodium sulfacetamide, hydroxypropyl methylcellulose, polysorbate 80, sodium thiosulfate, benzalkonium Cl 0.01%. Susp. Bot. 5 and 15 mL. *Rx.*
Use: Anti-infective, ophthalmic.
• **sulfamonomethoxine.** (SULL-fah-mahn-oh-meh-THOCK-seen) USAN.
Use: Anti-infective.
• **sulfamoxole.** (sull-fah-MOX-ole) USAN.
Use: Anti-infective.
p-sulfamoylbenzylamine hydrochloride. Sulfbenzamide.
Sulfamylon. (Bertek) Mafenide acetate 5%. Packets containing 50 g of ster-

ile mafenide acetate to be reconstituted in 1000 mL of sterile water for irrigation or 0.9% Sodium Chloride Irrigation. Top. Soln. Ctn. Pkt. 50 g, 5s. *Rx.*
Use: Burn therapy adjunct.
2-sulfanilamidopyridine. Sulfadiazine, *USP.*
Use: Anti-infective.
• **sulfanilate zinc.** (sull-FAN-ih-late) USAN.
Use: Anti-infective.
n-sulfanilylacetamide.
Use: Anti-infective.
See: Sulfacetamide.
sulfanilylbenzamide.
Use: Anti-infective.
See: Sulfabenzamide.
• **sulfanitran.** (SULL-fah-NYE-tran) USAN.
Use: Anti-infective.
• **sulfapyridine.** (sull-fah-PEER-ih-deen) *USP 28.*
Use: Dermatitic herpetiformis suppressant. [Orphan Drug]
• **sulfasalazine.** (SULL-fuh-SAL-uh-zeen) *USP 28. Formerly Salicylazosulfapyridine.*
Use: Anti-infective; antirheumatic.
See: Azulfidine.
Azulfidine EN-tabs.
Salicylazosulfapyridine.
Sulfapyridine.
sulfasalazine. (Various Mfr.) Sulfasalazine 500 mg. Tab. Bot. 50s, 100s, 500s, 1000s. *Rx.*
Use: Anti-infective; antirheumatic.
• **sulfasomizole.** (SULL-fah-SAHM-ih-zole) USAN.
Use: Antibacterial; anti-infective; sulfonamide.
sulfasymasine.
Use: Anti-infective sulfonamide.
Sulfa-10 Ophthalmic. (Maury) Sodium sulfacetamide 10%, hydroxyethylcellulose, sodium borate, boric acid, disodium edetate, sodium metabisulfite, sodium thiosulfate 0.2%, chlorobutanol 0.2%, methylparaben 0.015%. Bot. 15 mL. *Rx.*
Use: Anti-infective, ophthalmic.
Sulfa-Ter-Tablets. (A.P.C.) Trisulfapyrimidines. Tab. Bot. 1000s.
• **sulfathiazole.** (sull-fah-THIGH-ah-zole) *USP 28.*
Use: Anti-infective.
Sulfatrim. (Various Mfr.) Trimethoprim 40 mg, sulfamethoxazole 200 mg/5 mL Susp. Bot. 473 mL. *Rx.*
Use: Anti-infective.
Sulfatrim DS. (Ivax) Trimethoprim 800 mg, sulfamethoxazole 160 mg. Tab.

Bot. 100s, 500s. *Rx.*
Use: Anti-infective.
Sulfatrim SS. (Ivax) Trimethoprim
400 mg, sulfamethoxazole 80 mg. Tab.
Bot. 100s. *Rx.*
Use: Anti-infective.
Sulfa-Trip. (Major) Sulfathiazole 3.42%,
sulfacetamide 2.86%, sulfabenzamide
3.7%, urea 0.64%. Cream. Tube 82.5 g.
Rx.
Use: Anti-infective, vaginal.
Sulfa Triple No. 2. (Global Source) Sulfa-
diazine 162 mg, sulfamerizine 162 mg,
sulfamethazine 162 mg. Tab. Bot.
1000s. *Rx.*
Use: Anti-infective.
• **sulfazamet.** (sull-FAZE-ah-MET) USAN.
Use: Anti-infective.
Sulf-15. (Ciba Vision) Sodium sulfacet-
amide 15%. Soln. Bot. 5 mL, 15 mL.
Rx.
Use: Anti-infective, ophthalmic.
• **sulfinalol hydrochloride.** (SULL-FIN-ah-
lahl) USAN.
Use: Antihypertensive.
• **sulfinpyrazone.** (sull-fin-PEER-uh-zone)
USP 28.
Use: Uricosuric.
See: Anturane.
• **sulfisoxazole.** (sull-fih-SOX-uh-zole)
USP 28.
Tall Man: SulfiSOXAZOLE
Use: Anti-infective.
See: Gantrisin.
Soxa.
Sulfisoxazole.
Sulfizin.
W/Aminoacridine hydrochloride, allan-
toin.
See: Azo-Gantrisin.
Azo-Soxazole.
Azo-Sulfisoxazole.
sulfisoxazole. (Various Mfr.) Sulfisoxa-
zole 500 mg. Tab. Bot. 100s, 1000s.
Rx.
Use: Anti-infective.
• **sulfisoxazole, acetyl.** (sull-fih-SOX-uh-
zole, ASS-eh-till) *USP 28.*
Tall Man: SulfiSOXAZOLE
Use: Anti-infective.
W/Erythromycin Ethylsuccinate.
See: Pediazol.
sulfisoxazole diethanolamine. Sulfi-
soxazole Diolamine.
• **sulfisoxazole diolamine.** (sull-fih-SOX-
uh-zole die-OLE-ah-meen) *USP 28.*
Tall Man: SulfiSOXAZOLE
Use: Anti-infective.
See: Gantrisin.

Sulfoam. (Doak) Sulfur 2%, parabens.
Shampoo. Bot. 237 mL. *OTC.*
Use: Control dandruff.
sulfobromophthalein sodium. *USP 28.*
Use: Liver function test.
sulfocarbolates. Salts of Phenolsulfonic
Acid, Usually Ca, Na, K, Cu, Zn.
• **sulfocon B.** (sul-FOE-kon) USAN.
Use: Hydrophobic.
sulfocyanate.
See: Potassium Thiocyanate.
Sulfo-Ganic. (Marcen) Thioglycerol
20 mg, sodium citrate 5 mg, phenol
0.5%, benzyl alcohol 0.5%/mL. Inj. Vial
10 mL, 30 mL.
Use: Antiarthritic.
Sulfolax. (Major) Docusate calcium
240 mg. Parabens, sorbitol. Soft Gel
Cap. Bot. 100s. *OTC.*
Use: Laxative.
Sulfo-Lo. (Whorton Pharmaceuticals,
Inc.) Sublimed sulfur, freshly precipi-
tated polysulfides of zinc, potassium,
sulfate, and calamine in aqueous-alco-
holic suspension. **Lotion:** Bot. 4 oz,
8 oz. **Soap:** 3 oz. *OTC.*
Use: Dermatologic, acne.
• **sulfomyxin.** (SULL-foe-MIX-in) USAN.
Use: Anti-infective.
sulfonamides.
Use: Anticonvulsants.
See: Sulfacetamide Sodium.
Sulfadiazine.
Sulfamethizole.
Sulfamethoxazole.
Sulfisoxazole.
Sulfisoxazole Diolamine.
Zonisamide.
sulfonamides, triple.
See: Acet-Dia-Mer Sulfonamides.
Meth-Dia-Mer Sulfonamides.
sulfones.
See: Dapsone.
Glucosulfone Sodium.
• **sulfonterol hydrochloride.** (sull-FAHN-
teer-ole) USAN.
Use: Bronchodilator.
sulfonylureas.
See: Acetohexamide.
Chlorpropamide.
Glimepiride.
Glipizide.
Glyburide.
Tolazamide.
Tolbutamide.
Sulforcin. (Galderma) Sulfur 5%, resor-
cinol 2%, SD alcohol 40 11.65%, meth-
ylparaben. Lot. Bot. 120 mL. *OTC.*
Use: Dermatologic.
sulformethoxine. Name used for Sulfa-
doxine.

sulforthomidine. Name used for Sulfadoxine.
sulfosalicylate w/methenamine.
See: Hexalen.
sulfosalicylic acid. Salicylsulphonic acid.
sulfoxone sodium. *USP 28.*
Sulfoxyl Regular. (Stiefel) Benzoyl peroxide 5%, sulfur 2%, stearic acid, zinc laurate. Lot. Bot. 59 mL. *Rx.*
Use: Dermatologic, acne.
Sulfoxyl Strong. (Stiefel) Benzoyl peroxide 10%, sulfur 5%, stearic acid, zinc laurate. Lot. Bot. 59 mL. *Rx.*
Use: Dermatologic, acne.
Sulf-10. (Novartis Ophthalmic) Sodium sulfacetamide 10%. Bot. 15 mL; Dropperette 1 mL. *Rx.*
Use: Anti-infective, ophthalmic.
•**sulfur.**
Use: Antiseborrheic.
See: Sulfoam.
sulfurated lime topical solution.
Vleminckx Lotion.
Use: Scabicide; parasiticide.
sulfur combinations.
See: Acnaveen.
Acno.
Acnomel.
Acnotex.
Adult Acnomel.
Akne.
Akne Oral Kapsulets.
Antrocol
Avar.
Avar Green.
Bensulfoid.
Clearasil.
Clenia.
Fostex.
Fostex CM.
Hydro Surco.
Klaron.
Liquimat.
Neutrogena Disposables.
Pernox.
Plexion.
Plexion Cleansing Cloths.
Plexion SCT.
Plexion TS.
Rezamid.
Rosac.
SAStid Soap.
Sebulex.
Sulfacet-R.
Sulfo-lo.
Sulforcin.
Sulfur-8.
Sulpho-Lac.
Vancocin.
Xerac.

Zetacet.
Zetacet Wash.
•**sulfur dioxide.** (SULL-fer die-OX-ide) *NF 23.*
Use: Pharmaceutic aid (antioxidant).
Sulfur-8 Hair & Scalp Conditioner. (Schering-Plough) Sulfur 2%, menthol 1%, triclosan 0.1%. Cream. Jar 2 oz, 4 oz, 8 oz. *OTC.*
Use: Antiseborrheic.
Sulfur-8 Light Formula Hair & Scalp Conditioner. (Schering-Plough) Sulfur, triclosan, menthol. Cream. Jar 2 oz, 4 oz. *OTC.*
Use: Antiseborrheic.
Sulfur-8 Shampoo. (Schering-Plough) Triclosan 0.2%. Bot. 6.85 oz, 10.85 oz. *OTC.*
Use: Antiseborrheic.
•**sulfur hexafluoride.** USAN.
Use: Diagnostic aid (ultrasound).
•**sulfuric acid.** *NF 23.*
Use: Pharmaceutic aid (acidifying agent).
•**sulfuric acid/sulfonated phenolics.**
Use: Mouth and throat product.
See: Debacterol.
sulfur ointment.
Use: Scabicide; parasiticide.
•**sulfur, precipitated.** *USP 28.*
Use: Scabicide; parasiticide.
See: Bensulfoid.
SAStid Soap.
Sulfur Soap.
sulfur, salicyl diasporal. (Doak Dermatologics)
See: Diasporal.
sulfur soap. (Stiefel) Precipitated sulfur 10%, EDTA. Bulk 110 g. *OTC.*
Use: Dermatologic, acne.
•**sulfur, sublimed.** *USP 28.* Flowers of Sulfur.
Use: Parasiticide; scabicide.
sulfur, topical.
See: Thylox.
•**sulindac.** (sull-IN-dak) *USP 28.*
Use: Anti-inflammatory.
See: Clinoril.
sulindac. (sull-IN-dak) (Various Mfr.) Sulindac 150 mg, 200 mg. Tab. Bot. 100s, 500s, 1000s, UD 100s. *Rx.*
Use: Anti-inflammatory; NSAID.
•**sulisobenzone.** (sul-EYE-so-BEN-zone) USAN.
Use: Ultraviolet screen.
See: Uval.
Uvinul MS-40.
•**sulmarin.** (SULL-mah-rin) USAN.
Use: Hemostatic.

Sulmasque. (C & M Pharmacal) Sulfur 6.4%, isopropyl alcohol 15%, methylparaben. Mask 150 g. *OTC.*
Use: Dermatologic, acne.

Sulnac. (Alra) Sulfathiazole 3.42%, sulfacetamide 2.86%, sulfabenzamide 3.7%, urea 0.64% in cream base. Tube 2.75 oz. *Rx.*
Use: Anti-infective.

●**sulnidazole.** (sull-NIH-dah-zole) USAN.
Use: Antiprotozoal (trichomonas).

●**suloctidil.** (sull-OCK-tih-dill) USAN.
Use: Vasodilator (peripheral).

●**sulofenur.** (SUE-low-FEN-ehr) USAN.
Use: Antineoplastic.

●**sulopenem.** (sue-LOW-PEN-em) USAN.
Use: Anti-infective.

●**sulotroban.** (suh-LOW-troe-ban) USAN.
Use: Treatment of glomerulonephritis.

●**suloxifen oxalate.** (sull-OX-ih-fen OX-ah-late) USAN.
Use: Bronchodilator.

suloxybenzone. (Wyeth)
sulphabenzide.
See: Sulfabenzamide.

Sulpho-Lac Acne Medication. (Doak Dermatologics) Sulfur 5%, zinc sulfate 27%, Vleminckx's Soln. 53%. Cream. Tube 28.35 g, 50 g. *OTC.*
Use: Dermatologic, acne.

Sulpho-Lac Soap. (Doak Dermatologics) Sulfur 5%, a coconut and tallow oil soap base. Bar 85 g. *OTC.*
Use: Dermatologic, acne.

●**sulpiride.** (SULL-pih-ride) USAN.
Use: Antidepressant.

●**sulprostone.** (sull-PRAHST-ohn) USAN.
Use: Prostaglandin.

Sul-Ray Acne. (Last) Sulfur 2% in cream base. Cream. Jar 1.75 oz, 6.75 oz, 20 oz. *OTC.*
Use: Dermatologic, acne.

Sul-Ray Aloe Vera Analgesic Rub. (Last) Camphor 3.1%, menthol 1.25%. Bot. 4 oz, 8 oz. *OTC.*
Use: Analgesic, topical.

Sul-Ray Aloe Vera Skin Protectant. (Last) Zinc oxide 1%, allantoin 0.5%. Cream. Jar 1 oz. *OTC.*
Use: Dermatologic, protectant.

Sul-Ray Shampoo. (Last) Sulfur shampoo 2%. Bot. 8 oz. *OTC.*
Use: Antidandruff.

Sul-Ray Soap. (Last) Sulfur soap. Bar 3 oz. *OTC.*
Use: Dermatologic, acne.

Sulster. (Akorn) Sulfacetamide sodium 1%, prednisolone sodium phosphate. 0.25% Soln. Bot. 5 mL, 10 mL. *Rx.*
Use: Ophthalmic preparation.

●**sultamicillin.** (SULL-TAM-ih-sill-in) USAN.
Use: Anti-infective.

●**sulthiame.** (sull-THIGH-aim) USAN.
Use: Anticonvulsant.

●**sulukast.** (suh-LOO-kast) USAN.
Use: Antiasthmatic (leukotriene antagonist).

Sumacal. (Biosearch Medical Products) CHO 95 g, 380 Cal., Na 100 mg, chloride 210 mg, K < 39 mg, Ca 20 mg/100 g. Pow. Bot. 400 g. *OTC.*
Use: Glucose polymer.

●**sumarotene.** (sue-MAHR-oh-teen) USAN.
Use: Keratolytic.

●**sumatriptan succinate.** (SUE-muh-TRIP-tan SOOS-in-ate) USAN.
Use: Antimigraine, serotonin 5-HT$_1$ receptor agonist.
See: Imitrex.

Summer's Eve Disposable Douche. (C.B. Fleet) **Soln.:** Vinegar. 135 mL (1s, 2s). **Soln. Reg.:** Citric acid, sodium benzoate. **Soln. Scented:** Citric acid, sodium benzoate, octoxynol-9, EDTA. 135 mL (1s, 2s, 4s). *OTC.*
Use: Douche.

Summer's Eve Disposable Douche Extra Cleansing. (C.B. Fleet) Vinegar, sodium Cl, benzoic acid. Soln. 135 mL (1s, 2s, 4s). *OTC.*
Use: Douche.

Summer's Eve Feminine Bath. (C.B. Fleet) Ammonium laureth sulfate, EDTA. Liq. Bot. 45 mL, 345 mL. *OTC.*
Use: Vaginal preparation.

Summer's Eve Feminine Powder. (C.B. Fleet) Cornstarch, octoxynol-9, benzethonium chloride. Pow. Bot. 30 g, 210 g. *OTC.*
Use: Vaginal preparation.

Summer's Eve Feminine Wash. (C.B. Fleet) **Wipes:** Octoxynol-9, EDTA. Box 16s. **Liq.:** Ammonium laureth sulfate, PEG-75, lanolin, EDTA. Bot. 60 mL, 240 mL, 450 mL. *Rx.*
Use: Vaginal preparation.

Summer's Eve Medicated Disposable Douche. (C.B. Fleet) Contains povidone-iodide 0.3%. Single or twin 135 mL disposable units. *OTC.*
Use: Temporary relief of minor vaginal irritation and itching.

Summer's Eve Post Menstrual Disposable Douche. (C.B. Fleet) Sodium lauryl sulfate, parabens, monosodium and disodium phosphates, EDTA. Soln. 135 mL (2s). *OTC.*
Use: Douche.

Summit Extra Strength. (Pfeiffer) Acetaminophen 250 mg, aspirin 250 mg, caffeine 65 mg. Capl. Bot. 50s. *OTC.*
Use: Analgesic combination.

Sumycin '500'. (Par) Tetracycline hydrochloride 500 mg, mineral oil, lactose. Cap. Bot. 100s, 500s. *Rx.*
Use: Anti-infective; tetracycline.

Sumycin Syrup. (Par) Tetracycline hydrochloride 125 mg/5 mL, saccharin, sodium metabisulfite, sorbitol, sucrose, fruit flavor. Oral Susp. Bot. 473 mL. *Rx.*
Use: Anti-infective; tetracycline.

Sumycin '250'. (Par) Tetracycline hydrochloride 250 mg, mineral oil, lactose. Bot. 100s, 1000s. *Rx.*
Use: Anti-infective; tetracycline.

• **suncillin sodium.** (SUN-SILL-in SO-dee-uhm) USAN.
Use: Anti-infective.

Sundown. (Johnson & Johnson) A series of products marketed under the Sundown name including: **Moderate:** (SPF 4) Padimate O, oxybenzone. **Extra:** (SPF 6) Oxybenzone, padimate O. **Maximal:** (SPF 8) Oxybenzone, padimate O. **Ultra:** (SPF 15, 30) oxybenzone, padimate O, octyl methoxycinnamate. *OTC.*
Use: Sunscreen.

Sundown Sport Sunblock. (Johnson & Johnson) Titanium dioxide, zinc oxide. PABA free. Waterproof. SPF 15. Lot. 90 mL. *OTC.*
Use: Sunscreen.

Sundown Sunblock Cream Ultra SPF 24. (Johnson & Johnson) Padimate O, oxybenzone. *OTC.*
Use: Sunscreen.

Sundown Sunblock Stick SPF 15. (Johnson & Johnson) Octyl dimethyl PABA, oxybenzone. Stick 0.35 oz. *OTC.*
Use: Sunscreen.

Sundown Sunblock Stick SPF 20. (Johnson & Johnson) Octyl dimethyl PABA, octyl methoxycinnamate, oxybenzone, titanium dioxide. *OTC.*
Use: Sunscreen.

Sundown Sunblock Ultra Lotion 30 SPF. (Johnson & Johnson) Octyl methoxycinnamate, octyl salicylate, oxybenzone, titanium dioxide, cetyl alcohol, PABA free. Waterproof. Lot. Bot. 120 mL. *OTC.*
Use: Sunscreen.

Sundown Sunblock Ultra SPF 20. (Johnson & Johnson) Octyl dimethyl PABA, octyl methoxycinnamate, oxybenzone, titanium dioxide. *OTC.*
Use: Sunscreen.

Sundown Sunscreen Stick SPF 8. (Johnson & Johnson) Octyl dimethyl PABA, oxybenzone. Stick 0.35 oz. *OTC.*
Use: Sunscreen.

Sundown Sunscreen Ultra. (Johnson & Johnson) Octyl methoxycinnamate, octyl salicylate, oxybenzone, titanium dioxide, stearyl alcohol, cetyl alcohol, PABA free. Waterproof. SPF 15. Cream. Tube 60 g. *OTC.*
Use: Sunscreen.

• **sunepitron hydrochloride.** (soo-NE-pi-tron) USAN.
Use: Anxiolytic; antidepressant.

Sunice. (Citroleum) Allantoin 0.25%, menthol 0.25%, methyl salicylate 10%. Cream. Jar 3 oz. *OTC.*
Use: Burn therapy.

Sunkist Multivitamins Complete, Children's (Novartis) Fe 18 mg, vitamin A 5000 units, D_3 400 units, E 30 units, B_1 1.5 mg, B_2 1.7 mg, B_3 20 mg, B_5 10 mg, B_6 2 mg, B_{12} 6 mcg, C 60 mg, folic acid 400 mcg, Ca 100 mg, Cu, I, K, Mg, Mn, P, Zn 10 mg, biotin 40 mcg, K_1 10 mcg, sorbitol, aspartame, phenylalanine, tartrazine. Chew. Tab. Bot. 60s. *OTC.*
Use: Mineral, vitamin supplement.

Sunkist Multivitamins + Extra C, Children's. (Novartis) Vitamin A 2500 units, E 15 units, D_3 400 units, B_1 1.05 mg, B_2 1.2 mg, B_3 13.5 mg, B_6 1.05 mg, B_{12} 4.5 mcg, C 250 mg, folic acid 0.3 mg, vitamin K 5 mcg, sorbitol, aspartame, phenylalanine. Chew. Tab. Bot. 60s. *OTC.*
Use: Vitamin supplement.

Sunkist Vitamin C. (Novartis) Vitamin C (as ascorbic acid) 60 mg, 250 mg, 500 mg, fructose, sorbitol, sucrose, lactose, orange flavor. Chew. Tab. Bot. 11s (60 mg only), 60s (250 mg only), 75s (500 mg only). *OTC.*
Use: Vitamin supplement.

SUNPRuF 15. (C & M Pharmacal) Octyl methoxycinnamate 7.5%, benzophenone-3 5%. PABA free. Waterproof. SPF 15. Lot. Bot. 240 mL. *OTC.*
Use: Sunscreen.

SUNPRuF 17. (C & M Pharmacal) Octyl methoxycinnamate 7.8%, octyl salicylate 5.2%, oil-free, water-resistant. SPF 17. Lot. Bot. 120 g. *OTC.*
Use: Sunscreen.

Sunshine Chewable Tablets. (Fibertone) Fe 5 mg, vitamins A 5000 units, D 400 units, E 67 mg, B_1 15 mg, B_2 15 mg, B_3 25 mg, B_5 20 mg, B_6 15 mg, B_{12} 15 mcg, C 150 mg, folic acid 0.1 mg, Ca, Cu, Mn, Zn, K, iodide, bio-

tin, betaine, PABA, choline bitartrate, inositol, lecithin, hesperidin, rutin, bioflavonoids, sorbitol, aspartame, citrus flavor. Bot. 60s. *OTC.*
Use: Mineral, vitamin supplement.

Sunstick. (Rydelle) Lip and face protectant containing digalloyl trioleate 2.5% in emollient base. Stick Plas. swivel container 0.14 oz. *OTC.*
Use: Lip protectant.

SU-101.
Use: Malignant glioma. [Orphan Drug]

Supartz. (Smith & Nephew) Sodium hyaluronate 25 mg/2.5 mL. Soln. 2.5 prefilled syringes. *Rx.*
Use: Antiarthritic.

Super Aytinal. (Walgreen) Vitamins A 7000 units, B_1 5 mg, B_2 5 mg, B_5 10 mg, B_6 3 mg, B_{12} 9 mcg, C 90 mg, pantothenic acid 10 mg, D 400 units, E 30 units, niacin 30 mg, biotin 55 mcg, folic acid 0.4 mg, Fe 30 mg, Ca 162 mg, P 125 mg, I 150 mcg, Cu 3 mg, Mn 7.5 mg, Mg 100 mg, K 7.7 mg, Zn 24 mg, Cl 7 mg, Cr 15 mcg, Se 15 mcg, choline bitartrate 1000 mcg, inositol 1000 mcg, PABA 1000 mcg, rutin 1000 mcg, yeast 12 mg. Bot. 50s, 100s, 365s. *OTC.*
Use: Mineral, vitamin supplement.

Super-B. (Towne) Vitamins B_1 50 mg, B_2 20 mg, B_6 5 mg, B_{12} 15 mcg, C 300 mg, liver desiccated 100 mg, dried yeast 100 mg, niacinamide 25 mg, Ca pantothenate 5 mg, Fe 10 mg. Captab. Bot. 50s, 100s, 150s, 250s. *OTC.*
Use: Mineral, vitamin supplement.

Super Calicaps M-Z. (Nion Corp.) Ca 1200 mg, Mg 400 mg, Zn 15 mg, vitamins A 5000 units, D 400 units, Se 15 mcg. 3 Tabs. Bot. 90s. *OTC.*
Use: Mineral, vitamin supplement.

Super Calcium 1200. (Schiff Products/Weider Nutrition Intl.) Calcium carbonate 1512 mg (600 mg calcium). Cap. Bot. 60s, 120s. *OTC.*
Use: Mineral supplement.

Superdophilus. (NaTREN) *Lactobacillus acidophilus* strain DDS 1.2 billion/g Pow. 37.5 g, 75 g, 135 g. *OTC.*
Use: Antidiarrheal; nutritional supplement.

Super D Perles. (Pharmacia) Vitamins A 10,000 units, D 400 units. Cap. Bot. 100s. *OTC.*
Use: Vitamin supplement.

SuperEPA. (Advanced Nutritional Technology) Omega-3 polyunsaturated fatty acids 1200 mg. Cap. containing EPA 360 mg, DHA 240 mg. Bot. 60s, 90s. *OTC.*

Use: Nutritional supplement.

SuperEPA 2000. (Advanced Nutritional Technology) EPA 563 mg, DHA 312 mg, vitamin E 20 units. Cap. Bot. 30s, 60s, 90s. *OTC.*
Use: Nutritional supplement.

Supere-Pect. (Barth's) Alpha tocopherol 400 units, apple pectin 100 mg. Cap. Bot. 50s, 100s, 250s. *OTC.*
Use: Nutritional supplement.

Super Flavons. (Freeda) Citrus bioflavonoids and hesperidin complex 300 mg, sodium free. Tab. Bot. 250s. *OTC.*
Use: Vitamin supplement.

Super Flavons 300. (Freeda) Bioflavonoids 300 mg. Tab. Bot. 100s, 250s. *OTC.*
Use: Vitamin supplement.

Super Hi Potency. (Nion Corp.) Vitamins A 10,000 units, D 400 units, E 150 units, B_1 75 mg, B_2 75 mg, B_3 75 mg, B_5 75 mg, B_6 75 mg, B_{12} 75 mcg, C 250 mg, folic acid 0.4 mg, Zn 15 mg, betaine, biotin 75 mcg, Ca, Fe, hesperidin, I, K, Mg, Mn, Se. Tab. Bot. 100s. *OTC.*
Use: Mineral, vitamin supplement.

Super Hydramin Protein Powder. (Nion Corp.) Protein 41%, carbohydrate 21.8%, fat 1% in powder form. Can 1 lb. *OTC.*
Use: Nutritional supplement.

superinone. Tyloxapol.

Super Nutri-Vites. (Faraday) Vitamins A 36,000 units, D 400 units, B_1 25 mg, B_2 25 mg, B_6 50 mg, B_{12} 50 mcg, niacinamide 50 mg, Ca pantothenate 12.5 mg, choline bitartrate 150 mg, inositol 150 mg, betaine hydrochloride 25 mg, PABA 15 mg, glutamic acid 25 mg, desiccated liver 50 mg, C 150 mg, E 12.5 units, Mn gluconate 6.15 mg, bone meal 162 mg, Fe gluconate 50 mg, Cu gluconate 0.25 mg, Zn gluconate 2.2 mg, K iodide 0.1 mg, Ca 53.3 mg, P 24.3 mg, Mg gluconate 7.2 mg. Protein Coated Tab. Bot. 60s, 100s. *OTC.*
Use: Mineral, vitamin supplement.

superoxide dismutase (human, recombinant human).
Use: Protection of donor organ tissue. [Orphan Drug]

Super Plenamins Multiple Vitamins and Minerals. (Rexall Group) Vitamins A 8000 units, D_2 400 units, vitamins B_1 2.5 mg, B_2 2.5 mg, C 75 mg, niacinamide 20 mg, B_6 1 mg, B_{12} 3 mcg, biotin 20 mcg, E 10 units, pantothenic acid 3 mg, liver conc. 100 mg, Fe 30 mg, Ca 75 mg, P 58 mg, I 0.15 mg,

Cu 0.75 mg, manganese 1.25 mg, Mg 10 mg, Zn 1 mg. Tab. Bot. 36s, 72s, 144s, 288s, 365s. *OTC.*
Use: Mineral, vitamin supplement.
Superplex T. (Major) Vitamins B_1 15 mg, B_2 10 mg, B_3 100 mg, B_5 20 mg, B_6 5 mg, B_{12} 10 mcg, C 500 mg. Tab. Bot. 100s. *OTC.*
Use: Vitamin supplement.
Super Poli-Grip/Wernet's Cream. (Block Drug) Carboxymethylcellulose gum, ethylene oxide polymer, petrolatum-mineral oil base. Tube 0.7 oz, 1.4 oz, 2.4 oz. *OTC.*
Use: Denture adhesive.
Super Quints-50. (Freeda) Vitamins B_1 50 mg, B_2 50 mg, B_3 50 mg, B_5 50 mg, B_6 50 mg, B_{12} 50 mcg, folic acid 0.4 mg, PABA 30 mg, d-biotin 50 mcg, inositol 50 mg. Tab. Bot. 100s, 250s, 500s. *OTC.*
Use: Vitamin supplement.
Super Shade SPF-25. (Schering-Plough) Ethylhexyl p-methoxycinnamate, padimate O oxybenzone. SPF 25. Lot. Bot. 4 fl. oz. *OTC.*
Use: Sunscreen.
Super Shade Sunblock Stick SPF-25. (Schering-Plough) Ethylhexyl p-methoxycinnamate, oxybenzone, padimate O in stick. SPF 25. Tube 0.43 oz. *OTC.*
Use: Sunscreen.
Super Stress. (Towne) Vitamins C 600 mg, E 30 units, B_1 15 mg, B_2 15 mg, niacin 100 mg, B_6 5 mg, B_{12} 12 mcg, pantothenic acid 20 mg. Tab. Bot. 60s. *OTC.*
Use: Vitamin supplement.
Super Troche. (Weeks & Leo) Benzocaine 5 mg, cetalkonium Cl 1 mg. Loz. Bot. 15s, 30s. *OTC.*
Use: Mouth and throat preparation.
Super Troche Plus. (Weeks & Leo) Benzocaine 10 mg, cetalkonium Cl 2 mg. Loz. Bot. 12s. *OTC.*
Use: Mouth and throat preparation.
Super-T with Zinc. (Towne) Vitamins A 10,000 units, D 400 units, E 15 units, C 200 mg, B_1 10 mg, B_2 10 mg, B_6 5 mg, B_{12} 6 mcg, niacinamide 50 mg, Fe 18 mg, I 0.1 mg, Cu 2 mg, Mn 1 mg, Zn 15 mg. Cap. Bot. 130s. *OTC.*
Use: Mineral, vitamin supplement.
Supervim. (US Ethicals) Vitamins and minerals. Tab. Bot. 100s.
Use: Mineral, vitamin supplement.
Super Wernet's Powder. (Block Drug) Carboxymethylcellulose gum, ethylene oxide polymer. Bot. 0.63 oz, 1.75 oz, 3.55 oz. *OTC.*
Use: Denture adhesive.

Suplena. (Ross) A vanilla flavored liquid containing 29.6 g protein, 252.5 g carbohydrates, 95 g fat/L. With appropriate vitamins and minerals. Cans 240 mL. *OTC.*
Use: Nutritional supplement.
Suplical. (Parke-Davis) Calcium 600 mg/ Square. Bot. 30s, 60s. *OTC.*
Use: Mineral supplement.
Suppress. (Ferndale) Dextromethorphan HBr 7.5 mg. Loz. 1000s. *OTC.*
Use: Antitussive.
Supra Min. (Towne) Vitamins A 10,000 units, D 400 units, E 30 units, C 250 mg, folic acid 0.4 mg, B_1 10 mg, B_2 10 mg, niacin 100 mg, B_6 5 mg, B_{12} 6 mcg, pantothenic acid 20 mg, I 150 mcg, Fe 100 mg, Mg 2 mg, Cu 20 mg, Mn 1.25 mg. Tab. Bot. 130s. *OTC.*
Use: Mineral, vitamin supplement.
Suprane. (Ohmeda) Desflurane. 240 mL. Volatile Liq. Bot. *Rx.*
Use: Anesthetic, general.
Suprarenal. Dried, partially defatted and powdered adrenal gland of cattle, sheep, or swine.
Suprax. (Lupin Pharma) Cefixime. **Pow. for Oral Susp.:** 100 mg/5 mL. Sucrose. Strawberry flavored. 50 mL, 75 mL, 100 mL. *Rx.*
Use: Cephalosporin.
Suprazine. (Major) Trifluoperazine 1 mg, 2 mg, 5 mg, 10 mg. Tab. Bot. 100s, 250s, 1000s, UD 100s (2 mg only). *Rx.*
Use: Anxiolytic.
Suprins. (Towne) Vitamins A palmitate 10,000 units, D 400 units, B_1 10 mg, B_2 10 mg, B_6 5 mg, B_{12} 6 mcg, C 250 mg, calcium pantothenate 20 mg, niacinamide 100 mg, biotin 25 mcg, E 15 units, Ca 103 mg, P 80 mg, Fe 10 mg, I 0.1 mg, Cu 1.0 mg, Zn 20 mg, Mn 1.25 mg. Captab. Bot. 100s. *OTC.*
Use: Mineral, vitamin supplement.
•**suproclone.** (SUH-pro-klone) USAN.
Use: Sedative; hypnotic.
•**suprofen.** (sue-PRO-fen) *USP 28.*
Use: Anti-inflammatory.
See: Profenal.
•**suramin hexasodium.** (SOOR-ah-min hex-ah-SO-dee-uhm) USAN.
Use: Antineoplastic.
Surbex Filmtab. (Abbott) Vitamins B_1 6 mg, B_2 6 mg, B_3 30 mg, B_6 2.5 mg, B_5 10 mg, B_{12} 5 mcg. Filmtab. Bot. 100s. *OTC.*
Use: Mineral, vitamin supplement.
Surbex 750 with Iron. (Abbott) Vitamins B_1 15 mg, B_2 15 mg, B_6 25 mg, B_{12}

12 mcg, C 750 mg, B_5 20 mg, E 30 units, B_3 100 mg, Fe 27 mg, folic acid 0.4 mg. Tab. Bot. 50s. *OTC.*
Use: Mineral, vitamin supplement.

Surbex 750 with Zinc. (Abbott) B_1 15 mg, B_2 15 mg, B_6 20 mg, B_{12} 12 mcg, C 750 mg, E 30 units, B_5 20 mg, niacin 100 mg, folic acid 0.4 mg, Zn 22.5 mg. Tab. Bot. 50s. *OTC.*
Use: Mineral, vitamin supplement.

Surbex-T Filmtab. (Abbott) Vitamins B_1 15 mg, B_2 10 mg, B_3 100 mg, B_6 5 mg, B_{12} 10 mcg, B_5 20 mg, C 500 mg. Filmtab. Bot. 100s. *OTC.*
Use: Mineral, vitamin supplement.

Surbex with C Filmtabs. (Abbott) Vitamins B_1 6 mg, B_2 6 mg, B_3 30 mg, B_5 10 mg, B_6 2.5 mg, B_{12} 5 mg, C 500 mg. Film coated. Tab. Bot. 100s. *OTC.*
Use: Vitamin supplement.

Surbu-Gen-T. (Ivax) Vitamins B_1 15 mg, B_2 10 mg, B_3 100 mg, B_5 20 mg, B_6 5 mg, B_{12} 10 mcg, C 500 mg. Tab. Bot. 100s. *OTC.*
Use: Vitamin supplement.

SureCell HCG-Urine Test. (Kodak Dental) Polyclonal/monoclonal antibody sandwich-based ELISA to detect human chorionic gonadotropin in urine. Kit 10s, 25s, 100s.
Use: Diagnostic aid.

SureCell Herpes (HSV) Test. (Kodak Dental) Monoclonal antibody-based ELISA to detect HSV 1 & 2 antigens from lesions. Kit 10s, 25s.
Use: Diagnostic aid.

SureCell Strep A Test. (Kodak Dental) ELISA to detect group A streptococci. Kit 10s, 25s, 100s.
Use: Diagnostic aid.

SureLac. (Caraco) 3000 FCC lactase units, sorbitol, mannitol. Chew. Tab. Bot. 60s. *OTC.*
Use: Nutritional supplement.

surface active extract of saline lavage of bovine lungs.
Use: Respiratory failure in preterm infants. [Orphan Drug]

surfactant, natural lung.
Use: Surfactant replacement therapy in neonatal respiratory distress syndrome.
See: Survanta.

surfactant, synthetic lung.
Use: Surfactant replacement therapy in neonatal respiratory distress syndrome.
See: Exosurf Neonatal.

Surfak. (Pharmacia) Docusate calcium. 240 mg, sorbitol, parabens. Soft Gel Cap. Bot. 10s, 30s, 100s, 500s, UD

100s. *OTC.*
Use: Laxative.

•**surfilcon a.** (SER-FILL-kahn A) USAN.
Use: Hydrophilic contact lens material.

Surfol Post-Immersion Bath Oil. (Stiefel) Mineral oil, isopropyl myristate, isostearic acid, PEG-40, sorbitan peroleate. Bot. 8 oz. *OTC.*
Use: Dermatologic.

•**surfomer.** (SER-foe-mer) USAN.
Use: Hypolipidemic.

Surgasoap. (Wade) Castile vegetable oils. Bot. Qt., gal. *OTC.*
Use: Dermatologic, cleanser.

Surgel. (Ulmer Pharmacal) Propylene glycol, glycerin. Gel. Bot. 120 mL, 240 mL, gal. *OTC.*
Use: Lubricant.

Surgel Liquid. (Ulmer Pharmacal) Patient lubricant fluid. Bot. 4 oz, 8 oz, gal.
Use: Lubricant.

•**surgibone.** (SER-jih-bone) USAN. Bone and cartilage obtained from bovine embryos and young calves.
Use: Prosthetic aid (internal bone splint).

Surgical Simplex P. (Howmedica) Methyl methacrylate 20 mL poly 6.7 g, methyl methacrylate-styrene copolymer 33.3 g. **Pow.:** 40 g. **Liq.:** 20 mL. Bot.
Use: Bone cement.

Surgical Simplex P Radiopaque. (Howmedica) Methyl methacrylate 20 mL, poly 6 g, methyl methacrylate-styrene copolymer 30 g. **Pow.:** 40 g. **Liq.:** 20 mL. Bot.
Use: Bone cement.

Surgicel. (Johnson & Johnson) Sterile absorbable knitted fabric prepared by controlled oxidation of regenerated cellulose. Sterile strips 2 × 14, 4 × 8, 2 × 3, 0.5 × 2 inches. Surgical Nuknit: 1 × 1, 3 × 4, 6 × 9 inches. Box 1s.
Use: Hemostatic.

Surgidine. (Continental Consumer Products) Iodine 0.8% in iodine complex. Germicide. Bot. 8 oz, gal. Foot operated dispenser 8 oz, gal. *OTC.*
Use: Antiseptic.

Surgi-Kleen. (Sween) Bot. 2 oz, 8 oz, 16 oz, 21 oz, gal, 5 gal, 30 gal, 55 gal.
Use: Dermatologic, cleanser.

Surgilube. (E. Fougera) Sterile surgical lubricant. Foilpac 3 g, 5 g. Tube 5 g, 2 oz, 4.25 oz.
Use: Lubricant.

•**suricainide maleate.** (ser-ih-CANE-ide) USAN.
Use: Cardiovascular agent (antiarrhythmic).

●**suritozole.** (suh-RIH-tah-ZOLE) USAN.
Use: Antidepressant.

Surmontil. (Wyeth) Trimipramine maleate 25 mg, 50 mg, 100 mg, lactose. Cap. Bot. 100s, UD 100s (50 mg only). Redipaks. *Rx.*
Use: Antidepressant.

surofene. Hexachlorophene.

●**suronacrine maleate.** (SUE-row-NAH-kreen) USAN.
Use: Cholinergic; cholinesterase inhibitor.

Surpass. (Wrigley) Calcium carbonate 300 mg, aspartame, sorbitol, phenylalanine 3.9 mg, wintergreen flavor. Gum. Box. 10s. *OTC.*
Use: Antacid.

Surpass Extra Strength. (Wrigley) Calcium carbonate 450 mg, aspartame, sorbitol, phenylalanine 3.0 mg, fruit flavor. Gum. Box. 10s. *OTC.*
Use: Antacid.

Survanta. (Ross Labs) Beractant 25 mg/mL, sodium chloride solution 0.9%, triglycerides 0.5 to 1.75 mg, free fatty acids 1.4 to 3.5 mg, protein < 1 mg/mL. Susp. Single-use vial containing 8 mL suspension. *Rx.*
Use: Lung surfactant.

Suspen. (Circle) Penicillin V potassium 250 mg/5 mL. Bot. 100 mL. *Rx.*
Use: Anti-infective, penicillin.

●**suspension structured vehicle.** *NF 23.*
Use: Pharmaceutical vehicle.

Sustacal Basic. (Bristol-Myers Squibb) A vanilla, strawberry, or chocolate flavored liquid containing 36.6 g protein, 34.6 g fat, 145.8 g carbohydrate, 833 mg Na, 1583 mg K/L. 1.04 Cal/mL, with appropriate vitamin and mineral levels to meet 100% of the US RDAs. Liq. Can 240 ml. *OTC.*
Use: Nutritional supplement.

Sustacal HC. (Bristol-Myers Squibb) High calorie nutritionally complete food. Protein 16%, fat 34%, carbohydrate 50%. Can 8 oz. Vanilla, chocolate, or eggnog. *OTC.*
Use: Nutritional supplement.

Sustacal Plus. (Bristol-Myers Squibb) A vanilla, eggnog, or chocolate flavored liquid containing 61 g protein, 58 g fat, 190 g carbohydrate, 15.2 mg Fe, 850 mg Na, 1480 mg K, 1520 cal/L, with appropriate vitamin and mineral levels to meet 100% of the US RDAs. Liq. Bot. 237 mL, 960 mL. *OTC.*
Use: Nutritional supplement.

Sustacal Powder. (Bristol-Myers Squibb) Caloric distribution and nutritional value when added to milk are similar to that

of Sustacal liquid except lactose. Contains vanilla: Pow. 1.9 oz. packets 4s, 1 lb. can; Chocolate 1.9 oz. packets 4s. *OTC.*
Use: Nutritional supplement.

Sustacal Pudding. (Bristol-Myers Squibb) Ready-to-eat fortified pudding containing at least 15% of the US RDAs for protein, vitamins and minerals, in a 240 calorie serving. As a % of the calories, protein 11%, fat 36%, carbohydrate 53%. Flavors: Chocolate, vanilla, and butterscotch. Tins, 5 oz, 110 oz. *OTC.*
Use: Nutritional supplement.

Sustagen. (Bristol-Myers Squibb) High-calorie, high-protein supplement containing as a % of the calories, 24% protein, 8% fat, 68% carbohydrate. Contains all known essential vitamins and minerals. Prepared from nonfat milk, corn syrup solids, powdered whole milk, calcium caseinate, and dextrose. Vanilla: Can 1 lb, 5 lb. Chocolate: Can 1 lb. *OTC.*
Use: Nutritional supplement.

Sustain. (Zee Medical) Sodium chloride 220 mg, calcium carbonate 18 mg, potassium chloride 15 mg. Tab. 24s. *Rx.*
Use: Salt replacement.

Sustiva. (Bristol-Myers Squibb Oncology/Immunology) Efavirenz. **Cap:** 50 mg, 100 mg, 200 mg, lactose. Bot. 30s (except 200 mg), 90s (200 mg only). **Tab:** 600 mg, lactose. Bot 30s, UD blister 100s. *Rx.*
Use: Antiretroviral, non-nucleoside reverse transcriptase inhibitor.

●**suture, absorbable surgical.** *USP 28.*
Use: Surgical aid.

●**suture, nonabsorbable surgical.** *USP 28.*
Use: Surgical aid.

Su-Tuss DM. (Cypress) Dextromethorphan HBr 20 mg, guaifenesin 200 mg/5 mL, alcohol 5%, fruit flavor. Liq. Bot. 473 mL. *Rx.*
Use: Upper respiratory combination, antitussive, expectorant.

Su-Tuss HD. (Cypress) Hydrocodone bitartrate 2.5 mg, guaifenesin 100 mg, pseudoephedrine hydrochloride 30 mg/5 mL, alcohol 5%, fruit punch flavor. Elixir. Bot. 473 mL. *c-III.*
Use: Upper respiratory combination, antitussive, expectorant, decongestant.

Suvaplex. (Tennessee Pharmaceutic) Vitamins A 5000 units, D 500 units, B$_1$ 2.5 mg, B$_2$ 2.5 mg, B$_6$ 0.5 mg, B$_{12}$ 1 mcg, C 37.5 mg, Ca pantothenate 5 mg, niacinamide 20 mg, folic acid

0.1 mg. Tab. Bot. 100s. *OTC.*
Use: Mineral, vitamin supplement.

• **suxemerid sulfate.** (sux-EM-er-rid)
USAN.
Use: Antitussive.

swamp root. Compound of various organic roots in an alcohol base.
Use: Diuretic to the kidney.

Sween-A-Peel. (Sween) Wafer 4 x 4. Box
5s, 20s; Sheets 1212. Box 2s, 12s.
Use: Dermatologic, protectant.

Sween Cream. (Sween) Vitamin A and
D cream. Tube 0.5 oz, 2 oz, 5 oz. Jar
2 oz, 9 oz. *OTC.*
Use: Dermatologic.

Sween Kind Lotion. (Sween) Bot. 21 oz,
gal.
Use: Dermatologic, cleanser.

Sween Prep. (Sween) Box wipes 54s.
Dab-o-matic 2 oz. Spray Top 4 oz.
Use: Dermatologic, protectant, medicated.

Sween Soft Touch. (Sween) Bot. 2 oz,
16 oz, 21 oz, 32 oz, 1 gal., 5 gal.
Use: Dermatologic, protectant, medicated.

Sweeta. (Bristol-Myers Squibb) Saccharin sodium, sorbitol. Bot. 24 mL, 2 oz,
4 oz. *OTC.*
Use: Sweetening agent.

Sweetaste. (Purepac) Saccharin 0.25 g,
0.5 g, 1 g. Tab. w/Sodium bicarbonate.
Bot. 1000s. *OTC.*
Use: Sugar substitute.

sweetening agents.
See: Saccharin.
Sweetaste.

Swim-Ear. (E. Fougera) 2.75% boric acid
in isopropyl alcohol. Bot. 1 oz. *OTC.*
Use: Otic.

Swiss Kriss. (Modern Aids Inc.) Senna
leaves, herbs. Coarse cut mixture. Can
1.5 oz, 3.25 oz, Tab. 24s, 120s, 250s.
OTC.
Use: Laxative.

Syllact. (Wallace) Psyllium seed husks
3.3 g, 14 cal/rounded tsp, dextose,
parabens, fruit flavor, saccharin. Pow.
Bot. 284 g. *OTC.*
Use: Laxative.

Symax-SL. (Capellon) L-hyoscyamine
sulfate 0.125 mg. Sublingual Tab. Bot.
100s. *Rx.*
Use: Anticholinergic, antispasmodic,
belladonna alkaloid.

Symax-SR. (Capellon) L-hyoscyamine
sukfate 0.375 mg. SR Tab. Bot. 100s.
Rx.
Use: Anticholinergic, antispasmodic,
belladonna alkaloid.

Symbyax. (Eli Lilly) Olanzapine/fluoxetine hydrochloride 6 mg/25 mg; 6 mg/
50 mg; 12 mg/25 mg; 12 mg/50 mg.
Cap. 30s, 100s, 1000s, blister UD 100s.
Rx.
Use: Psychotherapeutic agent.

• **symclosene.** (SIM-kloe-seen) USAN.
Use: Anti-infective, topical.

• **symetine hydrochloride.** (SIM-eh-teen)
USAN.
Use: Antiamebic.

Symlin. (Amylin Pharmaceuticals, Inc.)
Pramlintide acetate 0.6 mg/mL. Metacresol 2.25 mg/mL as a preservative,
D-mannitol as a tonicity modifier, and
acetic acid and sodium acetate as pH
modifiers. Soln. for Inj. Vials. 5 mL. *Rx.*
Use: Antidiabetic agent.

Symmetrel. (Endo) Amantadine hydrochloride. **Tab:** 100 mg. Bot. 100s,
500s. **Syr:** 50 mg/5 mL, sorbitol, parabens. Bot. 480 mL. *Rx.*
Use: Antiviral; antiparkinsonian; treatment of drug-induced extrapyramidal symptoms.

sympatholytic agents.
See: Antiadrenergics/sympatholytics.

sympathomimetic agents.
See: Albuterol.
Bitolterol Mesylate.
Ephedrine Sulfate.
Epinephrine.
Formoterol Fumarate.
Isoetharine hydrochloride.
Isoproterenol hydrochloride.
Levalbuterol hydrochloride.
Metaproterenol Sulfate.
Pirbuterol Acetate.
Salmeterol.
Terbutaline Sulfate.

Syna-Clear. (Pruvo) Decongestant plus
Vitamin C. 25 mg. Tab. Bot. 12s, 30s.
Use: Decongestant.

Synacort. (Roche) Hydrocortisone
cream. **1%:** Tube 15 g, 30 g, 60 g.
2.5%: Tube 30 g. *Rx.*
Use: Corticosteroid, topical.

Synagis. (MedImmune) Palivizumab.
Inj.: 100 mg/mL. Histidine 4.7 mg, glycine 0.1 mg per mL. Preservative free.
Single-use vials. 1 mL. **Pow. for Inj.,
lyophilized:** 50 mg, 100 mg, histidine
47 mM, glycine 3 mM, mannitol 5.6%,
preservative free. Single-use vial
0.5 mL (50 mg), 1 mL (100 mg). *Rx.*
Use: Antibody.

Synalar. (Roche) Fluocinolone acetonide.
Cream: 0.01%: Tube 15 g, 30 g, 45 g,
60 g, 120 g. Jar 425 g. **0.025%:** Tube
15 g, 30 g, 60 g, 120 g. Jar 425 g.
Oint.: 0.025%: Tube 15 g, 30 g, 60 g,
120 g. Jar 425 g. **Soln. 0.01%:** Bot.

20 mL, 60 mL. *Rx.*
Use: Corticosteroid, topical.

Synalar-HP. (Roche) Fluocinolone acetonide 0.2% in water-washable aqueous base. Cream. Tube 12 g. *Rx.*
Use: Corticosteroid, topical.

Synalgos-DC. (Wyeth) Dihydrocodeine bitartrate 16 mg, aspirin 356.4 mg, caffeine 30 mg. Cap. Bot. 100s, 500s. *c-III.*
Use: Analgesic combination; narcotic.

Synarel. (Roche) Nafarelin acetate 2 mg/mL (as nafarelin base). Nasal solution. Bot. 10 mL with metered pump spray. *Rx.*
Use: Endometriosis.

SynBiotics-3. (NutraCea) *Bifidobacterium longum* 4.5 billion CFU, *Lactobacillus rhamnosus* A, *L. plantarum,* Saccharomyces boulardii, Maltodextrin. Cap. 60s, UD 200s. *OTC.*
Use: Nutritional supplement.

Syncaine.
See: Procaine Hydrochloride.

Syncort.
See: Desoxycorticosterone Acetate.

Syncortyl.
See: Desoxycorticosterone Acetate.

Synemol. (Roche) Fluocinolone acetonide 0.025% in water-washable aqueous emollient base. Tube 15 g, 30 g, 60 g, 120 g. *Rx.*
Use: Corticosteroid, topical.

Synercid. (Monarch) Quinupristin 150 mg, dalfopristin 350 mg/10 mL. Inj. lyophilized. Vial 10 mL. *Rx.*
Use: Streptogramin

synkonin.
See: Hydrocodone.

Synophylate. (Schwarz Pharma) Theophylline sodium glycinate. **Elix.:** Theophylline 165 mg/15 mL w/alcohol 20%. Bot. Pt, gal. **Tab.:** Theophylline 165 mg. Tab. Bot. 100s, 1000s. *Rx.*
Use: Bronchodilator.

Synophylate-GG. (Schwarz Pharma) Theophylline sodium glycinate 300 mg, guaifenesin 100 mg, alcohol 10%. Syr. Bot. Pt, gal. *Rx.*
Use: Bronchodilator.

Syn-Rx. (Medeva) **AM:** Pseudoephedrine hydrochloride 60 mg, guaifenesin 600 mg. CR Tab. Bot. 28s. **PM:** Guaifenesin 600 mg. CR Tab. Bot. 28s. In 14-day treatment regimen of 56 tablets. *Rx.*
Use: Upper respiratory combination, decongestant, expectorant.

Synsorb Pk.
Use: Verocytotoxogenic *E. coli* infections. [Orphan Drug]

Synthaloids. (Buffington) Benzocaine, calcium-iodine complex. Loz. Salt free. Bot. 100s, 1000s. Unit boxes 8s, 16s. Box 24s. *Dispens-a-Kit* 500s. *Aidpaks* 100s. *Medipaks* 200s. *OTC.*
Use: Sore throat relief.

synthetic conjugated estrogens, a.
Use: Estrogen.
See: Cenestin.

•**synthetic conjugated estrogens, b.** (ES-troe-jens) USAN.
Use: Hormone replacement therapy

synthetic lung surfactant.
See: Exosurf Neonatal.

synthoestrin.
See: Diethylstilbestrol.

Synthroid. (Abbott) Sodium levothyroxine 0.025 mg, 0.05 mg, 0.075 mg, 0.088 mg, 0.1 mg, 0.112 mg, 0.125 mg, 0.137 mg, 0.15 mg, 0.175 mg, 0.2 mg, 0.3 mg, sugar, lactose. Tab. Bot. 100s, 1000s, UD 100s (0.05 mg, 0.075 mg, 0.1 mg, 0.125 mg, 0.15 mg, 0.2 mg). *Rx.*
Use: Hormone, thyroid.

Synthroid Injection. (Abbott) Lyophilized sodium levothyroxine 200 mcg, 500 mcg. Vial. 10 mL (100 mcg/mL when reconstituted.) *Rx.*
Use: Hormone, thyroid.

Synvisc. (Wyeth) Sodium hyaluronate/hylan G-F 20 16 mg/2 mL. Glass syringe 2 mL with 3 disposable syringes. *Rx.*
Use: Antiarthritic.

Syphilis (FTA-ABS) Fluoro Kit. (Clinical Sciences)
Use: Test for syphilis.

Syprine. (Merck & Co.) Trientine hydrochloride 250 mg. Cap. Bot. 100s. *Rx.*
Use: Chelating agent.

Syracol CF. (Roberts) Dextromethorphan HBr 15 mg, guaifenesin 200 mg. Tab. Bot. 500s. *OTC.*
Use: Antitussive; expectorant.

Syroxine. (Major) Sodium levothyroxine 0.1 mg, 0.2 mg, 0.3 mg. Tab. Bot. 100s, 250s, 1000s, UD 100s. (3 mg 1000s). *Rx.*
Use: Hormone, thyroid.

Syrpalta. (Emerson) Syr. containing comb. of fruit flavors. Bot. Pt, gal.
Use: Pharmaceutical aid.

•**syrup.** *NF 23.*
Use: Pharmaceutic aid (flavor).

Syrvite. (Various Mfr.) Vitamins A 2500 units, D 400 units, E 15 mg, B_1 1.05 mg, B_2 1.2 mg, B_3 13.5 mg, B_6 1.05 mg, B_{12} 4.5 mcg, C 60 mg/5 mL Liq. Bot. 480 mL. *OTC.*
Use: Vitamin supplement.

T

TA. (C & M Pharmacal) Triamcinolone acetonide 0.025%, 0.05%. Cream. Jar 2 oz, 8 oz, 1 lb. *Rx.*
Use: Corticosteroid, topical.

TA. (Wampole) Antithyroid antibodies by IFA. Test 48s.
Use: Diagnostic aid, thyroid.

Tabasyn. (Freeport) Chlorpheniramine maleate 2 mg, phenylephrine hydrochloride 10 mg, acetaminophen 5 g, salicylamide 5 g. Tab. Bot. 1000s. *Rx.*
Use: Analgesic, antihistamine, decongestant.

Tab-A-Vite. (Major) Vitamins A 5000 units, D 400 units, E 30 units, B_1 1.5 mg, B_2 1.7 mg, B_3 20 mg, B_5 10 mg, B_6 2 mg, B_{12} 6 mcg, C 60 mg, FA 0.4 mg. Tab. Bot. 30s, 100s, 250s, 1000s, UD 100s. *OTC.*
Use: Mineral, vitamin supplement.

Tab-A-Vite + Iron. (Major) Fe 18 mg, vitamins A 5000 units, D 400 units, E 30 units, B_1 1.5 mg, B_2 1.7 mg, B_3 20 mg, B_5 10 mg, B_6 2 mg, B_{12} 6 mcg, C 60 mg, FA 0.4 mg, tartrazine. Tab. Bot. 100s. *OTC.*
Use: Mineral, vitamin supplement.

Tabloid. (GlaxoSmithKline) Thioguanine 40 mg. Lactose. Tab. 25s. *Rx.*
Use: Antineoplastic.

Tacaryl. (Bristol-Myers Squibb) Methdilazine 3.6 mg. Chew. Tab. Bot. 100s. *Rx.*
Use: Antipruritic.

●**tacedinaline.** (ta-see-DYE-na-leen) USAN.
Use: Cancer agent.

Tac-40. (Parnell) Triamcinolone acetonide 40 mg/mL. Inj. Susp. Vial 5 mL. *Rx.*
Use: Corticosteroid.

tachysterol.
See: Dihydrotachysterol.

Tacitin. (Novartis) Under study. Benzoctamine, B.A.N.

●**taclamine hydrochloride.** (TACK-lah-meen) USAN.
Use: Anxiolytic.

●**tacrine hydrochloride.** (TACK-reen) USAN.
Use: Cognition adjuvant.
See: Cognex.

●**tacrolimus.** (tack-CROW-lih-muss) USAN.
Use: Immunomodulator, topical; immunologic agent; immunosuppressive.
See: Prograf.
Protopic.

Tac-3. (Allergan) Triamcinolone acetonide 3 mg/mL. Susp. Vial 5 mL. *Rx.*
Use: Corticosteroid.

●**tadalafil.** (tah-DA-la-fil) USAN.
Use: Erectile dysfunction.
See: Cialis.

Tagamet. (SK-Beecham) Cimetidine. Tab. **300 mg:** Bot. 100s. **400 mg:** Bot. 60s. **800 mg:** Bot. 30s. *Rx.*
Use: Histamine H_2 antagonist.

Tagamet HB 200. (SmithKline Beecham) Cimetidine 200 mg. Tab. Bot. 30s, 50s. *OTC.*
Use: Histamine H_2 antagonist.

Talacen Caplets. (Sanofi-Synthelabo) Pentazocine hydrochloride 25 mg, acetaminophen 650 mg. Tab. Bot. 100s. UD 250s. (10 × 25s). *c-IV.*
Use: Analgesic combination, narcotic.

●**talactoferrin alfa.** (ta-LAK-toe-FEH-in) USAN.
Use: Anti-infective.

●**talampicillin hydrochloride.** (TAL-AM-pih-sill-in) USAN.
Use: Anti-infective.

●**talaporfin sodium.** (tal-a-PORE-fin) USAN.
Use: Photosensitizer.

●**talc.** *USP 28.* A native hydrous magnesium silicate.
Use: Dusting powder, pharmaceutic aid (tablet/capsule lubricant).

talc powder, sterile.
Use: Antineoplastic.
See: Sclerosol.

●**taleranol.** (TAL-ehr-ah-nole) USAN.
Use: Enzyme inhibitor (gonadotropin).

●**talisomycin.** (tal-EYE-so-MY-sin) USAN.
Formerly Tallysomycin A.
Use: Antineoplastic.

●**talizumab.** (tal-IZ-ue-mab) USAN.
Use: Anaphylaxis.

●**talmetacin.** (TAL-MET-ah-sin) USAN.
Use: Analgesic, antipyretic, anti-inflammatory.

●**talniflumate.** (tal-NYE-FLEW-mate) USAN.
Use: Anti-inflammatory, analgesic.

●**talopram hydrochloride.** (TAY-low-pram) USAN.
Use: Potentiator (catecholamine).

●**talosalate.** (TAL-oh-SAL-ate) USAN.
Use: Analgesic, anti-inflammatory.

●**talsaclidine fumarate.** (tale-SACK-lih-deen) USAN.
Use: Alzheimer disease treatment (muscarinic M_1-agonist).

●**taltobulin.** (tal-toe-BUE-lin) USAN.
Use: Antineoplastic.

Talwin. (Abbott Hospital Products) Pentazocine lactate 30 mg/mL. Inj. **Vials:** With acetone sodium bisulfite 2 mg and methylparaben 1 mg/mL. 10 mL. **Uni-Amps:** 1 mL. **Uni-Nest amps:** 1 mL. **Carpujects:** With acetone sodium bisulfite 1 mg. 1 mL, 2 mL. *c-iv.*
Use: Narcotic agonist-antagonist analgesic.

Talwin Compound. (Sanofi-Synthelabo) Pentazocine hydrochloride 12.5 mg, aspirin 325 mg. Tab. Bot. 100s. *c-iv.*
Use: Analgesic, narcotic.

Talwin NX. (Sanofi-Synthelabo) Pentazocine hydrochloride 50 mg, naloxone 0.5 mg. Tab. Bot. 100s, UD 250s. *c-iv.*
Use: Analgesic, narcotic.

Tambocor. (3M Pharm) Flecainide acetate 50 mg, 100 mg, 150 mg. Tab. Bot. 100s, UD 100s (except 150 mg). *Rx.*
Use: Antiarrhythmic agent.

•**tametraline hydrochloride.** (tah-MET-rah-leen) USAN.
Use: Antidepressant.

Tamiflu. (Roche) Oseltamivir phosphate. **Cap.:** 75 mg. Blister pack 10s. **Pow. for Oral Susp.:** 12 mg/mL after reconstitution, sorbitol, saccharin, tutti-frutti flavor. Bot. 100 mg w/bottle adapter and oral dispenser. *Rx.*
Use: Antiviral.

•**tamoxifen citrate.** (ta-MOX-ih-fen) *USP 28.*
Use: Treatment of mammary carcinoma, antiestrogen.
See: Nolvadex.

tamoxifen citrate. (Various Mfr.) Tamoxifen citrate 10 mg, 20 mg. Tab. Bot. 60s, 180s, 500s, 1000s, UD 100s (10 mg only); 30s, 90s, 100s, 500s, 1000s, UD 100s (20 mg only). *Rx.*
Use: Antineoplastic, antiestrogen.

•**tampramine fumarate.** (TAM-prah-MEEN) USAN.
Use: Antidepressant.

Tamp-R-Tel. (Wyeth) A tamper-resistant package for narcotic drugs which includes the following: **Codeine phosphate:** 30 mg, 60 mg/mL. **Hydromorphone hydrochloride:** 1 mg, 2 mg, 3 mg, 4 mg/*Tubex.* **Meperidine hydrochloride:** 25 mg/mL. **Promethazine hydrochloride:** 25 mg/mL, 2 mL. **Meperidine hydrochloride:** 25 mg/mL, 50 mg/mL, 75 mg/mL, 100 mg/mL. **Morphine Sulfate:** 2 mg, 4 mg, 8 mg, 10 mg, 15 mg/mL. **Pentobarbital, Sodium:** 100 mg/2 mL. **Phenobarbital, Sodium:** 30 mg, 60 mg, 130 mg/mL. **Secobarbital, Sodium:** 100 mg/2 mL.

•**tamsulosin hydrochloride.** USAN.
Use: Benign prostatic hyperplasia therapy; antiadrenergic.
See: Flomax.

Tanac Gel. (Del) Dyclonine hydrochloride 1%, allantoin 0.5%, petrolatum, lanolin. Tube 9.45 mL. *OTC.*
Use: Cold sores, fever blisters, moisturizer.

Tanac Liquid. (Del) Benzalkonium Cl 0.12%, benzocaine 10%, tannic acid 6%. Saccharin. Bot. 13 mL. *OTC.*
Use: Mouth and throat preparation.

Tanac Stick. (Del) Benzocaine 7.5%, tannic acid 6%, octyl dimethyl PABA 0.75%, allantoin 0.2%, benzalkonium Cl. 7.5%. Saccharin. Stick 0.1 oz. *OTC.*
Use: Cold sores, fever blisters, moisturizer.

Tanadex. (Del) Tannic acid 2.86%, phenol 1.05%, benzocaine 0.47%. Liq. Bot. 3 oz. *OTC.*
Use: Throat preparation.

Tan-a-Dyne. (Archer-Taylor) Tannic acid compound w/iodine. Liq. Bot. 4 oz., pt., gal. *OTC.*
Use: Gargle.

Tanafed DMX. (First Horizon) Dextromethorphan tannate 25 mg, dexchlorpheniramine tannate 2.5 mg, pseudoephedrine tannate 75 mg/5 mL, methylparaben, saccharin, sucrose, cotton candy flavor. Susp. 20 mL, 118 mL, 473 mL. *Rx.*
Use: Antitussive combination.

Tanafed DP. (First Horizon) Pseudoephedrine tannate 75 mg, dexchlorpheniramine tannate 2.5 mg/5 mL, methylparaben, saccharin, sucrose, strawberry-banana flavor. Susp. 20 mL, 118 mL, 473 mL. *Rx.*
Use: Decongestant and antihistamine.

•**tanaproget.** (tan-a-PRO-jet) USAN.
Use: Contraceptive.

tanbismuth.
See: Bismuth tannate.

•**tandamine hydrochloride.** (TAN-dah-meen) USAN.
Use: Antidepressant.

•**tandospirone citrate.** (tan-DOE-spy-rone) USAN.
Use: Anxiolytic.

•**tandutinib.** (tan-doo-TYE-nib) USAN.
Use: Cardiovascular agent.

•**tannic acid.** *USP 28.* Gallotannic acid. Glycerite. Tannin.
Use: Astringent.
See: Zilactin Medicated.
W/Benzocaine, phenol, thymol iodide, ephedrine hydrochloride, zinc oxide, peru balsam.

See: Clysodrast.
W/Boric acid, salicylic acid, isopropyl alcohol.
See: Sal Dex Boro.
W/Cyanocobalamin, zinc acetate, glutathione, phenol.
See: Depinar.
Tannic Spray. (Gebauer) Tannic acid 4.5%, chlorobutanol 1.3%, menthol < 1%, benzocaine < 1%, propylene glycol 33%, ethanol 60%. Liq. Bot. 2 oz. 4 oz. *OTC.*
Use: Relief of sunburn and other minor burns.
Tannic-12 Suspension. (Cypress) Carbetapentane tannate 30 mg, chlorpheniramine tannate 4 mg, phenylephrine tannate 5 mg/5 mL, methylparaben, saccharin, glucose, strawberry flavor. Susp. Bot. 473 mL. *Rx.*
Use: Upper respiratory combination, antitussive, antihistamine, decongestant.
Tannic-12 Tablets. (Cypress) Carbetapentane tannate 60 mg, chlorpheniramine tannate 5 mg, dye free. Tab. Bot. 100s. *Rx.*
Use: Upper respiratory combination, antitussive, antihistamine.
•**tanomastat.** (ta-NOE-ma-stat) USAN.
Use: Osteoarthritis; oncology.
Tanoral. (Pharmed) Phenylephrine tannate 25 mg, chlorpheniramine tannate 8 mg, pyrilamine tannate 25 mg. Tab. Bot. 100s. *Rx.*
Use: Antihistamine, decongestant.
tanphetamin.
See: Dextroamphetamine tannate.
Tapan. (Warner Chilcott) Acetaminophen 325 mg. Tab. Bot. 100s. *OTC.*
Use: Analgesic.
Tapazole. (Eli Lilly) Methimazole 5 mg, 10 mg. Tab. Bot. 100s. *Rx.*
Use: Hyperthyroidism.
•**tape, adhesive.** *USP 28.*
Use: Surgical aid.
Ta-Poff. (Ulmer Pharmacal) Adhesive tape remover. Liq. Bot. 1 pt. Aerosol. Can 6 oz. *OTC.*
Tapuline. (Wesley) Activated attapulgite 600 mg, pectin 60 mg, homatropine methylbromide 0.5 mg. Chew. Tab. Bot. 100s, 1000s. *OTC.*
Use: Antidiarrheal.
tar.
See: Coal Tar.
Tarabine PFS. (Adria) Cytarabine 20 mg/mL, preservative free. Inj. Single vial 5 mL, bulk package vial 50 mL. *Rx.*
Use: Antimetabolite.

Taraphilic. (Medco) Coal tar distillate 1%, stearyl alcohol, petrolatum, parabens. Oint. 454 g. *OTC.*
Use: Dermatologic.
Tarceva. (Genentech/OSI) Erlotinib 25 mg, 100 mg, 150 mg. Lactose. Film coated. Tab. 30s. *Rx.*
Use: Epidermal growth factor receptor inhibitor.
tar-containing products.
Use: Dermatologic.
See: Balnetar.
  Cutar Emulsion.
  Doak Tar Oil.
  Estar.
  Fototar.
  Medotar.
  MG 217 Medicated Tar.
  Oxipor VHC.
  Packer's Pine Tar.
  Polytar.
  PsoriGel.
  Taraphilic.
tar derivatives, shampoo.
Use: Dermatologic.
See: Creamy Tar.
  DHS Tar.
  Doak Tar.
  Ionil T Plus.
  MG 217 Medicated Tar.
  Neutrogena T/Gel Original.
  Polytar.
  Zetar.
Targretin. (Ligand) Bexarotene. **Soft Gelatin Cap.:** 75 mg. Bot. 100s. **Gel:** 1%, dehydrated alcohol. Tube 60 g. *Rx.*
Use: Rexinoid.
•**tariquidar.** (tar-I-kwi-dar) USAN.
Use: Chemotherapeutic aid.
Tarka. (Abbott) Trandolapril maleate 2 mg, verapamil hydrochloride 180 mg, or trandolapril 1 mg, verapamil hydrochloride 240 mg, or trandolapril 2 mg, verapamil 240 mg, or trandolapril 4 mg, verapamil 240 mg. Tab. Bot. 100s. *Rx.*
Use: Antihypertensive.
Tarnphilic. (Medco Lab) Coal tar 1%, polysorbate 0.5% in aquaphilic base. Jar 16 oz. *OTC.*
Use: Dermatologic.
Tarpaste. (Doak Dermatologics) Coal tar distilled 5% in zinc paste. Tube 1 oz, Jar 4 oz, w/Hydrocortisone 0.5%. Tube 1 oz. *OTC.*
Use: Dermatitis.
Tarsum Shampoo/Gel. (Summers) Coal tar 10%, salicylic acid 5% in shampoo base. Bot. 4 oz. *OTC.*
Use: Antiseborrheic, dermatologic, hair, and scalp.

tartar emetic.
See: Antimony Potassium Tartrate, USP.

•**tartaric acid.** *NF 23.*
Use: Pharmaceutic aid (buffering agent).
W/Sodium Bicarbonate.
See: Baros.

Tashan. (Block Drug) Skin Cream. Vitamins A palmitate, D_2, D-panthenol, E. Tube 1 oz. *OTC.*
Use: Emollient.

Tasmar. (Roche) Tolcapone 100 mg, 200 mg, lactose. Tab. Bot. 90s. *Rx.*
Use: Antiparkinson agent.

•**tasosartan.** (tass-OH-sahr-tan) USAN.
Use: Antihypertensive.

Taste Function Test, Accusens T. (Westport Pharmaceuticals, Inc.) Tastant 60 mL. Kit. 15 Bot.
Use: Diagnostic aid.

Ta-Verm. (Table Rock) Piperazine citrate 100 mg/mL Syr. Bot. 1 pt, 1 gal. 500 mg Tab. Bot. 100s, 500s. *Rx.*
Use: Anthelmintic.

Tavilen Plus. (Table Rock) Liver solution 1 g, ferric pyrophosphate soluble 500 mg, vitamins B_1 6 mg, B_2 7.2 mg, B_6 3 mg, B_{12} 24 mcg, panthenol 3 mg, niacinamide 60 mg, l-lysine hydrochloride 300 mg, 5% alcohol/mL. Bot. 16 oz., 1 gal. *OTC.*
Use: Hematinic.

Tavist. (Novartis) Clemastine fumarate. **Tab.:** 2.68 mg. Bot. 100s. **Syrup:** 0.67 mg/5 mL. Bot. 118 mL. *Rx.*
Use: Antihistamine.

Tavist Allergy. (Novartis Consumer Health) Clemastine fumarate 1.34 mg, lactose.Tab. Pkg. 8s. *OTC.*
Use: Antihistamine, nonselective ethanolamine.

Tavist Allergy/Sinus/Headache. (Novartis) Pseudoephedrine hydrochloride 30 mg, clemastine fumarate 0.335 mg, acetaminophen 500 mg, methylparaben. Tab. Bot. 24s, 48s. *OTC.*
Use: Upper respiratory combination, decongestant, antihistamine, analgesic.

Tavist ND. (Novartis) Loratadine 10 mg, lactose. Tab. 30s. *OTC.*
Use: Antihistamine, peripherally selective piperidine.

Tavist Sinus Maximum Strength. (Novartis) Pseudoephedrine hydrochloride 30 mg, acetaminophen 500 mg, lactose, dextrose, methylparaben. Tab. Pkg. 24s. *OTC.*
Use: Upper respiratory combination, decongestant, analgesic.

taxoids.
Use: Antimitotic.
See: Docetaxel.
Paclitaxel.

Taxol. (Bristol-Myers Squibb) Paclitaxel 6 mg/mL, polyoxyethylated castor oil (*Cremophor EL*) 527 mg/mL, dehydrated alcohol 49.7%. Inj. Multiple-dose Vial 5 mL, 16.7 mL, 50 mL. *Rx.*
Use: Antineoplastic; antimitotic, taxoid.

Taxotere. (Aventis) Docetaxel 20 mg/ 0.5 mL, 80 mg/2 mg, polysorbate 80 1040 mg/mL, ethanol 13%. Inj. Single-dose vial with 1.5 mL diluent (20 mg only) and 6 mL diluent (80 mg only). *Rx.*
Use: Antimitotic, taxoid.

•**tazadolene succinate.** (TAZZ-ah-DOE-leen) USAN.
Use: Analgesic.

•**tazarotene.** (tazz-AHR-oh-teen) USAN.
Use: Antiacne, antipsoriatic, retinoid.
See: Tazorac.

Tazicef. (GlaxoSmithKline; Bristol-Myers Squibb) Ceftazidime 500 mg, 1 g, 2 g, 6 g. Pow. for Inj. Vial 10 mL (500 mg only), 100 mL (6 g only); *ADD-Vantage* vials 20 mL (1 g only), 50 mL (2 g only), 100 mL (1 g and 2 g only); *Faspaks* (1 g and 2 g only). *Rx.*
Use: Anti-infective, cephalosporin.

Tazidime. (Eli Lilly) Ceftazidime. **Inj.:** 1 g, 2 g. *Galaxy* cont. **Pow. for Inj.:** 1 g, 2 g, 6 g. Vial, *ADD-Vantage* vials, piggy-back vials. Bulk pkg. (6 g only). *Rx.*
Use: Anti-infective, cephalosporin.

•**tazifylline hydrochloride.** (TAY-zih-FIH-lin) USAN.
Use: Antihistamine.

•**tazobactam.** (TAZZ-oh-BACK-tam) USAN.
Use: Inhibitor (beta-lactamase).

•**tazobactam sodium.** (TAZZ-oh-BACK-tam) USAN.
Use: Inhibitor (beta-lactamase).

tazobactam sodium/piperacillin sodium.
See: Piperacillin sodium, sterile w/tazobactam.

•**tazofelone.** (TAY-zah-feh-lone) USAN.
Use: Suppressant (inflammatory bowel disease).

•**tazolol hydrochloride.** (TAY-zoe-lole) USAN.
Use: Cardiotonic.

•**tazomeline citrate.** (tazz-OH-meh-leen SIH-trate) USAN.
Use: Alzheimer disease treatment (cholinergic agonist).

Tazorac. (Allergan) Tazarotene. **Cream:** 0.05%, 0.1%, benzyl alcohol 1%, EDTA, medium chain triglycerides,

mineral oil. Cream. Tube 15 g, 30 g, 60 g. **Gel:** 0.05%, 0.1%, benzyl alcohol 1%, EDTA. Tube. 30 g, 100 g. *Rx.*
Use: Antiacne, antipsoriatic, retinoid.

Taztia XT. (Andrx) Diltiazem hydrochloride 120 mg, 180 mg, 240 mg, 300 mg, 360 mg. ER Cap. 30s, 90s. *Rx.*
Use: Calcium channel blocker.

TBA-Pred. (Keene Pharmaceuticals) Prednisolone tebutate 10 mg/mL Susp. Vial 10 mL. *Rx.*
Use: Corticosteroid.

TC Suspension. (Aventis) Aluminum hydroxide 600 mg, magnesium hydroxide 300 mg/5 mL, sorbitol, sodium 0.8 mg/5 mL. Liq. In UD 15 mL, 30 mL (100s). *OTC.*
Use: Antacid.

T/Derm Tar Emollient. (Neutrogena) Neutar solubilized coal tar extract 5% in oil base. Bot. 4 oz. *OTC.*
Use: Antipsoriatic, antipruritic.

T-Dry. (Jones Pharma) Pseudoephedrine hydrochloride 120 mg, chlorpheniramine maleate 12 mg. SR Cap. Bot. 100s. *Rx.*
Use: Antihistamine, decongestant.

T-Dry Jr. (Jones Pharma) Pseudoephedrine hydrochloride 60 mg, chlorpheniramine maleate 4 mg. SR Cap. Bot. 100s. *OTC.*
Use: Antihistamine, decongestant.

TDX Cortisol. (Abbott Diagnostics) Fluorescence polarization immunoassay for the quantitative determination of cortisol in serum, plasma, or urine.
Use: Diagnostic aid.

TDX Thyroxine. (Abbott Diagnostics) Automated assay for quantitation of unsaturated thyroxine-binding sites in serum or plasma.
Use: Diagnostic aid.

TDX Total Estriol. (Abbott Diagnostics) Fluorescence polarization immunoassay for the quantitative determination of total estriol in serum, plasma, or urine.
Use: Diagnostic aid.

TDX Total T3. (Abbott Diagnostics) Automated assay for quantitation of total circulating triiodothyronine (T3) in serum or plasma.
Use: Diagnostic aid.

TDX T-Uptake. (Abbott Diagnostics) Automated assay for the determination of thyroxine-binding capacity in serum or plasma.
Use: Diagnostic aid.

Te Anatoxal Berna. (Berna) Tetanus toxoid adsorbed, 10 Lf units/0.5 mL. Vial 5 mL, Syringe. 0.5 mL. *Rx.*
Use: Immunization.

Tear Drop. (Parmed Pharmaceuticals, Inc.) Benzalkonium Cl 0.01%, polyvinyl alcohol, NaCl, EDTA. Soln. Drops. Bot. 15 mL. *OTC.*
Use: Artificial tears.

TearGard. (KM Lee) Hydroxyethyl cellulose, sorbic acid 0.25%, EDTA 0.1%. Soln. Bot. 15 mL. *OTC.*
Use: Lubricant, ophthalmic.

Teargen. (Ivax) Benzalkonium Cl 0.01%, EDTA, NaCl, polyvinyl alcohol. Soln. Bot. 15 mL. *OTC.*
Use: Artificial tears.

Teargen II. (Ivax) Hydroxypropyl methylcellulose 0.3%, dextran 70 0.1%, benzalkonium Cl 0.01%, EDTA 0.05%. Bot. 15 mL. *OTC.*
Use: Artificial tears.

Tearisol. (Novartis Ophthalmic) Hydroxypropyl methylcellulose 0.5%, chloride di sodium, benzalkonium chloride 0.01%, boric acid, potassium chloride. Bot. 15 mL. *OTC.*
Use: Artificial tears.

Tears Naturale. (Alcon) Dextran 70 0.1%, benzalkonium Cl 0.01%, hydroxypropyl methylcellulose 0.3%, sodium Cl, EDTA, hydrochloric acid, sodium hydrochloride, potassium Cl. Soln. Bot. 15 mL, 30 mL. *OTC.*
Use: Artificial tears.

Tears Naturale Forte. (Alcon) Dextran 70 1%, hydroxypropyl methylcellulose 0.3%, glycerin 0.2%, polyquaternium-1 0.001%, NaCl, KCl, sodium borate. Soln. 15 mL, 30 mL. *OTC.*
Use: Artificial tears.

Tears Naturale Free. (Alcon) Hydroxypropyl methylcellulose 2910 0.3%, dextran 70 0.1%, NaCl, KCl, sodium borate. Soln. Single-use containers 0.6 mL. *OTC.*
Use: Artificial tears.

Tears Naturale II. (Alcon) Dextran 70 0.1%, hydroxypropyl methylcellulose 2910 0.3%, polyquaternium-1 0.001%, sodium Cl, potassium Cl, sodium borate. Soln. *Drop-tainer* 15 mL, 30 mL. *OTC.*
Use: Artificial tears.

Tears Plus. (Allergan) Polyvinyl alcohol 1.4%, NaCl, povidone 0.6%, chlorobutanol 0.5%. *OTC.*
Use: Artificial tears.

Tears Renewed Ointment. (Akorn) White petrolatum, light mineral oil. Ophth. Tube 3.5 g. *OTC.*
Use: Lubricant, ophthalmic.

Tears Renewed Solution. (Akorn) Dextran 70 0.1%, sodium chloride, hydroxypropyl methylcellulose 2906, benzalkonium chloride 0.01%, EDTA. Soln. Bot. 2 mL, 15 mL, 30 mL. *OTC.* *Use:* Artificial tears.

tear test strips. *Use:* Ophthalmic diagnostic product. *See:* Schirmer Tear Test.

tea tree oil. (Metabolic Prod.) Australian oil of *Melaleuca alternifolia* 100% pure. Bot. 1 oz, 4 oz, 8 oz, 16 oz. **Cream:** Bot. 8 oz. **Oint.:** Tube 1 oz, 3 oz. *OTC.* *Use:* Antiseptic, antifungal, topical.

Tebamide. (G & W Labs) Trimetho-benzamide hydrochloride. **Pediatric Supp.:** 100 mg. Benzocaine 2%. Box. 10s. **Adult Supp.:** 200 mg. Benzocaine 2%. Box. 10s, 50s. *Rx.* *Use:* Antiemetic/antivertigo agent.

• **tebanicline tosylate.** (te-BAN-i-kleen) USAN. *Use:* Analgesic.

• **tebufelone.** (teh-BYOO-feh-LONE) USAN. *Use:* Analgesic, anti-inflammatory.

• **tebuquine.** (TEH-buh-KWIN) USAN. *Use:* Antimalarial.

T.E.C. (Invenex) Zn 1 mg, Cu 0.4 mg, Cr 4 mcg, Mn 0.1 mg. Vial 10 mL. *Rx.* *Use:* Trace element supplement.

• **tecadenoson.** (tek-a-DEN-o-son) USAN. *Use:* Cardiovascular agent.

• **tecalcet hydrochloride.** (TE-kal-set) USAN. *Use:* Hyperparathyroidism.

• **tecastemizole.** (tek-a-STEM-mi-zole) USAN. *Use:* Antihistamine.

• **teceleukin.** (teh-see-LOO-kin) USAN. *Use:* Immunostimulant.

Techneplex. (Bristol-Myers Squibb) Technetium Tc 99m penetate kit. 10 vials/kit. *Use:* Radiopaque agent.

TechneScan MAA. (Mallinckrodt) Aggregated albumin (human). *Use:* Preparation of Tc 99m Aggregated Albumin (Human).

• **technetium Tc 99m albumin aggregated injection.** (tek-NEE-shee-uhm Tc 99m al-BYOO-min AGG-reh-GAY-tuhd) *USP 28.* *Use:* Diagnostic aid (lung imaging), radioactive agent.

• **technetium Tc 99m albumin colloid injection.** (tek-NEE-shee-uhm Tc 99m al-BYOO-min) *USP 28.* *Use:* Radiopharmaceutical.

• **technetium Tc 99m albumin injection.** (tek-NEE-shee-uhm Tc 99m al-BYOO-min) *USP 28.* *Use:* Radiopharmaceutical.

• **technetium Tc 99m albumin microaggregated.** (tek-NEE-shee-uhm Tc 99m al-BYOO-min) USAN. *Use:* Radiopharmaceutical.

technetium Tc 99m antimelanoma murine monoclonalantibody. *Use:* Diagnostic aid. [Orphan Drug]

• **technetium Tc 99m antimony trisulfide colloid.** (tek-NEE-shee-uhm) USAN. *Use:* Radiopharmaceutical.

• **technetium Tc 99m apcitide.** (tek-NEE-shee-uhm APP-sih-tide) *USP 28.* *Use:* Radiopharmaceutical.

• **technetium Tc 99m arcitumomab injection.** USAN. *Use:* Radiopharmaceutical.

• **technetium Tc 99m bicisate.** (tek-NEE-shee-uhm Tc 99m bye-SIS-ate) USAN. *Use:* Diagnostic aid (brain imaging), radiopharmaceutical.

• **technetium Tc 99m depreotide injection.** (tek-NEE-shee-uhm) *USP 28.* *Use:* Radiopharmaceutical.

• **technetium Tc 99m disofenin injection.** (tek-NEE-shee-uhm) *USP 28.* *Use:* Radiopharmaceutical; diagnostic aid (hepatobiliary function determination).

• **technetium Tc 99m etidronate injection.** (tek-NEE-shee-uhm) *USP 28.* *Use:* Radiopharmaceutical.

• **technetium Tc 99m exametazime injection.** (tek-NEE-shee-uhm Tc 99m ex-ah-MET-ah-zeem) *USP 28.* *Use:* Radiopharmaceutical.

• **technetium Tc 99m fanolesomab.** (tek-NEE-shee-uhm fa-noe-LES-oh-mab) USAN. *Use:* Diagnostic aid (polymorphonuclear neutrophil accumulation); radiopharmaceutical.

technetium Tc 99m ferpentetate injection. *Use:* Radiopharmaceutical.

• **technetium Tc 99m furifosmin.** (tek-NEE-shee-uhm Tc 99m fyoor-ih-FOSS-min) USAN. *Use:* Diagnostic aid (radioactive, cardiac disease), radiopharmaceutical.

technetium Tc 99m generator solution. (New England Nuclear) Pertechnetate sodium Tc 99m. *Use:* Radiopharmaceutical, radiopaque agent.

• **technetium Tc 99m glucepate injection.** (tek-NEE-shee-uhm) *USP 28.* Formerly *Technetium Tc 99m Sodium Gluceptate.* *Use:* Radiopharmaceutical.

•**technetium Tc 99m lidofenin injection.** (tek-NEE-shee-uhm) *USP 28.*
Use: Radiopharamceutical.

•**technetium Tc 99m mebrofenin injection.** (tek-NEE-shee-uhm) *USP 28.*
Use: Radiopharmaceutical.

•**technetium Tc 99m medronate disodium.** (tek-NEE-shee-uhm) USAN.
Use: Radiopharmaceutical.

•**technetium Tc 99m medronate injection.** (tek-NEE-shee-uhm) *USP 28.*
Use: Diagnostic aid (skeletal imaging), radiopharmaceutical.
See: Macrotec.

•**technetium Tc 99m mertiatide injection.** (tek-NEE-shee-uhm Tc 99m MEER-TIE-ah-tide) *USP 28.*
Use: Diagnostic aid (renal function); radiopharmaceutical.

technetium Tc 99m murine monoclonal antibody (IgG2a) to BCE.
Use: Diagnostic aid. [Orphan Drug]

technetium Tc 99m murine monoclonal antibody to hCG.
Use: Diagnostic aid. [Orphan Drug]

technetium Tc 99m murine monoclonal antibody to human afp.
Use: Diagnostic aid. [Orphan Drug]

•**technetium Tc 99m nitridocade.** (tek-NEE-shee-uhm Tc 99m nye-TRID-oh-kade) USAN.
Use: Diagnostic aid (coronary artery disease); radlopharmaceutical.

•**technetium Tc 99m nofetumomab merpentan injection.** (tek-NEE-shee-uhm Tc 99m no-fe-TUE-mo-mab) *USP 28.*
Use: Radiopharmaceutical.

•**technetium Tc 99m oxidronate injection.** (tek-NEE-shee-uhm) *USP 28.*
Use: Diagnostic aid (skeletal imaging), radiopharmaceutical.

•**technetium Tc 99m pentetate calcium trisodium.** (tek-NEE-shee-uhm KAL-see-uhm try-so-dee-uhm) USAN.
Use: Radiopharmaceutical.

•**technetium Tc 99m pentetate injection.** (tek-NEE-shee-uhm) *USP 28. Formerly Technetium Tc 99m Pentetate Sodium.*
Use: Radiopharmaceutical.

•**technetium Tc 99m (pyro- and trimetra-) phosphates injection.** (tek-NEE-shee-uhm) *USP 28.*
Use: Radiopharmaceutical.

•**technetium Tc 99m pyrophosphate injection.** (tek-NEE-shee-uhm) *USP 28.*
Use: Radiopharmaceutical.

•**technetium Tc 99m red blood cells injection.** (tek-NEE-shee-uhm) *USP 28.*

Use: Radiopharmaceutical.

•**technetium Tc 99m sestamibi.** (tek-NEE-shee-uhmTc 99 m SESS-tah-MIH-bih) *USP 28.*
Use: Diagnostic aid (radiopaque medium, cardiac perfusion); radiopharmaceutical.

•**technetium Tc 99m siboroxime.** (tek-NEE-shee-uhm Tc 99m sih-boe-ROX-eem) USAN.
Use: Diagnostic aid (brain imaging), radiopharmaceutical.

•**technetium Tc 99m succimer injection.** (tek-NEE-shee-uhm) *USP 28.*
Use: Radiopharmaceutical, diagnostic aid (renal function determination).

•**technetium Tc 99m sulfur colloid injection.** (tek-NEE-shee-uhm) *USP 28.*
Use: Radiopharmaceutical.

technetium Tc 99m sulfur colloid kit.
Use: Radiopharmaceutical.
See: Tesuloid.

•**technetium Tc 99m teboroxime.** (tek-NEE-shee-uhm Tc 99m teh-boe-ROX-eem) USAN.
Use: Diagnostic aid (radiopaque medium, cardiac perfusion), radiopharmaceutical.

teclosine. Under study.
Use: Amebicide.

•**teclozan.** (TEH-kloe-zan) USAN.
Use: Antiamebic.
See: Falmonox

Tecnu Outdoor Skin Cleanser. (Tec Labs) Deodorized mineral spirits, propylene glycol, octylphenoxypolyethoxyethanol, mixed fatty acid soap. Lot. 118 mL, 355 mL. *OTC.*
Use: Poison ivy prevention

•**tecogalan sodium.** (TEE-koe-gay-lan) USAN.
Use: Antineoplastic adjunct.

Teczem. (Hoechst) Enalapril maleate 5 mg, diltiazem maleate 180 mg, sucrose. ER Tab. Unit-of-use 100s. *Rx.*
Use: Antihypertensive.

Tedral. (Parke-Davis) **Elix.:** Theophylline 32.5 mg, ephedrine hydrochloride 6 mg, phenobarbital 2 mg/5 mL. Alcohol 15%. Pediatric. Bot. Pt. **Tab.:** Theophylline 118 mg, ephedrine hydrochloride 24 mg, phenobarbital 8 mg. Tab. Bot. 24s, 100s, 1000s. UD 100s. **Susp. (Pediatric Pharmaceuticals):** Theophylline 65 mg, ephedrine hydrochloride 12 mg, phenobarbital 4 mg/5 mL. Bot. 8 oz. *Rx.*
Use: Antiasthmatic.

Tedral-SA. (Parke-Davis) Theophylline 180 mg, ephedrine hydrochloride

48 mg, phenobarbital 25 mg. SA Tab. Bot. 100s, 1000s. *Rx.*
Use: Antiasthmatic.

Tedrigen. (Ivax) Theophylline 120 mg, ephedrine hydrochloride 22.5 mg, phenobarbital 7.5 mg. Tab. Bot. 100s, 1000s. *OTC.*
Use: Antiasthmatic.

•**teduglutide.** (te-DUE-gloo-tide) USAN.
Use: Gastrointestinal disease.

Teebacin. (CMC) Sod. p-aminosalicylate. **Tab.:** 0.5 g Bot. 1000s. **Pow.:** Bot. lb. *Rx.*
Use: Antituberculosal.

Teebaconin. (CMC) Isoniazid 50 mg, 100 mg, 300 mg. Tab. Bot. 100s, 1000s. *Rx.*
Use: Antituberculosal.

Teebaconin w/Vitamin B₆. (CMC) Isoniazid 100 mg, 10 mg pyridoxine hydrochloride. Tab. Bot. 100s, 500s, 1000s. Isoniazid 300 mg, 30 mg pyridoxine hydrochloride. Tab. Bot. 100s, 1000s. *Rx.*
Use: Antituberculosal.

Teen Midol. (Bayer Corp. (Consumer Div.)) Acetaminophen 400 mg, pamabrom 25 mg. Cap. Bot. 16s. *OTC.*
Use: Analgesic combination.

Teev. (Keene Pharmaceuticals) Estradiol valerate 4 mg, testosterone enanthate 90 mg/mL. Inj. Vial 10 mL. *Rx.*
Use: Androgen, estrogen combination.

•**tefibazumab.** (tef-ee-BA-zoo-mab) USAN.
Use: Anti-infective.

•**teflurane.** (TEH-flew-rane) USAN.
Use: Anesthetic, general.

tegacid.
See: Glyceryl monostearate.

•**tegafur.** (TEH-gah-fer) USAN.
Use: Antineoplastic.

Tegamide. (G & W) Trimethobenzamide hydrochloride 100 mg, 200 mg. Supp. Box. 10s, 50s. *Rx.*
Use: Antiemetic.

•**tegaserod maleate.** (teg-a-SER-od) USAN.
Use: Gastrointestinal motility disorders.
See: Zelnorm.

Tegretol. (Novartis) Carbamazepine **Tab.:** 200 mg. Bot. 100s, 1000s. UD 100s. **Chew. Tab.:** 100 mg. Sucrose. Bot. 100s. UD 100s; **Susp.:** 100 mg/ 5 mL. Sorbitol, sucrose. Citrus/vanilla flavor. Bot. 450 mL. *Rx.*
Use: Anticonvulsant.

Tegretol-XR. (Novartis) Carbamazepine 100 mg, 200 mg, 400 mg, mannitol. ER Tab. Bot. 100s. *Rx.*

Use: Anticonvulsant.

Tegrin. (Block Drug) Allantoin 2%, coal tar extract 5% in cream base. Cream. Tube 2 oz, 4.4 oz. *OTC.*
Use: Antipsoriatic.

T.E.H. Compound. (Various Mfr.) Theophylline 130 mg, ephedrine sulfate 25 mg, hydroxyzine hydrochloride 10 mg. Tab. Bot. 100s, 500s. *Rx.*
Use: Antiasthmatic.

•**teicoplanin.** (teh-kah-PLAN-in) USAN.
Use: Anti-infective.

Telachlor TD Caps. (Major) Chlorpheniramine maleate 8 mg, 12 mg. TD Tab. Bot. 1000s. *Rx.*
Use: Antihistamine.

•**telavancin hydrochloride.** (tel-a-VAN-sin) USAN.
Use: Antibacterial agent.

•**telbivudine.** (tel-BI-vyoo-deen) USAN.
Use: Antiviral (hepatitis B infection).

Teldrin Maximum Strength Spansules. (GlaxoSmithKline) Chlorpheniramine maleate 12 mg. Cap. Pkg. 12s, 24s, 48s. *OTC.*
Use: Antihistamine.

Teldrin 12-Hour Allergy Relief. (GlaxoSmithKline) Chlorpheniramine 8 mg, pseudoephedrine hydrochloride 75 mg. Cap. Pkg. 12s, 24s. Bot. 48s. *OTC.*
Use: Antihistamine, decongestant.

Telepaque. (Nycomed Amersham) Iopanoic acid 500 mg, iodine 333.4 mg. Tab. Pkg. 6s. *Rx.*
Use: Radiopaque agent, oral cholecystographic agent.

•**telinavir.** (teh-LIN-ah-veer) USAN.
Use: Antiviral.

telithromycin.
Use: Anti-infective.
See: Ketek.

•**telmisartan.** (tell-mih-SAHR-tan) USAN.
Use: Angiotensin II receptor antagonist; antihypertensive.
See: Micardis.
W/Hydrochlorothiazide.
See: Micardis HCT.

•**teloxantrone hydrochloride.** (teh-LOX-an-trone) USAN.
Use: Antineoplastic.

•**teludipine hydrochloride.** (teh-LOO-dih-peen) USAN.
Use: Antihypertensive, calcium channel antagonist.

•**temafloxacin hydrochloride.** (teh-mah-FLOX-ah-SIN) USAN.
Use: Anti-infective (microbial DNA topoisomerase inhibitor).

●**tematropium methylsulfate.** (teh-mah-TROE-pee-UHM METH-ill-SULL-fate) USAN.
Use: Anticholinergic.

●**temazepam.** (tem-AZE-uh-pam) *USP 28.*
Use: Sedative/hypnotic, nonbarbiturate.
See: Restoril.

temazepam. (Various Mfr.) Temazepam 15 mg, 30 mg. Cap. 100s, 500s, UD 100s. *c-ɪv.*
Use: Sedative/hypnotic, nonbarbiturate.

●**temelastine.** (teh-mell-ASS-teen) USAN.
Use: Antihistamine.

●**temocapril hydrochloride.** (teh-MOE-cap-RILL) USAN.
Use: Antihypertensive.

●**temocillin.** (TEE-moe-SIH-lin) USAN.
Use: Anti-infective.

Temodar. (Schering Plough) Temozolomide 5 mg, 20 mg, 100 mg, 250 mg. Cap. Bot. 5s, 20s. *Rx.*
Use: Antineoplastic.

●**temoporfin.** (teh-moe-PORE-fin) USAN.
Use: Antineoplastic.

Temovate. (GlaxoSmithKline) **Cream:** Clobetasol propionate 0.05%. Tube 15 g, 30 g, 45 g. **Emollient:** Clobetasol propionate 0.05%. Tube 15 g, 30 g, 60 g. **Gel:** Clobetasol propionate 0.05%. Tube 15 g, 30 g, 60 g. **Oint.:** Clobetasol propionate 0.05%. Tube 15 g, 30 g, 45 g. *Rx.*
Use: Corticosteroid, topical.

Temovate Scalp. (GlaxoSmithKline) **Oint.:** Clobetasol propionate 0.05%, white petrolatum base. 15 g, 30 g, 45 g. **Cream:** Clobetasol propionate 0.03%, 15 g, 30 g, 45 g. **Scalp application:** Clobetasol propionate 0.05%, carbomer 934P. 25 mL, 50 mL. *Rx.*
Use: Corticosteroid, topical.

●**temozolomide.** USAN.
Use: Antineoplastic.
See: Temodar.

Tempo. (Thompson Medical) Calcium carbonate 414 mg, aluminum hydroxide 133 mg, magnesium hydroxide 81 mg, simethicone 20 mg. Chew. Tab. Bot. 10s, 30s, 60s. *OTC.*
Use: Antacid, antiflatulent.

Temporary Punctal/Canalicular Collagen Implant. (Eagle Vision) 0.2 mm, 0.3 mm, 0.4 mm, 0.5 mm, 0.6 mm. Box 72s. *Rx.*
Use: Collagen implant, ophthalmic.

Tempra. (Bristol-Myers Squibb) Acetaminophen. **Drops:** Grape flavor. 80 mg/0.8 mL. Bot. w/dropper 15 mL. **Syrup:** Cherry flavor. 160 mg/5 mL. Bot. 4 oz. **Tab.:** 80 mg. Bot 30s.

160 mg. *OTC.*
Use: Analgesic.

Temp Tab. (National Vitamin) Chloride (as sodium and potassium chloride) 287 mg, sodium (as chloride) 180 mg, potassium (as chloride) 15 mg. Tab. Preservative-free. 100s. *OTC.*
Use: Electrolyte.

●**temsirolimus.** (TEM-sir-OH-li-mus) USAN.
Use: Antineoplastic.

●**temurtide.** (teh-MER-TIDE) USAN.
Use: Vaccine adjuvant.

Tencet. (Roberts) Acetaminophen 500 mg, butalbital 50 mg, caffeine 40 mg. Cap. Bot. 100s, UD 1000s. *Rx.*
Use: Analgesic, hypnotic, sedative.

Tencon. (International Ethical Labs) Acetaminophen 650 mg, butalbital 50 mg. Tab. Bot. 100s. *Rx.*
Use: Analgesic, hypnotic, sedative.

●**tenecteplase.** (teh-NECK-teh-place) USAN.
Use: Thrombolytic agent, tissue plasminogen activator.
See: TNKase.

●**teneliximab.** (ten-el-IKS-i-mab) USAN.
Use: Monoclonal antibody.

Tenex. (Wyeth) Guanfacine hydrochloride 1 mg, 2 mg. Tab. Bot. 100s, 500s (1 mg only), UD 100s (1 mg only). *Rx.*
Use: Antihypertensive.

●**teniposide.** (TEN-ih-POE-side) USAN.
Use: Antineoplastic. [Orphan Drug]
See: Vumon.

●**tenivastatin calcium.** (te-NI-va-sta-tin) USAN.
Use: Antihyperlipidemic; HMG-CoA reductase inhibitor.

Ten-K. (Novartis) Potassium Cl 750 mg (10 mEq). CR Cap. Bot. 100s, 500s. UD, blister pak 100s. *Rx.*
Use: Electrolyte supplement.

●**tenofovir.** USAN.
Use: Antiviral.

●**tenofovir disoproxil fumarate.** USAN.
Use: Antiretroviral, nucleotide analog reverse transcriptase inhibitor.
See: Viread.
W/Emtricitabine.
See: Truvada.

Tenol. (Vortech Pharmaceuticals) **Liq.:** Acetaminophen 120 mg, NAPA alcohol 7%/5 mL. Bot. 3 oz, 4 oz, gal. **Tab.:** Acetaminophen 325 mg. Bot. 1000s. *OTC.*
Use: Analgesic.

Tenol-Plus. (Vortech Pharmaceuticals) Acetaminophen 250 mg, aspirin 250 mg, caffeine 65 mg. Tab. Bot.

1000s. *OTC.*
Use: Analgesic.

Tenoretic. (AstraZeneca) Tab. **50 mg:** Atenolol 50 mg, chlorthalidone 25 mg. Bot. 100s. **100 mg:** Atenolol 100 mg, chlorthalidone 25 mg. Bot. 100s. *Rx.*
Use: Antihypertensive, diuretic.

Tenormin. (AstraZeneca) Atenolol. **Tab.:** 25 mg, 50 mg, 100 mg. Bot. 100s, 1000s (50 mg only), UD 100s (except 25 mg). **Inj.:** 5 mg/10 mL. Amp. 10 mL. *Rx.*
Use: Antiadrenergic/sympatholytic, beta-adrenergic blocker.

• **tenoxicam.** (ten-OX-ih-kam) USAN.
Use: Anti-inflammatory.

Tensilon. (AstraZeneca) Edrophonium chloride. **Vial:** 10 mg/mL, w/phenol 0.45%, sodium sulfite 0.2% 10 mL. **Amp.:** 10 mg/mL, w/sodium sulfite 0.2%. 1 mL.
Use: Diagnostic aid, myasthenia gravis.

Tensive Conductive Adhesive Gel. (Parker) Nonflammable conductive adhesive electrode gel, eliminates tape and tape irritation. Tube 60 g.
Use: Therapeutic aid.

Tensocaine. (Sanofi-Synthelabo) Acetaminophen. Tab. *OTC.*
Use: Analgesic.

Tensolate. (Apco) Phenobarbital 0.25 g, hyoscyamine sulfate 0.1037 mg, atropine sulfate 0.0194 mg, hyoscine HBr 0.0065 mg. Tab. Bot. 100s. *Rx.*
Use: Antispasmodic.

Tensolax. (Sanofi-Synthelabo) Chlormezanone. Tab. *Rx.*
Use: Muscle relaxant.

Tensopin. (Apco) Phenobarbital 0.25 g, homatropine methylbromide 2.5 mg. Tab. Bot. 100s. *Rx.*
Use: Antispasmodic.

Tenuate. (Aventis) Diethylpropion hydrochloride 25 mg, lactose. Tab. Bot. 100s. *c-iv.*
Use: CNS stimulant, anorexiant.

Tenuate Dospan. (Aventis) Diethylpropion hydrochloride 75 mg, mannitol. CR Tab. Bot. UD 100s, 250s. *c-iv.*
Use: CNS stimulant, anorexiant.

T.E.P. (Geneva) Phenobarbital 8 mg, theophylline 130 mg, ephedrine hydrochloride 24 mg. Tab. Bot. 100s. *Rx.*
Use: Antiasthmatic combination.

Tepanil. (3M) Diethylpropion hydrochloride 25 mg. Tab. Bot. 100s. *c-iv.*
Use: Anorexiant.

Tepanil Ten-Tab. (3M) Diethylpropion 75 mg. Tab. Bot. 30s, 100s, 250s. *c-iv.*
Use: Anorexiant.

• **tepoxalin.** (teh-POX-ah-lin) USAN.
Use: Antipsoriatic.

• **teprotide.** (TEH-pro-tide) USAN.
Use: Angiotensin-converting enzyme inhibitor.

Tequin. (Bristol-Myers Squibb) Gatifloxacin. **Tab.:** 200 mg, 400 mg. Bot. 30s (200 mg only), 50s (400 mg only), blister pack 100s, *Teq-Paqs* (3 × 5 tablets) (400 mg only). **Inj., Conc.:** 400 mg, preservative free. Single-use vial 40 mL, dextrose 5%. **Inj. premix:** 200 mg, 400 mg, preservative free. Flexible Cont. 100 mL (200 mg only), 200 mL (400 mg only) w/dextrose 5%. **Pow. for Oral Susp.:** 200 mg per 5 mL (after reconstitution). Phenylalanine 168 mg per 5 mL, aspartame, parabens, sucrose. Fruit flavor. 1 g, 2 g, 3 g, 4 g (25 mL, 50 mL, 75 mL, 100 mL bottles). *Rx.*
Use: Anti-infective, fluoroquinolone.

tequinol sodium. Name used for Actinoquinol Sodium.

Tera-Gel. (Geritrex) Coal tar 0.5%. EDTA, parabens. Shampoo. 114 mL. *OTC.*
Use: Photochemotherapy.

Terak. (Akorn) Polymyxin B sulfate 10,000 units/g, oxytetracycline hydrochloride 5 mg/g, white and liquid petrolatum. Ophth. Oint. Tube 3.5 g. *Rx.*
Use: Anti-infective, ophthalmic.

Terazol 7. (Ortho-McNeil) Terconazole 0.4%, cetyl alcohol, stearyl alcohol. Vag. Cream. Tube 45 g w/1 measured-dose applicator. *Rx.*
Use: Antifungal, vaginal.

Terazol 3. (Ortho-McNeil) **Cream, vaginal:** Terconazole 0.8%. Tube 20 g with 1 measured-dose applicator. **Supp., vaginal:** Terconazole 80 mg, coconut oil/palm kernel oil. 2.5 g. 3s. *Rx.*
Use: Antifungal, vaginal.

• **terazosin hydrochloride.** (ter-AZE-oh-sin) *USP 28.*
Use: Antihypertensive, antiadrenergic.
See: Hytrin.

terazosin hydrochloride. (Geneva) Terazosin 1 mg, 2 mg, 5 mg, 10 mg (as base). Tab. Bot. 100s, 1000s. *Rx.*
Use: Antiadrenergic.

terazosin hydrochloride. (Various Mfr.) Terazosin hydrochloride 1 mg, 2 mg, 5 mg, 10 mg (as base), may contain lactose. Cap. Bot. 100s, 500s. *Rx.*
Use: Antiadrenergic.

• **terbinafine.** (TER-bin-ah-feen) USAN.
Use: Antifungal.
See: Lamisil AT.

terbinafine hydrochloride.
Use: Antifungal, allylamine.
See: DesenexMax.
Lamisil.
Lamisil AT.
●**terbutaline sulfate.** (ter-BYOO-tuh-leen)
USP 28.
Use: Bronchodilator, sympathomimetic.
See: Brethine.
Bricanyl.
terbutaline sulfate. (American Pharmaceutical Partners) Terbutaline sulfate
1 mg/mL. Inj. Vials. 1 mL single-use.
Rx.
Use: Bronchodilator, sympathomimetic.
terbutaline sulfate. (Global) Terbutaline
sulfate 2.5 mg, 5 mg. Tab. Bot. 100s.
Rx.
Use: Bronchodilator, sympathomimetic.
Tercodryl. (Health for Life Brands) Codeine phos. 0.75 g, pyrilamine maleate
25 mg/fl. oz. Bot. 4 oz. *c-v.*
Use: Antihistamine, antitussive.
●**terconazole.** (ter-CONE-uh-zole) USAN.
Formerly triaconazole.
Use: Antifungal.
See: Terazol 3.
Terazol 7.
Zazole.
terconazole. (Various Mfr.) Terconazole
0.4%, 0.8%. Alcohols. Vaginal cream.
Tubes. 20 g (0.8 only), 45 g (0.4 only).
Rx.
Use: Vaginal antifungal agent.
Terg-A-Zyme. (Alconox) Detergent with
enzyme action. Box 4 lb Ctn. 9 × 4 lb,
25 lb, 50 lb, 100 lb, 300 lb. *OTC.*
Use: Biodegradable detergent and wetting agent.
Teridol Jr. (Health for Life Brands) Terpin hydrate, cocillana, potassium
guaiacol sulfonate, ammonium chloride. Bot. 3 oz. *OTC.*
Use: Expectorant.
●**teriparatide.** (ter-i-PAR-a-tide) USAN.
Use: Bone resorption inhibitor, osteoporosis therapy adjunct, diagnostic aid,
thyroid function. [Orphan Drug]
teriparatide.
Use: Parathyroid hormone.
See: Forteo.
●**terlakiren.** (ter-lah-KIE-ren) USAN.
Use: Antihypertensive.
terlipressin.
Use: Treatment of bleeding esophageal
varices. [Orphan Drug]
See: Glypressin.
●**terodiline hydrochloride.** (TEH-row-
DIE-leen) USAN.
Use: Vasodilator, coronary.

●**teroxalene hydrochloride.** (ter-OX-ah-
leen) USAN.
Use: Antischistosomal.
●**teroxirone.** (TER-OX-ih-rone) USAN.
Use: Antineoplastic.
Terpex Jr. (Health for Life Brands) d-
Methorphan 25 mg, terpin hydrate, potassium guaiacol sulfonate, cocillana,
ammonium chloride. Bot. 4 oz. *OTC.*
Use: Expectorant.
Terphan. (Pal-Pak, Inc.) Terpin hydrate
85 mg, dextromethorphan hydrobromide 10 mg/5 mL w/alcohol 40% Elix.
Bot. Gal. *OTC.*
Use: Antitussive, expectorant.
●**terpin hydrate and codeine oral solution.** (TER-pin) *USP 28.*
Use: Expectorant, antitussive.
●**terpin hydrate oral solution.** (TER-pin)
USP 28.
Use: Expectorant.
Terra-Cortril. (Pfizer) Hydrocortisone
1.5%, oxytetracycline hydrochloride
0.5%. Ophth. Susp. Bot. 5 mL. *Rx.*
Use: Anti-infective, corticosteroid, ophthalmic.
Terramycin. (Roerig/Pfizer) Oxytetracycline 50 mg/mL, 125 mg/mL, lidocaine
2%. Inj. Amps. 2 mL single dose. Vials.
10 mL multidose (50 mg/mL only). *Rx.*
Use: Anti-infective, tetracycline.
Terramycin w/Polymyxin B Sulfate.
(Pfizer) Polymyxin B sulfate
10,000 units/g, oxytetracycline hydrochloride 5 mg/g, white and liquid petrolatum. Ophth. Oint. Tube 3.5 g. *Rx.*
Use: Anti-infective.
Terrell. (Minrad) Isoflurane. Liq. for Inh.
100 mL, 250 mL. *Rx.*
Use: General anesthetic.
Tersaseptic. (Doak Dermatologics) DEA-
lauryl sulfate, lauramide DEA, propylene glycol, ethoxydiglycol, PEG-12 distearate, EDTA, triclosan, citric acid/
Shampoo/cleanser. Soapless. 473 mL.
OTC.
Use: Dermatologic, acne.
tersavid.
Use: Monoamine oxidase inhibitor.
tertiary amyl alcohol.
See: Amylene Hydrate.
●**tesicam.** (TESS-ih-kam) USAN.
Use: Anti-inflammatory.
●**tesimide.** (TESS-ih-mide) USAN.
Use: Anti-inflammatory.
Teslac. (Bristol-Myers Squibb) Testolactone 50 mg, lactose. Tab. Bot. 100s.
c-III.
Use: Antineoplastic; sex hormone, androgen.

Teslascan. (Nycomed Amersham) Mangafodipir trisodium 37.9 mg (50 mcmol/mL), preservative free. Inj. Vial 10 mL. *Rx.*
Use: Diagnostic aid, parenteral.

Tesogen. (Sigma-Tau) Testosterone 25 mg, estrone 2 mg/mL. Vial 10 mL. *c-III.*
Use: Androgen.

Tesogen L.A. (Sigma-Tau) Testosterone enanthate 180 mg, 90 mg, 50 mg, estradiol valerate 8 mg, 4 mg, 2 mg, respectively/mL. Vial 10 mL. *Rx.*
Use: Androgen, estrogen combination.

Tesone. (Sigma-Tau) Testosterone 25 mg, 50 mg, 100 mg/mL. Vial 10 mL. *c-III.*
Use: Androgen.

Tesone L.A. (Sigma-Tau) Testosterone enanthate 200 mg/mL. Vial 10 mL. *c-III.*
Use: Androgen.

tespa.
Use: Antineoplastic.
See: Thiotepa.

Tessalon. (Forest) Benzonatate 200 mg, parabens. Cap. Bot. 100s, 500s. *Rx.*
Use: Antitussive.

Tessalon Perles. (Forest) Benzonatate 100 mg. Cap. Bot. 100s, 500s. *Rx.*
Use: Antitussive.

Testamone. (Oxypure) Testosterone 100 mg/mL. Inj. Vial 10 mL. *c-III.*
Use: Androgen.

Testex. (Taylor Pharmaceuticals) Testosterone propionate 50 mg, 100 mg/mL in sesame oil. Vial 10 mL. *c-III.*
Use: Androgen.

Testim. (Auxilium Pharm) Testosterone 1%, ethanol 74%, glycerin. Gel. 5 g. *c-III.*
Use: Sex hormone, androgen.

Testoject. (Merz) Testosterone cypionate 100 mg/mL. Vial 10 mL. *c-III.*
Use: Androgen.

Testoject-50. (Merz) Testosterone 50 mg/mL. Vial 10 mL. *c-III.*
Use: Androgen.

Testoject-LA. (Merz) Testosterone cypionate 200 mg/mL in oil. Vial 10 mL. *c-III.*
Use: Androgen.

•**testolactone.** (TESS-toe-LAK-tone) *USP 28.*
Use: Antineoplastic; sex hormone, androgen.
See: Teslac.

Testolin. (Taylor Pharmaceuticals) Testosterone suspension 25 mg, 50 mg, 100 mg/mL. Vial 10 mL 25 mg/mL. Vial 30 mL. *c-III.*
Use: Androgen.

Testopel. (Bartor Pharmacal) Testosterone 75 mg, stearic acid 0.2 mg, polyvinylpyrrolidone 2 mg/pellet. 1 Pellet/Vial. Box 3s, 10s, 100s. *c-III.*
Use: Sex hormone, androgen.

•**testosterone.** (tess-TAHS-ter-ohn) *USP 28.*
Use: Androgen.
See: Androderm.
    AndroGel 1%.
    Andronaq.
    Depotest.
    Homogene-S.
    Malotrone.
    Tesone.
    Testim.
    Testolin.
    Testopel.

testosterone. 2%. Oint.
Use: Vulvar dystrophies. [Orphan Drug]

testosterone, buccal.
Use: Androgen.
See: Striant.

testosterone cyclopentane propionate.
    Testosterone Cypionate.

•**testosterone cypionate.** (tess-TAHS-ter-ohn) *USP 28.*
Use: Androgen.
See: Andro-Cyp 100.
    Andro-Cyp 200.
    Depotest.
    Depo-Testosterone.
    Dep-Test.
    D-Test 100, 200.
    Durandro.
    Testoject.
    W/Combinations.
See: Depo-Testadiol.
    Depotestogen.
    Menoject LA.
    TE Ionate PA.

testosterone cypionate. (Watson) Testosterone cypionate 200 mg/mL. Benzyl alcohol, cottonseed oil. Inj. Multidose vials. 10 mL. *c-III.*
Use: Sex hormone.

testosterone cypionate. (Various Mfr.) Testosterone cypionate 100 mg/mL, 200 mg/mL. Inj. Vial 10 mL.
Use: Androgen.

•**testosterone enanthate.** (tess-TAHS-ter-ohn) *USP 28.*
Use: Sex hormone, androgen.
See: Andryl.
    Arderone 100, 200.
    Delatest.
    Delatestryl.
    Tesone L.A.
    Testate.
    Testrin-P.A.

W/Chlorobutanol.
See: Andro L.A. 200.
Anthatest.
Delatestryl.
Durathate-200.
W/Estradiol valerate.
See: Everone 200.
See: Valertest No. 1.
testosterone enanthate. (Various Mfr.)
Testosterone enanthate 100 mg/mL,
200 mg/mL. Inj. Vial 10 mL.
Use: Androgen.
testosterone heptanoate.
Use: Androgen.
See: Testosterone enanthate.
•**testosterone ketolaurate.** (tess-TAHS-
ter-ohn KEY-toe-LORE-ate) USAN.
Use: Androgen.
•**testosterone phenylacetate.** (tess-
TAHS-ter-ohn fen-ill-ASS-ah-tate)
USAN. Perandren phenylacetate.
Use: Androgen.
•**testosterone propionate.** (tess-TAHS-
ter-ohn) *USP 28.*
Use: Androgen.
•**testosterone undecanoate.** (tess-TAHS-
ter-ohn un-DEK-a-NOE-ate) USAN.
Use: Androgen.
testosterone w/combinations.
See: Andesterone.
Angen.
Depo-Testadiol.
Tesogen.
Testred. (Valeant) Methyltestosterone
10 mg. Cap. Bot. 100s. *c-III.*
Use: Sex hormone, androgen.
Testred Cypionate 200. (AstraZeneca)
Testosterone cypionate 200 mg/mL.
Vial 10 mL. *c-III.*
Use: Androgen.
Testrin-P.A. (Taylor Pharmaceuticals)
Testosterone enanthate 200 mg/mL, in
sesame oil with chlorobutanol. Vial
10 mL. *c-III.*
Use: Androgen.
Testuria. (Wyeth) Combination kit con-
taining 5 × 20 sterile dip strips and
5 × 20 culture trays of trypticase soy
agar.
Use: Diagnostic aid.
Tesuloid. (Bristol-Myers Squibb) Techne-
tium Tc 99m sulfur colloid. 5 Vials. Kit.
Use: Radiopaque agent.
•**tetanus and diphtheria toxoids adsorbed for adult use.** (TET-ah-nus and
diff-THEER-ee-uh TOX-oyds) *USP 28.*
Use: Immunization.
See: Decavac.
**tetanus and diphtheria toxoids ad-
sorbed purogenated.** (Wyeth) Tetanus

and diphtheria toxoids adsorbed puro-
genated. Adult *Lederject* disposable
syringe 10 × 0.5 mL. Vial 5 mL, new
package. *Rx.*
Use: Immunization.
**tetanus, diphtheria, and pertussis vac-
cine.**
Use: Immunization.
See: Certiva.
Daptacel.
Diphtheria and Tetanus Toxoids and
Whole Cell Pertussis Vaccine.
Infanrix.
TriHIBit.
Tri-Immunol.
Tripedia.
**tetanus, diphtheria toxoids, and alumi-
num phosphate adsorbed.** (Wyeth)
Tetanus, diphtheria toxoids, and aluminum phosphate adsorbed. Inj. Vial
5 mL, *Tubex* 0.5 mL. *Rx.*
Use: Immunization.
•**tetanus immune globulin.** (TET-ah-nus
ih-MYOON GLAH-byoo-lin) *USP 28.*
*Formerly Tetanus Immune Human
Globulin.* Gamma globulin fraction of
the plasma of persons who have been
hyperimmunized with tetanus toxoid,
16.5%. Vial 250 units.
Use: Prophylaxis of injured, against
tetanus (passive immunizing agent).
See: BayTet.
tetanus immune globulin, human. Tetanus immune globulin, human 250 units/
Tubex, 1 mL dissolved in glycine
0.3 M; thimerosal 0.01%. *Rx.*
Use: Immunization.
See: Baytet.
•**tetanus toxoid.** (TET-n-us TOX-oyd)
USP 28.
Use: Immunization.
tetanus toxoid. (Aventis Pasteur) Tetanus 4 Lf units/0.5 mL dose, thimerosal.
Inj. Vial 7.5 mL. *Rx.*
Use: Active immunization.
•**tetanus toxoid, adsorbed.** (TET-n-us
TOX-oyd) *USP 28.*
Use: Immunization.
tetanus toxoid, adsorbed. (Aventis Pasteur) Tetanus 5 Lf units/0.5 mL dose,
aluminum potassium sulfate, thimerosal. Inj. Vial 5 mL. *Rx.*
Use: Immunization.
**tetanus toxoid, adsorbed, puroge-
nated.** (Lederle) Tetanus toxoid adsorbed purogenated 5 Lf units/0.5 mL
dose, aluminum phosphate, thimerosal.
Inj. Vial 5 mL. Disposable syringe
0.5 mL. *Rx.*
Use: Immunization.

tetanus toxoid, aluminum phosphate adsorbed. *Rx.*
Use: Immunization.
See: Tetanus toxoid, aluminum phosphate adsorbed. Vial 5 mL 10s. *Lederject* Disp. Syr. 10 0.5 mL.

tetanus toxoid, fluid purogenated. (Wyeth) Tetanus toxoid, fluid purogenated. Vial 7.5 mL *Lederject* disposable syringe. 0.5 mL. Box 10s, 100s. *Rx.*
Use: Immunization.

tetanus toxoid purified, fluid. (Wyeth) Tetanus toxoid purified, fluid. Vial 7.5 mL, *Tubex* 0.5 mL. *Rx.*
Use: Immunization.

tetiothalein sodium.
See: Iodophthalein Sodium.

Tetrabead. (Abbott Diagnostics) Solid phase radioimmunoassay for the quantitative measurement of total circulating serum thyroxine.
Use: Diagnostic aid.

Tetrabead-125. (Abbott Diagnostics) T-3 uptake radioassay for the measurement of thyroid function by indirectly determining the degree of saturation of serum thyroxine binding globulin (TBG).
Use: Diagnostic aid.

●**tetracaine.** (TEH-trah-cane) *USP 28.*
Use: Anesthetic (topical).
See: Pontocaine.
Viractin.

tetracaine and menthol ointment.
Use: Anesthetic, local.

●**tetracaine hydrochloride.** *USP 28.*
Use: Anesthetic, injectable local ester.
See: Pontocaine Hydrochloride.
W/Benzocaine, butyl aminobenzoate.
See: Cetacaine.

tetracaine hydrochloride 0.5%. (Alcon) Tetracaine hydrochloride 0.5%. 1 mL *Drop-Tainer*, Ophth. 15 mL Steri-Unit, 2 mL (Ciba Vision) *Dropperettes* 1 mL in 10s. *Rx.*
Use: Anesthetic; ophthalmic.

Tetracap. (Circle) Tetracycline hydrochloride 250 mg. Cap. Bot. 100s. *Rx.*
Use: Anti-infective, tetracycline.

●**tetrachlorethylene.** *USP 28.* Perchlorethylene, tetrachlorethylene.
Use: Anthelmintic (hookworms and some trematodes).

Tetracon. (Professional Pharmacal) Tetrahydrozoline hydrochloride 0.5 mg, disodium edetate 1 mg, boric acid 12 mg, benzalkonium Cl 0.1 mg, sodium Cl 2.2 mg, sodium borate 0.5 mg/mL w/water. Liq. Bot. 15 mL. *OTC.*
Use: Anti-irritant; ophthalmic.

tetracyclic compounds.
Use: Antidepressant.
See: Maprotiline Hydrochloride.
Mirtazapine.

●**tetracycline and amphotericin B.** (teh-truh-SIGH-kleen) *USP 28.*

●**tetracycline hydrochloride.** (teh-trah-SIGH-kleen) *USP 28.*
Use: Anti-infective; antiamebic; antirickettsial.
See: Achromycin.
Bicycline.
Centet 250.
Cyclopar.
G-Mycin.
Maso-Cycline.
Panmycin.
Scotrex.
Sumycin.
Tetracap 250.
Tetracyn.
Tetram.
W/Nystatin.
See: Achromycin V.

tetracycline hydrochloride. (Various Mfr.) Tetracycline hydrochloride 250 mg. 500 mg. Cap. Bot. 100s, 1000s, UD 100s. *Rx.*
Use: Anti-infective, antiamebic, antirickettsial.

tetracycline hydrochloride and nystatin capsules.
Use: Anti-infective, tetracycline.

tetracycline oral suspension.
Use: Anti-infective, tetracycline.

●**tetracycline phosphate complex.** (teh-truh-SIGH-kleen FOSS-fate) *USP 28.*
Use: Anti-infective.

tetracyclines.
See: Demeclocycline hydrochloride.
Doxycycline.
Minocycline.
Oxytetracycline.
Tetracycline hydrochloride.

tetracycline w/n-acetyl-para-aminophenol, phenyltoloxamine citrate. (Roberts) Paltet, Cap.
Use: Anti-infective, tetracycline.
See: Telrex.

Tetracyn. (Pfizer) Tetracycline hydrochloride. Cap. **250 mg:** Bot. 1000s. **500 mg:** Bot. 100s. *Rx.*
Use: Anti-infective, tetracycline.

tetradecyl sulfate, sodium.
Use: Sclerosing agent.
See: Sotradecol.

tetraethyl ammonium bromide (teab).
Use: Diagnostic & therapeutic agent in peripheral vascular disorders. Diagnostic in hypertension.

tetraethylammonium chloride.
Use: Ganglionic blocking.
tetraethylthiuram disulfide.
See: Disulfiram.
●**tetrafilcon a.** (teh-trah-FILL-kahn) USAN.
Use: Contact lens material (hydrophilic).
Tetra-Formula. (Reese Pharm) Dextromethorphan HBr 10 mg, benzocaine 15 mg, sucrose, glucose, dextrose. Loz. Pkg. 10s. *OTC.*
Use: Antitussive.
tetrahydroaminoacridine.
Use: Cholinergic agent for Alzheimer disease.
See: Cognex.
tetrahydrophenobarbital calcium.
See: Cyclobarbital Calcium.
tetrahydroxyquinone. Name used for totroquinone.
●**tetrahydrozoline hydrochloride.** (teh-trah-high-DRAHZ-ah-leen) *USP 28.*
Use: Adrenergic (vasoconstrictor); nasal decongestant, imidazoline.
See: Collyrium Fresh Eye Drops.
　Geneye Extra.
　Mallazine Eye Drops.
　Murine Plus.
　Optigene 3.
　Soothe.
　Tetrasine.
　Tyzine.
　Tyzine Pediatric.
　Visine.
tetraiodophenolphthalein sodium.
See: Iodophthalein Sodium.
tetraiodophthalein sodium.
See: Iodophthalein Sodium.
tetramethylene dimethanesulfonate.
Busulfan.
tetramethylthiuram disulfide. Thiram.
Use: Anti-infective; antifungal.
●**tetramisole hydrochloride.** (teh-TRAM-ih-sole) USAN.
Use: Anthelmintic.
Tetraneed. (Hanlon) Pentaerythritol tetranitrate 80 mg. Time Cap. Bot. 100s. *Rx.*
Use: Antianginal.
tetrantoin.
Use: Anticonvulsant.
Tetrasine. (Optopics) Tetrahydrozoline hydrochloride 0.05%. Bot. 15 mL, 22.5 mL. *OTC.*
Use: Ophthalmic vasoconstrictor/mydriatic.
Tetrasine Extra. (Optopics) Polyethylene glycol 400 1%, tetrahydrozoline hydrochloride 0.05%. Bot. 15 mL. *OTC.*
Use: Mydriatic; vasoconstrictor.
Tetratab. (Freeport) Pentaerythritol tetranitrate 10 mg. Tab. Bot. 1000s. *Rx.*

Use: Antianginal.
Tetratab No. 1. (Freeport) Pentaerythritol tetranitrate 20 mg. Tab. Bot. 1000s. *Rx.*
Use: Antianginal.
●**tetraxetan.** (te-TRAX-e-tan) USAN.
Use: Chelating agent.
●**tetrazolast meglumine.** (teh-TRAZZ-ohlast meh-GLUE-meen) USAN.
Use: Antiallergic; antiasthmatic.
Tetrazyme. (Abbott Diagnostics) Test kit 100s, 500s.
Use: Enzyme immunoassay for quantitative measurement of total circulating serum thyroxine (free and protein bound).
●**tetrofosmin.** (teh-troe-FOSS-min) USAN.
Use: Diagnostic aid.
●**tetroquinone.** (TEH-troe-kwih-NOHN) USAN.
Use: Treat keloids, keratolytic (systemic).
●**tetroxoprim.** (tet-ROX-oh-prim) USAN.
Use: Anti-infective.
●**tetrydamine.** (teh-TRID-ah-meen) USAN.
Use: Analgesic; anti-inflammatory.
Tetterine. (Shuptrine) **Oint.:** Antifungal agents in green petrolatum base. Tin oz.; Antifungal agents in white petrolatum base. Tube oz. **Pow.:** Fungicide, germicide formula powder for heat and diaper rash. Can 2.25 oz. **Soap:** Bar 3.25 oz.
Use: Dermatologic; counterirritant.
Teveten. (Biovail) Esprosartan mesylate 600 mg. Lactose. Tab. Bot. 100s. *Rx.*
Use: Antihypertensive.
Teveten HCT. (Biovail) Eprosartan 600 mg/hydrochlorothiazide 12.5 mg, eprosartan 600 mg/hydrochlorothiazide 25 mg. Lactose. Tab. 100s. *Rx.*
Use: Antihypertensive.
Tev-Tropin. (Gate) Somatropin 5 mg (≈ 15 units), mannitol 30 mg. Pow. for Inj., lyophilized. Vials w/5 mL diluent (bacteriostatic sodium chloride 0.9% for injection). *Rx.*
Use: Growth hormone.
Texacort Scalp. (Medicis) Hydrocortisone 1%, alcohol 33%. Lipid free. Lot. Dropper Bot. 1 fl. oz. *Rx.*
Use: Corticosteroid.
tezacitabine.
Use: Antineoplastic.
tezosentan.
Use: Dual endothelin receptor antagonist.

T-Fluoride. (Tennessee Pharmaceutic) Sodium fluoride 2.21 mg. Tab. Bot. 100s, 1000s. *Rx.*
Use: Dental caries preventative.

T4.
See: levothyroxine sodium.

T4 endonuclease v, liposome encapsulated.
Use: Xeroderma pigmentosum. [Orphan Drug]

T-4 RIA (PEG). (Abbott Diagnostics) Diagnostic kit 50s, 100s, 500s. *Rx.*
Use: For quantitative measurement of total circulating serum thyroxine.

T4, soluble, human recombinant. (Biogen) Phase I/II HIV.
Use: Antiviral.

TG.
Use: Antineoplastic.
See: Thioguanine.

T/Gel Scalp. (Neutrogena) Neutar coal tar extract 2%, salicylic acid 2%. Soln. Bot. 2 oz. *OTC.*
Use: Antipsoriatic; antiseborrheic.

T/Gel Therapeutic Conditioner. (Neutrogena) Neutar coal tar extract 1.5% in oil free conditioner base. Liq. Bot. 1.4 oz. *OTC.*
Use: Antipsoriatic; antiseborrheic.

T/Gel Therapeutic Shampoo. (Neutrogena) Neutar coal tar extract 2% in mild shampoo base. Bot. 4.4 oz., 8.5 oz. *OTC.*
Use: Antipsoriatic; antiseborrheic.

T-Gen. (Goldline) Trimethobenzamide hydrochloride. **Adult Supp.:** 200 mg. Benzocaine 2%. Box 10s, 50s. **Pediatric Supp.:** 100 mg. Benzocaine 2%. Box 10s. *Rx.*
Use: Antiemetic/antivertigo agent.

T-Gesic. (T.E. Williams Pharmaceuticals) Hydrocodone bitartrate 5 mg, acetaminophen 500 mg. Cap. Bot. 100s. *c-III.*
Use: Analgesic combination; narcotic; hypnotic; sedative.

•**thalidomide.** (the-LID-oh-mide) USAN.
Use: Anti-infective; hypnotic; sedative; immunomodulator.
See: Thalomid.

Thalitone. (Horus Therapeutics, Inc.) Chlorthalidone 15 mg, 25 mg, lactose. Tab. Bot. 100s. *Rx.*
Use: Diuretic.

•**thallous chloride Tl 201 injection.** (THAL-uhs) *USP 28.*
Use: Diagnostic aid (radiopaque medium); radioactive agent.

Thalomid. (Celgene) Thalidomide 50 mg, 100 mg, 200 mg. Cap. Blister packs. 28s, 84s (200 mg only), 140s (100 mg only), 280s (50 mg only). *Rx.*

Use: Immunomodulator.

Tham. (Abbott) Tromethamine 18 g, acetic acid 2.5 g single-dose container. Soln. *Rx.*
Use: Nutritional supplement.

Tham-E. (Abbott) Tromethamine 36 g, NaCl 30 mEq/L, KCl 5 mEq/L, Cl 35 mEq/L. Total osmolarity 367 mOsm/L. Single-dose container 150 mL. *Rx.*
Use: Nutritional supplement.

THC.
Use: Antiemetic; antivertigo.
See: Marinol.

theamin. Monoethanolamine salt of theophylline.
W/Amobarbital.
See: Monotheamin.

thenalidine tartrate.
Use: Antihistamine; antipruritic.

thenyldiamine hydrochloride.
Use: Antihistamine.

•**theobroma oil.** *NF 23.* Cocoa Butter.
Use: Pharmaceutical aid; suppository base.

theobromine sodium acetate. Theobromine calcium salt mixture with calcium salicylate.
Use: Diuretic; muscle relaxant.

theobromine sodium salicylate.
W/Cal. lactate, phenobarbital.
See: Doan's Pills.

theobromine with phenobarbital combinations.
See: Harbolin.

Theochron. (Forest) Theophylline. **TR Tab.200 mg:** 200 mg, 300 mg. Bot. 100s, 500s, 1000s (200 mg only). **ER Tab. (12 to 24 hours):** 450 mg. 100s, 500s, 1000s. *Rx.*
Use: Bronchodilator.

Theochron. (Various Mfr.) Theophylline anhydrous 100 mg, 200 mg, 300 mg. ER Tab. 100s, 500s, 1000s. *Rx.*
Use: Bronchodilator.

Theocolate. (Rosemont) Theophylline 150 mg, guaifenesin 90 mg/15 mL Liq. Bot. Pt., gal. *Rx.*
Use: Antiasthmatic.

Theodrine. (Rugby) Theophylline 120 mg, ephedrine hydrochloride 22.5 mg. Tab. Bot. 1000s. *OTC.*
Use: Antiasthmatic.

•**theofibrate.** (THEE-oh-FIH-brate) USAN.
Use: Antihyperlipoproteinemic.

Theogen. (Sigma-Tau) Conjugated estrogens 2 mg/mL. Vial 10 mL, 30 mL. *Rx.*
Use: Estrogen.

Theogen I.P. (Sigma-Tau) Estrone 2 mg, potassium estrone sulfate 1 mg/mL. Inj. Vial 10 mL. *Rx.*
Use: Estrogen.

Theolate. (Various Mfr.) Theophylline 150 mg, guaifenesin 90 mg/15 mL. Liq. Bot. 118 mL, pt., gal. *Rx.*
Use: Antiasthmatic.

Theomax DF. (Various Mfr.) Theophylline 97.5 mg, ephedrine sulfate 18.75 mg, alcohol 5%, hydroxyzine hydrochloride 7.5 mg/15 mL. Syr. Bot. Pt., gal. *Rx.*
Use: Antiasthmatic.

Theo-Organidin. (Wallace) Theophylline anhydrous 120 mg, iodinated glycerol 30 mg/15 mL w/alcohol 15%, saccharin. Bot. Pt., gal. *Rx.*
Use: Antiasthmatic.

Theophenyllin. (H.L. Moore Drug Exchange) Theophylline 130 mg, ephedrine hydrochloride 24 mg, phenobarbital 8 mg. Tab. Bot. 1000s. *Rx.*
Use: Antiasthmatic.

● **theophylline.** (thee-AHF-ih-lin) *USP 28.*
Use: Bronchodilator; coronary vasodilator, diuretic; pharmaceutic necessity for Aminophylline Injection.
See: Accurbron.
　Aerolate.
　Bronkodyl.
　Elixicon.
　Elixophyllin.
　Elixophyllin SR.
　Lodrane.
　Quibron-T Dividose.
　Quibron-T/SR Dividose.
　Slo-Phyllin.
　Theochron.
　Uniphyl.

theophylline. (Able) Theophylline 300 mg, 400 mg, 450 mg, 600 mg. ER Tab. 30s, 100s, 500s, 1000s. *Rx.*
Use: Bronchodilator.

theophylline. (Various Mfr.) Theophylline 100 mg, 125 mg, 200 mg, 300 mg. ER Cap. Bot. 100s. *Rx.*
Use: Bronchodilator.

theophylline aminoisobutanol. Theophylline w/2-amino-2-methyl-1-propanol.
See: Butaphyllamine.

theophylline and 5% dextrose. (Abbott) Theophylline and dextrose 5%. Inj.
200 mg/Cont.: 50 mL, 100 mL.
400 mg/Cont.: 100 mL, 250 mL, 500 mL, 1000 mL. **800 mg/Cont.:** 250 mL, 500 mL, 1000 mL.
Use: Bronchodilator.

theophylline and guaifenesin capsules.
Use: Bronchodilator; expectorant.

theophylline and guaifenesin oral solution.
Use: Bronchodilator; expectorant.

theophylline choline salt.
See: Choledyl.

● **theophylline, 8-chloro, diphenhydramine.** *USP 28.* Dimenhydrinate.
See: Dramamine.

theophylline, ephedrine hydrochloride, and phenobarbital tablets.
Use: Bronchodilator; sedative.

theophylline ethylenediamine.
See: Aminophylline.

theophylline extended-release. (Dey) Theophylline 100 mg, 200 mg, 300 mg. ER Tab. Bot. 100s, 500s, 1000s. *Rx.*
Use: Bronchodilator.

theophylline extended-release. (Sidmak) Theophylline anhydrous 450 mg, lactose. ER Tab. Bot. 100s, 250s, 500s. *Rx.*
Use: Bronchodilator.

theophylline extended-release capsules.
Use: Bronchodilator.

theophylline KI. (Various Mfr.) Theophylline 80 mg, potassium iodide 130 mg/15 mL. Elix. 480 mL, gal. *Rx.*
Use: Antiasthmatic combination.

theophylline olamine. Theophylline compound with 2-amino-ethanol (1:1).
Use: Bronchodilator.

theophylline reagent strips. (Bayer Corp. (Consumer Div.)) Seralyzer reagent strip. Bot. 25s.
Use: Diagnostic aid; theophylline.

● **theophylline sodium glycinate.** (thee-AHF-ih-lin so-dee-uhm) *USP 28.*
Use: Bronchodilator.
See: Synophylate.
W/Guaifenesin.
See: Synophylate-GG.
W/Phenobarbital.
See: Synophylate w/Phenobarbital.
W/Potassium iodide.
See: TSG-KI.

theophylline with combinations.
See: B.A. Prods.
　Bronkaid.
　Co-Xan.
　Elixophyllin-KI.
　Marax DF.
　Quibron.
　Quibron Plus.
　Quibron-300.
　Slo-Phyllin GG.
　Synophylate.
　Tedral SA.
　Theo-Organidin.

theophylline with phenobarbital combinations.
See: Ceepa.

Theophyl-SR. (Ortho-McNeil) Theophylline 125 mg. Bot. 100s. *Rx.*

Use: Bronchodilator.

Theotal. (Major) Theophylline 125 mg, ephedrine hydrochloride 25 mg, phenobarbital 8 mg, lactose. Tab. Bot. 1000s. *Rx.*
Use: Antiasthmatic combination.

Theo-Time. (Major) Theophylline. **SR Tab.:** 100 mg, 200 mg, 300 mg. Bot. 100s, 500s. **TR Tab.:** 100 mg, 200 mg, 300 mg. Bot. 100s, 500s. *Rx.*
Use: Bronchodilator.

Theo-24. (UCB) Theophylline anhydrous. CR Cap. **100 mg:** Bot. 100s. UD 100s. **200 mg:** Bot. 100s, 500s. UD 100s. **300 mg:** Bot. 100s, 500s. UD 100s. *Rx.*
Use: Antiasthmatic; bronchodilator.

Thera Bath. (Walgreen) Mineral oil 90%. Bot. 16 oz. *OTC.*
Use: Emollient.

Thera Bath with Vitamin E. (Walgreen) Mineral oil 91%, Vit. E 2000 units/ 16 oz. *OTC.*
Use: Emollient.

Therabid. (Mission Pharmacal) Vitamins C 500 mg, B_1 15 mg, B_2 10 mg, B_3 100 mg, B_5 20 mg, B_6 10 mg, B_{12} 5 mcg, A 5000 units, D 200 units, E 30 mg. Tab. Bot. 60s. *OTC.*
Use: Mineral, vitamin supplement.

Therabrand. (Health for Life Brands) Vitamins A 25,000 units, D 1000 units, B_1 10 mg, B_2 10 mg, niacinamide 100 mg, C 200 mg, B_6 5 mg, calcium pantothenate 20 mg, B_{12} 5 mcg. Cap. Bot. 100s, 1000s. *OTC.*
Use: Mineral, vitamin supplement.

Therabrand-M. (Health for Life Brands) Vitamins A 25,000 units, D 1000 units, C 200 mg, B_1 10 mg, B_2 10 mg, B_6 5 mg, niacinamide 100 mg, calcium pantothenate 20 mg, E 5 units, B_{12} 5 mcg, I 0.15 mg, Fe 15 mg, Cu 1 mg, Ca 125 mg, Mn 1 mg, Mg 6 mg, Zn 1.5 mg. Cap. Bot. 100s, 1000s. *OTC.*
Use: Mineral, vitamin supplement.

Theracap. (Arcum) Vitamins A 10,000 units, D 400 units, B_1 10 mg, B_2 5 mg, niacinamide 150 mg, C 150 mg. Cap. Bot. 100s, 1000s. *OTC.*
Use: Vitamin supplement.

Thera-Combex H-P. (Parke-Davis) Vitamins C 500 mg, B_1 25 mg, B_2 15 mg, B_{12} 5 mcg, niacinamide 100 mg, panthenol 20 mg. Cap. Bot. 100s. *OTC.*
Use: Vitamin supplement.

TheraCys. (Aventis Pasteur) BCG, intravesical 10.5 ± 8.7 × 10^8 CFU (equivalent to ≈ 81 mg dry weight), msg. Pow. for Susp., lyophilized. Vial 81 mg w/3 mL diluent vial. *Rx.*
Use: Antineoplastic; biological response modifier.

TheraFlu Cold & Cough Night Time. (Novartis Consumer Healthcare) Dextromethorphan HBr 20 mg, chlorpheniramine maleate 4 mg, pseudoephedrine hydrochloride 60 mg, acetaminophen 650 mg, sucrose, lemon flavor. Pow. Pkt. 6s. *OTC.*
Use: Upper respiratory combination, antitussive, antihistamine, decongestant, analgesic.

TheraFlu Flu and Chest Congestion Non-Drowsy Powder. (Novartis) Dextromethorphan HBr 30 mg, guaifenesin 400 mg, pseudoephedrine hydrochloride 60 mg, acetaminophen 1000 mg, aspartame, phenylalanine 25 mg, sucrose, honey lemon flavor. Pow. Pkt. 6s. *OTC.*
Use: Upper respiratory combination, antitussive, expectorant, decongestant, analgesic.

TheraFlu Flu & Cold Medicine for Sore Throat, Maximum Strength. (Novartis Consumer Healthcare) Pseudoephedrine hydrochloride 60 mg, chlorpheniramine maleate 4 mg, acetaminophen 1000 mg, sucrose, aspartame, phenylalanine 20 mg, apple cinnamon flavor. Pow. Pkt. 6s. *OTC.*
Use: Upper respiratory combination, decongestant, antihistamine, analgesic.

TheraFlu, Flu & Cold Medicine Original Formula. (Novartis Consumer Healthcare) Pseudoephedrine hydrochloride 60 mg, chlorpheniramine maleate 4 mg, acetaminophen 650 mg, sucrose. Pow. Pks. 6s. *OTC.*
Use: Upper respiratory combination, analgesic, antihistamine, decongestant.

TheraFlu Flu & Cough Night Time, Maximum Strength. (Novartis Consumer Healthcare) Dextromethorphan HBr 30 mg, chlorpheniramine maleate 4 mg, pseudoephedrine hydrochloride 60 mg, acetaminophen 1000 mg, acesulfame K, aspartame, phenylalanine 26 mg, saccharin, sucrose, cherry flavor. Pow. Pkt. 6s. *OTC.*
Use: Upper respiratory combination, antitussive, antihistamine, decongestant, analgesic.

TheraFlu Flu & Sore Throat, Maximum Strength. (Novartis Consumer Healthcare) Pseudoephedrine hydrochloride 60 mg, chlorpheniramine maleate 4 mg, acetaminophen 1000 mg, acesulfame K, aspartame, sorbitol, sucrose. Pow. Pkt. 6s. *OTC.*
Use: Upper respiratory combination, decongestant, antihistamine, analgesic.

TheraFlu Flu & Sore Throat Night Time, Maximum Strength. (Novartis Consumer Healthcare) Pseudoephedrine hydrochloride 60 mg, chlorpheniramine maleate 4 mg, acetaminophen 1000 mg, acesulfame K, aspartame, phenylalanine 25 mg, sucrose, apple cinnamon flavor, alcohol free. Pow. Pkt. 6s. OTC.
Use: Upper respiratory combination, decongestant, antihistamine, analgesic.

TheraFlu Flu, Cold & Cough & Sore Throat, Maximum Strength. (Novartis Consumer Healthcare) Dextromethorphan HBr 30 mg, chlorpheniramine maleate 4 mg, pseudoephedrine hydrochloride 60 mg, acetaminophen 1000 mg, aspartame, acesulfame K, phenylalanine, sucrose, cherry flavor. Pow. Pkt. 6s. OTC.
Use: Upper respiratory combination, antitussive, antihistamine, decongestant, analgesic.

TheraFlu Flu, Cold & Cough Night Time, Maximum Strength. (Novartis Consumer Healthcare) Dextromethorphan HBr 30 mg, chlorpheniramine maleate 4 mg, pseudoephedrine hydrochloride 60 mg, acetaminophen 1000 mg, sucrose, lemon flavor. Tab. Pow. Pack. 6s, 12s. OTC.
Use: Upper respiratory combination, antitussive, antihistamine, decongestant, analgesic.

TheraFlu Maximum Strength Flu, Cold, & Cough. (Novartis) Dextromethorphan HBr 30 mg, guaifenesin 400 mg, pseudoephedrine hydrochloride 60 mg, acetaminophen 1000 mg, aspartame, phenylalanine, sucrose, honey lemon flavor, alcohol free. Pow. Pkt. 6s. OTC.
Use: Upper respiratory combination, antitussive, expectorant, decongestant, analgesic.

TheraFlu Maximum Strength Time Formula Flu, Cold & Cough Medicine. (Novartis Consumer Healthcare) Dextromethorphan HBr 15 mg, chlorpheniramine maleate 2 mg, pseudoephedrine hydrochloride 30 mg, acetaminophen 500 mg, lactose. Tab. Pkg. 12s, 24s. OTC.
Use: Upper respiratory combination, antitussive, antihistamine, decongestant, analgesic.

TheraFlu Non-Drowsy Flu, Cold & Cough Maximum Strength. (Novartis Consumer Healthcare) Pseudoephedrine hydrochloride 60 mg, dextromethorphan HBr 30 mg, acetaminophen 1000 mg, sucrose, lemon flavor. Pow.

Pkt. 6s, 12s. OTC.
Use: Upper respiratory combination, analgesic, antitussive, decongestant.

TheraFlu Non-Drowsy Formula, Maximum Strength. (Novartis Consumer Healthcare) Pseudoephedrine hydrochloride 30 mg, dextromethorphan HBr 15 mg, acetaminophen 500 mg, lactose, methylparaben. Pkg. 12s, 24s. OTC.
Use: Upper respiratory combination, antitussive, decongestant, analgesic.

Thera-Flur. (Colgate Oral) Fluoride 0.5% (from sod. fluoride 1.1%). pH 4.5. Gel-Drops. Bot. 24 mL, 60 mL. Rx.
Use: Dental caries agent.

Thera-Flur-N. (Colgate Oral) Neutral sodium fluoride 1.1% Liq. Bot. 24 mL, 60 mL. Rx.
Use: Dental caries agent

TheraFlu Severe Cold & Congestion Night Time, Maximum Strength. (Novartis Consumer Healthcare) Dextromethorphan HBr 30 mg, chlorpheniramine maleate 4 mg, pseudoephedrine hydrochloride 60 mg, acetaminophen 1000 mg, sucrose, lemon flavor. Pow. Pkt. 6s. OTC.
Use: Upper respiratory combination, antitussive, antihistamine, decongestant, analgesic.

TheraFlu Severe Cold & Congestion Non-Drowsy, Maximum Strength. (Novartis Consumer Healthcare) Dextromethorphan HBr 30 mg, pseudoephedrine hydrochloride 60 mg, acetaminophen 1000 mg, acesulfame K, aspartame, phenylalanine 17 mg, sucrose, lemon flavor. Pow. Pkt. 6s. OTC.
Use: Upper respiratory combination, antitussive, decongestant, analgesic.

TheraFlu Thin Strips Long Acting Cough. (Novartis) Dextromethorphan hydrobromide 15 mg. Alcohol (less than 5%), sorbitol sucralose. Cherry flavor. Orally Disintegrating Strips. 12. OTC.
Use: Nonnarcotic antitussive.

TheraFlu Thin Strips Multi Symptom. (Novartis) Diphenhydramine hydrochloride 25 mg. Alcohol (less than 5%), sorbitol, sucralose. Cherry flavor. Orally Disintegrating Strips. 12s. OTC.
Use: Nonnarcotic antitussive.

TheraFlu Vapor Stick. (Novartis) Camphor 4.8%, menthol 2.6%, cetyl alcohol, eucalyptus oil, parabens. Stick. 51 g. OTC.
Use: Upper respiratory combination, topical.

TheraFlu Vapor Stick Cough & Muscle Aches. (Novartis) Camphor 4.8%, men-

thol 2.6%, cetyl alcohol, eucalyptus oil, parabens. Stick. 51 g. *OTC.*
Use: Upper respiratory combination, topical.

Therafortis. (General Vitamin) Vitamins A 12,500 units, D 1000 units, B_1 5 mg, B_2 5 mg, B_6 1 mg, B_{12} 3 mcg, niacinamide 50 mg, pantothenic acid salt 10 mg, C 150 mg, folic acid 0.5 mg. Cap. Bot. 100s, 1000s. *OTC.*
Use: Vitamin supplement.

Theragenerix. (Ivax) Vitamins A 5500 units, D 400 units, E 30 mg, B_1 3 mg, B_2 3.4 mg, B_3 30 mg, B_5 10 mg, B_6 3 mg, B_{12} 9 mcg, C 120 mg, folic acid 0.4 mg, biotin 15 mcg, beta-carotene 2500 units. Tab. Bot. 130s, 1000s. *OTC.*
Use: Vitamin supplement.

Theragenerix-H. (Ivax) Fe 66.7 mg, vitamins A 8333 units, D 133 units, E 5 units, B_1 3.3 mg, B_2 3.3 mg, B_3 33.3 mg, B_5 11.7 mg, B_6 3.3 mg, B_{12} 50 mcg, C 100 mg, folic acid 0.33 mg, Cu, Mg. Tab. Bot. 100s, 1000s. *OTC.*
Use: Mineral, vitamin supplement.

Theragenerix-M. (Ivax) Fe 27 mg, vitamins A 5000 units, D 400 units, E 30 mg, B_1 3 mg, B_2 3.4 mg, B_3 30 mg, B_5 10 mg, B_6 3 mg, B_{12} 9 mcg, C 120 mg, folic acid 0.4 mg, Ca, Cl, Cr, Cu, I, K, biotin 15 mcg, Mg, Mn, Mo, P, Se, Zn 15 mg, beta-carotene 2500 units. Tab. Bot. 130s, 1000s. *OTC.*
Use: Mineral, vitamin supplement.

Thera-Gesic. (Mission Pharmacal) Methyl salicylate, menthol. Balm. Tube 90 g, 150 g. *OTC.*
Use: Analgesic, topical.

Theragran. (Bristol-Myers Squibb) **Capl.:** Vitamins A 5000 units, D 400 units, E 30 units, B_1 3 mg, B_2 3.4 mg, B_3 20 mg, B_5 10 mg, B_6 3 mg, B_{12} 9 mcg, C 90 mg, folic acid 0.4 mg, biotin 30 mcg. Bot. 100s. **Liq.:** Vitamins A 5000 units, D 400 units, B_1 10 mg, B_2 10 mg, B_3 100 mg, B_5 21.4 mg, B_6 4.1 mg, B_{12} 5 mcg, C 200 mg/5 mL. Liq. Bot. 120 mL. *OTC.*
Use: Vitamin supplement.

Theragran AntiOxidant. (Bristol-Myers Squibb) Vitamins A 5000 units, C 250 mg, E 200 units, Mn, Cu, Zn, Se. Softgel Cap. Bot. 50s. *OTC.*
Use: Mineral, vitamin supplement.

Theragran Jr. with Iron. (Bristol-Myers Squibb) Fe 18 mg, vitamins A 5000 units, D 400 units, E 30 mg, B_1 1.5 mg, B_2 1.7 mg, B_3 20 mg, B_6 2 mg, B_{12} 6 mcg, C 60 mg, folic acid 0.4 mg w/tartrazine. Tab. Bot. 75s. *OTC.*

Use: Mineral, vitamin supplement.

Theragran Stress Formula. (Bristol-Myers Squibb) Fe 27 mg, vitamins E 30 units, B_1 15 mg, B_2 15 mg, B_3 100 mg, B_5 20 mg, B_6 25 mg, B_{12}12 mcg, C 600 mg, folic acid 0.4 mg, biotin 45 mcg. Tab. Bot. 75s. *OTC.*
Use: Mineral, vitamin supplement.

Thera Hematinic. (Major) Fe 66.7 mg, A 8333 units, D 133 units, E 5 units, B_1 3.3 mg, B_2 3.3 mg, B_3 33.3 mg, B_5 11.7 mg, B_6 3.3 mg, B_{12} 50 mcg, C 100 mg, folic acid 0.33 mg, Cu, Mg. Tab. Bot. 250s, 1000s. *OTC.*
Use: Mineral, vitamin supplements.

Thera-Hist. (Major) Pseudoephedrine hydrochloride 60 mg, chlorpheniramine maleate 4 mg, acetaminophen 500 mg, sucrose. Pow. Pks. 6. *OTC.*
Use: Analgesic; antihistamine; decongestant.

Thera-Hist Cold & Allergy. (Major) Pseudoephedrine hydrochloride 15 mg, chlorpheniramine maleate 1 mg/5 mL, sorbitol, sucrose. Syr. Bot. 118 mL. *OTC.*
Use: Upper respiratory combination, decongestant, antihistamine.

Thera-Hist Cold & Cough. (Major) Pseudoephedrine hydrochloride 15 mg, chlorpheniramine maleate 1 mg, dextromethorphan HBr 5 mg/5 mL, sorbitol, sucrose, cherry flavor. Syr. Bot. 118 mL. *OTC.*
Use: Upper respiratory combination, decongestant, antihistamine, antitussive.

Thera-Hist Expectorant Chest Congestion. (Major) Pseudoephedrine hydrochloride 15 mg, guaifenesin 50 mg/5 mL, EDTA, sorbitol, sucrose, citrus flavor. Liq. Bot. 118 mL. *OTC.*
Use: Upper respiratory combination, decongestant, expectorant.

Thera-M. (Various Mfr.) Vitamins A 5000 units, B_1 3 mg, B_2 3.4 mg, B_3 20 mg, B_5 10 mg, B_6 3 mg, B_{12} 9 mcg, C 90 mg, D 400 units, E 30 units, Fe 27 mg, folic acid 0.4 mg, biotin 30 mcg, P, Ca, Cu, Cr, Se, Mo, K, Cl, I, Mg, Mn, Zn 15 mg. Tab. Bot. 130s, 1000s. *OTC.*
Use: Mineral, vitamin supplement.

Thera Multi-Vitamin. (Major) Vitamins A 10,000 units, D 400 units, B_1 10 mg, B_2 10 mg, B_3 100 mg, B_5 21.4 mg, B_6 4.1 mg, B_{12} 5 mcg, C 200 mg/5 mL. Liq. Bot. 118 mL. *OTC.*
Use: Vitamin supplement.

Theraneed. (Hanlon) Vitamins A 16,000 units, B_1 10 mg, B_2 10 mg, B_6 2 mg, C 300 mg, calcium pantothenate

10 mg, niacinamide 10 mg, B$_{12}$ 10 mcg. Cap. Bot. 100s. *OTC.*
Use: Mineral, vitamin supplement.

Therapals. (Faraday) Vitamins A 25,000 units, D 400 units, B$_1$ 10 mg, B$_2$ 5 mg, niacinamide 150 mg, B$_6$ 0.5 mg, E 5 units, C 150 mg, B$_{12}$10 mcg, Ca 103 mg, cobalt 0.1 mg, Cu 1 mg, K 0.15 mg, Mg 6 mg, Mn 1 mg, Mo 0.2 mg, P 80 mg, K 5 mg, Zn 1.2 mg. Tab. Bot. 100s, 250s, 1000s. *OTC.*
Use: Mineral, vitamin supplement.

TheraPatch Cold Sore. (LecTec) Lidocaine 4%, camphor 0.5%, aloe vera, eucalyptus oil, glycerin. Patch. Box 21s. *OTC.*
Use: Anesthetic, local.

TheraPatch Vapor Patch for Kids Cough Suppressant. (LecTec Corp.) Camphor 4.7%, menthol 2.0%, glycerin, cherry scent. Patch. Box. 7s. *OTC.*
Use: Upper respiratory combination, topical.

Therapeutic. (Ivax) Vitamins A 5000 units, D 400 units, E 30 units, B$_1$ 3 mg, B$_2$ 3.4 mg, B$_3$ 20 mg, B$_5$ 10 mg, B$_6$ 3 mg, B$_{12}$ 9 mcg, C 90 mg, folic acid 0.4 mg, d-biotin 30 mcg. Tab. Bot. 100s, 130s. *OTC.*
Use: Vitamin supplement.

Therapeutic B Complex with Vitamin C. (Upsher-Smith) Vitamins B$_1$ 15 mg, B$_2$ 10.2 mg, B$_3$ 50 mg, B$_5$ 10 mg, B$_6$ 5 mg, C 300 mg. Cap. Bot. UD 100s. *OTC.*
Use: Vitamin supplement.

Therapeutic-H. (Ivax) Fe 66.7 mg, A 8333 units, D 133 units, E 5 units, B$_1$ 3.3 mg, B$_2$ 3.3 mg, B$_3$ 33.3 mg, B$_5$ 11.7 mg, B$_6$ 3.3 mg, B$_{12}$ 50 mcg, C 100 mg, folic acid 0.33 mg, Cu, Mg. Tab. Bot. 100s. *OTC.*
Use: Mineral, vitamin supplement.

Therapeutic-M. (Ivax) Fe 27 mg, vitamins A 5000 units, D 400 units, E 30 units, B$_1$ 3 mg, B$_2$ 3.4 mg, B$_3$ 20 mg, B$_5$ 10 mg, B$_6$ 3 mg, B$_{12}$ 9 mcg, C 90 mg, folic acid 0.4 mg, Ca, Cl, Cr, Cu, I, K, Mg, Mn, Mo, P, Se, Zn 15 mg, biotin 30 mcg. Tab. Bot. 1000s. *OTC.*
Use: Mineral, vitamin supplement.

Therapeutic Mineral Ice. (Bristol-Myers Squibb) Menthol 2%, ammonium hydroxide, carbomer 934, cupric sulfate, isopropyl alcohol, magnesium sulfate, thymol. Gel. Tube 105 mL, 240 mL, 480 mL. *OTC.*
Use: Liniment.

Therapeutic V & M. (Whiteworth Towne) Vitamins A 10,000 units, D 400 units, B$_1$ 10 mg, B$_2$ 10 mg, B$_6$ 5 mg, B$_{12}$

5 mcg, niacinamide 100 mg, calcium pantothenate 20 mg, C 200 mg, E 15 units, I 0.15 mg, Fe 12 mg, Cu 2 mg, Mn 1 mg, Mg 60 mg, Zn 1.5 mg. Tab. *OTC.*
Use: Mineral, vitamin supplement.

Theraphon. (Health for Life Brands) Vitamins A 25,000 units, D 1000 units, B$_1$ 10 mg, B$_2$ 5 mg, C 150 mg, niacinamide 150 mg. Cap. Bot. 100s, 1000s. *OTC.*
Use: Vitamin supplement.

TheraTears. (Advanced Vision Research) Carboxymethylcellulose sodium 1%, KCl, sodium bicarbonate, NaCl, sodium phosphate. Gel. UD 28s. *OTC.*
Use: Artificial tears.

Theravee Hematinic Vitamin. (Vangard Labs, Inc.) Fe 66.7 mg, A 8333 units, D 133 units, E 5 units, B$_1$ 3.3 mg, B$_2$ 3.3 mg, B$_3$ 33.3 mg, B$_5$ 11.7 mg, B$_6$ 3.3 mg, B$_{12}$ 50 mcg, C 100 mg, folic acid 0.33 mg, Cu, Mg. Tab. Bot. UD 100s. *OTC.*
Use: Mineral, vitamin supplement.

Theravee-M. (Vangard Labs, Inc.) Fe 27 mg, vitamins A 5000 units, D 400 units, E 30 units, B$_1$ 3 mg, B$_2$ 3.4 mg, B$_3$ 30 mg, B$_5$ 10 mg, B$_6$ 3 mg, B$_{12}$ 9 mcg, C 120 mg, folic acid 0.4 mg, Ca, Cl, Cr, Cu, K, I, Mg, Mn, Mo, Se, Zn 15 mcg, biotin 15 mcg, beta-carotene 2500 units. Tab. Bot. 100s, 1000s, UD 100s. *OTC.*
Use: Mineral, vitamin supplement.

Theravee Vitamin. (Vangard Labs, Inc.) Vitamins A 5500 units, D 400 units, E 30 units, B$_1$ 3 mg, B$_2$ 3.4 mg, B$_3$ 30 mg, B$_5$ 10 mg, B$_6$ 3 mg, B$_{12}$ 9 mcg, C 120 mg, folic acid 0.4 mg, biotin 15 mcg. Tab. Bot. 100s. UD 100s. *OTC.*
Use: Vitamin supplement.

Theravim. (NBTY) Vitamins A 5000 units, D 400 units, E 30 units, B$_1$ 3 mg, B$_2$ 3.4 mg, B$_3$ 30 mg, B$_5$ 10 mg, B$_6$ 3 mg, B$_{12}$ 9 mcg, C 90 mg, folic acid 0.4 mg, beta-carotene 1250 units, biotin 35 mcg. Tab. Bot. 130s. *OTC.*
Use: Vitamin supplement.

Theravim-M. (NBTY) Fe 27 mg, vitamins A 5000 units, D 400 units, E 30 mg, B$_1$ 3 mg, B$_2$ 3.4 mg, B$_3$ 20 mg, B$_5$ 10 mg, B$_6$ 3 mg, B$_{12}$ 9 mcg, C 90 mg, folic acid 0.4 mg, Ca, Cl, Cr, Cu, I, K, Mg, Mn, Mo, P, Se, Zn 15 mg, biotin 30 mcg. Tab. Bot. 130s. *OTC.*
Use: Mineral, vitamin supplement.

Theravite. (Alra) Vitamins A 10,000 units, D 400 units, B$_1$ 10 mg, B$_2$ 10 mg, B$_3$ 100 mg, B$_5$ 21.4 mg, B$_6$ 4.1 mg, B$_{12}$ 5 mcg, C 200 mg/5 mL. Liq. Bot. 118 mL. *OTC.*

Use: Vitamin supplement.

Therems. (Rugby) Vitamins A 5000 units, D 400 units, E 30 mg, B$_1$ 3 mg, B$_2$ 3.4 mg, B$_3$ 30 mg, B$_5$ 10 mg, B$_6$ 3 mg, B$_{12}$ 9 mcg, C 120 mg, folic acid 0.4 mg, beta-carotene 1250 units, biotin 15 mcg. Tab. Bot. 130s, 1000s. *OTC.*
Use: Vitamin supplement.

Therems-M. (Rugby) Fe 27 mg, vitamins A 5500 units, D 400 units, E 30 mg, B$_1$ 3 mg, B$_2$ 3.4 mg, B$_3$ 20 mg, B$_5$ 10 mg, B$_6$ 3 mg, B$_{12}$ 9 mcg, C 90 mg, folic acid 0.4 mg, Ca, Cl, Cr, Cu, I, K, Mg, Mn, Mo, P, Se, Zn 15 mg, biotin 30 mcg. Tab. Bot. 90s, 100s, 1000s. *OTC.*
Use: Mineral, vitamin supplement.

Therevac. (Jones Pharma) Docusate potassium 283 mg, benzocaine 20 mg w/soft soap in PEG 400 and glycerin base. Unit 4 mL, Cap. Pkgs. 4s, 12s, 50s. *OTC.*
Use: Bowel evacuant.

Therevac Plus. (Jones Pharma) Docusate sodium 283 mg, benzocaine 20 mg, glycerin 275 mg in a base of soft soap, polyethylene glycol, per 4 mL ampule. Disposable enema. Box 50s, UD 30s. *OTC.*
Use: Laxative.

Therevac-SB. (Jones Pharma) Docusate sodium 283 mg in a base of soft soap, polyethylene glycol, glycerin 275 mg per 4 mL ampule. Disposable enema. UD 30s. *OTC.*
Use: Laxative.

Therex-M. (Halsey Drug) Vitamins A 10,000 units, D 400 units, E 15 units, C 200 mg, B$_1$ 10 mg, B$_2$ 10 mg, niacinamide 100 mg, B$_6$ 5 mg, B$_{12}$ 5 mcg, calcium pantothenate 20 mg, I 150 mcg, Fe 12 mg, Mg 65 mg, Cu 2 mg, Zn 1.5 mg, Mn 1 mg. Tab. Bot. 100s. *OTC.*
Use: Mineral, vitamin supplement.

Therex No. 1. (Halsey Drug) Vitamins A 10,000 units, D 400 units, E 15 units, C 200 mg, B$_1$ 10 mg, B$_2$ 10 mg, niacinamide 100 mg, B$_6$ 5 mg, B$_{12}$ 5 mcg, calcium pantothenate 20 mg. Tab. Bot. 100s. *OTC.*
Use: Vitamin, mineral supplement.

Therex-Z. (Halsey Drug) Vitamins A 10,000 units, D 400 units, E 15 units, C 200 mg, B$_1$ 10 mg, B$_2$ 10 mg, niacinamide 100 mg, B$_{12}$ 5 mcg, B$_6$ 5 mg, Ca pantothenate 20 mg, I 150 mcg, Cu 2 mg, Fe 12 mg, Zn 22.5 mg. Tab. Bot. 100s. *OTC.*
Use: Mineral, vitamin supplement.

Therma-Kool. (Nortech Laboratories) Compresses in following sizes: 3" × 5", 4" × 9", 8.5" × 10.5".

Use: Cold, hot compress.

Thermazene. (Sherwood Davis & Geck) Silver sulfadiazine 1% in white petrolatum. Cream. Tube 50 g, 400 g, 1000 g. *Rx.*
Use: Burn therapy.

Thermodent. (Mentholatum Co.) Strontium Cl 10%. Tube. *OTC.*
Use: Dentrifice.

Theroal. (Vangard Labs, Inc.) Theophylline 24 mg, ephedrine hydrochloride 24 mg, phenobarbital 8 mg. Tab. Bot. 100s, 1000s. *Rx.*
Use: Antiasthmatic combination.

Theroxide Wash. (Medicis) Benzoyl peroxide 10%. Liq. Bot. 120 mL. *Rx.*
Use: Dermatologic, acid.

ThexForte. (KM Lee) Vitamins B$_1$ 25 mg, B$_2$ 15 mg, B$_3$ 100 mg, B$_5$ 10 mg, B$_6$ 5 mg, C 500 mg. Cap. Bot. 75s. *OTC.*
Use: Vitamin supplement.

Thia. (Sigma-Tau) Thiamine hydrochloride 100 mg/mL. Inj. Vial 30 mL. *Rx.*
Use: Vitamin supplement.

•**thiabendazole.** (THIGH-uh-BEND-uh-zole) *USP 28.*
Use: Anthelmintic.
See: Mintezol.

thiacetarsamide sodium. Sodium mercaptoacetate S, S-diester with p-carbamoyl dithiobenzene arsonous acid.
Use: Antitrichomonal.

Thia-Dia-Mer-Sulfonamides. Sulfadiazine w/sulfamerazine & sulfathiazole.

thialbarbital.
See: Kemithal.

Thiamilate. (Tyson) Thiamin (B$_1$) 20 mg. EC Tab. Bot. 100s. *OTC.*
Use: Vitamin supplement.

thiamin (B$_1$).
Use: Vitamin.
See: Thiamilate.
  Thiamine Hydrochloride.

•**thiamine hydrochloride.** (THIGH-uh-min) *USP 28.*
Use: Enzyme co-factor vitamin.
See: Apatate.
  Betalin S.
  Thia.

thiamine hydrochloride. (THIGH-uh-min high-droe-KLOR-ide) (Various Mfr.) Thiamin (B$_1$). **Tab.:** 50 mg, 100 mg, 250 mg. Bot. 100s, 250s; 1000s, UD 100s (100 mg only). **Inj.:** 100 mg/mL, benzyl alcohol ≤ 9 mg. *Tubex* 1 mL, multiple-dose Vial 2 mL. *Rx-OTC.*
Use: Vitamin supplement.

•**thiamine mononitrate.** (THIGH-uh-min) *USP 28.*
Use: Enzyme cofactor vitamin.

●**thiamiprine.** (thigh-AM-ih-preen) USAN.
Use: Antineoplastic.
●**thiamphenicol.** (THIGH-am-FEN-ih-kahl)
USAN.
Use: Anti-infective.
●**thiamylal.** (thigh-AM-ih-lahl) *USP 28.*
Use: Anesthetic (intravenous).
●**thiamylal sodium, for injection.** (thigh-
AM-ih-lahl) *USP 28.*
Use: Anesthetic (intravenous).
thiazesim.
Use: Antidepressant.
●**thiazesim hydrochloride.** (thigh-AZE-
eh-sim) USAN.
Use: Antidepressant.
●**thiazinamium chloride.** (THIGH-ah-ZIN-
am-ee-uhm) USAN.
Use: Antiallergic.
thiazolidinedione.
Use: Antidiabetic.
See: Pioglitazone Hydrochloride.
Rosiglitazone Maleate.
thiethylene thiophosphoramide.
See: Thiotepa.
●**thiethylperazine.** (THIGH-eth-ill-PURR-
ah-zeem) USAN.
Use: CNS depressant; antiemetic.
●**thiethylperazine maleate.** (THIGH-eth-
ill-PURR-ah-zeen MAL-ee-ate) *USP 28.*
Use: Antiemetic.
●**thiethylperazine maleate.** *USP 28.*
Use: Antiemetic.
See: Torecan.
thihexinol methylbromide.
Use: Anticholinergic.
●**thimerfonate sodium.** (thigh-MER-foe-
nate) USAN.
Use: Anti-infective, topical.
●**thimerosal.** (thigh-MER-oh-sal) *USP 28.*
Use: Anti-infective, topical; pharmaceu-
tic aid (preservative).
See: Aeroaid.
Merphol Tincture 1:1000.
Mersol.
W/Trifluridine.
See: Merthiolate.
See: Viroptic.
thiocarbanidin. Under study.
Use: Tuberculosis.
thiocyanate sodium. Sodium thiocya-
nate.
Use: Antihypertensive.
thiodinone. Name used for Nifuratel.
thiodiphenylamine.
See: Phenothiazine.
thioglycerol.
W/Sodium citrate, phenol, benzyl
alcohol.
See: Sulfo-ganic.

●**thioguanine.** (THIGH-oh-GWAHN-een)
USP 28.
Use: Antineoplastic.
See: Tabloid.
thiohexamide.
Use: Blood sugar-lowering compound.
thioisonicotinamide. Under study.
Use: Antituberculosal.
Thiola. (Mission Pharmacal) Tiopronin
100 mg. Tab. Bot. 100s. *Rx.*
Use: Anticholelithiasis.
●**thiopental sodium.** (thigh-oh-PEN-tahl)
USP 28.
Use: Anesthetic (intravenous); anticon-
vulsant.
See: Pentothal Sodium.
thiopental sodium. (I.M.S., Ltd.) Thio-
pental sodium. Pow. for Inj. **20 mg/mL:**
400 mg *Min-I-Mix* vial w/injector.
25 mg/mL: 250 mg, 500 mg *Min I Mix*
vials w/injector; 500 mg, 1 g, 2.5 g, 5 g,
10 g kits. *Rx.*
Use: Anesthetic, general.
thiophosphoramide.
See: Thiotepa.
Thioplex. (Amgen) Thiotepa 15 mg.
Powd. for Inj. Vials. *Rx.*
Use: Antineoplastic.
thiopropazate hydrochloride.
Use: Anxiolytic.
thioproperazine mesylate.
Use: CNS depressant; antiemetic.
●**thioridazine.** (THIGH-oh-RID-uh-zeen)
USP 28.
Use: Antipsychotic; hypnotic; sedative.
See: Mellaril.
●**thioridazine hydrochloride.** (THIGH-oh-
RID-ah-zeen) *USP 28.*
Use: Antipsychotic; hypnotic; sedative.
**thioridazine hydrochloride concen-
trate.** (Various Mfr.) Thioridazine hydrochloride. **30 mg/mL:** Bot. 120 mL.
100 mg/mL: Bot. 120 mL, 3.4 mL
(UD 100s). *Rx.*
Use: Antipsychotic.
thioridazine hydrochloride tablets.
(Various Mfr.) Thioridazine hydrochloride 10 mg, 15 mg, 25 mg, 50 mg,
100 mg, 150 mg, 200 mg. Bot. 60s (except 15 mg, 150 mg, 200 mg), 100s,
1000s, UD 100s (except 150 mg,
200 mg). *Rx.*
Use: Antipsychotic.
●**thiosalan.** (THIGH-oh-sal-AN) USAN.
Use: Disinfectant.
●**thiotepa.** (thigh-oh-TEP-uh) *USP 28.*
Use: Antineoplastic.
See: Thioplex.
thiotepa. (Bedford) Thiotepa 15 mg. Pow.
for Inj, lyophilized. Single-dose vial. *Rx.*

Use: Antineoplastic.
thiotepa. (thigh-oh-TEP-uh) (Wyeth)
Thiotepa powder 15 mg, sodium chloride 80 mg, sodium bicarbonate 50 mg.
Vial. Pow. for Recon. Vial 15 mg. *Rx.*
Use: Antineoplastic.
•**thiothixene.** (THIGH-oh-THIX-een)
USP 28.
Use: Antipsychotic.
See: Navane.
Navane Concentrate.
thiothixene. (Various Mfr.) Thiothixene
1 mg, 2 mg, 5 mg, 10 mg. Cap. Bot.
100s, 1000s, UD 100s (2 mg, 5 mg
only). *Rx.*
Use: Antipsychotic.
•**thiothixene hydrochloride.** (THIGH-oh-
THIX-een) *USP 28.*
Use: Antipsychotic.
See: Navane.
thiouracil. 2-Thiouracil.
Use: Treatment of hyperthyroidism, antianginal, congestive heart failure.
thioxanthene derivatives.
See: Thiothixene.
•**thiphenamil hydrochloride.** (thigh-FEN-
ah-mill) USAN.
Use: Muscle relaxant.
•**thiphencillin potassium.** (thigh-fen-
SILL-in) USAN.
Use: Anti-infective.
•**thiram.** (THIGH-ram) USAN.
Use: Antifungal.
Thixo-Flur. (Colgate Oral) Acidulated
phosphate sodium fluoride in gel base
1.2%. Gel. Bot. 4 oz, 8 oz., 32 oz.
Use: Dental caries agent.
•**thonzonium bromide.** (thahn-ZOE-nee-
uhm) *USP 28.*
Use: Detergent.
W/Colistin base, neomycin base, hydrocortisone acetate, polysorbate 80, acetic acid, sodium acetate.
See: Coly-Mycin-S.
Cortisporin-TC.
W/Isoproterenol.
See: Nebair.
•**thonzylamine hydrochloride.** USAN.
Use: Antihistamine.
Thorazine. (GlaxoSmithKline) Chlorpromazine hydrochloride. **Tab.:** 25 mg,
50 mg, 100 mg, 200 mg. Lactose,
parabens. Bot. 100s. **Supp.:** Chlorpromazine base 100 mg. 12s. **Inj.:**
25 mg/mL. 1 and 2 mL amps (sodium
bisulfite, sodium sulfite). *Rx.*
Use: Antiemetic; antipsychotic.
Thorets. (Buffington) Benzocaine lozenge. *Dispens-A-Kits* 500s. Sugar, lactose, and salt free. *OTC.*

Use: Sore throat relief.
Thor-Prom. (Major) Chlorpromazine
10 mg, 25 mg, 50 mg, 100 mg, 200 mg.
Tab. Bot. 100s, 1000s (except
200 mg). Tab. Bot. 250s, 1000s
(200 mg only). *Rx.*
Use: Antiemetic; antipsychotic.
•**thozalinone.** (thoe-ZAL-ah-nohn) USAN.
Use: Antidepressant.
357 HR Magnum. (BDI) Caffeine 200 mg.
Tab. Bot. 36s, 100s, 500s. *OTC.*
Use: CNS stimulant, analeptic.
•**threonine.** (THREE-oh-neen) *USP 28.*
Use: Amino acid; antispasmodic.
[Orphan Drug]
See: Threostat.
l-threonine.
Use: Antispasmodic.
threonine. (Various Mfr.) Threonine
500 mg. **Cap.:** 60s, 100s. **Tab.:** 100s,
250s. *OTC.*
Use: Nutritional supplement.
Threostat. (Tyson) *Rx.*
Use: Antispasmodic.
See: Threonine.
Throat Discs. (GlaxoSmithKline) Capsicum, peppermint, mineral oil, sucrose.
Box 60s. *OTC.*
Use: Throat preparation.
Throat-Eze. (Faraday) Cetylpyridinium
chloride 1:3000, cetyl dimethylbenzyl
ammonium chloride 1:3000, benzocaine
10 mg. Wafer. Loz., foil wrapped. Vial
15. *OTC.*
Use: Anesthetic, local.
Thrombate III. (Bayer Corp. (Allergy
Div.)) Antithrombin III (human)
500 units, 1000 units. Pow. for Inj., lyophilized. Single-use vial w/10 mL
(500 mL units only), 20 mL (1000 units
only). Sterile water for injection. *Rx.*
Use: Antithrombin.
•**thrombin.** (THRAHM-bin) *USP 28.*
Thrombin, topical, mammalian origin.
Use: Hemostatic.
See: Thrombinar.
Thrombogen.
Thrombostat.
Thrombinar. (Jones Pharma) Thrombin
topical. 1000 units: 50% mannitol, 45%
NaCl. 5000 units: 50% mannitol, 45%
NaCl, sterile water for injection.
50,000 units: 50% mannitol, 45% NaCl.
Pow. Vial. Preservative free. *Rx.*
Use: Hemostatic, topical.
thrombin inhibitor.
Use: Anticoagulant.
See: Argatroban.
Bivalirudin.
Desirudin.

Lepirudin.

Thrombogen. (Johnson & Johnson) Thrombin 1000 units. 5000 units: With isotonic saline diluent and transfer needle. 10,000 units, 20,000 units: Isotonic saline diluent, benzethonium chloride, and transfer needle. Inj. Vial. *Rx.*
Use: Hemostatic, topical.

thrombolytic agents.
See: Alteplase, Recombinant.
Drotrecogin Alfa (Activated).
Recombinant Human Activated Protein C.
Reteplase, Recombinant.
Streptokinase.
Tenecteplase.
Tissue Plasminogen Activators.
Thrombolytic Enzymes.

thrombolytic enzymes.
See: Streptokinase.
Urokinase.

thromboplastin.
Use: Diagnostic aid (prothrombin estimation).

Thrombostat. (Parke-Davis) Prothrombin is activated by tissue thromboplastin in the presence of calcium chloride. **1000 U.S. (N.I.H.) units:** Vial 10 mL. **5000 U.S. units:** Vial 10 mL, 5 mL diluent. **10,000 U.S. units:** Vial 20 m, 10 mL diluent. **20,000 U.S. units:** Vial 30 mL, 20 mL diluent. *Rx.*
Use: Hemostatic.

Thylox. (C.S. Dent & Co.) Medicated bar soap w/absorbable sulfur. Bar 3.4 oz. *OTC.*
Use: Cleanser.

•**thymalfasin.** (thigh-MAL-fah-sin) USAN. *Formerly Thymosin.*
Use: Antineoplastic; vaccine enhancement; hepatitis, infectious disease treatment.

Thymoglobulin. (SangStat) Antithymocyte globulin (rabbit) 25 mg, glycine 50 mg, mannitol 50 mg, sodium chloride 10 mg. Pow. for Inj., lyophilized. Vial 7 mL w/diluent vial 5 mL. *Rx.*
Use: Immune globulin.

•**thymol.** (THIGH-mole) *NF 23.*
Use: Antifungal; anti-infective; anesthetic, local; antitussive; decongestant; pharmaceutic aid (stabilizer).
See: Vicks Regular & Wild Cherry Medicated Cough Drops.
Vicks Vaporub.
W/Combinations.
See: Listerine Antiseptic.
Listerine, Natural Citrus.
Listerine, Tartar Control.

thymol. (Various Mfr.) Thymol 0.25 lb, 1 lb.

Use: Antifungal; anti-infective; anesthetic, local; antitussive; decongestant; pharmaceutic aid (stabilizer).

thymol iodide.
Use: Antifungal; anti-infective.

•**thymopentin.** (THIGH-moe-PEN-tin) USAN. *Formerly Thymopoietin 32-36.*
Use: Immunoregulator.

thymosin alpha-1.
Use: Antiviral, hepatitis B. [Orphan Drug]

thyodatil. Name used for nifuratel.

Thyro-Block. (Wallace) Potassium iodide 130 mg. Tab. 14s. *Rx.*
Use: Antithyroid.

Thyrogen. (Genzyme) Thyrotropin alfa 1.1 mg (≥ 4 units)/ vial, mannitol 36 mg, sodium phosphate 5.1 mg, sodium chloride 2.4 mg. Pow. for Inj., lyophilized. Kit of two thyrotropin alfa single-use vials 1.1 mg and two diluent vials 10 mL. *Rx.*
Use: In vivo diagnostic aid, thyroid function test.

•**thyroid.** (THIGH-royd) *USP 28.*
Use: Hormone, thyroid.
See: Arco Thyroid.
S-P-T.

thyroid combinations.
See: Henydin.

thyroid desiccated. (THIGH-royd DESS-ih-KATE-uhd)
Use: Hormone, thyroid.
See: Armour Thyroid.
Bio-Thyroid.
Nature Thyroid.
Thyroid USP.
Westhroid.

thyroid function test.
Use: In vivo diagnostic aid.
See: Sodium Iodide I-123.
Thypinone.
Thyrogen.
Thyrotropin Alfa.
Thytropar.

thyroid hormones.
See: Levothyroxine Sodium.
Liothyronine Sod.
Liotrix.
Thyroid Dessicated.

thyroid preparations.
See: Thyrar.
Thyroxin.

Thyroid USP. (Various Mfr.) Thyroid desiccated 32.5 mg (½ gr), 65 mg (1 gr), 130 mg (2 gr), 195 mg (3 gr). Tab. Bot. 100s, 1000s. *Rx.*
Use: Hormone, thyroid.

Thyrolar. (Forest) Liotrix 0.25 gr, 0.5 gr, 1 gr, 2 gr, 3 gr, lactose. Tab. Bot. 100s. *Rx.*

Use: Hormone, thyroid.
•**thyromedan hydrochloride.** (thigh-ROW-meh-dan) USAN.
Use: Thyromimetic.
thyropropic acid. (Warner Chilcott) Triopron.
Use: Anticholesteremic.
Thyro-Tabs. (Lloyd) Levothyroxine sodium 0.025 mg, 0.05 mg, 0.075 mg, 0.088 mg, 0.1 mg, 0.112 mg, 0.125 mg, 0.15 mg, 0.175 mg, 0.2 mg, 0.3 mg. Tab. Bot. 100s, 1000s. *Rx.*
Use: Hormone, thyroid.
thyrotropic hormone.
Use: In vivo diagnostic aid.
See: Thytropar.
thyrotropic principle of bovine anterior pituitary glands.
See: Thytropar.
thyrotropin.
Use: Diagnostic aid.
See: Thytropar.
•**thyrotropin alfa.** USAN.
Use: Thyroid-stimulating hormone; in vivo diagnostic aid, thyroid function test.
See: Thyrogen.
thyrotropin-releasing hormone.
Use: Diagnostic aid.
See: Thypinone.
•**thyroxine I 131.** (thigh-ROX-een) USAN.
Use: Radiopharmaceutical.
•**thyroxine I 125.** (thigh-ROX-een) USAN.
Use: Radiopharmaceutical.
thyrozyme-II A. (Abbott Diagnostics) T-4 diagnostic kit. 100, 500 test units.
Use: Diagnostic aid, thyroid.
Thytropar. (Centeon) Thyrotropin from bovine anterior pituitary glands. Thyrotropin. Vial 10 units.
Use: Thyroid agent.
•**tiacrilast.** (TIE-ah-KRILL-ast) USAN.
Use: Antiallergic.
•**tiacrilast sodium.** (TIE-ah-KRILL-ast) USAN.
Use: Antiallergic.
tiagabine. (Abbott)
Use: Antiepileptic.
•**tiagabine hydrochloride.** (tye-AG-a-been) USAN.
Use: Anticonvulsant.
See: Gabitril.
Tiamate. (Hoechst Marion Roussel) Diltiazem hydrochloride 120 mg, 180 mg, 240 mg, sucrose. ER Tab. Bot. UD 30s. *Rx.*
Use: Calcium channel blocker.
•**tiamenidine.** (TIE-ah-MEN-ih-DEEN) USAN.
Use: Antihypertensive.

•**tiamenidine hydrochloride.** (TIE-ah-MEN-ih-DEEN) USAN.
Use: Antihypertensive.
•**tiapamil hydrochloride.** (tie-APP-ah-mill) USAN.
Use: Calcium antagonist.
•**tiaramide hydrochloride.** (TIE-ar-ah-MIDE) USAN.
Use: Antiasthmatic.
Tiazac. (Forest) Diltiazem hydrochloride 120 mg, 180 mg, 240 mg, 300 mg, 360 mg, 420 mg, sucrose. ER Cap. Bot. 7s, 30s, 90s, 1000s. *Rx.*
Use: Calcium channel blocker.
•**tiazofurin.** (TIE-AZE-oh-few-rin) USAN.
Use: Antineoplastic.
TI-Baby Natural. (Fischer) Titanium dioxide 5%. SPF 16. Lot. Bot. 120 mL. *OTC.*
Use: Sunscreen.
•**tibenelast sodium.** (TIE-ben-ell-ast) USAN.
Use: Antiasthmatic; bronchodilator.
•**tibolone.** (TIH-bole-ohn) USAN.
Use: Menopausal symptoms suppressant.
•**tibric acid.** (TIE-brick) USAN.
Use: Antihyperlipoproteinemic.
•**tibrofan.** (TIE-broe-fan) USAN.
Use: Disinfectant.
•**ticabesone propionate.** (tie-CAB-eh-sone) USAN.
Use: Corticosteroid, topical.
Ticar. (GlaxoSmithKline) Ticarcillin disodium 3 g. Pow. for Inj. Vial 3 g. *Rx.*
Use: Anti-infective.
•**ticarbodine.** (tie-CAR-boe-deen) USAN.
Use: Anthelmintic.
ticarcillin and clavulanate potassium.
Use: Penicillin.
See: Timentin.
•**ticarcillin cresyl sodium.** (tie-CAR-SIH-lin KREH-sill) USAN.
Use: Anti-infective.
•**ticarcillin disodium.** (tie-CAR-SIH-lin) *USP 28.*
Use: Anti-infective.
See: Ticar.
ticarcillin disodium and clavulanate potassium, sterile.
Use: Anti-infective; inhibitor (β-lactamase).
See: Timentin.
•**ticarcillin monosodium.** (tie-CAR-SIH-lin) *USP 28.*
Use: Anti-infective.
TICE BCG. (Organon Teknika) BCG, intravesical Tice strain (1 to 8 × 10^8 CFU (equivalent to ≈ 50 mg), lactose, preservative free. Pow. for Susp.,

lyophilized. Vial 2 mL. *Rx.*
Use: Antineoplastic; biological response modifier.
•**ticlatone.** (TIE-klah-tone) USAN.
Use: Anti-infective; antifungal.
Ticlid. (Roche) Ticlopidine hydrochloride 250 mg. Tab. Bot. 30s, 60s, 500s. *Rx.*
Use: Antiplatelet.
•**ticlopidine hydrochloride.** (tie-KLOE-pih-DEEN) USAN.
Use: Platelet inhibitor.
See: Ticlid.
ticlopidine hydrochloride. (Various Mfr.) Ticlopidine hydrochloride 250 mg. Tab. Bot. 30s, 60s, 100s, 500s, 1000s. *Rx.*
Use: Platelet inhibitor.
•**ticolubant.** (tih-kahl-YOU-bant) USAN.
Use: Antipsoriatic.
ticon. (Hauck) Trimethobenzamide hydrochloride 100 mg/mL, phenol. Inj. Vial 20 mL. *Rx.*
Use: Antiemetic; antivertigo.
ticonazole.
Use: Antifungal, vaginal.
See: Vagistat-1.
•**ticrynafen.** (TIE-krin-ah-fen) USAN.
Use: Diuretic; uricosuric; antihypertensive.
•**tidembersat.**
Use: Antimigraine.
Tidex. (Allison) Dextroamphetamine sulfate 5 mg. Tab. Bot. 100s, 1000s. *c-II.*
Use: Antiobesity agent.
Tidexsol. (Sanofi-Synthelabo) Acetaminophen. Tab. *OTC.*
Use: Analgesic.
•**tifurac sodium.** (TIE-fyoor-ak) USAN.
Use: Analgesic.
Tigan. (Monarch) Trimethobenzamide hydrochloride. **Cap.:** 300 mg. Bot. 100s. **Inj.:** 100 mg/mL. Amps (with methyl- and propylparabens). 2 mL. Vials (with phenol). 20 mL. Syringe (with phenol and EDTA). 2 mL. **Adult Supp.:** 200 mg. Benzocaine 2%. Box 10s, 50s. **Pediatric Supp.:** 100 mg. Benzocaine 2%. Box 10s. *Rx.*
Use: Antiemetic.
•**tigecycline.** (tye-ge-SYE-kleen) USAN.
Use: Anti-infective, glycylcycline.
See: Tygacil.
•**tigemonam dicholine.** (TIE-jem-OH-nam die-KOE-leen) USAN.
Use: Antimicrobial.
•**tigestol.** (tie-JESS-tole) USAN.
Use: Hormone, progestin.
Tigo. (Burlington) Polymyxin B sulfate 5000 units, zinc bacitracin 400 units, neomycin sulfate 5 mg/g Oint. Tube 0.5 oz. *OTC.*

Use: Anti-infective, topical.
Tihist-DP. (Vita Elixir) Dextromethorphan HBr 10 mg, pyrilamine maleate 16 mg, sodium citrate 3.3 g/5 mL. *OTC.*
Use: Antitussive; antihistamine.
Tihist Nasal Drops. (Vita Elixir) Pyrilamine maleate 0.1%, phenylephrine hydrochloride 0.25%, sodium bisulfite 0.2%, methylparaben 0.02%, propylparaben 0.01%/30 mL. Bot. *OTC.*
Use: Antihistamine; decongestant.
Tija. (Vita Elixir) Oxytetracycline hydrochloride. **Syr.:** 125 mg/5 mL. **Tab.:** 250 mg. *Rx.*
Use: Anti-infective, tetracycline.
Tikosyn. (Pfizer) Dofetilide 125 mcg, 250 mcg, 500 mcg. Cap. Bot. 14s, 60s, UD 40s. *Rx.*
Use: Antiarrhythmic.
Tilade. (Monarch) Nedocromil sodium 1.75 mg per actuation. Aerosol Can. 16.2 g with mouthpiece. *Rx.*
Use: Respiratory; anti-inflammatory; antiasthmatic.
•**tiletamine hydrochloride.** (tie-LET-ah-meen) *USP 28.*
Use: Anesthetic; anticonvulsant.
•**tilidine hydrochloride.** (TIl l-lih-DEEN) USAN.
Use: Analgesic.
Ti-lite. (Fischer) Ethylhexyl p-methoxycinnamate 7.5%, titanium dioxide 2%, cetyl alcohol, phenethyl alcohol, parabens, EDTA. Cream 60 g. *OTC.*
Use: Sunscreen.
•**tilmacoxib.** (til-ma-KOX-ib) USAN.
Use: Cox-2 inhibitor.
•**tilomisole.** (TILL-oh-mih-sahl) USAN.
Use: Immunoregulator.
•**tilorone hydrochloride.** (TIE-lore-ohn) USAN.
Use: Antiviral.
•**tiludronate disodium.** (tie-LOO-droe-nate) USAN.
Use: Bisphosphonate.
See: Skelid.
•**timefurone.** (tie-MEH-fyoor-OHN) USAN.
Use: Antiatherosclerotic.
Time-Hist. (MCR American) Pseudoephedrine hydrochloride 120 mg, chlorpheniramine maleate 8 mg. SR Cap. Bot. 100s. *Rx.*
Use: Upper respiratory combination, decongestant, antihistamine.
Timentin. (GlaxoSmithKline) **Pow. for Inj.:** Ticarcillin disodium 3 g, clavulanic acid (as potassium salt) 0.1 g, sodium 4.75 mEq, potassiam 0.15 mEq/g. Vials 3.1 g. Piggyback bot., *ADD-Vantage* vial, Pharmacy Bulk Pkg. 31 g (ticarcillin

disodium 30 g, clavulanic acid 1 g). **Inj. Soln.:** Ticarcillin disodium 3 g, clavulanic acid (as potassium salt) 0.1 g, sodium 18.7 mEq, potassium 0.5 mEq/100 mL. Premixed, frozen *Galaxy* Cont. 100 mL. *Rx.*
Use: Anti-infective.

•**timobesone acetate.** (tie-MOE-behsone) USAN.
Use: Adrenocortical steroid, topical.

Timolide 10-25. (Merck & Co.) Timolol maleate 10 mg, hydrochlorothiazide 25 mg. Tab. Bot. 100s. *Rx.*
Use: Antihypertensive.

•**timolol.** (TI-moe-lahl) USAN.
Use: Antiadrenergic (β-receptor).
See: Betimol.

•**timolol maleate.** (TI-moe-lahl) *USP 28.*
Use: Agent for glaucoma; antiadrenergic/sympatholytic, beta-adrenergic blocker.
See: Blocadren.
Betimol.
Istalol.
Timoptic.
Timoptic-XE.

timolol maleate. (TI-moe-lahl) (Falcon Ophthalmics) Timolol maleate 0.25%, 0.5%. Gel-forming Soln. Bot. 2.5 mL, 5 mL. *Rx.*
Use: Agent for glaucoma; beta-adrenergic blocker.

timolol maleate. (TI-moe-lahl) (Various Mfr.) Timolol maleate **Ophth. Soln.:** 0.25%, 0.5%. Bot. 2.5 mL, 5 mL, 10 mL, 15 mL. **Tab.:** 5 mg, 10 mg, 20 mg. Bot. 100s. *Rx.*
Use: Agent for glaucoma; antiadrenergic/sympatholytic; beta-adrenergic blocker.

timolol maleate and hydrochlorothiazide.
Use: Antihypertensive combination.
Tab.
See: Timolide.

timolol maleate ophthalmic. (Various Mfr.) Timolol maleate 3.4 mg/0.25 mL and 6.8 mg/0.5 mL. Soln. Bot. 2.5 mL, 5 mL, 10 mL, 15 mL. *Rx.*
Use: Antiglaucoma agent.

Timoptic. (Merck & Co.) Timolol maleate 0.25%, 0.5%. Ophth. Soln. *Ocumeter* 2.5 mL, 5 mL, 10 mL, 15 mL; *Ocudose* UD 60s. *Rx.*
Use: Antiglaucoma agent; beta-adrenergic blocker.

Timoptic-XE. (Merck & Co.) Timolol maleate 0.25%, 0.5%. Gel-forming Soln. *Ocumeter* 2.5 mL, 5 mL. *Rx.*
Use: Antiglaucoma agent; beta-adrenergic blocker.

•**tinabinol.** (tie-NAB-ih-NOLE) USAN.
Use: Antihypertensive.

Tinactin. (Schering-Plough) **Soln. 1%:** Tolnaftate (10 mg/mL) w/butylated hydroxytoluene, in nonaqueous homogeneous PEG 400. Plastic squeeze bot. 10 mL. **Cream 1%:** Tolnaftate (10 mg/g) in homogeneous, nonaqueous vehicle of PEG-400, propylene glycol, carboxypolymethylene, monoamylamine, titanium dioxide, butylated hydroxytoluene. Tube 15 g, 30 g, UD 0.7 g. **Pow. 1%:** Tolnaftate w/corn starch, talc. Plastic container 45 g, 90 g. **Aerosol Pow. 1%:** Tolnaftate w/butylated hydroxytoluene, talc, polyethylene-polypropylene glycol monobutyl ether, denatured alcohol and inert propellant of isobutane. Spray Can 100 g. **Aerosol Liq. 1%:** Tolnaftate w/butylated hydroxytoluene, polyethylene-polyproplyene glycol monobutyl ether, 36% alcohol, and inert propellant of isobutane. Spray Can 120 mL. *OTC.*
Use: Antifungal.

Tinastat. (Vita Elixir) Sodium hyposulfite, benzethonium Cl/2 oz. *OTC.*
Use: Keratolytic.

Tinaval. (Pal-Pak, Inc.) Tolnaftate 1%. Pow. Bot. 45 g. *OTC.*
Use: Antifungal for jock itch, athlete's foot.

Tindamax. (Presutti) Tinidazole 250 mg, 500 mg. Film-coated. Tab. 20s (500 mg only), 40s (250 mg only), 60s (500 mg only), 100s (250 mg only). *Rx.*
Use: Antiprotozoal.

tine test, old tuberculin. (Wyeth) Box of 25, 100, 250 test applicators.
See: Tuberculin Tine Test.

tine test, purified protein derivative. (Wyeth) Box of 25 or 100 test applicators.
See: Tuberculin Tine Test.

•**tin fluoride.** *USP 28.* Stannous Fluoride.

Ting. (Heritage) Miconazole nitrate 2%, SD alcohol 40 10%, aloe vera gel. Spray Pow. Bot. 85 g. *OTC.*
Use: Anti-infective, antifungal, topical.

•**tinidazole.** (tie-NIH-dah-zole) USAN.
Use: Antiprotozoal.
See: Tindamax.

Tinset. (Janssen) Oxatomide.
Use: Antiallergic; antiasthmatic.

Tinver. (PBH Wesley Jessen) Sodium thiosulfate 25%, salicylic acid 1%, isopropyl alcohol 10%, propylene glycol, menthol, disodium edetate, colloidal alumina. Lot. Bot. 4 oz., 6 oz. *Rx.*
Use: Dermatologic.

•**tinzaparin sodium.** (tin-ZAP-ah-rin) USAN.
Use: Anticoagulant; low molecular weight heparin.
See: Innohep.

•**tioconazole.** (TIE-oh-KOE-nah-zole) *USP 28.*
Use: Antifungal.
See: Monistat 1.
Vagistat-1.

•**tiodazosin.** (TIE-oh-DAY-zoe-sin) USAN.
Use: Antihypertensive.

•**tiodonium chloride.** (TIE-oh-doe-nee-uhm) USAN.
Use: Anti-infective.

•**tioperidone hydrochloride.** (tie-oh-PURR-ih-dohn) USAN.
Use: Antipsychotic.

•**tiopinac.** (tie-OH-pin-ACK) USAN.
Use: Anti-inflammatory; analgesic, antipyretic.

tiopronin.
Use: Homozygous cystinuria. [Orphan Drug]
See: Thiola.

•**tiospirone hydrochloride.** (tie-OH-spih-rone) USAN.
Use: Antipsychotic.

•**tiotidine.** (TIE-OH-tih-deen) USAN.
Use: Antiulcerative.

tiotropium bromide.
Use: Bronchodilator, anticholinergic.
See: Spiriva.

•**tioxidazole.** (tie-OX-ih-DAH-zole) USAN.
Use: Anthelmintic.

•**tipentosin hydrochloride.** (TIE-pin-toe-SIN) USAN.
Use: Antihypertensive.

•**tipifarnib.** (tip-ee-FAR-nib) USAN.
Use: Cancer.

Tipramine Tabs. (Major) Imipramine. Tab. **10 mg:** Bot. 250s. **25 mg, 50 mg:** Bot. 250s, 1000s. *Rx.*
Use: Antidepressant.

•**tipranavir disodium.** (tip-RA-na-veer) USAN.
Use: Antiretroviral treatment for HIV.
See: Aptivus.

•**tipredane.** (tie-PRED-ANE) USAN.
Use: Adrenocortical steroid, topical.

•**tiprenolol hydrochloride.** (tie-PREH-no-lole) USAN.
Use: Antiadrenergic (β-receptor).

•**tiprinast meglumine.** (TIE-prih-nast meh-GLUE-meen) USAN. Under study.
Use: Antiallergic.

•**tipropidil hydrochloride.** (TIE-PRO-pih-dill) USAN.
Use: Vasodilator.

•**tiqueside.** (TIE-kweh-side) USAN.
Use: Antihyperlipidemic.

•**tiquinamide hydrochloride.** (tie-KWIN-ah-mide) USAN.
Use: Anticholinergic (gastric).

•**tirapazamine.** (tie-rah-PAZZ-ah-meen) USAN.
Use: Antineoplastic.

tiratricol.
Use: Antineoplastic. [Orphan Drug]

•**tirilazad mesylate.** (tie-RIH-lah-zad MEH-sih-late) USAN.
Use: Antioxidant.
See: Freedox.

tirofiban.
Use: Antiplatelet.
See: Aggrastat.

•**tirofiban hydrochloride.** (tie-rah-FIE-ban) USAN.
Use: Antiplatelet, glycoprotein IIb/IIIa inhibitor.
See: Aggrastat.

TI-Screen. (Pedinol Pharmacal) **Gel:** SPF 20+, ethylhexyl p-methoxycinnamate 7.5%, oxybenzone 5%, 2-ethylhexyl salicylate 5%, SD alcohol 40 71%. 120 g. **Lip Balm:** SPF 8+, ethylhexyl p-methoxycinnamate 7.5%, oxybenzone 5%, petrolatum. 4.5 g. **Lot.: SPF 8:** Ethylhexyl p-methoxycinnamate 6%, oxybenzone 2%. Bot. 120 mL **SPF 15:** Ethylhexyl p-methoxycinnamate 7.5%, oxybenzone 5%. Bot. 120 mL. **SPF 30:** Octyl methoxycinnamate 7.5%, octyl salicylate 5%, oxybenzone 6%, octocrylene 7.5%. Bot. 120 mL. *OTC.*
Use: Sunscreen.

TI-Screen Natural. (Pedinol Pharmacal) Titanium dioxide 5%. Lot. Bot. 120 mL. *OTC.*
Use: Sunscreen.

TI-Screen Sunless. (Pedinol Pharmacal) Octyl methoxycinnamate 7.5%, benzophene-3 3%, mineral oil, alcohols, PEG-100, parabens. SPF 17 or 23. Cream. Tube 118 mL. *OTC.*
Use: Sunscreen.

•**tisilfocon a.** (tih-sill-FOE-kahn) USAN.
Use: Contact lens material (hydrophobic).

Tisit. (Pfeiffer) **Gel:** Pyrethrins 0.3%, piperonyl butoxide 3%. 30 mL. **Lot.:** Pyrethrins 0.3%, piperonyl butoxide 2% (petroleum distillate and piperonyl butoxide equiv. to 1.6% ether). 59 mL, 118 mL. **Shampoo:** Pyrethrins 0.33%, piperonyl butoxide 4%. Bot. 59 mL, 118 mL. With comb. *OTC.*
Use: Pediculicide.

TiSol. (Parnell) Benzyl alcohol 1%, menthol 0.04%, isotonic sodium chloride 0.9%, sorbitol, EDTA. Soln. Bot. 237 mL. *OTC.*
Use: Throat preparation.

tissue fixative and wash solution. (Wampole) A modified Michel's tissue fixative and buffered wash solution.
Use: Tissue specimen fixative.

tissue plasminogen activator.
See: Alteplase, Recombinant.
Reteplase, Recombinant.
Tenecteplase.

tissue respiratory factor (trf). (International Hormone) RSF, SRF, LYCD, PCO, Procytoxid marketed as 2000 units. Supplied as bulk liquid concentrate. *Rx.*
Use: Promotion of cellular oxidation.

Tis-U-Sol. (Baxter PPI) Pentalyte irrigation containing NaCl 800 mg, KCl 40 mg, magnesium sulfate 20 mg, sodium phosphate 8.75 mg, 6.25 mg monobasic potassium phosphate/ 100 mL. Bot. 250 mL, 1000 mL. *Rx.*
Use: Irrigant.

Titan. (PBH Wesley Jessen) EDTA 2%, nonionic cleaner buffers, potassium sorbate 0.13%. Soln. Bot. 30 mL. *OTC.*
Use: Contact lens care.

•**titanium dioxide.** (tie-TANE-ee-uhm die-OX-ide) *USP 28.*
Use: Solar ray protectant, topical.

Titralac. (3M) Calcium carbonate 420 mg, saccharin, Na 0.3 mg. Chew. Tab. Bot. 40s, 100s, 1000s. *OTC.*
Use: Antacid.

Titralac Extra Strength. (3M) Calcium carbonate 750 mg, saccharin, Na 0.6 mg. Chew. Tab. Bot. 100s. *OTC.*
Use: Antacid.

Titralac Plus. (3M) **Chew. Tab.:** Calcium carbonate 420 mg, simethicone 21 mg, saccharin, sodium 1.1 mg. Bot. 100s. **Liq.:** Calcium carbonate 500 mg, simethicone 20 mg, saccharin, sorbitol, sodium 0.15 mg. Bot. 360 mL. *OTC.*
Use: Antacid.

•**tixanox.** (TIX-ah-nox) *USAN.*
Use: Antiallergic.

•**tixocortol pivalate.** (tix-OH-kahr-tole PIH-vah-late) *USAN.*
Use: Anti-inflammatory, topical.

•**tizanidine hydrochloride.** (tie-ZAN-ih-deen) *USAN.*
Use: Antispasmodic. [Orphan Drug]

tizanidine hydrochloride. (Various Mfr.) Tizanidine hydrochloride (as base) 2 mg, 4 mg. Tab. 150s, 300s, 1000s (4 mg only). *Rx.*

Use: Antispasmodic.
tizanidine hydrochloride.
Use: Antispasmodic.
See: Zanaflex.

t-lymphotropic virus type III gp 160 antigens. *Rx.*
Use: Treatment for AIDS. [Orphan Drug]
See: Vaxsyn HIV-1.

TMP-SMZ. *Rx.*
Use: Anti-infective.
See: Proloprim.
Trimethoprim.
Trimpex.

TNKase. (Genentech) Tenecteplase 50 mg. L-arginine 0.55 g, phosphoric acid 0.17 g, polysorbate 20 4.3 mg. Pow. for Inj., lyophilized. Vial w/one 10-mL vial of Sterile Water for Injection and syringe. *Rx.*
Use: Thrombolytic agent; tissue plasminogen activator.

TOBI. (PathoGenesis) Tobramycin 300 mg, NaCl 11.25 g/5 mL. Soln for Inhalation. Single-use Amp. *Rx.*
Use: Cystic fibrosis.

•**toborinone.** (toe-BORE-ih-nohn) *USAN.*
Use: Cardiotonic.

Tobrades. (Alcon) Dexamethasone 0.1%, tobramycin 0.3%, thimerosal 0.001%, alcohol 0.5%, propylene glycol, polyoxyethylene, polyoxypropylene. Susp. 2.5 mL, 5 mL. *Rx.*
Use: Anti-infective; corticosteroid.

TobraDex. (Alcon) **Ophth. Oint.:** Dexamethasone 0.1%, tobramycin 0.3%, chlorobutanol 0.5%, mineral oil, white petrolatum. 3.5 g. **Ophth. Susp.:** Tobramycin 0.3%, dexamethasone 0.1%, benzalkonium chloride 0.01%, EDTA, hydroxyethyl cellulose, sodium chloride, sodium hydroxide tyloxapol. *Drŏp-Tainers* 2.5 mL, 5 mL, 10 mL. *Rx.*
Use: Anti-infective; corticosteroid; ophthalmic.

•**tobramycin.** (TOE-bruh-MY-sin) *USP 28.* An antibiotic obtained from cultures of *Streptomyces tenebrarius.*
Use: Anti-infective, ophthalmic. [Orphan Drug]
See: TOBI.
Tobrex.

tobramycin. (TOE-bruh-MY-sin) (Bausch & Lomb) Tobramycin 0.3%, benzalkonium Cl 0.01%, boric acid. Soln. 5 mL. *Rx.*
Use: Anti-infective, ophthalmic.

tobramycin and dexamethasone ophthalmic ointment.
Use: Anti-infective, ophthalmic.

• **tobramycin sulfate.** (TOE-bruh-MY-sin) *USP 28.*
Use: Anti-infective; aminoglycoside.

tobramycin sulfate. (American Pharmaceutical Partners) Tobramycin sulfate 1.2 g (40 mg/mL after reconstitution). Preservative free. Pow. for Inj. Pharmacy bulk package vial. 50 mL. *Rx.*
Use: Parenteral aminoglycoside.

tobramycin sulfate. (Various Mfr.) Tobramycin sulfate 40 mg/mL. Inj. Syringes: 1.5 mL, 2 mL. Vial 2 mL. Pediatric Inj. 10 mg/mL. Vial 2 mL. *Rx.*
Use: Aminoglycoside; anti-infective.

Tobrex. (Alcon) Tobramycin. **Ophth. Oint.:** 0.3% in sterile ointment base. Tube 3.5 g. **Ophth. Soln.:** 0.3%. Bot. 5 mL *Drop-Tainer. Rx.*
Use: Anti-infective, ophthalmia.

• **tocamphyl.** (toe-KAM-fill) USAN.
Use: Choleretic.

• **tocilizumab.** (toe-si-LIZ-oo-mab) USAN.
Use: Immune globulin.

• **tocladesine.** (toe-CLA-de-seen) USAN.
Use: Antineoplastic; immunomodulator.

• **tocopherols excipient.** (toe-KAHF-ehr-ols) *NF 23.*
Use: Pharmaceutic aid (antioxidant).

• **tocophersolan.** (toe-KAHF-ehr-SO-lan) USAN.
Use: Vitamin supplement.

dl-alpha tocopheryl. Vitamin E.
See: Aquasol E.
Denamone.
Ecofrol.
Epsilan M.
Myopone.

dl-alpha tocopheryl acetate. (toe-KAHF-ehr-ol) Vitamin E
See: Aquasol E.
Tocopher.
Vitamins E.

Tocosamine. (Trent) Sparteine sulfate 150 mg, sodium chloride 4.5 mg/mL. Amps. 1 mL. Box 12s, 100s. *Rx.*
Use: Oxytocic.

• **tofenacin hydrochloride.** (tah-FEN-ah-sin) USAN.
Use: Anticholinergic.

• **tofimilast.** (toe-FIM-i-last) USAN.
Use: Chronic obstructive disease; asthma.

tofranazine. (Novartis) Combination of imipramine and promazine. Pending release.

Tofranil. (Novartis) Imipramine hydrochloride 10 mg, 25 mg, 50 mg. Tab. Bot. 100s. *Rx.*
Use: Antidepressant; antienuretic.

Tofranil-PM. (Novartis) Imipramine pamoate 75 mg, 100 mg, 125 mg, 150 mg, parabens. Cap. Bot. 30s, 100s. *Rx.*
Use: Antidepressant.

Tolamide Tabs. (Major) Tolazamide. Tab. **100 mg:** Bot. 100s. **250 mg:** Bot. 200s, 500s. **500 mg:** Bot. 100s, 500s *Rx.*
Use: Antidiabetic.

• **tolamolol.** (tahl-AIM-oh-lahl) USAN.
Use: Beta-adrenergic receptor blocker; coronary vasodilator; cardiovascular agent (antiarrhythmic).

• **tolazamide.** (tole-AZE-uh-mid) *USP 28.*
Tall Man: TOLAZamide
Use: Hypoglycemic; antidiabetic.
See: Tolinase.

tolazamide. (Various Mfr.) Tolazamide. Tab. **100 mg:** Bot. 250s. **250 mg:** Bot. 100s, 200s, 500s. **500 mg:** Bot. 250s, 500s. *Rx.*
Use: Antidiabetic.

• **tolbutamide.** (tole-BYOO-tuh-mide) *USP 28.*
Tall Man: TOLBUTamide
Use: Hypoglycemic; antidiabetic.
See: Orinase.

tolbutamide. (Various Mfr.) Tolbutamide 500 mg. Tab. 100s, 500s. *Rx.*
Use: Antidiabetic.

• **tolbutamide sodium.** (tole-BYOO-tuh-mide) *USP 28.*
Tall Man: TOLBUTamide
Use: In vivo diagnostic aid (diabetes).
See: Orinase Diagnostic.

• **tolcapone.** (TOLE-kah-pone) USAN. Investigational.
Use: Antiparkinsonian.
See: Tasmar.

• **tolciclate.** (tole-SIGH-klate) USAN.
Use: Antifungal.

Tolectin 600. (McNeil) Tolmetin sodium 600 mg, sodium 54 mg. Tab. Bot. 100s, 500s. *Rx.*
Use: Analgesic, NSAID.

Tolectin 200. (McNeil) Tolmetin sodium 200 mg, sodium 18 mg. Tab. Bot. 100s. *Rx.*
Use: Analgesic, NSAID.

Tolerex. (Procter & Gamble) Protein 20.6 g, carbohydrate 226.3 g, fat 1.45 g, Na 468 mg, K 1172 mg, mOsm/Kg H_2O 550, cal/mL 1, vitamins A, B_1, B_2, B_3, B_5, B_6, B_{12}, C, D, E, K, folic acid, biotin, choline, Ca, P, I, Fe, Mg, Cu, Zn, Mn, Se, Mo, Cr. Assorted flavors Pow. Pkts. 80 g. *OTC.*
Use: Mineral, vitamin supplement.

• **tolevamer sodium.** (toe-LEV-a-mer) USAN.

Use: Antidiarrheal.

●**tolfamide.** (TAHL-fah-MIDE) USAN.
Use: Enzyme inhibitor (urease).

Tolfrinic. (B.F. Ascher) Ferrous fumarate 200 mg, vitamins B_{12} 25 mcg, C 100 mg. Tab. Bot. 100s. *OTC.*
Use: Mineral, vitamin supplement.

●**tolgabide.** (TOLE-gah-bide) USAN.
Use: Antiepileptic (control of abnormal movements).

●**tolimidone.** (TAHL-IH-mih-dohn) USAN.
Use: Antiulcerative.

Tolinase. (Pharmacia) Tolazamide 250 mg. Tab. Bot. 200s, 1,000s, UD 100s. *Rx.*
Use: Antidiabetic.

●**tolindate.** (TOLE-in-DATE) USAN.
Use: Antifungal.

●**tolmetin.** (TOLE-meh-tin) USAN.
Use: Anti-inflammatory.

●**tolmetin sodium.** (TOLE-meh-tin) *USP 28.*
Use: Anti-inflammatory.
See: Tolectin 600.
    Tolectin 200.

tolmetin sodium. (Various Mfr.) Tolmetin sodium. **Tab.:** 200 mg, 600 mg. Bot. 100s, 500s (600 mg only), UD 100s (600 mg only). **Cap.:** 400 mg. Bot. 100s, 500s, 1000s, UD 100s. *Rx.*
Use: Anti-inflammatory.

●**tolnaftate.** (tahl-NAFF-tate) *USP 28.*
Use: Antifungal.
See: Blis-To-Sol.
    Breezee Mist Antifungal.
    Dr. Scholl's.
    Tinactin.

●**tolofocon a.** (TOE-low-FOE-kahn A) USAN.
Use: Contact lens material (hydrophobic).

toloxychlorinal.
Use: Sedative.

●**tolpovidone I 131.** (tahl-POE-vih-dohnl 131) USAN.
Use: Diagnostic aid (hypoalbuminemia); radiopharmaceutical.

●**tolpyrramide.** (tahl-PIHR-ah-mid) USAN.
Use: Oral hypoglycemic; antidiabetic.

●**tolterodine.** (tole-TEH-roe-deen) USAN.
Use: Treatment of urinary incontinence.

tolterodine tartrate.
Use: Anticholinergic.
See: Detrol.
    Detrol LA.

●**tolu balsam.** (toe-LOO BALL-sam) *USP 28.*
Use: Pharmaceutic necessity for Compound Benzoin Tincture; expectorant.

See: Vicks Regular & Wild Cherry Medicated Cough Drops.

tolu balsam. (Eli Lilly) Syr. Bot. 16 fl. oz.
Use: Vehicle.

●**tolu balsam tincture.** *NF 23.*
Use: Flavor.

toluidine blue o chloride.
See: Blutene Chloride.

Tolu-Sed. (Scherer) Codeine phosphate 10 mg, guaifenesin 100 mg/5 mL w/alcohol 10%. Sugar free. Bot. 4 oz., pt. *c-v.*
Use: Antitussive; expectorant.

Tolu-Sed DM. (Scherer) Dextromethorphan HBr 10 mg, guaifenesin 100 mg/5 mL, alcohol 10%. Liq. Bot. 118 mL *OTC.*
Use: Upper respiratory combination, antitussive, expectorant.

●**tolvaptan.** (TOLE-vap-tan) USAN.
Use: Congestive heart failure; hyponatremia.

●**tomelukast.** (tah-MELL-you-KAST) USAN.
Use: Antiasthmatic (leukotriene antagonist).

Tomocat. (Mallinckrodt) Barium sulfate 5%, simethicone, sorbitol, strawberry flavor. Conc. Susp. Bot. 145 mL (480 mL for dilution), 225 mL (1000 mL for dilution); enema kit in 110 mL with 480 mL bot. for dilution with flexible tubing, clamp, and enema tip. *Rx.*
Use: Radiopaque agent, GI contrast agent.

Tomocat 1000. (Lafayette) Barium sulfate suspension concentrate 5% w/v. Bot. for dilution to 1.5% w/v at time of use. Bot. 225 mL w/1000 mL dilution Bot. Case 24 Bot. and 2 Dilution Bot.
Use: Radiopaque medium used to mark the GI tract during CT scans.

tomoxetine hydrochloride. (TOE-MOX-eh-teen)
See: Atomoxetine Hydrochloride.

Tom's of Maine Natural Cough & Cold Rub Cough Suppressant. (Tom's of Maine) Camphor 4.8%, menthol 2.6%. Rub. Tube 92.4 g. *OTC.*
Use: Upper respiratory combination, topical.

Tonavite-M. (Ivax) Elix. Bot. 12 oz, pt., gal.
Use: Dietary supplement.

●**tonazocine mesylate.** (tone-AZE-oh-SEEN) USAN.
Use: Analgesic.

Tono-B Pediatric. (Pal-Pak, Inc.) Fe 5 mg, thiamine hydrochloride 0.167 mg, riboflavin 0.133 mg. Tab. Bot. 1000s.

OTC.
Use: Mineral, vitamin supplement.
Tonopaque. (Mallinckrodt) Barium sulfate 95%, simethicone, sorbitol, cherry flavor. Pow. for Susp. UD 180 g. Bot. 1200 g. Cont. 25 lb. *Rx.*
Use: Radiopaque agent, GI contrast agent.
Toothache Gel. (Roberts) Benzocaine, oil of cloves, benzyl alcohol, propylene glycol. Tube 15 g. *OTC.*
Use: Anesthetic, local.
Toothache Relief-3 in 1. (C.S. Dent & Co.) Toothache gum, toothache drops, benzocaine. Lot. *OTC.*
Use: Analgesic, topical.
Topamax. (Ortho-McNeil) Topiramate **Tab.:** 25 mg, 50 mg, 100 mg, 200 mg, lactose. Dot 60s. **Sprinkle Cap.:** 15 mg, 25 mg, sucrose. Bot. 60s. *Rx.*
Use: Anticonvulsant.
Top Brass ZP-11. (Revlon) Zinc pyrithione 0.5% in cream base. *OTC.*
Use: Antidandruff.
Top Care LiquiCaps Nite Time Multi-Symptom Cold/Flu Relief. (Topco Assoc.) Dextromethorphan HBr 10 mg, doxylamine succinate 6.25 mg, pseudoephedrine hydrochloride 30 mg, acetaminophen 250 mg, sorbitol. Cap. Pkg. 20s. *OTC.*
Use: Upper respiratory combination, antitussive, antihistamine, decongestant, analgesic.
Top Care Maximum Strength Flu, Cold & Cough Medicine Night Time. (Topco Assoc.) Dextromethorphan HBr 30 mg, chlorpheniramine maleate 4 mg, pseudoephedrine hydrochloride 60 mg, acetaminophen 1000 mg, sucrose, lemon flavor. Pow. Pkt. 6s. *OTC.*
Use: Upper respiratory combination, antitussive, antihistamine, decongestant, analgesic.
Top Care Maximum Strength Soothing Cough & Head Congestion Relief D. (Topco Assoc.) Dextromethorphan HBr 10 mg, pseudoephedrine hydrochloride 20 mg/5 mL, alcohol 5%, corn syrup, saccharin, cherry flavor. Liq. Bot. 118 mL. *OTC.*
Use: Upper respiratory combination, antitussive, decongestant.
Top Care Multi-Symptom Pain Relief Cold. (Topco. Assoc.) Dextromethorphan HBr 15 mg, pseudoephedrine hydrochloride 30 mg, acetaminophen 325 mg. Tab. Pkg. 24s. *OTC.*
Use: Upper respiratory combination, antitussive, decongestant, analgesic.

Top Care Multi-Symptom Pain Relief Cold. (Topco Assoc.) Dextromethorphan HBr 15 mg, chlorpheniramine maleate 2 mg, pseudoephedrine hydrochloride 30 mg, acetaminophen 325 mg. Tab. Pkg. 24s. *OTC.*
Use: Upper respiratory combination, antitussive, antihistamine, decongestant, analgesic.
Top-Form. (Colgate Oral) Topical form-fitting gel applicators. Disposable trays for topical fluoride office treatments, plus permanent trays for topical fluoride home self-treatments. Box 100s. *Rx.*
Use: Topical fluoride applications in home or office.
Topic. (Roche) 5% benzyl alcohol in greaseless gel base containing camphor, menthol, w/30% Isopropyl alcohol. Tube 2 oz. *OTC.*
Use: Antipruritic.
topical anesthetics, miscellaneous.
See: Ethyl Chloride.
Fluro-Ethyl.
Topical Fluoride. (Pacemaker) Acidulated phosphate fluoride. Flavors: Orange, bubble gum, lime, raspberry, grape, cinnamon. Liq. Bot. 4 oz, pt. *Rx.*
Use: Corticosteroid, topical.
Topicort. (Taro) **Cream:** Desoximetasone 0.25% emollient cream consisting of isopropyl myristate, cetyl stearyl alcohol, white petrolatum, mineral oil, lanolin alcohol, purified water. Tube 15 g, 60 g, 120 g. **Gel:** Desoximetasone 0.05% in gel base. 20% alcohol. Tube 15 g, 60 g. **Oint.:** Desoximetasone 0.25% in ointment base. Tube 15 g, 60 g. *Rx.*
Use: Corticosteroid, topical.
Topicort LP. (Medicis Dermatologics) Desoximetasone 0.05%. Cream. Tube 15 g, 60 g. *Rx.*
Use: Corticosteroid, topical.
•**topiramate.** (toe-PIRE-ah-MATE) USAN.
Use: Anticonvulsant.
See: Topamax.
•**topixantrone.** (toe-PIX-an-trone) USAN.
Use: Antineoplastic.
Toposar. (Gensia Sicor) Etoposide 20 mg, benzyl alcohol 30 mg, alcohol 30.5%/mL. Inj. 5 mL, 10 mL, 25 mL. *Rx.*
Use: Antineoplastic.
•**topotecan hydrochloride.** (toe-poe-TEE-kan) USAN.
Use: Antineoplastic (DNA topoisomerase I inhibitor).
See: Hycamtin.
Toprol XL. (AstraZeneca) Metoprolol succinate 23.75 mg (equivalent to

metoprolol tartrate 25 mg), 47.5 mg (equivalent to metoprolol tartrate 50 mg), 95 mg (equivalent to metoprolol tartrate 100 mg), 190 mg (equivalent to metoprolol tartrate 200 mg). ER Tab. Bot. 100s. *Rx.*
Use: Antihypertensive; antiadrenergic/ sympatholytic, beta-adrenergic blocker.

•**topterone.** (TOP-ter-ohn) USAN.
Use: Antiandrogen.

•**toquizine.** (TOE-kwih-zeen) USAN.
Use: Anticholinergic.

Toradol. (Roche) Ketorolac tromethamine. **Tab.:** 10 mg, lactose. Bot. 100s. **Inj.:** 15 mg/mL (alcohol 10%, sodium chloride 6.68 mg in sterile water), 30 mg/mL. 15 mg/mL in 1 mL *Tubex* syringes, single-use Vial 1 mL; 30 mg/ mL in 1 mL (alcohol 10%, sodium chloride 4.35 mg in sterile water) and 2 mL (alcohol 10%, sodium chloride 8.7 mg in sterile water) *Tubex* syringes, single-use Vial 1 mL, 2 mL. *Rx.*
Use: Analgesic, NSAID.

•**toralizumab.** (toe-ra-LYE-zyoo-mab) USAN.
Use: Monoclonal antibody.

•**torapsel.** (tore-AP-sel) USAN.
Use: Hematologic agent.

•**torcetrapib.** (tore-SET-ra-pib) USAN.
Use: Cardiovascular agent.

•**torcitabine.** (tore-SITE-a-been) USAN.
Use: Polymerase inhibitor (hepatitis B).

Torecan. (Boehringer Ingelheim) Thiethylperazine. **Amp.:** 10 mg/2 mL (w/sod. metabisulfite 0.5 mg, ascorbic acid 2 mg, sorbitol 40 mg, q.s. carbon dioxide). *Rx.*
Use: Antiemetic; antinauseant.

toremifene.
Use: Antineoplastic. [Orphan Drug]
See: Estrinex.

•**toremifene citrate.** (TORE-EM-ih-feen SIH-trate) USAN.
Use: Antiestrogen; antineoplastic.
See: Fareston.

Tornalate. (Elan) **Aer.:** Bitolterol mesylate 0.8% (0.37 mg/actuation). Metered dose inhaler 15 mL (≥ 300 inhalations). **Soln. for Inh.:** Bitolterol mesylate 0.2%, alcohol 25%, propylene glycol. Bot. 10 mL, 30 mL, 60 mL w/dropper. *Rx.*
Use: Bronchodilator, sympathomimetic.

•**torsemide.** (TORE-suh-MIDE) *USP 28.*
Use: Diuretic.
See: Demadex.

torsemide. (Teva) Torsemide 5 mg, 10 mg, 20 mg, 100 mg, lactose. Tab.

100s. *Rx.*
Use: Diuretic.

torula yeast, dried. Obtained by growing *Candida (torulopsis) utilis* yeast on wood pulp wastes (Nutritional Labs) Conc. 100 lb drums.
Use: Natural source of protein and Vitamin B-complex vitamins.

•**tosagestin.** (TOE-sa-jes-tin) USAN.
Use: Hormone replacement therapy.

•**tosifen.** (TOE-sih-fen) USAN.
Use: Antianginal.

tositumomab and iodine ^{131}**I-tositumomab.**
Use: Antineoplastic.
See: Bexxar.

•**tosufloxacin.** (toe-SUE-FLOX-ah-sin) USAN.
Use: Anti-infective.

Totacillin. (GlaxoSmithKline) Ampicillin trihydrate equivalent to: **Cap.:** 250 mg, 500 mg. Bot. 500s. **Pow. for Oral Susp.:** 125 mg/5 mL, 250 mg/5 mL. Bot. 100 mL, 200 mL. *Rx.*
Use: Anti-infective, penicillin.

Total. (Allergan) Polyvinyl alcohol, edetate disodium, benzalkonium chloride in a sterile, buffered, isotonic solution. Soln. Bot. 60 mL, 120 mL. *OTC.*
Use: Contact lens care.

Total Eclipse Cooling Alcohol. (Novartis) Padimate O, oxybenzone, glyceryl PABA, alcohol 77%. SPF 15. Lot. Bot. 120 mL. *OTC.*
Use: Sunscreen.

Total Eclipse Moisturizing. (Novartis) Padimate O, oxybenzone, octyl salicylate. Moisturizing base. SPF 15. Lot. Bot. 120 mL. *OTC.*
Use: Sunscreen.

Total Eclipse Oil & Acne Prone Skin Sunscreen. (Novartis) Padimate O, oxybenzone, glyceryl PABA, alcohol 77%. SPF 15. Lot. Bot. 120 mL. *OTC.*
Use: Sunscreen.

Total Formula. (Vitaline) Fe 20 mg, vitamins A 10,000 units, D 400 units, E 30 units, B_1 15 mg, B_2 15 mg, B_3 25 mg, B_5 25 mg, B_6 25 mg, B_{12} 25 mcg, C 100 mg, folic acid 0.4 mg, Ca, Cr, Cu, I, K, Mg, Mn, Mo, P, Se, Si, V, vitamin K, biotin 300 mcg, Zn 30 mg, choline, bioflavonoids, hesperidin, inositol, PABA, rutin. Tab. Bot. 90s, 100s. *OTC.*
Use: Mineral, vitamin supplement.

Total Formula-2. (Vitaline) Fe 20 mg, vitamins A 10,000 units, D 400 units, E 30 units, B_1 15 mg, B_2 15 mg, B_3 25 mg, B_5 25 mg, B_6 25 mg, B_{12}

25 mcg, C 100 mg, folic acid 0.4 mg, Ca, Cr, Cu, I, K, Mg, Mn, Mo, P, Se, Si, V, vitamin K, biotin 300 mcg, Zn 30 mg, choline, bioflavonoids, hesperidin, inositol, PABA, rutin. Tab. with boron. Bot. 60s. *OTC.*
Use: Mineral, vitamin supplement.

Total Solution. (Allergan) Isotonic, buffered soln. of polyvinyl alcohol, benzalkonium chloride, EDTA. Soln. Bot. 60 mL, 120 mL. *OTC.*
Use: Ophthalmic.

totaquine. Alkaloids from *Cinchona* bark, 7% to 12% quinine anhydrous, 70% to 80% total alkaloids (cinchonidine, cinchonine, quinidine & quinine).

•**totomycin hydrochloride.** *USP 28.* Tetracycline.

Touro A & D. (Dartmouth) Chlorpheniramine maleate 4 mg, phenyltoloxamine citrate 50 mg, phenylephrine hydrochloride 20 mg. SR Cap. Bot. 100s. *Rx.*
Use: Antihistamine; decongestant.

Touro Allergy. (Dartmouth) Brompheniramine maleate 5.75 mg, psuedoephedrine hydrochloride 60 mg, sucrose. SR Cap. Bot. 100s. *Rx.*
Use: Upper respiratory combination, decongestant, antihistamine.

Touro CC. (Dartmouth) Guaifenesin 575 mg, pseudoephedrine hydrochloride 60 mg, dextromethorphan HBr 30 mg, dye free. SR Tab. Bot. 100s. *Rx.*
Use: Upper respiratory combination, decongestant, antitussive, expectorant.

Touro DM. (Dartmouth) Dextromethorphan HBr 30 mg, guaifenesin 575 mg. SR Tab. Bot. 100s. *Rx.*
Use: Upper respiratory combination, antitussive, expectorant.

Touro LA. (Dartmouth) Pseudoephedrine hydrochloride 120 mg, guaifenesin 525 mg. SR Tab. Bot. 100s. *Rx.*
Use: Upper respiratory combination, decongestant, expectorant.

Toxo. (Wampole) *Toxoplasma* antibody test system. Tests 120s.
Use: An IFA test system for the detection of antibodies to *Toxoplasma gondii.*

toxoid, diphtheria.
Use: Immunization.
See: Diphtheria and Tetanus Toxoids, Acellular Pertussis and Haemophilus Influenzae Type B Conjugate Vaccine.
Diphtheria and Tetanus Toxoids, Adult.
Diphtheria and Tetanus Toxoids, and Acellular Pertusis Adsorbed, Hepatitis B (Recombinant) and Inacti-

vated Poliovirus Vaccine Combined.
Diphtheria and Tetanus Toxoids, and Acellular Pertussis Vaccine Adsorbed.
Diphtheria and Tetanus Toxoids, Pediatric.
Tetanus and Diphtheria Toxoids (Adult Strength).

toxoid, tetanus. *Rx.*
Use: Immunization.
See: Diphtheria and Tetanus Toxoids, Acellular Pertussis and Haemophilus Influenzae Type B Conjugate Vaccine.
Diphtheria and Tetanus Toxoids, Adult.
Diphtheria and Tetanus Toxoids, and Acellular Pertusis Adsorbed, Hepatitis B (Recombinant) and Inactivated Poliovirus Vaccine Combined.
Diphtheria and Tetanus Toxoids and Acellular Pertussis Vaccine, Adsorbed.
Diphtheria and Tetanus Toxoids, Pediatric.
Diphtheria and Tetanus Toxoids Pertussis Vaccine Adsorbed.
Tetanus and Diphtheria Toxoids (Adult Strength).
Tetanus Toxoid.
Tetanus Toxoid, Adsorbed.
Tetanus Toxoid, Adsorbed, Purogenated.

toxoid, tetanus adsorbed.
Use: Immunization.

toxoplasmosis test.
Use: Diagnostic aid.
See: TPM Test.

t-PA.
Use: Tissue plasminogen activator.
See: Activase.

T-Phyl. (Purdue) Theophylline 200 mg. Tab. Bot. 100s. *Rx.*
Use: Bronchodilator.

TPM-Test. (Wampole) Indirect hemagglutination test for the qualitative and quantitative determination of antibodies to *Toxoplasma gondii* in serum. Kit 120s.
Use: Diagnostic aid, toxoplasmosis.

TPN Electrolytes. (Hospira) Na^+ 35 mEq, K^+ 20 mEq, Ca^{++} 4.5 mEq, Mg^{++} 5 mEq, Cl^- 35 mEq, acetate 29.5 mEq/20 mL, osmolarity 6220 mOsm/L. Soln. Pharmacy bulk packaging vial 100 mL. *Rx.*
Use: Intravenous nutritional therapy, intravenous replenishment solution.

TPN Electrolytes III. (Hospira) Na 25 Eq, K 40.6 mEq, Ca 5 mEq, Mg 8 mEq, Cl 33.5 mEq, acetate 40.6 mEq, gluconate 5 mEq/20 mL, osmolarity 7520 mOsm/L. Soln. Pharmacy bulk pkg. Vial

100 mL. *Rx.*
Use: Intravenous nutritional therapy, intravenous replenishment solution.

TPN Electrolytes II. (Hospira) Na 18 mEq, K 18 mEq, Ca 4.5 mEq, Mg 5 mEq, Cl 35 mEq, acetate 10.5 mEq/ 20 mL, osmolarity 4320 mOsm/L. Soln. Single-dose and additive syr. 20 mL *Rx.*
Use: Intravenous nutritional therapy, intravenous replenishment solution.

•**tracazolate.** (track-AZE-oh-late) USAN.
Use: Sedative; hypnotic.

•**trabectedin.** (tra-BEK-te-din) USAN.
Use: Antineoplastic.

Trace. (Young Dental) Erythrosine conc. soln. Squeeze Bot. 30 mL, 60 mL. Dispenser Packets 200s. *OTC.*
Use: Diagnostic aid, disclose dental plaque.

trace elements.
Use: Mineral supplement.
See: Carbonyl Iron.
    Complex Zinc Carbonates.
    Ferrous Fumarate.
    Ferrous Gluconate.
    Ferrous Sulfate.
    Ferrous Sulfate Exsiccated (Dried).
    Fluoride.
    Iron.
    Iron and Liver Combinations.
    Iron, Dextran.
    Iron Sucrose.
    Iron with Vitamin B_{12} and Intrinsic Factor.
    Iron with Vitamin C.
    Iron with Vitamins.
    Manganese.
    Polysaccharide-Iron Complex.
    Sodium Ferric Gluconate Complex.
    Zinc Acetate.
    Zinc Combinations.
    Zinc Gluconate.
    Zinc Sulfate.
    Zinc Supplements.

Traceplex. (Enzyme Process) Fe 30 mg, I 0.1 mg, Cu 0.5 mg, Mg 40 mg, Zn 10 mg, B_{12} 5 mcg/4 Tabs. Bot. 100s, 250s. *OTC.*
Use: Mineral supplement.

Tracer bG. (Boehringer Mannheim) Reagent strips. Kit. 25s, 50s.
Use: Diagnostic aid.

Trace 28. (Young Dental) **Liq.:** FD&C Red No. 28 in aqueous soln. Bot. 30 mL, 60 mL. **Tab.:** FD&C Red No. 28. Box 30s, 180s, 700s. *OTC.*
Use: Diagnostic aid, disclose dental plaque.

Tracleer. (Actelion Pharm) Bosentan 62.5 mg, 125 mg. Tab. Bot. 60s. *Rx.*

Use: Vasodilator, endothelin receptor antagonist.

Tracrium Injection. (GlaxoSmithKline) Atracurium besylate 10 mg/mL Amp. 5ml. Box 10s; 10 mL MDV. Box 10s. *Rx.*
Use: Muscle relaxant.

Trac Tabs 2X. (Hyrex) Atropine sulfate 0.06 mg, hyoscyamine sulfate 0.03 mg, methenamine 120 mg, methylene blue 6 mg, phenyl salicylate 30 mg, benzoic acid 7.5 mg. Tab. Bot. 100s, 1000s. *Rx.*
Use: Anti-infective, urinary.

•**trafermin.** (trah-FUR-min) USAN.
Use: Treatment of stroke and coronary artery disease.

•**tragacanth.** (TRAG-ah-kanth) *NF 23.*
Use: Pharmaceutic aid (suspending agent).

•**tralonide.** (TRAY-low-nide) USAN.
Use: Corticosteroid, topical.

tramadol. (Various Mfr.) Tramadol hydrochloride 50 mg. Tab. 100s, 500s, 1,000s. *Rx.*
Use: Opioid analgesic.

•**tramadol hydrochloride.** (TRAM-uh-dole) USAN.
Use: Opioid analgesic.
See: Ultram.
W/Acetaminophen.
See: Ultracet.

•**tramazoline hydrochloride.** (tram-AZE-oh-leen) USAN.
Use: Adrenergic.

Trandate. (Faro Pharmaceuticals) Labetalol hydrochloride. **Inj.:** 5 mg/mL, EDTA 0.1 mg, methylparaben 0.8 mg, propylparaben 0.1 mg. Multidose vial 20 mL, 40 mL. **Tab.:** 100 mg, 200 mg, 300 mg. Bot. 100s, 500s, UD 100s. *Rx.*
Use: Antiadrenergic/sympatholytic, alpha/beta-adrenergic blocker.

trandolapril.
Use: Antihypertensive.
See: Mavik.
W/Verapamil.
See: Tarka.

•**tranexamic acid.** (tran-ex-AM-ik) USAN.
Use: Hemostatic. [Orphan Drug]
See: Cyklokapron.

•**tranilast.** (TRAN-ill-ast) USAN.
Use: Antiasthmatic.

tranquilizers.
See: Atarax.
    Compazine.
    Equanil.
    Fenarol.
    Haldol.
    Librium.

Loxitane.
Mellaril.
Meprobamate.
Miltown.
Permitil.
Prolixin.
Stelazine.
Thorazine hydrochloride.
Trancopal.
Tranxene.
Trilafon.
Valium.
Vesprin.
Vistaril.

Tranquils. (Halsey Drug) **Cap.:** Pyrilamine maleate 25 mg. Bot. 30s. **Tab.:** Acetaminophen 300 mg, pyrilamine maleate 25 mg. Bot. 30s. *OTC.*
Use: Sleep aid.

•**transcainide.** (trans-CANE-ide) USAN.
Use: Antiarrhythmic, cardiovascular agent.

Transderm-Nitro. (Summit) Nitroglycerin 12.5 mg, 25 mg, 50 mg, 75 mg, 100 mg. Patch. Box 30s, UD 30s (except 75 mg), 100s (except 75 mg, 100 mg). *Rx.*
Use: Antianginal.

Transderm-Scop. (Baxter) Scopolamine 1.5 mg (delivers scopolamine ≈ 1 mg over 3 days). Transdermal Patch. 10s, 24s. *Rx.*
Use: Antiemetic/antivertigo agent.

transforming growth factor-beta 2. (Celtrix)
Use: Immunomodulator. [Orphan Drug]

Transthyretin EIA. (Abbott Diagnostics) Test kits 100s.
Use: Diagnostic aid.

Trans-Ver-Sal AdultPatch. (Doak Dermatologics) Salicylic acid 15%. Transdermal patch. 6 mm, 12 mm. 40s. Securing tape and cleaning file. *OTC.*
Use: Keratolytic.

Trans-Ver-Sal PediaPatch. (Doak Dermatologics) Salicylic acid 15%. Transdermal patch. 6 mm. 20s. Securing tape and cleaning file. *OTC.*
Use: Keratolytic.

Trans-Ver-Sal PlantarPatch. (Doak Dermatologics) Salicylic acid 15%. Transdermal patch. 20 mm patches, 25s. Securing tapes, cleaning file. *OTC.*
Use: Dermatologic, wart therapy.

Tranxene-SD. (Abbott) Clorazepate dipotassium 22.5 mg. Lactose. ER Tab. Bot. 100s. *c-iv.*
Use: Anxiolytic.

Tranxene-SD Half Strength. (Abbott) Clorazepate dipotassium 11.25 mg. Lactose. ER Tab. Bot. 100s. *c-iv.*

Use: Anxiolytic.

Tranxene T-tab. (Ovation) Clorazepate dipotassium 3.75 mg, 7.5 mg, 15 mg. Tab. 100s, 500s, UD 100s. *c-iv.*
Use: Anxiolytic.

tranylcypromine sulfate. (tran-ill-SIP-row-meen) *USP 28.*
Use: Antidepressant.
See: Parnate.

trastuzumab.
Use: Antineoplastic; monoclonal antibody.
See: Herceptin.

Trasylol. (Bayer Corp. (Consumer Div.)) Aprotinin 1.4 mg/mL. Inj. Vial 100 mL, 200 mL. *Rx.*
Use: Antihemophilic.

T-Rau. (Tennessee Pharmaceutic) Rauwolfia serpentina 50 mg or 100 mg. Tab. Bot. 100s, 1000s. *Rx.*
Use: Hypotensive.

TraumaCal. (Bristol-Myers Squibb) Nutritionally complete formula for traumatized patients. Can 8 oz. Vanilla flavor. *OTC.*
Use: Specific for nitrogen and energy needs in a limited volume for multiple trauma and major burns.

Travamulsion 10% Intravenous Fat Emulsion. 1.1 kcal/mL 270 mOsm/L. Bot. 500 mL. *Rx.*
Use: Nutritional supplement, parenteral.

Travamulsion 20% Intravenous Fat Emulsion. (Baxter PPI) 2 kcal/mL 300 mOsm/L. Bot. 500 mL. *Rx.*
Use: Nutritional supplement, parenteral.

Travasol. (Baxter PPI) Crystalline L-amino acids injection 5.5%, 8.5% (with or without electrolytes). IV Bot. 500 mL, 1000 mL, 2000 mL. *Rx.*
Use: Nutritional supplement, parenteral.

Travasol 10%. (Baxter PPI) Crystalline L-amino acids 10%. Inj. Bot. 200 mL, 500 mL, 1000 mL, 2000 mL. *Rx.*
Use: Nutritional supplement, parenteral.

Travasol 3.5% M Injection with Electrolyte #45. (Baxter PPI) Crystalline L-amino acids 3.5% Soln. Bot. IV 500 mL, 1000 mL. *Rx.*
Use: Nutritional supplement, parenteral.

Travasol 3.5% w/Electrolytes. (Clintec Nutrition) Amino acid concentration 3.5%, nitrogen 0.591 g/100 mL, 500 mL, 1000 mL. *Rx.*
Use: Nutritional supplement, parenteral.

Travasorb HN Peptide Diet. (Baxter PPI) High-nitrogen defined peptide 333 kcal. Pkt. 6 pkt. Carton. *OTC.*
Use: Nutritional supplement.

Travsorb MCT Liquid Diet. (Baxter PPI) Digestible protein medium-chain triglyc-

eride diet. 89 g packets. *OTC.*
Use: Nutritional supplement.
Travasorb MCT Powder Diet. (Baxter PPI) Digestible protein medium-chain triglyceride diet 400 kcal. Pkt. 6 pkt. Carton. *OTC.*
Use: Nutritional supplement.
Travasorb Renal Diet. (Baxter PPI) 467 kcal. Pkt. 6 pkt. Carton. 112 g packets. *OTC.*
Use: Nutritional supplement.
Travasorb Standard Diet. (Baxter PPI) Defined peptide diet, 333 kcal. pkt. 6 packets. Ctn. *OTC.*
Use: Nutritional supplement.
Travasorb STD. (Clintec Nutrition) Enzymatically hydrolyzed lactalbumin 10 g, glucose oligosaccharides 63.3 g, MCT (fractioned coconut oil) 4.5 g, sunflower oil 4.5 g, Na 307 mg, K 390 mg, mOsm/560 Kg, H_2O, cal 333.3/mL, vitamins A, B_1, B_2, B_3, B_5, B_6, B_{12}, C, D, E, K, Ca, Cl, Cu, Fe, I, Mg, Mn, P, Zn. Gluten free. Pow. Pkts. 83.3 g. *OTC.*
Use: Nutritional supplement.
Travasorb Whole Protein Liquid Diet. (Baxter PPI) Lactose free complete nutrition 250 kcal. Can. 8 oz. *OTC.*
Use: Nutritional supplement.
Travatan. (Alcon) Travoprost 0.004%, benzalkonium chloride 0.015%/mL, EDTA. Soln. *Drop-Tainer* 2.5 mL. *Rx.*
Use: Antiglaucoma; prostaglandin agonist.
Travel Aids. (Faraday) Dimenhydrinate 50 mg. Tab. Bot. 30s. *OTC.*
Use: Antiemetic; antivertigo.
Travel-Eze. (Health for Life Brands) Pyrilamine maleate 25 mg, hyoscine hydrobromide 0.325 mg. Tab. Pkg. 20s. *OTC.*
Use: Antiemetic; antivertigo.
Travel Sickness. (Walgreen) Dimenhydrinate 50 mg. Tab. Bot. 24s. *OTC.*
Use: Antiemetic; antivertigo.
Traveltabs. (Armenpharm Ltd.) Dimenhydrinate 50 mg. Tab. Bot. 100s. *OTC.*
Use: Antiemetic; antivertigo.
Travert. (Baxter PPI) Invert sugar injection 10% in water or saline. Plastic Bot. 500 mL, 1000 mL, electrolyte No. 2 Bot. 500 mL, 1000 mL, electrolyte No. 4 Bot. 250 mL, 500 mL Soln. (10%). *Rx.*
Use: Fluid, electrolyte replacement.
5% Travert and Electrolyte No. 2. (Baxter PPI) Invert sugar 50 g/L, calories 196 Cal/L, Na 56 mEq/L, K 25 mEq/L, Mg 6 mEq/L, Cl 56 mEq/L, phosphate 12.5 mEq/L, lactate 25 mEq/L, osmolarity 449 mOsm/L. 1000 mL. *Rx.*
Use: Nutritional supplement, parenteral.

10% Travert and Electrolyte No. 2. (Baxter PPI) Invert sugar 100 g/L, calories 384 Cal/L, Na 56 mEq/L, K 25 mEq/L, Mg 6 mEq/L, Cl 56 mEq/L, phosphate 12.5 mEq/L, lactate 25 mEq/L, osmolarity 726 mOsm/L. 1000 mL. *Rx.*
Use: Nutritional supplement, parenteral.
travoprost.
Use: Antiglaucoma; prostaglandin agonist.
See: Travatan.
●**trazodone hydrochloride.** (TRAY-zoe-dohn) *USP 28.*
Use: Antidepressant.
See: Desyrel.
　Desyrel Dividose.
trazodone hydrochloride. (Barr) Trazodone hydrochloride 300 mg. Tab. Bot. 100s. *Rx.*
Use: Antidepressant.
trazodone hydrochloride. (Various Mfr.). Trazodone hydrochloride. Tab. **50 mg:** Bot. 50s, 500s, 1000s, UD 100s, *Robot Ready* 25s. **100 mg:** Bot. 50s, 500s, 1000s, UD 100s, *Robot Ready* 25s. **150 mg:** Bot. 100s, 250s, unit-of-use 30s. *Rx.*
Use: Antidepressant.
●**trebenzomine hydrochloride.** (TRAY-BEN-zoe-meen) USAN.
Use: Antidepressant.
Trecator S.C. (Wyeth) Ethionamide 250 mg. Tab. Bot. 100s. *Rx.*
Use: Antituberculosal.
●**trecovirsen sodium.** (treh-koe-VEER-sin) USAN.
Use: Antiviral.
●**trefentanil hydrochloride.** (treh-FEN-tah-nill) USAN.
Use: Analgesic.
●**treloxinate.** (trell-OX-ih-nate) USAN.
Use: Antihyperlipoproteinemic.
Trelstar Depot. (Pharmacia) Triptorelin pamoate equivalent to 3.75 mg triptorelin peptide base, mannitol. Microgranules for Inj., lyophilized. Single-dose vial. *Rx.*
Use: Hormone; gonadotropin-releasing hormone analog.
Trelstar LA. (Pharmacia) Triptorelin pamoate equivalent to 11.25 mg triptorelin peptide base, mannitol. Microgranules for Inj., lyophilized. Single-dose vial. *Rx.*
Use: Hormone; gonadotropin-releasing hormone analog.
Trental. (Hoechst) Pentoxifylline 400 mg. CR Tab. Bot. 100s. UD 100s. *Rx.*
Use: Hemorrheologic.

Treo. (Biopharmaceutics) **SPF 8:** Octocrylene, octyl methoxycinnamate, benzophenone-3, octyl salicylate, isostearyl alcohol, diazolidinyl urea, propylparabens, citronella oil 0.05% (as insect repellant). Lot. Bot. 118 mL. **SPF 15:** Octocrylene, octyl methoxycinnamate, benzophenone-3, octyl salicylate, isostearyl alcohol, diazolidinyl urea, propylparaben, citronella oil 0.05% (as insect repellant). Lot. Bot. 118 mL. **SPF 30:** Octocrylene, octyl methoxycinnamate, benzophenone-3, octyl salicylate, isostearyl alcohol, diazolidinyl urea, propylparaben, citronella oil 0.05% (as insect repellant). Lot. Bot. 118 mL. *OTC.*
Use: Sunscreen.

Iruusulfan.
Use: Antineoplastic. [Orphan Drug]
See: Ovastat.

•**trepipam maleate.** (TREH-pih-pam MAL-ee-ate) USAN. *Formerly Trimopam Maleate.*
Use: Sedative; hypnotic.

•**treprostinil sodium.** (treh-PRAHST-in-ill SO-dee-uhm) USAN.
Use: Antiplatelet agent.
See: Remodulin.

•**trestolone acetate.** (TRESS-toe-lone) USAN.
Use: Antineoplastic; androgen.

trethocanoic acid.
Use: Anticholesteremic.

•**tretinoin.** (TREH-tih-NO-in) *USP 28.*
Use: Retinoid.
See: Avita.
   Retin-A.
   Renova.
   Vesanoid.
W/Combinations.
See: Tri-Luma.

tretinoin. (Alpharma, Spear Dermatology) Tretinoin 0.025%, may contain stearyl alcohol. Cream. Tube. 20 g, 45 g. *Rx.*
Use: Retinoid.

tretinoin. (Spear Dermatology.) Tretinoin. **Cream:** 0.05%, 0.1%, stearyl alcohol. Tube. 20 g, 45 g. **Gel:** 0.01%, 0.025%, alcohol. Tube. 15 g, 45 g. *Rx.*
Use: Retinoid.

tretinoin lf, iv. (Argus)
Use: Antineoplastic. [Orphan Drug]

Trexall. (Barr) Methotrexate 5 mg, 7.5 mg, 10 mg, 15 mg, lactose. Film coated. Tab. Bot. 30s, 60s, 100s. *Rx.*
Use: Antipsoriatic; antirheumatic; antimetabolite.

Trexan. (DuPont) Naltrexone hydrochloride 50 mg. Tab. Bot. 50s. *Rx.*
Use: Opioid antagonist.

Triac. (Eon Labs) Triprolidine hydrochloride 2.5 mg, pseudoephedrine hydrochloride 60 mg. Tab. Bot. 100s, 1000s. *Rx.*
Use: Antihistamine; decongestant.

Triacet. (Teva) Triamcinolone acetonide 0.1%. Cream. Tube 15 g, 80 g. *Rx.*
Use: Corticosteroid, topical.

•**triacetin.** (try-ah-SEE-tin) *USP 28. Formerly glyceryl triacetate.*
Use: Antifungal, topical.
See: Fungacetin.

Triacin-C Cough. (Alpharma) Pseudoephedrine hydrochloride 30 mg, triprolidine hydrochloride 1.25 mg, codeine phosphate 10 mg/5 mL, alcohol 4.3%, methylparaben, caramel flavor. Syr. Bot. 118 mL, 473 mL. *Rx.*
Use: Upper respiratory combination, antihistamine, antitussive, decongestant.

Triact. (Sanofi-Synthelabo) Aluminum, magnesium hydroxide, simethicone. Liq., Tab. *OTC.*
Use: Antacid; antiflatulent.

Triacting. (Various Mfr.) Pseudoephedrine hydrochloride 15 mg, guaifenesin 50 mg/5 mL, may contain EDTA, sorbitol, sucrose. Liq. Bot. 118 mL. *OTC.*
Use: Upper respiratory combination, decongestant, expectorant.

Triacting Cold & Allergy. (Amerisource-Bergen) Pseudoephedrine hydrochloride 15 mg, chlorpheniramine maleate 1 mg/5 mL, sorbitol, sucrose, orange flavor, alcohol free. Liq. Bot. 118 mL. *OTC.*
Use: Upper respiratory combination, decongestant, antihistamine.

Tri-Acting Cold & Allergy. (Topco) Pseudoephedrine hydrochloride 15 mg, chlorpheniramine maleate 1 mg/5 mL, sorbitol, sucrose, orange flavor, alcohol free. Syr. Bot. 118 mL. *OTC.*
Use: Upper respiratory combination, decongestant, antihistamine.

Tri-Acting Cold & Cough. (Topco) Pseudoephedrine hydrochloride 15 mg, chlorpheniramine maleate 1 mg, dextromethorphan HBr 5 mg/5 mL, sorbitol, sucrose, cherry flavor, alcohol free. Syr. Bot. 118 mL. *OTC.*
Use: Upper respiratory combination, decongestant, antihistamine, antitussive.

Triad. (Forest) Butalbital 50 mg, acetaminophen 325 mg, caffeine 40 mg. Cap. Bot. 100s. *Rx.*
Use: Analgesic; hypnotic; sedative.

•**triafungin.** (TRY-ah-FUN-jin) USAN.
Use: Antifungal.
Trial AG. (Zee Medical) Aluminum hydroxide 200 mg, magnesium hydroxide 200 mg, simethicone 25 mg. Sucrose, mannitol. Lemon flavor. Tab. 20s. *OTC.*
Use: Antacid.
Trial Antacid. (Zee Medical) Calcium carbonate 420 mg. Sorbitol. Spearmint flavor. Tab. 24s. *OTC.*
Use: Antacid.
Triam-A. (Hyrex) Triamcinolone acetonide 40 mg/mL. Inj. Vial 5 mL. *Rx.*
Use: Corticosteroid.
•**triamcinolone.** (TRY-am-SIN-oh-lone) *USP 28.*
Use: Corticosteroid, topical.
See: Aristocort.
Aristospan.
•**triamcinolone acetonide.** (TRY-am-SIN-oh-lone ah-SEE-toe-nide) *USP 28.*
Use: Corticosteroid, topical; anti-inflammatory, topical; respiratory inhalant, corticosteroid.
See: Aristocort.
Aristogel.
Azmacort.
Delta-Tritex.
Flutex.
Kenalog.
Kenonel.
Nasacort AQ.
Triacet.
Triderm.
Tri-Kort.
Tri-Nasal.
W/Neomycin, gramicidin, Nystatin.
See: Mycolog.
triamcinolone acetonide. (Various Mfr.) Triamcinolone acetonide. **Cream: 0.025%, 0.1%:** Tube 15 g, 80 g, 454 g. **0.5%:** 15 g. **Lot.:** 0.025%, 0.1%. Bot. 60 mL. **Oint.: 0.025%, 0.1%:** Tube 15 g, 80 g, 454 g. **0.5%:** Tube 15 g. **Paste:** 0.1%.
Use: Corticosteroid, topical; anti-inflammatory, topical.
•**triamcinolone acetonide sodium phosphate.** (TRY-am-SIN-oh-lone ah-SEE-toe-nide) USAN.
Use: Costicosteroid, topical.
•**triamcinolone diacetate.** (try-am-SIN-oh-lone try-ASS-ah-tate) *USP 28.*
Use: Corticosteroid, topical.
See: Amcort.
Aristocort Diacetate Forte.
Aristocort Diacetate Intralesional.
Triam Forte.

•**triamcinolone hexacetonide.** (TRY-am-SIN-ole-ohn HEX-ah-SEE-tone-ide) *USP 28.*
Use: Costiscosteroid, topical.
See: Aristospan.
triamcinolone-16,17-acetonide.
See: Triamcinolone acetonide.
Triam Forte. (Hyrex) Triamcinolone diacetate 40 mg/mL. Vial 5 mL. *Rx.*
Use: Corticosteroid.
Triaminic Allerchews. (Novartis) Loratadine 10 mg. Mannitol. Orally Disintegrating Tab. 8s. *OTC.*
Use: Antihistamine.
Triaminic Allergy Congestion. (Novartis) Pseudoephedrine hydrochloride. **Chew. Tab.:** 15 mg, orange flavor. Pkg. 18s. **Liq.:** 15 mg/5 mL, EDTA, sucrose, sorbitol. Bot. 118 mL. *OTC.*
Use: Nasal decongestant, arylalkylamine.
Triaminic AM Cough and Decongestant Formula. (Novartis) Pseudoephedrine hydrochloride 15 mg, dextromethorphan HBr 7.5 mg/5 mL, sorbitol, sucrose, orange flavor. Alcohol and dye free. Liq. Bot. 118 mL, 237 mL. *OTC.*
Use: Antitussive; decongestant.
Triaminic AM Decongestant Formula. (Novartis) Pseudoephedrine hydrochloride 15 mg/5 mL, sorbitol, sucrose, orange flavor, alcohol and dye free. Syr. Bot. 118 mL, 237 mL. *OTC.*
Use: Decongestant.
Triaminic AM Non-Drowsy Cough & Decongestant. (Novartis) Pseudoephedrine hydrochloride 15 mg, dextromethorphan HBr 7.5 mg/5 mL, EDTA, sorbitol, sucrose, orange/strawberry flavor. Liq. Bot. 118 mL. *OTC.*
Use: Upper respiratory combination, decongestant, antitussive.
Triaminic Chest & Nasal Congestion Liquid. (Novartis) Pseudoephedrine hydrochloride 15 mg, guaifenesin 50 mg/mL, EDTA, sorbitol, sucrose, citrus flavor. Liq. Bot. 118 mL. *OTC.*
Use: Upper respiratory combination, decongestant, expectorant.
Triaminic Cold, Allergy, Sinus Medicine. (Novartis) Pseudoephedrine hydrochloride 60 mg, chlorpheniramine maleate 4 mg, acetaminophen 650 mg, lactose, methylparaben. Tab. Pkg. 24s. *OTC.*
Use: Upper respiratory combination, decongestant, antihistamine, analgesic.
Triaminic Cold & Allergy. (Novartis) Pseudoephedrine hydrochloride 15 mg, chlorpheniramine maleate 1 mg/5 mL, sorbitol, sucrose, orange flavor, alcohol

free. Liq. Bot. 118 mL, 147 mL. *OTC.*
Use: Upper respiratory combination, decongestant, antihistamine.
Triaminic Cold & Cough. (Novartis)
Pseudoephedrine hydrochloride 15 mg, chlorpheniramine maleate 1 mg, dextromethorphan HBr 5 mg/5 mL, sorbitol, sucrose, cherry flavor, alcohol free. Liq. Bot. 118 mL. *OTC.*
Use: Upper respiratory combination, decongestant, antihistamine, antitussive.
Triaminic Cold & Cough Softchews.
(Novartis) Pseudoephedrine hydrochloride 15 mg, chlorpheniramine maleate 1 mg, dextromethorphan HBr 5 mg, aspartame, mannitol, phenylalanine 17.7 mg, sucrose, cherry flavor. Chew Tab. Pkg. 18s. *OTC.*
Use: Upper respiratory combination, decongestant, antihistamine, antitussive.
Triaminic Cough. (Novartis) Liq.:
Pseudoephedrine hydrochloride 15 mg, dextromethorphan hydrobromide 7.5 mg/5 mL. Sorbitol, sucrose. Cherry flavor. 118 mL. **Softchew Tab.:**
Pseudoephedrine hydrochloride 15 mg, chlorpheniramine maleate 1 mg, dextromethorphan HBr 5 mg, aspartame, sucrose, phenylalanine 22.5 mg, mannitol, strawberry flavor. Pkg. 18s. *OTC.*
Use: Upper respiratory combination, decongestant, antihistamine, antitussive.
Triaminic Cough & Sore Throat. (Novartis) Pseudoephedrine hydrochloride 15 mg, dextromethorphan HBr 7.5 mg, acetaminophen 160 mg/5 mL, EDTA, sucrose, grape flavor, alcohol free. Liq. Bot. 118 mL, 237 mL. *OTC.*
Use: Upper respiratory combination, decongestant, antitussive, analgesic.
Triaminic Flu, Cough & Fever. (Novartis) Pseudoephedrine hydrochloride 15 mg, chlorpheniramine maleate 1 mg, dextromethorphan HBr 7.5 mg, acetaminophen 160 mg/5 mL, acesulfame K, EDTA, sucrose, bubble gum flavor. Liq. Bot. 118 mL. *OTC.*
Use: Upper respiratory combination, decongestant, antihistamine, antitussive, analgesic.
Triaminic Infant Oral Decongestant Drops. (Novartis) Pseudoephedrine hydrochloride 7.5 mg/0.8 mL, sorbitol, sucrose, EDTA, alcohol free, grape flavor. Liq. Dropper Bot. 15 mL. *OTC.*
Use: Decongestant.
Triaminic Night Time Cough & Cold.
(Novartis) Pseudoephedrine hydro-

chloride 15 mg, chlorpheniramine maleate 1 mg, dextromethorphan HBr 7.5 mg/5 mL, sorbitol, sucrose, grape flavor, alcohol free. Liq. Bot. 118 mL. *OTC.*
Use: Upper respiratory combination, decongestant, antihistamine.
Triaminic Nite Light Liquid. (Novartis) Pseudoephedrine 15 mg, chlorpheniramine maleate 1 mg, dextromethorphan HBr 7.5 mg/5 mL. Bot. 120 and 240 mL. *OTC.*
Use: Antihistamine; antitussive; decongestant.
Triaminic Softchews. (Novartis) Pseudoephedrine hydrochloride 15 mg, chlorpheniramine maleate 1 mg, phenylalanine 17.5 mg, aspartame, mannitol, sucrose, orange flavor. Tab. Pkg. 18s. *OTC.*
Use: Upper respiratory combination, decongestant, antihistamine.
Triaminic Softchews Allergy Sinus & Headache. (Novartis) Pseudoephedrine hydrochloride 15 mg, acetaminophen 160 mg, phenylalanine 11.2 mg, aspartame, mannitol, sorbitol, sucrose, fruit-punch flavor. Tab. Pkg. 18s. *OTC.*
Use: Upper respiratory combination, decongestant, analgesic.
Triaminic Softchews Cold & Sore Throat. (Novartis) Pseudoephedrine hydrochloride 15 mg, dextromethorphan hydrobromide 5 mg, acetaminophen 160 mg. Aspartame, phenylalanine 28.1 mg, mannitol, sucrose, sorbitol. Grape flavor. Chew. Tab. 18s. *OTC.*
Use: Pediatric antitussive.
Triaminic Sore Throat Formula. (Novartis) Pseudoephedrine hydrochloride 15 mg, dextromethorphan HBr 7.5 mg, acetaminophen 160 mg/5 mL, EDTA, sucrose, alcohol free. Liq. Bot. 240 mL. *OTC.*
Use: Antitussive; analgesic; decongestant.
Triaminic Sore Throat Spray. (Novartis Consumer Health) Phenol 0.5%. Alcohol free, sugar free. Saccharin, sorbitol. Grape flavor. Throat Spray. 118 mL. *OTC.*
Use: Mouth and throat product.
Triaminic Thin Strips Cough & Runny Nose. (Novartis) Diphenhydramine hydrochloride 12.5 mg. Alcohol (less than 5%), sorbitol, sucralose. Grape flavor. Orally Disintegrating Strips. 16s. *OTC.*
Use: Nonnarcotic antitussive.
Triaminic Thin Strips Long Acting Cough. (Novartis) Dextromethorphan hydrobromide 7.5 mg. Alcohol (less

than 5%), sorbitol, sucralose. Cherry flavor. Orally Disintegrating Strips. 16. *OTC.*
Use: Nonnarcotic antitussive.

Triaminic Throat Pain & Cough Softchews. (Novartis) Acetaminophen 160 mg, pseudoephedrine hydrochloride 15 mg, dextromethorphan HBr 5 mg, aspartame, mannitol, phenylalanine 28.1 mg, grape flavor. Chew. Tab. Box. 18s. *OTC.*
Use: Upper respiratory combination, analgesic, decongestant, antitussive.

Triaminic Vapor Patch for Cough. (Novartis) Camphor 4.7%, menthol 2.6%, glycerin, cherry and menthol scents. Patch. Box. 6s *OTC.*
Use: Upper respiratory combination, topical.

Triamolone 40. (Forest) Triamcinolone diacetate 40 mg/mL. Vial 5 mL. *Rx.*
Use: Corticosteroid.

Triamonide 40. (Forest) Triamcinolone acetonide 40 mg/mL. Vial 5 mL. *Rx.*
Use: Corticosteroid.

• **triampyzine sulfate.** (TRY-AM-pih-zeen SULL-fate) USAN.
Use: Anticholinergic.

• **triamterene.** (try-AM-tur-een) *USP 28.*
Use: Diuretic.
See: Dyrenium.

triamterene and hydrochlorothiazide.
Use: Diuretic. Cap.
See: Dyazide.

triamterene/hydrochlorothiazide. (Various Mfr.) **Cap.:** Triamterene 37.5 mg, 50 mg, hydrochlorothiazide 25 mg, may contain lactose. Bot. 100s, 1000s. **Tab.:** Triamterene 37.5 mg, hydrochlorothiazide 25 mg. Bot. 100s, 500s, 1000s; triamterene 75 mg, hydrochlorothiazide 50 mg. Bot. 100s, 250s, 500s, 1000s. *Rx.*
Use: Diuretic combination.

Trianide. (Seatrace) Triamcinolone acetonide 40 mg/mL. Vial 5 mL. *Rx.*
Use: Corticosteroid.

Tri-A-Vite F. (Major) F_1 0.5 mg, vitamins A 1500 units, D 400 units, C 35 mg/mL Drops. Bot. 50 mL. *Rx.*
Use: Vitamin supplement.

Triaz. (Medicis) Benzoyl peroxide. **Gel:** 3%, 6%, 9%. Glycerin (except 9%), zinc lactase, EDTA, cetyl stearyl alcohol (except 3%), glycolic acid (9% only). Tube 42.5 g. **Lot.:** 3%, 6%, 10%. Glycerin, glycolic acid, petrolatum, menthol, zinc lactate. 85.1 g (10% only), 170.3 g, 340.2 g (except 10%). *Rx.*
Use: Antiacne.

triazenes.
Use: Alkylating agents.
See: Dacarbazine.

• **triazolam.** (try-AZE-oh-lam) *USP 28.*
Use: Sedative/hypnotic, nonbarbiturate.
See: Halcion.

triazolam. (Various Mfr.) Triazolam 0.125 mg, 0.25 mg. Tab. Bot. 10s, 100s, 500s, UD 100s. *c-IV.*
Use: Sedative/hypnotic, nonbarbiturate.

triazole antifungals.
Use: Antifungal agents.
See: Fluconazole.
Itraconazole.
Voriconazole.

Triban. (Great Southern) Trimethobenzamide hydrochloride 200 mg, benzocaine 2%. Adult Supp. Pkg. 10s, 50s. *Rx.*
Use: Antiemetic/antivertigo agent.

• **tribenoside.** (try-BEN-oh-SIDE) USAN. Not available in US.
Use: Sclerosing agent.

Tri-Biozene. (Reese) Polymyxin B sulfate 10,000 units, neomycin 3.5 mg, bacitracin zinc 500 units, pramoxine hydrochloride 10 mg/g, white petrolatum. Oint. Tube 15 g. *OTC.*
Use: Anti-infective, antibiotic, topical.

tribromoethanol.
Use: Anesthetic (inhalation).

tribromomethane. Bromoform.

• **tribromsalan.** (try-BROME-sah-lan) USAN.
Use: Disinfectant.

tricalcium phosphate.
Use: Electrolytes, mineral supplement.
See: Posture.

• **tricetamide.** (TRY-see-tam-id) USAN.
Use: Hypnotic; sedative.

Tri-Chlor. (Gordon Laboratories) Trichloroacetic acid 80%. Bot. 15 mL. *Rx.*
Use: Cauterizing agent.

trichlorfon.
See: Metrifonate.

• **trichlormethiazide.** (try-klor-meth-EYE-ah-zide) *USP 28.*
Use: Antihypertensive; diuretic.
See: Metahydrin.
Naqua.

trichloroacetic acid. Acetic acid, trichloro.
Use: Topical, as a caustic.

trichlorobutyl alcohol.
See: Chlorobutanol.

• **trichloromonofluoromethane.** (try-klor-oh-mahn-oh-flure-oh-METH-ane) *NF 23.*
Use: Pharmaceutic aid (aerosol propellant).

tricholine citrate.
See: Choline citrate.

trichomonas test.
See: Isocult for *Trichomonas vaginalis*.

Trichotine. (Schwarz Pharma) **Pow.**: Sodium lauryl sulf., sod. perborate, monohydrate silica. Pkg. 150 g, 360 g. **Liq.**: Sodium lauryl sulfate, sodium borate, SD alcohol 40 8%, SD alcohol 23-A, EDTA. Bot. 120 mL, 240 mL. *OTC.*
Use: Feminine hygiene.

●**triciribine phosphate.** (TRY-SIH-bean FOSS-fate) USAN. *Formerly Phosphate Salt of Tricyclic Nucleoside.*
Use: Antineoplastic.

●**tricitrates oral solution.** (TRY-SIH-trates) *USP 28.*
Use: Alkalizer (systemic, urinary); antiurolithic (cystine calculi, uric acid calculi), buffer (neutralizing).

triclobisonium. (Roche) Triburon, Oint.

triclobisonium chloride.
Use: Anti-infective, topical.

●**triclocarban.** (TRY-kloe-CAR-ban) USAN.
Use: Disinfectant.
W/Clofulcarban.
See: Artra Beauty Ban.

●**triclofenol piperazine.** (TRY-kloe-FEE-nole pih-PURR-ah-zeen) USAN.
Use: Anthelmintic.

●**triclofos sodium.** (TRY-kloe-foss) USAN.
Use: Hypnotic; sedative.

●**triclonide.** (TRY-kloe-nide) USAN.
Use: Anti-inflammatory.

●**triclosan.** (TRY-kloe-san) *USP 28.*
Use: Anti-infective; disinfectant.
See: Ambi 10.
ASC Lotionized.
Clearasil Daily Face Wash.
Clearasil Soap.
Oxy ResiDon't.
Stridex Face Wash.

Tricodene Cough and Cold. (Pfeiffer) Pyrilamine maleate 12.5 mg, codeine phosphate 8.2 mg/5 mL. Liq. Bot. 120 mL. *c-v.*
Use: Upper respiratory combination, antihistamine, antitussive.

Tricodene Liquid. (Pfeiffer) Chlorpheniramine maleate 0.5 mg, dextromethorphan HBr 10 mg, ammonium Cl 90 mg, sodium citrate, sorbitol, mannitol/5 mL. Liq. Bot. 120 mL. *OTC.*
Use: Antihistamine; antitussive; expectorant.

Tricodene Sugar Free. (Pfeiffer) Chlorpheniramine maleate 2 mg, dextromethorphan HBr 10 mg/5 mL, menthol,

saccharin, sorbitol, mannitol, alcohol free. Liq. Bot. 120 mL. *OTC.*
Use: Upper respiratory combination, antihistamine, antitussive.

Tricodene Syrup. (Pfeiffer) Pyrilamine maleate 4.17 mg, codeine phosphate 8.1 mg, terpin hydrate, menthol/5 mL. Syr. Bot. 120 mL. *c-v.*
Use: Antihistamine; antitussive.

Tricor. (Abbott) Fenofibrate 48 mg, 145 mg, lactose, sucrose. Tab. Bot. 90s. *Rx.*
Use: Antihyperlipidemic; fibric acid derivatives.

Tricosal. (Invamed) Choline magnesium trisalicylate 500 mg, 750 mg, 1000 mg. Tab. Bot. 100s, 500s. *Rx.*
Use: Salicylate.

tricyclic compounds.
Use: Antidepressant.
See: Amitriptyline Hydrochloride.
Amoxapine.
Clomipramine Hydrochloride.
Desipramine Hydrochloride.
Doxepin Hydrochloride.
Imipramine Hydrochloride.
Imipramine Pamoate.
Nortriptyline Hydrochloride.
Protriptyline Hydrochloride.
Trimipramine Maleate.

Triderm. (Del-Ray) Triamcinolone acetonide 0.1%. Cream. Tube 30 g, 90 g. *Rx.*
Use: Corticosteroid.

Tridesilon. (Bayer) Desonide 0.05% in vehicle buffered to the pH range of normal skin w/glycerin, methylparaben, sodium lauryl sulfate, aluminum sulfate, calcium acetate, cetyl stearyl alcohol, synthetic bees wax, white petrolatum, mineral oil. Cream. Tube 15 g, 60 g. *Rx.*
Use: Corticosteroid.

Tridesilon Otic. (Bayer Corp. (Consumer Div.)) Desonide 0.05%, acetic acid 2% in vehicle. Bot. 10 mL. *Rx.*
Use: Otic.

Tridrate Bowel Cleansing System. (Lafayette) Magnesium citrate 19 g. Bisacodyl tablets 5 mg each (3s). Bisacodyl suppository 10 mg (1s). Kit. *OTC.*
Use: Laxative.

●**trientine hydrochloride.** (TRY-en-TEEN) *USP 28.*
Use: Chelating agent; Wilson disease therapy adjunct.
See: Cuprid.
Syprine.

triethanolamine.
See: Trolamine.

triethanolamine polypeptide oleate condensate.
See: Cerumenex.

triethanolamine salicylate.
See: Aspercreme.
Myoflex.
triethanolamine trinitrate biphosphate.
Trolnitrate Phosphate.
●**triethyl citrate.** *NF 23.*
Use: Pharmaceutic aid (plasticizer).
triethylenemelamine. Tretamine TEM.
Use: Antineoplastic.
triethylenethiophosphoramide.
See: Thiotepa.
Trifed-C. (Geneva) Pseudoephedrine hydrochloride 30 mg, triprolidine hydrochloride 1.25 mg, codeine phosphate 10 mg/5 mL, alcohol 4.3%. Syr. Bot. Pt., gal. *c-v.*
Use: Antihistamine; antitussive; decongestant.
●**trifenagrel.** (try-FEN-ah-GRELL) USAN.
Use: Antithrombotic.
●**triflocin.** (try-FLOW-sin) USAN.
Use: Diuretic.
Tri-Flor-Vite with Fluoride. (Everett) Fluoride 0.25 mg, vitamins A 1500 units, D 400 units, C 35 mg/mL. Drops. 50 mL. *Rx.*
Use: Fluoride, vitamin supplement.
●**triflubazam.** (try-FLEW-bah-zam) USAN.
Use: Anxiolytic.
●**triflumidate.** (try-FLEW-mih-DATE) USAN.
Use: Anti-inflammatory.
●**trifluoperazine hydrochloride.** (try-flew-oh-PURR-uh-zeen) *USP 28.*
Use: Antipsychotic; anxiolytic; hypnotic; sedative.
trifluoperazine hydrochloride. (Various Mfr.) Trifluoperazine hydrochloride 1 mg, 2 mg, 5 mg, 10 mg. Tab. Bot. 100s, 500s, 1000s, UD 100s. *Rx.*
Use: Antipsychotic.
n-trifluoroacetyladriamycin-14-valerate. (Anthra)
Use: Antineoplastic. [Orphan Drug]
trifluorothymidine. *Rx.*
Use: Ophthalmic.
See: Viroptic.
●**trifluperidol.** (TRY-flew-PURR-ih-dahl) USAN.
Use: Antipsychotic.
●**trifluridine.** (try-FLEW-RIH-deen) *USP 28.*
Use: Antiviral used to treat herpes simplex eye infections.
See: Viroptic Ophth.
trifluridine. (Falcon Ophthalmics) Trifluridine 1%, in aqueous solution with NaCl, thimerosal 0.001%. Ophth. Soln. Bot. 7.5 mL. *Rx.*
Use: Antiviral.

Triglide. (First Horizon) Fenofibrate 50 mg, 160 mg. Lactose. Tab. 90s. *Rx.*
Use: Antihyperlipidemic agent.
triglyceride reagent strip. (Bayer Corp. (Consumer Div.)) Seralyzer reagent strip. Bot. 25s.
Use: Diagnostic aid, triglycerides.
triglycerides, medium chain.
Use: Nutritional supplement.
See: MCT.
Trihexane. (Rugby) Trihexyphenidyl 2 mg. Tab. Bot. 100s, 1000s. *Rx.*
Use: Anticholinergic; antiparkinsonian.
Trihexidyl. (Schein) Trihexyphenidyl 2 mg. Tab. Bot. 100s, 1000s. *Rx.*
Use: Anticholinergic; antiparkinsonian.
Trihexy-5. (Geneva) Trihexyphenidyl 5 mg. Tab. Bot. 100s, 1000s. *Rx.*
Use: Anticholinergic; antiparkinsonian.
●**trihexyphenidyl hydrochloride.** (try-hex-ee-FEN-in-dill) *USP 28.*
Use: Anticholinergic; antiparkinsonian.
trihexyphenidyl hydrochloride. (VersaPharm) Trihexyphenidyl hydrochloride 2 mg per 5 mL. Alcohol 5%, parabens, sorbitol. Lime-peppermint flavor. Elix. 473 mL. *Rx.*
Use: Antiparkinson agent.
Trihexy-2. (Geneva) Trihexyphenidyl 2 mg. Tab. Bot. 100s, 1000s. *Rx.*
Use: Anticholinergic; antiparkinsonian.
TriHIBit. (Aventis Pasteur) *Haemophilus influenzae* type b purified capsular polysaccharide 10 mcg conjugated to inactivated tetanus toxoid 24 mcg, diphtheria toxoid 6.7 Lf, tetanus toxoid 5 Lf, pertussis antigens 46.8 mcg/0.5 mL, sucrose, thimerosal. Inj. Supplied as *ActHIB* with *Tripedia*. *ActHIB* single-dose vials of dry lyophilized powder for reconstitution with 0.6 mL single-use vials of *Tripedia*). *Rx.*
Use: Immunization.
Tri-Histin. (Recsei) **Cap.:** Bot. 100s, 500s, 1000s. **Liq.:** Pyrilamine maleate 5 mg, chlorpheniramine maleate 0.5 mg/5 mL. Bot. Pt., gal. **SA Cap.: 100 mg:** Pyrilamine maleate 40 mg, pheniramine maleate 25 mg. **Tab.: 25 mg :** Pyrilamine maleate 10 mg, chlorpheniramine maleate 1 mg. Bot. 100s, 500s, 1000s. **50 mg:** Pyrilamine maleate 20 mg, methapyrilene hydrochloride 15 mg, chlorpheniramine maleate 2 mg. Bot. 1000s. *Rx-OTC.*
Use: Antihistamine combination.
W/Benzyl alcohol, chlorobutanol and isopropyl alcohol.
See: Derma-Pax.
W/Ephedrine hydrochloride, aminophylline, mephobarbital.

See: Asmasan.
Tri-Hydroserpine. (Rugby) Hydrochloro-
thiazide 15 mg, reserpine 0.1 mg, hy-
dralazine hydrochloride 25 mg. Tab.
Bot. 100s, 1000s. *Rx.*
Use: Antihypertensive combination.
Trihydroxyestrine. Trihydroxyestrin.
Trihydroxyethylamine. Triethanolamine.
•**l-triiodothyronine sodium.**
Use: Hormone, thyroid.
See: Cytomel.
Liothyronine sodium.
Tri-K. (Century) Potassium acetate 0.5 g,
potassium bicarbonate 0.5 g, potas-
sium citrate 0.5 g/fl. oz. Saccharin. Bot.
Pt., gal. *Rx.*
Use: Electrolyte supplement.
•**trikates oral solution.** (TRY-kates)
USP 28.
Use: Replenisher (electrolyte).
Tri-Kort. (Keene Pharmaceuticals) Tri-
amcinolone acetonide suspension
40 mg/mL. Vial 5 mL. *Rx.*
Use: Corticosteroid, topical.
Trilafon. (Schering) Perphenazine.
Conc.: 16 mg/5 mL. Alcohol, sorbitol.
118 mL w/dropper. **Tab.:** 2 mg, 4 mg,
8 mg, 16 mg. Bot. 100s, 500s. **Inj.:**
5 mg/mL, sodium bisulfite. Amp. 1 mL.
Rx.
Use: Antiemetic/antivertigo agent.
Trileptal. (Novartis) Oxcarbazepine.
Tab.: 150 mg, 300 mg, 600 mg. Bot.
100s, 1000s, UD 100s. **Susp.:** 300 mg/
5 mL, saccharin, sorbitol, ethanol. Bot.
250 mL with dosing syr. and adapter.
Rx.
Use: Anticonvulsant.
Tri-Levlen. (Berlex) **Phase 1:** Levonorgestrel 0.05 mg, ethinyl estradiol
30 mcg (6 brown tablets). **Phase 2:**
Levonorgestrel 0.075 mg, ethinyl estra-
diol 40 mcg (5 white tablets). **Phase
3:** Levonorgestrel 0.125 mg, ethinyl
estradiol 30 mcg (10 light yellow tablets). Lactose. Slidecase Dispenser 28s.
Rx.
Use: Sex hormone, contraceptive
hormone.
Trilog. (Roberts) Triamcinolone aceto-
nide 40 mg/mL. Vial 5 mL. *Rx.*
Use: Corticosteroid.
Trilone. (Century) Triamcinolone diacetate. Susp. Amp. 10 mL. *Rx.*
Use: Corticosteroid.
Trilone. (Roberts) Triamcinolone diace-
tate 40 mg/mL. Vial 5 mL. *Rx.*
Use: Corticosteroid.
•**trilostane.** (TRY-low-stane) USAN.
Use: Adrenocortical suppressant.

Tri-Luma. (Galderma) Fluocinolone ace-
tonide 0.01%, hydroquinone 4%, tretin-
oin 0.05%, cetyl alcohol, glycerin, para-
bens, sodium metabisulfite, stearyl al-
cohol. Cream. Tube 30 g. *Rx.*
Use: Treatment of melasma.
Trimahist. (Tennessee Pharmaceutic)
Phenylephrine hydrochloride 5 mg, pro-
phenpyridamine maleate 12.5 mg, l-
menthol 1 mg, alcohol 5%/5 mL. Elix.
Bot. Pt., gal. *Rx.*
Use: Antihistamine; decongestant.
Trimax. (Sanofi-Synthelabo) Aluminum,
magnesium hydroxide, simethicone.
Gel. Tab. *OTC.*
Use: Antacid; antiflatulent.
Trimazide. (Major) Trimethobenzamide
hydrochloride. **Adult Supp.:** 200 mg.
Box. 10s. **Pediatric Supp.:** 100 mg.
10s. Rx.
Use: Antiemetic/antivertigo agent.
trimazinol.
Use: Anti-inflammatory.
•**trimazosin hydrochloride.** (try-MAY-
zoe-sin) USAN.
Use: Antihypertensive.
•**trimegestone.** (try-meh-JESS-tone)
USAN.
Use: Hormone, progestin.
•**trimeprazine tartrate.** (trye-MEP-ra-
zeen) USAN.
Use: Antipruritic.
trimetamide. Trimethamide.
trimethamide.
Use: Antihypertensive.
trimethobenzamide. (Various Mfr.) Trimethobenzamide hydrochloride. **Cap.:**
300 mg. Bot. 100s, 250s, 500s,
1,000s, UD 30s, UD 60s. **Supp., Adult:**
200 mg. Box 10s, 50s. **Supp., Pediatric:** 100 mg. Box 10s. *Rx.*
Use: Antiemetic/antivertigo agent.
•**trimethobenzamide hydrochloride.** (try-
meth-oh-BEN-zuh-mide) *USP 28.*
Use: Antiemetic.
See: Pediatric Triban.
Tebamide.
T-Gen.
Tigan.
Triban.
Trimazide.
trimethobenzamide hydrochloride.
(Various Mfr.) Trimethobenzamide hydrochloride 100 mg/mL. Amp. 2 mL. Vials. 20 mL. *Rx.*
Use: Antiemetic/antivertigo agent.
**trimethobenzamide hydrochloride and
benzocaine suppositories.**
Use: Antiemetic.
See: Pediatric Triban.

Triban.

•**trimethoprim.** (try-METH-oh-prim) *USP 28.*
Use: Anti-infective.
See: Proloprim.
Trimpex.
W/Polymyxin B Sulfate.
See: Polytrim Ophth.
W/Sulfamethoxazole.
See: Bactrim.
Septra.
Septra DS.

trimethoprim and sulfamethoxazole. (Various Mfr.) **Tab.:** Trimethoprim 80 mg, sulfamethoxazole 400 mg. Bot. 100s, 500s. **Susp.:** Trimethoprim 40 mg, sulfamethoxazole 200 mg/5 mL. Bot. 150 mL, 200 mL, 480 mL. **Inj.:** Sulfamethoxazole 80 mg/mL, trimethoprim 16 mg/mL. 5 mL. *Rx.*
Use: Anti-infective combination.

trimethoprim and sulfamethoxazole DS. (Various Mfr.) Trimethoprim 160 mg, sulfamethoxazole 800 mg. Tab. Bot. 100s, 500s. *Rx.*
Use: Anti-infective combination.

trimethoprim hydrochloride.
Use: Anti-infective.
See: Primsol.

•**trimethoprim sulfate.** (try-METH-oh-prim SULL-fate) USAN.
Use: Anti-infective.

trimethoprim sulfate and polymyxin b sulfate ophthalmic. (Various Mfr.) Trimethoprim 1 mg, polymyxin B sulfate 10,000 units/mL. Soln. Bot. 10 mL. *Rx.*
Use: Anti-infective, ophthalmic.

trimethylene. Cyclopropane.

•**trimetozine.** (try-MET-oh-zeen) USAN.
Use: Hypnotic; sedative.

•**trimetrexate.** (TRY-meh-TREK-sate) USAN.
Use: Antineoplastic.
See: Neutrexin.

•**trimetrexate glucuronate.** (TRY-meh-TREK-sate glue-CURE-uh-nate) USAN.
Use: Antineoplastic. [Orphan Drug]

•**trimipramine.** (TRY-MIH-prah-meen) USAN.
Use: Antidepressant.

•**trimipramine maleate.** (TRY-MIH-prah-meen) USAN.
Use: Antidepressant.
See: Surmontil.

Trimixin. (Hance) Bacitracin 200 units, polymyxin B sulfate 4000 units, neomycin sulfate 3 mg/g Oint. Tube 0.5 oz. *OTC.*
Use: Anti-infective, topical.

•**trimoprostil.** (TRY-moe-PRAHS-till) USAN.
Use: Gastric antisecretory.

Trimo-San. (Milex) Oxyquinoline sulfate 0.025%, boric acid 1%, sodium borate 0.7%, sodium lauryl sulfate 0.1%, glycerin, methylparaben. Jelly. 120 g w/applicator, 120 g refill. *OTC.*
Use: Vaginal agent.

Trimox. (Apothecon) Amoxicillin trihydrate. **Cap.:** 250 mg, 500 mg. Bot. 30s, 100s, 500s, UD 100s. **Chew. Tab.:** 125 mg, 250 mg, mannitol, sucrose. Bot. 60s (125 mg only), 100s (250 mg only), 500s (250 mg only). **Oral Susp.:** 125 mg/5 mL, 250 mg/5 mL, sucrose. Bot. 80 mL, 100 mL, 150 mL. *Rx.*
Use: Anti-infective, penicillin.

•**trimoxamine hydrochloride.** (TRY-MOX-am-een) USAN.
Use: Antihypertensive.

Trimox Pediatric Drops. (Apothecon) Amoxicillin trihydrate 50 mg/mL when reconstituted, sucrose. Pow. for Oral Susp. Bot. 15 mL. *Rx.*
Use: Anti-infective, penicillin.

Trimpex. (Roche) *Tel-E-Dose* 100s. *Rx.*
Use: Anti-infective, urinary.

Trim-Qwik. (Columbia) Powder-based meal food supplement. Can 10 oz. *OTC.*
Use: Nutritional supplement.

Trimstat. (Laser) Phendimetrazine tartrate 35 mg. Tab. Bot. 100s, 1000s. *c-III.*
Use: Anorexiant.

Trim-Sulfa. *Rx.*
Use: Anti-infective.
See: Proloprim.
Trimethoprim.
Trimpex.

Trim Sulf D/S. (Lexis Laboratories) Sulfamethoxazole 800 mg, trimethoprim 160 mg. Tab. Bot. 100s, 500s. *Rx.*
Use: Anti-infective.

Trim Sulf S/S. (Lexis Laboratories) Sulfamethoxazole 400 mg, trimethoprim 80 mg. Tab. Bot. 100s, 500s. *Rx.*
Use: Anti-infective.

Tri-Nasal. (Muro) Triamcinolone acetonide 50 mcg/spray, EDTA, benzalkonium chloride 0.01%. Spray. Bot. 15 mL with triamcinolone acetonide 7.5 mg/bot. (120 metered sprays) with nasal applicator. *Rx.*
Use: Respiratory inhalant, intranasal steroid.

Trinate. (Cypress) Ca 200 mg, Fe 28 mg, vitamin A 3000 units, D 400 units, E (dl-alpha tocopheryl acetate) 22 mg, B_1 1.8 mg, B_2 4 mg, B_3 20 mg, B_6 25 mg,

B_{12} 12 mcg, C 120 mg, folic acid 1 mg, Zn 25 mg, Cu, Mg. Tab. Bot. 100s. *Rx*.
Use: Mineral, vitamin, supplement.

•**trinecol.** (TRI-ne-kol) USAN. (Pullus)
Use: Oral tolerance therapy.

TriNessa. (Watson) **Phase 1:** Norgestimate 0.18 mg, ethinyl estradiol 35 mcg. **Phase 2:** Norgestimate 0.215 mg, ethinyl estradiol 35 mcg. **Phase 3:** Norgestimate 0.25 mg, ethinyl estradiol 35 mcg.Tab. 28s. 7 inert tablets. *Rx*.
Use: Oral contraceptive.

trinitrin tablets.
See: Nitroglycerin tablets.

trinitrophenol.
See: Picric Acid.

Tri-Norinyl. (Watson) **Phase 1:** Norethindrone 0.5 mg, ethinyl estradiol 35 mcg (7 blue tablets) **Phase 2:** Norethindrone 1 mg, ethinyl estradiol 35 mcg (9 yellow-green tablets). **Phase 3:** Norethindrone 0.5 mg, ethinyl estradiol 35 mcg (5 blue tablets). Lactose. *Wallette* 28s. *Rx*.
Use: Sex hormone, contraceptive hormone.

Trinotic. (Forest) Secobarbital 65 mg, amobarbital 40 mg, phenobarbital 25 mg. Tab. Bot. 1000s. *c-II*.
Use: Hypnotic.

Trinsicon. (UCB) Liver-stomach concentrate 240 mg, Fe 110 mg, vitamin C 75 mg, folic acid 0.5 mg, B_{12} 15 mcg. Cap. Bot. 60s, 500s, UD 100s. *Rx*.
Use: Nutritional supplement.

Triofed. (Alra) Pseudoephedrine hydrochloride 30 mg, triprolidine hydrochloride 1.25 mg/5 mL. Syr. Bot. 118 mL, 473 mL. *OTC*.
Use: Antihistamine, decongestant.

•**triolein I 131.** (TRY-oh-leen) USAN.
Use: Radiopharmaceutical.

•**triolein I 125.** (TRY-oh-leen) USAN.
Use: Radiopharmaceutical.

Trionate. (Breckenridge Pharm) Carbetapentane tannate 60 mg, chlorpheniramine tannate 5 mg. Tab. Bot. 100s. *Rx*.
Use: Upper respiratory combination, antitussive, antihistamine.

Triostat. (Monarch) Liothyronine sodium 10 mcg/mL, w/ammonia 2.19 mg/mL, alcohol 6.8%. Inj. Vial 1 mL. *Rx*.
Use: Hormone, thyroid.

Triotann. (Various Mfr.) Phenylephrine tannate 25 mg, chlorpheniramine tannate 8 mg, pyrilamine tannate 25 mg. Tab. Bot. 100s, 500s. *Rx*.
Use: Antihistamine; decongestant.

Triotann Pediatric. (Prasco Laboratories) Phenylephrine tannate 5 mg, chlorpheniramine tannate 2 mg, pyrilamine tannate 12.5 mg/5 mL, saccharin, sucrose, methylparaben, strawberry-blackberry-currant flavor. Susp. Bot. 473 mL. *Rx*.
Use: Upper respiratory combination, antihistamine, decongestant.

Triotann-S Pediatric. (Duramed) Phenylephrine tannate 5 mg, chlorpheniramine tannate 2 mg, pyrilamine tannate 12.5 mg/5 mL, methylparaben, saccharin, sucrose, strawberry-blackberry-currant flavor. Susp. Unit of use 118 mL. *Rx*.
Use: Upper respiratory combination, decongestant, antihistamine.

Tri-Otic. (Pharmics) Chloroxylenol 1 mg, pramoxine hydrochloride 10 mg, hydrocortisone 10 mg/mL. Drops. Vial 10 mL. *Rx*.
Use: Otic.

trioxane.
See: Trioxymethylene.

•**trioxifene mesylate.** (TRY-OX-ih-feen) USAN.
Use: Antiestrogen.

trioxymethylene. Name is incorrectly used to denote paraformaldehyde in some pharmaceuticals.
See: Paraformaldehyde.
W/Sodium oleate, triethanolamine, docusate sodium, stearic acid, and aluminum silicate.
See: Ooopor Crome.

Tri-Pain. (Ferndale) Acetaminophen 162 mg, aspirin 162 mg, salicylamide 162 mg, caffeine 16.2 mg. Tab. Bot. 100s. *OTC*.
Use: Analgesic combination.

•**tripamide.** (TRIP-ah-mide) USAN.
Use: Antihypertensive; diuretic.

Tripedia. (Aventis Pasteur) Diphtheria 6.7 Lf units, tetanus 5 Lf units and acellular pertussis antigens 46.8 mcg/ 0.5 mL (pertussis toxin and hemagglutinin ≈ 23.4 mcg each), gelatin, thimerosal. Inj. Preservative-free single-dose vial, multidose vial 7.5 mL (also contains polysorbate 80). *Rx*.
Use: Immunization.

•**tripelennamine citrate.** (trih-pell-EN-au-meen SIH-trate) *USP 28*.
Use: Antihistamine.

•**tripelennamine hydrochloride.** (trih-pell-EN-au-meen) *USP 28*.
Use: Antihistamine.
See: PBZ.
Pyribenzamine Hydrochloride.

triphasic oral contraceptives.
See: Estrostep Fe.

Estrostep 21.
Ortho-Novum 7/7/7.
Ortho Tri-Cyclen.
Tri-Levlen.
TriNessa.
Tri-Norinyl.
Triphasil.
Tri-Sprintec.
Trivora-28.

Triphasil. (Wyeth Labs) **Phase 1:** Levonorgestrel 0.05 mg, ethinyl estradiol 30 mcg (6 brown tablets). **Phase 2:** Levonorgestrel 0.075 mg, ethinyl estradiol 40 mcg (5 white tablets). **Phase 3:** Levonorgestrel 0.125 mg, ethinyl estradiol 30 mcg (10 light yellow tablets). Lactose. Dispenser 21s, 28s. *Rx.*
Use: Sex hormone, contraceptive hormone.

triphenylmethane dyes.
See: Fuchsin.
   Methylrosaniline Chloride.

triphenyltetrazolium chloride. TTC.

tripiperazine dicitrate, hydrous.
See: Piperazine Citrate.

triple antibiotic. Various Mfr. Polymyxin B sulfate 5000 units, neomycin 3.5 mg, bacitracin zinc 400 units/g. Oint. Tube 15 g, 30 g, 454 g. *OTC.*
Use: Anti-infective, antibiotic, topical.

triple antibiotic ophthalmics. (Various Mfr.) Polymyxin B sulfate 10,000 units/g, neomycin sulfate 3.5 mg/g, bacitracin 400 units. Oint. 3.5 g. *Rx.*
Use: Anti-infective; ophthalmic.

triple barbiturate elixir. (CMC) Phenobarbital 0.25 g, butabarbital 0.125 g, pentobarbital g/5 mL. Bot. Pt., gal. *c-II.*
Use: Sedative.

Triple Dye. (Kerr Drug) Gentian violet, proflavine, hemisulfate, brilliant green in water. Dispensing Bot. 15 mL. Single-Use *Dispos-A-Swab* 0.65 mL. Box 10s. Case 10 × 50 Box.
Use: Antiseptic.

Triple Dye. (Xttrium) Brilliant green 2.29 mg, proflavine hemisulfate 1.14 mg, gentian violet 2.29 mg/mL. Bot. 30 mL.
Use: Disinfectant.

Triple-Gen. (Ivax) Hydrocortisone 1%, neomycin sulfate 0.35%, polymyxin B sulfate 10,000 units/mL, benzalkonium chloride, cetyl alcohol, glyceryl monostearate, polyoxyl 40 stearate, propylene glycol, mineral oil. Susp. Bot. 7.5 mL. *Rx.*
Use: Anti-infective; corticosteroid; ophthalmic.

Triplen. (Henry Schein) Tripelennamine hydrochloride 50 mg. Tab. Bot. 100s,

1000s. *Rx.*
Use: Antihistamine.

•**triple sulfa.** *USP 28.* Sulfathiazole, sulfacetamide, and sulfabenzamide.
Use: Anti-infective.

Triple Sulfoid. (Pal-Pak, Inc.) Sulfadiazine 167 mg, sulfamerazine 167 mg, sulfamethazine 167 mg/5 mL. **Liq.:** Bot. Pt., 2 oz. 12s. **Tab.:** Bot. 100s, 1000s. *Rx.*
Use: Anti-infective, sulfonamide.

triple sulfonamide. Dia-Mer-Thia Sulfonamides. Meth-Dia-Mer Sulfonamides.
Use: Anti-infective, sulfonamide.

Triple Vita. (Rosemont) Vitamins A 1500 units, D 400 units, C 35 mg/mL, alcohol free. Drops. Bot. 50 mL. *OTC.*
Use: Vitamin supplement.

Triple Vita-Flor. (Rosemont) Fluoride 0.5 mg, vitamins A 1500 units, D 400 units, C 35 mg/mL, alcohol free. Drops. Bot. 50 mL. *Rx.*
Use: Dental caries agent; vitamin supplement.

Triple Vitamin ADC w/Fluoride. (Nilor Pharm) Fluoride 0.5 mg, vitamins A 1500 units, D 400 units, C 35 mg/mL. Drops. Bot. 50 mL. *Rx.*
Use: Mineral, vitamin supplement; dental caries agent.

Triple Vitamins w/Fluoride. (Major) Vitamin A 2500 units, D 400 units, C 60 mg, fluoride 1 mg, dextrose, sucrose. Chew. Tab. Bot. 100s. *Rx.*
Use: Vitamin supplement; dental caries agent.

Triplevite w/Fluoride. (Geneva) Fluoride. **0.25 mg/mL:** Vitamins A 1500 units, D 400 units, C 35 mg, alcohol free. Drops. Bot. 50 mL. **0.5 mg/mL:** Vitamins A 1500 units, D 400 units, C 35 mg/mL, alcohol free, cherry flavor. Drops. Bot. 50 mL. *Rx.*
Use: Dental caries agent; vitamin supplement.

Tripodrine. (Schein) Pseudoephedrine hydrochloride 60 mg, triprolidine hydrochloride 2.5 mg. Tab. Bot. 100s, UD 100s. *Rx.*
Use: Antihistamine; decongestant.

Triposed Syrup. (Halsey Drug) **Syr.:** Triprolidine hydrochloride 1.25 mg, pseudoephedrine hydrochloride 30 mg/5 mL. Bot. 120 mL, 240 mL, 473 mL, gal. **Tab.:** Triprolidine hydrochloride 2.5 mg, pseudoephedrine hydrochloride 60 mg. Bot. 100s, 1000s. *OTC.*
Use: Antihistamine; decongestant.

tripotassium citrate. *USP 28.*
See: Potassium Citrate.

Tri-Previfem. (Teva) **Phase 1:** Norgestimate 0.18 mg, ethinyl estradiol 35 mcg. **Phase 2:** Norgestimate 0.215 mg, ethinyl estradiol 35 mcg. **Phase 3:** Norgestimate 0.25 mg, ethinyl estradiol 35 mcg. Lactose. Tab. *Rx.*
Use: Sex hormone.

•**triprolidine.** (try-PRO-lih-deen) *USP 28.*
Use: Antihistamine, nonselective alkylamine.
See: Zymine.

triprolidine hydrochloride and pseudoephedrine hydrochloride. (Various Mfr.) Triprolidine hydrochloride 1.25 mg, pseudoephedrine hydrochloride 30 mg/5 mL. Syr. Bot. 118 mL. *OTC.*
Use: Upper respiratory combination; antihistamine, decongestant.

•triprolidine hydrochloride and pseudoephedrine hydrochloride. *USP 28.*
Use: Upper respiratory combination, antihistamine, decongestant.
See: Actifed Cold & Allergy.
Allerfrim.
Aprodine.
Atridine.
Cenafed Plus.
Genac.
Silafed.
Sudafed Sinus Nighttime Maximum Strength.

triprolidine hydrochloride, codeine phosphate, and pseudoephedrine hydrochloride.
Use: Upper respiratory combination, antihistamine, antitussive, decongestant.
See: Triacin-C Cough.

Triptifed. (Weeks & Leo) Triprolidine hydrochloride 2.5 mg, pseudoephedrine hydrochloride 60 mg. Tab. Bot. 36s, 100s. *Rx.*
Use: Antihistamine; decongestant.

Triptone Caplets. (Del) Dimenhydrinate 50 mg. Tab. Bot. 12s. *OTC.*
Use: Antiemetic; antivertigo.

•**triptorelin.** (TRIP-toe-RELL-in) USAN.
Use: Antineoplastic.

triptorelin pamoate.
Use: Antineoplastic; hormone, gonadotropin-releasing hormone analog.
See: Trelstar Depot.
Trelstar LA.

trisaccharides a and b.
Use: Hemolytic disease of the newborn. [Orphan Drug]

Trisenox. (Cell Therapeutics) Arsenic trioxide 1 mg/mL, preservative free. Inj. Box 10s. *Rx.*
Use: Antineoplastic.

trisodium citrate concentration.
Use: Leukapheresis procedures.
[Orphan Drug]

Trisol. (Buffington) Borax, sodium Cl, boric acid. Irrig. Bot. oz, 4 oz. *OTC.*
Use: Artificial tears.

Tri-Sprintec. (Barr) **Phase 1:** Norgestimate 0.18 mg, ethinyl estradiol 35 mcg. **Phase 2:** Norgestimate 0.215 mg, ethinyl estradiol 35 mcg. **Phase 3:** Norgestimate 0.25 mg, ethinyl estradiol 35 mcg. Lactose. Tab. 28s. 7 inert tablets. *Rx.*
Use: Oral contraceptive.

Tri-Statin. (Rugby) Triamcinolone acetonide 0.1%, neomycin sulfate 0.25%, gramicidin 0.25 mg, nystatin 100,000 units/g Cream. Tube 15 g, 30 g, 60 g, 120 g, 480 g. *Rx.*
Use: Anti-infective; corticosteroid, topical.

Tri-Statin II. (Rugby) Triamcinolone acetonide 0.1%, 100,000 units nystatin per g, white petrolatum, parabens. Cream. Tube 15 g, 30 g, 60 g, 120 g, 480 g. *Rx.*
Use: Antifungal; corticosteroid, topical.

Tristoject. (Merz) Triamcinolone diacetate 40 mg/mL. Vial 5 mL. *Rx.*
Use: Corticosteroid.

trisulfapyridmines.
Use: Anti-infective, sulfonamide.
See: Triple Sulfa No. 2.

•**trisulfapyrimidines oral suspension.** (try-SULL-fah-peer-II-mih-deenz) *USP 28.*
Use: Anti-infective.
See: Meth-Dia-Mer Sulfonamides.

Tri-Super Flavons 1000. (Freeda) Bioflavonoids 1000 mg. Tab. Bot. 100s, 250s, 500s. *OTC.*
Use: Vitamin supplement.

Tritan. (Eon Labs) Phenylephrine tannate 25 mg, chlorpheniramine tannate 8 mg, pyrilamine tannate 25 mg. Tab. Bot. 100s, 250s, 1000s. *Rx.*
Use: Antihistamine; decongestant.

Tri-Tannate. (Rugby) Phenylephrine tannate 25 mg, chlorpheniramine tannate 8 mg, pyrilamine tannate 25 mg. Tab. Bot. 100s, 250s. *Rx.*
Use: Antihistamine; decongestant.

Tri-Tannate Pediatric. (Rugby) Phenylephrine tannate 5 mg, chlorpheniramine tannate 2 mg, pyrilamine tannate 12.5 mg. Susp. Bot. 473 mL. *Rx.*
Use: Antihistamine; decongestant.

Tri-Tannate Plus Pediatric Suspension. (Rugby) Phenylephrine tannate 5 mg, ephedrine tannate 5 mg, chlorpheniramine tannate 4 mg, carbetapentane

tannate 30 mg/5 mL. Bot. 480 mL. *Rx.*
Use: Antihistamine; antitussive; decongestant.

• **tritiated water.** (TRISH-ee-at-ehd water) USAN.
Use: Radiopharmaceutical.

Tri-Tinic. (Vortech Pharmaceuticals) Liver desiccated 75 mg, stomach 75 mg, Vitamins B$_{12}$ 15 mcg, Fe 110 mg, folic acid 1 mg, ascorbic acid 75 mg. Cap. Bot. 100s. *Rx.*
Use: Mineral, vitamin supplement.

Tritussin Cough. (Towne) Pyrilamine maleate 40 mg, pheniramine maleate 20 mg, citric acid 100 mg, codeine phosphate 58 mg/fl. oz. w/menthol and glycerin in flavored base. Syr. Bot. 4 oz. *c-v.*
Use: Antihistamine; antitussive; expectorant.

Tri-Vert. (T.E. Williams Pharmaceuticals) Dimenhydrinate 25 mg, niacin 50 mg, pentylenetetrazol 25 mg. Cap. Bot. 100s. *OTC.*
Use: Motion sickness.

Tri-Vi-Flor 1.0 mg. (Bristol-Myers Squibb) Fluoride 1 mg, vitamins A 2500 units, D 400 units, C 60 mg, sucrose. Tab. Bot. 100s, 1000s. *Rx.*
Use: Dental caries agent; nutritional supplement.

Tri-Vi-Flor 0.5 mg. (Bristol-Myers Squibb) Fluoride 0.5 mg, vitamins A 1500 units, D 400 units, C 35 mg/mL. Drops. Bot. 50 mL. *Rx.*
Use: Dental caries agent; nutritional supplement.

Tri-Vi-Flor 0.25 mg. (Bristol-Myers Squibb) Fluoride 0.25 mg, vitamins A 1500 units, D 400 units, C 35 mg/1 mL. Drops. Bot. 50 mL. *Rx.*
Use: Dental caries agent; nutritional supplement.

Tri-Vi-Flor 0.25 mg with Iron. (Bristol-Myers Squibb) Fluoride 0.25 mg, vitamins A 1500 units, D 400 units, C 35 mg, Fe 10 mg/1 mL. Drops. Bot. 50 mL. *Rx.*
Use: Dental caries agent; nutritional supplement.

Tri-Vi-Sol. (Bristol-Myers Squibb) Vitamin A 1500 units, D 400 units, C 35 mg/1 mL. Drops. Bot. 50 mL with calibrated safety-dropper. *OTC.*
Use: Vitamin supplement.

Tri-Vi-Sol with Iron. (Bristol-Myers Squibb) Vitamins A 1500 units, C 35 mg, D 400 units, Fe 10 mg/mL. Drops. Bot. 50 mL. *OTC.*
Use: Mineral, vitamin supplement.

Trivitamin Fluoride. (Schein) **Drops:** Fluoride 0.25 mg or 0.5 mg, vitamins A 1500 units, D 400 units, C 35 mg/mL. Bot. 50 mL. **Chew. Tab.:** Fluoride 0.5 mg, vitamins A 2500 units, D 400 units, C 60 mg, sucrose. Bot. 100s. *Rx.*
Use: Fluoride, vitamin supplement; dental caries agent.

Tri-Vitamin with Fluoride. (Rugby) Fluoride 0.5 mg, Vitamins A 1500 units, D 400 units, C 35 mg/mL Drops. Bot. 50 mL. *Rx.*
Use: Mineral, vitamin supplement.

Tri-Vite. (Foy Laboratories) Thiamine hydrochloride 100 mg, pyridoxine hydrochloride 100 mg, cyanocobalamin 1000 mcg/mL. Vial 10 mL. *Rx.*
Use: Vitamin supplement.

Tri Vit w/Fluoride 0.5 mg. (Alra) Fluoride 0.5 mg, vitamins A 1500 units, D 400 units, C 35 mg/mL. Drops. Bot. 50 mL. *Rx.*
Use: Mineral, vitamin supplement; dental caries agent.

Tri Vit w/Fluoride 0.25 mg. (Alra) Fluoride 0.25 mg, vitamins A 1500 units, D 400 units, C 35 mg/mL. Drops. Bot. 50 mL. *Rx.*
Use: Mineral, vitamin supplement; dental caries agent.

Trivora. (Watson) **Phase 1:** Levonorgestrel 0.5 mg, ethinyl estradiol 30 mcg (6 blue tablets). **Phase 2:** Levonorgestrel 0.075 mg, ethinyl estradiol 40 mcg (5 white tablets). **Phase 3:** Levonorgestrel 0.125 mg, ethinyl estradiol 30 mcg (10 pink tablets). Lactose. Pack. 28s. *Rx.*
Use: Sex hormone, contraceptive hormone.

Trizivir. (GlaxoSmithKline) Abacavir sulfate 300 mg, lamivudine 150 mg, zidovudine 300 mg. Tab. Bot. 60s. *Rx.*
Use: Antiretroviral, nucleoside analog reverse transcriptase inhibitor combination.

Trobicin. (Upjohn) Spectinomycin hydrochloride 400 mg/mL when reconstituted. Pow. for Inj. Vial 2 g w/diluent 3.2 mL (w/0.9% benzyl alcohol). *Rx.*
Use: Anti-infective.

Trocaine. (Roberts) Benzocaine 10 mg. Loz. UD 4s, 500s. *OTC.*
Use: Dietary aid.

Trocal. (Textilease) Dextromethorphan HBr 7.5 mg, cherry flavor. Loz. 10s, 50s, 500s. *OTC.*
Use: Antitussive.

• **troclosene potassium.** (TROE-kloeseen) USAN.
Use: Anti-infective, topical.

•**trodusquemine.** (troe-DOO-skwe-meen) USAN.
Use: Obesity.

•**troglitazone.** (TROE-glih-tazz-ohn) USAN.
Use: Antidiabetic.

•**trolamine.** (TROLE-ah-meen) *NF 23.*
Formerly Triethanolamine.
Use: Pharmaceutic aid (alkalizing agent), analgesic.
See: Ortho-iodobenzoic.

trolamine salicylate.
Use: Rub and liniment.
See: Flex-Power Performance Sports.

tromal.
Use: Analgesic; antidepressant agent.

•**tromethamine.** (TROE-meth-ah-meen) *USP 28.*
Use: Alkalizer.
W/Combinations.
See: Prohance.
Ultravist.

Tronolane. (Ross) **Cream:** Pramoxine hydrochloride 1% in cream base. Tube 30 g, 60 g. **Supp.:** Zinc oxide 11%, hard fat 95%. Pkg. 10s, 20s. *OTC.*
Use: Anorectal preparation.

Tronothane hydrochloride. (Abbott) Pramoxine hydrochloride 1%, cetyl alcohol, glycerin, parabens. Cream. 28.4 g. *OTC.*
Use: Anesthetic, local.

Tropamine. (NeuroGenesis/Matrix Tech.) Vitamins D 250 mg, l-phenylalanine, l-tyrosine 150 mg, l-glutamine 50 mg, B_1 1.67 mg, B_2 2.5 mg, B_3 16.7 mg, B_5 15 mg, B_6 3.3 mg, B_{12} 5 mcg, folic acid 0.067 mg, C 100 mg, Ca 25 mg, Cr 0.01 mg, Fe 1.5 mg, Mg 25 mg, Zn 5 mg, yeast and preservative free. Cap. Bot. 42s, 180s. *OTC.*
Use: Nutritional supplement.

•**tropanserin hydrochloride.** (trope-ANE-ser-IN) USAN.
Use: Seratonin receptor antagonist (specific in migraine).

TrophAmine Injection. (McGaw) Nitrogen 4.65 g, amino acids 30 g, protein 29 g/500 mL. Bot. 500 mL IV infusion. *OTC.*
Use: Nutritional supplement.

Troph-Iron. (GlaxoSmithKline) Vitamins B_{12} 25 mcg, B_1 10 mg, Fe 20 mg/5 mL. Saccharin. Bot. 4 fl. oz. *OTC.*
Use: Mineral, vitamin supplement.

Trophite (Iron). (Menley & James Labs, Inc.) Fe 60 mg, B_1 30 mg, B_{12} 75 mcg. Liq. Bot. 120 mL. *OTC.*
Use: Mineral, vitamin supplement.

Tropicacyl. (Akorn) Tropicamide solution 0.5%. 15 mL. 1% tropicamide. 2 mL, 15 mL. *Rx.*
Use: Cycloplegic; mydriatic.

Tropical Blend. (Schering-Plough) A series of products is marketed under the *Tropical Blend* name including: Hawaii Blend Oil SPF 2 (Bot. 8 oz.); Hawaii Blend Lotion SPF 2 (Bot. 8 oz.); Rio Blend Oil SPF 2 (Bot. 8 oz.); Rio Blend Lotion SPF 2 (Bot. 8 oz.); Jamaica Blend Oil SPF 2 (Bot. 8 oz.); Jamaica Blend Lotion SPF 2 (Bot. 8 oz.). All contain homosalate in various oil and lotion bases. *OTC.*
Use: Sunscreen.

Tropical Blend Dark Tanning. (Schering-Plough) **SPF 2:** Homosalate. **Oil:** Padimate O, oxybenzone. Bot. 180 mL, 240 mL. **Lot.:** Bot. 240 mL. **SPF 4:** Ethylhexyl p-methoxycinnamate, oxybenzone. Bot. 240 mL. *OTC.*
Use: Sunscreen.

Tropical Blend Dry Oil. (Schering-Plough) Homosalate, oxybenzone. Oil. Bot. 180 mL. *OTC.*
Use: Sunscreen.

Tropical Blend Tan Magnifier. (Schering-Plough) Triethanolamine salicylate. Oil. Bot. 240 mL. *OTC.*
Use: Sunscreen.

Tropical Gold Dark Tanning Lotion. (Ivax) SPF 4. Ethylhexyl p-methoxycinnamate, oxybenzone, benzyl alcohol, parabens, aloe extract, jojoba oil, vitamin E, EDTA, PABA free. Waterproof Lot. Bot. 240 mL. *OTC.*
Use: Sunscreen.

Tropical Gold Dark Tanning Oil. (Ivax) SPF 2. Ethylhexyl p-methoxycinnamate, octyldimethyl PABA, mineral oil, coconut oil, cocoa butter, aloe, lanolin, eucalyptus oil, oils of plumeria, manako (mango), kuawa (guava), mikara (papaya), liliko (passion fruit), taro, kukui. Oil. Bot. 240 mL. *OTC.*
Use: Sunscreen.

Tropical Gold Sport Sunblock. (Ivax) SPF 15. Ethylhexyl p-methoxycinnamate, oxybenzone, diazolidinyl urea, parabens, aloe extract, jojoba oil, vitamin E, EDTA. PABA free. Perspiration-proof. Lot. Bot. 180 mL. *OTC.*
Use: Sunblock.

Tropical Gold Sunblock. (Ivax) **Lot: SPF 15:** Ethylhexyl p-methoxycinnamate, oxybenzone, vegetable oil, benzyl alcohol, parabens, imidazolidinyl urea, vitamin E, aloe extract, jojoba oil, EDTA. PABA free. Waterproof. Bot. 118 mL. **SPF 17:** Ethylhexyl p-methoxycinnamate, 2-ethylhexyl salicylate,

homosalate, oxybenzone, aloe extract, vitamin E, vegetable and jojoba oils, benzyl alcohol, imidazolidinyl urea, parabens, EDTA. PAPA free. Waterproof. Bot. 118 mL. **SPF 30:** Ethylhexyl p-methoxycinnamate, 2-ethylhexyl salicylate, homosalate, oxybenzone, aloe extract, vitamin E, vegetable and jojoba oils, benzyl alcohol, imidizolidinyl urea, parabens, EDTA. PABA free. Waterproof. 118 mL. *OTC.*
Use: Sunblock.

Tropical Gold Sunscreen. (Ivax) SPF 8. Ethylhexyl p-methoxycinnamate, oxybenzone, benzyl alcohol, parabens, aloe extract, jojoba oil, vitamin E, EDTA. PABA free. Waterproof. Lot. Bot. 118 mL. *OTC.*
Use: Sunscreen.

•**tropicamide.** (TROP-ik-ah-mid) *USP 28.*
Use: Anticholinergic (ophthalmic).
See: Mydriacyl.
Opticyl.
Tropicacyl.

tropicamide. (Various Mfr.) Tropicamide 0.5%, 1%. Soln. Bot. 2 mL (0.5%), 15 mL.
Use: Anticholinergic (ophthalmic).

tropine benzhydryl ester methanesulfonate. Also named benztropine methane-sulfonate.

•**trospectomycin.** (TROE-speck-toe-MY-sin) USAN.
Use: Anti-infective.

•**trospium chloride.** (TROSE-pee-um) USAN.
Use: Urinary incontinence.
See: Sanctura.

Trovit. (Sigma-Tau) Vitamins B_2 0.3 mg, B_6 1 mg, choline Cl 25 mg, panthenol 2 mg, dl-methionine 10 mg, inositol 20 mg, niacinamide 50 mg, vitamins B_{12} 10 mcg/mL. Vial 30 mL. *Rx.*
Use: Vitamin B supplement.

T.R.U.E. Test. (GlaxoSmithKline) Allergen-containing patches. Test in multipak cartons (5s). *Rx.*
Use: Diagnostic aid, allergic.

Truphylline. (G & W) Aminophylline 250 mg (equiv. to theophylline 198 mg). Supp. UD 10s, 25s. *Rx.*
Use: Bronchodilator.

Trusopt. (Merck) Dorzolamide (as base) 2%. Benzalkonium chloride 0.0075%, hydroxyethylcellulose, sodium hydroxide, mannitol. Soln. *Ocumeters.* 5 mL, 10 mL. *Rx.*
Use: Antiglaucoma.

Truvada. (Gilead) Emtricitabine 200 mg/ tenofovir disoproxil fumarate 300 mg (equiv. to tenofovir disoproxil 245 mg). Film coated. Tab. 30s. *Rx.*
Use: Antiretroviral.

Trycet. (Tryon Laboratories) Propoxyphene napsylate 100 mg, acetaminophen 325 mg. Lactose. Film coated. Tab. 100s. *c-iv.*
Use: Narcotic analgesic.

trypan blue.
Use: Ophthalmic surgery aid.
See: VisionBlue.

•**trypsin, crystallized.** (TRIP-sin) *USP 28.*
Use: Proteolytic enzyme.
W/Castor oil.
See: Granulex.

•**tryptizol hydrochloride.** *USP 28.* Amitriptyline hydrochloride.

•**tryptophan.** (TRIP-toe-FAN) *USP 28.*
Use: Amino acid.

T/Scalp. (Neutrogena) Hydrocortisone 1%. Liq. Greaseless. Bot. 60 mL, 105 mL. *OTC.*
Use: Antipruritic; corticosteroid, topical.

TSPA.
Use: Antineoplastic.
See: Thiotepa.

TTC. Triphenyltetrazolium Chloride.

T-3 RIAbead. (Abbott Diagnostics) Test kit 50s, 100s.
Use: Diagnostic aid, thyroid.

•**tuaminoheptane sulfate.** *USP 28.*
Use: Adrenergic.

•**tuberculin.** (too-BURR-kyoo-lin) *USP 28.*
Use: Diagnostic aid (dermal reactivity indicator).
See: Aplisol.
Aplitest.
Tubersol.

Tuberculin, Mono-Vacc Test. (Lincoln Diagnostics) Mono-Vacc test is a sterile, disposable multiple puncture scarifier with liquid Old Tuberculin on the points. Box 25 tests. *Rx.*
Use: Diagnostic aid.

Tuberculin, Old Monovacc Test. (Wyeth) 5 TU activity test. Soln. of Old Tuberculin containing acacia 7%, lactose 8.5%. Test. Kits 25s, 100s, 250s. *Rx.*
Use: Diagnostic aid.

Tuberculin, Old, Tine Test. (Wyeth) 5 TY activity per test. Soln. of Old Tuberculin, containing acacia 7%, lactose 8.5%. Test. Kits 25s, 100s, 250s.
Use: Diagnostic aid.

tuberculin purified protein derivative.
Use: Diagnostic aid.
See: Aplisol.
Tubersol.

tuberculin tests.
Use: Diagnostic aid.
See: Aplisol.
Aplitest.
Tine Test PPD.
Tuberculin, Old Mono Vacc Test.
Tuberculin, Old, Tine Test.
Tubersol.
tuberculin tine test. (Wyeth) **Old Tuberculin (OT):** Each disposable test unit consists of a stainless steel disc, with 4 tines (or prongs) 2 mm long, attached to a plastic handle. The tines have been dip-dried with antigenic material. The entire unit is sterilized by ethylene oxide gas. The test has been standardized by comparative studies, utilizing 0.05 mg US Standard Old Tuberculin 5 units or 0.0001 mg US Standard 5 units by the Mantoux technique. Reliability appears to be comparable to the standard Mantoux. Tests in a jar 25s. Package 100s. Bin Package 250s. **Purified Protein Derivative (PPD):** Equivalent to or more potent than 5 TU PPD Mantoux test. Tests in a jar 25s. Package 100s.
Use: Diagnostic aid.
tuberculosis vaccine.
Use: Immunization.
See: TICE BCG.
Tubersol. (Aventis Pasteur) Tuberculin purified protein derivative (Mantoux) 5 TU/0.1 mL, potassium and sodium phosphates, phenol 0.35%, polysorbate 80. Vial 1 mL (10 tests), 5 mL (50 tests). *Rx.*
Use: Diagnostic aid, tuberculosis.
Tubex. (Wyeth) The following drugs are available in various *Tubex* sizes: Ativan, Bicillin C-R, Bicillin C-R 900/300, Bicillin Long-Acting, Codeine Phosphate, Cyanocobalamin, Digoxin, Dimenhydrinate, Diphenhydramine hydrochloride, Diphtheria and Tetanus Toxoids Adsorbed (Pediatric Pharmaceuticals), Epinephrine, Furosemide, Heparin Flush Kits, Heparin Lock Flush, Heparin Sodium Solution, Hydromorphone hydrochloride, Hydroxyzine hydrochloride, Influenza Virus Vaccine, Trivalent, Mepergan, Meperidine hydrochloride, Morphine Sulfate, Naloxone Injection, Naloxone Injection, Neonatal, Oxytocin, Pentobarbital Sodium, Phenergan, Phenobarbital Sodium, Prochlorperazine Edisylate, Secobarbital Sodium, Sodium Chloride, Bacteriostatic, Tetanus and Diphtheria Toxoids Adsorbed, Adult, Tetanus Immune Globulin, Human, Tetanus Toxoid

Alum Phos Ad.; Tetanus Toxoid, Fluid; Thiamine Hydrochloride; Wycillin. *Rx.*
• **tubocurarine chloride.** (too-boe-cure-AHR-een) *USP 28.*
Use: Neuromuscular blocker.
tubocurarine chloride, dimethyl. Dimethylether of d-tubocurarine chloride.
• **tubocurarine chloride hydrochloride pentahydrate.** (too-boe-cure-AHR-een) Tubocurarine Chloride.
tubocurarine iodide, dimethyl. Dimethyl ether of d-tubocurarine iodide.
Use: Muscle relaxant.
See: Metubine.
• **tubulozole hydrochloride.** (too-BYOO-lah-ZAHL) USAN.
Use: Antineoplastic (microtubule inhibitor).
Tucks Take-Alongs. (Parke-Davis) Nonwoven wipes saturated with solution of witch hazel 50%, glycerine 10%, benzalkonium chloride 0.003%. Box 12s. *OTC.*
Use: Anorectal preparation.
Tuinal. (Eli Lilly) Equal parts Seconal Sod. & Amytal Sod. Pulvule. 100 mg, 200 mg. Bot. 100s. *c-II.*
Use: Hypnotic; sedative.
tumor necrosis factor-binding protein I and II. Serono *Rx.*
Use: Treatment of AIDS. [Orphan Drug]
Tums. (GlaxoSmithKline Consumer) Calcium carbonate 500 mg (elemental calcium 200 mg), sucrose, talc, assorted fruit and peppermint flavors. Chew. Tab. Bot. 75s, 150s. *OTC.*
Use: Antacid; mineral, calcium.
Tums Calcium for Life Bone Health. (GlaxoSmithKline Consumer) Calcium carbonate 1250 mg (elemental calcium 500 mg). Chew. Tab. Bot. 90s. *OTC.*
Use: Mineral, calcium.
Tums Calcium for Life PMS. (GlaxoSmithKline Consumer) Calcium carbonate 750 mg (elemental calcium 300 mg), sucrose, strawberry flavor. Chew. Tab. Bot. 120s. *OTC.*
Use: Mineral, calcium.
Tums E-X. (GlaxoSmithKline Consumer) Calcium carbonate 750 mg (elemental calcium 300 mg), sucrose, talc, mixed berry, assorted fruit and sugar free orange flavors (aspartame, phenylalanine < 1 mg, sorbitol). Chew. Tab. Bot. 96s. *OTC.*
Use: Antacid, mineral, calcium.
Tums Plus. (GlaxoSmithKline) Calcium carbonate 500 mg, (elemental calcium 200 mg), simethicone 20 mg, sucrose, sodium, assorted fruit and mint flavors.

Chew. Tab. Bot. 48s. *OTC.*
Use: Antacid.

Tums Smooth Dissolve. (GlaxoSmith-Kline) Calcium carbonate 750 mg (elemental calcium 300 mg), sorbitol, dextrose, sucrose (2 g sugar), peppermint and assorted fruit flavors. Tab. 45s. *OTC.*
Use: Mineral.

Tums Ultra. (GlaxoSmithKline Consumer) Calcium carbonate 1000 mg (elemental calcium 400 mg), sucrose, talc, mint flavor. Chew. Tab. Bot. 86s. *OTC.*
Use: Mineral, calcium.

Tur-Bi-Kal Nasal Drops. (Emerson) Phenylephrine hydrochloride in a saline solution. Drops. Bot. oz., 12s. *OTC.*
Use: Decongestant.

Turbinaire.
See: Decadron Phosphate.

Turbinaire Decadron Phosphate. (Merck & Co.) Each metered spray delivers dexamethasone sodium phosphate equivalent to dexamethasone ≈ 84 mcg (170 sprays per cartridge), alcohol 2%. Aerosol. 12.6 g w/adapter or 12.6 g refill. *Rx.*
Use: Corticosteroid, topical.

turpentine oil w/combinations.
See: Sloan's Liniment.

Tusibron. (Kenwood) Guaifenesin 100 mg/5 mL, alcohol 3.5%. Liq. Bot. 118 mL. *OTC.*
Use: Expectorant.

Tussabar. (Tennessee Pharmaceutic) Acetaminophen 400 mg, salicylamide 500 mg, potassium guaiacolsulfonate 120 mg, pyrilamine maleate 30 mg, ammonium chloride 500 mg, sodium citrate 500 mg, phenylephrine hydrochloride 30 mg/oz. Bot. Pt., gal. *Rx.*
Use: Analgesic; antihistamine; decongestant; expectorant.

Tussabid. (ION Laboratories, Inc.) Guaifenesin 200 mg, dextromethorphan HBr 30 mg. Cap. Bot. 24s, 100s. *OTC.*
Use: Antihistamine; expectorant.

Tussafed. (Everett) Dextromethorphan HBr 15 mg, pseudoephedrine hydrochloride 60 mg, carbinoxamine maleate 4 mg/5 mL, menthol, grape flavor, alcohol free. Syr. Bot. 120 mL, 480 mL. *Rx.*
Use: Upper respiratory combination, antihistamine, antitussive, decongestant.

Tussafed. (Everett) Carbinoxamine maleate 2 mg, pseudoephedrine hydrochloride 25 mg, dextromethorphan HBr 4 mg/mL. Drops. Bot. 30 mL with calibrated dropper. *Rx.*
Use: Antihistamine; antitussive; decongestant.

Tussafed EX. (Everett) Dextromethorphan HBr 30 mg, guaifenesin 200 mg, phenylephrine hydrochloride 10 mg/5 mL, EDTA, saccharin, sorbitol, cherry-vanilla flavor, alcohol free. Syr. Bot. 473 mL. *Rx.*
Use: Upper respiratory combination, antitussive, expectorant, decongestant.

Tussafed HC. (Everett) Hydrocodone bitartrate 2.5 mg, phenylephrine hydrochloride 7.5 mg, guaifenesin 50 mg/5 mL, alcohol free. Syr. Bot. 473 mL. *c-III.*
Use: Upper respiratory combination, decongestant, antitussive, expectorant.

Tussafed LA. (Everett) Guaifenesin 600 mg, pseudoephedrine hydrochloride 60 mg, dextromethorphan HBr 30 mg, dye free. SR Tab. Bot. 100s. *Rx.*
Use: Upper respiratory combination, expectorant, decongestant, antitussive.

Tussafin Expectorant. (Rugby) Pseudoephedrine hydrochloride 60 mg, hydrocodone bitartrate 5 mg, guaifenesin 200 mg/5 mL, alcohol 2.5%. Liq. Bot. 480 mL. *c-III.*
Use: Antitussive; decongestant; expectorant.

Tussanil DH. (Edwards) Phenylephrine hydrochloride 10 mg, chlorpheniramine maleate 4 mg, hydrocodone bitartrate 2.5 mg/5 mL w/alcohol 5%. Syr. Bot. Pt. *c-III.*
Use: Antihistamine; antitussive; decongestant.

Tussanil Expectorant. (Edwards) Hydrocodone bitartrate 2.5 mg, phenylephrine hydrochloride 10 mg, guaifenesin 100 mg/5 mL w/alcohol 5%. Syr. Bot. Pt. *c-III.*
Use: Antitussive; decongestant; expectorant.

Tussanol. (Tyler) Pyrilamine maleate ¾ g, codeine phosphate 1 g, ammonium chloride 7.5 g, sodium citrate 5 g, menthol g/fl. oz. Bot. 4 fl. oz, pt, gal. *c-v.*
Use: Antihistamine; antitussive; expectorant.

Tussanol with Ephedrine. (Tyler) Ephedrine sulfate 2 g, pyrilamine maleate 0.75 g, codeine phosphate 1 g, ammonium chloride 7.5 g, sodium citrate 5 g, menthol g/30 mL. Bot. 16 fl. oz. *c-v.*
Use: Bronchodilator; antihistamine; antitussive; expectorant.

Tussar DM. (Aventis) Dextromethorphan HBr 15 mg, chlorpheniramine maleate 2 mg, phenylephrine hydrochloride 5 mg/5 mL w/methylparaben 0.1% Bot. 4 oz., pt. *Rx.*
Use: Antihistamine; antitussive; expectorant.

Tussar SF. (Aventis) Codeine phosphate 10 mg, guaifenesin 100 mg, pseudoephedrine hydrochloride 30 mg/5 mL, alcohol 2.5%. Bot. 120 mL, 473 mL. *c-v.*
Use: Antitussive; decongestant; expectorant.

Tussar-2. (Aventis) Codeine phosphate 10 mg, guaifenesin 100 mg, pseudoephedrine hydrochloride 30 mg/5 mL, alcohol 2.5%. Syr. Bot. 473 mL. *c-v.*
Use: Antitussive; expectorant; decongestant.

Tuss-DM. (Hyrex) Dextromethorphan HBr 10 mg, guaifenesin 200 mg. Tab. Bot. 100s, 1000s, UD 50s. *Rx.*
Use: Upper respiratory combination, antitussive, expectorant.

Tussend. (Monarch) **Syr.:** Hydrocodone bitartrate 2.5 mg, pseudoephredrine hydrochloride 30 mg, chlorpheniramine maleate 2 mg/5 mL, alcohol 5%, corn syrup, parabens, saccharin, sucrose, banana flavor. Bot. 473 mL. **Tab.:** Hydrocodone bitartrate 5 mg, chlorpheniramine maleate 4 mg, pseudoephedrine hydrochloride 60 mg, lactose. Bot. 100s. *c-iii.*
Use: Upper respiratory combination, antitussive, antihistamine, decongestant.

Tussgen. (Ivax) Pseudoephedrine hydrochloride 60 mg, hydrocodone bitartrate 5 mg/5 mL. Liq. Bot. 100s, 1000s. *c-iii.*
Use: Antitussive; decongestant.

Tussi-bid. (Capellon) Dextromethorphan HBr 60 mg, guaifenesin 1200 mg. SR Tab. Bot. 100s. *Rx.*
Use: Upper respiratory combination, antitussive, expectorant.

Tussigon. (Daniels) Hydrocodone bitartrate 5 mg, homatropine methylbromide 1.5 mg. Tab. Bot. 100s, 500s. *c-iii.*
Use: Upper respiratory combination, antispasmodic, anticholinergic, antitussive.

Tussionex. (Medeva) Hydrocodone (as polistirex) 10 mg, chlorpheniramine 8 mg. Liq. Bot. 473 mL, 900 mL. *c-iii.*
Use: Antihistamine; antitussive.

Tussionex Pennkinetic. (CellTech) Hydrocodone polistirex 10 mg, chlorpheniramine polistirex 8 mg/5 mL, parabens, sucrose, corn syrup, alcohol free. ER Susp. Bot. 473 mL. *c-iii.*

Use: Upper respiratory combination, antitussive, antihistamine.

Tussi-Organidin-DM NR. (Wallace) Dextromethorphan HBr 10 mg, guaifenesin 100 mg/5 mL, saccharin, sorbitol, raspberry flavor. Liq. Bot. 473 mL. *Rx.*
Use: Upper respiratory combination, antitussive, expectorant.

Tussi-Organidin NR. (Wallace) Codeine phosphate 10 mg, guaifenesin 100 mg/5 mL, saccharin, sorbitol, raspberry flavor. Liq. Bot. 473 mL. *c-v.*
Use: Upper respiratory combination, antitussive, expectorant.

TUSSI-PRES. (Kramer-Novis) Dextromethorphan hydrobromide 15 mg, guaifenesin 200 mg, phenylephrine hydrochloride 5 mg per 5 mL. Phenylalanine 14 mg, aspartame, parabens. Cherry flavor. Liq. 237 mL. *Rx.*
Use: Antitussive and expectorant.

Tussirex. (Scot-Tussin) Phenylephrine hydrochloride 4.17 mg, pheniramine maleate 13.3 mg, codeine phosphate 10 mg, sodium citrate 83.3 mg, sodium salicylate 83.3 mg, caffeine citrate 25 mg/5 mL, menthol 0.17 mg, alcohol and dye free. Syr. Bot. 473 mL, 3.8 L. *c-v.*
Use: Upper respiratory combination, antihistamine, antitussive, decongestant, expectorant.

Tussirex Sugar Free. (Scot-Tussin) Codeine phosphate 10 mg, pheniramine maleate 13.33 mg, phenylephrine hydrochloride 4.17 mg, sodium citrate 83.33 mg, sodium salicylate 83.33 mg, caffeine citrate 25 mg/5 mL, menthol 0.17 mg, alcohol and dye free. Liq. Bot. 30 mL, 473 mL, 3.8 L. *c-v.*
Use: Upper respiratory combination, analgesic, antihistamine, antitussive, decongestant, expectorant.

Tussi-12. (Wallace) **Susp.:** Carbetapentane tannate 30 mg, chlorpheniramine tannate 4 mg, phenylephrine tannate 5 mg/mL, glycerin, methylparaben, saccharin, sucrose. Bot. Pt. **Tab.:** Carbetapentane tannate 60 mg, chlorpheniramine tannate 5 mg. Bot. 100s. *Rx.*
Use: Upper respiratory combination, antihistamine, antitussive, decongestant.

Tussi-12 D. (Wallace) Carbetapentane tannate 60 mg, pyrilamine tannate 40 mg, pheyleprhine tannate 10 mg. Tab. 100s. *Rx.*
Use: Antitussive combination.

Tussi-12D S. (Wallace) Carbetapentane tannate 30 mg, pyrilamine tannate

30 mg, phenylephrine tannate 5 mg/ 5 mL, tartrazine, methylparaben, saccharin, sucrose, strawberry-currant flavor. Susp. 120 mL w/oral syringe. *Rx.*
Use: Antitussive combination.

Tussi-12 S. (Wallace) Chlorpheniramine tannate 4 mg, carbetapentane tannate 30 mg/5 mL, methylparaben, saccharin, sucrose, tartrazine, strawberry-currant flavor. Susp. Bot. 118 mL with syr. *Rx.*
Use: Upper respiratory combination, antihistamine, antitussive.

Tussizone-12 RF. (Mallinckrodt) **Susp.:** Carbetapentane tannate 30 mg, chlorpheniramine tannate 4 mg/5 mL, tartrazine, methylparaben, saccharin, sucrose, strawberry currant flavor. 118 mL. **Tab.:** Carbetapentane tannate 60 mg, chlorpheniramine tannate 5 mg. 100s. *Rx.*
Use: Antitussive combination.

Tuss-LA. (Hyrex) Pseudoephedrine hydrochloride 120 mg, guaifenesin 500 mg. LA Tab. Bot. 100s. *Rx.*
Use: Decongestant; expectorant.

Tusso-DM. (Everett) Dextromethorphan HBr 10 mg, iodinated glycerol 30 mg, alcohol free. Liq. Bot. 473 mL. *Rx.*
Use: Cough preparation.

Tuss-Tan. (Econolab) Carbetapine tannate 60 mg, chlorpheniramine tannate 5 mg, ephedrine tannate 10 mg, phenylephrine tannate 10 mg. Tab. 100s. *Rx.*
Use: Antitussive; antihistamine; decongestant.

Tuss-Tan Pediatric. (Econolab) Carbetapentane tannate 30 mg, chlorpheniramine tannate 4 mg, ephedrine tannate 5 mg, phenylephrine tannate 5 mg/ 5 mL, methylparaben, saccharin, sucrose. Susp. Bot. 473 mL. *Rx.*
Use: Antitussive; antihistamine; decongestant.

Tusstat. (Century) Diphenhydramine hydrochloride 12.5 mg/5 mL, alcohol 5%. Syr. Bot. 30 mL, 118 mL, 473 mL, 3.8 L. *Rx.*
Use: Antihistamine, nonselective ethanolamine; antitussive.

Tusstat Expectorant. (Century) Diphenhydramine hydrochloride 80 mg, ammonium chloride 12 g, sodium citrate 5 g, menthol 0.13 g, alcohol 5%/oz. Bot. 4 fl. oz, pt, gal. *Rx.*
Use: Antihistamine; expectorant.

•**tuvirumab.** (tuh-VIE-roo-mab) USAN.
Use: Monoclonal antibody (antiviral).

T-Vites. (Freeda) Vitamins B$_1$ 25 mg, B$_2$ 25 mg, B$_3$ 150 mg, B$_5$ 25 mg, B$_6$ 25 mg, C 100 mg, biotin 30 mcg, PABA, K, Mg, Mn carbonate 2 mg, Zn gluconate 20 mg. Tab. Bot. 100s. *OTC.*
Use: Mineral, vitamin supplement.

tween 20, 40, 60, 80. *NF 23.* (AstraZeneca) Polysorbates.
Use: Surface active agents.

12-Hour Antihistamine Nasal Decongestant. (United Research Laboratories) Pseudoephedrine sulfate 120 mg, dexbrompheniramine maleate 6 mg, sugar, sucrose. SR Tab. Bot. 10s. *OTC.*
Use: Decongestant.

12-Hour Cold. (Ivax) Dexbrompheniramine maleate 6 mg, pseudoephedrine sulfate 120 mg. SR Tab. Pkg. 10s, 20s. *OTC.*
Use: Antihistamine; decongestant.

12 Hour Nasal. Various Mfr. Oxymetazoline hydrochloride 0.05%. Soln. Spray Bot. 15 mL. *OTC.*
Use: Nasal decongestant, imidazoline.

Twelve Resin-K. (Key Company) Vitamin B$_{12}$ 1,000 mcg on resin. Tab. 60s, 250s, 1000s. *OTC.*
Use: Vitamin.

20% ProSol. (Baxter Healthcare) Amino acids 20 g, total nitrogen 3.21 g/ 100 mL, lysine acetate, glacial acetic acid. Sulfite free. Inj. *Vialflex* Cont. 500 mL, 1000 mL, 2000 mL. *Rx.*
Use: Nutritional therapy, intravenous.

20-20. (BDI) Caffeine 200 mg. Tab. Bot. 100s, 500s. *OTC.*
Use: CNS stimulant, analeptic.

Twice-a-Day 12-Hour Nasal. (Major) Oxymetazoline 0.05%, EDTA, benzalkonium chloride, benzyl alcohol. Soln. Spray bot. 15 mL, 30 mL. *OTC.*
Use: Nasal decongestant, imidazoline.

Twilite. (Pfeiffer) Diphenhydramine hydrochloride 50 mg. Tab. 20s. *OTC.*
Use: Sleep aid.

Twin-K. (Knoll) Potassium ions 20 mEq/ 15 mL. Liq. Bot. Pt. *Rx.*
Use: Treatment of hypokalemia.

Twinrix. (GlaxoSmithKline) Inactivated hepatitis A ≥ 720 ELU, recombinant HBsAg protein 20 mcg/mL, thimerosal (mercury < 1 mcg). Inj. Single-dose vial 1s, 10s, single-dose prefilled syr. 5s. *Rx.*
Use: Active immunization, viral vaccine.

TwoCal HN High Nitrogen Liquid Nutrition. (Ross) High-nitrogen liquid nutrition (2 calories/mL). 1900 calories (1 quart), provides 100% US RDA for vitamins and minerals for adults and children over 4 yrs. Can 8 fl. oz. *OTC.*
Use: Nutritional supplement.

2-Tone Disclosing Solution. (Young Dental) Dropper Bot. 2 oz.
Use: Disclosing solution.

•**tybamate.** (TIE-bam-ate) USAN.
Use: Anxiolytic.

Ty-Cold. (Major) 30 mg pseudoephedrine, 2 mg chlorpheniramine maleate, 15 mg dextromethorphan HBr, 325 mg acetaminophen. Tab. Pkg. 24s. *OTC.*
Use: Analgesic; antihistamine; antitussive; decongestant.

Tygacil. (Wyeth) Tigecycline 50 mg. Pow. for Inj., lyophilized. Single-dose vial 5 mL. *Rx.*
Use: Anti-infective, glycylcycline.

Tylenol Allergy Complete Multi-Symptom. (McNeil Consumer) Pseudoephedrine hydrochloride 30 mg, chlorpheniramine maleate 2 mg, acetaminophen 500 mg. Tab. Pkg. 24s, 48s. Geltab, Gelcap. Parabens, EDTA. Pkg. 24s, 48s. *OTC.*
Use: Upper respiratory combination, decongestant, antihistamine, analgesic.

Tylenol Allergy Complete Multi-Symptom Day & Night. (McNeil Consumer) **Day Formula:** Pseudoephedrine hydrochloride 30 mg, chlorpheniramine maleate 4 mg, acetaminophen 500 mg. Tab. 12s. **Night Formula:** Pseudoephedrine hydrochloride 30 mg, diphenhydramine hydrochloride 25 mg, acetaminophen 500 mg. Tab. 12s. *OTC.*
Use: Decongestant, antihistamine, analgesic.

Tylenol Allergy Complete NightTime. (McNeil Consumer) Pseudoephedrine hydrochloride 30 mg, diphenhydramine hydrochloride 25 mg, acetaminophen 500 mg. Tab. Pkg. 24s *OTC.*
Use: Upper respiratory combination, decongestant, antihistamine, analgesic.

Tylenol Arthritis. (McNeil Consumer) Acetaminophen 650 mg. ER Tab. Bot. 100s. *OTC.*
Use: Analgesic.

Tylenol Children's. (McNeil Consumer) **Chew. Tab.:** Acetaminophen 80 mg. Bot. 30s, 48s. Blisters 2s. Hospital pack 250s. **Elix.:** Acetaminophen 160 mg/ 5 mL. Elix. Bot. 60 mg, 120 mL. **Susp.:** Acetaminophen 160 mg/5 mL. Butylparaben, corn syrup, sorbitol. Alcohol free. Bot. 60 mL. *OTC.*
Use: Analgesic.

Tylenol Children's Cold. (McNeil Consumer) **Chew. Tab.:** Pseudoephedrine hydrochloride 7.5 mg, chlorpheniramine maleate 0.5 mg, acetaminophen 80 mg, aspartame, mannitol, phenylalanine 6 mg, grape flavor. Pkg. 24s.

Liq.: Pseudoephedrine hydrochloride 15 mg, chlorpheniramine maleate 1 mg, acetaminophen 160 mg/15 mL, sorbitol, sucrose, grape flavor, alcohol free. Bot. 120 mL. *OTC.*
Use: Upper respiratory combination, decongestant, antihistamine, analgesic.

Tylenol Children's Cold Plus Cough. (McNeil) **Chew. Tab.:** Pseudoephedrine hydrochloride 7.5 mg, chlorpheniramine maleate 0.5 mg, dextromethorphan HBr 2.5 mg, acetaminophen 80 mg, aspartame, mannitol, phenylalanine 4 mg, cherry flavor. Pkg. 24s. **Susp.:** Pseudoepedrine hydrochloride 15 mg, chlorpheniramine maleate 1 mg, dextromethorphan HBr 5 mg, acetaminophen 160 mg/5 mL, acesulfame K, butylparaben, corn syrup, sorbitol, cherry flavor, alcohol free. Bot. 120 mL. *OTC.*
Use: Upper respiratory combination, decongestant, antihistamine, antitussive, analgesic.

Tylenol Children's Flu. (McNeil) Pseudoephedrine hydrochloride 15 mg, chlorpheniramine maleate 1 mg, dextromethorphan HBr 7.5 mg, acetaminophen 160 mg/5 mL, acesulfame K, butylparaben, corn syrup, sorbitol, bubble gum flavor, alcohol free. Susp. Bot. 120 mL. *OTC.*
Use: Upper respiratory combination, decongestant, antihistamine, antitussive, analgesic.

Tylenol Children's Plus Cold. (McNeil Consumer) Pseudoephedrine hydrochloride 15 mg, acetaminophen 160 mg/5 mL, acesulfame K, butylparaben, corn syrup, sorbitol, fruit flavor. Susp. Bot. 118 mL. *OTC.*
Use: Upper respiratory combination, decongestant, analgesic.

Tylenol Cold & Flu Medication. (McNeil Consumer) Pseudoephedrine hydrochloride 60 mg, chlorpheniramine maleate 4 mg, dextromethorphan HBr, acetaminophen 650 mg, aspartame, sucrose, phenylalanine 11 mg, lemon flavor. Pow. Pks. 6s, 12s. *OTC.*
Use: Analgesic; antihistamine; decongestant.

Tylenol Cold, Children's. (McNeil Consumer) **Chew. Tab.:** Pseudoephedrine hydrochloride 7.5 mg, chlorpheniramine maleate 0.5 mg, acetaminophen 80 mg, aspartame, sucrose, phenylalanine 4 mg. Grape flavor. Bot. 24s. **Liq.:** Pseudoephedrine 15 mg, chlorpheniramine maleate 1 mg, acetaminophen 160 mg/5 mL, sorbitol, sucrose, alcohol

free, grape flavor. Bot. 120 mL. *OTC.*
Use: Analgesic; antihistamine; decongestant.

Tylenol Cold Complete Formula. (McNeil Consumer) Dextromethorphan HBr 15 mg, chlorpheniramine maleate 2 mg, pseudoephedrine hydrochloride 30 mg, acetaminophen 325 mg. Tab. Pkg. 24s. *OTC.*
Use: Upper respiratory combination, antitussive, antihistamine, decongestant, analgesic.

Tylenol Cold Multi-Symptom Plus Cough, Children's. (McNeil Consumer) Acetaminophen 160 mg, dextromethorphan HBr 5 mg, chlorpheniramine maleate 1 mg, pseudoephedrine 15 mg/5 mL. Liq. Bot. 120 mL. *OTC.*
Use: Antihistamine; antitussive; decongestant.

Tylenol Cold Non-Drowsy Formula. (McNeil Consumer) Pseudoephedrine hydrochloride 30 mg, dextromethorphan HBr 15 mg, acetaminophen 325 mg. Tab. Bot. 24s. Gelcap. Parabens. Bot. 24s. *OTC.*
Use: Upper respiratory combination, analgesic, antitussive, decongestant.

Tylenol Cold Severe Congestion. (McNeil Consumer) Dextromethorphan HBr 15 mg, guaifenesin 200 mg, pseudoephedrine hydrochloride 30 mg, acetaminophen 325 mg. Tab. Pkg. 24s. *OTC.*
Use: Upper respiratory combination, antitussive, expectorant, decongestant, analgesic.

Tylenol Cough w/Decongestant. (McNeil Consumer) Pseudoephedrine hydrochloride 15 mg, dextromethorphan HBr 7.5 mg, acetaminophen 250 mg, alcohol 10%, saccharin, sobitol, sucrose. Liq. Bot. 120 mL, 240 mL. *OTC.*
Use: Analgesic; antitussive; decongestant.

Tylenol 8 Hour. (McNeil) Acetaminophen 650 mg, benzyl alcohol, parabens, castor oil, EDTA. **Caplets:** 24s, 50s, 100s, 150s. **Geltabs:** 20s, 40s, 80s. *OTC.*
Use: Analgesic.

Tylenol Extended Relief. (McNeil Consumer) Acetaminophen 650 mg. ER Capl. 100s. *OTC.*
Use: Analgesic.

Tylenol Extra Strength. (McNeil Consumer) Acetaminophen 500 mg. **Gel Cap.:** Bot. 24s, 50s, 100s. **Gel Tab.:** Bot. 24s, 50s, 100s. **Tab.:** Bot. 30s, 60s, 100s, 200s. **Capl.:** Bot. 24s, 50s, 100s, 175s. *OTC.*
Use: Analgesic.

Tylenol Extra Strength Adult. (McNeil Consumer) Acetaminophen 1000 mg/30 mL w/alcohol 8.5%. Liq. Bot. 8 oz. Hosp. 8 oz. *OTC.*
Use: Analgesic.

Tylenol Flu, Maximum Strength. (McNeil) Pseudoephedrine hydrochloride 30 mg, diphenhydramine hydrochloride 25 mg, acetaminophen 500 mg. Benzyl alcohol, castor oil, parabens. Gelcaps. 12s. *OTC.*
Use: Decongestant, antihistamine, analgesic.

Tylenol Flu Maximum Strength Non-Drowsy. (McNeil Consumer) Pseudoephedrine hydrochloride 30 mg, dextromethorphan HBr 15 mg, acetaminophen 500 mg, parabens. Gelcap. Pkg. 24s. *OTC.*
Use: Upper respiratory combination, analgesic, antitussive, decongestant.

Tylenol Flu Night Time Maximum Strength. (McNeil Consumer) **Gelcap:** Pseudoephedrine hydrochloride 30 mg, diphenhydramine hydrochloride 25 mg, acetaminophen 500 mg, parabens. Pkg. 24s. **Liq.:** Dextromethorphan HBr 5 mg, doxylamine succinate 2.1 mg, pseudoephedrine hydrochloride 10 mg, acetaminophen 167 mg/5 mL, corn syrup, saccharin, sorbitol. Bot. 237 mL. *OTC.*
Use: Upper respiratory combination.

Tylenol Infant's. (McNeil Consumer) Acetaminophen 80 mg/0.8 mL. Butylparaben, corn syrup, sorbitol. Alcohol free. Drops. Bot. w/dropper 7.5 mL, 15 mL. *OTC.*
Use: Analgesic.

Tylenol Infant's Drops Plus Cold. (McNeil) Pseudoephedrine hydrochloride 9.375 mg, acetaminophen 100 mg/mL, saccharin, corn syrup, bubble gum flavor, alcohol free. Conc. Drops. Bot. 15 mL with dropper. *OTC.*
Use: Upper respiratory combination, decongestant, analgesic.

Tylenol Junior Strength. (McNeil Consumer) Acetaminophen 160 mg, aspartame (6 mg phenylalanine). Chew. Tab. 24s. *OTC.*
Use: Analgesic.

Tylenol Junior Strength Swallowable Tablets. (McNeil Consumer) 160 mg. Tab. Box. 30s. Hosp. 250 × 1. *OTC.*
Use: Analgesic.

Tylenol Maximum Strength Allergy Sinus. (McNeil Consumer) Pseudoephedrine hydrochloride 30 mg, chlorpheniramine maleate 2 mg, acetaminophen 500 mg. **Capl.:** Bot. 24s, 50s.

Gelcap: Bot. 20s, 40s. *OTC.*
Use: Analgesic; antihistamine; decongestant.

Tylenol Maximum Strength Sinus Medication. (McNeil Consumer) Acetaminophen 500 mg, pseudoephedrine hydrochloride 30 mg. Tab., Capl. Bot. 24s, 50s. *OTC.*
Use: Analgesic; decongestant.

Tylenol Multi-Symptom Hot Medication. (McNeil Consumer) Pseudoephedrine hydrochloride 60 mg, chlorpheniramine maleate 4 mg, dextromethorphan HBr 30 mg, acetaminophen 650 mg. Pow. Pkt. 6s. *OTC.*
Use: Analgesic; antihistamine; antitussive; decongestant.

Tylenol No Drowsiness Cold. (McNeil Consumer) Pseudoephedrine hydrochloride 30 g, dextromethorphan HBr 15 mg, acetaminophen 325 mg. Cap. Bot. 24s, 50s. *OTC.*
Use: Analgesic; antitussive; decongestant.

Tylenol Plus Cold & Cough Infants'. (McNeil) Pseudoephedrine hydrochloride 9.375 mg, dextromethorphan HBr 3.125 mg, acetaminophen 100 mg/mL, acesulfame K, corn syrup, cherry flavor, alcohol free. Conc. Drops. Bot. 15 mL with dropper. *OTC.*
Use: Upper respiratory combination, decongestant, antitussive, analgesic.

Tylenol PM, Extra Strength. (McNeil Consumer) Acetaminophen 500 mg, diphenhydramine 25 mg. Tab. Bot. 24s, 50s, 100s, 150s. Gelcap. Parabens. Bot. 50s. Geltab. Parabens. Bot. 50s, 100s. *OTC.*
Use: Upper respiratory combination, analgesic, antihistamine.

Tylenol Regular Strength. (McNeil Consumer) Acetaminophen 325 mg. **Tab.:** Tin 12s. Vial 12s. Bot. 24s, 50s, 100s, 200s. **Capl.:** Bot. 24s, 50s. *OTC.*
Use: Analgesic.

Tylenol Severe Allergy. (McNeil Consumer) Diphenhydramine hydrochloride 12.5 mg, acetaminophen 500 mg. Tab. Pkg. 24s. *OTC.*
Use: Upper respiratory combination, analgesic, antihistamine.

Tylenol Sinus Night Time, Maximum Strength. (McNeil Consumer) Pseudoephedrine hydrochloride 30 mg, doxylamine succinate 6.25 mg, acetaminophen 500 mg. Tab. Pkg. 24s. *OTC.*
Use: Upper respiratory combination, decongestant, antihistamine, analgesic.

Tylenol Sinus Non-Drowsy Maximum Strength. (McNeil) Pseudoephedrine

hydrochloride 30 mg, acetaminophen 500 mg. Tab. Pkg. 24s. Gelcap, Geltab. Bot. 24s, 48s, 60s. *OTC.*
Use: Upper respiratory combination, decongestant, analgesic.

Tylenol Sinus Severe Congestion. (McNeil) Pseudoephedrine hydrochloride 30 mg, guaifenesin 200 mg, acetaminophen 325 mg. Tab. 24s. *OTC.*
Use: Decongestant, expectorant.

Tylenol with Codeine. (Ortho-McNeil) **Tab.:** Acetaminophen 300 mg with codeine phosphate. **No. 2:** Codeine phosphate 15 mg. Bot. 100s, 500s. **No. 3:** Codeine phosphate 30 mg. Bot. 100s, 500s, 1000s, UD 100s. **No. 4:** Codeine phosphate 60 mg. Bot. 100s, 500s, UD 500s. *c-III.*
Use: Analgesic combination; narcotic.

Tylenol with Codeine. (Ortho-McNeil) Acetaminophen 120 mg, codeine phosphate 12 mg/5 mL w/alcohol 7%. Elix. Bot. 480 mL. *c-V.*
Use: Analgesic combination; narcotic.

Tylosterone. (Eli Lilly) Diethylstilbestrol 0.25 mg, methyltestosterone 5 mg. Tab. Bot. 100s. *Rx.*
Use: Androgen, estrogen combination.

Tylox. (Ortho-McNeil) Oxycodone hydrochloride 5 mg, acetaminophen 500 mg. Cap. Bot. 100s, UD 100s. *c-II.*
Use: Analgesic combination; narcotic.

•**tyloxapol.** (till-OX-ah-pahl) *USP 28.*
Use: Detergent, ophthalmic; cystic fibrosis. [Orphan Drug]
See: Enuclene.

Tympagesic. (Pharmacia) Phenylephrine hydrochloride 0.25%, antipyrine 5%, benzocaine 5%, in propylene glycol. Liq. Bot. w/dropper 13 mL. *Rx.*
Use: Antihistamine, otic.

Typhim Vi. (Aventis Pasteur) Typhoid purified Vi polysaccharide vaccine 25 mcg/ 0.5 mL, sodium chloride 4.15 mg, disodium phosphate 0.065 mg, monosodium phosphate 0.023 mg, Sterile Water for Injection 0.5 mL. Inj. Syringes 0.5 mL, vial 20 dose, 50 dose. *Rx.*
Use: Immunization, typhoid.

•**typhoid vaccine.** (TIE-foyd) USAN.
Use: Immunization.
See: Vivotif Berna.

•**typhoid vi polysaccharide vaccine.** USAN.
Use: Immunization.
See: Typhim Vi.

Tyrex-2. (Ross) Protein 30 g, fat 15.5 g, carbohydrates 30 g, Na 880 mg, K 1370 mg, Cal 410/100 g. With appropriate vitamins and minerals. Phenylala-

nine and tyrosine free. Pow. Can 325 g. *OTC.*
Use: Nutritional supplement.

Tyrodone. (Major) Hydrocodone bitartrate 5 mg, pseudoephedrine hydrochloride 60 mg/5 mL, alcohol 5%. Liq. Bot. 473 mL. *c-III.*
Use: Antitussive; decongestant.

Tyromex-1. (Ross) Protein 15 g, fat 23.9 g, carbohydrates 46.3 g, linoleic acid 1800 mg, Fe 9 mg, Na 190 mg, K 675 mg, Cal 480/100 g. With appropriate vitamins and minerals. Phenylalanine, tyrosine, and methionine free. Pow. Can 350 g. *OTC.*
Use: Nutritional supplement.

•**tyropanoate sodium.** (TIE-row-PAN-oh-ate) *USP 28.*
Use: Diagnostic aid (radiopaque medium, cholecystographic).

tyropaque caps. (Sanofi-Synthelabo) Tyropanoate sodium. *Rx.*
Use: Oral cholecystographic medium.

•**tyrosine.** (TIE-row-SEEN) *USP 28.* L-Tyrosine.
Use: Amino acid.

tyrosine hydroxylase inhibitor.
Use: Antihypertensive.
See: Demser.

Tyrosum Skin Cleanser. (Summers) Isopropanol 50%, polysorbate 80 2%, and acetone 10%. Bot. 120 mL, pt. Towelettes 24s, 50s. *OTC.*
Use: Dermatologic, cleanser.

Tyzine. (Kenwood) Tetrahydrozoline hydrochloride 0.1%, benzalkonium chloride, EDTA. Soln. Bot. 30 mL with dropper. Spray bot. 15 mL. *Rx.*
Use: Nasal decongestant, imidazoline.

Tyzine Pediatric. (Kenwood) Tetrahydrozoline hydrochloride 0.05%, benzalkonium chloride, EDTA. Soln. Dropper bot. 15 mL. *Rx.*
Use: Nasal decongestant, imidazoline.

U

UAA. (Econo Med Pharmaceuticals) Methenamine 40.8 mg, phenyl salicylate 18.1 mg, methylene blue 5.4 mg, benzoic acid 4.5 mg, atropine sulfate 0.03 mg, hyoscyamine 0.03 mg. Tab. Bot. 100s, 1000s. *Rx.*
Use: Anti-infective, urinary.

UAD Cream. (Forest) Clioquinol 3%, hydrocortisone 1%, ceresin, glyceryl oleate, propylene glycol, parabens, mineral oil, pramoxine Cream. Tube. hydrochloride. 15 g. *Rx.*
Use: Corticosteroid; anesthetic, local.

UAD Lotion. (Forest) Clioquinol 0.75%, hydrocortisone 0.25%, cetyl alcohol, glyceryl stearate, lanolin, parabens, mineral oil, pramoxine hydrochloride, propylene glycol. Lot. Bot. 20 mL. *Rx.*
Use: Corticosteroid; anesthetic, local.

UAD Otic. (Forest) Hydrocortisone 1%, neomycin sulfate 5 mg, polymyxin B sulfate 10,000 units/mL, thimersol 0.01%, cetyl alcohol, propylene glycol, polysorbate 80. Susp. Bot. 10 mL w/dropper. *Rx.*
Use: Corticosteroid, otic.

•**ubidecarenone.** *NF 23.*
Use: Dietary supplement.

UBT. (Biomerica) For detection of blood in the urine.
Use: Diagnostic aid.

UCG-Beta Slide Monoclonal II. (Wampole) Two-minute latex agglutination inhibition slide test for the qualitative detection of B-hCG/hCG (sensitivity 0.5 units hCG/mL) in urine. Kit 50s, 100s, 300s.
Use: Diagnostic aid.

UCG-Beta Stat. (Wampole) One-hour passive hemagglutination inhibition tube test for the qualitative detection and quantitative determination of B-hCG/hCG (sensitivity 0.2 units hCG/mL) in urine. Kit 50s, 300s.
Use: Diagnostic aid.

UCG-Lyphotest. (Wampole) One-hour passive hemagglutination inhibition tube test for the qualitative or quantitative determination of human chorionic gonadotropin (sensitivity 0.5-1 units hCG/mL) in urine. Kit 10s, 50s, 300s.
Use: Diagnostic aid.

UCG-Slide Test. (Wampole) Rapid latex agglutination inhibition slide test for the qualitative detection of human chorionic gonadotropin (Sensitivity: 2 units hCG/mL) in urine. Kit 30s, 100s, 300s, 1000s.
Use: Diagnostic aid.

UCG-Test. (Wampole) Two-hour hemagglutination inhibition tube test for the determination of human chorionic gonadotropin (sensitivity 0.5 units hCG/mL undiluted specimen; 1.5 units hCG/mL 1:3 diluted specimen) in urine and serum. Kit 10s, 25s, 100s, 300s.
Use: Diagnostic aid.

UCG-Titration Set. (Wampole) Two-hour hemagglutination inhibition tube test for the determination of human chorionic gonadotropin (sensitivity 1 units hCG/mL) in urine or serum. Kit 45s.
Use: Diagnostic aid.

U-cort. (Taro) Hydrocortisone acetate 1%. Urea 10%, alcohol, EDTA. Cream. 28.35 g, 7 g. *Rx.*
Use: Anti-inflammatory.

Uendex. Dextran sulfate, inhaled, aerosolized.
Use: Cystic fibrosis treatment. [Orphan Drug]

Ulcerease. (Med-Derm) Liquified phenol 0.6%, glycerin, sugar free. Liq. Bot. 180 mL. *OTC.*
Use: Anesthetic, local.

Ulcerin. (Sanofi-Synthelabo) Aluminum hydroxide. Tab. *OTC.*
Use: Antacid.

Ulcerin P. (Sanofi-Synthelabo) Aluminum hydroxide. Tab. *OTC.*
Use: Antacid.

•**uldazepam.** (uhl-DAY-zeh-pam) USAN.
Use: Hypnotic; sedative.

Ulpax. (Roche) Ablukast sodium.
Use: Antiasthmatic (leukotriene antagonist).

Ultane. (Abbott) Sevoflurane. Bot. 250 mL. *Rx.*
Use: Anesthetic, general, volatile liquid.

Ultiva. (Abbott) Remifentanil hydrochloride (as base) 1 mg (3 mL vials), 2 mg (5 mL vials), 5 mg (10 mL vials), preservative free. Glycine 15 mg. Pow. for Inj. *c-ii.*
Use: Opioid analgesic.

Ultrabex. (Health for Life Brands) Vitamins B, 20 mg, C 50 mg, B_2 2 mg, B_6 0.5 mg, niacinamide 35 mg, calcium pantothenate 0.5 mg, wheat germ oil 30 mg, B_{12} 20 mcg, liver desiccated 150 mg, iron 11.58 mg, calcium 29 mg, phosphorus 23 mg, dicalcium phosphate 100 mg, magnesium 1.11 mg, manganese 1.3 mg, potassium 2.24 mg, zinc 0.68 mg, choline 25 mg, inositol 25 mg, pepsin 32.5 mg, diastase 32.5 mg, hesperidin 25 mg, biotin 20 mcg, hydrolyzed yeast 81.25 mg, protein digest 47.04 mg, amino acids 34.21 mg. Cap. Bot. 50s, 100s, 1000s.

OTC.
Use: Mineral, vitamin supplement.
Ultra B-50. (NBTY) Vitamins B$_1$ 50 mg,
B$_2$ 50 mg, B$_3$ 50 mg, B$_5$ 50 mg, B$_6$
50 mg, B$_{12}$ 50 mcg, folic acid 0.1 mg,
PABA 50 mg, inositol 50 mg, biotin
50 mcg, choline 50 mg, lecithin 50 mg.
Tab. Bot. 60s, 180s. *OTC.*
Use: Vitamin supplement.
Ultra B-100. (NBTY) Vitamins B$_1$ 100 mg,
B$_2$ 100 mg, B$_3$ 100 mg, B$_5$ 100 mg, B$_6$
100 mg, B$_{12}$ 100 mcg, folic acid
0.1 mg, PABA 100 mg, inositol 100 mg,
biotin 100 mcg, choline bitartrate
100 mg. TR Tab. Bot. 50s. *OTC.*
Use: Vitamin supplement.
ULTRAbrom. (WE Pharmaceuticals)
Brompheniramine maleate 12 mg,
pseudoephedrine hydrochloride
120 mg. ER Cap. Bot. 100s, dispenser
pack 10s. *Rx.*
Use: Upper respiratory combination, antihistamine, decongestant.
ULTRAbrom PD. (WE Pharmaceuticals)
Brompheniramine maleate 6 mg,
pseudoephedrine 60 mg. ER Cap. Bot.
100s. *Rx.*
Use: Upper respiratory combination, antihistamine, decongestant.
Ultracal. (Bristol-Myers Squibb) Protein
44 g, carbohydrate 123 g, fat 45 g, Na
930 mg, K 1610 mg, mOsm 310 kg
H$_2$O, 1.06 cal/mL, vitamins A, B$_1$, B$_2$,
B$_3$, B$_5$, B$_6$, B$_{12}$, C, D, E, K, folic acid,
choline, biotin, Ca, P, I, Fe, Mg, Cu,
Zn, Mn, Cl, Se, Cr, Mo. Liq. Can. 8 oz.
OTC.
Use: Nutritional supplement.
Ultra Cap. (Weeks & Leo) Acetaminophen 300 mg, guaifenesin 100 mg,
chlorpheniramine maleate 4 mg,
phenylephrine hydrochloride 10 mg,
dextromethorphan HBr 6 mg. Cap. Vial
18s. *Rx.*
Use: Analgesic; antihistamine; antitussive; decongestant; expectorant.
Ultra-Care. (Allergan) **Disinfecting
Soln.:** Hydrogen peroxide 3%, sodium
stannate, sodium nitrate, phosphate
buffer. Bot. 120 mL, 360 mL. **Neutralizer Tab.:** Catalase, hydroxypropyl
methylcellulose, buffering agents. Pkg.
12s, 36s w/cup. *OTC.*
Use: Contact lens care.
Ultracet. (Ortho-McNeil) Tramadol hydrochloride 37.5 mg, acetaminophen
325 mg. Tab. Bot. 20s, 100s, 500s, UD
100s. *Rx.*
Use: Nonnarcotic analgesic combination.

Ultracortinol. (Novartis) Agent to suppress overactive adrenal glands. Pending release.
Ultra Freeda. (Freeda) Vitamins A
4166 units, D 133 units, E 66.7 mg, B$_1$
16.7 mg, B$_2$ 16.7 mg, B$_3$ 33 mg, B$_5$
33 mg, B$_6$ 16.7 mg, B$_{12}$ 33 mcg, C
333 mg, folic acid 0.27 mg, iron 2 mg,
calcium 27 mg, zinc 1.1 mg, choline,
inositol, bioflavonoids, PABA, biotin
100 mcg, Cr, I, K, Mg, Mn, Mo, Se. Tab.
Bot. 90s, 180s, 270s. *OTC.*
Use: Mineral, vitamin supplement.
Ultra Freeda Iron Free. (Freeda) Vitamins A 4166 units, D 133 units, E$_2$
66.7 mg, B$_1$ 16.7 mg, B$_2$ 16.7 mg, B$_3$
33 mg, B$_5$ 33 mg, B$_6$ 16.7 mg, B$_{12}$
33 mcg, C 333 mg, FA 0.27 mg, Ca
27 mg, Zn 1.1 mg, choline, inositol, bioflavonoids, PABA, biotin 100 mcg, Cr,
I, K, Mg, Mn, Mo, Se. Tab. Bot. 90s,
180s, 270s. *OTC.*
Use: Mineral, vitamin supplement.
Ultragesic. (Stewart-Jackson Pharmacal) Acetaminophen 500 mg, hydrocodone bitartrate 5 mg. Cap. Bot. 100s.
c-III.
Use: Analgesic combination; narcotic.
Ultralan. (Elan) Protein 60 g, fat 50 g,
carbohydrates 202 g, Na 1.035 g, K
1.755 g/L. Lactose free. With appropriate vitamins and minerals. Liq. In
1000 mL *New Pak* systems w/and w/o
ColorCheck. OTC.
Use: Nutritional supplement.
ultralente insulin.
See: Iletin.
Ultram. (Ortho-McNeil) Tramadol hydrochloride 50 mg, lactose. Film coated.
Tab. Bot. 100s, 500s, UD 100s. *Rx.*
Use: Opioid analgesic.
Ultra Mide 25. (Baker Cummins Dermatologicals) Bot. 8 oz. *OTC.*
Use: Emollient.
Ultra-Natal. (Ethex) Iron (carbonyl iron)
90 mg, iodine (potassium iodide)
150 mg, calcium citrate 200 mg, cupric oxide 2 mg, zinc oxide 25 mg, folic
acid 1 mg, vitamins A 2700 units, D$_3$
400 units, E 30 units, C 120 mg, B$_1$
3 mg, B$_2$ 3.4 mg, B$_6$ 20 mg, B$_{12}$ 12 mcg,
niacinamide 20 mg, docusate sodium,
dye free. Tab. UD 100s. *Rx.*
Use: Vitamin, mineral supplement.
Ultra-NatalCare. (Ethex) Ca 200 mg, Fe
(as carbonyl iron) 90 mg, vitamin A
2700 units, D$_3$ 400 units, E (dl-alpha-
tocopheryl acetate) 30 units, B$_1$ 3 mg,
B$_2$ 3.4 mg, B$_3$ 20 mg, B$_6$ 20 mg, B$_{12}$
12 mcg, C 120 mg, folic acid 1 mg, Zn
25 mg, Cu, I, docusate sodium 50 mg.
Tab. UD 100s. *Rx.*

Use: Vitamin, mineral supplement.

Ultrapred. (Horizon) Prednisolone acetate 1%. Susp. Bot. 5 mL. *Rx.*
Use: Corticosteroid, ophthalmic.

Ultrase. (Axcan Scandipharm) Lipase 4500 units, amylase 20,000 units, protease 25,000 units, sugar. Cap. Bot. 100s. *Rx.*
Use: Digestive enzyme.

Ultrase MT 18. (Axcan Scandipharm) Lipase 18,000 units, protease 58,500 units, amylase 58,500 units. Cap. Bot. 100s. *Rx.*
Use: Digestive enzyme.

Ultrase MT 12. (Axcan Scandipharm) Lipase 12,000 units, amylase 39,000 units, protease 39,000 units. Cap. Bot. 100s. *Rx.*
Use: Digestive enzyme.

Ultrase MT 20. (Axcan Scandipharm) Lipase 20,000 units, protease 65,000 units, amylase 65,000 units. Cap. Bot. 100s, 500s. *Rx.*
Use: Digestive enzyme.

Ultrasone. (Gordon Laboratories) Ultrasound aid. Bot. qt, gal. Plastic Bot. 8 oz.
Use: Ultrasound contact cream.

Ultra Tears. (Alcon) Hydroxypropyl methylcellulose 2910 1%, benzalkonium Cl 0.01%, NaCl. Bot. 15 mL. *OTC.*
Use: Artificial tears.

Ultravate. (Bristol-Myers Squibb) Halobetasol propionate. *Rx.*
Use: Corticosteroid, topical.

Ultravist 150. (Berlex) Iopromide 311.7 mg, iodine 150 mg/mL, EDTA. Inj. Vial 50 mL. *Rx.*
Use: Radiopaque, parenteral.

Ultravist 300. (Berlex) Iopromide 623.4 mg, iodine 300 mg/mL, EDTA. Inj. Vial 50 mL, 100 mL, 150 mL. *Rx.*
Use: Radiopaque, parenteral.

Ultravist 370. (Berlex) Iopromide 768.86 mg, iodine 370 mg/mL, EDTA. Inj. Vial 50 mL, 100 mL, 150 mL. 200 mL fill in 250 mL vial. *Rx.*
Use: Radiopaque, parenteral.

Ultravist 240. (Berlex) Iopromide 498.72 mg, iodine 240 mg/mL, EDTA. Inj. Vial 50 mL, 100 mL fill in 250 mL vial. *Rx.*
Use: Radiopaque, parenteral.

Ultra Vitamin A & D. (NBTY) Vitamins A 25,000 units, D 1000 units. Tab. Bot. 100s. *OTC.*
Use: Vitamin supplement.

Ultra Vita Time. (NBTY) Iron 6 mg, vitamins A 10,000 units, D 400 units, E 13 units, B_1 25 mg, B_2 25 mg, B_3

50 mg, B_5 12.5 mg, B_6 15 mg, B_{12} 50 mcg, C 150 mg, folic acid 0.4 mg, B, Ca, Cr, Cu, I, K, Mg, Mn, Mo, P, Se, Zn 5 mg, biotin 1 mg, bioflavonoids, bone meal, PABA, choline bitartrate, betaine, inositol, lecithin, desiccated liver, rutin. Tab. Bot. 100s. *OTC.*
Use: Mineral, vitamin supplement.

Ultrazyme Enzymatic Cleaner. (Allergan) Subtilisin A, effervescing, buffering, and tableting agents for dilution in hydrogen peroxide 3%. Tab. Pkg. 5s, 10s, 15s, 20s. *OTC.*
Use: Contact lens care.

Ultrum. (Towne) Vitamins A 5000 units, E 30 units, C 90 mg, folic acid 400 mcg, B_1 2.25 mg, B_2 2.6 mg, niacinamide 20 mg, B_6 3 mg, B_{12} 9 mcg, biotin 45 mcg, D 400 units, pantothenic acid 10 mg, calcium 162 mg, phosphorus 125 mg, iodine 150 mcg, iron 27 mg, magnesium 100 mg, copper 3 mg, manganese 7.5 mg, potassium 7.5 mg, zinc 22.5 mg. Tab. Bot. 100s. *OTC.*
Use: Mineral, vitamin supplement.

Ultrum with Selenium. (Towne) Vitamins A 5000 units, E 30 units, C 90 mg, folic acid 2.25 mg, B_1 2.25 mg, B_2 2.6 mg, niacinamide 20 mg, B_6 3 mg, B_{12} 9 mcg, D 400 units, biotin 45 mcg, pantothenic acid 10 mg, calcium 162 mg, phosphorus 125 mg, iodine 150 mcg, iron 27 mg, magnesium 100 mg, copper 3 mg, manganese 7.5 mg, potassium 7.7 mg, chloride 7 mg, molybdenum 15 mcg, selenium 15 mcg, zinc 22.5 mg. Tab. Bot. 130s. *Rx.*
Use: Mineral, vitamin supplement.

Umecta. (JSJ) Urea. **Emulsion:** 40%. Helianthus annuus oil, EDTA. 113.5 g. **Top. Susp.:** 40%. Helianthus annuus oil, EDTA. 283.4 g. *Rx.*
Use: Emollient.

UN-Aspirin, Extra Strength. (Zee Medical) Acetaminophen 500 mg. Tab. 24s. *OTC.*
Use: Analgesic.

Unasyn. (Roerig) Ampicillin sodium 1 g, sulbactam sodium 0.5 g; ampicillin sodium 2 g, sulbactam sodium 1 g; ampicillin sodium 10 g, sulbactam sodium 5 g. Pow. for Inj. Vial, bottles. *ADD-Vantage* vial (except 10 g), bulk pkg. (10 g only). *Rx.*
Use: Anti-infective, penicillin.

• **undecanoate.** (un-DEK-a-NOE-ate) USAN.
Use: Antifungal.

• **10-undecenoic acid.** *USP 28.* Undecylenic Acid.
Use: Antifungal, topical.
• **10-undecenoic acid, zinc (2+) salt.** *USP 28.* Zinc Undecylenate.
Use: Antifungal, topical.
undecoylium chloride-iodine. (Ruson) Virac, Preps.
Use: Anti-infective, topical.
• **undecylenic acid.** (un-deh-sill-EN-ik) *USP 28.*
Use: Antifungal, topical.
See: Desenex.
Elon Dual Defense Antifungal Formula.
Gordochom.
W/Dichlorophene.
See: Fungicidal Talc.
Onychomycetin.
W/Salicylic acid.
See: Fungicidal.
W/Zinc undecylenate.
See: Desenex.
undecylenic acid salts. Calcium, copper, zinc.
Undelenic Ointment. (Gordon Laboratories) Undecylenic acid 5%, zinc undecylenate 20%. Jar, lb. *OTC.*
Use: Antifungal, topical.
Undelenic Tincture. (Gordon Laboratories) Undecylenic acid 10%, chloroxylenol 0.5%. Brush Bot. oz. Bot. pt. *OTC.*
Use: Antifungal, topical.
Unguentine Maximum Strength. (Lee) Benzocaine 5%, resorcinol 2%. Alcohols, methylparaben, mineral oil. Cream. 28.3 g. *OTC.*
Use: Local anesthetic, topical.
Unguentine Ointment "Original Formula". (Mentholatum Co.) Phenol 1% in ointment base. Tube oz. *OTC.*
Use: Dermatologic; counterirritant.
Unguentine Plus First Aid Cream. (Mentholatum Co.) Parachlorometaxylenol 2%, lidocaine hydrochloride 2%, phenol 0.5% in a moisturizing cream base. Tube 0.5 oz, 1 oz, 2 oz. *OTC.*
Use: Dermatologic; counterirritant.
Uni-Ace. (United Research Laboratories) Acetaminophen 100 mg/mL, alcohol free. Liq. Bot. 15 mL with dropper. *OTC.*
Use: Analgesic.
Unibase. (Parke-Davis) Water-absorbing oint. base. Jar lb. *Rx.*
Use: Pharmaceutical aid; ointment base.
Unicap. (Pharmacia) **Cap.:** Vitamins A 5000 units, D 400 units, E 30 units, B_1 1.5 mg, B_2 1.7 mg, B_3 20 mg, B_6 2 mg, B_{12} 6 mcg, C 60 mg, FA 0.4 mg. Bot. 120s. **Tab.:** Vitamins A 5000 units, D

400 units, E 15 units, B_1 1.5 mg, B_2 1.7 mg, B_3 20 mg, B_6 2 mg, B_{12} 6 mcg, C 60 mg, FA 0.4 mg. Tab. Bot. 120s. *OTC.*
Use: Vitamin supplement.
Unicap Jr. Chewable. (Pharmacia) Vitamins A 5000 units, D 400 units, E 15 units, C 60 mg, folic acid 400 mcg, B_1 1.5 mg, B_2 1.7 mg, B_3 20 mg, B_6 2 mg, B_{12} 6 mcg. Tab. Bot. 120s. *OTC.*
Use: Vitamin supplement.
Unicap M. (Pharmacia) Iron 18 mg, vitamins A 5000 units, D 400 units, E 30 units, B_1 1.5 mg, B_2 1.7 mg, B_3 20 mg, B_5 10 mg, B_6 2 mg, B_{12} 6 mcg, C 60 mg, folic acid 0.4 mg, Ca, Cu, I, K, Mn, P, Zn 15 mg, tartrazine. Tab. Bot. 120s. *OTC.*
Use: Mineral, vitamin supplement.
Unicap Plus Iron. (Pharmacia) Vitamins A 5000 units, D 400 units, E 30 units, C 60 mg, folic acid 0.4 mg, B_1 1.5 mg, B_2 1.7 mg, B_3 20 mg, B_5 10 mg, B_6 2 mg, B_{12} 6 mcg, iron 22.5 mg, Ca. Tab. Bot. 120s. *OTC.*
Use: Mineral, vitamin supplement.
Unicap Sr. (Pharmacia) Iron 10 mg, vitamins A 5000 units, D 200 units, E 15 units, B_1 1.2 mg, B_2 1.4 mg, B_3 16 mg, B_5 10 mg, B_6 2.2 mg, B_{12} 3 mcg, C 60 mg, folic acid 0.4 mg, Ca, Cu, I, K, Mg, Mn, P, Zn 15 mg. Tab. Bot. 120s. *OTC.*
Use: Mineral, vitamin supplement.
Unicap T. (Pharmacia) Iron 18 mg, vitamins A 5000 units, D 400 units, E 30 units, B_1 10 mg, B_2 20 mg, B_3 100 mg, B_5 25 mg, B_6 6 mg, B_{12} 18 mcg, C 500 mg, folic acid 0.4 mg, Cu, I, K, Mn, Se, Zn 15 mg, tartrazine. Tab. Bot. 60s. *OTC.*
Use: Mineral, vitamin supplement.
Unicomplex-M. (Rugby) Iron 18 mg, vitamins A 5000 units, D 400 units, E 15 units, B_1 1.5 mg, B_2 1.7 mg, B_3 20 mg, B_5 10 mg, B_6 2 mg, B_{12} 6 mcg, C 60 mg, folic acid 0.4 mg, Ca, Cu, I, K, Mn, Zn. Tab. Bot. 90s, 1000s. *OTC.*
Use: Mineral, vitamin supplement.
Unicomplex-T & M. (Rugby) Iron 18 mg, vitamins A 5000 units, D 400 units, E 30 mg, B_1 10 mg, B_2 10 mg, B_3 100 mg, B_5 25 mg, B_6 6 mg, B_{12} 18 mcg, C 500 mg, FA 0.4 mg, Ca, Cu, I, K, Mn, Zn 15 mg. Tab. Bot. 60s. *OTC.*
Use: Mineral, vitamin supplement.
Unicomplex-T with Minerals. (Rugby) Iron 10 mg, vitamins A 5000 units, D 400 units, E 15 units, B_1 10 mg, B_2 10 mg, B_3 100 mg, B_5 20 mg, B_6 2 mg, B_{12} 4 mcg, C 300 mg, folic acid

0.4 mg, Ca, Cu, I, K, Mg, Mn. Tab. Bot. 60s. *OTC.*
Use: Mineral, vitamin supplement.
Unifed. (Altaire) Pseudoephedrine hydrochloride 30 mg per 5 mL. Methylparaben, glycerin, sorbitol, sucrose. Liq. 118 mL. *OTC.*
Use: Nasal decongestant.
Unifiber. (Niche) Powdered cellulose. Pow. Bot. 150 g, 270 g, 480 g. *OTC.*
Use: Laxative.
•**unifocon a.** (you-nih-FOE-kahn A) USAN.
Use: Contact lens material (hydrophic).
Uniphyl. (Purdue) Theophylline. CR Tab. **200 mg:** Bot. 60s, 100s, UD 100s. **400 mg:** Bot. 60s, 100s, 500s, UD 100s. **600 mg:** Bot. 100s. *Rx.*
Use: Bronchodilator.
Uniretic. (Schwarz Pharma) Moexipril hydrochloride 7.5 mg/hydrochlorothiazide 12.5 mg, moexipril hydrochloride 15 mg/hydrochlorothiazide 12.5 mg, moexipril hydrochloride 15 mg/hydrochlorothiazide 25 mg, lactose. Tab. Bot. 100s. *Rx.*
Use: Antihypertensive.
Unisol. (Alcon) Buffered isotonic solution with sodium Cl, boric acid, sodium borate. Bot. 15 mL (25s), 120 mL (2s, 3s). *OTC.*
Use: Contact lens care.
Unisol 4 Sterile Saline. (Alcon) Buffered isotonic solution with sodium Cl, boric acid, sodium borate. Bot. 120 mL. *OTC.*
Use: Contact lens care.
Unisol Plus. (Alcon) Buffered isotonic solution w/NaCl, boric acid, sodium borate. Aerosol Bot. 240 mL, 360 mL. *OTC.*
Use: Contact lens care.
Unisom Nighttime Sleep-Aid. (Pfizer) Doxylamine succinate 25 mg. Tab. Blister Pack 8s, 16s, 32s, 48s. *OTC.*
Use: Sleep aid.
Unisom with Pain Relief. (Pfizer) Acetaminophen 650 mg, diphenhydramine hydrochloride 50 mg. Tab. Blister Pack 16s. *OTC.*
Use: Analgesic; sleep aid.
Unithroid. (Lannett) Levothyroxine sodium 0.025 mg, 0.05 mg, 0.075 mg, 0.088 mg, 0.1 mg, 0.112 mg, 0.125 mg, 0.15 mg, 0.175 mg, 0.2 mg, 0.3 mg, lactose. Tab. Bot. 100s, 1000s. *Rx.*
Use: Hormone, thyroid.
Uni-Tussin DM. (United Research Laboratories) Dextromethorphan HBr 10 mg, guaifenesin 100 mg/5 mL. Syr. Bot. 118 mL. *OTC.*
Use: Antitussive; expectorant.

Univasc. (Schwarz Pharma) Moexipril hydrochloride 7.5 mg, 15 mg, lactose. Film-coated. Tab. Bot. 100s, unit-of-use 90s. *Rx.*
Use: Antihypertensive; renin angiotensin system antagonist; angiotensin-converting enzyme inhibitor.
unna's boot.
See: Zinc Gelatin.
Unproco Capsules. (Solvay) Dextromethorphan HBr 30 mg, guaifenesin 200 mg. Cap. Bot. 100s. *OTC.*
Use: Antitussive; expectorant.
Uplex. (Arcum) Vitamins A 5000 units, D 400 units, B_1 3 mg, B_2 3 mg, B_6 1 mg, B_{12} 2.5 mcg, nicotinamide 20 mg, calcium pantothenate 5 mg, C 50 mg. Cap. Bot. 100s, 1000s. *OTC.*
Use: Mineral, vitamin supplement.
Uplex No. 2. (Arcum) Vitamins A palmitate 10,000 units, D 400 units, B_1 5 mg, B_2 5 mg, C 100 mg, B_6 2 mg, B_{12} 3 mcg, E 2.5 units, niacinamide 25 mg, calcium pantothenate 5 mg. Cap. Bot. 100s, 1000s. *OTC.*
Use: Mineral, vitamin supplement.
upper respiratory combinations.
See: Analgesic and Antihistamine Combinations.
  Analgesic and Decongestant Combinations.
  Analgesic, Antihistamine, and Decongestant Combinations.
  Analgesic, Antihistamine, Antitussive, and Decongestant Combinations.
  Analgesic, Antitussive, Decongestant, and Expectorant Combinations.
  Anticholinergic, Antihistamine, and Decongestant Combinations.
  Anticholinergic, Antihistamine, Antitussive, and Decongestant Combinations.
  Antihistamine and Decongestant Combinations.
  Antihistamine, Antitussive, and Decongestant Combinations.
  Antihistamine, Antitussive, Decongestant, and Expectorant Combinations.
  Antihistamine, Decongestant, and Expectorant Combinations.
  Antitussive and Expectorant Combinations.
  Antitussive, Decongestant, and Expectorant Combinations.
  Decongestant and Expectorant Combinations.
Urabeth Tabs. (Major) Bethanechol 5 mg, 10 mg, 25 mg, 50 mg. Tab. **5 mg:** Bot. 100s. **10 mg:** Bot. 250s. **25 mg:** Bot. 250s, 1000s. **50 mg:** Bot. 100s, UD

100s. *Rx.*
Use: Genitourinary.
Uracid. (Wesley) dl-Methionine 0.2 g.
Cap. Bot. 100s, 1000s. *Rx.*
Use: Diaper rash preparation.
•**uracil.** (YOUR-ah-sil) USAN.
Use: Potentiator in tegafur therapy.
uradal.
See: Carbromal.
•**urea.** (you-REE-ah) *USP 28.*
Use: Topically for dry skin; diuretic.
See: Aquacare.
Aquacare-HP.
Artra Ashy Skin.
Calmurid.
Carmol.
Carmol 40.
Carmol Ten.
Elaqua 10% or 20%.
Gormel.
Keralac.
Keralac Nail Gel.
Nutraplus.
Rea-lo.
Umecta.
Vanamide.
W/Benzocaine, benzyl alcohol, p-chloro-m-xylenol, propylene glycol.
See: Carmol-HC.
W/Glycerin.
See: Akne Drying Lotion.
W/Papain.
See: Accuzyme.
Ethezyme 830.
Gladase.
Gladase-C.
Panafil.
urea. (Hi-Tech) Urea. **Cream:** 40%. Mineral oil, petrolatum, cetyl alcohol. 28.35 g, 198.6 g. **Lot.:** 40%. Mineral oil, petrolatum, cetyl alcohol. 236.6 mL. *Rx.*
Use: Emollient.
•**urea.** (River's Edge) Urea 35%. Cetyl alcohol, EDTA, lactic acid. Lot. 207 mL, 325 mL. *Rx.*
Use: Emollient.
•**urea C 14.** (yoor-EE-a) *USP 28.*
Ureacin-10. (Pedinol Pharmacal) Urea 10%. Lot. Bot. 8 oz. *OTC.*
Use: Emollient.
Ureacin-20 Creme. (Pedinol Pharmacal) Urea 20%. Cream. Jar 2.5 oz. *OTC.*
Use: Emollient.
•**urea C 13.** (yoor-EE-a) *USP 28.*
urea peroxide.
See: Gly-Oxide.
Proxigel.
Ureaphil. (Abbott Hospital Products) Sterile urea 40 g, citric acid 1 mg/

150 mL. Bot. 150 mL. *Rx.*
Use: Diuretic.
Urecholine. (Odyssey) Bethanechol chloride 25 mg, lactose. Tab. 100s. *Rx.*
Use: Urinary cholinergic.
•**uredepa.** (YOU-ree-DEH-pah) USAN.
Use: Antineoplastic.
See: Avinar.
ureides.
Use: Sedative/hypnotic, nonbarbiturate.
See: Acetylcarbromal.
p-ureidobenzenearsonic acid.
See: Carbarsone.
Urelief. (Rocky Mtn.) Methenamine 2 g, salol 0.5 g, methylene blue 1/10 g, benzoic acid g, hyoscyamine sulfate g, atropine sulfate g. Tab. Bot. 100s. *Rx.*
Use: Anti-infective, urinary.
Urelle. (Pharmelle) Methenamine 81 mg, sodium phosphate monobasic 40.8 mg, phenyl salicylate 32.4 mg, methylene blue 10.8 mg, hyoscyamine sulfate 0.12 mg, sugar, mineral oil. Tab. 90s. *Rx.*
Use: Anti-infective, urinary.
Urese. (Roerig)
See: Benzthiazide.
urethan. Ethyl Carbamate, Ethyl Urethan, Urethane.
Use: Antineoplastic.
Uretron D/S. (Marin) Methenamine 120 mg, sodium biphosphonate 40.8 mg, phenyl salicylate 36.2 mg, methylene blue 10.8 mg, hyoscyamine sulfate 0.12 mg, parabens, sucrose. Tab. 100s. *Rx.*
Use: Anti-infective, urinary.
Urex. (3M) Methenamine hippurate 1 g. Tab. Bot. 100s. *Rx.*
Use: Anti-infective, urinary.
Uric Acid Reagent Strips. (Bayer Corp. (Consumer Div.)) Seralyzer reagent strip. For uric acid in serum or plasma. Bot. 25s.
Use: Diagnostic aid.
uricosuric agents.
See: Anturane.
Benemid.
Uricult. (Orion) Urine culture test to detect bacteria and identify uropathogens. Bot. 10s.
Use: Diagnostic aid.
uridine, 2-deoxy-5-iodo. *USP 28.* Idoxuridine.
Uridon Modified. (Rugby) Methenamine 40.8 mg, phenyl salicylate 18.1 mg, atropine sulfate 0.03 mg, hyoscyamine 0.03 mg, benzoic acid 4.5 mg, methylene blue 5.4 mg. Tab. Bot. 100s, 1000s. *Rx.*
Use: Anti-infective, urinary.

Urifon-Forte. (T.E. Williams Pharmaceuticals) Sulfamethizole 450 mg, phenazopyridine hydrochloride 50 mg. Cap. Bot. 100s, 1000s. *Rx.*
Use: Anti-infective, urinary.

Urigen. (Fellows) Calcium mandelate 0.2 g, methenamine 0.2 g, phenazopyridine hydrochloride 50 mg, sodium phosphate 80 mg. Cap. Bot. 100s, 1000s. *Rx.*
Use: Anti-infective, urinary.

Urimar-T. (Marnel) Methenamine 81.6 mg, sodium biphosphate 40.8 mg, phenyl salicylate 36.2 mg, methylene blue 10.8 mg, hyoscyamine sulfate 0.12 mg. Tab. Bot. 100s. *Rx.*
Use: Anti-infective, urinary.

Urimax. (Integrity) Methenamine 81.6 mg, sodium biphosphate 40.8 mg, phenyl salicylate 36.2 mg, methylene blue 10.8 mg, hyoscyamine sulfate 0.12 mg. Tab. Bot. 100s. *Rx.*
Use: Urinary tract agent.

Urinary Antiseptic #3 S.C.T. (Teva) Atropine sulfate 0.06 mg, hyoscyamine sulfate 0.03 mg, methenamine 120 mg, methylene blue 6 mg, phenyl salicylate 30 mg, benzoic acid 7.5 mg. Tab. Bot. 100s, 1000s. *Rx.*
Use: Anti-infective, urinary.

Urinary Antiseptic #2. (Various Mfr.) Atropine sulfate 0.03 mg, hyoscyamine 0.03 mg, methenamine 40.8 mg, methylene blue 5.4 mg, phenyl salicylate 18.1 mg, benzoic acid 4.5 mg. Tab. Bot. 100s, 1000s. *Rx.*
Use: Anti-infective, urinary.

Urinary Antiseptic #2 S.C.T. (Teva) Atropine sulfate 0.03 mg, hyoscyamine sulfate 0.03 mg, methenamine 40.8 mg, methylene blue 5.4 mg, phenyl salicylate 18.1 mg, benzoic acid 4.5 mg. Tab. Bot. 100s, 1000s. *Rx.*
Use: Anti-infective, urinary.

urinary cholinergics.
See: Bethanechol Chloride.
Neostigmine Methylsulfate.

urine.
See: Diagnostic Agents.

urine glucose tests.
See: Biotel Diabetes.
Chemstrip uG.
Clinistix.
Clinitest.
Diastix.
Test Tape.

urine sugar test.
See: Clinistix.

urine tests, miscellaneous.
See: Answer One-Step Pregnancy Test.
Nitrazine Paper.

Urin-Tek. (Bayer Corp. (Consumer Div.)) Tubes, plastic caps, adhesive labels, collection cups, and disposable tube holder. Package 100 × 5.

Urisan-P. (Sandia) Atropine sulfate 0.03 mg, hyoscyamine 0.03 mg, gelsemium 6.1 mg, methenamine 40.8 mg, salol 18.1 mg, benzoic acid 4.5 mg, methylene blue 5.4 mg, phenylazo diamino pyridine hydrochloride 100 mg. Tab. Bot. 100s, 1000s. *Rx.*
Use: Anti-infective, urinary.

Urised. (PolyMedica) Atropine sulfate 0.03 mg, hyoscyamine 0.03 mg, methenamine 40.8 mg, methylene blue 5.4 mg, benzoic acid 4.5 mg, phenyl salicylate 18.1 mg. Tab. Bot. 100s, 500s. *Rx.*
Use: Anti-infective, urinary.

Urisedamine. (PolyMedica) Methenamine mandelate 500 mg, l-hyoscyamine 0.15 mg. Tab. Bot. 100s. *Rx.*
Use: Anti-infective, urinary.

Uriseptic. (SDA Labs) Methenamine 40.8 mg, phenyl salicylate 18.1 mg, methylene blue 5.4 mg, benzoic acid 4.5 mg, atropine sulfate 0.03 mg, hyoscyamine sulfate 0.03 mg. Tab. 100s. *Rx.*
Use: Anti-infective, urinary.

Urispas. (ALZA) Flavoxate hydrochloride 100 mg, castor oil. Tab. Bot. 100s, UD 100s. *Rx.*
Use: Anticholinergic.

Uristix. (Bayer Corp. (Consumer Div.)) Urine test for glucose and protein. Reagent strips. 100s.
Use: Diagnostic aid.

Uristix 4 Reagent Strips. (Bayer Corp. (Consumer Div.)) Urinalysis reagent strip test for glucose, protein, nitrite, leukocytes. Bot. 100s.
Use: Diagnostic aid.

Uristix Reagent Strips. (Bayer Corp. (Consumer Div.)) Urinalysis reagent strip test for protein and glucose. Bot. 100s.
Use: Diagnostic aid.

UriSym. (Vindex) Methenamine 100 mg, phenyl salicylate 40 mg, sodium bisphosphate 40.8 mg, methylene blue 10.8 mg, hyoscyamine sulfate 0.12 mg. Cap. 100s. *Rx.*
Use: Urinary tract infections, prophylaxis, suppression/eliminiation.

Uritact DS. (Cypress) Hyoscyamine sulfate 0.06 mg, methenamine 81.6 mg, phenyl salicylate 36.2 mg, atropine sulfate 0.06 mg, methylene blue 10.8 mg, benzoic acid 9 mg, alcohol and sugar free. Tab. 100s. *Rx.*

Use: Anti-infective, urinary.

Uritin. (Global Source) Methenamine 40.8 mg, atropine sulfate 0.03 mg, hyoscyamine sulfate 0.03 mg, salol 18.1 mg, benzoic acid 4.5 mg, methylene blue 5.4 mg, gelsemium 6.1 mg. Tab. Bot. 1000s. *Rx.*
Use: Anti-infective, urinary.

Uritin Formula. (Various Mfr.) Atropine sulfate 0.03 mg, hyoscyamine 0.03 mg, methenamine 40.8 mg, methylene blue 5.4 mg, phenyl salicylate 18.1 mg, benzoic acid 4.5 mg. Tab. Bot. 1000s. *Rx.*
Use: Anti-infective, urinary.

Urobak. (Shire US) Sulfamethoxazole 500 mg. Tab. Bot. 100s, 1000s. *Rx.*
Use: Anti-infective, sulfonamide.

Uro Blue. (R.A. McNeil) Methenamine 120 mg, sodium phosphate monobasic 40.8 mg, phenyl salicylate 36.2 mg, methylene blue 10.8 mg, hyoscyamine sulfate 0.12 mg, sugar. Tab. 100s. *Rx.*
Use: Anti-infective, urinary.

Urocit-K. (Mission Pharmacal) Potassium citrate 540 mg, 10 mEq. Tab. Bot. 100s. *Rx.*
Use: Genitourinary.

• **urofollitropin.** (YOUR-oh-fahl-ih-TROE-pin) USAN.
Use: Sex hormone, ovulation stimulant.
See: Bravelle.

urogastrone. (Chiron Vision)
Use: Corneal transplant surgery.
[Orphan Drug]

Urogesic. (Edwards) Phenazopyridine hydrochloride 100 mg, hyoscyamine HBr 0.12 mg, atropine sulfate 0.08 mg, scopolamine HBr 0.003 mg. Tab. Bot. 100s, 500s. *Rx.*
Use: Analgesic, urinary.

Urogesic Blue. (Edwards) Methenamine 81.6 mg, sodium biphosphate 40.8 mg, phenyl salicylate 36.2 mg, methylene blue 10.8 mg, hyoscyamine (as sulfate) 0.12 mg. Tab. Bot. 100s. *Rx.*
Use: Anti-infective, urinary.

urography agents.
See: Iodohippurate Sodium.
Iodopyracet.
Iodopyracet Compound.
Methiodal.
Renografin.
Renovist.
Renovue.
Sodium Acetrizoate.
Sodium Iodomethamate.

• **urokinase.** (YOUR-oh-KIN-ace) USAN.
Use: Plasminogen activator; thrombolytic agent; thrombolytic enzyme.
See: Abbokinase.

• **urokinase alfa.** (YOUR-oh-KIN-ace) USAN.
Use: Thrombolytic (plasminogen activator).

Uro-KP-Neutral. (Star) Phosphorus 250 mg, potassium 49.4 mg, sodium 250.5 mg. Tab. Bot. 100s. *Rx.*
Use: Mineral supplement.

Urolene Blue. (Star) Methylene blue 65 mg. Tab. Bot. 100s, 1000s. *Rx.*
Use: Anti-infective, urinary.

Urologic Sol G. (Abbott Hospital Products) Bot. 1000 mL.
Use: Irrigant, ophthalmic.
See: Thiosulfil.

Uro-Mag. (Blaine) Magnesium oxide 140 mg (elemental Mg 84.5 mg). Cap. Bot. 100s, 1000s, UD 100s. *OTC.*
Use: Mineral.

uronal.
See: Barbital.

Uro-Phosphate. (ECR) Sodium biphosphate 434.78 mg, methenamine 300 mg. Film coated Tab. Bot. 100s. *Rx.*
Use: Anti-infective, urinary.

Uroplus DS. (Shire US) Trimethoprim 160 mg, sulfamethoxazole 800 mg. Tab. Bot. 100s, 500s. *Rx.*
Use: Anti-infective.

Uroplus SS. (Shire US) Trimethoprim 80 mg, sulfamethoxazole 800 mg. Tab. Bot. 100s, 500s. *Rx.*
Use: Anti-infective.

Uroquid-Acid No. 2. (Beach) Methenamine mandelate 500 mg, sodium acid phosphate monohydrate 500 mg. Tab. Bot. 100s. *Rx.*
Use: Anti-infective, urinary.

urotropin new. (Various Mfr.) Methenamine anhydromethylene citrate.

Urovist Cysto. (Berlex) Diatrizoate meglumine 300 mg, edetate calcium disodium 0.05 mg/mL. Dilution Bot. 500 mL w/300 mL. *Rx.*
Use: Radiopaque agent.

Urovist Cysto Pediatric. (Berlex) Diatrizoate meglumine 300 mg, edetate calcium disodium 0.1 mg/mL. Dilution bot. 300 mL w/100 mL soln. *Rx.*
Use: Radiopaque agent.

Urovist Meglumine DIU/CT. (Berlex) Diatrizoate meglumine 300 mg, edetate calcium disodium 0.05 mg/mL. Soln. Bot. 300 mL. Ctn. 10s. *Rx.*
Use: Radiopaque agent.

Urovist Sodium 300. (Berlex) Diatrizoate sodium 500 mg, edetate calcium disodium 0.1 mg/mL. Soln. Vial 50 mL, Box 10s. *Rx.*
Use: Radiopaque agent.

Uroxatral. (Sanofi-Syntholabo) Alfuzosin hydrochloride 10 mg, mannitol. ER Tab. 30s, 100s, UD 100s. *Rx.*
Use: Antihypertensive, antiadrenergic.
Ursinus Inlay-Tabs. (Novartis) Pseudoephedrine hydrochloride 30 mg, aspirin 325 mg. Tab. Bot. 24s. *OTC.*
Use: Decongestant; analgesic.
URSO. (Novartis) Ursodiol.
Use: Management and treatment of primary biliary cirrhosis. [Orphan Drug]
ursodeoxycholic acid.
Use: Primary biliary cirrhosis. [Orphan Drug]
•ursodiol. (ERR-so-DIE-ole) *USP 28.* Ursodeoxycholic acid.
Use: Anticholelithogenic; urolithic. Management and treatment of primary biliary cirrhosis, gallstone solubilizing agent.
See: Actigall.
URSO.
ursodiol. (Watson) Ursodiol 300 mg. Cap. 100s. *Rx.*
Use: Anticholelithogenic; urolithic; gallstone solubilizing agent.
Urso Forte. (Axcan Pharma) Ursodiol 500 mg. Film coated. Tab. 100s, 500s. *Rx.*
Use: Gallstone solubilizing agent.
Urso 250. (Axcan Pharma) Ursodiol 250 mg. Film coated. Tab. 100s, 500s.

Rx.
Use: Gallstone solubilizing agent.
uterine-active agents.
See: Abortifacients.
Cervical Ripening, Agents for.
Oxytocics.
Uterine Relaxant.
uterine relaxant.
See: Ritodrine Hydrochloride.
uterine stimulants.
See: Ergonovine Maleate.
Methylergonovine Maleate.
Utimox. (Parke-Davis) Amoxicillin trihydrate. **Cap.:** 250 mg Bot. 100s, 500s, UD 100s; 500 mg Bot. 100s, UD 100s.
Oral Susp.: 125 mg or 250 mg/5 mL Bot. 80 mL, 100 mL, 150 mL, 200 mL. *Rx.*
Use: Anti-infective, penicillin.
Uvadex. (Therakos) Methoxsalen 20 mcg/mL, alcohol 0.05 mL. Soln. Vial 10 mL. *Rx.*
Use: Cutaneous T-cell lymphoma; sclerosis treatment; cardiac allograft rejection prevention; psoralens.
Uvasal. (Sanofi-Synthelabo) Sodium bicarbonate, tartaric acid. Pow. Bot. *OTC.*
Use: Antacid.
uva ursi. (Sherwood Davis & Geck) Leaves. Fluid extract. Bot. pt, gal.
Uvinul MS-40. (General Aniline & Film)
See: Sulisobenzone.

V

vaccine, adenovirus. *Rx.*
Use: Immunization.
See: Adenovirus Vaccine.
vaccine, anthrax. *Rx.*
Use: Immunization.
See: Anthrax Vaccine.
vaccine, BCG. *Rx.*
Use: Immunization.
See: BCG Vaccine.
TheraCys.
Tice BCG.
vaccine, Haemophilus b conjugate. *Rx.*
Use: Immunization. ·
See: ActHIB.
HibTITER.
Liquid PedvaxHIB.
W/Hepatitis B.
See: Comvax.
vaccine, hepatitis A. *Rx.*
Use: Immunization.
See: Havrix.
Vaqta.
vaccine, hepatitis B. *Rx.*
Use: Immunization.
See: Engerix-B.
Recombivax HB.
vaccine, influenza A & B. *Rx.*
Use: Immunization.
See: Fluogen.
FluShield.
Fluvirin.
Fluzone.
vaccine, Japanese encephalitis. *Hx.*
Use: Immunization.
See: JE-Vax.
vaccine, measles. *Rx.*
Use: Immunization.
See: Attenuvax.
W/Mumps and rubella vaccines.
See: M-M-R II.
W/Rubella vaccine.
See: M-R II.
vaccine, meningococcal polysaccha-ride. *Rx.*
Use: Immunization.
See: Menomune A/C/Y/W-135.
vaccine, mumps. Mumps Virus Vaccine
Live.
Use: Immunization.
See: Mumpsvax.
vaccine, pertussis. Pertussis Vaccine.
Use: Immunization.
See: Acel-Imune.
ActHIB/DTP, Set of DTwP vial plus
Hib.
Diphtheria and Tetanus Toxoids with
Pertussis Vaccine.
Tetramune.
Tri-Immunol.

Tripedia.
vaccine, plague.
Use: Immunization.
See: Plague vaccine.
vaccine, pneumococcal polyvalent.
Use: Immunization.
See: Pneumovax 23.
Pnu-Imune 23.
**vaccine, pneumococcal 7-valent
conjugate.**
Use: Immunization.
See: Prevnar.
vaccine, poliovirus.
Use: Immunization.
See: IPOL.
Orimune.
Poliovirus vaccine.
vaccine, rabies. Rabies Vaccine.
Use: Immunization.
See: Imovax Rabies.
RabAvert.
Rabies Vaccine Adsorbed.
vaccines, bacterial.
Use: Immunization.
See: BCG Vaccine.
Haemophilus b Conjugate Vaccine.
Haemophilus b Conjugate Vaccine
with Hepatitis B Vaccine.
Meningococcal Vaccine.
Pneumococcal 7-Valent Conjugate
Vaccine.
Pneumococcal Vaccine, Polyvalent.
Typhoid Vaccine.
vaccine, smallpox. Smallpox Vaccine.
Use: Immunization.
See: Dryvax
vaccine, typhoid.
Use: Immunization.
See: Typhim Vi.
Vivotif Berna.
vaccine, varicella.
Use: Immunization.
See: Varivax.
vaccine, viral.
Use: Immunization.
See: Hepatitis A, Inactivated and Hepa-titis B, Recombinant Vaccine.
Hepatitis A Vaccine, Inactivated.
Hepatitis B Vaccine, Recombinant.
Influenza Virus Vaccine.
Poliovirus Vaccine, Inactivated.
Smallpox Vaccine.
Varicella Virus Vaccine.
vaccine, whooping cough. Pertussis
Vaccine.
Use: Immunization.
See: Acel-Imune.
ActHIB/DTP, Set of DTwP vial plus
Hib.
Diphtheria and Tetanus Toxoids with
Pertussis Vaccine.

Tetramune.
Tri-Immunol.
Tripedia.
vaccine, yellow fever.
Use: Immunization.
See: YF-Vax.
•**vaccinia immune globulin intravenous.**
(vax-IN-ee-ah) *USP 28. Formerly Vaccinia Immune Human Globulin.*
Use: Immunization.
vaccinia immune globulin intravenous (human). (Dynport Vaccine Company LLC) Vaccinia immue globulin 50 mcg/mL (immunoglobulin 2,500 mg/vial). Sucrose 5%, albumin (human) 1%. Soln. for Inj. Vials. *Rx.*
Use: Immunization.
vacocin. Under study.
Use: Anti-infective.
Vademin-Z. (Roberts) Vitamin A 12,500 units, D 50 units, E 50 mg, B_1 10 mg, B_2 5 mg, B_3 25 mg, B_5 10 mg, B_6 2 mg, C 150 mg, Zn 2.6 mg, Mg, Mn. Cap. Bot. 60s. *OTC.*
Use: Mineral, vitamin supplement.
Vagifem. (Novo Nordisk) Estradiol hemihydrate 25.8 mcg, lactose. Film-coated. Vaginal Tab. 8s, 15s, 18s. *Rx.*
Use: Estrogen.
Vagi-Gard Advanced Sensitive Formula. (Lake Consumer) Benzocaine 5%, resorcinol, methylparaben, sodium sulfite, EDTA, mineral oil. Cream. Tube 45 g. *OTC.*
Use: Vaginal agent.
Vagi-Gard Maximum Strength. (Lake Consumer) Benzocaine 20%, resorcinol 3%, methylparaben, sodium sulfite, EDTA, mineral oil. Cream. Tube 45 g. *OTC.*
Use: Vaginal agent.
vaginal antifungal agents.
See: Butoconazole Nitrate.
Clotrimazole.
Miconazole Nitrate.
Nystatin.
Terconazole.
Tioconazole.
vaginal preparations.
See: Butoconazole Nitrate.
Clindamycin Phosphate.
Clotrimazole.
Metronidazole.
Miconazole Nitrate.
Miscellaneous Anti-Infectives.
Nystatin.
Sulfonamides.
Terconazole.
Tioconazole.
Vaginal Antifungal Agents.

Vaginex. (Durex) Tripelennamine hydrochloride. Cream. Tube 30 g, 300 g. *OTC.*
Use: Vaginal agent.
Vagisec Plus. (Durex) Polyoxyethylene nonylphenol 5.25 mg, sodium edetate 0.66 mg, docusate sodium 0.07 mg, aminoacridine hydrochloride 6 mg. Supp. Box 28s. *Rx.*
Use: Vaginal agent.
Vagisil. (Combe) Benzocaine and resorcin with lanolin alcohol, parabens, trisodium HEDTA, mineral oil, sodium sulfite. Cream. 30 g, 60 g. *OTC.*
Use: Vaginal agent.
Vagisil Powder. (Combe) Cornstarch, aloe, mineral oil, benzethonium chloride, magnesium stearate, silica, fragrance. Pow. 198 g, 312 g. *OTC.*
Use: Vaginal agent.
Vagistat-1. (Bristol-Myers Squibb) Tioconazole 6.5%, white petrolatum. Vaginal Oint. Prefilled single-dose applicator 300 mg. *OTC.*
Use: Antifungal; vaginal.
Valacet. (Pal-Pak, Inc.) Hyoscyamus 10.8 mg, aspirin 259.2 mg, caffeine anhydrous 16.2 mg, gelsemium extract 0.6 mg. Tab. Cap. Bot. 100s, 1000s, 5000s. *Rx.*
Use: Analgesic; anticholinergic; antispasmodic.
•**valacyclovir hydrochloride.** (val-lay-SIGH-kloe-vihr) USAN.
Use: Antiviral, antiherpes virus agent.
See: Valtrex.
Valcyte. (Roche) Valganciclovir hydrochloride 450 mg. Tab. Bot. 60s. *Rx.*
Use: Antiviral.
Valentine. (BDI) Caffeine 200 mg. Tab. Bot. 100s, 500s. *OTC.*
Use: CNS stimulant, analeptic.
Valergen 20. (Hyrex) Estradiol Valerate in oil 20 mg/mL, castor oil, benzyl benzoate, benzyl alcohol. Inj. Multi-dose vial 10 mL. *Rx.*
Use: Estrogen.
•**valerian.** (va-LAR-ee-an) *NF 23.*
Use: Dietary supplement.
valerian. (Eli Lilly) Tincture, alcohol 68%. Bot. 4 fl oz, 16 fl oz.
•**valerian extract, powdered.** (va-LAR-ee-an) *NF 23.*
Use: Pharmaceutical vehicle.
Valertest. (Hyrex) **No. 1:** Estradiol valerate 4 mg, testosterone enanthate 90 mg/mL. Vial 10 mL. **No. 2:** Double strength. Vial 10 mL. Amp. 2 mL, 10s. *Rx.*
Use: Androgen, estrogen combination.

valethamate bromide.
Use: Anticholinergic.

• **valganciclovir hydrochloride.** (val-gan-SIGH-kloe-veer) USAN.
Use: Antiviral.
See: Valcyte.

• **valine.** (VAY-leen) *USP 28.*
Use: Amino acid.

valine, isoleucine, and leucine.
Use: Hyperphenylalaninemia. [Orphan Drug]
See: VIL.

Valisone. (Schering-Plough) Betamethasone valerate. **Cream:** 1 mg hydrophilic cream of water, mineral oil, petrolatum, polyethylene glycol 1000 monocetyl ether, cetostearyl alcohol, monobasic sodium phosphate, phosphoric acid, 4-chloro-m-cresol as preservative. Tube 15 g, 45 g, 110 g. Jar 430 g. **Oint.:** 1 mg/g base of liquid and white petrolatum and hydrogenated lanolin. Tube 15 g, 45 g. **Lot.:** 1 mg/g w/isopropyl alcohol 47.5%, water slightly thickened w/carboxyvinyl polymer, pH adjusted w/sodium hydroxide. Bot. 20 mL, 60 mL. **Reduced Strength Cream 0.01%:** Hydrophilic cream of water, mineral oil, petrolatum, polyethylene glycol 1000 monocetyl ether, cetostearyl alcohol, monobasic sodium phosphate, phosphoric acid, 4-chloro-m-cresol as preservative. Tube 15 g, 60 g. *Rx.*
Use: Corticosteroid, topical.

Valium. (Roche) Diazepam 2 mg, 5 mg, 10 mg. Lactose. Tab. Bot. 100s, 500s. *c-iv.*
Use: Anxiolytic; anticonvulsant.

Valium Injection. (Roche) Diazepam 5 mg/mL, propylene glycol 40%, ethyl alcohol 10%, sodium benzoate 5%, benzoic acid, benzyl alcohol 1.5%. Amp. 2 mL. Vial 10 mL. *Tel-E-Ject.* (Disposable syringe) 2 mL. *c-iv.*
Use: Anxiolytic; anticonvulsant.

vallergine.
See: Promethazine hydrochloride.

Valnac Cream. (Alra) Betamethasone valerate 0.1%. Cream. Oint. Tube 15 g, 45 g. *Rx.*
Use: Corticosteroid, topical.

• **valnoctamide.** (val-NOCK-tah-mid) USAN.
Use: Anxiolytic.

• **valomaciclovir stearate.** (val-oh-ma-SYE-kloe-veer) USAN.
Use: Herpes zoster (inhibitor of DNA polymerase).

• **valproate sodium.** (VAL-pro-ate) USAN.
Use: Anticonvulsant.

valproate sodium. (Bedford) Valproic acid (as valproate sodium) 100 mg/mL. Preservative free. Inj. Single-dose vials. 5 mL. *Rx.*
Use: Anticonvulsant.

• **valproic acid.** (VAL-pro-ik) *USP 28.*
Use: Anticonvulsant; antimigraine.
See: Depacon.
　Depakene.
　Depakote.
　Depakote ER.

valproic acid. (Various Mfr.) **Cap.:** Valproic acid 250 mg. Bot. 10s, 30s, 31s, 100s. **Syrup:** Sodium valproate 250 mg/5 mL. Bot. 473 mL. *Rx.*
Use: Anticonvulsant.

• **valrocemide.** (val-ROE-se-mide) USAN.
Use: Antiepileptic, anticonvulsant.

• **valsartan.** (VAL-sahr-tan) USAN.
Use: Antihypertensive.
See: Diovan.
W/Hydrochlorothiazide.
See: Diovan HCT.

• **valspodar.** (VAL-spoh-dar) USAN.
Use: Antineoplastic; multidrug resistance inhibitor.

• **valtorcitabine dihydrochloride.** (val-tore-SITE-ah-been) USAN.
Use: Antifungal.

Valtrex. (GlaxoSmithKline) Valacyclovir hydrochloride 500 mg, 1 g. Tab. Bot. 21s (1 g only); 30s, UD 100s (500 mg only). *Rx.*
Use: Antiviral, antiherpes virus agent.

Valuphed. (H.L. Moore Drug Exchange) Pseudoephedrine hydrochloride 60 mg, triprolidine hydrochloride 2.5 mg. Tab. Pkg. 24s. *OTC.*
Use: Antihistamine, decongestant.

Vamate. (Major) Hydroxyzine pamoate 50 mg. Cap. Bot. 100s, 250s, 500s, UD 100s. *Rx.*
Use: Anxiolytic.

Vanadryx TR. (Vangard Labs, Inc.) Dexbrompheniramine maleate 6 mg, pseudoephedrine sulfate 120 mg. Tab. Bot. 100s, 500s. *Rx.*
Use: Antihistamine, decongestant.

Vanamide. (Dermik) Urea 40%, light mineral oil, cetyl alcohol, petrolatum. Cream. 85 g, 199 g. *Rx.*
Use: Emollient.

Vancocin. (Eli Lilly) Vancomycin. **Pulvules:** 125 mg, 250 mg. *Identi-Dose* 20s. **Pow. for Oral Soln.:** 1 g, 10 g, Bot. **Pow. for Inj.:** 500 mg, 1 g, 10 g. Vials 10 mL, *ADD-Vantage* Vial 15 mL (500 mg only); Vials 20 mL *ADD-Vantage* Vials 15 mL (1 g only); Vial 100 mL (10 g only). *Rx.*

Use: Anti-infective.

Vancoled. (Wyeth) Vancomycin 500 mg, 1 g, 5 g. Vial (500 mg, 1 g only). Bulk pkg. (5 g only). *Rx.*
Use: Anti-infective.

• **vancomycin.** (van-koe-MY-sin) *USP 28.*
Use: Anti-infective.

• **vancomycin hydrochloride.** (van-koe-MY-sin) *USP 28.* An antibiotic from *Streptomyces orientalis.*
Use: (IV) Gram-positive (staph.) infection; anti-infective.
See: Vancocin.
Vancoled.

vancomycin hydrochloride. (Various Mfr.) Vancomycin. **Pow. for Oral Soln.:** 1 g. Bot. **Pow. for Inj.:** 500 mg, 1 g, 5 g, 10 g. Vial. 100 mL Vial (5 g only). *Rx.*
Use: Anti-infective.

Vancor Intravenous. (Pharmacia) Vancomycin hydrochloride 500 mg, 1 g. Pow. for Inj. Vials.
Use: Anti-infective.

Vanex Expectorant. (Jones Pharma) Pseudoephedrine hydrochloride 30 mg, hydrocodone bitartrate 2.5 mg, guaifenesin 100 mg/5 mL, alcohol 5%, glucose, saccharin, sorbitol, sucrose, tartrazine. Tropical fruit punch flavor. Liq. Bot. 473 mL. *c-III.*
Use: Antitussive, decongestant, expectorant.

Vanex HD. (Abana) Phenylephrine hydrochloride 5 mg, chlorpheniramine maleate 2 mg, hydrocodone bitartrate 1.7 mg/5 mL, dye free, cherry flavor. Liq. Bot. 480 mL. *c-III.*
Use: Upper respiratory combination; antihistamine, anticholinergic, antitussive, decongestant.

Vanicream. (Pharmaceutical Specialties) Oil in water vanishing cream containing white petrolatum, cetearyl alcohol, ceteareth-20, sorbitol, propylene glycol, simethicone, glyceryl monostearate, polyethylene glycol monostearate, sorbic acid. Oint. 1 lb. *OTC.*
Use: Pharmaceutical aid; ointment base.

• **vanilla.** (va-NIL-a) *NF 23.*
Use: Pharmaceutic aid (flavor).

vanillal.
See: Ethyl Vanillin.

• **vanilla tincture.** (va-NIL-a) *NF 23.*
Use: Pharmaceutic aid (flavor).

• **vanillin.** (vah-NILL-in) *NF 23.*
Use: Pharmaceutical aid (flavor).

Vaniqa. (Women First Healthcare) Eflornithine hydrochloride monohydrate 150 mg/g, parabens, cetearyl alcohol, mineral oil, stearyl alcohol. Cream. Tube 30 g, 2 × 30 g. *Rx.*
Use: Reduce unwanted facial hair.

vanirome.
See: Ethyl Vanillin.

Vanocin. (ViroPharma) Sodium sulfacetamide 10%, sulfur 5%, benzyl alcohol, cetyl alcohol, EDTA, parabens, stearyl alcohol. Lot. Bot. 30 g, 60 g. *Rx.*
Use: Anti-infective.

Vanos. (Medicis) Fluocinonide 0.1%. Cream. 30 g, 60 g. *Rx.*
Use: Anti-inflammatory agent, topical corticosteroid.

Vanoxide-HC. (Dermik) Hydrocortisone alcohol 0.5%, benzyl peroxide 5%, mineral oil, propylene glycol, EDTA, parabens. Lot. 25 mL. *Rx.*
Use: Dermatologic, acne.

Vanquish. (Bayer Corp. (Consumer Div.)) Aspirin 227 mg, acetaminophen 194 mg, caffeine 33 mg, aluminum hydroxide 25 mg, magnesium hydroxide 50 mg. Capl. Bot. 60s, 100s. *OTC.*
Use: Analgesic combination; antacid.

Vantas. (Valeras) Histrelin acetate 50 mg. Implant. In carton with implantation kit. *Rx.*
Use: Treatment of advanced prostate cancer.

Vantin. (Pharmacia) Cefpodoxime proxetil, lactose. **Tab.:** 100 mg, 200 mg. Bot. 20s, 100s, UD 100s. **Gran. for Susp.:** 50 mg/5 mL, 100 mg/5 mL. Sucrose, lemon creme flavor. Bot. 50 mL, 75 mL, 100 mL. *Rx.*
Use: Anti-infective.

• **vapiprost hydrochloride.** (VAP-ih-prahst) USAN.
Use: Antagonist (thromboxane A₂).

Vapocet. (Major) Hydrocodone 5 mg, acetaminophen 500 mg. Tab. Bot. 100s. *c-III.*
Use: Analgesic combination; narcotic.

Vaponefrin. (Medeva) A 2.25% solution of bioassayed racemic epinephrine as hydrochloride, chlorobutanol 0.5%. Soln. Vial 7.5 mL, 15 mL, 30 mL. *OTC.*
Use: Bronchodilator.

Vaporizer in a Bottle. (Columbia) Wick-dispensed medicated vapors.
Use: Cough, cold, sinus, hayfever preparation.

Vapor Lemon Sucrets. (GlaxoSmithKline) Dyclonine hydrochloride 2 mg, corn syrup, sucrose. Loz. Pkg. 18s. *OTC.*
Use: Mouth and throat preparation.

VapoRub. (Procter & Gamble)
See: Vicks Vaporub.

Vaposteam. (Procter & Gamble)
See: Vicks Vaposteam.
• **vapreotide.** (vap-REE-oh-tide) USAN.
Use: Antineoplastic.
Vaqta. (Merck & Co.) **Adult:** Hepatitis A antigen 50 U/mL. **Pediatric/Adolescent:** Hepatitis A antigen 25 U/0.5 mL, Inj. Single-dose vial, prefilled syr. *Rx.*
Use: Active immunization agent, viral vaccine.
• **vardenafil dihydrochloride.** (var-DEN-a-fil) USAN.
Use: Erectile dysfunction.
vardenafil hydrochloride.
Use: Impotence agent.
See: Levitra.
• **varenicline tartrate.** (var-e-NI-kleen) USAN.
Use: Smoking cessation.
• **varespladib.** (va-res-PLA-dib) USAN.
Use: Sepsis.
varicella virus vaccine.
Use: Immunization, viral vaccine.
See: Varivax.
varicella-zoster IgG IFA test system. (Wampole) Test for the qualitative or semi-qualitative detection of VZ IgG antibody in human serum. Test kit 100s.
Use: Diagnostic aid.
• **varicella-zoster immune globulin.** *USP 28.*
Use: Immunization.
varicella-zoster immune globulin, human. (American Red Cross) Varicella-zoster immune globulin (human) sterile 10% to 18% solution of the globulin fraction of human plasma, primarily IgG, glycine 0.3 M, preservative free, solvent/detergent treated. Inj. Single dose vial containing 125 units of varicella-zoster virus antibody in ≈ 1.25 mL and 625 units in ≈ 6.25 mL. *Rx.*
Use: Immunization.
Vari-Flavors. (Ross) Flavor packets to provide flavor variety for patients on liquid diets. Dextrose, artificial flavor, artificial color. Packet 1 g, Ctn. 24s. *Rx.*
Use: Flavoring.
Variplex-C. (NBTY) Vitamins B_1 15 mg, B_2 10 mg, B_3 100 mg, B_5 20 mg, B_6 5 mg, B_{12} 10 mcg, C 500 mg. Tab. Bot. 100s. *OTC.*
Use: Vitamin supplement.
Varivax. (Merck & Co.) Varicella virus vaccine. 1350 PFU of Oka/Merck varicella virus (live), sucrose. Pow. for Inj. Single-dose vials 1s, 10s. *Rx.*
Use: Immunization, viral vaccine.
Vascunitol. (Apco) Mannitol hexanitrate 0.5 g. Tab. Bot. 100s. *Rx.*

Use: Vasodilator.
Vascused. (Apco) Mannitol hexanitrate 0.5 g, phenobarbital 0.25 g. Tab. Bot. 100s. *Rx.*
Use: Vasodilator.
Vaseline Dermatology Formula Cream. (Chesebrough-Ponds USA) Petrolatum, mineral oil, dimethicone. Jar 3 oz, 5.25 oz. *OTC.*
Use: Emollient.
Vaseline Dermatology Formula Lotion. (Chesebrough-Ponds USA) Petrolatum, mineral oil, dimethicone. Bot. 5.5 oz, 11 oz, 16 oz. *OTC.*
Use: Emollient.
Vaseline First Aid Carboxylated Petroleum Jelly. (Chesebrough-Ponds USA) Petrolatum, chloroxylenol. Plastic Jar 1.75 oz, 3.75 oz. Plastic Tube 1 oz, 2.5 oz. *OTC.*
Use: Medicated anti-infective.
Vaseline Intensive Care Active Sport. (Chesebrough-Ponds USA) Ethylhexyl p-methoxycinnamate, oxybenzone. PABA free. **SPF 8:** Lot. Bot. 120 mL. **SPF 15:** Lot. Bot. 120 mL. *OTC.*
Use: Sunscreen.
Vaseline Intensive Care Baby SPF 15. (Chesebrough-Ponds USA) Titanium dioxide. PABA free. Waterproof. Lot. Bot. 120 mL. *OTC.*
Use: Sunscreen.
Vaseline Intensive Care Baby SPF 30. (Chesebrough-Ponds USA) Ethylhexyl p-methoxycinnamate, oxybenzone, 2-ethylhexyl salicylate, titanium dioxide, C12-15 alkyl benzoate, glycerin, aloe vera gel, vitamin E, cetyl alcohol, parabens, EDTA. Lot. Bot. 118 mL. *OTC.*
Use: Sunscreen.
Vaseline Intensive Care Blockout SPF 40+. (Chesebrough-Ponds USA) Padimate O, ethylhexyl p-methoxycinnamate, oxybenzone, 2-ethylhexyl salicylate, titanium dioxide. Waterproof. Lot. Bot. 120 mL. *OTC.*
Use: Sunscreen.
Vaseline Intensive Care Blockout SPF 30. (Chesebrough-Ponds USA) Ethylhexyl p-methoxycinnamate, oxybenzone, 2-ethylhexyl salicylate, titanium dioxide. Waterproof. Lot. Bot. 120 mL. *OTC.*
Use: Sunscreen.
Vaseline Intensive Care Moisturizing Sunscreen. (Chesebrough-Ponds USA) Ethylhexyl p-methoxycinnamate, oxybenzone, C12-15 alkyl octanoate, glycerin, aloe vera gel, cetyl alcohol, petrolatum, vitamin E, parabens, EDTA. SPF 4, SPF 8: Lot. Bot. 117 mL. *OTC.*

Use: Sunscreen.

Vaseline Intensive Care No Burn No Bite SPF 8. (Chesebrough-Ponds USA) Ethylhexyl p-methoxycinnamate, oxybenzone. PABA free. Waterproof. Lot. Bot. 180 mL. *OTC.*
Use: Sunscreen.

Vaseline Intensive Care Sport Sunblock. (Chesebrough-Ponds USA) Ethylhexyl p-methoxycinnamate, oxybenzone, C12-15 alkyl benzoate, aloe vera gel, vitamin E, EDTA. Lot. Bot. 118 mL. *OTC.*
Use: Sunscreen.

Vaseline Intensive Care Sunblock. (Chesebrough-Ponds USA) Ethylhexyl p-methoxycinnamate, 2-ethylhexyl salicylate. PABA free. Waterproof. **SPF 4:** Lot. Bot. 180 mL; **SPF 8:** Lot. Bot. 120 mL, 180 mL; **SPF 15:** Lot. Bot. 120 mL, 180 mL; **SPF 25:** Lot. Bot. 120 mL, 180 mL. *OTC.*
Use: Sunscreen.

Vaseline Intensive Care Ultra Violet Daily Defense. (Chesebrough-Ponds USA) Ethylhexyl p-methoxycinnamate, oxybenzone, vitamin E, cetyl alcohol, acetylated lanolin, alcohol, parabens, EDTA. SPF 15. Lot. Bot. 118 mL. *OTC.*
Use: Sunscreen.

Vaseline Pure Petroleum Jelly Skin Protectant. (Chesebrough-Ponds USA) White petrolatum. Tube 1 oz, 2.5 oz. Jar 1.75 oz, 3.75 oz, 7.75 oz, 13 oz. *OTC.*
Use: Dermatologic; counterirritant.

Vaseretic 5-12.5. (Biovail) Enalapril maleate 5 mg, hydrochlorothiazide 12.5 mg, lactose. Tab. Bot. 100s. *Rx.*
Use: Antihypertensive.

Vaseretic 10-25. (Biovail) Enalapril maleate 10 mg, hydrochlorothiazide 25 mg. Tab. Bot. 100s. *Rx.*
Use: Antihypertensive.

Vasimid.
See: Tolazoline hydrochloride.

vasoactive intestinal polypeptide. (Research Triangle Pharmaceuticals)
Use: Treatment of acute esophageal food impaction. [Orphan Drug]

Vasocidin Ophthalmic Solution. (Novartis) Prednisolone sodium phosphate 0.25%, sulfacetamide sodium 10%. Bot. 5 mL, 10 mL. *Rx.*
Use: Anti-infective; corticosteroid; ophthalmic.

VasoClear. (Novartis Ophthalmics) Naphazoline hydrochloride 0.02%. Bot. 15 mL. *OTC.*
Use: Mydriatic; vasoconstrictor.

VasoClear A. (Novartis Ophthalmics) Naphazoline hydrochloride 0.02%. Bot. 15 mL. *OTC.*
Use: Mydriatic, vasoconstrictor.

Vasocon-A Ophthalmic Solution. (Novartis Ophthalmics) Naphazoline hydrochloride 0.05%, antazoline phosphate 0.5%. Bot. 15 mL. *Rx.*
Use: Mydriatic; vasoconstrictor.

Vasocon Regular. (Ciba Vision) Naphazoline hydrochloride 0.1%. Bot. 15 mL. *Rx.*
Use: Mydriatic; vasoconstrictor.

Vasoderm. (Taro) Fluocinonide 0.05%, anhydrous glycerin base. Cream. Tube 15 g, 30 g, 60 g. *Rx.*
Use: Corticosteroid, topical.

Vasoderm-E. (Taro) Fluocinonide 0.05%, emollient mineral oil and white petrolatum base. Cream. Tube 15 g, 30 g, 60 g, 120 g. *Rx.*
Use: Corticosteroid, topical.

Vasodilan. (Bristol-Myers Squibb) Isoxsuprine hydrochloride 10 mg, 20 mg. Tab. **10 mg:** Bot. 100s, 1000s, UD 100s. **20 mg:** Bot. 100s, 500s, 1000s, UD 100s. *Rx.*
Use: Vasodilator.

•**vasodilator combinations, peripheral.**
See: Lipo-Nicin.

vasodilators.
See: Amyl Nitrite.
   Bosentan.
   Endothelin Receptor Antagonists.
   Epoprostenol Sodium.
   Erythrityl Tetranitrate.
   Ethaverine Hydrochloride.
   Glyceryl Trinitrate Preps.
   Human B-Type Natriuretic Peptides.
   Hydralazine Hydrochloride.
   Iloprost.
   Isosorbide Dinitrate.
   Isosorbide Mononitrate.
   Isoxsuprine Hydrochloride.
   Mannitol Hexanitrate.
   Minoxidil.
   Nesiritide.
   Nitrates.
   Nitroglycerin.
   Papaverine Hydrochloride.
   Peripheral Vasodilators.
   Prostacyclin Analog.
   Sodium Nitrate.
   Tolazoline Hydrochloride.

vasodilators, coronary.
See: Glyceryl Trinitrate.
   Isordil.
   Khellin.
   Papaverine.
   Pentaerythritol Tetranitrate.
   Peritrate.

vasodilators, peripheral.
See: Epoprostenol Sodium.
Ethaverine Hydrochloride.
Hydralazine Hydrochloride.
Isoxsuprine Hydrochloride.
Minoxidil.
Papaverine Hydrochloride.
Tolazoline Hydrochloride.
Vasodilator Combinations, Peripheral.
Vasoflo. (Roberts) Papaverine hydrochloride 150 mg. Cap. Bot. 100s. *Rx.*
Use: Vasodilator.
Vasolate. (Parmed Pharmaceuticals, Inc.) Pentaerythritol tetranitrate 30 mg. Cap. Bot. 100s, 1000s. *Rx.*
Use: Antianginal.
Vasolate-80. (Parmed Pharmaceuticals, Inc.) Pentaerythritol tetranitrate 80 mg. Cap. Bot. 100s, 1000s. *Rx.*
Use: Antianginal.
•**vasopressin.** (VAY-so-PRESS-in) *USP 28.*
Use: Posterior pituitary hormone.
See: Pitressin.
vasopressin. (Various Mfr.) Vasopressin 20 pressor units/mL, chlorobutanol 0.5%. Inj. Vial. 0.5 mL, 1 mL, 10 mL. *Rx.*
Use: Posterior pituitary hormone.
vasopressors.
See: Dobutamine.
Dopamine Hydrochloride.
Ephedrine.
Epinephrine.
Isoproterenol Hydrochloride.
Metaraminol.
Methoxamine Hydrochloride.
Midodrine Hydrochloride.
Norepinephrine Bitartrate.
Phenylephrine Hydrochloride.
Vasosulf. (Ciba Vision) Sulfacetamide sodium 15%, phenylephrine hydrochloride 0.125%. Bot. 5 mL, 15 mL. *Rx.*
Use: Anti-infective; decongestant; ophthalmic.
Vasotec. (Biovail) Enalapril maleate 2.5 mg, 5 mg, 10 mg, 20 mg, lactose. Tab. Bot. 100s, 1000s, 10,000s, unit-of-use 90s, UD 100s. *Rx.*
Use: Antihypertensive.
Vasotus. (Sheryl) Codeine phosphate ⅙ g, phenylephrine hydrochloride, prophenpyridamine maleate. Liq. Bot. 473 mL. *c-v.*
Use: Antihistamine, antitussive, decongestant.
Vaxsyn HIV-1. (MicroGeneSys) T-Lymphotropic Virus Type III GP 160 Antigen.
Use: AIDS. [Orphan Drug]

VaZol. (WraSer) Brompheniramine tannate 2 mg/5 mL. Bubble gum flavor. Liq. 472 mL. *Rx.*
Use: Antihistamine.
Vazosan. (Sandia) Papaverine hydrochloride 150 mg. Tab. Bot. 100s, 1000s. *Rx.*
Use: Vasodilator.
VCF. (Apothecus) Contraceptive film: nonoxynol-9 28%, glycerin, and polyvinyl alcohol. Pkg. 3s, 6s, 12s. *OTC.*
Use: Contraceptive; spermicide.
V-Cillin K. (Eli Lilly) Penicillin V potassium 125 mg, 250 mg, 500 mg. Tab. **125 mg:** Bot. 100s. **250 mg:** Bot. 100s, 500s. **500 mg:** Bot. 24s, 100s, 500s. *Rx.*
Use: Anti-infective; penicillin.
V-Cillin K for Oral Solution. (Eli Lilly) Penicillin V potassium 125 mg, 250 mg/5 mL, 125 mg: Bot. 100 ml 150 mL, 200 mL, UD 5 mL. **250 mg:** Bot. 100 mL, 150 mL, 200 mL. *Rx.*
Use: Anti-infective; penicillin.
V-Dec-M. (Seatrace) Pseudoephedrine hydrochloride 120 mg, guaifenesin 500 mg. SR Tab. Bot. 12s, 100s. *Rx.*
Use: Upper respiratory combination; decongestant, expectorant.
VDRL Antigen. (Laboratory Diagnostics) VDRL antigen with buffered saline. Blood test in diagnosis of syphilis. **Vial:** Sufficient for 500 tests. **Amp.:** 10 × 0.5 mL sufficient for 500 tests.
Use: Diagnostic aid.
VDRL Slide Test. (Laboratory Diagnostics) VDRL antigen. Slide flocculation and spinal fluid test for syphilis. Vial 5 mL Complete kit, reactive control, nonreactive control, 5 mL.
Use: Diagnostic aid.
Vectrin. (Warner Chilcott) Minocycline 50 mg, 100 mg. Cap. Bot. 50s (100 mg only), 100s (50 mg only), 1000s. *Rx.*
Use: Anti-infective.
•**vecuronium bromide.** (veh-CUE-row-nee-uhm) *USP 28.*
Use: Neuromuscular blocker.
vecuronium bromide. (Marsam) Vecuronium bromide 10 mg, 20 mg. Inj. Vial 10 mL (with and without diluent), 20 mL (without diluent). *Rx.*
Use: Neuromuscular blocker.
vecuronium bromide. (Various Mfr.) Vecuronium bromide 10 mg, 20 mg. May contain mannitol. Pow. for Inj. Vials. 10 mL (10 mg only), 20 mL (20 mg only). *Rx.*
Use: Neuromuscular blocker.
Veetids. (Geneva) Penicillin-V. **Pow. for Oral Soln.:** 125 mg/5 mL, 250 mg/5 mL, DL-menthol, saccharin, sucrose.

Bot. 100 mL, 200 mL. **Tab.:** 250 mg, 500 mg, lactose. Bot. 100s, 1000s. *Rx.*
Use: Anti-infective; penicillin.
VE-400. (Western Research) Vitamin E 400 units. Cap. Bot. 1008s. *OTC.*
Use: Vitamin supplement.
•**vegetable oil, hydrogenated.** *NF 23.*
Use: Pharmaceutical aid (tablet/capsule lubricant).
vehicle/n and vehicle/n mild. (Neutrogena) Topical vehicle system for compounding. Appliderm Applicator Bot. oz. *OTC.*
Use: Pharmaceutical aid.
velacycline.
Use: Anti-infective; tetracycline.
Velban. (Lilly) Vinblastine sulfate 10 mg. Pow. for Inj. Vial. *Rx.*
Use: Antineoplastic.
Velcade. (Millenium) Bortezomib 3.5 mg, mannitol 35 mg. Preservative free. Pow. for Inj., lyophilized. Single-dose vials. *Rx.*
Use: Proteasome inhibitor.
Velivet. (Barr) **Phase 1:** Desogestrel 0.1 mg, ethinyl estradiol 25 mcg. 7 tabs. **Phase 2:** Desogestrel 0.125 mg, ethinyl estradiol 25 mcg. 7 tabs. **Phase 3:** Desogestrel 0.15 mg, ethinyl estradiol 25 mcg. 7 tabs. *Rx.*
Use: Triphasic oral contraceptive.
•**velnacrine maleate.** (VELL-NAH-kreen) USAN.
Use: Inhibitor (cholinesterase).
Velosef. (Bristol-Myers Squibb) Cephradine. **Pow. for Oral Susp.:** 125 mg, 250 mg/5 mL, sucrose, fruit flavor. Bot. 100 mL. **Cap.:** 250 mg, 500 mg. *Rx.*
Use: Anti-infective; cephalosporin.
Velvachol. (Galderma) Hydrophilic ointment base petrolatum, mineral oil, cetyl alcohol, cholesterol, parabens, stearyl alcohol, purified water, sodium lauryl sulfate. Jar lb. *OTC.*
Use: Pharmaceutical aid; ointment base.
venesetic.
See: Amobarbital Sodium.
venlafaxine.
Use: Antidepressant.
See: Effexor.
Effexor XR.
•**venlafaxine hydrochloride.** (VEN-lah-fax-EEN) USAN.
Use: Antidepressant.
See: Effexor.
Effexor XR.
Venofer. (American Regent Labs) Elemental iron 20 mg/mL, preservative free, sucrose 300 mg/mL w/v. Inj.

Single-dose Vial 5 mL. *Rx.*
Use: Trace element.
Venomil. (Bayer Corp. (Consumer Div.)) Freeze-dried venom or venom protein. Vials of 12 mcg or 120 mcg for honey bee, white-faced hornet, yellow hornet, yellow jacket, or wasp. Vials of 36 mcg or 360 mcg for mixed vespids (white-faced hornet, yellow hornet, yellow jacket). Diagnostic 1 mcg/mL. Maintenance 100 mcg/mL. Individual patient kit. *Rx.*
Use: Antivenin.
Venstat. (Seatrace) Brompheniramine maleate 10 mg/mL. Vial 10 mL. *Rx.*
Use: Antihistamine.
Ventavis. (CoTherix) Iloprost 20 mcg. Inhalation Soln. Single-use ampules. 2 mL. *Rx.*
Use: Treatment of pulmonary arterial hypertension.
Ventolin. (GlaxoSmithKline) Albuterol. **Syr.:** Albuterol sulfate 2 mg/5 mL, saccharin, strawberry flavor. Bot. 480 mL. **Tab.:** Albuterol sulfate 2 mg, 4 mg. Bot. 100s, 500s. *Rx.*
Use: Bronchodilator, sympathomimetic.
Ventolin HFA. (GlaxoSmithKline) Albuterol sulfate 90 mcg/actuation. Aerosol. Can. 18 g (200 inhalations). Contains no CFCs. *Rx.*
Use: Bronchodilator, sympathomimetic.
Ventolin Inhalation Solution. (GlaxoSmithKline) Albuterol sulfate 0.5%. Bot. 20 mL w/calibrated dropper. *Rx.*
Use: Bronchodilator.
Ventolin Nebules. (GlaxoSmithKline) Albuterol sulfate 0.083%, sulfuric acid. Soln. for Inh. In 3 mL unit-dose nebules. *Rx.*
Use: Bronchodilator.
Ventolin Rotacaps. (GlaxoSmithKline) Microfine albuterol sulfate 200 mg, lactose. Cap. for Inh. Bot. 100s, UD 24s. For use with the *Rotahaler* inhalation device. *Rx.*
Use: Bronchodilator.
VePesid. (Bristol-Myers Squibb Oncology/Virology) Etoposide. **Vial:** 100 mg. **Cap.:** 50 mg. Bot. 20s. *Rx.*
Use: Antineoplastic.
•**veradoline hydrochloride.** (VEER-aid-OLE-een) USAN.
Use: Analgesic.
•**verapamil.** (veh-RAP-ah-mill) USAN.
Use: Vasodilator (coronary).
•**verapamil hydrochloride.** (veh-RAP-ah-mill) *USP 28.*
Use: Antianginal, antiarrhythmic, antihypertensive, calcium channel blocker.

See: Calan.
Calan SR.
Covera-HS.
Isoptin SR.
Verelan.
Verelan PM
W/Trandolapril.
See: Tarka.
verapamil hydrochloride. (Various Mfr.)
Verapamil hydrochloride. **40 mg. Tab.:**
Bot. 30s, 100s, 500s, 1000s. **80 mg,
120 mg. Tab.:** 100s, 250s, 500s, 1000s,
4000s (120 mg only), 7000s (80 mg
only), UD 100s (120 mg only). **120 mg,
180 mg, 240 mg. ER Tab.:** 100s, 500s
(except 120 mg). **2.5 mg/mL. Inj.:**
2 mL, 4 mL vials, amps, and syringes;
single-use 2 mL fills; *Carpuject* syringe
2 mL; 2 mL fill in single-use 2 mL .
Carpuject Interlink syringe. Rx.
Use: Antianginal; antiarrhythmic; antihypertensive.
verapamil hydrochloride ER. (Various
Mfr.) Verapamil hydrochloride 120 mg,
180 mg, 240 mg. ER Cap. Bot. 100s,
500s, UD 80s (240 mg only), 100s (except 240 mg). *Rx.*
Use: Antianginal; antiarrhythmic; antihypertensive.
verapamil hydrochloride SR. (Schein)
Verapamil hydrochloride 120 mg,
180 mg, 240 mg, 360 mg, parabens.
SR Cap. Bot. 100s. *Rx.*
Use: Antianginal; antiarrythmic; antihy-
pertensive.
veratrum alba.
See: Protoveratrines A and B.
Verazeptol. (Femco) Chlorothymol, euca-
lyptol, menthol, phenol, boric acid, zinc
sulfate. Pow. Bot. 3 oz, 6 oz, 10 oz.
OTC.
Use: Vaginal agent.
Verazinc. (Forest) Zinc sulfate 220 mg.
Cap. Bot. 100s, 1000s. *OTC.*
Use: Mineral supplement.
Verelan. (Schwarz Pharma) Verapamil
hydrochloride 120 mg, 180 mg,
240 mg, 360 mg, sugar, parabens. SR
Cap. Bot. 100s. *Rx.*
Use: Calcium channel blocker.
Verelan PM. (Schwarz Pharma) Verapa-
mil hydrochloride 100 mg, 200 mg,
300 mg, sugar. ER Cap. Bot. 100s. *Rx.*
Use: Calcium channel blocker.
Vergo. (Daywell Laboratories, Inc.) Cal-
cium pantothenate 8%, ascorbic acid
2%, starch. Oint. Tube 0.5 oz. *Rx.*
Use: Keratolytic.
●**verilopam hydrochloride.** (veh-RILL-
OH-pam) USAN.
Use: Analgesic.

●**verlukast.** (ver-LOO-kast) USAN.
Use: Antiasthmatic (leukotriene antago-
nist).
Verluma. (NeoRx; DuPont) Nofetu-
momab merpentan 10 mg for conjuga-
tion w/technetium 99m. Kit. *Rx.*
Use: Radioimmunoscintigraphy agent.
Vermox. (Janssen) Mebendazole
100 mg. Tab. Box 12s. *Rx.*
Use: Anthelmintic.
vernamycins. Under study.
Use: Anti-infective.
vernolepin. A sesquiterpene dilactone.
Under study.
Use: Antineoplastic.
●**verofylline.** (VER-OH-fill-in) USAN.
Use: Antiasthmatic; bronchodilator.
veronal sodium.
See: Barbital Sodium.
Versacaps. (Seatrace) Pseudoephedrine
hydrochloride 60 mg, guaifenesin
300 mg, benzyl alcohol, EDTA, para-
bens, sucrose. SR. Cap. Bot. 100s. *Rx.*
Use: Upper respiratory combination;
decongestant, expectorant.
Versal. (Suppositoria Laboratories, Inc.)
Bismuth subgallate, balsam peru, zinc
oxide, benzyl benzoate. Supp. Box
12s, 100s, 1000s. *OTC.*
Use: Anorectal preparation.
versenate, calcium disodium.
See: Calcium Disodium Versenate.
versenate disodium.
See: Disodium Versenate.
●**versetamide.** (ver-SET-ah-mide) USAN.
Use: Pharmaceutical aid.
Versiclear. (Hope) Sodium thiosulfate
25%, salicylic acid 1%, isopropyl al-
cohol 10%, propylene glycol, menthol,
EDTA. Lot. 120 mL. *Rx.*
Use: Anti-infective, topical.
versidyne.
Use: Analgesic.
Verstran. (Parke-Davis) Prazepam.
Use: Anxiolytic.
●**verteporfin.** (ver-teh-PORE-fin) USAN.
Use: Antineoplastic; ophthalmic pho-
totherapy.
See: Visudyne.
Verukan-20. (Syosset Laboratories Co.,
Inc.) Salicylic acid 16.7%, lactic acid
in flexible collodion 16.7%. Bot. 15 mL.
OTC.
Use: Keratolytic.
Verv Alertness. (A.P.C.) Caffeine
200 mg. Cap. Vial 15s. *OTC.*
Use: CNS stimulant.
Vesanoid. (Roche) Tretinoin 10 mg. Cap.
Bot. 100s. *Rx.*
Use: Antineoplastic; retinoid.

Vesicare. (GlaxoSmithKline) Solifenacin succinate 5 mg, 10 mg. Film coated. Tab. 30s, 90s, UD 100s. *Rx.*
Use: Anticholinergic.

•**vesnarinone.** (VESS-nah-rih-NOHN) USAN.
Use: Cardiovascular agent.

•**vestipitant mesylate.** (ves-tee-PIT-ant) USAN.
Use: CNS agent.

Vexol. (Alcon) Rimexolone 1%. Ophth. Susp. *Drop-Tainers.* 2.5 mL, 5 mL, 10 mL. *Rx.*
Use: Corticosteroid, ophthalmic.

Vfend. (Roerig) Voriconazole. **Tab.:** 50 mg, 200 mg, lactose. Bot. 30s. **Pow. for Inj., lyophilized:** 200 mg, sulfobutyl ether beta-cyclodextrin sodium 3200 mg. Single-use vials. **Pow. for Oral Susp.:** 45 g (40 mg/mL after reconstitution). Sucrose. Orange flavor. 100 mL high-density polyethylene bottles w/a 5 mL oral dispenser and a press-in bottle adaptor. *Rx.*
Use: Antifungal.

Viacaps. (Manne) Vitamins A (soluble) 45,000 units, C 500 mg. Cap. Bot. 60s, 120s, 1000s. *OTC.*
Use: Vitamin supplement.

Viadur. (Alza) Leuprolide acetate 72 mg. Implant. Single-dose Kit. *Rx.*
Use: Hormone; gonadotropin-releasing hormone analog.

Viagra. (Pfizer) Sildenafil citrate 25 mg, 50 mg, 100 mg (except 25 mg), lactose. Tab. Bot. 30s, 100s. *Rx.*
Use: Anti-impotence.

Vianain. (Genzyme) Ananain, comosain.
Use: Burn treatment. [Orphan Drug]

vi antigen.
Use: Immunization.
See: Typhim Vi.

vibesate. Polvinate 9.3%, molrosinol 3.1% with propellant.

Vibramycin. (Pfizer) **Cap.:** Doxycycline hyclate 50 mg, 100 mg. Bot. 50s. **Pow. for Oral Susp.:** Doxycycline monohydrate 25 mg/5 mL, paragbens, sucrose, raspberry flavor. Bot. 60 mL. **Syr.:** Doxycycline calcium 50 mg/5 mL, parabens, sodium metabisulfite, sorbitol, apple-raspberry flavor. Bot. 473 mL. *Rx.*
Use: Anti-infective; tetracycline.

Vibramycin IV. (Roerig) Doxycycline (as hyclate) 200 mg. Powder for Inj. Vial. *Rx.*
Use: Anti-infective; tetracycline.

Vibra-Tabs. (Pfizer) Doxycycline hyclate 100 mg. Tab. Bot. 50s. *Rx.*
Use: Anti-infective; tetracycline.

Vicam Injection. (Keene Pharmaceuticals) Vitamins B_1 50 mg, B_2 5 mg, B_3 125 mg, B_5 6 mg, B_6 5 mg, B_{12} 1000 mcg, C 50 mg/mL. Vial 10 mL. *Rx.*
Use: Vitamin supplement.

Vicam IV. (Keene Pharmaceuticals) Vitamins B_1 50 mg, B_2 5 mg, B_{12} 1000 mcg, B_6 5 mg, dexpanthenol 6 mg, niacinamide 125 mg, C 50 mg/mL, benzyl alcohol 1% as preservative in water for injection. Vial, multiple-dose. *Rx.*
Use: Nutritional supplement; parenteral.

Vicks Children's Chloraseptic Lozenges. (Procter & Gamble) Benzocaine 5 mg, corn syrup, sucrose. Grape flavor. Loz. Pkg. 18s. *OTC.*

Vicks Children's Chloraseptic Spray. (Procter & Gamble) Phenol 0.5%, saccharin, sorbitol. Alcohol free. Spray. Bot. 177 mL. *OTC.*
Use: Anesthetic; antiseptic.

Vicks Children's NyQuil Cold/Cough Relief. (Procter & Gamble) Pseudoephedrine hydrochloride 10 mg, dextromethorphan HBr 5 mg, chlorpheniramine maleate 0.67 mg/5 mL, alcohol free, sucrose. Bot. 118 mL. *OTC.*
Use: Upper respiratory combination; antihistamine, antitussive, decongestant.

Vicks Chloraseptic Mouthrinse/Gargle. (Procter & Gamble) Phenol 1.4%, saccharin. Alcohol free. Liq. 355 mL. *OTC.*
Use: Antiseptic.

Vicks Chloraseptic Sore Throat. (Procter & Gamble) Benzocaine 6 mg, menthol 10 mg. Loz. Pkg. 18s. *OTC.*
Use: Anesthetic.

Vicks Cough Drops. (Procter & Gamble) Menthol. **Menthol flavor:** Benzyl alcohol, camphor, eucalyptus oil, tolu balsam, corn syrup, sucrose, thymol. **Cherry flavor:** Corn syrup, sucrose, citric acid. Box 14. Bag 40. *OTC.*
Use: Mouth and throat preparation.

Vicks DayQuil LiquiCaps. (Procter & Gamble) Dextromethorphan HBr 10 mg, pseudoephedrine hydrochloride 30 mg, acetaminophen 250 mg, guaifenesin 100 mg. Softgel Cap. Pkg. 12s, 20s. *OTC.*
Use: Analgesic, antitussive, decongestant, expectorant.

Vicks DayQuil LiquiCaps Multi-Symptom Cold/Flu Relief. (Procter & Gamble) Dextromethorphan HBr 10 mg, pseudoephedrine hydrochloride 30 mg, acetaminophen 250 mg, sorbitol. Cap. Pkg. 12s, 20s, 36s. *OTC.*
Use: Upper respiratory combination; antitussive, decongestant, analgesic.

Vicks DayQuil Liquid. (Procter & Gamble) Pseudoephedrine hydrochloride 60 mg, guaifenesin 200 mg, acetaminophen 650 mg, dextromethorphan HBr 20 mg/30 mL. Bot. 6 oz. *OTC.*
Use: Analgesic, antitussive, decongestant, expectorant.

Vicks DayQuil Multi-Symptom Cold/Flu Relief. (Procter & Gamble) Dextromethorphan HBr 3.3 mg, pseudoephedrine hydrochloride 10 mg, acetaminophen 108.3 mg/5 mL, saccharin, sucrose. Liq. Bot. 177 mL. *OTC.*
Use: Upper respiratory combination; antitussive, decongestant, analgesic.

Vicks DayQuil Sinus Pressure & Pain Relief. (Procter & Gamble) Pseudoephedrine hydrochloride 30 mg, acetaminophen 500 mg. Cap. Pkg. 24s. *OTC.*
Use: Analgesic, decongestant

Vicks Dry Hacking Cough. (Procter & Gamble) Dextromethorphan HBr 30 mg/10 mL, alcohol 10%, invert sugar. Liq. Bot. 4 oz, 8 oz w/Vicks *AccuTip* Dispenser. *OTC.*
Use: Antitussive.

Vicks 44 Cough Relief. (Procter & Gamble) Dextromethorphan HBr 10 mg/5 mL, alcohol 5%, corn syrup, saccharin. Liq. Bot. 118 mL. *OTC.*
Use: Antitussive.

Vicks 44D Cough & Decongestant Liquid. (Procter & Gamble) Pseudoephedrine hydrochloride 20 mg, dextromethorphan HBr 10 mg/5 mL, alcohol 10%, saccharin, sucrose. Bot. 120 mL, 240 mL. *OTC.*
Use: Antitussive, decongestant.

Vicks 44D Cough & Head Congestion Relief. (Procter & Gamble) Dextromethorphan 10 mg, pseudoephedrine hydrochloride 20 mg/5 mL, alcohol 5%, saccharin, corn syrup. Liq. Bot. 118 mL, 236 mL. *OTC.*
Use: Upper respiratory combination; antitussive, decongestant.

Vicks 44D Dry Hacking-Cough & Head Congestion, Pediatric. (Procter & Gamble) Dextromethorphan HBr 15 mg, pseudoephedrine hydrochloride 3 mg/15 mL, alcohol free, sorbitol, sucrose, cherry flavor. Liq. Bot. 120 mL. Vicks *AccuTip* Dispenser. *OTC.*
Use: Upper resriratory combination; antitussive, decongestant.

Vicks 44D Pediatric Cough & Decongestant Liquid. (Procter & Gamble) Pseudoephedrine hydrochloride 10 mg, dextromethorphan HBr 5 mg/5 mL, alcohol free. Bot. 120 mL. *OTC.*
Use: Antitussive, decongestant.

Vicks 44E Cough & Chest Congestion Relief. (Procter & Gamble) Dextromethorphan HBr 6.67 mg, guaifenesin 66.7 mg/5 mL, alcohol 5%, corn syrup, saccharin. Bot. 118 mL, 236 mL. *OTC.*
Use: Upper respiratory combination; antitussive, expectorant.

Vicks 44E Pediatric Liquid. (Procter & Gamble) Dextromethorphan HBr 10 mg, guaifenesin 100 mg/5 mL, sorbitol, sucrose. Alcohol free. Bot. 120 mL w/Vicks *AccuTip* Dispenser. *OTC.*
Use: Antitussive, expectorant.

Vicks 44M Cold, Flu & Cough LiquiCaps. (Procter & Gamble) Dextromethorphan HBr 10 mg, pseudoephedrine hydrochloride 30 mg, chlorpheniramine maleate 2 mg, acetaminophen 250 mg. Cap. Pkg. 12s. *OTC.*
Use: Analgesic, antihistamine, antitussive, decongestant.

Vicks 44M Cough, Cold, & Flu. (Procter & Gamble) Dextromethorphan HBr 30 mg, pseudoephedrine hydrochloride 60 mg, chlorpheniramine maleate 4 mg, acetaminophen 650 mg/20 mL, alcohol 10%. Liq. Bot. 4 oz, 8 oz w/Vicks *AccuTip* Dispenser. *OTC.*
Use: Analgesic, antihistamine, antitussive, decongestant.

Vicks 44M Cough, Cold & Flu Relief. (Procter & Gamble) Dextromethorphan HBr 7.5 mg, chlorpheniramine maleate 1 mg, pseudoephedrine hydrochloride 15 mg, acetaminophen 162.5 mg/5 mL, alcohol 10%, corn syrup, saccharin. Liq. Bot. 236 mL. *OTC.*
Use: Upper respiratory combination; antitussive, antihistimine, decongestant, analgesic.

Vicks 44 Non-Drowsy Cold & Cough LiquiCaps. (Procter & Gamble) Dextromethorphan HBr 30 mg, pseudoephedrine hydrochloride 60 mg. Cap. Pkg. 10s. *OTC.*
Use: Antitussive, decongestant.

Vicks NyQuil Cough. (Procter & Gamble) Dextromethorphan HBr 5 mg, doxylamine succinate 2.1 mg/5 mL, alcohol, corn syrup, saccharin, cherry flavor. Syr. Bot. 177 mL. *OTC.*
Use: Upper respiratory combination; antitussive, antihistamine.

Vicks NyQuil LiquiCaps. (Procter & Gamble) Acetaminophen 250 mg, pseudoephedrine hydrochloride 30 mg, dextromethorphan HBr 10 mg, doxylamine succinate 6.25 mg. Pkg. 12s, 20s. *OTC.*

Use: Analgesic, antihistamine, antitussive, decongestant.

Vicks NyQuil Liquid Multi-Symptom Cold/Flu Relief. (Procter & Gamble) Acetaminophen 1000 mg, doxylamine succinate 12.5 mg, pseudoephedrine hydrochloride 60 mg, dextromethorphan HBr 30 mg/30 mL, alcohol 10%. Regular and cherry flavors. Regular contains FD&C Yellow No. 6. Bot. 6 oz, 10 oz, 14 oz. *OTC.*
Use: Analgesic, antihistamine, antitussive, decongestant.

Vicks NyQuil Multi-Symptom Cold & Flu Relief LiquiCaps. (Procter & Gamble) Dextromethorphan HBr 10 mg, doxylamine succinate 6.25 mg, pseudoephedrine hydrochloride 30 mg, acetaminophen 250 mg, sorbitol. Cap. Pkg. 12s, 20s, 36s. *OTC.*
Use: Upper respiratory combination; antitussive, antihistamine, decongestant, analgesic.

Vicks NyQuil Multi-Symptom Cold/Flu Relief. (Procter & Gamble) Pseudoephedrine hydrochloride 10 mg, doxylamine succinate 2.1 mg, dextromethorphan HBr 5 mg, acetaminophen 167 mg/5 mL, alcohol 10%, corn syrup, saccharin, regular and cherry flavor. Liq. Bot. 180 mL, 300 mL, 420 mL. *OTC.*
Use: Upper respiratory combination; analgesic, antihistamine, antitussive, decongestant.

Vicks Pediatric 44E Cough & Chest Congestion Relief. (Procter & Gamble) Dextromethorphan HBr 3.3 mg, guaifenesin 33.3 mg/5 mL, corn syrup, saccharin, cherry flavor. Liq. Bot. 118 mL. *OTC.*
Use: Upper respiratory combination; antitussive, expectorant.

Vicks Pediatric 44M Cough & Cold Relief. (Procter & Gamble) Pseudoephedrine hydrochloride 10 mg, chlorpheniramine maleate 0.67 mg, dextromethorphan HBr 5 mg/5 mL, corn syrup, saccharin, cherry flavor, alcohol free. Liq. Bot. 115 mL. *OTC.*
Use: Upper respiratory combination; decongestant, antihistamine, antitussive.

Vicks Sinex. (Procter & Gamble) Phenylephrine hydrochloride 0.5%, camphor, menthol, eucalyptol, EDTA, benzalkonium chloride, tyloxapol. Soln. Spray Bot. 14.7 mL. *OTC.*
Use: Nasal decongestant, arylalkylamine.

Vicks Sinex 12-Hour. (Procter & Gamble) Oxymetazoline hydrochloride 0.05%, camphor, menthol, eucalyptol, EDTA, benzylkonium chloride, chlorhexidine, gluconate, sodium chloride, tyloxapol. Soln. Spray Bot. 15 mL. *OTC.*
Use: Nasal decongestant, imidazoline.

Vicks Sinex 12-Hour Ultra Fine Mist for Sinus Relief. (Procter & Gamble) Oxymetazoline hydrochloride 0.05%, aromatic vapors (camphor, eucalyptus, menthol), tyloxapol, EDTA, benzalkonium chloride, sodium chloride. Soln. Spray Bot. 15 mL. *OTC.*
Use: Nasal decongestant, imidazoline.

Vicks Vapor Inhaler. (Procter & Gamble) Levmetamfetamine 50 mg, menthol, camphor, lavender oil. Inhaler. Single plastic inhaler. *OTC.*
Use: Nasal decongestant, imidazoline.

Vicks VapoRub. (Procter & Gamble) Camphor 5.2%, menthol 2.8%, eucalyptus oil 1.2%. **Oint.:** Mineral oil, petrolatum. **Cream:** EDTA, glycerin, cetyl alcohol, parabens, stearyl alcohol. Jar 56 g. *OTC.*
Use: Upper respiratory combination; decongestant; vaporizing agent.

Vicks Vaposteam. (Procter & Gamble) Eucalyptus oil 1.5%, camphor 6.2%, menthol 3.2%, alcohol 74%, cedar leaf oil, nutmeg oil. Bot. 4 oz, 8 oz. *OTC.*
Use: Antitussive, decongestant.

Vicks Vitamin C Drops. (Procter & Gamble) Vitamin C 25 mg (as sodium ascorbate and ascorbic acid), sucrose, corn syrup, orange flavor. Loz. Pkg. 20s. *OTC.*
Use: Vitamin supplement.

Vicodin. (Abbott) Hydrocodone bitartrate 5 mg, acetaminophen 500 mg. Tab. Bot. 100s, 500s, UD 100s. *c-III.*
Use: Analgesic combination; narcotic.

Vicodin ES. (Abbott) Hydrocodone bitartrate 7.5 mg, acetaminophen 750 mg. Tab. Bot. 100s, UD 100s. *c-III.*
Use: Analgesic combination; narcotic.

Vicodin HP. (Abbott) Hydrocodone bitartrate 10 mg, acetaminophen 660 mg. Tab. Bot. 100s, 500s. *c-III.*
Use: Analgesic combination; narcotic.

Vicon-C. (UCB) Vitamins B_1 17.9 mg, B_2 10 mg, B_3 95 mg, B_5 22 mg, B_6 4 mg, C 300 mg, Mg, zinc 15.9 mg. Cap. Bot. 60s. *OTC.*
Use: Mineral, vitamin supplement.

Vicon Forte. (UCB) Vitamins A 8000 units, E 50 units, C 150 mg, B_3 25 mg, B_1 10 mg, B_5 10 mg, B_2 5 mg, B_6 2 mg, B_{12} 10 mcg, folic acid 1 mg, zinc sulfate 18 mg, Mg, Mn, lactose. Cap. Bot. 60s, 500s, UD 100s. *Rx.*

Use: Mineral, vitamin supplement.

Vicon Plus. (UCB) Vitamins A 4000 units, E 50 units, C 150 mg, B_3 25 mg, B_1 10 mg, B_5 10 mg, B_2 5 mg, zinc sulfate 18 mg, Mg, Mn, lactose, B_6 2 mg. Cap. Bot. 60s. *OTC.*
Use: Mineral, vitamin supplement.

Vicoprofen. (Abbott) Hydrocodone bitartrate 7.5 mg, ibuprofen 200 mg. Tab. Bot. 100s, 500s, UD 100s. *c-III.*
Use: Analgesic; narcotic.

Victors. (Procter & Gamble) Special Vicks Medication (menthol, eucalyptus oil) in a soothing Vicks sugar base. Regular or Cherry flavor drops. Stick-Pack 10s, Bag 40s. *OTC.*
Use: Anesthetic, local.

• **vidarabine.** (vih-DAR-ah-BEAN) *USP 28.*
Use: Antiviral.

• **vidarabine sodium phosphate** (vih-DAR-ah-BEAN) USAN.
Use: Antiviral.

Vi-Daylin ADC Drops. (Ross) Vitamins A 1500 units, C 35 mg, D 400 units/mL. Bot. 30 mL, 50 mL w/dropper. *OTC.*
Use: Vitamin supplement.

Vi-Daylin ADC Vitamin + Iron Drops. (Ross) Vitamins A 1500 units, C 35 mg, D 400 units, Fe 10 mg/mL, methylparaben, Bot. 50 mL. *OTC.*
Use: Mineral, vitamin supplement.

Vi-Daylin Chewable. (Ross) Vitamins A 2500 units, D 400 units, E 15 units, C 60 mg, folic acid 0.3 mg, B_1 1.05 mg, B_2 1.2 mg, niacin 13.5 mg, B_6 1.05 mg, B_{12} 4.5 mcg. Tab. Bot. 100s. *OTC.*
Use: Vitamin supplement.

Vi-Daylin Chewable w/Fluoride. (Ross) Fluoride 1 mg, vitamins B_1 1.05 mg, B_2 1.2 mg, niacinamide 13.5 mg, B_6 1.05 mg, C 60 mg, A 2500 units, B_{12} 4.5 mcg, E 15 units, folic acid 0.3 mg, D 400 units. Tab. Bot. 100s. *Rx.*
Use: Dental caries agent; mineral, vitamin supplement.

Vi-Daylin Drops. (Ross) Vitamins A 1500 units, D 400 units, E 5 units, C 35 mg, B_1 0.5 mg, B_2 0.6 mg, niacin 8 mg, B_6 0.4 mg, B_{12} 1.5 mcg/mL. Bot. 50 mL. *OTC.*
Use: Vitamin supplement.

Vi-Daylin/F ADC + Iron Drops. (Ross) Vitamins A 1500 units, C 35 mg, D 400 units, Fe 10 mg, fluoride 0.25 mg/mL, methylparaben. Bot. 50 mL. *Rx.*
Use: Dental caries agent; mineral, vitamin supplement.

Vi-Daylin/F ADC Vitamins Drops. (Ross) Vitamins A 1500 units, D 400 units, C 35 mg, fluoride 0.25 mg/mL. Alcohol ≈ 0.3%, parabens. Bot. 50 mL. *Rx.*

Use: Dental caries agent; vitamin supplement.

Vi-Daylin/F Drops. (Ross) Vitamins A 1500 units, D 400 units, E 5 units, C 35 mg, B_1 0.5 mg, B_2 0.6 mg, B_3 8 mg, B_6 0.4 mg, fluoride 0.25 mg/mL, methylparaben. Bot. 50 mL. *Rx.*
Use: Dental caries agent; vitamin supplement.

Vi-Daylin/F Multivitamin + Iron. (Ross) Fluoride 0.25 mg, vitamins A 1500 units, D 400 units, E 4.1 mg, B_1 0.5 mg, B_2 0.6 mg, B_3 8 mg, B_6 0.4 mg, C 35 mg, Fe 10 mg/mL, alcohol < 0.1%, methylparaben. Drops. Bot. 50 mL. *Rx.*
Use: Dental caries agent; mineral, vitamin supplement.

Vi-Daylin Liquid. (Ross) Vitamins A 2500 units, B_1 1.05 mg, B_2 1.2 mg, B_6 1.05 mg, B_{12} 4.5 mcg, C 60 mg, D 400 units, E 20.4 mg (as d-alpha tocopheryl acetate); niacin 13.5 mg/5 mL. Bot. 8 oz, 473 mL. *OTC.*
Use: Vitamin supplement.

Vi-Daylin Multivitamin Drops. (Ross) Vitamins A 1500 units, D 400 units, E 5 mg, B_1 0.5 mg, B_2 0.6 mg, B_3 8 mg, B_6 0.4 mg, B_{12} 1.5 mcg, C 35 mg/mL, < 0.5% alcohol. Bot. 50 mL. *OTC.*
Use: Vitamin supplement.

Vi-Daylin Multivitamin Liquid. (Ross) Vitamins A 2500 units, D 400 units, E 15 mg, B_1 1.05 mg, B_2 1.2 mg, B_3 13.5 mg, B_6 1.05 mg, B_{12} 4.5 mcg, C 60 mg/5 mL, < 0.5% alcohol. Bot. 240 mL, 480 mL. *OTC.*
Use: Vitamin supplement.

Vi-Daylin Multivitamin Plus Iron Chewable. (Ross) Vitamins A 2500 units, D 400 units, E 15 mg, C 60 mg, folic acid 0.3 mg, B_1 1.05 mg, B_2 1.2 mg, B_3 13.5 mg, B_6 1.05 mg, B_{12} 4.5 mcg, iron 12 mg. Tab. Bot. 100s. *OTC.*
Use: Mineral, vitamin supplement.

Vi-Daylin Multivitamin + Iron Drops. (Ross) Fe 10 mg, vitamins A 1500 units, D 400 units, E 5 mg, B_1 0.5 mg, B_2 0.6 mg, B_3 8 mg, B_6 0.4 mg, C 35 mg, < 0.5% alcohol, methylparaben. Bot. 50 mL. *OTC.*
Use: Mineral, vitamin supplement.

Vi-Daylin Multivitamin Plus Iron Liquid. (Ross) Vitamins A 2500 units, D 400 units, C 60 mg, E 15 units, B_1 1.05 mg, B_2 1.2 mg, B_3 13.5 mg, B_6 1.05 mg, B_{12} 4.5 mcg, Fe 10 mg/tsp. ≤ 0.5% alcohol, glucose, sucrose, parabens. 237 mL, 473 mL. *OTC.*
Use: Mineral, vitamin supplement.

Vidaza. (Pharmion) Azacitidine 100 mg. Mannitol 100 mg. Pow. for Inj., lyophilized. Single-use vials. *Rx.*
Use: Antineoplastic.

Videcon. (Vita Elixir) Vitamin D 50,000 units. Cap. *Rx.*
Use: Vitamin supplement.

Vi-Derm Soap. (Arthrins) Extract of Amaryllis 10%. Cake. Pkg. 1s. Bar 3.5 oz. *OTC.*
Use: Dermatologic; cleanser.

Videx. (Bristol-Myers Squibb) Didanosine. **Tab.:** 25 mg, 50 mg, 100 mg, 200 mg, aspartame, sorbitol, magnesium stearate, phenylalanine, orange flavor. Buffered, chewable/dispersible Tab. (Buffered w/calcium carbonate, magnesium hydroxide.) Bot. 60s. **Pow. for Oral Soln., buffered:** 100 mg, 250 mg, sodium 1380 mg/packet, sucrose. Buffered with dibasic sodium phosphate, sodium citrate, citric acid. Single-dose packet. **Pow. for Oral Soln., pediatric:** 2 g, 4 g. Bot. 4 oz (2 g), 8 oz (4 g). *Rx.*
Use: Antiretroviral, nucleoside reverse transcriptase inhibitor.

Videx EC. (Bristol-Myers Squibb) Didanosine 125 mg, 200 mg, 250 mg, 400 mg. DR Cap. (with enteric coated beadlets) Bot. 30s, 60s. *Rx.*
Use: Antiretroviral, nucleoside reverse transcriptase inhibitor.

•**vifilcon a.** (vie-FILL-kahn A) USAN.
Use: Contact lens material (hydrophilic).

•**vifilcon b.** (vie-FILL-kahn B) USAN.
Use: Contact lens material (hydrophilic).

Vifluorineed. (Hanlon) Vitamins A 5000 units, D 400 units, C 75 mg, B_1 2 mg, B_2 3 mg, niacinamide 20 mg, fluoride 1 mg. Chew. Tab. Bot. 100s. *Rx.*
Use: Mineral, vitamin supplement.

•**vigabatrin.** (vie-GAB-at RIN) USAN.
Use: Anticonvulsant (tardive dyskinesia).

Vigamox. (Alcon) Moxifloxacin hydrochloride 0.5% (5 mg/mL), boric acid, sodium chloride, purified water. Soln. *Drop-Tainer* 3 mL. *Rx.*
Use: Antibiotic, ophthalmic.

Vigomar Forte. (Marlop) Fe 12 mg, vitamins A 10,000 units, D 400 units, E 15 units, B_1 10 mg, B_2 10 mg, B_3 100 mg, B_5 20 mg, B_6 5 mg, B_{12} 5 mcg, C 200 mg, I, Mg, Mn, Cu, Zn 1.5 mg. Tab. Bot. 100s. *OTC.*
Use: Mineral, vitamin supplement.

Vigortol. (Rugby) Vitamins B_1 0.8 mg, B_2 0.4 mg, B_3 8.3 mg, B_5 1.7 mg, B_6 0.2 mg, B_{12} 0.2 mcg, Fe 0.3 mg, Zn 0.3 mg, choline, I, Mg, Mn, alcohol 18%, sugar, methylparaben. Liq. Bot. 473 mL. *OTC.*
Use: Mineral, vitamin supplement.

VIL. (Leas Research)
Use: Hyperphenylalaninemia. [Orphan Drug]

Vilex. (Oxypure) Vitamin B_1 100 mg, riboflavin phosphate sodium 1 mg, B_6 10 mg, panthenol 5 mg, niacinamide 100 mg/mL. Amp. 30 mL. *Rx.*
Use: Vitamin supplement.

Viliva. (Vita Elixir) Ferrous fumarate 3 g. *OTC.*
Use: Mineral supplement.

•**viloxazine.** (vih-LOX-ah-zeen) USAN.
Use: Antidepressant.
See: Catatrol.

Viminate. (Various Mfr.) Vitamins B_1 2.5 mg, B_2 1.25 mg, B_3 25 mg, B_5 5 mg, B_6 0.5 mg, B_{12} 0.5 mcg, Fe 7.5 mg, Zn 1 mg, choline, I, Mg, Mn 5 mL, alcohol 18%. Liq. Bot. 480. *OTC.*
Use: Mineral, vitamin supplement.

Vi-Min-for-All. (Barth's) Vitamins A 3 mg, D 10 mcg, C 120 mg, B_1 35 mg, B_{12} 15 mcg, biotin, niacin 2.33 mg, E 30 units, B_6, pantothenic acid, Ca 375 mg, P 180 mg, Fe 20 mg, I 0.1 mg, rutin 10 mg, hesperidin-lemon bioflavonoid complex 10 mg, choline, inositol 2.4 mg, Cu 10 mcg, Mn 2 mg, Zn 110 mcg, silicone 210 mcg. Tab. Bot. 100s, 500s. *OTC.*
Use: Mineral, vitamin supplement.

Vinactane Sulfate. (Novartis) Viomycin Sulfate.

•**vinafocon a.** (VIE-nah-FOE-kahn A) USAN.
Use: Contact lens material (hydrophobic).

Vinate Good Start Chewable Prenatal Formula. (Breckenridge) Ca 200 mg, Fe 29 mg, vitamin A 1000 units, D 400 units, E 30 units, B_1 3 mg, B_2 3 mg, B_3 15 mg, B_5 7 mg, B_6 20 mg, B_{12} 12 mcg, C 100 mg, folic acid 1 mg, Zn 20 mg. Chew. Tab. 100s. *Rx.*
Use: Prenatal vitamin.

Vinate GT. (Breckenridge) Ca 200 mg, Fe 90 mg, vitamin A 2700 units, D_3 400 units, E 10 units, B_1 3 mg, B_2 3.4 mg, B_3 20 mg, B_5 6 mg, B_6 20 mg, B_{12} 12 mcg, C 120 mg, folic acid 1 mg, biotin 30 mcg, docusate sodium 50 mg, Zn 15 mg, Cu, Mg. Tab. UD 90s. *Rx.*
Use: Vitamin supplement.

vinbarbital.
Use: Hypnotic, sedative.

vinbarbital sodium.
Use: Hypnotic, sedative.

- **vinblastine sulfate.** (vin-BLAST-een) *USP 28.* Vincaleukoblastine. Alkaloid extracted from *Vinca rosea* Linn.
Tall Man: VinBLAStine
Use: Antineoplastic.
See: Velban.

vinblastine sulfate. (Various Mfr.) Vinblastine sulfate. **Pow. for Inj.:** 10 mg. Vial. **Inj.:** 1 mg/mL, benzyl alcohol 0.9%. Vial 10 mL, 25 mL. *Rx.*
Use: Antineoplastic.

vinca alkaloids.
Use: Antimitotic agent.
See: Vinblastine Sulfate.
Vincristine Sulfate.
Vinorelbine Tartrate.

vincaleukoblastine, 22-oxo-sulfate (1:1) (salt). Vincristine Sulfate.

Vincasar PFS. (Gensia Sicor) Vincristine sulfate 1 mg/mL. Vial 1 mL. *Rx.*
Use: Antineoplastic.

- **vincofos.** (VIN-koe-foss) USAN.
Use: Anthelmintic.

- **vincristine sulfate.** (vin-KRISS-teen) *USP 28.*
Tall Man: VinCRIStine
Use: Antineoplastic.
See: Oncovin.
Vincasar PFS.

- **vindesine.** (VIN-deh-seen) USAN.
Use: Antineoplastic.

- **vindesine sulfate.** (VIN-deh-seen) USAN.
Use: Antineoplastic.

- **vinepidine sulfate.** (VIN-eh-pih-DEEN) USAN.
Use: Antineoplastic.

- **vinglycinate sulfate.** (vin-GLIE-sin-ate) USAN.
Use: Antineoplastic.

- **vinleurosine sulfate.** (vin-LOO-row-seen) USAN. Sulfate salt of an alkaloid extracted from *Vinca rosea* Linn. Also see Vinblastine.
Use: Antineoplastic.

- **vinorelbine tartrate.** (vih-NORE-ell-bean) USAN. Sulfate salt of an alkaloid extracted from *Vinca rosea* Linn.
Use: Antineoplastic.
See: Navelbine.

vinorelbine tartrate. (Gensia Sicor) Vinorelbine tartrate 10 mg/mL. Inj. Vials. 1 mL, 5 mL. *Rx.*
Use: Antineoplastic.

- **vinpocetine.** (VIN-poe-SEH-teen) USAN.
Use: Antineoplastic.

- **vinrosidine sulfate.** (vin-ROW-sih-deen) USAN. Sulfate salt of an alkaloid extracted from *Vinca rosea* Linn.
Use: Antineoplastic.

See: Vinblastine.
vinylacetate-polyvinylpyrrolidone.
See: Ivy-Rid Spray.
vinyl ether. *USP 28.*
Use: Anesthetic, general.
vinyzene. Bromchlorenone.
Use: Fungicide.

- **vinzolidine sulfate.** (VIN-ZOLE-ih-deen) USAN.
Use: Antineoplastic.

Vio-Bec. (Solvay) Vitamins B_1 25 mg, B_2 25 mg, niacinamide 100 mg, calcium pantothenate 40 mg, B_6 25 mg, C 500 mg. Cap. Bot. 100s. *OTC.*
Use: Mineral, vitamin supplement.

Viodo HC. (Alra) Iodochlorhydroxyquin 3%, hydrocortisone 1% in cream base. Tube 20 g. *OTC.*
Use: Antifungal; corticosteroid, topical.

Viogen-C. (Ivax) Vitamins D_1 20 mg, D_2 10 mg, B_3 100 mg, B_5 20 mg, B_6 5 mg, C 300 mg, Mg, zinc sulfate 50 mg, tartrazine. Cap. Bot. 100s. *OTC.*
Use: Mineral, vitamin supplement.

Viokase. (Axcan Scandipharm) **8:** Lipase 8000 units, protease 30,000 units, amylase 30,000 units, lactose. Tab. Bot. 100s, 500s. **16:** Lipase 16,000 units, protease 60,000 units, amylase 60,000 units, lactose. Tab. Bot. 100s, 500s. **Pow.:** Lipase 16,800 units, protease 70,000 units, amylase 70,000 units, lactose. Bot. 227 g. *Rx.*
Use: Digestive enzyme.

Viosterol w/Halibut Liver Oil. Vitamins A 50,000 units, D 10,000 units/g. (Abbott Laboratories) Bot. 5 mL, 20 mL, 50 mL. Cap.: Vitamins A 5000 units, D 1000 units (Ives) Cap.: Vitamins A 5000 units, D 1700 units. *OTC.*
Use: Vitamin supplement.

- **viprostol.** (vie-PRAHST-ole) USAN.
Use: Hypotensive; vasodilator.

Virac. (Ruson) Undecoylium Cl-iodine. Iodine complexed with a cationic detergent. Surgical Soln. Bot. 2 oz, 8 oz, 1 gal. *OTC.*
Use: Antiseptic.

Viracept. (Agouron) Nelfinavir mesylate. **Tab.:** 250 mg. Bot. 270s, 300s. **Pow.:** 50 mg, aspartame (11.2 mg phenylanine), sucrose. Multi-dose bottles. 144 g Pow. w/1 g scoop. *Rx.*
Use: Antiviral.

Viracil. (Health for Life Brands) Phenylephrine hydrochloride 5 mg, hesperidin 50 mg, thenylene hydrochloride 12.5 mg, pyrilamine maleate 12.5 mg, vitamin C 50 mg, salicylamide 2.5 g, caffeine 0.5 g, sodium salicylate 1.25 g. Cap. Bot. 16s, 36s. *OTC.*

Use: Analgesic, antihistamine, decongestant, vitamin supplement.

Viractin. (J.B. Williams Company)
See: Cēpacol Viractin.

Viramisol. (Seatrace) Adenosine phosphate 25 mg/mL. Vial 10 mL. *OTC.*
Use: Relief of varicose vein complications.

Viramune. (Boehringer Ingelheim) Nevirapine. **Tab.:** 200 mg. Lactose. Bot. 60s, 100s, UD 100s. **Oral Susp.:** 50 mg/5 mL (as nevirapine hemihydrate), parabens, sorbitol, sucrose. 240 mL. *Rx.*
Use: Antiviral.

Viranol. (Aventis) Salicylic acid in collodion gel w/lactic acid, camphor, pyroxylin, ethyl alcohol, ethyl acetate. Gel. Tube 8 g. *OTC.*
Use: Dermatologic; wart therapy.

Viravan-DM. (PediaMed) **Chew. Tab.:** Dextromethorphan tannate 25 mg, pyrilamine tannate 30 mg, phenylephrine tannate 25 mg. Sugar, sucralose. Dye-free. Grape flavor. 100s. **Susp.:** Dextromethorphan tannate 25 mg, pyrilamine tannate 30 mg, phenylephrine tannate 12.5 mg/5 mL. Methylparaben, sucralose, sucrose. Grape flavor. 473 mL. *Rx.*
Use: Pediatric antitussive.

Viravan-S. (PediaMed) Phenylephrine tannate 12.5 mg, pyrilamine tannate 30 mg/5 mL, grape flavor. Susp. 118 mL, 473 mL. *Rx.*
Use: Decongestant and antihistamine.

Viravan-T. (PediaMed) Phenylephrine tannate 25 mg, pyrilamine tannate 30 mg, sugar, saccharin, dye free, grape flavor. Chew. Tab. 100s. *Rx.*
Use: Decongestant and antihistamine.

Virazole. (ICN) Ribavirin 6 g/100 mL. Contains 20 mg/mL when reconstituted w/300 mL sterile water. Lyophilized Pow. for Aerosol Reconstitution. Vial. *Rx.*
Use: Antiviral.

Viread. (Gilead Sciences) Tenofovir disoproxil fumarate 300 mg (equivalent to tenofovir disoproxil 245 mg), lactose. Film-coated. Tab. Bot. 30s. *Rx.*
Use: Antiretroviral, nucleoside analog reverse transcriptase inhibitor.

•**virginiamycin.** (vihr-JIH-nee-ah-MY-sin) USAN. An antibiotic produced by *Streptomyces virgina.*
Use: Anti-infective.

•**viridofulvin.** (vih-RID-oh-FULL-vin) USAN.
Use: Antifungal.

Virilon. (Star) Methyltestosterone 10 mg. Cap. Bot. 100s, 1000s. *c-iii.*
Use: Sex hormone, androgen.

Virilon IM. (Star) Methyltestosterone 200 mg/mL in cottonseed oil with benzyl benzoate 20%, benzyl alcohol 0.9%. Inj. Vial 1 mL, multiple dose vial 10 mL. *c-iii.*
Use: Sex hormone, androgen.

Virogen Herpes Slide Test. (Wampole) Latex agglutination slide test for the detection of herpes simplex virus antigens directly from lesions or cell culture. Test kit 100s.
Use: Diagnostic aid.

Virogen Rotatest. (Wampole) Latex agglutination slide test for the qualitative detection of rotavirus in fecal specimens. Test kit 50s.
Use: Diagnostic aid.

Virogen Rubella Microlatex Test. (Wampole) Latex agglutination microlatex test for the detection of rubella virus antibody in serum. Test kit 500s, 5000s.
Use: Diagnostic aid.

Virogen Rubella Slide Test. (Wampole) Latex agglutination slide test for the detection of rubella virus antibody in serum. Test kit 100s, 500s, 5000s.
Use: Diagnostic aid.

Virogen Rubella Slide Test with Fast Trak Slides. (Wampole) Latex agglutination slide test for the detection of rubella virus antibody in serum.
Use: Diagnostic aid.

Viroptic. (Monarch) Trifluridine 1%, thimerosal 0.001%. Soln. Drop-Dose 7.5 mL. *Rx.*
Use: Antiviral; ophthalmic.

•**viroxime.** (vie-ROX-eem) USAN.
Use: Antiviral.

Virozyme Injection. (Marcen) Sodium nucleate 2.5%, phenol 0.5%, protein hydrolysate 2.5%, benzyl alcohol 0.2%. Vial 5 mL, 10 mL. *Rx.*
Use: Immunomodulator.

Virugon. Under study. Anhydro bis-(beta-hydroxyethyl) biguanide derivative.
Use: Treatment of influenza, mumps, measles, chickenpox, and shingles.

Viscoat. (Alcon) Sodium chondroitin sulfate 40 mg, sodium hyaluronate 30 mg, sodium dihydrogen phosphate hydrate 0.45 mg, disodium hydrogen phosphate 2 mg, sodium Cl 4.3 mg/mL. Soln. Disposable Syr. 0.5 mL. *Rx.*
Use: Viscoelastic.

viscum album, extract. Visnico.
Use: Vasodilator.

Visicol. (InKine Pharmaceutical) Sodium phosphate monobasic monohydrate

1.102 g, sodium phosphate dibasic anhydrous 0.398 g. Tab. Bot. 40s. *Rx.*
Use: Bowel cleansing agent.
●**visilizumab.** (vye-si-loo-zoo-mab) USAN.
Use: Treatment of organ transplantation rejection and other T lymphocyte-mediated diseases and disorders.
Visine Allergy Relief. (Pfizer) Tetrahydrozoline hydrochloride 0.05%. Bot. 15 mL, 30 mL. *OTC.*
Use: Mydriatic, vasoconstrictor.
Visine L.R. (Pfizer) Oxymetazoline hydrochloride 0.025%. Soln. Bot. 15 mL, 30 mL. *OTC.*
Use: Mydriatic; vasoconstrictor.
Visine Moisturizing. (Pfizer) Polyethylene glycol 400 1%, tetrahydrozoline hydrochloride 0.05%. Drop Bot. 15 mL, 30 mL. *OTC.*
Use: Mydriatic; vasoconstrictor.
Visine Pure Tears. (Pfizer Consumer) Glycerin 0.2%, hypromellose 0.2%, polyethylene glycol 400 1%. Drops. Single-drop dispenser. 9.5 mL. *OTC.*
Use: Artificial tears.
Visine Tears. (Pfizer Consumer) Glycerin 0.2%, hypromellose 0.2%, polyethylene glycol 400 1%. Drops. 15 mL, 30 mL. *OTC.*
Use: Artificial tears.
Visine Tears Preservative Free. (Pfizer Consumer) Glycerin 0.2%, hypromellose 0.2%, polyethylene glycol 400 1%. Preservative free. Drops. Single-use containers. 0.4 mL. *OTC.*
Use: Artificial tears.
VisionBlue. (Dutch Ophthalmic) Trypan blue 0.06%. Ophthalmic Soln. 0.5 mL in 2.25 mL single-use *Luer Lok* syringe. *Rx.*
Use: Ophthalmic surgery aid
Vision Care Enzymatic Cleaner. (Alcon) Highly purified pork pancreatin to be diluted in saline solution. Tab. Pkg. 24s. *OTC.*
Use: Contact lens care.
Visipaque 320. (Nycomed Amersham) Iodixanol 652 mg, iodine 320 mg/mL, EDTA. Inj. Vial 50 mL. Bot. 50 mL, 100 mL, 200 mL, 150 mL fill in 200 mL bot. Flexible containers 100 mL, 150 mL, 200 mL. *Rx.*
Use: Radiopaque agent, parenteral.
Visipaque 270. (Nycomed Amersham) Iodixanol 550 mg, iodine 270 mg/mL, EDTA. Inj. Vial 50 mL. Bot. 50 mL, 100 mL, 200 mL, 150 mL fill in 200 mL bot. Flexible containers 100 mL, 150 mL, 200 mL. *Rx.*
Use: Radiopaque agent, parenteral.

Visken. (Novartis) Pindolol 5 mg, 10 mg. Tab. Bot. 100s. *Rx.*
Use: Antihypertensive; antiadrenergic/sympatholytic, beta-adrenergic blocker.
Vistacon. (Roberts) Hydroxyzine hydrochloride 50 mg/mL. Inj. 25 mg/mL, 50 mg/mL, benzyl alcohol. Vial 10 mL; UD Vial 1 mL, 2 mL (50 mg/mL only). *Rx.*
Use: Antihistamine; anxiolytic.
Vistaril. (Pfizer) Hydroxyzine pamoate equivalent to hydroxyzine hydrochloride. **Cap.:** 25 mg, 50 mg, 100 mg. Bot. 100s, 500s, UD 100s. **Oral Susp.:** 25 mg/5 mL, sorbitol, lemon flavor. Bot. 120 mL, 480 mL. **Inj.:** 25 mg/mL. Benzyl alcohol. Vials. 10 mL. *Rx.*
Use: Anxiolytic; antihistimine, nonselective piperazine.
Vistaril I.M. (Roerig) Hydroxyzine hydrochloride, benzyl alcohol. **25 mg/mL:** Vial 10 mL. **50 mg/mL:** Vial 10 mL. Vial 1 mL, 2 mL. *Rx.*
Use: Anxiolytic; antihistamine, nonselective piperazine.
Vistide. (Gilead Sciences) Cidofovir 75 mg/ml , preservative free. Inj. Single-use vial 5 mL. *Rx.*
Use: Antiviral.
Visual-Eyes. (Optopics) Sodium Cl, sodium phosphate mono- and dibasic, benzalkonium Cl, EDTA. Soln. Bot. 120 mL. *OTC.*
Use: Irrigant; ophthalmic.
Visudyne. (QLT Phototherapeutics/Novartis Ophthalmics) Verteporfin 15 mg (reconstituted to 2 mg/mL), egg phosphatidylglycerol. Lyophilized Cake for Inj. Single-use Vial. *Rx.*
Use: Opthalmic phototherapy.
Vita-Bee with C Caplets. (Rugby) Vitamins B_1 15 mg, B_2 10.2 mg, B_3 50 mg, B_5 10 mg, B_6 5 mg, C 300 mg. TR Cap. Bot. 100s, 1000s. *OTC.*
Use: Vitamin supplement.
Vitabix. (Spanner) Vitamins B_1 100 mg, B_2 2 mg, B_6 5 mg, B_{12} 30 mcg, niacinamide 100 mg, panthenol 10 mg/mL. Vial 10 mL. Multiple-dose vial 30 mL. *Rx.*
Use: Vitamin supplement.
Vita-Bob Softgel Capsules. (Scot-Tussin) Vitamins A 5000 units, D 400 units, E 30 mg, B_1 1.5 mg, B_2 1.7 mg, B_3 20 mg, B_6 2 mg, B_{12} 6 mcg, C 60 mg, folic acid 0.4 mg. Cap. Bot. 100s. *OTC.*
Use: Vitamin supplement.
Vita-C. (Freeda) Ascorbic acid 1000 mg/ 0.25 tsp. Crystals. Can. 120 g, 1 lb. *OTC.*

Use: Vitamin supplement.

Vitacarn. (McGaw) L-carnitine 1 g/10 mL. UD Box 50s, 100s. *Rx.*
Use: L-carnitine supplement.

Vit-A-Drops. (Vision Pharmaceuticals) Vitamin A 5000 units, polysorbate 80. Bot. 10 mL, 15 mL. *OTC.*
Use: Lubricant; ophthalmic.

Vitadye. (AstraZeneca) FD&C yellow No. 5, FD&C red No. 40, FD&C blue No. 1 dyes and dihydroxyacetone 5%. Bot. 0.5 oz, 2 oz. *OTC.*
Use: Cosmetic for hyperpigmentation.

Vitafol Caplets. (Everett) Fe 65 mg, vitamins A 6000 units, D 400 units, E 30 mg, B_1 1.1 mg, B_2 1.8 mg, B_3 15 mg, B_6 2.5 mg, B_{12} 5 mcg, C 60 mg, folic acid 1 mg, calcium. Tab. Bot. 100s, 1000s. *Rx.*
Use: Mineral, vitamin supplement.

Vitafol-PN. (Everett) Ca 125 mg, Fe 65 mg, vitamins A 1700 units, D 400 units, C 60 mg, E 30 units, folic acid 1 mg, B_1 1.6 mg, B_2 1.8 mg, B_6 2.5 mg, B_{12} 5 mcg, B_3 15 mg, Mg 25 mg, Zn 15 mg. Tab. UD 100s. *Rx.*
Use: Mineral, vitamin supplement.

Vitafol Syrup. (Everett) Fe 90 mg, B_3 39.9 mg, B_6 6 mg, B_{12} 25.02 mcg, folic acid 0.75 mg. Bot. 473 mL. *Rx.*
Use: Mineral, vitamin supplement.

Vita-Iron Formula. (Barth's) Fe 120 mg, vitamins B_1 5 mg, B_2 10 mg, C 20 mg, niacin 2 mg, B_{12} 25 mcg, lysine, desiccated liver 200 mg, bromelains. Tab. Bot. 100s, 500s. *OTC.*
Use: Mineral, vitamin supplement.

Vita-Kaps Filmtabs. (Abbott) Vitamins A 5000 units, D 400 units, B_1 3 mg, B_2 2.5 mg, nicotinamide 20 mg, B_6 1 mg, C 50 mg, B_{12} 3 mcg. Bot. 100s, 1000s. *OTC.*
Use: Vitamin supplement.

Vitakaps-M. (Abbott) Vitamins A 5000 units, D 400 units, B_1 3 mg, B_2 2.5 mg, nicotinamide 20 mg, B_6 1 mg, B_{12} 3 mcg, C 50 mg, Fe 10 mg, Cu 1 mg, I 0.15 mg, Mn 1 mg, Zn 7.5 mg. Filmtab. Bot. 100s. *OTC.*
Use: Mineral, vitamin supplement.

Vita-Kid Chewable Wafers. (Solgar) Vitamins A 10,000 units, D 400 units, E 10 mg, B_1 2 mg, B_2 2 mg, B_3 10 mg, B_6 2 mg, B_{12} 5 mcg, C 100 mg, FA 0.3 mg, orange flavor. Bot. 50s, 100s. *OTC.*
Use: Vitamin supplement.

Vitalax. (Vitalax) Candy base, gumdrop flavor. Pkg. 20s. *OTC.*
Use: Laxative.

Vital B-50. (Ivax) Vitamins B_1 50 mg, B_2 50 mg, B_3 50 mg, B_5 50 mg, B_6 50 mg, B_{12} 50 mcg, folic acid 0.1 mg, biotin 50 mcg, PABA, choline bitartrate, inositol. TR Tab. Bot 60s. *OTC.*
Use: Vitamin supplement.

Vitalets. (Freeda) Fe 10 mg, vitamins A 5000 units, D 400 units, E 5 mg, B_1 2.5 mg, B_2 0.9 mg, B_3 20 mg, B_5 3 mg, B_6 2 mg, B_{12} 5 mcg, C 60 mg, biotin 25 mcg, Mn, Ca. Chew. Tab. Bot 100s, 250s. *OTC.*
Use: Mineral, vitamin supplement.

VitalEyes. (Allergan) Vitamins A 10,000 units, C 200 mg, E 100 units, Zn 40 mg, Cu, Se, Mn. Cap. Bot. 60s. *OTC.*
Use: Mineral, vitamin supplement.

Vital High Nitrogen. (Ross) Amino acids, partially hydrolyzed whey, meat, and soy, hydrolyzed corn starch, sucrose, safflower oil, MCT mono- and diglycerides, soy lecithin, vitamins A, B_1, B_2, B_3, B_5, B_6, B_{12}, C, D, E, K, folic acid, biotin, choline, Ca, P, Mg, Fe, Cu, Zn, Mn, I, Cl. Packet 80 g. *OTC.*
Use: Nutritional supplement.

Vitalize SF. (Scot-Tussin) Fe 66 mg, B_1 30 mg, B_6 15 mg, B_{12} 75 mcg, l-lysine 300 mg. Liq. Bot. 120 mL. *OTC.*
Use: Mineral, vitamin supplement.

Vitamel with Iron. (Eastwood) Drops 50 mL. Chew. Tab. Bot. 100s. *OTC.*
Use: Mineral, vitamin supplement.

•**vitamin A.** (VYE-ta-min) *USP 28.* Formerly Oleovitamin A.
Use: Antixerophthalmic vitamin; emollient.
See: Aquasol A.
Palmitate-A 5000.
W/Combinations.
See: Advanced Formula Zenate.
Advera.
Bonamil Infant Formula with Iron.
Boost.
Choice dm.
Fosfree.
Neocate One +.
Nepro.
Ocuvite.
Ocuvite Extra.
Ocuvite PreserVision.
Oncovite.
Ondrox.
Prenatal H.P.
Prenatal Plus.
Prenatal Plus w/Beta-Carotene.
Prenatal Rx.
Prenatal Z Advanced Formula.
Stuartnatal Plus.
Theragran AntiOxidant.
Tri-Flor-Vite with Flouride.

vitamin A. Vitamin A 10,000 units, 15,000 units, 25,000 units. Cap. Bot. 100s, 250s (except 25,000 units), 500s (10,000 units only). *Rx-OTC.* *Use:* Antixerophthalmic vitamin; emollient.

vitamin A acid. *See:* Tretinoin.

vitamin A, alphalin. (Eli Lilly) Vitamin A 50,000 units. Gelseal. Bot. 100s. *Rx.* *Use:* Vitamin supplement.

vitamin A, water miscible or soluble. Water-miscible vitamin A. *Use:* Vitamin supplement.

vitamin B₁. Thiamine hydrochloride. *Use:* Vitamin supplement. *See:* Thiamilate. Thiamine hydrochloride.

vitamin B₁ mononitrate. Thiamine mononitrate. *Use:* Vitamin supplement.

vitamin B₁ w/thyroid. *See:* T & T.

vitamin B₂. Riboflavin. *Use:* Vitamin supplement. *See:* Riboflavin.

vitamin B₃. Niacinamide, Nicotinamide. *Use:* Vitamin supplement. *See:* Niacor. Nicotinex. Nicotinic Acid (Niacin). Slo-Niacin.

vitamin B₅. Calcium Pantothenate. *Use:* Vitamin supplement. *See:* Calcium Pantothenate.

vitamin B₆. Pyridoxine hydrochloride. *Use:* Vitamin supplement. *See:* Aminoxin. Nestrex. Pyridoxine hydrochloride. Vitelle.

vitamin B₆. (Various Mfr.) Vitamin B₆ 50 mg, 100 mg, 250 mg, 500 mg. Tab. Bot. 100s, 250s (50 mg, 100 mg only), 1000s (50 mg only). *OTC.* *Use:* Vitamin supplement.

vitamin B₈. *See:* Adenosine phosphate.

vitamin B₁₂. Cyanocobalamin. Cobalamine. Vial. Amp. *See:* Bedoce. Betalin-12. Big Shot B-12. Cabadon-M. Cobadoce Forte. Crysto-Gel. Cyano-Gel. Dodex. Nascobal. Rubramin. Ruvite 1000.

Sigamine. Twelve Resin-K. Vi-Twel. W/Ferrous sulfate, ascorbic acid, folic acid. *See:* Intrin. W/Folic acid, niacinamide, liver. *See:* Hepfomin 500. W/Thiamine. *See:* Cobalin. Cyamine. W/Thiamine, vitamin B₆. *See:* Orexin.

vitamin B12. (Freeda) Vitamin B₁₂ 50 mcg, sorbitol, mannitol. Loz. Bot. 100s. *OTC.* *Use:* Vitamin supplement.

vitamin B₁₂. (Various Mfr.) Cyanocobalamin crystalline. **100 mcg/mL:** Vials 30 mL. **1000 mcg/ml** ⋅ Multidose vials 10 mL, 30 mL. *Rx.* *Use:* Vitamin supplement.

vitamin B₁₂. (Various Mfr.). Cyanocobalamin, oral (B₁₂). **Tab.:** 100 mcg, 500 mcg, 1000 mcg. Bot. 100s. **Loz.:** 50 mcg (sorbitol, mannitol), 100 mcg, 250 mcg, 500 mcg. Bot. 100s, 250s (250 mcg and 500 mcg only). *OTC.* *Use:* Vitamin supplement.

vitamin B₁₂ a & b. *See:* Hydroxocobalamin.

vitamin B₁₅. *Use:* Alleged to increase oxygen supply in blood. Not approved by FDA as a vitamin or drug. Illegal to sell Vitamin B₁₅.

vitamin Bc. *See:* Folic Acid.

vitamin B combinations. *Use:* Nutritional products. *See:* Calafol. Cardiotek Rx. ComBgen. DexFol. Folpace. W/Vitamin C. *See:* Dialyvite 3000. Full Spectrum B.

vitamin B complex. Concentrated extract of dried brewer's yeast and extract of corn processed w/*Clostridium acetobutylicum.* *See:* Becotin. Betalin Complex.

Vitamin B Complex, Betalin Complex, Elixir. (Eli Lilly) Vitamins B₁ 2.7 mg, B₂ 1.35 mg, B₁₂ 3 mcg, B₆ 0.555 mg, pantothenic acid 2.7 mg, niacinamide 6.75 mg, liver fraction 500 mg/5 mL, alcohol 17%. Bot. 16 oz. *OTC.* *Use:* Vitamin supplement.

Vitamin B Complex, Betalin Complex Pulvules. (Eli Lilly) Vitamins B_1 1 mg, B_2 2 mg, B_6 0.4 mg, pantothenic acid 3.333 mg, niacinamide 10 mg, B_{12} 1 mcg. Cap. Bot. 100s. *OTC.*
Use: Vitamin supplement.
See: Advanced Formula Zenate.
　Advera.
　B-C-Bid.
　Bonamil Infant Formula with Iron.
　Boost.
　Choice dm.
　Fosfree.
　Neocate One +.
　Nephplex RX.
　Nephron FA.
　Nepro.
　Ocuvite Extra.
　Oncovite.
　Prenatal HP.
　Prenatal Plus.
　Prenatal Plus w/Beta-Carotene.
　Prenatal Rx.
　Prenatal Z Advanced Formula.
　Stuartnatal Plus.
Vitamin B Complex No. 104. (Century) Vitamins B_1 100 mg, B_2 2 mg, B_6 2 mg, d-panthenol 10 mg, niacinamide 125 mg. Vial, benzyl alcohol 1%, gentisic acid ethanolamide 2.5%. Vial 30 mL. *Rx.*
Use: Vitamin supplement.
Vitamin B complex 100. (McGuff) Vitamin B_1 100 mg, B_2 2 mg, B_3 100 mg, B_5 2 mg, B_6 2 mg/mL. Inj. Vial 10 mL, 30 mL. *Rx.*
Use: Vitamin supplement.
Vitamin B Complex w/Vitamin C. (Century) Vitamins B_1 25 mg, B_2 5 mg, B_6 5 mg, niacinamide 50 mg, panthenol 5 mg, Ca 50 mg, propethylene glycol 300 10%, gentisic acid ethanolamide 2.5%, benzyl alcohol 2%. Vial 30 mL. *Rx.*
Use: Mineral, vitamin supplement.
vitamin C. (Various Mfr.). Ascorbic acid, sodium ascorbate, calcium ascorbate.
See: Ascorbic Acid Preps.
　Calcium Ascorbate.
　Cecon.
　Cenolate.
　Cevi-Bid.
　Chew-C.
　Dull-C.
　N'ice Vitamin C Drops.
　Vita-C.
W/Combinations.
See: Advanced Formula Zenate.
　Advera.
　Allbee C-800.
　Allbee-T.

　Allbee with C.
　Antiox.
　Bonamil Infant Formula with Iron.
　Boost.
　Chewable Vitamin C.
　Choice dm.
　Chromagen FA.
　Chromagen Forte.
　C-Max.
　Fosfree.
　Fruit C 100.
　Fruit C 500.
　Fruit C 200.
　Neocate One +.
　Nephplex Rx.
　Nephron FA.
　Nepro.
　Nialexo-C.
　Ocuvite.
　Ocuvite Extra.
　Ocuvite Lutein.
　Ocuvite PreserVision.
　Oncovite.
　Prenatal HP.
　Prenatal Plus.
　Prenatal Plus w/Beta-Carotene.
　Prenatal Rx.
　Protegra Softgels.
　Stuartnatal Plus.
　SunKist Vitamin C.
　Theragran Antioxidant.
　Thex.
　Thex Forte.
　Tri-Flor-Vite with Flouride.
　Vicks Vitamin C Drops.
　Vicon-C.
　Vicon Forte.
　Vicon Plus.
　Vi-Zac.
　Z-BEC.
vitamin C, cevalin. (Eli Lilly) Ascorbic acid 250 mg, 500 mg. Tab. Bot. 100s. *OTC.*
Use: Vitamin supplement.
vitamin D. Cholecalciferol.
Use: Vitamin D supplement.
W/Combinations.
See: Advanced Formula Zenate.
　Advera.
　Bonamil Infant Formula with Iron.
　Boost.
　Caltrate Plus.
　Caltrate 600 + D.
　Choice dm.
　Desert Pure Calcium.
　Fosfree.
　Neocate One +.
　Nepro.
　Oesto-Mins.
　Oncovite.
　Ondrox.

Prenatal Plus.
Prenatal Plus w/Beta-Carotene.
Prenatal Rx.
Stuartnatal Plus.
Tri-Flor-Vite with Flouride.
Vitamin D. (Various Mfr.) Ergocalciferol
(D_2) 50,000 units. Cap. Bot. 100s,
1000s. *Rx.*
Use: Vitamin supplement.
vitamin D-1.
See: Dihydrotachysterol.
vitamin D_2. Activated ergasterol, Ergo-
calciferol.
See: Calciferol.
Drisdol.
Viosterol.
vitamin D_3.
See: Delta-D.
Vitamin D_2.
vitamin D_3. (Freeda) Cholecalciferol (D_3)
1000 units. Tab. Bot. 100s, 500s. *OTC.*
Use: Vitamin supplement.
vitamin D-3-cholesterol. Compound of
crystalline vitamin D-3 and cholesterol.
vitamin D-4.
See: Dihydrotachysterol.
vitamin D, synthetic.
See: Activated 7-Dehydro cholesterol
Calciferol.
• **vitamin E.** (VYE-ta-min) *USP 28.*
Use: Vitamin E supplement.
See: d'ALPHA E 400 Softgels.
d'ALPHA E 1000 Softgels.
Dry E 400.
Lactinol-E.
Mixed E 400 Softgels.
One-A-Day Extras Vitamin E.
Soft Sense.
Tocopher.
Tocopherol.
Vitamin E with Mixed Tocopherols.
Vita-Plus E.
Wheat Germ Oil.
W/Combinations.
See: Advanced Formula Zenate.
Advera.
Antiox.
Bonamil Infant Formula with Iron.
Boost.
Choice dm.
Neocate One +.
Nepro.
Ocuvite.
Ocuvite Extra.
Ocuvite Lutein.
Ocuvite PreserVision.
Oncovite.
Ondrox.
Prenatal Plus.
Prenatal Plus w/Beta-Carotene.
Stuartnatal Plus.

Theragran AntiOxidant.
vitamin E. (Various Mfr.) Vitamin E. **Tab.:**
d-alpha tocopherol 100 units, 200 units,
400 units, 500 units, 800 units. Bot.
100s, 250s (except 800 units), 500s
(200 units, 400 units only). **Cap.:**
100 units, 200 units, 400 units,
1000 units. Bot. 50s (1000 only), 100s,
250s (400 units only). **Liq.:** (Freeda)
15 units/30 mL. Bot. 30 mL, 60 mL,
120 mL. *OTC.*
Use: Vitamin supplement.
vitamin E, eprolin. (Eli Lilly) Alpha-
tocopherol 100 units. Gelseal. Bot.
100s. *OTC.*
Use: Vitamin supplement.
• **vitamin E polyethylene glycol succinate.** *NF 23.*
Use: Vitamin supplement.
vitamin E with mixed tocopherols.
(Freeda) Vitamin E 100 units, 200 units,
400 units. Tab. Bot. 100s, 250s, 500s
(400 units only). *OTC.*
Use: Vitamin supplement.
vitamin, fat-soluble.
See: Fat-soluble vitamins.
vitamin G.
See: Riboflavin.
vitamin K.
See: AquaMEPHYTON.
Menadiol, Sodium Diphosphate.
Menadione.
Menadione Sodium Bisulfite.
Mephyton.
Phytonadione.
W/Combinations.
See: Advera.
Bonamil Infant Formula with Iron.
Choice dm.
Neocate One +.
vitamin K-1.
See: Phytonadione.
vitamin K oxide. Not available, but usu-
ally K-1 is desired.
vitamin K-3.
See: Menadione.
vitamin M.
See: Folic Acid.
vitamin, maintenance formula.
See: Stuart Formula.
vitamin-mineral-supplement liquid.
(Morton Grove) Vitamins B_1 0.83 mg,
B_2 0.42 mg, B_3 8.3 mg, B_5 1.67 mg, B_6
0.17 mg, B_{12} 0.17 mcg, I, Fe 2.5 mg,
Mg, Zn 0.3 mg, Mn, choline, alcohol
18%. Liq. 473 mL. *OTC.*
Use: Mineral, vitamin supplement.
vitamin P. Bioflavonoids.
See: Amino-Opti-C.
Bio-Flavonoid Compounds).
C Factors "1000" Plus.

Ester-C Plus 500 mg Vitamin C.
Ester-C Plus 1000 mg Vitamin C.
Ester-C Plus Multi-Mineral.
Flavons.
Hesperidin Preps.
Pan C Ascorbate.
Pan C-500.
Peridin-C.
Quercetin.
Rutin.
Span C.
Super Flavons.
Super Flavons 300.
Tri-Super Flavons 1000.
vitamins: stress formula.
See: Probec-T.
StressForm "605" w/Iron.
Stress Formula with Iron.
Stresstabs 600.
Thera-combex Kap.
vitamins w/liver & lipotropic agents.
See: Metheponex.
vitamin T. Sesame seed factor, termite factor.
Use: Claimed to aid proper blood coagulation and promote formation of blood platelets. Not approved by FDA as an active vitamin.
vitamin U. Present in cabbage juice.
Vita Natal. (Scot-Tussin) Folic acid 1 mg. Tab. Bot. 100s. *Rx.*
Use: Vitamin supplement.
Vitaneed. (Biosearch Medical Products) P-beef, Ca and Na caseinates, CHO-maltodextrin. F-partially hydrogenated soy oil, mono- and diglycerides, soy lecithin. Protein 35 g, CHO 125 g, fat 40 g, Na 500 mg, K 1250 mg/L, 1 Cal/mL, 375 mOsm/kg H_2O. Liq. Ready-to-use 250 mL. *OTC.*
Use: Nutritional supplement.
Vitaon. (Vita Elixir) Vitamin B_{12} 25 mcg, thiamine hydrochloride 10 mg, ferric pyrophosphate 250 mg/5 mL. *OTC.*
Use: Vitamin supplement.
Vita-Plus B12. (Scot-Tussin) Vitamin B_{12} 1000 mcg/mL. Inj. *Rx.*
Use: Vitamin supplement.
Vita-Plus E. (Scot-Tussin) Vitamin E 400 units as d-alpha tocopheryl acetate. Cap. Bot. 50s. *OTC.*
Use: Vitamin supplement.
Vita-Plus G . (Scot-Tussin) Vitamins A 10,000 units, D 400 units, E_2 2 mg, B_1 5 mg, B_2 2.5 mg, B_3 40 mg, B_6 1 mg, B_{12} 2 mcg, pantothenic acid 4 mg, C 75 mg, Fe, Ca, Zn 0.5 mg, K, Mg, Mn, P. Softgel Cap. Bot. 100s. *OTC.*
Use: Mineral, vitamin supplement.
Vita-Plus H Liquid Sugar Free. (Scot-Tussin) Vitamins B_1 30 mg, l-lysine

monohydrochloride 300 mg, B_{12} 75 mcg, B_6 15 mg, iron pyrophosphate soluble 100 mg/5 mL. Bot. 4 oz, 8 oz, pt, gal. *OTC.*
Use: Mineral, vitamin supplement.
Vita-Plus H Softgel. (Scot-Tussin) Fe 13.4 mg, vitamins A 5000 units, D 400 units, E 3 units, B_1 3 mg, B_2 2.5 mg, B_3 20 mg, B_5 5 mg, B_6 1.5 mg, B_{12} 2.5 mcg, C 50 mg, Ca, K, Mg, Mn, P, Zn 1.4 mg. Cap. Bot. 100s. *OTC.*
Use: Mineral, vitamin supplement.
Vita-PMS. (Bajamar Chemical) Vitamins A 2083 units, E 16.7 units, D_3 16.7 units, folic acid 33 mcg, B_1 4.2 mg, B_2 4.2 mg, B_3 4.2 mg, B_5 4.2 mg, B_6 50 mg, B_{12} 10.4 mcg, biotin, C 250 mg, Ca, Mg, I, Fe, Cu, Zn 4.2 mg, Mn, K, Se, Cr, betaine. Tab. Bot. 100s. *OTC.*
Use: Mineral, vitamin supplement.
Vita-PMS Plus. (Bajamar Chemical) Vitamins A 667 units, E 16.7 units, D_3 16.7 units, folic acid 33 mcg, B_1 4.2 mg, B_2 4.2 mg, B_3 4.2 mg, B_5 4.2 mg, B_6 16.7 mg, B_{12} 10.4 mcg, biotin, C 250 mg, Mg, I, Ca, Fe, Cu, Zn 4.2 mg, Mn, K, Se, Cr, betaine. Tab. Bot. 100s. *OTC.*
Use: Mineral, vitamin supplement.
Vita-Ray Creme. (Gordon Laboratories) Vitamins E 3000 units, A 200,000 units/oz w/aloe 10%. Jar 0.5 oz, 2.5 oz. *OTC.*
Use: Emollient.
Vitarex. (Taylor Pharmaceuticals) Vitamins A 10,000 units, D 200 units, B_1 15 mg, B_2 10 mg, B_6 5 mg, B_{12} 5 mcg, C 250 mg, B_3 100 mg, B_5 20 mg, E 15 mg, Fe 15 mg, Ca, Cu, I, K, Mg, Mn, P, Zn 10 mg. Tab. Bot. 100s. *OTC.*
Use: Mineral, vitamin supplement.
Vitazin. (Mesemer) Ascorbic acid 300 mg, niacinamide 100 mg, thiamine mononitrate 20 mg, d-calcium pantothenate 20 mg, riboflavin 10 mg, pyridoxine hydrochloride 5 mg, magnesium sulfate 70 mg, Zn 25 mg. Cap. Bot. 100s. *OTC.*
Use: Mineral, vitamin supplement.
Vita-Zoo. (Towne) Vitamins A 2500 units, D 400 units, E 15 units, C 60 mg, folic acid 0.3 mg, B_1 1.05 mg, B_2 1.2 mg, niacin 13.5 mg, B_6 1.05 mg, B_{12} 4.5 mcg. Tab. Bot. 100s. *OTC.*
Use: Vitamin supplement.
Vita-Zoo Plus Iron. (Towne) Vitamins A 2500 units, D 400 units, E 15 units, C 60 mg, folic acid 0.3 mg, B_1 1.05 mg, B_2 1.2 mg, niacin 13.5 mg, B_6 1.05 mg, B_{12} 4.5 mcg, Fe 15 mg. Tab. Bot. 100s. *OTC.*
Use: Mineral, vitamin supplement.

Vitec. (Pharmaceutical Specialties) Dl-alpha tocopheryl acetate in a vanishing cream base. Cream. 120 g. *OTC.*
Use: Emollient.

Vitelle Irospan. (Fielding) Iron 65 mg (from ferrous sulfate exsiccated), ascorbic acid 150 mg. Sugar. Cap. 60s. *OTC.*
Use: Vitamin and mineral supplement.

Vitelle Lurline PMS. (Fielding) Acetaminophen 500 mg, pamabrom 25 mg, pyridoxine hydrochloride 50 mg. Tab. Bot 50s. *OTC.*
Use: Analgesic combination.

Vitelle Nesentials. (Fielding) Vitamin A 5000 units, D_2 400 units, E 30 units, B_1 3 mg, B_2 3 mg, B_3 25 mg, B_6 2 mg, B_{12} 6 mcg, C 120 mg, Ca, P, Zn. Tab. Bot. 60s. *OTC.*
Use: Vitamin, mineral supplement.

Vitelle Nestabs OTC. (Fielding) Vitamins A 5000 units, C 120 mg, D 400 units, E 30 units, thiamin 3 mg, riboflavin 3 mg, niacinamide 20 mg, B_6 3 mg, folic acid 800 mcg, B_{12} 8 mcg, Ca 200 mg, Fe 29 mg, I, Zn 15 mg. Tab. Bot. 100s. *OTC.*
Use: Vitamin, mineral supplement.

Vitelle Nestrex. (Fielding) Pyridoxine hydrochloride 25 mg, dextrose. Tab. Bot. 100s. *OTC.*
Use: Vitamin supplement.

Vitrase. (ISTA Pharmaceutical) Hyaluronidase (ovine source). **Pow. for Inj., lyophilized:** 6,200 units. Lactose 5 mg. Preservative free. Single-use 5 mL vials with 1 mL syringe and 5 mcg filter needle. **Soln. for Inj.:** 200 units/mL. Lactose 0.93 mg. Preservative free. Single-use 2 mL vials. *Rx.*
Use: Physical adjunct.

Vitrasert. (Chiron Vision) Ganciclovir 4.5 mg (released over 5 to 8 months). Intravitreal implant. Box 1. *Rx.*
Use: Antiviral; cytomegalovirus.

Vitravene. (Novartis Ophthalmics) Fomivirsen sodium 6.6 mg/mL, sodium bicarbonate, sodium chloride, sodium carbonate. Inj. Single-use vial 0.25 mL. Preservative free. *Rx.*
Use: Antiviral; ophthalmic.

Vitron-C. (Heritage Consumer Products) Iron (from ferrous fumarate) 66 mg, ascorbic acid 125 mg. Tab. Bot. 60s. *OTC.*
Use: Mineral and vitamin supplement.

Vitussin. (Cypress) Hydrocodone bitartrate 5 mg, guaifenesin 100 mg/5 mL, cherry flavor, alcohol and dye free. Syr. Bot. 473 mL. *c-III.*
Use: Upper respiratory combination; antitussive, expectorant.

Vivactil. (Merck & Co.) Protriptyline hydrochloride 5 mg, 10 mg, lactose. Tab. Bot. 100s, UD 100s (10 mg only). *Rx.*
Use: Antidepressant.

Viva-Drops. (Vision Pharmaceuticals) Polysorbate 80, sodium Cl, EDTA, retinyl palmitate, mannitol, sodium citrate, pyruvate. Soln. Bot. 10 mL, 15 mL. *OTC.*
Use: Artificial tears.

Vivarin. (GlaxoSmithKline) Caffeine 200 mg, dextrose. Tab. Bot. 16s, 24s, 40s, 80s. *OTC.*
Use: CNS stimulant, analeptic.

Vivelle. (Novartis) Estradiol 3.28 mg (0.0375 mg/day), 4.33 mg (0.05 mg/day), 6.57 mg (0.075 mg/day), 8.66 mg (0.1 mg/day). Transdermal system. Calendar pack (8 and 24 [except 2.17 mg] systems). *Rx.*
Use: Estrogen.

Vivelle-Dot. (Novartis) Estradiol 0.39 mg (0.025 mg/day), 0.585 mg (0.0375 mg/day), 0.78 mg (0.05 mg/day), 1.17 mg (0.075 mg/day), 1.56 mg (0.1 mg/day). Transdermal system. Calendar pack (8 and 24 [0.025 mg only] systems). *Rx.*
Use: Estrogen.

Vivikon. (AstraZeneca) Vitamins B_1 5 mg, B_2 2 mg, B_6 10 mg, d-panthenol 5 mg, niacinamide 10 mg, procaine hydrochloride 2%/mL. 100 mL. *OTC.*
Use: Vitamin supplement.

Vivonex Flavor Packets. (Procter & Gamble) Nonnutritive flavoring for *Vivonex* diets when consumed orally. Orange-pineapple, lemon-lime, strawberry, and vanilla. Pkg. 60s. *OTC.*
Use: Flavoring.

Vivonex, Standard. (Procter & Gamble) Free amino acid/complete enteral nutrition. Six packets provide kcal 1800, available nitrogen 5.88 g as amino acids 37 g, fat 2.61 g, carbohydrate 407 g, and full day's balanced nutrition. Calorie:nitrogen ratio is 300:1. Unflavored pow. Packet 80 g. Pkg. 6s. *OTC.*
Use: Nutritional supplement.

Vivonex T.E.N. (Procter & Gamble) Free amino acid, high nitrogen/high branched chain amino acid complete enteral nutrition. Ten packets provide kcal 3000, available nitrogen 17 g, amino acids 115 g, fat 8.33 g, carbohydrate 617 g, and full day's balanced nutrition. Calorie:nitrogen ratio is 175:1. Unflavored pow. Packet 80 g. Pkg. 10s. *OTC.*
Use: Nutritional supplement.

Vivotif Berna. (Berna) Typhoid vaccine (oral). *Salmonella typhi* Ty21a (viable)

2 to 6 × 10^9 colony-forming units and *S. typhi* Ty21a (non-viable) 5 to 50 × 10^9 colony-forming units, sucrose 26 to 130 mg, ascorbic acid 1 to 5 mg, amino acid mixture 1.4 to 7 mg, lactose 100 to 180 mg, magnesium stearate 3.6 to 4.4 mg. EC Cap. Blister pack 4s. *Rx.*
Use: Immunization.

Vi-Zac. (UCB) Vitamins A 5,000 units, E 50 units, C 500 mg, Zn 18 mg, lactose. Bot. 60s. *OTC.*
Use: Mineral, vitamin supplement.

Vlemasque. (Dermik) Sulfurated lime topical solution 6% (Vleminck's Soln.), alcohol 7% in drying clay mask. Jar 4 oz. *OTC.*
Use: Dermatologic, acne.

VM. (Last) Vitamins B_1 6 mg, B_2 4 mg, niacinamide 40 mg, Fe 100 mg, Ca 188 mg, P 188 mg, Mn 4 mg, alcohol 12%. Bot. 16 oz. *OTC.*
Use: Mineral, vitamin supplement.

•**vofopitant dihydrochloride.** (voe-FOE-pi-tant) USAN.
Use: Antimetic.

volatile liquids.
Use: Anesthetic, general.
See: Sevoflurane.
Ultane.

•**volazocine.** (voe-LAY-zoe-SEEN) USAN. Under study.
Use: Analgesic.

Volitane. (Trent) Parethoxycaine 0.2%, hexachlorophene 0.025%, dichlorophene 0.025%. Aerosol spray can 3 oz. *OTC.*
Use: Counterirritant; antiseptic.

Voltaren. (Novartis Pharmaceuticals) Diclofenac sodium. **DR Tab.:** 25 mg, 50 mg, 75 mg, lactose. Bot. 60s, 100s, 1000s (except 25 mg), UD 100s. **Soln.:** 0.1%. EDTA 1 mg/mL, boric acid, polyoxyl 35 castor oil, sorbic acid 2 mg/mL, tromethamine. Bot. 2.5 mL, 5 mL w/dropper. *Rx.*
Use: NSAID; ophthalmic.

Voltaren-XR. (Novartis) Diclofenac sodium 100 mg, sucrose, cetyl alcohol. ER Tab. Bot. 100s, UD 100s. *Rx.*
Use: Analgesic; NSAID.

vonedrine hydrochloride. Vonedrine (phenylpropylmethylamine) hydrochloride. *OTC.*
Use: Decongestant.

von Willebrand factor complex/anti-hemophilic factor.
Use: Antihemophilic agent.

See: Humate-P.

Vopac. (Athlon) Codeine phosphate 30 mg, acetaminophen 650 mg. Tab. 100s, 500s. *c-III.*
Use: Narcotic analgesic.

•**voriconazole.** (voe-ri-CONE-a-zole) USAN.
Use: Antifungal.
See: Vfend.

•**vorozole.** (VORE-oh-zole) USAN.
Use: Antineoplastic.

VoSpire ER. (Odyssey) Albuterol (as sulfate) 4 mg, 8 mg. ER Tab. 100s. *Rx.*
Use: Bronchodilator.

•**votumumab.** (vah-TOOM-uh-mab) USAN.
Use: Monoclonal antibody.

Voxsuprine. (Major) Isoxsuprine hydrochloride 10 mg, 20 mg. Tab. Bot. 100s, 250s, 1000s, UD 100s. *Rx.*
Use: Vasodilator.

V-Tuss Expectorant. (Vangard Labs, Inc.) Hydrocodone bitartrate 5 mg, pseudoephedrine hydrochloride 60 mg, guaifenesin 200 mg/5 mL, alcohol 12.5%. *c-III.*
Use: Antitussive, decongestant, expectorant.

Vumon. (Bristol-Myers Squibb Oncology/Virology) Teniposide 50 mg (10 mg/mL), benzyl alcohol 30 mg, *Cremophor EL* (polyoxyethylated castor oil), dehydrated alcohol 42.7 %. Inj. Amp. 5 mL. *Rx.*
Use: Antineoplastic.

Vytone. (Dermik) Hydrocortisone 1%, iodoquinol 1%, greaseless base. Cream. Bot. 30 g. *Rx.*
Use: Anti-infective; corticosteroid, topical.

Vytorin. (Merck/Schering-Plough) Ezetimibe/simvastatin 10 mg/10 mg, 10 mg/20 mg, 10 mg/40 mg, 10 mg/80 mg. Lactose. Tab. 30s, 90s, 500s (10 mg/40 mg, 10 mg/80 mg only), 1,000s (10 mg/10 mg, 10 mg/20 mg only), UD 50s (10 mg/40 mg, 10 mg/80 mg only), UD 100s (10 mg/10 mg, 10 mg/20 mg only). *Rx.*
Use: Antihyperlipidemic.

VZIG. (American Red Cross; Mass. Public Health Bio. Lab.) Varicella-Zoster Immune Globulin Human Globulin fraction of human plasma, primarily IgG 10% to 18% in single-dose vials containing 125 units varicella-zoster virus antibody in 2.5 mg or less. Inj.
Use: Immunization.

W

Wade Gesic Balm. (Wade) Menthol 3%, methyl salicylate 12%, petrolatum base. Tube oz, Jar lb. *OTC.*
Use: Analgesic, topical.

Wade's Drops. Compound Benzoin Tincture.

Wakespan. (Weeks & Leo) Caffeine 250 mg. TR Cap. Pkg. 15s. *Rx.*
Use: CNS stimulant.

Wal-Finate Allergy. (Walgreen) Chlorpheniramine maleate 4 mg. Tab. Bot. 50s. *OTC.*
Use: Antihistamine.

Wal-Finate Decongestant. (Walgreen) Chlorpheniramine maleate 4 mg, pseudoephedrine sulfate 60 mg. Tab. Bot. 50s. *OTC.*
Use: Antihistamine, decongestant.

Wal-Formula Cough Syrup with D-Methorphan. (Walgreen) Dextromethorphan HBr 15 mg, doxylamine succinate 7.5 mg, sodium citrate 500 mg/10 mL. Syr. Bot. 6 oz, 8 oz. *OTC.*
Use: Antihistamine, antitussive, expectorant.

Wal-Formula M Cough Syrup. (Walgreen) Dextromethorphan HBr 30 mg, pseudoephedrine hydrochloride 60 mg, guaifenesin 200 mg, acetaminophen 500 mg/20 mL. Syr. Bot. 8 oz. *OTC.*
Use: Analgesic, antitussive, decongestant, expectorant.

Wal-Frin Nasal Mist. (Walgreen) Phenylephrine hydrochloride 0.5%, pheniramine maleate 0.2%. Soln. Bot. 0.5 oz. *OTC.*
Use: Antihistamine, decongestant.

Walgreen Artificial Tears. (Walgreen) Hydroxypropyl methylcellulose 0.5%. Soln. Bot. 0.5 oz. *OTC.*
Use: Artificial tears.

Walgreen's Finest Iron. (Walgreen) Iron 30 mg. Tab. Bot. 100s. *OTC.*
Use: Mineral supplement.

Walgreen's Finest Vit B₆. (Walgreen) Pyridoxine hydrochloride 50 mg. Tab. Bot. 100s. *OTC.*
Use: Vitamin supplement.

Walgreen Soda Mints. (Walgreen) Sodium bicarbonate 300 mg. Tab. Bot. 100s, 200s. *OTC.*
Use: Antacid.

Wal-Phed. (Walgreen) Pseudoephedrine hydrochloride. **Syr.:** 30 mg/5 mL. Bot. 4 oz. **Tab.:** 30 mg. Bot. 50s, 100s. *OTC.*
Use: Decongestant.

Wal-Phed Plus. (Walgreen) Pseudoephedrine hydrochloride 60 mg, chlorpheniramine maleate 4 mg. Tab. Bot.

50s. *OTC.*
Use: Antihistamine, decongestant.

Wal-Tussin. (Walgreen) Guaifenesin 100 mg/5 mL. Bot. 4 oz. *OTC.*
Use: Expectorant.

Wampole One-Step hCG. (Wampole) For in vitro detection of hCG in serum and urine. Test. In 3, 24, 96, 500 test kits.
Use: Diagnostic aid, pregnancy.

• **warfarin sodium.** (WORE-fuh-rin) *USP 28.*
Use: Anticoagulant.
See: Coumadin.
Jantoven.

warfarin sodium. (Various Mfr.) Warfarin sodium 1 mg, 2 mg, 2.5 mg, 3 mg, 4 mg, 5 mg, 6 mg, 7.5 mg, 10 mg. Tab. Bot. 100s, 1000s (except 10 mg). *Rx.*
Use: Anticoagulant.

Wart Fix. (Last) Castor oil 100%. Bot. 0.3 fl oz. *OTC.*
Use: Dermatologic; wart therapy.

Wart-Off. (Pfizer) Salicylic acid 17% in flexible collodion, alcohol 20.5%, ether 54.2%. Bot. 0.5 oz. *OTC.*
Use: Keratolytic.

wasp vemon.
Use: Immunization.
See: Albay.
Pharmalgen.
Venomil.

• **water.** *USP 28.*
Use: Pharmaceutic aid.

Water Babies Little Licks by Coppertone. (Schering-Plough) SPF 30, ethylhexyl p-methoxycinnamate, oxybenzone, 2-ethylhexyl salicylate, cherry flavor. Lot. Tube 4.8 g. *OTC.*
Use: Sunscreen.

Water Babies UVA/UVB SPF 15 Sunblock. (Schering-Plough) Ethylhexyl-p-methoxycinnamate, oxybenzone in lotion base. Lot. Bot. 120 mL. *OTC.*
Use: Sunscreen.

Water Babies UVA/UVB SPF 45 Sunblock. (Schering-Plough) Ethylhexyl p-methoxycinnamate, 2-ethylhexyl salicylate, otocrylene oxybenzone, benzyl alcohol. PABA free, waterproof. Lot. Bot. 120 mL. *OTC.*
Use: Sunscreen.

Water Babies UVA/UVB SPF 30 Sunblock. (Schering-Plough) Ethylhexyl p-methoxycinnamate, 2-ethylhexyl salicylate, homosalate, oxybenzone, benzyl alcohol. PABA free, waterproof. Lot. Bot. 120 mL, 240 mL. *OTC.*
Use: Sunscreen.

Water Babies SPF 25 Sunblock. (Schering-Plough) Ethylhexyl p-methoxycinna-

mate, 2-ethylhexyl salicylate, homo-salate, oxybenzone, benzyl alcohol. PABA free, waterproof. Cream. Bot. 90 g. *OTC.*
Use: Sunscreen.

•**water for hemodialysis.** *USP 28.*
Use: Hemodialysis.

•**water for injection.** *USP 28.*
Use: Pharmaceutic aid (solvent).

watermelon seed extract.
See: Citrin.
W/Phenobarbital, theobromine.
See: Cithal.

•**water, purified.** *USP 28.*
Use: Pharmaceutic aid (solvent).

water-soluble vitamins.
Use: Vitamin supplement.
See: Aminobenzoate Potassium.
Ascorbic Acid.
Ascorbic Acid Combinations.
Bioflavonoids (Vitamin P).
Calcium Ascorbate.
Cyanocobalamin (B_{12}).
Folic Acid and Derivatives.
Leucovorin Calcium.
Hydroxocobalamin.
Niacin (B_3; Nicotinic Acid).
Niacinamide (Nicotinamide).
Parenteral Liver Preparations.
Pyridoxine Hydrochloride (B_6).
Riboflavin (B_2).
Sodium Ascorbate.
Thiamin (B_1).
Vitamin B_{12}.
Vitamin C (Ascorbic Acid).

•**wax, carnauba.** *NF 23.*
Use: Pharmaceutic aid (tablet coating agent).

•**wax, emulsifying.** *NF 23.*
Use: Pharmaceutic aid (emulsifying, stiffening agent).

•**wax, microcrystalline.** *NF 23.*
Use: Pharmaceutic aid (stiffening, tablet coating agent).

Waxsol. Docusate Sodium.

•**wax, white.** *NF 23.*
Use: Pharmaceutic aid (stiffening agent).

•**wax, yellow.** *NF 23.*
Use: Pharmaceutic aid (stiffening agent).

Wayds. (Wayne) Docusate sodium 100 mg. Cap. Bot. 100s. *OTC.*
Use: Laxative.

Wayds-Plus. (Wayne) Docusate w/casanthranol. Cap. Bot. 50s. *OTC.*
Use: Laxative.

Wayne-E. (Wayne) Vitamin E. Cap.
100 units, 200 units: Bot. 1000s.
400 units: Bot. 100s. *OTC.*

Use: Vitamin supplement.

Wehless. (Roberts) Phendimetrazine tartrate 35 mg. Cap. Bot. 100s. *c-iii.*
Use: Anorexiant.

Wehless-105 Timecelles. (Roberts) Phendimetrazine tartrate 105 mg. SA Cap. Bot. 100s. *c-iii.*
Use: Anorexiant.

Wehydryl. (Roberts) Diphenhydramine hydrochloride 50 mg/mL. Vial 10 mL. *Rx.*
Use: Antihistamine.

Welchol. (Sankyo Pharma) Colesevelam hydrochloride 625 mg. Tab. Bot. 24s, 180s. *Rx.*
Use: Antihyperlipidemic; bile acid sequestrant.

Welders Eye. (Weber) Tetracaine, potassium Cl, boric acid, camphor, glycerin, disodium edetate, benzalkonium Cl as preservatives. Lot. Bot. oz. *OTC.*
Use: Burn therapy.

Wellbutrin. (GlaxoSmithKline) Bupropion hydrochloride 75 mg, 100 mg, 200 mg, film-coated. Tab. Bot. 100s. *Rx.*
Use: Antidepressant.

Wellbutrin SR. (GlaxoSmithKline) Bupropion hydrochloride 100 mg, 150 mg, 200 mg, film-coated. SR Tab. Bot. 60s. *Rx.*
Use: Antidepressant.

Wellbutrin XL. (GlaxoSmithKline) Bupropion hydrochloride 150 mg, 300 mg. ER Tab. 30s. *Rx.*
Use: Antidepressant.

Wernet's Adhesive Cream. (Block Drug) Carboxymethylcellulose gum, ethylene oxide polymer, petrolatum in mineral oil base. Cream. Tube 1.5 oz. *OTC.*
Use: Denture adhesive.

Wernet's Powder. (Block Drug) Karaya gum, ethylene oxide polymer. Bot. 0.63 oz, 1.75 oz, 3.55 oz. *OTC.*
Use: Denture adhesive.

Wes-B/C. (Western Research) Vitamins B_1 15 mg, B_2 10 mg, B_6 5 mg, niacinamide 50 mg, calcium pantothenate 10 mg, C 300 mg. Cap. Bot. 1000s. *OTC.*
Use: Mineral, vitamin supplement.

Wesmatic Forte Tablets. (Wesley) Phenobarbital 1/8 g, ephedrine sulfate 0.25 g, chlorpheniramine maleate 2 mg, guaifenesin 100 mg. Tab. Bot. 100s, 1000s. *Rx.*
Use: Antihistamine, decongestant, expectorant, hypnotic, sedative.

Westcort. (Bristol-Myers Squibb) Hydrocortisone valerate 0.2% in a hydrophilic base with white petrolatum. **Cream:** Tube. 15 g, 45 g, 60 g, 120 g. **Oint.:**

Mineral oil. Tube. 15 g, 45 g, 60 g. *Rx.*
Use: Corticosteroid, topical.

Westhroid. (Western Research Labs) Thyroid desiccated 32.4 mg (½ grain), 64.8 mg (1 grains), 129.6 mg (2 grains), 194.4 mg (3 grains). Tab. Bot. 100s. *Rx.*
Use: Hormone, thyroid.

Wesvite. (Western Research) Vitamins B_1 10 mg, B_2 5 mg, B_6 2 mg, pantothenic acid 10 mg, niacinamide 30 mg, B_{12} 3 mcg, C 100 mcg, E 5 units, A 10,000 units, D 400 units, Fe 15 mg, Cu 1 mg, I 0.15 mg, Mn 1 mg, Zn 1.5 mg. Tab. Bot. 1000s. *OTC.*
Use: Mineral, vitamin supplement.

Wet-N-Soak. (Allergan) Borate buffered. WSCP 0.006%, hydroxyethylcellulose. Soln. Bot. 15 mL. *OTC.*
Use: Contact lens care.

Wet-N-Soak Plus. (Allergan) Polyvinyl alcohol, edetate disodium, benzalkonium Cl 0.003%. Soln. Bot. 120 mL, 180 mL. *OTC.*
Use: Contact lens care.

Wetting and Soaking. (Bausch & Lomb) Chlorhexidine gluconate 0.006%, EDTA 0.05%, cationic cellulose derivative polymer. Soln. Bot. 118 mL. *OTC.*
Use: Contact lens care.

Wetting and Soaking. (PBH Wesley Jessen) Buffered, isotonic. Chlorhexidine gluconate 0.005%, NaCl, octylphenoxy (oxyethylene) ethanol, povidone, polyvinyl alcohol, propylene glycol, hydroxyethylcellulose. Soln. Bot. 120 mL. *OTC.*
Use: Contact lens care.

Wetting Solution. (PBH Wesley Jessen) Polyvinyl alcohol, benzalkonium Cl 0.004%, EDTA 0.02%. Soln. Bot. 60 mL. *OTC.*
Use: Contact lens care.

wheat germ oil. (Various Mfr.)
Use: Vitamin supplement
See: Natural Viobin Wheat Germ Oil.
Natural Wheat Germ Oil.
Tocopherol.

wheat germ oil concentrate. (Thurston) Wheat germ oil concentrate. Perles. 6 min. Bot. 100s. *OTC.*
Use: Cardiovascular agent.

whey protein concentrate (bovine).
See: Bovine Whey Protein Concentrate.

WHF Lubricating Gel. (Lake Consumer) Chlorehexidine gluconate, methylparaben, glycerin. Gel. Tube 113.4 g. Ind. packets 3 g. *OTC.*
Use: Vaginal dryness relief.

Whirl-Sol. (Sween) Moisturizing bath additive. Bot. 2 oz, 8 oz, 16 oz, 21 oz, gal,

5 gal, 30 gal, 55 gal. *OTC.*
Use: Emollient.

white-faced hornet venom.
Use: Immunization.
See: Albay.
Pharmalgen.
Venomil.

white lotion. Lotio Alba.
Use: Astringent.
See: Zinc Sulfide Topical Suspension.

white precipitate.
See: Ammoniated Mercury.

Whitfield's Ointment. (Various Mfr.) Benzoic acid 6%, salicylic acid 3%. Oint. Tube. *OTC.*
Use: Antiinfective, topical.

•**whooping cough vaccine.** *USP 28.*
See: Acel-Imune.
ActHIB/DTP, Set of DTwP vial plus Hib.
Diphtheria and Tetanus Toxoids with Pertussis Vaccine.
Infanrix.
Pertussis Vaccine.
Tetramune.
Tri-Immunol.
Tripedia.

Whorto's Calamine Lotion. (Whorton Pharmaceuticals, Inc.) Calamine, zinc oxide, glycerin (U.S.P. strength) in carboxymethylcellulose lotion vehicle. Lot. Bot. 4 oz, gal. *OTC.*
Use: Dermatologic; counterirritant.

Wibi. (Galderma) Purified water, SD alcohol 40, glycerin, PEG-4, PEG-6-32 stearate, PEG-6-32, glycol stearate, carbomer 940, PEG-75, methylparaben, propylparaben, triethanolamine, menthol, fragrance. Lot. Bot. 8 oz, 16 oz. *OTC.*
Use: Emollient.

widow spider species antivenin (Latrodectus mactans). (Merck & Co.) Antivenin, *Lactrodectus mactans.*
Use: Immunization.

wild cherry.
Use: Flavored vehicle.

Wilpor-Clear. (Foy Laboratories) Phentermine hydrochloride 30 mg. Cap. Bot. 1000s. *c-iv.*
Use: Anorexiant.

Wilpowr. (Foy Laboratories) Phentermine hydrochloride 30 mg. Cap. Bot. 100s, 500s, 1000s. *c-iv.*
Use: Anorexiant.

WinRho SDF. (NABI) $RH_o(D)$ immune globulin IV human 600 units, 1500 units, 5000 units, glycine 0.1 M, sodium chloride 0.04 M, polysorbate 80 0.01%, preservative free, solvent/detergent treated, sodium chloride injection dilu-

ent 0.9% 2.5 mL (600 units, 1500 units only), 8.5 mL (5000 units). Pow. for Inj., freeze-dried. Single-dose vial. *Rx.*
Use: Immune globulin.

Wintergreen Sucrets. (GlaxoSmithKline) Dyclonine hydrochloride 0.1%, alcohol 10%, sorbitol. Spray. Bot. 90 mL. *OTC.*
Use: Mouth and throat preparation.

•**witch hazel.** *USP 28.*
Use: Astringent.

witch hazel. (Various Mfr.) Hamamelis water (witch hazel). Bot. 120 mL, 240 mL, 280 mL, 480 mL, 960 mL, gal.
Use: Astringent.

Within. (Bayer Corp. (Consumer Div.)) Vitamins A 5000 units, E 30 units, C 60 mg, folic acid 0.4 mg, $B_1$1.5 mg, B_2 1.7 mg, niacin 20 mg, B_6 2 mg, B_{12} 6 mcg, pantothenic acid 10 mg, D 400 units, Fe 27 mg, Ca 450 mg, Zn 15 mg. Tab. Bot. 60s, 100s. *OTC.*
Use: Mineral, vitamin supplement.

WNS. (Sanofi-Synthelabo) Sulfamylon hydrochloride. Supp. *Rx.*
Use: Anorectal preparation.

Women's Gentle Laxative. (Goldline Consumer) Bisacodyl 5 mg, lactose, sugar. EC Tab. Pkg. 30s. *OTC.*
Use: Laxative.

Women's Tylenol Multi-Symptom Menstrual Relief. (McNeil Consumer) Acetaminophen 500 mg, pamabrom 25 mg. Tab. Bot. 24s. *OTC.*
Use: Analgesic.

Wonderful Dream. (Kondon) Phenylmercuric nitrate 1:5000, oils of tar, turpentine, olive and linseed, rosin, burgundy pitch, camphor, beeswax, mutton tallow. Salve. 34 g. *OTC.*
Use: Topical.

Wonder Ice. (Pedinol Pharmacal) Menthol in a specially formulated base. Gel. Tube 113 mL. *OTC.*
Use: Liniment.

Wondra. (Procter & Gamble) Petrolatum, lanolin acid, glycerin, stearyl alcohol, cyclomethicone, EDTA, hydrogenated vegetable glycerides phosphate, cetyl alcohol, isopropyl palmitate, stearic acid, PEG-100 stearate, carbomer 934, dimethicone, titanium dioxide, imidazolidinyl urea, parabens. Lot. Bot. 180 mL, 300 mL, 450 mL. *OTC.*
Use: Emollient.

wood charcoal. (Cowley) Wood charcoal. 5 g, 10 g. Tab. Bot. 1000s. *OTC.*

wood creosote.
See: Creosote.

wool fat. Lanolin, Anhydrous.

Wyanoids Relief Factor. (Wyeth) Cocoa butter 79%, shark liver oil 3%, corn oil, EDTA, parabens, tocopherol. Supp. 12s. *OTC.*
Use: Anorectal preparation.

Wydase Lyophilized. (Wyeth) Purified bovine testicular hyaluronidase. Vial 150 units/mL, 1500 units/10 mL with lactose and thimerosal. *Rx.*
Use: Absorption facilitator; hypodermoclysis; urography.

Wydase Stabilized Solution. (Wyeth) Purified bovine testicular hyaluronidase 150 units/mL in sterile saline soln. with sodium Cl, EDTA, thimerosal. Vial 1 mL, 10 mL. *Rx.*
Use: Absorption facilitator; hypodermoclysis; urography.

Wymox. (Wyeth-Ayerst) Amoxicillin trihydrate. **Cap.:** 250 mg Bot. 100s, 500s; 500 mg Bot. 50s, 500s. **Pow. for Oral Susp.:** 125 mg/5 mL (as trihydrate) when reconstituted; 250 mg/ 5 mL (as trihydrate) when reconstituted. Bot. 100 mL, 150 mL. Sucrose. *Rx.*
Use: Anti-infective, penicillin.

Wytensin. (Wyeth) Guanabenz acetate 4 mg, 8 mg, 16 mg. Tab. Bot. 100s; 500s, *Redipak* 100s (4 mg only). *Rx.*
Use: Antihypertensive.

X

Xalatan. (Pfizer) Latanoprost 0.005%, benzalkonium chloride 0.02%, sodium chloride. Soln. In 2.5 mL fill dropper bottles. *Rx.*
Use: Agent for glaucoma.

• **xaliproden.** (ZAL-ip-roe-den) USAN.
Use: Nootrope.

• **xamoterol.** (ZAM-oh-ter-ole) USAN.
Use: Cardiovascular agent.

• **xamoterol fumarate.** (ZAM-oh-ter-ole FEW-mah-rate) USAN.
Use: Cardiovascular agent.

Xanax. (Pfizer) Alprazolam 0.25 mg, 0.5 mg, 1 mg, 2 mg. Lactose. Tab. 100s, 500s, 1000s (except 2 mg), UD 100s (0.25 mg, 0.5 mg only). *c-iv.*
Use: Anxiolytic.

Xanax XR. (Pfizer) Alprazolam 0.5 mg, 1 mg, 2 mg, 3 mg. Lactose. ER Tab. 60s. *c-iv.*
Use: Anxiolytic.

• **xanomeline.** (zah-NO-meh-leen) USAN.
Use: Cholinergic agonist (for Alzheimer disease).

• **xanomeline tartrate.** (zah-NO-meh-leen TAR-trate) USAN.
Use: Cholinergic agonist (for Alzheimer disease).

• **xanoxate sodium.** (ZAN-ox-ate SO-dee-uhm) USAN.
Use: Bronchodilator.

• **xanthan gum.** *NF 23.*
Use: Pharmaceutic aid, suspending agent.

xanthine derivatives.
See: Caffeine
Theobromine.
Theophylline.

• **xanthinol niacinate.** (ZAN-thih-nahl NYE-ah-SIN-ate) USAN.
Use: Vasodilator, peripheral.

xanthiol hydrochloride.
Use: Antinauseant.

xanthotoxin. Methoxsalen.

Xeloda. (Roche) Capecitabine 150 mg, 500 mg, lactose. Tab. Bot. 60s (150 mg only), 120s, 240s (500 mg only). *Rx.*
Use: Antimetabolite, pyrimidine analog.

• **xemilofiban hydrochloride.** (zem-ih-LOW-fih-ban) USAN.
Use: Treatment of unstable angina; prevention of post-recanalization reocclusion of coronary vessels.

• **xenalipin.** (ZEN-ah-LIH-pin) USAN.
Use: Hypolipidemic.

• **xenbucin.** (ZEN-BYOO-sin) USAN.
Use: Antihyperlipidemic.

Xenical. (Roche) Orlistat 120 mg. Cap. Bot. 90s. *Rx.*
Use: Antiobesity agent; lipase inhibitor.

• **xenon Xe 133.** (ZEE-nahn) *USP 28.*
Use: Radiopharmaceutical.

• **xenon Xe 127.** (ZEE-nahn) *USP 28.*
Use: Diagnostic aid; medicinal gas; radiopharmaceutical.

Xerac AC. (Person and Covey) Aluminum Cl hexahydrate 6.25% in anhydrous ethanol 96%. Bot 35 mL, 60 mL. *Rx.*
Use: Dermatologic, acne.

Xeroform 3%. (Various Mfr.) Pow. 0.25 lb, 1 lb. Jar 1 lb, 5 lb.
Use: Wound care.

Xero-Lube. (Scherer) Monobasic potassium phosphate, dibasic potassium phosphate, magnesium Cl, potassium Cl, calcium Cl, sodium Cl, sodium fluoride, sorbitol, sodium carboxymethylcellulose, methylparaben. Soln. Bot. 6 oz. *OTC.*
Use: Mouth and throat preparation.

Xibrom. (Bausch & Lomb) Bromfenac 0.09%. Benzalkonium chloride 0.05 mg/mL, EDTA 0.2 mg/mL, povidone 20 mg/mL, sodium hydroxide. Soln. Dropper bottles. 5 mL. *Rx.*
Use: Nonsteroidal anti-inflammatory drug, ophthalmic.

Xifaxan. (Salix) Rifaximin 200 mg. EDTA. Film-coated. Tab. 30s. *Rx.*
Use: Anti-infective.

Xigris. (Eli Lilly) Drotrecogin alfa (activated) 5 mg (sodium chloride 40.3 mg), 20 mg (sodium chloride 158.1 mg), preservative free, sucrose. Pow. for Infusion. lyophilized. Single-use vials. *Rx.*
Use: Thrombolytic agent, recombinant human activated protein C.

• **xilobam.** (ZIE-low-bam) USAN.
Use: Muscle relaxant.

• **ximelagatran.** (zye-mel-a-GAT-ran) USAN.
Use: Investigational antithrombotic.

• **xipamide.** (ZIP-ah-mide) USAN.
Use: Antihypertensive; diuretic.

Xolair. (Genentech) Omalizumab 129.6 mg (75 mg/0.6 mL after reconstitution, sucrose 93.1 mg), 202.5 mg (150 mg/1.2 mL after reconstitution, sucrose 145.5 mg), preservative free. Lyophilized Pow. for Inj. Single-use 5 mL vials. *Rx.*
Use: Monoclonal antibody.

Xopenex. (Sepracor) Levalbuterol. **Soln. for Inhalation:** 0.31 mg/3 mL (as base), 0.63 mg/3 mL (as base), 1.25 mg/3 mL

(as base), preservative free, sulfuric acid. UD Vial 3 mL. **Soln. for Inhalation, concentrate:** 1.25 mg/0.5 mL (as base). Preservative free. In 0.5 mL UD vials. *Rx.*
Use: Bronchodilator, sympathomimetic.
●**xorphanol mesylate.** (ZAHR-fan-ahl MEH-sih-LATE) USAN.
Use: Analgesic.
X-Prep. (Gray) Senna extract, parabens, sugar 50 g, alcohol free. Liq. Bot. 74 mL. *OTC.*
Use: Laxative.
X-Prep Bowel Evacuant Kit-1. (Gray) **X-Prep:** Liq. 74 mL (extract of senna concentrate, sugar 50 g, sucrose, parabens, alcohol free). **Senokot-S:** Tab (2) (standardized senna concentrate, docusate sodium 50 mg, lactose). **Rectolax:** Supp. (1) (Bisacodyl 10 mg). *OTC.*
Use: Laxative.
X-Ray Contrast Media.
See: Iodine Products, Diagnostic.
X-Seb. (Norton) Salicylic acid 4%, coal tar soln. 10% in a blend of surface-active agents. Shampoo. Bot. 4 oz. *OTC.*
Use: Antiseborrheic.
X-Seb Plus. (Norton) Pyrithionic zinc 1%, salicylic acid 2%. Shampoo. Bot. 120 mL. *OTC.*
Use: Antiseborrheic.
X-Seb T. (Norton) Coal tar soln. 10%, salicylic acid 4%. Soln. Bot. 4 oz. *OTC.*
Use: Antiseborrheic.
X-Seb T Plus. (Norton) Coal tar solution 10%, salicylic acid, menthol 1%. Shampoo. Bot. 120 mL. *OTC.*
Use: Antiseborrheic.
Xtracare. (Sween) Bot. 2 oz, 4 oz, 8 oz, 21 oz, gal. *OTC.*
Use: Emollient.
Xtra-Vites. (Barth's) Vitamins A 10,000 units, D 400 units, C 150 mg, B₁ 5 mg, B₂ 1 mg, niacin 3.33 mg, pantothenic acid 183 mcg, B₆ 250 mcg, B₁₂ 215 mcg, E 15 units, rutin 20 mg, citrus bioflavonoid complex 15 mg, choline 6.67 mg, inositol 10 mg, folic acid 50 mcg, biotin, aminobenzoic acid. Tab. Bot. 30s, 90s, 180s, 360s. *OTC.*
Use: Vitamin supplement.
X-Trozine. (Shire US) Phendimetrazine tartrate 35 mg. Cap. Tab. Bot. 1000s. *c-III.*
Use: Anorexiant.
X-Trozine S.R. (Shire US) Phendimetrazine tartrate 105 mg. Cap. Bot. 100s, 200s, 1000s. *c-III.*
Use: Anorexiant.

●**xylamidine tosylate.** (zie-LAM-ih-deen TAH-sill-ate) USAN.
Use: Serotonin inhibitor.
●**xylazine hydrochloride.** (ZIE-lih-zeen) USAN.
Use: Analgesic.
●**xylitol.** (ZIE-lih-tahl) *NF 23.*
Use: Pharmaceutic aid, vehicle, sweetened.
Xylocaine. (AstraZeneca) Lidocaine hydrochloride 2%. Parabens. Gel. 5 mL, 30 mL. *Rx.*
Use: Topical local anesthetic.
Xylocaine Hydrochloride for Spinal Anesthesia. (AstraZeneca) Lidocaine hydrochloride 1.5%, 5%, glucose 7.5%, sodium hydroxide to adjust pH. Specific gravity 1.028-1.034. Amp. 2 mL. Box 10s. *Rx.*
Use: Anesthetic, local.
Xylocaine Hydrochloride IV for Cardiac Arrhythmias. (Astra) Lidocaine 2% (20 mg/mL). Inj. (for direct IV administration). Amp 5 mL. *Rx.*
Use: Antiarrhythmic agent.
Xylocaine Hydrochloride 4%. (Astra-Zeneca) Lidocaine 4%. Soln. Bot. 50 mL. *Rx.*
Use: Anesthetic, local topical.
Xylocaine Hydrochloride w/Dextrose. (AstraZeneca) Lidocaine hydrochloride 1.5%, dextrose 7.5%. Inj. Amp. 2 mL. *Rx.*
Use: Anesthetic, local.
Xylocaine Hydrochloride w/Epinephrine. (AstraZeneca) Lidocaine hydrochloride 2% w/epinephrine 1:200,000. Amp. w/sodium metabisulfite 20 mL. Inj. Single dose vials w/sodium metabisulfite. 20 mL. *Rx.*
Use: Anesthetic, local.
Xylocaine Hydrochloride w/Glucose. (AstraZeneca) Lidocaine hydrochloride 5%, glucose 7.5%. Inj. Amp. 2 mL. *Rx.*
Use: Anesthetic, local.
Xylocaine Injection. (AstraZeneca) Lidocaine 0.5%, 1%, 2%, methylparaben. Multidose vials 10 mL, 20 mL (except 0.5%); 50 mL. Cartridge 1.8 mL (2% only). Lidocaine 0.5% epinephrine 1:200,000, methylparaben. Multidose vial 50 mL. Lidocaine 1%, epinephrine 1:100,000, methylparaben. Multidose vials 10 mL, 20 mL, 50 mL. Lidocaine 2% epinephrine 1:50,000, sodium metabisulfite. Dental Cart. 1.8 mL. Lidocaine 2%, epinephrine 1:100,000. Multidose vials 10 mL, 20 mL, 50 mL, methylparaben, sodium metabisulfite. Cart 1.8 mL, sodium metabisulfite.

Lidocaine 1.5%, dextrose 7.5%. Amp. 2 mL. *Rx.*
Use: Anesthetic, local amide.

Xylocaine Jelly. (AstraZeneca) Lidocaine hydrochloride 2% in sodium carboxymethylcellulose with parabens. Jelly. Tube 5 mL, 30 mL. *Rx.*
Use: Anesthetic, local amide.

Xylocaine MPF. (AstraZeneca) Lidocaine. **0.5%:** Single-dose vial 50 mL. **1%:** Amp. 2 mL, 5 mL, 30 mL. *PolyAmp DuoFit* 10 mL, 20 mL. Single-dose vial 2 mL, 5 mL, 10 mL, 30 mL. **1.5%:** Amp. 20 mL. *PolyAmp DuoFit* 10 mL, 20 mL. Single-dose vial 5 mL, 10 mL. **2%:** Amp. 2 mL, 10 mL. *PolyAmp DuoFit* 10 mL. Single-dose vial 2 mL, 5 mL, 10 mL. **4%:** Amp. 5 mL. Syr. 5 mL w/laryngotracheal cannula. **1% w/epinephrine 1:200,000:** Amp. 30 ml Single-dose vial 5 mL, 10 mL, 30 mL, sodium metabisulfite. **1.5% w/epinephrine 1:200,000:** Amp. 5 mL, 30 mL. Single-dose vial 5 mL, 10 mL, 30 mL, sodium metabisulfite. **2% w/epinephrine 1:200,000:** Amp. 20 mL. Single-dose vial 5 mL, 10 mL, 20 mL, sodium metabisulfite. **1.5% w/dextrose 7.5%:** Amp. 2 mL. **5% w/dextrose 7.5%:** Amp. 2 mL. *Rx.*
Use: Anesthetic, local amide.

Xylocaine Ointment. (AstraZeneca) Lidocaine 2.5%, water soluble carbowaxes. Oint. Tube 35 g *OTC.*
Use: Anesthetic, local.

Xylocaine Viscous. (AstraZeneca) Lidocaine hydrochloride 2%, sodium carboxymethylcellulose, parabens. Bot. 20 mL (25s), 100 mL, 450 mL and UD 20 mL. *Rx.*
Use: Anesthetic, local.

•**xylofilcon a.** (ZILE-oh-FILL-kahn A) USAN.
Use: Contact lens material (hydrophilic).

•**xylometazoline hydrochloride.** (zie-low-met-AZZ-oh-leen) *USP 28.*
Use: Adrenergic (vasoconstrictor).
See: Long Acting Neo-Synephrine.
Natru-Vent.
Otrivin.
Otrivin Pediatric Nasal.
Rhinall L.A.
Sinu-Off.
Vicks Sinex Long Acting.

•**xylose.** (ZIE-lohs) *USP 28.*
Use: Diagnostic aid, intestinal function determination.

Xyrem. (Orphan Medical) Sodium oxybate 500 mg/mL. Sodium ≥ 83 mg/mL. Oral Soln. 180 mL with syringe and dosing cups. *c-III.*
Note: Available only through the *Xyrem* Success Program. Call 1–866–997–3688 for more information.
Use: Psychotherapeutic agent, miscellaneous.

Y

Yager's Liniment. (Yager) Oil of turpentine and camphor w/clove oil fragrance, emulsifier, emollient, ammonium oleate (less than 0.5% free ammonia) penetrant base. *OTC.*
Use: Rubefacient.

Yasmin. (Berlex) Ethinyl estradiol 30 mcg, drospirenone 3 mg, lactose. Tab. Blister pack 28s. *Rx.*
Use: Sex hormone, contraceptive hormone.

yatren.
See: Chiniofon.

YDP Lice. (Youngs Drug) Synthetic pyrethroid in aerosol. Spray. Can. 5 oz. *OTC.*
Use: Pediculicide, inanimate objects.

yeast adenylic acid. An isomer of adenosine 5-monophosphate, has been found inactive.
See: Adenosine 5-Monophosphate.

yeast, dried.
Use: Protein and vitamin B Complex source.

Yeast-Gard. (Lake Consumer) Pulsatilla 28x, *Candida albicans*: 28x. Supp. 10s w/applicator. *OTC.*
Use: Vaginal agent.

Yeast-Gard Medicated Disposable Douche. (Lake Consumer) Povidone-iodine 0.3% when reconstituted. Soln. 180 mL twin-pack w/two 5.4 mL medicated douche concentrate packets. *OTC.*
Use: Douche.

Yeast-Gard Medicated Disposable Douche Premix. (Lake Consumer) Octoxynol 9, lactic acid, sodium lactate, sodium benzoate, aloe vera. Soln. 180 mL twin-pack. *OTC.*
Use: Douche.

Yeast-Gard Medicated Douche. (Lake Consumer) Povidone-iodine 10%. Soln. Concentrate. 240 mL. *OTC.*
Use: Douche.

yeast tablets, dried.
Use: Supplementary source of B complex vitamins.
See: Brewer's Yeast.

yeast, torula.
See: Torula Yeast.

yeast w/iron.
See: Natural Super Iron Yeast Powder.

Yeast-X. (C.B. Fleet) Pulsatilla 28x. Supp. Pkg. 12s w/applicator. *OTC.*
Use: Vaginal agent.

Yelets. (Freeda) Iron 20 mg, vitamins A 10,000 units, D 400 units, E 10 units, B₁ 10 mg, B₂ 10 mg, B₃ 25 mg, B₅ 10 mg, B₆ 10 mg, B₁₂ 10 mcg, C 100 mg, folic acid 0.1 mg, PABA, lysine, glutamic acid, Ca, I, Mg, Mn, Se, Zn 4 mg. Tab. Bot. 100s, 250s. *OTC.*
Use: Mineral, vitamin supplement.

yellow enzyme.
See: Riboflavin.

•**yellow fever vaccine.** *USP 28.*
Use: Immunization.
See: YF-Vax.

yellow hornet venom.
Use: Desensitizing agent.
See: Albay.
Pharmalgen.
Venomil.

yellow jacket venom.
Use: Desensitizing agent.
See: Albay.
Pharmalgen.
Venomil.

yellow mercuric oxide 1%. (Various Mfr.) Yellow mercuric oxide 1% Oint. Tube 3.5, 3.75, 30 g. *OTC.*
Use: Antiseptic.

yellow mercuric oxide 2%. (Various Mfr.) Yellow mercuric oxide 2%. Oint. Tube 3.5, 3.75, 30 g. *OTC.*
Use: Antiseptic.
See: Stye.

yellow ointment.
Use: Pharmaceutic aid. (ointment base).

yellow wax.
Use: Pharmaceutic aid. (stiffening agent).

YF-Vax. (Aventis Pasteur) Yellow fever vaccine. Inj. Vial 1 dose, 5 dose, 20 dose with diluent. *Rx.*
Use: Immunization.

Yocon. (Glenwood) Yohimbine hydrochloride 5.4 mg. Tab. Bot. 100s, 1000s. *Rx.*
Use: Anti-impotence agent.

Yodora Deodorant. (GlaxoSmithKline) Cream. Jar 2 oz. *OTC.*
Use: Deodorant.

Yodoxin. (Glenwood) Iodoquinol. **Pow.:** Bot. 25 g. **Tab.:** 210 mg, 650 mg. Bot. 100s, 1,000s. *Rx.*
Use: Amebicide.

•**yohimbine hydrochloride.** *USP 28.*
Use: Yohimbine has no FDA sanctioned indications.
See: Aphrodyne.
Yokon.

yohimbine hydrochloride. (Various Mfr.) Indolalkylamine alkaloid. 5.4 mg. Tab. Bot. 100s, 500s, 1000s. *Rx.*
Use: Yohimbine has no FDA sanctioned indications.
W/Methyltestosterone.

See: Nux Vomica Extract.
Yohimex. (Kramer) Yohimbine hydrochloride 5.4 mg. Tab. Bot. 100s. *Rx.*
Use: Antiimpotence agent.
Your Choice Non-Preserved Saline Solution. (Amcon) Buffered, isotonic soln. w/NaCl, boric acid, sodium borate. Bot. 360 mL. *OTC.*
Use: Contact lens care.
Your Choice Sterile Preserved Saline Solution. (Amcon) Isotonic. Sorbic acid 0.1%, EDTA, NaCl, boric buffer. Bot. 60 mL, 360 mL. *OTC.*
Use: Contact lens care.
ytterbium Yb 169 pentetate injection.
Use: Radiopharmaceutical.

•**yttrium y 90 epratuzumab.** (IT-ree-um e-pra-TOO-zoo-mab) USAN.
Use: Radiopharmaceutical.
•**yttrium y 90 ibritumomab.** (IT-ree-um ib-ri-TYOO-mo-mab) *USP 28.*
Use: Radiopharmaceutical.
•**yttrium y 90 labetuzumab.** (IT-ree-um la-be-TOO-zoo-mab) USAN.
Use: Radiopharmaceutical.
•**yttrium y 90 tacatuzumab.** (IT-ree-um tak-a-TUE-zoo-mab) USAN.
Use: Radiopharmaceutical.
Yutopar. (AstraZeneca) Ritodrine hydrochloride 10 mg/mL. Amp. 5 mL. 15 mg/mL. Vial 10 mL, Inj. syringe 10 mL. *Rx.*
Use: Uterine relaxant.

Z

zacopride hydrochloride. (ZAK-oh-pride) USAN.
Use: Antiemetic; stimulant (peristaltic).

Zaditor. (Novartis Ophthalmics) Ketotofen fumarate 0.025%, glycerol, sodium hydroxide/hydrochloric acid, purified water, benzalkonium chloride 0.01%. Soln. Bot. 5 mL, 7.5 mL. *Rx.*
Use: Antiallergic.

zafirlukast. (zah-FEER-loo-kast) USAN.
Use: Antiasthmatic (leukotriene antagonist).
See: Accolate.

Zagam. (Bertek) Sparfloxacin 200 mg. Tab. Bot. 55s, Blister packs of 11. *Rx.*
Use: Fluoroquinolone.

zalcitabine. (zal-SITE-ah-bih-EEN)
USP 28.
Use: Antiretroviral.
See: Hivid.

zaleplon. (ZAL-eh-plahn) USAN.
Use: Hypnotic; sedative.
See: Sonata.

zalospirone hydrochloride. (zal-OH-spy-rone) USAN.
Use: Anxiolytic.

zaltidine hydrochloride. (ZAHL-tih-deen) USAN.
Use: Antiulcerative.

Zanaflex. (Acorda Therapeutics) Tizanidine hydrochloride. **Cap.:** 2 mg, 4 mg, 6 mg. Sugar spheres. 150s. **Tab.:** 2 mg, 4 mg, lactose. Bot. 150s. *Rx.*
Use: Skeletal muscle relaxant.

zanamivir. (zan-AM-ih-veer) USAN.
Use: Antiviral; influenza virus neuraminidase inhibitor.
See: Relenza.

Zanfel. (Zanfel Labs) Polyethylene granules, nonoxynol-9, disodium EDTA, triethanolamine. Cream. Tube. 30 g. *OTC.*
Use: Dermatitis.

Zanfel Wash. (Zanfel Labs) Polyethylene granules, sodium lauroyl sarcosinate, nonoxynol-9, EDTA, triethanolamine. Wash. 30 mL. *OTC.*
Use: Poison ivy treatment.

zankiren hydrochloride. (zan-KIE-ren) USAN.
Use: Antihypertensive.

Zanosar. (Gensia Sicor) Streptozocin 1 g (100 mg/mL). Pow. for Inj. Vial. *Rx.*
Use: Antineoplastic.

zanoterone. (zan-OH-ter-ohn) USAN.
Use: Antiandrogen.

Zantac. (GlaxoSmithKline) Ranitidine hydrochloride (as base). **Inj.:** 1 mg/mL, sodium chloride 0.45%, preservative free. Premixed single-dose plastic containers. 50 mL. 25 mg/mL. Vials. 2 mL, 6 mL with phenol. **Syrup:** 15 mg/mL, alcohol 7.5%, saccharin, sorbitol, parabens. Peppermint flavor. Bot. 480 mL. **Tab.:** 150 mg, 300 mg. Film coated. 30s (300 mg only), 60s (150 mg only), 180s (150 mg only), 250s (300 mg only), 500s (150 mg only), 1,000s (150 mg only), UD 100s. *Rx.*
Use: Histamine H_2 antagonist.

Zantac EFFERdose. (GlaxoSmithKline) Ranitidine hydrochloride (as base).
Granules: 150 mg. Aspartame, phenylalanine 16.84 mg. 1.44 g packets (30s, 60s). **Effervescent Tab:** 25 mg (phenylalanine 2.81 mg, sodium 30.52 mg per tablet), 150 mg (phenylalanine 16.84 mg, sodium 183.12 mg per tablet). Aspartame. 60s. *Rx.*
Use: Histamine H_2 antagonist.

Zantac 150. (Pfizer Consumer) Ranitidine hydrochloride (as base) 150 mg. Tab. 8s, 24s, 50s, 65s. *OTC.*
Use: Histamine H_2 antagonist.

Zantac 75. (Warner-Lambert) Ranitidine hydrochloride (as base) 75 mg. Tab. Pkg. 4s, 10s, 20s, 30s, 60s, 80s. *OTC.*
Use: Histamine H_2 antagonist.

Zantine. (Lexis Laboratories) Dipyridamole 25 mg, 50 mg, 75 mg. Tab. Bot. 1000s. *Rx.*
Use: Coronary vasodilator.

Zarontin. (Parke-Davis) Ethosuximide. **Cap.:** 250 mg. Bot. 100s. **Syr.:** 250 mg/5 mL. Bot. Pt. *Rx.*
Use: Anticonvulsant.

Zaroxolyn. (Medeva) Metolazone 2.5 mg, 5 mg, 10 mg. Tab. Bot. 100s, 500s, 1000s, UD 100s. *Rx.*
Use: Diuretic.

zatosetron maleate. (ZAT-oh-SEH-trahn) USAN.
Use: Antimigraine.

Zavesca. (Actelion) Miglustat 100 mg. Sodium starch glucollate, gelatin. Cap. 90s, blister card 18s. *Rx.*
Use: Gaucher disease.

Zazole. (PharmaDerm) Terconazole 0.8%. Alcohols. Vaginal Cream. 20 g tube with measured-dose applicator. *Rx.*
Use: Vaginal antifungal agent.

Z-Bec. (Wyeth) Vitamins E 45 mg, C 600 mg, B_1 15 mg, B_2 10.2 mg, B_3 100 mg, B_6 10 mg, B_{12} 6 mcg, pantothenic acid 25 mg, Zn 22.5 mg. Tab. Bot. 60s, 100s, 500s. *OTC.*
Use: Mineral, vitamin supplement.

Z-Cof DM. (Zyber Pharmaceuticals) Dextromethorphan HBr 15 mg, guaifenesin

200 mg, pseudoephedrine hydrochloride 40 mg/5 mL, grape flavor, alcohol free. Syr. Bot. 473 mL. *Rx.*
Use: Upper respiratory combination, antitussive, expectorant, deongestant.

Z-Cof HC. (Zyber Pharmaceuticals) Hydrocodone bitartrate 3.5 mg, chlorpheniramine maleate 2.5 mg, phenylephrine hydrochloride 10 mg/5 mL, saccharin sorbitol, raspberry flavor, alcohol free. Syr. Bot. 473 mL. *c-III.*
Use: Upper respiratory combination, antitussive, antihistamine, deongestant.

Z-Cof LA. (Zyber Pharmaceuticals) Dextromethorphan HBr 30 mg, guaifenesin 650 mg. SR Tab. 100s. *Rx.*
Use: Upper respiratory combination, antitussive, expectorant.

Zeasorb. (Stiefel) Talc, microporous cellulose, supersorb carbohydrate acrylic copolymer. Pow. Sifter-top Can 2.5 oz, 8 oz. *OTC.*
Use: Dermatologic.

Zeasorb-AF. (Stiefel) Miconazole nitrate 2%. Pow. Can 70 g. *OTC.*
Use: Antifungal, topical.

Zebeta. (Barr) Bisoprolol fumarate 5 mg, 10 mg. Tab. Bot. 30s. *Rx.*
Use: Antiadrenergic/sympatholytic, beta-adrenergic blocker.

Ze Caps. (Everett) Vitamin E 200 mg, Zn 9.6 mg as gluconate. Cap. Bot. 60s. *OTC.*
Use: Mineral, vitamin supplement.

Zee-Seltzer. (Zee Medical) Aspirin 325 mg, citric acid 1000 mg, sodium bicarbonate 1916 mg, sodium 524 mg. Effervescent Tab. 12s. *OTC.*
Use: Antacid.

Zefazone. (Pharmacia) Cefmetazole sodium. **Pow. for Inj.:** 1 g, 2 g (2 mEq sodium/g). Vial. **Inj.:** 1 g/50 mL, 2 g/ 50 mL (2.7 mEq sodium/g) in frozen iso-osmotic, premixed solution in single-dose plastic container. *Rx.*
Use: Anti-infective.

Zegerid. (Santarus) Omeprazole 20 mg, 40 mg. Sucrose, sucralose, sodium bicarbonate (460 mg sodium per dose), xanthan gum. Pow. for Oral Susp. 30 unit-dose packets. *Rx.*
Use: Proton Pump Inhibitor.

•**zein.** (ZEE-in) *NF 23.*
Use: Pharmaceutic aid (coating agent).

Zelnorm. (Norvatis) Tegaserod maleate 2 mg, 6 mg, lactose. Tab. 60s (6 mg only), 500s (6 mg only), UD 60s. *Rx.*
Use: Gastric motility disorders.

Zemaira. (Aventis) Alpha₁-proteinase inhibitor (human) 1000 mg. Sodium mannitol. Preservative-free. Pow. for Inj.,

lyophilized. Single-dose vial with 20 mL diluent. *Rx.*
Use: Respiratory enzyme.

Zemalo. (Alra) Sulfur, zinc oxide, camphor, titanium oxide. Bot. 4 oz, pt, gal. *OTC.*
Use: Dermatologic, counterirritant.

Zemplar. (Abbott) Paricalcitol 5 mcg/mL Inj. Single-dose fliptop vials, 1 mL, 2 mL. *Rx.*
Use: Hyperparathyroidism.

Zemuron. (Organon) Rocuronium bromide 10 mg/mL. Inj. Multidose vials. 5 mL, 10 mL. *Rx.*
Use: Muscle relaxant.

Zenapax. (Roche) Daclizumab 25 mg/ 5 mL. Preservative free. Inj. Single-use vials. *Rx.*
Use: Prevent organ rejection; immunosuppressant.

Zenate.
See: Advanced Formula Zenate.

•**zenazocine mesylate.** (zen-AZE-oh-seen MEH-sih-late) USAN.
Use: Analgesic.

Zendium. (Oral-B) Sodium fluoride 0.22%. Tube 0.9 oz, 2.3 oz.
Use: Dental caries agent.

•**zeniplatin.** (zen-ih-PLAT-in) USAN.
Use: Antineoplastic.

Zephiran. (Sanofi-Synthelabo) **Aqueous soln.:** Benzalkonium Cl 1:750. Bot. 240 mL, gal. **Disinfectant concentrate:** 17% in 120 mL, gal. **Tincture:** 1:750 in gal. **Tincture spray:** 1:750 in 30 g, 180 g, gal. *OTC.*
Use: Antiseptic; antimicrobial.

Zephiran Towelettes. (Sanofi-Synthelabo) Moist paper towels with soln. of zephiran Cl 1:750. Box 20s, 100s, 1000s. *OTC.*
Use: Antiseptic; antimicrobial.

Zephrex. (Sanofi-Synthelabo) Pseudoephedrine hydrochloride 60 mg, guaifenesin 400 mg. Tab. Bot. 100s. *Rx.*
Use: Decongestant, expectorant.

Zephrex LA. (Sanofi-Synthelabo) Pseudoephedrine hydrochloride 120 mg, guaifenesin 600 mg. ER Tab. Bot. 100s. *Rx.*
Use: Decongestant, expectorant.

Zepine. (Foy Laboratories) Reserpine alkaloid 0.25 mg. Tab. Bot. 100s, 500s, 1000s. *Rx.*
Use: Antihypertensive.

•**zeranol.** (ZER-ah-nole) USAN.
Use: Anabolic.

Zerit. (BMS Virology) Stavudine. **Cap.:** 15 mg, 20 mg, 30 mg, 40 mg, lactose. Bot. 60s. **Pow. for Oral Soln.:** 1 mg/

mL, sucrose, parabens, dye free, fruit flavor. Bot. 200 mL. *Rx.*
Use: Antiretroviral, nucleoside reverse transcriptase inhibitor.
Zerit XR. (BMS Virology) Stavudine 37.5 mg, 50 mg, 75 mg, 100 mg, lactose. ER Cap. Bot. 30s. *Rx.*
Use: Antiretroviral, nucleoside reverse transcriptase inhibitor.
Zestoretic. (AstraZeneca) Lisinopril 10 mg, hydrochlorothiazide 12.5 mg. Lisinopril 20 mg, hydrochlorothiazide 12.5 mg. Lisinopril 20 mg, hydrochlorothiazide 25 mg. Tab. Bot. 100s. *Rx.*
Use: Antihypertensive.
Zestril. (AstraZeneca) Lisinopril 2.5 mg, 5 mg, 10 mg, 20 mg, 30 mg, 40 mg, mannitol. Tab. 100s, UD 100s (5 mg, 10 mg, 20 mg only). *Rx.*
Use: Antihypertensive.
Zetacet. (Stiefel) Sulfur 5%, sodium sulfacetamide 10%, cetyl alcohol, benzyl alcohol, EDTA. Top. Susp. 30 g. *Rx.*
Use: Dermatologic, acne.
Zetacet Wash. (Stiefel) Sulfur 5%, sodium sulfacetamide 10%. Alcohols, EDTA, parabens, white petrolatum. Wash. 170.1 g, 340.2 g. *Rx.*
Use: Dermatologic, acne.
Zetar. (Dermik) Coal tar 1%. Shampoo. Bot. 177 mL. *OTC.*
Use: Antiseborrheic.
Zetia. (Merck/Schering-Plough) Ezetimibe 10 mg, lactose. Tab. Bot. 30s, 90s, 500s, UD 100s. *Rx.*
Use: Antihyperlipidemic.
Zevalin. (IDEC) Ibritumomab tiuxetan 3.2 mg, preservative free. Inj. Vial 2 mL. In-111 ibritumomab tiuxetan and Y-90 ibritumomab tiuxetan kits w/50 mM sodium acetate vial, formulation buffer vial, reaction vial, and identification labels. *Rx.*
Use: Monoclonal antibody.
Ziac. (Barr) Bisoprolol fumarate 2.5 mg, 5 mg, 10 mg; hydrochlorothiazide 6.25 mg. Tab. Bot. 30s, 100s (except 10 mg). *Rx.*
Use: Antihypertensive.
Ziagen. (GlaxoSmithKline) Abacavir sulfate. **Tab.:** 300 mg. Bot. 60s, UD blister packs of 60s. **Oral Soln.:** 20 mg/mL, parabens, saccharin, sorbitol, strawberry-banana flavor. Bot. 240 mL. *Rx.*
Use: Antiviral, nucleoside reverse transcriptase inhibitor.
• **ziconotide.** (zi-KOE-noe-tide) USAN.
Use: Analgesic.
See: Prialt.
• **zidometacin.** (ZIE-doe-MEH-tah-sin) USAN.

Use: Anti-inflammatory.
• **zidovudine.** (zie-DOE-view-DEEN) *USP 28.* Formerly azidothymidine, AZT.
Use: Antiviral; AIDS; HIV infection.
See: Retrovir.
W/Abacavir sulfate, lamivudine.
See: Trizivir.
W/Lamivudine.
See: Combivir.
• **zifrosilone.** (zih-FROE-sih-lone) USAN.
Use: Acetylcholinesterase inhibitor.
Ziks. (Nodum) Methyl salicylate 12%, menthol 1%, capsaicin 0.025%, cetyl alcohol. Cream. Tube. 60 g. *OTC.*
Use: Analgesic.
Zilactin-B Medicated. (Zila) Benzocaine 10%, alcohol 76%. Gel. Tube. 7.5 g. *OTC.*
Use: Anesthetic, local.
Zilactin-L. (Zila) Lidocaine 2.5%, alcohol 79.3%. Liq. Bot. 7.5 mL. *OTC.*
Use: Anesthetic, local.
Zilactin Medicated. (Zila) Tannic acid 7%, suspended in alcohol 80.8%. Gel. Tube. 0.25 oz. *OTC.*
Use: Cold sores.
ZilaDent. (Zila) Benzocaine 6%, alcohol 74.9%. Gel. Tube. 7.5 g, single packs. *OTC.*
Use: Anesthetic, local.
• **zilantel.** (ZILL-an-tell) USAN.
Use: Anthelmintic.
• **zileuton.** (ZIE-loo-tone) *USP 28.*
Use: Inhibitor (5-lipoxygenase).
See: Zyflo.
• **zimeldine hydrochloride.** (zie-MELL-ih-deen) USAN. Formerly Zimelidine Hydrochloride.
Use: Antidepressant.
Zinacef. (GlaxoSmithKline) Cefuroxime 750 mg, 1.5 g, 7.5 g as sodium. Pow. for Inj. 750 mg, 1.5 g (as sodium). Inj. **Pow. for Inj.: 750 mg, 1.5 g:** Vials and infusion pack. **7.5 g:** Pharmacy bulk Pkg. **Inj.: 750 mg, 1.5 g, premixed:** 50 mL. *Rx.*
Use: Anti-infective, cephalosporin.
• **zinc acetate.** (zingk) *USP 28.* Acetic acid, zinc salt, dihydrate.
Use: Pharmaceutic necessity for zinc-eugenol cement; topical poison ivy product; Wilson disease.
See: Benadryl Itch Relief.
Benadryl Itch Relief, Children's.
Benadryl Itch Relief, Maximum Strength.
Benadryl Itch Stopping Children's Formula.
Benadryl Itch Stopping Maximum Strength.

Caladryl Clear.
Galzin.
Ivy-Dry.
Ivy-Super Dry.
Nasal•Ease with Zinc.
W/Combinations.
See: Anti-Itch.
Zinca-Pak. (SoloPak Pharmaceuticals, Inc.) Zinc 1 mg, 5 mg/mL. Inj. **1 mg:** Vial 10 mL, 30 mL. **5 mg:** Vial 5 mL. *Rx.*
Use: Nutritional supplement, parenteral.
Zincate. (Paddock) Zinc sulfate 220 mg (elemental zinc 50 mg). Cap. Bot. 100s, 1000s. *OTC.*
Use: Mineral supplement.
•**zinc bacitracin.** *USP 28.* Bacitracin Zinc.
Use: Anti-infective.
•**zinc carbonate.** *USP 28.*
Use: Antiseptic, topical; astringent.
•**zinc chloride.** *USP 28.*
Use: Astringent; dentin desensitizer.
W/Formaldehyde.
See: Forma Z Concentrate.
•**zinc chloride Zn 65.** USAN.
Use: Radiopharmaceutical.
zinc citrate.
See: Zinc Lozenges.
zinc-eugenol cement. *USP 28.*
Use: Dental protectant.
Zincfrin. (Alcon) Zinc sulfate 0.25%, phenylephrine hydrochloride 0.12%. Soln. *Drop-Tainer* 15 mL, 30 mL. *OTC.*
Use: Astringent, decongestant, ophthalmic.
•**zinc gelatin.** *USP 28.*
Use: Topical protectant.
Zinc-Glenwood. (Glenwood) Zinc sulfate 220 mg. Cap. Bot. 100s. *OTC.*
Use: Mineral supplement.
•**zinc gluconate.** *USP 28.*
Use: Supplement, trace mineral.
See: Nasal•Ease with Zinc Gluconate.
Zinc Lozenges.
zinc insulin.
See: Insulin Zinc.
Zinc Lozenges. (Ivax) Zinc citrate 23 mg, zinc gluconate, fructose, sorbitol. Bot. 30s. *OTC.*
Use: Mineral supplement.
Zincon. (Medtech) Pyrithione zinc 1%, propylene glycol. Shampoo. Bot. 118 mL, 240 mL. *OTC.*
Use: Antiseborrheic.
•**zinc oxide.** *USP 28.* Flowers of zinc.
Use: Astringent; topical protectant.
See: Calamine.
W/Combinations.
See: Akne.
Anusol.

Anusol-HC.
Balmex.
Blis-To-Sol.
Bonate.
Calamatum.
Columbia Antiseptic Powder.
Desitin.
Dr. Smith's Adult Care.
Dr. Smith's Diaper.
Elder Diaper Rash.
Hemorrhoidal.
Hydro Surco.
Medicated Foot Powder.
Medicated Powder.
Mexsana.
Pazo.
Rectal Medicone HC.
RVPaque.
Saratoga.
Schamberg.
Sebasorb.
Taloin.
Unguentine "Original Formula".
Versal.
Wyanoids.
Xylocaine.
zinc phenolsulfonate.
Use: Astringent.
W/Belladonna leaf extract, kaolin, pectin, sodium carboxymethylcellulose.
See: Diastay.
W/Bismuth subsalicylate, salol, methyl salicylate.
See: Pepto-Bismol.
W/Kaolin, pectin.
See: Pectocel.
W/Opium, bismuth subgallate, pectin, kaolin.
See: Bismuth, Pectin & Paregoric.
zinc pyrithione.
Use: Bactericide, fungicide, antiseborrheic.
See: Zincon.
•**zinc stearate.** *USP 28.* Octadecanoic acid, zinc salt.
Use: Dusting powder; pharmaceutic aid (tablet/capsule lubricant).
zinc sulfanilate. Zinc sulfanilate tetrahydrate. Nizin, Op-Isophrin-Z, Op-Isophrin-Z-M (Broemmel).
Use: Anti-infective.
•**zinc sulfate.** *USP 28.* Sulfuric acid, zinc salt (1:1), heptahydrate.
Use: Astringent, ophthalmic.
See: Op-Thal-Zin.
Zinc-Glenwood.
Zin-Cora.
W/Boric acid, phenylephrine hydrochloride.
See: Phenylzin.
W/Calcium lactate.

See: Zinc-220.
W/Menthol, methyl salicylate, alum, boric acid, oxyquinoline citrate.
See: Maso pH.
W/Phenylephrine hydrochloride, polyvinyl alcohol.
See: Prefrin-Z.
W/Piperocaine hydrochloride, boric acid, potassium Cl.
See: M-Z.
W/Sodium Cl.
See: Bromidrosis Crystals.
W/Vitamins.
See: Vicon-C.
Vicon Forte.
Vicon Plus.
Vi-Zac.
Z-Bec.
zinc sulfate. (Various Mfr.) Zinc 5 mg/ mL (as sulfate 21.95 mg). Inj. Vial 5, 10 mL.
Use: Nutritional supplement, parenteral.
zinc sulfate. (Various Mfr.) **Cap.:** Zinc sulfate 220 mg, lactose, gelatin. Bot. 100s. **Inj.:** Zinc 1 mg/mL (as sulfate 4.39 mg). Vial 10, 30 mL. *Rx-OTC.*
Use: Nutritional supplement, parenteral.
•**zinc sulfide topical suspension.** (zingk) *USP 28. Formerly White Lotion.* Synonym Lotio alba.
Use: Astringent.
zinc-10-undecenoate.
See: Zinc Undecylenate.
zinc trace metal additive. (I.M.S., Ltd.) Zinc 4 mg/mL. Inj. Vial. 10 mL. *Rx.*
Use: Nutritional supplement, parenteral.
Zinc-220. (Alto) Zinc sulfate 220 mg. Cap. Bot. 100s, 1000s, UD 100s. *OTC.*
Use: Mineral supplement.
•**zinc undecylenate.** (zingk uhn-deh-SILL-en-ate) *USP 28.*
Use: Antifungal.
See: Blis-To-Sol.
W/Benzocaine, hexachlorophene.
See: Decyl-Cream LBS.
W/Caprylic acid, sodium propionate.
See: Deso-Cream.
Deso-Talc.
W/Undecylenic acid.
See: Cruex Cream.
Desenex.
Quinsana.
Zincvit. (Kenwood) Vitamin A 5000 units, D_3 50 units, E 50 units, B_1 10 mg, B_2 5 mg, B_6 2 mg, C 300 mcg, B_3 25 mg, Zn 40 mg, Mg 9.7 mg, Mn 1.3 mg, folic acid 1 mg. Cap. Bot. 60s. *Rx.*
Use: Mineral, vitamin supplement.
•**zindotrine.** (ZIN-doe-TREEN) USAN.
Use: Bronchodilator.

Zinecard. (Pfizer) Dexrazoxane 250 mg, 500 mg (10 mg/mL when reconstituted). Pow. for Inj., lyophilized. Single-use vial with vial 25 mL (250 mg), 50 mL (500 mg) sodium lactate injection. *Rx.*
Use: Antineoplastic; antidote; cytoprotective agent.
•**zinoconazole hydrochloride.** (zih-no-KOE-nah-zole) USAN.
Use: Antifungal.
•**zinostatin.** (ZEE-no-STAT-in) USAN. *Formerly neocarzinostatin.*
Use: Antineoplastic.
•**zinterol hydrochloride.** (ZIN-ter-ole) USAN.
Use: Bronchodilator.
•**zinviroxime.** (zin-VIE-rox-eem) USAN.
Use: Antiviral.
•**ziprasidone hydrochloride.** (zih-PRAY-sih-dohn) USAN.
Use: Antipsychotic, benzisoxazole derivative.
See: Geodon.
•**ziprasidone mesylate.** (zih-PRAY-sih-dohn MEH-sih-LATE) USAN.
Use: Antipsychotic.
zirconium carbonate or oxide.
See: Dermanene.
W/Benzocaine, Menthol, Camphor.
See: Rhuli.
W/Benzocaine, Menthol, Camphor, Calamine, Isopropyl Alcohol.
See: Rhuli.
W/Benzocaine, Menthol, Camphor, Calamine, Pyrilamine Maleate.
See: Ivarest.
Zithromax. (Pfizer) Azithromycin. **Tab.:** 250 mg, 500 mg, 600 mg as dihydrate, lactose. Bot. 30s, UD 50s (except 600 mg). Z-Pak 6s (250 mg only), TRI-PAK 3s (500 mg only). **Pow. for Inj.:** 500 mg, sucrose. Lyophilized vials 10 mL, vials 10 mL with 1 *Vial-Mate* adapter. **Pow. for Oral Susp.:** 100 mg/ 5 mL (as dihydrate) when reconstituted, sucrose. Bot. 300 mg. 200 mg/ 5 mL (as dihydrate) when reconstituted, sucrose. Bot. 600 mg, 900 mg, 1200 mg. 1 g/packet as dihydrate, sucrose. Single-dose pack, 3s, 10s. *Rx.*
Use: Anti-infective, macrolide.
ZNG. (Western Research) Zinc gluconate 35 mg. Tab. *Handicount* 28s (36 bags of 28 tab.). *OTC.*
Use: Mineral supplement.
ZNP Bar. (Stiefel) Zinc pyrithione 2%, corn starch, glycerin, hydrogenated castor oil, mineral oil, cetostearyl alcohol. Soap. 119 g. *OTC.*

Use: Antiseborrheic.
ZN-Plus Protein. (Miller Pharmacal Group) Zinc in a zinc-protein complex made with isolated soy protein 15 mg. Tab. Bot. 100s. *OTC.*
Use: Mineral supplement.
Zocor. (Merck) Simvastatin 5 mg, 10 mg, 20 mg, 40 mg, 80 mg, lactose. Film-coated. Tab. Bot. 1000s, 10,000s (10 mg, 20 mg only), UD 100s, unit-of-use 30s, 60s (except 10 mg). *Rx.*
Use: Antihyperlipidemic, HMG-CoA reductase inhibitor.
Zodeac-100. (Econo Med Pharmaceuticals) Fe 60 mg, vitamins A 8000 units, D 400 units, E 30 units, B_1 1.7 mg, B_2 2 mg, B_3 20 mg, B_5 11 mg, B_6 4 mg, B_{12} 8 mcg, C 120 mg, folic acid 1 mg, biotin 300 mcg, Ca, Cu, I, Mg, Zn 15 mg. Tab. Bot. 100s. *Rx.*
Use: Mineral, vitamin supplement.
Zoderm. (Doak) Benzoyl peroxide.
  Cleanser: 4.5%, 6.5%, 8.5%. Alcohols, EDTA, glycerin, urea. 400 mL. **Cream:** 4.5%, 6.5%, 8.5%. Alcohols, EDTA, urea. 125 mL. **Gel.:** 4.5%, 6.5%, 8.5%. EDTA, glycerin, urea. 125 mL. *Rx.*
  Use: Anti-infective.
• **zofenoprilat arginine.** (zoe-FEN-oh-PRILL-at AHR-jih-neen) USAN.
  Use: Antihypertensive.
• **zofenopril calcium.** (zoe-FEN-oh-PRILL) USAN.
  Use: Enzyme inhibitor (angiotensin-converting).
Zofran. (GlaxoSmithKline) Ondansetron hydrochloride. **Tab.:** 4 mg, 8 mg, 24 mg, lactose. Bot. 30s, UD 100s, 1 × 3 UD pack (4 mg, 8 mg only); 1 × 1 daily UD pack (24 mg only). **Inj.:** 2 mg/mL, 32 mg/50 mL (premixed), parabens (2 mg/mL only); preservative free, with dextrose 2500 mg, citric acid 26 mg, sodium citrate 11.5 mg (32 mg/50 mL only). Single-dose vial 2 mL, multidose vial 20 mL (2 mg/mL); single-dose cont. 50 mL. **Oral Soln.:** 4 mg/5 mL, sorbitol, strawberry flavor. Bot. 50 mL. *Rx.*
Use: Antiemetic; antivertigo.
Zofran ODT. (GlaxoSmithKline) Ondansetron 4 mg, 8 mg, phenylalanine < 0.03 mg, aspartame, mannitol, parabens, strawberry flavor. Orally Disintegrating Tab. UD 10s (8 mg only), UD 30s. *Rx.*
Use: Antiemetic; antivertigo.
Zoladex. (AstraZeneca) Goserelin acetate 3.6 mg, 10.8 mg. Implant. Preloaded Syringes. *Rx.*
Use: Hormone, gonadotropin-releasing hormone analog.

• **zolamine hydrochloride.** (zoe-lah-meen) USAN.
  Use: Antihistamine; anesthetic, topical.
• **zolazepam hydrochloride.** (zole-AZE-eh-pam) USAN.
  Use: Hypnotic; sedative.
• **zoledronate disodium.** (ZOE-leh-droe-nate) USAN.
  Use: Bone resorption inhibitor; osteoporosis treatment and prevention.
• **zoledronate trisodium.** (ZOE-leh-droe-nate) USAN.
  Use: Bone resorption inhibitor; osteoporosis treatment and prevention.
• **zoledronic acid.** (ZOE-leh-drah-nik) USAN.
  Use: Calcium regulator; osteoporosis treatment and prevention; bisphosphonate.
  See: Zometa.
• **zolertine hydrochloride.** (ZOE-ler-teen) USAN.
  Use: Antiadrenergic; vasodilator.
Zolicef. (Apothecon) Cefazolin sodium 1 g. Sodium 1.2 mEq/g. Pow. for Inj. Vials. 10 mL. *Rx.*
Use: Anti-infective, cephalosporin.
• **zolimomab aritox.** (zah-LIM-ah-mab a-rih-TOX) USAN.
  Use: Monoclonal antibody (antithrombotic).
• **zolmitriptan.** (zohl-mi-TRIP-tan) USAN.
  Use: Antimigraine, serotonin 5-HT$_1$ receptor agonist.
  See: Zomig.
    Zomig ZMT.
Zoloft. (Pfizer) Sertraline hydrochloride. **Tab.:** 25 mg, 50 mg, 100 mg. Film-coated. Bot. 50s, (25 mg only); 100s, 500s, 5000s, UD 100s (50 mg and 100 mg only). **Oral Conc.:** 20 mg/mL, menthol, alcohol 12%. Bot. 60 mL. Dropper dispenser contains dry natural rubber. *Rx.*
Use: Antidepressant, SSRI.
• **zolpidem tartrate.** (ZOLE-pih-dem) USAN.
  Use: Hypnotic; sedative.
  See: Ambien.
• **zomepirac sodium.** (ZOE-mih-PEER-ack) USAN.
  Use: Analgesic; anti-inflammatory.
Zometa. (Novartis) Zoledronic acid monohydrate 4.264 mg equiv. to zoledronic acid anhydrous 4 mg, mannitol 220 mg, sodium citrate 24 mg. Pow. for Inj. Vial. *Rx.*
Use: Bisphosphonate.
• **zometapine.** (zoe-MET-ah-peen) USAN.
  Use: Antidepressant.

Zomig. (MedPointe) Zolmitriptan. **Nasal Spray:** 5 mg. 100 mcL unit-dose spray device. 6s. **Tab.:** 2.5 mg, 5 mg, lactose. Blister pack 6s (2.5 mg), 3s (5 mg). *Rx.*
Use: Antimigraine, serotonin 5-HT$_1$ receptor agonist.

Zomig ZMT. (MedPointe) Zolmitriptan 2.5 mg, phenylalanine 2.81 mg, mannitol, aspartame, orange flavor. Orally disintegrating tab. Blister pack 6s. *Rx.*
Use: Antimigraine, serotonin 5-HT$_1$ receptor agonist.

Zonalon. (Medicis Dermatologics) Doxepin hydrochloride 5%, cetyl alcohol, petrolatum, benzyl alcohol, titanium dioxide. Cream. Tube. 30 g. *Rx.*
Use: Antihistamine, topical.

● **zonampanel.** (zon-AM-pa-nel) USAN.
Use: Ischemic stroke.

Zone-A Forte. (Forest) Hydrocortisone 2.5%, pramoxine hydrochloride in a hydrophilic base containing stearic acid 1%, forlan-L, glycerin, triethanolamine, polyoxyl 40 stearate, di-isopropyl adipate, povidone, silicone fluid-200. Paraben free. Lot. Bot. 60 mL. *Rx.*
Use: Corticosteroid; anesthetic, local.

Zone-A Lotion. (Forest) Hydrocortisone acetate 1%, pramoxine hydrochloride 1%. Bot. 2 oz. *Rx.*
Use: Corticosteroid; anesthetic, local.

Zonegran. (Eisai) Zonisamide 25 mg, 50 mg, 100 mg. Cap. Bot. 100s. *Rx.*
Use: Anticonvulsant.

● **zoniclezole hydrochloride.** (zoe-NIH-klih-ZOLE) USAN.
Use: Anticonvulsant.

● **zoniporide mesylate.** (zon-i-POR-ide) USAN.
Use: Cardioprotective agent.

● **zonisamide.** (zoe-NISS-ah-MIDE) USAN.
Use: Anticonvulsant.
See: Zonegran.

Zonite Liquid Douche Concentrate. (Menley & James Labs, Inc.) Benzalkonium Cl 0.1%, menthol, thymol, EDTA in buffered soln. Bot. 240 mL, 360 mL. *OTC.*
Use: Vaginal agent.

● **zopolrestat.** (zoe-PAHL-reh-STAT) USAN.
Use: Antidiabetic; aldose reductase inhibitor.

● **zorbamycin.** (ZAHR-bah-MY-sin) USAN.
Use: Anti-infective.

Zorbtive. (Serono) Somatropin 4 mg (≈ 12 units), 5 mg (≈ 15 units), 6 mg (≈ 18 units), 8.8 mg (≈ 26.4 units). Su-crose, benzyl alcohol (8.8 mg only). Pow. for Inj. Single-use vials with diluents. 7s (except 8.8 mg). 10 mL multidose vial with diluent. 1s (8.8 mg only). *Rx.*
Use: Hormone, growth.

ZORprin. (Knoll) Aspirin 800 mg. SR Tab. Bot. 100s. *Rx.*
Use: Analgesic.

● **zorubicin hydrochloride.** (zoe-ROO-bih-sin) USAN.
Use: Antineoplastic.

Zostrix. (Rodlen Laboratories) Capsaicin 0.025%. Cream. Tube. 45 g. *Rx.*
Use: Analgesic, topical.

Zostrix-HP. (Rodlen Laboratories) Formerly called Axsain, formerly marketed by Galen.

● **zosuquidar trihydrochloride.** (zoe-SOO-kwi-dar) USAN.
Use: Treatment of multidrug resistance.

Zosyn. (Wyeth) Piperacillin sodium/tazobactam sodium. **Inj.:** 2 g/0.25 g (sodium 5.7 mEq) , 3 g/0.375 g (sodium 8.6 mEq), 4 g/0.5 g (sodium 11.4 mEq). *Galaxy* containers. **Pow. for Inj., lyophilized:** 2 g/0.25 g (sodium 4.69 mEq), 3 g/0.375 mg (sodium 7.04 mEq), 4 g/0.5 g (sodium 9.39 mEq), 36 g/4.5 g (sodium 84.5 mEq). Vials, *ADD-Vantage* vials (except 36g/4.5 g). Bulk vials (36 g/4.5 g only). Preservative free. *Rx.*
Use: Anti-infective, penicillins.

Zoto-HC. (Horizon) Chloroxylenol 1%, pramoxine hydrochloride 10%, hydrocortisone 10%/mL in non-aqueous vehicle with 3% propylene glycol diacetate. Otic Drops. Vial 10 mL. *Rx.*
Use: Otic.

Zovia 1/50E. (Watson) Ethinyl estradiol 50 mcg, ethynodiol diacetate 1 mg, lactose. Tab. Pkg. 21s, 28s. *Rx.*
Use: Sex hormone, contraceptive hormone.

Zovia 1/35E. (Watson) Ethinyl estradiol 35 mcg, ethynodiol diacetate 1 mg, lactose. Tab. Pkg. 21s, 28s. *Rx.*
Use: Sex hormone, contraceptive hormone.

Zovirax. (GlaxoSmithKline) Acyclovir. **Cap.:** 200 mg. May contain parabens. Bot. 100s, UD 100s. **Tab.:** 400 mg, 800 mg. Bot. 100s, UD 100s (800 mg only). **Cream:** 5% in aqueous cream base, cetostearyl alcohol, mineral oil, white petrolatum. 2 g. **Pow. for Inj., lyophilized:** 500 mg. Sodium 49 mg. Vials. 10 mL. **Susp.:** 200 mg/5 mL. Bot. 473 mL. *Rx.*
Use: Antiviral.

Z-Pak.
See: Zithromax.

Z-Pro-C. (Person and Covey) Zinc sulfate 200 mg (elemental zinc 45 mg), ascorbic acid 100 mg. Tab. Bot. 100s. *OTC.*
Use: Mineral, vitamin supplement.

ZTuss Expectorant. (Huckaby Pharmacal) Hydrocodone bitartrate 2.5 mg, guaifenesin 100 mg, pseudoephedrine hydrochloride 15 mg, chlorpheniramine maleate 2 mg/5 mL, phenylalanine. Liq. Bot. 473 mL. *c-III.*
Use: Upper respiratory combination, antitussive, expectorant, decongestant, antihistamine.

• **zucapsaicin.** (zoo-cap-SAY-sin) USAN.
Use: Analgesic, topical.

• **zuclomiphene.** (zoo-KLOE-mih-FEEN) USAN. *Formerly transclomiphene.*

Zurinol. (Major) Allopurinol. Tab. **100 mg:** Bot. 100s, 500s, 1000s, UD 100s. **300 mg:** Bot. 100s, 500s, UD 100s. *Rx.*
Use: Antigout agent.

Z-Xtra. (Magna) Pyrilamine maleate 2.07 mg, benzocaine 2.08 mg, zinc oxide 41.35 mg/mL, apple blossom, silicone, lanolin, and Wysteria oils, isopropanol, camphor, menthol, parabens. Lot. Bot. 118 mL. *OTC.*
Use: Antihistamine, topical.

Zyban. (GlaxoSmithKline) Bupropion hydrochloride 150 mg, film-coated. SR Tab. Bot. 60s. *Rx.*
Use: Smoking deterrent.

Zyderm I. (Inamed) Highly purified bovine dermal collagen 35 mg/mL implant. Sterile syringe 0.1 mL, 0.5 mL, 1 mL, 2 mL.
Use: Collagen implant.

Zyderm II. (Inamed) Highly purified bovine dermal collagen 65 mg/mL implant. Syringe 0.75 mL.
Use: Collagen implant.

Zydone. (DuPont) Hydrocodone bitartrate 5 mg, 7.5 mg, 10 mg, acetaminophen 400 mg. Cap. Bot. 100s, 500s, UD 100s. *c-III.*
Use: Analgesic combination, narcotic.

Zyflo. (Abbott) Zileuton 600 mg. Tab. Bot. 120s. *Rx.*
Use: Antiasthmatic.

Zyloprim. (GlaxoWellcome) Allopurinol 100 mg, 300 mg. Lactose. Tab. Bot. 100s, 500s (300 mg only). *Rx.*
Use: Antigout agent; antimetabolite; purine analog.

Zymacap. (Pharmacia) Vitamins A 5000 units, D 400 units, E 15 mg, C

90 mg, folic acid 400 mcg, B_1 2.25 mg, B_2 2.6 mg, niacin 30 mg, B_6 3 mg, B_{12} 9 mcg, pantothenic acid 15 mg. Cap. Bot. 90s, 240s. *OTC.*
Use: Vitamin supplement.

Zymar. (Allergan) Gatifloxacin 0.3% (3 mg/mL), EDTA, benzalkonium chloride 0.005%. Soln. Dropper Bot. 2.5 mL, 5 mL. *Rx.*
Use: Antibiotic, ophthalmic.

Zymine. (Vindex Pharmaceuticals) Triprolidine hydrochloride 1.25 mg/ 5 mL, apple flavor. Liq. Bot. 15 mL, 473 mL. *Rx.*
Use: Antihistamine, nonselective alkylamine.

Zyprexa. (Eli Lilly) Olanzapine 2.5 mg, 5 mg, 7.5 mg, 10 mg, 15 mg, 20 mg, lactose. Tab. Bot. 60s, 1000s, UD blister 100s. *Rx.*
Use: Antipsychotic, dibenzapine derivative.

Zyprexa IntraMuscular. (Eli Lilly) Olanzapine 10 mg. Pow. for Inj. Vials. *Rx.*
Use: Antipsychotic.

Zyprexa Zydis. (Eli Lilly) Olanzapine 5 mg, 10 mg, 15 mg, 20 mg; aspartame; parabens; mannitol; phenylalanine 0.34 mg (5 mg only), 0.45 mg (10 mg only), 0.67 mg (15 mg only), 0.9 mg (20 mg only). Orally disintegrating tab. Dose pack 30s. *Rx.*
Use: Antipsychotic, dibenzapine derivative.

Zyrtec. (Pfizer) Cetirizine. **Chew. Tab.:** 5 mg, 10 mg. Lactose. Grape flavor. 30s. **Tab.:** 5 mg, 10 mg. Lactose. Film coated. Bot. 100s. **Syr.:** 5 mg/5 mL. Parabens, sugar, banana-grape flavor. Bot. 120 mL, 473 mL. *Rx.*
Use: Antihistamine, peripherally-selective piperazine.

Zyrtec-D 12 Hour. (Pfizer) Pseudoephedrine hydrochloride 120 mg, cetirizine hydrochloride 5 mg, lactose. ER Tab. Bot. 100s. *Rx.*
Use: Upper respiratory combination, decongestant, antihistamine.

Zyvox. (Pharmacia) Linezolid. **Tab.:** 400 mg, 600 mg, sodium 0.1 mEq. Bot. 20s, 100s, UD 30s. **Pow. for Oral Susp.:** 100 mg/5 mL, sodium 0.4 mEq/ 5 mL, sucrose, aspartame, mannitol, phenylalanine 20 mg, orange flavor. Bot. 115 mL fill in 240 mL. **Inj.:** 2 mg/ mL, sodium 0.38 mg/mL, sodium citrate. Single-use, ready-to-use bag 100 mL, 200 mL, 300 mL. *Rx.*
Use: Oxalodinone.

Standard Medical Abbreviations

Abbreviation	Meaning
≈	approximately equals
Δ	delta
ε	epsilon; molar absorption coefficient
Ω	omega; ohm
5-HIAA	5-hydroxyindoleacetic acid
5-HT	5-hydroxytryptamine (serotonin)
6-MP	6-mercaptopurine
17-OHCS	17-hydroxycorticosteroids
α	alpha
A	ampere(s)
Å	angstrom(s)
aa.	of each (ana)
āā.	of each (ana)
AA	Alcoholics Anonymous; amino acid
AACP	American Association of Clinical Pharmacy; American Association of Colleges of Pharmacy
AARP	American Association of Retired Persons
Ab	antibody
ABGs	arterial blood gases
abs feb	when fever is absent *(absente febre)*
ABVD	Adriamycin (doxorubicin), bleomycin, vinblastine, (and) dacarbazine
ac	before meals or food *(ante cibum)*
ACCP	American College of Clinical Pharmacy
ACD	acid-citrate-dextrose
ACE	angiotensin-converting enzyme
ACEI	angiotensin-converting enzyme inhibitor
ACh	acetylcholine
ACIP	Advisory Committee on Immunization Practices
ACLS	advanced cardiac life support
ACPE	American Council on Pharmaceutical Education
ACS	American Chemical Society
ACT	activated clotting time
ACTH	adrenocorticotropic hormone
a.d.	right ear *(aurio dextra)*
ad to;	to; up to *(ad)*
ADE	adverse drug experience
ADH	antidiuretic hormone
adhib	to be administered *(adhibendus)*

Abbreviation	Meaning
ad lib	as desired, at pleasure *(ad libitum)*
ADLs	activities of daily living
ADME	absorption, distribution, metabolism, and elimination
admov	apply *(admove)*
ADP	adenosine diphosphate
ADR	adverse drug reaction
ADRRS	Adverse Drug Reaction Reporting System
ad sat	to saturation *(ad saturatum, ad saturandum)*
adst feb	when fever is present *(adstante febre)*
ad us.	for external use *(ad usum externum)*
adv	against *(adversum)*
aer	aerosol
Ag	antigen; silver *(argentum)*
agit. Ante us.	shake before using *(agita ante usum)*
agit. Bene.	shake well *(agita bene)*
AHA	American Hospital Association
AID	artificial insemination donor
AIDS	acquired immunodeficiency syndrome
AJHP	American Journal of Hospital Pharmacy
ala	alanine
ALL	acute lymphocytic leukemia
ALT	alanine aminotransferase serum (previously SGPT)
alt hor	every other hour *(alternis horis)*
A.M.	before noon; morning *(ante meridiem)*
AMA	American Medical Association
AML	acute myelogenous leukemia
AMP	adenosine monophosphate
ANA	antinuclear antibody(ies)
ANC	acid neutralizing capacity
ANDA	abbreviated new drug application
ANOVA	analysis of variance
ANUG	acute necrotizing ulcerative gingivitis
APA	antipernicious anemia
APAP	acetaminophen
APC	antigen presenting cell(s)
APhA	American Pharmaceutical Association

Abbreviation	Meaning
aPTT	activated partial thromboplastin time
aq.	water *(aqua)*
aq. dest	distilled water *(aqua destillata)*
ARC	AIDS-related complex
ARDS	adult respiratory distress syndrome
ARF	acute renal failure
Arg	arginine
ARV	AIDS-related virus
as	left ear *(aurio sinister)*
ASA	American Society of Anesthesiologists; aspirin
ASHD	arteriosclerotic heart disease
ASHP	American Society of Hospital Pharmacists
Asn	asparagine
Asp	aspartic acid
AST	aspartate aminotransferase, serum (previously SGOT)
atm	standard atmosphere
ATN	acute tubular necrosis
ATP	adenosine triphosphate
ATPase	adenosine triphosphatase
ATPD	ambient temperature and pressure, saturated
at wt	atomic weight
au	both ears *(aures utrae)*
AU	gold *(aurum)*
AUC	area under the plasma concentration-time curve
AV	atrioventricular
A-V	arteriovenous; atrioventricular (block, bundle, conduction, dissociation, extrasystole)
AW	atomic weight
AWP	average wholesale price
ax.	axis
β	beta
BAC	blood-alcohol concentration
BADL	basic activities of daily life
BBB	blood brain barrier
BC	blood culture
BDZ	benzodiazepine
bib	drink *(bibe)*
bid	twice daily; two times a day *(bis in die)*
bm	bowel movement
BMR	basal metabolic rate
bp.	boiling point
BP	blood pressure

Abbreviation	Meaning
BPH	benign prostatic hypertrophy
bpm	beats per minute
BSA	body surface area
BT	bleeding time
BUN	blood urea nitrogen
C	centigrade
C.	*clostridium*
c	gallon *(cong)*
c̄	with *(cum)*
°C	degrees Celsius
Ca	calcium
CA	cancer; carcinoma; cardiac arrest; chronologic age; croup-associated
CAD	coronary artery disease
Cal	Calorie (kilocalorie)
cAMP	cyclic adenosine monophosphate
caps	capsule *(capsula)*
CAS	Chemical Abstracts Service
CAT	computerized axial tomography
cath	catheterize
CBA	cost-benefit analysis
CBC	complete blood count
CC	chief complaint
cc	cubic centimeter
CCBs	calcium channel blockers
CCU	coronary care unit; critical care unit
CD4	T-helper lymphocytes and macrophages
CDC	Centers for Disease Control and Prevention
CEA	cost effectiveness analysis
CF	cystic fibrosis
CFC	chlorofluorocarbon
CFU	colony-forming units
CHD	coronary heart disease
CHF	congestive heart failure
Ci	curie
CK	creatinine kinase
Cl	chlorine
Cl_{cr}	creatinine clearance
cm	centimeter
Cm	curium
cm^2	square centimeter(s)
cm^3	cubic centimeter
CMA	Certified Medical Assistant
CMC	carpometacarpal
CMI	cell-mediated immunity

Abbreviation	Meaning
CML	chronic myelocytic leukemia
C_{max}	maximum effective plasma concentration
C_{min}	minimum effective plasma concentration
CMT	Certified Medical Transcriptionist
CMV	cytomegalovirus I
CMVIG	cytomegalovirus immune globulin
CN	cranial nerve
CNM	Certified Nurse Midwife
CNS	central nervous system
CO	cardiac output
CO_2	carbon dioxide
CoA	coenzyme A
COG	center of gravity
comp	compound (compositus)
COMT	catecholamine-o-methyl transferase
cont rem	let the medicine be continued (continuetur remedium)
COPD	chronic obstructive pulmonary disease
CPAP	continuous positive airway pressure
CPK	creatine phosphokinase
CPR	cardiopulmonary resuscitation
CQI	continuous quality improvement
Cr	creatinine, chromium
CrCl	creatinine clearance
CRD	chronic respiratory disease
CRF	chronic renal failure
CRH	corticotropin-releasing hormone
crm	cream
CRNA	Certified Registered Nurse Anesthetist
C&S	culture and sensitivity
CSA	Controlled Substances Act; cyclosporin A
CSF	cerebrospinal fluid; colony-stimulating factors
CSP	cellulose sodium phosphate
ct	clotting time
CT	computerized tomography
CTZ	chemoreceptor trigger zone
cu	cubic
Cu	copper (cuprum)
CV	cardiovascular
CVA	cerebrovascular accident
CVP	central venous pressure
CXR	chest x-ray

Abbreviation	Meaning
cyl	cylinder; cylindrical (lens)
cys	cysteine
d	day (dies)
D5W	Dextrose 5% in Water Solution
D10W	Dextrose 10% in Water Solution
D&C	dilation and curettage; designation applied to dyes permitted for use in drugs and cosmetics
D&E	dilation and evacuation
DC	Doctor of Chiropratic
DDS	Doctor of Dental Surgery
DEA	Drug Enforcement Administration
deglut	swallow (degluttiatur)
DERM	dermatologic
det	give (detur)
DHHS	Department of Health and Human Services
DIC	disseminated intravascular coagulation
dieb alt	every other day (diebus alternis)
dil	dilute (dilue)
dim	one-half (dimidius)
dir prop	with proper direction (directione propria)
div in par aeq	divide into equal parts (divide in partes aequales)
DIS	drug information source
disp	dispense (dispensa)
div	divide
DJD	degenerative joint disease
DKA	diabetic ketoacidosis
dL	deciliter (100 mL)
DMD	Doctor of Dental Medicine
DMSO	dimethyl sulfoxide
DNA	deoxyribonucleic acid
DNR	do not resuscitate
DNS	Director of Nursing Service; Doctor of Nursing Services
DO	Doctor of Osteopathy
DOA	dead on arrival
DP	Doctor of Podiatry
DPH	Doctor of Public Health; Doctor of Public Hygiene
DPI	dry powder inhaler
DPM	Doctor of Physical Medicine; Doctor of Podiatric Medicine
DPS	disintegrations per second
DRG	diagnosis-related groups
DRI	Dietary Reference Intakes
drp	drop(s)

Abbreviation	Meaning
DrPh.	Doctor of Public Health; Doctor of Public Hygiene
DRR	Drug Regimen Review
DT	delirium tremens
dtd	give of such a dose *(dentur tales doses)*
DTP	diphtheria, tetanus toxoids & pertussis vaccine
DTRs	deep tendon reflexes
DUB	dysfunctional uterine bleeding
DUE	Drug Usage Evaluations
DUR	Drug Utilization Review
dur dol	while pain lasts *(durante dolore)*
DVA	Department of Veterans Affairs
DVM	Doctor of Veterinary Medicine
DVT	deep venous thrombosis
E.	*Enterococcus;Escherichia*
EBV	Epstein-Barr virus
EC	enteric coated
ECG	electrocardiogram
ECT	electroconvulsive therapy
ed.	editor
ED	emergency department; effective dose
ED_{50}	median-effective dose
EDTA	ethylenediamine tetraacetic acid
EEG	electroencephalogram
EENT	eye, ear, nose, and throat
EF	ejection fraction
eg.	for example *(exempli gratia)*
EIA	enzyme immunoassay
EKG	electrocardiogram
el	elixir
ELISA	enzyme-linked immunosorbent assay
elix	elixir
EMIT	enzyme-multiplied immunoassay test
emp	as directed
ENL	erythema nodosum leprosum
ENT	ear, nose, throat
EPA	Environmental Protection Agency
EPAP	expiratory positive airway pressure
EPO	erythropoietin
EPS	extrapyramidal syndrome (or symptoms)
ER	emergency room; estrogen receptor; extended release; endoplasmic reticulum

Abbreviation	Meaning
ESR	erythrocyte sedimentation rate; electron spin resonance
ESRD	end-stage renal disease
et	and
ET	via endotracheal tube
et al.	for 3 or more coauthors or co-workers *(et alii)*
ex aq	in water
ext rel	extended release
F	fluorine
f	make; let be made *(fac, fiat, fiant)*
°F	degress Fahrenheit
Fab.	fragment of immunoglobulin G involved in antigen binding
FAO	Food and Agriculture Organizations
FAS	fetal alcohol syndrome
FBS	fasting blood sugar
FDA	Food and Drug Administration
FD&C	designation applied to dyes permitted for use in foods, drugs, and cosmetics; Food, Drug and Cosmetic Act
Fe	iron *(ferrum)*
FEF	forced expiratory flow
FET	forced expiratory time
FEV_1	forced expiratory volume in 1 second
fl oz	fluid ounce(s)
Fru	fructose
FSH	follicle-stimulating hormone
ft.	foot (feet)
ft^2	square foot (feet)
FTC	Federal Trade Commission
FTI	free-thyroxine index
FUO	fever of unknown origin
FVC	forced vital capacity
γ.	gamma
g.	gram *(gramma)*
G-6-P	glucose-6-phosphate
G-6-PD	glucose-6-phosphate dehydrogenase
GABA	gamma-aminobutyric acid
Gal	galactose
gal	gallon
G-CSF	granulocyte colony-stimulating factor
GERD	gastroesophageal reflux disease
GFR	glomerular filtration rate
GGTP	gamma glutamyl transpeptidase

Abbreviation	Meaning
GH	growth hormone
GHRF	growth hormone-releasing factor
GHRH	growth hormone-releasing hormone
GI	gastrointestinal
GLC	gas-liquid chromatography
gln	glutamine
glu	glutamic acid; glutamyl
gly	glycine
Gm	gram *(gramma)*
gr	grain *(granum)*
grad	gradually *(gradatim)*
gran	granule(s)
GRAS	generally regarded as safe
gtt	a drop *(gutta)*
GU	genitourinary
Gyn	gynecology
H.	*Haemophilus;Helicobacter*
h.	hour *(hora)*
H$_2$	histamine 2
H$_2$O	water
HA	hyaluronic acid
Hb	hemoglobin
HbF	fetal hemoglobin
HBIG	hepatitis B immune globulin
HCFA	Health Care Financing Administration
HCG	human chorionic gonadotropin
HCl	hydrochloride
HCN	hydrogen cyanide
Hct	hematocrit
hd.	bedtime *(hora decubitus)*
HDL	high-densitiy lipoprotein
HEMA	hematologic
HEME	hematologic
hep	hepatic
HEPA	high efficiency particulate air
Hg	mercury *(hydragyrum)*
Hgb	hemoglobin
HGH	human pituitary growth hormone
Hib.	*Haemophilus influenzae*
His..	*Haemophilus influenzae* type b
HIV	human immunodeficiency virus
HLA	human leukocyte antigen
HMG-CoA	3-hydroxy-3-methylglutaryl coenzyme A
HMO	health maintenance organization
hor decub	at bedtime *(hora decubitus)*
hor som	at bedtime *(hora somni)*

Abbreviation	Meaning
HPA	hypothalamic-pituitary-adrenocortical (axis)
HPLC	high performance liquid chromatography
HPLC/MS	high performance liquid chromatography/mass spectrometry
HPMC	hydroxypropylmethylcellulose
HPV	human papillomavirus
HR	heart rate
hr	hour
hs	at bedtime *(hora somni)*
HSA	human serum albumin
HSV-1	herpes simplex virus type 1
HSV-2	herpes simplex virus type 2
Hz	hertz
I	iodine
IADL	instrumental activities of daily living
I/O	intake/output
IBW	ideal body weight
IC	intracoronary
ICD	International Classification of Diseases of the World Health Organization
ICF	intracellular fluid
ICP	intracranial pressure
ID	intradermal; infective dose
IDDM	insulin-dependent diabetes mellitus (type 1 diabetes)
IDU	idoxuridine
IFN	interferon
Ig	immunoglobulin
IL	interleukin
Ile	isoleucine
IM	intramuscular
in	inch(es)
in^2	square inch(es)
IND	Investigational New Drug
in d	daily *(in dies)*
INDA	Investigational New Drug Application
Inh	inhaled
INH	isoniazid
Inhal	inhalation
Inj	injection
INR	International Normalized Ratio
int cib	between meals *(inter cibos)*
IOP	intraocular pressure
IP	intraperitoneal(ly)

Abbreviation	Meaning
IPA	International Pharmaceutical Abstracts
IPPB	intermittent positive pressure breathing
IPV	poliovirus vaccine inactivated
IQ	intelligence quotient
ISA	intrinsic sympathomimetic activity
ISF	interstitial fluid
ISI	Institute for Scientific Information
ISO	International Organization for Standardization
IT	intrathecal(ly)
IU	international unit(s)
IUD	intrauterine device
IV	intravenous
IVF	intravascular fluid
IVP	intravenous piggyback
J	joule(s)
JCAH	Joint Commission on Accreditation of Hospitals
JCAHO	Joint Commission on Accreditation of Healthcare Organizations
K	potassium (kalium); kelvin
kcal	kilocalorie(s)
keV	kiloelectronvolt(s)
kg	kilogram
kJ	kilojoule(s)
Kleb.	Klebsiella
KVO	keep vein open
L	liter
L.	Legionella; Listeria
lb	pound
LBW	low body weight
LD	lethal dose
LD-50	a dose lethal to 50% of the specified animals or microorganisms
LDH	lactate dehydrogenase
LDL	low-density lipoprotein
LE	lupus erythematosus
Leu	leucine
LFT	liver function test
LH	luteinizing hormone
liq	liquid (liquor)
LM	Licentiate in Midwifery
LOC	level of consciousness
Lot	lotion
LPN	Licensed Practical Nurse

Abbreviation	Meaning
Lr	lawrencium
LSD	lysergic acid diethylamide
LTCF	long-term care facility
LTM	long-term memory
LUQ	left upper quadrant (of abdomen)
LVEDP	left ventricular end-diastolic pressure
LVET	left ventricular ejection time
LVF	left ventricular function
LVN	Licensed Visiting Nurse; Licensed Vocational Nurse
LVP	large-volume parenterals
Lw	former symbol for lawrencium (see Lr)
Lys	lysine
μm	micrometer
μg	microgram
m	meter
M	mix (misce); molar (strength of a solution)
M.	Moraxella; Mycobacterium; Mycoplasma
m^2	square meter (of body surface area)
m^3	cubic meter(s)
MA	mental age
MAC	maximum allowable cost
MADD	Mothers Against Drunk Driving
man pr	early morning; first thing in the morning (mane primo)
MAO	monoamine oxidase
MAOI	monoamine oxidase inhibitor
MAP	mean arterial pressure
max	maximum
MBC	minimum bactericidal concentration
MBD	mimimal brain dysfunction
mcg	microgram
MCH	mean corpuscular hemoglobin
MCHC	mean corpuscular hemoglobin concentration
mCi	millicurie
MCT	medium-chain triglyceride
MCV	mean corpuscular volume
MD	Doctor of Medicine (Medicinae Doctor)
MDI	metered-dose inhaler
m dict	as directed (more dictor)
MDR	minimum daily requirements
MEC	minimum effective concentration

Abbreviation	Meaning
MEDLARS	Medical Literature Analysis and Retrieval System
MEDLINE	National Library of Medicine medical database
mEq	milliequivalent
Met.	methionine
MeV	megaelectronvolt(s)
Mg	magnesium
mg	milligram
MHC	major histocompatibility complex
MI.	myocardial infarction
MIA	metabolite bacterial inhibition assay
MIC	minimum inhibitory concentration
MID	minimal inhibitory dose
min	minute; minimum
MIP	maximum inspiratory pressure
mixt	a mixture (mixtura)
MJ	mejajoule(s)
mL	milliliter
mm.	millimeter
mm²	square millimeter(s)
mm³	cubic millimeter(s)
mmHg	millimeters of mercury
mmol	millimole
MMR	measles, mumps and rubella virus vaccine, live
MMWR	Morbidity and Mortality Weekly Report
Mn	manganese
Mo	molybdenum
mo	month
mol	mole(s)
mor dict	in the manner stated (more dicto)
mor sol	as usual; as customary (more solito)
mOsm	milliosmole
MPH	Master of Public Health
MRI	magnetic resonance imaging
mRNA	messenger RNA
MS	mass spectrometry; mitral stenosis; multiple sclerosis
MW	molecular weight
N	normal (strength of a solution)
N.	Neisseria
NA	sodium (natrium)
NABP	National Association of Boards of Pharmacy
NABPLEX	National Association of Boards of Pharmacy Licensing Exam
NAD	nicotinamide-adenine dinucleotide phosphate
NADH	reduced form of nicotine adenine dinucleotide
NADP	nicotinamide-adenine dinucleotide phosphate
NADPH	nicotinamide-adenine dinucleotide phosphate (reduced form)
NAPA	N-acetyl procainamide
NARD	National Association of Retail Druggists - Now NCPA; National Asssociation of Community Pharmacists
nb.	note well (nota bene)
nCi	nanocurie(s)
NCPA	National Association of Community Pharmacists
ND	Doctor of Naturopathic Medicine
NDA	new drug application
NF	National Formulary'
ng.	nanogram
NG	nasogastric
NK	natural killer (cells); killer T cells
NIDDM	non-insulin-dependent diabetes mellitus (type 2 diabetes)
NIH.	National Institutes of Health
NLM	National Library of Medicine
nm	nanometer(s)
NMS.	neuroleptic malignant syndrome
NMT.	not more than (on prescriptions)
no.	number (numerus)
noc.	in the night (nocturnal)
noc maneq	at night and in the morning (nocte maneque)
non rep	do not repeat; no refills (non repetatur)
NPN	nonprotein nitrogen
NPO.	nothing by mouth
NS	normal saline (as in solution)
NSAIA	nonsteroidal antiinflammatory agent
NSAID	nonsteroidal antiinflammatory drug
NTD	neural tube defect
O	a pint (octarius)
OB/GYN	obstetrics and gynecology
OBRA.	Omnibus Budget Reconciliation Act of 1990
OBS	organic brain syndrome

Abbreviation	Meaning
OC	Oral contraceptive
Oct	a pint *(octarius)*
od	right eye *(oculus dexter)*
OD	Doctor of Optometry; overdose
Oint	ointment
ol	left eye *(oculus laevus)*
omn hor	at every hour *(omni hora)*
Ophth	ophthalmic
os	left eye *(oculus sinister)*
OSHA	Occupational Safety and Health Administration
OT	occupational therapy
otc	over-the-counter (nonprescription)
OPV	oral polioviurs vaccine, live
ou	each eye *(oculo uterque)*
o/w	oil-in-water (emulsion)
oz	ounce
P	phosphorus
P	probability
P&T	pharmacy and therapeutics (committee)
Pa	pascal(s)
PA	Physician Assistant; Physician's Assistant
PABA	para-aminobenzoic acid
PAC	premature atrial contraction
$PaCO_2$	arterial plasma partial pressure of carbon dioxide
PAD	premature atrial depolarization
PAF	platelet-activating factor
PaO_2	partial alveolar oxygen
part aeq	equal parts/amounts *(partes aequales)*
part vic	in divided doses *(partitis vicibus)*
PAS	para-aminosalicylic acid
PAW	pulmonary arterial wedge
PAWP	pulmonary arterial wedge pressure
Pb	lead *(plumbum)*
PBP	penicillin-binding protein
pc	after meals *(post cibum; post cibos)*
PCA	patient-controlled analgesia
pCO_2	plasma partial pressure of carbon dioxide
PCP	phencyclidine
PCR	polymerase chain reaction
PDGF	platelet-derived growth factor

Abbreviation	Meaning
PDLL	poorly differentiated lymphocytic lymphoma
PE	pulmonary embolism
PEEP	positive and expiratory pressure
PEG	polyethylene glycol
PERLA	pupils equal, react to light and accommodation
PET	positron emission tomography
pg	picograms(s)
PG	prostaglandin
PGA	prostaglandin A
PGB	prostaglandin B
PGE	prostaglandin E
PGF	prostaglandin F
pH	the negative logarithm of the hydrogen ion concentration
PharmD	Doctor of Pharmacy *(Pharmaciae Doctor)*
PhD	Doctor of Philosophy *(Philosophiae Doctor)*
Phe	phenylalanine
PhG	German Pharmacopeia *(Pharmacopoeia Germanica)*
PHS	Public Health Service
pKa	the negative logarithm of the dissociation constant
PKU	phenylketonuria
PMA	Pharmaceutical Manufacturers Association
PMH	past medical history
PMI	posterior myocardial infarction
PMN	polymorphonuclear leukocyte
PMR	patient medication record
PMS	premenstrual syndrome
PND	paroxysmal nocturnal dyspnea
po	by mouth; orally *(per os)*
pO_2	oxygen pressure (tension)
POR	problem-oriented medical record
POS	point of service
post cib	after meals *(post cibos)*; pc
PPD	purified protein derivative of tuberculin
PPI	patient package insert
ppm	parts per million
PPO	preferred provider organization
pr	per rectum
Pr.	*Proteus*
prn	as needed; when required *(pro re nata)*
Pro	proline

Abbreviation	Meaning
pro rat. Aet.	According to patient's age (pro ratione aetatis)
Ps.	Pseudomonas
PSA	prostate-specific antigen
PSP	phenolsulfonphthalein
PSVT	paroxysmal supraventricular tachycardia
pt	pint
PT	prothrombin time; pharmacy and therapeutics; physical therapy
PTH	parathyroid hormone
PTT	partial thromboplastin time
PUD	peptic ulcer disease
pulv	a powder (pulvis)
PUVA	oral administration of psoralen and subsequent exposure to ultraviolet light of A wave-lenghts (UVA)
PVC	premature ventricular contraction; polyvinyl chloride
PVD	peripheral vascular disease; premature ventricular depolarizations
pwdr	powder
q.	every
Q	volume of blood flow
QA	quality assurance
qad.	every other day (quoque alternis die)
QC	quality control
qd.	every day (quaque die)
qh.	every hour (quaque hora)
q hr	every hour
qid	four times daily (quarter in die)
ql	as much as desired (quantum libet)
qod.	every other day
q 2 hr	every 2 hours
qs	a sufficient quantity (quantum sufficiat); as much as is enough (quantum satis)
qs ad	a sufficient quantity to make
qt	quart
qv	as much as you wish (quam volueris)
R&D	research and development
RA	rheumatoid arthritis
RAI	radioactive iodine
RAS	renin-angiotension system; reticular-activating system
RAST	radioallergosorbent test
RBC	red blood (cell) count

Abbreviation	Meaning
RDA	Recommended Dietary (Daily) Allowance
RDS	respiratory distress
RDW	red-cell distribution width
RE	reticuloendothelial
rem	radio equivalent man
REM	rapid eye movement
rep	let it be repeated (repetatur)
RES	reticuloendothelial system
RF	releasing factor
Rh	Rhesus (RH blood group)
RIA	radioimmunoassay
RN	Registered Nurse
RNA	ribonucleic acid
ROM	range of motion
RPh	registered pharmacist
rpm	revolutions per minute
rps	revolutions per second
RR	respiratory rate
RT₃U	total serum thyroxine concentration
RUL	right upper lobe (of lung)
RUQ	right upper quadrant (of abdomen)
Rx	prescription only; take; a recipe (recipe)
S	Salmonella; Serratia
s	second; without (sine)
s̄	without (sine)
S&S	signs and symptoms
S-A	sinoatrial
sa	according to art (secundum artem)
sat	saturated (sataratus)
Sb	antimony (stibium)
SBE	self breast examination; subacute bacterial endocarditis
SC	subcutaneous(ly)
S_cr	serum creatinine
SD	standard deviation; streptodornase
Se	selenium
sec	second
Ser	serine
sf	sugar free
SGGT	serum gamma-glutamyl transferase
SGOT	(see AST)
SGPT	(see ALT)
Sh	Shigella

Abbreviation	Meaning
SIADH	syndrome of inappropriate secretion of antidiuretic hormone
SIDS	sudden infant death syndrome
Sig	label; let it be printed (signa)
SI units	International System of Units
SK	streptokinase
SL	sublingual(ly)
SLE	systemic lupus erythematosus
SMA	sequential multiple analysis
Sn	tin (stannum)
SNF	skilled nursing facility
sol	solution (solutio)
soln	solution
solv	dissolve
sp	species
SPECT	single photon emission computerized tomography
sp gr	specific gravity
SPF	sun protection factor
sq	square
SR	sedimentation rate; sustained release
ss	one-half (semis)
s̄s̄	one-half (semis)
SSRI	selective serotonin reuptake inhibitors
Staph.	Staphylococcus
stat	immediately; at once (statim)
STM	short-term memory
STP	standard temperature and pressure
Str.	Streptococcus
STD	sexually transmitted disease
supp	suppository (suppositorium)
suppl	supplement(s)
susp	suspension
SV	stroke volume
syr	syrup (syrupus)
$t_{1/2}$	half-life
T_3	triiodothyronine
T_4	thyroxine
tab	tablet (tabella)
tal	such
tal dos	such doses
TB	tuberculosis
TBC	thyroxine-binding globulin
TBP	thyroxine-binding proteins
TBPA	thyroxine-binding pre-albumin
TBW	total body weight

Abbreviation	Meaning
TCA	tricyclic antidepressant
TD_{50}	median toxic dose
TEEC	transesophageal echocardiography
TEN	toxic epidermal necrolysis
TENS	transcutaneous electrical nerve stimulation
TG	total triglycerides
THC	tetrahydrocannabinol
Thr	threonine
TIA	transient ischemic attack
tid	three times daily (ter in die)
tbsp	tablespoonful
tinct	tincture
TLC	total lung capacity; thin layer chromatography
T_{max}	time to maximum concentration
TMJ	temporomandibular joint
TNF	tumor necrosis factor
TNM	tumor, node, metastasis (tumor staging)
top	topical(ly)
TOPV	trivalent oral polio vaccine
tPA	tissue plasminogen activator
TPN	total parenteral nutrition
TPR	temperature, pulse, respirations
TQM	total quality management
tr	tincture
trit	triturate (tritura)
tRNA	transfer RNA
Trp	tryptophan
TSA	tumor-specific antigens
TSH	thyroid-stimulating hormone
tsp	teaspoonful
TSS	toxic shock syndrome
TSTA	tumor-specific transplantation antigen
TT	thrombin time
TV	tidal volume
Tyr	tyrosine
U	unit
ud	as directed
UD	unit-dose package
UK	United Kingdom
ung	ointment (unguentum)
URI	upper respiratory infection
USAN	United States Adopted Name(s)
USP	United States Pharmacopeia
USPHS	United States Public Health Service

Abbreviation	Meaning
ut dict	as directed *(ut dictum)*
UTI	urinary tract infection
UVA	ultraviolet A wave
V	volt
VA	Veterans Administration
vag	vaginal(ly)
Val	valine
var	variety
VC	vital capacity
V_c	volume of distribution of the central compartment
V_d	volume of distribution (one compartment)
$V_{d\beta}$	volume of distribution of the β phase
V_{dss}	steady-state apparent volume of distribution
VHDL	very high-density lipoprotein
VLDL	very low-density lipoprotein
VMA	vanillylmandelic acid
vol	volume

Abbreviation	Meaning
VS	vital signs
v/v	volume in volume
v/w	volume in weight
wa	while awake
WBC	white blood (cell) count
WBCT	whole blood clotting time
WDLL	well-differentiated lymphocytic lymphoma
WFI	water for injection
WHO	World Health Organization
wk	week
WNL	within normal limits
w/o	water in oil
wt	weight
w/v	weight in volume
w/w	weight in weight
y/o	years old
yr	year
ZE	Zollinger-Ellison
Zn	zinc

Calculations

To calculate milliequivalent weight:

$$mEq = \frac{\text{gram molecular weight/valence}}{\text{valence}}$$

$$mEq = \frac{mg}{\text{eq wt}} \qquad \text{equivalent weight or eq wt} = \frac{\text{gram molecular weight}}{\text{valence}}$$

Commonly Used mEq Weights			
Chloride	35.5 mg = 1 mEq	Magnesium	12 mg = 1 mEq
Sodium	23 mg = 1 mEq	Potassium	39 mg = 1 mEq
Calcium	20 mg = 1 mEq		

To convert temperature:

Fahrenheit to Celsius: (°F − 32) × 5/9 = °C

Celsius to Fahrenheit: (°C × 9/5) = °F

Celsius to Kelvin: °C + 273 = °K

Temperature Equivalents
°C = 5 ÷ sec × (°F − 32)
°F = 9÷5 × (°C) + 32
°K = °C + 273

To calculate creatinine clearance (Ccr) from serum creatinine (mL/min):

Male: $Ccr = \dfrac{\text{weight (kg)} \times (140 - \text{age})}{72 \times \text{serum creatinine (mg/dL)}}$ Female: Ccr = 0.85 × calculation for males

---

To calculate ideal body weight (IBW) (kg) in adults:

IBW (kg) (Males) = 50 + (2.3 × Height in inches over 60 inches)

IBW (kg) (Females) = 45.5 kg + (2.3 × Height in inches over 60 inches)

To calculate absolute neutrophil count (ANC):

$WBC \times (\% \text{ Segs} + \% \text{ Bands})$

To calculate aninon gap:

$Na^+ - (Cl^- \ HCo_3^-)$

Elevated anion gap usually indicates unmeasured anions in the extracellular fluid due to any of the following: methanol, uremia, diabetes, paraldehyde, ischemia, ethylene glycol, salicylates.

To calculate daily fluid requirements (based on patient's weight):

Weight from 0 to 10 kg: 100 kg
Weight from 10 to 20 kg: 50 mL/kg
Weight > 20 kg: 20 mL/kg

To calculate cholesterol calculations:

$LDL_{chol} = (Total_{chol} - HDL_{chol}) - [\text{Triglycerides (must be} < 400)/5]$

To calculate volume status:

BUN: Serum Creatine ratio

* If > 20:1, Patient is volume depleted and requires fluid replacement.

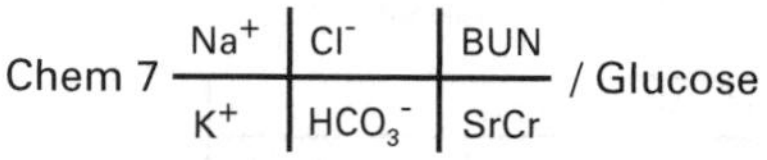

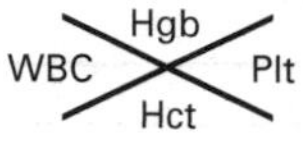

$$\text{Chem 7} \quad \frac{Na^+ \quad | \quad Cl^- \quad | \quad BUN}{K^+ \quad | \quad HCO_3^- \quad | \quad SrCr} \, / \, \text{Glucose} \qquad WBC \diagcross{\overset{Hgb}{\underset{Hct}{}}} Plt$$

* Glucose: add 1.6 mEq/L Na^+ for every 100 mg/dL glucose is above normal.

To calculate total calcium corrected for albumin:

[Normal albumin – patient's albumin] $\times$ 0.8 patient's calcium = corrected calcium

---

Common Systems of Weights and Measures

The listing of common systems of weights and measures is included to aid the practitioner in calculating dosages.

METRIC SYSTEM

Metric Weight			Metric Liquid Measure		
1 femtogram (fg)	= 0.001	pg	1 femtoliter (fL)	= 0.001	pL
1 picogram (pg)	= 0.001	ng	1 picoliter (pL)	= 0.001	nL
1 nanogram (ng)	= 0.001	mcg	1 nanoliter (nL)	= 0.001	μL
1 microgram* (μg [mcg])	= 0.001	mg	1 microliter (μL)	= 0.001	mL
1 milligram (mg)	= 0.001	g	1 milliliter (mL)	= 0.001	L
1 centigram (cg)	= 0.01	g	1 centiliter (cL)	= 0.01	L (= 10 mL)
1 decigram (dg)	= 0.1	g	1 deciliter (dL)	= 0.1	L (= 100 mL)
1 gram (g)	= 1.0	g	1 liter (l)	= 1.0	L (= 1000 ml)
1 dekagram (dag)	= 10.0	g	1 dekaliter (daL)	= 10.0	L
1 hectogram (hg)	= 100.0	g	1 hectoliter (hL)	= 100.0	L
1 kilogram (kg)	= 1000.0	g	1 kiloliter (kL)	= 1000.0	L

* The abbreviation μg or mcg is used for microgram in pharmacy rather than gamma (γ) as in biology.

APOTHECARY SYSTEM*

Apothecary Weight Equivalents			Apothecary Volume Equivalents		
1 grain† (gr)	= 1 gr		1 minim (♏.)	= 1 ♏.	
1 scruple (Э)	= 20 gr		1 fluidram (fl ʒ)	= 60 ♏.	= 8 fl ʒ
1 dram (ʒ)	= 60 gr	= 3 Э	1 fluid ounce (fl ʒ)	= 480 ♏.	= 8 fl ʒ
1 ounce (ʒ)	= 480 gr	= 8 ʒ	1 pint (pt or O)	= 7680 ♏.	= 16 fl ʒ
1 pound (lb)	= 5760 gr	= 12 ʒ	1 quart (qt)	= 15630 ♏.	= 32 fl ʒ
			1 gallon (gal or cong)	= 61440 ♏.	= 128 fl ʒ

* Used in preparation of pharmaceuticals.

† The grain in each of the above systems has the same value, and thus serves as a basis for the interconversion of the other units.

AVOIRDUPOIS SYSTEM*

Avoirdupois Equivalents		
1 ounce (oz)	= 437.5 grains (gr)	
1 pound (lb)	= 16 ounces (oz)	= 7000 grains (gr)

* Used by manufacturers and wholesalers.

Approximate Practical Equivalents

The listing of approximate practical equivalents is included to aid the practitioner in calculating and converting dosages among the various systems.

Weight Equivalents

1 grain	=	1 gr	=	65 milligrams
1 milligram	=	1 mg	=	0.017 grains
1 gram	=	1 g	=	15.432 grains
1 gram	=	1 g	=	0.035 ounces
1 ounce avoirdupois	=	1 oz	=	28.35 grams
1 ounce apothecary	=	1 ʒ	=	31.1 grams
1 pound avoirdupois	=	1 lb	=	454.0 grams
1 pound avoirdupois	=	1 lb	=	0.45 kilograms
1 kilogram	=	1 kg	=	2.20 pounds avoirdupois (lb)

Measure Equivalents

1 milliliter	=	1 mL	=	16.23 minims (♏.)
1 cubic centimeter*	=	1 cc	=	1.0 mL
1 fluidram†	=	1 f ʒ	=	3.4 mL
1 teaspoonful†	=	1 tsp	=	5.0 mL
1 tablespoonful	=	1 tbsp	=	15.0 mL
1 fluid ounce	=	1 fl ʒ	=	29.57 mL
1 wineglassful	=	2 fl ʒ	=	60.0 mL
1 teacupful	=	4 fl ʒ	=	120.0 mL
1 tumblerful	=	8 fl ʒ	=	240.0 mL
1 pint	=	1 pt or O or Oct	=	473.0 mL
1 quart	=	1 qt	=	946.0 mL
1 liter	=	1 L	=	33.8 fluid ounces (fl ʒ)
1 gallon	=	1 gal or C or Cong	=	3785.0 mL

* Cubic centimeter and milliliter are equivalent.

† On prescription a fluidram is assumed to contain a teaspoonful, which is 5 mL.

Weight to Volume Equivalents

1 mg/dL	=	10 μ/mL
1 mg/dL	=	1 mg %
1% solution	=	10 mg per mL
1 ppm	=	1 mg/L

Linear Equivalents

1 millimeter	=	1 mm	=	0.04 inches
1 inch	=	1 in	=	25.4 millimeters
1 inch	=	1 in	=	2.54 centimeters
1 meter	=	1 meter	=	39.37 inches
1 inch	=	1 in	=	0.025 meters

International System Of Units

The *Système international d 'unités* (International System of Units) or *SI* is a modernized
version of the metric system. The primary goal of the conversion to SI units is to
revise the present confused measurement system and to improve test-result
communications.

The SI has 7 basic units from which other units are derived:

Base Units of SI		
Physical quantity	Base unit	SI symbol
length	meter	m
mass	kilogram	kg
time	second	s
amount of substance	mole	mol
thermodynamic temperature	kelvin	K
electric current	ampere	A
luminous intensity	candela	cd

Combinations of these base units can express any property, although, for simplicity,
special names are given to some of these derived units.

Representative Derived Units		
Derived unit	Name and symbol	Derivation from base units
area	square meter	m^2
volume	cubic meter	m^3
force	newton (N)	$kg•m•s^{-2}$
pressure	pascal (Pa)	$kg•m^{-1}•s^{-2}(N/m^2)$
work, energy	joule (J)	$kg•m^2•s^{-2}(N•m)$
mass density	kilogram per cubic meter	kg/m^3
frequency	hertz (Hz)	1 cycles/s^{-1}
temperature degree	Celsius (°C)	°C = °K − 273.15
concentration		
mass	kilogram/liter	kg/L
substance	mole/liter	mol/L
molality	mole/kilogram	mol/kg
density	kilogram/liter	kg/L

Prefixes to the base unit are used in this system to form decimal multiples and submultiples. The preferred multiples and submultiples listed below change the quantity by increments of 10^3 or 10^{-3}. The exceptions to these recommended factors are within the middle rectangle.

Prefixes and Symbols for Decimal Multiples and Submultiples		
Factor	Prefix	Symbol
10^{18}	exa	E
10^{15}	peta	P
10^{12}	tera	T
10^{9}	giga	G
10^{6}	mega	M
10^{3}	kilo	k
10^{2}	hecto	h
10^{1}	deka	da
10^{-1}	deci	d
10^{-2}	centi	c
10^{-3}	milli	m
10^{-6}	micro	μ
10^{-9}	nano	n
10^{-12}	pico	p
10^{-15}	femto	f
10^{-18}	atto	a

To convert drug concentrations to or from SI units:

Conversion factor (CF) = $1000/\text{mol wt}$

Conversion *to* SI units: μg/mL × CF = μmol/L

Conversion *from* SI units: μmol/L ÷ CF = μg/mL

Normal Laboratory Values

In the following tables, normal reference values for commonly requested laboratory tests are listed in traditional units and in SI units. The tables are a guideline only. Values are method dependent and "normal values" may vary between laboratories.

Blood, Plasma or Serum		
	Reference Value	
Determination	Conventional units	SI units
Alpha-fetoprotein	Adult: < 15 ng/mL Pregnant (16-18 wk): 38-45 ng/mL	Adult: < 15 mcg/L Pregnant (16-18 wk): 38-45 mcg/L
Ammonia (NH_3) - diffusion	20-120 mcg/dL	12-70 mcmol/L
Ammonia nitrogen	15-45 µg/dL	11-32 µmol/L
Amylase	20-100 units/dL	37-185 U/L
Anion gap ($Na^+ - [Cl^- + HCO_3^-]$) (P)	7-16 mEq/L	7-16 mmol/L
Antinuclear antibodies	negative at 1:10 dilution of serum	negative at 1:10 dilution of serum
Antithrombin III (AT III)	80-120 U/dL	800-1200 U/L
Bicarbonate: Arterial Venous	21-28 mEq/L 22-29 mEq/L	21-28 mmol/L 22-29 mmol/L
Bilirubin: Conjugated (direct) Total	≤ 0.2 mg/dL 0.1-1 mg/dL	≤ 4 mcmol/L 2-18 mcmol/L
Calcitonin: Female Male	≤ 20 pg/mL ≤ 40 pg/mL	≤ 20 ng/L ≤ 40 ng/L
Calcium: Total Ionized	8.6-10.3 mg/dL 4.4-5.1 mg/dL	2.2-2.74 mmol/L 1-1.3 mmol/L
Carbon dioxide content (plasma)	21-32 mmol/L	21-32 mmol/L
Carcinoembryonic antigen	< 3 ng/mL	< 3 mcg/L
Chloride	95-110 mEq/L	95-110 mmol/L
Coagulation screen: Bleeding time Prothrombin time Partial thromboplastin time (activated) Protein C Protein S	3-9.5 min 10-13 sec 22-37 sec 0.7-1.4 µ/mL 0.7-1.4 µ/mL	180-570 sec 10-13 sec 22-37 sec 700-1400 U/ml 700-1400 U/mL
Copper, total	70-160 mcg/dL	11-25 mcmol/L
Corticotropin (ACTH [adrenocorticotropic hormone]) - 0800 hr	< 60 pg/mL	< 13.2 pmol/L
Cortisol: 0800 hr 1800 hr 2000 hr	5-30 mcg/dL 2-15 mcg/dL ≤ 50% of 0800 hr	138-810 nmol/L 50-410 nmol/L ≤ 50% of 0800 hr
Creatine kinase: Female Male	20-170 IU/L 30-220 IU/L	0.33-2.83 mckat/L 0.5-3.67 mckat/L
Creatinine kinase isoenzymes, MB fraction	0-12 IU/L	0-0.2 mckat/L
Creatinine	0.5-1.7 mg/dL	44-150 mcmol/L
Fibrinogen (coagulation factor I)	150-360 mg/dL	1.5-3.6 g/L
Follicle-stimulating hormone (FSH): Female Midcycle Male	2-13 mIU/mL 5-22 mIU/mL 1-8 mIU/mL	2-13 IU/L 5-22 IU/L 1-8 IU/L
Glucose, fasting	65-115 mg/dL	3.6-6.3 mmol/L

Glucose tolerance test (oral)	mg/dL		mmol/L	
	Normal	Diabetic	Normal	Diabetic
Fasting	70-105	> 140	3.9-5.8	> 7.8
60 min	120-170	≥ 200	6.7-9.4	≥ 11.1
90 min	100-140	≥ 200	5.6-7.8	≥ 11.1
120 min	70-120	≥ 140	3.9-6.7	≥ 7.8

(γ) - Glutamyltransferase (GGT): Male Female	9-50 units/L 8-40 units/L	9-50 units/L 8-40 units/L
Haptoglobin	44-303 mg/dL	0.44-3.03 g/L

Blood, Plasma or Serum		
	Reference Value	
Determination	Conventional units	SI units
Hematologic tests:		
Fibrinogen	200-400 mg/dL	2-4 g/L
Hematocrit (Hct), female	36%-44.6%	0.36-0.446 fraction of 1
male	40.7%-50.3%	0.4-0.503 fraction of 1
Hemoglobin A_{1C}	4%-6%	0.053-0.075
Hemoglobin (Hb), female	12-16 g/dL	7.49-9.9 mmol/L
male	14-18 g/dL	8.7-11.2 mmol/L
Leukocyte count (WBC)	3800-9800/mcL	$3.8\text{-}9.8 \times 10^9$/L
Erythrocyte count (RBC), female	$3.5\text{-}5.5 \times 10^6$/mcL	$3.5\text{-}5.5 \times 10^{12}$/L
male	$4.3\text{-}5.9 \times 10^6$/mcL	$4.3\text{-}5.9 \times 10^{12}$/L
Mean corpuscular volume (MCV)	80-97.6 mcm^3	80-97.6 fl
Mean corpuscular hemoglobin (MCH)	27-33 pg/cell	1.66-2.09 fmol/cell
Mean corpuscular hemoglobin concentrate (MCHC)	33-36 g/dL	20.3-22 mmol/L
Erythrocyte sedimentation rate (sedrate, ESR)	≤ 30 mm/hr	≤ 30 mm/hr
Erythrocyte enzymes:		
Glucose-6-phosphate dehydrognase (G-6-PD)	250-5000 units/10^6 cells	250-5000 mcunits/cell
Ferritin	10-300 ng/mL	10-300 pmol/L
Folic acid: normal	> 3.1-12.4 ng/mL	7-28.1 nmol/L
Platelet count	$150\text{-}450 \times 10^3$/mcL	$150\text{-}450 \times 10^9$/L
Reticulocytes	0.5%-1.5% of erythrocytes	0.005-0.015
Vitamin B_{12}	223-1132 pg/mL	165-835 pmol/L
Iron: Female	30-160 mcg/dL	5.4-31.3 mcmol/L
Male	45-160 mcg/dL	8.1-31.3 mcmol/L
Iron binding capacity	220-420 mcg/dL	39.4-75.2 mcmol/L
Isocitrate dehydrogenase	1.2-7 units/L	1.2-7 units/L
Isoenzymes		
Fraction 1	14%-26% of total	0.14-0.26 fraction of total
Fraction 2	29%-39% of total	0.29-0.39 fraction of total
Fraction 3	20%-26% of total	0.20-0.26 fraction of total
Fraction 4	8%-16% of total	0.08-0.16 fraction of total
Fraction 5	6%-16% of total	0.06-0.16 fraction of total
Lactate dehydrogenase	100-250 IU/L	1.67-4.17 mckat/L
Lactic acid (lactate)	6-19 mg/dL	0.7-2.1 mmol/L
Lead	≤ 20 mcg/dL	≤ 2.41 mcmol/L
Lipase	10-150 IU/L	10-150 IU/L
Lipids:		
Total Cholesterol		
Desirable	< 200 mg/dL	< 5.2 mmol/L
Borderline-high	200-239 mg/dL	< 5.2-6.2 mmol/L
High	> 239 mg/dL	> 6.2 mmol/L
LDL		
Desirable	< 130 mg/dL	< 3.36 mmol/L
Borderline-high	130-159 mg/dL	3.36-4.11 mmol/L
High	> 159 mg/dL	> 4.11 mmol/L
HDL		
Low	< 40 mg/dL	
High	≥ 60 mg/dL	
Triglycerides		
Desirable	< 150 mg/dL	
Borderline-high	150-199 mg/dL	
High	200-499 mg/dL	
Very high	> 500 mg/dL	
Magnesium	1.3-2.2 mEq/L	0.65-1.1 mmol/L
Osmolality	280-300 mOsm/kg	280-300 mmol/kg
Oxygen saturation (arterial)	94%-100%	0.94-1 fraction of 1
PCO_2, arterial	35-45 mm Hg	4.7-6 kPa

Blood, Plasma or Serum		
	Reference Value	
Determination	Conventional units	SI units
pH, arterial	7.35-7.45	7.35-7.45
PO₂, arterial: Breathing room air[1] On 100% O₂	80-105 mm Hg > 500 mm Hg	10.6-14 kPa
Phosphatase (acid), total at 37°C	0.13-0.63 IU/L	2.2-10.5 IU/L or 2.2-10.5 mckat/L
Phosphatase alkaline[2]	20-130 IU/L	20-130 IU/L or 0.33-2.17 mckat/L
Phosphorus, inorganic,[3] (phosphate)	2.5-5 mg/dL	0.8-1.6 mmol/L
Potassium	3.5-5 mEq/L	3.5-5 mmol/L

Progesterone
Female
  Follicular phase
  Luteal phase
Male
	
	0.1-1.5 ng/mL
	0.1-1.5 ng/mL
	2.5-28 ng/mL
	< 0.5 ng/mL
		
		0.32-4.8 nmol/L
		0.32-4.8 nmol/L
		8-89 nmol/L
		< 1.6 nmol/L

Prolactin	1.4-24.2 ng/mL	1.4-24.2 mcg/L
Prostate specific antigen	0-4 ng/mL	0-4 ng/mL

Protein: Total
  Albumin
  Globulin
	6-8 g/dL
	3.6-5 g/dL
	2.3-3.5 g/dL
		60-80 g/L
		36-50 g/L
		23-35 g/L

Rheumatoid factor	< 60 IU/mL	< 60 kIU/L
Sodium	135-147 mEq/L	135-147 mmol/L
Testosterone: Female Male	6-86 ng/dL 270-1070 ng/dl	0.21-3 nmol/L 9.3-37 nmol/L
Thyroid Hormone Function Tests: Thyroid-stimulating hormone (TSH) Thyroxine-binding globulin capacity Total triiodothyronine (T₃) Total thyroxine by RIA (T₄) T₃ resin uptake	 0.35-6.2 mcU/mL 10-26 mcg/dL 75-220 ng/dL 4-11 mcg/dL 25%-38%	 0.35-6.2 mU/L 100-260 mcg/L 1.2-3.4 nmol/L 51-142 nmol/L 0.25-0.38 fraction of 1
Transaminase, AST (aspartate amino-transferase, SGOT)	11-47 IU/L	0.18-0.78 mckat/l
Transaminase, ALT (alanine aminotrans-ferase, SGPT)	7-53 IU/L	0.12-0.88 mckat/L
Transferrin	220-400 mg/dL	2.20-4.00 g/L
Urea nitrogen (BUN)	8-25 mg/dL	2.9-8.9 mmol/L
Uric acid	3-8 mg/dL	179-476 mcmol/L
Vitamin A (retinol)	15-60 mcg/dl	0.52-2.09 mcmol/L
Zinc	50-150 mcg/dL	7.7-23 mcmol/L

[1] Age dependent
[2] Infants and adolescents up to 104 U/L
[3] Infants in the first year up to 6 mg/dL

Urine		
	Reference value	
Determination	Conventional units	SI units
Calcium[1]	50-250 mcg/day	1.25-6.25 mmol/day
Catecholamines: Epinephrine Norepinephrine	< 20 mcg/day < 100 mcg/day	< 109 nmol/day < 590 nmol/day
Catecholamines, 24-hr	< 110 µg	< 650 nmol
Copper[1]	15-60 mcg/day	0.24-0.95 mcmol/day
Creatinine: Child	8-22 mg/kg	71-195 µmol/kg
Adolescent	8-30 mg/kg	71-265 µmol/kg
Female	0.6-1.5 g/day	5.3-13.3 mmol/day
Male	0.8-1.8 g/day	7.1-15.9 mmol/day
pH	4.5-8	4.5-8
Phosphate[1]	0.9-1.3 g/day	29-42 mmol/day
Potassium[1]	25-100 mEq/day	25-100 mmol/day
Protein		
Total	1-14 mg/dL	10-140 mg/L
At rest	50-80 mg/day	50-80 mg/day
Protein, quantitative	< 150 mg/day	< 0.15 g/day
Sodium[1]	100-250 mEq/day	100-250 mmol/day
Specific gravity, random	1.002-1.030	1.002-1.030
Uric acid, 24-hr	250-750 mg	1.48-4.43 mmol

[1] Diet Dependent

	Drug Levels*	
	Reference value	
Drug determination	Conventional units	SI units
Aminoglycosides		
Amikacin		
(trough)	1-8 mcg/mL	1.7-13.7 mcmol/L
(peak)	20-30 mcg/mL	34-51 mcmol/L
Gentamicin		
(trough)	0.5-2 mcg/mL	1-4.2 mcmol/L
(peak)	6-10 mcg/mL	12.5-20.9 mcmol/L
Kanamycin		
(trough)	5-10 mcg/mL	nd[1]
(peak)	20-25 mcg/mL	nd
Netilimicin		
(trough)	0.5-2 mcg/mL	nd
(peak)	6-10 mcg/mL	nd
Streptomycin		
(trough)	< 5 mcg/mL	nd
(peak)	20-30 mcg/mL	nd
Tobramycin		
(trough)	0.5-2 mcg/mL	1.1-4.3 mcmol/L
(peak)	6-10 mcg/mL	12.8-21.8 mcmol/L
Antiarrhythmics		
Amiodarone	0.5-2.5 mcg/mL	1.5-4 mcmol/L
Bretylium	0.5-1.5 mcg/mL	nd
Digitoxin	9-25 mcg/L	11.8-32.8 nmol/L
Digoxin	0.8-2 ng/mL	0.9-2.5 nmol/L
Disopyramide	2-8 mcg/mL	6-18 mcmol/L
Flecainide	0.2-1 mcg/mL	nd
Lidocaine	1.5-6 mcg/mL	4.5-21.5 mcmol/L
Mexiletine	0.5-2 mcg/mL	nd
Procainamide	4-8 mcg/mL	17-34 mcmol/mL
Propranolol	50-100 ng/mL	190-390 nmol/L
Quinidine	2-6 mcg/mL	4.6-9.2 mcmol/L
Tocainide	5-12 mcg/mL	22-52 mcmol/L
Verapamil	50-200 ng/mL	100-420 nmol/L
Anticonvulsants		
Carbamazepine	4-12 mcg/mL	17-51 mcmol/L
Phenobarbital	10-40 mcg/mL	43-172 mcmol/L
Phenytoin	10-20 mcg/mL	40-80 mcmol/L
Primidone	5-15 mg/mL	23-69 mcmol/L
Valproic Acid	50-100 mcg/L	346-693 mcmol/L
Antidepressants		
Amitriptyline	110-250 ng/mL[2]	500-900 nmol/L
Amoxapine	200-500 ng/mL	637-1594 nmol/L
Bupropion	50-100 ng/mL	nd
Clomipramine	80-100 ng/mL	nd
Desipramine	115-300 ng/mL	281-1125 nmol/L
Doxepin	30-250 ng/mL	107-537 nmol/L
Imipramine	100-300 ng/mL	nd
Maprotiline	200-300 ng/mL	nd
Nortriptyline	50-150 ng/mL	190-665 nmol/L
Protriptyline	70-250 ng/mL	266-950 nmol/L
Trazodone	800-1600 ng/mL	nd

Drug Levels*		
	Reference value	
Drug determination	Conventional units	SI units
Antipsychotics		
Chlorpromazine	50-300 ng/mL	157-942 nmol/L
Fluphenazine	5-20 ng/mL	nd
Haloperidol	5-20 ng/mL	10-30 nmol/L
Perphenazine	2-6 ng/mL	nd
Thiothixene	2-57 ng/mL	nd
Miscellaneous		
Amantadine	300 ng/mL	nd
Amrinone	3.7 mcg/mL	nd
Chloramphenicol	10-20 mcg/mL	31-62 mcmol/L
Cyclosporine[3]	250-800 ng/mL (whole blood, RIA)	nd
	50-300 ng/mL (plasma, RIA)	nd
Ethanol[4]	0 mg/dL	0 mmol/L
Hydralazine	100 ng/mL	nd
Lithium	0.6-1.2 mEq/L	0.6-1.2 mmol/L
Salicylate	100-300 mg/L	724-2172 mcmol/L
Sulfonamide	5-15 mg/dL	nd
Theophylline	10-20 mcg/mL	55-110 mcmol/L
Vancomycin		
(trough)	5-15 ng/mL	nd
(peak)	20-40 mcg/mL	nd

* The values given are generally accepted as desirable for treatment without toxicity for most patients. However, exceptions are not uncommon.
[1] nd = No data available.
[2] Parent drug plus N-desmethyl metabolite.
[3] 24-hour trough values.
[4] Toxic: 50-100 mg/dL (10.9–21.7 mmol/L).

The following table is adopted from the Sixth Report of the Joint National Committee on Prevention, Detection, Evaluation, and Treatment of High Blood Pressure, National Institutes of Health.

Classification of Blood Pressure*				
	Reference value			
Category	Systolic (mm Hg)		Diastolic (mm Hg)	
Optimal[1]	< 120	and	< 80	
Normal	< 130	and	< 85	
High-normal	130-139	or	85-89	
Hypertension[2]				
Stage 1	140-159	or	90-99	
Stage 2	160-179	or	100-109	
Stage 3	≥ 180	or	≥ 110	

* For adults age 18 and older who are not taking antihypertensive drugs and not acutely ill. When systolic and diastolic blood pressures fall into different categories, the higher category should be selected to classify the individual's blood pressure status. In addition to classifying stages of hypertension on the basis of average blood pressure levels, clinicians should specify presence or absence of target organ disease and additional risk factors.
[1] Optimal blood pressure with respect to cardiovascular risk is below 120/88 mm Hg. However, unusually low readings should be evaluated for clinical significance.
[2] Based on the average of two or more readings taken at each of two or more visits after an initial screening.

FDA Pregnancy Categories

The rational use of any medication requires a risk vs benefit assessment. Among the myriad of risk factors which complicate this assessment, pregnancy is one of the most perplexing.

The FDA has established five categories to indicate the potential of a systemically absorbed drug for causing birth defects. The key differentiation among the categories rests upon the degree (reliability) of documentation and the risk vs benefit ratio. Pregnancy Category X is particularly notable in that if any data exists that may implicate a drug as a teratogen and the risk vs benefit ratio does not support use of the drug, the drug is contraindicated during pregnancy. These categories are summarized below:

FDA Pregnancy Categories	
Pregnancy Category	**Definition**
A	Controlled studies show no risk. Adequate, well-controlled studies in pregnant women have failed to demonstrate risk to the fetus.
B	No evidence of risk in humans. Either animal findings show risk, but human findings do not; or if no adequate human studies have been done, animal findings are negative.
C	Risk cannot be ruled out. Human studies are lacking, and animal studies are either positive for fetal risk or lacking. However, potential benefits may justify the potential risks.
D	Positive evidence of risk. Investigational or postmarketing data show risk to the fetus. Nevertheless, potential benefits may outweigh the potential risks. If needed in a life-threatening situation or a serious disease, the drug may be acceptable if safer drugs cannot be used or are ineffective.
X	Contraindicated in pregnancy. Studies in animals or humans, or investigational or post-marketing reports have shown fetal risk that clearly outweighs any possible benefit to the patients.

Regardless of the designated pregnancy category or presumed safety, no drug should be administered during pregnancy unless it is clearly needed and potential benefits outweigh potential hazards to the fetus.

Controlled Substances

The Controlled Substances Act of 1970 regulates the manufacturing, distribution, and dispensing of drugs that have abuse potential. The Drug Enforcement Administration (DEA) within the US Department of Justice is the chief federal agency responsible for enforcing the act.

DEA schedules: Drugs under jurisdiction of the Controlled Substances Act are divided into five schedules based on their potential for abuse and physical and psychological dependence. All controlled substances listed in *American Drug Index* are identified by schedule as follows:

Schedule I *(c-i)*: High abuse potential and no accepted medical use (eg, heroin, marijuana, LSD).

Schedule II *(c-ii)*: High abuse potential with severe dependence liability (eg, narcotics, amphetamines, dronabinol, some barbiturates).

Schedule III *(c-iii)*: Less abuse potential than schedule II drugs and moderate dependence liability (eg, nonbarbiturate sedatives, nonamphetamine stimulants, limited amounts of certain narcotics)

Schedule IV *(c-iv)*: Less abuse potential than III drugs and limited dependence liability (eg, some sedatives, antianxiety agents, nonnarcotic analgesics).

Schedule V *(c-v)*: Limited abuse potential. Primarily small amounts of narcotics (codeine) used as antitussives or antidiarrheals. Under federal law, limited quantities of certain *c-v* drugs may be purchased without a prescription directly from a pharmacist if allowed under state statutes. The purchaser must be at least 18 years of age and must furnish suitable identification. All such transactions must be recorded by the dispensing pharmacist.

Registration: Prescribing physicians and dispensing pharmacies must be registered with the DEA, PO Box 28083, Central Station, Washington, DC 20005.

Inventory: Separate records must be kept of purchases and dispensing of controlled substances. An inventory of controlled substances must be made every 2 years.

Prescriptions: Prescriptions for controlled substances must be written in ink and include: Date; name and address of the patient; name, address and DEA number of the physician. Oral prescriptions must be promptly committed to writing. Controlled substance prescriptions may not be dispensed or refilled more than 6 months after the date issued or be refilled more than 5 times. A written prescription signed by the physician is required for schedule II drugs. In case of emergency, oral prescriptions for schedule II substances may be filled; however, the physician must provide a signed prescription within 72 hours. Schedule II prescriptions cannot be refilled. A triplicate order form is necessary for the transfer of controlled substances in schedule II. Forms are available for the individual prescriber at no charge from the DEA.

State Laws: In many cases, state laws are more restrictive than federal laws and therefore impose additional requirements (eg, triplicate prescription forms).

Medical Terminology Glossary

abduction – the act of drawing away from a center.

abstergent – a cleansing application or medicine.

acaricide – an agent lethal to mites.

achlorhydria – the absence of hydrochloric acid from gastric secretions.

acidifier, systemic – a drug used to lower internal body fluid pH in patients with systemic alkalosis.

acidifier, urinary – a drug used to lower the pH of the urine.

acidosis – an accumulation of acid in the body.

acne – an inflammatory disease of the skin accompanied by the eruption of papules or pustules.

active immunity – see Immunity, Active.

acute – a short-term, intense health effect.

acute Hepatitis C – newly acquired symptomatic hepatitis C virus (HCV) infection.

Addison disease – a condition caused by adrenal gland destruction.

adduction – the act of drawing toward a center.

adenitis – a gland or lymph node inflammation.

adjuvant – an agent added to a product formulation that complements or accentuates the active ingredient.

adrenergic – a sympathomimetic drug that activates organs innervated by the sympathetic branch of the autonomic nervous system.

adrenocortical steroid, anti-inflammatory – an adrenal cortex hormone that participates in regulation of organic metabolism and inhibits the inflammatory response to stress; a glucocorticoid.

adrenocortical steroid, salt-regulating – an adrenal cortex hormone that maintains sodium-potassium electrolyte balance by stimulating and regulating sodium retention and potassium excretion by the kidneys.

adrenocorticotropic hormone – an anterior pituitary hormone that stimulates and regulates secretion of the adrenocortical steroids.

adsorbent – an agent that binds chemicals to its surface, thus reducing the bioavailability of toxic substances.

adverse events – undesirable experiences occurring after immunization that may or may not be related to the vaccine.

alkalizer, systemic – a drug that raises internal body fluid pH in patients with systemic acidosis.

allergen – a specific substance that causes an unwanted reaction in the body.

amblyopia – pertaining to a dimness of vision.

amebiasis – an infection with a pathogenic amoeba.

amenorrhea – an abnormal discontinuance of the menses.

amphiarthrosis – a joint in which the surfaces are connected by discs of fibrocartilage.

anabolic – an agent that promotes conversion of a simple substance into more complex compounds; a constructive process for the organism.

analeptic – a potent central nervous system stimulant used to maintain vital functions during severe central nervous system depression.

analgesic – a drug that selectively suppresses pain perception without inducing unconsciousness.

ancyclostomiasis – a disease characterized by the presence of hookworms in the intestine.

androgen – a hormone that stimulates and maintains male secondary sex characteristics.

anemia – a deficiency of red blood cells.

anesthetic, general – a drug that eliminates pain perception by inducing unconsciousness.

anesthetic, local – a drug that eliminates pain perception in a limited area by local action on sensory nerves; a topical anesthetic.

angina pectoris – a sharp chest pain starting in the heart, often spreading down the left arm. A symptom of coronary artery disease.

angiography – visualization of blood vessels upon x-ray following an injection of contrast media.

anhidrotic – a drug that checks perspiration flow from sweat glands; an antidiaphoretic.

anodyne – a drug that acts on the sensory nervous system, either centrally or peripherally, to produce relief from pain.

anorexiant – a drug that reduces appetite.

anorexigenic – an agent that promotes appetite reduction.

antacid – a drug that locally neutralizes excess gastric acid secretions.

antiadrenergic – a drug that prevents response to sympathetic nervous system stimulation and adrenergic drugs; a sympatholytic or sympathoplegic drug.

antiamebic – a drug that kills or inhibits the pathogenic protozoan *Entamoeba histolytica*, the causative agent of amebic dysentery.

antianemic – an agent that treats or prevents anemia.

antiasthmatic – an agent that relieves the symptoms of asthma.

antibacterial – a drug that kills or inhibits pathogenic bacteria, the causative agents of many systemic gastrointestinal and superficial infections.

antibiotic – an agent produced by or derived from living cells of molds, bacteria, or other plants that destroy or inhibit the growth of microbes.

antibody – a protein found in the blood that is produced in response to foreign substances (eg, bacteria or viruses) invading the body. Antibodies protect the body from disease by binding to these organisms and destroying them.

anticholesteremic – a drug that lowers blood cholesterol levels.

anticholinergic – a drug that prevents response to parasympathetic nervous system stimulation and cholinergic drugs; a parasympatholytic or parasympathoplegic drug.

anticoagulant – a drug that inhibits blood clotting.

anticonvulsant – a drug that selectively prevents epileptic seizures.

antidepressant – a psychotherapeutic drug that induces mood elevation, useful in treating depressive neuroses and psychoses.

antidiabetic – a drug used to lower blood sugar or counteract diabetes.

antidote – a drug that prevents or counteracts the effects of poisons or drug overdoses by adsorption in the gastrointestinal tract (general antidotes) or by specific systemic action (specific antidotes).

antieczematic – a topical drug that aids in the control of exudative inflammatory skin lesions.

antiemetic – a drug that prevents or controls vomiting.

antifibrinolytic – a drug that decreases fibrin breakdown.

antifilarial – a drug that kills or inhibits pathogenic filarial worms of the superfamily *Filarioidea*, the causative agents of diseases such as loaiasis.

antiflatulent – an agent that inhibits the excessive formation of gas in the stomach or intestines.

antifungal – a drug that kills or inhibits pathogenic fungi; antimycotic.

antigens – foreign substances (eg, bacteria or viruses) in the body that are capable of causing disease. The presence of antigens in the body triggers an immune response, usually the production of antibodies.

antihelmintic – a drug that kills or expels worm infestations such as pinworms and tapeworms (eg, nematodes, cestodes, trematodes).

antihemophilic – a blood derivative containing the clotting factors absent in the hereditary disease hemophilia.

antihistaminic – a drug that prevents response to histamine, including histamine released by allergic reactions.

antihypercholesterolemic – a drug that lowers blood cholesterol levels, especially elevated levels sometimes associated with cardiovascular disease.

antihypertensive – a drug that lowers blood pressure.

anti-infective, local – a drug that kills a variety of pathogenic microorganisms and is suitable for sterilizing the skin or wounds.

anti-inflammatory – a drug that counteracts or suppresses inflammation.

antileishmanial – a drug that kills or inhibits pathogenic protozoa of the genus *Leishmania*, the causative agents of diseases such as kala azar.

antileprotic – an agent used against leprosy.

antilipemic – an agent that reduces the amount of circulating lipids.

antimalarial – a drug that prevents malaria or inhibits the causative agent (ie, malarial parasites).

antimetabolite – a substance that competes with or replaces a certain metabolite.

antimethemoglobinemic – an agent that reduces the production of methemoglobin.

antimycotic – an agent that inhibits the growth of fungi.

antinauseant – a drug that suppresses nausea.

antineoplastic – a drug that is selectively toxic to rapidly multiplying cells and is useful in destroying malignant tumors.

antioxidant – an agent used to reduce decay or transformation of a material from oxidation.

antiperiodic – a drug that prevents the regular recurrence of a disease or symptom.

antiperistaltic – a drug that inhibits intestinal motility, especially for the treatment of diarrhea.

antipruritic – a drug that prevents or relieves itching.

antipyretic – a drug used to reduce fever; antifebrile; febrifugal.

antirheumatic – a drug that suppresses symptoms of rheumatic disease (eg, reduces the inflammation of rheumatic arthritis).

antirickettsial – a drug that kills or inhibits pathogenic microorganisms of the genus *Rickettsia*, the causative agents of diseases such as typhus (eg, chloramphenicol).

antischistosomal – a drug that kills or inhibits pathogenic flukes of the genus *Schistosoma*, the causative agents of schistosomiasis.

antiseborrheic – a drug that aids in the control of seborrheic dermatitis ("dandruff"); prevents or relieves excessive sebum secretion.

antiseptic – a substance that prevents the growth and development of microorganisms that may lead to infection.

antisialagogue – a drug that diminishes the flow of saliva.

antispasmodic – an agent used to quiet the spasms of voluntary and involuntary muscles; calmative; antihysteric.

antisyphilitic – a remedy used in the treatment of syphilis.

antitoxin – a biological drug containing antibodies against the toxic principles of a pathogenic microorganism, used for passive immunization against the associated disease.

antitrichomonal – a drug that kills or inhibits the pathogenic protozoan *Trichomonas vaginalis*, the causative agent of trichomonal vaginitis.

antitrypanosomal – a drug that kills or inhibits pathogenic protozoa of the genus *Trypanosoma*, the causative agents of diseases such as West African trypanosomiasis.

antitussive – a drug that suppresses coughing; antibechic.

antivenin – a biological drug containing antibodies against the venom of a poisonous animal or insect; an antidote for a venomous bite.

antiviral – literally "against virus;" any medicine capable of destroying or weakening a virus.

anxiety – a feeling of apprehension, uncertainty and fear.

aperient – a mild laxative.

aphasia – the inability to use or understand written and spoken words due to language center injuries in the brain.

aphonia – loss of voice due to disease of the larynx or its innervation.

apnea – the absence of breathing.

areola – a pigmented/depigmented zone surrounding a neoplasm.

arsenical – an agent containing arsenic.

arteriosclerosis – a hardening of the arteries.

arthritis – the inflammation of a joint.

ascariasis – a condition caused by roundworms in the intestine.

ascaricide – an agent that kills roundworms of the genus *Ascaris*.

Aspergillus – a genus of fungi.

astasia – the inability to stand up without help.

asthma – a disease characterized by recurring breathing difficulty due to bronchial muscle constriction.

astringent – an agent that causes tissue contraction, arrests secretion, or controls bleeding.

ataractic – an agent that has a quieting, tranquilizing effect.

ataxia – incoordination, especially of gait.

atheroma – lipid deposits on the inner surface of arteries; a characteristic of atherosclerosis.

atrophy – a wasting away.

avitaminosis – a pathologic state or dysfunction resulting in the body lacking one or more vitamins.

axilla – the armpit.

bacteria – tiny one-celled organisms present throughout the environment that require a microscope to be seen. While not all bacteria are harmful, some cause disease. Examples of bacterial disease include diphtheria, pertussis, tetanus, *Haemophilus influenzae*, and pneumococcus (pneumonia).

bacteriostatic – an agent that inhibits the growth of bacteria.

Basedow disease – a form of hyperthyroidism, also known as Grave disease and Parry disease.

biliary colic – a sharp pain in the upper right side of the abdomen due to a gallstone impaction.

bilirubin – a red bile pigment.

biliuria – the presence of bile in the urine.

blood calcium regulator – a drug that maintains the blood level of ionic calcium, especially by regulating its metabolic disposition elsewhere.

blood volume supporter – an intravenous solution whose solutes are retained in the vascular system to supplement the osmotic activity of plasma proteins.

bradycardia – a slow heart rate.

Bright disease – a disease of the kidneys, including the presence of edema and excessive urine protein formation.

bromidrosis – foul-smelling perspiration.

bronchitis – an inflammation of the bronchi.

bronchodilator – a drug that dilates the bronchus or bronchial tubes (air passages of the lung).

bruit – an abnormal arterial sound audible with a stethoscope.

Buerger disease – a thromboanglitis obliterans inflammation of the walls and surrounding rise of the veins and arteries.

bursitis – an inflammation of the bursa.

callus – a tissue mass that develops at bone fracture sites.

calmative – a sedative.

candidiasis – an infection by the yeastlike genus *Candida*, especially *Candida albicans*.

carbonic anhydrase inhibitor – an enzyme inhibitor, the therapeutic effects of which are diuresis and reduced formation of intraocular fluid.

carcinoma – a malignant growth.

cardiac depressant – a drug that depresses myocardial function so as to suppress rhythmic irregularities characterized by fast heart rate; antiarrhythmic.

cardiac stimulant – a drug that increases the contractile force of the myocardium, especially in weakened conditions such as congestive heart failure; cardiotonic.

cardiopathy – a disease of the heart.

caries – the decay of the teeth.

carminative – an aromatic or pungent drug that mildly irritates the gastrointestinal tract and is useful in the treatment of flatulence and colic. Peppermint Water is a common carminative.

carrier – a person or animal that harbors a specific infectious agent without visible symptoms of the disease. A carrier acts as a potential source of infection.

caruncle – a small, fleshy projection on the skin.

cathartic – an agent having purgative action.

caudal – pertains to the distal end or tail.

caustic – an agent whose effect resembles that of a burn; used to remove abnormal skin growths.

central depressant – a drug that reduces the functional state of the central nervous system and with increasing dosage may induce sedation, hypnosis, and general anesthesia; degree of respiratory suppression is agent dependent.

central stimulant – a drug that increases the functional state of the central nervous system and with increasing dosage may induce restlessness, insomnia, disorientation, and convulsions; degree of respiratory suppression is agent dependent.

cerebrum – the parts of the brain relating to the telecephalon and includes mainly the cerebral cortex and basal ganglia.

cerumen – earwax.

childhood immunizations – a series of immunizations that are given to prevent disease that pose a threat to children. The immunizations in the United States currently include: hepatitis B, diphtheria, tetanus, acellular pertussis, *Haemophilus influenzae* type b, inactivated polio, pneumococcal conjugate, measles, mumps, rubella, varicella, and hepatitis A.

chloasma – a skin discoloration.

cholagogue – a drug that stimulates the emptying of the gallbladder and the flow of bile into the duodenum.

cholecystitis – an inflammation of the gallbladder.

cholecystokinetic – an agent that promotes emptying of the gallbladder.

cholelithiasis – the presence of calculi (stones) in the gallbladder.

choleretic – a drug that increases the production and secretion of bile by the liver.

chorea – a disorder, usually of childhood, characterized by uncontrolled spasmotic muscle movements; sometimes referred to as St. Vitus' dance.

chronic health condition – a health-related state that lasts for a long period of time (eg, multiple sclerosis, asthma).

chronic hepatitis C – liver inflammation in patients with chronic HCV infection; characterized by abnormal levels of liver enzymes.

chymotrypsin – a proteinase in the gastrointestinal tract; its proposed use has been the treatment of edema and inflammation.

cirrhosis – widespread disruption of normal liver structure (scarring of the liver).

claudication – limping.

climacteric – a time period in women just preceding menopause.

clonus – movements noted by rapid muscle contraction then relaxation.

coagulant – an agent that stimulates or accelerates blood clotting.

coccidiostat – a drug used in the treatment of coccidal (protozoal) infections in animals, especially birds; used in veterinary medicine.

colitis – an inflammation of the colon.

colloid – a disperse system of particles larger than those of true solutions but smaller than those of suspensions (1 to 100 millimicrons in size).

collyrium – an eyewash.

colostomy – the surgical formation of a cutaneous opening into the colon.

combination vaccine – two or more vaccines combined and administered at once in order to reduce the number of shots given. For example, the MMR (measles, mumps, rubella) vaccine.

communicable – capable of spreading disease. Also known as infectious.

contagious – capable of being transmitted from one person to another by contact or close proximity.

corticoid – a term applied to hormones of the adrenal cortex or any substance, natural or synthetic, having similar activity.

corticosteroid – a steroid produced by the adrenal cortex.

coryza – acute rhinitis.

counterirritant – an agent (irritant) that causes irritation of the part to which it is applied, and draws blood away from a deep-seated area.

cranial – pertaining to the skull.

crepitation – a crackling sound.

cryptitis – an inflammation of a follicle or glandular tubule, usually in the rectum.

Cryptococcus – a genus of fungi that does not produce spores, but reproduces by budding.

cryptorchidism – the failure of one or both testes to descend.

cutaneous – pertaining to the skin.

cyanosis – a blue or purple skin discoloration due to oxygen deficiency.

cycloplegia – the loss of light accommodation due to loss of control in the eye 's ciliary muscle.

cycloplegic – a drug that paralyzes accommodation of the eye.

cystitis – an inflammation of the bladder.

cystourethography – the examination by x-ray of the bladder and urethra.

cytostasis – a slowing of the movement of blood cells at an inflamed area, sometimes causing capillary blockage.

debridement – the cutting away of dead or excess skin from a wound.

decongestant – a drug that reduces congestion.

decubitus – the patient's position in bed; the act of lying down.

demulcent – an agent generally used internally to sooth and protect mucous membranes.

dermatitis – an inflammation of the skin.

dermatomycosis – a fungal skin infection caused by dermatophytes, yeasts, and other fungi.

detergent – a cleansing or purging agent; an emulsifying agent useful for cleansing wounds and ulcers as well as the skin.

dextrocardia – a condition when the heart is located on the right side of the chest.

diagnostic Aid – a drug used to determine the functional state of a body organ or the presence of a disease.

diaphoretic – a drug used to increase perspiration; hydroticorsudorfice.

diarrhea – an abnormally frequent defecation of semisolid or fluid fecal matter from the bowels.

digestive enzyme – an enzyme used in digestion.

digitalization – the administration of digitalis to obtain a desired tissue level of drug.

diplopia – double vision.
disease – symptomatic sickness, illness, or loss of health.
disinfectant – an agent that destroys pathogenic microorganisms on contact and is suitable for sterilizing inanimate objects.
distal – farthest from a point of reference.
diuretic – a drug that promotes renal excretion of electrolytes and water, thereby increasing urine volume.
dysarthria – a difficulty in speech articulation.
dysmenorrhea – pertaining to painful menstruation.
dysphagia – a difficulty in swallowing.
dyspnea – a difficulty in breathing.
ecbolic – a drug used to stimulate the gravid uterus to the expulsion of the fetus, or to cause uterine contraction; oxytocic.
eclampsia – a toxic disorder occurring late in pregnancy involving hypertension, edema, and renal dysfunction.
ectasia – pertaining to distension or stretching.
ectopic – out of place; not in normal position.
eczema – an inflammatory disease of the skin with infiltrations, watery discharge, scales, and crust.
effervescent – a bubbling; sparkling; giving off gas bubbles.
embolus – a plug (typically a thrombus, bacteria mass, or foreign body) lodged in a vessel; may obstruct circulation.
emetic – a drug that induces vomiting, either locally by gastrointestinal irritation or systemically by stimulation of receptors in the central nervous system.
emollient – a topical drug, especially an oil or fat, used to soften the skin and make it more pliable.
endemic – the continual, low-level presence of disease in a community.
endometrium – the uterine mucous membrane.
enteralgia – an intestinal pain.
enterobiasis – a pinworm infestation.
enuresis – an involuntary urination, as in bedwetting.
epidemic – the occurrence of disease within a specific geographical area or population that is in excess of what is normally expected.
epidemiology – the study of the spread of diseases. Epidemiologists are often sent to investigate outbreaks.
epidermis – the outermost layer of the skin.
episiotomy – a surgical incision of the vulva when deemed necessary during childbirth.
epistaxis – a nosebleed.
erythema – redness.
erythrocyte – a red blood cell.
escharotic – corrosive.
estrogen – a hormone that stimulates and maintains female secondary sex characteristics and functions in the menstrual cycle to promote uterine gland proliferation.

etiology – the cause of a disease.
euphoria – an exaggerated feeling of well-being.
eutonic – a normal muscular tone.
exfoliation – a scaling of the skin.
exophthalmos – a protrusion of the eyeballs.
expectorant – a drug that increases secretion of respiratory tract fluid by lowering its viscosity and promoting its ejection.
extension – the movement of a joint that increases the angle between the bones of the limb at the joint.
exteroceptors – the receptors on the exterior of the body.
fasciculations – the visible twitching movements of muscle bundles.
fibroid – a tumor of fibrous tissue, resembling fibers.
filariasis – the condition of having roundworm parasites reproducing in the body tissues.
fistula – an abnormal opening between one epithelialized surface to another epithelialized body cavity.
flexion – the movement of a joint that decreases the angle between the bones of the limb at the joint.
fulminant – occurring suddenly, with lightning-like rapidity, and with great intensity or severity.
fungistatic – the inhibition of the growth of fungi.
furunculosis – a condition marked by the presence of boils.
gallop rhythm – a heart condition where three separate beats are heard instead of two.
gastralgia – a stomach pain.
gastritis – an inflammation of the stomach lining.
gastrocele – a hernial protrusion of the stomach.
gastrodynia – a pain in the stomach, a stomach ache.
geriatrics – a branch of medicine caring for medical problems of the aged.
germicidal – an agent that kills germs or other pathogenic microorganisms.
gingivitis – an inflammation of the gums.
glaucoma – a disease of the eye evidenced by an increase in intraocular pressure and resulting in hardness of the eye, atrophy of the retina, and eventual blindness.
glossitis – an inflammation of the tongue.
glucocorticoid – a corticoid that increases gluconeogenesis, thereby raising the concentration of liver glycogen and blood sugar.
glycosuria – an abnormal quantity of glucose and carbohydrates in the urine.
gout – a disorder that is characterized by a high uric acid level and sudden onset of recurrent arthritis.
granulation – the formation of small round fleshy granules on a wound as part of the healing process.
Guillain-Barré syndrome – an inflammation of the nerves of unknown cause characterized especially by muscle weakness and paralysis.

hematemesis – the vomiting of blood.

hematinic – an agent that improves blood quality by increasing the hemoglobin concentration and/or the number of red blood cells.

hematopoietic – a drug that stimulates formation of blood cells.

hemiplegia – a condition in which one side of the body is paralyzed.

hemophilia – a sex-linked hereditary blood defect that occurs almost exclusively in males and is characterized by delayed clotting of the blood and consequent difficulty in controlling hemorrhage even after minor injuries.

hemoptysis – the coughing-up of blood.

hemorrhage – an escape of blood through vessel walls; to bleed.

hemostatic – a locally-acting drug that arrests hemorrhage by promoting clot formation or by serving as a mechanical matrix for a clot.

hepatitis – an inflammation of the liver.

hepatitis A – a liver disease caused by the hepatitis A virus (HAV). HAV does not cause a chronic (long-lasting) illness. The virus is transmitted through close intimate contact with an infected person or through ingestion of contaminated food or water.

hepatitis B – a liver disease caused by the hepatitis B virus (HBV). HBV is found in the blood of infected persons and is most commonly transmitted through unprotected sex.

hepatitis B core antibody (anti-HBc) – appears at the onset of symptoms in acute hepatitis B and persists for life. The presence of anti-HBc indicates previous or ongoing infection with HBV.

hepatitis B e antigen (HBeAg) – a secreted product of the nucleocapsid gene of HBV and is found in serum during acute and chronic hepatitis B. Its presence indicated that the virus is replicating and the infected individual is potentially infectious.

hepatitis B immune globulin (HBIG) – a product available for prophylaxis against hepatitis B virus infection. HBIG is prepared from plasma containing high titers of anti-HBs and provides short-term protection (3 to 6 months).

hepatitis B surface antibody (anti-HBs) – the presence of anti-HBs is generally interpreted as indicating recovery and immunity from HBV infection.

hepatitis B surface antigen (HBsAg) – a serologic marker on the surface of HBV. It can be detected in high levels in serum during acute or chronic hepatitis. The body normally produces antibodies to surface antigen as part of the normal immune response to infection.

hepatitis C – a liver disease caused by the hepatitis C virus (HCV), which is found in the blood of persons who have the disease. HCV is spread by contact with the blood of an infected person, most commonly through injection drug use.

hepatitis D – a liver disease caused by hepatitis delta virus (HDV). HDV is a defective virus that needs HBV to exist. HDV is found in the blood of persons infected with the virus and is transmitted in much the same way as HBV is transmitted; however, the case fatality rate with HDV infection is higher than with hepatitis B.

hepatitis E – a disease of the liver caused by the hepatitis E virus (HEV). HEV is transmitted in much the same way as HAV. Hepatitis E, however, does not often originate in the United States. Mortality is high among pregnant women who have hepatitis E.

hepatocellular carcinoma (HCC) – the most common primary malignant liver tumor.

high-risk group – a group in the community with an elevated risk of disease.

histoplasmosis – a lung infection caused by the inhalation of fungus spores, often resulting in pneumonitis.

HIV – human immunodeficiency virus.

Hodgkin disease – a disease marked by chronic lymph node enlargement that may also include spleen and liver enlargement.

hydrocholeresis – the puffing out of a thinner, more watery bile.

hypercholesterolemia – the condition of having an abnormally large amount of cholesterol in the plasma and cells of circulating blood.

hyperemia – an excess of blood in any part of the body.

hyperesthesia – an increase in sensitivity to sensory stimuli.

hyperglycemic – a drug that increases blood glucose levels, especially for the treatment of hypoglycemic states.

hypertension – blood pressure above the normally accepted limits; high blood pressure.

hypertriglyceridemia – an increased level of triglycerides in the blood.

hypnotic – an agent that promotes sleep.

hypodermoclysis – a subcutaneous injection with a solution.

hypoesthesia – a diminished sensation of touch.

hypoglycemic – a drug that lowers blood glucose levels; useful in the control of diabetes mellitus.

hypokalemia – an abnormally small concentration of potassium ions in the blood.

hyposensitize – to reduce the sensitivity to an agent, referring to allergies.

hypotensive – a drug that diminishes tension or pressure to lower blood pressure.

ichthyosis – an inherited skin disease characterized by dryness and scales.

idiopathic – the denoting of a disease of unknown cause.

IDU – injection drug user.

IgM anti-HBc – detected at onset of acute hepatitis B and persists for 3 to 12 months if the disease resolves. In patients who develop chronic hepatitis B, IgM anti-HBc persists at low levels as long as viral replication persists.

ileostomy – the establishment of an opening from the ileum to the outside of the body.

immune globulin (IG) – proteins found in the blood that function as antibodies that fight infection. Previously known as gamma globulin.

immune serum – a biological drug containing antibodies for a pathogenic microorganism, useful for passive immunization against the associated disease.

immune system – the complex system in the body responsible for fighting disease. Its primary function is to identify foreign substances in the body (bacteria, viruses, fungi, or parasites) and develop a defense against them. This defense is known as the immune response. It involves production of protein molecules called antibodies to eliminate foreign organisms that invade the body.

Immunity – protection against a disease. There are two types of immunity, passive and active. Immunity is indicated by the presence of antibodies in the blood and can usually be determined with a laboratory test. See Immunity, Active and Passive.

immunity, active – resistance developed in response to an antigen (infecting agent or vaccine) and usually characterized by the presence of antibody produced by the host.

immunity, passive – immunity conferred by an antibody produced in another host. This type of immunity can be acquired naturally by an infant from its mother or artificially by administration of an antibody-containing preparation (antiserum or immune globulin).

immunization – the process by which a person or animal becomes protected against a disease.

immunizing agent, active – an antigenic preparation (toxoid or vaccine) used to induce formation of specific antibodies against a pathogenic microorganism that provides delayed but permanent protection against the associated disease.

immunizing agent, passive – a biological preparation (antitoxin, antivenin, or immune serum) containing specific antibodies against a pathogenic microorganism that provides immediate but temporary protection against the associated disease.

immunoprophylaxis – preventing the spread of disease by providing physiological immunity.

immunosuppression – when the immune system is unable to protect the body from disease. This condition can be caused by disease (like AIDS) or by certain drugs (like those used in chemotherapy). Individuals whose immune systems are compromised should not receive live, attenuated vaccines.

impetigo – a contagious inflammatory skin infection with isolated pustules, most commonly occurring on the face of young children.

incidence – the number of new disease cases reported in a population over a certain period of time.

incubation period – the time from contact with infectious agents (bacteria or viruses) to onset of disease.

infection – an invasion of an organism by a pathogen such as bacteria or viruses. Some infections lead to disease.

infectious – capable of spreading disease. Also known as communicable.

infectious agents – organisms capable of spreading disease (eg, bacteria or viruses).

insulin – a hormone that promotes use of glucose, protein synthesis, and the formation and storage of neutral lipids; used in the treatment of diabetes mellitus.

inversion – a turning inward.

irrigating solution – a solution for washing wounds or various body cavities.

jaundice – a yellowing of the skin, whites of the eyes, tissues, and certain body fluids, which can result from certain liver diseases, including hepatitis C, or from excessive breakdown of red blood cells due to internal hemorrhage or various other conditions.

keratitis – an inflammation of the cornea.

keratolytic – a topical drug that softens the superficial keratin-containing layer of the skin to promote exfoliation.

lacrimal – pertaining to tears.

laxative – a gentle purgative medicine; mild cathartic.

leishmaniasis – infections transmitted by sand flies.

leukocyte – a white blood cell.

leukocytopenia – a decrease in the number of white blood cells.

leukocytosis – an increased white blood cell count.

leukoderma – an absence of pigment from the skin.

libido – sexual desire.

lipoma – a benign fatty tumor.

lipotropic – a drug, especially one supplementing a dietary factor, that prevents the abnormal accumulation of fat in the liver.

lochia – a vaginal discharge of mucus, blood, and tissue after childbirth.

lues – a plague; specifically syphilis.

macrocyte – a large red blood cell.

malaise – a general feeling of illness.

mastitis – an inflammation of the breast.

melasma – a darkening of the skin.

melena – black feces or black vomit from altered blood in the higher GI tract.

meninges – the membranes covering the brain and spinal cord.

metastasis – the shifting of a disease or its symptoms from one part of the body to another.

microbes – tiny organisms (including viruses and bacteria) that can only be seen with a microscope.

miotics – agents that constrict the pupil of the eye; a myotic.

moniliasis – an infection with any of the species of monilia types of fungi (*Candida*).

morbidity – any departure, subjective or objective, from a state of physiological or psychological well-being.

mortality – the number of deaths in a given time or place.

mucolytic – an agent that can destroy or dissolve mucous membrane secretions.

myalgia – a pain in the muscles.

myasthenia gravis – a chronic progressive muscular weakness caused by myoneural conduction, usually spreading from the face and throat.

myelocyte – an immature white blood cell in the bone marrow.

myelogenous – originating in bone marrow.

myoclonus – involuntary, sudden, rapid, unpredictable jerks.

mydriatic – a drug that dilates the pupil of the eye, usually by anticholinergic or adrenergic mechanisms.

myoneural – pertaining to muscle and nerve.

myopia – nearsightedness.

narcotic – a drug with effects similar to opium and derivatives that produces analgesic effects and has the potential for dependence and tolerance.

neonatal – pertaining to the first four weeks of life.

neoplasm – an abnormal tissue that grows more rapidly than normal and shows a lack of structural organization.

nephritis – an inflammation of the kidney.

nephrosclerosis – a hardening of the kidney tissue.

neuralgia – a pain extending along the course of one or more nerves.

neurasthenia – a condition accompanying or following depression that is characterized by vague fatigue.

neuroglia – the supporting elements of the nervous system.

neuroleptic – a psychotropic drug used to treat psychosis.

neurosis – a psychological or behavioral disorder characterized by anxiety.

NIH – National Institutes of Health.

nocturia – urination at night.

normocytic – erythrocytes that are normal in size, shape, and color.

nosocomial – referring to an infection acquired by a patient while in a hospital.

nuchal – the back of the neck.

nystagmus – a rhythmic oscillation of the eyes.

oleaginous – oily or greasy.

omphalitis – an inflammation of the navel and surrounding area.

onychomycosis – a fungal infection of the nails.

ophthalmic – pertaining to the eye.

oral – pertaining to the mouth.

organism – any living thing. Organisms include humans, animals, plants, bacteria, protozoa, and fungi.

orthopnea – a discomfort in breathing when lying flat.

ossification – a formation of, or conversion to, bone.

osteomyelitis – an inflammation of the marrow of the bone.

osteoporosis – a reduction in bone quantity; skeletal atrophy.

otalgia – pain in the ear; earache.

otitis – inflammation of the ear.

otomycosis – an ear infection caused by fungus.

otorrhea – a discharge from the ear.

outbreak – sudden appearance of a disease in a specific geographic area (eg, neighborhood or community) or population (eg, adolescents).

oxytocic – a drug that selectively stimulates uterine motility and is useful in obstetrics, especially in the control of postpartum hemorrhage.

Paget disease – a skeletal disease in which bone resorption and formation are increased leading to thickening and softening of bones; a disease characterized by lesions around the nipple and areola found in elderly women.

pallor – paleness.

palpitations – an awareness of one's heart action.

pandemic – an epidemic occuring over a very large area.

parasites – any organism that lives in or on another organism without benefiting the host organism; commonly refers to pathogens, most commonly in reference to protozoans and helminths.

parasympatholytic – See Anticholinergic.

parasympathomimetic – See Cholinergic.

parenteral – pertaining to the administration of a drug by means other than through the intestinal tract; subcutaneous, intramuscular, or intravenous drug administration.

parkinsonism – a group of neurological disorders caused by dopamine deficiency marked by hypokinesia, tremor, and muscular rigidity.

paroxysm – a sharp spasm or convulsion.

passive immunity – see Immunity, Passive.

pathogenic – causing an abnormality or disease.

pathogens – bacteria, viruses, parasites, or fungi that can cause disease.

pediatrics – a branch of medicine caring for the medical problems of children from birth through adolescence.

pediculicide – an agent used to kill lice.

pediculosis – an infestation with lice.

pellagra – characterized by GI disturbances, mental disorders, skin redness, and scaling due to niacin deficiency.

pernicious – particularly dangerous or harmful.

phlebitis – an inflammation of a vein.

pleurisy – an inflammation of the membrane surrounding the lungs and the thoracic cavity.

pneumonia – an infection of the lungs.

poikilocytosis – a condition in which pointed or irregularly shaped red blood cells are found in the blood.

polydipsia – excessive thirst.

posology – the science of dosage.

posterior pituitary hormone(s) – a hormone with oxytocic, vasoconstrictor, antidiuretic, and intestinal stimulant properties.

post-exposure prophylaxis (PEP) – prevention or treatment of disease after a possible exposure.

prevalance – the number of disease cases (new and existing) within a population at a given time.

progestin – a hormone that functions in the menstrual cycle and during pregnancy to promote uterine gland secretion and to reduce uterine motility.

pronation – the body's position when lying face downward; rotation of the forearm so the palm on the hand faces backward when the arm is in anatomical position.

prophylactic – a remedy that tends to prevent disease.

protectant – a topical drug that remains on the skin and serves as a physical, protective barrier to the environment.

proteolytic enzyme – an enzyme used to liquify fibrinous or purulent exudates.

psoriasis – an inflammatory skin disease accompanied by itching.

psychotherapy – therapy utilizing communication and interventions with the patient instead of chemical or physical treatments.

ptosis – a drooping or sagging of a muscle or organ, such as the eyelid.

pulmonary – pertaining to the lungs.

purulent – containing or forming pus.

pyelitis – a local inflammation of renal and pelvic cells due to bacterial infection.

pylorospasm – a spasmodic muscle contraction of the pyloric portion of the stomach.

pyoderma – any fever-producing skin infection.

quarantine – to isolate an individual who has or is suspected of having a disease, in order to prevent spreading the disease to others; alternatively, to isolate a person who does not have a disease during a disease outbreak, in order to prevent that person from catching the disease (this is called reverse isolation). Quarantine can be voluntary or ordered by public health officials in times of emergency.

radiopaque medium – a diagnostic drug, opaque to x-rays, whose retention in a body organ or cavity makes x-ray visualization possible.

Raynaud phenomenon – spasms of the digital arteries with blanching and numbness precipitated by cold temperature.

reflex stimulant – a mild irritant suitable for application to the nasopharynx to induce reflex respiratory stimulation.

rheumatoid – resembling rheumatoid arthritis.

rhinitis – an inflammation of the mucous membrane of the nose.

risk – the likelihood that an individual will experience a certain event.

rubefacient – a topical drug that induces mild skin irritation with erythema, sometimes used to relieve the discomfort of deep-seated inflammation.

rubeola/measles – not to be confused with rubella.

saprophytic – receiving nourishment from dead material.

sarcoma – a malignant tumor derived from connective tissue.

scabicide – an insecticide suitable for the erradication of itch mite infestations in humans (scabies).

schistosomacide – an agent that destroys schistosomes; destructive to the trematodic parasites or flukes.

schistosomiasis – an infection with *Schistosoma haematobium*.

scintillation – a visual sensation manifested by an emission of sparks.

sclerosing agent – an irritant suitable for injection into varicose veins to induce their fibrosis and obliteration.

scotomata – an area of varying size and shape within the visual field in which vision is absent or depressed.

seborrhea – a condition arising from an excess secretion of sebum.

sebum – the fatty secretions of sebaceous glands.

sedative – a drug that calms nervous excitement.

seroconversion – development of antibodies in the blood of an individual who previously did not have detectable antibodies.

serology – measurement of antibodies, and other immunological properties, in the blood serum.

side effect – undesirable reaction resulting from immunization or other medication, treatment, etc.

sinusitis – an inflammation of a sinus membrane lining.

skeletal muscle relaxant – a drug that inhibits contraction of voluntary muscles, usually by interfering with their innervation.

smooth muscle relaxant – a drug that inhibits contraction of involuntary (eg, visceral) muscles, usually by action upon their contractile elements.

sociopath – a person designated to have an antisocial personality disorder.

spasmolytic – an agent that relieves spasms and involuntary contractions of a muscle; antispasmodic.

sputum – expectorated mucus.

STD – sexually transmitted disease.

stenosis – the narrowing of the lumen of a blood vessel.

stomachic – a drug that is used to stimulate the appetite and gastric secretion.

stomatitis – an inflammation of the mucous membranes of the mouth.

subcutaneous – underneath the skin.

sudorific – causing perspiration.

superacidity – excessive acidity.

supination – the body 's position when lying face upwards; rotation of the forearm so the palm on the hand faces forward when the arm is in anatomical position.

suppressant – a drug useful in the control, rather than the cure, of a disease; an agent that stops secretion, excretion, or normal discharge.

surfactant – a surface active agent that decreases the surface tension between two miscible liquids; used to prepare emulsions, act as a cleansing agent, etc.

susceptible – unprotected against a certain disease.

synarthrosis (fibrous joint) – a joint in which the bony elements are united by continuous fibrous tissue.

syncope – fainting; loss of consciousness.

synovia – a clear fluid that lubricates the joints; joint oil.

systole – the ventricular contraction phase of a heartbeat.

tachycardia – a rapid contraction rate of the heart.

taeniacide – an agent used to kill tapeworms.

taeniafuge – an agent used to expel tapeworms.

therapeutic – a treatment of disease.

thoracic – pertaining to the chest.

thyroid hormone – a drug containing one or more of the iodinated amino acids that stimulate and regulate the metabolic rate and functional state of body tissues.

thyroid inhibitor – a drug that reduces excessive thyroid hormone production, usually by blocking hormone synthesis.

tics – a repetitive twitching of muscles, often in the face and upper trunk.

tinea – a fungal infection of the skin, hair, or nails.

tonic – continuous muscular contraction.

tonometry – the measurement of tension in some part of the body.

topical – the local external application of a drug to a particular place.

toxoid – a modified toxin, less toxic than the original form, used to induce active immunity to bacterial pathogens.

tranquilizer – a psychotherapeutic drug that promotes tranquility without significant sedation, useful in treating certain neuroses and psychoses.

tremors – involuntary rhythmic tremulous movements.

trichomoniasis – an infection with parasitic flagellate protozoa of the genus *Trichomonas*.

trypanosomiasis – any disease caused by *Trypanosomatidae*.

uricosuric – a drug that promotes renal uric acid excretion; used to treat gout.

urolithiasis – a condition marked by the formation of stones in the urinary tract.

urticaria – a rash or hives.

vaccination – injection of a killed or weakened infectious organism in order to prevent the disease.

vaccine – the preparation of live attenuated or dead pathogenic microorganisms, used to induce active immunity.

vaccine schedule – a chart or plan of vaccinations that are recommended for specific ages and/or circumstances.

vasoconstrictor – an agent used to narrow blood vessels; to constrict blood vessels and reduce tissue congestion in the nose.

vasodilator – a drug that relaxes vascular smooth muscles, especially for the purpose of improving peripheral or coronary blood flow.

vasopressor – an adrenergic drug used systemically to constrict blood vessels and raise blood pressure.

verruca – a wart.

vertigo – dizziness.

vesicant – an agent that, when applied to the skin, causes blistering and the formation of vesicles; an epispastic.

virus – a tiny organism that multiplies within cells and causes disease such as chickenpox, measles, mumps, rubella, pertussis, and hepatitis. Viruses are not affected by antibiotics, the drugs used to kill bacteria.

visceral – pertaining to the internal organs.

vitamin – an organic chemical essential in small amounts for normal body metabolism, used therapeutically to supplement the naturally occurring counterpart in foods.

WHO – World Health Organization.

Oral Dosage Forms That Should Not
Be Crushed or Chewed

The purpose of this feature is to alert health care professionals about medications that should not be crushed or chewed because of their special pharmaceutical formulations or characteristics. Oral dosage forms that are sustained release (slow release) comprise the vast majority of this designation. Crushing or chewing such products may substantially alter their intended pharmacokinetics. Additional reasons for not chewing or crushing drugs include poor taste, irritant properties, or carcinogenic potential. Alternative liquid forms of these products are listed if available. Refer to the end of the table for a complete explanation of references.

It is important to understand that the inability to crush or chew drugs with slow-release properties does not always mean the dosage form cannot be divided or halved. Some newer slow-release dosage forms (eg, *Toprol XL*) are commercially available as scored tablets. This reference addresses those drugs that cannot be crushed or chewed.

Anyone who visits any acute- or long-term care facility can observe personnel meticulously grinding tablets or the contents of capsules in a mortar and pestle. Their rationale is well intentioned: they have an order to administer medication to a patient with an nasogastric tube or who cannot swallow solids and have to incorporate the drug into a liquid vehicle. However, they do so at the risk of changing the pharmacokinetics of the solid dosage formulation. Examples of special formulations include sublingual or buccal, enteric-coated, and extended-release tablets or capsules. Products containing extended-release dosage forms frequently have an abbreviation affixed to their brand name that serves as a clue that crushing may affect the formulation (Table 1). In addition, some medications are inherently corrosive to the oral mucosa and/or upper gastrointestinal tract, remarkably bitter to the taste, or capable of staining the oral mucosa and teeth.

Finally, several medications are potentially carcinogenic and require limited handling by medical personnel. Crushing or breaking of products that have carcinogenic/teratogenic potential (ie, antineoplastics) may not alter the dosage form or delivery mechanisms but may cause aerosolization of particles, exposing health care workers who handle these products. The reader is encouraged to review the American Society of Health-System Pharmacists' (previously the American Society of Hospital Pharmacists) bulletin on handling cytotoxic and hazardous drugs.

A more detailed description of the dosage forms mentioned above has been published in previous versions of this article and is summarized in Table 2.

Alternatives to Crushing

For patients who cannot swallow whole tablets or capsules, the most logical approach is to use liquid suspension forms of the same medication. Table 3 identifies examples of medications that have a liquid form commercially available. In some cases, there must be a dosage adjustment when the liquid is substituted. This is especially true if the tablet or capsule is an extended-release medication. If a liquid or suspension is not commercially available, the pharmacist should be consulted to determine if a liquid formulation could be extemporaneously prepared.

Occasionally, it is possible to substitute the injectable form of the medication by placing the appropriate amount of injection in some suitable fluid, such as juice. This should be done, however, only after consultation with a pharmacist to ensure that there are no problems regarding compatibility, stability, or changes in absorption of the drug. Another alternative is to use a chemically different but clinically similar medication that is available in a liquid form. Some medications that cannot be crushed may be admin-

istered in other ways, such as administering the contents of a capsule in soft food. This
type of information is provided in Table 3 and indexed in the footnote.

Updates to List

Inherent with a listing of this type is the difficulty in keeping such lists current. The author en-
courages manufacturers, pharmacist, nurses, and other health professionals to notify
us of any changes or updates.

References

1. American Society of Hospital Pharmacists. ASHP technical assistance bulletin on handling cytotoxic and hazardous drugs. *Am J Hosp Pharm.* 1990;47:1033-1049.
2. Mitchell JF. Oral dosage forms that should not be crushed: 2000 update. *Hosp Pharm.*
2000;35:553-567.

Table 1: Common Abbreviations for Extended-Release Products

CD	controlled dose
CR	controlled release
CRT	controlled release tablet
LA	long acting
SA	sustained action
SR	sustained release
TR	time release
TD	time delay
XL	extended release
XR	extended release

Table 2: Summary of Drug Formulations that Preclude Crushing

Type	Reason(s) for the formulation
Enteric coated	Designed to pass through the stomach intact with drug being released in the intestines to:
	(1) prevent destruction of drug by stomach acids
	(2) prevent stomach irritation
	(3) delay onset of action
Extended release	Designed to release drug over an extended period of time. Such products include:
	(1) multiple-layered tablets releasing drug as each layer is dissolved
	(2) mixed release pellets that dissolve at different time intervals
	(3) special matrixes that are themselves inert, but slowly release drug from the matrix
Sublingual	Designed to dissolve quickly in oral fluids for rapid absorption by the abundant blood supply of the mouth.
Miscellaneous	Drugs that:
	(1) produce oral mucosa irritation
	(2) are extremely bitter
	(3) contain dyes or inherently could stain teeth and mucosal tissue
	(4) drugs that, if handled without adequate protec-tion, are potentially carcinogenic

Table 3: Medications that Should Not Be Crushed or Chewed

Drug Product	Dosage Form	Reason/Comments
Aciphex	Tablet	Slow release
Accuhist	Tablet	Slow release[6]
Accutane	Capsule	Mucous membrane irritant
Adalat CC	Tablet	Slow release
Aggrenox	Capsule	Slow release Note: Capsule may be opened. Contents include an aspirin tablet that may be chewed and dipyridamole pellets that may be sprinkled.
Adderall XR	Capsule	Slow release[2]
Advicor	Tablet	Slow release
AeroHist Plus	Tablet	Slow release[6]
Afeditab CR	Tablet	Slow release
Alavert Allergy Sinus 12 Hour	Tablet	Slow release
Allegra D	Tablet	Slow release
Altocor	Tablet	Slow release
Arthritis Bayer Time Release	Capsule	Slow release
Arthrotec	Tablet	Enteric coated
ASA Enseals	Tablet	Enteric coated
Asacol	Tablet	Slow release
Ascriptin A/D	Tablet	Enteric coated
Ascriptin Extra Strength	Tablet	Enteric coated
Augmentin XR	Tablet	Slow release[1,6]
Avinza	Capsule	Slow release[2] (not pudding)
Avodart	Capsule	Teratogenic potential[7]
Azulfidine EN-tabs	Tablet	Enteric coated
Bayer Enteric-Coated	Caplet	Enteric coated
Bayer Low Adult 81 mg	Tablet	Enteric coated
Bayer Regular Strength 325 mg	Caplet	Enteric coated
Bellahist-D LA	Tablet	Slow release
Biaxin-XL	Tablet	Slow release
Biltricide	Tablet	Taste[6]
Biohist LA	Tablet	Slow release[6]
Bisacodyl	Tablet	Enteric coated[5]
Bontril-SR	Capsule	Slow release
Bromafed PD	Capsule	Slow release
Bromafed SR	Capsule	Slow release
Budeprion SR	Tablet	Slow release
Calan SR	Tablet	Slow release[6]
Carbatrol	Capsule	Slow release[2]
Cardene SR	Capsule	Slow release
Cardizem	Tablet	Slow release
Cardizem CD	Capsule	Slow release[2]
Cardizem LA	Tablet	Slow release
Cardizem SR	Capsule	Slow release[2]
Carter's Little Pills	Tablet	Enteric coated
Cartia XT	Capsule	Slow release
Ceclor CD	Tablet	Slow release

Drug Product	Dosage Form	Reason/Comments
Ceftin	Tablet	Taste[1] Note: Use suspension for children
CellCept	Capsule, Tablet	Teratogenic potential[7]
Charcoal Plus	Tablet	Enteric coated
Chloral Hydrate	Capsule	Note: Product is in liquid form within a special capsule[1]
Chlor-Trimeton 12-Hour	Tablet	Slow release[1]
Cipro	Tablet	Taste[4]
Cipro XR	Tablet	Slow release
Claritin-D 12 Hour	Tablet	Slow release
Claritin-D 24 Hour	Tablet	Slow release
Colace	Capsule	Taste[4]
Colestid	Tablet	Slow release
Comhist LA	Capsule	Slow release[2]
Compazine Spansule	Capsule	Slow release[1]
Concerta	Tablet	Slow release
Commit	Lozenge	Note: Integrity compromised by chewing or crushing
Contac 12-Hour	Capsule	Slow release[1,2]
Cotazym-S	Capsule	Enteric coated[2]
Covera-HS	Tablet	Slow release
Creon 5, 10, 20	Capsule	Enteric coated[2]
Crixivan	Capsule	Taste Note: Capsule may be opened and mixed with fruit puree (eg, banana).
Cytovene	Capsule	Skin irritant
Cytoxan	Tablet	Note: Drug may be crushed, but manufacturer recommends injection
Dallergy	Capsule	Slow release
Dallergy-JR	Capsule	Slow release
Deconamine SR	Capsule	Slow release[1]
Defen-LA	Tablet	Slow release[6]
Depakene	Capsule	Slow release, mucous membrane irritant[1]
Depakote	Capsule	Enteric coated
Depakote ER	Tablet	Slow release
Desoxyn	Tablet	Slow release
Desyrel	Tablet	Taste[4]
Detrol LA	Capsule	Slow release
Dexedrine Spansule	Capsule	Slow release
Diamox Sequels	Capsule	Slow release
Dilacor XR	Capsule	Slow release
Dilatrate-SR	Capsule	Slow release
Diltia XT	Capsule	Slow release
Ditropan XL	Tablet	Slow release
Dolobid	Tablet	Irritant
Donnatal Extentab	Tablet	Slow release[1]
Drisdol	Capsule	Liquid filled[8]
DriHist SR	Tablet	Slow release[6]

Drug Product	Dosage Form	Reason/Comments
Drixoral	Tablet	Slow release[1]
Drixoral Plus	Tablet	Slow release
Drixoral Sinus	Tablet	Slow release
Dulcolax	Tablet	Enteric coated[5]
Dulcolax	Capsule	Liquid filled
DuraHist	Tablet	Slow release[6]
Duratuss G, GP	Tablet	Slow release[6]
Dynabac	Tablet	Enteric coated
DynaCirc CR	Tablet	Slow release
Easprin	Tablet	Enteric coated
EC-Naprosyn	Tablet	Enteric coated
Ecotrin Adult Low Strength	Tablet	Enteric coated
Ecotrin Maximum Strength	Tablet	Enteric coated
Ecotrin Regular Strength	Tablet	Enteric coated
E.E.S. 400	Tablet	Enteric coated[1]
Effexor XR	Capsule	Slow release
Efidac/24	Tablet	Slow release
Efidac/24 Pseudoephedrine	Tablet	Slow release
E-Mycin	Tablet	Enteric coated
Entex LA	Tablet	Slow release[1]
Entex PSE	Tablet	Slow release
Entocort EC	Capsule	Enteric coated[2]
Ergomar	Tablet	Sublingual form[9]
Eryc	Capsule	Enteric coated[2]
Ery-Tab	Tablet	Enteric coated
Erythrocrin Stearate	Tablet	Enteric coated
Erythromycin Base	Tablet	Enteric coated
Eskalith CR	Tablet	Slow release
Evista	Tablet	Taste; teratogenic potential[7]
Extendryl JR	Capsule	Slow release
Extendryl SRC	Capsule	Slow release[1]
Feldene	Capsule	Mucous membrane irritant
Feosol	Tablet	Enteric coated[1]
Feratab	Tablet	Enteric coated[1]
Fergon	Capsule	Slow release[2]
Fero-Grad 500 mg	Tablet	Slow release
Ferro-Sequels	Tablet	Slow release
Flagyl ER	Tablet	Slow release
Flomax	Capsule	Slow release
Fosamax	Tablet	Mucous membrane irritant
Fumatinic	Capsule	Slow release
Geocillin	Tablet	Taste
GFN/PSE/DM	Tablet	Slow release
Gleevec	Tablet	Taste[6] Note: May be dissolved in mineral oil or apple juice.
Glucophage XR	Tablet	Slow release
Glucotrol XL	Tablet	Slow release

Drug Product	Dosage Form	Reason/Comments
Gris-PEG	Tablet	Note: Crushing may result in precipitation as larger particles
Guiafed	Capsule	Slow release
Guiafed-PD	Capsule	Slow release
Guaifenex DM	Tablet	Slow release[6]
Guaifenex LA	Tablet	Slow release[6]
Guaifenex PSE	Tablet	Slow release[6]
Guaifenex-Rx DM	Tablet	Slow release
Guaimax-D	Tablet	Slow release
Hista-Vent DA	Tablet	Slow release[6]
Humibid DM	Tablet	Slow release
Humibid LA	Tablet	Slow release
Iberet Filmtab	Tablet	Slow release[1]
Iberet 500	Tablet	Slow release[1]
Iberet-Folic	Tablet	Slow release
ICaps Time Release	Tablet	Slow release
Imdur	Tablet	Slow release[6]
Inderal LA	Capsule	Slow release
Inderide LA	Capsule	Slow release
Indocin SR	Capsule	Slow release[1,2]
Innopran XL	Capsule	Slow release
Ionamin	Capsule	Slow release
Isoptin SR	Tablet	Slow release
Isordil Sublingual	Tablet	Sublingual form[9]
Isosorbide Dinitrate Sublingual	Tablet	Sublingual form[9]
Isosorbide SR	Tablet	Slow release
K + 8	Tablet	Slow release[1]
K + 10	Tablet	Slow release[1]
Kadian	Capsule	Slow release[2]
Kaon Cl	Tablet	Slow release[1]
K-Dur	Tablet	Slow release
Klor-Con	Tablet	Slow release[1]
Klor-Con M	Tablet	Slow release[1]
Klotrix	Tablet	Slow release[1]
K-Lyte	Tablet	Effervescent tablet[3]
K-Lyte CL	Tablet	Effervescent tablet[3]
K-Lyte DS	Tablet	Effervescent tablet[3]
K-Tab	Tablet	Slow release[1]
Lescol XL	Tablet	Slow release
Levbid	Tablet	Slow release[6]
Levsinex Timecaps	Capsule	Slow release
Lexxel	Tablet	Slow release
Lipram 4500	Capsule	Enteric coated[2]
Lipram CR, PN, UL	Capsule	Enteric coated[2]
Lipram (all)	Capsule	Slow release[2]
Liquibid-D 1200	Tablet	Slow release[6]
Liquibid-PD	Tablet	Slow release[6]
Lithobid	Tablet	Slow release

Drug Product	Dosage Form	Reason/Comments
Lodine XL	Tablet	Slow release
Lodrane LD	Capsule	Slow release[2]
Mag-Tab SR	Tablet	Slow release
Maxifed	Tablet	Slow release
Maxifed DM	Tablet	Slow release
Maxifed G	Tablet	Slow release
Medent-DM	Tablet	Slow release
Medent LD	Tablet	Slow release
Mestinon Timespan	Tablet	Slow release[1]
Metadate CD	Capsule	Slow release[2]
Metadate ER	Tablet	Slow release
Methylin ER	Tablet	Slow release
Micro K	Capsule	Slow release[1,2]
Motrin	Tablet	Taste[4]
MS Contin	Tablet	Slow release[1]
Mucinex	Tablet	Slow release
Muco-Fen-DM	Tablet	Slow release[6]
Myfortic	Tablet	Slow release
Naprelan	Tablet	Slow release
Nasatab LA	Tablet	Slow release[6]
Nexium	Capsule	Slow release[2]
Niaspan	Tablet	Slow release
Nicotinic Acid	Capsule, Tablet	Slow release
Nifediac CC	Tablet	Slow release
Nitrostat	Tablet	Sublingual form[9]
Norflex	Tablet	Slow release
Norpace CR	Capsule	Slow release form within a special capsule
Ondrox	Tablet	Slow release
Optilets 500	Tablet	Enteric coated
Optilets-M 500	Tablet	Enteric coated
Oramorph SR	Tablet	Slow release[1]
Oruvail	Capsule	Slow release
OxyContin	Tablet	Slow release
Palgic-D Extended Release	Tablet	Slow release[6]
Pancrease	Capsule	Enteric coated[2]
Pancrease MT	Capsule	Enteric coated[2]
Pancrecarb MS	Capsule	Enteric coated[2]
PanMist Jr, LA	Tablet	Slow release[6]
PanMist DM	Tablet	Slow release[6]
Pannaz	Tablet	Slow release[6]
Papaverine Sustained Action	Capsule	Slow release
Paxil CR	Tablet	Slow release
Pentasa	Tablet	Slow release
Perdiem	Granules	Wax coated
Phena Vent D	Tablet	Slow release
Pre-Hist-D	Tablet	Slow release[6]
Plendil	Tablet	Slow release

Drug Product	Dosage Form	Reason/Comments
Prelu-2	Capsule	Slow release
Prevacid	Capsule	Slow release
Prevacid Suspension	Suspension	Slow release Note: Contains enteric coated granules.
Prilosec	Capsule	Slow release
Procainamide HCl SR	Tablet	Slow release
Procanbid	Tablet	Slow release
Procardia	Capsule	Delays absorption[1,4]
Procardia XL	Tablet	Slow release Note: AUC is unaffected
Profen II	Tablet	Slow release[6]
Profen II DM	Tablet	Slow release[6]
Profen Forte DM	Tablet	Slow release
Pronestyl SR	Tablet	Slow release
Propecia	Tablet	Note: Women who are or may become pregnant should not handle crushed or broken tablets
Proscar	Tablet	Note: Women who are or may become pregnant should not handle crushed or broken tablets
Protonix	Tablet	Slow release
Protuss DM	Tablet	Slow release
Pytest	Capsule	Note: Radiopharmaceutical
QDALL	Capsule	Slow release
Quibron-T SR	Tablet	Slow release[1]
Quinidex Extentabs	Tablet	Slow release
Rescon JR	Tablet	Slow release
Rescon MX	Tablet	Slow release
Respa-1st	Tablet	Slow release[6]
Respa-DM	Tablet	Slow release[6]
Respahist	Capsule	Slow release[2]
Respaire 120 SR	Capsule	Slow release
Ritalin SR	Tablet	Slow release
Rondec TR	Tablet	Slow release[1]
R-Tanna	Tablet	Slow release
Rythmol SR	Capsule	Slow release
Sinemet CR	Tablet	Slow release
Singlet for Adults	Tablet	Slow release
SINUtuss DM CR	Tablet	Slow release[6]
SINUvent PE	Tablet	Slow release[6]
Slo-Niacin	Tablet	Slow release[6]
Slow-K	Tablet	Slow release[1]
Slow-Mag	Tablet	Slow release
Somnote	Capsule	Liquid filled
Sudafed 12 hour	Capsule	Slow release[1]
Sudal 60/500	Tablet	Slow release
Sular	Tablet	Slow release
Symax SR	Tablet	Slow release
Taztia XT	Capsule	Slow release
Tegretol-XR	Tablet	Slow release

Drug Product	Dosage Form	Reason/Comments
Temodar	Capsule	Note: If capsules are accidentally opened or damaged, rigorous precautions should be taken to avoid inhalation or contact of contents with the skin or mucous membranes.[7]
Tessalon Perles	Capsule	Slow release
Theo-24	Tablet	Slow release[1]
Theochron	Tablet	Slow release
Theo-Time SR	Tablet	Slow release
Tiazac	Capsule	Slow release
Topamax	Tablet	Taste
Topamax	Capsule	Taste[2]
Touro CC	Tablet	Slow release
Touro EX	Tablet	Slow release
Touro LA	Tablet	Slow release
Trental	Tablet	Slow release
Triptone	Tablet	Slow release
Tussafed LA	Tablet	Slow release
Tylenol Arthritis	Tablet	Slow release
Tylenol 8 Hour	Tablet	Slow release
Ultrace	Capsule	Enteric coated[2]
Ultrace MT	Capsule	Enteric coated[2]
Uniphyl	Tablet	Slow release
Urocit-K	Tablet	Wax coated
Verelan	Capsule	Slow release[2]
Videx EC	Capsule	Slow release
Voltaren XR	Tablet	Slow release
Vospire ER	Tablet	Slow release
Wellbutrin SR, XL	Tablet	Slow release
Xanax XR	Tablet	Slow release
Z-Cof LA	Tablet	Slow release[6]
Zephrex LA	Tablet	Slow release
ZORprin	Tablet	Slow release
Zyban	Tablet	Slow release

1 Liquid dosage forms of the product are available; however, dose, frequency of administration, and manufacturers may differ from that of the solid dosage form.

2 Capsule may be opened and the contents taken without crushing or chewing; soft food such as applesauce or pudding may facilitate administration; contents may generally be administered via nasogastric tube using an appropriate fluid, provided entire contents are washed down the tube.

3 Effervescent tablets must be dissolved in the amount of diluent recommended by the manufacturer.

4 The taste of this product in a liquid form would likely be unacceptable to the patient; administration via nasogastric tube should be acceptable.

5 Antacids and/or milk may prematurely dissolve the coating of the tablet.

6 Tablet is scored and may be broken in half without affecting release characteristics.

7 Skin contact may enhance tumor production; avoid direct contact.

8 Capsule may be opened and the liquid contents removed for administration.

9 Tablets are made to disintegrate under the tongue.

Revised by John F. Mitchell, PharmD, FASHP, from an article that originally appeared in *Hosp Pharm*. 1996;1:27–37.

Drug Names That Look Alike and Sound Alike

This list has been prepared to sensitize health professionals and their support personnel for the need to properly communicate when writing, speaking, reading, and hearing drug names.

No drug name is without problems. Any name can be written or spoken poorly enough so that it can be mistaken for another.

Listed in the accompanying table are drug names that can look and/or sound alike. Some are dangerously close, whereas others require incomplete prescribing information, poor communications skills, poor listening, and/or lack of knowledge about the drugs for an error to result. Brand names are italicized in the table.

To reduce errors, practitioners must share the common goal of drug name safety with pharmaceutical manufacturers, the Food and Drug Administration (FDA), the World Health Organization (WHO), the United States Adopted Name Council (USANC), and the United States Pharmacopeia (USP).

The potential errors can be reduced by:

- Pretesting proposed names for error potential
- Careful selection of brand names and generic names by manufacturers, FDA, WHO, and USANC
- Legible handwriting
- Clear oral communications
- Writing complete drug orders
- Specifying the dosage form (eg, tablet)
- Specifying the drug strength (eg, 100 mg)
- Specifying directions (eg, take one daily with breakfast)
- Specifying the purpose/indication (eg, take one daily with breakfast to control blood pressure)
- Printing orders for new or rarely prescribed drugs
- Using computer-generated orders
- For those involved in drug dispensing and administration, being aware of the drugs that are available, paying careful attention to the work at hand, and minimize distractions.
- Knowing the patient's condition/problems, to ascertain if the drug name which has been read or heard is indicated
- Double-checking completed prescriptions in the pharmacy
- Educating patients about their drug regimens (this serves as another final check that the prescription was properly read and dispensed)

Proprietary names are capitalized; other names are in lower case letters.

Accolate	Accupril	acetohexamide	acetazolamide
Accolate	Aclovate	acetylcholine	acetylcysteine
Accupril	Accolate	acetylcysteine	acetylcholine
Accupril	Accutane	Aciphex	Accupril
Accupril	Aciphex	Aciphex	Aricept
Accurbron	Accutane	Aclovate	Accolate
Accutane	Accupril	Acular	Ocular
Accutane	Accurbron	Adderall	Inderal
acetazolamide	acetohexamide	Adeflor M	Aldoclor

Adriamycin	Aredia
Adriamycin	Idamycin
Afrin	aspirin
Aggrastat	Aggrenox
Aggrastat	argatroban
Aggrenox	Aggrastat
Akarpine	atropine
Albutein	albuterol
albuterol	Albutein
albuterol	atenolol
Alcaine	Alcare
Alcare	Alcaine
Aldactazide	Aldactone
Aldactone	Aldactazide
Aldara	Alora
Aldoclor	Adeflor M
Aldoclor	Aldoril
Aldoril	Aldoclor
Alesse	Aleve
Aleve	Alesse
Alfenta	Sufenta
alfentanil	Anafranil
alfentanil	fentanyl
alfentanil	sufentanil
Alkeran	Leukeran
Alor 5/500	Alora
Alora	Aldara
Alora	Alor 5/500
alprazolam	lorazepam
alprazolam	alprostadil
alprostadil	alprazolam
Altace	alteplase
Altace	Artane
alteplase	Altace
Alupent	Atrovent
Amaryl	Amerge
Ambien	Amen
Amen	Ambien
Amerge	Amaryl
Amicar	amikacin
Amicar	Amikin
amikacin	Amicar
Amikin	Amicar
amiloride	amiodarone
amiloride	amlodipine
aminophylline	amitriptyline
aminophylline	ampicillin
amiodarone	amiloride
amitriptyline	aminophylline

amitriptyline	nortriptyline
amlodipine	amiloride
amoxapine	amoxicillin
amoxicillin	amoxapine
ampicillin	aminophylline
Anafranil	alfentanil
Anafranil	enalapril
Anafranil	nafarelin
Anaprox	Anaspaz
Anaspaz	Anaprox
Anaspaz	Antispas
Ancobon	Oncovin
Antispas	Anaspaz
Antivert	Axert
Anturane	Artane
Anusol	Anusol-HC
Anusol	Aplisol
Anusol	Aquasol
Anusol-HC	Anusol
Aplisol	Anusol
Aplisol	Atropisol
Apresazide	Apresoline
Apresoline	Apresazide
Aquasol	Anusol
Aranesp	Aricept
Aredia	Adriamycin
argatroban	Aggrastat
argatroban	Orgaran
Aricept	Aciphex
Aricept	Aranesp
Aricept	Ascriptin
Artane	Altace
Artane	Anturane
Asacol	Os-Cal
Ascriptin	Aricept
Asendin	aspirin
asparaginase	pegaspargase
aspirin	Afrin
aspirin	Asendin
Atarax	Ativan
Atarax	Marax
atenolol	albuterol
atenolol	timolol
Atgam	Ativan
Ativan	Atarax
Ativan	Atgam
Ativan	Avitene
atropine	Akarpine
Atropisol	Aplisol

Atrovent	Alupent
Avalide	Avandia
Avandia	Avalide
Avandia	Coumadin
Avandia	Prandin
Avelox	Avonex
Aventyl	Bentyl
Avinza	Invanz
Avitene	Ativan
Avonex	Avelox
Axert	Antivert
azatadine	azathioprine
azathioprine	azatadine
azathioprine	azidothymidine
azathioprine	Azulfidine
azidothymidine	azathioprine
azithromycin	erythromycin
Azulfidine	azathioprine
bacitracin	Bactrim
bacitracin	Bactroban
baclofen	Bactroban
Bactrim	bacitracin
Bactrim	Bactroban
Bactroban	bacitracin
Bactroban	baclofen
Bactroban	Bactrim
Benadryl	benazepril
Benadryl	Bentyl
Benadryl	Benylin
benazepril	Benadryl
Benoxyl	Brevoxyl
Benoxyl	Peroxyl
Bentyl	Aventyl
Bentyl	Benadryl
Benylin	Benadryl
Benylin	Ventolin
benztropine	bromocriptine
bepridil	Prepidil
Betadine	betaine
Betagan	Betagen
Betagen	Betagan
betaine	Betadine
betaxolol	bethanechol
bethanechol	betaxolol
Betoptic	Betoptic S
Betoptic S	Betoptic
Bicillin	Wycillin
Brethaire	Brethine
Brethine	Brethaire

Brevoxyl	Benoxyl
bromocriptine	benztropine
bupivacaine	mepivacaine
bupropion	buspirone
buspirone	bupropion
butabarbital	Butalbital
Butalbital	butabarbital
Cafergot	Carafate
Caladryl	calamine
calamine	Caladryl
Calan	Colace
calcifediol	calcitriol
calciferol	calcitriol
calcitonin	calcitriol
calcitriol	calcifediol
calcitriol	calcitonin
calcium glubionate	calcium gluconate
calcium gluconate	calcium glubionate
camphorated tincture of opium (paregoric)	opium tincture
Capastat	Cepastat
Capitrol	Captopril
Captopril	Capitrol
Carafate	Cafergot
Carbatrol	Cartrol
Carbex	Surbex
Carboplatin	Cisplatin
Cardene	Cardura
Cardene	codeine
Cardene SR	Cardizem SR
Cardizem CD (LA, SR)	Cardizem SR (CD, LA)
Cardizem SR	Cardene SR
Cardura	Cardene
Cardura	Cordarone
Cardura	Coumadin
Cardura	K-Dur
carteolol	carvedilol
Cartrol	Carbatrol
carvedilol	carteolol
Catapres	Cetapred
Catapres	Combipres
cefamandole	cefmetazole
cefazolin	cefprozil
cefmetazole	cefamandole
Cefobid	cefonicid

Cefol .Cefzil
cefonicid. . . . . .Cefobid
Cefotan . . . . .Ceftin
cefotaxime . . . . .cefoxitin
cefotaxime . . . . .ceftizoxime
cefotaxime . . . . .cefuroxime
cefotetan . . . . .cefoxitin
cefoxitin . . . . .cefotaxime
cefoxitin . . . . .cefotetan
cefoxitin . . . . .Cytoxan
cefprozil . . . . .cefazolin
ceftazidime. . . . . .ceftizoxime
Ceftin . . . . .Cefotan
Ceftin . . . . .Cefzil
ceftizoxime. . . . . .cefotaxime
ceftizoxime. . . . . .ceftazidime
cefuroxime . . . . .cefotaxime
cefuroxime . . . . .deferoxamine
Cefzil . . . . .Cefol
Cefzil . . . . .Ceftin
Cefzil . . . . .Kefzol
Celebrex. . . . . .Cerebyx
Cepastat. . . . . .Capastat
cephapirin . . . . .cephradine
cephradine. . . . . .cephapirin
Cerebyx . . . . .Celebrex
Cerebyx . . . . .Cerezyme
Ceredase . . . . .Cerezyme
Cerezyme. . . . . .Cerebyx
Cerezyme. . . . . .Ceredase
Cetaphil . . . . .Cetapred
Cetapred . . . . .Catapres
Cetapred . . . . .Cetaphil
Chenix . . . . .Cystex
chlorambucil. . . . . .Chloromycetin
Chloromycetin . . . . .chlorambucil
chlorpromazine. . . . . .chlorpropamide
chlorpromazine. . . . . .clomipramine
chlorpromazine. . . . . .prochlorperazine
chlorpropamide . . . . .chlorpromazine
Cidex . . . . .Lidex
Ciloxan. . . . . .cinoxacin
Ciloxan. . . . . .Cytoxan
cimetidine. . . . . .simethicone
cinoxacin . . . . .Ciloxan
Cisplatin. . . . . .Carboplatin
Citracal. . . . . .Citrucel
Citrucel. . . . . .Citracal
Clarinex . . . . .Claritin

Claritin . . . . .Clarinex
Clinoril . . . . .Clozaril
clofazimine. . . . . .clozapine
clomiphene. . . . . .clomipramine
clomiphene. . . . . .clonidine
clomipramine . . . . .chlorpromazine
clomipramine . . . . .clomiphene
clonazepam . . . . .lorazepam
clonidine. . . . . .clomiphene
clonidine. . . . . .quinidine
clotrimazole . . . . .co-trimoxazole
clozapine . . . . .clofazimine
Clozaril. . . . . .Clinoril
Clozaril. . . . . .Colazal
co-trimoxazole . . . . .clotrimazole
codeine . . . . .Cardene
codeine . . . . .Lodine
Colace . . . . .Calan
Colazal. . . . . .Clozaril
Combipres . . . . .Catapres
Combivent . . . . .Combivir
Combivir. . . . . .Combivent
Compazine. . . . . .Copaxone
Comvax . . . . .Recombivax HB
Copaxone. . . . . .Compazine
Cordarone . . . . .Cordran
Cordarone . . . . .Cardura
Cordran . . . . .Cordarone
Cort-Dome . . . . .Cortone
Cortef. . . . . .Lortab
Cortone . . . . .Cort-Dome
Coumadin. . . . . .Avandia
Coumadin. . . . . .Cardura
Coumadin. . . . . .Kemadrin
Covera HS . . . . .Provera
Cozaar . . . . .Zocor
cyclobenzaprine . . . . .cycloserine
cyclobenzaprine . . . . .cyproheptadine
cyclophosphamide . . . . .cyclosporine
cycloserine. . . . . .cyclobenzaprine
cycloserine. . . . . .cyclosporine
cyclosporine. . . . . .cyclophospha-
mide
cyclosporine. . . . . .cycloserine
cyclosporine. . . . . .Cyklokapron
Cyklokapron . . . . .cyclosporine
cyproheptadine. . . . . .cyclobenzaprine
Cystex . . . . .Chenix
Cytadren . . . . .cytarabine

cytarabine	Cytadren
cytarabine	vidarabine
CytoGam	Cytoxan
Cytosar U	Cytovene
Cytosar U	Cytoxan
Cytotec	Cytoxan
Cytovene	Cytosar U
Cytoxan	cefoxitin
Cytoxan	Ciloxan
Cytoxan	CytoGam
Cytoxan	Cytosar U
Cytoxan	Cytotec
dacarbazine	Dicarbosil
dacarbazine	procarbazine
Dacriose	Danocrine
dactinomycin	daptomycin
dactinomycin	daunorubicin
dactinomycin	doxorubicin
Dalmane	Demulen
Dalmane	Dialume
Danocrine	Dacriose
Dantrium	Daraprim
dapsone	Diprosone
daptomycin	dactinomycin
Daranide	Daraprim
Daraprim	Dantrium
Daraprim	Daranide
Darvocet-N	Darvon-N
Darvon	Diovan
Darvon-N	Darvocet-N
daunorubicin	dactinomycin
daunorubicin	doxorubicin
daunorubicin	idarubicin
deferoxamine	cefuroxime
Delsym	Desyrel
Demerol	Demulen
Demerol	Dymelor
Demulen	Dalmane
Demulen	Demerol
Depo-Estradiol	Depo-Testadiol
Depo-Medrol	Solu-Medrol
Depo-Testadiol	Depo-Estradiol
Dermatop	Dimetapp
desipramine	disopyramide
desipramine	imipramine
desoximetasone	dexamethasone
Desoxyn	digoxin
Desyrel	Delsym
Desyrel	Zestril

dexamethasone	desoximetasone
Dexedrine	Dextran
Dexedrine	Excedrin
Dextran	Dexedrine
DiaBeta	Zebeta
Dialume	Dalmane
Diamox	Trimox
diazepam	diazoxide
diazepam	Ditropan
diazoxide	diazepam
diazoxide	Dyazide
Dicarbosil	dacarbazine
dichloroacetic acid	trichloracetic acid
diclofenac	Diflucan
diclofenac	Duphalac
dicyclomine	doxycycline
dicyclomine	dyclonine
Diflucan	diclofenac
Diflucan	disulfiram
digoxin	Desoxyn
digoxin	doxepin
Dilantin	Dilaudid
Dilaudid	Dilantin
dimenhydrinate	diphenhydramine
Dimetane	Dimetapp
Dimetapp	Dermatop
Dimetapp	Dimetane
Diovan	Darvon
diphenhydramine	dimenhydrinate
Diprivan	Ditropan
Diprosone	dapsone
dipyridamole	disopyramide
disopyramide	desipramine
disopyramide	dipyridamole
disulfiram	Diflucan
dithranol	Ditropan
Ditropan	diazepam
Ditropan	Diprivan
Ditropan	dithranol
dobutamine	dopamine
Dolobid	Slo-bid
donepezil	doxepin
dopamine	dobutamine
dopamine	Dopram
Dopar	Dopram
Dopram	dopamine
Dopram	Dopar

doxacurium . . . . .doxapram
doxacurium . . . . .doxorubicin
doxapram. . . . . .doxacurium
doxapram. . . . . .doxazosin
doxapram. . . . . .doxepin
doxapram. . . . . .doxorubicin
doxazosin. . . . . .doxapram
doxazosin. . . . . .doxepin
doxazosin. . . . . .doxorubicin
doxepin . . . . .digoxin
doxepin . . . . .donepezil
doxepin . . . . .doxapram
doxepin . . . . .doxazosin
doxepin . . . . .Doxidan
Doxidan . . . . .doxepin
Doxil. .Doxy
Doxil. .Paxil
doxorubicin. . . . . .dactinomycin
doxorubicin. . . . . .daunorubicin
doxorubicin. . . . . .doxacurium
doxorubicin. . . . . .doxapram
doxorubicin. . . . . .doxazosin
doxorubicin. . . . . .idarubicin
Doxy. .Doxil
doxycycline . . . . .dicyclomine
doxycycline . . . . .doxylamine
doxylamine. . . . . .doxycycline
dronabinol . . . . .droperidol
droperidol. . . . . .dronabinol
Duphalac . . . . .diclofenac
Dyazide . . . . .diazoxide
dyclonine . . . . .dicyclomine
Dymelor . . . . .Demerol
Dynabac. . . . . .Dynacin
Dynabac. . . . . .DynaCirc
Dynacin . . . . .Dynabac
Dynacin . . . . .DynaCirc
DynaCirc . . . . .Dynabac
DynaCirc . . . . .Dynacin
Ecotrin . . . . .Edecrin
Edecrin. . . . . .Ecotrin
Efidac. . . . . .Efudex
Efudex . . . . .Efidac
Elavil .Equanil
Elavil .Mellaril
Eldepryl . . . . .enalapril
Eldopaque Forte . . . . .Eldoquin Forte
Eldoquin Forte . . . . .Eldopaque Forte
Elmiron. . . . . .Imuran

Emcyt. .Eryc
enalapril . . . . .Anafranil
enalapril . . . . .Eldepryl
Enduronyl Forte . . . . .Inderal 40 mg
enflurane . . . . .isoflurane
Entex .Tenex
ephedrine. . . . . .epinephrine
epinephrine . . . . .ephedrine
Epogen . . . . .Neupogen
Equanil. . . . . .Elavil
Eryc . . . . .Emcyt
Erythrocin. . . . . .Ethmozine
erythromycin. . . . . .azithromcyin
erythromycin. . . . . .Ethmozine
Esimil .Ismelin
Estraderm . . . . .Testoderm
ethambutol . . . . .Ethmozine
Ethamolin. . . . . .ethanol
ethanol . . . . .Ethamolin
ethanol . . . . .Ethyol
Ethmozine . . . . .Erythrocin
Ethmozine . . . . .erythromycin
Ethmozine . . . . .ethambutol
ethosuximide . . . . .methsuximide
Ethyol. . . . . .ethanol
etidronate. . . . . .etomidate
etomidate . . . . .etidronate
Eurax .Evoxac
Eurax .Serax
Eurax .Urex
Evoxac. . . . . .Eurax
Excedrin. . . . . .Dexedrine
Factrel . . . . .Sectral
Faslodex . . . . .Fosamax
Femara . . . . .Femhrt
Femhrt . . . . .Femara
Femiron . . . . .Femring
Femring . . . . .Femiron
fentanyl . . . . .alfentanil
Feosol . . . . .Fer-in-Sol
Fer-in-Sol . . . . .Feosol
Feridex . . . . .Fertinex
Fertinex . . . . .Feridex
Fioricet . . . . .Fiorinal
Fiorinal. . . . . .Fioricet
Fiorinal. . . . . .Florinef
flecainide . . . . .fluconazole
Flexeril . . . . .Floxin
Flexon . . . . .Floxin

Flomax................Fosamax
Flomax................Volmax
Florinef...............Fiorinal
Florvite................Flovite
Floxin.................Flexeril
Floxin.................Flexon
fluconazole............flecainide
Fludara................FUDR
Flumadine.............flunisolide
Flumadine.............flutamide
flunisolide.............Flumadine
flunisolide.............fluocinonide
fluocinolone...........fluocinonide
fluocinonide...........flunisolide
fluocinonide...........fluocinolone
fluoxetine.............fluvastatin
flutamide.............Flumadine
fluvastatin............fluoxetine
folic acid..............folinic acid
folinic acid............folic acid
Folvite................Florvite
Foradil................Toradol
Fosamax..............Fasudex
Fosamax..............Flomax
fosinopril.............lisinopril
FUDR..................Fludara
Fulvicin...............Furacin
Furacin................Fulvicin
furosemide............Torsemide
Furoxone..............Fuzeon
Fuzeon................Furoxone
Genpril...............Genprin
Genprin...............Genpril
Glaucon...............glucagon
glimepiride............glipizide
glipizide...............glimepiride
glipizide...............glyburide
glucagon..............Glaucon
Glucotrol..............glyburide
glutethimide...........guanethidine
glyburide..............glipizide
glyburide..............Glucotrol
GoLYTELY.............NuLytely
guanabenz.............guanadrel
guanabenz.............guanfacine
guanadrel.............guanabenz
guanethidine...........glutethimide
guanethidine...........guanidine
guanfacine............guaifenesin

guanfacine............guanabenz
guanfacine............guanidine
guanidine.............guanethidine
guanidine.............guanfacine
halcinonide............Halcion
Halcion................halcinonide
Halcion................Haldol
Halcion................Healon
Haldol.................Halcion
Haldol.................Halog
Halog.................Haldol
Halotestin.............halothane
halothane.............Halotestin
Healon................Halcion
heparin...............Hespan
Hespan...............hoparin
Humalog..............Humulin
Humulin...............Humalog
Hycodan..............Vicodin
hydralazine............hydroxyzine
hydrochlorothiazide.........hydroflumethia-
                          zide
hydrocodone...........hydrocortisone
hydrocortisone..........hydrocodone
hydrocortisone..........hydroxychloro-
                          quine
hydroflumethiazide.........hydrochlorothi-
                          azide
Hydrogesic............hydroxyzine
hydromorphone..........morphine
hydroxychloroquine........hydrocortisone
hydroxyprogesterone........medroxypro-
                          gesterone
hydroxyurea...........hydroxyzine
hydroxyzine...........hydralazine
hydroxyzine...........Hydrogesic
hydroxyzine...........hydroxyurea
Hygroton..............Regroton
Hyperstat.............Nitrostat
Hytone................Vytone
Idamycin..............Adriamycin
idarubicin.............daunorubicin
idarubicin.............doxorubicin
Iletin.................Lente
Imdur.................Imuran
imipramine............desipramine
Imodium..............Indocin
Imodium..............Ionamin
Imovax...............Imovax I.D.
Imovax I.D............Imovax

Imuran	Elmiron
Imuran	Imdur
Imuran	Inderal
indapamide	iopamidol
indapamide	Iopidine
Inderal	Adderall
Inderal	Imuran
Inderal	Inderide
Inderal	Isordil
Inderal 40 mg	Enduronyl Forte
Inderide	Inderal
Indocin	Imodium
Indocin	Vicodin
interferon 2	interleukin 2
interferon alfa-2a	interferon alfa-2b
interferon alfa-2b	interferon alfa-2a
interleukin 2	interferon 2
interleukin 2	interleukin 11
interleukin 11	interleukin 2
Intropin	Isoptin
Invanz	Avinza
iodine	Iopidine
iodine	Lodine
iodipamide	Iopidine
Ionamin	Imodium
iopamidol	indapamide
Iopidine	iodipamide
Iopidine	iodine
Iopidine	Lodine
Ismelin	Esimil
Ismelin	Isuprel
isoflurane	enflurane
Isoptin	Intropin
Isopto Carbachol	Isopto Carpine
Isopto Carpine	Isopto Carbachol
Isordil	Inderal
Isordil	Isuprel
Isuprel	Ismelin
Isuprel	Isordil
K-Dur	Cardura
K-Lor	Kaochlor
K-Phos Neutral	Neutra-Phos-K
Kaochlor	K-Lor
Kefzol	Cefzil
Kemadrin	Coumadin
Klaron	Klor-Con
Klor-Con	Klaron
lactose	lactulose
lactulose	lactose

Lamictal	Lamisil
Lamictal	Lomotil
Lamisil	Lamictal
lamivudine	lamotrigine
lamotrigine	lamivudine
Lanoxin	Levsinex
Lanoxin	Lonox
Lantus	Lente
Lasix	Lidex
Lasix	Luvox
Lasix	Luxiq
Lente	Iletin
Lente	Lantus
Leukeran	Alkeran
Leukeran	Leukine
Leukine	Leukeran
Leustatin	lovastatin
Levatol	Lipitor
Levbid	Lithobid
Levbid	Lorabid
Levitra	Lexiva
Lexiva	Levitra
levothyroxine	liothyronine
Levsinex	Lanoxin
Librax	Librium
Librium	Librax
Lidex	Cidex
Lidex	Lasix
Lioresal	lisinopril
liothyronine	levothyroxine
Lipitor	Levatol
lisinopril	fosinopril
lisinopril	Lioresal
Lithobid	Levbid
Lithobid	Lithostat
Lithobid	Lithotabs
Lithonate	Lithostat
Lithostat	Lithobid
Lithostat	Lithonate
Lithostat	Lithotabs
Lithotabs	Lithobid
Lithotabs	Lithostat
Livostin	lovastatin
Lodine	codeine
Lodine	iodine
Lodine	Iopidine
Lomotil	Lamictal
Loniten	Lotensin
Lonox	Lanoxin

Lonox	Loprox
Loprox	Lonox
Lorabid	Levbid
Lorabid	Lortab
lorazepam	alprazolam
lorazepam	clonazepam
Lortab	Cortef
Lortab	Lorabid
Lotensin	Loniten
Lotensin	lovastatin
Lotrimin	Lotrisone
Lotrisone	Lotrimin
lovastatin	Leustatin
lovastatin	Livostin
lovastatin	Lotensin
Luminal	Tuinal
Lupron	Nuprin
Luvox	Lasix
Luxiq	Lasix
Maalox	Maolate
Maalox	Marax
magnesium sulfate	manganese sulfate
manganese sulfate	magnesium sulfate
Maolate	Maalox
Maranox	Marax
Marax	Atarax
Marax	Maalox
Marax	Maranox
Maxidex	Maxzide
Maxzide	Maxidex
Mebaral	Medrol
Mebaral	Mellaril
Medrol	Mebaral
medroxyprogesterone	hydroxyprogesterone
medroxyprogesterone	methylprednisolone
medroxyprogesterone	methyltestosterone
Mellaril	Elavil
Mellaril	Mebaral
melphalan	Mephyton
mephenytoin	Mephyton
mephenytoin	phenytoin
mephobarbital	methocarbamol
Mephyton	melphalan
Mephyton	mephenytoin
mepivacaine	bupivacaine

Mesantoin	Mestinon
Mestinon	Mesantoin
Mestinon	Metatensin
Metadate CD (CR, ER)	Metadate CR (CD, ER)
metaproterenol	metipranolol
metaproterenol	metoprolol
Metatensin	Mestinon
methazolamide	metolazone
methenamine	methionine
methionine	methenamine
methocarbamol	mephobarbital
methsuximide	ethosuximide
methylprednisolone	medroxyprogesterone
methyltestosterone	medroxyprogesterone
metipranolol	metaproterenol
metolazone	methiazolamine
metolazone	metoprolol
metoprolol	metaproterenol
metoprolol	metolazone
metyrapone	metyrosine
metyrosine	metyrapone
Mevacor	Mivacron
miconazole	Micronase
miconazole	Micronor
Micro-K	Micronase
Micronase	miconazole
Micronase	Micro-K
Micronase	Micronor
Micronor	miconazole
Micronor	Micronase
Midrin	Mydfrin
Mifeprex	Mirapex
mifepristone	misoprostol
Minocin	Mithracin
Minocin	niacin
MiraLax	Mirapex
Mirapex	Mifeprex
Mirapex	MiraLax
misoprostol	mifepristone
Mithracin	Minocin
Mivacron	Mevacor
Moban	Mobidin
Mobidin	Moban
Modane	Mudrane
Monopril	Monurol
Monurol	Monopril

morphine	hydromorphone
Mudrane	Modane
Myambutol	Nembutal
Mycelex	Myoflex
Mydfrin	Midrin
Mylanta	Mynatal
Myleran	Mylicon
Mylicon	Myleran
Mynatal	Mylanta
Myoflex	Mycelex
nafarelin	Anafranil
Naldecon	Nalfon
Nalfon	Naldecon
naloxone	naltrexone
naltrexone	naloxone
Narcan	Norcuron
Nasarel	Nizoral
Navane	Norvasc
Navane	Nubain
Nembutal	Myambutol
Nephro-Calci	Nephrocaps
Nephrocaps	Nephro-Calci
Neumega	Neupogen
Neupogen	Epogen
Neupogen	Neumega
Neupogen	Nutramigen
Neurontin	Neutrexin
Neurontin	Noroxin
Neutra-Phos-K	K-Phos Neutral
Neutrexin	Neurontin
niacin	Minocin
nicardipine	nifedipine
Nicorette	Nordette
nifedipine	nicardipine
nifedipine	nimodipine
Nilstat	Nitrostat
Nilstat	Nystatin
nimodipine	nifedipine
nitroglycerin	nitroprusside
Nitrol	Nizoral
nitroprusside	nitroglycerin
Nitrostat	Hyperstat
Nitrostat	Nilstat
Nitrostat	Nystatin
Nizoral	Nasarel
Nizoral	Nitrol
Norcuron	Narcan
Nordette	Nicorette
Norgesic #40	Norgesic Forte
Norgesic Forte	Norgesic #40
Noroxin	Neurontin
nortriptyline	amitriptyline
Norvasc	Navane
Norvasc	Vascor
Nubain	Navane
NuLytely	GoLYTELY
Nuprin	Lupron
Nutramigen	Neupogen
Nystatin	Nilstat
Nystatin	Nitrostat
Occlusal-HP	Ocuflox
OctreoScan	octreotide
OctreoScan	OncoScint
octreotide	OctreoScan
Ocufen	Ocuflox
Ocuflox	Occlusal-HP
Ocuflox	Ocufen
Ocular	Acular
olanzapine	olsalazine
olsalazine	olanzapine
OncoScint	OctreoScan
Oncovin	Ancobon
Ophthaine	Ophthetic
Ophthetic	Ophthaine
opium tincture	camphorated tincture of opium (paregoric)
opium tincture, camphorated (paregoric)	opium tincture
Optiray	Optival
Optivar	Optiray
Organan	argatroban
Ortho-Cept	Ortho-Cyclen
Ortho-Cyclen	Ortho-Cept
Os-Cal	Asacol
oxybutynin	OxyContin
OxyContin	oxybutynin
oxymetazoline	oxymetholone
oxymetholone	oxymetazoline
oxymetholone	oxymorphone
oxymorphone	oxymetholone
paclitaxel	paroxetine
paclitaxel	Paxil
Panadol	pindolol
pancuronium	pipecuronium
Paraplatin	Platinol
paregoric	Percogesic

Parlodel	.pindolol
paroxetine	.paclitaxel
paroxetine	.pyridoxine
Patanol.	.Platinol
Pathocil	.Placidyl
Paxil.	.Doxil
Paxil.	.paclitaxel
Paxil.	.Plavix
Paxil.	.Taxol
pegaspargase	.asparaginase
penicillamine	.penicillin
penicillin.	.penicillamine
penicillin G	penicillin G
potassium.	procaine
penicillin G	penicillin G
procaine.	potassium
pentobarbital	.phenobarbital
pentosan	.pentostatin
pentostatin	.pentosan
Pentrax	.Permax
Percocet.	.Percodan
Percodan	.Percocet
Percodan	.Percogesic
Percogesic.	.paregoric
Percogesic.	.Percodan
Perdiem	.Pyridium
Peridex.	.Precedex
Permax	.Pentrax
Permax	.Pernox
Pernox	.Permax
Peroxyl.	.Benoxyl
phenobarbital	.pentobarbital
phentermine.	.phentolamine
phentolamine	.phentermine
phenytoin	.mephenytoin
pHisoDerm.	.pHisoHex
pHisoHex	.pHisoDerm
Phos-Flur	.PhosLo
PhosChol	.PhosLo
PhosChol	.Phosphocol P32
PhosLo.	.Phos-Flur
PhosLo.	.PhosChol
Phosphocol P32.	.PhosChol
physostigmine	.Prostigmin
physostigmine	.pyridostigmine
pindolol	.Panadol
pindolol	.Parlodel
pindolol	.Plendil
pipecuronium	.pancuronium
Pitocin	.Pitressin

Pitressin	.Pitocin
Placidyl	.Pathocil
Platinol.	.Paraplatin
Platinol.	.Patanol
Plavix.	.Paxil
Plendil	.pindolol
Plendil	.Pletal
Pletal	.Plendil
Polocaine	.prilocaine
pralidoxime.	.Pramoxine
pralidoxime.	.pyridoxine
Pramoxine	.pralidoxime
Prandin	.Avandia
Pravachol.	.Prevacid
Pravachol.	.propranolol
PreCare	.Precose
Precedex	.Peridex
Precose	.PreCare
prednisolone.	.prednisone
prednisone	.prednisolone
prednisone	.primidone
Premarin	.Primaxin
Premarin	.Remeron
Premphase.	.Prempro
Prempro.	.Premphase
Prepidil.	.bepridil
Prevacid.	.Pravachol
Prevacid.	.Prevpac
Preven	.Prevnar
Prevnar	.Preven
Prevpac	.Prevacid
prilocaine	.Polocaine
prilocaine	.Prilosec
Prilosec	.prilocaine
Prilosec	.Prinivil
Prilosec	.Prozac
Primaxin.	.Premarin
primidone	.prednisone
Prinivil	.Prilosec
Prinivil	.Proventil
ProAmatine	.protamine
probenecid	.Procanbid
Procanbid.	.probenecid
procarbazine	.dacarbazine
prochlorperazine	.chlorpromazine
Profen II.	.Profen LA
Profen LA.	.Profen II
Proloprim	.Protropin
propranolol	.Pravachol

propylthiouracil. . . . . .Purinethol
Proscar . . . . .ProSom
Proscar . . . . .Prozac
Proscar . . . . .Psorcon
ProSom . . . . .Proscar
ProSom . . . . .Prozac
ProSom . . . . .Psorcon
Prostigmin . . . . .physostigmine
protamine. . . . . .ProAmatine
protamine. . . . . .Protopam
protamine. . . . . .Protropin
Protonix . . . . .Protopic
Protopam . . . . .protamine
Protopam . . . . .Protropin
Protopic . . . . .Protonix
Protropin . . . . .Proloprim
Protropin . . . . .protamine
Protropin . . . . .Protopam
Proventil. . . . . .Prinivil
Provera . . . . .Covera HS
Prozac. . . . . .Prilosec
Prozac. . . . . .Proscar
Prozac. . . . . .ProSom
Psorcon . . . . .Proscar
Psorcon . . . . .ProSom
Purinethol. . . . . .propylthiouracil
Pyridium. . . . . .Peridiem
Pyridium. . . . . .pyridoxine
pyridostigmine . . . . .physostigmine
pyridoxine. . . . . .paroxetine
pyridoxine. . . . . .pralidoxime
pyridoxine. . . . . .Pyridium
quinidine. . . . . .clonidine
quinidine. . . . . .quinine
quinine . . . . .quinidine
ranitidine . . . . .rimantadine
ranitidine . . . . .ritodrine
Recombivax. . . . . .Comvax
Recombivax HB . . . . .Comvax
Reglan. . . . . .Regonol
Reglan. . . . . .Renagel
Regonol . . . . .Reglan
Regonol . . . . .Regroton
Regonol . . . . .Renagel
Regranex . . . . .Repronex
Regroton . . . . .Hygroton
Regroton . . . . .Regonol
Remeron . . . . .Premarin
Remicade. . . . . .Renacidin

Reminyl . . . . .Robinul
Renacidin. . . . . .Remicade
Renagel . . . . .Reglan
Renagel . . . . .Regonol
Reno-M-60. . . . . .Renografin-60
Renografin-60 . . . . .Reno-M-60
Repronex . . . . .Regranex
reserpine . . . . .risperidone
Restasis. . . . . .Retavase
Restoril. . . . . .Vistaril
Restoril. . . . . .Zestril
Retavase . . . . .Restasis
Retrovir . . . . .ritonavir
Revex. . . . . .ReVia
ReVia. . . . . .Revex
Ribavirin. . . . . .riboflavin
riboflavin. . . . . .Ribavirin
rifabutin . . . . .rifampin
Rifadin . . . . .Rifater
Rifadin . . . . .Ritalin
Rifamate. . . . . .rifampin
rifampin . . . . .rifabutin
rifampin . . . . .Rifamate
rifampin . . . . .rifapentine
rifapentine . . . . .rifampin
Rifater . . . . .Rifadin
rimantadine . . . . .ranitidine
risperidone . . . . .reserpine
Ritalin. . . . . .Rifadin
Ritalin LA . . . . .Ritalin SR
Ritalin SR. . . . . .Ritalin LA
ritodrine . . . . .ranitidine
ritonavir . . . . .Retrovir
Robinul. . . . . .Reminyl
Roxanol . . . . .Roxicet
Roxicet. . . . . .Roxanol
Rynatan . . . . .Rynatuss
Rynatuss . . . . .Rynatan
Sandimmune . . . . .Sandoglobulin
Sandimmune . . . . .Sandostatin
Sandoglobulin . . . . .Sandimmune
Sandoglobulin . . . . .Sandostatin
Sandostatin . . . . .Sandimmune
Sandostatin . . . . .Sandoglobulin
saquinavir. . . . . .Sinequan
Sarafem . . . . .Serophene
Sectral . . . . .Factrel
selegiline . . . . .Stelazine
Serax .Eurax

Serax	Xerac
Serentil	Serevent
Serentil	sertraline
Serevent	Serentil
Serophene	Sarafem
Seroquel	Serzone
sertraline	Serentil
sertraline	Soriatane
Serzone	Seroquel
simethicone	cimetidine
Sinequan	saquinavir
Slo-bid	Dolobid
Slow FE	Slow-K
Slow-K	Slow FE
Solu-Medrol	Depo-Medrol
somatrem	somatropin
somatropin	somatrem
somatropin	sumatriptan
Soriatane	sertraline
sotalol	Stadol
Stadol	sotalol
Stelazine	selegiline
Sufenta	Alfenta
Sufenta	Survanta
sufentanil	alfentanil
sulfadiazine	sulfasalazine
sulfamethizole	sulfamethoxazole
sulfamethoxazole	sulfamethizole
sulfasalazine	sulfadiazine
sulfasalazine	sulfisoxazole
sulfisoxazole	sulfasalazine
sumatriptan	somatropin
Surbex	Carbex
Surbex	Surfak
Surfak	Surbex
Survanta	Sufenta
Synagis	Synalgos-DC
Synalgos-DC	Synagis
t-PA	TNKase
Taxol	Paxil
Taxol	Taxotere
Taxotere	Taxol
Tazicef	Tazidime
Tazidime	Tazicef
Tegretol	Toradol
Tegretol	Trental
Ten-K	Tenex
Tenex	Entex
Tenex	Ten-K

Tenex	Xanax
Tequin	Ticlid
terbinafine	terbutaline
terbutaline	terbinafine
terbutaline	tolbutamide
terconazole	tioconazole
Testoderm	Estraderm
testolactone	testosterone
testosterone	testolactone
Thera-Flur	TheraFlu
TheraFlu	Thera-Flur
thiamine	Thorazine
thioridazine	thiothixene
thioridazine	Thorazine
thiothixene	thioridazine
Thorazine	thiamine
Thorazine	thioridazine
tiagabine	tizanidine
Tiazac	Ziac
Ticlid	Tequin
timolol	atenolol
Timoptic	Viroptic
tioconazole	terconazole
tizanidine	tiagabine
TNKase	t-PA
TobraDex	Tobrex
tobramycin	Trobicin
Tobrex	TobraDex
tolazamide	tolbutamide
tolbutamide	terbutaline
tolbutamide	tolazamide
tolnafate	Tornalate
Topamax	Toprol XL
Toprol XL	Topamax
Toradol	Foradil
Toradol	Tegretol
Toradol	Torecan
Toradol	tramadol
Torecan	Toradol
Tornalate	tolnaftate
Torsemide	furosemide
Tracleer	Tricor
tramadol	Toradol
tramadol	Trandate
tramadol	trazodone
Trandate	tramadol
Trandate	Trental
Travatan	Xalatan
trazodone	tramadol

Trental	Tegretol
Trental	Trandate
tretinoin	trientine
Trexall	Trexan
Trexan	Trexall
Triaminic	TriHemic
triamterene	trimipramine
trichloracetic acid	dichlotoacetic acid
trientine	tretinoin
trifluoperazine	triflupromazine
triflupromazine	trifluoperazine
TriHemic	Triaminic
trimipramine	triamterene
Trimox	Diamox
Trimox	Tylox
Trobicin	tobramycin
Tronolane	Tronothane
Tronothane	Tronolane
Tuinal	Luminal
Tuinal	Tylenol
Tylenol	Tuinal
Tylenol	Tylox
Tylox	Trimox
Tylox	Tylenol
Ultane	Ultram
Ultram	Ultane
Urex	Eurax
Urised	Urispas
Urispas	Urised
Vaginex	Vigamox
Valcyte	Valium
Valium	Valcyte
valsartan	Valstar
Valstar	valsartan
Vaniqa	Viagra
Vantin	Ventolin
Vascor	Norvasc
Vasocidin	Vasodilan
Vasodilan	Vasocidin
Vasosulf	Velosef
Velosef	Vasosulf
Ventolin	Benylin
Ventolin	Vantin
VePesid	Versed
Verelan	Virilon
Verelan	Vivarin
Verelan	Voltaren
Versed	VePesid
Vexol	VoSol
Viagra	Vaniqa
Vicodin	Hycodan
Vicodin	Indocin
vidarabine	cytarabine
Vigamox	Vaginex
Vigamox	Vigomar
Vigomar	Vigamox
vinblastine	vincristine
vinblastine	vinorelbine
vincristine	vinblastine
vinorelbine	vinblastine
Vioxx	Zyvox
Virilon	Verelan
Viroptic	Timoptic
Visine	Visken
Visken	Visine
Vistaril	Restoril
Vivarin	Verelan
Volmax	Flomax
Voltaren	Verelan
VoSol	Vexol
Vytone	Hytone
Wellbutrin	Wellferon
Wellbutrin SR	Wellbutrin XL
Wellbutrin XL	Wellbutrin SR
Wellferon	Wellbutrin
Wycillin	Bicillin
Xalatan	Travatan
Xanax	Tenex
Xanax	Xopenex
Xanax	Zantac
Xeloda	Xenical
Xenical	Xeloda
Xerac	Serax
Xopenex	Xanax
Zagam	Zyban
Zantac	Xanax
Zantac	Zofran
Zantac	Zyrtec
Zarontin	Zaroxolyn
Zaroxolyn	Zarontin
Zebeta	DiaBeta
Zestril	Desyrel
Zestril	Restoril
Zestril	Zetia
Zestril	Zostrix
Zetia	Zestril

Ziac . . . . .Tiazac	Zyban. . . . . .Zagam
Zocor .Cozaar	Zyloprim . . . . .ZORprin
Zofran . . . . .Zantac	Zymar. . . . . .Zymine
Zofran . . . . .Zosyn	Zymine . . . . .Zymar
ZORprin . . . . .Zyloprim	Zyprexa . . . . .Zyrtec
Zostrix . . . . .Zestril	Zyrtec. . . . . .Zantac
Zostrix . . . . .Zovirax	Zyrtec. . . . . .Zyprexa
Zosyn. . . . . .Zofran	Zyvox .Vioxx
Zosyn. . . . . .Zyvox	Zyvox .Zosyn
Zovirax. . . . . .Zostrix	Zyvox .Zovirax
Zovirax. . . . . .Zyvox	

This list was compiled by Neil M. Davis, MS, PharmD, FASHP, President, Safe Medication Practices Consulting, Inc., Huntingdon Valley, PA. The list was originally developed by Benjamin Teplitsky, retired Chief Pharmacist of Veterans Administration Hospitals in Albany, NY and Brooklyn, NY.

New Therapeutic Agents Marketed January-August 2005

Generic name	Trade name	Manufacturer	Therapeutic classification	Route of administration	FDA classification*
Acamprosate calcium	Campral	Forest	Agent for alcohol dependence	Oral	1-P
Clofarabine	Clolar	Genzyme	Antineoplastic agent	Intravenous	1-P, H, O
Darifenacin hydrobromide	Enablex	Novartis	Agent for overactive bladder	Oral	1-S
Entecavir	Baraclude	Bristol-Myers Squibb	Antiviral agent	Oral	1-P
Eszopiclone	Lunesta	Sepracor	Hypnotic	Oral	1-S
Exenatide	Byetta	Amylin; Lilly	Antidiabetic agent	Subcutaneous	1-S
Galsulfase	Naglazyme	BioMarin	Agent for mucopolysac- charidosis	Intravenous	P, O
Ibandronate sodium	Boniva	GlaxoSmith- Kline; Roche	Agent for osteo- porosis	Oral	1-S
Iloprost	Ventavis	CoTherix	Agent for pulmo- nary arterial hy- pertension	Inhalation	1-P, O
Nepafenac	Nevanac	Alcon	Anti-inflamma- tory agent	Ophthalmic	1-P
Palifermin	Kepivance	Amgen	Agent for oral mucositis	Intravenous	1-P
Pegaptanib sodium	Macugen	Eyetech; Pfizer	Agent for macu- lar degeneration	Intravitreous	1-P
Pramlintide acetate	Symlin	Amylin	Antidiabetic agent	Subcutaneous	1-S
Ramelteon	Rozerem	Takeda	Hypnotic	Oral	1-S
Solifenacin succinate	Vesicare	GlaxoSmith- Kline; Yaman- ouchi	Agent for over- active bladder	Oral	1-S
Tigecycline	Tygacil	Wyeth	Antibiotic	Intravenous	1-P
Tipranavir	Aptivus	Boehringer Ingelheim	Antiviral agent	Oral	1-P
Ziconotide	Prialt	Elan	Analgesic	Intrathecal	1-P

* FDA classification of new drugs: 1 = new molecular entity; P = priority review; S = standard review; H = accelerated approval; O = designated orphan drug.

This list was compiled by Daniel A. Hussar, PhD, Remington Professor of Pharmacy, Philadelphia College of Pharmacy, University of the Sciences in Philadelphia, for publication in *The Drug Advisor*.

Discontinued Drugs

The following is a list of products no longer available in the United States because they were discontinued by the manufacturer or withdrawn from the market.

AccuHist Pediatric Drops
Aci-jel Vaginal Gel
Actisite
Activella Tablets
Adeflor M Tablets
AK-Trol Ophthalmic Ointment
AK-Trol Ophthalmic Suspension
Alkets, Extra Strength Antacid, Chewable
  Tablets
Allercreme Skin Lotion
Allercreme Ultra Emollient Cream
Almora Tablets
Alpha-Keri Moisturizing Soap Bar
Alphatrex Cream
Americaine Otic Solutions
Amitone Antacid Chewable Tablets
Ancef Injection
Ancef Powder for Injection
Andehist Drops
Andehist Syrup
Andehist-DM Syrup
Anemagen Capsules
Antiminth Oral Suspension
Apatate Tablets
AquaMEPHYTON Injection
Aquaphyllin Syrup
AquaSite Solution
Arduan Powder for Injection
Arfonad
Argesic Cream
Aristocort Forte Injection
Atarax
Atuss EX Syrup
Auroto Otic Solution
Barbidonna Tablets
Barbidonna #2 Tablets
B-C Bid Tablets
Benadryl Maximum Strength Cream
Benadryl Maximum Strength Solution
  (Spray)
Bengay SPA Cream
Benzthiazide
Bepridil Hydrochloride
Bextra Tablets
Bonine Chewable Tablets
Borofax Skin Protectant

Calcifediol
Calciferol Injection
Carbinoxamine Compound Drops
  (Pediatric)
Carbinoxamine Compound Syrup
Cardizem SR Capsules
Cefadyl
Cefamandole Nafate
Cefonicid Sodium
Cenogen-OB Capsules
Cephalexin Hydrochloride Monohydrate
Cephapirin Sodium
Cerumenex Drops (Solution)
Chloroptic S.O.P. Ointment
Choledyl SA Tablets
Clearplan Easy Kit
Clofazimine
Colfosceril Palmitate
Conceive Ovulation Predictor Cassettes
Cortizone•5 Cream
Cysto-Conray
Cysto-Conray II
Cystospaz-M Capsules
Cytosar-U Powder for Injection
Danocrine Capsules
Daranide
Dayalets Filmtabs Tablets
Dazamide Tablets
Defen-LA Tablets
Demecarium Bromide
Derma Viva Lotion
Dexacine Ophthalmic Ointment
Diamox Tablets
Dical-D Wafers
Dichlorphenamide
Didronel IV Injection
Dilor Elixir
Dilor Injection
Diucardin Tablets
Doxacurium Chloride
Duadacin Extra Strength Cold and Flu
  Tablets
Duradryl JR Capsules
Dyclone
Dyclonine Hydrochloride
Dyline-GG Liquid

Endal (Nasal Decongestant) Tablets
Epifrin Solution
Erygel 2% Gel
Estar Gel 5%
Ethaquin
Ethatab
Ethaverine
Ethavex-100
Exna Tablets
Exosurf Neonatal
Femiron Multivitamin and Iron Tablets
Ferumoxsil
Flovent Aerosol
Floxin Injection
Fluori-Methane Spray
Fostril Lotion 2%
Gamimune N Injection
GastroMARK
Gerivite Tablets
Glaucon Solution
Glutethimide
Griseofulvin Microsize
Guaifenex G Tablets (Sustained-release)
Guaifenex LA Tablets (Extended-release)
Guiatuss CF Syrup
Guiatuss PE Liquid
Halfan Tablets
Halofantrine Hydrochloride
Halog Cream 0.025%
Halotestin Tablets
Halotussin AC Liquid
Halotussin DAC Syrup
Human Albumin Microspheres
Humibid DM Tablets
Humorsol
Hydergine LC Capsules
Hydergine LC Liquid
Hydroflumethiazide
Hytakerol Capsules
Imuran Injection
Intropin Injection
Iothalamate Meglumine 17.2%
Iothalamate Meglumine 43% Injection
Isordil Tembid Tablets
Kay Ciel Liquid
Keftab
Keri Crème Cream
Keri Light Lotion
K-Lease Capsules

K-Norm Capsules
Kutapressin Injection
Lamprene
Levocabastine Hydrochloride Ophthalmic
    Suspension
Levomethadyl Acetate Hydrochloride
Liver Derivative Complex
Livostin
Loniten Tablets
Lubriderm Bath Oil
Lubriderm Cream
Lucidex Tablets
Lufyllin Elixir
Lufyllin Injection
Lunelle Injection
Maginex DS Powder
Maginex Tablets, Enteric-coated
Mallamint Chewable Tablets
Maltsupex Liquid
Maltsupex Tablets
Mandol
Maxivate Lotion
MD-Gastroview Solution
MED-DM Tablets
Medicone Suppositories
Medroxyprogesterone Acetate/Estradiol
    Cypionate (MPA/E2C)
Mellaril (all products)
Mephentermine
Mephenytoin
Mescolor Tablets
Mesoridazine Besylate
Metoclopramide Intensol Concentrated
    Solution
Moctanin Infusion
Monocid
Monoctanoin
MouthKote P/R (all products)
Mucosil-10 Solution
Mucosil-20 Solution
Mytrex (all products)
Natalizumab
Nephro-Vite + Fe Tablets
Netilmicin Sulfate
Nicosyn Lotion
Nitroglyn Capsules
Nitrong Tablets
Nupercainal Cream
Nuromax Injection

Ocupress Solution 1%
Ony-Clear Solution 1%
Optison
ORLAAM
OvuGen Kit
OvuKIT Self-Test Kit
OvuQuick Self-Test Kit
P_1E_1 Solution
P_2E_1 Solution
P_4E_1 Solution
P_6E_1 Solution
Pacis Powder for Suspension
Panatuss DX Liquid
Pediatric Bear-E-Bag
Perchloracap
pHisoDerm Cleansing Bar
Pilocarpine and Epinephrine Solutions
    (Ophthalmic Agents for Glaucoma)
Pipecuronium Bromide
Pnu-Imune 23 Injection
Polysporin Powder
Polythiazide Potassium Perchlorate
Predalone 50 Injection
Prenatal Plus w/Betacarotene
Prenate GT Tablets
Protirelin
Protropin Powder for injection
Protuss DM Tablets
Protuss Liquid
Protuss-D Liquid
Proventil Repetabs Tablets
P-Tanna 12 Suspension
Purge Liquid (95% castor oil)
QTest Ovulation Kit
Quinidex Extentabs Tablets
Relefact RTH
Renese Tablets
Replens Gel
Rescula Solution
Respbid Tablets
Rheaban Maximum Strength Tablets
Rinade-B.I.D. Capsules
Rofecoxib
R-Tannic-S A/D Suspension
Rulox #1 Tablets
Rulox #2 Tablets
Ryna Liquid
Ryna-C Liquid
Serentil Tablets

Serzone Tablets
Sinequan Oral Concentrate
Slo-Phyllin GG Capsules
Slo-Phyllin GG Syrup
Slo-Phyllin Gyrocaps Capsules
Slow-K Tablets
SLT Lotion
Sno Strips Test
Sofenol 5 Lotion
Somatrem
Sorbitrate Chewable Tablets
Sorbitrate Sublingual Tablets
Sorbitrate Tablets
Spectrocin Plus Ointment
Stadol NS Solution
Sudal 60/500 Tablets
Sulfoil Liquid
Supprelin Injections
Suprax Tablets
Susano Elixir
Sustaire Tablets
Syntest DS Tablets
Syntest HS Tablets
Synthroid Powder for Injection
Tencon Capsules
Testoderm Transdermal System
Tetracycline Hydrochloride Fiber
Theobid Duracaps Capsules
Theoclear-80 Syrup
Theoclear L.A. Capsules
Theolair Solution
Theolair S.R. Tablets
Theo-Sav Tablets
Theovent Capsules
Theo-X Tablets
Therac Lotion
Theragran-M Caplets
Thypinone
Thyrel TRH
Tocainide Hydrochloride
Tolazoline Hydrochloride
Tolectin DS Capsules
Tonocard Tablets
Touro EX Tablets
Triavil Tablets
Tridil Injection
Trimethaphan Camsylate
Trinalin Repetabs Tablets
Trovafloxacin Mesylate/Alatrofloxacin
    Mesylate

Trovan
T-Stat Pads
T-Stat Solution
Tubocurarine Chloride Injection
Tucks Clear Gel
Tucks Pads
Tussex Cough Syrup
Tussi-Organidin-S NR Liquid
Tysabri Injection
Ultra Derm Bath Oil
Ultra Derm Lotion
Unoprostone Isopropyl
Valdecoxib
Valrubicin

Valstar Solution
Vascor Tablets
Velosulin BR (rDNA) Injection
Venoglobulin-S Powder for Injection
Versed Injection
Versed Syrup
Vidarabine
Vioxx Suspension
Vioxx Tablets
Vira-A Ointment
VoSol Solution
Wigraine Tablets
Wyamine Sulfate
Wygesic Tablets

Common Abbreviations of Chemotherapy Regimens

5 + 2

Use: Acute myelocytic leukemia (AML; reinduction). *Cycle:* 7 days. Regimen given once after an induction regimen has been used.

Regimen: Cytarabine 100 to 200 mg/m^2/day continuous IV infusion, days 1 through 5
with
Daunorubicin 45 mg/m^2 IV, days 1 and 2
or
Mitoxantrone 12 mg/m^2 IV, days 1 and 2

References: •Amadori S, Ceci A, Comelli A, et al. Treatment of acute myelogenous leukemia in children: results of the Italian Cooperative Study AIEOP/LAM 8204. *J Clin Oncol.* 1987;5:1356-1363.
•Arlin Z, Case DC Jr, Moore J, et al. Randomized multicenter trial of cytosine arabinoside with mitoxantrone or daunorubicin in previously untreated adult patients with acute nonlymphocytic leukemia. *Leukemia.* 1990;4:177-183.

7 + 3

Use: Acute myelocytic leukemia (AML; induction). *Cycle:* 7 days. Give 1 cycle only.

Regimen: Cytarabine 100 to 200 mg/m^2/day continuous IV infusion, days 1 through 7
with
Daunorubicin 30 or 45 mg/m^2/day IV, days 1 through 3
or
Idarubicin 12 mg/m^2/day IV, days 1 through 3
or
Mitoxantrone 12 mg/m^2/day IV, days 1 through 3

References: •Bow EJ, Kilpatrick MG, Scott BA, Clinch JJ, Cheang MS. Acute myeloid leukemia in Manitoba: the consequences of standard "7 + 3" remission-induction therapy followed by high dose cytarabine postremission consolidation for myelosuppression, infectious morbidity, and outcome. *Cancer.* 1994;74:52-60.
•MacCallum PK, Rohatiner AZS, Davis CL, et al. Mitoxantrone and cytosine arabinoside as treatment for acute myeloblastic leukemia in older patients. *Ann Hematol.* 1995;71:35-39.
•Paciucci PA, Dutcher JP, Cuttner J, Strauman JJ, Wiernik PH, Holland JF. Mitoxantrone and Ara-C in previously treated patients with acute myelogenous leukemia. *Leukemia.* 1987;1:565-567.
•Vogler WR, Velez-Garcia E, Omura G, Raney M. A phase-three trial comparing daunorubicin or idarubicin combined with cytosine arabinoside in acute myelogenous leukemia. *Semin Oncol.* 1989;16(suppl 2):21-24.
•Yates J, Glidewell O, Wiernik P, et al. Cytosine arabinoside with daunorubicin or adriamycin for therapy of acute myelocytic leukemia: a CALGB study. *Blood.* 1982;60:454-462.

7 + 3 + 7

Use: Acute myelocytic leukemia (AML; induction—adult). *Cycle*: 21 days. Give 1 cycle. If patient has persistent leukemia at day 21, give 1 to 2 additional cycles.

Regimen: Cytarabine 100 mg/m^2/day continuous IV infusion, days 1 through 7
Daunorubicin 50 mg/m^2/day IV, days 1 through 3
Etoposide 75 mg/m^2/day IV, days 1 through 7

Reference: •Bishop JF, Lowenthal RM, Joshua D, et al. Etoposide in acute nonlymphocytic leukemia. *Blood.* 1990;75:27-32.

"8 in 1"

Use: Brain tumors (pediatric). *Cycle*: 14 days

Regimen: Methylprednisolone 300 mg/m^2/dose PO every 6 hours for 3 doses, day 1, starting at hour 0
Vincristine 1.5 mg/m^2 (2 mg maximum dose) IV, day 1, hour 0
Lomustine 100 mg/m^2 PO, day 1, hour 0
Procarbazine 75 mg/m^2 PO, day 1, hour 1
Hydroxyurea 3,000 mg/m^2 PO, day 1, hour 2
Cisplatin 90 mg/m^2 IV, day 1, starting at hour 3 (6-hour infusion)
Cytarabine 300 mg/m^2 IV, day 1, hour 9
Dacarbazine 150 mg/m^2 IV, day 1, hour 12

References: •Finlay JF, Boyett JM, Yates AJ, et al. Randomized phase III trial in childhood high-grade astrocytoma comparing vincristine, lomustine, and prednisone with the eight-drugs-in-1-day regimen. *J Clin Oncol.* 1995;13:112-123.
•Pendergrass TW, Milstein JM, Geyer JR, et al. Eight drugs in one day chemotherapy for brain tumors: experience in 107 children and rationale for preradiation chemotherapy. *J Clin Oncol.* 1987;5:1221-1231.

ABV

Use: Kaposi sarcoma. *Cycle*: 28 days

Regimen: Doxorubicin 40 mg/m^2 IV, day 1
Bleomycin 15 units IV, days 1 and 15
Vinblastine 6 mg/m^2 IV, day 1

Reference: •Laubenstein LJ, Krigel RL, Odajnyk CM, et al. Treatment of epidemic Kaposi's sarcoma with etoposide or a combination of doxorubicin, bleomycin, and vinblastine. *J Clin Oncol.* 1984;2:1115-1120.

Use: Kaposi sarcoma. *Cycle*: 28 days

Regimen: Doxorubicin 10 mg/m^2 IV, days 1 and 15
Bleomycin 15 units IV, days 1 and 15
Vincristine 1 mg (dose is not in mg/m^2) IV, days 1 and 15

Reference: •Gill PS, Wernz J, Scadden DT, et al. Randomized phase III trial of liposomal daunorubicin versus doxorubicin, bleomycin, and vincristine in AIDS-related Kaposi's sarcoma. *J Clin Oncol.* 1996;14:2353-2364.

ABVD

Use:	Lymphoma (Hodgkin). *Cycle*: 28 days
Regimen:	Doxorubicin 25 mg/m^2 IV, days 1 and 15 Bleomycin 10 units/m^2 IV, days 1 and 15 Vinblastine 6 mg/m^2 IV, days 1 and 15 *with* Dacarbazine 375 mg/m^2 IV, days 1 and 15 *or* Dacarbazine 150 mg/m^2/day IV, days 1 through 5

References: •Bonadonna G, Valagussa P, Santoro A. Alternating non-cross-resistant combination chemotherapy or MOPP in stage IV Hodgkin's disease. *Ann Intern Med.* 1986;104:739-746.
•Bonadonna G, Zucali R, Monfardini S, DeLena M, Uslenghi C. Combination chemotherapy of Hodgkin's disease with adriamycin, bleomycin, vinblastine, and imidazole carboxamide versus MOPP. *Cancer.* 1975;36:252-259.

AC (CY/A)

Use:	Breast cancer. *Cycle*: 21 days
Regimen:	Doxorubicin 60 mg/m^2 IV, day 1 Cyclophosphamide 600 mg/m^2 IV, day 1

Reference: •Fisher B, Brown AM, Dimitrov NV, et al. Two months of doxorubicin-cyclophosphamide with and without interval reinduction therapy compared with 6 months of cyclophosphamide, methotrexate, and fluorouracil in positive-node breast cancer patients with tamoxifen-nonresponsive tumors: results from the National Surgical Adjuvant Breast and Bowel Project B-15. *J Clin Oncol.* 1990;8:1483-1496.

Use:	Sarcoma (bone). *Cycle*: 21 to 28 days
Regimen:	Doxorubicin 30 mg/m^2/day continuous IV infusion, days 1 through 3 Cisplatin 100 mg/m^2 IV, day 4

References: •Ettinger LJ, Douglass HO, Mindell ER, et al. Adjuvant adriamycin and cisplatin in newly diagnosed, nonmetastatic osteosarcoma of the extremity. *J Clin Oncol.* 1986;4:353-362.
•Pathak AB, Advani SH, Iyer RS, et al. Adjuvant chemotherapy for osteogenic sarcoma of the extremity with sequential adriamycin and cisplatin. *J Surg Oncol.* 1993;52:181-184.

Use:	Neuroblastoma (pediatrics). *Cycle*: 21 to 28 days
Regimen:	Cyclophosphamide 150 mg/m^2/day PO, days 1 through 7 Doxorubicin 35 mg/m^2 IV, day 8

Reference: •Nitschke R, Smith EI, Altshuler G, et al. Postoperative treatment of nonmetastatic visible residual neuroblastoma: a Pediatric Oncology Group study. *J Clin Oncol.* 1991;9:1181-1188.

AC/Paclitaxel, Dose Dense

Use: Breast cancer. *Cycle*: 14 days. Give 4 cycles of Treatment A followed by
            4 cycles of Treatment B.

Regimen: **Treatment A** (cycles 1 through 4)
             Doxorubicin 60 mg/m^2 IV, day 1
             Cyclophosphamide 600 mg/m^2 IV, day 1
             Filgrastim 5 mcg/kg/day subcutaneously (rounded to 300 or 480 mcg),
                days 3 through 10
             Treatment B (cycles 5 through 8)
             Paclitaxel 175 mg/m^2 IV, day 1 for 4 cycles
             Filgrastim 5 mcg/kg/day subcutaneously (rounded to 300 or 480 mcg),
                days 3 through 10

Reference: •Citron ML, Berry DA, Cirrincione C, et al. Randomized trial of dose-dense
             versus conventionally scheduled and sequential versus concurrent combi-
             nation chemotherapy as postoperative adjuvant treatment of node-positive
             primary breast cancer: first report of Intergroup trial C9741/Cancer and
             Leukemia Group B trial 9741. *J Clin Oncol*. 2003;21:1431-1439.

AC/Paclitaxel, Sequential

Use: Breast cancer. *Cycle*: 21 days

Regimen: Give 4 cycles of AC regimen for breast cancer
             followed by
             Paclitaxel 175 mg/m^2 IV, day 1 for 4 cycles

Reference: •Henderson IC, Berry D, Demetri G, et al. Improved disease-free and over-
             all survival from the addition of sequential paclitaxel but not from the esca-
             lation of doxorubicin dose level in the adjuvant therapy of patients with
             node-positive primary breast cancer [abstract]. *Proc ASCO*. 1998;17:101a.
             Abstract 390A.

ACE (CAE)

Use: Lung cancer (small cell). *Cycle*: 21 to 28 days

Regimen: Cyclophosphamide 1,000 mg/m^2 IV, day 1
             Doxorubicin 45 mg/m^2 IV, day 1
             Etoposide 50 mg/m^2/day IV, days 1 through 5

Reference: •Aisner J, Whitacre M, Abrams J, Propert K. Doxorubicin, cyclophospha-
             mide, etoposide and platinum, doxorubicin, cyclophosphamide, and etopo-
             side for small-cell carcinoma of the lung. *Semin Oncol*. 1986;13(3 suppl
             3):54-62.

ACe

Use: Breast cancer. *Cycle*: 21 to 28 days

Regimen: Cyclophosphamide 200 mg/m^2/day PO, days 3 through 6
             Doxorubicin 40 mg/m^2 IV, day 1

Reference: •Jones SE, Durie BG, Salmon SE. Combination chemotherapy with adria-
             mycin and cyclophosphamide for advanced breast cancer. *Cancer*.
             1975;36:90-97.

AD

Use: Sarcoma (soft tissue or bone). *Cycle*: 21 days

Regimen: Doxorubicin 45 to 60 mg/m^2 IV, day 1
Dacarbazine 200 to 250 mg/m^2/day IV, days 1 through 5
or
Doxorubicin 15 mg/m^2/day continuous IV infusion, days 1 through 4
Dacarbazine 250 mg/m^2/day continuous IV infusion, days 1 through 4

References: •Antman K, Crowley J, Balcerzak P, et al. An intergroup phase III randomized study of doxorubicin and dacarbazine with or without ifosfamide and mesna in advanced soft tissue and bone sarcomas. *J Clin Oncol.* 1993;11:1276-1285.
•Baker LH, Frank J, Fine G, et al. Combination chemotherapy using adriamycin, DTIC, cyclophosphamide, and actinomycin D for advanced soft tissue sarcomas: a randomized comparative trial. *J Clin Oncol.* 1987;5:851-861.
•Borden EC, Amato DA, Rosenbaum C, et al. Randomized comparison of three adriamycin regimens for metastatic soft tissue sarcomas. *J Clin Oncol.* 1981;5:840-850.

Advanced Stage Burkitt or B-Cell ALL Pediatric Protocol

Use: Lymphoma (Burkitt or B-cell ALL—pediatrics). *Cycle*: 18 to 25 days, based on hematologic recovery. Give Treatment A, then follow with Treatment B after hematologic recovery; repeat alternating treatments a total of 4 times over 5 to 6 months.

Regimen: **Treatment A**
Methotrexate 10 mg/m^2 intrathecal, hours 0 and 72 for first cycle; then hour 0 only of subsequent cycles
Cytarabine 50 mg/m^2 intrathecal, hours 0 and 72 for first cycle; then hour 0 only of subsequent cycles
Cyclophosphamide 300 mg/m^2/dose IV, every 12 hours for 6 doses, given at hours 0, 12, 24, 36, 48, and 60
Vincristine 1.5 mg/m^2 IV, hour 72 (first cycle only: an additional dose at day 11)
Doxorubicin 50 mg/m^2 IV, hour 72
Treatment B (give after hematologic recovery)
Methotrexate 12 mg/m^2 intrathecal, hour 0
Methotrexate 200 mg/m^2 IV, hour 0 (on day 1)
then
Methotrexate 800 mg/m^2/day continuous IV infusion over 24 hours, begin hour 0 (on day 1)
Cytarabine 50 mg/m^2 intrathecal, hour 24 (on day 2, give at end of methotrexate infusion)
Cytarabine 200 mg/m^2/day continuous IV infusion, days 2 and 3 for first cycle.
Increase to 400 mg/m^2/day continuous IV infusion, days 2 and 3 for second cycle; 800 mg/m^2/day continuous IV infusion, days 2 and 3 for third cycle; and 1,600 mg/m^2/day continuous IV infusion, days 2 and 3 for final cycle.
Leucovorin 30 mg/m^2/dose IV, every 6 hours for 2 doses at hours 36 and 42
then
Leucovorin 3 mg/m^2/dose IV, every 12 hours for 3 doses at hours 54, 66, and 78

Advanced Stage Burkitt or B-Cell ALL Pediatric Protocol (cont.)

Reference: •Murphy SB, Bowman WP, Abromowitch M, et al. Results of treatment of advanced-stage Burkitt's lymphoma and B-cell (SIg+) acute lymphoblastic leukemia with high-dose fractionated cyclophosphamide and coordinated high-dose methotrexate and cytarabine. *J Clin Oncol.* 1986;4:1732-1739.

AP

Use: Ovarian, endometrial cancer. *Cycle:* 21 to 28 days

Regimen: Doxorubicin 50 to 60 mg/m^2 IV, day 1
Cisplatin 50 to 60 mg/m^2 IV, day 1

References: •Deppe G, Malviya VK, Malone JM, Christensen CW, Saunders D. Treatment of recurrent and metastatic endometrial carcinoma with cisplatin and doxorubicin. *Eur J Gynaecol Oncol.* 1994;15:263-266.
•Homesley HD, Harry DS, O'Toole RV, et al. Randomized comparison of cisplatin plus epirubicin or doxorubicin for advanced epithelial ovarian carcinoma. *Am J Clin Oncol.* 1992;15:129-134.

ARAC-DNR

Use: Acute myelocytic leukemia (AML). *Cycle:* 14 days. Give 1 cycle. If patient has persistent leukemia on day 14, give 1 to 2 additional cycles as described below.

Regimen: Cytarabine 100 mg/m^2/day continuous IV infusion, days 1 through 7
Daunorubicin 30 or 45 mg/m^2/day IV, days 1 through 3
If leukemia is persistent on day 14, additional doses are given: cytarabine on days 1 through 5, daunorubicin on days 1 and 2

Reference: •Yates J, Glidewell O, Wiernik P, et al. Cytosine arabinoside with daunorubicin or adriamycin for therapy of acute myelocytic leukemia: a CALGB study. *Blood.* 1982;60:454-462.

AT

Use: Breast cancer. *Cycle:* 21 days for up to 8 cycles

Regimen: Doxorubicin 50 mg/m^2 IV, day 1
Paclitaxel 220 mg/m^2 IV over 3 hours, day 2 (given 24 hours after doxorubicin)

Reference: •Jassem J, Pienkowski T, Pluzanska A, et al. Doxorubicin and paclitaxel versus fluorouracil, doxorubicin, and cyclophosphamide as first-line therapy for women with metastatic breast cancer: final results of a randomized phase II multicenter trial. *J Clin Oncol.* 2001;19:1707-1715.

ATRA + CT—see DA + ATRA

B-CAVe

Use: Lymphoma (Hodgkin). *Cycle:* 28 days

Regimen: Bleomycin 5 units/m^2 IV, days 1, 28, and 35
Lomustine 100 mg/m^2 PO, day 1
Doxorubicin 60 mg/m^2 IV, day 1
Vinblastine 5 mg/m^2 IV, day 1

Reference: •Harker WG, Kushlan P, Rosenberg SA. Combination chemotherapy for advanced Hodgkin's disease after failure of MOPP: ABVD and B-CAVe. *Ann Intern Med.* 1984;101:440-446.

BCVPP (BVCPP)

Use: Lymphoma (Hodgkin). *Cycle*: 28 days

Regimen: Carmustine 100 mg/m² IV, day 1
Cyclophosphamide 600 mg/m² IV, day 1
Vinblastine 5 mg/m² IV, day 1
Procarbazine 50 mg/m² PO, day 1
Procarbazine 100 mg/m²/day PO, days 2 through 10
Prednisone 60 mg/m²/day PO, days 1 through 10

Reference: •Bakemeier RF, Anderson JR, Costello W, et al. BCVPP chemotherapy for advanced Hodgkin's disease: evidence for greater duration of complete remission, greater survival, and less toxicity than with a MOPP regimen. *Ann Intern Med.* 1984;101:447-456.

BEACOPP

Use: Lymphoma (Hodgkin). *Cycle*: 21 days

Regimen: Bleomycin 10 units/m² IV, day 8
Etoposide 100 mg/m²/day IV, days 1 through 3
Doxorubicin 25 mg/m² IV, day 1
Cyclophosphamide 650 mg/m² IV, day 1
Vincristine 1.4 mg/m² (2 mg maximum dose) IV, day 1
Procarbazine 100 mg/m²/day PO, days 1 through 7
Prednisone 40 mg/m²/day PO, days 1 through 14
Filgrastim 300 to 480 mcg/day subcutaneously, starting on day 8, give for 3 days or more or until leukocytes exceed 2,000 cells/mm³ for 3 days

References: •Diehl V, Franklin J, Hasenclever D, et al. BEACOPP: a new regimen for advanced Hodgkin's disease. *Ann Oncol.* 1998;9:143-148.
•Tesch H, Diehl V, Lathan B, et al. Moderate dose escalation for advanced stage Hodgkin's disease using the bleomycin, etoposide, adriamycin, cyclophosphamide, vincristine, procarbazine, and prednisone scheme and adjuvant radiotherapy: a study of the German Hodgkin's Lymphoma Study Group. *Blood.* 1998;92:4560-4567.

BEP

Use: Testicular cancer, germ cell tumors. *Cycle*: 21 days

Regimen: Bleomycin 30 units IV, days 2, 9, and 16
Etoposide 100 mg/m²/day IV, days 1 through 5
Cisplatin 20 mg/m²/day IV, days 1 through 5

Reference: •Williams SD, Birch R, Einhorn LH, Irwin L, Greco FA, Loehrer PJ. Treatment of disseminated germ-cell tumors with cisplatin, bleomycin, and either vinblastine or etoposide. *N Engl J Med.* 1987;316:1435-1440.

Bicalutamide + LHRH-A

Use: Prostate cancer. *Cycle*: ongoing

Regimen: Bicalutamide 50 mg PO, daily
with
Goserelin acetate 3.6 mg/dose implant subcutaneously, every 28 days
or
Leuprolide depot 7.5 mg/dose IM, every 28 days

Reference: •Schellhammer P, Sharifi R, Block N, et al. A controlled trial of bicalutamide versus flutamide, each in combination with luteinizing hormone-releasing hormone analogue therapy, in patients with advanced prostate cancer. *Urology.* 1995;45:745-752.

Bio-Chemotherapy—see Interleukin 2-Interferon alfa 2

BIP

Use: Cervical cancer. *Cycle*: 21 days

Regimen: Bleomycin 30 units/day continuous IV infusion over 24 hours, day 1
Cisplatin 50 mg/m^2 IV, day 2
Ifosfamide 5,000 mg/m^2/day continuous IV infusion over 24 hours, day 2
Mesna 6,000 mg/m^2/cycle continuous IV infusion over 36 hours, day 2
(start with ifosfamide)

Reference: •Buxton EJ, Meanwell CA, Hilton C, et al. Combination bleomycin, ifosfamide, and cisplatin chemotherapy in cervical cancer. *J Natl Cancer Inst.* 1989;81:359-361.

BOMP

Use: Cervical cancer. *Cycle*: 6 weeks

Regimen: Bleomycin 10 units IM, days 1, 8, 15, 22, 29, and 36
Vincristine 1 mg/m^2 (2 mg maximum dose) IV, days 1, 8, 22, and 29
Cisplatin 50 mg/m^2 IV, days 1 and 22
Mitomycin 10 mg/m^2 IV, day 1

Reference: •Vogl SE, Moukhtar M, Calanog A, Greenwald EH, Kaplan BH. Chemotherapy for advanced cervical cancer with bleomycin, vincristine, mitomycin C, and cis-diamminedichloroplatinum (II) (BOMP). *Cancer Treat Rep.* 1980;64:1005-1007.

C-MOPP—see COPP

CA

Use: Acute myelocytic leukemia (AML; induction—pediatric). *Cycle*: 7 days. Give 2 cycles. If patient has persistent blasts at day 15, give a third cycle.

Regimen: Cytarabine 3,000 mg/m^2/dose IV every 12 hours for 4 doses, days 1 and 2
Asparaginase 6,000 units/m^2 IM, at hour 42

References: •Capizzi RL, Davis R, Powell B, et al. Synergy between high-dose cytarabine and asparaginase in the treatment of adults with refractory and relapsed acute myelogenous leukemia: a Cancer and Leukemia Group B study. *J Clin Oncol.* 1988;6:499-508.
•Woods WG, Kobrinsky N, Buckley JD. Timed-sequential induction therapy improves postremission outcome in acute myeloid leukemia: a report from the Children's Cancer Group. *Blood.* 1996;87:4979-4989.

CA-VP16 (AVE)

Use: Lung cancer (small cell). *Cycle*: 21 days

Regimen: Cyclophosphamide 1,000 mg/m^2 IV, day 1
Doxorubicin 45 mg/m^2 IV, day 1
Etoposide 80 mg/m^2/day, days 1 through 3

Reference: •Klastersky J, Sculier JP, Dumont JP, et al. Combination chemotherapy with adriamycin, etoposide, and cyclophosphamide for small cell carcinoma of the lung. *Cancer.* 1985;56:71-75.

CABO

Use: Head and neck cancer. *Cycle*: 21 days

Regimen: Cisplatin 50 mg/m^2 IV, day 4
Methotrexate 40 mg/m^2 IV, days 1 and 15
Bleomycin 10 units/dose IV, days 1, 8, and 15
Vincristine 2 mg/dose (dose is not in mg/m^2) IV, days 1, 8, and 15

CABO (cont.)

Reference: •Clavel M, Vermorken JB, Cognetti F, et al. Randomized comparison of cisplatin, methotrexate, bleomycin and vincristine (CABO) versus cisplatin and 5-fluorouracil (CF) versus cisplatin (C) in recurrent or metastatic squamous cell carcinoma of the head and neck. *Ann Oncol.* 1994;5:521-526.

CAE—see ACE

CAF

Use: Breast cancer. *Cycle*: 28 days

Regimen: Cyclophosphamide 100 mg/m^2/day PO, days 1 through 14
Doxorubicin 30 mg/m^2 IV, days 1 and 8
Fluorouracil 500 mg/m^2 IV, days 1 and 8

Reference: •Bull JM, Tormey DC, Li S-H, et al. A randomized comparative trial of adriamycin versus methotrexate in combination drug therapy. *Cancer.* 1978;41:1649-1657.

Use: Breast cancer. *Cycle*: 21 days

Regimen: Cyclophosphamide 500 mg/m^2 IV, day 1
Doxorubicin 50 mg/m^2 IV, day 1
Fluorouracil 500 mg/m^2 IV, day 1

Reference: •Smalley RV, Carpenter J, Bartolucci A, Vogel C, Krauss S. A comparison of cyclophosphamide, adriamycin, 5-fluorouracil (CAF) and cyclophosphamide, methotrexate, 5-fluorouracil, vincristine, prednisone (CMFVP) in patients with metastatic breast cancer. *Cancer.* 1077;10;625-632

CAL-G

Use: Acute lymphocytic leukemia (ALL; induction—adult). *Cycle*: 4 weeks. Give 1 cycle only.

Regimen: Cyclophosphamide 1,200 mg/m^2 IV, day 1
Daunorubicin 45 mg/m^2/day IV, days 1 through 3
Vincristine 2 mg/dose (dose is not in mg/m^2) IV, days 1, 8, 15, and 22
Prednisone 60 mg/m^2/day PO or IV, days 1 through 21
with
Asparaginase 6,000 units/m^2/day subcutaneously, days 5, 8, 11, 15, 18, and 22

Reference: •Larson RA, Dodge RK, Burns CP, et al. A five-drug remission induction regimen with intensive consolidation for adults with acute lymphoblastic leukemia: Cancer and Leukemia Group B study 8811. *Blood.* 1995;85:2025-2037.

CAMP

Use: Lung cancer (non-small cell). *Cycle*: 28 days

Regimen: Cyclophosphamide 300 mg/m^2 IV, days 1 and 8
Doxorubicin 20 mg/m^2 IV, days 1 and 8
Methotrexate 15 mg/m^2 IV, days 1 and 8
Procarbazine 100 mg/m^2/day PO, days 1 through 10

Reference: •Bitran JD, Desser RK, DeMeester TR, et al. Cyclophosphamide, adriamycin, methotrexate, and procarbazine (CAMP)—effective four-drug combination chemotherapy for metastatic non-oat cell bronchogenic carcinoma. *Cancer Treat Rep.* 1976;60:1225-1230.

CAP

Use: Lung cancer (non-small cell). *Cycle*: 28 days

Regimen: Cyclophosphamide 400 mg/m^2 IV, day 1
Doxorubicin 40 mg/m^2 IV, day 1
Cisplatin 60 mg/m^2 IV, day 1

Reference: •Eagan RT, Frytak S, Creagan ET, Ingle JN, Kvols LK, Coles DT. Phase II study of cyclophosphamide, adriamycin, and cis-dichlorodiammineplatinum (II) by infusion in patients with adenocarcinoma and large cell carcinoma of the lung. *Cancer Treat Rep.* 1979;63:1589-1591.

Capecitabine-Docetaxel

Use: Breast cancer. *Cycle*: 21 days

Regimen: Capecitabine 1,250 mg/m^2/dose PO twice daily, days 1 through 14
Docetaxel 75 mg/m^2 IV, day 1

Reference: •O'Shaughnessy J, Miles D, Vukelja S, et al. Superior survival with capecitabine plus docetaxel combination therapy in anthracycline-pretreated patients with advanced breast cancer: phase III trial results. *J Clin Oncol.* 2002;20:2812-2823.

CAPIRI

Use: Colorectal cancer. *Cycle*: 21 days

Regimen: Capecitabine 1,000 mg/m^2/dose PO twice daily, days 1 through 14
Irinotecan 80 to 100 mg/m^2 IV, days 1 and 8

References: •Grothey A, Jordan K, Kellner C, et al. Capecitabine/irinotecan (CapIri) and capecitabine/oxaliplatin (CapOx) are active second-line protocols in patients with advanced colorectal cancer (ACRC) after failure of first-line combination therapy: results of a randomized phase II study [abstract 3354]. *J Clin Oncol.* 2004;22(14S):253a.
•Grothey A, Jordan K, Kellner C, et al. Randomized phase II trial of capecitabine plus irinotecan (CapIri) vs. capecitabine plus oxaliplatin (CapOx) as first-line therapy of advanced colorectal cancer (ACRC) [abstract 1022]. *Proc ASCO.* 2003;22:255a.

Carboplatin-Fluorouracil—see CF

Carbo-Tax (see also CaT)

Use: Ovarian cancer. *Cycle*: 21 days

Regimen: Paclitaxel 175 mg/m^2 IV over 3 hours, day 1
Carboplatin IV dose by Calvert equation to AUC 7.5 mg/mL/min, day 1 (after paclitaxel)
or
Paclitaxel 185 mg/m^2 IV over 3 hours, day 1
Carboplatin IV dose by Calvert equation to AUC 6 mg/mL/min, day 1 (after paclitaxel)

References: •Meerpohl H, du Bois A, Kuhnle H, et al. Paclitaxel combined with carboplatin in the first-line treatment of advanced ovarian cancer. *Semin Oncol.* 1995;22(6 suppl 15):7-12.
•Ozols RF. Combination regimens of paclitaxel and the platinum drugs as first-line regimens for ovarian cancer. *Semin Oncol.* 1995;22(6 suppl 15): 1-6.

Carbo-Tax (see also CaT) (cont.)

Use: Adenocarcinoma (unknown primary). *Cycle:* 21 days for up to 8 cycles

Regimen: Paclitaxel 200 mg/m^2 IV over 3 hours, day 1 (after carboplatin)
Carboplatin IV dose by Calvert equation to AUC 6 mg/mL/min, day 1
Filgrastim 300 mcg/day subcutaneously, days 5 to 12

Reference: •Briasoulis E, Kalofonos H, Bafaloukos D, et al. Carboplatin plus paclitaxel in unknown primary carcinoma: a phase II Hellenic Cooperative Oncology Group study. *J Clin Oncol.* 2000;18:3101-3107.

CaT (see also Carbo-Tax)

Use: Adenocarcinoma (unknown primary), lung cancer (non-small cell), ovarian cancer. *Cycle:* 21 days

Regimen: Carboplatin IV dose by Calvert equation to AUC 7.5 mg/mL/min, day 1 or 2 (give after paclitaxel infusion)
with
Paclitaxel 175 mg/m^2 IV over 3 hours, day 1
or
Paclitaxel 135 mg/m^2/day continuous IV infusion over 24 hours, on day 1

References: •Bookman MA, McGuire WP III, Kilpatrick D, et al. Carboplatin and paclitaxel in ovarian carcinoma: a phase I study of the Gynecologic Oncology Group. *J Clin Oncol.* 1996;14:1895-1902.
•Langer CJ, Leighton JC, Comis RL, et al. Paclitaxel by 24- or 1-hour infusion in combination with carboplatin in advanced non-small cell lung cancer: the Fox Chase Cancer Center experience. *Semin Oncol.* 1995;22 (4 suppl 9):18-29.

Use: Lung cancer (non-small cell). *Cycle:* 21 days

Regimen: Carboplatin IV dose by Calvert equation to AUC 6 mg/mL/min, day 1 (give after paclitaxel)
Paclitaxel 225 mg/m^2 IV over 3 hours, day 1

Reference: •Schiller JH, Harrington D, Belani CP, et al. Comparison of four chemotherapy regimens for advanced non-small-cell lung cancer. *N Engl J Med.* 2002;346:92-98.

CAV (VAC)

Use: Lung cancer (small cell). *Cycle:* 21 days

Regimen: Cyclophosphamide 1,000 mg/m^2 IV, day 1
Doxorubicin 40 to 50 mg/m^2 IV, day 1
Vincristine 1 to 1.4 mg/m^2 (2 mg maximum dose) IV, day 1

References: •Comis RL. Clinical trials of cyclophosphamide, etoposide, and vincristine in the treatment of small-cell lung cancer. *Semin Oncol.* 1986;13(3 suppl 3):40-44.
•Greco FA, Richardson RL, Schulman SF, Stroup S, Oldham RK. Treatment of oat cell carcinoma of the lung: complete remissions, acceptable complications, and improved survival. *BMJ.* 1978;2:10-11.

CAV/EP

Use:	Lung cancer (small cell). *Cycle*: 42 days for 3 cycles
Regimen:	Cyclophosphamide 1,000 mg/m^2 IV, day 1
	Doxorubicin 50 mg/m^2 IV, day 1
	Vincristine* 1.2 mg/m^2 IV, day 1
	Etoposide 100 mg/m^2/day IV, days 22 through 24
	Cisplatin 25 mg/m^2/day IV, days 22 through 24
	*Note: The vincristine dose is not capped in this protocol. Consult the prescriber if there is any question about the intended vincristine dose.
Reference:	•Murray N, Livingston RB, Shepard FA, et al. Randomized study of CODE versus alternating CAV/EP for extensive-stage small-cell lung cancer: an intergroup study of the National Cancer Institute of Canada Clinical Trials Group and the Southwest Oncology Group. *J Clin Oncol.* 1999;17:2300-2308.

CAVE

Use:	Lung cancer (small cell). *Cycle*: 21 days
Regimen:	Cyclophosphamide 1,000 mg/m^2 IV, day 1
	Doxorubicin 50 mg/m^2 IV, day 1
	Vincristine 2 mg (dose is not in mg/m^2) IV, day 1
	Etoposide 100 mg/m^2/day IV, days 2 through 4
Reference:	•Tummarello D, Graziano F, Mari D, et al. Small cell lung cancer (SCLC): a randomized trial of cyclophosphamide, adriamycin, vincristine plus etoposide (CAV-E) or teniposide (CAV-T) as induction treatment, followed in complete responders by alfa-interferon or no treatment, as maintenance therapy. *Anticancer Res.* 1994;14:2221-2227.

CC

Use:	Ovarian cancer. *Cycle*: 28 days
Regimen:	Cyclophosphamide 600 mg/m^2 IV, day 1
	Carboplatin 300 to 350 mg/m^2 IV, day 1
References:	•Meerpohl HG, Sauerbrei W, Kühnle H, Schumacher M, Pfleiderer A. Randomized study comparing carboplatin/cyclophosphamide and cisplatin/cyclophosphamide as first-line treatment in patients with stage III/IV epithelial ovarian cancer and small volume disease. *Gynecol Oncol.* 1997;66:75-84.
	•Swenerton K, Jeffrey J, Stuart G, et al. Cisplatin-cyclophosphamide versus carboplatin-cyclophosphamide in advanced ovarian cancer: a randomized phase III study of the National Cancer Institute of Canada Clinical Trials Group. *J Clin Oncol.* 1992;10:718-726.

CDB

Use:	Melanoma. *Cycle*: 21 days
Regimen:	Cisplatin 25 mg/m^2/day IV, days 1 through 3
	Dacarbazine 220 mg/m^2/day IV, days 1 through 3
	Carmustine 150 mg/m^2 IV, day 1 of odd-numbered cycles only (eg, cycle 1, 3, 5)
Reference:	•Creagan ET, Suman VJ, Dalton RJ, et al. Phase III clinical trial of the combination of cisplatin, dacarbazine, and carmustine with or without tamoxifen in patients with advanced malignant melanoma. *J Clin Oncol.* 1999;17:1884-1890.

CDB + Tamoxifen (Dartmouth regimen)

Use: Melanoma. *Cycle*: 21 days

Regimen: Tamoxifen 10 mg PO twice daily, continuously, started 1 week prior to cytotoxic chemotherapy
Cisplatin 25 mg/m^2/day IV, days 1 through 3
Dacarbazine 220 mg/m^2/day IV, days 1 through 3
Carmustine 150 mg/m^2 IV, day 1 of odd-numbered cycles only (eg, cycle 1, 3, 5), given before cisplatin and dacarbazine

Reference: •Chapman PB, Einhorn LH, Meyers ML, et al. Phase III multicenter randomized trial of the Dartmouth regimen versus dacarbazine in patients with metastatic melanoma. *J Clin Oncol.* 1999;17:2745-2751.

CDDP/VP-16

Use: Brain tumors (pediatrics). *Cycle*: 21 days

Regimen: Cisplatin 90 mg/m^2 IV, day 1
Etoposide 150 mg/m^2/day IV, days 3 and 4

Reference: •Kovnar EH, Kellie SJ, Horowitz ME, et al. Preirradiation cisplatin and etoposide in the treatment of high-risk medulloblastoma and other malignant embryonal tumors of the central nervous system: a phase II study. *J Clin Oncol.* 990;8:330-336.

CDE

Use: Lymphoma (HIV-related, non-Hodgkin—adult). *Cycle*: 28 days

Regimen: Cyclophosphamide 200 mg/m^2/day continuous IV infusion, days 1 through 4
Doxorubicin 12.5 mg/m^2/day continuous IV infusion, days 1 through 4
Etoposide 60 mg/m^2/day continuous IV infusion, days 1 through 4
Filgrastim 5 mcg/kg/day subcutaneously starting on day 6, at least 24 hours after the end of the continuous infusions, and ending when the absolute neutrophil count (ANC) Is 10,000 cells/mm^3 or higher

Reference: •Sparano JA, Wiernik PH, Hu X, et al. Pilot trial of infusional cyclophosphamide, doxorubicin, and etoposide plus didanosine and filgrastim in patients with human immunodeficiency virus-associated non-Hodgkin's lymphoma. *J Clin Oncol.* 1996;14:3026-3035.

CEF (see also FEC)

Use: Breast cancer. *Cycle*: 28 days

Regimen: Cyclophosphamide 75 mg/m^2/day PO, days 1 through 14
Epirubicin 60 mg/m^2 IV, days 1 and 8
Fluorouracil 500 mg/m^2 IV, days 1 and 8
Cotrimoxazole 2 tablets PO twice daily, days 1 through 28

Reference: •Levine MN, Bramwell VH, Pritchard KI, et al. Randomized trial of intensive cyclophosphamide, epirubicin, and fluorouracil chemotherapy compared with cyclophosphamide, methotrexate, and fluorouracil in premenopausal women with node-positive breast cancer. *J Clin Oncol.* 1998;16:2651-2658.

CEPP(B)

Use:	Lymphoma (non-Hodgkin). *Cycle*: 28 days
Regimen:	Cyclophosphamide 600 to 650 mg/m^2 IV, days 1 and 8 Etoposide 70 to 85 mg/m^2/day IV, days 1 through 3 Prednisone 60 mg/m^2/day PO, days 1 through 10 Procarbazine 60 mg/m^2/day PO, days 1 through 10 *may or may not give with* Bleomycin 15 units/m^2 IV, days 1 and 15
Reference:	•Chao NJ, Rosenberg SA, Horning SJ. CEPP(B): an effective and well-tolerated regimen in poor-risk, aggressive non-Hodgkin's lymphoma. *Blood.* 1990;76:1293-1298.

CEV

Use:	Lung cancer (small cell). *Cycle*: 21 days
Regimen:	Cyclophosphamide 1,000 mg/m^2 IV, day 1 Etoposide 50 mg/m^2 IV, day 1 Etoposide 100 mg/m^2/day PO, days 2 through 5 Vincristine 1.4 mg/m^2 (2 mg maximum dose) IV, day 1
References:	•Comis RL. Clinical trials of cyclophosphamide, etoposide, and vincristine in the treatment of small-cell lung cancer. *Semin Oncol.* 1986;13(3 suppl 3): 40-44. •Hong WK, Nicaise C, Lawson R, et al. Etoposide combined with cyclophosphamide plus vincristine compared with doxorubicin plus cyclophosphamide plus vincristine and with high-dose cyclophosphamide plus vincristine in the treatment of small-cell carcinoma of the lung: a randomized trial of the Bristol Lung Cancer Study Group. *J Clin Oncol.* 1989;7:450-456.

CF

Use:	Adenocarcinoma, head and neck cancer. *Cycle*: 21 to 28 days
Regimen:	Cisplatin 100 mg/m^2 IV, day 1 Fluorouracil 1,000 mg/m^2/day continuous IV infusion, days 1 through 4 or days 1 through 5
References:	•De Andrés L, Brunet J, López-Pousa A, et al. Randomized trial of neoadjuvant cisplatin and fluorouracil versus carboplatin and fluorouracil in patients with stage IV-M0 head and neck cancer. *J Clin Oncol.* 1995;13:1493-1500. •Kish JA, Ensley JF, Jacobs J, Weaver A, Cummings G, Al-Sarraf M. A randomized trial of cisplatin (CACP) + 5-fluorouracil (5-FU) infusion and CACP + 5-FU bolus for recurrent and advanced squamous cell carcinoma of the head and neck. *Cancer.* 1985;56:2740-2744. •Rowland KM Jr, Taylor SG IV, Spiers AS, et al. Cisplatin and 5-FU infusion chemotherapy in advanced, recurrent cancer of the head and neck: an Eastern Cooperative Oncology Group Pilot study. *Cancer Treat Rep.* 1986;70:461-464.

CF (cont.)

Use:	Head and neck cancer. *Cycle*: 21 to 28 days
Regimen:	Carboplatin 400 mg/m^2 IV, day 1
	Fluorouracil 1,000 mg/m^2/day continuous IV infusion, days 1 through 4 or days 1 through 5
References:	•De Andrés L, Brunet J, López-Pousa A, et al. Randomized trial of neoadjuvant cisplatin and fluorouracil versus carboplatin and fluorouracil in patients with stage IV-M0 head and neck cancer. *J Clin Oncol.* 1995;13:1493-1500.
	•Gregoire V, Beauduin M, Humblet Y, et al. A phase I-II trial of induction chemotherapy with carboplatin and fluorouracil in locally advanced head and neck squamous cell carcinoma: a report from the UCL-Oncology Group, Belgium. *J Clin Oncol.* 1991;9:1385-1392.

CFM—see CNF

CHAMOCA (Modified Bagshawe)

Use:	Gestational trophoblastic neoplasm. *Cycle*: 18 days or longer, as toxicity permits
Regimen:	Hydroxyurea 500 mg/dose PO every 6 hours for 4 doses, day 1 (start at 6 am)
	Dactinomycin 0.2 mg/day (dose is not in mg/m^2) IV, days 1 through 3 (give at 7 pm)
	Vincristine 1 mg/m^2 IV (2 mg maximum dose), day 2 (give at 7 am)
	Methotrexate 100 mg/m^2 IV push, day 2 (give at 7 pm)
	Methotrexate 200 mg/m^2 IV over 12 hours, day 2 (give after IV push dose)
	Leucovorin 14 mg/dose IM every 6 hours for 6 doses, days 3 through 5 (begin at 7 pm on day 3)
	Cyclophosphamide 500 mg/m^2 IV, days 3 and 8 (give at 7 pm)
	Dactinomycin 0.5 mg/day (dose is not in mg/m^2) IV, days 4 and 5 (give at 7 pm)
	Doxorubicin 30 mg/m^2 IV, day 8 (give at 7 pm)
Reference:	•Weed JC, Barnard DE, Currie JL, Clayton LA, Hammond CB. Chemotherapy with the modified Bagshawe protocol for poor prognosis metastatic trophoblastic disease. *Obstet Gynecol.* 1982;59:377-380.

CHAP

Use:	Ovarian cancer. *Cycle*: 28 days
Regimen:	Cyclophosphamide 150 mg/m^2/day PO, days 2 through 8
	or
	Cyclophosphamide 400 mg/m^2 IV, day 1
	with
	Doxorubicin 30 mg/m^2 IV, day 1
	Cisplatin 50 to 60 mg/m^2 IV, day 1
	Altretamine 150 mg/m^2/day PO, days 2 through 8
References:	•Bruckner HW, Cohen CJ, Deppe G, et al. Treatment of chemotherapy-resistant advanced ovarian cancer with a combination of cyclophosphamide, hexamethylmelamine, adriamycin, and *cis*-diamminedichloroplatinum (CHAP). *Gynecol Oncol.* 1981;12:150-153.
	•Edmonson JH, McCormack GW, Fleming TR, et al. Comparison of cyclophosphamide plus cisplatin versus hexamethylmelamine, cyclophosphamide, doxorubicin, and cisplatin in combination as initial chemotherapy for stage III and IV ovarian carcinomas. *Cancer Treat Rep.* 1985;69:1243-1248.

ChlVPP

Use:	Lymphoma (Hodgkin). *Cycle*: 28 days
Regimen:	Chlorambucil 6 mg/m²/day (10 mg/day maximum dose) PO, days 1 through 14

Regimen: Chlorambucil 6 mg/m²/day (10 mg/day maximum dose) PO, days 1 through 14
Vinblastine 6 mg/m² (10 mg/day maximum dose) IV, days 1 and 8
Procarbazine 100 mg/m²/day (150 mg/day maximum dose) PO, days 1 through 14
Prednisone 40 to 50 mg/day PO, days 1 through 14*
*Note: Prednisolone is recommended in the British literature. In the United States, prednisone is the preferred corticosteroid. The doses of these 2 corticosteroids are equivalent (ie, prednisone 40 mg PO = prednisolone 40 mg PO).

References: •Radford JA, Crowther D, Rohatiner AZS, et al. Results of a randomized trial comparing MVPP chemotherapy with a hybrid regimen, ChlVPP/EVA, in the initial treatment of Hodgkin's disease. *J Clin Oncol.* 1995;13:2379-2385.
•Selby P, Patel P, Milan S, et al. ChlVPP combination chemotherapy for Hodgkin's disease: long term results. *Br J Cancer.* 1990;62:279-285.

ChlVPP/EVA

Use: Lymphoma (Hodgkin). *Cycle*: 28 days

Regimen: Chlorambucil 10 mg/day PO, days 1 through 7
Vinblastine 10 mg (dose is not in mg/m²) IV, day 1
Procarbazine 150 mg/day PO, days 1 through 7
Prednisone 50 mg/day PO, days 1 through 7*
with
Etoposide 200 mg/m² IV, day 8
Vincristine 2 mg (dose is not in mg/m²) IV, day 8
Doxorubicin 50 mg/m² IV, day 8
*Note: Prednisolone is recommended in the British literature. In the United States, prednisone is the preferred corticosteroid. The doses of these 2 corticosteroids are equivalent (ie, prednisone 40 mg PO = prednisolone 40 mg PO).

Reference: •Radford JA, Crowther D, Rohatiner AZS, et al. Results of a randomized trial comparing MVPP chemotherapy with a hybrid regimen, ChlVPP/EVA, in the initial treatment of Hodgkin's disease. *J Clin Oncol.* 1995;13:2379-2385.

CHOP

Use: Lymphoma (non-Hodgkin), HIV-related lymphoma. *Cycle*: 21 to 28 days

Regimen: Cyclophosphamide 750 mg/m² IV, day 1
Doxorubicin 50 mg/m² IV, day 1
Vincristine 1.4 mg/m² (2 mg maximum dose) IV, day 1
Prednisone 100 mg/day PO, days 1 through 5

References: •Armitage JO, Dick FR, Corder MP, Garneau SC, Platz CE, Slymen DJ. Predicting therapeutic outcome in patients with diffuse histiocytic lymphoma treated with cyclophosphamide, adriamycin, vincristine, and prednisone (CHOP). *Cancer.* 1982;50:1695-1702.
•McKelvey EM, Gottlieb JA, Wilson HE, et al. Hydroxyldaunomycin (adriamycin) combination chemotherapy in malignant lymphoma. *Cancer.* 1976;38:1484-1493.
•Weiss R, Huhn D, Mitrou P, et al. HIV-related non-Hodgkin's lymphoma: CHOP induction therapy and interferon-alpha-2b/zidovudine maintenance therapy. *Leuk Lymphoma.* 1998;29:103-118.

CHOP (cont.)

Use: Lymphoma (non-Hodgkin; induction and consolidation—pediatric)

Regimen: **Induction**. *Cycle*: Give 1 cycle only (6 weeks)
Cyclophosphamide 750 mg/m^2 IV, days 1 and 22
Doxorubicin 40 mg/m^2 IV, days 1 and 22
Vincristine 1.5 mg/m^2 (2 mg maximum dose) IV weekly, weeks 1 through 6
Prednisone 40 mg/m^2/day PO, days 1 through 28
may be used in conjunction with
Radiation therapy

Consolidation therapy. *Cycle*: 21 days
Cyclophosphamide 750 mg/m^2 IV, day 1
Doxorubicin 40 mg/m^2 IV, day 1
Vincristine 1.5 mg/m^2 (2 mg maximum dose) IV, day 1
Prednisone 40 mg/m^2/day PO, days 1 through 5
Note: CHOP refers to induction and consolidation phase. Protocol also includes maintenance and central nervous system prophylaxis.

Reference: •Link MP, Donaldson SS, Berard CW, Shuster JJ, Murphy SB. Results of treatment of childhood localized non-Hodgkin's lymphoma with combination chemotherapy with or without radiotherapy. *N Engl J Med*. 1990;322:1169-1174.

CHOP-BLEO

Use: Lymphoma (non-Hodgkin). *Cycle*: 21 to 28 days

Regimen: **Add to CHOP:** Bleomycin 15 units/day IV, days 1 through 5

Reference: •Rodriguez V, Cabanillas F, Burgess MA, et al. Combination chemotherapy ("CHOP-Bleo") in advanced (non-Hodgkin) malignant lymphoma. *Blood*. 1977;49:325-333.

CHOP + Rituximab (R-CHOP)

Use: Lymphoma (B-cell). *Cycle*: 21 days for up to 8 cycles

Regimen: **Add to CHOP:** Rituximab 375 mg/m^2 IV, day 1

References: •Coiffier B, Lepage E, Briere J, et al. CHOP chemotherapy plus rituximab compared with CHOP alone in elderly patients with diffuse large-B-cell lymphoma. *N Engl J Med*. 2002;346:235-242.
•Czuczman MS, Grillo-López AJ, White CA, et al. Treatment of patients with low-grade B-cell lymphoma with the combination of chimeric anti-CD20 monoclonal antibody and CHOP chemotherapy. *J Clin Oncol*. 1999;17:268-276.

CISCA

Use: Bladder cancer. *Cycle*: 21 to 28 days

Regimen: Cyclophosphamide 650 mg/m^2 IV, day 1
Doxorubicin 50 mg/m^2 IV, day 1
Cisplatin 100 mg/m^2 IV, day 2

Reference: •Sternberg JJ, Bracken RB, Handel PB, Johnson DE. Combination chemotherapy (CISCA) for advanced urinary tract carcinoma. *JAMA*. 1977;238:2282-2287.

CISCA II/VB IV

Use: Germ cell tumors. *Cycle*: Individualized based on duration of myelosuppression

Regimen: Cyclophosphamide 500 mg/m^2/day IV, days 1 and 2
Doxorubicin 40 to 45 mg/m^2/day IV, days 1 and 2
Cisplatin 100 to 120 mg/m^2 IV, day 3
alternating with
Vinblastine 3 mg/m^2/day continuous IV infusion, days 1 through 5
Bleomycin 30 units/day continuous IV infusion, days 1 through 5

References: •Logothetis CJ, Samuels ML, Selig DE, et al. Cyclic chemotherapy with cyclophosphamide, doxorubicin, and cisplatin plus vinblastine and bleomycin in advanced germinal tumors. *Am J Med.* 1986;81:219-228.
•Logothetis CJ, Samuels ML, Selig D, Swanson D, Johnson DE, von Eschenbach AC. Improved survival with cyclic chemotherapy for nonseminomatous germ cell tumors of the testis. *J Clin Oncol.* 1985;3:326-335.

Cisplatin-Docetaxel

Use: Bladder cancer.*Cycle*: Every 7 days for 8 weeks

Regimen: Cisplatin 30 mg/m^2 IV, day 1
Docetaxel 40 mg/m^2 IV, day 4
used in conjunction with
Radiation therapy

Reference: •Varveris H, Delakas D, Anezinis P, et al. Concurrent platinum and docetaxel chemotherapy and external radical radiotherapy in patients with invasive transitional cell bladder carcinoma. *Anticancer Res.* 1997;17(6D):4771-4780.

Use: Bladder cancer. *Cycle*: 21 days

Regimen: Cisplatin 75 mg/m^2 IV, day 1
Docetaxel 75 mg/m^2 IV, day 1

Reference: •Sengeløv L, Kamby C, Lund B, Engelholm SA. Docetaxel and cisplatin in metastatic urothelial cancer: a phase II study. *J Clin Oncol.* 1998;16:3392-3397.

Cisplatin-Fluorouracil

Use: Cervical cancer. *Cycle*: 21 days

Regimen: Cisplatin 75 mg/m^2 IV, day 1
followed by
Fluorouracil 1,000 mg/m^2/day continuous IV infusion, days 1 through 4
  (for 96 hours total)
used in conjunction with
Radiation therapy

Reference: •Morris M, Eifel PJ, Lu J, et al. Pelvic radiation with concurrent chemotherapy compared with pelvic and para-aortic radiation for high-risk cervical cancer. *N Engl J Med.* 1999;340:1137-1143.

Use: Cervical cancer. *Cycle*: 28 days

Regimen: Cisplatin 50 mg/m^2 IV, day 1 starting 4 hours *before* external beam radiotherapy
Fluorouracil 1,000 mg/m^2/day continuous IV infusion, days 2 through 5

Reference: •Whitney CW, Sause W, Bundy BN, et al. Randomized comparison of fluorouracil plus cisplatin versus hydroxyurea as an adjunct to radiation therapy in stage IIB-IVA carcinoma of the cervix with negative para-aortic lymph nodes: a Gynecologic Oncology Group and Southwest Oncology Group study. *J Clin Oncol.* 1999;17:1339-1348.

Cisplatin-Vinorelbine (see also Vinorelbine-Cisplatin)

Use: Cervical cancer. *Cycle*: 21 days

Regimen: Cisplatin 80 mg/m² IV, day 1
Vinorelbine 25 mg/m² IV, days 1 and 8

Reference: •Pignata S, Silvestro G, Ferrari E, et al. Phase II study of cisplatin and vinorelbine as first-line chemotherapy in patients with carcinoma of the uterine cervix. *J Clin Oncol.* 1999;17:756-760.

CLD-BOMP

Use: Cervical cancer. *Cycle*: 21 days

Regimen: Bleomycin 5 units/day continuous IV infusion, days 1 through 7
Cisplatin 10 mg/m²/day IV, days 1 through 7
Vincristine* 0.7 mg/m² IV, day 7
Mitomycin 7 mg/m² IV, day 7
*Note: The vincristine dose is not capped in this protocol. Consult the prescriber if there is any question about the intended vincristine dose.

Reference: •Shimuzu Y, Akiyama F, Umezawa S, Ishiya T, Utsugi K, Hasumi K. Combination of consecutive low-dose cisplatin with bleomycin, vincristine, and mitomycin for recurrent cervical carcinoma. *J Clin Oncol.* 1998;16:1869-1878.

CMF

Use: Breast cancer. *Cycle*: 28 days

Regimen 1:   Patients 65 years of age and younger:
Methotrexate 40 mg/m² IV, days 1 and 8
Fluorouracil 600 mg/m² IV, days 1 and 8
with
Cyclophosphamide 100 mg/m²/day PO, days 1 through 14
or
Cyclophosphamide 750 mg/m² IV, day 1

Regimen 2:   Patients older than 65 years of age:
Methotrexate 30 mg/m² IV, days 1 and 8
Fluorouracil 400 mg/m² IV, days 1 and 8
Cyclophosphamide 100 mg/m²/day PO, days 1 through 14

References: •Bonadonna G, Brusamolino E, Valagussa P, et al. Combination chemotherapy as an adjuvant treatment in operable breast cancer. *N Engl J Med.* 1976;294:405-410.
•Canellos GP, Pocock SJ, Taylor SG III, Sears ME, Klaasen DJ, Band PR. Combination chemotherapy for metastatic breast carcinoma. *Cancer.* 1976;38:1882-1886.
•Fisher B, Brown AM, Dimitrov NV, et al. Two months of doxorubicin-cyclophosphamide with and without interval reinduction therapy compared with 6 months of cyclophosphamide, methotrexate, and fluorouracil in positive-node breast cancer patients with tamoxifen-nonresponsive tumors: results from the National Surgical Adjuvant Breast and Bowel Project B-15. *J Clin Oncol.* 1990;8:1483-1496.

CMF-IV

Use: Breast cancer. *Cycle*: 21 days

Regimen: Cyclophosphamide 600 mg/m² IV, day 1
Methotrexate 40 mg/m² IV, day 1
Fluorouracil 600 mg/m² IV, day 1

Reference: •Moliterni A, Bonadonna G, Valagussa P, Ferrari L, Zambetti M. Cyclophosphamide, methotrexate, and fluorouracil with and without doxorubicin in the adjuvant treatment of resectable breast cancer with one to three positive axillary nodes. *J Clin Oncol.* 1991;9:1124-1130.

CMFP

Use: Breast cancer. *Cycle*: 28 days

Regimen: Cyclophosphamide 100 mg/m²/day PO, days 1 through 14
Methotrexate 30 to 40 mg/m² IV, days 1 and 8
Fluorouracil 400 to 600 mg/m² IV, days 1 and 8
Prednisone 40 mg/m²/day PO, days 1 through 14

Reference: •Marschke RF, Ingle JN, Schaid DJ, et al. Randomized clinical trial of CFP versus CMFP in women with metastatic breast cancer. *Cancer.* 1989;63:1931-1937.

CMFVP

Use: Breast cancer. *Cycle*: 28 days

Regimen: Cyclophosphamide 400 mg/m² IV, day 1
Methotrexate 30 mg/m² IV, days 1 and 8
Fluorouracil 400 mg/m² IV, days 1 and 8
Vincristine 1 mg (dose is not in mg/m²) IV, days 1 and 8
Prednisone 80 mg/day PO, days 1 through 7

Reference: •Smalley RV, Carpenter J, Bartolucci A, Vogel C, Krauss S. A comparison of cyclophosphamide, adriamycin, 5-fluorouracil (CAF) and cyclophosphamide, methotrexate, 5-fluorouracil, vincristine, prednisone (CMFVP) in patients with metastatic breast cancer. *Cancer.* 1977;40:625-632.

CMV

Use: Bladder cancer. *Cycle*: 21 days

Regimen: Cisplatin 100 mg/m² IV, day 2 (at least 12 hours after methotrexate)
Methotrexate 30 mg/m² IV, days 1 and 8
Vinblastine 4 mg/m² IV, days 1 and 8

Reference: •Harker WG, Meyers FJ, Freiha FS, et al. Cisplatin, methotrexate, and vinblastine (CMV): an effective chemotherapy regimen for metastatic transitional cell carcinoma of the urinary tract: a Northern California Oncology Group study. *J Clin Oncol.* 1985;3:1463-1470.

CNF

Use: Breast cancer. *Cycle*: 21 days

Regimen: Cyclophosphamide 500 mg/m² IV, day 1
Mitoxantrone 10 mg/m² IV, day 1
Fluorouracil 500 mg/m² IV, day 1

Reference: •Bennett JM, Muss HB, Doroshow JH, et al. A randomized multicenter trial comparing mitoxantrone, cyclophosphamide, and fluorouracil with doxorubicin, cyclophosphamide, and fluorouracil in the therapy of metastatic breast carcinoma. *J Clin Oncol.* 1988;6:1611-1620.

CNOP

Use: Lymphoma (non-Hodgkin). *Cycle*: 21 to 28 days

Regimen: Cyclophosphamide 750 mg/m^2 IV, day 1
Mitoxantrone 12 mg/m^2 IV, day 1
Vincristine 1.4 mg/m^2 (2 mg maximum dose) IV, day 1
Prednisone 50 mg/m^2/day PO, days 1 through 5

Reference: •Brusamolino E, Bertini M, Guidi S, et al. CHOP versus CNOP (N=mitoxantrone) in non-Hodgkin's lymphoma: an interim report comparing efficacy and toxicity. *Haematologica.* 1988;73:217-222.

COB

Use: Head and neck cancer. *Cycle*: 21 days

Regimen: Cisplatin 100 mg/m^2 IV, day 1
Vincristine 1 mg (dose is not in mg/m^2) IV, days 2 and 5
Bleomycin 30 units/day continuous IV infusion, days 2 through 5

References: •Drelichman A, Cummings G, Al-Sarraf M. A randomized trial of the combination of cis-platinum, oncovin and bleomycin (COB) versus methotrexate in patients with advanced squamous cell carcinoma of the head and neck. *Cancer.* 1983;52:399-403.
•Peppard SB, Al-Sarraf M, Powers WE, Loh JK, Weaver AW. Combination of cis-platinum, oncovin, and bleomycin (COB) prior to surgery and/or radiotherapy in advanced untreated epidermoid cancer of the head and neck. *Laryngoscope.* 1980;90:1273-1280.

CODE

Use: Lung cancer (small cell). *Cycle*: 9-week regimen

Regimen: Cisplatin 25 mg/m^2 IV, every week for 9 weeks
Vincristine 1 mg/m^2 (2 mg maximum dose) IV weekly, weeks 1, 2, 4, 6, and 8
Doxorubicin 40 mg/m^2 IV weekly, weeks 1, 3, 5, 7, and 9
Etoposide 80 mg/m^2 IV, day 1 of weeks 1, 3, 5, 7, and 9
Etoposide 80 mg/m^2/day PO, days 2 and 3 of weeks 1, 3, 5, 7, and 9
used in conjunction with
Prednisone 50 mg PO daily for 5 weeks, then alternate days until chemotherapy completion, then taper over 2 weeks

References: •Fukuoka M, Masuda N, Negoro S, et al. CODE chemotherapy with and without granulocyte colony-stimulating factor in small-cell lung cancer. *Br J Cancer.* 1997;75:306-309.
•Murray N, Shah A, Osoba D, et al. Intensive weekly chemotherapy for the treatment of extensive-stage small-cell lung cancer. *J Clin Oncol.* 1991;9:1632-1638.

CODOX-M/IVAC*

Use: Lymphoma (advanced B-cell). *Cycle:* Give 4 cycles as myelosuppression permits. Give next cycle when granulocyte count is above 1,000 cells/mm^3 and platelet count is above 50,000 cells/mm^3.

Regimen: **Treatment A**—CODOX-M (cycles 1 and 3)
Cyclophosphamide 800 mg/m^2 IV, day 1
Cyclophosphamide 200 mg/m^2/day IV, days 2 through 5
Vincristine 1.5 mg/m^2 (2 mg maximum dose) IV, days 1 and 8
Doxorubicin 40 mg/m^2 IV, day 1
Methotrexate 1,200 mg/m^2 IV over 1 hour, day 10
Methotrexate 240 mg/m^2/hour continuous IV infusion over 23 hours, day 10 (begin after 1,200 mg/m^2 dose)
Leucovorin 192 mg/m^2 IV, day 11, given 36 hours after the start of the methotrexate infusion
Leucovorin 12 mg/m^2/dose IV every 6 hours, day 11, beginning 42 hours after the start of the methotrexate infusion and continued until the methotrexate concentration is below 0.05 microMol/L
Cytarabine 70 mg intrathecal, days 1 and 3
Methotrexate 12 mg intrathecal, day 15
Filgrastim 5 mcg/kg/day subcutaneously, starting on day 13 and continuing until granulocyte count is above 1,000 cells/mm^3
Treatment B—IVAC (cycles 2 and 4)
Ifosfamide 1,500 mg/m^2/day IV, days 1 through 5
Mesna 1,500 mg/m^2/day continuous IV infusion, days 1 through 5
Etoposide 60 mg/m^2/day IV, days 1 through 5
Cytarabine 2,000 mg/m^2/dose IV every 12 hours for 4 doses, days 1 and 2
Methotrexate 12 mg intrathecal, day 5
Filgrastim 5 mcg/kg/day subcutaneously, starting on day 7 and continuing until granulocyte count is above 1,000 cells/mm^3
*Note: These two regimens are normally used in combination with each other and are rarely given alone. Patients with malignant pleocytosis receive additional intrathecal drugs:
Cycle 1 (CODOX-M) cytarabine 70 mg intrathecal on day 5 and methotrexate 12 mg intrathecal on day 15
Cycle 2 (IVAC) cytarabine 70 mg intrathecal on days 7 and 9

References: •Adde M, Shad A, Venzon D, et al. Additional chemotherapy agents improve treatment outcome for children and adults with advanced B-cell lymphomas. *Semin Oncol.* 1998;25(2 suppl 4):33-39.
•Magrath I, Adde M, Shad A, et al. Adults and children with small noncleaved cell lymphoma have a similar excellent outcome when treated with the same chemotherapy regimen. *J Clin Oncol.* 1996;14:925-934.
•Mead GM, Sydes MR, Walewski J, et al. An international evaluation of CODOX-M and CODOX-M alternating with IVAC in adult Burkitt's lymphoma: results of United Kingdom Lymphoma Group LY06 study. *Ann Oncol.* 2002;13:1264-1274.
•Wang ES, Straus DJ, Teruya-Feldstein J, et al. Intensive chemotherapy with cyclophosphamide, doxorubicin, high-dose methotrexate/ifosfamide, etoposide, and high-dose cytarabine (CODOX-M/IVAC) for human immunodeficiency virus-associated Burkitt lymphoma. *Cancer.* 2003;98:1196-1205.

COMLA

Use: Lymphoma (non-Hodgkin). *Cycle*: 78 to 85 days

Regimen: Cyclophosphamide 1,500 mg/m^2 IV, day 1
Vincristine 1.4 mg/m^2 (2 mg maximum dose) IV, days 1, 8, and 15
Methotrexate 120 mg/m^2 IV, days 22, 29, 36, 43, 50, 57, 64, and 71
Leucovorin 25 mg/m^2/dose PO every 6 hours for 4 doses, beginning
24 hours after each methotrexate dose
Cytarabine 300 mg/m^2 IV, days 22, 29, 36, 43, 50, 57, 64, and 71

References: •Berd D, Cornog J, DeConti RC, Levitt M, Bertino JR. Long-term remission
in diffuse histiocytic lymphoma treated with combination sequential chemotherapy. *Cancer.* 1975;35:1050-1054.
•Gaynor ER, Ultmann JE, Golomb HM, Sweet DL. Treatment of diffuse histiocytic lymphoma (DHL) with COMLA (cyclophosphamide, oncovin, methotrexate, leucovorin, cytosine arabinoside): a 10-year experience in a single
institution. *J Clin Oncol.* 1985;3:1596-1604.
•Sweet DL, Golomb HM, Ultmann JE, et al. Cyclophosphamide, vincristine,
methotrexate with leucovorin rescue, and cytarabine (COMLA) combination
sequential chemotherapy for advanced diffuse histiocytic lymphoma. *Ann
Intern Med.* 1980;92:785-790.

COMP

Use: Lymphoma (non-Hodgkin—pediatric)

Regimen: **Induction.** *Cycle:* Give 1 cycle only
Cyclophosphamide 1,200 mg/m^2 IV, day 1
Vincristine 2 mg/m^2 (2 mg maximum dose) IV, days 3, 10, 17, and 24
Methotrexate 300 mg/m^2 IV, day 12 or 17
Prednisone 60 mg/m^2/day (60 mg/day maximum dose) PO in 4 divided
doses, days 3 through 30, then taper for 7 to 10 days
used in conjunction with
Intrathecal chemotherapy
Maintenance therapy. *Cycle:* 28 days for 15 cycles
Cyclophosphamide 1,000 mg/m^2 IV, day 1
Vincristine 1.5 mg/m^2 (2 mg maximum dose) IV, days 1 and 15
Methotrexate 300 mg/m^2 IV, day 15
Prednisone 60 mg/m^2/day (60 mg/day maximum dose) PO in 4 divided
doses, days 1 through 5, cycles 2 through 15
used in conjunction with
Intrathecal chemotherapy

References: •Nachman J. Therapy for childhood non-Hodgkin's lymphomas, nonlym-
phoblastic type. *Am J Pediatr Hematol Oncol.* 1990;12:359-366.
•Sposto R, Meadows AT, Chilcote RR, et al. Comparison of long-term outcome of children and adolescents with disseminated non-lymphoblastic
non-Hodgkin lymphoma treated with COMP or daunomycin-COMP: a report form the Children's Cancer Group. *Med Pediatr Oncol.* 2001;37:432-
441.

Cooper Regimen

Use:　　Breast cancer. *Cycle*: 36 weeks

Regimen:　Cyclophosphamide 2 mg/kg/day PO, weeks 1 through 36
Methotrexate 0.7 mg/kg IV weekly, weeks 1 through 8
Methotrexate 0.7 mg/kg IV every other week, weeks 10, 12, 14, 16, 18, 20, 22, 24, 26, 28, 30, 32, 34, and 36
Fluorouracil 12 mg/kg IV weekly, weeks 1 through 8
Fluorouracil 12 mg/kg IV every other week, weeks 10, 12, 14, 16, 18, 20, 22, 24, 26, 28, 30, 32, 34, and 36
Vincristine* 0.035 mg/kg IV weekly, weeks 1 through 5
Vincristine* 0.035 mg/kg IV monthly, weeks 8, 12, 16, 20, 24, 28, 32, and 36
Prednisone 0.75 mg/kg/day PO, days 1 through 10, then taper off over next 40 days
*Note: The vincristine dose is not capped in this protocol. Consult the prescriber if there is any question about the intended vincristine dose.

Reference:　•Cooper RG, Holland JF, Glidewell O. Adjuvant chemotherapy of breast cancer. *Cancer.* 1979;44:793-798.

COP

Use:　　Lymphoma (non-Hodgkin). *Cycle*: 14 to 28 days

Regimen:　Cyclophosphamide 800 to 1,000 mg/m^2 IV, day 1
Vincristine 2 mg (dose is not in mg/m^2) IV, day 1
Prednisone 60 mg/m^2/day (or 100 mg/day) PO, days 1 through 5, then taper off over next 3 days

References:　•Luce JK, Gamble JF, Wilson HE, et al. Combined cyclophosphamide, vincristine, and prednisone therapy of malignant lymphoma. *Cancer.* 1971;28:306-317.
•Rodriguez V, Cabanillas F, Burgess MA, et al. Combination chemotherapy ("CHOP-Bleo") in advanced (non-Hodgkin) malignant lymphoma. *Blood.* 1977;49:325-333.

COPE

Use:　　Lung cancer (small cell). *Cycle*: 21 days

Regimen:　Cyclophosphamide 750 mg/m^2 IV, day 1
Vincristine 2 mg (dose is not in mg/m^2) IV, day 14
Cisplatin 50 mg/m^2 IV, day 2
Etoposide 100 mg/m^2/day IV, days 1 through 3

Reference:　•Collins C, Higano CS, Livingston RB, Griffin BR, Keppen MD, Miller TP. Cyclophosphamide, vincristine, cisplatin, VP-16 and radiation therapy in extensive small-cell lung cancer. *Cancer Chemother Pharmacol.* 1989;24:128-132.

COPE (Baby Brain I)

Use: Brain tumors (pediatric). *Cycle*: 28 days

Regimen: Alternate cycles AABAAB.
Cycle A: Vincristine 0.065 mg/kg (1.5 mg maximum dose) IV, days 1 and 8
Cyclophosphamide 65 mg/kg IV, day 1
Cycle B: Cisplatin 4 mg/kg IV, day 1
Etoposide 6.5 mg/kg/day IV, days 3 and 4

Reference: •Duffner PK, Horowitz ME, Krischer JP, et al. Postoperative chemotherapy and delayed radiation in children less than three years of age with malignant brain tumors. *N Engl J Med*. 1993;328:1725-1731.

COPP (C-MOPP)

Use: Lymphoma (non-Hodgkin or Hodgkin). *Cycle*: 28 days

Regimen: Cyclophosphamide 450 to 650 mg/m^2 IV, days 1 and 8
Vincristine 1.4 to 2 mg/m^2 (2 mg maximum dose) IV, days 1 and 8
Procarbazine 100 mg/m^2/day PO, days 1 through 14
Prednisone 40 mg/m^2/day PO, cycles 1 and 4,* days 1 through 14
*Note: Some clinicians give prednisone with every cycle of COPP. The original clinical trials gave prednisone only with the first and fourth cycles.

References: •DeVita VT Jr, Canellos GP, Chabner B, Schein P, Hubbard SP, Young RC. Advanced diffuse histiocytic lymphoma, a potentially curable disease. *Lancet*. 1975;1:248-250.
•Liang R, Todd D, Chan TK, Chiu E, Lie A, Ho F. COPP chemotherapy for elderly patients with intermediate and high grade non-Hodgkin's lymphoma. *Hematol Oncol*. 1993;11:43-50.

CP

Use: Chronic lymphocytic leukemia (CLL). *Cycle*: 14 days

Regimen: Chlorambucil 30 mg/m^2/day PO, day 1
Prednisone 80 mg/day PO, days 1 through 5

Reference: •Raphael B, Anderson JW, Silber R, et al. Comparison of chlorambucil and prednisone versus cyclophosphamide, vincristine, and prednisone as initial treatment for chronic lymphocytic leukemia: long-term follow-up of an Eastern Cooperative Oncology Group randomized clinical trial. *J Clin Oncol*. 1991;9:770-776.

Use: Ovarian cancer. *Cycle*: 21 to 28 days

Regimen: Cyclophosphamide 600 to 1,000 mg/m^2 IV, day 1
Cisplatin 60 to 80 mg/m^2 IV, day 1

References: •Edmonson JH, McCormack GW, Fleming TR, et al. Comparison of cyclophosphamide plus cisplatin versus hexamethylmelamine, cyclophosphamide, doxorubicin, and cisplatin in combination as initial chemotherapy for stage III and IV ovarian carcinomas. *Cancer Treat Rep*. 1985;69:1243-1248.
•McGuire WP, Hoskins WJ, Brady MF, et al. Cyclophosphamide and cisplatin compared with paclitaxel and cisplatin in patients with stage III and stage IV ovarian cancer. *N Engl J Med*. 1996;334:1-6.
•Meerpohl HG, Sauerbrei W, Kühnle H, Schumacher M, Pfleiderer A. Randomized study comparing carboplatin/cyclophosphamide and cisplatin/cyclophosphamide as first-line treatment in patients with stage III/IV epithelial ovarian cancer and small volume disease. *Gynecol Oncol*. 1997;66:75-84.
•Swenerton K, Jeffrey J, Stuart G, et al. Cisplatin-cyclophosphamide versus carboplatin-cyclophosphamide in advanced ovarian cancer: a randomized phase III study of the National Cancer Institute of Canada Clinical Trials Group. *J Clin Oncol*. 1992;10:718-726.

CT

Use:	Ovarian cancer. *Cycle*: 21 days
Regimen:	Cisplatin 75 mg/m² IV, day 1 or 2 (given immediately after paclitaxel infusion) *with*
	Paclitaxel 175 mg/m² IV infusion over 3 hours, day 1
	or
	Paclitaxel 135 mg/m²/day continuous IV infusion over 24 hours, on day 1

References: •McGuire WP, Hoskins WJ, Brady MF, et al. Cyclophosphamide and cisplatin compared with paclitaxel and cisplatin in patients with stage III and stage IV ovarian cancer. *N Engl J Med.* 1996;334:1-6.
•Nejit JP, Engleholm SA, Tuxen MK, et al. Exploratory phase II study of paclitaxel and cisplatin versus paclitaxel and carboplatin in advanced ovarian cancer. *J Clin Oncol.* 2000;18:3084-3092.

Use:	Lung cancer (non-small cell). *Cycle*: 21 days
Regimen:	Cisplatin 75 mg/m² IV, day 2 (given after paclitaxel)
	Paclitaxel 135 mg/m²/day continuous IV infusion over 24 hours, day 1

Reference: •Schiller JH, Harrington D, Belani CP, et al. Comparison of four chemotherapy regimens for advanced non-small-cell lung cancer. *N Engl J Med.* 2002;346:92-98.

CVD

Use:	Malignant melanoma. *Cycle*: 21 days
Regimen:	Cisplatin 20 mg/m²/day IV, days 2 through 5
	Vinblastine 1.6 mg/m²/day IV, days 1 through 5
	Dacarbazine 800 mg/m² IV, day 1

Reference: •Legha SS, Ring S, Papadopoulos N, Plager C, Chawla S, Benjamin R. A prospective evaluation of a triple-drug regimen containing cisplatin, vinblastine, and dacarbazine (CVD) for metastatic melanoma. *Cancer.* 1989;64:2024-2029.

CVD + IL-2I

Use:	Malignant melanoma. *Cycle*: 21 days
Regimen:	Cisplatin 20 mg/m²/day IV, days 1 through 4
	Vinblastine 1.6 mg/m²/day IV, days 1 through 4
	Dacarbazine 800 mg/m² IV, day 1
	Aldesleukin 9 million units/m²/day continuous IV infusion, days 1 through 4
	Interferon alfa 5 million units/m²/day subcutaneously, days 1 through 5, 7, 9, 11, and 13

Reference: •Legha SS, Ring S, Eton O, et al. Development of a biochemotherapy regimen with concurrent administration of cisplatin, vinblastine, dacarbazine, interferon alfa, and interleukin-2 for patients with metastatic melanoma. *J Clin Oncol.* 1998;16:1752-1759.

CVI (VIC)

Use: Lung cancer (non-small cell). *Cycle*: 28 days

Regimen: Carboplatin 300 to 350 mg/m^2 IV, day 1
Etoposide 60 to 100 mg/m^2 IV, days 1, 3, and 5
Ifosfamide 1,500 mg/m^2 IV, days 1, 3, and 5
Mesna 400 mg/m^2 IV before ifosfamide given, days 1, 3, and 5
Mesna 1,600 mg/m^2/day continuous IV infusion, days 1, 3, and 5 (give after mesna bolus)

Reference: •van Zandwijk N, ten Bokkel Huinink WW, Wanders J, et al. Dose-finding studies with carboplatin, ifosfamide, etoposide, and mesna in non-small cell lung cancer. *Semin Oncol.* 1990;17(1 suppl 2):16-19.

CVP

Use: Lymphoma (non-Hodgkin), chronic lymphocytic leukemia (CLL). *Cycle*: 21 days

Regimon: Cyclophosphamide 300 to 400 mg/m^2/day PO, days 1 through 5
Vincristine 1.2 to 1.4 mg/m^2 (2 mg maximum dose) IV, day 1
Prednisone 40 to 100 mg/m^2/day PO, days 1 through 5

References: •Bagley CM Jr, Devita VT, Berard CW, Canellos GP. Advanced lymphosarcoma: intensive cyclical combination chemotherapy with cyclophosphamide, vincristine, and prednisone. *Ann Intern Med.* 1972;76:227-234.
•Hagenbeek A, Carde P, Meerwaldt JH, et al. Maintenance of remission with human recombinant interferon alfa-2a in patients with stages III and IV low-grade malignant non-Hodgkin's lymphoma. *J Clin Oncol.* 1998;16:41-47.
•Raphael B, Anderson JW, Silber R, et al. Comparison of chlorambucil and prednisone versus cyclophosphamide, vincristine, and prednisone as initial treatment for chronic lymphocytic leukemia: long-term follow-up of an Eastern Cooperative Oncology Group randomized clinical trial. *J Clin Oncol.* 1991;9:770-776.

CVPP

Use: Lymphoma (Hodgkin). *Cycle*: 28 days

Regimen: Lomustine 75 mg/m^2 PO, day 1
Vinblastine 4 mg/m^2 IV, days 1 and 8
Procarbazine 100 mg/m^2/day PO, days 1 through 14
Prednisone 40 mg/m^2/day PO, cycles 1 and 4, days 1 through 14

Reference: •Cooper MR, Pajak TF, Nissen NI, et al. A new effective four-drug combination of CCNU (1-]-3-cyclohexyl-1-nitrosourea) (NSC-79038), vinblastine, prednisone, and procarbazine for the treatment of advanced Hodgkin's disease. *Cancer.* 1980;46:654-662.

CY/A—see AC

Cyclophosphamide-Fludarabine

Use: Chronic lymphocytic leukemia (CLL). *Cycle*: 28 days

Regimen: Cyclophosphamide 250 mg/m^2/day IV, days 1 through 3
Fludarabine 25 to 30 mg/m^2/day IV, days 1 through 3

References: •Frewin R, Turner D, Tighe M, Davies S, Rule S, Johnson S. Combination therapy with fludarabine and cyclophosphamide as salvage treatment in lymphoproliferative disorders. *Br J Haematol.* 1999;104:612-613.
•Hallek M, Schmitt B, Wilhelm M, et al. Fludarabine plus cyclophosphamide is an efficient treatment for advanced chronic lymphocytic leukaemia (CLL): results of a phase II study of the German CLL study group. *Br J Haematol.* 2001;114:342-348.

CYVADIC

Use: Sarcoma (bony or soft tissue). *Cycle*: 21 days

Regimen: Cyclophosphamide 500 mg/m^2 IV, day 1
Vincristine 1 mg/m^2 (2 mg maximum dose) IV, days 1 and 5
Doxorubicin 50 mg/m^2 IV, day 1
Dacarbazine 250 mg/m^2/day IV, days 1 through 5

References: •Bramwell V, Rouesse J, Steward W, et al. Adjuvant CYVADIC chemo-therapy for adult soft tissue sarcoma—reduced local recurrence but no im-provement in survival: a study of the European Organization for Research and Treatment of Cancer Soft Tissue and Bone Sarcoma Group. *J Clin On-col.* 1994;12:1137-1149.
•Wilbur JR, Sutow WW, Sullivan MP, Gottlieb JA. Chemotherapy of sarco-mas. *Cancer.* 1975;36:765-769.

DA

Use: Acute myelocytic leukemia (AML; induction—pediatrics)

Regimen: Daunorubicin 45 to 60 mg/m^2/day IV, days 1 through 3
Cytarabine 100 mg/m^2/day continuous IV infusion, days 1 through 7

References: •Rowe JM. What is the best induction regimen for acute myelogenous leu-kemia? *Leukemia.* 1998;12(suppl 1):S16-S19.
•Yates J, Glidewell O, Wiernik P, et al. Cytosine arabinoside with dauno-rubicin or adriamycin for therapy of acute myelocytic leukemia: a CALGB study. *Blood.* 1982;60:454-462.

DA + ATRA (ATRA + CT)

Use: Acute promyelocytic leukemia (APL; induction and consolidation)

Regimen: Tretinoin 45 mg/m^2/day PO, days 1 through 90, or until complete remission, whichever occurs earlier
Induction. *Cycle:* Give 1 induction cycle followed by 2 consolidation cycles after hematologic recovery.
    Daunorubicin 60 mg/m^2/day IV, days 3 through 5
    Cytarabine 200 mg/m^2/day continuous IV infusion, days 3 through 9
First consolidation. *Cycle:* Give 1 cycle.
    Daunorubicin 60 mg/m^2/day IV, days 1 through 3
    Cytarabine 200 mg/m^2/day continuous IV infusion, days 1 through 7
Second consolidation. *Cycle:* Give 1 cycle. Do not give to elderly patients.
    Daunorubicin 45 mg/m^2/day IV, days 1 through 3
    Cytarabine 1,000 mg/m^2/dose IV every 12 hours for 8 doses, days 1 through 4

Reference: •Fenaux P, Chastang C, Chevret S, et al. A randomized comparison of all transretinoic acid (ATRA) followed by chemotherapy and ATRA plus che-motherapy and the role of maintenance therapy in newly diagnosed acute promyelocytic leukemia. *Blood.* 1999;94:1192-1200.

Dartmouth Regimen—see CDB + Tamoxifen

DAT

Use:	Acute myelocytic leukemia (AML; induction—pediatrics). *Cycle*: 14 to 21 days
Regimen:	Cytarabine 100 mg/m^2/dose IV every 12 hours for 14 doses, days 1 through 7 Thioguanine 100 mg/m^2/dose PO, every 12 hours for 14 doses, days 1 through 7 Daunorubicin 60 mg/m^2/day continuous IV infusion, days 5 through 7
Reference:	•Gale RP, Cline MJ. High remission-induction rate in acute myeloid leukemia. *Lancet*. 1977;1:497-499.

Use:	Acute myelocytic leukemia (AML; induction—pediatrics)
Regimen:	**Remission induction.** *Cycle:* Give 1 cycle only Daunorubicin 45 mg/m^2/day IV, days 1 through 3 Cytarabine 100 mg/m^2/day continuous IV infusion, days 1 through 7 Thioguanine 100 mg/m^2/day PO, days 1 through 7 **Second induction.** *Cycle*: Give a single cycle 14 days after initial remission induction course, delay until hematologic recovery in patients with remission or with hypoplastic marrow. Daunorubicin 45 mg/m^2/day IV, days 1 and 2 Cytarabine 100 mg/m^2/day continuous IV infusion, days 1 through 5 Thioguanine 100 mg/m^2/day PO, days 1 through 5 *used in conjunction with* Intrathecal chemotherapy
Reference:	•Ravindranth Y, Steuber CP, Krischer J, et al. High-dose cytarabine for intensification of early therapy of childhood acute myeloid leukemia: a Pediatric Oncology Group study. *J Clin Oncol*. 1991;9:572-580.

DAV

Use:	Acute myelocytic leukemia (AML; induction—pediatrics). *Cycle*: Give a single cycle
Regimen:	Cytarabine 100 mg/m^2/day continuous IV infusion, days 1 through 2 Cytarabine 100 mg/m^2/dose IV every 12 hours for 12 doses, days 3 through 8 Daunorubicin 60 mg/m^2/day IV, days 3 through 5 Etoposide 150 mg/m^2/day IV, days 6 through 8
Reference:	•Creutzig U, Ritter J, Schellong G. Identification of two risk groups in childhood acute myelogenous leukemia after therapy intensification in study AML-BFM-83 as compared with study AML-BFM-78. *Blood*. 1990;75:1932-1940.

DCT

Use:	Acute myelocytic leukemia (AML; induction—adults). *Cycle*: 7 days. Give once. May be given a second time based on individual response. Time between cycles not specified.
Regimen:	Daunorubicin 40 mg/m^2/day IV, days 1 through 3 Cytarabine 100 mg/m^2/dose IV every 12 hours for 14 doses, days 1 through 7 Thioguanine 100 mg/m^2/dose PO every 12 hours for 14 doses, days 1 through 7
Reference:	•Leoni F, Ciolli S, Patriarchi S, Morfini M, Ferrini PR. Etoposide in remission induction of adult acute myeloid leukemia. *Acta Haematol*. 1990;83:82-85.

DHAOx

Use: Lymphoma (non-Hodgkin). *Cycle:* 21 days

Regimen: Oxaliplatin 130 mg/m^2 IV, day 1
Dexamethasone 40 mg/day PO or IV, days 1 through 4
Cytarabine 2,000 mg/m^2/dose IV every 12 hours for 2 doses (total dose 4,000 mg/m^2), day 2
Filgrastim 5 mcg/kg/day subcutaneously, starting on day 3 and continued until granulocyte count is above 500 cells/mm^3

References: •Chau I, Webb A, Cunningham D, et al. An oxaliplatin-based chemotherapy in patients with relapsed or refractory intermediate and high-grade non-Hodgkin's lymphoma. *Br J Haematol.* 2001;115:786-792.
•Machover D, Delmas-Marsalet B, Misra SC, et al. Dexamethasone, high-dose cytarabine, and oxaliplatin (DHAOx) as salvage treatment for patients with initially refractory or relapsed non-Hodgkin's lymphoma. *Ann Oncol.* 2001;12:1439-1443.

DHAP

Use Lymphoma (non-Hodgkin). *Cycle:* 21 to 28 days

Regimen: Cisplatin 100 mg/m^2/day continuous IV infusion, day 1
Dexamethasone 40 mg/day PO or IV, days 1 through 4
Cytarabine 2,000 mg/m^2/dose IV every 12 hours for 2 doses (total dose, 4,000 mg/m^2), day 2

Reference: •Velasquez WS, Cabanillas F, Salvador P, et al. Effective salvage therapy for lymphoma with cisplatin in combination with high-dose ara-c and dexamethasone (DHAP). *Blood.* 1988;71:117-122.

DI

Use: Sarcoma (soft-tissue). *Cycle:* 21 days

Regimen: Doxorubicin 50 mg/m^2 IV, day 1
Ifosfamide 5,000 mg/m^2/day continuous IV infusion, day 1 (after doxorubicin given)
Mesna 600 mg/m^2 IV bolus before ifosfamide infusion, day 1
Mesna 2,500 mg/m^2/day continuous IV infusion over 36 hours, day 1 (give after mesna bolus)

Reference: •Schütte J, Mouridsen HT, Steward W, et al. Ifosfamide plus doxorubicin in previously untreated patients with advanced soft-tissue sarcoma. *Cancer Chemother Pharmacol.* 1993;31(suppl 2):S204-S209.

Docetaxel-Cisplatin

Use: Lung cancer (non-small cell). *Cycle:* 21 days

Regimen: Docetaxel 75 mg/m^2 IV, day 1
Cisplatin 75 mg/m^2 IV, day 1 (after docetaxel)

Reference: •Zalcberg J, Millward M, Bishop J, et al. Phase II study of docetaxel and cisplatin in advanced non-small-cell lung cancer. *J Clin Oncol.* 1998;16:1948-1953.

Docetaxel-Estramustine

Use: Prostate cancer. *Cycle:* 21 days (6 cycles maximum)

Regimen: Estramustine 280 mg/dose PO every 6 hours for 5 doses, day 1
              Docetaxel 70 mg/m^2 IV, day 1 (given 12 hours after first estramustine dose)

Reference: •Sinibaldi VJ, Carducci MA, Moore-Cooper S, Laufer M, Zahurak M, Eisenberger MA. Phase II evaluation of docetaxel plus one-day oral estramustine phosphate in the treatment of patients with androgen independent prostate carcinoma. *Cancer.* 2002;94:1457-1465.

Dox ➡ CMF, Sequential

Use: Breast cancer. *Cycle:* 21 days

Regimen: Doxorubicin 75 mg/m^2 IV, day 1 for 4 cycles
              followed by
              CMF-IV for 8 cycles

Reference: •Bonadonna G, Zambetti M, Valagussa P. Sequential or alternating doxorubicin and CMF regimens in breast cancer with more than three positive nodes: ten-year results. *JAMA.* 1995;273:542-547.

DTIC/Tamoxifen

Use: Malignant melanoma. *Cycle:* 21 days

Regimen: Dacarbazine 250 mg/m^2/day IV, days 1 through 5
              Tamoxifen 20 mg/m^2/day PO, days 1 through 5

Reference: •Cocconi G, Bella M, Calabresi F, et al. Treatment of metastatic malignant melanoma with dacarbazine plus tamoxifen. *N Engl J Med.* 1992;327:516-523.

DVP

Use: Acute lymphocytic leukemia (ALL; induction—pediatrics). *Cycle:* 35 days. Give a single cycle.

Regimen: Daunorubicin 25 mg/m^2 IV, days 1, 8, and 15
              Vincristine 1.5 mg/m^2 (2 mg maximum dose) IV, days 1, 8, 15, and 22
              Prednisone 60 mg/m^2/day PO, days 1 through 28 then taper over next 14 days
              used in conjunction with
              Intrathecal chemotherapy

Reference: •Belasco JB, Luery N, Scher C. Multiagent chemotherapy in relapsed acute lymphoblastic leukemia in children. *Cancer.* 1990;66:2492-2497.

EAP

Use: Gastric, small bowel cancer. *Cycle:* 21 to 28 days

Regimen: Etoposide 100 to 120 mg/m^2/day IV, days 4 through 6
              Doxorubicin 20 mg/m^2 IV, days 1 and 7
              Cisplatin 40 mg/m^2 IV, days 2 and 8

References: •Preusser P, Wilke H, Achterrath W, et al. Phase II study with the combination etoposide, doxorubicin, and cisplatin in advanced measurable gastric cancer. *J Clin Oncol.* 1989;7:1310-1317.
              •Wilke M, Preusser P, Fink U, et al. Preoperative chemotherapy in locally advanced and nonresectable gastric cancer: a phase II study with etoposide, doxorubicin, and cisplatin. *J Clin Oncol.* 1989;7:1318-1326.

EC

Use: Lung cancer. *Cycle:* 21 to 28 days

Regimen: Etoposide 100 to 120 mg/m^2/day IV, days 1 through 3
Carboplatin 300 to 350 mg/m^2 IV, day 1
or
Carboplatin IV dose by Calvert equation to AUC 6 mg/mL/min, day 1

References: •Bardet E, Riviere A, Charloux A, et al. A phase II trial of radiochemotherapy with daily carboplatin, after induction chemotherapy (carboplatin and etoposide), in locally advanced nonsmall-cell lung cancer: final analysis. *Int J Radiat Oncol Biol Phys.* 1997;38:163-168.
•Birch R, Weaver CH, Hainsworth JD, Bobo C, Greco FA. A randomized study of etoposide and carboplatin with or without paclitaxel in the treatment of small cell lung cancer. *Semin Oncol.* 1997;24(4 suppl 12):S12-135–S12-137.
•Kosmidis PA, Samantas E, Fountzilas G, Pavlidis N, Apostolopoulou F, Skarlos D. Cisplatin/etoposide versus carboplatin/etoposide chemotherapy and irradiation in small cell lung cancer: a randomized phase III study. *Semin Oncol.* 1994;21(3 suppl 6):23-30.
•Smith IE. Carboplatin in small cell lung cancer: the Royal Marsden Hospital experience. *Semin Oncol.* 1992;19:(1 suppl 2):24-27.

ECF

Use: Gastric cancer. *Cycle:* 21 days for up to 8 cycles

Regimen: Epirubicin 50 mg/m^2 IV, day 1
Cisplatin 60 mg/m^2 IV, day 1
Fluorouracil 200 mg/m^2/day continuous IV infusion, days 1 through 180

References: •Ross P, Nicolson M, Cunningham D, et al. Prospective randomized trial comparing mitomycin, cisplatin, and protracted venous-infusion fluorouracil (PVI 5-FU) with epirubicin, cisplatin, and PVI 5-FU in advanced esophagogastric cancer. *J Clin Oncol.* 2002;20:1996-2004.
•Waters JS, Norman A, Cunningham D, et al. Long-term survival after epirubicin, cisplatin, and fluorouracil for gastric cancer: results of a randomized trial. *Br J Cancer.* 1999;80:269-272.

EFP

Use: Gastric, small bowel cancer. *Cycle:* 21 to 28 days

Regimen: Etoposide 80 to 100 mg/m^2 IV, days 1, 3, and 5
Fluorouracil 800 to 900 mg/m^2/day continuous IV infusion, days 1 through 5
Cisplatin 20 mg/m^2/day IV, days 1 through 5

References: •Ajani JA, Ota DM, Jackson DE. Current strategies in the management of locoregional and metastatic gastric carcinoma. *Cancer.* 1991;67:260-265.
•Ajani JA, Roth JA, Ryan B, et al. Evaluation of pre- and postoperative chemotherapy for resectable adenocarcinoma of the esophagus or gastroesophageal junction. *J Clin Oncol.* 1990;8:1231-1238.
•Ryoo BY, Kang YK, Im YH, et al. Adjuvant (cisplatin, etoposide, and 5-fluorouracil) chemotherapy after curative resection of gastric adenocarcinomas involving the esophagogastric junction. *Am J Clin Oncol.* 1999;22:253-257.

ELF

Use: Gastric cancer. *Cycle*: 21 to 28 days

Regimen: Etoposide 120 mg/m²/day IV, days 1 through 3
Leucovorin 300 mg/m²/day IV, days 1 through 3
Fluorouracil 500 mg/m²/day IV, days 1 through 3 (after leucovorin)

References: •Ajani JA, Ota DM, Jackson DE. Current strategies in the management of locoregional and metastatic gastric carcinoma. *Cancer*. 1991;67:260-265.
•Wilke H, Preusser P, Stahl M, et al. Etoposide, folinic acid, and 5-fluorouracil in carboplatin-pretreated patients with advanced gastric cancer. *Cancer Chemother Pharmacol*. 1991;29:83-84.

EMA 86

Use: Acute myelocytic leukemia (AML; induction—adults). *Cycle*: Give a single cycle.

Regimen: Mitoxantrone 12 mg/m²/day IV, days 1 through 3
Etoposide 200 mg/m²/day continuous IV infusion, days 8 through 10
Cytarabine 500 mg/m²/day continuous IV infusion, days 1 through 3 and days 8 through 10

Reference: •Archimbaud E, Fenaux P, Reiffers J, et al. Granulocyte-macrophage colony-stimulating factor in association to timed-sequential chemotherapy with mitoxantrone, etoposide, and cytarabine for refractory acute myelogenous leukemia. *Leukemia*. 1993;7:372-377.

EM-V—see Estramustine/Vinblastine

EP

Use: Testicular cancer. *Cycle*: 21 days

Regimen: Etoposide 100 mg/m²/day IV, days 1 through 5
Cisplatin 20 mg/m²/day IV, days 1 through 5

Reference: •Motzer RJ, Sheinfeld J, Mazumdar M, et al. Etoposide and cisplatin adjuvant therapy for patients with pathologic stage II germ cell tumors. *J Clin Oncol*. 1995;13:2700-2704.

Use: Lung cancer, adenocarcinoma. *Cycle*: 21 to 28 days

Regimen: Etoposide 80 to 120 mg/m²/day IV, days 1 through 6
Cisplatin 80 to 100 mg/m² IV, day 1

References: •Goldhirsch A, Joss RA, Cavalli F, Sonntag RW, Brunner KW. Cis-dichlorodiammineplatinum (II) and VP 16-213 combination chemotherapy for non-small cell lung cancer. *Med Pediatr Oncol*. 1981;9:205-208.
•Greco FA, Johnson DH, Hainsworth JD. Etoposide/cisplatin-based chemotherapy for patients with metastatic poorly differentiated carcinoma of unknown primary site. *Semin Oncol*. 1992;19(6 suppl 13):14-18.
•Perng RP, Chen YM, Ming-Liu J, et al. Gemcitabine versus the combination of cisplatin and etoposide in patients with inoperable non-small-cell lung cancer in a phase II randomized study. *J Clin Oncol*. 1997;15:2097-2102.
•Veslemes M, Polyzos A, Latsi P, et al. Optimal duration of chemotherapy in small cell lung cancer: a randomized study of 4 versus 6 cycles of cisplatin-etoposide. *J Chemother*. 1998;10:136-140.

EPOCH

Use: Lymphoma (non-Hodgkin). *Cycle*: 21 days

Regimen: Etoposide 50 mg/m^2/day continuous IV infusion, days 1 through 4
Prednisone 60 mg/m^2/day PO, days 1 through 6
Vincristine* 0.4 mg/m^2/day continuous IV infusion, days 1 through 4[†]
Cyclophosphamide 750 mg/m^2 IV, day 5
Doxorubicin 10 mg/m^2/day continuous IV infusion, days 1 through 4[†]
Cotrimoxazole double-strength (160/800) 1 tablet PO twice daily, given for 3 consecutive days each week
*Note: The vincristine dose is not capped in this protocol. Consult the prescriber if there is any question about the intended vincristine dose.
[†]Note: Vincristine and doxorubicin may be mixed and administered in the same infusion bag, if diluted with 0.9% Sodium Chloride. Etoposide is usually infused in a separate line.

References: •Gutierrez M, Chabner BA, Pearson D, et al. Role of a doxorubicin-containing regimen in relapsed and resistant lymphomas: an 8-year follow-up study of EPOCH. *J Clin Oncol.* 2000;18:3633-3642.
•Wilson WH, Bryant G, Bates S, et al. EPOCH chemotherapy: toxicity and efficacy in relapsed and refractory non-Hodgkin's lymphoma. *J Clin Oncol.* 1993;11:1573-1582.

EPOCH-R

Use: Lymphoma (B-cell, mantle cell). *Cycle*: 21 days for at least 6 cycles, delay subsequent cycles until hematologic recovery.

Regimen: Rituximab 375 mg/m^2 IV, day 1
Etoposide 50 mg/m^2/day continuous IV infusion, days 1 through 4
Vincristine* 0.4 mg/m^2/day continuous IV infusion, days 1 through 4[†]
Doxorubicin 10 mg/m^2/day continuous IV infusion, days 1 through 4[†]
Prednisone 60 mg/m^2/day PO, days 1 through 5
Cyclophosphamide 750 mg/m^2 IV, day 5
Filgrastim 5 mcg/kg/day subcutaneously, starting on day 6 and continued until granulocyte count exceeds 5,000 cells/mm^3
Cotrimoxazole double-strength (160/800) 1 tablet PO twice daily, given on Monday, Wednesday, and Friday of each week
*Note: The vincristine dose is not capped in this protocol. Consult the prescriber if there is any question about the intended vincristine dose.
[†]Note: Vincristine and doxorubicin may be mixed and administered in the same infusion bag, if diluted with 0.9% Sodium Chloride. Etoposide is usually infused in a separate line.

References: •Dunleavy KM, Little RF, Grant N, White T, Wright G, Janik J. Rituximab is associated with late onset neutropenia (LON) when administered with doxorubicin-based chemotherapy for the initial treatment of aggressive B-cell lymphomas [abstract]. Presented at the American Society of Hematology Meeting, 2003. Abstract 1443.
•Wilson WH, Gutierrez M, O'Connor P, et al. The role of rituximab and chemotherapy in aggressive B-cell lymphoma: a preliminary report of dose-adjusted EPOCH-R. *Semin Oncol.* 2002;29(1 suppl 2):41-47.

ESHAP

Use: Lymphoma (non-Hodgkin). *Cycle*: 21 to 28 days

Regimen: Methylprednisolone 250 to 500 mg/day IV, days 1 through 4 or 1 through 5
Etoposide 40 to 60 mg/m^2/day IV, days 1 through 4
Cytarabine 2,000 mg/m^2 IV, day 5 (after etoposide and cisplatin are completed)
Cisplatin 25 mg/m^2/day continuous IV infusion, days 1 through 4

References: •Rodriguez MA, Cabanillas FC, Velasquez W, et al. Results of a salvage treatment program for relapsing lymphoma: MINE consolidated with ESHAP. *J Clin Oncol.* 1995;13:1734-1741.
•Velasquez WS, McLaughlin P, Tucker S, et al. ESHAP—an effective chemotherapy regimen in refractory and relapsing lymphoma: a 4 year follow-up study. *J Clin Oncol.* 1994;12:1169-1176.

Estramustine/Vinblastine (EM-V)

Use: Prostate cancer. *Cycle*: 8 weeks

Regimen: Vinblastine 4 mg/m^2 IV weekly, weeks 1 through 6
with
Estramustine 10 mg/kg/day PO given in 3 divided doses, days 1 through 42
or
Estramustine 600 mg/m^2/day PO given in 2 to 3 divided doses, days 1 through 42

References: •Hudes G, Einhorn L, Ross E, et al. Vinblastine versus vinblastine plus oral estramustine phosphate for patients with hormone refractory prostate cancer: a Hoosier Oncology Group and Fox Chase Network phase III trial. *J Clin Oncol.* 1999;17:3160-3166.
•Seidman AD, Scher HI, Petrylak D, Dershaw DD, Curley T. Estramustine and vinblastine: use of prostate specific antigen as a clinical trial end point for hormone refractory prostatic cancer. *J Urol.* 1992;147:931-934.

EVA

Use: Lymphoma (Hodgkin). *Cycle*: 28 days

Regimen: Etoposide 100 mg/m^2/day IV, days 1 through 3
Vinblastine 6 mg/m^2 IV, day 1
Doxorubicin 50 mg/m^2 IV, day 1

Reference: •Canellos GP, Petroni GR, Barcos M, Duggan DB, Peterson BA. Etoposide, vinblastine, and doxorubicin: an active regimen for the treatment of Hodgkin's disease in relapse following MOPP. *J Clin Oncol.* 1995;13:2005-2011.

F-CL (FU/LV)

Use: Colorectal cancer. *Cycle*: 4 to 8 weeks

Regimen: Leucovorin 500 mg/m^2 IV, weekly for 6 weeks, then 2-week rest period
Fluorouracil 600 mg/m^2 IV, weekly for 6 weeks (after starting leucovorin), then 2-week rest period
or
Leucovorin 20 mg/m^2/day IV, days 1 through 5
Fluorouracil 370 to 425 mg/m^2/day IV, days 1 through 5 (after starting leucovorin)
or
Leucovorin 200 mg/m^2/day IV, days 1 through 5
Fluorouracil 370 mg/m^2/day IV, days 1 through 5 (after starting leucovorin)

F-CL (FU/LV) (cont.)

References: •Buroker TR, O'Connell MJ, Wieand HS, et al. Randomized comparison of two schedules of fluorouracil and leucovorin in the treatment of advanced colorectal cancer. *J Clin Oncol.* 1994;12:14-20.

•Poon MA, O'Connell MJ, Moertel CG, et al. Biochemical modulation of fluorouracil: evidence of significant improvement of survival and quality of life in patients with advanced colorectal carcinoma. *J Clin Oncol.* 1989;7:1407-1417.

•Poon MA, O'Connell MJ, Wieand HS, et al. Biochemical modulation of fluorouracil with leucovorin: confirmatory evidence of improved therapeutic efficacy in advanced colorectal cancer. *J Clin Oncol.* 1991;9:1967-1972.

FAC

Use: Breast cancer. *Cycle*: 21 to 28 days

Regimen: Fluorouracil 500 mg/m^2 IV, days 1 and 8
Doxorubicin 50 mg/m^2 IV, day 1
Cyclophosphamide 500 mg/m^2 IV, day 1

References: •Legha SS, Buzdar AU, Smith TL, et al. Complete remissions in metastatic breast cancer treated with combination drug therapy. *Ann Intern Med.* 1979;91:847-852.

•Swenerton KD, Legha SS, Smith T, et al. Prognostic factors in metastatic breast cancer treated with combination chemotherapy. *Cancer Res.* 1979;39:1552-1562.

FAM

Use: Adenocarcinoma, gastric cancer. *Cycle*: 8 weeks

Regimen: Fluorouracil 600 mg/m^2 IV, days 1, 8, 29, and 36
Doxorubicin 30 mg/m^2 IV, days 1 and 29
Mitomycin 10 mg/m^2 IV, day 1

References: •Butler TP, MacDonald JS, Smith FP, Smith LF, Woolley PV, Schein PS. 5-Fluorouracil, adriamycin, and mitomycin-c (FAM) chemotherapy for adenocarcinoma of the lung. *Cancer.* 1979;43:1183-1188.

•MacDonald JS, Woolley PV, Smythe T, Ueno W, Hoth D, Schein PS. 5-Fluorouracil, adriamycin, and mitomycin-c (FAM) combination chemotherapy in the treatment of advanced gastric cancer. *Cancer.* 1979;44:42-47.

FAMTX

Use: Gastric cancer. *Cycle*: 28 days

Regimen: Methotrexate 1,500 mg/m^2 IV, day 1
Fluorouracil 1,500 mg/m^2 IV, day 1 (give after methotrexate)
Leucovorin 15 mg/m^2/dose PO every 6 hours for 8 doses (start 24 hours after methotrexate); increase dose to 30 mg/m^2/dose PO every 6 hours for 16 doses if 24-hour methotrexate level is 2.5 mol/L or higher.
Doxorubicin 30 mg/m^2 IV, day 15

References: •Wils J, Bleiberg H, Dalesio O, et al. An EORTC gastrointestinal group evaluation of the combination of sequential methotrexate and 5-fluorouracil, combined with adriamycin in advanced measurable gastric cancer. *J Clin Oncol.* 1986;4:1799-1803.

•Wils JA, Klein HO, Wagener DJ, et al. Sequential high-dose methotrexate and fluorouracil combined with doxorubicin—a step ahead in the treatment of advanced gastric cancer: a trial of the European Organization for Research and Treatment of Cancer Gastrointestinal Tract Cooperative Group. *J Clin Oncol.* 1991;9:827-831.

FAP

Use: Gastric cancer. *Cycle*: 5 weeks

Regimen: Fluorouracil 300 mg/m²/day IV, days 1 through 5
Doxorubicin 40 mg/m² IV, day 1
Cisplatin 60 mg/m² IV, day 1

Reference: •Cullinan SA, Moertel CG, Wieand S, et al. Controlled evaluation of three drug combination regimens versus fluorouracil alone for the therapy of advanced gastric cancer. *J Clin Oncol.* 1994;12:412-416.

FEC (see also CEF)

Use: Breast cancer. *Cycle*: 21 days

Regimen: Fluorouracil 500 mg/m² IV, day 1
Cyclophosphamide 500 mg/m² IV, day 1
Epirubicin 100 mg/m² IV, day 1

References: •Bonneterre J, Roché H, Bremond A, et al. Results of a randomized trial of adjuvant chemotherapy with FEC 50 vu FEC 100 in high risk node-positive breast cancer patients [abstract 473]. *Proc ASCO.* 1998;17:124a.
•The French Epirubicin Study Group. Epirubicin-based chemotherapy in metastatic breast cancer patients: role of dose-intensity and duration of treatment. *J Clin Oncol.* 2000;18:3115-3124.

FED

Use: Lung cancer (non-small cell). *Cycle*: 21 days

Regimen: Cisplatin 100 mg/m² IV, day 1
Fluorouracil 960 mg/m²/day continuous IV infusion, days 2 through 4
Etoposide 80 mg/m²/day IV, days 2 through 4

Reference: •Sridhar KS, Thurer RJ, Markoe AM, et al. Multidisciplinary approach to the treatment of locally and regionally advanced non-small cell lung cancer. *Semin Surg Oncol.* 1993;9:114-119.

FL

Use: Prostate cancer. *Cycle*: Ongoing

Regimen: Flutamide 250 mg/dose PO every 8 hours
with
Leuprolide acetate 1 mg subcutaneously daily
or
Leuprolide depot 7.5 mg/dose IM, every 28 days
or
Leuprolide depot 22.5 mg/dose IM, every 3 months

References: •Lupron. [package insert]. Deerfield, IL: TAP Pharmaceuticals Inc.; April 1996.
•Lupron Depot-3. [package insert]. Deerfield, IL: TAP Pharmaceuticals Inc.; March 1997.
•McLeod DG, Schellhammer PF, Vogelzang NJ, et al. Exploratory analysis on the effect of race on clinical outcome inpatients with advanced prostate cancer receiving bicalutamide or flutamide, each in combination with LHRH analogues. *Prostate.* 1999;40:218-224.

FLAG

Use: Acute myelocytic leukemia (AML; remission induction). *Cycle*: Give a single cycle

Regimen: Filgrastim 300 mcg/day subcutaneously, day 1 until neutropenia resolves
Fludarabine 30 mg/m^2/day IV, days 2 through 6
Cytarabine 2,000 mg/m^2/day IV, days 2 through 6 (begin 4 hours after starting fludarabine)

References: •Clavio M, Carrara P, Miglino M, et al. High efficacy of fludarabine-containing therapy (FLAG-FLANG) in poor risk acute myeloid leukemia. *Haematologica*. 1996;81:513-520.
•Virchis A, Koh M, Rankin P, et al. Fludarabine, cytosine arabinoside, granulocyte-colony stimulating factor with or without idarubicin in the treatment of high risk acute leukemia or myelodysplastic syndromes. *Br J Haematol*. 2004;124:26-32.

FLAG-Ida

Use: Acute myelocytic leukemia (AML; remission induction). *Cycle*: Give a single cycle. May be given a second time based on individual response. Time between cycles not specified.

Regimen: Filgrastim 300 mcg/day subcutaneously, day 1 until neutropenia resolves
Fludarabine 30 mg/m^2/day IV, days 2 through 6
Cytarabine 2,000 mg/m^2/day IV, days 2 through 6 (begin 4 hours after starting fludarabine)
Idarubicin 8 mg/m^2/day IV, days 2 through 4

References: •Byrne JL, Dasgupta E, Pallis M, et al. Early allogeneic transplantation for refractory or relapsed acute leukemia following remission induction with FLAG. *Leukemia*. 1999;13:786-791.
•Jackson G, Taylor P, Smith GM, et al. A multicentre, open, non-comparative phase II study of a combination of fludarabine phosphate, cytarabine and granulocyte colony stimulating factor in relapsed and refractory acute myeloid leukaemia and *de novo* refractory anaemia with excess of blasts in transformation. *Br J Haematol*. 2001;112:127-137.
•Pawson P, Postter MN, Theocharous P, et al. Treatment of relapse after allogenic bone marrow transplantation with reduced intensity conditioning (FLAG +/− Ida) and second allogenic stem cell transplant. *Br J Haematol*. 2001;115:622-629.

Fle

Use: Colorectal cancer. *Cycle*: 1 year

Regimen: Fluorouracil 450 mg/m^2/day IV, days 1 through 5
Fluorouracil 450 mg/m^2/week IV, weeks 5 through 52
Levamisole 50 mg/dose PO every 8 hours, days 1 through 3 of every other week for 1 year

Reference: •Moertel CG, Fleming TR, MacDonald JS, et al. Levamisole and fluorouracil for adjuvant therapy of resected colon carcinoma. *N Engl J Med*. 1990;322:352-358.

Fludarabine-Cyclophosphamide

Use: Chronic lymphocytic leukemia (CLL). *Cycle:* 4 to 6 weeks based on recovery of myelosuppression

Regimen: Fludarabine 30 mg/m²/day IV, days 1 through 3
Cyclophosphamide 300 mg/m²/day IV, days 1 through 3

Reference: •O'Brien SM, Kantarjian HM, Cortes J, et al. Results of the fludarabine and cyclophosphamide combination regimen in chronic lymphocytic leukemia. *J Clin Oncol.* 2001;19:1414-1420.

FMD—see FND

FNC—see CNF

FND (FMD)

Use: Lymphoma (non-Hodgkin). *Cycle:* 28 days for up to 8 cycles

Regimen: Fludarabine 25 mg/m²/day IV, days 1 through 3
Mitoxantrone 10 mg/m² IV, day 1
Dexamethasone 20 mg/day IV or PO, days 1 through 5
Cotrimoxazole double-strength (160/800) 2 tablets PO daily for 2 consecutive days each week (usually given every Saturday and Sunday)

References: •Crawley CR, Foran JM, Gupta RK, et al. A phase II study to evaluate the combination of fludarabine, mitoxantrone and dexamethasone (FMD) in patients with follicular lymphoma. *Ann Oncol.* 2000;11:861-865.
•McLaughlin P, Hagemeister FB, Rodriguez MA, et al. Safety of fludarabine, mitoxantrone, and dexamethasone combined with rituximab in the treatment of stage IV indolent lymphoma. *Semin Oncol.* 2000;27(6 suppl 12):37-41.
•McLaughlin P, Hagemeister FB, Romaguera JE, et al. Fludarabine, mitoxantrone, and dexamethasone: an effective new regimen for indolent lymphomas. *J Clin Oncol.* 1996;14:1262-1268.
•Tsimberdou AM, McLaughlin P, Younes A, et al. Fludarabine, mitoxantrone, dexamethasone (FND) compared with an alternating triple therapy (ATT) regimen in patients with stage IV indolent lymphoma. *Blood.* 2002;100:4351-4357.

FND + Rituximab, Concurrent (FND-R)

Use: Lymphoma (non-Hodgkin). *Cycle:* 28 days for up to 8 cycles

Regimen: Fludarabine 25 mg/m²/day IV, days 2 through 4
Mitoxantrone 10 mg/m² IV, day 2
Dexamethasone 20 mg/day IV or PO, days 2 through 4
Rituximab 375 mg/m² IV, days 1 and 8 for first cycle only; then rituximab 375 mg/m² IV, day 1 for cycles 2 through 5
Cotrimoxazole double-strength (160/800) 1 tablet PO twice daily for 2 consecutive days each week (usually given every Saturday and Sunday)

References: •McLaughlin P, Hagemeister FB, Rodriguez MA, et al. Safety of fludarabine, mitoxantrone, and dexamethasone combined with rituximab in the treatment of stage IV indolent lymphoma. *Semin Oncol.* 2000;27(6 suppl 12):37-41.
•McLaughlin P, Rodriguez MA, Hagemeister FB, et al. Stage IV indolent lymphoma: a randomized study of concurrent vs. sequential use of FND chemotherapy (fludarabine, mitoxantrone, dexamethasone) and rituximab (R) monoclonal antibody therapy, with interferon maintenance [abstract]. *Proc ASCO.* 2003;22:564. Abstract 2269.

FOLFIRI

Use:	Colorectal cancer. *Cycle*: 14 days
Regimen:	Leucovorin 400 mg/m^2 IV, day 1 Irinotecan 180 mg/m^2 IV, day 1 (begin with leucovorin) *then* Fluorouracil 400 mg/m^2 IV bolus, day 1 *then* Fluorouracil 2,400 mg/m^2/dose continuous IV infusion over 46 hours for 2 cycles, starting on day 1. Increase to 3,000 mg/m^2/dose for remaining cycles if tolerated.
References:	•Douillard JY, Sobrero A, Carnaghi C, et al. Metastatic colorectal cancer: integrating irinotecan into combination and sequential chemotherapy. *Ann Oncol*. 2003;14(suppl 2):ii7-ii12. •Tournigand C, Andre T, Achille E, et al. FOLFIRI followed by FOLFOX6 or the reverse sequence in advanced colorectal cancer: a randomized GER-COR study. *J Clin Oncol*. 2004;22:229-237.

FOLFOX-2

Use:	Colorectal cancer. *Cycle*: 14 days
Regimen:	Oxaliplatin 100 mg/m^2 IV, day 1 (begin with leucovorin) Leucovorin 500 mg/m^2/day IV, days 1 and 2 *then* Fluorouracil 1,500 mg/m^2/dose continuous IV infusion over 22 hours, days 1 and 2, for 2 cycles. Increase to 2,000 mg/m^2/dose for remaining cycles if toxicity was below WHO grade 2 during first 2 cycles.
Reference:	•de Gramont A, Vignoud J, Tournigand C, et al. Oxaliplatin with high-dose leucovorin and 5-fluorouracil 48-hour continuous infusion in pretreated metastatic colorectal cancer. *Eur J Cancer*. 1997;33:214-219.

FOLFOX-3

Use:	Colorectal cancer. *Cycle*: 14 days
Regimen:	Oxaliplatin 85 mg/m^2 IV, day 1 (begin with leucovorin) Leucovorin 500 mg/m^2/day IV, days 1 and 2 *then* Fluorouracil 1,500 mg/m^2/dose continuous IV infusion over 22 hours, days 1 and 2, for 2 cycles. Increase to 2,000 mg/m^2/dose for remaining cycles if toxicity was below WHO grade 2 during first 2 cycles.
Reference:	•Andre T, Louvet C, Raymond E, et al. Bimonthly high-dose leucovorin, 5-fluorouracil infusion and oxaliplatin (FOLFOX3) for metastatic colorectal cancer resistant to the same leucovorin and 5-fluorouracil regimen. *Ann Oncol*. 1998;9:1251-1253.

FOLFOX-4

Use:	Colorectal cancer. *Cycle*: 14 days
Regimen:	Oxaliplatin 85 mg/m^2 IV, day 1 (begin with leucovorin) Leucovorin 200 mg/m^2/day IV, days 1 and 2 *then* Fluorouracil 400 mg/m^2/day IV bolus, days 1 and 2 *then* Fluorouracil 600 mg/m^2/dose continuous IV infusion over 22 hours, days 1 and 2

FOLFOX-4 (cont.)

References: •Eloxatin. (oxaliplatin for injection) [package insert]. New York, NY: Sanofi-Synthelabo; August 2002.

•Gilles-Amar V, Garcia ML, Sebille A, et al. Evolution of severe sensory neuropathy with oxaliplatin combined to the bimonthly 48 hour leucovorin (LV) and 5-fluorouracil (5FU) regimens (FOLFOX) in metastatic colorectal cancer [abstract]. *Proc ASCO.* 1999;18-19.

•Manga GP, Garcia-Alfonso P, Calvo FA, et al. Neoadjuvant oxaliplatin + 5FU (FOLFOX 4) in primary uT3-4NxM0 rectal cancer: clinical and endorectal ultrasound response assessment [abstract]. *Proc ASCO.* 2002;21. Abstract 2291.

FOLFOX-6

Use: Colorectal cancer. *Cycle*: 14 days

Regimen: Leucovorin 400 mg/m^2 IV, day 1
Oxaliplatin 100 mg/m^2 IV, day 1 (begin with leucovorin)
then
Fluorouracil 400 mg/m^2 IV bolus, day 1
then
Fluorouracil 2,400 mg/m^2/dose continuous IV infusion over 46 hours for 2 cycles, starting on day 1. Increase to 3,000 mg/m^2/dose for remaining cycles if tolerated.

References: •Douillard JY, Sobrero A, Carnaghi C, et al. Metastatic colorectal cancer: integrating irinotecan into combination and sequential chemotherapy. *Ann Oncol.* 2003;14(suppl 2):ii7-ii12.

•Tournigand C, Andre T, Achille E, et al. FOLFIRI followed by FOLFOX6 or the reverse sequence in advanced colorectal cancer: a randomized GERCOR study. *J Clin Oncol.* 2004;22:229-237.

FOLFOX-7

Use: Colorectal cancer. *Cycle*: 14 days

Regimen: Leucovorin 400 mg/m^2 IV, day 1
Oxaliplatin 130 mg/m^2 IV, day 1 (begin with leucovorin)
then
Fluorouracil 400 mg/m^2 IV bolus, day 1
then
Fluorouracil 2,400 mg/m^2/dose continuous IV infusion over 46 hours, starting on day 1

Reference: •Maindrault-Goebel F, de Gramont A, Louvet C, et al. High-dose intensity oxaliplatin added to the simplified bimonthly leucovorin and 5-fluorouracil regimen as second-line therapy for metastatic colorectal cancer (FOLFOX 7). *Eur J Cancer.* 2001;37:1000-1005.

FU/LV—see F-CL

FU/LV/CPT-11

Use: Metastatic colorectal cancer.* *Cycle*: 42 days

Regimen: Fluorouracil 500 mg/m^2 IV, days 1, 8, 15, and 22
Leucovorin 20 mg/m^2 IV, days 1, 8, 15, and 22
Irinotecan 125 mg/m^2 IV, days 1, 8, 15, and 22
*Note: A recent study analysis found an increased risk of early deaths (within 60 days of initiating treatment) with use of this regimen. Specific risk factors that may have contributed to death were not identified. Intensive patient monitoring and dosage modification are recommended to reduce the risk of severe adverse effects.

FU/LV/CPT-11 (cont.)

References: •Saltz LB, Cox JV, Blanke C, et al. Irinotecan plus fluorouracil and leucovorin for metastatic colorectal cancer. *N Engl J Med.* 2000;343:905-914.
•Sargent DJ, Niedzwiecki D, O'Connell MJ, Schilsky RL. Recommendation for caution with irinotecan, fluorouracil, and leucovorin for colorectal cancer. *N Engl J Med.* 2001;345:144-145.

Use:	Metastatic colorectal cancer. *Cycle*: 14 days
Regimen:	Fluorouracil 400 mg/m^2 IV bolus, day 1

then

Fluorouracil 600 mg/m^2/dose continuous IV infusion over 22 hours, day 1
Leucovorin 200 mg/m^2/day IV, days 1 and 2
Irinotecan 180 mg/m^2 IV, day 1
or
Fluorouracil 2,300 mg/m^2/day continuous IV infusion, days 1 and 8
Leucovorin 500 mg/m^2 IV, days 1 and 8
Irinotecan 80 mg/m^2 IV, days 1 and 8

Reference: •Douillard JY, Cunningham D, Roth AD, et al. Irinotecan combined with fluorouracil compared with fluorouracil alone as first-line treatment for metastatic colorectal cancer: a multicentre randomised trial. *Lancet.* 2000;355:1041-1047.

FUP

Use: Gastric cancer. *Cycle*: 28 days

Regimen: Fluorouracil 1,000 mg/m^2/day continuous IV infusion, days 1 through 5
Cisplatin 100 mg/m^2 IV, day 2

Reference: •Vanhoefer U, Rougier P, Wilke H, et al. Final results of a randomized phase III trial of sequential high-dose methotrexate, fluorouracil, and doxorubicin versus etoposide, leucovorin, and fluorouracil versus infusional fluorouracil and cisplatin in advanced gastric cancer: a trial of the European Organization for Research and Treatment of Cancer Gastrointestinal Tract Cancer Cooperative Group. *J Clin Oncol.* 2000;18:2648-2657.

FZ

Use: Prostate cancer. *Cycle*: Ongoing

Regimen: Flutamide 250 mg/dose PO every 8 hours
with
Goserelin acetate 3.6 mg/dose implant subcutaneously every 28 days
or
Goserelin acetate 10.8 mg/dose implant subcutaneously every 12 weeks

References: •McLeod DG, Schellhammer PF, Vogelzang NJ, et al. Exploratory analysis on the effect of race on clinical outcome in patients with advanced prostate cancer receiving bicalutamide or flutamide, each in combination with LHRH analogues. *Prostate.* 1999;40:218-224.
•Zoladex. [package insert]. Wilmington, DE: Zeneca Pharmaceuticals; April 1996.

G + V (see also Gemcitabine-Vinorelbine)

Use: Lung cancer (non-small cell). *Cycle:* 21 days for up to 6 cycles

Regimen: Gemcitabine 1,200 mg/m^2 IV, days 1 and 8
Vinorelbine 30 mg/m^2 IV, days 1 and 8

Reference: •Frasci G, Lorusso V, Panza N, et al. Gemcitabine plus vinorelbine versus vinorelbine alone in elderly patients with advanced non-small cell lung cancer. *J Clin Oncol.* 2000;18:2529-2536.

Gemcitabine-Capecitabine

Use: Pancreatic cancer. *Cycle*: 21 days for 6 cycles

Regimen: Capecitabine 650 mg/m^2/dose PO twice daily, days 1 through 14
Gemcitabine 1,000 mg/m^2 IV, days 1 and 8

Reference: •Hess V, Saltzberg M, Borner M, et al. Combining capecitabine and gemcitabine in patients with advanced pancreatic carcinoma: a phase I/II trial. *J Clin Oncol.* 2003;21:66-68.

Gemcitabine-Carboplatin

Use: Lung cancer (non-small cell). *Cycle*: 28 days

Regimen: Gemcitabine 1,000 or 1,100 mg/m^2 IV, days 1 and 8
Carboplatin IV dose by Calvert equation to AUC 5 mg/mL/min, day 8

Reference: •Iaffaioli RV, Tortoriello A, Facchini G, et al. Phase I-II study of gemcitabine and carboplatin in stage IIIB-IV non-small-cell lung cancer. *J Clin Oncol.* 1999;17:921-926.

Gemcitabine-Cis

Use: Lung cancer (non-small cell). *Cycle*: 28 days

Regimen: Gemcitabine 1,000 to 1,200 mg/m^2 IV, days 1, 8, and 15
Cisplatin 100 mg/m^2 IV, day 15*
*Note: Some references state that a single dose of cisplatin may be given on day 1, 2, or 15 of each cycle. However, the best results are seen when cisplatin is given on day 15.

References: •Abratt RP, Sandler A, Crino L, et al. Combined cisplatin and gemcitabine for non-small cell lung cancer: influence of scheduling on toxicity and drug delivery. *Semin Oncol.* 1998;25(suppl 9):35-43.
•Anton A, Fernández ND, González JL, et al. Phase II trial assessing the combination of gemcitabine and cisplatin in advanced non-small cell lung cancer (NSCLC). *Lung Cancer.* 1998;22:139-148.

Gemcitabine-Cisplatin

Use: Metastatic bladder cancer. *Cycle*: 28 days for up to 6 cycles

Regimen: Gemcitabine 1,000 mg/m^2 IV, days 1, 8, and 15
Cisplatin 70 mg/m^2 IV, day 2

Reference: •von der Maase H, Hansen SW, Roberts JT, et al. Gemcitabine and cisplatin versus methotrexate, vinblastine, doxorubicin, and cisplatin in advanced or metastatic bladder cancer: results of a large, randomized, multinational, multicenter phase III study. *J Clin Oncol.* 2000;18:3068-3077.

Gemcitabine-Irinotecan

Use: Pancreatic cancer. *Cycle*: 21 days

Regimen: Gemcitabine 1,000 mg/m^2 IV, days 1 and 8
Irinotecan 100 mg/m^2 IV, days 1 and 8 (after gemcitabine)

Reference: •Rocha Lima CMS, Savarese D, Bruckner H, et al. Irinotecan plus gemcitabine induces both radiographic and CA 19-9 tumor marker responses in patients with previously untreated advanced pancreatic cancer. *J Clin Oncol.* 2002;20:1182-1191.

Gemcitabine-Vinorelbine (see also G + V)

Use: Lung cancer (non-small cell). *Cycle*: 28 days for up to 6 cycles

Regimen: Gemcitabine 800 or 1,000 mg/m^2 IV, days 1, 8, and 15
              Vinorelbine 20 mg/m^2 IV, days 1, 8, and 15

References: •Chen YM, Perng RP, Yang KY, et al. A multicenter phase II trial of vinorel-
              bine plus gemcitabine in previously untreated (Stage IIIB/IV) non-small cell
              lung cancer. *Chest.* 2000;117:1583-1589.
              •Hainsworth JD, Burris HA, Litchy S, et al. Gemcitabine and vinorelbine in
              the second-line treatment of nonsmall cell lung carcinoma patients. *Cancer.*
              2000;88:1353-1358.

HDCA (High-dose cytarabine)—see professional monograph for Cytarabine
HDMTX

Use: Sarcoma (bone). *Cycle*: 1 to 4 weeks

Regimen: Methotrexate 8,000 to 12,000 mg/m^2 (20,000 mg maximum dose) IV, day 1
              Leucovorin 15 mg/m^2/dose PO or IV every 6 hours for 10 doses, beginning
              20 to 30 hours after beginning of methotrexate infusion

References: •Bacci G, Picci P, Ferrari S, et al. Primary chemotherapy and delayed sur-
              gery for nonmetastatic osteosarcoma of the extremities. *Cancer.*
              1993;72:3227-3238.
              •Camitta BM, Holcenberg JS. Safety of delayed leucovorin "rescue" follow-
              ing high-dose methotrexate in children. *Med Pediatr Oncol.* 1978;5:55-59.
              •Leung S, Marshall GM, Mahr MA, Tobias V, Lee DB, Hughes DO. Prog-
              nostic significance of chemotherapy dosage characteristics in children with
              osteogenic sarcoma. *Med Pediatr Oncol.* 1997;28:179-182.
              •Rosen G, Caparros B, Huvos AG, et al. Preoperative chemotherapy for os-
              teogenic sarcoma: selection of postoperative adjuvant chemotherapy
              based on the response of the primary tumor to preoperative chemotherapy.
              Cancer. 1982;49:1221-1230.

HEC

Use: Breast cancer. *Cycle*: 21 days for up to 8 cycles

Regimen: Epirubicin 100 mg/m^2 IV, day 1
              Cyclophosphamide 830 mg/m^2 IV, day 1

Reference: •Piccart MJ, Di Leo A, Beauduin M, et al. Phase III trial comparing two dose
              levels of epirubicin combined with cyclophosphamide, methotrexate, and
              fluorouracil in node-positive breast cancer. *J Clin Oncol.* 2001;19:3103-
              3110.

Hexa-CAF

Use: Ovarian cancer. *Cycle*: 28 days

Regimen: Altretamine 150 mg/m^2/day PO, days 1 through 14
              Cyclophosphamide 100 to 150 mg/m^2/day PO, days 1 through 14
              Methotrexate 40 mg/m^2 IV, days 1 and 8
              Fluorouracil 600 mg/m^2 IV, days 1 and 8

References: •Neijt JP, van der Burg MEL, Vriesendorp R, et al. Randomised trial com-
              paring two combination chemotherapy regimens (HEXA-CAF vs CHAP-5)
              in advanced ovarian carcinoma. *Lancet.* 1984;2:594-600.
              •Young RC, Chabner BA, Hubbard SP, et al. Advanced ovarian adenocar-
              cinoma: a prospective clinical trial of melphalan (L-PAM) versus combina-
              tion chemotherapy. *N Engl J Med.* 1978;299:1261-1266.

Hi-C DAZE

Use: Acute myelogenous leukemia (AML; induction—pediatrics). *Cycle*: Give a single cycle

Regimen: Daunorubicin 30 mg/m²/day IV, days 1 through 3
Cytarabine 3,000 mg/m²/dose IV every 12 hours, days 1 through 4 (total of 8 doses)
Etoposide 200 mg/m²/day IV, days 1 through 3 and days 6 through 8
Azacitidine 150 mg/m²/day IV, days 3 through 5 and days 8 through 10

Reference: •Grier HE, Gelber RD, Link MP, Camitta BP, Clavell LA, Weistein HJ. Intensive sequential chemotherapy for children with acute myelogenous leukemia: VAPA, 80-035, and HI-C-Daze. *Leukemia*. 1992;6:48-51.

HIDAC (High-dose cytarabine)—see professional monograph for Cytarabine

Hyper-CVAD/HD MTX Ara-C*

Use: Lymphoma (mantle cell). *Cycle*: 21 days, delay subsequent cycles until hematologic recovery. Give up to 4 cycles

Regimen: **Treatment A**—Hyper-CVAD (cycles 1 and 3)
Cyclophosphamide 300 mg/m²/dose IV every 12 hours for 6 doses, days 1 through 3
Doxorubicin 25 mg/m²/day continuous IV infusion, days 4 and 5
Vincristine 2 mg (dose is not in mg/m²) IV, day 4 (given 12 hours after last cyclophosphamide dose) and day 11
Dexamethasone 40 mg/day IV or PO, days 1 through 4 and days 11 through 14
Filgrastim 5 mcg/kg/day subcutaneously, starting on day 6 and continued until granulocyte count exceeds 4,500 cells/mm³
Treatment B—HD MTX Ara-C (cycles 2 and 4)
Methotrexate 200 mg/m² IV bolus, day 1
then
Methotrexate 800 mg/m²/day continuous IV infusion, day 1
Cytarabine 3,000 mg/m²/dose IV every 12 hours for 4 doses, days 2 and 3
Leucovorin 50 mg PO, day 3, given 24 hours after methotrexate infusion is completed
Leucovorin 15 mg/dose PO every 6 hours for 8 doses, days 3 through 5, starting 30 hours after methotrexate infusion is completed
Filgrastim 5 mcg/kg/day subcutaneously, starting on day 6 and continued until granulocyte count exceeds 4,500 cells/mm³
used in conjunction with
Autologous stem cell transplantation
*Note: These two regimens are normally used in combination with each other and are rarely given alone.

Reference: •Khouri IF, Romaguera J, Kantarjian H, et al. Hyper-CVAD and high-dose methotrexate/cytarabine followed by stem-cell transplantation: an active regimen for aggressive mantle cell lymphoma. *J Clin Oncol*. 1998;16:3803-3809.

Hyper-CVAD/HD MTX Ara-C* (cont.)

Use: Acute lymphocytic leukemia (ALL; induction—adults). *Cycle:* 21 days, delay subsequent cycles until hematologic recovery. Give 8 cycles.

Regimen: **Treatment A**—Hyper-CVAD (cycles 1, 3, 5, and 7)
Cyclophosphamide 300 mg/m^2/dose IV every 12 hours for 6 doses, days 1 through 3
Mesna 600 mg/m^2/day continuous IV infusion, days 1 through 3 (begin with cyclophosphamide)
Doxorubicin 50 mg/m^2 IV, day 4
Vincristine 2 mg (dose is not in mg/m^2) IV, days 4 and 11
Dexamethasone 40 mg/day IV or PO, days 1 through 4 and days 11 through 14
Filgrastim 10 mcg/kg/day subcutaneously, starting day 5 and continued until granulocyte count exceeds 3,000 cells/mm^3
Treatment B—HD MTX Ara-C (cycles 2, 4, 6, and 8)
Methotrexate 200 mg/m^2 IV bolus, day 1
then
Methotrexate 800 mg/m^2/day continuous IV infusion, day 1
Cytarabine 3,000 mg/m^2/dose IV every 12 hours for 4 doses, days 2 and 3
Leucovorin 15 mg PO or IV every 6 hours for 8 doses, beginning on day 3, starting 24 hours after methotrexate infusion finished and continued until methotrexate concentration is less than 0.1 microMol/L; increase dose to 50 mg/dose PO or IV every 6 hours if the methotrexate concentration is greater than 20 microMol/L at the end of the infusion or greater than 1 microMol/L 24 hours after the end of the infusion, or greater than 0.1 microMol/L 48 hours after the end of the infusion.
Methylprednisolone 50 mg/dose IV twice daily, days 1 through 3
Filgrastim 10 mcg/kg/day subcutaneously, starting day 4 and continued until granulocyte count exceeds 3,000 cells/mm^3
CNS prophylaxis: Given for cycle 1 and 2 for low-risk patients, cycle 1 through 4 for unknown risk, and all 8 cycles for high-risk patients.
Methotrexate 12 mg intrathecal, day 2
Cytarabine 100 mg intrathecal, day 8
used in conjunction with antimicrobial prophylaxis
Fluconazole 200 mg/day PO, continuously
plus
Ciprofloxacin 500 mg PO twice daily, continuously
or
Levofloxacin 500 mg/day PO, continuously
plus
Acyclovir 200 mg PO twice daily, continuously
or
Valacyclovir 500 mg/day PO, continuously
*Note: These two regimens are normally used in combination with each other and are rarely given alone.

Hyper-CVAD/HD MTX Ara-C* (cont.)

References: •Garcia-Manero G, Kantarjian HM. Advances in the treatment of adult acute lymphocytic leukemia. The Hyper-CVAD regimen in adult acute lymphocytic leukemia. *Hematol Oncol Clin North Am.* 2000;14:1381-1396.

•Kantarjian HM, O'Brien S, Smith TL, et al. Results of treatment with hyper-CVAD, a dose-intensive regimen, in adult acute lymphocytic leukemia. *J Clin Oncol.* 2000;18:547-561.

•Weiser MA, O'Brien S, Thomas DA, Pierce SA, Lam TP, Kantarjian HM. Comparison of two different treatment schedules of granulocyte-colony-stimulating-factor during treatment for acute lymphocytic leukemia with a Hyper-CVAD (cyclophosphamide, doxorubicin, vincristine, and dexamethasone) regimen. *Cancer.* 2002;94:285-291.

ICE—see MICE

ICE + Autologous Stem Cell Transplantation

Use: Lymphoma (non-Hodgkin—adults). *Cycle*: 14 days for 3 cycles

Regimen. Etoposide 100 mg/m²/day IV, days 1 through 3
Ifosfamide 5,000 mg/m²/day continuous IV infusion, day 2*
Mesna 5,000 mg/m²/day continuous IV infusion, day 2*
Carboplatin IV dose by Calvert equation to AUC 5 mg/mL/min (800 mg maximum dose), day 2
Filgrastim 5 mcg/kg/day subcutaneously, days 5 through 12; increased in third cycle to 10 mcg/kg/day subcutaneously, from day 5 until leukapheresis
used in conjunction with
Autologous stem cell transplantation
*Note: Ifosfamide and mesna may be mixed and administered in the same infusion bag.

References: •Kewalramani T, Zelenetz AD, Hedick EE, et al. High-dose chemotherapy and autologous stem cell transplantation for patients with primary refractory aggressive non-Hodgkin lymphoma: an intention-to-treat analysis. *Blood.* 2000;96:2399-2404.

•Moskowitz CH, Bertino JR, Glassman JR, et al. Ifosfamide, carboplatin, and etoposide: a highly effective cytoreduction and peripheral-blood progenitor-cell mobilization regimen for transplant-eligible patients with non-Hodgkin's lymphoma. *J Clin Oncol.* 1999;17:3776-3785.

ICE Protocol—see Idarubicin, Cytarabine, Etoposide

ICE-T

Use: Breast cancer, sarcoma, lung cancer (non-small cell). *Cycle*: 28 days

Regimen: Ifosfamide 1,250 mg/m²/day IV, days 1 through 3
Carboplatin 300 mg/m² IV, day 1
Etoposide 80 mg/m²/day IV, days 1 through 3
Paclitaxel 175 mg/m² IV over 3 hours, day 4
with
Mesna 20% of ifosfamide dose IV before, then mesna 40% of ifosfamide dose PO given 4 and 8 hours after ifosfamide, days 1 through 3
or
Mesna 1,250 mg/m²/day IV, days 1 through 3

Reference: •Chang AY, Boros L, Garrow GC, Asbury RF, Hui L. Ifosfamide, carboplatin, etoposide, and paclitaxel chemotherapy: a dose-escalation study. *Semin Oncol.* 1996;23(3 suppl 6):74-77.

IDA-based BF12—see Idarubicin, Cytarabine, Etoposide

Idarubicin, Cytarabine, Etoposide (ICE Protocol)

Use: Acute myelogenous leukemia (AML; induction—adults). *Cycle*: Give a single cycle

Regimen: Idarubicin 6 mg/m²/day IV, days 1 through 5
            Cytarabine 600 mg/m²/day IV, days 1 through 5
            Etoposide 150 mg/m²/day IV, days 1 through 3

Reference: •Carella AM, Carlier P, Pungolino E, et al. Idarubicin in combination with intermediate-dose cytarabine and VP-16 in the treatment of refractory or rapidly relapsed patients with acute myeloid leukemia. *Leukemia.* 1993;7:196-199.

Idarubicin, Cytarabine, Etoposide (IDA-based BF12)

Use: Acute myelogenous leukemia (AML; induction—adults). *Cycle*: Usually 1 cycle used. A second cycle may be considered for patients with partial response. Time between cycles not specified.

Regimen: Idarubicin 5 mg/m²/day IV, days 1 through 5
            Cytarabine 2,000 mg/m²/dose IV every 12 hours, days 1 through 5 (total of 10 doses)
            Etoposide 100 mg/m²/day IV, days 1 through 5

Reference: •Mehta J, Powles R, Singhal S, et al. Idarubicin, high-dose cytarabine, and etoposide for induction of remission in acute leukemia. *Semin Hematol.* 1996;33:18-23.

IDMTX

Use: Acute lymphocytic leukemia (ALL; intensification—pediatrics). *Cycle*: 14 days, for 12 cycles

Regimen: Methotrexate 1,000 mg/m²/day continuous IV infusion, day 1 (24-hour infusion)
            Mercaptopurine 1,000 mg/m² IV over 6 hours following methotrexate, day 2
            Leucovorin 5 mg/m²/dose IV over 6 hours for at least 5 doses, days 3 and 4, starting 48 hours after the start of the methotrexate infusion and continued until methotrexate concentration is less than 0.1 microMol/L
            Methotrexate 20 mg/m² IM, day 8
            Mercaptopurine 50 mg/m²/day PO, days 8 through 14

Reference: •Mahoney DH, Shuster J, Nitschke R, Lauer S, Steuber CP, Camitta B. Intensification with intermediate-dose intravenous methotrexate effective therapy for children with lower-risk B-precursor acute lymphoblastic leukemia: a Pediatric Oncology Group study. *J Clin Oncol.* 2000;18:1285-1294.

IDMTX/6-MP

Use: Acute lymphocytic leukemia (ALL; consolidation—pediatrics). *Cycle*: 2 weeks, up to 12 cycles

Regimen: **Week 1**: Methotrexate 200 mg/m² IV bolus, day 1
            Mercaptopurine 200 mg/m² IV bolus, day 1
            then
            Methotrexate 800 mg/m²/day continuous IV infusion, day 1
            Mercaptopurine 800 mg/m² IV over 8 hours, day 1
            Leucovorin 5 mg/m²/dose PO or IV every 6 hours for 5 to 13 doses, beginning 24 hours after methotrexate infusion is completed
            Week 2: Methotrexate 20 mg/m² IM, day 8
            Mercaptopurine 50 mg/m²/day PO, days 8 through 14

Reference: •Camitta B, Mahoney D, Leventhal B, et al. Intensive intravenous methotrexate and mercaptopurine treatment of higher-risk non-T, non-B acute lymphocytic leukemia: a Pediatric Oncology Group study. *J Clin Oncol.* 1994;12:1383-1389.

IE

Use: Sarcoma (soft-tissue). *Cycle*: 21 days

Regimen: Ifosfamide 1,800 mg/m²/day IV, days 1 through 5
Etoposide 100 mg/m²/day IV, days 1 through 5
with
Mesna 1,800 mg/m²/day IV, days 1 through 5
or
Mesna 20% of ifosfamide dose prior to, then 4 and 8 hours after ifosfamide, days 1 through 5

References: •Ben Arush MW, Stein ME, Kuten A, et al. Postsurgical etoposide-ifosfamide regimen in poor-risk nonmetastatic osteogenic sarcoma. *Am J Clin Oncol.* 1998;21:72-74.
•Mesnex. [package insert]. Princeton, NJ: Bristol-Myers Squibb Oncology/ Immunology Division; March 1998.

IFL + Bevacizumab

Use: Colorectal cancer. *Cycle*: 42 days

Regimen: Irinotecan 125 mg/m² IV, days 1, 8, 15, and 22
Fluorouracil 500 mg/m² IV, days 1, 8, 15, and 22
Leucovorin 20 mg/m² IV, days 1, 8, 15, and 22
Bevacizumab 5 mg/kg IV, days 1, 15, and 29

Reference: •Hurwitz H, Fehrenbacher L, Novotny W, et al. Bevacizumab plus irinotecan, fluorouracil, and leucovorin for metastatic colorectal cancer. *N Engl J Med.* 2004;350:2335-2342.

IfoVP

Use: Sarcoma (osteosarcoma—pediatrics). *Cycle*: 21 days

Regimen: Ifosfamide 1,800 mg/m²/day IV, days 1 through 5
Etoposide 100 mg/m²/day IV, days 1 through 5
Mesna 1,800 mg/m²/day IV, days 1 through 5

Reference: •Ben Arush MW, Stein ME, Kuten A, et al. Postsurgical etoposide-ifosfamide regimen in poor-risk nonmetastatic osteogenic sarcoma. *Am J Clin Oncol.* 1998;21:72-74.

Interferon-Cytarabine-Hydroxyurea

Use: Chronic myelogenous leukemia (CML). *Cycle*: 28 days

Regimen: Interferon alfa-2b 5 million units/day subcutaneously, continuously; adjust dose to white blood cell count
Hydroxyurea 50 mg/kg/day PO, continuously; adjust dose to white blood cell count
Cytarabine 20 mg/m²/day subcutaneously, days 15 through 24 (therapy modified based on white blood cell count and therapeutic response)

Reference: •Guilhot F, Chastang C, Michallet M, et al. Interferon alfa-2b, combined with cytarabine versus interferon alone in chronic myelogenous leukemia. *N Engl J Med.* 1997;337:223-229.

Interleukin 2-Interferon alfa 2

Use: Renal cell carcinoma. *Cycle*: 56 days

Regimen: Aldesleukin 20 million units/m²/dose subcutaneously 3 times weekly, weeks 1 and 4
Aldesleukin 5 million units/m²/dose subcutaneously 3 times weekly, weeks 2, 3, 5, and 6
Interferon alfa 6 million units/m²/dose subcutaneously once weekly, weeks 1 and 4
Interferon alfa 6 million units/m²/dose subcutaneously 3 times weekly, weeks 2, 3, 5, and 6

Reference: •Atzpodien J, Kirchner H, Hanninen EL, et al. European studies of interleukin-2 in metastatic renal cell carcinoma. *Semin Oncol.* 1993;20(6 suppl 9):22-26.

Use: Renal cell carcinoma

Regimen: **Remission induction.** *Cycle*: 11 days for 2 cycles
Aldesleukin 18 million units/m²/day continuous IV infusion, days 1 through 5
Interferon alfa-2a 6 million units/dose subcutaneously, days 1, 3, and 5
Maintenance. *Cycle*: 26 days for 4 cycles
Aldesleukin 18 million units/m²/day continuous IV infusion, days 1 through 5
Interferon alfa-2a 6 million units/dose subcutaneously, days 1, 3, and 5

Reference: •Negrier S, Escudier B, Lasset C, et al. Recombinant human interleukin-2, recombinant human interferon alfa-2a, or both in metastatic renal-cell carcinoma. *N Engl J Med.* 1998;338:1272-1278.

Interleukin 2-Interferon alfa 2-Fluorouracil

Use: Renal cell carcinoma. *Cycle*: 8 weeks

Regimen: Aldesleukin 20 million units/m²/dose subcutaneously 3 times weekly, weeks 1 and 4
Aldesleukin 5 million units/m²/dose subcutaneously 3 times weekly, weeks 2 and 3
Interferon alfa-2a 6 million units/m²/dose subcutaneously once weekly, weeks 1 and 4
Interferon alfa-2a 6 million units/m²/dose subcutaneously 3 times weekly, weeks 2 and 3
Interferon alfa-2a 9 million units/m²/dose subcutaneously 3 times weekly, weeks 5 through 8
Fluorouracil 750 mg/m²/dose IV bolus once weekly, weeks 5 through 8

References: •Atzpodien J, Kirchner H, Hanninen EL, et al. European studies of interleukin-2 in metastatic renal cell carcinoma. *Semin Oncol.* 1993;20(6):22-26.
•van Herpen CML, Jansen RLH, Kruit WHJ, et al. Immunochemotherapy with interleukin-2, interferon-α and 5-fluorouracil for progressive metastatic renal cell carcinoma: a multicenter phase II study. *Br J Cancer.* 2000;82(4):772-776.

Interleukin 2-Interferon alfa 2-Fluorouracil (cont.)

Use: Renal cell carcinoma. *Cycle*: 8 weeks for up to 3 cycles

Regimen: Aldesleukin 10 million units/m^2/dose subcutaneously twice daily, days 3 through 5, weeks 1 and 4

Aldesleukin 5 million units/m^2/day subcutaneously once daily, days 1, 3, and 5, weeks 2 and 3

Interferon alfa-2a 5 million units/m^2/dose subcutaneously, day 1, weeks 1 and 4

Interferon alfa-2a 5 million units/m^2/day subcutaneously, days 1, 3, and 5, weeks 2 and 3

Interferon alfa-2a 10 million units/m^2/day subcutaneously, days 1, 3, and 5, weeks 5 through 8

Fluorouracil 1,000 mg/m^2/dose IV, day 1, weeks 5 through 8

Reference: •Atzpodien J, Krichner H, Illiger HJ, et al. IL-2 combination with IFN-α and 5-FU versus tamoxifen in metastatic renal cell carcinoma: long-term results of a controlled randomized clinical trial. *Br J Cancer.* 2001;85(8):1130-1136.

IPA

Use: Hepatoblastoma (pediatrics). *Cycle*: 21 days

Regimen: Ifosfamide 500 mg/m^2 IV bolus, day 1

Ifosfamide 1,000 mg/m^2/day continuous IV infusion, days 1 through 3

Cisplatin 20 mg/m^2/day IV, days 4 through 8

Doxorubicin 30 mg/m^2/day continuous IV infusion, days 9 and 10

Reference: •von Schweinitz D, Byrd DJ, Hecker H, et al. Efficiency and toxicity of ifosfamide, cisplatin and doxorubicin in the treatment of childhood hepatoblastoma. *Eur J Cancer.* 1997;33:1243-1249.

Larson Regimen

Use: Acute lymphoblastic leukemia (ALL; adults)

Regimen: **Remission induction.** *Cycle*: 28 days. Give a single cycle.

Patients aged 60 years and younger.
Cyclophosphamide 1,200 mg/m^2 IV, day 1
Daunorubicin 45 mg/m^2/day IV, days 1 through 3
Vincristine 2 mg (dose is not in mg/m^2) IV, days 1, 8, 15, and 22
Prednisone 60 mg/m^2/day PO or IV, days 1 through 21
Asparaginase 6,000 units/m^2/dose subcutaneously, days 5, 8, 11, 15, 18, and 22

Patients older than 60 years of age:
Cyclophosphamide 800 mg/m^2 IV, day 1
Daunorubicin 30 mg/m^2/day IV, days 1 through 3
Vincristine 2 mg (dose is not in mg/m^2) IV, days 1, 8, 15, and 22
Prednisone 60 mg/m^2/day PO, days 1 through 7
Asparaginase 6,000 units/m^2/dose subcutaneously, days 5, 8, 11, 15, 18, and 22

Larson Regimen (cont.)

Regimen: **Early intensification.** *Cycle:* 28 days. Give 2 cycles.
Methotrexate 15 mg intrathecally, day 1
Cyclophosphamide 1,000 mg/m^2 IV, day 1
Mercaptopurine 60 mg/m^2/day PO, days 1 through 14
Cytarabine 75 mg/m^2/day subcutaneously, days 1 through 4 and days 8 through 11
Vincristine 2 mg (dose is not in mg/m^2) IV, days 15 and 22
Asparaginase 6,000 units/m^2/dose subcutaneously, days 15, 18, 22, and 25
CNS prophylaxis and interim maintenance. *Cycle:* 84 days. Give a single cycle.
Methotrexate 15 mg intrathecally, days 1, 8, 15, 22, and 29
Methotrexate 20 mg/m^2/dose PO, days 36, 43, 50, 57, and 64
Mercaptopurine 60 mg/m^2/day PO, days 1 through 70
used in conjunction with
Cranial irradiation
used in conjunction with antimicrobial prophylaxis*
Cotrimoxazole (either 80/400 or 160/800 strength) 1 tablet PO daily, continuously
or
Pentamidine 300 mg inhaled once monthly, continuously
Late intensification. *Cycle:* 56 days. Give a single cycle.
Doxorubicin 30 mg/m^2/dose IV, days 1, 8, and 15
Vincristine 2 mg (dose is not in mg/m^2) IV, days 1, 8, and 15
Dexamethasone 10 mg/m^2/day PO, days 1 through 14
Cyclophosphamide 1,000 mg/m^2 IV, day 29
Thioguanine 60 mg/m^2/day PO, days 29 through 42
Cytarabine 75 mg/m^2/dose subcutaneously, days 29 through 32 and days 36 through 39
used in conjunction with antimicrobial prophylaxis*
Cotrimoxazole (either 80/400 or 160/800 strength) 1 tablet PO daily, continuously
or
Pentamidine 300 mg inhaled once monthly, continuously
Prolonged maintenance. *Cycle:* 28 days, continue until 24 months after diagnosis.
Vincristine 2 mg (dose is not in mg/m^2) IV, day 1
Prednisone 60 mg/m^2/day PO, days 1 through 5
Methotrexate 20 mg/m^2/dose PO, days 1, 8, 15, and 22, for first cycle only
Mercaptopurine 60 mg/m^2/day PO, days 1 through 28, for first cycle only
used in conjunction with antimicrobial prophylaxis*
Cotrimoxazole (either 80/400 or 160/800 strength) 1 tablet PO daily, continuously
or
Pentamidine 300 mg inhaled once monthly, continuously
*Note: Antimicrobial prophylaxis doses not specified in original articles; the dose given here is derived from the Isada reference, a tertiary book.

Larson Regimen (cont.)

References: •Pneumocystis carinii. In: Isada CM, Kasten BL, Goldman MP, Gray LD, Aberg JA, eds. *Infectious Diseases Handbook*. 5th ed. Hudson, OH: Lexi-Comp; 2003:253-255.

•Larson RA, Dodge RK, Burns CP, et al. A five-drug remission induction regimen with intensive consolidation for adults with acute lymphoblastic leukemia: Cancer and Leukemia Group B study 8811. *Blood*. 1995;85:2025-2037.

Linker Protocol

Use: Acute lymphocytic leukemia (ALL; induction and consolidation)

Regimen: **Remission induction**. *Cycle*: Give 1 cycle only
Daunorubicin 50 mg/m²/day IV, days 1 through 3
Vincristine 2 mg (dose is not in mg/m²) IV, days 1, 8, 15, and 22
Prednisone 60 mg/m²/day PO, days 1 through 28
Asparaginase 6,000 units/m²/day IM, days 17 through 28
if residual leukemia in marrow on day 14:
  Daunorubicin 50 mg/m² IV, day 15
if residual leukemia in marrow on day 28:
  Daunorubicin 50 mg/m²/day IV, days 29 and 30
  Vincristine 2 mg (dose is not in mg/m²) IV, days 29 and 36
  Prednisone 60 mg/m²/day PO, days 29 through 42
  Asparaginase 6,000 units/m²/day IM, days 29 through 35
Consolidation therapy. *Cycle*: 28 days
Treatment A (cycles 1, 3, 5, and 7)
  Daunorubicin 50 mg/m²/day IV, days 1 and 2
  Vincristine 2 mg (dose is not in mg/m²) IV, days 1 and 8
  Prednisone 60 mg/m²/day PO, days 1 through 14
  Asparaginase 12,000 units/m² IM, days 2, 4, 7, 9, 11, and 14
Treatment B (cycles 2, 4, 6, and 8)
  Teniposide 165 mg/m² IV, days 1, 4, 8, and 11
  Cytarabine 300 mg/m² IV, days 1, 4, 8, and 11
Treatment C (cycle 9)
  Methotrexate 690 mg/m² IV over 42 hours
  Leucovorin 15 mg/m²/dose IV every 6 hours for 12 doses (start at end of methotrexate infusion)

Reference: •Linker CA, Levitt LJ, O'Donnell M, Forman SJ, Ries CA. Treatment of adult acute lymphoblastic leukemia with intensive cyclical chemotherapy: a follow-up report. *Blood*. 1991;78:2814-2822.

M-2

Use: Multiple myeloma. *Cycle*: 5 weeks

Regimen: Vincristine 0.03 mg/kg (2 mg maximum dose) IV, day 1
Carmustine 0.5 mg/kg IV, day 1
Cyclophosphamide 10 mg/kg IV, day 1
Prednisone 1 mg/kg/day PO, days 1 through 7, tapered over next 14 days
with
Melphalan 0.25 mg/kg/day PO, days 1 through 4
or
Melphalan 0.1 mg/kg/day PO, days 1 through 7 or days 1 through 10

Reference: •Case DC Jr, Lee BJ, Clarkson B. Improved survival times in multiple myeloma treated with melphalan, prednisone, cyclophosphamide, vincristine, and BCNU: M-2 protocol. *Am J Med*. 1977;63:897-903.

m-BACOD (see also M-BACOD)*

Use: Lymphoma (non-Hodgkin). *Cycle*: 21 days

Regimen: Bleomycin 4 units/m^2 IV, day 1
Doxorubicin 45 mg/m^2 IV, day 1
Cyclophosphamide 600 mg/m^2 IV, day 1
Vincristine 1 mg/m^2 (2 mg maximum dose) IV, day 1
Dexamethasone 6 mg/m^2/day PO, days 1 through 5
Methotrexate 200 mg/m^2 IV, days 8 and 15
Leucovorin 10 mg/m^2/dose PO every 6 hours for 8 doses, begin 24 hours after each methotrexate dose
Sargramostim 5 mcg/kg/day subcutaneously, days 4 through 13
used in conjunction with
Intrathecal chemotherapy
*Note: m-BACOD and M-BACOD differ in the dose and timing of the methotrexate. Leucovorin dose not specified in original articles; the dose given here is derived from the Wooldridge reference, a tertiary book.

References: •Kaplan LD, Straus DJ, Testa MA, et al. Low-dose compared with standard-dose m-BACOD chemotherapy for non-Hodgkin's lymphoma associated with human immunodeficiency virus infection. *N Engl J Med.* 1997;336:1641-1648.
•Shipp MA, Harrington DP, Klatt MM, et al. Identification of major prognostic subgroups of patients with large-cell lymphoma treated with m-BACOD or M-BACOD. *Ann Intern Med.* 1986;104:757-765.
•Wooldridge JE. Chemotherapy programs. In: Perry MC. *The Chemotherapy Source Book.* 3rd ed. Philadelphia, PA: Lippincott Williams & Wilkins; 2001:876-904.

m-BACOD (Reduced Dose)*

Use: Lymphoma (non-Hodgkin) associated with HIV infection. *Cycle*: 21 days

Regimen: Bleomycin 4 units/m^2 IV, day 1
Doxorubicin 25 mg/m^2 IV, day 1
Cyclophosphamide 300 mg/m^2 IV, day 1
Vincristine 1.4 mg/m^2 (2 mg maximum dose) IV, day 1
Dexamethasone 3 mg/m^2/day PO, days 1 through 5
Methotrexate 200 mg/m^2 IV, day 15
Sargramostim 5 mcg/kg/day subcutaneously, days 4 through 13 (added during subsequent cycles), for granulocyte count less than 500 cells/mm^3 at any time during the cycle or less than 1,000 cells/mm^3 on day 22 of any chemotherapy cycle
used in conjunction with
Intrathecal chemotherapy
*Note: m-BACOD (reduced dose) has decreased doses of cyclophosphamide and dexamethasone, and decreased number of methotrexate doses compared with m-BACOD.

Reference: •Kaplan LD, Straus DJ, Testa MA, et al. Low-dose compared with standard-dose m-BACOD chemotherapy for non-Hodgkin's lymphoma associated with human immunodeficiency virus infection. *N Engl J Med.* 1997;336:1641-1648.

M-BACOD (see also m-BACOD)*

Use: Lymphoma (non-Hodgkin). Cycle: 21 days

Regimen: Bleomycin 4 units/m^2 IV, day 1
Doxorubicin 45 mg/m^2 IV, day 1
Cyclophosphamide 600 mg/m^2 IV, day 1
Vincristine 1 mg/m^2 (2 mg maximum dose) IV, day 1
Dexamethasone 6 mg/m^2/day PO, days 1 through 5
Methotrexate 3,000 mg/m^2 IV, day 15
Leucovorin 10 mg/m^2/dose PO every 6 hours for 8 doses, begin 24 hours after methotrexate dose
Sargramostim 5 mcg/kg/day subcutaneously, days 4 through 13
*Notes: m-BACOD and M-BACOD differ in the dose and timing of the methotrexate. Leucovorin dose not specified in original articles; the dose given here is derived from the Wooldridge reference, a tertiary book.

References: •Shipp MA, Harrington DP, Klatt MM, et al. Identification of major prognostic subgroups of patients with large-cell lymphoma treated with m-BACOD or M-BACOD. Ann Intern Med. 1986;104:757-765.
•Wooldridge JE. Chemotherapy programs. In: Perry MC. The Chemotherapy Source Book. 3rd ed. Philadelphia, PA: Lippincott Williams & Wilkins; 2001:876-904.

M-VAC

Use: Bladder cancer. Cycle: 28 days

Regimen: Methotrexate 30 mg/m^2 IV, days 1, 15, and 22
Vinblastine 3 mg/m^2 IV, days 2, 15, and 22
Doxorubicin 30 mg/m^2 IV, day 2
Cisplatin 70 mg/m^2 IV, day 2

Reference: •Sternberg CN, Yagoda A, Scher HI, et al. Preliminary results of M-VAC (methotrexate, vinblastine, doxorubicin and cisplatin) for transitional cell carcinoma of the urothelium. J Urol. 1985;133:403-407.

MAC III

Use: Gestational trophoblastic neoplasm (high-risk). Cycle: 21 days

Regimen: Methotrexate 1 mg/kg IM, days 1, 3, 5, and 7
Leucovorin 0.1 mg/kg IM, days 2, 4, 6, and 8 (give 24 hours after each methotrexate dose)
Dactinomycin 0.012 mg/kg/day IV, days 1 through 5
Cyclophosphamide 3 mg/kg/day IV, days 1 through 5

Reference: •Berkowitz RS, Goldsteinn DP, Bernstein MR. Modified triple chemotherapy in the management of high-risk metastatic gestational trophoblastic tumors. Gynecol Oncol. 1984;19:173-181.

MACC

Use: Lung cancer (non-small cell). Cycle: 21 days

Regimen: Methotrexate 30 to 40 mg/m^2 IV, day 1
Doxorubicin 30 to 40 mg/m^2 IV, day 1 (total cumulative dose 550 mg/m^2)
Cyclophosphamide 400 mg/m^2 IV, day 1
Lomustine 30 mg/m^2/day PO, day 1

References: •Chahinian AP, Arnold DJ, Cohen JM, et al. Chemotherapy for bronchogenic carcinoma: methotrexate, doxorubicin, cyclophosphamide, and lomustine. JAMA. 1977;237:2392-2396.
•Chahinian AP, Mandel EM, Holland JF, Jaffrey IS, Teirstein AS. MACC (methotrexate, adriamycin, cyclophosphamide and CCNU) in advanced lung cancer. Cancer. 1979;43:1590-1597.

MACOP-B

Use: Lymphoma, (non-Hodgkin). *Cycle*: Give only a single cycle

Regimen: Methotrexate 400 mg/m^2 IV weekly, weeks 2, 6, and 10
Leucovorin 15 mg/dose PO every 6 hours for 6 doses, begin 24 hours after each methotrexate dose
Doxorubicin 50 mg/m^2 IV weekly, weeks 1, 3, 5, 7, 9, and 11
Cyclophosphamide 350 mg/m^2 IV weekly, weeks 1, 3, 5, 7, 9, and 11
Vincristine 1.4 mg/m^2 (2 mg maximum dose) IV weekly, weeks 2, 4, 6, 8, 10, and 12
Bleomycin 10 units/m^2 IV weekly, weeks 4, 8, and 12
Prednisone 75 mg/day PO for 12 weeks, tapered over last 2 weeks
used in conjunction with
Intrathecal chemotherapy
used in conjunction with antimicrobial prophylaxis
    Ketoconazole 200 mg/day PO, continuously
    Cotrimoxazole double-strength (160/800) 2 tablets PO twice daily, continuously

References: •Klimo P, Connors JM. MACOP-B chemotherapy for the treatment of diffuse large-cell lymphoma. *Ann Intern Med.* 1985;102:596-602.
•Klimo P, Connors JM. Updated clinical experience with MACOP-B. *Semin Hematol.* 1987;24(2 suppl 1):26-34.

MAID

Use: Sarcoma (soft-tissue, bony). *Cycle*: 21 days

Regimen: Mesna 2,000 mg/m^2/day continuous IV infusion, days 1 through 4*
Doxorubicin 15 mg/m^2/day continuous IV infusion, days 1 through 4
Ifosfamide 2,000 mg/m^2/day continuous IV infusion, days 1 through 3*
Dacarbazine 250 mg/m^2/day continuous IV infusion, days 1 through 4
*Note: Ifosfamide and mesna may be mixed and administered in the same infusion bag.

References: •Antman K, Crowley J, Balcerzak SP, et al. A Southwest Oncology Group and Cancer Leukemia Group B phase II study of doxorubicin, dacarbazine, ifosfamide, and mesna in adults with advanced osteosarcoma, Ewing's sarcoma, and rhabdomyosarcoma. *Cancer.* 1998;82:1288-1295.
•Antman K, Crowley J, Balcerzak SP, et al. An intergroup phase III randomized study of doxorubicin and dacarbazine with or without ifosfamide and mesna in advanced soft tissue and bone sarcomas. *J Clin Oncol.* 1993;11:1276-1285.

MBC

Use: Head and neck cancer. *Cycle*: 21 days

Regimen: Methotrexate 40 mg/m^2 IV, days 1 and 14
Bleomycin 10 units/m^2 IM or IV, days 1, 7, and 14
Cisplatin 50 mg/m^2 IV, day 4

Reference: •Villar A, Pera J, Arellano A, et al. Induction chemotherapy with cisplatin, bleomycin and methotrexate in advanced head and neck cancer—lack of therapeutic gain. *Radiother Oncol.* 1987;10:175-181.

MC

Use:	Acute myelocytic leukemia (AML; induction—adults). *Cycle*: Give a single cycle
Regimen:	Mitoxantrone 12 mg/m^2/day IV, days 1 through 3 Cytarabine 100 to 200 mg/m^2/day continuous IV infusion or IV, days 1 through 7
References:	•MacCallum PK, Rohatiner AZS, Davis CL, et al. Mitoxantrone and cytosine arabinoside as treatment for acute myeloblastic leukemia in older patients. *Ann Hematol*. 1995;71:35-39. •Paciucci PA, Dutcher JP, Cuttner J, Strauman JJ, Wiernik PH, Holland JF. Mitoxantrone and Ara-C in previously treated patients with acute myelogenous leukemia. *Leukemia*. 1987;1:565-567.

MCF

Use:	Gastric cancer. *Cycle*: 42 days for up to 4 cycles
Regimen:	Mitomycin 7 mg/m^2 (14 mg maximum dose) IV, day 1 Cisplatin 60 mg/m^2 IV, days 1 and 22 Fluorouracil 300 mg/m^2/day continuous IV infusion, days 1 through 180
Reference:	•Ross P, Nicolson M, Cunningham D, et al. Prospective randomized trial comparing mitomycin, cisplatin, and protracted venous-infusion fluorouracil (PVI 5-FU) with epirubicin, cisplatin, and PVI 5-FU in advanced esophagogastric cancer. *J Clin Oncol*. 2002;20:1996-2004.

MF

Use:	Breast cancer. *Cycle*: 28 days
Regimen:	Methotrexate 100 mg/m^2 IV, days 1 and 8 Fluorouracil 600 mg/m^2 IV, days 1 and 8, given 1 hour after methotrexate Leucovorin 10 mg/m^2/dose IV or PO every 6 hours for 6 doses, starting 24 hours after methotrexate
Reference:	•Fisher B, Dignam J, Mamounas EP, et al. Sequential methotrexate and fluorouracil for the treatment of node-negative breast cancer patients with estrogen receptor-negative tumors: eight-year results from National Surgical Adjuvant Breast and Bowel Project (NSABP) B-13 and first report of findings from NSABP B-19 comparing methotrexate and fluorouracil with conventional cyclophosphamide, methotrexate, and fluorouracil. *J Clin Oncol*. 1996;14:1982-1992.

MICE (ICE)

Use:	Sarcoma (adult), osteosarcoma (pediatric), lung cancer. *Cycle*: 21 to 28 days
Regimen:	Ifosfamide 1,250 to 1,500 mg/m^2/day IV, days 1 through 3 Carboplatin 300 to 635 mg/m^2 IV, once on day 1 or 3 Etoposide 80 to 100 mg/m^2/day IV, days 1 through 3 *with* Mesna 1,250 mg/m^2/day IV, days 1 through 3 *or* Mesna 20% of ifosfamide dose IV before, 4 hours after, and 8 hours after each ifosfamide infusion, days 1 through 3

MICE (ICE) (cont.)

References: •Cairo MS. The use of ifosfamide, carboplatin, and etoposide in children with solid tumors. *Semin Oncol.* 1995;22(3 suppl 7):23-27.
•Chang AY, Asbury RF, Boros L, Garrow GC, Hsieh S. Ifosfamide, carboplatin, etoposide chemotherapy in patients with metastatic non-small cell lung cancer. *Semin Oncol.* 1995;22:9-12.
•Kung FH, Desai SJ, Dickerman JD, et al. Ifosfamide/carboplatin/etoposide (ICE) for recurrent malignant solid tumors of childhood: a Pediatric Oncology Group Phase I/II study. *J Pediatr Hematol Oncol.* 1995;17:265-269.
•Mesnex. [package insert]. Princeton, NJ: Bristol-Myers Squibb Oncology/ Immunology Division; March 1998.

MINE

Use: Lymphoma (non-Hodgkin). *Cycle*: 21 days

Regimen: Mesna 1,330 mg/m^2/day IV, days 1 through 3, given with ifosfamide
Mesna 500 mg/dose PO, 4 hours after ifosfamide, days 1 through 3
Ifosfamide 1,330 mg/m^2/day IV, days 1 through 3
Mitoxantrone 8 mg/m^2 IV, day 1
Etoposide 65 mg/m^2/day IV, days 1 through 3

Reference: •Rodriguez MA, Cabanillas FC, Velasquez W, et al. Results of a salvage treatment program for relapsing lymphoma: MINE consolidated with ESHAP. *J Clin Oncol.* 1995;13:1734-1741.

MINE-ESHAP

Use: Lymphoma (non-Hodgkin). *Cycle*: 21 days

Regimen: Give MINE for 6 cycles, then give ESHAP for 3 to 6 cycles

References: •Cabanillas F. Experience with salvage regimens at MD Anderson Hospital. *Ann Oncol.* 1991;2(suppl 1):31-32.
•Rodriguez MA, Cabanillas FC, Velasquez W, et al. Results of a salvage treatment program for relapsing lymphoma: MINE consolidated with ESHAP. *J Clin Oncol.* 1995;13:1734-1741.

---

mini-BEAM

Use: Lymphoma (Hodgkin). *Cycle*: 4 to 6 weeks

Regimen: Carmustine 60 mg/m^2 IV, day 1
Etoposide 75 mg/m^2/day IV, days 2 through 5
Cytarabine 100 mg/m^2/dose IV every 12 hours for 8 doses, days 2 through 5
Melphalan 30 mg/m^2 IV, day 6

Reference: •Colwill R, Crump M, Couture F, et al. Mini-BEAM as salvage therapy for relapsed or refractory Hodgkin's disease before intensive therapy and autologous bone marrow transplantation. *J Clin Oncol.* 1995;13:396-402.

MOBP

Use: Cervical cancer. *Cycle*: 6 weeks

Regimen: Bleomycin 30 units/day continuous IV infusion, days 1 through 4
Vincristine* 0.5 mg/m^2 IV, days 1 and 4
Cisplatin 50 mg/m^2 IV, days 1 and 22
Mitomycin 10 mg/m^2 IV, day 2
*Note: The vincristine dose is not capped in this protocol. Consult the prescriber if there is any question about the intended vincristine dose.

MOBP (cont.)

References: •Alberts DS, Martimbeau PW, Surwit EA, Oishi N. Mitomycin-C, bleomycin, vincristine, and cis-platinum in the treatment of advanced, recurrent squamous cell carcinoma of the cervix. *Cancer Clin Trials.* 1981;4:313-316.
•Weiner SA, Aristizabal S, Alberts DS, Surwit EA, Deatherage-Deuser K. A phase II trial of mitomycin, vincristine, bleomycin, and cisplatin (MOBP) as neoadjuvant therapy in high-risk cervical carcinoma. *Gynecol Oncol.* 1988;30:1-6.

MOP

Use: Brain tumors (pediatric). *Cycle*: 28 days

Regimen: Mechlorethamine 6 mg/m^2 IV, days 1 and 8
Vincristine 1.5 mg/m^2 (2 mg maximum dose) IV, days 1 and 8
Procarbazine 100 mg/m^2/day PO, days 1 through 14

Reference: •Kretschmar CS, Tarbell NJ, Kupsky W, et al. Pre-irradiation chemotherapy for infants and children with medulloblastoma. *J Neurosurg.* 1989;71:820-825.

MOPP

Use: Lymphoma (Hodgkin—adults). *Cycle*: 28 days

Regimen: Mechlorethamine 6 mg/m^2 IV, days 1 and 8
Vincristine 1.4 mg/m^2 (2 mg maximum dose) IV, days 1 and 8
Procarbazine 100 mg/m^2/day PO, days 1 through 14
Prednisone 40 mg/m^2/day PO, cycles 1 and 4,* days 1 through 14
*Note: Some clinicians give prednisone with every cycle of MOPP. The original clinical trials gave prednisone only with the first and fourth cycles.

References: •Cooper MR, Pajak TF, Nissen NI, et al. A new effective four-drug combination of CCNU (1-]-3-cyclohexyl-1-nitrosourea) (NSC-79038), vinblastine, prednisone, and procarbazine for the treatment of advanced Hodgkin's disease. *Cancer.* 1980;46:654-662.
•DeVita VT Jr, Serpick AA, Carbone PP. Combination chemotherapy in the treatment of advanced Hodgkin's disease. *Ann Intern Med.* 1970;73:881-895.
•Wooldridge JE. Chemotherapy programs. In: Perry MC. *The Chemotherapy Source Book.* 3rd ed. Philadelphia, PA: Lippincott Williams & Wilkins; 2001:876-904.

Use: Lymphoma (Hodgkin—pediatrics). *Cycle*: 28 days

Regimen: Mechlorethamine 6 mg/m^2 IV, days 1 and 8
Vincristine 1.4 mg/m^2 (2 mg maximum dose) IV, days 1 and 8
Procarbazine 50 mg PO, day 1
Procarbazine 100 mg/m^2/day PO, days 2 through 14
Prednisone 40 mg/m^2/day PO, cycles 1 and 4,* days 1 through 14
*Note: Some clinicians give prednisone with every cycle of MOPP. The original clinical trials gave prednisone only with the first and fourth cycles.

References: •Gehan EA, Sullivan MP, Fuller LM, et al. The intergroup Hodgkin's disease in children: a study of stages I and II. *Cancer.* 1990;65:1429-1437.
•Wooldridge JE. Chemotherapy programs. In: Perry MC. *The Chemotherapy Source Book.* 3rd ed. Philadelphia, PA: Lippincott Williams & Wilkins; 2001:876-904.

MOPP (cont.)

Use: Brain cancer (medulloblastoma). *Cycle*: 28 days

Regimen: Mechlorethamine 3 mg/m^2 IV, days 1 and 8
Vincristine 1.4 mg/m^2 (2 mg maximum dose) IV, days 1 and 8
Prednisone 40 mg/m^2/day PO, days 1 through 10
Procarbazine 50 mg PO, day 1
Procarbazine 100 mg PO, day 2
Procarbazine 100 mg/m^2/day PO, days 3 through 10

Reference: •Kirscher JP, Ragab AH, Kun L, et al. Nitrogen mustard, vincristine, pro-carbazine, and prednisone as adjuvant chemotherapy in the treatment of medulloblastoma. *J Neurosurg*. 1991;74:905-909.

MOPP/ABV

Use: Lymphoma (Hodgkin). *Cycle*: 28 days

Regimen: Mechlorethamine 6 mg/m^2 IV, day 1
Vincristine 1.4 mg/m^2 (2 mg maximum dose) IV, day 1
Procarbazine 100 mg/m^2/day PO, days 1 through 7
Prednisone 40 mg/m^2/day PO, days 1 through 14
Doxorubicin 35 mg/m^2 IV, day 8
Bleomycin 10 units/m^2 IV, day 8
Vinblastine 6 mg/m^2 IV, day 8

Reference: •Conners JM, Klimo P. MOPP/ABV hybrid chemotherapy for advanced Hodgkin's disease. *Semin Hematol*. 1987;24:35-40.

MOPP/ABVD

Use: Lymphoma (Hodgkin). *Cycle*: 28 days

Regimen: Alternate MOPP and ABVD regimens every month

Reference: •Bonadonna G, Valagussa P, Santoro A. Alternating non-cross-resistant combination chemotherapy or MOPP in stage IV Hodgkin's disease. *Ann Intern Med*. 1986;104:739-746.

MP

Use: Multiple myeloma. *Cycle*: 21 to 28 days

Regimen: Melphalan 8 mg/m^2/day PO, days 1 through 4
Prednisone 60 mg/m^2/day PO, days 1 through 4

References: •Oken MM, Harrington DP, Abramson N, Kyle RA, Knospe W, Glick JH. Comparison of melphalan and prednisone with vincristine, carmustine, mel-phalan, cyclophosphamide, and prednisone in the treatment of multiple my-eloma. *Cancer*. 1997;79:1561-1567.
•Salmon SE, Haut A, Bonnet JD, et al. Alternating combination chemo-therapy and levamisole improves survival in multiple myeloma: a South-west Oncology Group Study. *J Clin Oncol*. 1983;1:453-461.

Use: Prostate cancer. *Cycle*: 21 days

Regimen: Mitoxantrone 12 mg/m^2 IV, day 1
Prednisone 5 mg/dose PO twice daily

Reference: •Tannock I, Osoba D, Stockler MR, et al. Chemotherapy with mitoxantrone plus prednisone or prednisone alone for symptomatic hormone-resistant prostate cancer: a Canadian randomized trial with palliative end points. *J Clin Oncol*. 1996;14:1756-1764.

MTX/6-MP

Use:	Acute lymphocytic leukemia (ALL; continuation—pediatric). *Cycle*: Ongoing, weeks 25 through 130
Regimen:	Methotrexate 20 mg/m^2 IM weekly Mercaptopurine 50 mg/m^2/day PO *used in conjunction with* Intrathecal therapy once every 12 weeks
Reference:	•Mahoney DH Jr, Shuster J, Nitschke R, et al. Intermediate-dose intravenous methotrexate with intravenous mercaptopurine is superior to repetitive low-dose oral methotrexate with intravenous mercaptopurine for children with lower-risk B-lineage acute lymphoblastic leukemia: a Pediatric Oncology Group phase III trial. *J Clin Oncol*. 1998;16:246-254.

MTX/6-MP/VP

Use:	Acute lymphocytic leukemia (ALL; continuation—pediatric). *Cycle*: Ongoing, 2 to 3 years
Regimen:	Methotrexate 20 mg/m^2/dose PO weekly Mercaptopurine 75 mg/m^2/day PO Vincristine* 1.5 mg/m^2 IV, once monthly Prednisone 40 mg/m^2/day PO for 5 days each month *Note: The vincristine dose is not capped in this pediatric protocol. Consult the prescriber if there is any question about the intended vincristine dose.
Reference:	•Bleyer WA, Sather HN, Nickerson HJ, et al. Monthly pulses of vincristine and prednisone prevent bone marrow and testicular relapse in low-risk childhood acute lymphoblastic leukemia: a report of the CCG-161 study by the Childrens Cancer Study Group. *J Clin Oncol*. 1991;9:1012-1021.

MTX-CDDPAdr

Use:	Osteosarcoma (pediatric). *Cycle*: 28 days
Regimen:	Methotrexate 12,000 mg/m^2 IV, days 1 and 8 Leucovorin 20 mg/m^2/dose IV every 3 hours for 8 doses then give PO every 6 hours for 8 doses (begin 16 hours after end of methotrexate infusion) Cisplatin 75 mg/m^2 IV, day 15 of cycles 1 through 7 Cisplatin 120 mg/m^2 IV, day 15 of cycles 8 through 10 Doxorubicin 25 mg/m^2/day IV, days 15 through 17 of cycles 1 through 7
Reference:	•Weiner MA, Harris MB, Lewis M, et al. Neoadjuvant high-dose methotrexate, cisplatin, and doxorubicin for the management of patients with nonmetastatic osteosarcoma. *Cancer Treat Rep*. 1986;70:1431-1432.

MV

Use:	Breast cancer. *Cycle*: 6 to 8 weeks
Regimen:	Mitomycin 20 mg/m^2 IV, day 1 Vinblastine 0.15 mg/kg IV, days 1 and 21
Reference:	•Konits PH, Aisner J, van Echo DA, Lichtenfeld K, Wiernik PH. Mitomycin C and vinblastine chemotherapy for advanced breast cancer. *Cancer*. 1981;48:1295-1298.

Use:	Acute myelocytic leukemia (AML; induction). *Cycle*: Give 1 cycle. Second cycle may be considered if complete response not achieved (ie, persistent blasts present on day 21).
Regimen:	Mitoxantrone 10 mg/m^2/day IV, days 1 through 5 Etoposide 100 mg/m^2/day IV, days 1 through 5

MV (cont.)

      Reference: •Ho AD, Lipp T, Ehninger G, et al. Combination of mitoxantrone and etoposide in refractory acute myelogenous leukemia—an active and well-tolerated regimen. *J Clin Oncol.* 1988;6:213-217.

MVP

      Use: Lung cancer (non-small cell). *Cycle*: 6 weeks

      Regimen: Mitomycin 8 mg/m^2 IV, day 1
                Vinblastine 6 mg/m^2 IV, days 1 and 22
                Cisplatin 50 mg/m^2 IV, days 1 and 22

      Reference: •Ellis PA, Nicolson MC, Tait D, Smith IE. MVP with moderate dose cisplatin: a pragmatic and effective chemotherapy for symptom relief in non-small cell lung cancer. *Br J Cancer.* 1994;69(suppl 21):14.

MVPP

      Use: Lymphoma (Hodgkin). *Cycle*: 6 weeks

      Regimen: Mechlorethamine 6 mg/m^2 (10 rng maximum dose) IV, days 1 and 8
                Vinblastine 4 to 6 mg/m^2 (10 mg maximum dose) IV, days 1 and 8
                Procarbazine 100 mg/m^2/day (150 mg maximum dose) PO, days 1 through 14
                Prednisone 40 mg/m^2/day (50 mg maximum dose) PO, cycles 1 and 4,*
                  days 1 through 14
                *Note: Some clinicians give prednisone with every cycle of MVPP. The original clinical trials gave prednisone only with the first and fourth cycles. Prednisolone is recommended in the British literature. In the United States, prednisone is the preferred corticosteroid. The doses of these 2 corticosteroids are equivalent (ie, prednisone 40 mg PO = prednisolone 40 mg PO).

      References: •Anderson H, Deakin DP, Wagstaff J, et al. A randomised study of adjuvant chemotherapy after mantle radiotherapy in supradiaphragmatic Hodgkin's disease PS IA-IIB: a report form the Manchester lymphoma group. *Br J Cancer.* 1984;49:695-702.
                •Cooper MR, Pajak TF, Nissen NI, et al. A new effective four-drug combination of CCNU (1-]-3-cyclohexyl-1-nitrosourea) (NSC-79038), vinblastine, prednisone, and procarbazine for the treatment of advanced Hodgkin's disease. *Cancer.* 1980;46:654-662.
                •Lister TA, Dorreen MS, Faux M, Jones AE, Wrigley PF. The treatment of stage IIIA Hodgkin's disease. *J Clin Oncol.* 1983;1:745-749.
                •Nicholson WM, Beard MEJ, Crowther D, et al. Combination chemotherapy in generalized Hodgkin's disease. *Br Med J.* 1970;3:7-10.
                •Radford JA, Crowther D, Rohatiner AZ, et al. Results of a randomized trial comparing MVPP chemotherapy with a hybrid regimen, ChlVPP/EVA, in the initial treatment of Hodgkin's disease. *J Clin Oncol.* 1995;13:2379-2385.

NA—see Vinorelbine-Doxorubicin

NFL

      Use: Breast cancer. *Cycle*: 21 days

      Regimen: Mitoxantrone 12 mg/m^2 IV, day 1
                Fluorouracil 350 mg/m^2/day IV, days 1 through 3 after leucovorin
                Leucovorin 300 mg/day IV, days 1 through 3
                or
                Mitoxantrone 10 mg/m^2 IV, day 1
                Fluorouracil 1,000 mg/m^2/day continuous IV infusion, days 1 through 3
                Leucovorin 100 mg/m^2/day IV, days 1 through 3, give before fluorouracil on
                  day 1

NFL (cont.)

References: •Hainsworth JD, Andrews MB, Johnson DH, Greco FA. Mitoxantrone, fluorouracil, and high-dose leucovorin: an effective, well-tolerated regimen for metastatic breast cancer. *J Clin Oncol.* 1991;9:1731-1735.

•Jones SE, Mennel RG, Brooks B, et al. Phase II study of mitoxantrone, leucovorin, and infusional fluorouracil for treatment of metastatic breast cancer. *J Clin Oncol.* 1991;9:1736-1739.

NOVP

Use: Lymphoma (Hodgkin). *Cycle*: 21 days

Regimen: Mitoxantrone 10 mg/m² IV, day 1
Vinblastine 6 mg/m² IV, day 1
Prednisone 100 mg/day PO, days 1 through 5
Vincristine 1.4 mg/m² (2 mg maximum dose) IV, day 8

Reference: •Meistrich ML, Wilson G, Mathur K, et al. Rapid recovery of spermatogenesis after mitoxantrone, vincristine, vinblastine, and prednisone chemotherapy for Hodgkin's disease. *J Clin Oncol.* 1997;15:3488-3495.

OPA

Use: Lymphoma (Hodgkin—pediatrics). *Cycle*: 15 days. Up to 2 cycles used. Time between cycles not specified.

Regimen: Vincristine 1.5 mg/m² (2 mg maximum dose) IV, days 1, 8, and 15
Prednisone 60 mg/m²/day PO in 3 divided doses, days 1 through 15
Doxorubicin 40 mg/m² IV, days 1 and 15

Reference: •Schellong G, Riepenhausen, Creutzig U, et al. Low risk of secondary leukemias after chemotherapy without mechlorethamine in childhood Hodgkin's disease. *J Clin Oncol.* 1997;15:2247-2253.

OPPA

Use: Lymphoma (Hodgkin—pediatrics). *Cycle*: 15 days. Up to 2 cycles used. Time between cycles not specified.

Regimen: **Add to OPA**: Procarbazine 100 mg/m²/day PO in 2 to 3 divided doses, days 1 through 15

Reference: •Schellong G, Riepenhausen M, Creutzig U, et al. Low risk of secondary leukemias after chemotherapy without mechlorethamine in childhood Hodgkin's disease. *J Clin Oncol.* 1997;15:2247-2253.

PA-CI

Use: Hepatoblastoma (pediatrics). *Cycle*: 21 days

Regimen: Cisplatin 90 mg/m² IV, day 1
Doxorubicin 20 mg/m²/day continuous IV infusion, days 2 through 5

References: •Ortega JA, Douglass EC, Feusner JH, et al. Randomized comparison of cisplatin/vincristine/fluorouracil and cisplatin/continuous infusion doxorubicin for treatment of pediatric hepatoblastoma: a report form the Children's Cancer Group and the Pediatric Oncology Group. *J Clin Oncol.* 2000;18:2665-2675.

•Ortega JA, Krailo MD, Haas JE, et al. Effective treatment of unresectable or metastatic hepatoblastoma with cisplatin and continuous infusion doxorubicin chemotherapy: a report from the Childrens Cancer Study Group. *J Clin Oncol.* 1991;9:2167-2176.

•von Schweinitz D, Byrd DJ, Hecker H, et al. Efficiency and toxicity of ifosfamide, cisplatin, and doxorubicin in the treatment of childhood hepatoblastoma. *Eur J Cancer.* 1997;33:1243-1249.

PAC

Use: Ovarian, endometrial cancer. *Cycle*: 28 days

Regimen: Cisplatin 50 mg/m^2 IV, day 1
             Doxorubicin 50 mg/m^2 IV, day 1
             Cyclophosphamide 500 mg/m^2 IV, day 1

Reference: •Burke TW, Gershenson DM, Morris M, et al. Postoperative adjuvant cis-platin, doxorubicin, and cyclophosphamide (PAC) chemotherapy in women with high-risk endometrial carcinoma. *Gynecol Oncol.* 1994;55:47-50.

PAC-I (Indiana Protocol)

Use: Ovarian cancer. *Cycle*: 21 days

Regimen: Cisplatin 50 mg/m^2 IV, day 1 (total cumulative dose 300 mg/m^2)
             Doxorubicin 50 mg/m^2 IV, day 1
             Cyclophosphamide 750 mg/m^2 IV, day 1

Reference: •Ehrlich CE, Einhorn L, Williams SD, Morgan J. Chemotherapy for stage III-IV epithelial ovarian cancer with cis-dichlorodiammineplatinum (II), adria-mycin, and cyclophosphamide. *Cancer Treat Rep.* 1979;63:281-288.

Paclitaxel-Carboplatin-Etoposide

Use: Adenocarcinoma (unknown primary), lung cancer (small cell). *Cycle*: 21 days

Regimen: Paclitaxel 200 mg/m^2 IV over 1 hour, day 1
             Carboplatin IV dose by Calvert equation to AUC 6 mg/mL/min, day 1 (give after paclitaxel)
             Etoposide 50 mg/day PO alternated with 100 mg/day PO, days 1 through 10

References: •Greco FA, Hainsworth JD. One-hour paclitaxel, carboplatin, and extended-schedule etoposide in the treatment of carcinoma of unknown primary site. *Semin Oncol.* 1997;24(6 suppl 19):S19-101-S19-105.
             •Hainsworth JD, Gray JR, Stroup SL, et al. Paclitaxel, carboplatin, and ex-tended-schedule etoposide in the treatment of small-cell lung cancer: com-parison of sequential phase II trials using different dose-intensities. *J Clin Oncol.* 1997;15:3464-3470.

Paclitaxel-Herceptin

Use: Breast cancer. *Cycle:* 7 days

Regimen: Paclitaxel 70 to 90 mg/m^2 IV over 1 hour, day 1 (give after trastuzumab)
             Trastuzumab 4 mg/kg IV, day 1 for first cycle only (loading dose); then tras-tuzumab 2 mg/kg IV, day 1 for subsequent cycles

Reference: •Chrisodoulou C, Klouvas G, Pateli A, Mellou S, Sgouros J, Skarlos DV. Prolonged administration of weekly paclitaxel and trastuzumab in patients with advanced breast cancer. *Anticancer Res.* 2003;23:737-744.

Paclitaxel-Vinorelbine

Use: Breast cancer. *Cycle*: 28 days

Regimen: Paclitaxel 135 mg/m^2 IV over 3 hours, day 1 (after vinorelbine infusion)
             Vinorelbine 30 mg/m^2 IV, days 1 and 8

Reference: •Acuna LR, Langhi M, Perez J, et al. Vinorelbine and paclitaxel as first-line chemotherapy in metastatic breast cancer. *J Clin Oncol.* 1999;17:74-81.

PC

Use:	Lung cancer (non-small cell). *Cycle*: 21 days
Regimen:	Paclitaxel 135 mg/m^2/day continuous IV infusion over 24 hours, day 1 Carboplatin IV dose by Calvert equation to AUC 7.5 mg/mL/min, day 2 (after paclitaxel)
Reference:	•Langer CJ, Leighton JC, Comis RL, et al. Paclitaxel by 24- or 1-hour infusion in combination with carboplatin in advanced non-small cell lung cancer: the Fox Chase Cancer Center experience. *Semin Oncol.* 1995;22 (4 suppl 9):18-29.

Use:	Lung cancer (non-small cell). *Cycle*: 21 days
Regimen:	Paclitaxel 175 mg/m^2 IV over 3 hours, day 1 Cisplatin 80 mg/m^2 IV, day 1 (after paclitaxel)
Reference:	•Giaccone G, Spliner TAW, Debruyne C, et al. Randomized study of paclitaxel-cisplatin versus cisplatin-teniposide in patients with advanced non-small-cell lung cancer. *J Clin Oncol.* 1998;16:2133-2141

Use:	Bladder cancer. *Cycle*: 21 days
Regimen:	Paclitaxel 200 or 225 mg/m^2 IV over 3 hours, day 1 Carboplatin IV dose by Calvert equation to AUC 5 to 6 mg/mL/min, day 1 (after paclitaxel)
References:	•Redman BG, Smith DC, Flaherty L, Du W, Hussain M. Phase II trial of paclitaxel and carboplatin in the treatment of advanced urothelial carcinoma. *J Clin Oncol.* 1998;16:1844-1848. •Vaughn DJ, Malkowicz SB, Zoltick B, et al. Paclitaxel plus carboplatin in advanced carcinoma of the urothelium: an active and tolerable outpatient regimen. *J Clin Oncol.* 1998;16:255-260.

PCV

Use:	Brain tumor. *Cycle*: 6 to 8 weeks
Regimen:	Lomustine 110 mg/m^2/day PO, day 1 Procarbazine 60 mg/m^2/day PO, days 8 through 21 Vincristine 1.4 mg/m^2 (2 mg maximum dose) IV, days 8 and 29
Reference:	•Levin VA, Silver P, Hannigan J, et al. Superiority of post-radiotherapy adjuvant chemotherapy with CCNU, procarbazine, and vincristine (PCV) over BCNU for anaplastic gliomas: NCOG 6G61 final report. *Int J Radiat Oncol Biol Phys.* 1990;18:321-324.

PE

Use:	Prostate cancer. *Cycle*: 21 days
Regimen:	Paclitaxel 30 mg/m^2/day continuous IV infusion over 24 hours, days 1 through 4 Estramustine 600 mg/m^2/day PO given in 2 to 3 divided doses (start 24 hours before first paclitaxel infusion)
Reference:	•Hudes GR, Nathan FE, Khater C, et al. Paclitaxel plus estramustine in metastatic hormone-refractory prostate cancer. *Semin Oncol.* 1995;22 (5 suppl 12):41-45.

PFL

Use:	Head and neck, gastric cancer. *Cycle*: 28 days
Regimen:	Cisplatin 25 mg/m^2/day continuous IV infusion, days 1 through 5
	Fluorouracil 800 mg/m^2/day continuous IV infusion, days 2 through 6
	Leucovorin 500 mg/m^2/day continuous IV infusion, days 1 through 6
Reference:	•Dreyfuss AI, Clark JR, Wright JE, et al. Continuous infusion high-dose leucovorin with 5-fluorouracil and cisplatin for untreated stage IV carcinoma of the head and neck. *Ann Intern Med.* 1990;112:167-172.

Use:	Head and neck, gastric cancer. *Cycle*: 21 days
Regimen:	Cisplatin 100 mg/m^2 IV, day 1
	Fluorouracil 600 to 800 mg/m^2/day continuous IV infusion, days 1 through 5
	Leucovorin 50 mg/m^2/dose PO every 4 to 6 hours, days 1 through 6
Reference:	•Vokes EE, Schilsky RL, Weichselbaum RR, et al. Cisplatin, 5-fluorouracil, and high-dose oral leucovorin for advanced head and neck cancer. *Cancer.* 1989;63:1048-1053.

POC

Use:	Brain tumors (pediatrics). *Cycle*: 6 weeks
Regimen:	Prednisone 40 mg/m^2/day PO, days 1 through 14
	Vincristine 1.5 mg/m^2 IV (2 mg maximum dose), days 1, 8, and 15
	Lomustine 100 mg/m^2/day PO, day 1
Reference:	•Finlay JF, Boyett JM, Yates AJ, et al. Randomized phase III trial in childhood high-grade astrocytoma comparing vincristine, lomustine, and prednisone with the eight-drugs-in-1-day regimen. *J Clin Oncol.* 1995;13:112-123.

ProMACE

Use:	Lymphoma (non-Hodgkin). *Cycle*: 28 days
Regimen:	Prednisone 60 mg/m^2/day PO, days 1 through 14
	Methotrexate 750 mg/m^2 IV, day 14
	Leucovorin 50 mg/m^2/dose IV every 6 hours for 5 doses, day 15 (start 24 hours after methotrexate)
	Doxorubicin 25 mg/m^2 IV, days 1 and 8
	Cyclophosphamide 650 mg/m^2 IV, days 1 and 8
	Etoposide 120 mg/m^2 IV, days 1 and 8
References:	•Fisher RI, DeVita VT Jr, Hubbard SM, et al. Diffuse aggressive lymphomas: increased survival after alternating flexible sequences for proMACE and MOPP chemotherapy. *Ann Intern Med.* 1983;98:304-309.
	•Nielsen H. Salvage therapy with PROMACE in relapsed non-Hodgkin malignant lymphoma. *Eur J Haematol.* 1991;46:123-124.

ProMACE/cytaBOM

Use: Lymphoma (non-Hodgkin). *Cycle*: 21 days

Regimen: Prednisone 60 mg/m²/day PO, days 1 through 14
Doxorubicin 25 mg/m² IV, day 1
Cyclophosphamide 650 mg/m² IV, day 1
Etoposide 120 mg/m² IV, day 1
Cytarabine 300 mg/m² IV, day 8
Bleomycin 5 units/m² IV, day 8
Vincristine 1.4 mg/m² (2 mg maximum dose) IV, day 8
Methotrexate 120 mg/m² IV, day 8
Leucovorin 25 mg/m²/dose PO every 6 hours for 4 doses (start 24 hours after methotrexate dose)
Cotrimoxazole double-strength (160/800) 2 tablets PO twice daily, days 1 through 21

Reference: •Longo DL, DeVita VT Jr, Duffey PL, et al. Superiority of ProMACE-cytaBOM over ProMACE-MOPP in the treatment of advanced diffuse aggressive lymphoma: results of a prospective randomized trial. *J Clin Oncol.* 1991;9:25-38.

ProMACE/MOPP

Use: Lymphoma (non-Hodgkin). *Cycle*: 28 days

Regimen: Prednisone 60 mg/m²/day PO, days 1 through 14
Doxorubicin 25 mg/m² IV, day 1
Cyclophosphamide 650 mg/m² IV, day 1
Etoposide 120 mg/m² IV, day 1
Mechlorethamine 6 mg/m² IV, day 8
Vincristine 1.4 mg/m² (2 mg maximum dose) IV, day 8
Procarbazine 100 mg/m²/day PO, days 8 through 14
Methotrexate 500 mg/m² IV, day 15
Leucovorin 50 mg/m²/dose PO every 6 hours for 4 doses (start 24 hours after methotrexate dose)

Reference: •Longo DL, DeVita VT Jr, Duffey PL, et al. Superiority of ProMACE-cytaBOM over ProMACE-MOPP in the treatment of advanced diffuse aggressive lymphoma: results of a prospective randomized trial. *J Clin Oncol.* 1991;9:25-38.

PVVM

Use: Neuroblastoma (pediatrics). *Cycle*: 21 to 28 days

Regimen: Cisplatin 90 mg/m² IV, day 1
Teniposide 100 mg/m² IV, day 3

References: •Castleberry RP, Shuster JJ, Altshuler G, et al. Infants with neuroblastoma and regional lymph node metastases have a favorable outlook after limited postoperative chemotherapy: a Pediatric Oncology Group study. *J Clin Oncol.* 1992;10:1299-1304.
•Nitschke R, Smith EI, Altshuler G, et al. Postoperative treatment of non-metastatic visible residual neuroblastoma: a Pediatric Oncology Group study. *J Clin Oncol.* 1991;9:1181-1188.

PVA

Use: Acute lymphocytic leukemia (ALL; induction—pediatrics).*Cycle*: 28 days. Give a single cycle.

Regimen: Prednisone 40 mg/m^2/day (60 mg maximum dose) PO, given in 3 divided doses, days 1 through 28
Vincristine 1.5 mg/m^2 (2 mg maximum dose) IV, days 1, 8, 15, and 22
with
Asparaginase 6,000 units/m^2/dose IM, 3 times weekly for 2 weeks (ie, days 2, 5, 7, 9, 12, and 14)
or
Asparaginase 6,000 units/m^2/dose IM, days 2, 5, 8, 12, 15, and 19
or
Asparaginase 5,000 units/m^2/dose IM, days 2, 5, 8, 12, 15, and 18
used in conjunction with
Intrathecal therapy

References: •Camitta B, Leventhal B, Lauer S, et al. Intermediate-dose intravenous methotrexate and mercaptopurine therapy for non-T, non-B acute lympho-cytic leukemia of childhood: a Pediatric Oncology Group study. *J Clin Oncol.* 1989;7:1539-1544.
•Mahoney DH Jr, Shuster J, Nitschke R, et al. Intermediate-dose intra-venous methotrexate with intravenous mercaptopurine is superior to repeti-tive low-dose oral methotrexate with intravenous mercaptopurine for chil-dren with lower-risk B-lineage acute lymphoblastic leukemia: a Pediatric Oncology Group phase III trial. *J Clin Oncol.* 1998;16:246-254.

PVB

Use: Testicular cancer, adenocarcinoma. *Cycle*: 21 days

Regimen: Cisplatin 20 mg/m^2/day IV, days 1 through 5
Vinblastine 0.15 mg/kg/day IV, days 1 and 2
Bleomycin 30 units IV, days 2, 9, and 16

Reference: •Williams SD, Birch R, Einhorn LH, Irwin L, Greco FA, Loehrer PJ. Treat-ment of disseminated germ-cell tumors with cisplatin, bleomycin, and either vinblastine or etoposide. *N Engl J Med.* 1987;316:1435-1440.

PVDA

Use: Acute lymphocytic leukemia (ALL; induction—pediatrics). *Cycle*: 28 days. Give a single cycle.

Regimen: Prednisone 40 mg/m^2/day PO, days 1 through 28
Vincristine 1.5 mg/m^2 (2 mg maximum dose) IV, days 1, 8, 15, and 22
Daunorubicin 25 mg/m^2 IV, days 1, 8, 15, and 22
Asparaginase 10,000 units/m^2 IM, 3 times weekly for 12 doses, beginning on day 1
used in conjunction with
  Intrathecal therapy
  Cotrimoxazole 5 mg/kg/day (as trimethoprim) PO in 2 divided doses, days 1 through 28

Reference: •Buchanan GR, Rivera GK, Boyett JM, Chauvenet AR, Crist WM, Vietti TJ. Reinduction therapy in 297 children with acute lymphoblastic leukemia in first bone marrow relapse: a Pediatric Oncology Group study. *Blood.* 1988;72:1286-1292.

PVDA (cont.)

> *Use:*   Acute lymphocytic leukemia (ALL; induction—pediatrics). *Cycle*: 28 days. Give a single cycle.
>
> *Regimen:*   Prednisone 40 mg/m^2/day PO, days 1 through 28
> Vincristine 1.5 mg/m^2 (2 mg maximum dose) IV, days 2, 8, 15, and 22
> Daunorubicin 25 mg/m^2 IV days 2, 8, 15, and 22
> Asparaginase 5,000 units/m^2/dose IM, days 2, 5, 8, 12, 15, 19
> *used in conjunction with*
> Intrathecal therapy
>
> *Reference:*   •Lauer SJ, Camitta BM, Leventhal BG, et al. Intensive alternating drug pairs for treatment of high-risk childhood acute lymphoblastic leukemia: a Pediatric Oncology Group pilot study. *Cancer*. 1993;71:2854-2861.

R-CHOP—see CHOP + Rituximab

Sequential AC/Paclitaxel—see AC/Paclitaxel, Sequential

Sequential Dox → CMF—see Dox → CMF, Sequential

SMF

> *Use:*   Pancreatic cancer. *Cycle*: 8 weeks
>
> *Regimen:*   Streptozocin 1,000 mg/m^2 IV, days 1, 8, 29, and 36
> Mitomycin 10 mg/m^2 IV, day 1
> Fluorouracil 600 mg/m^2 IV, days 1, 8, 29, and 36
>
> *References.*   •Kelsen D, Hudis C, Niedzwiecki D, et al. A phase III comparison trial of streptozotocin, mitomycin, and 5-fluorouracil with cisplatin, cytosine arabinoside, and caffeine in patients with advanced pancreatic carcinoma. *Cancer*. 1991;68:965-969.
> •Wiggans RG, Woolley PV, Macdonald JS, Smythe T, Ueno W, Scheil PS. Phase II trial of streptozotocin, mitomycin-C and 5-fluorouracil (SMF) in the treatment of advanced pancreatic cancer. *Cancer*. 1978;41:387-391.

Stanford V

> *Use:*   Lymphoma (Hodgkin). *Cycle*: 28 days
>
> *Regimen:*   Mechlorethamine 6 mg/m^2 IV, day 1
> Doxorubicin 25 mg/m^2 IV, days 1 and 15
> Vinblastine 6 mg/m^2 IV, days 1 and 15
> Vincristine 1.4 mg/m^2 (2 mg maximum dose) IV, days 8 and 22
> Bleomycin 5 units/m^2 IV, days 8 and 22
> Etoposide 60 mg/m^2/day IV, days 15 and 16
> Prednisone 40 mg/m^2/dose PO, every other day continually for 10 weeks, then taper off by 10 mg every other day for next 14 days
> *used in conjunction with antimicrobial prophylaxis*
> Cotrimoxazole double-strength (160/800) 2 tablets PO twice daily, continuously
> Ketoconazole 200 mg/day PO, continuously
> Acyclovir 200 mg PO 3 times daily, continuously
>
> *References:*   •Bartlett NL, Rosenberg SA, Hoppe RT, Hancock SL, Horning SJ. Brief chemotherapy, Stanford V, and adjuvant radiotherapy for bulky or advanced-stage Hodgkin's disease: a preliminary report. *J Clin Oncol*. 1995;13:1080-1088.
> •Horning SJ, Rosenberg SA, Hoppe RT. Brief chemotherapy (Stanford V) and adjuvant radiotherapy for bulky or advanced Hodgkin's disease: an update. *Ann Oncol*. 1996;7(suppl 4):S105-S108.

TAC

Use:	Breast cancer. *Cycle*: 21 days (up to 8 cycles)
Regimen:	Doxorubicin 50 mg/m^2 IV, day 1 Cyclophosphamide 500 mg/m^2 IV, day 1 (after doxorubicin) Docetaxel 75 mg/m^2 IV, day 1 (after cyclophosphamide) Ciprofloxacin 500 mg PO twice daily, days 5 through 15

References: •Nabholtz JM, Mackey JR, Smylie M, et al. Phase II study of docetaxel, doxorubicin, and cyclophosphamide as first-line chemotherapy for metastatic breast cancer. *J Clin Oncol.* 2001;19:314-321.

•Nabholtz JM, Pienkowski T, Mackey JR, et al. Phase III trial comparing TAC (docetaxel, doxorubicin, cyclophosphamide) with FAC (5-fluorouracil, doxorubicin, cyclophosphamide) in the adjuvant treatment of node positive breast cancer (BC) patients: interim analysis of the BCIRG 001 study [abstract]. *Proc ASCO.* 2002;21. Abstract 141.

TAD

Use:	Acute myelocytic leukemia (AML; induction—adults). *Cycle*: 21 days. Give 2 cycles.
Regimen:	Daunorubicin 60 mg/m^2/day IV, days 3 through 5 Cytarabine 100 mg/m^2/day continuous IV infusion, days 1 and 2 Cytarabine 100 mg/m^2/dose IV every 12 hours for 12 doses, days 3 through 8 Thioguanine 100 mg/m^2/dose PO every 12 hours for 14 doses, days 3 through 9

Reference: •Buchner T, Hiddemann W, Wormann B, et al. Double induction strategy for acute myeloid leukemia: the effect of high-dose cytarabine with mitoxantrone instead of standard-dose cytarabine with daunorubicin and 6-thioguanine: a randomized trial by the German AML Cooperative Group. *Blood.* 1999;93:4116-4124.

Tamoxifen-Epirubicin

Use:	Breast cancer. *Cycle*: 28 days for 6 cycles
Regimen:	Tamoxifen 20 mg PO daily, continuously for 4 years Epirubicin 50 mg/m^2 IV, on days 1 and 8

Reference: •Wils JA, Bliss JM, Marty M, et al. Epirubicin plus tamoxifen versus tamoxifen alone in node-positive postmenopausal patients with breast cancer: a randomized trial of the International Collaborative Cancer Group. *J Clin Oncol.* 1999;17:1988-1998.

TC

Use:	Gastric cancer. *Cycle*: 21 days (up to 8 cycles)
Regimen:	Docetaxel 85 mg/m^2 IV, day 1 Cisplatin 75 mg/m^2 IV, day 1 (after docetaxel)

Reference: •Roth AD, Maibach R, Martinelli G, et al. Docetaxel (Taxotere)-cisplatin (TC): an effective drug combination in gastric carcinoma. *Ann Oncol.* 2000;11:301-306.

TCF

Use:	Esophageal cancer. *Cycle*: 28 days
Regimen:	Paclitaxel 175 mg/m² IV over 3 hours, day 1
	Cisplatin 20 mg/m²/day IV, days 1 through 5 (give after paclitaxel)
	Fluorouracil 750 mg/m²/day continuous IV infusion, days 1 through 5
Reference:	•Ajani JA, Ilson D, Bhalla K, et al. Taxol, cisplatin, and 5-FU (TCF): a multi-institutional phase II study in patients with carcinoma of the esophagus [abstract]. *Proc ASCO*. 1995;14:203. Abstract 489.

TEC

Use:	Prostate cancer. *Cycle*: 28 days
Regimen:	Estramustine 10 mg/kg/day (840 mg maximum daily dose) PO given in 3 divided doses, start 2 days before chemotherapy and continue for 2 days after chemotherapy, 5 days total (days −1 to +3 of each cycle)
	Paclitaxel 100 mg/m² IV over 1 hour, days 1, 8, 15, and 22
	Carboplatin IV dose by Calvert equation to AUC 6 mg/mL/min (1,000 mg maximum dose), day 1
Reference:	•Kelly WK, Curley T, Slovin S, et al. Paclitaxel, estramustine phosphate, and carboplatin in patients with advanced prostate cancer. *J Clin Oncol*. 2001;19:44-53.

TIP

Use:	Head and neck, esophageal cancer. *Cycle*: 21 to 28 days
Regimen:	Paclitaxel 175 mg/m² IV over 3 hours, day 1
	Ifosfamide 1,000 mg/m²/day IV, days 1 through 3
	Mesna 400 mg/m²/day IV pre-ifosfamide, days 1 through 3
	Mesna 200 mg/m²/dose IV given 4 hours after ifosfamide, days 1 through 3
	Cisplatin 60 mg/m² IV, day 1 (give after paclitaxel infusion)
Reference:	•Shin DM, Glisson BO, Khuri FR, et al. Phase II trial of paclitaxel, ifosfamide, and cisplatin in patients with recurrent head and neck squamous cell carcinoma. *J Clin Oncol*. 1998;16:1325-1330.

Use:	Testicular cancer. *Cycle*: 21 days (4 cycles)
Regimen:	Paclitaxel 175 to 250 mg/m²/day continuous IV infusion over 24 hours, day 1
	Ifosfamide 1,200 mg/m²/day IV, days 2 through 6
	Cisplatin 20 mg/m²/day IV, days 2 through 6
	Mesna 400 mg/m²/dose IV prior to, then 4 and 8 hours after ifosfamide, days 2 through 6
Reference:	•Motzer RJ, Sheinfeld J, Mazumdar M, et al. Paclitaxel, ifosfamide, and cisplatin second-line therapy for patients with relapse testicular germ cell cancer. *J Clin Oncol*. 2000;18:2413-2418.

TIT

Use: Acute lymphocytic leukemia (ALL; CNS prophylaxis—pediatrics).

Regimen: Doses are based on patient's age. Give during weeks 1, 2, 3, 7, 13, 19, and 25 of intensification and every 12 weeks during maintenance.*

      Age 1 to 2 years:
        Methotrexate 8 mg intrathecal
        Cytarabine 16 mg intrathecal
        Hydrocortisone 8 mg intrathecal
      Age 2 to 3 years:
        Methotrexate 10 mg intrathecal
        Cytarabine 20 mg intrathecal
        Hydrocortisone 10 mg intrathecal
      Age 3 to 9 years:
        Methotrexate 12 mg intrathecal
        Cytarabine 24 mg intrathecal
        Hydrocortisone 12 mg intrathecal
      Age 9 years and older:
        Methotrexate 15 mg intrathecal
        Cytarabine 30 mg intrathecal
        Hydrocortisone 15 mg intrathecal

      *Note: All three drugs may be mixed and administered in a single syringe, if diluted with preservative-free 0.9% Sodium Chloride. Regimen used in combination with an induction/maintenance regimen.

References: •Camitta B, Mahoney D, Leventhal B, et al. Intensive intravenous methotrexate and mercaptopurine treatment of higher-risk non-T, non-B acute lymphocytic leukemia: a Pediatric Oncology Group study. *J Clin Oncol.* 1994;12:1383-1389.

        •Mahoney DH Jr, Shuster J, Nitschke R, et al. Intermediate-dose intravenous methotrexate with intravenous mercaptopurine is superior to repetitive low-dose oral methotrexate with intravenous mercaptopurine for children with lower-risk B-lineage acute lymphoblastic leukemia: a Pediatric Oncology Group phase III trial. *J Clin Oncol.* 1998;16:246-254.

Use: Acute lymphocytic leukemia (ALL; CNS prophylaxis—pediatrics).

Regimen: Doses are based on patient's age. Give on day 1 of induction, during weeks 1, 2, 3, 6, 11, 16, 21, and 26 of intensification, during week 31, and every 12 weeks during maintenance.*

      Age 1 year:
        Methotrexate 10 mg intrathecal
        Cytarabine 20 mg intrathecal
        Hydrocortisone 10 mg intrathecal
      Age 2 years:
        Methotrexate 12.5 mg intrathecal
        Cytarabine 25 mg intrathecal
        Hydrocortisone 12.5 mg intrathecal
      Age greater than 3 years:
        Methotrexate 15 mg intrathecal
        Cytarabine 30 mg intrathecal
        Hydrocortisone 15 mg intrathecal

      *Note: All three drugs may be mixed and administered in a single syringe, if diluted with preservative-free 0.9% Sodium Chloride. Regimen used in combination with an induction/maintenance regimen.

TIT (cont.)

Reference: •Lauer SJ, Camitta BM, Leventhal BG, et al. Intensive alternating drug pairs for treatment of high-risk childhood acute lymphoblastic leukemia: a Pediatric Oncology Group pilot study. *Cancer.* 1993;71:2854-2861.

Use: Acute lymphocytic leukemia (ALL; CNS prophylaxis—adults).

Regimen: Give on days 1 and 5 of week 1, day 1 of week 4, days 1 and 5 of week 7, day 1 of week 10, days 1 and 5 of week 13, and day 1 of week 16.
Methotrexate 15 mg intrathecal
Cytarabine 40 mg intrathecal
Dexamethasone 4 mg intrathecal*
*Note: No preservative-free product is available; dexamethasone 4 mg/mL injection contains benzyl alcohol 10 mg/mL, a preservative that is unsuitable for intrathecal injection. Because other intrathecal regimens are available that do not include benzyl alcohol-containing products, this regimen should be reserved for use when no other options are available and the benefit in the patient clearly outweighs the risk of benzyl alcohol toxicity. Regimen used in combination with an induction/maintenance regimen.

Reference: •Hoelzer D, Ludwig WD, Thiel E, et al. Improved outcome in adult B-cell acute lymphoblastic leukemia. *Blood.* 1996;87:495-508.

Topo/CTX

Use: Sarcomas (bone and soft-tissue—pediatrics). *Cycle*: 21 days

Regimen: Cyclophosphamide 250 mg/m^2/day IV, days 1 through 5
Topotecan 0.75 mg/m^2/day IV, days 1 through 5 after cyclophosphamide
Mesna 150 mg/m^2/dose IV before and 3 hours after each cyclophosphamide dose, days 1 through 5

Reference: •Saylors RL III, Stewart CF, Zamboni WC, et al. Phase I study of topotecan in combination with cyclophosphamide in pediatric patients with malignant solid tumors. a Pediatric Oncology Group study. *J Clin Oncol.* 1998;16:945-952.

Trastuzumab-Paclitaxel

Use: Breast cancer. *Cycle*: 21 days for at least 6 cycles

Regimen: Paclitaxel 175 mg/m^2/dose IV over 3 hours, day 1
Trastuzumab 4 mg/kg IV, day 1 first cycle only (loading dose)
Trastuzumab 2 mg/kg IV weekly, days 1, 8, and 15, except for day 1 of first cycle

References: •Herceptin. [package insert]. South San Francisco, CA: Genentech Inc; September 1998.
•Baselga J. Herceptin alone or in combination with chemotherapy in the treatment of HER2-positive metastatic breast cancer: pivotal trials. *Oncology.* 2001;61(suppl 2):14-21.

VAB-6

Use: Testicular cancer. *Cycle*: 21 to 28 days

Regimen: Cyclophosphamide 600 mg/m^2 IV, day 1
Dactinomycin 1 mg/m^2 IV, day 1
Vinblastine 4 mg/m^2 IV, day 1
Cisplatin 120 mg/m^2 IV, day 4
Bleomycin 30 units IV push, day 1 (omit from cycle 3)
then
Bleomycin 20 units/m^2/day continuous IV infusion, days 1 through 3 (omit from cycle 3)

VAB-6 (cont.)

References: •Bosl GJ, Gluckman R, Geller NL, et al. VAB-6: an effective chemotherapy regimen for patients with germ-cell tumors. *J Clin Oncol.* 1986;4:1493-1499.
•Vugrin D, Herr HW, Whitmore WF, Sogani PC, Golbey RB. VAB-6 combination chemotherapy in disseminated cancer of the testis. *Ann Intern Med.* 1981;95:59-61.

VAC Pediatric

Use: Sarcoma (pediatrics). *Cycle:* 21 days

Regimen: Vincristine 2 mg/m^2 IV (2 mg maximum dose), day 1
Dactinomycin 1 mg/m^2 IV, day 1
Cyclophosphamide 600 mg/m^2 IV, day 1

Reference: •Green DM. Evaluation of single-dose vincristine, actinomycin D, and cyclophosphamide in childhood solid tumors. *Cancer Treat Rep.* 1978;62:1517-1520.

VAC Pulse

Use: Sarcomas.

Regimen: Vincristine 2 mg/m^2 (2 mg maximum dose) IV weekly, for 12 weeks
Dactinomycin 0.015 mg/kg/day (0.5 mg/day maximum dose) continuous IV infusion, days 1 through 5, every 3 months for 5 courses
Cyclophosphamide 10 mg/kg/day IV or PO, days 1 through 7, every 6 weeks

Reference: •Wilbur JR, Sutow WW, Sullivan MP, Gottlieb JA. Chemotherapy of sarcomas. *Cancer.* 1975;36:765-769.

VAC Standard

Use: Sarcomas.

Regimen: Vincristine 2 mg/m^2 (2 mg maximum dose) IV weekly, for 12 weeks
Dactinomycin 0.015 mg/kg/day (0.5 mg/day maximum dose) continuous IV infusion, days 1 through 5, every 3 months for 5 courses
Cyclophosphamide 2.5 mg/kg/day PO, daily for 2 years

Reference: •Wilbur JR, Sutow WW, Sullivan MP, Gottlieb JA. Chemotherapy of sarcomas. *Cancer.* 1975;36:765-769.

VACAdr

Use: Sarcoma (bone and soft-tissue—pediatrics).

Regimen: Vincristine 1.5 mg/m^2 (2 mg maximum dose) IV, days 1, 8, 15, 22, 29, and 36
Cyclophosphamide 500 mg/m^2 IV, days 1, 8, 15, 22, 29, and 36
Doxorubicin 60 mg/m^2 IV, day 36
followed by 6-week rest period, then
Dactinomycin 0.015 mg/kg/day IV, days 1 through 5
Vincristine 1.5 mg/m^2 (2 mg maximum dose) IV, days 14, 21, 28, 35, and 42
Cyclophosphamide 500 mg/m^2 IV, days 14, 21, 28, 35, and 42
Doxorubicin 60 mg/m^2 IV, day 42 (give on day of final vincristine and cyclophosphamide doses)

Reference: •Nesbit ME Jr, Gehan EA, Burgert EO Jr, et al. Multimodal therapy for the management of primary, nonmetastatic Ewing's sarcoma of bone: a long-term follow-up of the first intergroup study. *J Clin Oncol.* 1990;8:1664-1674.

VAD

Use: Multiple myeloma. *Cycle*: 3 to 4 weeks

Regimen: Vincristine 0.4 mg/day (dose is not in mg/m^2) continuous IV infusion, days 1 through 4*

Doxorubicin 9 mg/m^2/day continuous IV infusion, days 1 through 4*

Dexamethasone 40 mg/day PO, days 1 through 4, days 9 through 12, and days 17 through 20[†]

*Note: Vincristine and doxorubicin may be mixed and administered in the same infusion bag, if diluted with 0.9% Sodium Chloride.

[†]Note: After completing the first 2 cycles of VAD, some clinicians give dexamethasone only on days 1 through 4 of each cycle to reduce the risk of infection. Antibiotic prophylaxis with cotrimoxazole also has been used for this purpose.

References: •Barlogie B, Smith L, Alexanian R. Effective treatment of advanced multiple myeloma refractory to alkylating agents. *N Engl J Med.* 1984;310:1353-1356.
•Gillin R, Greaves M, Proctor FE. Potential value of vincristine-adriamycin-dexamethasone combination chemotherapy (VAD) in refractory and rapidly progressive myeloma. *Eur J Haematol.* 1987;39:203-208.
•Mineur P, Menard JF, Loet XL, et al. VAD or VMBCP in multiple myeloma refractory to or relapsing after cyclophosphamide-prednisone therapy (protocol MY 85). *Br J Haematol.* 1998;103:512-517.

Use: Acute lymphocytic leukemia (ALL). *Cycle*: 24 to 28 days

Regimen: Vincristine 0.4 mg/day (dose is not in mg/m^2) continuous IV infusion, days 1 through 4*

Doxorubicin 9 to 12 mg/m^2/day continuous IV infusion, days 1 through 4*

Dexamethasone 40 mg/day PO, days 1 through 4, days 9 through 12, and days 17 through 20

*Note: Vincristine and doxorubicin may be mixed and administered in the same infusion bag, if diluted with 0.9% Sodium Chloride.

References: •Hovenga S, de Wolf J, Klip H, Vellenga E. Consolidation therapy with autologous stem cell transplantation in plasma cell leukemia after VAD, high-dose cyclophosphamide and EDAP courses: a report of three cases and a review of the literature. *Bone Marrow Transplant.* 1997;20:901-904.
•Kantarjian H, Walters RS, Keating MJ, et al. Results of the vincristine, doxorubicin, and dexamethasone regimen in adults with standard- and high-risk acute lymphocytic leukemia. *J Clin Oncol.* 1990;8:994-1004.

Use: Wilm tumor (pediatrics). *Cycle*: 1 year. Give 1 cycle only.

Regimen 1: Vincristine 1.5 mg/m^2 (2 mg maximum dose) IV, weekly for first 10 to 11 weeks then every 3 weeks for 15 more weeks
with
Dactinomycin 1.5 mg/m^2 IV every 6 weeks, starting week 1, for 9 doses
Doxorubicin 40 mg/m^2 IV every 6 weeks for 26 weeks, starting week 4, for 9 doses

Regimen 2: Vincristine 1.5 mg/m^2 (2 mg maximum dose) IV, given every 6 weeks for 6 to 15 months
Dactinomycin 0.015 mg/kg/day IV for 5 doses, given every 6 weeks for 6 to 15 months
or
Dactinomycin 0.06 mg/kg IV, given every 6 weeks for 6 to 15 months
may or may not give with
Doxorubicin 20 mg/m^2 IV, given every 6 weeks for 6 to 15 months

VAD (cont.)

References: •de Camargo B, Franco EL. A randomized clinical trial of single-dose versus fractionated-dose dactinomycin in the treatment of Wilms' tumor. *Cancer.* 1994;73:3081-3086.

•Pritchard J, Imeson J, Barnes J, et al. Results of the United Kingdom Children's Cancer Study Group first Wilms' tumor study. *J Clin Oncol.* 1995;13:124-133.

VAD/CVAD

Use: Acute lymphocytic leukemia (ALL; induction—adults). *Cycle*: Give 1 cycle only

Regimen: Vincristine 0.4 mg/day (dose is not in mg/m^2) continuous IV infusion, days 1 through 4 and days 24 through 27*

Doxorubicin 12 mg/m^2/day continuous IV infusion, days 1 through 4 and days 24 through 27*

Dexamethasone 40 mg/day PO, days 1 through 4, days 9 through 12, days 17 through 20, days 24 through 27, days 32 through 35, and days 40 through 43

Cyclophosphamide 1,000 mg/m^2 IV, day 24

*Note: Vincristine and doxorubicin may be mixed and administered in the same infusion bag, if diluted with 0.9% Sodium Chloride.

Reference: •Kantarjian HM, Walters RS, Keating MJ, et al. Results of the vincristine, doxorubicin, and dexamethasone regimen in adults with standard- and high-risk acute lymphocytic leukemia. *J Clin Oncol.* 1990;8:994-1004.

VAD-Liposomal (VLAD)

Use: Multiple myeloma. *Cycle*: 28 days

Regimen: Vincristine 2 mg (dose is not in mg/m^2) IV, day 1

Liposomal doxorubicin 30 to 40 mg/m^2 IV, day 1

Dexamethasone 40 mg/day PO, days 1 through 4, days 9 through 12, and days 17 through 20

References: •Dingeldein GC, Hoffman M, Huebner G, et al. Phase I/II study with liposomal-encapsulated doxorubicin in VAD-protocol for patients with multiple myeloma [abstract]. Presented at the American Society of Hematology Meeting, 2001. Abstract 4985.

•Tsiara SN, Kapsali E, Christou L, et al. Administration of a modified chemotherapeutic regimen containing vincristine, liposomal doxorubicin, and dexamethasone to multiple myeloma patients: preliminary data. *Eur J Haematol.* 2000;65:118-122.

VAD, Rapid Infusion

Use: Multiple myeloma. *Cycle*: 28 days

Regimen: Vincristine 0.4 mg/day (dose is not in mg/m^2) IV over 30 minutes, days 1 through 4*
Doxorubicin 9 mg/m^2/day IV over 30 minutes, days 1 through 4*
Dexamethasone 40 mg/day PO, days 1 through 4 of all cycles
Dexamethasone 40 mg/day PO, days 9 through 12, and days 17 through 20 of odd-numbered cycles only (eg, cycle 1, 3, 5)
used in conjunction with antimicrobial prophylaxis
Fluconazole 200 mg PO daily, continuously
Cotrimoxazole double-strength (160/800) PO twice daily, continuously
*Note: Vincristine and doxorubicin may be mixed and administered in the same infusion bag, if diluted with 0.9% Sodium Chloride.

References: •Segeren CM, Sonneveld P, van der Holt B, et al. Vincristine, doxorubicin and dexamethasone administered as rapid intravenous infusion for first-line treatment in untreated multiple myeloma. *Br J Haematol*. 1999;105:127-130.
•Segeren CM, Sonneveld P, van der Holt B, et al. Overall and event-free survival are not improved by the use of myeloablative therapy following intensified chemotherapy in previously untreated patients with multiple myeloma: a prospective randomized phase 3 study. *Blood*. 2003;101:2144-2151.

VATH

Use: Breast cancer. *Cycle*: 21 days

Regimen: Vinblastine 4.5 mg/m^2 IV, day 1
Doxorubicin 45 mg/m^2 IV, day 1
Thiotepa 12 mg/m^2 IV, day 1
Fluoxymesterone 30 mg/day PO in 3 divided doses, throughout entire course

Reference. •Hart RD, Perloff M, Holland JF. One-day VATH (vinblastine, adriamycin, thiotepa, and halotestin) therapy for advanced breast cancer refractory to chemotherapy. *Cancer*. 1981;48:1522-1527.

VBAP

Use: Multiple myeloma. *Cycle*: 21 days

Regimen: Vincristine 1 mg/m^2 (2 mg maximum dose) IV, day 1
Carmustine 30 mg/m^2 IV, day 1
Doxorubicin 30 mg/m^2 IV, day 1
Prednisone 60 mg/m^2/day PO, days 1 through 4

Reference: •Salmon SE, Haut A, Bonnet JD, et al. Alternating combination chemotherapy and levamisole improves survival in multiple myeloma: a Southwest Oncology Group study. *J Clin Oncol*. 1983;1:453-461.

VBMCP

Use: Multiple myeloma. *Cycle*: 35 days

Regimen: Vincristine 1.2 mg/m^2 (2 mg maximum dose) IV, day 1
Carmustine 20 mg/m^2 IV, day 1
Melphalan 8 mg/m^2/day PO, days 1 through 4
Cyclophosphamide 400 mg/m^2 IV, day 1
Prednisone 40 mg/m^2/day PO, days 1 through 7 of all cycles
with
Prednisone 20 mg/m^2/day PO, days 8 through 14 of first 3 cycles only

VBMCP (cont.)

Reference: •Oken MM, Harrington DP, Abramson N, Kyle RA, Knospe W, Glick JH. Comparison of melphalan and prednisone with vincristine, carmustine, melphalan, cyclophosphamide, and prednisone in the treatment of multiple myeloma. *Cancer.* 1997;79:1561-1567.

VC

Use: Lung cancer (non-small cell).

Regimen: Vinorelbine 30 mg/m^2 IV, weekly
Cisplatin 120 mg/m^2 IV, days 1 and 29, then give 1 dose every 6 weeks

Reference: •Le Chevalier T, Pujol JL, Douillard JY, et al. A three-arm trial of vinorelbine (navelbine) plus cisplatin, vindesine plus cisplatin, and a single-agent vinorelbine in the treatment of non-small cell lung cancer: an expanded analysis. *Semin Oncol.* 1994;21(5 suppl 10):28-34.

VCAP

Use: Multiple myeloma. *Cycle*: 21 days

Regimen: Vincristine 1 mg/m^2 (2 mg maximum dose) IV, day 1
Cyclophosphamide 125 mg/m^2/day PO, days 1 through 4
Doxorubicin 30 mg/m^2 IV, day 1
Prednisone 60 mg/m^2/day PO, days 1 through 4

Reference: •Salmon SE, Haut A, Bonnet JD, et al. Alternating combination chemotherapy and levamisole improves survival in multiple myeloma: a Southwest Oncology Group study. *J Clin Oncol.* 1983;1:453-461.

VCMP—see VMCP

VD

Use: Breast cancer. *Cycle*: 21 days

Regimen: Vinorelbine 25 mg/m^2 IV, days 1 and 8
Doxorubicin 50 mg/m^2 IV, day 1

Reference: •Hochster HS. Combined doxorubicin/vinorelbine (navelbine) therapy in the treatment of advanced breast cancer. *Semin Oncol.* 1995;22(2 suppl 5):55-60.

VeIP

Use: Genitourinary cancer, testicular cancer. *Cycle*: 21 days

Regimen: Vinblastine 0.11 mg/kg/day IV, days 1 and 2
Cisplatin 20 mg/m^2/day IV, days 1 through 5
Ifosfamide 1,200 mg/m^2/day IV, days 1 through 5
Mesna 1,200 mg/m^2/day continuous IV infusion, days 1 through 5

References: •Farhat F, Culine S, Theodore C, Bekradda M, Terrier-Lacombe MJ, Droz JP. Cisplatin and ifosfamide with either vinblastine or etoposide as salvage therapy for refractory or relapsing germ cell tumor patients. *Cancer.* 1996;77:1193-1197.
•Loehrer PJ, Lauer R, Roth BJ, Williams SD, Kalasinski LA, Einhorn LH. Salvage therapy in recurrent germ cell cancer: ifosfamide and cisplatin plus either vinblastine or etoposide. *Ann Intern Med.* 1988;109:540-546.
•Motzer RJ, Bajorin DF, Vlamis V, Weisen, Bosl GJ. Ifosfamide-based chemotherapy for patients with resistant germ cell tumors: the Memorial Sloan-Kettering Cancer Center experience. *Semin Oncol.* 1992;19(6 suppl 12):8-12.

VIC—see CVI

Vinorelbine-Cisplatin (see also Cisplatin-Vinorelbine)

Use: Lung cancer (non-small cell). *Cycle:* 42 days

Regimen: Vinorelbine 30 mg/m^2 IV, weekly
Cisplatin 120 mg/m^2 IV, days 1 and 29 for first cycle; then day 1 of subsequent cycles

Reference: •Smith TJ, Hillner BE, Neighbors DM, McSorley PA, Le Chevalier T. Economic evaluation of a randomized clinical trial comparing vinorelbine, vinorelbine plus cisplatin, and vindesine plus cisplatin for non-small-cell lung cancer. *J Clin Oncol.* 1995;13:2166-2173.

Vinorelbine-Doxorubicin

Use: Breast cancer. *Cycle:* 21 days

Regimen: Vinorelbine 25 mg/m^2 IV, days 1 and 8
Doxorubicin 50 mg/m^2 IV, day 1

Reference: •Spielmann M, Dorval T, Turpin F, et al. Phase II trial of vinorelbine/doxorubicin as first-line therapy of advanced breast cancer. *J Clin Oncol.* 1994;12:1764-1770.

Vinorelbine-Gemcitabine

Use: Lung cancer (non-small cell). *Cycle:* 28 days for up to 6 cycles

Regimen: Vinorelbine 20 mg/m^2 IV, days 1, 8, and 15
Gemcitabine 800 mg/m^2 IV, days 1, 8, and 15

Reference: •Chen YM, Perng RP, Yang KY, et al. A multicenter phase II trial of vinorelbine plus gemcitabine in previously untreated inoperable (Stage IIIB/IV) non-small cell lung cancer. *Chest.* 2000;117:1583-1589.

VIP

Use: Genitourinary cancer, testicular cancer. *Cycle:* 21 days

Regimen: Cisplatin 20 mg/m^2/day IV, days 1 through 5
Etoposide 75 mg/m^2/day IV, days 1 through 5
Ifosfamide 1,200 mg/m^2/day IV, days 1 through 5
Mesna 1,200 mg/m^2/day continuous IV infusion, days 1 through 5

References: •Farhat F, Culine S, Theodore C, Bekradda M, Terrier-Lacombe MJ, Droz JP. Cisplatin and ifosfamide with either vinblastine or etoposide as salvage therapy for refractory or relapsing germ cell tumor patients. *Cancer.* 1996;77:1193-1197.
•Loehrer PJ, Lauer R, Roth BJ, Williams SD, Kalasinski LA, Einhorn LH. Salvage therapy in recurrent germ cell cancer: ifosfamide and cisplatin plus either vinblastine or etoposide. *Ann Intern Med.* 1988;109:540-546.
•Motzer RJ, Bajorin DF, Vlamis V, Weisen, Bosl GJ. Ifosfamide-based chemotherapy for patients with resistant germ cell tumors: the Memorial Sloan-Kettering Cancer Center experience. *Semin Oncol.* 1992;19(6 suppl 12): 8-12.

VIP (cont.)

Use:	Lung cancer (small cell). *Cycle*: 21 to 28 days
Regimen:	Ifosfamide 1,200 mg/m²/day IV, days 1 through 4
	Cisplatin 20 mg/m²/day IV, days 1 through 4
	Mesna 120 to 300 mg/m² IV, day 1 (give before ifosfamide is started)
	Mesna 1,200 mg/m²/day continuous IV infusion, days 1 through 4 (after mesna bolus is given)
	with
	Etoposide 37.5 mg/m²/day PO, days 1 through 14
	or
	Etoposide 75 mg/m²/day IV, days 1 through 4

References: •Faylona EA, Loehrer PJ, Ansari R, Sandler AB, Gonin R, Einhorn LH. Phase II study of daily oral etoposide plus ifosfamide plus cisplatin for previously treated recurrent small-cell lung cancer: a Hoosier Oncology Group trial. *J Clin Oncol.* 1995;13:1209-1214.

•Loehrer PJ Sr, Ansari R, Gonin R, et al. Cisplatin plus etoposide with and without ifosfamide in extensive small-cell lung cancer: a Hoosier Oncology Group study. *J Clin Oncol.* 1995;13:2594-2599.

Use:	Lung cancer (non-small cell). *Cycle*: 28 days
Regimen:	Ifosfamide 1,000 to 1,200 mg/m²/day IV, days 1 through 3
	Cisplatin 100 mg/m² IV, days 1 and 8
	Etoposide 60 to 75 mg/m²/day IV, days 1 through 3
	with
	Mesna 300 mg/m²/dose IV every 4 hours, days 1 through 4
	or
	Mesna 20% of ifosfamide dose IV before, 4 and 8 hours after ifosfamide, days 1 through 4

References: •Mesnex. [package insert]. Princeton, NJ: Bristol-Myers Squibb Oncology/ Immunology Division; March 1998.

•Perez EA, Sowray PC, Gardner SL, Gandara DR. Phase I study of high-dose cisplatin, ifosfamide, and etoposide. *Cancer Chemother Pharmacol.* 1994;34:331-334.

VLAD (see VAD-Liposomal)

VM

Use:	Breast cancer. *Cycle*: 6 to 8 weeks
Regimen:	Mitomycin 10 mg/m² IV, days 1 and 28 for 2 cycles, then day 1 only
	Vinblastine 5 mg/m² IV, days 1, 14, 28, and 42 for 2 cycles, then days 1 and 21 only

Reference: •Garewal HS, Brooks RJ, Jones SE, Miller TP. Treatment of advanced breast cancer with mitomycin C combined with vinblastine or vindesine. *J Clin Oncol.* 1983;1:772-775.

VMCP (VCMP)

Use:	Multiple myeloma. *Cycle*: 21 days
Regimen:	Vincristine 1 mg/m² (2 mg maximum dose) IV, day 1
	Melphalan 6 mg/m²/day PO, days 1 through 4
	Cyclophosphamide 125 mg/m²/day PO, days 1 through 4
	Prednisone 60 mg/m²/day PO, days 1 through 4

Reference: •Salmon SE, Haut A, Bonnet JD, et al. Alternating combination chemotherapy and levamisole improves survival in multiple myeloma: a Southwest Oncology Group study. *J Clin Oncol.* 1983;1:453-461.

VP

Use:	Lung cancer (small cell). *Cycle*: 21 days
Regimen:	Etoposide 100 mg/m²/day IV, days 1 through 4 Cisplatin 20 mg/m²/day IV, days 1 through 4
Reference:	•Loehrer PJ Sr, Ansari R, Gonin R, et al. Cisplatin plus etoposide with and without ifosfamide in extensive small-cell lung cancer: a Hoosier Oncology Group study. *J Clin Oncol.* 1995;13:2594-2599.

V-TAD

Use:	Acute myelocytic leukemia (AML; induction). *Cycle*: 7 days. Give 1 cycle. Up to 3 cycles have been given, but time between cycles is not specified.
Regimen:	Etoposide 50 mg/m²/day IV, days 1 through 3 Thioguanine 75 mg/m²/dose PO every 12 hours for 10 doses, days 1 through 5 Daunorubicin 20 mg/m²/day IV, days 1 and 2 Cytarabine 75 mg/m²/day continuous IV infusion, days 1 through 5
Reference:	•Bigelow CL, Kopecky K, Files JC, et al. Treatment of acute myelogenous leukemia in patients over 50 years of age with V-TAD: a Southwest Oncology Group study. *Am J Hematol.* 1995;48:228-232.

XELOX

Use:	Colorectal cancer. *Cycle*: 21 days
Regimen 1:	Patients who have not received prior chemotherapy: Capecitabine 1,250 mg/m²/dose PO twice daily, days 1 through 14 Oxaliplatin 130 mg/m² IV, day 1
Regimen 2:	Patients who have received prior chemotherapy: Capecitabine 1,000 mg/m²/dose PO twice daily, days 1 through 14 Oxaliplatin 130 mg/m² IV, day 1
References:	•Borner MM, Dietrich D, Stupp R, et al. Phase II study of capecitabine and oxaliplatin in first- and second-line treatment of advanced or metastatic colorectal cancer. *J Clin Oncol.* 2002;20:1759-1766. •Cassidy J, Tabernero J, Twelves C, et al. XELOX (capecitabine plus oxaliplatin): active first-line therapy for patients with metastatic colorectal cancer. *J Clin Oncol.* 2004;22:2084-2091.

X + T—see Capecitabine-Docetaxel

Radio-Contrast Media

Generic Name	Doseform	Trade Name	Manufacturer
Barium Sulfate 650 mg	Tablet	Bar-Test	Glenwood
Barium Sulfate	Capsule	Sitzmarks	Konsyl
Barium Sulfate 72%	Liquid	Sol-O-Pake	E-Z-EM
Barium Sulfate 100%	Liquid	E-Z-AC	E-Z-EM
Barium Sulfate 100%	Liquid	Polibar	E-Z-EM
Barium Sulfate 105%	Liquid	E-Z-Dose	E-Z-EM
Barium Sulfate 105%	Liquid	Polibar Plus	E-Z-EM
Barium Sulfate 1.2%	Suspension	E-Z-Cat	E-Z-EM
Barium Sulfate 1.2%	Suspension	Readi-Cat	E-Z-EM
Barium Sulfate 1.5%	Suspension	Baro-Cat	Lafayette
Barium Sulfate 1.5%	Suspension	Bear-E-Yum CT	Lafayette
Barium Sulfate 1.5%	Suspension	Prepcat	Lafayette
Barium Sulfate 2%	Suspension	Readi-Cat 2	E-Z-EM
Barium Sulfate 2.2%	Suspension	Cheetah	Lafayette
Barium Sulfate 2.2%	Suspension	Mede-Scan	Lafayette
Barium Sulfate 5%	Suspension	Tomocat	Lafayette
Barium Sulfate 5%	Suspension	Tomocat 1000	Lafayette
Barium Sulfate 5%	Suspension	Enecat CT Enema Kit	Lafayette
Barium Sulfate 50%	Suspension	Entrobar	Lafayette
Barium Sulfate 50%	Suspension	Entrokit	Lafayette
Barium Sulfate 50%	Suspension	Entrokit/Catheter	Lafayette
Barium Sulfate 60%	Suspension	Bear-E-Yum GI	Lafayette
Barium Sulfate 60%	Suspension	Liquid Barosperse	Lafayette
Barium Sulfate 85%	Suspension	HD 85	Lafayette
Barium Sulfate 85%	Suspension	Enemark Rectal Marker	Lafayette
Barium Sulfate 85%	Suspension	Eneset 2	Lafayette
Barium Sulfate 95%	Suspension	Barosperse	Lafayette
Barium Sulfate 95%	Suspension	Tonojug	Lafayette
Barium Sulfate 95%	Suspension	Tonopaque	Lafayette
Barium Sulfate 95%	Suspension	Barobag Enema	Lafayette
Barium Sulfate 95%	Suspension	Barosperse Enema	Lafayette
Barium Sulfate 95%	Suspension	Pediatric Bear-E-Bag	Lafayette
Barium Sulfate 96%	Suspension	Digital HD	Lafayette
Barium Sulfate 98%	Suspension	Baricon	Lafayette
Barium Sulfate 98%	Suspension	HD 200 Plus	Lafayette
Barium Sulfate 100%	Suspension	Flo-Coat	Lafayette
Barium Sulfate 100%	Suspension	Imager AC	Lafayette
Barium Sulfate 100%	Suspension	Medebar Plus	Lafayette
Barium Sulfate 150%	Suspension	Epi-C	Lafayette
Barium Sulfate 210%	Suspension	Liqui-Coat HD	Lafayette
Barium Sulfate 250%	Suspension	E-Z-HD	E-Z-EM
Barium Sulfate	Powder	Barium Sulfate	Various
Barium Sulfate	Powder	E-Z-Paque	E-Z-EM

Generic Name	Doseform	Trade Name	Manufacturer
Barium Sulfate	Powder	Sol-O-Pake	E-Z-EM
Barium Sulfate	Powder	Ultra-R	E-Z-EM
Barium Sulfate 97%	Powder	Barium Sulfate	Various
Barium Sulfate 70%	Cream	E-Z-Paste	E-Z-EM
Barium Sulfate 70%	Paste	Intropaste	Lafayette
Barium Sulfate 100%	Paste	Anatrast	Lafayette
Diatrizoate meglumine & Iodipamide meglumine 52.7%/26.8%	Injection	Sinografin	Bracco
Diatrizoate meglumine & Diatrizoate sodium 52%/8%	Injection	Renografin-60	Bracco
Diatrizoate meglumine & Diatrizoate sodium 66%/10%	Injection	Hypaque-76	Amersham Health
Diatrizoate meglumine & Diatrizoate sodium 66%/10%	Injection	Reno-Cal-76	Bracco
Diatrizoate meglumine & Diatrizoate sodium 66%/10%	Solution	Gastrografin	Bracco
Diatrizoate meglumine & Diatrizoate sodium 66%/10%	Solution	MD-Gastroview	Mallinckrodt
Diatrizoate meglumine 18%	Injection	Cystografin-Dilute	Bracco
Diatrizoate meglumine 30%	Injection	Hypaque Meglumine	Amersham Health
Diatrizoate meglumine 30%	Injection	Reno-Dip	Bracco
Diatrizoate meglumine 60%	Injection	Hypaque Meglumine	Amersham Health
Diatrizoate meglumine 60%	Injection	Reno-60	Bracco
Diatrizoate meglumine 30%	Solution	Cystografin	Bracco
Diatrizoate meglumine 30%	Solution	Hypaque-Cysto	Amersham Health
Diatrizoate meglumine 30%	Solution	Hypaque-Cysto Pediatric	Amersham Health
Diatrizoate meglumine 30%	Solution	Reno-30	Bracco
Diatrizoate sodium 20%	Injection	Hypaque Sodium	Amersham Health
Diatrizoate sodium 25%	Injection	Hypaque Sodium	Amersham Health
Diatrizoate sodium 50%	Injection	Hypaque Sodium	Amersham Health
Diatrizoate sodium	Powder	Hypaque Sodium	Amersham Health
Ethiodized Oil		Ethiodol	Savage
Ferumoxides 11.2 mg FE/mL	Solution	Feridex IV	Berlex Imaging
Ferumoxsil 175 mcg/mL	Suspension	GastroMARK	Mallinckrodt
Iodipamide meglumine 52%	Injection	Cholografin Meglumine	Bracco
Iodixanol 270 mg/mL	Injection	Visipaque	Amersham Health
Iodixanol 320 mg/mL	Injection	Visipaque	Amersham Health
Iohexol 140 mg/mL	Injection	Omnipaque	Amersham Health
Iohexol 180 mg/mL	Injection	Omnipaque	Novaplus (PL)
Iohexol 180 mg/mL	Injection	Omnipaque	Amersham Health
Iohexol 180 mg/mL	Injection	Myelo-Kit	Amersham Health
Iohexol 210 mg/mL	Injection	Omnipaque	Amersham Health
Iohexol 240 mg/mL	Injection	Omnipaque	Novaplus (PL)
Iohexol 240 mg/mL	Injection	Myelo-Kit	Amersham Health
Iohexol 240 mg/mL	Injection	Omnipaque	Amersham Health

Generic Name	Doseform	Trade Name	Manufacturer
Iohexol 300 mg/mL	Injection	Omnipaque	Novaplus (PL)
Iohexol 300 mg/mL	Injection	Omnipaque	Amersham Health
Iohexol 300 mg/mL	Injection	Omnipaque	Various
Iohexol 350 mg/mL	Injection	Omnipaque	Novaplus (PL)
Iohexol 350 mg/mL	Injection	Omnipaque	Amersham Health
Iohexol 350 mg/mL	Injection	Omnipaque	Various
Iopamidol 26%	Injection	Isovue-128	Bracco
Iopamidol 41%	Injection	Isovue-200	Bracco
Iopamidol 41%	Injection	Isovue-M 200	Bracco
Iopamidol 51%	Injection	Isovue-250	Bracco
Iopamidol 61%	Injection	Isovue-300	Bracco
Iopamidol 61%	Injection	Isovue-M 300	Bracco
Iopamidol 76%	Injection	Isovue 370	Bracco
Iopamidol 41%	Solution	Isovue-200	Bracco
Iopamidol 61%	Solution	Isovue-300	Bracco
Iopanoic acid 500 mg	Tablet	Telepaque	Amersham Health
Iopromide 31% (150 mg/mL)	Injection	Ultravist	Hospira
Iopromide 50% (240 mg/mL)	Injection	Ultravist	Hospira
Iopromide 62% (300 mg/mL)	Injection	Ultravist	Hospira
Iopromide 77% (370 mg/mL)	Injection	Ultravist	Hospira
Iothalamate meglumine 17.2%	Injection	Cysto-Conray II	Mallinckrodt
Iothalamate meglumine 30%	Injection	Conray 30	Mallinckrodt
Iothalamate meglumine 43%	Injection	Conray 43	Mallinckrodt
Iothalamate meglumine 60%	Injection	Conray	Mallinckrodt
Iothalamate meglumine 60%	Solution	Conray	Mallinckrodt
Iothalamate sodium 0.1%	Injection	Glofil-125	Questcor
Iothalamate sodium 66.8%	Injection	Conray 400	Mallinckrodt
Ioversol 64%	Injection	Optiray 300	Mallinckrodt
Ioversol 74%	Injection	Optiray 350	Mallinckrodt
Ioxaglate meglumine & ioxaglate sodium 39.3%/19.6%	Injection	Hexabrix	Mallinckrodt
Tyropanoate sodium 750 mg	Capsule	Bilopaque	Amersham Health

Radio-Isotopes

Active Isotope	Generic Name	Doseform or Packaging	Trade Name	Manufacturer
18-F	Fluorine F-18	Injection	nd	Amersham Health
32-P	Chromic Phosphate P-32	Injection	Phosphocol P-32	Mallinckrodt
32-P	Sodium Phosphate P-32	Capsules	Sodium Phosphate P-32	Mallinckrodt
		Oral Solution	Sodium Phosphate P-32	Mallinckrodt
		Injection	Sodium Phosphate P-32	Mallinckrodt
51-Cr	Sodium Chromate Cr-51	Injection	Chromitope Sodium	Bracco Diagnostics
57-Co	Cyanocobalamin Co-57	Capsules	Cyanocobalamin Co-57	Mallinckrodt
		Capsules	Rubratrope-57	Bracco Diagnostics
57&58 Co	Cyanocobalamin Co-57 & Co-58	Injection	nd	Amersham Health
67-Ga	Gallium Citrate Ga-67	Injection	Gallium Citrate Ga 67	Mallinckrodt
89-Sr	Strontium Chloride Sr-89	Injection	Metastron	Amersham Health
99m-Tc	Technetium Tc-99m	Generator	nd	Amersham Health
		Generator	Ultra-TechneKow	Mallinckrodt
99m-Tc	Technetium-99m Macro-aggregated Albumin	Kit	AN Stannous Ag..	Benedict Nuclear
		Kit	Pulmolite	CIS-US
		Kit	TechneScan MAA	Mallinckrodt
		Kit	Lungaggregate Reagent	Amersham Health
		Kit	Macrotec	Bracco Diagnostics
99m-Tc	Technetium-99m Serum Albumin	Kit	nd	Amersham Health
99m-Tc	Technetium-99m Exametazime	Kit	Ceretec	Amersham Health
99m-Tc	Technetium-99m Fanolesomab	Kit	NeutroSpec	Palatin
99m-Tc	Technetium-99m Mebrofenin	Kit	Choletec	Bracco Diagnostics
99m-Tc	Technetium-99m Medronate	Kit	Amer-Scan MDP	Amersham Health
		Kit	Osteolite	CIS-US
		Kit	nd	Drax Image
		Kit	nd	Amersham Health
		Kit	TechneScan MDP	Mallinckrodt
		Kit	MDP-Bracco	Bracco Diagnostics
99m-Tc	Technetium-99m Mertiatide	Kit	TechneScan MAG3	Mallinckrodt
99m-Tc	Technetium-99m Oxidronate	Kit	TechneScan HDP	Mallinckrodt
		Injection	Gallium-67	Amersham Health

Active Isotope	Generic Name	Doseform or Packaging	Trade Name	Manufacturer
99m-Tc	Technetium-99m Pyro-phosphate	Injection	CIS-Pyro	CIS-US
99m-Tc	Technetium-99m Pentetate Sodium	Kit	AN-DTPA	CIS-US
		Kit	MPI DTPA Kit	Amersham Health
		Kit	TechneScan DTPA	Mallinckrodt
		Kit	Techneplex	Bracco Diagnostics
		Kit	nd	Drax Image
99m-Tc	Tc-99m Pyro- & Trimeta-Phosphates	Kit	Pyrolite	CIS-US
		Kit	TechneScan PYP	Mallinckrodt
		Kit	Tc-99m Poly-phosphate	Amersham Health
		Kit	Phosphotec	Bracco Diagnostics
		Kit	RBC-Scan	Cadema Med.
99m-Tc	Technetium-99m Red Blood Cell	Kit	UltraTag	Mallinckrodt
99m-Tc	Technetium-99m Glucep-tate	Kit	TechneScan Gluceptate	Mallinckrodt
99m-Tc	Technetium-99m Succimer	Kit	Tc-99m DMSA	Amersham Health
99m-Tc	Technetium-99m Sulfur Colloid	Kit	Cis-Sulfur Colloid	CIS-US
		Kit	TechneScan Sulfur Colloid	Mallinckrodt
		Kit	TSC	Amersham Health
99m-Tc	Technetium-99m Tebor-oxime	Kit	CardioTec	Bracco Diagnostics
99m-Tc	Technetium-99m Tetro-fosmin	Kit	Myoview	Amersham Health
		Injection	nd	Amersham Health
111-In	Indium-111 Capromab Pendetide	Kit	ProstaScint	Cytogen
111-In	Indium-111 Ibritumomab Tiuxetan	Kit	Zevalin	IDEC
111-In	Indium-111 Oxyquinoline Sodium (Oxine)	Solution	nd	Amersham Health
111-In	Indium-111 Pentetate Disodium	Injection	In-111 DTPA	Amersham Health
111-In	Indium-111 Pentetreotide	Kit	OctreoScan	Mallinckrodt
111-In	Indium-111 Satumomab Pentetide	Injection	OncoScint CR/OV	Cytogen
123-I	Sodium Iodide-123	Capsules	nd	Syncor
		Capsules	Sodium Iodide I-123 Diagnostic	Mallinckrodt
		Capsules	Sodium Iodide I-123	Amersham Health
125-I	Iothalamate Sodium I-125	Injection	Glofil-125	Iso-Tex

Active Isotope	Generic Name	Doseform or Packaging	Trade Name	Manufacturer
125-I	Iodinated Albumin I-125	Injection	Jeanatope 125-I	Iso-Tex
		Injection	Iodinated Albumin I-125	Mallinckrodt
131-I	Iodinated Albumin I-131	Injection	Megatope	Iso-Tex
		Injection	Sodium Chromate Cr-51	Mallinckrodt
131-I	Iodohippurate Sodium I-131	Injection	nd	CIS-US
131-I	Iodomethylnorcholesterol (NP-59)	Injection	nd	University of Michigan
131-I	Metaiodobenzylguanidine (MIBG)	Injection	nd	CIS-US
131-I	Sodium Iodide I-131	Capsules	nd	CIS-US
		Capsules	Sodium Iodide I 131 Diagnostic & Sodium Iodide I-131 Therapeutic	Mallinckrodt
		Capsules	Iodotope	Bracco Diagnostics
		Capsules	nd	Syncor
		Oral Solution	nd	CIS-US
		Oral Solution	Sodium Iodide I-131 Solution	Mallinckrodt
		Oral Solution	Iodotope	Bracco Diagnostics
		Oral Solution	nd	Syncor
131-I	Tositumomab	Injection	Bexxar	Corixa
133-Xe	Xenon Xe-133	Gas	nd	General Electric
		Gas	nd	Mallinckrodt
153-Sa	Samarium 153 Lexidroman	Injection	Quadramet	DuPont
201-Tl	Thallous Chloride Tl-201	Injection	Thallous Chloride Tl-201	Mallinckrodt
		Injection	nd	Amersham Health
		Injection	nd	Bracco Diagnostics

nd = No data available.

Manufacturer and Distributor Listing

00089, 55298, 55326
3M Personal Healthcare Prods.
3M Center Building 275-5W-05
St. Paul, MN 55144-1000
651-733-1110
800-364-3577
http://www.mmm.com

00089
3M Pharmaceuticals
3M Center Building 275-5W-05
St. Paul, MN 55144-1000
651-773-1110
800-364-3577
http://www.mmm.com

63801
7 Oaks Pharmaceutical Corp.
161 Harry Stanley Dr.
Easley, SC 29640
864-850-1700
877-723-6725
http://www.7oakspharma.com

A & D Medical
1555 McCandless Drive
Milpitas, CA 95035
408-263-5333
888-726-9966
http://www.andmedical.com

AAI Pharma (Headquarters)
2320 Scientific Park Drive
Wilmington, NC 28405
910-254-7350
800-575-4224
http://www.aaipharma.com

12463
Abana Pharmaceuticals, Inc.
See Jones Pharma Incorporated

Abbott Diabetes Care
1420 Harbor Bay Pkwy
Suite 290
Alameda, CA 94502
510-749-5400
http://www.therasense.com

Abbott Diagnostics
100 Abbott Park Rd.
Abbott Park, IL 60064-6154
800-323-9100

Abbott Hospital Products
100 Abbott Park Rd.
Abbott Park, IL 60064-6154
847-937-6100
800-615-0187

00074
Abbott Laboratories
   Pharmaceutical Division
200 Abbott Park Rd.
Abbott Park, IL 60064-6400
800-633-9110
http://www.abbott.com

Aber Pharmaceuticals, Inc.
See Atley Pharmaceuticals, Inc.

Able Laboratories, Inc.
600 Montrose Avenue
South Plainfield, NJ 07080
908-754-2253
800-982-2253
http://www.ablelabs.com

Abraxis Oncology
800-551-7176

Academic Pharmaceuticals, Inc.
21 N. Skokie Valley Highway
Suite G-3
Lake Bluff, IL 60044
847-735-1170

Access Pharmaceuticals
2000 Stemmons Freeway
Suite 176
Dallas, TX 75207-2107
214-905-5100
http://www.accesspharma.com

Acme United Corp.
1931 Black Rock Turnpike
Fairfield, CT 06825
203-332-7330
800-835-2263
http://www.acmeunited.com

Acorda Therapeutics
15 Skyline Drive
Hawthorne, NY 10532
914-347-4300

Actavis Pharma
2 Maria Louisa Blvd.
Sofia 1000
Bulgaria
02/9321 861
http://www.actavis.bg

Actelion Pharmaceuticals US, Inc.
601 Gateway Blvd.
Suite 100
South San Francisco, CA 94080
650-624-6900
866-228-3546
http://www.actelion.com

53014
Adams Laboratories, Inc.
14801 Sovereign Road
Fort Worth, TX 76155-2645
817-354-3858
800-770-5270
http://www.adamslabs.com

Adria Laboratories
See Pharmacia Corp.

Advance
2201-F 5th Avenue
Ronkonkoma, NY 11779
631-981-4600

00062
Advance Biofactures Corp.
   Biospecifics Technologies
35 Wilbur Street
Lynbrook, NY 11563
516-593-7000
http://www.biospecifics.com

10888
Advanced Nutritional Technology
6988 Sierra Ct.
Dublin, CA 94568
800-624-6543
http://www.antlab.com

Advanced Polymer Systems
See AP Pharma

Advanced Vision Research
12 Alfred St.
Suite 200
Woburn, MA 01801
781-932-8327
800-579-8327
http://www.theratears.com

Advancis Pharmaceutical
   Corporation
20425 Seneca Meadows Parkway
Germantown, MD 20876
301-944-6600

Aero Pharmaceuticals
3848 FAU Blvd, Suite 100
Boca Raton, FL 33431
800-223-6837
http://www.aeropharmaceuticals.com

63010
Agouron Pharmaceuticals
See Pfizer

A.H. Robins Consumer Products
See Whitehall-Robins Healthcare

00031
A.H. Robins, Inc.
See Whitehall-Robins Healthcare

Aid-Pack USA
See NutraMax Products, Inc.

17478
Akorn, Inc.
2500 Millbrook Dr.
Buffalo Grove, IL 60089
888-519-8384
800-535-7155
http://www.akorn.com

41383
AKPharma, Inc.
6840 Old Egg Harbor Rd.
Pleasantville, NJ 08232
800-994-4711
http://www.akpharma.com

Alamo Pharmaceuticals, LLC
8501 Wilshire Blvd., Suite 318
Beverly Hills, CA 90211-3119
310-859-7799

A.L. Labs
See Alpharma USPD, Inc.

Alberto Culver
2525 West Armitage Avenue
Melrose Park, IL 60160
708-450-3000
800-333-6666
http://www.alberto.com

00065, 00998
Alcon Laboratories, Inc.
6201 S. Freeway
Ft. Worth, TX 76134-2009
800-451-3937
800-862-5266
http://www.alconlabs.com

Aligen
2415 Jerusalem Avenue
N. Bellmore, NY 11710

Aligon Pharmaceuticals
1860 County Road 95
Helena, AL 35080
205-663-0521

Alimenterics Inc
301 American Road
Morris Plains, NJ 07950

ALK Abello
1700 Royston Lane
Round Rock, TX 78664
888-255-3744
800-325-7354
http://www.alk-abello.com

38697
ALK Laboratories, Inc.
See ALK Abello

00173
Allen & Hanburys
See GlaxoSmithKline, Inc.

Allendale Pharmaceuticals, Inc.
73 Franklin Turnpike
Allendale, NJ 07401
888-343-4499
http://www.allendalepharm.com

Allercreme
See Carme, Inc.

Allerderm Laboratories, Inc.
P.O. Box 5295
Phoenix, AZ 85010-5295
800-365-6868
http://www.allerderm.com

00023, 11980
Allergan, Inc.
2525 DuPont Dr.
Irvine, CA 92623-9534
714-246-4500
800-433-8871
http://www.allergan.com

Allergy Laboratories, Inc.
P.O. Box 348
Oklahoma City, OK 73101-0348
405-235-1451
800-654-3971
http://www.allergylabs.com

Allermed
7203 Convoy Court
San Diego, CA 92111
858-292-1060
800-221-2748
http://www.allermed.com

Alliance Pharmaceutical Corp.
6175 Lusk Blvd.
San Diego, CA 92121
858-410-5200
http://www.allp.com

Alliant Pharmaceuticals, Inc.
312 Maxwell Road, Suite 400
Alpharetta, GA 30004
770-817-4500

Allied Pharmacy
801 Stadium Dr.
Suite 111
Arlington, TX 76011
817-226-5050

54569
Allscripts, Inc.
2401 Commerce Dr.
Libertyville, IL 60048-4464
847-680-3515
800-654-0889
http://www.allscripts.com

Almay, Inc.
1501 Williamsboro St.
Oxford, NC 27565
919-603-2953
800-992-5629
http://www.almay.com

Alpha 1 Biomedicals, Inc.
See Arriva Pharmaceuticals

49669
Alpha Therapeutic Corp.
See Grifols

Alpharma Purepac Pharmaceuticals
200 Elmora Avenue
Elizabeth, NJ 07207
800-432-8534
http://www.alpharma.com
http://www.purepac.com

Alpharma USPD, Inc.
7205 Windsor Blvd.
Baltimore, MD 21244
410-298-1000
800-638-9096
http://www.alpharmaUSPD.com

51641
Alra Laboratories, Inc.
3850 Clearview Ct.
Gurnee, IL 60031
847-244-4238
800-248-2572

Altaire Pharmaceuticals, Inc.
P.O. Box 849
311 West Lane
Aquebogue, NY 11931
800-258–2471

Altana Inc.
See Fougera Company

AltaRex Corp.
8223 Roper Road NW
Edmonton, Canada T6E654
781-672-0138
780-944-9993
http://www.altarex.com

00731
Alto Pharmaceuticals, Inc.
P. O. Box 271150
Tampa, FL 33688-1150
800-330-2891

Alva-Amco Pharmacal Cos, Inc.
7711 Merrimac Avenue
Nile, IL 60714
800-792-2582
http://www.alva-amco.com

17314
Alza Corp.
1900 Charleston Rd.
Mountain View, CA 94039
650-564-5000
http://www.alza.com

Amarin Pharmaceuticals
See Valeant

AMBI Pharmaceuticals, Inc.
See Nutrition 21

10038
Ambix Laboratories
55 West End Road
Totowa, NJ 07512
973-890-9002
http://www.ambixlabs.com

89709, 90605
Amcon Laboratories
40 N. Rock Hill Rd.
St. Louis, MO 63119
314-961-5758
800-255-6161
http://www.amconlabs.com

Amend Drug and Chemical Corporation
See Ruger Chemical

51201
American Dermal Corp.
See Aventis Pharmaceuticals

American Generics, Inc.
No longer in business

American Health Packaging
2550 John Glenn Avenue A
Columbus, OH 43217
614-492-8177
800-707-4621
http://www.amerisourcebergen.com

American Home Products
See Wyeth Pharmaceuticals

American Lecithin Company
115 Hurley Rd., Unit 2B
Oxford, CT 06478
203-262-7100
800-364-4416
http://www.americanlecithin.com

11649
American Medical Industries
330 E. Third St., Suite 2
Dell Rapids, SD 57022
605-428-5501
http://www.ezhealthcare.com

American Pharmaceutical Co.
1340 N. Jefferson St.
Anaheim, CA 92807
714-579-7545

90000
American Pharmaceutical Partners, Inc.
11777 San Vincente Blvd.
Suite 550
Los Angeles, CA 90049
800-551-7176
http://www.appdrugs.com

52769
American Red Cross
1616 N. Ft. Myers Dr. 17th Floor
Arlington, VA 22209
800-446-8883
http://www.redcross.org/plasma

American Red Cross (National Headquarters)
431 18th Street, NW
Washington, DC 20006
202-303-4498
http://www.redcross.org

00517
American Regent Labs., Inc.
See Luitpold Pharmaceuticals, Inc.

Ameriderm Laboratories, Inc.
13 Kentucky Avenue
Paterson, NJ 07503
800-455-7211
http://www.ameriderm.com

Amerilab Technologies
3101 Louisiana Avenue North
New Hope, MN 55427
763-525-1262
http://www.amerilabtech.com

AmerisourceBergen
1300 Morris Dr.
Suite 100
Chesterbrook, PA 19087
800-829-3132
http://www.amerisourcebergen.com

Amerx Health Care Corp.
1150 Cleveland Avenue
Suite 410
Clearwater, FL 33755
727-443-0530
800-448-9599
http://www.amerigel.com

55513
Amgen Inc.
1 Amgen Center Dr.
Thousand Oaks, CA 91320
805-480-1299
800-772-6436
http://www.amgen.com

52152
Amide Pharmaceuticals, Inc.
See Actavis

Amkas Laboratories Inc.
4217 Commercial Way
Glenview, IL 60025
847-296-5075
866-235-2331

Amphastar Pharmaceutical, Inc.
11570 6th St.
Rancho Cucamonga, CA 91730
800-423-4136
http://www.amphastar.com

53926
AMSCO Scientific
See Steris Laboratories

Anabolic Inc.
17802 Gillette Avenue
Irvine, CA 92614
949-863-0340
800-445-6849
http://www.anaboliclabs.com

Anaquest
See Baxter

Andrew Jergens Company
2535 Spring Grove Ave.
Cincinnati, OH 45214
513-421-1400
800-742-8798
http://www.jergens.com

Andrulis Pharmaceutical Corp.
P.O. Box 2135
Bethesda, MD 20817
301-419-2400

Andrx Laboratories, Inc.
3040 Universal
Suite 150
Weston, FL 33331
800-331-2632
800-621-7143
954-306-7000
http://www.andrx.com

62037
Andrx Pharmaceuticals, Inc.
4001 S.W. 47th Ave.
Ft. Lauderdale, FL 33314
954-581-7500
800-621-7143
http://www.andrx.com

Angelini Pharmaceuticals, Inc.
50 Tice Blvd.
Woodcliff Lake, NJ 07677-7654
201-476-9000
201-489-4100
http://www.angelinipharmaceuticals.com

Ansell Healthcare, Inc.
200 Schulz Dr.
Red Bank, NJ 07701
732-345-5400
http://www.ansell.com

Antares Pharma
707 Eagleview Boulevard
Suite 111
Exton, PA 19341
610-458-6200

Anthra Pharmaceuticals, Inc.
103 Carnegie Center
Suite 102
Princeton, NJ 08540
http://www.anthra.com

Antibodies, Inc.
P.O. Box 1560
Davis, CA 95617
530-758-4400
800-824-8540
http://www.antibodiesinc.com

Antigenics Inc.
630 5th Ave.
Suite 2100
New York, NY 10111
212-994-8200
http://www.antigenics.com

48028
Aplicare Inc.
50 E. Industrial Rd.
Branford, CT 06405
800-760-3236
203-760-3226
http://www.aplicare.com

Apollon Inc.
1 Great Valley Parkway
Malvern, PA 19355

60505
Apotex Corp.
2400 N. Commerce Pkwy.
Suite 400
Weston, FL 33326
847-821-8005
800-706-5575
http://www.apotexcorp.com

Apotex USA
616 Heathrow Dr.
Lincolnshire, IL 60069
847-821-8005
800-706-5575
http://www.apotexcorp.com

Apothecary Products, Inc.
11750 12th Ave. S.
Burnsville, MN 55337
952-890-1940
800-328-2742
http://www.apothecaryproducts.com

00003, 00015
Apothecon, Inc. (Bristol-Myers Squibb)
P.O. Box 4500
Princeton, NJ 08540
609-897-2000
800-321-1335
800-332-2056
http://www.bms.com

48723
Apothecus, Inc.
220 Townsend Sq.
Oyster Bay, NY 11771
516-624-8200
800-227-2393
http://www.infoapothecus.com

Applied Analytical Industries
2320 Scientific Park Drive
Wilmington, NC 28405
877-263-6726
910-254-7000
800-575-4224

Applied Biotech, Inc.
10237 Flanders Ct.
San Diego, CA 92121
858-587-6771
800-257-9525
http://www.abiapogent.com

Applied Genetics Inc. Dermatics
205 Buffalo Ave.
Freeport, NY 11520
516-868-9026
http://www.agiderm.com

Applied Medical Research
308 15th Ave. N.
Nashville, TN 37203
615-327-0670

Approved Drug
See Health for Life Brands, Inc.

00275
Arco Pharmaceuticals, Inc.
See Natures Bounty, Inc.

00070
Arcola Laboratories
See Aventis

Armour Pharmaceutical
See Aventis Behring

Aronex Pharmaceuticals, Inc.
http://www.aronex.com
See Antigenics Inc.

Arrow International Corp. Headquarters
2400 Bernville Rd.
Reading, PA 19605
610-378-0131
800-523-8446
http://www.arrowintl.com

Asafi Pharmaceutical
P.O. Box 801764
Santa Clarita, CA 91380-1764
661-294-9509
http://www.asafi.com
http://www.home.aid.com

59439
Ascent Pediatrics, Inc.
See Medicis

AstraZeneca LP
1800 Concord Pike
Wilmington, DE 19850
800-456-3669
800-842-9920
800-237-8898
http://www.AstraZeneca-us.com

59075
Athena Neurosciences, Inc.
See Elan Pharmaceuticals

Athlon Pharmaceuticals, Inc.
301 Snow Drive
Birmingham, AL 35209
888-638-7605

59702
Atley Pharmaceuticals, Inc.
10511 Old Ridge Rd.
Ashland, VA 23005
804-227-2250
http://www.atley.com

Aurobindo Pharma USA, Inc.
2615 Route 130 South
Cranbury, NJ 08512
866-850-2876

AutoImmune, Inc.
1199 Madia St.
Pasadena, CA 91103
626-792-1235
http://www.autoimmuneinc.com

Auxilium Pharmaceuticals, Inc.
160 W. Germantown Pike
Suite D5
Norristown, PA 19401
610-278-6316
http://www.auxilium.com

00053
Aventis Behring L.L.C.
See ZLB Behring

44184
Aventis Pasteur
Discovery Drive
Swiftwater, PA 18370
800-822-2463
http://www.us.aventispasteur.com

Aventis Pharmaceuticals
300 Somerset Corporate Blvd.
Bridgewater, NJ 08807
800-633-1610
800-207-8049
http://www.aventis.com

Axcan Scandipharm
22 Inverness Center Pkwy.
Suite 310
Birmingham, AL 35242
800-472-2634
800-950-8085
http://www.axcanscandipharm.com

B. Braun Medical Inc.
1601 Wallace Drive
Suite 150
Carrollton, TX 75006
800-627-7867
800-854-6851
http://www.bbraunusa.com

Bajamar Chemical Co., Inc.
9609 Dielman Rock Island
St. Louis, MO 63132
314-997-3414
888-242-3414
http://www.vesselvite.com

58174
Baker Cummins Dermatologicals
See Baker Norton Pharmaceuticals

00575, 11414
Baker Norton Pharmaceuticals
4400 Biscayne Blvd.
Miami, FL 33137
800-327-4114
http://www.ivax.com

Ballard Medical Products
12050 S. Lone Peak Pkwy.
Draper, UT 84020
801-572-6800
800-528-5591
http://www.kchealthcare.com

Ballay Pharmaceuticals, Inc.
200 Stillwater
P.O. Box 1356
Wimberley, TX 78676
512-847-6458

Banner Pharmacaps
4125 Premiere Dr.
High Point, NC 27265
336-812-8700
800-447-1140
http://www.banpharm.com

Bard
See C.R. Bard

Barr/Duramed
See Barr Laboratories

00555
Barr Laboratories, Inc.
400 Chestnut Ridge Road
Woodcliff Lake, NJ 07677
845-362-1100
800-222-0190
http://www.barrlabs.com

10116
Bartor Pharmacal Co.
70 High St.
Rye, NY 10580
914-967-4219

58887
Basel Pharmaceuticals
See Novartis Pharmaceuticals

BASF Corporation
3000 Continental Drive North
Mount Olive, NJ 07828-1234
973-426-3786
973-426-2600
800-526-1072
http://www.basf.com/usa

10119
**Bausch & Lomb Personal Products
Division**
1400 N. Goodman St.
P.O. Box 450
Rochester, NY 14692-0450
800-344-8815
585-338-6000
800-553-5340
http://www.bausch.com

24208, 57782
Bausch & Lomb Pharmaceuticals
8500 Hidden River Pkwy.
Tampa, FL 33637
813-975-7770
800-323-0000
http://www.bausch.com

Bausch & Lomb Surgical
180 Via Verde
San Dimas, CA 91773
800-338-2020
http://www.bausch.com

Baxa Corporation
14445 Grasslands Dr.
Inglewood, CO 80112
303-690-4204
800-567-2292
http://www.baxa.com

00944
**Baxter Healthcare Corporation
Baxter Bioscience**
1627 Lake Cook Road
Deerfield, IL 60015
800-423-2090
http://www.baxter.com

Baxter Healthcare Corporation

Clintec Nutrition
One Baxter Pkwy.
Deerfield, IL 60015
800-422-2751
http://www.nutriforum.com

Baxter Healthcare Corporation
One Baxter Pkwy.
Deerfield, IL 60015
800-422-9837
888-229-0001
http://www.baxter.com

Baxter Healthcare Corporation

**Anesthesia Critical Care
Pharmaceuticals**
95 Spring Street
New Providence, NJ 07974
800-667-0959

Baxter Healthcare Corporation

Medication Delivery
Route 120 and Wilson Road
Round Lake, IL 60073
800-229-0001
http://www.baxter.com

Baxter Hyland Immuno
See Baxter Healthcare Corporation,
Baxter Bioscience

**Baxter Pharm. Prods., Inc.
(Baxter PPI)**
See Baxter Healthcare, Anesthesia
Critical Care Pharmaceuticals

00118
Bayer Allergy Products
See Hollister-Stier

Bayer Biological
See Bayer Corp.

12843, 16500
Bayer Consumer Care Division
36 Columbia Rd.
P.O. Box 1910
Morristown, NJ 07962
800-800-4793
800-331-4536
http://www.bayercare.com

00026, 00161, 00192
Bayer Corp.
400 Morgan Lane
West Haven, CT 06516
203-937-2000
800-288-8371
http://www.bayer.com

00193
Bayer Diagnostics
511 Benedict Ave.
Tarrytown, NY 10591
877-229-3711
800-248-2637
http://www.bayerdiag.com
http://www.glucometer.com

31280
BD (Becton Dickinson & Co.)
1 Becton Dr.
Franklin Lakes, NJ 07417
201-847-6800
800-631-7783
http://www.bd.com

00011
BD Biosciences
2350 Qume Drive
San Jose, CA 95131
877-232-8995
http://www.bdbiosciences.com

**BD Diagnostic Systems & Medical
Supplies**
7 Loveton Circle
Sparks, MD 21152
800-675-0908
410-316-4000
http://www.bd.com

BDI Marketing
9700 N. Michigan Road
Carmel, IN 46032
317-228-0000
800-428-1717
http://www.bdi-marketing.com

BDI Pharmaceuticals, Inc.
See BDI Marketing

00486
Beach Pharm.
5220 S. Manhattan Ave.
Tampa, FL 33611
800-322-8210

**Beckman Coulter Primary Care
Diagnostics**
4300 N. Harbor Blvd.
Fullerton, CA 92834
800-877-6242
http://www.beckmancoulter.com/pcd

Becton Dickinson & Co.
See BD

**Becton Dickinson Microbiology
Systems**
7 Loveton Circle
Sparks, MD 21152
410-316-4000
800-638-8663
http://www.bd.com

55390
Bedford Laboratories
300 Northfield Rd.
Bedford, OH 44146
440-232-3320
800-521-5169
800-562-4797
http://www.bedfordlabs.com

10356
Beiersdorf, Inc.
360 Martin Luther King Dr.
South Norwalk, CT 06856-5529
203-853-8008
800-233-2340
http://www.beiersdorf.com

Bergen Brunswig Drug Co.
4000 Metropolitan Dr.
Orange, CA 92868
714-385-4000
800-841-4662
http://www.amerisourcebergen.net

50419
Berlex Laboratories, Inc.
340 Changebridge Road
Montville, NJ 07045
973-694-4100
888-237-5394
http://www.berlex.com

58337
Berna Products Corp.
4216 Ponce De Leon Blvd.
Coral Gables, FL 33146
305-443-2900
800-533-5899
http://www.bernaproducts.com

Bertek Pharmaceuticals, Inc.
781 Chestnut Ridge Road
Morgantown, WV 26505
281-240-1000
800-231-3052
http://www.bertek.com

Best Generics
See Goldline Consumer, Inc.

Beta Dermaceuticals
P.O. Box 691106
San Antonio, TX 78269-1106
210-349-9326
800-434-2382
http://www.beta-derm.com

00283
Beutlich Pharmaceuticals
1541 Shields Dr.
Waukegan, IL 60085
847-473-1100
800-238-8542
http://www.beutlich.com

00225
B. F. Ascher and Co.
15501 West 109th St.
Lenexa, KS 66219
913-888-1880
800-324-1880
http://www.bfascher.com

Bi-Coastal Pharmaceutical Corp.
130 Maple Avenue
Red Bank, NJ 07701
732-530-6606
800-530-9317
http://www.bicoastalpharm.com

Biocare International, Inc.
2643 Grand Ave.
Bellmore, NY 11710
516-781-5800

Biocore Medical Technologies
11800 Tech Road
Suite 240
Silver Spring, MD 20904
888-689-5655
888-565-5243
http://www.biocore.com

00332
Biocraft Laboratories, Inc.
See Teva Pharmaceuticals USA

BioCryst Pharmaceuticals, Inc.
2190 Parkway Lake Dr.
Birmingham, AL 35244
205-444-4600
http://www.biocryst.com

Biofilm, Inc.
3225 Executive Ridge
Vista, CA 92081
760-727-9030
800-848-5900
http://www.astroglide.com

Biogen
See Biogen Idec

Biogen Idec
14 Cambridge Center
Cambridge, MA 02142
617-679-2000
800-262-4363
800-456-2255
http://www.biogenidec.com

BioGenex Laboratories
4600 Norris Canyon Rd.
Suite 400
San Ramon, CA 94583
925-275-0550
800-421-4149
http://www.biogenex.com

Bioglan Pharmaceuticals
7 Great Valley Parkway
Suite 301
Malvern, PA 19355
610-232-2000
888-246-4526
http://www.bioglan.com

Bioline Labs, Inc.
See Ivax Corporation

BioMarin Pharmaceutical Inc.
105 Digital Drive
Novato, CA 94949
415-506-6700

Biomedical Frontiers, Inc.
1095 10th Avenue, S.E.
Minneapolis, MN 55414
612-378-0228

Biomerica, Inc.
1533 Monrovia Ave.
Newport Beach, CA 92663
949-645-2111
800-854-3002
http://www.biomerica.com

Biomerieux
595 Anglum Road
Hazelwood, MO 63042
314-731-8500
800-634-7656
http://www.biomerieux.com

Biomira USA, Inc.
1002 East Park Blvd.
Newport Beach, CA 92663
609-655-5300
http://www.biomira.com

Biomolecular Sciences, Inc.
13428 Maxella Avenue 285
Marina del Ray, CA 90292
310-301-9439
800-260-3587
http://www.genomicwhey.com

Bionexus, Ltd.
30 Brown Road, NY 14850
607-266-9492
800-835-0869
http://www.bionexs.com

Bioniche Pharma Group
231 Dundas Street East
P.O. Box 1570
Belleville, Ontario K8N5J2
Canada
613-966-8058
800-265-5464
http://www.bioniche.com

Biopharmaceutics, Inc.
See Feminique Corp.

Biopharm Labs
2091 Hortel Street
Levittown, PA 19057
215-949-3711
http://www.biopharm.de/

Biopure Corp.
11 Hurley
Cambridge, MA 02141
617-234-6500
http://www.biopure.com

Bioscience Amersham
800 Centennial Avenue
Piscataway, NJ 08855-1327
732-457-8000
732-457-0557
http://www.amersham.com

53191
Biospecifics Technologies Corp.
35 Wilbur Street
Lynbrook, NY 11563
516-593-7000
http://www.biospecifics.com

BIO-TECH Pharmacal, Inc.
P.O. Box 1992
Fayetteville, AR 72702
479-443-9148
800-345-1199
http://www.bio-tech-pharm.com

Bio-Technology General Corp.
1 Tower Center
East Brunswick, NJ 08816
800-284-2480
http://www.btgc.com

Biotrol International
650 S. Taylor Avenue
Suite 20
Louisville, CO 80027
303-673-0341
800-822-8550
http://www.biotrol.com

BioVail Pharmaceuticals, Inc.
700 Rte 202-206 North
Bridgewater, NJ 08807
919-674-2600
877-357-4276
866-246-8245
http://www.biovail.com

BIRA Corp.
2525 Quicksilver
McDonald, PA 15057
724-796-1820
888-796-4832
http://www.hardtofindbrands.com

50289
Birchwood Laboratories, Inc.
7900 Fuller Rd.
Eden Prairie, MN 55344
952-937-7900
800-328-6156
http://www.birchlabs.com

12136
Bird Products Corp.
1100 Bird Center Dr.
Palm Springs, CA 92262
760-778-7200
800-328-4139
http://www.viasyscriticalcare.com

00165
Blaine Pharmaceuticals
1515 Production Dr.
Burlington, KY 41005
859-283-9437
800-633-9353
http://www.blainepharma.com

00154
Blair Laboratories
See Purdue Frederick Co.

50486
Blairex Labs, Inc.
1600 Brian Drive
Columbus, IN 47202
812-378-1864
800-252-4739
http://www.blairex.com

Blansett Pharmacal Co., Inc.
P.O. Box 638
14 Parkstone Circle N.
Little Rock, AR 72115
501-758-8635
http://www.blansett.com

10157
Blistex Inc.
1800 Swift Dr.
Oak Brook, IL 60523
630-571-2870
888-784-2472
http://www.blistex.com

10158
Block Drug Co., Inc.
See GlaxoSmithKline Consumer
  Healthcare, L.P.

10160
Bluco Inc.
28350 Schoolcraft
Livonia, MI 48150
734-513-4500
800-832-4464
http://www.blucoinc.com

Boca Pharmacal, Inc.
6601 Lyons Rd.
Coconut Creek, FL 33073
800-354-8460
http://www.bocamedicalproducts.com

00563
Bock Pharmacal Co.
See Sanofi Synthelabo Inc.

00597
**Boehringer Ingelheim
  Pharmaceuticals, Inc.**
900 Ridgebury Rd.
Ridgefield, CT 06877-0368
203-798-9988
800-542-6257
http://www.boehringer-ingelheim.com

53169
Boehringer Mannheim
See Roche Laboratories

Boericke & Tafel
See Nature's Way

Bone Care Center
1600 Aspen Commons
Middleton, WI 53562
608-662-7800
888-389-3300
http://www.bonecare.com

Bone Care International
1600 Aspen Commons
Middleton, WI 53562
888-389-4242
http://www.bonecare.com

Bonnie Bell
18519 Detroit Avenue
P.O. Box 770349
Lakewood, OH 44107
216-221-0800
800-321-1006
http://www.bonniebell.com

Boots Pharmaceuticals, Inc.
http://www.boots.co.uk/frontpage.html
See Abbott Laboratories

Botanical Laboratories
1441 W. Smith Rd.
Ferndale, WA 98248
360-384-5656
888-977-8008
http://www.botlab.com

00003
Bracco Diagnostics, Inc.
P.O. Box 52250
Princeton, NJ 08543
609-514-2200
800-631-5244
http://www.bdi.bracco.com

Bradley Pharmaceutical
383 Rt. 46 West
West Fairfield, NJ 07004
800-929-9300
http://www.bradpharm.com

52268
Braintree Laboratories, Inc.
P.O. Box 850929
Braintree, MA 02185-0929
781-843-2202
800-874-6756
http://www.braintreelabs.com

45617
Breath Asure, Inc.
http://www.breathasure.com
See Health Assure, Inc.

51991
Breckenridge Pharmaceutical, Inc.
1141 S. Rogers Circle
Suite 3
Boca Raton, FL 33487
561-367-8512
800-466-2700
http://www.breckenridgepharma.com

72363
Brimms Inc.
See Shield Manufacturing

Brioschi
19-01 Pollitt Drive
Fairlawn, NJ 07410
201-796-4226
http://www.brioschi-usa.com

Bristol-Myers Oncology/Virology
P.O. Box 4500
Princeton, NJ 08543
800-426-7644
http://www.bmsoncology.com

19810
Bristol-Myers Products
1350 Liberty Ave
Hillside, NJ 07205
800-468-7746
800-332-2056
http://www.bms.com

00003, 00015, 00087
Bristol-Myers Squibb Company
P.O. Box 4500
Princeton, NJ 08543
609-897-2000
800-321-1335
http://www.bms.com
http://www.bmsoncology.com

63256
Bryan Corporation
4 Plympton St.
Woburn, MA 01801
781-935-0004
800-343-7711
http://www.bryancorp.com

BSN, Jobst
5825 Carnegie Blvd.
Charlotte, NC 28209
800-221-7573
http://www.jobst.com

BTG Pharmaceutical Corporation
One Tower Center Blvd. 14th Floor
East Brunswick, NJ 08816
732-418-9300
800-284-2480
http://www.btgc.com

Burroughs Wellcome Co.
See GlaxoSmithKline

00398
C & M Pharmacal, Inc.
1721 Maple Lane Ave.
Hazel Park, MI 48030
248-548-7846
800-423-5173
http://www.genesispharm.com

Cag Nutrition
See ConAgra Functional Foods, Inc.

Cangene Corp.
104 Chancellor Matheson Rd.,
    Manitoba R3T 5Y3
Canada
204-275-4200
http://www.cangene.com

Calmoseptine, Inc.
16602 Burke Lane
Huntington Beach, CA 92647
800-800-3405
http://www.calmoseptineointment.com

Calwood Nutritionals, Inc.
500 McCormick Drive
Suite J
Glen Burnie, MD 21061
410-590-4890
800-479-9942
http://www.calwoodnutritionals.com

00147
Camall Co., Inc.
P.O. Box 989
Traverse City, MI 49685

Cambrex Bioscience
5901 East Lombard Street
Baltimore, MD 21224
410-563-9200
877-676-5888
http://www.cambrex.com

Cambridge NeuroScience
See Baxter Health Care

43656
Cambridge Nutraceuticals
See Baxter Nutrition

Can-Am Care Corp.
3780 Manfell Rd., Suite T50
Alpharetta, GA 30022
800-461-7448

64543
Capellon Pharmaceuticals, Ltd.
7509 Flagstone Street
Ft. Worth, TX 76118
817-595-5820
http://www.capellon.com

57664
**Caraco Pharmaceutical
    Laboratories Ltd.**
1150 Elijah McCoy Dr.
Detroit, MI 48202
313-871-8400
800-818-4555
http://www.caraco.com

Cardinal Health, Inc.
7000 Cardinal Place
Dublin, OH 43017
614-757-5000
800-234-8701
http://www.cardinal-health.com

Care Technologies, Inc.
10 Corbin Dr.
Darien, CT 06820
http://www.lice.com

Carma Labs, Inc.
5801 W. Airways Ave.
Franklin, WI 53132
414-421-7707
http://www.carma-labs.com

Carme, Inc.
620 Airpark Road
Napa, CA 94558
707-226-3900
http://www.senetekplc.net

Carnation
See Nestle Instant Nutrition

00086
Carnrick Laboratories
See Elan Pharmaceuticals

Cardinal Health
1430 Waukegan Road
McGaw Park, IL 60085
847-689-8410
800-964-5227
http://www.cardinal.com

46287
Carolina Medical Products
8026 US 264 Alternate
Farmville, NC 27828
252-753-7111
800-227-6637
http://www.carolinamedical.com

46287
Carolina Medical Products
8026 US 264 Alternate
Farmville, NC 27828
252-753-7111
800-227-6637
http://www.carolinamedical.com

Carolina Pharmaceuticals
8000 Regency Parkway, Suite 430
Cary, NC 27511
866-280-5755
http://www.carolinapharm.com

Carter Products
See Church & Dwight Co.

00164
Carter-Wallace, Inc.
See MedPointe

00132
C.B. Fleet Co., Inc.
4615 Murray Place
P.O. Box 11349
Lynchburg, VA 24502
434-522-8429
800-999-9711
http://www.cbfleet.com

CCA Industries, Inc.
East Rutherford, NJ 07073
800-524-2720
http://www.ccaindustries.com

Cebert Pharmaceuticals, Inc.
1200 Corporate Drive
Suite 370
Birmingham, AL 35242
205-981-0201
800-211-0589
http://www.cebert.com

Celestial Seasonings, Inc.
4600 Sleepytime Dr.
Boulder, CO 80301
303-530-5300
800-525-0347
http://www.celestialseasonings.com

Celgene Corp.
7 Powder Horn Dr.
Warren, NJ 07059
732-271-1001
800-890-4619
http://www.celgene.com

Cell Pathways
http://www.cellpathways.com
See OSI Pharmaceuticals

Cell Therapeutics
501 Elliott Ave. West
Suite 400
Seattle, WA 98119
206-272-4000
800-215-2355
http://www.ctiseattle.com

Cellcor, Inc.
800 Wells Avenue
Newton, MA 02159

Cellegy Pharmaceuticals, Inc.
349 Oyster Pointe Blvd.
Suite 200
South San Francisco, CA 94080
650-616-2200
http://www.cellegy.com

Celltech Pharmaceutical Co.
755 Jefferson Rd.
Rochester, NY 14623
585-475-9000
800-234-5535
http://www.celltechgroup.com

Celtrix Pharmaceuticals, Inc.
2033 Gateway Pl., Suite 600
San Jose, CA 95110
408-988-2500
http://www.bioportfolio.com

00053
Centeon
See Aventis Behring

Center Laboratories
See ALK Abello

00268
Center Pharmaceuticals, Inc.
See ALK Abello

Centers for Disease Control and Prevention
1600 Clifton Rd. N.E.
Atlanta, GA 30333
404-639-3670
404-639-3534
800-311-3435
http://www.cdc.gov

Centocor, Inc.
200 Great Valley Pkwy.
Malvern, PA 19355
610-651-6000
800-457-6399
http://www.centocor.com

00131
Central Pharmaceuticals, Inc.
See Schwarz Pharma

00436
Century Pharmaceuticals, Inc.
10377 Hague Rd.
Indianapolis, IN 46256-3399
317-849-4210
866-343-2576

Cephalon, Inc.
145 Brandywine Pkwy.
West Chester, PA 19380
610-344-0200
800-782-3656
http://www.cephalon.com

Cera Products
9017 Mendenhall Court
Columbia, MD 21045
301-490-4941
888-ceralyte
http://www.ceralyte.com

00173
Cerenex Pharmaceuticals
See GlaxoSmithKline

Cervical Cap Ltd.
430 Monterey Ave.
Suite 1B
Los Gatos, CA 95030
408-395-2100
http://www.cervcap.com

10223
Cetylite Industries, Inc.
9051 River Rd.
Pennsauken, NJ 08110
865-665-6111
800-257-7740
http://www.cetylite.com

Chantal Pharmaceutical
12121 Wilshire Blvd.
Suite 1120
Los Angeles, CA 90025

54429
Chase Laboratories
See Banner Pharmacaps

49447
Chattem Consumer Products
1715 W. 38th St.
Chattanooga, TN 37409
423-821-4571
800-366-6833
http://www.chattem.com

ChemTrak, Inc.
929 East Arques Avenue
Sunnyvale, CA 94086

Chesapeake Biological Labs., Inc.
1111 S. Paca St.
Baltimore, MD 21230
410-843-5000
800-441-4225
http://www.cblinc.com

00521
Chesebrough-Ponds USA, Inc.
See Unilever Home and Personal
Care USA

Cheshire Pharmaceutical Systems
6225 Shiloh Rd.
Alpharetta, GA 30005

Chester Labs
1900 Section Road
Suite A
Cincinnati, OH 45237

Chew-Rite Co.
265 S. Pioneer Blvd.
Springboro, OH 45066
937-746-5509

Chiesi Pharmaceuticals, Inc.
150 Danbury Rd.
Ridgefield, CT 06877

Childrens Hospital of Columbus
700 Childrens Dr.
Columbus, OH 43205
614-722-2000
http://www.columbuschildrens.com

Chilton Labs., Inc.
299B Fairfield Ave.
Fairfield, NJ 07004
973-575-1992

53905
Chiron Therapeutics
4560 Horton St.
Emeryville, CA 94608
510-655-8730
800-244-7668
http://www.chiron.com

Chiron Vision
See Bausch & Lomb Surgical

Chronimed Inc.
10900 Red Circle Dr.
Minnetonka, MN 55343
952-979-3600
800-444-5951
http://www.chronimed.com

Church & Dwight Co.
469 N. Harrison Street
Princeton, NJ 08543
800-833-9532
http://www.churchdwight.com

00083
Ciba-Geigy Pharmaceuticals
See Novartis Pharmaceuticals

00346
Ciba Vision Corporation
11460 Johns Creek Pkwy.
Duluth, GA 30097
770-476-3937
800-845-6585
http://www.cibavision.com

Cima Labs
10000 Valley View Road
Eden Prairie, MN 55344
952-947-8700
http://www.cimalabs.com

00677, 00725, 71114
Circa Pharmaceuticals, Inc.
See Watson Laboratories, Inc.

94503
Cirrus Healthcare Products, L.L.C.
60 Main St.
Cold Spring Harbor, NY 11724
631-692-7600
800-327-6151
http://www.cirrushealthcare.com

CIS-US, Inc.
10 DeAngelo Dr.
Bedford, MA 01730
781-275-7120
800-221-7554
http://www.cisusinc.com

Citra Anticoagulants
55 Messina Drive
Braintree, MA 02184
781-848-2174
800-299-3411

Claragen, Inc.
12300 Washington Avenue
Suite 200
Rockville, MD 20852
304-405-0742
http://www.claragen.com

45802
Clay-Park Labs, Inc.
1700 Bathgate Ave.
Bronx, NY 10457
718-901-2800
800-933-5550
http://www.claypark.com

Clear Technologies
See Care Technologies Inc.

55553
Clint Pharmaceuticals
629 Shute Lane
Old Hickory, TN 37138
615-882-0042
800-677-5022

Clintec Nutrition
See Baxter Healthcare Corporation,
  Baxter Health Care

Closure Medical Corp
5250 Greensdairy Road
Raleigh, NC 27616
919-876-7800
http://www.closuremed.com

57145
CNS, Inc.
7615 Smethand Ln.
Eden Prairie, MN 55344
952-229-1500
http://www.cns.com

Coats Aloe
2146 Merrit Drive
Garland, TX 75041
972-278-9651
800-486-ALOE
http://www.coatsaloe.com

Colgate Oral Pharmaceuticals
1 Colgate Way
Canton, MA 02021
781-821-2880
800-821-2880
http://www.colgateprofessional.com

Colgate-Palmolive Co.
300 Park Ave.
New York, NY 10022
212-310-2000
800-221-4607
http://www.colgate.com

Collagen Corp.
See INAMED Corp.

27280
CollaGenex Pharmaceuticals, Inc.
41 University Dr.
Suite 200
Newtown, PA 18940
215-579-7388
888-339-5678
http://www.collagenex.com

Coloplast
1955 West Oak Circle
Marietta, GA 30062
800-533-0464
http://www.us.coloplast.com

Colorado Biolabs
404 N Street
P.O. Box 125
Cozad, NE 69130
888-442-0067
http://www.coloradobiolabs.com

00837, 21406
Columbia Laboratories, Inc.
354 Eisenhower Parkway Plaza 1, 2nd
  Floor
Livingston, NJ 07039
973-994-3999
866-566-5636
http://www.columbialabs.com

11509
Combe, Inc.
1101 Westchester Ave.
White Plains, NY 10604
914-694-5454
800-431-2610
http://www.combe.com

**CompliMed Medical Research
Group**
1441 West Smith Rd.
Ferndale, WA 98248
360-384-5656
888-977-8008
http://www.complimed.com

ConAgra Functional Foods, Inc.
1218 E. Hartman Ave.
Omaha, NE 68110
402-455-0634
888-828-4242
http://www.culturelle.com

Conair Interplak Division
1 Cummings Point Rd.
Stamford, CT 06902
800-726-6247
http://www.conair.com

Con-Cise Contact Lens Co.
14450 Doolittle Dr.
San Leandro, CA 94577
510-483-9400
800-772-3911
http://www.con-cise.com

20254
Concord Laboratories
140 New Dutch Lane
Fairfield, NJ 07004
973-227-6757

11793, 49281, 50361
Connaught Labs
See Aventis Pasteur

00007
Connetics Corporation
3290 W. Bayshore Rd.
Palo Alto, CA 94303
650-843-2800
800-280-2879
http://www.connetics.com

43786
Consep Inc.
See Woodstream Corp.

00223
Consolidated Midland Corp.
20 Main St.
Brewster, NY 10509
845-279-6108

18149
Consumers Choice Systems, Inc.
2370 130th Ave. NE
Suite 101
Bellevue, WA 98005
425-883-6310

34044
Continental Consumer Products
770 Forest
Suite B
Birmingham, MI 48009
800-542-5903

33130
Continental Quest Research
220 W. Carmel Dr.
Carmel, IN 46032
317-843-2501
800-451-5773
http://www.continentalquest.com

Contract Pharmacal Corp.
135 Adams Ave.
Hauppauge, NY 11788
631-231-4610
http://www.cpchealth.com

00003
ConvaTec
P.O. Box 5254
Princeton, NJ 08543
908-904-2200
800-422-8811
http://www.convatec.com

Cooke Pharma, Inc.
See Unither Pharma

59426
CooperVision
370 Woodcliff Drive
Suite 200
Fairport, NY 14450
585-385-6810
800-538-7850
http://www.coopervisionhydron.com

38245
Copley Pharmaceutical
See Teva Pharmaceuticals USA

COR Therapeutics, Inc.
See Millennium Pharmaceuticals

Cord Labs
See Geneva Pharmaceuticals

Corixa
1900 9th Avenue
Suite 1100
Seattle, WA 98101
206-754-5711
http://www.corixa.com

Cornerstone BioPharma Inc.
2000 Regency Parkway
Cary, NC 27511
888-466-6505

C.R. Bard
730 Central Avenue
Murray Hill, NJ 07974
908-277-8000
http://www.crbard.com

08011
C.R. Bard, Inc. Urological Division
8195 Industrial Blvd.
Covington, GA 30014
770-784-6100
800-526-4455
http://www.crbard.com

Creomulsion
See Summit Industries, Inc.

C.S. Dent & Co Division
See Grandpa Brands Company

CTEX Pharmaceuticals Inc.
See Andrx Labs

Cubist Pharmaceuticals
65 Hayden Avenue
Lexington, MA 02421
781-860-8660
866-793-2786
http://www.cubist.com

Cumberland Swan, Inc.
One Swan Drive
Smyrna, TN 37167
615-459-8900
800-486-7926
http://www.cumberlandswan.com

55326
Curatek Pharmaceuticals
See 3M Pharmaceuticals

Cutis Pharma, Inc.
100 Cummings Ctr.
Suite 421C
Beverly, MA 01915
978-867-1010
http://www.cutispharma.com

Cutter Biologicals
See Bayer Corp.

Cyanotech Corp.
73-4460 Queen Kaahamanu Hwy.
Suite 102
Kailua-Kona, HI 96740
808-326-1353
800-395-1353
http://www.cyanotech.com

Cyclin Pharmaceuticals Inc.
1289 Demingy Way
Madison, WI 53717
800-558-7046
800-982-1186
http://www.womenshealth.com

Cygnus, Inc.
400 Penobscot Dr.
Redwood City, CA 94063
650-369-4300
http://www.cygn.com

54799
Cynacon/OCuSOFT
5311 Ave. North
Rosenburg, TX 77471
800-233-5469
http://www.ocusoft.com

Cypress Pharmaceutical, Inc.
135 Industrial Blvd.
Madison, MS 39110
601-856-4393
800-856-4393
http://www.cypressrx.com

Cypros Pharmaceutical Corp.
See Questcor Pharmaceuticals, Inc.

Cytogen Corporation
650 College Rd. East 3rd Floor
Princeton, NJ 08540
609-750-8200
800-833-3533
http://www.cytogen.com

23731
Cytosol Laboratories
55 Messina Dr.
Braintree, MA 02184
781-848-9386
800-288-3858
http://www.cytosol.com

Cytosol Ophthalmics
P.O. Box 1408
1325 William White Pl. NE
Lenoir, NC 28645
828-758-2343
800-234-5166
http://www.cytosol.com

CytRx Corp.
11726 San Vicente Blvd.
Suite 650
Los Angeles, CA 90049
310-826-5648
http://www.cytrx.com

Daiichi Pharm. Corp.
11 Philips Pkwy.
Montvale, NJ 07645-1810
201-573-7000
877-324-4244
http://www.daiichius.com

**Danbury Pharmacal (Watson
    Laboratories)**
1033 Stoneleigh Ave.
Carmel, NY 10512
914-767-2000
800-553-4044
http://www.watson.com

Danco Labs., LLC
P.O. Box 4816
New York, NY 10185
212-424-1950
877-432-7596
http://www.earlyoptionpill.com

D & K Healthcare Resources
8235 Forsyth Blvd.
St. Louis, MO 63105
888-727-3485
http://www.dkwd.com

00689
Daniels Pharmaceuticals, Inc.
See Jones Pharma Incorporated

58869
**Dartmouth Pharmaceuticals (Elan
    Pharmaceuticals)**
38 Church Ave.
Wareham, MA 02571
508-295-2200
800-414-3566
http://www.ilovemynails.com

00938
Davis and Geck Care Products
See Kendall Health Care Products

Davol, Inc.
100 Sockanossett Crossroad
Cranston, RI 02920
401-463-7000
800-556-6275
http://www.davol.com

52041
Dayton Laboratories
7760 NW 56th St.
Miami, FL 33166
305-594-0988
800-446-0255

Debio Pharmaceuticals S.A.
17, Rue des Terreaux Case Postale
  211 CH-1000
Lausanne 9, Switzerland
0041 21 321 0111
http://www.debio.com

Degussa Corp.
379 Enterpace Pkwy.
Parsippany, NJ 07054-0677
973-541-8000
877-273-2668
http://www.degussa.com

Deliz Pharmaceutical Corporation
P.O. Box 29765
San Juan, PR 00929-0765
787-272-2202

10310
Del Pharmaceuticals
565 Broad Hollow Rd.
Farmingdale, NY 11735
516-844-2020
800-645-9888
http://www.dellabs.com

00316
Del Ray Laboratories
349 Lasecox Drive
Johnson City, TN 37604
800-334-4286
http://www.delrayderm.com

48532
Delmont Laboratories, Inc.
P.O. Box 269
Swarthmore, PA 19081
610-543-3365
800-562-5541
http://www.delmont.com

Delta Pharmaceuticals
2 Davis Dr.
P.O. Box 12278
Research Triangle Park, NC 29063

Den-Mat Corporation
2727 Skyway Dr.
Santa Maria, CA 93455
805-922-8491
800-433-6628
http://www.den-mat.com

00295
Denison Labs., Inc.
P.O. Box 1305
Pawtucket, RI 02862
401-723-5500

49336
Dental Herb Co.
1000 Holland Dr., Suite 7
Boca Raton, FL 33487
561-241-4262
800-747-4372
http://www.dentalherbcompany.com

DepoTech Corp. (SkyePharma)
10450 Science Center
San Diego, CA 92121-1119
858-625-2424
http://www.skyepharma.com

Derma Science
214 Carnegie Center
Suite 100
Princeton, NJ 08540
609-514-4744
800-825-4325
http://www.dermasciences.com

Dermalogix Partners
P.O. Box 1510
Scarborough, ME 04070
207-883-4103
800-753-0047
http://www.dermalogix.com

Dermarite
3 East 26th Street
Paterson, NJ 07513
973-569-9000
800-337-6296
http://www.dermarite.com

00066
Dermik Laboratories, Inc. (Arcola)
1050 Westlake Dr.
Berwin, PA 19312
484-595-2700
800-666-6030
800-340-7502
http://www.dermik.com

DeRoyal Industries, Inc.
200 DeBusk Lane
Powell, TN 37849
423-938-7828
800-337-6925
800-251-9864
http://www.deroyal.com

DexGen Pharmaceuticals, Inc.
P.O. Box 675
Manasquan, NJ 08736
732-223-8811
877-339-4361
http://www.dexgen.com

49502
Dey Laboratories, Inc.
2751 Napa Valley Corporate Dr.
Napa, CA 94558
707-224-3200
800-755-5560
http://www.deyinc.com

DHS, Inc.
250 Hembree Park Drive
Suite 112
Roswell, GA 30076
770-751-1787

Diacrin Corp
Bldg. 96, 13th St.
Charlestown, MA 02129
617-242-9100
http://www.diacrin.com

Dial Corporation
15501 N. Dial Blvd.
Scottsdale, AZ 85260
480-754-3425
800-258-3425
http://www.dialcorp.com

DiaPharma Group, Inc.
8948 Beckett Rd.
West Chester, OH 45069-2939
513-860-9324
800-526-5224
http://www.diapharma.com

Diatide, Inc.
See Berlex Laboratories

Dickinson Brands, Inc.
31 East High Street
East Hampton, CT 06424
860-267-2279
888-860-2279
http://www.witchhazel.com

Digestive Care Inc.
1120 Win Dr.
Bethlehem, PA 18017
610-882-5950

Discovery Laboratories, Inc.
350 S Main St.
Suite 307
Doylestown, PA 18901
215-340-4699
http://www.discoverylabs.com

Discus Dental Inc.
8550 Higuera St.
Culver City, CA 90232
310-845-8200
800-273-2847
http://www.discusdental.com

00777
Dista Products Co.
See Eli Lilly and Co.

Dixon-Shane
256 Geiger Rd.
Philadelphia, PA 19115
215-673-3415
800-262-7770
http://www.dixonshane.com

DJ Pharma, Inc.
See BioVail

10337
Doak Dermatologics
See Bradley Pharmaceuticals

Dolisos America, Inc.
3014 Rigel Ave.
Las Vegas, NV 89102
800-365-4767
http://www.dolisos.com

25358
Donell DerMedex
See Donell Inc.

Donell Inc.
501 Fifth Avenue
Suite 1214
New York, NY 10017
212-682-0666
877-853-9605
http://www.cxproducts.com

Dover Pharmaceutical, Inc.
P.O. Box 809
Islington, MA 02090
800-777-6847

00514
Dow Hickam, Inc.
See Bertek Pharmaceuticals, Inc.

Dow Pharmaceutical Sciences
1330A Redwood Way
Petaluma, CA 94954
707-793-2600
http://www.dowpharm.com

Dreir Pharmaceuticals, Inc.
9602 N. 122nd Place
Scottsdale, AZ 85259
480-607-3584
800-541-4044
http://www.dreirpharmaceuticals.com

Dr. Reddys Laboratories, Inc.
One Park Way
Upper Saddle River, NJ 07458
908-203-4900
http://www.drreddys.com

Drug Abuse Sciences
25954 Eden Landing Rd.
Hayward, CA 94545
http://www.drugabusesciences.com

DSC Laboratories
1979 Latimer Dr.
Muskegon, MI 49442
800-492-5988
231-777-3012
http://www.dsclab.com

00094
DuPont Pharmaceuticals Co.
See Bristol-Myers Squibb

51479
Dura/Elan Pharmaceuticals
See Elan Pharmaceuticals

51285
Duramed Pharmaceuticals
See Barr Laboratories

Durex Consumer Products
3585 Engineering Dr.
Suite 200
Norcross, GA 30092
770-582-2222
888-566-3468
http://www.durex.com

Durham Pharmacal Corp.
See Steifel Consumer Healthcare

DUSA Pharmaceuticals, Inc.
25 Upton
Wilmington, MA 01887
978-657-7500
877-533-DUSA
http://www.dusapharma.com

DynaGen Inc.
See Able Laboratories, Inc.

Eagle Vision, Inc.
8500 Wolf Lake Dr.
Suite 110
P.O. Box 34877
Memphis, TN 38184
901-380-7000
800-222-7584
http://www.eaglevis.com

Eastman Kodak Co.
343 State St.
Rochester, NY 11650
585-724-4000
800-242-2424
http://www.kodak.com

Eaton Medical Corp.
1401 Heistan Place
Memphis, TN 38104
901-274-0000
800-253-5949
http://www.easyeyes.com

19458
Eckerd Drug Corp.
P.O. Box 4689
Clearwater, FL 33758
800-325-3737
http://www.eckerd.com

Ecological Formulas, Inc.
1061-B Shary Circle, Suite B
Concord, CA 94518
800-888-4585

38130
Econo Med Pharmaceuticals
4305 Sartin Rd.
Burlington, NC 27217-7522
336-226-1091
800-327-6007

55053
Econolab
See Breckenridge Pharmaceuticals

00095, 59010
ECR Pharmaceuticals
3969 Deep Rock Rd.
P.O. Box 71600
Richmond, VA 23255
804-527-1950
800-527-1955
http://www.ecrpharmaceuticals.com

Edwards Lifescience
6864 S. 300 West
Midvale, UT 84047
800-453-8432

00485
Edwards Pharmaceuticals, Inc.
111 Mulberry St.
Ripley, MS 38663
800-543-9560

55806
Effcon Laboratories
1800 Sandy Plains Pkwy.
Suite 102
P.O. Box 7499
Marietta, GA 30065-1499
770-428-7011
800-722-2428
http://www.effcon.com

00168
E. Fougera Co.
60 Baylis Rd.
Melville, NY 11747
800-432-6673
http://www.fougera.com

Eisai Inc.
500 Frank W. Burr Blvd.
Teaneck, NJ 07666
201-692-1100
http://www.eisai.com

Elan Pharmaceuticals
7475 Lusk Blvd.
San Diego, CA 92121
888-638-7605
800-859-8586
http://www.elan.com

00002, 59075
Eli Lilly and Co.
Lilly Corp. Center
Indianapolis, IN 46285
317-276-2000
800-545-5979
http://www.lilly.com

00641
Elkins-Sinn, Inc.
See Wyeth-Ayerst

EM Industries, Inc.
See EMD Chemicals, Inc.

EMD Chemicals, Inc.
480 S. Democrat Road
Gibbstown, NJ 08027
800-222-0342

00802
Emerson Laboratories
See Humco Holding Group, Inc.

Enamelon, Inc.
7 Cedar Brook Dr.
Cranbury, NJ 08512
888-432-3535
http://www.enamelon.com

60951
Endo Laboratories, Inc.
100 Painters Dr.
Chadds Ford, PA 19317
610-558-9800
800-462-3636
http://www.endo.com

Endurance Products Co.
9914 SW Tigard St.
P.O. Box 230489
Tigard, OR 97281
800-483-2532
http://www.endur.com

62333
EnviroDerm Pharmaceuticals, Inc.
46 Christa McAuliffe Blvd.
Plymouth, MA 02360
508-747-9601
800-991-DERM
http://www.enviroderm.com

57665
Enzon, Inc.
685 Route 202/206
Bridgewater, NJ 08854
908-541-8600
http://www.enzon.com

00185, 00536
Eon Labs Manufacturing, Inc.
227-15 N. Conduit Ave.
Laurelton, NY 11413
718-276-8600
800-526-0225
http://www.eonlabs.com

EPIEN Medical
4225 White Bear Pkwy, Ste 600
St. Paul, MN 55110–3389
651-653-3380
888-884-4675

Epitope Inc.
See OraSure Technologies

E.R. Squibb & Sons, Inc.
See Bristol-Myers Squibb Co.

00005, 59911
ESI Lederle Generics
See Wyeth Pharmaceuticals

ESP Pharma
2035 Lincoln Hwy.
Suite 2150
Edison, NJ 08817
866-437-7742
http://www.esppharma.com

58177
Ethex Corp.
10888 Metro Ct.
St. Louis, MO 63043-2413
314-567-3307
800-321-1705
http://www.ethex.com

Ethicon, Inc. (Johnson & Johnson)
US Route 22 West
Somerville, NJ 08876-0151
908-218-0707
800-255-2500
http://www.ethiconinc.com

Eurand America, Inc.
845 Center Dr.
Vandalia, OH 45377
937-898-9669
http://www.eurand.com

Eurand International S.P.A.
20060 Pessano con Bornagio
Milan, Italy
39-02-954281
http://www.eurand.com

Evans Vaccines Ltd.
Florey House The Oxford Science
Park
Oxford, UK OX 44GA
44 8547 451 500
http://www.evansvaccines.com

Evenflo Company, Inc.
1801 Commerce Drive
Piqua, OH 45356
800-223-5921
http://www.evenflo.com

00642
Everett Laboratories, Inc.
29 Spring St.
West Orange, NJ 07052
973-324-0200
http://www.everettlabs.com

Excellium Pharmaceutical
3-G Oak Road
Fairfield, NJ 07004
973-276-9600

Excelsior Medical Corporation
P.O. Box 299
Long Branch, NJ 07740
800-487-4276

Eye Care & Cure Corporation
1140 N. Rosemont Boulevard
Tucson, AZ 85712
520-321-1262
800-486-6169
http://www.eyecareandcure.com

E-Z-EM
717 Main St.
Westbury, NY 11590
516-333-8230
800-544-4624
http://www.ezem.com

Falcon Ophthalmics, Inc.
6201 S. Freeway
Fort Worth, TX 76134
817-551-8710
800-343-2133
http://www.alconlabs.com

Farmacon, Inc.
90 Grove St.
Suite 109
Ridgefield, CT 06877-4118

60976
Faro Pharmaceuticals, Inc.
Houston, TX 77043
877-994-3276
800-480-1985

99766
Faulding USA
See Mayne Pharma (USA) Inc.

The F. C. Sturtevant Company
P.O. Box 607
Bronxville, NY 10708
914-337-5131
888-871-5661
http://www.columbiapowder.com

11423
Female Health Co.
515 N. State St.
Suite 2225
Chicago, IL 60610
312-595-9123
800-884-1601
http://www.femalehealth.com

Feminique Corp.
990 Station Rd.
Bellport, NY 11713

00496
Ferndale Laboratories, Inc.
780 W. Eight Mile Rd.
Ferndale, MI 48220-1218
248-548-0900
888-548-0900
http://www.ferndalelabs.com

Ferraris Medical Ltd.
4 Harforde Court John Tate Road
Hertford, UK SG13 7NW
+44 (0) 1992 526300
http://www.ferrarismedical.com

Ferring Pharmaceuticals Inc.
400 Rella Blvd.
Suffern, NY 10901
845-770-2600
888-337-7464
http://www.ferringusa.com

FH Faulding & Co. Ltd.
See Mayne Group Limited

31795
Fibertone
See Naturally Vitamins Co.

Fidia Pharmaceutical Corporation
2000 K St. N.W. #700
Washington, DC 20006
http://www.fidiapharma.com

Fielding Pharmaceutical Co.
See Novavax, Inc.

First Horizon Pharmaceutical Corp.
6195 Shiloh Rd.
Alpharetta, GA 30005
770-442-9707
800-849-9707
http://www.firsthorizonpharm.com

First Quality Products
80 Cuttermill Road
Suite 500
Great Neck, NY 11021
516-929-3030
http://www.firstquality.com

First Scientific Inc.
Lake Forest Plaza 2222 Francisco Dr.,
  510-174
El Dorado Hills, CA 95762
916-491-5088
800-767-2208
http://www.freshcleanse.com

51687
Fischer Pharmaceuticals, Inc
7040 W. Palmetto Park Rd. #4
Suite 606
Boca Raton, FL 33433-3407
561-338-3338
800-782-0222
http://www.dr-fischer.com

Fiske Industries
50 Ramland Road
Orangeburg, NY 10962
845-398-3340
800-248-8033
http://www.cosmeticsolutions.com

00585
Fison Corp.
See Celltech Pharmaceutical Co.

54323
Flanders, Inc.
P.O. Box 80428
Charleston, SC 29416
843-571-3363
http://www.flandersbuttocksointment.com

00256
Fleming & Co.
1733 Gilsinn Lane
Fenton, MO 63026-2918
636-343-5206
800-343-0164
http://www.flemingcompany.com

Flents Products Company
5401 S. Graham Road
St. Charles, MI 48655
989-865-8221
800-262-8221
http://www.apothecaryproducts.com

Flex-Power
1563 Solano Avenue
Berkeley, CA 94706
866-FLEXPOWER
866-353-9769
http://www.flexpower.com

00288
Fluoritab Corp.
P.O. Box 507
Temperance, MI 48182-0507
734-847-3985

FNC Medical Corporation
5000 Everglades Units 11 & C
Ventura, CA 93003
805-644-7576
800-440-2888
http://www.fncmedical.com

Forest Laboratories, Inc.
909 Third Ave.
New York, NY 10022
212-421-7850
800-947-5227
http://www.frx.com
http://www.forestpharm.com

Forest Laboratories Ireland Ltd
See Forest Pharmaceutical, Inc.

00258, 00456, 00535
Forest Pharmaceutical, Inc.
13600 Shoreline
St. Louis, MO 63045
314-493-7000
800-678-1605
http://www.forestpharm.com

Forte Pharma
See Eon Labs Manufacturing, Inc.

Fougera
See E. Fougera Co.

Fournier Pharma
6 Capitol Drive
Parsippany, NJ 07054
973-683-0024
http://www.fournierpharma.com

Free Radical Sciences, Inc.
245 First St.
Cambridge, MA 02142

10432
Freeda Vitamins, Inc.
36 E. 41st St.
New York, NY 10017-6203
212-685-4980
800-777-3737
http://www.freedavitamins.com

**Fresenius Medical Care North
  America**
95 Hayden Avenue
Lexington, MA 02420
781-402-9000
http://www.fmcna.com

Fuisz Technologies, Ltd.
14555 Avion at Lakeside
Suite 250
Chantilly, VA 22151
703-803-3260

00469, 57317
Fujisawa Healthcare, Inc.
3 Parkway N.
Deerfield, IL 60015-2548
800-727-7003
800-888-7704
http://www.fujisawa.com

00713
G & W Laboratories
111 Coolidge St.
South Plainfield, NJ 07080-3895
908-753-2000
800-922-1038
http://www.gwlabs.com

Galagen Nutrition Medical, Inc.
See Hormel Healthlabs

00299
Galderma Laboratories, Inc.
14501 N. Freeway
Ft. Worth, TX 76177
817-961-5000
800-582-8225
http://www.galdermausa.com

Galen Pharma
22 Seagoe Industrial Estate
Craigavon, UK BT63 5QD
028 3833 4974
http://www.galen.co.uk

Gallipot, Inc.
2020 Silver Bell Rd.
St. Paul, MN 55120
651-681-9517
800-423-6967
http://www.gallipot.com

00254
Gambro, Inc.
10810 W. Collins Ave.
Lakewood, CO 80215-4498
303-232-6800
800-525-2623
http://www.gambro.com

57844
Gate Pharmaceuticals
1090 Horsham Rd.
North Wales, PA 19454-1090
215-591-3046
800-292-4283
http://www.gatepharma.com

00386
Gebauer Co.
9410 St. Catherine Ave.
Cleveland, OH 44104-5226
216-271-5252
800-321-9348
http://www.gebauerco.com

00028
Geigy Pharmaceuticals
See Novartis Pharmaceuticals

Geist Pharmaceutical, L.L.C.
20 N. Meridian St.
Suite 9500
Indianapolis, IN 46204
317-833-0700
888-644-3478
http://www.geistrx.com

Gel-Kam
P.O. Box 80009
Dallas, TX 75380
214-233-2800

Gel-Tech
http://www.zicam.com
See Matrix Initiatives, Inc.

Gen-King
See Kinray

52761
GenDerm Corp.
See Medicis Pharmaceutical Corp.

50242
Genentech, Inc.
1 DNA Way
S. San Francisco, CA 94080-4990
650-225-1000
800-551-2231
800-821-8590
http://www.gene.com

52584
General Injectables & Vaccines
U.S. Hwy. 52 South
P.O. Box 9
Bastian, VA 24314-0009
276-688-4121
800-521-7468
http://www.giv.com

00918
General Medical Corp.
See McKesson Medical-Surgical

General Nutrition Inc.
300 6th Ave.
Pittsburgh, PA 15222
412-288-4600
888-462-2548
http://www.gnc.com

98318
Genesis Nutrition
1816 Wall St.
Florence, SC 29501
843-665-6928
800-451-7933
http://www.genesisnutrition.com

Genesis Pharmaceuticals
9 Campus Drive, Suite 7
Parsippany, NJ 07054
800-459-8663
http://www.genesispharm.com

Genetic Therapy, Inc.
938 Clopper Rd.
Gaithersburg, MD 20878
301-590-2626

Genetics Institute
35 Cambridge Park Dr.
Cambridge, MA 02140
617-503-7332
888-446-3344
http://www.genetics.com

Geneva Pharmaceutical
  Technology Corporation
2400 Route 130N
Dayton, NJ 08810
732-274-2400
http://www.genevarx.com

00781
Geneva Pharmaceuticals
See Sandoz

GenpharmInternational, Inc.
See Medarex, Inc.

00703
Gensia Sicor Pharmaceuticals, Inc.
19 Hughes
Irvine, CA 92618
800-331-0124
800-729-9991
http://www.gensiasicor.com

GenVec, Inc.
65 W. Watkins Mill Rd.
Gaithersburg, MD 20878
240-632-0740
http://www.genvec.com

58468
Genzyme Corp.
One Kendall Square Building 1400
Cambridge, MA 02139
617-252-7500
800-326-7002
800-868-8208
http://www.genzyme.com

Genzyme Transplant
500 Kendall Street
Cambridge, MA 02142
888-764-7828
800-326-7002

Geodesic MediTech, Inc.
2921 Sandy Pointe No. 3
Del Mar, CA 92014
858-792-1100
888-357-9399
http://www.geodesicmrditech.com

Gerber Products Company
445 State St.
Fremont, MI 49413-0001
800-443-7237
http://www.gerber.com

Geriatric Pharmaceutical Corp.
See Roberts Pharmaceutical Corp.

Geri-Care Products
250 Moonachie Avenue
Moonachie, NJ 07074-1897
201-440-0409
800-654-8322
geri-careproducts.com

Geritrex Corporation
144 Kingsbridge Road East
East Mount Vernon, NY 10550
914-668-4003
800-736-3437
http://www.geritrex.com

Gilead Sciences
333 Lakeside Dr.
Foster City, CA 94404
650-574-3000
800-445-3235
800-403-3945
http://www.gilead.com

59366
Glades Pharmaceuticals
6340 Sugarloaf Parkway, Suite 400
Duluth, GA 30097
866-436-0318
888-445-2337
http://www.glades.com

GlaxoSmithKline
1 Franklin Plaza
Philadelphia, PA 19102
215-751-4000
888-825-5249
http://www.gsk.com

GlaxoSmithKline Consumer
  Healthcare, L.P.
100 Beecham Dr.
Pittsburgh, PA 15205
800-245-1040
http://www.gsk.com

GlaxoSmithKline Pharm.
1 Franklin Plaza
Philadelphia, PA 19101
888-825-5249
http://www.gsk.com

00081, 00173
GlaxoWellcome, Inc.
See GlaxoSmithKline

00516
Glenwood, Inc.
111 Cedar Land
P.O. Box 5419
Englewood, NJ 07631
201-569-0050
800-542-0772
http://www.glenwood-llc.com

00115
Global Pharmaceuticals, Inc.
3735 Castor Avenue
Philadelphia, PA 19124
215-289-2220
http://www.globalphar.com

Global Source
5371 Hiatus Rd.
Sunrise, FL 33351
954-747-8977
http://www.globalvitamin.com

GM Pharmaceutical
P.O. Box 150312
Arlington, TX 76015

GML Industries, LLC
51 Monarch Dr.
P.O. Box 1973
Denison, TX 75020
903-463-7321
877-828-4633
http://www.gml-industries.com

60429
Golden State Medical Supply
1799 Eastman Avenue
Ventura, CA 93003
805-477-9866
800-284-8633
http://www.gsms.us

Goldline Consumer
See Ivax Corporation

00182
Goldline Laboratories, Inc.
See Ivax Pharmaceuticals

74684
Goody's Manufacturing Corp.
See GlaxoSmithKline Consumer
   Healthcare, L.P.

10481
Gordon Laboratories
6801 Ludlow St.
Upper Darby, PA 19082-2408
610-734-2011
800-356-7870
http://www.gordonlabs.com

12165
Graham Field Health Products Inc.
2935 NE Parkway
Atlanta, GA 30360
800-347-5678
http://www.grahamfield.com

Grandpa Brands Company
1820 Airport Exchange Blvd.
Erlanger, KY 41018
859-647-0777
800-684-1468
http://www.grandpabrands.com

00152
Gray Pharmaceutical Co.
See Purdue Frederick Co.

Great American Nutrition
2002 S. 5070 West
Salt Lake City, UT 84104
800-223-5326
http://www.weider.com

51301
Great Southern Laboratories
10863 Rockley Rd.
Houston, TX 77099
281-530-3077

Green Turtle Bay Vitamin Co.
56 High St.
P.O. Box 642
Summit, NJ 07901
800-877-2849
800-887-8535
http://www.energywave.com

59762
Greenstone Limited
See Pfizer, Inc.

22840
Greer Laboratories, Inc.
P.O. Box 800
Lenoir, NC 28645-0800
828-754-5327
800-378-3906
http://www.greerlabs.com

Grifols USA, Inc.
2410 Lillyvale Avenue
Los Angeles, CA 90032
888-GRIFOLS (888-474-3657)
800-421-0008
http://www.grifolsusa.com

Guardian Drug Company
P.O. Box 915
Dayton, NJ 08810
609-860-2600
http://www.guardiandrug.com

Guardian Laboratories
230 Marcus Blvd.
P.O. Box 18050
Hauppauge, NY 11788
631-273-0900
800-645-5566
http://www.u-g.com

Guilford Pharmaceuticals, Inc.
6611 Tributary St.
Baltimore, MD 21224
410-631-6300
800-453-3746
866-405-9038
http://www.guilfordpharm.com

Gum-Tech Industries, Inc.
See Matrix Initiatives, Inc.

Gynetics
3371 Route One
Suite 200
Lawrenceville, NJ 08648
609-919-1931
800-311-7378
http://www.gynetics.com

Halocarbon Products Corporation
887 Kinderkamack Rd.
P.O. Box 661
River Edge, NJ 07661
201-262-8899
http://www.halocarbon.com

00879
Halsey Drug Co. (Watson)
695 N. Perryville Rd.
Rockford, IL 61107
815-399-2060
800-336-2750
http://www.halseydrug.com

Hannan Ophthalmic Marketing
   Services, Inc.
34 Sherrill Rd.
Nashville, MA 02050
781-834-8111

52512
Harmony Laboratories
1109 S. Main
P.O. Box 39
Landis, NC 28088
704-857-0707
800-245-6284
http://www.harmonylabs.com

Hart Health & Safety
P.O. Box 94044
Seattle, WA 98124
800-234-4278
http://www.harthealth.com

Harvard Drug Corp.
31778 Enterprise Drive
Livonia, MI 48150
800-875-0123
http://www.harvarddrugs.com

Harvest Pharmaceuticals Inc.
1881 Grove Avenue
P.O. Box 3586
Radford, VA
800-455-5525
540-633-7976
http://www.harvestpharmaceuticals.com

52637
Hauser Pharmaceutical Inc.
4401 E. U.S. Hwy. 30
Valparaiso, IN 46383
800-441-2309
http://www.hauserpharmaceutical.com

63717
Hawthorn Pharmaceuticals Inc.
See Cypress Pharmaceutical, Inc.

HDC Corporation
628 Gibraltar Ct.
Milpitas, CA 95035
408-942-7340
800-227-8162
http://www.hdccorp.com

Health & Medical Techniques
See Graham Field Health Products
Inc.

Health Assure, Inc.
26635 West Agoura Road
Suite 205
Calabasas, CA 91302
800-548-8680
http://www.healthassure.com

50383
Health Care Products
369 Bayview Ave.
Amityville, NY 11701
631-789-8455
800-899-3116
http://www.diabeticproducts.com

Health Enterprises
90 George Leven Drive
N. Attleboro, MA 02760
508-695-0727
800-633-4243
http://www.healthenterprises.com

00598
Health for Life Brands, Inc.
1643 E. Genessee St.
Syracuse, NY 13210
315-478-6303
800-448-5255

Health-Mark Diagnostics
3341 S.W. 15th St.
Pompano Beach, FL 33069
954-984-8881

Health Products Corp.
1060 Nepper Han
Yonkers, NY 10703
914-423-2900

Healthcare Direct Services
15424 N. Nebraska Ave.
Lutz, FL 33549
813-948-3005
800-729-8446
800-844-8345
http://www.hcdsales.com

51662
Healthfirst Corp.
22316 70th Ave. W., Unit A
Mountlake Terrace, WA 98043-2184
425-771-5733
800-331-1984
http://www.healthfirstcorp.com

00064
Healthpoint Medical
3909 Hulen St.
Ft. Worth, TX 76107
817-900-4105
800-441-8227
http://www.healthpoint.com

Heel Inc.
11025 LH Lafontaine
Anjou, QC H1J 2Z4
514-353-4335
888-879-4335

Helena Laboratories
1530 Lindbergh Dr.
Beaumont, TX 77707
409-842-3714
800-231-5663
http://www.helena.com

Hemacare Corp.
21101 Oxnard St.
Woodland Hills, CA 91367
877-310-0717
http://www.hemacare.com

Hemagen Diagnostics, Inc.
9033 Red Branch Rd.
Columbia, MD 21045
443-367-5500
800-495-2180
http://www.hemagen.com

Hemispherex Biopharma
1 Penn Center
1617 John F. Kennedy Blvd.
Suite 660
Philadelphia, PA 19103
215-988-0080
http://www.hemispherx.net

HemispheRx Biopharma, Inc.
1 Penn Center
1617 John F. Kennedy Blvd.
Suite 660
Philadelphia, PA 19103
215-988-0080
http://www.hemispherx.net

Hemotec Medical Products, Inc.
P.O. Box 19255
Johnston, RI 02919
401-934-2571

Henry Schein, Inc.
135 Duryea Rd.
Melville, NY 11747
631-843-5500
800-472-4346
http://www.henryschein.com

Herald Pharmacal Inc.
See Allergan, Inc.

Herbert Laboratories
See Allergan, Inc.

Heritage Consumer Products, LLC.
141 South Ave.
Suite 2
Fanwood, NJ 07023
800-344-7239

50383
Hi-Tech Pharmacal Co. Inc.
369 Bayview Ave.
Amityville, NY 11701
631-789-8228
http://www.hitechpharm.com

28105
Hill Dermaceuticals, Inc.
2650 S. Mellonville Ave.
Sanford, FL 32773
800-344-5707
http://www.hillderm.com

Hillestad Pharmaceuticals
178 U.S. Highway 51 N
P.O. Box 1700
Wooddruff, WI 54568-1700
800-535-7742
http://www.hillestadlabs.com

17808
Himmel Pharmaceuticals, Inc.
P.O. Box 5479
Lake Worth, FL 33466
561-585-0070
800-535-3823

Hisamitsu America
3528 Torrance Boulevard
Suite 112
Torrance, CA 90503
310-540-1408
http://www.salonpas-usa.com

00839
H.L. Moore Drug Exchange, Inc.
See Moore Medical Corp.

00039, 00068, 00088
Hoechst-Marion Roussel
See Aventis Pharmaceuticals

Hoffman-LaRoche
See Roche Laboratories

58573
Hogil Pharmaceutical Corp.
2 Manhattansville Rd.
Purchase, NY 10577
914-696-7600
http://www.hogil.com

47992
Holles Laboratories, Inc.
30 Forest Notch
Cohasset, MA 02025-1198
781-383-0005
800-356-4015

Hollister-Stier
3525 N. Regal
Spokane, WA 99220
800-992-1120
http://www.hollister-stier.com

Home Access Health Corporation
2401 W. Hassell Rd.
Suite 1510
Hoffman Estates, IL 60195-5200
847-781-2500
800-448-8378
http://www.homeaccess.com

Home Diagnostics
51 James Way
Eatontown, NJ 07724

Hope Pharmaceuticals
8260 E. Gelding Dr.
Suite 104
Scottsdale, AZ 85260
480-607-1970
800-755-9595
http://www.hopepharm.com

59630
Horizon Pharmaceutical Corp.
See First Horizon Pharmaceutical
   Corp.

Hormel Healthlabs
1 Hormel Place
Austin, MN 55912
800-866-7757
http://www.hormelhealthlabs.com

Hospak Unit Dose Products
5910 Creekside Lane
Rockford, IL 61114
815-877-6480
815-636-8829
http://www.hospakrockford.com

Hospira
275 N. Field Dr.
Lake Forest, IL 60045
877-946-7747
800-615-0187
http://www.hospira.com

58407
Houba (Halsey Drug Co.)
16235 State Rd. 17
Culver, IN 46511
574-842-3305

Huckaby Pharmacal, Inc.
11802 Brinley Ave.
Suite 201
Louisville, KY 40243
502-243-4000
888-206-5525
http://www.huckabypharmacal.com

Humanicare International
9 Elkins Road
East Brunswick, NJ 08816
732-613-9000
800-631-5270
http://www.humanicare.com

00395
Humco Holding Group, Inc.
7400 Alumax
Texarkana, TX 75501
903-831-7808
800-662-3435
http://www.humco.com

Humphreys Pharmacal
31 East High Street
East Hampton, CT 06424
201-933-7744

Hybritech (Beckman Coulter)
7330 Carroll Rd.
San Diego, CA 92121
858-578-9800
http://www.beckmancoulter.com

Hyland Immuno
See Baxter Healthcare Corporation,
   Baxter Bioscience

Hyland Laboratories, Inc.
See Standard Homeopathic Co.

Hyland Therapeutics
See Baxter Hyland Immuno

Hynson, Westcott & Dunning
See Becton Dickinson Microbiology
   Systems

Hyperion Medical, Inc.
1100 Celebration Boulevard
Celebration, FL 34747
http://www.hyperionmedical.com

Hypoguard USA, Inc.
7301 Ohms Lane
Suite 200
Edina, MN 55439
952-646-3200
800-818-8877
http://www.hypoguard.com

00314
Hyrex Pharmaceuticals
3494 Democrat Rd.
Memphis, TN 38118
901-794-9050
800-238-5282

Iatric Corp.
2330 S. Industrial Park Ave.
Tempe, AZ 85282

ICI Pharmaceuticals
See AstraZeneca L.P.

ICN Canada Ltd.
Montreal, Quebec
Canada

ICN Pharmaceuticals
See Valeant Pharmaceutical

IDEC Pharmaceuticals
See Biogen Idec

Ilex Oncology Inc.
4545 Horizon Hill Blvd.
San Antonio, TX 78229
210-949-8200
http://www.ilexonc.com

Immucell Corp.
56 Evergreen Dr.
Portland, ME 04103
207-878-2770
800-466-8235
http://www.immucell.com

00205, 58406
Immunex Corp.
See Amgen, Inc.

54129
**Immuno U.S., Inc. (Baxter
   Healthcare Corp.)**
1200 Parkdale Rd.
Rochester, MI 48307-1744
http://www.baxter.com

Immunobiology Research Inst.
Route 22 East
P.O. Box 999
Annandale, NJ 08801-0999

ImmunoGen
128 Sidney St.
Cambridge, MA 02139
617-995-2500
http://www.immunogen.com

Immunomedics Inc.
300 American Rd.
Morris Plains, NJ 07950
973-605-8200
http://www.immunomedics.com

Immunotec Research Ltd.
292 Adrien Patenaude
Vandreuil-Dorion, QC J7V 5V5
450-424-9992
888-917-7779
http://www.immunotec.com

Impax Laboratories, Inc.
30831 Huntwood Ave.
Hayward, CA 94544
510-476-2000
http://www.impaxlabs.com

00548
I.M.S., Ltd.
See Celltech Pharmaceutical Co.

IMX Pharmaceuticals, Inc.
2295 Corporate Blvd.
Boca Raton, FL 33431

INAMED Corporation
5540 Ekwill Drive
Santa Barbara, CA 93111
805-683-6761
800-722-2007
800-766-0171
http://www.inamed.com

Inbrand
1169 Canton Road
Marietta, GA 30066
770-422-3036

Indevus Pharmaceuticals, Inc.
99 Hayden Ave.
Suite 200
Lexington, MA 02421
781-861-8444
http://www.indevus.com

InKine Pharmaceutical Company, Inc.
1787 Sentry Pkwy. West
Bldg. 18, Suite 440
Blue Bell, PA 19422
215-283-6850
http://www.inkine.com

Inner Health Group
6203 Woodlake Ctr.
San Antonio, TX 78244
210-661-9257
800-381-4697
http://www.michaelshealth.com

Innovite, Inc.
See Endurance Products Company

InnoZen, Inc.
6429 Independence Avenue
Woodland Hills, CA 91367
818-593-4880
800-599-8892

INO Therapeutics, Inc.
6th State Route 173
Clinton, NJ 08809
908-238-6600
877-566-9466
http://www.inotherapeutics.com

Insource
P.O. Box 39
Bland, VA 24315
276-688-0211
800-366-3829
http://www.insourceonline.com

Inspire Pharmaceuticals, Inc.
4222 Emperor Blvd.
Suite 200
Durham, NC 27703
919-941-9777
877-800-4536
http://www.inspirepharm.com

Integrated Therapeutics
9755 S.W. Commerce Circle
Suite B2
Wilsonville, OR 97070
800-869-9705
800-931-1709
503-682-9755
http://www.integrativeinc.com

Integrity Pharmaceutical Corporation
9084 Technology Drive
Suite 600
Fishers, IN 46038
317-558-2820
800-823-6878
http://www.integritypharma.com

Interchem Corp.
120 Route 17 N., Suite 115
P.O. Box 1579
Paramus, NJ 07653
201-261-7333
800-261-7332
http://www.interchem.com

Intercure, Inc.
400 Kelby Street, Parker Plaza 12th
Floor
Fort Lee, NJ 07024
201-720-7750
http://www.intercure.com

Interferon Sciences
See Hemispherex Biopharma

Intermax Pharmaceuticals, Inc.
228 Sherwood Ave.
Farmingdale, NY 11735
631-777-3318

InterMune Pharmaceuticals, Inc.
3280 Bayside Blvd.
Bayshore, CA 94005
415-466-2200
http://www.intermune.com

11584
International Ethical Labs
Reparto Metropolitano Avenue
Americo Miranda #1021
Rio Piedras, PR 00921
787-765-3510

International Laboratory Technology Corp.
3389 Sheridan St.
Suite 149
Hollywood, FL 33021
http://www.germsafe.com

International Labs
2350 31st Street South
St. Petersburg, FL 33712
727-327-4094
http://www.internationallabs.com

International Medications Systems, Ltd.
1886 Santa Anita Ave.
South El Monte, CA 91733
800-423-4136
http://www.ims-limited.com

Interneuron Pharmaceuticals, Inc.
See Indevus Pharmaceuticals, Inc.

Interpharm Ltd.
99b Cobbold Road Unit 1
Willesden, London NW 10 9SL
UK
020 8830 0803
http://www.interpharm.co.uk

00814
Interstate Drug Exchange
See Henry Schein, Inc.

Intramed Corp
4333 Orange St., #3610
Riverside, CA 92501

52189
Invamed, Inc.
See Geneva Pharmaceuticals

Inveresk Research, Inc.
11000 Weston Pkwy.
Suite 100
Cary, NC 27513
919-460-9005
800-988-9845
http://www.inveresk.com

Inverness Medical Innovations
51 Sawyer Rd.
Suite 200
Waltham, MA 02453
781-647-3900
800-899-7353
http://www.invernessmedical.com

00258
Inwood Laboratories
See Forest Laboratories

Iolab Pharmaceuticals
See Ciba Vision Corp.

61646
Iomed
See IoPharm

IOP, Inc.
3151 Airway Ave.
Suite I-1
Costa Mesa, CA 92626
714-549-1185
800-535-3545
http://www.iopinc.com

IoPharm
7509 Flagstone Street
Ft. Worth, TX 76118
817-595-5820

54921
IPR Pharmaceuticals, Inc.
P.O. Box 1967
Carolina, PR 00984
787-750-5353
800-477-6385

Isis Pharmaceuticals
2292 Faraday Ave.
Carlsbad, CA 92008
760-931-9200
http://www.isispharm.com

50914
Iso-Tex Diagnostics, Inc.
1511 County Rd. 129
P.O. Box 909
Friendswood, TX 77546
281-482-1231
http://www.isotexdiagnostics.com

Ivax Corporation
4400 Biscayne Blvd.
9th Floor
Miami, FL 33137-3212
305-575-6000
800-455-9871
http://www.ivaxpharmaceuticals.com

Ivax Pharmaceuticals, Inc.
4400 Biscayne Blvd.
Miami, FL 33137
305-575-6000
800-327-4114
http://www.ivaxpharmaceuticals.com

Ivy Corporation
P.O. Box 596
W. Caldwell, NJ 07006
800-443-8856

16837
J & J Merck Consumer Pharm. Co.
7050 Camp Hill Rd.
Ft. Washington, PA 19034
215-273-7000
800-523-3484
http://www.jnj-merck.com

49938
Jacobus Pharmaceutical Co.
37 Cleveland Lane
P.O. Box 5290
Princeton, NJ 08540
609-921-7447

Jamol Labs
13 Ackerman Avenue
Emerson, NJ 07630
201-262-6363

50458
Janssen Pharmaceutica
1125 Trenton-Harbourton Rd.
Titusville, NJ 08560-0200
609-730-2000
800-526-7736
http://www.janssen.com

J.B. Williams Company, Inc.
65 Harristown Rd.
Glen Rock, NJ 07452-3317
201-251-8100
800-254-8656

Jergens
See The Andrew Jergens Company

Jerome Stevens
Pharmaceuticals, Inc.
60 Da Vinci Drive
Bohemia, NY 11234
516-567-1113

00304
J.J. Balan, Inc.
5725 Foster Ave.
Brooklyn, NY 11234
800-552-2526
http://www.jjbalan.com

JMI-Canton Pharmaceuticals
See Jones Pharma Incorporated

00137
Johnson & Johnson
One Johnson & Johnson Plz.
New Brunswick, NJ 08933
732-524-0400
http://www.jnj.com

Johnson & Johnson Consumers
Products Company
199 Grandview Rd.
Skillman, NJ 08558-9418
732-524-0400
800-526-3967
http://www.jnj.com

56091
Johnson & Johnson Medical
2500 E. Arbrook Blvd.
Arlington, TX 76014
800-423-5850
http://www.jnjmedical.com

00252, 52604, 00689
Jones Pharma Incorporated
See King Pharmaceuticals, Inc.

88395
J. R. Carlson Laboratories
15 College Dr.
Arlington Heights, IL 60004-1985
847-255-1600
888-234-5656
http://www.carlsonlabs.com

10106
J.T. Baker, Inc.
See Mallinckrodt-Baker, Inc.

KabiVitrum, Inc.
See Pharmacia Corp.

Kanetta Pharmacal
90 Park Ave.
New York, NY 10016
212-907-2690
800-372-6634

00588
Keene Pharmaceuticals, Inc.
303 South Mockingbird
P.O. Box 7
Keene, TX 76059-0007
817-645-8083
800-541-0530

28851
Kendall Health Care Products
15 Hampshire St.
Mansfield, MA 02048
508-261-8000
800-962-9888
http://www.kendallhq.com

Kendall-McGaw Labs, Inc.
See B. Braun Medical Inc.

00482
Kenwood Laboratories
See Bradley Pharmaceuticals

(The) Key Company
1313 West Essex
St. Louis, MO 63122
314-965-6699
800-325-9592
http://www.thekeycompany.com

00085
Key Pharmaceuticals
See Schering-Plough Corp.

Kiel Laboratories, Inc.
2225 Centennial
Gainesville, GA 30504
770-534-0079
http://www.kielpharm.com

Kimberly-Clark
351 Phelps Drive
Irving, TX 75038
972-281-1200
http://www.kimberly-clark.com

60793
King Pharmaceuticals, Inc.
501 Fifth St.
Bristol, TN 37620
423-989-8000
800-776-3637
http://www.kingpharm.com

55299
Kingswood Laboratories, Inc.
10375 Hague Rd.
Indianapolis, IN 46256
317-849-9513
800-968-7772

Kinray
152-35 10th Ave.
Whitestone, NY 11357
718-767-1234
800-854-6729

58223
Kirkman Laboratories, Inc.
6400 SW Rosewood
Lake Oswego, OR 97035
503-694-1600
800-245-8282
http://www.kirkmanlabs.com

31600
Kiwi Brands, Inc. (Sara Lee
Household & Body Care)
447 Old Swede Rd.
Douglassville, PA 19518
610-385-3041

KLI Corp.
1119 Third Ave. S.W.
Carmel, IN 46032
317-846-7452
800-308-7452
888-301-0751
http://www.entertainers-secret.com

00044, 00048, 00524
Knoll Pharmaceuticals
See Abbott Laboratories

Kodak Dental
343 State St.
Rochester, NY 14650
716-724-5631
800-933-8031
http://www.kodak.com

(Eastman) Kodak Co.
343 State St.
Rochester, NY 14650
585-724-4000
http://www.kodak.com

Konec, Inc.
3840 East 44th Street
Suite 609
Tucson, AZ 85713
520-671-0119
http://www.konec-inc.com

00224
Konsyl Pharmaceuticals
10 Killmer Road
Edison, NJ 08818
817-763-8011
800-356-6795
800-356-6795
http://www.konsyl.com

Kos Pharmaceutics, Inc.
1001 Brickell Bay Dr. 25th Floor
Miami, FL 33131
305-577-3464
888-564-2772
http://www.kospharm.com

55505
Kramer Laboratories, Inc.
8778 S.W. 8th St.
Miami, FL 33174-9990
302-223-1287
800-824-4894
http://www.kramerlabs.com

Kramer-Novis
PO Box 191775
San Juan, PR 00919–1775
787-767-2072

Kremers Urban
P.O. Box 427
Mequon, WI 53092
414-238-5205
800-625-5710

K-Tech USA, Inc.
80 S. W. 8th Street
Miami, FL 33130
305-373-8248

K.V. Pharmaceutical Co.
2503 S. Hanley Rd.
St. Louis, MO 63144
314-645-6600
http://www.kvpharmaceutical.com

La Haye Laboratories, Inc.
See U.S. Neutraceuticals, LLC

Labcorp
840 Research Way
Oklahoma City, OK 73104
405-290-4000
800-634-9330
http://www.labcorp.com

Lacrimedics, Inc.
P.O. Box 1209
Eastsound, WA 98245
360-376-7095
800-367-8327
http://www.lacrimedics.com

41383
Lactaid, Inc.
7050 Camp Hill Rd.
Ft. Washington, PA 19034
215-273-7000
800-522-8243
http://www.lactaid.com

59081
Lafayette Pharmaceuticals, Inc.
See Mallinckrodt-Baker, Inc.

Lake Consumer Products
1 Pharmacol Way
Jackson, WI 53037
262-677-5007
800-537-8658
http://www.lakeconsumer.com

L.A.M. Pharmaceutical Corp.
736 Center Street Unit 5
Lewiston, NY 14092
716-754-2002
877-526-7717
http://www.lampharm.com

Lane Labs
25 Commerce Drive
Allendale, NJ 07401
201-236-9090
800-526-3005
http://www.lanelabs.com

00527
Lannett Co., Inc.
9000 State Rd.
Philadelphia, PA 19136
215-333-9000
800-325-9994
http://www.lannett.com

Lansinoh Laboratories
333 North Fairfax Street
Suite 400
Alexandria, VA 22314
703-299-1100
http://www.lansinoh.com

Lantiseptic
See Summit Industries, Inc.

Larken Laboratories
148 Weisenberger Road
Madison, WI 38119
601-605-5275

00277
Laser, Inc.
2200 W. 97th Place
P.O. Box 905
Crown Point, IN 46307
219-663-1165
800-325-0925

10651
Lavoptik Co., Inc.
661 Western Ave.
St. Paul, MN 55103

Layton Bioscience, Inc.
709 E. Evelyn Ave.
Sunnyvale, CA 94086
408-616-1000
http://www.laytonbio.com

LecTec Corporation
10701 Red Circle Dr.
Minnetonka, MN 55343
952-933-2291
800-777-2291
http://www.lectec.com

Lederle Consumer Health
See Wyeth Consumer Health

Lederle Labs
See Wyeth

Lederle Pharmaceutical Division
See Wyeth-Ayerst Labs

Lederle-Praxis Biologicals (Wyeth)
555 East Lancaster Avenue
St. Davids, PA 19087
914-272-7000
800-999-9384

23558
Lee Pharmaceuticals
1434 Santa Anita Ave.
South Elmonte, CA 91733
800-950-5337
http://www.leepharmaceuticals.com

Leeming
See Pfizer US Pharmaceutical Group

25332
Legere Pharmaceuticals, Inc.
7326 E. Evans Rd.
Scottsdale, AZ 85260
480-991-4033
800-528-3144

19200
Lehn & Fink
See Reckitt & Colman

Leiner Health Products
901 East 233rd St.
Carson, CA 90745
310-835-8400
800-421-1168
http://www.leiner.com

Leiras Pharmaceuticals, Inc.
2345 Waukegan Rd.
Suite N-135
Bannockburn, IL 60015
http://www.lieras.com

Lek Pharmaceuticals, Inc.
115 North 3rd Street
Suite 301
Wilmington, NC 28401
910-362-0021
866-542-4360
http://www.lek.si

00093, 00332
Lemmon Co.
See Teva Pharmaceuticals USA

Liberty Medical Supply
10045 South Federal Highway
Port St. Lucie, FL 34952
http://www.libertymedical.com

Liberty Pharmaceutical
8881 Liberty Lane
Port St. Lucie, FL 34952
866-738-9419
800-615-0721
866-836-9936
http://www.libertymedical.com

Life Cycle Ventures, Inc.
220 Lake Dr.
Newark, DE 19702

Lifescan, Inc.
1000 Gibraltar
Milpitas, CA 95035-6312
408-263-9789
800-524-7226
800-227-8862
http://www.lifescan.com

LifeSign LLC
71 Veronica Ave.
P.O. Box 218
Somerset, NJ 08875-0218
908-246-3366
800-526-2125
http://www.lifesignmed.com

LifeStyle
1800 Route 34 North
Suite 401
Walltownship, NJ 07719
800-622-7376
732-972-9205

Ligand Pharmaceuticals, Inc.
10275 Science Center Dr.
San Diego, CA 92121
858-550-7500
800-964-5836
http://www.ligand.com

00002, 59075
Lilly and Co.
See Eli Lilly and Co.

Lilly France S.A.
F-67640
Fegersheim, France

Lincoln Diagnostics
P.O. Box 1128
Decatur, IL 62525
217-877-2531
800-537-1336
http://www.lincolndiagnostics.com

Line One Laboratories
Pasadena, CA 91107
818-886-2288
818-886-2818
http://www.lineonelabsusa.com

Lipha Pharmaceuticals, Inc.
9 West 57th St.
Suite 3825
New York, NY 10019
800-547-4299

60799
Liposome Co.
See Elan Pharmaceuticals

Liverite Products Inc.
15405 Redhill Avenue
Suite C
Tustin, CA 92780
888-425-5483
http://www.liverite.com

Llorens Pharmaceutical
P.O. Box 720008
Miami, FL 33172
866-595-5598
http://www.llorenspharm.com

LNK International, Inc.
60 Arkay Dr.
Hauppauge, NY 11788

**Lobana Laboratories (Ulmer
    Pharmacal)**
1614 Industry Ave.
P.O. Box 408
Park Rapids, MN 56470
612-559-0601
800-848-5637
http://www.lobanaproducts.com

Lobob Laboratories
1440 Atteberry Lane
San Jose, CA 95131
408-432-0580
800-835-6262
http://www.loboblabs.com

Loch Pharmaceuticals
See Bedford Laboratories

Logimedix
1675 N. Commerce Parkway
Weston, FL 33326
800-821-0047
http://www.logimedix.com

Loma Lux Laboratories
P.O. Box 702418
Tulsa, OK 74170-2418
918-664-9882
800-316-9636
http://www.lomalux.com

L'Oreal Suncare Research
575 Fifth Avenue 26th Floor
New York, NY 10017
212-984-4109
800-322-2036
http://www.lorealparisusa.com

00273
Lorvic Corp.
See Young Dental Mfg.

59417
Lotus Biochemical Corporation
See New River Pharma

LSI America Corporation
4732 Twin Valley Dr.
Austin, TX 78731-3537
512-451-3738
800-720-5936
http://www.ondrox.com

Luitpold Pharmaceuticals, Inc.
1 Luitpold Dr.
Shirley, NY 11967
631-924-4000
800-645-1706
http://www.luitpold.com

Lunsco
Route 2, Box 62
Pulaski, VA 24301
540-980-4358

Lupin Pharma
Harborplace Tower, 111 S. Calvert St.
21st Floor
Baltimore, MD 21202
410-576-2000

Luyties Pharmacal Co.
P.O. Box 8080
Richford, VT 05476
800-325-8080
http://www.1800homeopathy.com

00374
Lyne Laboratories
10 Burke Dr.
Brockton, MA 02301
508-583-8700
800-525-0450
http://www.lyne.com

MAGNA Pharmaceuticals, Inc.
11802 Brinley Avenue
Suite 201
Louisville, KY 40243
502-254-5552
888-206-5525
http://www.magnaweb.com

**Magno-Humphries Laboratories,
    Inc.**
8800 S.W. Commercial St.
Tigard, OR 97223
503-684-5464
http://www.magno-humphries.com

Majestic Drug
4996 Main Street Route 42
South Fallsburg, NY 12779
845-436-0011
800-238-0220
http://www.majesticdrug.com

00904
Major Pharmaceuticals, Inc.
31778 Enterprise Dr.
Livonia, MI 48150
734-525-8700
800-688-9696
http://www.harvarddrugs.com

10106
Mallinckrodt Baker, Inc.
222 Red School Lane
Phillipsburg, NJ 08865
908-859-2151
800-582-2537
http://www.jtbaker.com

00406
Mallinckrodt Chemical
2nd St.
St. Louis, MO 63042
314-539-1216
800-325-8888
http://www.mallinckrodt.com

00019
Mallinckrodt, Inc.
675 McDonnell Blvd.
Hazelwood, MO 63042
314-654-2000
800-554-5343
800-325-8888
http://www.mallinckrodt.com

Manloe Labs, Inc. (New Horizons Distributing)
6320 S. Sandhill Rd
Suite 10
Las Vegas, NV 89120
702-449-7154
800-777-4876

10706
Manne
P.O. Box 825
Johns Island, SC 29457
800-517-0228

Marathon Biopharmaceuticals
See Cambrex Bioscience

Marin Pharmaceuticals
1730 N.W. 79th Avenue
Miami, FL 33126
305-593-5333

Marion Merrell Dow
9300 Ward Parkway
P.O. Box 8480
Kansas City, MO 64114

Marlex Pharmaceuticals, Inc.
50 McCullough Dr. Southgate Center
New Castle, DE 19720
302-328-3355
http://www.marlexpharm.com

Marlin Industries
P.O. Box 560
Grover City, CA 93483-0560
805-473-2743
800-423-5926

12939
Marlop Pharmaceuticals, Inc.
230 Marshall St.
Elizabeth, NJ 07206
908-355-8854

10712
Marlyn Nutraceuticals, Inc.
4404 E. Ellwood
Phoenix, AZ 85040
480-991-0200
888-766-4406
http://www.naturally.com

00682
Marnel Pharmaceuticals, Inc.
206 Luke St.
Lafayette, LA 70506
337-232-1396

00209
Marsam Pharmaceuticals, Inc.
See Watson Pharmaceuticals, Inc.

52555
Martec Pharmaceutical, Inc.
1800 N. Topping Avenue
Box 33510
Kansas City, MO 64120-3510
816-241-4144
800-822-6782
http://www.martec-kc.com

12758
Mason Pharmaceuticals, Inc.
4425 Jamboree/Suite 250
Newport Beach, CA 92660
949-851-6860
800-366-2454

11845
Mason Vitamins, Inc.
5105 N.W. 159th St.
Miami Lakes, FL 33014-6370
305-624-5557
800-327-6005
http://www.masonvitamins.com

14362
Mass. Public Health Bio. Lab.
305 South St.
Jamaica Plains, MA 02130-3597
617-983-6400

Matrix Initiatives, Inc.
2375 Camelback
Suite 500
Phoenix, AZ 85016
602-387-5353
800-808-4866
http://www.zicam.com

Matrix Laboratories, Inc.
See Chiron

Mayer Laboratories
646 Kennedy Street Building C
Oakland, CA 94606
510-437-8989
http://www.mayerlabs.com

99766
Mayne Pharma (USA) Inc.
650 From Rd.
Mack-Cali Centre II Second Floor
Paramus, NJ 07652
201-225-5500
888-606-2245
866-594-8420
http://www.maynepharma.com/us

Mayo Foundation
200 1st St. S.W.
Rochester, MN 55905
507-284-2511
http://www.mayo.edu

00259
Mayrand, Inc.
See Merz Pharmaceuticals

00264
McGaw, Inc.
See B. Braun Medical Inc.

49072
McGuff Pharmaceuticals, Inc.
2921 W. MacArthur Blvd., Suite 141
Santa Ana, CA 92704
877-444-1133
800-854-7220
http://www.mcguff.com

McKesson Drug Co.
1 Post St.
San Francisco, CA 94104
415-983-8300
800-482-3784
http://www.mckesson.com

McKesson Medical-Surgical
8741 Landmark Rd.
Richmond, VA 23228
804-264-7500
http://www.mckgenmed.com

00045
McNeil Consumer & Specialty Pharmaceuticals
7050 Camp Hill Rd. Mail Stop 278
Ft. Washington, PA 19034-2292
215-273-7000
800-962-5357
http://www.tylenol.com

McNeil Pharmaceutical
See Ortho-McNeil

MCR American Pharmaceuticals
16206 Flight Path Dr.
Brooksville, FL 34604
352-754-8587
http://www.mcramerican.com

MD Pharmaceutical
3130 S. Harbor Blvd. #320
Santa Ana, CA 92704
714-755-4400

Mead Johnson Laboratories
See Bristol-Myers Squibb

00087
Mead Johnson Nutritionals
2400 W. Lloyd Expressway
Evansville, IN 47721-7189
812-429-5000
http://www.meadjohnson.com

Mead Johnson Oncology
See Bristol-Myers Oncology/Virology

45565
Med-Derm Pharmaceuticals
P.O. Box 1166
Johnson City, TN 37605
423-926-4413
800-334-4286
800-877-8869
http://www.delrayderm.com

53978
Med-Pro, Inc.
210 E. 4th St.
Lexington, NE 68850
308-324-4571
800-447-6060
http://www.med-pro-inc.com

Medac GmbH c/o Princeton
Regulatory Assoc
116 Village Blvd., Suite 200
Princeton, NJ 08540
609-951-9596

Medarex, Inc.
707 State Rd.
Princeton, NJ 08540
609-430-2880
http://www.medarex.com

Medchem Products
160 New Boston St.
Woburn, MA 01801

11940
Medco Lab, Inc.
P.O. Box 864
Sioux City, IA 51102-5333
712-255-8770
http://www.medcolabs.com

Medcon Biolab Technologies, Inc.
50 Brigham Hill Road
Grafton, MA 01519-0196
508-839-4203
800-443-6332
http://www.ilexpaste.com

Medco Research, Inc.
See King Pharmaceuticals Inc.

00585
Medeva Pharmaceuticals
See Celltech Pharmaceutical Co.

Medi Aid Corp.
See Baxa Corporation

Medi-Plex Pharm., Inc.
See ECR Pharmaceuticals

Medical Action Industries
800 Prime Place
Hauppauge, NY 11788
631-231-4600
800-645-7042
http://www.medical-action.com

Medical Nutrition
10 West Forest Avenue
Englewood, NJ 07531
201-569-1188
http://www.pbsnutrition.com

00576
Medical Products Panamericana
647 W. Flagler St.
Miami, FL 33130
305-545-6524

(The) Medicines Company
8 Campus Drive
Parsippany, NJ 07054
917-225-0099
800-264-4662
http://www.angiomax.com

Medicis Dermatologics, Inc.
See Medicis Pharmaceutical Corp.

99207
Medicis Pharmaceutical Corp.
8125 N. Hayden Dr.
Scottsdale, AZ 85258
602-808-8800
800-550-5115
http://www.medicis.com

Medicore Inc.
2337 W. 76th St.
Hialeah, FL 33016
305-558-4000

60574
MedImmune, Inc.
One Medimmune Way
Gaithersburg, MD 20878
877-633-4411
http://www.medimmune.com

Mediniche
167 Lamp & Lantern Village/PMB 300
Chesterfield, MO 63017
314-542-9539
800-711-4303
http://www.mediniche.com

Medique Products Co.
4159 Shoreline Drive
St. Louis, MO 63045
630-694-4100
800-634-7680
http://www.greenguard.com

Medisca Inc.
661 Route 3, Unit C
Plattsburgh, NY 12901
518-561-0109
800-932-1039
http://www.medisca.com

MediSense, Inc.
See Abbott

Medix Pharmaceuticals Americas,
Inc. (MPA)
12505 Starkey Rd.
Suite M
Largo, FL 33773
888-242-3463
800-672-7811
http://www.biafine.com

Med Pointe Healthcare, Inc.
265 Davidson Ave., Suite 300
Somerset, NJ 08873-4147
732-564-2200
http://www.medpointeinc.com

00348, 75137
Medtech Laboratories, Inc.
3510 N. Lake Creek
Jackson, WY 83001-1108
914-524-6810
800-803-4471
800-443-4908
http://www.medtechinc.com

58281
Medtronic Inc.
710 Medtronic Pkwy.
Minneapolis, MN 55432
763-514-4000
800-328-0810
http://www.medtronic.com

MedVantx, Inc.
9171 Towne Center Drive/Suite 100
San Diego, CA 92122-6231
858-625-2990
http://www.medvantx.com

Meijer
2929 Walker Avenue N.W.
Grand Rapids, MI 49544
616-453-6711
http://www.meijer.com

Melville Biologics (Precision
Pharma Services)
155 Duryea Rd.
Melville, NY 11747
631-752-7320
http://www.precisionpharma.com

Menicon America
1840 Gateway Dr. 2nd Floor
San Mateo, CA 94404
650-378-1424
800-MENICON
http://www.menicon.com

22200
Mennen Co.
See Colgate-Palmolive Co.

Menper Distributors, Inc.
6500 N.W. 35th Ave.
Miami, FL 33147
305-551-7204

10742
Mentholatum Co., Inc.
707 Sterling Dr.
Orchard Park, NY 14127
716-677-2500
800-688-7660
http://www.mentholatum.com

Mentor Urology
201 Mentor Drive
Santa Barbara, CA 93111
805-879-6000
800-525-0245
http://www.mentorcorp.com

00006
Merck & Co., Inc.
1 Merck Dr.
White House Station, NJ 08889-1000
908-423-1000
800-672-6372
http://www.merck.com

Merck Human Health (a division of Merck & Co)
770 Sumneytown Pike
West Point, PA 19486-0004
215-652-5000

Meretek Diagnostics, Inc.
2655 Crescent Dr./Suite C
Lafayette, CO 80026
720-479-6400
800-MERETEK
http://www.meretek.com

00394
Mericon Industries, Inc.
8819 N. Pioneer Rd.
Peoria, IL 61615
309-693-2150
800-242-6464
http://www.mericon-industries.com

Meridian Chemical & Equipment
1316 Commerce Dr.
Decatur, AL 35601
256-350-1297
800-687-7850
http://www.letcoinc.com

Meridian Medical Technologies
10240 Old Columbian Rd.
Columbia, MD 21046
410-309-6830
800-638-8093
http://www.meridianmeds.com

Merieux Institute, Inc.
See Aventis

30727
Merit Pharmaceuticals
2611 San Fernando Rd.
Los Angeles, CA 90065
323-227-4831
800-421-9657
http://www.meritpharms.com

Merkle GmBh Omnibusverkehr
Ulmer Weg 28/ 89558
Bohmenkirch, Germany
07332/922133
http://www.merkle-reisen.de/

Merrell-Dow
See Aventis

Merz Pharmaceuticals
4215 Tudor Lane
Greensboro, NC 27410
336-856-2003
800-335-0514
888-MERZ-USA (888-637-9872)
http://www.merzusa.com

Methapharm, Inc. (Corporate Office)
131 Clarence St.
Brantford, Ontario N3T2V6
Canada
800-287-7686
http://www.methapharm.com

Methapharm, Inc. (Head Office)
11772 West Sample Road
Suite 101
Coral Springs, FL 33065
519-751-3602
800-287-7686
888-431-4276
http://www.methapharm.com

Metrika, Inc.
510 Oakmead Pkwy.
Sunnyvale, CA 94085
408-524-2255
877-212-4968
http://www.A1cNow.com

Met-Rx USA
6111 Broken Sound Parkway, N.W.
Boca Raton, FL 33487
800-556-3879
http://www.met-rx.com

MGI Pharma, Inc.
5775 W. Old Shakopee Rd./Suite 100
Bloomington, MN 55437-3714
952-346-4700
800-562-5580
http://www.mgipharma.com

Michigan Department of Health
320 S. Walnut
Lansing, MI 48913
517-373-3740

MicroGeneSys, Inc.
1000 Research Pkwy.
Meriden, CT 06450-7159
203-686-0800
800-488-7099

Micron Technology, Inc.
8000 S. Federal Way
Boise, ID 83707
208-368-4000

Midlothian Laboratories
5323 Perimeter Parkway Ct.
Montgomery, AL 36116–5125
334-288-8661

00682, 46672
Mikart, Inc.
1750 Chattahoochee Ave.
Atlanta, GA 30318
404-354-4510
800-4MIKART
http://www.mikart.com

Miles, Inc.
See Bayer Corp.

00396, 34567
Milex Products, Inc.
4311 N. Normandy
Chicago, IL 60634
773-736-5500
800-621-1278
http://www.milexproducts.com

Millennium Pharmaceuticals, Inc.
75 Sidney St.
Cambridge, MA 02139
617-679-7000
800-589-9005
http://www.millennium.com

17204
Miller Pharmacal Group, Inc.
350 Randy Rd., Suite #2
Carol Stream, IL 60188
630-871-9557
800-323-2935
http://www.millerpharmacal.com

Minrad Inc.
3950 Schelden Circle
Bethlehem, PA 18017
716-855-1068
800-832-3303
http://www.minrad.com

00276
Misemer Pharmaceuticals, Inc.
See Edwards Pharmaceuticals, Inc.

00178
Mission Pharmacal Company
P.O. Box 786099
San Antonio, TX 78278-6099
210-696-8400
800-531-3333
http://www.missionpharmacal.com

Miza Pharmaceuticals
4950 Younge St.
Suite 2001
P.O. Box 118
Toronto, Ontario M2N 6K1
Canada
416-927-0600

Miza Pharmaceuticals USA
40 Main St.
P.O. Box 210
Fairton, NJ 08320-0210

Molnlycke Healthcare
826 Newtown-Yardley Road
Newtown, PA 18940
267-685-2000
800-882-4582
http://www.molnlyckehc.com

Monaghan Medical Corporation
5 Latour Ave.
Suite 1600
P.O. Box 2805
Plattsburgh, NY 12901
518-561-7330
800-833-9653
http://www.monaghanmed.com

53169
Monarch Pharmaceuticals
501 5th St.
Bristol, TN 37620
423-989-8000
800-776-3637
888-840-5370
http://www.monarchpharm.com

Monticello Drug Co.
1604 Stockton Co.
Jacksonville, FL 32204
904-384-3666
800-735-0666
http://www.monticellocompanies.com

Moore Medical Corp.
389 John Downey Dr.
P.O. Box 2740
New Britain, CT 06050-1500
800-234-1464
http://www.mooremedical.com

Morepen Laboratories Limited
4th Floor
Antriksh Bhawan
22 Kasturba Gandhi Marg
New Delhi 110001
India
+91-11-23324443
http://www.morepen.com

00426, 00832, 60432
Morton Grove Pharmaceuticals, Inc.
6451 W. Main St.
Morton Grove, IL 60053
847-967-5600
800-346-6854
http://www.mgp-online.com

Morton International
100 Independence Mall West
Philadelphia, PA 19106
215-592-3000
http://www.rohmhaas.com

Morton Salt
123 N. Wacker Dr.
Chicago, IL 60606
312-807-2000
http://www.mortonsalt.com

MotherSOY International, Inc.
424 S. Kentucky Ave.
Evansville, IN 47714
812-424-5432
888-769-0769
http://www.mothersoy.com

Mount Sinai Medical Ctr.
1 Gustave L. Levy Place
New York, NY 10029-6574
212-241-6500
http://www.mountsinai.org

Mova Pharmaceutical Corp.
Villa Blanca Industrial Park
State Road #1, KM.34.8
Capuas, Puerto Rico 00726
787-746-8500
800-468-5201

Movo Pharmaceuticals
P.O. Box 8639
Caguas, PR 00726
787-746-8500
800-468-5201

MPM Medical Inc.
2301 Crown Ct.
Irving, TX 75038
972-893-4090
800-232-5512
http://www.mpmmedicalinc.com

MSD
See Merck & Co.

MTI Biotech
2625 North Loop Drive/Suite 2150
Ames, IA 50010
877-465-8836
http://www.mtibiotech.com

54964
Murdock, Madaus, Schwabe
See Natures Way

00451
Muro Pharmaceutical, Inc.
890 East St.
Tewksbury, MA 01876-1496
978-851-5981
800-225-0974
http://www.muropharm.com

00150
Murray Drug Corp.
1103 Northwood Dr.
Murray, KY 42071
270-753-6654

53489
Mutual Pharmaceutical Co., Inc.
(United Research Laboratories)
1100 Orthodox St.
Philadelphia, PA 19124
215-288-6500
800-523-3684
http://www.urlmutual.com

00378
Mylan Pharmaceuticals, Inc.
130 Seventh Street
1030 Century Building
Pittsburgh, PA 15222
304-599-2595
800-796-9526
http://www.mylan.com

05973
Nabi
5800 Park of Commerce Blvd. NW
Boca Raton, FL 33487
561-989-5800
800-635-1766
http://www.nabi.com

05745
Nastech Pharmaceutical Co., Inc.
3450 Montevilla Pkwy.
Bothell, WA 98021
425-908-3600
http://www.nastech.com

National Medical Products, Inc.
57 Parker St.
Irvine, CA 92618-1605
949-768-1147
http://www.jtip.com

National Vitamin Co., Inc.
2075 West Scranton Ave.
Porterville, CA 93257-8358
559-781-8871
800-538-5828
http://www.nationalvitamin.com

53983
NATREN, Inc.
3180 Willow Lane
Suite 100
Westlake Village, CA 91361
805-371-4737
800-992-3323
http://www.natren.com

Natrol, Inc.
21411 Prairie St.
Chatsworth, CA 91311
800-262-8765
http://www.natrol.com

Naturally Vitamins Co.
4404 E. Elwood St.
Phoenix, AZ 85040
480-991-0200
888-766-4406
http://www.naturallyvitamins.com

Nature Smart
1500 East 128th Ave.
Thornton, CO 80241

Natures Best
550 N. Kingsbury St.
Unit 514
Chicago, IL 60610
800-584-8544
http://www.naturesbestenzyme.com

25077
Natures Bounty, Inc.
P.O. Box 801612
Boca Raton, FL 33481
631-567-9500
800-433-2990
http://www.naturesbounty.com

Natures Sunshine Products, Inc.
75 East 1700 South
Provo, UT 84606
801-342-4300
800-223-8225
http://www.naturessunshine.com

Natures Way
10 Mountain Springs Pkwy.
Springville, UT 84663
801-489-1500
800-926-8883
http://www.naturesway.com

74312
NBTY, Inc.
See Natures Bounty, Inc.

Neil Labs
55 Lake Drive
East Windsor, NJ 08520
609-448-5500
http://www.neillabs.com

Nellson Neutraceutical (formerly NCI Medical Foods)
5801 Ayala Avenue
Irwindale, CA 91706
626-812-6522
800-869-1515

NeoRx Corp.
300 Elliot Ave. West, Suite 500
Seattle, WA 98119
206-281-7001
http://www.neorx.com

Nephro-Tech, Inc.
P.O. Box 16106
Shawnee, KS 66203
785-883-4108
800-879-4755
http://www.nephrotech.com

00487
Nephron Pharmaceuticals Corp.
4121 SW 34th St.
Orlando, FL 32811-5459
407-246-1389
800-443-4313
http://www.nephronpharm.com

Nestle Clinical Nutrition
3 Parkway N.
Suite 500
Deerfield, IL 60015
847-317-2800
877-463-7853
http://www.nestleclinicalnutrition.com

Nestle Infant Nutrition
P.O. Box AW
Wilkes-Barre, PA 18703
800-628-2229
800-284-9488
http://www.verybestbaby.com

Neurex Pharmaceuticals
See Elan Pharmaceuticals

NeuroGenesis
120 Park Ave.
League City, TX 77573
800-345-8912
http://www.neurogenesis.com

10812, 70501
Neutrogena Corporation
5760 W. 96th St.
Los Angeles, CA 90045-5595
310-642-1150
800-582-4048
http://www.neutrogena.com

Neutron Technology Corp.
See Micron Technology, Inc.

New Halsey Drug Co., Inc.
See Halsey Drug Co.

New River Pharma
See Harvest Pharmaceuticals

New World Trading Corp.
P.O. Box 952
DeBary, FL 32713

56146
NeXstar Pharmaceuticals, Inc.
See Gilead Sciences

NF Formulas
9755 S.W. Commerce Circle/Suite B2
Wilsonville, OR 97070
503-682-9755
800-931-1709
http://www.integrativeinc.com

59016
Niche Pharmaceuticals, Inc.
209 N. Oak St.
Roanoke, TX 76262
817-491-2770
800-677-0355
http://www.niche-inc.com

Nion Corp.
15501 E. First St.
Irwindale, CA 91706

Nnodum Corporation
1761 Tennessee Ave
Suite D
Cincinnati, OH 45229
513-861-2329
888-301-0457
http://www.zikspain.com

Nolco Pharmaceuticals
Villas Del Senorial, Apt 1203
San Juan, PR
00926

51801
Nomax, Inc.
40 N. Rock Hill Rd.
St. Louis, MO 63119
314-961-2500
800-397-0012
http://www.nomax.com

Noramco Inc.
1440 Olympic Dr.
Athens, GA 30601
706-353-4400
http://www.noramco.com

Norcliff Thayer
See GlaxoSmithKline

10118
Norstar Consumer Products Co., Inc.
5517 95th Ave.
Kenosha, WI 53144
262-652-8505
888-282-5164
http://www.norstarcpc.com

North American Biologicals, Inc.
See Nabi

North American Vaccine, Inc.
See Baxter

Northern Research Laboratories, Inc.
See EPIEN Medical

Novartis Consumer Health
200 Kimball Dr.
Parsippany, NJ 07054-0622
973-503-8000
http://www.novartis.com

Novartis Nutrition
1600 Utica Ave. S.
Suite 600
Minneapolis, MN 55416
800-999-9978
800-333-3785
952-848-6000
http://www.novartisnutrition.com

Novartis Ophthalmics, Inc.
11695 Johns Creek Parkway
Duluth, GA 30097-1556
866-393-6336
http://www.novartisophthalmics.com

Novartis Pharma AG
CH 4402
Basale, Switzerland
41613241111
http://www.novartis.com

00028, 00067, 00083, 58887
Novartis Pharmaceuticals Corp.
59 Route 10
East Hanover, NJ 04936
973-781-8300
888-669-6682
http://www.pharma.us.novartis.com

Novavax, Inc.
8320 Guilford Road, Suite C
Columbia, MD 21046
301-854-3900
http://www.novavax.com

Noven Pharmaceuticals
11960 SW 144th St.
Miami, FL 33186
305-253-5099
888-253-5099
http://www.noven.com

00169
Novo Nordisk Pharmaceuticals
100 College Rd. West
Princeton, NJ 08540
609-987-5800
http://www.novonordisk-us.com

00362
Novocol
See Septodont, Inc.

55953
Novopharm USA, Inc.
165 E. Commerce Dr., Suite 100
Schaumburg, IL 60173
800-727-6500
http://www.novopharm-us.com

NuGyn, Inc.
1633 County Hwy 10 NE
Suite 15
Spring Lake Park, MN 55432
763-398-0108
877-774-1442
http://www.eros-therapy.com

55499
Numark Laboratories, Inc.
164 Northfield Avenue
Edison, NJ 08818
732-417-1870
800-338-8079
http://www.numarklabs.com

NutraCea
1261 Hawk's Flight Court
El Dorado Hills, CA 95762
877-723-1700
www.nutracea.com

Nutraceutical Solutions
6704 Ranger Avenue
Corpus Christi, TX 78415
800-856-7040
http://www.eliquidsolutions.com

NutraMax Laboratories, Inc.
2208 Lakeside Blvd.
Edgewood, MD 21040
410-776-4000
800-925-5187
http://www.nutramaxlabs.com

NutraMax Products
51 Blackburn Dr.
Gloucester, MA 01930
978-282-1800
http://www.nutramax.com

Nutri Vention
6203 Woodlake Center, TX 78244
210-661-8589
800-390-7940

NutriSoy International, Inc.
See MotherSOY International, Inc.

Nutrition 21
4 Manhattanville Road
Suite 202
Purchase, NY 10577
914-701-4500
http://www.nutrition21.com

Nutrition Medical, Inc.
See Hormel Healthlabs

Nutro Laboratories
See NBTY, Inc

00407
Nycomed Amersham
See Bioscience Amersham

10797
Oakhurst Co.
3000 Hempstead Turnpike
Levittown, NY 11756
516-731-5380
800-831-1135
http://www.omedicine.com

55515
Oclassen Pharmaceuticals, Inc.
See Watson Pharm

O'Connor, Inc.
See Columbia Laboratories, Inc.

Octopharma USA, Inc.
13800 Coppermine Road
Herndon, VA 20170
800-827-6905

51944
Ocumed, Inc.
119 Harrison Ave.
Roseland, NJ 07068
973-226-2330
http://www.ocumedgroupinc.com

Odyssey Pharmaceuticals, Inc.
72 Eagle Rock Ave.
East Hanover, NJ 07936
877-427-9068
http://www.odysseypharm.com

OHM Laboratories, Inc.
1385 Ohm Labs
New Brunswick, NJ 08902
732-418-2235
800-527-6481
http://www.ohmlabs.com

10019
Ohmeda Pharmaceuticals
See Baxter Healthcare

Omnii Oral Pharmaceuticals
1500 N. Florida Mango Rd.
Suite 1
West Palm Beach, FL 33409
561-689-1140
800-445-3386
http://www.4oralcare.com

ONY, Inc.
1576 Sweet Home Rd.
Amherst, NY 14228
716-636-9096
877-274-4669

Optics Laboratory, Inc.
9480 Telstar Ave. #3
El Monte, CA 91731
626-350-1926
800-968-6788
http://www.opticslab.com

Optikem International
2172 S. Jason St.
Denver, CO 80223
303-936-1137
800-525-1752

50520
Optimox Corp.
P.O. Box 3378
Torrance, CA 90510
310-618-9370
800-223-1601
http://www.optimox.com

52238
Optopics Laboratories Corp.
See Miza Pharmaceuticals USA

00041
Oral-B Laboratories
1 Gillette Park
South Boston, MA 02127-1096
800-446-7252
http://www.oral-b.com

OraPharma, Inc.
732 Louis Dr.
Warminster, PA 18974
215-956-2200
http://www.orapharm.com

Orasure Technologies
220 East First Street
Bethlehem, PA 18015
610-882-1820
800-869-3538
http://www.orasure.com

Organogenesis Inc.
150 Dan Rd.
Canton, MA 02021
781-575-0775
http://www.organogenesis.com

00052
Organon, Inc.
375 Mt. Pleasant Ave.
West Orange, NJ 07052
973-325-4500
800-631-1253
http://www.organon-usa.com

Organon Teknika Corp.
See Biomerieux

Orion Corp.
Koivumankkaantie 6 Ovi 73 02200
Espoo
Finland
358-9-429-2745

Orion Diagnostica
See Lifesign

Orphan Medical, Inc.
13911 Ridgedale Dr.
Suite 250
Minnetonka, MN 55305
888-867-7426
http://www.orphan.com

Orphan Pharmaceuticals USA
See Rare Disease Therapeutics

59676
Ortho Biotech Products, L.P.
430 Route 22 East
P.O. Box 6914
Bridgewater, NJ 08807-0914
800-325-7504
900-541-4000
http://www.orthobiotech.com

Ortho-Clinical Diagnostics
100 Indigo Creek Dr.
Rochester, NY 14626
800-828-6316
585-453-3390
http://www.orthoclinical.com

00062
Ortho-McNeil Pharmaceutical
1000 Route 202 South
P.O. Box 300
Raritan, NJ 08869
908-218-6000
800-631-5273
http://www.ortho-mcneil.com

Ortho Neutrogena
199 Grandview Rd.
Skillman, NJ 08558
800-426-7762
http://www.orthonetrogena.com

Oscient Pharmaceuticals
100 Beaver Street
Waltham, MA 02154
781-398-2300

OSI Pharmaceuticals
58 South Service Road
Suite 110
Melville, NY 11747
631-962-2000
800-572-1932
http://www.osip.com

Otis Clapp & Sons Inc.
115 Shawmut Rd.
Canton, MA 02021
800-777-6847
781-821-5400
http://www.otisclapp.com

59148
**Otsuka America Pharmaceutical,
Inc.**
2440 Research Blvd.
Suite 250
Rockville, MD 20850
301-417-0900
800-562-3974
http://www.otsuka.com

Ovation Pharmaceuticals, Inc.
Four Parkway North
Deerfield, IL 60015
888-514-5204
847-282-1000
http://www.ovationpharma.com

Owen/Galderma
See Galderma Laboratories, Inc.

Owen Mumford Inc.
1755 A West Oak Commons Ct.
Marietta, GA 30062
770-977-2226
800-421-6936
http://www.owenmumford.com

**Oxford Pharmaceutical
Services, Inc.**
1 US Highway 46 West
Totowa, NJ 07512
973-256-0600
877-284-9120
http://www.oxfordpharm.com

Oxis International
6040 N. Cutter Circle
Suite 317
Portland, OR 97217
503-283-3911
800-547-3686
http://www.oxisresearch.com

Oxypure Inc.
3550 Morris St. N.
St. Petersburg, FL 33713
888-216-8930

00574
P & S Laboratories, Inc.
See Standard Homeopathic

Paddock Laboratories
3490 Quebec Ave. N.
Minneapolis, MN 55427
763-546-4676
800-328-5113
http://www.paddocklabs.com

53159
Palisades Pharmaceuticals, Inc.
See Glenwood, Inc.

Pamlab, LLC
P.O. Box 8950
Mandeville, LA 70470-8950
985-893-4097
http://www.pamlab.com

Pan American Laboratories
P.O. Box 8950
Mandeville, LA 70470-8950
985-893-4097
http://www.panamericanlabs.com

49884
Par Pharmaceutical, Inc.
300 Tice Blvd., 3rd Floor
Woodcliff Lake, NJ 07677
201-802-4000
800-828-9393
http://www.parpharm.com

Parenta Pharmaceuticals, Inc.
Three Southern Ct.
West Columbia, SC 29169
803-461-5500
800-898-9948
http://www.parentarx.com

00071
**Parke-Davis
A Pfizer Company**
235 E. 42nd St.
New York, NY 10017
800-438-1985

Parkedale Pharmaceuticals
501 5th St.
Bristol, TN 37620
800-776-3637
800-336-7783

Parker Laboratories, Inc.
286 Eldridge Rd.
Fairfield, NJ 07004
973-276-9500
800-631-8888
http://www.parkerlabs.com

50930
Parnell Pharmaceuticals, Inc.
1525 Francisco Blvd., Suite 15
San Rafael, CA 94901
415-256-1800
800-457-4276
http://www.parnellpharm.com

10865
Parthenon Co., Inc.
3311 W. 2400 S.
Salt Lake City, UT 84119
801-972-5184
800-453-8898
http://www.parthenoninc.com

00418
Pasadena Research Labs
See Taylor Pharmaceuticals

Pascal Co., Inc.
2929 N.E. Northrup Way
P.O. Box 1478
Bellevue, WA 98009-1478
425-827-4694

11793, 49281, 50361
Pasteur-Merieux-Connaught Labs
See Aventis

PathoGenesis Corp.
See Chiron Therapeutics

PBM Pharmaceuticals
Linney House
204 N. Main St.
Cordonovillo, VA 22942
800-485-9828

PD-RX Pharmaceuticals, Inc.
727 N. Ann Arbor Ave.
Oklahoma City, OK 73127
405-942-3040
800-299-7379
http://www.pdrx.com

PediaMed Pharmaceuticals, Inc.
7310 Turfway Road
Suite 490
Florence, KY 41042
859-282-8582
866-543-6337
http://www.pediamedpharma.com

Pediatric Pharmaceuticals
120 Wood Ave. S., Suite 300
Iselin, NJ 08830
732-603-7708
http://www.pediatricpharm.com

00884
Pedinol Pharmacal, Inc.
30 Banfi Plaza N.
Farmingdale, NY 11735
631-293-9500
800-733-4665
http://www.pedinol.com

10974
Pegasus Laboratories, Inc.
8809 Ely Rd.
Pensacola, FL 32514
850-478-2770
http://www.pegasuslabs.com

Penederm, Inc.
See Bertek

Pentech Pharmaceuticals, Inc.
3315 Algonquin Rd., Suite 310
Rolling Meadows, IL 60008
847-255-0303
http://www.pentechinc.com

Pennex Pharmaceutical, Inc.
See Morton Grove Pharmaceuticals,
Inc.

Permeable Technologies, Inc.
See LifeStyle

Perrigo Company
515 Eastern Ave.
Allegan, MI 49010
269-673-8451
800-719-9260
http://www.perrigo.com

00096
Person and Covey, Inc.
616 Allen Ave.
Glendale, CA 91201
818-240-1030
800-423-2341
http://www.personandcovey.com

Personal Care
225 Summit Ave.
Montvale, NJ 07645-1574
201-573-5633
800-816-5742

Personal Products Company
199 Grandview Rd.
Skillman, NJ 08558
800-582-6097
http://www.jnj.com

00927
Pfeiffer Co.
71 University Aveune SW
Atlanta, GA 30315
404-614-0255
800-342-6450
http://www.pfeifferpharmaceuticals.com

Pfipharmecs
See Pfizer US Pharmaceutical Group

Pfizer Consumer Health
235 E. 42nd St.
New York, NY 10017
800-223-0182
http://www.pfizer.com

00069, 00663, 74300
Pfizer US Pharmaceutical Group
235 E. 42nd St.
New York, NY 10017
800-438-1985
http://www.pfizer.com

Pharma 21
503-494-8474

Pharma Medica
966 Pantera Drive, Unit 31
Mississauga, Ontario L4W2S1
Canada
877-742-7621
905-624-9115
http://www.pharmamedica.com

Pharma Pac
513 Sandydale Dr.
Nipomo, CA 93444
805-929-1333
800-841-5554
http://www.pharmapac.com

Pharma-Tek, Inc.
See X-Gen Pharmaceuticals

Pharmaderm
4126 Steve Reynolds Blvd.
Norcross, GA 30093
866-337-6457
678-287-1500
http://www.pharmaderm.com

00121
Pharmaceutical Associates, Inc.
201 Delaware St.
Greenville, SC 29605
864-277-7282
800-845-8210
http://www.pa-inc.net

Pharmaceutical Basics, Inc.
See Rosemont Pharmaceutical Corp.

51655
**Pharmaceutical Corp of America
(PCA)**
6210 Technology Center Dr.
Indianapolis, IN 46278
317-616-4498
800-722-0722

21659
Pharmaceutical Labs, Inc.
See Nutraceutical Solutions, Inc.

45334
Pharmaceutical Specialties, Inc.
P.O. Box 6298
Rochester, MN 55903-6298
507-288-8500
800-325-8232
http://www.psico.com

00013, 00016
**Pharmacia Corp.
A Division of Pfizer**
235 E. 42nd St.
New York, NY 10017
800-323-4204
http://www.pnu.com

Pharmacia & Upjohn Consumer Healthcare
A division of Pfizer
7000 Portage Rd.
Kalamazoo, MI 49001
269-833-9599
800-717-2824

Pharmadigm, Inc.
2401 Foothill Dr.
Salt Lake City, U I 84109
801-464-6100
http://www.pharmadigm.com

Pharmafair
See Bausch & Lomb Pharmaceuticals

55422
Pharmakon Labs
6050 Jet Port Industrial Blvd.
Tampa, FL 33634
813-886-3216
800-888-4045
http://www.pharmakonlabs.com

Pharmanex
75 West Center
Provo, UT 84601
801-345-9800
800-487-1000
http://www.pharmanex.com

Pharmascience Lab
6111 Royal Mount Ave.
Suite 100
Montreal, Quebec H4 P2 T4
514-340-9735
800-340-9735
http://www.pharmascience.com

00813
Pharmavite
P.O. Box 9606
Mission Hills, CA 91346-9606
800-423-2405
http://www.naturemade.com

Pharmedix
3281 Whittel Road
Union City, CA 94587
800-486-1811
http://www.pharmedixrx.com

Pharmelle
890 N. Lafayette St.
St. Louis, MO 63031
314-830-4950
877-577-2577
http://www.pharmelle.com

Pharmics, Inc.
2702 S. 3600 West, Suite H
Salt Lake City, UT 84119
801-966-4138
800-456-4138
http://www.pharmics.com

Pharmion Corporation
2525 28th Street
Suite 200
Boulder, CO 80301
720-564-9100
866-742-7646
http://www.pharmion.com

PharmPak, Inc.
1221 Andersen Dr. Ste. B
San Rafael, CA 94901
415-455-9981
800-541-6315
http://www.pharmpakinc.com

Phillips Gulf Corporation
See Healthcare Direct Services

Phoenix Laboratories
140 Lauman Ln.
Hicksville, NY 11801
516-822-1230
800-517-7965

Physicians Total Care
5415 S. 125th East Ave.
Suite 205
Tulsa, OK 74146
918-254-2273
800-759-3650
http://www.physicianstotalcare.com

PhytoPharmica, Inc.
See Integrated Therapeutics

Plan B
2 Quaker Road
Pomona, NY 10970
845-362-1100
800-222-0190

Playtex Co.
75 Commerce Dr.
Allendale, NJ 07401-1600
201-785-8000
800-816-5742
http://www.playtex.com

Pliva
72 Eagle Rock Ave.
P.O. Box 371
East Hanover, NJ 07936
973-386-5566
800-922-0547
http://www.plivainc.com

Plough, Inc.
See Schering-Plough HealthCare
   Products

Poly Pharmaceuticals, Inc.
200 N Archusa Avenue
Quitman, MS 39355
800-882-1041
601-776-3497

00998
PolyMedica Corporation
11 State Street
Woburn, MA 01801
781-933-2020
800-886-4050
http://www.polymedica.com

47144
Polymer Technology Corp.
100 Research Dr.
Wilmington, MA 01887
978-658-6111

Portal Pharmaceutical
67E Mendez Vigo
Myaguez, PR 00680
787-832-6645

Porton Product Limited
See Speywood Pharmaceuticals, Inc.

Powderject Vaccines
8551 Research Way
Middleton, WI 53562
608-824-3730

**Praecis Pharmaceuticals
   Incorporated**
830 Winter Street
Waltham, MA 02451-1420
877-PRAECIS
877-772-3247

Prasco Laboratories
7155 E. Kemper Rd.
Cincinnati, OH 45249
513-618-3333
866-525-0688
http://www.prascolabs.com

59012
Pratt Pharmaceuticals
See Pfizer

Premier
See A P Pharma

**Press Chemical & Pharmceutical
   Laboratories, Inc.**
4231 Donlyn Ct.
Columbus, OH 43232
614-863-2802

Prestige Brands International
90 N Broadway
Irvington, NY 10533
800-803-4471
http://www.prestigebrands.com

00684
Primedics Laboratories
14131 S. Avalon
Los Angeles, CA 90061
323-770-3005

Primus Pharmaceuticals, Inc.
4725 N. Scottsdale Rd, Suite 200
Scottsdale, AZ 85251
480-483-1410

Princeton Pharm. Products
See Bristol-Myers Squibb Co.

Priority Healthcare
250 Technology Park, Suite 124
Lake Mary, FL 32746
407-804-6700
866-474-8326
http://www.priorityhealthcare.com

37000
Procter & Gamble Pharmaceuticals
8500 Governors Hill Dr.
Cincinnati, OH 45249
800-448-4878
http://www.pg.com

ProCyte Corporation
P.O. Box 808
Redmond, WA 98052-0808
425-869-1239
800-848-3668
http://www.procyte.com

ProEthic Pharmaceuticals, Inc.
5531 Perimeter Pkwy. Ct.
Mongomery, AL 36116
334-288-1288
866-776-3844
http://www.proethic.com

Prometheus Laboratories, Inc.
5739 Pacific Center Blvd.
San Diego, CA 92121-4203
858-824-0895
888-423-5227
http://www.prometheuslabs.com

ProMetic Pharma USA, Inc.
5436 W. 78th St.
Indianapolis, IN 46368

Propharma
7760 N.W. 56 St.
Miami, FL 33166
305-592-9216
800-446-0255

Propst Pharmaceuticals
130 Vintage Dr.
Huntsville, AL 35811
256-704-6394

Protein Design Labs, Inc.
34801 Campus Dr.
Fremont, CA 94555
510-574-1400
http://www.pdl.com

Protein Sciences Corp.
1000 Research Pkwy.
Meriden, CT 06450-7159
203-686-0800
800-488-7099
http://www.proteinsciences.com

Protherics Inc.
5214 Maryland Way
Suite 405
Brentwood, TN 37027
615-327-1027
http://www.protherics.com

PRX Pharm
See Par Pharmaceuticals

Psychemedics Corp.
1280 Massachusetts Ave.
Cambridge, MA 02138
617-868-7455
800-628-8073
http://www.psychemedics.com

PTS Laboratories, Inc.
8100 Secura Way
Santa Fe Springs, CA 90670
562-907-3607

PTS Labs International, Inc.
4342 West 12th St.
Houston, TX 77055
713-680-2291
http://www.ptslabs.com

Purdue Frederick Co.
One Stamford Forum
201 Tressor Blvd.
Stamford, CT 06091-3431
203-588-8000
800-877-5666
http://www.purduepharma.com

00228
Purepac Pharmaceutical Co.
14 Commerce Drive
Suite 301
Cranford, NJ 07016
800-432-8534
http://www.purepac.com

Purilens, Inc.
See The LifeStyle Company, Inc.

Puritans Pride
1233 Montauk Hwy.
P.O. Box 9001
Oakdale, NY 11769-9001
800-645-9584
http://www.puritanspride.com

Q-Pharma, Inc.
120 W. Dayton
Suite C-7
Edmonds, WA 98020

QLT, Inc.
887 Great Northern Way
Vancouver, BC V5T 4T5
Canada
604-707-7000
800-663-5486
http://www.qltinc.com

00603
Qualitest Pharmaceuticals
See Qualitest Products

Qualitest Products
130 Vintage Dr.
Huntsville, AL 35811
256-859-4011
800-444-4011

Quality Care Pharm, Inc.
3000 W. Warner Ave.
Santa Ana, CA 92704
714-754-5800

Quality Care Products, LLC
7560 Lewis Ave.
Temperance, MI 48182
734-847-3847

Questcor Pharmaceuticals, Inc.
3260 Whipple Rd.
Union City, CA 94587
510-400-0700
800-411-3065
http://www.questcor.com

Quidel Corp.
10165 McKellar Ct.
San Diego, CA 92121
858-552-1100
800-874-1517
http://www.quidel.com

Quigley Corp.
470 Park Avenue S.
New York, NY 10016
212-725-4500
http://www.quigleyco.com

Quintessa Corporation
P.O. Box 808
Lancaster, CA 93584
661-940-5600

54391
R & D Laboratories, Inc.
See Watson

R & R Registrations
P.O. Box 262069
San Diego, CA 92196
858-586-0751

R.A. McNeil Company
1210 East Dallas Rd.
Chattanooga, TN 37405
423-265-8240
800-755-3038

Ranbaxy Pharmaceuticals Inc.
Suite 2100
600 College Rd. E.
Princeton, NJ 08540
609-720-9200
888-726-2299
http://www.ranbaxy.com

30103
Randob Laboratories, Ltd.
6 Walnut St.
P.O. Box 440
Cornwall, NY 12518
845-534-2197

Rare Disease Therapeutics
1101 Kermit Dr., Suite 608
Nashville, TN 37217
615-399-0700
http://www.raretx.com

Reckitt & Colman
See Reckitt Benckiser Pharm

10952
Reckitt Benckiser Pharmaceuticals
10710 Midlothien Turnpike
Suite 430
Richmond, VA 23235
804-379-1090
800-444-7599

Recsei Laboratories
330 S. Kellogg
Building M
Goleta, CA 93117-3875
805-964-2912

48028
Redi-Products Labs, Inc.
See Aplicare, Inc.

00021
Reed & Carnrick
See Schwarz Pharma

10956
Reese Pharmaceutical Co., Inc.
10617 Frank Ave.
Cleveland, OH 44106-0157
216-231-6441
800-321-7178
http://www.reesepharmaceutical.com

Regeneron Pharmaceuticals
777 Old Saw Mill River Rd.
Tarrytown, NY 10591
914-345-7400
http://www.regeneron.com

Regent Labs, Inc.
700 W. Hillsboro Blvd. #2-206
Deerfield Beach, FL 33441
800-872-1525
954-426-4403
http://www.regentlabs.com

Reid Rowell
See Solvay Pharmaceuticals

Reliant Pharmaceuticals
110 Allen Rd.
Liberty Corner, NJ 07938
908-580-1200
http://www.reliantrx.com

Remel, Inc.
12076 Santa Fe Dr.
Lenexa, KS 66215
913-888-0939
800-255-6730
http://www.remel.com

Repligen Corp.
41 Seyon Street
Suite 100
Waltham, MA 02453
781-250-0111
800-622-2259
http://www.repligen.com

10961
Requa, Inc.
540 Barnum Building 2
Bridgeport, CT 06608
800-321-1085
http://www.requa.com

Research Industries Corp.
See Edwards Lifesciences

Research Triangle Institute
P.O. Box 12194
Research Triangle Park, NC
27709-2194
919-541-6000
http://www.rti.org

60575
Respa Pharmaceuticals, Inc.
P.O. Box 88222
Carol Stream, IL 60188
630-543-3333

Resperonics
1001 Murray Ridge Lane
Murrysville, PA 15668
800-345-6443
724-387-5200
http://www.respironics.com

Rexall Group
851 Broken Sound Pkwy. NW
Boca Raton, FL 33487
800-255-7399

00122
Rexall Sundown, Inc.
851 Broken Sound Pkwy. NW
Boca Raton, FL 33487
561-241-9400
800-327-0908
http://www.rexallsundown.com

Rgene Therapeutics, Inc.
2170 Buckthorne Pl.
Suite 170
Houston, TX 77380
713-367-5443

RH Pharmaceuticals, Inc.
See Cangene Corp.

Rhone-Poulenc Rorer Consumer, Inc.
See Aventis Pharmaceuticals

00075, 00083
Rhone-Poulenc Rorer Pharmaceuticals, Inc.
See Aventis Pharmaceuticals

Ribi
See Corixa Corporation

Richardson-Vicks, Inc.
See Procter & Gamble Co.

12071
Richie Pharmacal, Inc.
119 State Ave.
P.O. Box 460
Glasgow, KY 42141
502-651-6159
800-627-0250
http://www.richiepharmacal.com

Richmond Pharmaceuticals
3510 Mayland Court
Richmond, VA 23233
804-270-4498

Ricola USA, Inc.
51 Gibraltar Dr.
Morris Plains, NJ 07950
973-984-6811
http://www.ricolausa.com

54807
R.I.D., Inc.
609 N. Mednik Ave.
Los Angeles, CA 90022-1326
323-268-0635

R.I.J. Pharmaceutical Corp.
40 Commercial Ave.
Middletown, NY 10941
845-692-5799

Rising Pharm
411 Sette Drive, #N3
Paramus, NJ 07652
201-262-4200

Rite Aid Corp.
30 Hunter Ln.
Camp Hill, PA 17011
717-761-2633
http://www.riteaid.com

River's Edge Pharmaceutical
Suwanee, GA 30024
866-507-4837

54092
Roberts Pharmaceutical Corp.
See Shire

Roche Diagnostic Systems, Inc.
9115 Hague Road
Indianapolis, IN 46250
317-521-2000
800-428-5074
http://www.rocheusa.com

00004, 00033, 00140, 18393, 42987
Roche Laboratories
340 Kingsland St.
Nutley, NJ 07110-1199
973-235-5000
800-526-6367
http://www.rocheusa.com

Rodlen Laboratories
100 Fairway Drive, Suite 134
Vernon Hills, IL 60061
847-362-8200

00049
Roerig
See Pfizer

Romark Laboratories
3000 Bay Point
Suite 200
Tampa, FL 33607-8146
813-282-8544
http://www.romarklabs.com

00832
Rosemont Pharmaceutical Corp.
301 S. Cherokee St.
Denver, CO 80223
800-445-8091

00074
Ross Products Division, Abbott Labs
625 Cleveland
Columbus, OH 40214
800-986-8510
http://www.ross.com

00054
Roxane Laboratories, Inc.
1809 Wilson Road
Columbus, OH 43216
800-962-8364
614-276-4000
http://www.roxane.com

51875
Royce Laboratories, Inc.
See Watson Laboratories

R P Scherer Cardinal Health
14 Schoolhouse Road
Somerset, NJ 08873
732-537-6200

00536
Rugby Labs, Inc.
See Watson Pharmaceuticals

RX Flite
1404 N. Main St.
Suite 200
Meridian, ID 83642
208-288-5550
800-414-1901
http://www.rxelite.com

46500
Rydelle Laboratories
See S.C. Johnson

Rystan, Inc.
47 Center Ave.
P.O. Box 214
Little Falls, NJ 07424-0214
973-256-3737

65649
Salix Pharmaceuticals, Inc.
3600 W. Bayshore Rd.
Palo Alto, CA 94303
650-849-5900

00043
Sandoz Consumer
506 Carnegie Center Dr., Suite 400
Princeton, NJ 08540
800-525-8747
609-627-8500
http://www.us.sandoz.com

00212
Sandoz Nutrition Corp.
Sandoz Consumer
506 Carnegie Center Dr., Suite 400
Princeton, NJ 08540
800-525-8747
609-627-8500
http://www.us.sandoz.com

00078
Sandoz Pharmaceuticals
Sandoz Consumer
506 Carnegie Center Dr., Suite 400
Princeton, NJ 08540
800-525-8747
609-627-8500
http://www.us.sandoz.com

SangStat Medical Corp.
See Genzyme Transplant

Sankyo Pharma
Parsippany, NJ 07054-1296
973-359-2600
http://www.sankyopharma.com

00024
Sanofi-Synthelabo, Inc.
90 Park Ave.
New York, NY 10016
212-551-4000
800-223-1062
http://en.sanofi-aventis.com

Santen, Inc.
555 Gateway Rd.
Napa, CA 94558
707-254-1750
800-611-2011
http://www.santeninc.com

00281
Savage Laboratories
60 Baylis Rd.
Melville, NY 11747-2006
631-454-9071
800-231-0206
http://www.savagelabs.com

Savient Pharmaceuticals, Inc.
70 Wood Avenue
South Iselin, NJ 08830
723-632-8800

S C Johnson
1525 Howe Street
Racine, WI 53403-5011
800-494-4855
http://www.scjohnson.com

Scandinavian Formulas, Inc.
140 E. Church Street
Sellersville, PA 18960
215-453-2507
800-288-2844
http://www.scandinavianformulas.com

11012
Schaffer Laboratories
3128 Pacific Coast Hwy #98
Torrance, CA 90505
800-231-ORAL
310-325-4200
http://www.schafferlabs.com

00364, 00591
Schein Pharmaceutical, Inc.
See Watson

00274, 00032
Scherer Laboratories, Inc.
84 Church Street
Suite C
Marietta, GA 30060
800-310-5357
770-514-1333

00085, 11017, 41100, 54092
Schering-Plough Corp.
2000 Galloping Hill Rd.
Kenilworth, NJ 07033-0530
908-298-4000
http://www.sch-plough.com

00085, 11017, 41000, 41100
Schering-Plough HealthCare Products
Three Connell Drive
Berkeley Heights, NJ 07922
800-070-1010
800-842-4090
http://www.sphcp.com

00234
Schmid Products Co.
See Durex Consumer Products

Scholl, Inc.
See Schering-Plough HealthCare Products

00021, 00091, 00131, 62175
Schwarz Pharma
P.O. Box 2038
Milwaukee, WI 53201
800-558-5114
http://www.schwarzusa.com

Schwarzkopf & Dep Inc.
2101 E. Via Arado
Rancho Dominguez, CA 90220
310-604-0777
800-326-2855
http://www.henkel.com

SciClone Pharmaceuticals, Inc.
901 Mariners Island Blvd.
Suite 205
San Mateo, CA 94404
650-358-3456
http://www.sciclone.com

Scios Inc.
6500 Paseo Padre Parkway
Fremont, CA 94555
510-248-2500
http://www.sciosinc.com

00372
Scot-Tussin Pharmacal, Inc.
32 West Hamden Road
Cranston, RI 02920-0217
401-942-8555
800-638-7268
http://www.scot-tussin.com

SDA Laboratories
280 Railroad Ave.
Greenwich, CT 06830
203-861-0005

SDR Pharmaceuticals, Inc.
27 Mountain View Drive
Andover, NJ 07821
973-786-7996
http://www.sdrpharma.com

00014, 00025
Searle
See Pharmacia Corp.

00551
Seatrace Pharmaceuticals
P.O. Box 7200
Gadsden, AL 35906

Sepracor
84 Waterford Drive
Marlboro, MA 01752
508-481-6700
800-245-5961
http://www.sepracor.com

Septodont, Inc.
245 C Quigley Blvd.
New Castle, DE 19720
302-328-1102
800-872-8305
http://www.septodontinc.com

61471
Sequus Pharmaceuticals, Inc.
See Alza Corp.

50694
Seres Laboratories
3331B Industrial Dr.
Santa Rosa, CA 95403
707-526-4526
http://www.sereslabs.com

44087
Serono Laboratories, Inc.
One Technology Place
Rockland, MA 02370
800-283-8088
781-982-9000
http://www.seronousa.com

Seyer Pharmatec, Inc.
413 St. George St.
San Juan, Puerto Rico 00936
787-728-7044
787-728-7055

Shaklee Corp.
4747 Willow Rd.
Pleasanton, CA 94588
925-924-2000
800-928-0327
http://www.shaklee.com

Sheffield Laboratories
170 Broad St.
New London, CT 06320
860-442-4451
800-222-1087
http://www.sheffield-labs.com

08884
Sherwood Davis & Geck
See Kendall Health Care Products

08884
Sherwood Medical
See Kendall Health Care Products

Shield Manufacturing, Inc.
425 Fillmore Ave.
Tonawanda, NY 14150
800-828-7669
http://www.shieldsports.com

Shinogi Qualicaps, Inc.
6505 Frunz Warner Parkway
Whitsett, NC 27377-9215
336-449-3900
800-227-7853
http://www.qualicaps.com

58521
Shire US, Inc.
One Riverfront Place
Newport, KY 41071
859-669-8000
800-828-2088
http://www.shire.com

SHS North America
P.O. Box 117
Rockville, MD 20884-0117
301-795-2300
800-636-2283
http://www.SHSNA.com

50111
Sidmak Laboratories, Inc.
See Pliva

54482
Sigma-Tau Pharmaceuticals
800 S. Frederick Ave.
Suite 300
Gaithersburg, MD 20877-4150
301-948-1041
800-447-0169
http://www.sigmatau.com

54838
Silarx Pharmaceuticals, Inc.
19 West St.
Spring Valley, NY 10977
845-352-4020
888-9SILARX
http://www.silarx.com

Similisan
1745 Shea Center
Suite 380
Highlands Ranch, CO 80129
303-539-4060
800-240-9780
http://www.healthyrelief.com

Sirius Laboratories, Inc.
100 Fairway Dr.
Suite 130
Vernon Hills, IL 60061
847-968-2424
866-968-2425

SkinMedica, Inc.
5909 Sea Lion Place, Ste. H
Carlsbad, CA 92008
760-448-3600
866-867-0110
http://www.skinmedica.com

SkyePharma Inc.
10 East 63rd Street
New York, NY 10021
212-753-5780
http://www.skyepharma.com

Slim Fast Foods Co.
777 S. Flagler Dr.
West Tower Suite 1400
P.O. Box 3625
West Palm Beach, FL 33402
561-833-9920
877-754-6111
877-754-6777

Smith & Nephew Ortho
1450 Brooks Rd.
Memphis, TN 38116
800-821-5700
901-396-2121
http://www.smithnephew.com

Smith & Nephew Inc. Endoscopy
150 Minuteman Road
Andover, MA 01810
978-749-1000

08026
**Smith & Nephew Wound
  Management**
11775 Starkey Road
Largo, FL 33773
721-392-1261
http://www.snwmd.com

00766
**SmithKline Beecham Consumer
  Healthcare**
1500 Littleton Rd.
Parsippany, NJ 07084
973-889-2100
http://www.sb.com

Snuva, Inc.
715 South Boulevard
Oak Park, IL 60302-2978
708-725-3783
800-250-4258
http://www.snuva.com

33984
Solgar Co., Inc.
500 Willow Tree Rd.
Leonia, NJ 07605
201-944-2311
800-645-2246
http://www.solgar.com

00032
Solvay Pharmaceuticals
901 Fawyer Rd.
Marietta, GA 30062-2224
770-578-9000
800-241-1643
http://www.solvaypharmaceuticals.com

39506
Somerset Pharmaceuticals
2202 N.W. Shore Blvd.
Suite 450
Tampa, FL 33607
813-288-0040
800-892-8889
http://www.somersetpharm.com

Southwest Technologies
1746 Levee Road
North Kansas City, MO 64116
816-221-2442
800-247-9951
http://www.elastogel.com

Southwood Pharmaceuticals
60 Empire Drive
Lake Forest,, CA 92630
800-442-4443
http://www.southwoodpharm.com

Sovereign Pharmaceuticals
7590 Sand St.
Ft. Worth, TX 76118
817-284-0429
http://www.sovpharm.com

Sparta Pharmaceuticals
905 Louis Drive
Warminster, PA 18974
215-442-1700

Spear Dermatology Products
1247 Sussex Turnpike, Suite 120
Randolph, NJ 07869
973-895-6447
866-507-7327
http://www.speardermatology.com

Specialty Medical Supplies
3882 NW 124th Street
Coral Spring, FL 33065
954-752-5603
http://www.specialtymedicalsupplies.com

38137
Spectrum Chemical Mfg. Corp.
14422 S. San Pedro St.
Gardena, CA 90248-9985
310-516-8000
800-772-8786
http://www.spectrumchemical.com

Spenco Medical Corporation
P.O. Box 2501
Waco, TX 76702
520-325-1554
254-772-6000
800-877-3626
254-772-6000
http://www.spenco.com

55688
Speywood Pharmaceuticals, Inc.
7114 Springbrook Terrace
Suite 200
Spotsylvania, VA 22553
818-879-2200

S.S.S. Company
71 University Avenue S.W.
P.O. Box 4447
Atlanta, GA 30315
404-521-0857
800-237-3843
http://www.ssspharmaceuticals.com

St. Jude Medical, Inc.
1 Lillehei Plaza
St. Paul, MN 55117-9913
651-483-2000
800-328-9634

Stada Pharmaceuticals, Inc.
5 Cedar Brook Dr.
Cranbury, NJ 08512
609-409-5999
800-542-6682
http://www.stadausa.com

Stanback Co. (GlaxoSmithKline)
200 North 16th St.
Philadelphia, PA 19101
http://www.gsk.com

53385
**Standard Drug Co. & Family
   Pharmacy**
1279 N. 7th St.
Riverton, IL 62561
217-629-9884

**Standard Homeopathic Co. &
   Hylands**
210 W. 131st St.
P.O. Box 61067
Los Angeles, CA 90061
310-768-0700
800-624-9659
http://www.hylands.com

00076
Star Pharmaceuticals, Inc.
1990 N.W. 44th St.
Pompano Beach, FL 33064-8712
954-971-9704
800-845-7827
http://www.starpharm.com

51318
Stellar Pharmacal Corp.
1881 W. State Road 84
Suite 101
Ft. Lauderdale, FL 33315
954-759-3436
800-845-7827
http://www.starpharm.com

Stephan Company
1850 W. McNab Rd.
Ft. Lauderdale, FL 33309
954-971-0600
800-327-4963

Stericycle
28161 N. Keith Drive
Lake Forest, IL 60045
800-643-0240
847-367-9493
http://www.stericycle.com

00402
Steris Corp.
5960 Heisley Road
Mentor, OH 44060-1834

Sterling Health
15070 Beltwood Pkwy.
Addison, TX 75001-3715
972-991-9293
http://www.sterlinghealthcenter.com

Sterling Winthrop
See Sanofi-Synthelabo

Stewart-Jackson Pharmacal
4587 Damascus Rd.
Memphis, TN 38118
800-367-1395

Stiefel Consumer Healthcare
Route 145
Oak Hill, NY 12460
518-239-4195
888-438-7426
http://www.stiefel.com

00145
Stiefel Laboratories, Inc.
6340 Sugarloaf Parkway, Suite 400
Duluth, GA 30097
800-633-7647
888-784-3335
http://www.stiefel.com

57706
Storz
See Bausch & Lomb Surgical

58980
Stratus Pharmaceuticals, Inc.
14377 S.W. 142nd St.
Miami, FL 33186-6727
305-254-6793
800-442-7882
http://www.stratuspharmaceuticals.com

Stuart Pharmaceuticals
See AstraZeneca L.P.

Sugen Inc. (Informagen, Inc.)
375 Little Bay Rd.
Newington, NH 03801
http://www.informagen.com

Summa Rx Laboratories
2940 FM 3028
Mineral Wells, TX 76067
940-325-0771
http://www.summalabs.com

11086
Summers Laboratories, Inc.
103 G.P. Clement Dr.
Collegeville, PA 19426-2044
888-774-7546
800-533-7546
http://www.sumlab.com

Summit Industries, Inc.
2901 W. Lawrence Ave.
Chicago, IL 60625
773-588-2444
800-729-9729
http://www.summitindustries.net

57267
Summit Pharmaceuticals
See Novartis Pharmaceuticals Corp.

Sunrise Medical HHG, Inc.
240 Motor Parkway
Hauppauge, NY 11788
631-435-1515
800-782-0282
http://www.sunriselab.com

SuperGen, Inc.
4140 Dublin Blvd.
Suite 200
Dublin, CA 94568
925-560-0100
800-353-1075
http://www.supergen.com

Superior Pharmaceutical Co.
1385 Kemper Meadow Dr.
Cincinnati, OH 45240
800-826-5035
http://www.superiorpharm.com

11704
Survival Technical, Inc.
See Meridian Medical Technologies

Swiss-American Products, Inc.
4641 Nall Rd.
Dallas, TX 75244
972-385-2900
800-633-8872
http://www.elta.net

Swiss Bioceutical
2533 N. Carson St., Ste. 3573
Carson City, NV 89706
775-841-7020

Syncom Pharmaceuticals, Inc.
66 Hanover Rd.
Florham Park, NJ 07932
973-822-9222
800-400-0056
http://www.sycom.com

Synergen, Inc.
See Amgen Inc.

00033, 18393, 42987
Syntex Laboratories
See Roche Laboratories

Synthon Pharmaceuticals, Ltd.
6330 Quadrangle Drive
Suite 305
Chapel Hill, NC 27517
800-576-4459
http://www.synthon-usa.com

Syva Co.
1717 Deerfield Rd.
Deerfield, IL 60015
847-267-5300
800-241-0420

Takeda Chemical Industries, Ltd.
1-1 Doshomachi 4-Chome Chuo-Ku
Osaka
Japan

Takeda Pharmaceuticals America, Inc.
475 Half Day Rd., Suite 500
Lincolnshire, IL 60069
847-383-3000
http://www.tpna.com

Tambrands, Inc.
777 Westchester Avenue
White Plains,, NY
914-696-6000

Tanning Research Labs, Inc.
1190 U.S. 1 N.
Ormond Beach, FL 32174
386-677-9559
800-874-4844
http://www.htropic.com

Tanox Inc.
10301 Stella Link
Houston, TX 77025-5497
713-664-2288
http://www.tanox.com

00300
TAP Pharmaceuticals
2355 Waukegan Rd.
Deerfield, IL 60015
800-621-1020
http://www.tap.com

Targeted Genetics Corp.
1100 Olive Way, Ste. 100
Seattle, WA 98101
206-623-7612
http://www.targen.com

51672
Taro Pharmaceuticals USA, Inc.
5 Skyline Dr.
Hawthorne, NY 10532-9998
914-345-9001
800-544-1449
http://www.taropharma.com

Taylor Pharmacal (Akorn)
2500 Millbrook Dr.
Buffalo Grove, IL 60089
847-279-6100
800-932-5676
http://www.akorn.com

00418
Taylor Pharmaceuticals (Akorn)
2500 Millbrook Dr.
Buffalo Grove, IL 60089
847-279-6100
800-223-9851

TEAMM Pharmaceuticals, Inc.
3000 Aerial Center Parkway
Suite 110
Morrisville, NC 27560
919-481-9020
866-481-9020
http://www.teammpharma.com

83926
Tec Laboratories, Inc.
7100 Tec Labs Way SW
Albany, OR 97321-0512
541-926-4577
800-482-4464
http://www.teclabsinc.com

Teikoku Seiyaku Co. Ltd.
567 Sanbonmatsu Ochi Cho Kagawa
Ohkawa Gun 7692695
Japan

Telluride Pharm. Corp.
300 Valley Road
Hillsborough, NJ 08844-4059
908-369-1800
908-369-1331
http://www.tellpharm.com

Tel-Test, Inc.
P.O. Box 1421
Friendswood, TX 77546
281-482-2762
800-631-0600
http://www.tel-test.com

Terumo Medical Corporation
2101 Cottontail Lane
Somerset, NJ 08873
732-302-4900
800-283-7866
http://www.terumomedical.com

TestPak, Inc.
125 Algonquin Parkway
Whippany, NJ 07981
973-887-4440
973-887-9098
http://www.testpak.com

Teva Marion Partners
10236 Marion Park Dr.
P.O. Box 9627
Kansas City, MO 64134
800-362-7466

00093, 00332
Teva Pharmaceuticals USA
1090 Horsham Rd.
P.O. Box 1090
North Wales, PA 19454-1090
215-591-3000
800-545-8800
http://www.tevausa.com

49158
Thames Pharmacal, Inc.
See Taro

Ther-Rx Corporation
4080 Wedgeway Ct.
I Arth City, MO 63010
314-209-1517
877-567-7676
http://www.kvph.com

Therakos, Inc.
437 Creameryway
Exton, PA 19341
610-280-1000
http://www.therakos.com

Therapeutic Antibodies, Inc.
See Protherics

Therasense
See Abbott Diabetes Care

11290
Thompson Medical Co., Inc.
See Chattem Consumer Products

T/I Pharmaceuticals, Inc.
See Fischer Pharmaceuticals, Inc.

49483
Time-Cap Labs, Inc.
7 Michael Avenue
Farmingdale, NY 11735
631-753-9090
http://www.timecaplabs.com

Tishcon Corp.
30 New York Ave.
Westbury, NY 11590
516-333-3050
800-848-8442
http://www.tishcon.com

Toms of Maine, Inc.
302 Lafayette Center
Kennebunk, ME 04043
207-985-2944
800-775-2388
http://www.tomsofmaine.com

Topco Assoc. LLC
7711 Gross Point Rd.
Skokie, IL 60077
847-676-3030
http://www.topco.com

Topix Pharmaceuticals
5200 New Horizons Blvd.
North Amityville, NY 11701-1144
800-445-2595

Transdermal Technologies, Inc.
1368 North Killian Drive
Lake Park, FL 33403
561-848-2345
800-282-5511
http://www.transdermaltechnologies.com

Trask Industries, Inc.
163 Farrell Street
Somerset, NJ 08873
800-579-3131

Tri-Med Laboratories
68 Veronica Ave.
Somerset, NJ 08873
732-249-6363

Tri Tec Laboratories
1000 Robins Rd.
Lynchburg, VA 24504-3558
804-845-7073

Triage Pharmaceuticals
See Health for Life Brands, Inc.

Trigen Laboratories, Inc.
207 Kiley Drive
Salisbury, MD 21802
410-860-8500
http://www.trigenlabs.com

Trimen, Inc.
P.O. Box 309
New Oxford, PA 17350
717-624-4770

Trinity Technologies
572 Washington Street
Wellesley, MA 02482-6418
781-235-2223
http://www.trinitytechnologies.com

79511
Triton Consumer Products, Inc.
561 W. Golf Rd.
Arlington Heights, IL 60005-3904
847-228-7650
800-942-2009
http://www.mg217.com

Truxton
136 Harding Avenue
P.O. Box 1081
Bellmawr, NJ 08099
856-933-2333

Tryon Laboratories
27368 Via Industria
Temecula, CA 92590
951-719-1104

Tweezerman
2 Tri-Harbo Ct.
Port Washington, NY 11050
516-676-7772
800-645-3340
http://www.tweezerman.com

Twinlab Corp.
150 Motor Pkwy.
Hauppauge, NY 11788
631-467-3140
800-645-5626
http://www.twinlab.com

Tyler, Inc.
See Integrated Therapies Inc.

53335
Tyson Nutraceuticals
12832 S. Chadron Ave.
Hawthorne, CA 90250-5525
310-675-1080
800-799-3233
http://www.tysonnutraceuticals.com

UAD Laboratories, Inc.
See Forest Pharmaceutical, Inc.

UCB Pharmaceuticals, Inc.
1950 Lake Park Dr.
Smyrna, GA 30080
770-970-7500
800-477-7877
http://www.ucbpharma.com

51079
UDL Laboratories, Inc.
1718 Northrock Ct.
Rockford, IL 61103
815-282-1201
800-435-5272
http://www.udllabs.com

00127
Ulmer Pharmacal Co.
1011 Industry Ave
P.O. Box 408
Park Rapids, MN 56470
218-732-2656
800-848-5637
http://www.lobanaproducts.com

Ultimed
287 East Sixth St.
St. Paul, MN 55101
651-291-7909
http://www.diabetes-care.com

Unico Holdings, Inc.
1830 2nd Ave. N.
Lake Worth, FL 33461
800-367-4477

Unigen Pharmaceuticals, Inc.
1221 Tech Court
Westminster, MD 21157
410-751-2108
http://www.unigenpharma.com

Unilever Home and Personal Care USA
33 Benedict Place
Greenwich, CT 06836
203-661-2000
800-243-5320
http://www.unilever.com

41785
Unimed Pharmaceuticals
4 Parkway North
Deerfield, IL 60015
847-282-5400
800-742-7366
http://www.solvay.com

Unipath Diagnostics Co.
47 Hulfish St.
Suite 400
Princeton, NJ 08542
609-430-2727
800-321-3279
http://www.unipath.com

00327
United Guardian Laboratories
P.O. Box 18050
Hauppauge, NY 11788
631-273-0900
800-645-5566
http://www.u-g.com

00677
United Research Laboratories (URL)
See Mutual Pharmaceutical Company

Unither Pharma (United Therapeutics Corp.)
1110 Spring St.
Silver Spring, MD 20910
301-608-9292
888-808-6838
http://www.unitedtherapeutics.com

Univax Biologics
See Nabi

00009
Upjohn Co.
See Pfizer

00245
Upsher-Smith Labs, Inc.
14905 23rd Ave. N.
MN 55447-4709
612-473-4412
800-328-3344
http://www.upsher-smith.com

Upstate Pharma, LLC
Rochester, NY 14623
800-234-5535

URL
See Mutual Pharmaceutical Company

Urocare Products, Inc.
2735 Melbourne Avenue
Pomona, CA 91767-1931
909-621-6013
800-423-4441
http://www.urocare.com

UroCor, Inc.
See Labcorp

Urologix
14405 21st Ave. N.
Minneapolis, MN 55447
763-475-1400
800-475-1403
888-229-0772
http://www.urologix.com

Urometrics, Inc.
2022 Ferry Street
Suite 3125
Anoka, MN 55303
877-774-1442
http://www.urometrics.com

58178
US Bioscience
100 Front St.
Suite 400
West Conshohocken, PA 19428
215-832-4553
800-447-3969
http://www.usbio.com

US DenTek Corp.
307 Excellence Way
Maryville, TN 37801
865-983-1300
800-433-6835
http://www.usdentek.com

US Dermatologics
133 Franklin Corner Rd.
Lawrenceville, NJ 08648
609-406-7900
877-873-3762
http://www.usderm.com

U.S. Neutraceuticals, LLC
2751 Nutra Lane
Eustis, FL 32726
352-357-2004
877-729-7256
http://www.usnutra.com

52747
US Pharmaceutical Corp.
2401-C Mellon Ct.
Decatur, GA 30035
770-987-4745
http://www.uspco.com

US Surgical Corp.
150 Glover Ave.
Norwalk, CT 06856
203-845-1000
800-722-8772
http://www.ussurg.com

USA Nutritionals
513 Commack Rd.
Deerpark, NY 11729
631-643-0600
800-722-7570
http://www.USANutritionals.com

Valeant Pharmaceuticals International
Valeant Plaza
3300 Hyland Avenue
Costa Mesa, CA 92626
714-545-0100
800-548-5100

ValMed, Inc.
221 Spring Street
Shewsbury, MA 01545
508-845-3438

Value in Pharmaceuticals
3000 Alt Blvd.
Grand Island, NY 14072
716-773-4600
800-724-3784
http://www.vippharm.com

Van Den Bergh Foods Company (Unilever Home and Personal Care USA)
75 Merritt Blvd.
Trumbull, CT 06611
203-381-3500

Vangard Labs, Inc.
P.O. Box 1268
Glasgow, KY 42142-1268
800-825-4123

Ventana Medical Systems, Inc.
1910 Innovation Park Drive
Tucson, AZ 85737
520-887-2155
800-227-2155

Ventlab Corporation
155 Boyce Drive
Mocksville, NC 27028
336-753-5000
800-593-4654
http://www.ventlab.com

Veracity Pharmaceuticals Inc.
6601 Lyons Road, Suite E-7
Coconut Creek, FL 33073
954-426-4199

VersaPharm Inc.
1775 W. Oak Pkwy.
Suite 800
Marietta, GA 30062-2260
770-499-8100
800-548-0700
http://www.versapharm.com

Vertex Pharmaceuticals, Inc.
130 Waverly St.
Cambridge, MA 02139-4211
617-576-3111
http://www.vpharm.com

Verum Pharmaceuticals
See Victory Pharmaceuticals

Vetco Inc.
105 Baylis Rd.
Melville, NY 11747
631-755-1155
800-754-8853

53258
VHA Inc.
220 E. Las Colinas Blvd.
Irving, TX 75039
972-830-0000
800-842-7587
http://www.vha.com

23900
Vicks Health Care Products
See Procter & Gamble Co.

25866
Vicks Pharmacy Products
See Procter & Gamble Co.

Victory Pharmaceuticals
12707 High Bluff Drive
Suite 200
San Diego, CA 92130
858-350-4217
866-427-6819

Viratek
See Valeant

Virco Pharmaceuticals Inc.
P.O. Box 11117
Blacksburg, VA 24062
810 663 1008

ViroPharma, Inc.
397 Eagleview Blvd.
Exton, PA 19341
610-458-7300

54891
Vision Pharmaceuticals, Inc.
1022 N. Main Street
Mitchell, SD 57301-0400
605-996-3356
800-325-6789
http://www.visionpharm.com

VistaPharm
2224 Cahaba Valley Dr.
Suite B-3
Birmingham, AL 35242
205-981-1387
877-437-8567
http://www.vistapharm.com

Vita-Rx Corp
P.O. Box 8229
Columbus, GA 31908
706-568-1881

Vital Care Group
8935 NW 27 St.
Miami, FL 33172
305-620-4007
http://www.vitalcare.com

54022
Vitaline Corp. (Integrated Therapeutics, Inc.)
9725 Southwest Commerce Cir.
Suite B-2
Wilsonville, OR 97070
541-482-9231
800-648-4755
http://www.vitaline.com

Vitality Inc.
8935 NW 27 St.
Miami, FL 33172
305-620-4007

Vital Signs Inc.
20 Campus Road
Totowa, NJ 07512
800-932-0760
http://www.vital-signs.com

Vitamin Research Product, Inc.
3579 Hwy. 50 E.
Carson City, NV 89701
775-884-1300
775-884-8210
800-877-2447
http://www.vrp.com

Vitamin Science Inc.
914 Westwood Blvd.
Los Angeles, CA 90024
310-443-9952
800-480-VITE
http://www.vitaminscience.com

Vivus Inc.
1172 Castro Street
Mountainview, CA 94040
650-934-5200
888-345-6873
http://www.vivus.com

59310
Wakefield Pharmaceuticals, Inc.
See Ivax Pharmaceuticals, Inc.

Wal-Med, Inc.
11302 164th Street East
Puyallup, WA 98374
877-542-3688
http://www.wallace-medical.com

00037
Wallace Laboratories (Carter Wallace)
Half Acre Rd.
Cranbury, NJ 08512-0181
800-526-3840
http://www.wallacelabs.com

Wallace Pharmaceuticals
See Med Pointe Healthcare, Inc.

00017
Wampole Laboratories
2 Research Way
Princeton, NJ 08540
609-627-8000
800-257-9525
http://www.wampolelabs.com

00047, 00430
Warner Chilcott Laboratories
100 Enterprise Dr.
Rockaway, NJ 07866
800-521-8813
973-442-3200
http://www.warnerchilcott.com

11370, 12546, 12547, 00071, 00501
Warner Lambert
See Pfizer

Warner Lambert Consumer Healthcare
See Pfizer

59930
Warrick Pharmaceutical, Corp. (Schering Plough Corp.)
12125 Moya Blvd.
Reno, NV 89506
800-547-3869

Watson Laboratories
1033 Stoneleigh Avenue
Carmel, NY 10512
914-767-2000
800-553-4044
http://www.watsonpharm.com

00047, 52544, 51875, 55515
Watson Pharmaceuticals
311 Bonnie Circle Dr.
Corona, CA 92880
800 103 8300
800-272-5525
http://www.watsonpharm.com

W. E. Bassett
100 Trap Falls Road
Shelton, CT 06484-4647
203-929-8483
http://www.trim.com

50106
WE Pharmaceuticals, Inc.
P.O. Box 1142
Ramona, CA 92065
619-788-9155
800-262-9555
http://www.wepharma.com

Weider Nutrition International, Inc.
2002 S. 5070 W.
Salt Lake City, UT 84104
801-975-5000
800-453-9542
http://www.weider.com

Weleda
175 North Rt. 9W
P.O. Box 249
Congers, NY 10920
845-268-8572
800-265-2615
http://www.usa.weleda.com

Wellspring Pharmaceutical
1430 Route 34
Neptune, NJ 07753
732-938-5885
http://www.wellspringpharm.com

Wendt Laboratories
P.O. Box 1142
Belle Plaine, MN 56011
800-328-5890

00917
Wesley Pharmacal, Inc.
114 Railroad Dr.
Ivyland, PA 18974
215-953-1680

59591
West Point Pharma
See Endo Laboratories, Inc.

Western Research Laboratories
21602 N. 21st Ave.
Phoenix, AZ 85027
623-879-8535
877-797-7997
http://www.wrlonline.com

00003, 00072
West-Ward Pharmaceutical Corp.
465 Industrial Way W.
Eatontown, NJ 07724
732-542-1191
800-631-2174

**Westwood Squibb Pharmaceuticals
(Bristol-Myers Squibb)**
100 Forest Ave.
Buffalo, NY 14213
716-887-7667
800-333-0950
http://www.westwoodsquibb.com

W. F. Young
302 Benton Drive
East Longmeadow, MA 06484-4674
800-628-9653
http://www.absorbine.com

11444
W.F. Young, Inc.
P.O. Box 1990
Springfield, MA 01028-5990
413-737-0201
800-628-9653
http://www.absorbine.com

50474
Whitby Pharmaceuticals, Inc.
See UCB Pharmaceuticals, Inc.

00031, 00573
Whitehall-Robins Healthcare
See Wyeth Consumers Health

White Labs, Inc.
7564 Trade Street
San Diego, CA 92121
858-693-3441
http://www.whitelabs.com

Willen Pharmaceuticals
See Baker Norton Pharmaceuticals

William Labs
P.O. Box 101
Oradell, NJ 07649
973-772-4004

Wintec
4280 Technology Drive
Fremont, CA 94538
510-360-6300
http://www.wintecind.com

Winthrop Consumer
See Bayer Consumer Care Division

Winthrop Pharmaceuticals
See Sanofi-Synthelabo

12120
Wisconsin Pharmacal Co.
1 Pharmcal Way
P. O. Box 198
Jackson, WI 53037
262-677-4121
800-558-6614
http://www.wispharm.com

Wm. Wrigley Jr. Co.
410 N. Michigan Ave.
Chicago, IL 60611
312-644-2121
866-787-7277
http://www.wrigley.com

Women First Healthcare Inc.
12220 El Camino Real
Suite 400
San Diego, CA 92130
858-509-1171
http://www.womenfirst.com

Womens Capital Corp.
See Plan B

Woodside Biomedical Inc.
1915 Aston Ave., Suite 102
Carlsbad, CA 92008
760-804-6900
888-297-9728
http://www.woodsidebiomedical.com

Woodward Laboratories, Inc.
125-B Columbia
Aliso Viejo, CA 92656-1458
949-362-4600
http://www.woodwardlabs.com

Wraser Pharmaceuticals
P.O. Box 1699
Madison, MS 39130
601-605-0664
http://www.wraser.com

Wyeth-Ayerst Laboratories
P.O. Box 8299
Philadelphia, PA 19101
610-688-4400
800-934-5556
http://www.wyeth.com

Wyeth Consumer Health
5 Giralda Farms
Madison, NJ 07940
973-660-5100
800-322-3129

00008, 00031
Wyeth
Wyeth Arcola Road
Collegeville, PA 19426
610-902-1200
http://www.wyeth.com

X-Gen Pharmaceuticals, Inc.
P.O. Box 445
Big Flats, NY 14814
607-732-4411
866-390-4411
http://www.x-gen.us.com

50962
Xactdose, Inc.
See Alpharma USPD, Inc.

Xanodyne Pharmaceuticals, Inc.
7300 Turfway Road
Suite 300
Florence, KY 41042
877-926-6396
http://www.xanodyne.com

Xcel Pharmaceuticals
6363 Greenwich Drive
Suite 100
San Diego, CA 92122
858-202-2700
877-361-2719
http://www.xcelpharmaceuticals.com

Xoma LLC/Xoma Ltd.
2910 Seventh St.
Berkeley, CA 94710
510-644-1170
800-544-9662
http://www.xoma.com

00116
Xttrium Laboratories, Inc.
415 W. Pershing Rd.
Chicago, IL 60609
773-268-5800
800-587-3721
http://www.xttrium.com

York Pharmaceuticals, Inc.
1201 Douglas Avenue
Kansas City, KS 66103
913-321-1070

64855
Young Again Products
3608-B Oleander Dr. #310
Wilmington, NC 28403
910-392-6775

60077, 00273
Young Dental Mfg.
13705 Shoreline Ct. E.
Earth City, MO 63045
314-344-0010
800-325-1881
http://www.youngdental.com

Zee Medical, Inc.
22 Corporate Park
Irvine, CA 92606
800-841-8417
http://www.zeemedical.com

00310, 00163, 00187
Zeneca Pharmaceuticals
See AstraZeneca PLC

00172, 00182
Zenith Goldline Pharmaceuticals
See Ivax Pharmaceutical

Zenith Laboratories
140 LeGrand Ave.
Northvale, NJ 07647-2403

51284
Zila Pharmaceuticals, Inc.
5227 N. 7th St.
Phoenix, AZ 85014
602-266-6700
800-922-7887
http://www.zila.com

ZLB Behring
P.O. Box 61501
1020 First Avenue
King of Prussia, PA 19406
800-683-1288
http://www.zlbusa.com

ZLB Bioplasma
See ZLB Behring

Zoetica Pharmaceutical Group
214 Carnegie Center
Suite 106
Princeton, NJ 08540

Zonagen, Inc.
2408 Timberloch Pl., B-4
The Woodlands, TX 77381
281-719-3456
http://www.zonagen.com

Zyber Pharmaceuticals, Inc.
P.O. Box 40
Gonzales, LA 70707
225-647-3002
800-793-2145
http://www.zyberphar.com

ZymeTx, Inc.
655 Research Parkway
Suite 554
Oklahoma City, OK 73104
405-271-1314
888-817-1314
http://www.zymetx.com

Zymogenetics, Inc.
1201 Eastlake Ave. E.
Seattle, WA 98102-3702
206-442-6600
http://www.zymogenetics.com